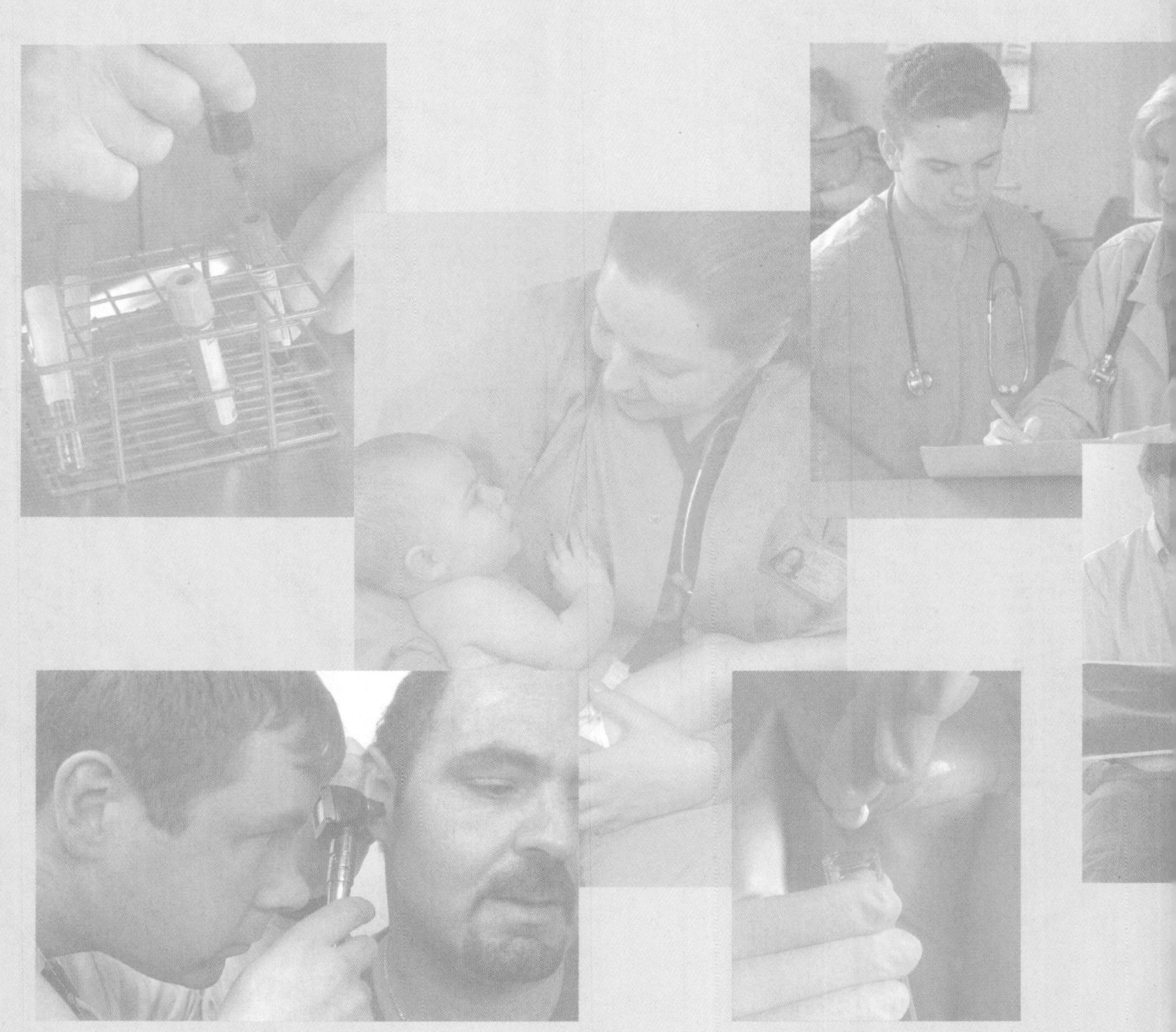

MOSBY'S

Clinical Skills for Medical Assistants

FOURTH EDITION

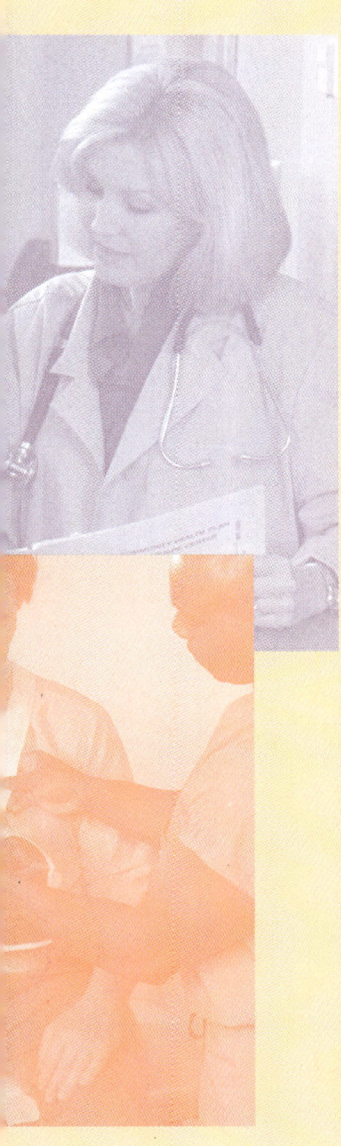

Sharron M. Zakus, RN, BA, MS, CMA

Educator, Health Science Department
City College of San Francisco, San Francisco, California
Formerly Director and Instructor, Medical Assistant Program,
College of California Medical Affiliates, San Francisco, California

with more than 800 illustrations

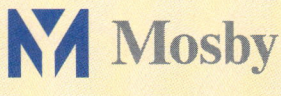 **Mosby**

A Harcourt Health Sciences Company

St. Louis   London   Philadelphia   Sydney   Toronto

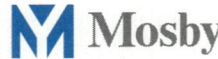

Editor-in-Chief: Andrew Allen
Acquisitions Editor: Adrianne Williams
Developmental Editor: Sarahlynn Lester
Project Manager: John Rogers
Project Specialist: Beth Hayes
Book Design Manager: Judi Lang
Designer: Michael Warrell

FOURTH EDITION

Mosby Inc.
A Harcourt Health Sciences Company
11830 Westline Industrial Drive
St. Louis, Missouri 63146

Printed in the United States of America

Library of Congress Cataloging in Publication Data

Zakus, Sharron M., 1942-
    Mosby's clinical skills for medical assistants / Sharron M. Zakus.—4th ed.
        p. ; cm.
    Rev. ed. of: Clinical procedures for medical assistants. 3rd ed. c1995.
    Includes bibliographical references and index.
    ISBN 0-323-00766-X
        1. Physicians' assistants.   2. Clinical medicine.   I. Title: Clinical skills for medical
assistants.   II. Zakus, Sharron M., 1942- Clinical procedures for medical assistants.   III.
Title.
        [DNLM: 1. Physician Assistants.   2. Clinical Competence.   3. Patient Care.   W 21.5 Z21c 2001]
R697.P45 Z35 2001
610.69′53—dc21   00-066999

01   02   03   04   05   GW/KPT   9 8 7 6 5 4 3 2 1

To
Mom *and* **Dad**
Donn, Joseph, *and* **Jude**
and to the memory of **Nana**

■

Thank you for so much—
small words, but filled with meanings and feelings

Preface

New techniques and developments in the medical field have a direct influence on the medical assistant's professional duties and responsibilities. Because the educational standards of each medically oriented professional career continue to escalate, each assumes new functions, roles, and responsibilities. With the increasing demands of modern medical practice on members of the medical profession, physicians are turning more and more to trained medical assistants to help administer their offices and perform routine clinical duties.

The **intent** of this book is to help medical assistants attain the knowledge and skills required to meet the increasing demands of their profession and enable them to function as major contributing individuals in the health care field.

A textbook should expose the student to new ideas, thoughts, and concepts. It should motivate the student or reader, and above all, it should teach. To achieve these goals, this book presents in a concise, clear, and readable style up-to-date, accurate information about clinical assisting and skills, theory, and related medical information that the medical assistant must understand in order to contribute to quality health care services and education for patients.

The **chief objective** is to aid the student and the teacher in the learning/teaching process. I have attempted to create a book that students will want to pick up and enjoy because it stimulates them, and thus a book from which they will learn eagerly and easily. I have also tried to make this book one that will excite teachers and in turn help make their teaching tasks easier (an instructor's manual, a video series, and a student workbook to accompany the fourth edition are available).

This book is designed to provide knowledge of effective and efficient techniques in contemporary patient care and assisting for beginning medical assistants. Moreover, it supplies current reference material for those assistants actively employed in a medical setting and serves as an information source for the principles and techniques underlying clinical assisting for individuals who wish to reenter the employment field. Actively employed medical assistants who have previous editions of this book in their office and/or home library say that they refer to it frequently when performing their daily work duties. The objectives at the beginning of each chapter and the case studies, vocabulary review, critical thinking skills review, and performance tests given as a study guide at the end of each chapter are particularly helpful for individuals preparing to take the national certification examination(s) administered by the American Association of Medical Assistants and/or by the American Medical Technologists.

To achieve this goal, the cognitive and competency-based terminal performance objectives and materials in each chapter meet the requirements of the national curriculum certification outlines and areas of competency as determined by both credentialing agencies, the American Association of Medical Assistants (AAMA) and the American Medical Technologists (AMT).

Successful completion and mastering of the objectives and related materials will prepare and provide the student with the knowledge, skills, qualifications, and professionalism needed to succeed as a professional medical assistant. This will also prepare the student to pass either certification examination administered by the above associations that award the credential "CMA"—Certified Medical Assistant, from the American Association of Medical Assistants, or "RMA"—Registered Medical Assistant, from the American Medical Technologists.

The scope of this book meets the growing need for a comprehensive and effective textbook that deals with:

- Routine clinical skills and assisting techniques with related information required of the medical assistant.
- Patient procedures that may be performed satisfactorily by the medical assistant.
- Patient procedures in which the medical assistant may be required to assist the physician.
- Tests and procedures that the medical assistant must know to provide the patient with accurate preparatory information.
- Information necessary to understand the procedures, the medical techniques and their underlying principles, and the functions of other professionals who provide health care.
- Quality patient care as the medical assistant's primary goal based on the development of a positive attitude toward individual responsibilities and a commitment to the other members of the health care team.
- Quality patient education.
- Critical thinking skills.
- The most current theoretic information available, with an emphasis on practical application.

Acquiring clinical skills and assisting techniques is best accomplished when learning experiences are organized and the learner is provided with opportunities to acquire knowledge and to practice with professionals in settings that enhance learning. For example, in a skills laboratory, which is a simulation of a joblike environment, learners can practice new skills with each other; or in a clinical setting, which is a working experience, the learners may work under direct supervision.

This book *also* introduces the medical assistant to the nature and purpose of many procedures, both diagnostic and therapeutic, used by the various medical specialties and related medical fields, such as the changing and ever-expanding specialties of nuclear medicine, diagnostic medical imaging, radiation oncology, physical therapy, and laboratory technology, so that the medical assistant can anticipate and prepare the patient for procedures in these fields. Although the medical assistant is only indirectly involved with these specialties, it is essential to become knowledgeable of these fields of medical practice.

The *fourth edition* of this book has been expanded and Chapters 2 through 5 have been renumbered. To meet the requests of some instructors, Chapter 2 is now "Infection Control." The depth of the text remains. *Every chapter* incorporates *new* and the most up-to-date information available on clinical procedures and related theory.

More new and updated color photographs and illustrations have been added to reinforce content, to keep the text lively and engaging, and to enhance the student's visualization and understanding of the theory, procedures, and equipment presented. A glossary of the vocabulary terms from each chapter and Appendix A remain. The Patients' Bill of Rights is on page xv in the *fourth edition*. These are valuable assets and reference sources for the student. Emphasis is on helping the students learn to perform the tasks, acquire the skills of their profession, use the related basic scientific and technical knowledge, acquire the capabilities for critical thinking and problem-solving (i.e., making reliable decisions related to their tasks and adapting to new situations), and treat the patient as a whole individual and not merely as a condition or as a diseased body part.

The organization in the chapters of the fourth edition remains the same as that of the first three editions, because this has proven to be educationally effective for the learning and teaching process. Each chapter contains the following:

- Cognitive- and competency-based terminal performance objectives targeting the main ideas and skills to be mastered
- Vocabulary lists with pronunciation keys
- Specific procedures, related information, and charting examples
- Patient education "Health Matters" boxes

To help reinforce learning, each chapter also includes:

- Reviews of vocabulary (most of which use medical reports as examples)
- Thought-provoking critical thinking skills reviews relating to both theory and skills mastered, many with practical application to an on-the-job situation
- Performance tests

MAJOR CONTENT REVISION FOR THE FOURTH EDITION

The major content changes are summarized as follows:

- **New:** Increased emphasis on patient education in **all** chapters, featuring new boxes called "Health Matters—Keeping Your Patients Informed."
- **New:** CDC and HICPAC revised guidelines for isolation precautions and infection control—"Standard Precautions" and "Transmission-Based Precautions."
- **New:** Graphic icons placed with each procedure as a visual reminder of the protocols required by Standard and Transmission-Based Precautions.
- **New:** Lists of health care hotlines, agencies, associations, and departments (including telephone numbers) to enable the medical assistant to locate community and national resources and disseminate this information to patients, as well as use it for his or her own professional growth.
- **New:** References for resources on the World Wide Web are provided for each chapter.
- **New:** Occupational exposure to HIV; follow-up that should be done if an exposure occurs; risks of infection after exposure; new tests for HIV infection; and confidential vs. anonymous testing.
- **New:** Information and a table on hepatitis A, B, C, D, and E.
- **New:** Important facts about vaccines for older adults.
- **New:** Diseases for which the CDC has issued immunization guidelines for health care providers.
- **New:** Immunization recommendations for adults.
- **New:** The latest classification of blood pressure, hypertension, recommendations for referral for treatment, and patient education on lifestyle modifications for prevention and management of hypertension.
- **New:** Patient's rights and responsibilities under managed care.
- **New:** Section on communication skills—verbal and nonverbal.
- **New:** Cultural considerations in health assessment and health care. Guidelines for relating to patients from different cultures.
- **New:** Information on pain and how it should be assessed.
- **New:** How to provide patient education. Guidelines for patient teaching. Teaching patients how to keep records of symptoms and treatment.
- **New:** How to work with patients regarding compliance issues.
- **New:** Durable power of attorney for health care: Who makes health care decisions for incapacitated patients?
- **New:** Medical reports documenting a patient's history, care, and treatment.
- **New:** Clinical preventive services recommended for normal-risk adults.
- **New:** Foot care guidelines for patients with diabetes.
- **New:** Testicular self-examination.
- **New:** The latest CDC Vaccine Information Statements, immunization schedules, and what to do if a child has discomfort after being vaccinated.
- **New:** Information on lead poisoning and screening children for blood levels of lead.
- **New:** Asthma—diagnosis, treatment, and management.
- **New:** Tests to measure the adequacy of ventilation and oxygenation: oximetry, spirometry, and peak expiratory flow rates.
- **New:** Table on birth control methods.
- **New:** Protocol for accidental needlestick and occupational exposure to blood.
- **New:** Infection control and TB precautions for the medical office.
- **New:** Clinical Laboratory Improvement Amendments (CLIA) classifications and requirements for laboratory testing. Examples of waived tests.

- **New:** "Be an organ donor . . . It's the chance of a lifetime."
- **New:** Laboratory tests for selected sexually transmitted diseases and other conditions and diseases.
- **New:** Blood donation process and eligibility guidelines.
- **New:** Work-related musculoskeletal disorders; ergonomics for the office; bad computer habits to break; and stretching exercises.
- **New:** Portable automated external defibrillators (AED).
- **New:** Dietary Guidelines for Americans, Year 2000; cultural guide to good eating; vegetarian diets; how to judge reports on food and nutrition research findings; food facts and quick tips.
- **New:** Tables have been added in many chapters.
- **Expanded:** Coverage and updates on vocabulary, blood pressure, gynecologic and obstetric examinations, Pap smears, physical examinations, eye examinations and vision problems, immunizations, pediatric injections, care of instruments and sterilization procedures, minor surgical procedures, drug administration, drug classifications, drug dosages and calculations, testing for tuberculosis, quality control for laboratory procedures, diagnostic studies, laboratory tests, physical therapy modalities, common heart rhythms and electrocardiograms, common emergencies and first aid, and various diseases and disorders, including sexually transmitted diseases, HIV, AIDS, allergies, cancer, diabetes, carpal tunnel syndrome, stroke, urinary incontinence, and many more.

The organization and careful selection ensure a relevant and complete resource for students, teachers, and practicing medical assistants, enhancing the competency level in each responsibility.

The reading level of the text was given special attention. Improved readability has resulted without compromising high educational standards and professionalism.

TEXTBOOK SUPPLEMENTS for this edition include a **new *Student Mastery Manual,*** a series of twelve **video cassettes** addressing specific chapters and procedures, and a new **instructor's resource CD-ROM.**

A **CD-ROM** ("Virtual Medical Office Challenge") is enclosed at the back of the book. Through the use of case studies, the program allows students to practice the application of information provided in the textbook, and to use problem-solving, decision-making, and critical thinking skills. In addition, for specific clinical competencies, the learner's ability to use critical thinking and priority-setting skills during a clinical procedure can be challenged.

The new and expanded *Student Mastery Manual* is an extremely valuable companion to the textbook. Using the manual will assist the student in further developing the following:

- The knowledge needed to work as a professional medical assistant
- Problem-solving and critical thinking skills
- Communication skills
- Patient-teaching skills, verbal and nonverbal

- Charting skills for recording and documenting information on a patient's medical chart or record and other clinical records

Highlights of the new *Student Mastery Manual* include the following:

- **Critical thinking skills activities** including problem solving on-the-job situations to decide what should be done, where, why, when, and how
- **Practice charting and documenting information**
- **Small-group exercises** to enhance the ability to work in a team setting
- **Patient teaching experiences** providing health education and promotion, advising, instructing, and referrals to the patients
- **Critical thinking skills review** of the chapter material that includes a variety of the following:
  - Fill-in-the-blank questions
  - Short-answer questions
  - Multiple-choice questions
  - Matching questions
  - True-or-false questions
  - Labeling diagrams
- **Review of the vocabulary using crossword puzzles**
- **A general introduction to anatomy and physiology with practice exercises**
- **Medical Ethics** are discussed in a unique appendix
- **Summary of studies used for diagnosing conditions affecting body organs and systems**
- **Summary of pediatric immunization recommendations**
- **Common Medical Terminology/Combining Word Parts**
- **Performance tests** to test skills and ensure total competencies
- **Performance checklists.** Possible points for each step are given to emphasize the importance of each step. Students can use these to test their own skills and knowledge and that of others before being tested by the instructor. The checklists should be kept as a permanent record in each student's file to verify their competency levels.
- **Evaluations** of the student's techniques and patient interactions

The successful completion of each chapter's objectives and procedures will demonstrate competency levels as required by the American Association of Medical Assistants (AAMA), the American Medical Technologists (AMT), and future employers.

The new **Instructor's Resource CD-ROM** provides the most critical teaching tools in one place. The CD-ROM includes an updated and expanded version of the instructor's manual, an electronic test bank with over 1000 questions, and a 500-image PowerPoint slide show presentation.

The instructor's manual portion of this ancillary is entirely updated for this new edition. Additional information has also been added, including performance checklists with relative point values weighting each step. A more thorough description of this feature is detailed in the discussion of the new *Student Mastery Manual.*

The test bank has sample test questions and answers for all 18 chapters, plus two additional "final exam" style tests.

The PowerPoint portion of the instructor's CD contains 350 photos from the text and 170 text slides, including outlines of the chapters, which are useful for facilitating class interactions and discussions, lectures, and practicing skills and techniques.

This is more than just a how-to book, it is also a why, when, where, who, and what book. Included are explanations of the physician's actions during a patient examination or a procedure in which the medical assistant is participating. In addition, **this book** contains:

- Revised tables for hematology, blood chemistry, serology, and other blood tests with normal values and the significance of the results.
- A table of urine examinations with the type of specimen required, the normal values for the results, and the significance of the results.
- Tables of x-ray and nuclear medicine procedures, with the time period required for each, an indication of when special patient preparation is required, and samples of patient preparation.
- A table of patient conditions that benefit from physical therapy and the common modalities used.
- Guidelines for assisting with the patient history/interview.
- Complete chapters dedicated to Standard/Universal Precautions and Nutrition.
- Expanded coverage on the health care and examinations for the obstetric and the hypertensive patient.
- Actual forms such as medical reports, case histories, and discharge summaries to allow the student to see how the vocabulary terms presented in the chapter are used in an actual report, how the contents of the chapter relate to medical reports, and how health care providers document information obtained about a patient.
- Performance tests and checklists that may be used by the students and adapted for teacher use in the instructor's manual and *Student Mastery Manual.*
- Charting examples for the assistant to use when recording the completion and results of procedures and tests.

To aid the learning process for beginning students, vocabulary boxes are included with pronunciation of difficult terms as they are introduced. It will be helpful for the teacher to give the correct pronunciation of the term and then have the students repeat it.

In the chapters on physical therapy and common emergencies and first aid, students are given the opportunity to design procedural steps, performance checklists, and instructions to be given to the patient to use at home.

Information offered in each chapter is written with the assumption that the medical assistant student has a background in or is currently studying basic anatomy, physiology, and microbiology. Thus detailed explanations pertaining to these subjects are omitted. The teacher of the class for clinical procedures is encouraged to review the theoretic aspects pertaining to these subjects as they relate to each skill the student will be expected to perform.

The chapter on anatomy and physiology is found in the *Student Mastery Manual* for this edition.

All procedures (skills and tasks) are presented in a concise, step-by-step format. When necessary, explanations of the physician's role, specific notes on patient care, and notes stressing the rationale behind a step are offered. The procedures are written to assist the student in the learning process. Sometimes the ideas or procedure steps are included in another procedure or chapter to reinforce the ideas presented. The student should analyze the facts and try to place them in a meaningful order.

It should be remembered that frequently different methods and techniques may be used in a medical procedure. *This book presents one method of performing a procedure.* When there are regional differences of opinion, teachers are encouraged to teach the skill in the fashion most suitable for their area of practice.

This book is written with procedures that may be performed by medical assistants nationwide as identified by the American Association of Medical Assistants and the American Medical Technologists; however, because of various state laws, some procedures may not be considered a duty of the medical assistant. Nevertheless, it is hoped that the information provided helps medical assistants understand the nature and purpose of all procedures presented.

With these facets in mind, it is my hope that educators, students, and medical assistants will use this textbook with the enthusiasm and thirst for knowledge equal to my own as I researched, compiled, and wrote it. I also hope that this book challenges the student to develop a permanent interest in the medical field and a desire for continued growth and knowledge.

Sharron M. Zakus

Acknowledgments

This book could not have been compiled without the encouragement, support, inspiration, and assistance of many friends, colleagues, and other specialists in the medical field. I am deeply indebted to each one of them.

The completion of the fourth edition of this book also gives me the opportunity to thank all the educators and students who responded so positively to the previous editions.

My very special gratitude is extended to Donn R. Harris for his unlimited support, understanding, faith, and encouragement throughout the writing of the complete manuscript and for his valuable assistance in various stages of preparation.

I am especially grateful for the dedicated and invaluable assistance of Ann A. Gunderson, RN, California Pacific Medical Center, Pacific Campus, San Francisco, for continuous consultations and review of numerous areas in this book and for a valued friendship.

To Kate Charlton, RN, Faculty, Medical Assisting Program, City College of San Francisco, special thanks and words of appreciation for her time and the comprehensive review and feedback on the third edition of this book and accompanying workbook.

With pleasure, I gratefully acknowledge the following practicing professionals who offered special area consultations and reviews. I am deeply indebted to each of them for the time, energy, and knowledge that he or she so willingly contributed. In alphabetical order they are:

- Helen Archer-Dusté, RN, MS, CNA, Director, Pediatric Services, Kaiser Foundation Hospital, San Francisco, California
- Rita Arriaga, MS, PT, Assistant Clinical Professor, UCSF/SFSU Graduate program in Physical Therapy, San Francisco, California
- Patricia Barrow, RN, Pediatric Services, Family Health Center, California Pacific Medical Center, San Francisco, California
- Marlene Bonham, RPT, Physical Therapy, Education Coordinator, Pacific Medical Center, San Francisco, California
- Louise Brown, LVN, Pediatric Services, Kaiser Foundation Hospital, San Francisco, California
- Ruth Berry Hanley Bultman, RN, Kaiser Hospital Clinic, San Francisco, California
- Virginia Caen, MA, Specialty Services, California Pacific Family Health Center, San Francisco, California

- Nora Chan, Pharm D, Clinical Coordinator, Pharmacy Technician Program, City College of San Francisco, California
- Cecile M. Dawydiak, RN, MA, Department Chair, RN Nursing Dept., City College of San Francisco, California
- Barbara DeBaun, RN, BSN, CIC, Infection Control Coordinator, Infection Control Services, California Pacific Medical Center, San Francisco, California
- William Delameter, MT(ASCP), Children's Hospital of San Francisco, California
- Sarah L. Dunmeyer, EdD, Health Care Consulting Services, San Francisco, California
- Anne Emmons, MA, Gynecology, Obstetric, and Neurology Clinic Specialties, California Pacific Medical Center, California Campus, San Francisco, California
- Diane R. Garcia, RT(R) (CT), Faculty, Diagnostic Medical Imaging, City College of San Francisco, California
- Fred Schalit, BS, RP, MS (Pharmacology), San Francisco, California
- Elise Stone, MS, Health Education Coordinator, San Francisco Regional Poison Control Center, San Francisco General Hospital, San Francisco, California
- Sara Syer, MS, PA-C, Clinical Instructor in Stanford Primary Care Associate Program, Palo Alto, California
- Martin Walsh OTR/CHT, Davies Medical Center, San Francisco, California
- William B. Wolfe, CRT, San Francisco, California
- Les Yim, BS, CRT, Department Chair, Radiology Programs, City College of San Francisco, California
- Pat Zachary, RN, Pediatric Services, Unit Manager, Kaiser Foundation Hospital, San Francisco, California

I am indebted to the following professionals, who have provided continuing support and expertise:

- Julia Ender, MT(ASCP), San Francisco, California
- John M. Gunning, Mobile Intensive Care Paramedic, San Francisco, California
- Marilyn Jordan, RN, MPH, Nurse Epidemiologist, Hospital Infection Control Unit, Medical Center at The University of California, San Francisco, California
- Elizabeth C. Lee, CRT, San Francisco, California
- Deborah Leeds, PharmD, Director of Pharmacy Services, Shield Healthcare Center, Berkeley, California

- Louisa Lo, RPT, Senior Physical Therapist, Outpatient Services, Pacific Medical Center, San Francisco, California
- Ann McCabe, MT, BA, Microbiology, SmithKline Beecham Clinical Laboratory, San Francisco, California
- Dennis McDevitt, Mobile Intensive Care Paramedic, San Francisco, California
- William C. McDill, RPT, Director, Physical Therapy Services, San Francisco, California
- Bonnie Miller, DSN, OB-GYN Clinic RN, San Francisco, California
- James Mochizuki, CNMT, Nuclear Medicine Technologist, California Pacific Medical Center, San Francisco, California
- Joseph I. Musallam, BSc, Senior Medical Technologist, California Pacific Medical Center, California Campus, San Francisco, California
- Robert Navarro, Mobile Intensive Care Paramedic, San Francisco, California
- James Pritchard, MT(ASCP), San Francisco, California
- The School of Behavioral and Social Sciences, City College of San Francisco, California

I thank the authors and publishers for their kind permission to use some of the illustrations from their books and all the firms and their representatives who cooperated with me in supplying illustrations and descriptive literature of their products. They are given appropriate credit throughout the book.

I am grateful to Nick Kaufman Productions for their work in taking numerous photographs for this edition.

Many physicians; other laboratory, pharmaceutical, and medical personnel; and hospitals contributed medical reports and other special reference material and provided the facilities for taking many photographs.

To Dorothy Bush, a very special thank you and words of appreciation for her assistance and excellence in preparing many parts of the manuscript by spending endless hours at the computer, and for her encouragement and friendship.

I want to sincerely thank the members of Harcourt Health Sciences for all their assistance in the production of this book, and express very special words of appreciation to my excellent editorial team, Adrianne Williams, Senior Editor, Sarahlynn Lester, Developmental Editor, and Andrea Bold and Ellen Wurm, editorial assistants, for their consideration of my ideas and requests, and for their support, interest, assistance, and innovative ideas and contributions. A special thanks and words of appreciation to Michael S. McConnell, Production Editor at Graphic World Publishing Services, for his excellence in editing and work in the final stages of production, as well as Beth Hayes, Project Specialist at Harcourt Health Sciences.

Finally, I wish to acknowledge all my past and present students whom I have had the privilege of knowing and working with in the classroom, and to many other colleagues, friends, and family for their continued interest and support.

Sharron M. Zakus

To the Student

You are about to enter the professional area of clinical medical assisting, an interesting and challenging field. When you have mastered the knowledge and skills presented in this book, you will be able to enhance patient care, and increase your value to the physician, co-workers, and related health specialists.

Always keep in mind that you are an important member of the medical team and it is only through dedicated professional teamwork that quality and appropriate medical care can be provided and accomplished. Never underestimate your value in the field of medical care.

Points to keep in mind as you are studying and practicing procedures and assisting the physician include the following:

- The importance of being exact (precise) in all that you do
- The great service that you are rendering to the patient and to the physician/employer
- The influence that your attitude (positive or negative) can have on your performance and subsequent relationship with patients
- The legal implications of your actions
- That the career you are learning can be extremely rewarding and intellectually stimulating when you apply yourself and continually strive for improvement and continuing educational endeavors
- The importance of understanding and practicing according to the principles and codes of *Medical Ethics*
- Understanding how required workplace skills are integrated into your program of study and recognizing the transferable nature of these skills. Transferable skills that are needed in school and on the job include the ability to:
  - Communicate clearly
  - Organize
  - Plan
  - Manage time
  - Problem solve
  - Develop and use critical thinking skills and find creative solutions
  - Be flexible and adaptable
  - Develop and use leadership and management skills
  - Work as a team member
  - Get along with other people and co-workers

Numerous studies show that the top traits employers look for in employees are the ability to work well with others and the ability to communicate well. Employers want people who are dependable, have the proper and a positive attitude, are capable of being good team members, and, *then,* have the specialized knowledge needed for top performance.

You must develop and practice the following:

- Positive and clear communication skills
- The ability to work with multicultural and diverse populations and have awareness and sensitivity to all
- The ability to work as a team member
- Time management skills
- Strategies to identify and prioritize patient needs
- The ability to provide clear and understandable patient education

For each chapter in this book, read and master the objectives and vocabulary listed. Test yourself and a study companion with the critical thinking skills review and performance checklists provided in the text and the workbook. When you think that you can perform a particular skill, have your instructor give you the performance test. Written and oral testing may also be given to you at the discretion of your instructor.

Samples of patients' records are provided for vocabulary review in the chapters and to allow you to see how medical personnel record information for a patient's permanent medical record. These records will stimulate your interest, enhance learning, and help you relate your studies to actual on-the-job experiences. Read each report carefully and relate its contents to the current and previous chapters of study.

Inherent in the performance of all clinical skills are basic principles that you should recall and integrate:

1. Use and understand the standards and techniques of the federal guidelines for Universal/Standard Precautions at *all* times.
2. Always check and follow the physician's orders.
3. Obtain and prepare the equipment necessary for the procedure. This involves knowledge of the procedure.
4. Thoroughly wash your hands before and after each procedure and patient contact.
5. Prepare and assist the patient both mentally and physically.

   Mental preparation involves an adequate but simple explanation of the situation. Patients are more relaxed and cooperative when they know what to expect during an examination or procedure. To explain effectively, you must know medical terminology and be prepared to translate that language into terms that the patient can readily understand. Provide reassurance and support while maintaining a supportive, empathetic (not sympathetic) attitude.

   Physical preparation involves positioning the patient correctly for the procedure, draping appropriately, and offering assistance as needed, always providing for the patient's comfort and safety.

6. Perform or assist the physician with the procedure.
7. Record the procedure and findings accurately.
8. Dispose of waste and used equipment correctly.
9. Clean and ready the treatment room and equipment for reuse.

As you begin your studies, I wish you success and happiness in a most rewarding professional career and share with you a poem (see below) that I have shared with many of my former students and graduates. Think about it as you begin this program of study and periodically throughout your new career.

Sharron M. Zakus

TAKE TIME

Take time to think—thoughts are the source of power.

Take time to play—play is the secret of perpetual youth.

Take time to read—reading is the fountain of wisdom.

Take time to pray—prayer can be a rock of strength in time of trouble.

Take time to love—loving is what makes living worthwhile.

Take time to be friendly—friendships give life a delicious flavor.

Take time to laugh—laughter is the music of the soul.

Take time to give—any day of the year is too short for selfishness.

Take time to do your work well—pride in your work, no matter what it is, nourishes the ego and the spirit.

Take time to show appreciation—"thanks" is the frosting on the cake of life.

Author unknown

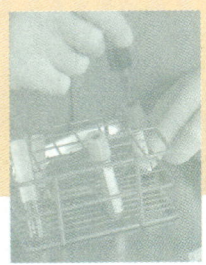

Standard Precaution Icons for Clinical Procedures

The consistent use of standard or standard and transmission-based precautions is required by all health care professionals in all health care settings as a method of infection control. It is assumed that these precautions are used in all clinical procedures as required. Review Chapter 1 if you have any questions on the details of the methods to use, as these will not be repeated in detail in the procedures in each chapter. To assist you, **graphic icons** are placed at the beginning of a procedure as a visual reminder to identify the protocols required by Standard and Transmission-Based Precautions. The icons are illustrated below with their descriptions.

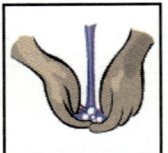

WASH HANDS (Plain soap)

Wash after touching **blood, body fluids, secretions, excretions,** and **contaminated items.** Wash before gloving and immediately **after gloves are removed** and **between patient contacts.** Avoid transfer of microorganisms to other patients or environments.

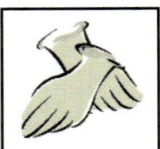

WEAR GLOVES

Wear gloves when touching **blood, body fluids, secretions, excretions,** and **contaminated items.** Put on **clean** gloves just before **touching mucous membranes** and **nonintact skin.** **Change gloves** between tasks and procedures on the same patient after contact with material that may contain high concentrations of microorganisms. **Remove gloves promptly** after use, before touching noncontaminated items and environmental surfaces, and before going to another patient, and **wash hands immediately** to avoid transfer of microorganisms to other patients or environments.

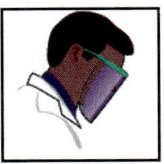

WEAR MASK AND EYE PROTECTION OR FACE SHIELD

Protect mucous membranes of the eyes, nose, and mouth during procedures and patient-care activities that are likely to generate **splashes** or **sprays** of **blood, body fluids, secretions,** or **excretions.**

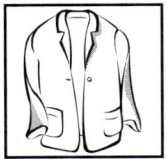

WEAR GOWN, BUTTONED LABORATORY COAT, OR APRON

Protect skin and prevent soiling of clothing during procedures that are likely to generate **splashes** or **sprays** of **blood, body fluids, secretions,** or **excretions.** Remove a soiled gown as promptly as possible and **wash hands** to avoid transfer of microorganisms to other patients or environments.

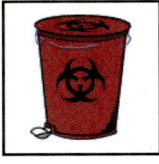

BIOHAZARD CONTAINERS

Place infectious waste in containers that are **leakproof** (i.e., one lined with a strong plastic or vinyl bag or one that is rigid and **puncture resistant**), **closable,** and **suitable** for containing the waste during handling, transport, shipping, or storage. These containers must be **color-coded** or bear the **biohazard symbol** and the legend "biohazard." The container's cover must be closed or tied closed before removal.

Place used disposable syringes and needles, scalpel blades, and other sharp items in **puncture-resistant sharps containers** located as close as practical to the area in which the items were used, and place reusable syringes and needles in a puncture-resistant container for transport to the reprocessing area.

PATIENTS' BILL OF RIGHTS

1. The patient has the right to considerate and respectful care.

2. The patient has the right to obtain from his or her physician complete current information concerning his or her diagnosis, treatment, and prognosis in terms the patient can be reasonably expected to understand.

3. The patient has the right to receive from his or her physician information necessary to give informed consent before the start of any procedure and/or treatment. . . . Where medically significant alternatives for care or treatment exist, or when the patient requests information concerning medical alternatives, the patient has the right to such information and to know the name of the person responsible for the procedures and treatment.

4. The patient has the right to refuse treatment to the extent permitted by law, and to be informed of the medical consequences of his or her action.

5. The patient has the right to every consideration of his or her privacy concerning his or her own medical care program.

6. The patient has the right to expect that all communications and records pertaining to his or her care be treated as confidential.

7. The patient has the right to expect that, within its capacity, a hospital must make reasonable response to his or her request for services.

8. The patient has the right to obtain information concerning any relationship of his or her hospital to other health care and educational institutions insofar as his or her care is concerned and any professional relationships among individuals, by name, who are treating him or her.

9. The patient has the right to be advised if the hospital proposes to engage in or perform human experimentation affecting his or her care or treatment and has the right to refuse to participate.

10. The patient has the right to expect reasonable continuity of care.

11. The patient has the right to examine and receive an explanation of his or her bill, regardless of the source of payment.

12. The patient has the right to know what hospital rules and regulations apply to his or her conduct as a patient.

Adapted from American Hospital Association, *Nurs Outlook* 24:29, 1976.

Contents

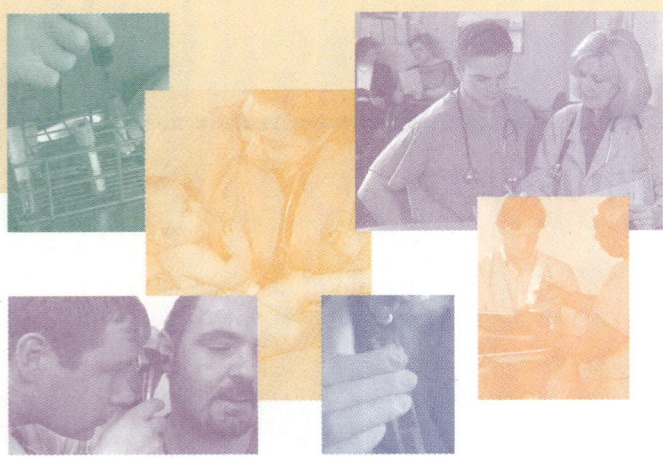

Universal and Standard Body Substance Precautions

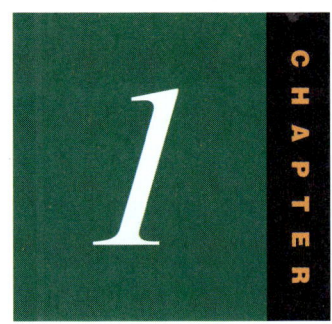

1

■ **Cognitive Objectives**

On completion of Chapter 1, the medical assistant student should be able to:

1. Define, spell, and pronounce the vocabulary terms.
2. State the primary purpose of infection control systems.
3. State why Body Substance Precautions (BSP) or Universal Precautions and Standard Precautions provide protection for all patients and health care providers.
4. Explain the three types of Transmission-Based Precautions used to control infection.
5. List at least 12 situations when handwashing must occur.
6. State the most important function of handwashing.
7. State the purpose of wearing gloves. List at least seven situations when they should be worn by the health care provider. State when gloves should be changed.
8. Discuss the steps to follow if the glove(s) you are wearing is/are accidentally torn or damaged.
9. Describe situations when masks or face shields and protective eyewear should be worn by the health care provider.
10. List three situations when a health care provider should wear a gown or a long-sleeved laboratory coat and state the reason for why it should be worn.
11. Describe 12 procedures recommended for discarding and disposing of used needles and other sharps.
12. Describe and discuss eight procedures and techniques to follow for handling and transporting laboratory specimens. Include a description of how these specimens should be labeled.
13. Explain what to do with reusable equipment after use.
14. Explain how to dispose of broken glassware.
15. List at least five substances or items that should be treated as infectious waste. Discuss how these substances should be handled for disposal.
16. Describe how you should dispose of other waste materials such as paper towels and moist waste materials.
17. Explain how work and environmental surfaces should be cleaned and/or decontaminated.
18. Discuss what should be done with clothing and laundry that has been soiled with body secretions.
19. State the types of labels and signs that must be used to indicate areas and materials that would contain potentially infectious materials.
20. Discuss the appropriate actions to take and whom to contact in an emergency involving blood or other potentially infectious materials.
21. Explain the procedure to follow if an *exposure incident* occurs, including the method of reporting the incident and the medical follow-up that is made available.
22. Discuss the *postexposure evaluation* follow-up that is provided to the employee after an exposure incident.
23. Identify the labels and color coding used to identify a *biohazardous waste*.
24. State the cause, signs and symptoms, stages of infection, diseases that may develop, means of transmission, diagnostic tests, and therapy used for the human immunodeficiency virus (HIV) disease.
25. Differentiate between being HIV positive and having acquired immunodeficiency syndrome (AIDS).
26. Become familiar with agencies that can provide up-to-date information on HIV disease.
27. Differentiate between confidential and anonymous testing.
28. State the cause and signs and symptoms of hepatitis.
29. Differentiate among the six types of hepatitis.
30. Discuss the vaccination for hepatitis B, stating for whom it is recommended and how many doses are given.
31. Discuss the vaccines available for hepatitis A.

■ **Terminal Performance Objectives**

On completion of Chapter 1, the medical assistant student should be able to:

1. Demonstrate the correct procedures for following and adhering to the federal standards, Standard Precautions, and Universal Precautions as outlined in this chapter.
2. Dispose of equipment and specimens according to federal, state, and local standards.

3. Use equipment according to federal, state, and local standards.

4. Provide instructions and patient education that is within the professional scope of a medical assistant's training and responsibilities as assigned.

The student is expected to perform these objectives with 100% accuracy before proceeding past this chapter.

VOCABULARY

For the purposes of this chapter, the following definitions apply according to the Centers for Disease Control and Prevention (CDC) and the Occupational Safety and Health Administration (OSHA).

acquired immunodeficiency syndrome (AIDS)—The most severe manifestation of infection with the human immunodeficiency virus (HIV). The CDC lists numerous opportunistic infections and neoplasms (cancers) that, in the presence of HIV infection, constitute an AIDS diagnosis. In addition, a CD4+ T-cell count below 200 per cubic millimeter of blood in the presence of HIV infection constitutes an AIDS diagnosis.

aerosol—Dispersion of fine particles into the air.

AIDS—Acquired (not born with) immune (body's defense system) deficiency (not working properly or defective) syndrome (a group of signs and symptoms).

antibodies—Molecules in the blood or secretory fluids that tag, destroy, or neutralize bacteria, viruses, or other harmful toxins. They are members of a class of proteins known as immunoglobulins, which are produced and secreted by B lymphocytes in response to stimulation by antigens. An antibody is specific to an antigen.

antigen—A substance that, when introduced into the body, is capable of inducing the production of a specific antibody.

assay—Another word for test.

bloodborne pathogens—Pathogenic microorganisms that are present in human blood and can cause disease in humans. These pathogens include but are not limited to hepatitis B virus (HBV), hepatitis C virus, and HIV.

body substance—Any fluid or substance produced by the body that can carry infectious agents (for example, blood, urine, sputum, and stool).

Body Substance Precautions (BSP)—Same as, and used interchangeably with, Universal Precautions. A system focusing on the cautious handling of potentially infectious body substances by using barrier precautions (for example, gloves, masks).

CD4 (T4) or CD4+ cells—White blood cells killed or disabled during HIV infection. These cells normally orchestrate the immune response, signaling other cells in the immune system to perform their special functions. Also known as T helper cells.

Centers for Disease Control and Prevention (CDC)—The federal agency responsible for assessing the status and characteristics of the HIV/AIDS epidemic and many other diseases and conditions in the United States of America.

clinical laboratory—A workplace where diagnostic or other screening procedures are performed on blood or other potentially infectious materials.

contaminated—The presence or reasonably anticipated presence of blood or other potentially infectious materials on an item or surface.

contaminated laundry—Laundry that has been soiled with blood or other potentially infectious materials or may contain sharps.

contaminated sharps—Any contaminated object that can penetrate the skin, including but not limited to needles, scalpels, broken glass, and broken capillary tubes.

decontamination—The use of physical or chemical means to remove, inactivate, or destroy bloodborne pathogens on a surface or item to the point at which they are no longer capable of transmitting infectious particles and the surface or item is rendered safe for handling, use, or disposal.

detergents—Chemicals used for cleaning purposes, sometimes used in combination with germicides (for example, LpH and Staphene).

EIA or ELISA (enzyme immunoassay or enzyme-linked immunosorbent assay)—Assay used to detect antibodies to HIV in the blood, urine, or oral samples. An assay based on antigen-antibody interactions, it uses enzymes attached to an antibody to measure the reaction.

engineering controls—Controls (for example, sharps disposal containers, self-sheathing needles) that isolate or remove the bloodborne pathogens hazard from the workplace.

enzyme—A protein that accelerates a specific chemical reaction without altering itself.

exposure incident—A specific eye, mouth, other mucous membrane, nonintact skin, or parenteral contact with blood or other potentially infectious materials that results from the performance of an employee's duties.

HAV—Hepatitis A virus.

HBV—Hepatitis B virus.

HCV—Hepatitis C virus.

HDV—Hepatitis D virus.

HEV—Hepatitis E virus.

HGV—Hepatitis G virus.

HICPAC—Hospital Infection Control Practices Advisory Committee.

HIV—Human immunodeficiency virus. The retrovirus isolated and recognized as a cause of immune suppression and/or AIDS.

nosocomial infection—An infection acquired at least 72 hours after admission to a hospital.

occupational exposure—Reasonably anticipated skin, eye, mucous membrane, or parenteral contact with blood or other potentially infectious materials that may result from the performance of an employee's duties.

VOCABULARY—cont'd

OSHA—The Department of Labor's Occupational Safety and Health Administration.

potentially infectious materials

1. Blood—human blood, human blood components, and products made from human blood.
2. The following human body fluids: semen, vaginal secretions, cerebrospinal fluid, synovial fluid, pleural fluid, pericardial fluid, peritoneal fluid, amniotic fluid, saliva in dental procedures, any body fluid that is visibly contaminated with blood, and all body fluids in situations in which it is difficult or impossible to differentiate between body fluids.
3. Any unfixed tissue or organ (other than intact skin) from a human (living or dead).
4. HIV-containing cell or tissue cultures, organ cultures, and HIV- or HBV-containing culture medium or other solutions.

regulated waste—Liquid or semiliquid blood or other potentially infectious materials, contaminated items that would release blood or other potentially infectious materials in a liquid or semi-liquid state if compressed, items that are caked with dried blood or other potentially infectious materials and capable of releasing these materials during handling, contaminated sharps, and pathologic and microbiologic wastes containing blood or other potentially infectious materials.

Standard Precautions—Part of a system that incorporates features of Universal Blood and Body Fluid Precautions and Body Substance Isolation Precautions to be used for **all** patient care. **When referring to infection control systems, the term "Standard Precautions" is now used by most health care agencies and practitioners rather than "Universal Precautions." However, those who still use the term "Universal Precautions" do so with the intent of including all body fluids, regardless of whether they contain visible blood or not** (see page 5 and Figure 1-2).

sterilize—The use of a physical or chemical procedure to destroy all microbial life, including highly resistant bacterial endospores.

Universal Precautions—Same as, and used interchangeably with, Body Substance Precautions (BSP). An approach to infection control. According to the concept of Universal Precautions, all human blood and certain human body fluids are treated as if known to be infectious for HIV, HBV, and other bloodborne pathogens. Also, use of uniform infection control procedures with **all** patients and in **all** work situations, on the basis of the degree of exposure risk to body substances, not diagnosis.

waste

1. *Medical waste* (formerly referred to as infectious waste).

NOTE: The terminology may vary from state to state and even from county to county. Check with your local agencies for the terms that they use most often.

   a. Laboratory wastes, including cultures of etiologic agents (disease-producing microorganisms) that pose a substantial threat to health because of volume and virulence.
   b. Pathologic specimens, including human tissue, blood elements, excrement, and secretions that contain etiologic agents and attendant disposable fomites (disposable substances that can absorb and transport infectious microorganisms).
   c. Surgical specimens, including human parts and tissue removed surgically or at autopsy, which in the opinion of the attending physician contain etiologic agents and attendant disposable fomites.
   d. Sharps (needles, sharp disposable instruments, and glass slides). Sharps means any device having acute rigid corners, edges, or protuberances capable of cutting or piercing.
   e. Liquid body substances such as blood, urine, bile, vomitus, other secretions or excretions, and stool.

NOTE: The Environmental Protection Agency (EPA) estimates that about 15% of all medical waste is infectious. Infectious waste is defined as any waste capable of producing an infectious disease.

2. *Contaminated* waste is all moist waste, including products that have been in contact with the patient's body fluids or wastes that might attract vermin (for example, tongue blades; diapers; urine cups; moist, blood-stained dressings; nonsharp disposable instruments; and food wastes).
3. *Other* wastes are paper material and other office materials.

OR

4. *Nonmedical* waste. Waste not defined as "medical/biohazardous" (items such as paper towels, paper products, articles containing nonfluid blood, and other medical solid waste products commonly found in medical facilities).
   a. Most patient care clinic and surgery waste such as dressings, disposable diapers, intravenous tubing and bags, surgical drapes, and ventilator circuits.
   b. Office and nonpatient care department waste.
   c. Kitchen waste.

The nature and severity of certain infectious diseases (namely, HIV, AIDS, and hepatitis B virus (HBV) have led to the formulation and adoption by medical personnel of what are commonly referred to as the Universal Precautions (also known as the BSP) and now the Standard Precautions. Over the years the terms have changed, but **all** are approaches to *infection control*. The intent is the same, that is, to minimize the transmission of infection—to protect the patient *and* the health care provider.

These standards, first recommended by the CDC, are a vital component and responsibility of many health care providers' everyday activities. The key to all Standard and Universal Precautions is to handle all blood and body fluids and substances as if known to be infected.

Universal/Standard Precautions against transmission of bloodborne pathogens in the health care workplace are no longer just recommended—**they are law.** OSHA issued a federal standard on December 2, 1991.

The regulations covered by this standard apply to employees of facilities where a worker could be "reasonably anticipated" to come in contact with blood or other potentially infectious materials, including body fluids, saliva, and tissue. When it is difficult or impossible to differentiate between body fluid types, all body fluids shall be considered potentially infectious materials.

All health care facilities had to comply with the new bloodborne pathogen standard by July 6, 1992.

Each state must develop its own law, using these standards as guidelines. The federal regulation requires the following:

- A written infection control plan with a policies and procedures manual must be developed by every health care facility. It must be updated annually and made accessible to employees. This exposure control plan must also describe workplace risks, workers at risk, and how workers are trained and protected.
- Training and education in Universal/Standard Precautions must be provided annually for employees.
- Hepatitis B vaccinations must be offered within 10 days of employment to all employees who have occupational exposure at no cost to the employee. If employees decline the vaccinations, they must sign a form that indicates this decision (Figure 1-1). The vaccination must be made available to the employees at no cost if they decide to receive it at a later date.
- Records must be kept on each employee's training, occupational injuries, and vaccinations for at least 30 years.
- Personal protective equipment must be provided at no cost to the employee. Examples of protective equipment include gloves, masks, and gowns.
- Engineering controls such as puncture-resistant containers for used needles must be in place.
- Work practice controls such as handwashing must be enforced.
- Biohazard signs must be posted.
- Warning labels must be used.
- Medical treatment and counseling must be made available to exposed employees (see Figure 1-10).

Since the incorporation of these new guidelines, some considerable local variations have been seen in the interpretation of Universal Precautions and Body Substance Isolation (BSI). There was lack of agreement about the importance of handwashing when gloves were used; the need for additional precautions beyond BSI to prevent airborne, droplet, and contact transmission; and failure of some hospitals to implement appropriate guidelines for preventing transmission of tuberculosis.

FIGURE 1-1 Hepatitis B vaccination refusal form that is to be signed by an employee if he or she refuses to have the vaccination while employed by the health care facility.

RECORD OF HEPATITIS "B" VACCINE DECLINATION

Date _____

I understand that due to my occupational exposure to blood or other potentially infectious materials, I may be at risk of acquiring hepatitis B virus (HBV) infection. I have been given the opportunity to be vaccinated with hepatitis B vaccine, at no charge to me. However, I decline hepatitis B vaccination at this time. I understand that by declining this vaccine, I continue to be at risk of acquiring hepatitis B, a serious disease. If in the future, I continue to have occupational exposure to blood or other potentially infectious materials and I want to be vaccinated with hepatitis B vaccine, I can receive the vaccination series at no charge to me.

Employee Name _____

Employee Signature _____

Social Security No. _____

Employer Representative _____

Bloodborne Pathogens Standard, OSHA.

In view of these and other concerns, the CDC and the **Hospital Infection Control Practices Advisory Committee** (HICPAC) believed that a synthesis of the various systems was needed to provide a guideline with feasible recommendations for preventing the many infections that occur in hospitals through diverse modes of transmission. Thus the "Guidelines for Isolation Precautions in Hospitals" were revised to meet the following objectives:

1. To be epidemiologically sound
2. To recognize the importance of **all** body fluids, secretions, and excretions in the transmission of nosocomial pathogens
3. To contain adequate precautions for infections transmitted by the airborne, droplet, and contact routes of transmission
4. To be as simple and user friendly as possible
5. To use new terms to avoid confusion with existing infection control and isolation systems

Gaps still exist in the knowledge of epidemiology and modes of transmission of some diseases; thus disagreement with some of the recommendations is expected. HICPAC recognizes that the goal of preventing transmission of infections in hospitals can be accomplished by multiple means and that hospitals will modify the recommendations according to their needs and circumstances and as directed by federal, state, or local regulations. Modification of the recommendations is encouraged if (1) the principles of epidemiology and disease transmission are maintained and (2) precautions are included to interrupt spread of infection by all routes that are likely to be encountered in the hospital. The new guideline supersedes previous CDC recommendations for isolation precautions in hospitals.

HICPAC ISOLATION PRECAUTIONS

The revised guideline contains two tiers of precautions. In the *first,* and most important, tier are those precautions designed for **all** patients in hospitals, regardless of their diagnosis or presumed infection status. Implementation of these **"Standard Precautions"** is the primary strategy for successful nosocomial infection control. In the *second* tier are precautions designed only for the care of specified patients. These additional **"Transmission-Based Precautions"** are for patients known or suspected to be infected by epidemiologically important pathogens spread by airborne or droplet transmission or by contact with dry skin or contaminated surfaces.

Standard Precautions

Standard Precautions synthesize the major features of Universal Precautions (Blood and Body Fluids Precautions; designed to reduce the risk of transmission of **bloodborne** pathogens) and Body Substance Isolation (BSI) (designed to reduce the risk of transmission of pathogens from moist body substances) and apply them to all patients receiving care in hospitals, regardless of their diagnosis or presumed infection status. **Standard Precautions apply to** (1) blood; (2) **all** body fluids, secretions, and excretions *except* sweat, regardless of whether they contain visible blood; (3) nonintact skin; and (4) mucous membranes. Standard Precautions are designed to reduce the risk of transmission of microorganisms from both recognized and unrecognized sources of infection in hospitals. Standard Precautions, or the equivalent, should be used for the care of **all** patients (Figure 1-2).

Transmission-Based Precautions

Transmission-Based Precautions are designed for patients documented or suspected to be infected with highly transmissible or epidemiologically important pathogens for which additional precautions beyond Standard Precautions are necessary to interrupt transmission in hospitals. *There are three types of Transmission-Based Precautions:* Airborne Precautions, Droplet Precautions, and Contact Precautions (Figure 1-3). They may be combined for diseases that have multiple routes of transmission. **When used either singularly or in combination, they are to be used in addition to Standard Precautions.**

Airborne precautions

In addition to Standard Precautions, use Airborne Precautions, or the equivalent, for patients known or suspected to be infected with microorganisms transmitted by airborne droplet nuclei.

Airborne Precautions are designed to reduce the risk of airborne transmission of infectious agents. Airborne transmission occurs by dissemination of either airborne droplet nuclei (small-particle residue [5 µm or smaller] of evaporated droplets that may remain suspended in the air for long periods) or dust particles containing the infectious agent. Microorganisms carried in this manner can be dispersed widely by air currents and may become inhaled by or deposited on a susceptible host within the same room or over a longer distance from the source patient, depending on environmental factors; therefore special air handling and ventilation are necessary to prevent airborne transmission. Airborne Precautions apply to patients known or suspected to be infected with epidemiologically important pathogens that can be transmitted by the airborne route. Microorganisms transmitted by airborne transmission include *Mycobacterium tuberculosis* and the rubeola (measles) and varicella (chickenpox) viruses (see Figure 1-3, *A*).

Droplet precautions

In addition to Standard Precautions, use Droplet Precautions, or the equivalent, for a patient known or suspected to be infected with microorganisms transmitted by droplets (large-particle droplets).

Droplet Precautions are designed to reduce the risk of droplet transmission of infectious agents. Droplet transmission involves contact of the conjunctivae or the mucous membranes of the nose or mouth of a susceptible person with large-particle droplets (larger than 5 µm) containing microorganisms generated from a person who has a clinical disease or who is a carrier of the microorganism. Droplets are generated from the source person primarily during coughing, sneezing, or talking and during the performance of certain procedures, such as suctioning and bronchoscopy. Transmission via large-particle droplets requires close contact between source and recipient

FIGURE 1-2 Standard Precautions. (Courtesy Brevis Corporation, Salt Lake City, Utah.)

STANDARD PRECAUTIONS

FOR INFECTION CONTROL

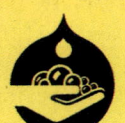

Wash Hands (Plain soap)
Wash after touching **blood**, **body fluids**, **secretions**, **excretions**, and **contaminated items**. Wash immediately **after gloves are removed** and **between patient contacts**. Avoid transfer of microorganisms to other patients or environments.

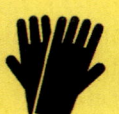

Wear Gloves
Wear when touching **blood**, **body fluids**, **secretions**, **excretions**, and **contaminated items**. Put on **clean** gloves just **before touching mucous membranes** and **nonintact skin**. Change gloves between tasks and procedures on the same patient after contact with material that may contain high concentrations of microorganisms. Remove gloves promptly after use, before touching noncontaminated items and environmental surfaces, and before going to another patient, and wash hands immediately to avoid transfer of microorganisms to other patients or environments.

Wear Mask and Eye Protection or Face Shield
Protect mucous membranes of the eyes, nose and mouth during procedures and patient–care activities that are likely to generate **splashes** or **sprays** of **blood**, **body fluids**, **secretions**, or **excretions**.

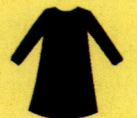

Wear Gown
Protect skin and prevent soiling of clothing during procedures that are likely to generate **splashes** or **sprays** of **blood**, **body fluids**, **secretions**, or **excretions**. Remove a soiled gown as promptly as possible and wash hands to avoid transfer of microorganisms to other patients or environments.

Patient-Care Equipment
Handle used patient–care equipment soiled with **blood**, **body fluids**, **secretions**, or **excretions** in a manner that prevents skin and mucous membrane exposures, contamination of clothing, and transfer of microorganisms to other patients and environments. Ensure that reusable equipment is not used for the care of another patient until it has been appropriately cleaned and reprocessed and single use items are properly discarded.

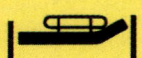

Environmental Control
Follow hospital procedures for routine care, cleaning, and disinfection of environmental surfaces, beds, bedrails, bedside equipment and other frequently touched surfaces.

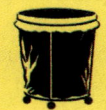

Linen
Handle, transport, and process used linen soiled with **blood**, **body fluids**, **secretions**, or **excretions** in a manner that prevents exposures and contamination of clothing, and avoids transfer of microorganisms to other patients and environments.

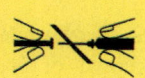

Occupational Health and Bloodborne Pathogens
Prevent injuries when using needles, scalpels, and other sharp instruments or devices; when handling sharp instruments after procedures; when cleaning used instruments; and when disposing of used needles.

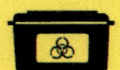

Never recap used needles using both hands or any other technique that involves directing the point of a needle toward any part of the body; rather, use either a one-handed "scoop" technique or a mechanical device designed for holding the needle sheath.

Do not remove used needles from disposable syringes by hand, and do not bend, break, or otherwise manipulate used needles by hand. Place used disposable syringes and needles, scalpel blades, and other sharp items in puncture–resistant sharps containers located as close as practical to the area in which the items were used, and place reusable syringes and needles in a puncture–resistant container for transport to the reprocessing area.

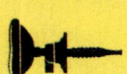

Use **resuscitation devices** as an alternative to mouth–to–mouth resuscitation.

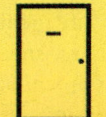

Patient Placement
Use a **private room** for a patient who contaminates the environment or who does not (or cannot be expected to) assist in maintaining appropriate hygiene or environmental control. Consult Infection Control if a private room is not available.

The information on this sign is abbreviated from the HICPAC Recommendations for Isolation Precautions in Hospitals.

Form No. **SPR**   BREVIS CORP., 3310 S 2700 E, SLC, UT 84109   © 1996 Brevis Corp.

FIGURE 1-3 Transmission-Based Precautions **A,** Airborne Precautions; **B,** Droplet Precautions. (Courtesy Brevis Corporation, Salt Lake City, Utah.)

AIRBORNE PRECAUTIONS
(in addition to Standard Precautions)

VISITORS: Report to nurse before entering.

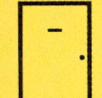

Patient Placement
Use **private room** that has:
  Monitored negative air pressure,
  6 to 12 air changes per hour,
  Discharge of air outdoors or HEPA filtration if recirculated.
Keep room door closed and patient in room.

Respiratory Protection
Wear an **N95 respirator** when entering the room of a patient with known or suspected infectious pulmonary **tuberculosis.**
Susceptible persons should not enter the room of patients known or suspected to have **measles** (rubeola) or **varicella** (chickenpox) if other immune caregivers are available. If susceptible persons must enter, they should wear an **N95 respirator.** (Respirator or surgical mask not required if immune to measles and varicella.)

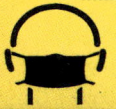

Patient Transport
Limit transport of patient from room to essential purposes only.
Use **surgical mask** on patient during transport.

Form No. **APR**   BREVIS CORP., 3310 S 2700 E, SLC, UT 84109   © 1996 Brevis Corp.

A

DROPLET PRECAUTIONS
(in addition to Standard Precautions)

VISITORS: Report to nurse before entering.

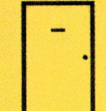

Patient Placement
Private room, if possible. Cohort or maintain spatial separation of **3 feet** from other patients or visitors if private room is not available.

Mask
Wear mask when working within **3 feet** of patient (or upon entering room).

Patient Transport
Limit transport of patient from room to essential purposes only.
Use **surgical mask** on patient during transport.

Form No. **DPR**   BREVIS CORP., 3310 S 2700 E, SLC, UT 84109   © 1996 Brevis Corp.

B

FIGURE 1-3—cont'd   **C,** Contact Precautions. (Courtesy Brevis Corporation, Salt Lake City, Utah.)

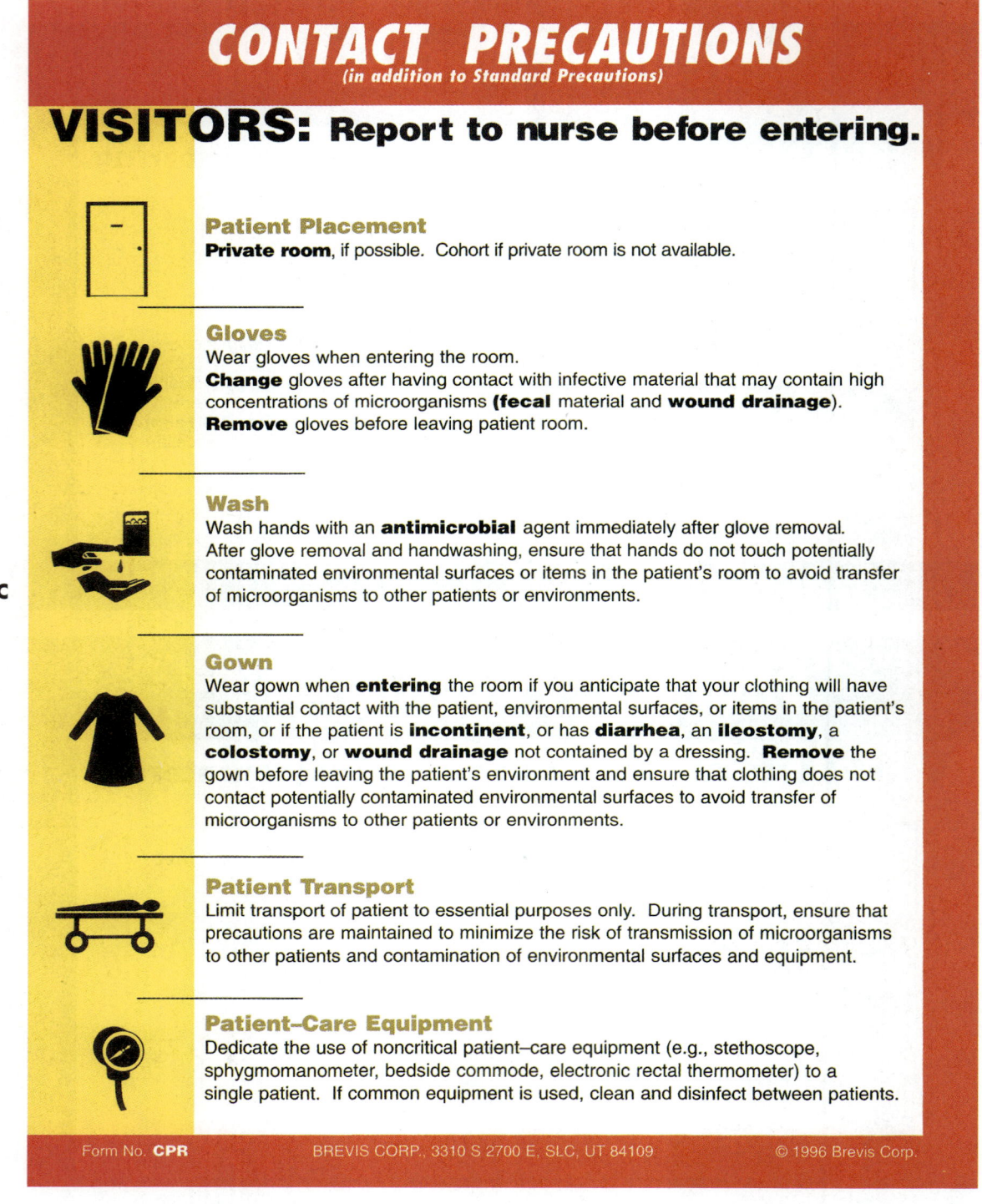

persons because droplets do not remain suspended in the air and generally travel only short distances, usually 3 feet or less, through the air. Because droplets do not remain suspended in the air, special air handling and ventilation are not necessary to prevent droplet transmission. Droplet Precautions apply to any patient known or suspected to be infected with epidemiologically important pathogens that can be transmitted by infectious droplets (see Figure 1-3, *B*). Illnesses transmitted by this route include diphtheria, influenza, rubella, pertussis, and mumps.

Contact precautions

In addition to Standard Precautions, use Contact Precautions, or the equivalent, for specified patients known or suspected to be infected or colonized with epidemiologically important microorganisms that can be transmitted by direct or indirect contact with the patient.

Contact Precautions are designed to reduce the risk of transmission of epidemiologically important microorganisms by direct or indirect contact. **Direct-contact transmission** involves skin-to-skin contact and physical transfer of microorganisms to a susceptible host from an infected or colonized person, such as occurs when personnel turn patients, bathe patients, or perform other patient care activities that require physical contact. Direct-contact transmission also can occur between two patients (for example, by hand contact), with one serving as the source of infectious microorganisms and the other as a susceptible host. **Indirect-contact transmission** involves contact of a susceptible host with a contaminated intermediate object, usually inanimate, in the patient's environment. Contact Precautions apply to specified patients known or suspected to be infected or colonized (presence of microorganisms in or on the patient but without clinical signs and symptoms of infection) with epidemiologically important microorganisms that can be transmitted by direct or indirect contact (see Figure 1-3, *C*).

Contact Precautions apply to patients who are actively infected or colonized with multidrug-resistant bacteria, such as vancomycin-resistant enterococci (VRE) and methicillin/nafcillin–resistant *Staphylococcus aureus* (MRSA); enteric infections with a low ineffective dose or prolonged survival in the environment, such as *Clostridium difficile;* and skin infections that are highly contagious, such as scabies, major abscesses, impetigo, herpes simplex, and herpes zoster. **Handwashing remains the single most important step to reduce the transmission of infectious agents from person to person or from one site to another.**

The aforementioned recommendations are all categorized as Category IB, which means that they are strongly recommended for all hospitals and reviewed as effective by experts in the field even though definitive scientific studies have not been done. Other types of health care facilities, such as clinics and physician's offices, are encouraged to adopt these new standards. **On the other hand, many facilities are continuing to use the terms and standards of Universal Precautions and Body Substance Isolation (BSI).**

Everyone has a responsibility to make these regulations work. The employer must provide the information and equipment, and the employee must use it.

The **Infection Precautions** (*Standard Precautions and Universal Precautions*), standards, and guidelines are presented in the beginning of this textbook because they are an integral part of many procedures and activities that are discussed in other chapters. It is vital to understand these principles, adhere to them at all times, and practice them until they become second nature. The Universal Precautions, or BSP, or Standard Precautions are to protect you and the patient against infectious conditions that could prove fatal. Their importance to you as a member of the health care team cannot be overemphasized.

Read this chapter *very carefully,* making sure that you understand it completely, and practice and follow these guidelines diligently throughout your program of study and in your future

career. There is an old saying: "The life you save may be your own." Keep this in mind as you practice these principles and precautions. Doing so may help you realize the significance and role they play in combating the spread of infectious disease. It may also influence your habits and techniques if you are ever tempted to take shortcuts or use easier, less time-consuming techniques.

The spread and nature of infectious disease, the causative microorganisms, the body's defenses against disease and infection, immunity, immunizations, infection control, and the principles and techniques of medical asepsis and sterilization procedures are discussed in Chapter 2. Presenting the standards and guidelines at the beginning of this book will help you relate to the principles and rationales for many of the procedures in other chapters.

INFECTION CONTROL SYSTEMS

Infection control systems are designed to prevent health care providers from transferring infections to patients and from acquiring infections themselves. Infection precautions previously used were based on diagnosis. Universal Precautions and Standard Precautions improve on the traditional systems because they protect workers during the period before a patient's diagnosis is known. Sometimes it is not possible to tell by looking if a patient is infectious; also, it is not practical to test all patients for all possible infections, nor is it timely because exposure would occur before test results are obtained. Pathologic agents may be present in body substances, even if they are not known to be present, and they may be transmitted from ostensibly clinically healthy individuals.

Universal/Standard Precautions are designed for use with all patients, not just those who are identified as infected. They are based on the knowledge of how diseases are transmitted, of how disease transmission is prevented, and on degree of exposure risk to blood and other body substances rather than on diagnosis; precautions should be based on the degree of risk.

Universal/Standard Precautions should always include routine use of appropriate barrier precautions to prevent skin and mucous membrane exposure when contact with the patient's blood or other body substances is anticipated. Because all patients and laboratory specimens are considered possibly infected, Universal/Standard Precautions provide protection not only from known infected cases but also from unrecognized cases, therefore protecting patients and health care providers alike.

Health care providers who have weeping dermatitis or exudative lesions should not take part in direct patient care and should not handle patient care equipment until the condition is resolved.

The following text is in accordance with recommendations from the U.S. Public Health Service, CDC, and OSHA.

BARRIER PRECAUTIONS

The following barrier precautions should be used (see Figures 1-2 and 1-3).

Handwashing

Body substances that may contain disease microorganisms easily contaminate health care providers' hands. If these microorganisms enter an opening in the body (for example, the mouth), infection can occur. **Handwashing is one of the most effective means of infection control.**

Handwashing should occur:

- Before eating or preparing food, drinking, smoking, applying cosmetics or lip balm, or handling contact lenses
- Before performing clean or sterile invasive procedures
- Before and after performing a clinical procedure
- Before and after assisting a physician with a clinical procedure
- Before and after touching wounds or other drainage
- After coming in contact with blood or body fluids, mucous membranes, secretions, or excretions such as saliva, urine, and feces
- After handling soiled linen or waste
- After handling devices or equipment soiled with body substances (for example, urine collection containers)
- *Immediately* after removing gloves or other personal protective equipment such as masks, goggles, face shields, gowns, aprons, and caps
- After using the toilet
- After nose blowing or coughing into the hands
- Between each patient contact

The most important function of handwashing is to remove infectious organisms. No handwashing product on the market kills all disease-causing organisms. Physical removal (that is, washing soil and organisms down the drain) is the most effective practice for removing infectious organisms. Soap-impregnated towelettes should be used *only* in the field, where handwashing facilities are not available; towelettes should not be substituted for soap and water in the office or clinic except during an internal disaster. Other chemicals such as alcohol or bleach should not be used for handwashing; they may damage skin and cause open or chapped areas, which are more easily infected.

Skin can become dry and chapped with frequent handwashing. Lotion used after handwashing helps replace the oils removed during handwashing. Hands must always be washed before using lotion. Using a lotion bottle while hands are dirty is likely to contaminate the lotion container and thereafter each user's hands. Claims that medicated lotions control this problem have proven less than satisfactory in test data. Each health care provider should use his or her own bottle of lotion, which can be left in a locker or other convenient location, and the user should be aware if the lotion becomes contaminated. Community lotion bottles should not be left in staff bathrooms (see the procedure for handwashing on p. 49).

OSHA's federal regulations state that employers must provide handwashing facilities that are readily accessible to the employees. They must also ensure that employees wash their hands and any other skin with soap and water or flush mucous membranes with water immediately or as soon as feasible after contact of body areas with blood or other potentially infectious materials.

Personal Protective Equipment

Gloves

Gloves give the health care provider additional protection beyond that of intact skin and handwashing. Gloves should be worn whenever contact with blood or other body fluids or tissue is expected. Vinyl, other synthetic materials, and latex gloves are suitable for patient care activities, and each has a 95% effectiveness rate. All gloves tear with heavy or prolonged use. Torn gloves should be replaced as soon as patient safety permits.

Hypoallergenic gloves, and other nonlatex gloves, glove liners, powderless gloves, or other similar alternatives must be readily accessible for employees who are allergic to the gloves normally provided.

According to the Food and Drug Administration (FDA), an alarming number of health care providers (approximately 17% to 25%) have developed latex sensitivity or allergies as a result of the increased use of latex products in health care settings. Health care providers should be told that wearing latex gloves agrees with most people but that some people have a reaction to them. Gloves can be even more hazardous when used with powder because the airborne particles absorb latex proteins and are inadvertently inhaled. Hypersensitive persons may experience local reactions, such as contact dermatitis or contact urticarial syndrome (hives), flushing, itching, teary eyes, runny nose, and even asthma. Some develop more severe contact and systemic reactions and may react anaphylactically. (Anaphylactic shock is a severe and sometimes fatal systemic hypersensitivity reaction to a sensitizing substance. It is commonly marked by vascular collapse and respiratory distress, which can occur seconds or minutes after exposure to the allergen. Other symptoms may include nausea, diarrhea, hypotension, laryngeal edema, arrhythmia, respiratory congestion, and shock.) If the health care provider experiences any of these symptoms, vinyl gloves should be worn. Some hypoallergenic gloves on the market still have a moderate amount of antigen content, which could cause a reaction in a person. If the health care provider starts to have a reaction, he or she must see the Employee Health Practitioner or the physician in the medical office or clinic, who will give advice on how to proceed. A physician from the Mayo clinic in Rochester, Minnesota, advises that any person who has a severe hypersensitivity to latex wear a medical identification tag indicating this fact (see Chapter 19, "MedicAlert") because in emergency situations rescue personnel may be wearing latex gloves. Determining what component of latex triggers the allergy is a problem. Additional studies are being conducted by the CDC in Atlanta.

Gloves should be worn for the following procedures:

- When touching blood and body fluids, mucous membranes, or nonintact skin of all patients.

HEALTH MATTERS

KEEPING YOUR PATIENTS INFORMED

As of September 1998, the FDA required manufacturers to include warning labels on all products and medical devices containing natural rubber latex that could directly contact human tissue. The labels would identify the product as containing natural rubber latex, which may cause allergic reactions.

The guidelines also prohibit companies from claiming products as hypoallergenic, because the term erroneously implies that people allergic or sensitive to latex can use the product safely.

PRODUCTS CONTAINING LATEX

A wide variety of products contain latex, including medical supplies, personal protective equipment, and numerous household objects. Most people who encounter latex products only through their general use in society have no health problems from the use of these products. Workers who repeatedly use latex products are the focus of this alert. The following are examples of products that may contain latex:

Emergency Equipment	Oral and nasal airways	Electrode pads
Blood pressure cuffs	Endotracheal tubes	**Office Supplies**
Stethoscope tubing	Tourniquets	Rubber bands
Disposable gloves	Intravenous tubing	Erasers
	Disposable syringes	

Hospital Supplies
Anesthesia masks
Catheters
Wound drains
Injection ports
Rubber tops of multidose vials
Dental dams
Adhesive tape
Elastic bandages

Personal Protective Equipment
Gloves
Surgical masks
Goggles
Respirators
Rubber aprons

Household Objects
Automobile tires
Motorcycle and bicycle handgrips

Carpeting
Swimming goggles
Racquet handles
Shoe soles
Tennis balls
Expandable fabrics (waistbands)
Dishwashing gloves
Hot water bottles
Condoms
Diaphragms
Balloons
Pacifiers
Baby bottle nipples
Disposable diapers

Individuals who already have a latex allergy should be aware of latex-containing products that may trigger an allergic reaction. Some of the listed products are available in latex-free forms.

To reduce the chance of a reaction to latex gloves, *do not* use oil-based hand creams or lotions (which can cause glove deterioration) unless they have been shown to reduce latex-related problems and maintain glove barrier protection, wash you hands with a mild soap, and dry thoroughly after removing latex gloves.

- When handling items or surfaces moist with blood or body fluids and substances.
- When performing venipuncture or other vascular access procedures.
- When working with blood or specimens containing blood, body fluids, excretions, and secretions.
- When cleansing reusable instruments and equipment wear heavy rubber gloves over disposable gloves; a plastic apron or gown; and safety glasses, goggles, or personal glasses with solid side shields added when involved in decontamination activities of instruments and equipment.
- When decontaminating areas contaminated with body substances.
- When cleaning up blood spills and other contaminated areas. Small spills should be wiped up with disposable absorbent towels; any broken glass should be scooped up with several paper towels and disposed of in a red sharps container; and finally, the area should be mopped with a disinfectant. Large blood spills also should be mopped up with a disinfectant.
- **Sterile gloves** should be worn for all sterile procedures to protect both the patient and the health care provider.
- **Nonsterile** gloves can be worn for nonsterile patient care procedures when worker protection is needed.

- **Finger cots or gloves** should be worn while working to cover cuts, abrasions, rashes, or minor infections on the hands.
- If a glove is torn or punctured by a needlestick or other accident, the damaged glove should be removed, hands rewashed, and a new glove put on as promptly as patient safety permits.
- If gloves are contaminated, the health care provider should not touch telephone receivers, other uncontaminated surfaces, or other areas of the same patient's body that may be uncontaminated.
- **Care providers must change gloves between patients and wash hands immediately after glove removal.**
- Gloves always should be removed when answering the telephone, opening a door or drawer, handling a record book or worksheet, and performing other clean procedures.
- **Handwashing remains the most effective infection control procedure.** Glove use, as described, is used to augment the barrier provided by intact skin against infectious agents. However, gloves can transport infectious agents from one person to another or to the mouth as easily as ungloved hands; therefore these policies are *not* to be interpreted as replacing the need for handwashing.

FIGURE 1-4   Wearing protective eyewear and face masks. **A,** Goggles; **B,** safety glasses; **C,** face shield; **D,** face mask.

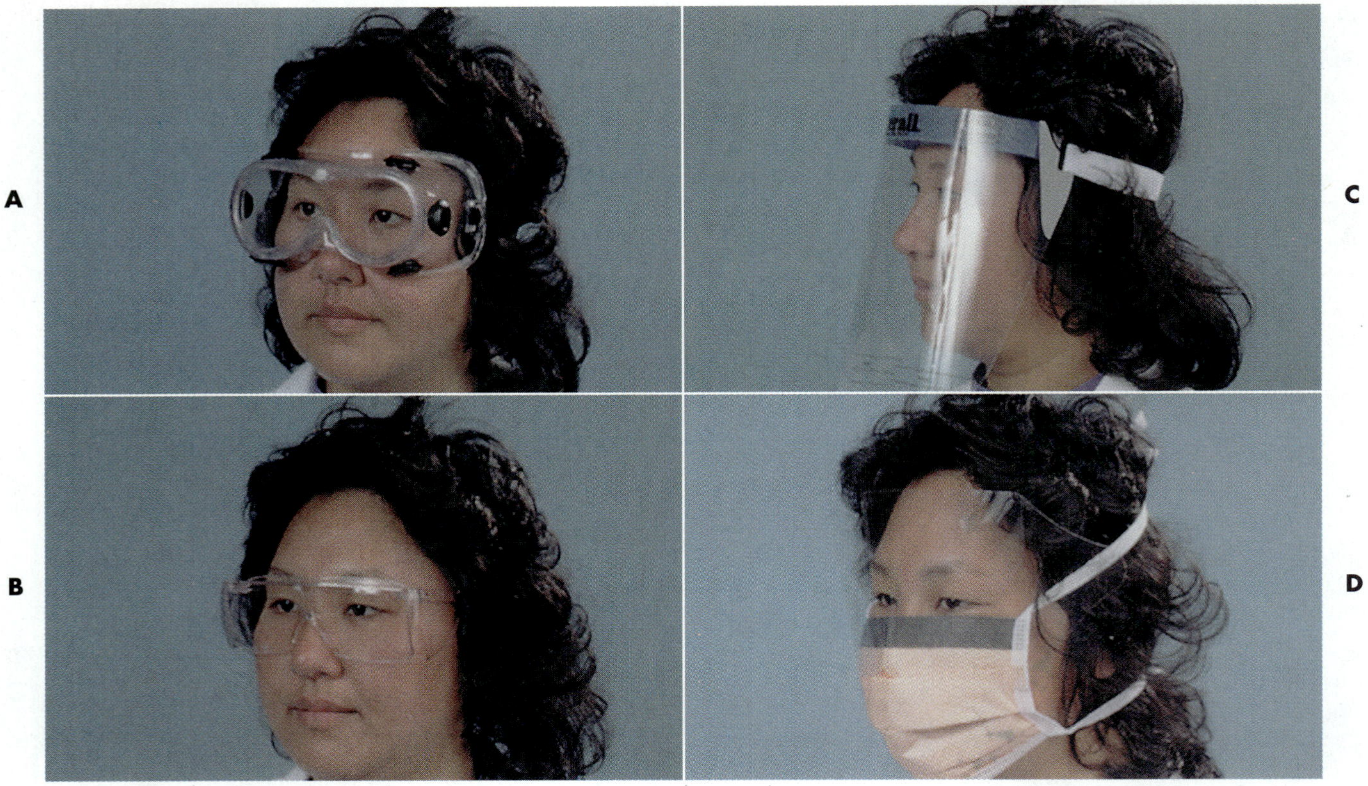

- Disposable gloves (single-use gloves) must not be washed or decontaminated for reuse.
- Utility gloves may be decontaminated for reuse if the integrity of the glove is not compromised. However, they must be discarded if they are cracked, peeling, torn, or punctured; if they exhibit other signs of deterioration; or when their ability to function as a barrier is compromised.

Masks and Protective Eyewear

Masks and protective eyewear should be worn (1) to prevent exposure of the care provider's mucous membranes of the mouth, nose, and eyes during procedures that are likely to generate aerosol droplets or splashes of blood or other body fluids and (2) when cleaning equipment that may have disease-producing microorganisms on it. Masks should cover both the nose and the mouth and fit close to the face so that air can be breathed only through the mask. Care providers should not loosen the mask. Over time, a mask becomes impregnated with moisture from the breath, and it is harder to breathe through the mask. When this occurs, the mask should be changed—not loosened. Masks should be discarded after each use or when they become damp. They are treated as regular, not infectious, waste.

Protective eyewear, such as personal glasses (with solid side shields added), goggles, safety glasses, or face shields, should be worn to protect the face from any splashes (Figure 1-4). Procedures in which eyewear might be needed include certain diagnostic procedures such as endoscopies, any invasive surgical procedure, and when cleaning and decontaminating reusable instruments and equipment. Face shields are best suited for nonpatient care activities such as sorting laundry. After use, undamaged eyewear must be washed with soap and water and then dried before being used again.

Gowns, Aprons, and Laboratory Coats

A gown, apron, or laboratory coat should be worn to protect the arms and clothes during all procedures that are likely to generate splashes or soiling from blood or body fluids. The care provider should wear a gown when cleaning noncontaminated equipment, when cleaning and decontaminating reusable instruments and equipment, and when performing procedures involving contact with large amounts of patient substances. When performing laboratory procedures, the care provider should wear either a long-sleeved gown with a closed front or a long-sleeved laboratory coat buttoned shut. The gown or laboratory coat should be removed when leaving the laboratory area. Care providers should change a gown or laboratory coat immediately if it becomes contaminated with blood or body fluids and at other appropriate periods to ensure cleanliness. Contaminated gowns and laboratory coats should be placed in a biohazard bag for sending to the appropriate laundry as arranged by the facility. If laboratory gowns or coats are contaminated with a microbiologic agent because of a laboratory accident, the gown or coat should be sterilized in the steam sterilizer before it is sent to the laundry.

FIGURE 1-5 Ambu bag and special face shields or pocket masks should be available on all crash carts. These should be used in preference to mouth-to-mouth resuscitation on all patients to prevent direct contact with a person's mouth and saliva. (**B, C,** Courtesy Rondex Products, Inc. USA.)

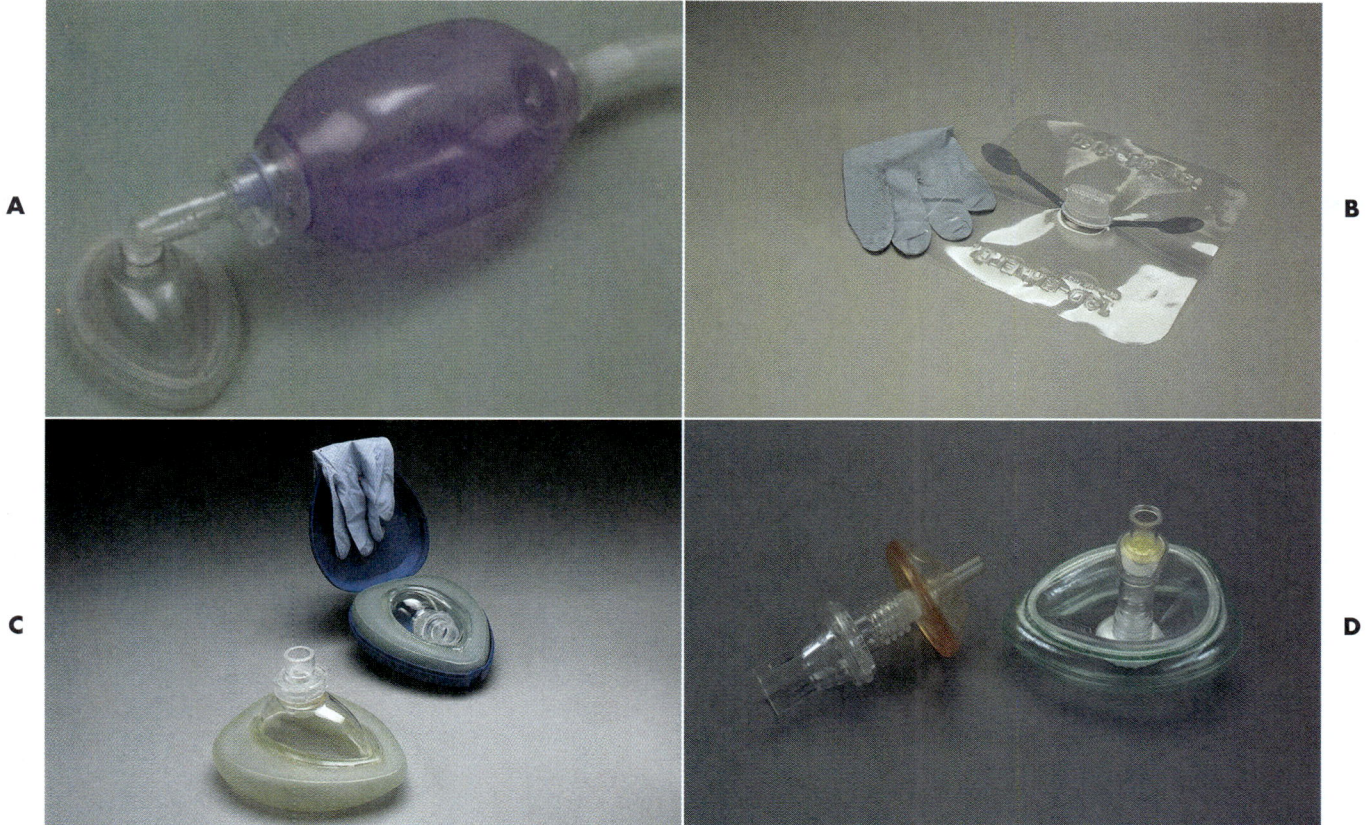

Disposable plastic aprons should be worn if a significant probability exists that blood or body fluids may be splashed. After the task is completed, the disposable apron, if contaminated, should be discarded in a biohazard container or sterilized in the steam sterilizer before it is discarded as ordinary waste. Used laboratory wear should never be stored with street clothes.

Ventilation Devices

Mouthpieces, resuscitation bags, pocket masks, or other ventilation devices should be available to use in areas where the need for resuscitation is predictable. These devices should be used instead of mouth-to-mouth resuscitation on all patients (Figure 1-5).

HANDLING OF EQUIPMENT, SUPPLIES, AND WASTE

Specific procedures have been designed for handling equipment, supplies, and waste taken from patient care areas and the laboratory and for caring for environmental surfaces.

Needles and Other Sharps

Needles, scalpel blades, and any other sharps that can easily puncture the skin must be handled with extreme caution to pre-

vent infection with HIV and hepatitis. Most needlesticks happen when used needles are not handled properly. Broken skin or mucous membrane contact and a needlestick or other blood-to-blood accident can transmit infection. The following procedures must be carried out to prevent any undue infection:

1. Place used disposable needles and syringes, scalpel blades, and other sharp items in a **rigid, puncture-resistant** disposable container with a lid (needle container) that is easily recognized (for example, a red container) and clearly marked as a **biohazard** (Figure 1-6). Preferably, the container should be made of rigid plastic and must be leakproof on the sides and bottom. Do not use cardboard or paper containers. Never put needles or sharps in the trash or linen. This is dangerous to others.
2. Locate puncture-resistant containers as close as practical to the area where needles and other sharps are used. The sharps containers should be located in each treatment room, at each laboratory table, and at any other area where syringes, needles, and slides are used in the office or clinic.
3. Keep needle containers upright throughout use and at a level where the top opening can be seen. Needles should not project from the top of the container.
4. **Never** try to take anything out of a needle box. If a needle will not go in easily and the box is not full, use a large

FIGURE 1-6 Samples of easily recognized rigid, puncture-resistant disposable containers with a lid and clearly marked as a biohazard.

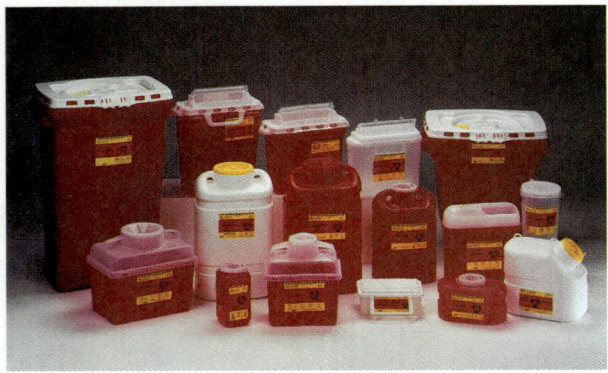

syringe to dislodge it. Do not push or force items with your hands. If the box is full, arrange to have it replaced.

5. Place the cover to close and seal the sharps container when it is three-fourths full and dispose of the container as infectious waste. No additional protective garb is necessary for handling these containers. One method of disposing of full sharps containers is to place the full container in a brown cardboard box labeled "Infectious Waste and Biohazard" and marked with the biohazard symbol. This box is lined with plastic sheeting or a strong, red plastic bag marked "Biohazardous Material." The disposal box should be located in a centralized, authorized area. A contract scavenger company should then pick up the sealed boxes and deliver them to an incineration company on a weekly basis.

6. Pick up improperly discarded needles with extreme caution and dispose of them in the nearest sharps container. Do not attempt to cap the needle. Wash your hands after you dispose of the needle. Use tongs or forceps to pick up the sharps.

7. *Never* purposely bend or break by hand a used needle. *Never* recap a used needle unless absolutely necessary or in approved special circumstances (for example, in drawing blood for blood gases). To recap Vacutainer needles, put the cap on the table and slide the needle into it without holding the cap. Then tighten the cap at the needle hub (see Figure 7-24).

8. *Never* remove a used needle from a used disposable syringe (*except* as discussed in No. 10).

9. *Never* put a used needle into your pocket.

10. Wear gloves when doing laboratory work in which a needle needs to be removed from a syringe. Discard the gloves immediately if they become contaminated with blood. It is preferable to use a needle disposal container that has an integral device for removing needles without necessitating touching the needles with your hands.

11. Discard Vacutainer sleeves in the sharps container at the end of each day or when they are soiled with blood.

12. Place *reusable sharps* in a suitable puncture-resistant container after use and take them to the decontamination area, where they are cleaned and disinfected or sterilized. Wear

protective garb such as gowns, aprons, gloves, and face protection while cleaning up.

Laboratory Specimens

To control the spread of infection and to protect the health of employees, patients, and the public, all laboratory specimens should be handled and transported according to the following procedures:

1. Specimens of blood or other potentially infectious materials must be placed in a container that prevents leakage during collection, handling, processing, storage, transport, or shipping.

2. Laboratory specimens should be contained for transport. Special secure, stiff, impermeable containers such as the Igloo-type containers should be used by messenger service personnel when transporting blood and other body fluids from the office or clinic to a laboratory. Specimen containers may be placed in test tube racks, then in the secure transport container. Some facilities also demand that the specimen be placed in a Ziploc or other hand-sealed plastic bag and sealed shut before being placed in the secure transport container for delivery to the laboratory. If the specimen container is too large to fit in a sealable plastic bag, the cap can be secured with tape and the entire item enclosed in a plastic bag with a twist tie. The laboratory work slip should be attached by rubber band or tape to the *outside* of the bag.

    Specimen mailers must have a metal inner container and a rigid outer container to comply with CDC regulations (see Figures 11-2 and 11-3).

3. The container for storage, transport, or shipping must be labeled or color coded according to federal standards and closed before being stored, transported, or shipped.

4. If outside contamination of the primary container occurs, the primary container must be placed within a second container that prevents leakage during handling, processing, storage, transport, or shipping and is labeled or color coded according to the requirements of OSHA standards.

5. All blood or body fluid specimens must be centrifuged in carriers with safety domes. The carrier and dome must be decontaminated according to the manufacturer's direction. Human tissue, blood, body secretions and excretions, or other specimens and cultures should be autoclaved before they are disposed of in a sanitary landfill.

6. Gloves should be used for handling laboratory specimens when contamination of the hands is anticipated. Care must be taken when collecting specimens to avoid contamination of the outside of the container or the laboratory slip. Disposable gloves should be worn and urine specimens disposed of in a toilet or utility sink and feces disposed of into toilets that empty into a sewer system. Sinks should then be rinsed thoroughly and toilets flushed. (To avoid cross-contamination, this sink should *not* be used for other activities such as preparing clean supplies or supplying drinking water. Other sinks should be used for routine handwashing.) Specimen containers and gloves should be disposed of in a closed waste container lined with a strong plastic or vinyl bag marked "Biohazardous Waste."

7. Hands must be washed after handling all specimens and after removing gloves. Hands and other skin surfaces contaminated with blood or other body fluids must be washed immediately and thoroughly. When procedures have been completed or if a specimen is spilled, laboratory work surfaces must be decontaminated with a disinfectant such as a 1:10 dilution of sodium hypochlorite (household bleach) or Staphene germicide solution.

8. All potentially contaminated materials used in laboratory tests should be decontaminated, preferably by steam sterilization, before disposal or reprocessing. All infectious laboratory waste should be treated by steam sterilization, incineration, or disinfection before disposal to render the waste harmless.

Promptly contact your supervisor when you have been exposed to blood or other body fluids.

Reusable Equipment

As soon as possible, if appropriate, all used reusable equipment not classified as sharps should be placed in an Environmental Protection Agency (EPA)–registered and approved detergent/disinfectant/germicide and transported to the decontamination area. Items that require sterilization or high-level disinfection first must be thoroughly cleaned and decontaminated. Cleaning and decontamination should be done by personnel wearing gloves, gown, and face protection. Each facility must develop cleaning and decontamination procedures appropriate to its needs.

Blood pressure equipment, scales, and other reusable room equipment should be decontaminated with a disinfectant solution at the end of each day. Stethoscope earpieces must be cleaned after each use with an alcohol swab. Tonometers must be disinfected with alcohol swabs, rinsed thoroughly in clean water, and then left to air-dry or be dried with a clean nonlint material after *each* use. When visibly soiled or at least weekly, centrifuges should be cleaned with 70% alcohol swabs or disposable cloths soaked in 70% alcohol or other EPA-registered solution mixed according to the product's directions. Tourniquets can be soaked in a 1:10 dilution of 5% sodium hypochlorite solution for 15 minutes. Bloodstained tourniquets must be discarded. After each use, goggles and heavy rubber gloves used during decontamination procedures must be decontaminated with alcohol. After each use, brushes and buckets or basins used for decontamination procedures must be decontaminated with a detergent solution, rinsed, and then placed in an area specifically designated for such supplies. This equipment should be sterilized weekly.

Broken Glassware

Broken glassware that might be contaminated must not be picked up directly with the hands. It must be cleaned up, using mechanical means such as a brush and dust pan, tongs, or forceps, and then disposed of in a puncture-resistant container that is labeled or color coded to indicate that it is for contaminated sharps.

Tissues, Body Fluids, and Cultures

- Patient specimens and the containers that hold them should be collected and treated as infectious waste.

- Cultures and the containers that hold them should be collected and treated as infectious waste.
- Human tissues or body parts should be treated as infectious waste.
- Large volumes of blood or drainage such as that from suction machines should be flushed down the sewer or disposed of in collection containers and treated as infectious waste.
- Used disposable dialysis equipment should be treated as infectious waste.
- Large volumes of urine, stool, or dialysate should be flushed down the sewer with appropriate precautions to guard against spillage.

Before being transported for disposal, infectious waste must be held in covered or bagged, leakproof waste containers. It must be collected in identifiable containers or bags for transportation to a separate disposal site. If disposal cans without working lids are used, moist trash must be bagged before it is placed in an open can. All trash containers must have a liner thick enough to withstand necessary handling, and they must be tied closed when disposed. Waste containers should be cleaned weekly with a disinfectant solution.

Other Waste

All other waste such as paper towels and packaging materials should be placed in regular waste containers lined with plastic or vinyl liners strong or thick enough to withstand necessary handling. For convenience, small items such as contaminated cotton balls may be disposed of in the sharps container. Other disposable moist waste generated by clinics or offices should be collected in *covered* foot-operated cans that are lined with moisture-proof bags. When removed, the bags should be closed, not emptied, and disposed of as ordinary waste.

Each waste container liner must be removed as a single unit and tied shut without turning the container upside down to consolidate waste. Waste containers must be strong enough to resist tears and leaks under normal handling. Final disposal of waste is by approval of the local health officers and includes incineration, autoclaving, sewer system, or sanitary landfill.

Surfaces

- When body fluids are spilled, the visible material should be removed from surfaces followed by decontamination processes with an approved disinfectant, such as a 1:10 dilution of sodium hypochlorite (household bleach) or Bytech solution. Gloves must be worn for this process.
- Spills should be cleaned up promptly. Large spills should be cleaned up by a gloved employee, using paper towels, which should be placed in an infectious waste container (Figure 1-7). Then 5.25% sodium hypochlorite (household bleach) diluted 1:10 should be used to disinfect the area. Sodium hypochlorite should not be placed directly on large amounts of protein matter (for example, urine, stool, blood, sputum) to protect the employee from noxious fumes. A 1:10 dilution of bleach may be ordered for the office or clinic from a hospital pharmacy.
- Laboratory work surfaces should be decontaminated with a disinfectant such as a 1:10 dilution of sodium

FIGURE 1-7   Spills of body fluids must be cleaned up by a gloved employee, using paper towels, which should then be placed in an infectious waste container. Afterward, 5.25% sodium hypochlorite (household bleach) diluted 1:10 should be used to disinfect the area.

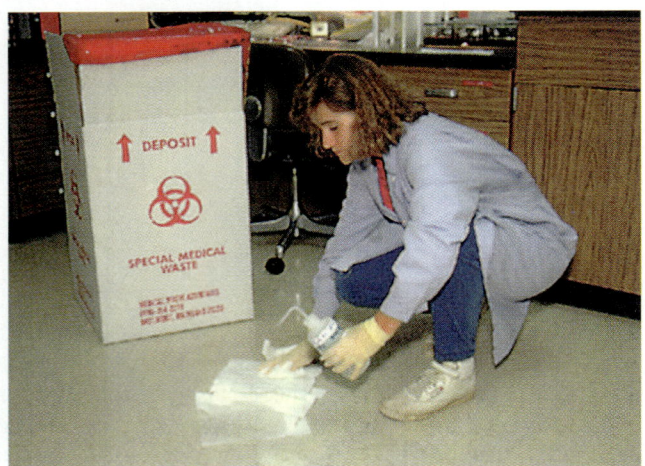

FIGURE 1-8   Contaminated laundry should be placed and transported in bags or containers labeled or color-coded.

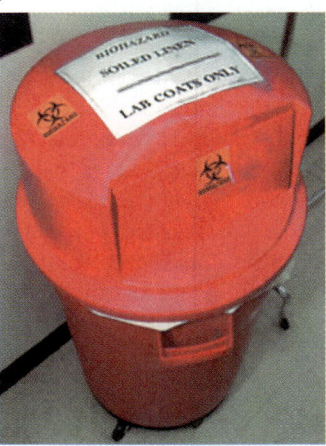

hypochlorite or Staphene germicide solution at the completion of work activities or in the event of a specimen spill.

- Regular cleaning of diapering areas is recommended because of the potential for fecal-orally transmitted agents.
- Environmental surfaces in patient care areas should be cleaned with an approved disinfectant weekly and as needed.
- Periodic cleaning of the clinic or office environment is good housekeeping rather than an infection control concern.
- Materials used for cleanup should be disposed of in a covered, moist-infectious-waste container.
- Covers on examination tables and Mayo stands must be changed after each patient.
- At the end of the day, examination tables, counters, Mayo stands, and other equipment should be decontaminated with a disinfectant solution (for example, LpH or other EPA-registered solution).
- Supply closets should be dusted and cleaned at least monthly, using a rag saturated with 70% alcohol to wipe the shelves, then allowing the shelves to air-dry. The door to the room should be left open while this procedure is in progress to avoid any side effects from fumes.
- Janitorial staff must be taught how to handle and dispose of ordinary, contaminated, and infectious waste.

Universal Spills

Blood and body substances and rebag or collection vessels containing potentially virulent body fluids spilled on floors or work surfaces necessitate quick action. A universal spill kit or treatment system gives medical assistants quick access to protection and containment of the spill. It should contain fog-free goggles and clear safety glasses with side shields, gowns, masks, antimicrobial towels, and disposal bags. Liquid treatment systems may use microencapsulated technology that converts the liquid spill into a solid treated waste product that can be incinerated or disposed of in landfills. They are biodegradable, nontoxic, and nonflammable. All supplies should be in a readily accessible location and replenished promptly after use.

Mercury Spills

Uncontained mercury (Hg) emits dangerous mercury vapors. A broken mercury sphygmomanometer or thermometer must be quickly and safely cleaned up to prevent toxic vapor contamination. A mercury spill kit includes sponges, towels, liquid, or wipes containing a powder coating that consumes its own weight in mercury and is used to decontaminate an area after a mercury spill and to amalgamate small mercury droplets. The resulting amalgam will not emit dangerous mercury vapors. The powder also converts elemental mercury on work surfaces, cracks, and other hard-to-reach areas in a mercury amalgam. For detecting mercury presence, a mercury indicator powder changes color overnight (for example, yellow to brown), when it comes in contact with mercury metal or vapor. It is sprinkled over surfaces suspected to contain mercury droplets and reduces the concentration of mercury vapor remaining in inaccessible areas after cleanup of spills. Gloves, eyewear, and personal protection equipment, including a mercury vapor chlorine respirator to protect against mercury vapor concentrations, are other important considerations in ensuring proper handling of mercury. A mercury recovery disposal bag safely contains the mercury and everything used to safely clean up mercury spills.

To avoid possible hazardous mercury spills, electronic/digital and tympanic clinical thermometers or aneroid sphygmomanometers can replace the mercurial type.

UNIFORMS AND CLOTHING

Uniforms and clothing that are soiled with body secretions should be cleaned with soap and cool water and washed, following normal laundering procedures. Clothing with large amounts of contaminates or that has been penetrated should be changed immediately or as soon as possible.

LAUNDRY

1. Contaminated laundry should be handled as little as possible, with a minimum of agitation.

TABLE 1–1   Labeling Requirements

Item	No Label Needed		Biohazard Label		Red Container
Regulated waste bags			X	and	X
Sharp containers (disposable and/or reusable)			X		
Refrigerator/freezer holding blood or other potentially infectious material			X		
Containers used for storage, transport, or shipping of blood or OPIM			X	or	X
Blood/blood products for clinical use	No labels required				
Individual specimen containers of blood or other potentially infectious materials remaining in facility	X*	or	X	or	X
Contaminated equipment needing service (e.g., dialysis equipment, suction apparatus)			X		
			Plus a label specifying where the contamination exists		
Specimens and regulated waste shipped from the primary facility to another facility for service or disposal			X		
Contaminated laundry	X*	or	X	or	X
Contaminated laundry sent to another facility that does not use Universal/Standard Precautions			X	or	X

*No label needed if Universal/Standard Precautions are used and specific use of container or item is known to all employees.

OPIM, Other potentially infectious material.

a. Contaminated laundry should be bagged or container-ized without sorting or rinsing it at the location where it was used.

b. Contaminated laundry should be placed and transported in labeled or color-coded bags or containers (Figure 1-8). When a facility uses Universal/Standard Precautions in the handling of all soiled laundry, alternative labeling or color coding may be used if all employees recognize the containers as complying with Universal/Standard Precautions.

c. Whenever contaminated laundry is wet and presents a reasonable likelihood of soaking through or leaking from the bag or container, the laundry should be placed and transported in bags or containers that prevent leakage.

2. The employer must ensure that employees who have contact with contaminated laundry wear protective gloves and other appropriate personal protective equipment.

3. When a facility ships contaminated laundry off-site to a second facility that does not use Universal/Standard Precautions in all laundry handling, the facility generating the contaminated laundry must place such laundry in labeled or color-coded bags or containers.

COMMUNICATION OF HAZARDS TO EMPLOYEES

Labels (Table 1-1)

- Warning labels must be affixed to containers of regulated waste; refrigerators and freezers containing blood or other potentially infectious material; and other containers used

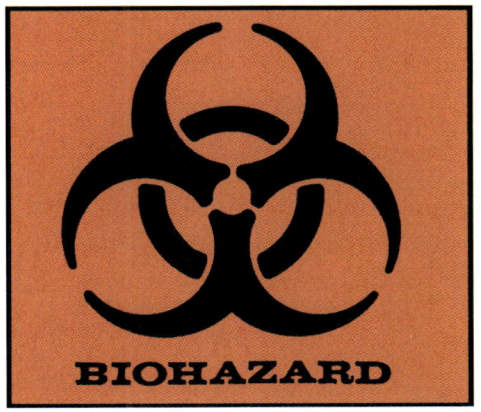

FIGURE 1-9   Biohazard label.

to store, transport, or ship blood or other potentially infectious materials, except as stated below.

- Labels required by this standard must include the legend "BIOHAZARD" (Figure 1-9).
- The labels must be fluorescent orange or orange-red or predominantly so, with lettering or symbols in a contrasting color.
- Labels required must be affixed as close as feasible to the container by string, wire, adhesive, or other method that prevents their loss or unintentional removal.
- Red bags or red containers may be substituted for labels.
- Individual containers of blood or other potentially infectious materials that are placed in a labeled container during storage, transport, shipment, or disposal are exempt from the labeling requirement.

- Labels necessary for contaminated equipment must be in accordance with this paragraph and must also state which portion of the equipment remains contaminated.
- Regulated waste that has been decontaminated does not need to be labeled or color coded.

Signs

- The employer must post signs at the entrance of work areas specified as HIV and HBV Research Laboratory and Production Facilities. These signs must bear the legend "BIOHAZARD" and state the name of the infectious agent; the special requirements for entering the area; and the name and telephone number of the laboratory director or other responsible person.
- These signs must be fluorescent orange-red or predominately so, with lettering or symbols in a contrasting color.

Disposal

In the physician's office or clinic, a registered hazardous waste company picks up waste containers for proper disposal according to the standards set by the law. A qualified company can be found by asking another employee or looking in the yellow pages of your telephone book under "WASTE DISPOSAL—MEDICAL AND INFECTIOUS." Methods of treatment of medical waste are specified by law. Biohazardous waste cannot be disposed of without prior treatment, which is both costly and complicated.

COMPLIANCE

Universal/Standard Precautions must be observed to prevent contact with blood or other potentially infectious materials. Under circumstances in which it is difficult or impossible to differentiate between body fluid types, all body fluids must be considered potentially infectious materials.

EMPLOYEE HEALTH ISSUES

Needlesticks, Mucous Membrane, or Conjunctival Exposure to Body Fluids From All Patients

All needlesticks and other exposures to body fluids from patients must be reported to the physician and to the Employee Health Service if working at a hospital clinic. An accident report should be filled out. The employee is evaluated for hepatitis B and C and HIV exposure and treated accordingly. Hepatitis B immune globulin (HBIG) and the hepatitis B vaccine (unless contraindicated for medical reasons) are given as a part of this protocol. An employee with exposure must receive counseling by the physician or Employee Health Service and information regarding the availability of antibody testing and postexposure prophylaxis (see also Chapter 7) for those who wish it (Figure 1-10).

FIGURE 1-10   OSHA's hepatitis B postexposure follow-up procedures. This form could be adapted for a health care facility's procedural manual.

OSHA's hepatitis B postexposure follow-up procedures. This form could be adapted for a health care facility's procedural manual.

Postexposure Evaluation and Follow-up

All exposure incidents shall be reported, investigated, and documented. When the employee incurs an exposure incident, it shall be reported to (list who has responsibility for investigating exposure incident): _____.

Following a report of an exposure incident, the exposed employee shall immediately receive a confidential medical evaluation and follow-up, including at least the following elements:

   a.   Documentation of the route of exposure, and the circumstances under which the exposure incident occurred;

   b.   Identification and documentation of the source individual, unless it can be established that the identification is infeasible or prohibited by state or local law. (Employers may need to modify this in accordance with applicable local laws on this subject. Modifications should be listed here: _____)

   c.   The source individual's blood shall be tested as soon as feasible and after consent is obtained, in order to determine Bloodborne Pathogens infectivity. If consent is not obtained, the (insert name of position/person) _____ shall establish that legally required consent is not required by law, the source individual's blood, if available, shall be tested and the results documented.

   d.   When the source individual is already known to be infected with HBV or HIV, testing for the source individual's known HBV or HIV status need not be repeated.

FIGURE 1-10—cont'd   OSHA's hepatitis B postexposure follow-up procedures. This form could be adapted for a health care facility's procedural manual.

e.   Results of the source individual's testing shall be made available to the exposed employee, and the employee shall be informed of applicable laws and regulations concerning disclosure of the identity and infectious status of the source individual.

Collection and testing of blood for HBV and HIV serological status will comply with the following:

a.   The exposed employee's blood shall be collected as soon as feasible and tested after consent is obtained;

b.   The employee will be offered the option of having their blood collected for testing for HIV/HBV serological status. The blood sample will be preserved for up to 90 days to allow the employee to decide if the blood should be tested for HIV serological status.

All employees who incur an exposure incident will be offered postexposure evaluation and follow-up in accordance with the state's OSHA standard. All postexposure follow-up will be performed by (insert name of clinic, physician, department) _____.

Information Provided to the Health Care Professional

The (insert name of position/person) _____ shall ensure that the health care professional responsible for the employee's hepatitis B vaccination and evaluating an employee after an exposure incident is provided the following additional information:

a.   A copy of OSHA's Bloodborne Pathogens Standard (while the standard outlines the confidentiality requirements of the health care professional, it might be helpful for the employer to remind that individual of these requirements).

b.   A written description of the exposed employee's duties as they relate to the exposure incident;

c.   Written documentation of the route of exposure and circumstances under which exposure occurred;

d.   Results of the source individuals blood testing, if available; and

e.   All medical records relevant to the appropriate treatment of the employee including vaccination status.

Health Care Professional's Written Opinion

The (insert name of position/person) _____ shall obtain and provide the employee with a copy of the evaluating health care professional's written opinion within 15 days of the completion of the evaluation.

The health care professional's written opinion for HBV vaccination and postexposure follow-up shall be limited to the following information:

a.   Whether vaccination is indicated for the employee and if the employee has received such vaccination;

b.   A statement that the employee has been informed of the results of the evaluation; and

c.   A statement that the employee has been told about any medical conditions resulting from exposure to blood or other potentially infectious materials that require further evaluation or treatment.

Note: All other findings or diagnoses shall remain confidential and shall not be included in the written report.

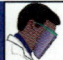

PROCEDURE 1-1

PRECAUTIONS FOR OTHER DISEASES THAT *MAY* BE SEEN IN AIDS PATIENTS

PROCEDURE	RATIONALE
Cytomegalovirus (CMV)	
1. Women trying to become pregnant should use very good personal hygiene (handwashing and gloves) with any body secretions from any patient.	*Many AIDS patients excrete CMV. Because CMV may cause birth defects, it is advisable for pregnant women not to have direct contact with known excretors. Although good hygiene has been shown to prevent acquisition of CMV, pregnant women should be extremely cautious in the care of any patient because not all CMV excretors are identified. Handwashing is extremely important after any patient or body fluid contact.*
Opportunistic and Other Infections	
1. Masks (worn by others in the room when the patient cannot wear a mask) when the patient has an undiagnosed pulmonary process and is coughing and when others have sustained close contact (until tuberculosis is excluded).	*Until the patient's respiratory illness is diagnosed, others need to be protected from diseases spread by the respiratory route. Immunocompetent persons need protection from Mycobacterium tuberculosis. Immunocompromised persons need protection from Mycobacterium avium and Pneumocystis. Although some AIDS patients have CMV in their lungs, it is not known if CMV can be transmitted by the respiratory route.*
2. Other precautions should be as usual for the particular disease. See an Infection Control Manual for guidance.	*There is no evidence that the AIDS virus is spread by the respiratory route. However, because tuberculosis is a cause of pulmonary disease in a small percentage of cases, masks are a prudent precaution until tuberculosis is excluded.*

Individuals With Immunosuppression

Individuals with immunosuppression as a result of disease or therapy should evaluate, with their personal physicians, their own risk of working in a hospital environment. If these individuals think they are at risk, they should provide a letter from their physician to their supervisor indicating their ability to work and outlining any patient care areas in which they should not work.

Employees With AIDS

Employees with AIDS should be handled on a case-by-case basis by an Employee Health physician in consultation with an AIDS Clinic physician. The final decision regarding work assignment is made by the Infection Control Committee using advice from Employee Health and AIDS Clinic physicians on a case-by-case basis, taking into account the safety of all employees and patients. Generally, asymptomatic office, clinic, or hospital employees with AIDS who have recovered from an intercurrent illness may return to work. They should be instructed about health care precautions such as handwashing and wearing gloves for contact with mucous membranes or nonintact skin of patients. Any employee with exudative or weeping (that is, moist) skin lesions should be reassigned to nonpatient care areas. Evaluation of such employees is by the physician or the Employee Health Service of the hospital.

In situations in which it is not advisable for employees with AIDS to return to their clinical assignment, reassignment to another area should be coordinated with their supervisors.

Cardiopulmonary Resuscitation

Devices to protect employees from mucous membrane contact with blood and other secretions during any resuscitation should be made readily available. Ambu bags (see Figure 1-5), face masks, or pocket masks should be located on all crash carts and are to be used in preference to mouth-to-mouth resuscitation on all patients.

Cardiopulmonary resuscitation (CPR) recertification standards should be maintained. Because studies have shown that low levels of HIV can be found in oral fluids, especially when visible blood is present, employees with AIDS should not participate in manikin CPR training. For the protection of all CPR participants, in two-person CPR, the second rescuer simulates ventilation, and a solution of bleach is used to decontaminate the manikin's face and mouth between all participants.

NOTE: Precautions beyond those recommended should be avoided because their use does not afford additional protection and may interfere with patient care. Health care providers should be well informed about the ways in which HIV and other infectious diseases are transmitted and follow precautions appropriate for their protection. Use of excessive precautions by health care providers conveys misinformation to patients and other employees about the mode of transmission and appropriate precautions.

HEALTH MATTERS

OCCUPATIONAL EXPOSURE TO HIV*

Health care workers are at risk for occupational exposure to the human immunodeficiency virus (HIV). Exposures occur through needlesticks or cuts from other sharp instruments (percutaneous exposures) contaminated with an infected patient's blood or through contact of the eye, nose, mouth (mucous membrane), or skin with a patient's blood.

Most exposures do not result in infection. The risk of infection varies with the type of exposure and factors, such as:

- The amount of blood involved in the exposure
- The amount of virus in the patient's blood at the time of exposure
- Whether postexposure treatment was taken

Your employer should have in place a system for reporting exposures to *quickly* evaluate the risk of infection from the exposure, counsel you about recommendations for treatments available to prevent infection, monitor you for side effects of treatments, and determine if infection occurs. This may involve testing your blood and that of the source patient and offering appropriate postexposure treatment. (See Figure 1-10; see also Figures 7-25 and 7-26.)

IF AN EXPOSURE TO BLOOD OCCURS

1. Immediately following an exposure to blood:
- **Needlesticks and cuts** should be washed with soap and water.
- Splashes to the **nose, mouth,** or **skin** should be flushed with water.
- **Eyes** should be irrigated with clean water, saline, or sterile irrigants.

No scientific evidence shows that the use of antiseptics for wound care or squeezing the wound will reduce the risk of transmission of HIV. The use of a caustic agent such as bleach is not recommended.

2. Following any blood exposure you should:
- Report the exposure to the department (for example, occupational health, infection control) responsible for managing exposures. **Prompt reporting is essential because, in some cases, HIV postexposure treatment may be recommended and it should be started as soon as possible—preferably within 1 to 2 hours.**
- *In addition to HIV, discuss the possible risks of acquiring hepatitis B and hepatitis C with your health care provider.* You should have already received hepatitis B vaccine, which is extremely safe and effective in preventing hepatitis B.

RISK OF INFECTION AFTER EXPOSURE

Although the risk is very low, it is not zero. HIV infection has been reported after occupational exposures to HIV-infected blood through needlesticks or cuts; splashes in the eyes, nose, or mouth; and skin contact.

- Exposures from **needlesticks** or **cuts** cause most infections. The average risk of HIV infection after a needlestick or cut exposure to HIV-infected blood is 0.3% (that is, three-tenths of 1%, or about 1 in 300). Stated another way, 99.7% of needlestick or cut exposures do **not** lead to infection.
- The risk after exposure of the **eye, nose,** or **mouth** to HIV-infected blood is estimated to be, on average, 0.1% (1 in 1000).
- The risk after exposure of the **skin** to HIV-infected blood is estimated to be less than 0.1%. A small amount of blood on intact skin probably poses no risk at all. There have been no cases of HIV transmission documented as caused by an exposure involving a small amount of blood on intact skin. The risk may be higher if the skin is damaged (for example, by a recent cut) or if the contact involves a large area of skin or is prolonged.

Risk from all exposures is probably increased if the exposure involves a larger volume of blood or a higher amount of HIV in the patient's blood. (Source patients near death with AIDS or patients with symptoms of acute HIV infection usually have higher amounts of HIV in their blood.)

EXPOSURES TO BLOOD FOR WHICH THE HIV STATUS OF THE SOURCE PATIENT IS UNKNOWN

If the source individual cannot be identified or tested, decisions regarding follow-up should be based on the exposure risk and whether the source is likely to be a person who is HIV positive. Follow-up HIV testing should be available to all workers who are concerned about possible HIV infection through occupational exposure.

Treatments Available

Studies suggest that postexposure treatment with certain antiviral drugs may prevent infection with HIV. Several new antiviral drugs have been licensed for use in the United States. The Public Health Service recommendations are continually reviewed and may be modified, taking into account the availability of additional drugs. However, postexposure treatment will probably not prevent all cases of infection transmission.

Follow-up That Should Be Done After Exposure

- You should be tested for HIV antibody as soon as possible after exposure (baseline) and periodically for at least 6 months after the exposure (for example, at 6 weeks, 12 weeks, and 6 months).
- If you take antiviral drugs for postexposure treatment, you should be checked for drug toxicity, including a complete blood count and kidney and liver function tests, just before starting treatment and 2 weeks after starting treatment.
- You should report any sudden or severe flulike illness that occurs during the follow-up period, especially if it involves fever,

*U. S. Department of Health and Human Services, Public Health Service, CDC.

HEALTH MATTERS—continued

rash, muscle aches, tiredness, malaise, or swollen glands. Such an illness or symptoms may suggest HIV infection, drug reaction, or other medical conditions.

- You should contact your health care provider if you have any questions or problems during the follow-up period.

Precautions That Should Be Taken During the Follow-up Period

During the follow-up period, especially the first 6 to 12 weeks when most infected persons are expected to show signs of infection, you should follow recommendations for preventing transmission of HIV. These include refraining from blood, semen, or organ donation and abstaining from sexual intercourse. If you choose to have sexual intercourse, using a latex condom consistently and correctly may reduce the risk of HIV transmission. In addition, women should not breastfeed infants during the follow-up period to prevent exposing their infants to HIV in breast milk.

HIV OCCUPATIONAL EXPOSURE REGISTRY

Because information is limited about the side effects or toxicity of antiviral drugs in uninfected people, the Centers for Disease Control and Prevention, Glaxo Wellcome Inc., and Merck & Co., Inc., have begun the **HIV Postexposure Prophylaxis (PEP) Registry** to collect information about the safety, tolerability, and outcome of taking antiviral drugs for postexposure treatment.

If you give permission, your health care provider will provide information to the Registry about the exposure, the antiviral drugs taken, and abnormal laboratory findings and physical symptoms associated with the use of these drugs. **Participation is voluntary and confidential. No information that would identify you will be collected.**

Ask your health care provider; he or she can obtain information about the Registry by calling toll-free: 1-888-PEP4HIV (1-888-737-4448).

HIV INFECTION/HIV DISEASE/AIDS

The CDC first defined AIDS in 1982. With incomplete scientific understanding at the time, AIDS was thought of as an immune disorder of unknown origin that led to the development of certain life-threatening opportunistic diseases. As time went on, other diseases were added to the initial list, and a distinction was made between the more and less severe conditions. As research continued, the HIV was isolated, and researchers described the life cycle of the virus, including the latency period during which infection caused by the HIV progresses silently. This led to a critical change in how the scientific community thought of and referred to AIDS. AIDS is now referred to as the later stage of *HIV disease*; the designations *asymptomatic seropositive, symptomatic HIV disease,* and *AIDS* are stages of HIV infection and *not* totally different entities. The new definition of AIDS is clearly associated to the direct role of the HIV in the development of disease(s). Attention is now on the direct effects of the virus on the immune system health rather than on the physical manifestations of these effects. Disease starts at the time of infection, and the virus is active, even if symptoms are not apparent. Because viral activity is better understood, medical treatment can be started earlier. Early intervention has been shown to slow viral activity and disease progression. Early intervention is defined as starting therapy before any symptoms appear and definitely before the onset of AIDS. This prolongs survival and *quality,* symptom-free and disease-free time for HIV-infected people.

HIV Disease

HIV disease is caused by the virus known as human immunodeficiency virus. When the virus gets into a person's bloodstream, the person is HIV infected. The body produces antibodies in response to this invasion and then can be referred to as HIV antibody positive. HIV disease attacks several types of

cells in a person's immune system, especially the T cells. The immune system is the body system that helps protect the body against disease by producing antibodies against foreign substances (antigens) (see also Figure 2-3, page 38). When the immune system is weakened, the body loses its ability to fight common infections. Some illnesses can become life threatening and may even be fatal.

HIV disease refers to all stages of HIV infection

1. *Asymptomatic HIV disease.* This is the earliest stage of infection. The only indication of this stage of HIV infection is a positive HIV antibody blood test. Antibodies to the HIV can be found in the bloodstream usually from 3 to 6 months from the time the person was infected with the HIV. The person is presumed to be infected with the virus when antibodies are present. It is also assumed that the person can pass the virus on to others through the usual routes of transmission. Most people show no signs of illness at this time.
2. *Symptomatic HIV disease.* This is the middle stage of infection. Many people in this stage experience mild to severe physical symptoms that can't be explained by any other illness. Examples include swollen lymph glands at two or more sites in the body, persistent fever, diarrhea, and skin problems.
3. *AIDS.* This is the later stages of the disease when the immune system has been severely damaged by the HIV and can no longer fight some infections. People in this stage may develop one or more opportunistic infections, life-threatening diseases, or other diseases listed in the following paragraphs.

It is very important to understand the difference between being HIV antibody positive and having AIDS. The **incubation**

period for both stages 2 and 3 could be from several months to 10 years and as long as 15 years.

Broadened Definition of AIDS

CDC revised the definition of AIDS in 1985 and 1987 and now again to include the following:

1. People who are HIV positive **and** who have at least one of the 26 reportable opportunistic diseases or other serious diseases. These diseases include:
   a. Kaposi's sarcoma (KS): A sarcoma (cancer) affecting tissues beneath the skin and the mucus-secreting surfaces of the gastrointestinal tract, lymph nodes, and lungs.
   b. *Pneumocystis carinii* pneumonia (PCP): A pneumonia caused by a protozoan.
   c. Cryptococcosis: A fungal infection that may attack the brain, lungs, liver, intestinal tract, and skin.
   d. Non-Hodgkin's lymphoma: A cancer affecting the lymph nodes.
   e. Candidiasis: A yeast infection that may be seen in the mouth, anus, genital region, and other areas of the body.
   f. Herpes simplex: A viral infection that may cause blisters or eruptions on the face, buttocks, anus, or genitals.
   g. Cytomegalovirus (CMV): A viral infection that often has symptoms similar to infectious mononucleosis or may produce no symptoms at all. In the person with AIDS, it can lead to serious infections, including pneumonia.
   h. Toxoplasmosis: A parasitic infection that may involve the brain and cause central nervous system disorders. It commonly shows symptoms of malaise and the flu.
   i. HIV dementia: HIV infection of the brain that may cause personality disintegration, confusion, disorientation, deterioration of intellectual capacity and function, and impairment of memory and judgment.
   j. Progressive multifocal leukoencephalopathy (PML): This affects the coating of the nerve cells in the brain.
   k. *Mycobacterium avium* complex (MAC): A bacterial infection.
   l. HIV-related wasting syndrome.
   m. Pulmonary tuberculosis: An infection of the lung(s).
   n. Recurrent pneumonia: An infection in the lung(s).
   o. Invasive cervical cancer: Seen in females.
2. **All** people who are HIV positive with fewer than 200 T cells per cubic millimeter of blood *even if they do not have an opportunistic infection.*

Physicians consider a T-cell level of less than 200 to be a danger sign for getting an AIDS-related disease, so it is included in the definition of AIDS. The T cells (also called a T4 cell, a CD4 cell, or a helper cell) help the body fight infections. In a person who is HIV positive, the HIV virus gets into the person's T cells and destroys them. The normal range for T cells is thought to be above 500 cells per cubic millimeter of blood. A *T-cell count* is only one of several important tests that can help the physician determine the health of a person who has been diagnosed as HIV positive. Three other tests are available to help measure immune health or reflect the progress of HIV infection. One is the *beta-2 microglobulin test*, which measures the rate at which cells are dying and being replaced by new ones. The higher the number, the greater the degree of cell death. As HIV disease progresses to AIDS, this number goes up. A normal beta-2 number is around 2. A beta-2 number of 4 or 5 is typical of a person who is nearing or already has the diagnosis of AIDS.

A second test is the *p24 antigen test,* which measures the level of the protein p24 in the blood. This protein is produced by HIV. People who have been infected for a long time usually have significant levels of p24 and are thought to be at a greater risk of progressing to AIDS, but this is not always the case. Some people with AIDS never test positive to p24 because in the first few months it may be masked by the presence of HIV antibodies; thus this test does not always predict what will occur in an individual. The p24 test is used to test donated blood because it appears in the early stages of infection.

A third test that can be used to determine *immune health* is the *p24 antibody test.* Having a considerable level of p24 antibody is considered a good sign that the virus is more or less under control, thereby slowing down the action of the HIV. When levels of the p24 antibody drop, it is thought to be a sign that the person is moving closer to AIDS and that the virus is becoming more active.

Despite the new broadened definition of AIDS, many believe that it still *does not* give us a total picture of the size of the epidemic because it still does not include some of the serious diseases that HIV-positive women and children can get.

HIV Transmission

A person can become infected with HIV in the following ways:

1. Having unprotected vaginal, anal, or oral sexual intercourse with a person infected with HIV. The virus can be transmitted through semen or vaginal fluids.
2. Sharing an intravenous drug needle with an HIV-infected person. The virus can be transmitted to the needle user, injecting infected blood into the bloodstream.
3. Mother-to-child transmission. An HIV-positive woman can transmit the virus to the unborn baby through the placenta; to the baby during birth; or after birth, through infected breast milk.

   NOTE: Infants born to HIV-infected mothers will test positive for the HIV *antibodies.* About 25% to 30% of these infants are actually HIV infected; the others have only their mother's antibodies, *not* the virus. The antibodies from the mother will disappear from the infant's blood by about 15 months of age. Special tests can be done to identify which children actually have HIV infection. If these tests are not available, some physicians recommend medical treatment for all antibody-positive infants.

HEALTH MATTERS

KEEPING YOUR PATIENTS INFORMED

TESTING THE BLOOD SUPPLY

Q. **What is the risk of contracting HIV-1 from the U.S. blood supply? Is there a way to get 100% safe blood?**

A. The American Red Cross uses both an HIV-1/HIV-2 "combination" antibody EIA and a HIV p24 antigen screening test for all donated blood. The risk of contracting HIV-1 from the U.S. blood supply is between 1 in 450,000 units to 1 in 660,000 units. The only way to ensure 100% safe blood is for persons to bank their own for future use.

For more information, contact:
American Association of Blood Banks
8101 Glenbrook Road
Bethesda, MD 20814
(301) 907-6977

American Red Cross
Blood Donation Hotline
1-800-GIVE-BLOOD

CDC National AIDS Clearinghouse.

Clinical trials using zidovudine (AZT) for reducing perinatal HIV transmission indicated a two-thirds decrease in mother-to-fetus transmission rates.

4. Transfusions with infected blood or blood products. However, since late spring of 1985, all blood donations have been screened for HIV antibodies, and donors are also screened for risk factors to ensure that this method of transmission does not occur. **No one can get HIV by donating blood.**

5. Accidental contact with HIV-contaminated blood or body fluids by health care providers as discussed previously.

HIV DISEASE IS NOT TRANSMITTED THROUGH CASUAL CONTACT SUCH AS CLOSE PROXIMITY, TOUCHING, OR SNEEZING.

Signs and Symptoms of HIV Disease

The following are signs and symptoms that an HIV-positive person may experience, *but* they also could be signs and symptoms of diseases totally unrelated to HIV disease. Therefore it is imperative that a person see a physician for an accurate diagnosis and treatment for any troublesome condition.

A person can experience some or all of these signs and symptoms in any order:

1. Easy bruising, bleeding gums, or nose bleeds
2. Fevers greater than 100° F for 10 or more days
3. Dry cough
4. Memory, concentration, speech, or coordination problems
5. Painful, swollen lymph glands
6. Persistent diarrhea
7. Persistent headaches, numbness, or tingling in the feet or hands
8. Persistent skin problems
9. Persistent vaginal infections
10. Recurrent, drenching night sweats
11. Shortness of breath
12. Sores or unusual blemishes or patches on the tongue or in the mouth

13. Unexplained fatigue that interferes with normal activities
14. Unintentional weight loss of greater than 10 pounds

Many women who are HIV positive have chronic gynecologic problems. These often appear as the first signs of immune suppression. However, *none* of the following conditions are unique to HIV-positive women. Two of the most common conditions in these women are vaginal yeast infections and pelvic inflammatory disease (PID). Other common problems include:

• Unusually heavy or painful, irregular, or stopped menstrual periods
• Abnormal Pap smears
• Genital warts (condylomata)
• Frequent and severe occurrences of genital herpes
• Cervical dysplasia, which may lead to cancerous growths (carcinomas)

Doctors recommend that HIV-positive women have pelvic examinations and Pap smears done every 6 months so that any gynecologic change or problem can be detected early.

Diagnosis of HIV Infection

Blood tests

A blood test commonly referred to as the *HIV or AIDS antibody test* is used to determine if a person has been infected with HIV. The technical name for this test is the **enzyme-linked immunosorbent assay (ELISA),** which is used as the screening test. If the test results are positive, the person is said to be HIV positive or HIV antibody positive. A person who is HIV positive has HIV disease. Another test, the **Western blot test**, can be performed to confirm the results of the ELISA test.

The Western blot test is a specific test that looks for three different proteins that would be present in abundance if the person is HIV positive. When used together, the results from these two tests have greater than 99% accuracy. When people develop antibodies to HIV, they "seroconvert" (that is, there is a change in blood serum tests from negative to positive as antibodies develop in reaction to an infection or vaccine) from antibody negative to antibody positive. Depending on the circumstances of infection, the estimated time for development of antibodies to HIV is between 2 weeks to 6 months. During this interval, sometimes referred to as the "window period," a person may test HIV antibody negative and yet be infected with the virus. This is because his or her immune system has not produced enough antibodies for the test to detect.

HIV oral fluid tests*

The oral HIV antibody enzyme immunoassay (EIA) and the oral HIV antibody Western blot test are alternatives to blood testing for HIV-1 antibody. The tests can be used on a single oral sample, so no needles or skin puncturing are necessary in any of the steps to detect the presence of HIV-1 antibody. A follow-up HIV antibody EIA for blood is not needed to confirm the results of the oral HIV antibody EIA. A correctly performed oral HIV antibody EIA is as accurate as the HIV antibody EIA for blood. The **OraSure HIV-1 Antibody Testing System** is used for these tests.

The oral sample being collected is known as **mucosal transudate,** which comes from the cheek and gums; **it is not a sample of saliva.** Saliva comes from the salivary glands.

Mucosal transudate contains large amounts of immunoglobulin G (IgG), the type of antibody used to detect HIV. These proteins can pass through the thin lining of the mouth and gums from blood vessels located close to the surface of the mouth. The collection pad, which looks like an ordinary cotton swab, encourages the flow of these proteins, which are then drawn into the pad. Therefore the oral HIV antibody EIA gives results that are essentially equivalent to that of a blood test for HIV antibodies.

This test **detects HIV antibody,** a type of protein present in oral specimens—not the virus itself. Previous studies have shown that low levels of HIV can be found in oral fluids, especially when visible blood is present. However, no cases of HIV transmission have been clearly attributed to oral fluids.

Oral conditions, diseases, medications, and non–HIV-related medical conditions *will not* affect the accuracy of the OraSure test. Persons who are tested for HIV antibody with this oral test should be given the same considerations as those taking any other HIV test. They must consent to being tested and receive appropriate pretest and posttest counseling. All test results should be kept confidential. A diagnosis of HIV infection can be made with an oral HIV antibody EIA after confirmation with the licensed *OraSure oral HIV-1 antibody Western blot kit.* Studies have shown that the OraSure system is more than 99% accurate (see also Chapter 11 for the OraSure test).

Confidential and anonymous testing

For anyone who is getting tested for HIV, the confidentiality policies of the testing center are important to understand. Individuals should ask the testing counselor how results are pro-

tected. Most counseling and testing centers follow either a confidential or anonymous policy, and some facilities follow both.

Confidential testing.   The confidential testing site records the person's name with the test result. Records are kept secret from everyone except medical personnel or, in some states, the state health department. Individuals should ask who will know the results and how the record will be stored. If the HIV antibody test is done confidentially, a release form can be signed to have the test results sent to the individual's physician. However, at some centers, such as doctors' offices or clinics, information about the test result may become part of the individual's medical record and may be seen by health care providers, insurers, or employers. The individual's status may become known to the insurance company if he or she makes a claim for health insurance benefits or applies for life insurance or disability insurance. If any health care provider proposes to test someone for HIV antibodies, the reasons and the potential benefits should be discussed before deciding whether to take the test.

Anonymous testing.   No name is given with the anonymous policy. The person being tested is the only one who can tell anyone else his or her test results. As of March 1996, anonymous testing was available in 41 states, the District of Columbia, and Puerto Rico.

The CDC supports the availability of anonymous counseling and testing in states where such services are permissible by state law or regulation and provides funding to states to provide these services.

Drug and alternative therapies

Research and studies continue in the search for successful treatments and cures, aspiring for the eventual elimination of HIV infection and AIDS. Currently a variety of drugs are used in the treatment for HIV-positive patients and AIDS patients. These drugs are *not* a cure, but they do help to slow down the progression of HIV in the body by disrupting the life cycle of the virus. Three groups of drugs currently being used include the following:

- **Antiretroviral agents**—These drugs are used to decrease the amount of virus in the body. At present, 11 different drugs are included in this group, one type being the protease inhibitors.
- **Antiinfective agents**—These drugs are used to target any infection that the immune system is unable to fight. This group includes over 20 antiviral, antifungal, and antibiotic drugs.
- **Immunomodulators (immunotherapies, such as interleukin therapy)**—These are immune-based therapies used to boost the immune system to make the fight against *any* infection more successful.

Drug studies for developing a vaccine are also being done. For information about the vaccine, call VAXGEN at (650) 225-3701. **Additional information on the treatment of AIDS can be obtained from the following:**

---

*U.S. Department of Health and Human Services, CDC.

HEALTH MATTERS

KEEPING YOUR PATIENTS INFORMED

HOME BLOOD COLLECTION SYSTEMS FOR HIV SELF-TESTING

Q. What is in a kit?

A. Materials included in the different brands of kits vary. In general, each kit contains a counseling pamphlet on HIV/AIDS and the materials needed to obtain a sample of your blood and mail it to the testing facility. This is not like a home pregnancy test kit: individuals are not able to perform the actual test or see the results at home.

Q. How do people get the blood sample and where does the sample go?

A. Consumers prick a finger with a lancet provided in the kit, then apply three drops of blood to a card. The card is then put in a special, preaddressed, leakproof package and mailed. Several days later, the person can make a toll-free call to get the results, using an identification number contained in the kit.

Q. Who gives the results?

A. If the results are negative, a recording will give the results and advise individuals about HIV prevention methods. If the results are positive, a counselor will come on the line immediately. In addition to explaining the results, the counselor will refer HIV-positive callers to doctors, counselors, and other services in the area.

Q. How accurate is the home kit?

A. According to the Food and Drug Administration, clinical studies showed that *Confide* was able to correctly identify negative samples 99.95% of the time based on evaluations of over 3940 samples. The test also correctly identified 100% of 150 positive samples.

Q. How will people get the kit?

A. There are currently two brands of kits available in the United States: *Confide* and *Home Access*. Kits are now sold in drugstores, college health centers, and clinics. Consumers are also able to order kits by mail through a toll-free number. **Contact the CDC National AIDS Clearinghouse at 1-800-458-5231 for these phone numbers.** This requires giving an address and a credit card number.

- AIDS Treatment Data Network: M-F 10 AM–6 PM EST (800) 734-7104
- AIDS Treatment Information Service (ATIS): M-F 9 AM–7 PM EST (800) 448-0440

Combinations of drugs are showing promising results in improving the quality and length of an HIV-positive person's life.

In addition to drug therapy, an increase has been seen in the use of alternative/integrative therapies, such as nutrition, homeopathy, acupuncture, reflexology, hydrotherapy, and aromatherapy. **More information on alternative/integrative therapies can be obtained from the National Institutes of Health Office of Alternative Medicine at (888) 644-6226.**

WORLD AIDS DAY

In 1988 the World Health Organization (WHO) established an annual event to take place on December 1 worldwide. On this special day, called "World AIDS Day," people around the world take special note of the AIDS pandemic. The purpose of this event is to increase public awareness of AIDS, promote participation in prevention efforts, and disseminate information about the disease. According to the American Association for World Health, at least 10 to 12 million people have been infected with HIV since the pandemic began. *Each person must fight this disease and the ignorance surrounding it by becoming an informational and educational resource for his or her own community.* **Information can be obtained from the following agencies.**

- Association of Nurses in AIDS Care, 704 Stony Hill Rd., Ste. 106, Yardley, PA 19067

- National AIDS hotline: (800) 342-AIDS
- Spanish AIDS hotline: (800) 344-SIDA
- Hearing-impaired AIDS hotline: (800) 243-7889
- National AIDS Information Clearinghouse: (800) 458-5231
- AIDS Clinical Trials Information Center: (800) TRIALS-A
- Project Inform (information on experimental AIDS drugs): (800) 822-7422
- Drug abuse hotline: (800) 662-HELP
- National Centers for Disease Control and Prevention voice information system: (404) 332-4555
- Women and AIDS Resource Network: (718) 596-6007
- National Pediatric HIV Resource Center: (800) 362-0071
- National HIV Telephone Service Consultation Service: (800) 933-3413

HEPATITIS (Table 1-2)

Another big threat to health care providers is hepatitis, especially hepatitis B and hepatitis C. Hepatitis is an inflammatory process and infection of the liver caused by a virus. There are several forms of this disease because new strains of the virus have appeared in the past 15 years. Blood tests are used to confirm a diagnosis of hepatitis A through D, but no tests are available to diagnose hepatitis E and G.

Hepatitis A

Hepatitis A is caused by the hepatitis A virus (HAV). It is usually transmitted by fecal contamination of food and water. HAV can also be passed from person to person during oral or anal sex. The incubation period is 15 to 50 days. Hepatitis A *does not* lead to chronic hepatitis or cirrhosis. Most people recover

TABLE 1–2   The ABCs of Hepatitis

	Hepatitis A (HAV)	Hepatitis B (HBV)	Hepatitis C (HCV)	Hepatitis D (HDV)	Hepatitis E (HEV)
What is it?	HAV is a virus that causes inflammation of the liver. It does not lead to chronic disease.	HBV is a virus that causes inflammation of the liver. The virus can cause liver cell damage, leading to cirrhosis and cancer.	HCV is a virus that causes inflammation of the liver. This infection can lead to cirrhosis and cancer.	HDV is a virus that causes inflammation of the liver. It only infects those persons with HBV.	HEV is a virus that causes inflammation of the liver. It is rare in the Untied States. There is no chronic state.
Incubation period	15 to 50 days. Average 30 days.	4 to 25 weeks. Average 8 to 12 weeks.	2 to 25 weeks. Average 7 to 9 weeks.	4 to 26 weeks.	2 to 9 weeks. Average 40 days.
How is it spread?	Transmitted by fecal/oral route, through close person-to-person contact, or by ingestion of contaminated food and water.	Contact with infected blood, seminal fluid, and vaginal secretions. Sex contact, contaminated needles, tattoo/body piercing, and other sharp instruments. Infected mother to newborn. Human bite.	Contact with infected blood, contaminated IV needles, razors, tattoo/body piercing, and other sharp instruments. Infected mother to newborn. It is **not easily** transmitted through sex.	Contact with infected blood, contaminated needles. Sexual contact with HDV-infected person.	Transmitted through fecal/oral route. Outbreaks associated with contaminated water supply in other countries.
Symptoms	May have no symptoms. Adults may have light stools, dark urine, fatigue, fever, nausea, vomiting, abdominal pain, and jaundice.	May have no symptoms. Some persons have mild flu-like symptoms, dark urine, light stools, jaundice, fatigue, and fever.	Same as HBV.	Same as HBV.	Same as HBV.
Treatment of chronic disease	Not applicable.	Interferon is effective in up to 35% to 45% of those treated; antivirals.	Interferon and combination therapies with varying success.	Interferon with varying success.	Not applicable.
Vaccine	Two doses of vaccine to anyone over the age of 2.	Three doses may be given to persons of any age.	None	HBV vaccine prevents HDV infection.	None
Who is at risk?	Household or sex contact with an infected person or living in an area with HAV outbreak. Travelers to developing countries, homosexual men, and IV drug users.	Infant born to infected mother, having sex with infected person or multiple partners, IV drug users, emergency responders and health care providers, homosexual men, and hemodialysis patients.	Anyone who had a blood transfusion before 1992; health care providers, IV drug users, hemodialysis patients, infants born to infected mother, and multiple sex partners.	IV drug users, homosexual men, and those having sex with a HDV infected person.	Travelers to developing countries.
Prevention	Immune globulin within 2 weeks of exposure. Vaccination. Washing hands with soap and water after going to the toilet. Use household bleach to clean surfaces contaminated with feces, such as changing tables. Safe sex.	Immune globulin within 2 weeks of exposure. Vaccination provides protection for 18 years. Safe sex. Clean up infected blood with bleach and wear protected gloves. Do not share razors, toothbrushes, needles.	Safe sex. Clean up spilled blood with bleach. Wear gloves when touching blood. Do not share razors, toothbrushes, or needles with anyone.	Hepatitis B vaccine to prevent HBV infection. Safe sex.	Avoid drinking or using potentially contaminated water.

Courtesy of the Hepatitis Foundation International, 30 Sunrise Terrace, Cedar Grove, NJ 07009 800-891-0707.

within 6 to 10 weeks, whereas some may take 6 to 12 months to recover completely. Once a person has had hepatitis A, he or she will never get the disease again. Immune (gamma) globulin, used in the past for passive immunity before vaccines were available, still plays a role in preventing hepatitis in people who have been in close personal contact with someone who has acute hepatitis A. In this case, contacts should be given an injection of immune globulin within 2 weeks after exposure. This approach helps to prevent hepatitis A from developing or at least reduces the severity or length of time of the disease for someone that has been exposed. Hepatitis A vaccine should be given at the same time.

The vaccine "Havrix" has been available since the spring of 1995. Two doses of the drug are recommended—an initial inoculation plus a booster dose in 6 to 12 months. This vaccination provides protection 2 weeks after it is administered and is expected to provide immunity for at least 20 years and maybe forever.

The second hepatitis A vaccine currently licensed in the United States is called "Vaqta." Adults should be given two doses, with the second dose administered 6 months later. For children and adolescents (ages 2 to 17 years), two doses are given, with the second dose administered 6 to 18 months after the first dose. People can be considered to be protected 4 weeks after receiving the initial vaccine dose.

Those who should *not* receive this vaccination include people who have had hepatitis A and therefore are naturally immune and people who may be hypersensitive to its components (this would have to be checked with a physician). Pregnant and lactating women should receive this vaccination *only* when it is clearly needed. It is thought that the vaccine poses *no danger* to people who have depressed immune systems (also see the section on immunity in Chapter 2).

Hepatitis B

Hepatitis B, caused by the hepatitis B virus (HBV), is a potentially fatal disease. It is transmitted through contaminated blood, by contaminated needles, and also by other body fluids, including semen, saliva, vaginal secretions, and breast milk. This disease is of particular concern because of its association with the spread of the HIV infection leading to AIDS. The incubation period averages 60 to 90 days.

Signs and symptoms.   Signs and symptoms for both hepatitis A and hepatitis B are similar, but they are sometimes more severe for hepatitis B. They may include fever, chills, headache, generalized aches, loss of appetite, nausea, vomiting, dark yellow urine that may have a brownish tinge, diarrhea, clay-colored stools, enlarged and tender liver, and jaundice. If jaundice develops, it is usually first seen in the whites of the eyes and then in the skin.

Diagnosis.   Diagnosis is based on identifying the virus or the antibodies to the virus or through liver biopsy.

Treatment.   Generally, treatment consists of rest and a high-protein diet until the disease runs its course. Treatment is more difficult for hepatitis B, which generally has a more serious prognosis and increased potential for relapse and remission.

Postexposure management.   Hepatitis B vaccine is recommended as part of the therapy used to prevent hepatitis B infection after exposure to HBV. The first dose should be given along with hepatitis B immune globulin (HBIG). See Summary of Pediatric Immunization Recommendations in the *Student Mastery Manual*.

Prevention.   A presumably safe and effective vaccine is available for use in the *prevention* of hepatitis B.

Immunization against hepatitis B is recommended for those individuals considered to be at high risk for the disease (for example, health care practitioners, intravenous drug abusers, people who have many sexual partners, people who require regular blood transfusions, and kidney dialysis patients). A series of three doses is given, the second and third doses administered 1 to 1½ and 6 months after the first dose. The dosage used varies with the age and health status of the person. Health officials and the CDC recommend that all infants and adolescents be vaccinated for *hepatitis B* to prevent the disease in the future, which is *100 times more contagious than HIV*. The recommendation states that infants receive the first dose of HBV vaccine at birth and the next two doses during their regular immunization schedules.

Children and adolescents who have not been vaccinated against hepatitis B in infancy may begin the series during any visit. Those who have not previously received three doses of hepatitis B vaccine should initiate or complete the series during the 11- to 12-year-old visit. Unvaccinated older adolescents should be vaccinated whenever possible. The second dose should be administered at least 1 month after the first dose, and the third dose should be administered at least 4 months after the first dose and at least 2 months after the second dose.

Hepatitis B vaccine should be administered *only* in the deltoid muscle of adults and children or in the anterolateral thigh muscle of newborns and infants; the immunogenicity of the vaccine for adults is substantially lower when injections are administered in the buttock (see Appendix D).

At this time the immunization appears to persist for 18 years or more. A booster dose *may* be required for immunized children *at a later date*. The CDC estimates that approximately 300,000 Americans are infected with HBV each year. Some may develop acute hepatitis and even die from it; about 10% become chronically infected carriers who can pass the disease on to others; some develop liver cancer or cirrhosis and die many years after first becoming infected. It is also estimated that over 1 million people in the United States are carriers of the HBV.

Hepatitis C

Hepatitis C, caused by the hepatitis C virus (HCV) and traditionally called *non-A, non-B hepatitis,* is the third type of hepatitis identified to date. Symptoms and treatment follow similar patterns to the other forms of the disease. This form of hepatitis accounts for 85% to 90% of the new cases of hepatitis each year.

Because of the high incidence of hepatitis C, a federal Blood Safety Advisory Committee recommended in the summer of 1997 that anyone who had received a blood transfusion *before* 1992 be identified and tested for HCV. The current test used for screening for the virus was not available until 1992. This test is also being used to screen blood in blood donor settings. Hepatitis C may result from exposure to blood or body fluids that contain HCV. People at increased risk of acquiring this disease include injecting-drug users, health care providers with occupational exposure to blood, hemodialysis patients, and transfusion recipients. Doctors have also reported a higher prevalence of hepatitis C among people who have gotten tattoos. Hepatitis C has been transmitted between sex partners; *however, the degree of this risk is still unknown and questioned by many.* Those who acquire hepatitis C may never fully recover and may carry the virus for the rest for their lives. More than half of these people suffer some liver damage and may eventually develop cirrhosis, liver cancer, and liver failure. Hepatitis C is believed to be the leading reason for liver transplants in the United States (see Table 1-2).

Hepatitis D

Hepatitis D or *delta hepatitis virus* (HDV) infects only people who have hepatitis B. Experts believe that this type of hepatitis may have more serious health consequences than any other type. It may progress to cirrhosis and chronic hepatitis and has a high mortality rate. The symptoms are usually more severe than those seen in the other forms of hepatitis. Hepatitis D is most commonly spread through intimate sexual contact with infected persons and through blood-contaminated needles. Again, treatment consists of rest and a high-protein diet. Interferon is used with varying success. Antibiotics may be used to resist bacterial infections that could cause additional problems. The HBV vaccine prevents HDV.

Hepatitis E

Hepatitis E is transmitted by ingesting food or water that is contaminated with human feces. Hepatitis E is among the leading causes of acute viral hepatitis in young to middle-aged adults in developing countries. People at greatest risk for acquiring hepatitis E are those exposed to unsanitary conditions in which they may eat and drink contaminated food and water. Epidemics of hepatitis E have been reported in Asia, India, the Middle East, North Africa, and Mexico.

Hepatitis G

Hepatitis G, caused by the hepatitis G virus (HGV) is transmitted through contaminated blood. This virus had been found in approximately 1% to 2% of blood donors in the United States. The infection can persist for up to 16 years. More research is necessary to determine any long-term effects. At present, infection with HGV appears to be uneventful, and very few people develop elevated liver enzymes. Currently, no screening test is available for detecting the presence of the virus in the blood supply.

Infectious Periods

The infectious period for hepatitis A usually ends a week after symptoms subside. A person with hepatitis B can transmit the infection as long as the blood tests show that the antigen is still in the blood. This duration is usually 20 weeks for people who *do not* become chronic carriers. The infectious period for hepatitis C is the same as that for hepatitis B. Infectious periods for hepatitis D, E, and G are unknown at this time.

Other sexually transmitted diseases are discussed in Chapter 11 and Table 11-1.

CONCLUSION

The importance of understanding and always adhering to the standards and guidelines given cannot be overemphasized. These standards **must** be used in all aspects of work and practice. Refer to this chapter often for review and as a reminder of the significance of disease prevention and precautions.

REVIEW OF VOCABULARY

The following are recommendations for prevention of infections in health care personnel as stated by The Hospital Infection Control Practices Advisory Committee, CDC, Public Health Service, U.S. Department of Health and Human Services. After reading these, you should be able to discuss the contents with your instructor. Be prepared to define and explain the medical terms that are in italics. A medical dictionary, other reference books, and information given in other chapters of this book may be used as references for obtaining definitions or explanations of the contents of these recommendations.

Elements of a Personnel Health Service for Infection Control
Placement evaluation

1. Before personnel begin duty or are given a new work assignment, conduct health inventories. The inventories should include the following: (a) *immunization* status or history of *vaccine-preventable* diseases (for example, *chickenpox, measles, mumps, rubella, hepatitis B*) and (b) history of any conditions that may predispose personnel toward acquiring or transmitting infectious diseases.

2. Perform directed physical and laboratory examinations on personnel, as indicated by the results of the *health inventory*. Include examinations to detect conditions that might increase the likelihood of *transmitting disease* to patients or cause unusual *susceptibility* to *infection* and examinations to serve as a baseline for determining whether any future problems are work related.

3. Conduct personnel health assessments other than placement evaluations on an as-needed basis (for example, as required to evaluate work-related illness or *exposures* to *infectious diseases*).

4. Do not perform routine cultures on personnel (for example, cultures of the nose, throat, or stool) as part of the placement evaluation.

5. Conduct *routine screening* for *tuberculosis (TB)* by using the intradermal *(Mantoux),* intermediate-strength (5 tuberculin units) *PPD test* on personnel who have potential for exposure to TB.

6. Conduct routine *serologic* screening for some *vaccine-preventable diseases,* such as *hepatitis B, measles, mumps, rubella,* or *varicella,* if deemed to be cost effective to the hospital and beneficial to the health care personnel.

Personnel health and safety education

1. Provide personnel, annually and whenever the need arises, with in-service training and education on infection control appropriate and specific for their work assignments so that personnel can maintain accurate and up-to-date knowledge about the essential elements of infection control. Ensure that the following topics are included in the initial training on *infection control:* (a) handwashing; (b) modes of transmission of infection and importance of complying with *Standard and Transmission-Based Precautions;* (c) importance of reporting certain illnesses or conditions (whether work related or acquired outside the hospital), such as *generalized rash* or skin lesions that are vesicular, pustular, or weeping, *jaundice,* illnesses that do not resolve within a designated period (for example, a cough that persists for *more than 2 weeks, gastrointestinal illness,* or *febrile* illness with *fever of greater than 103° F lasting more than 2 days),* and *hospitalizations* resulting from febrile or other *contagious diseases;* (d) tuberculosis control; (e) importance of complying with *Standard Precautions* and reporting exposure to blood and body fluids to prevent transmission of *bloodborne pathogens;* (f) importance of cooperating with infection control personnel during outbreak investigations; and (g) importance of *personnel screening and immunization programs.*

Prophylaxis and Follow-up After Exposure— General Recommendations

1. Ensure that when personnel are offered necessary *prophylactic treatment* with drugs, *vaccines,* or *immune globulins,* they are informed of (a) options for *prophylaxis,* (b) the

risk (if known) of infection when treatment is not accepted, (c) the degree of protection provided by the therapy, and (d) the potential *side effects* of therapy.

2. Ensure that when personnel are exposed to particular *infectious agents,* they are informed of (a) the recommended *postexposure management* that is based on current knowledge about the *epidemiology* of the infection; (b) the risk (if known) of transmitting the infection to patients, other personnel, or other contacts; and (c) *the methods of preventing transmission of the infection* to other persons.

Prevention of *Nosocomial* Transmission of Selected *Infections*

1. **Bloodborne pathogens—general recommendation**
   Ensure that health care personnel are familiar with precautions to prevent *occupational transmission of bloodborne pathogens.*

   Follow state and federal guidelines and strategies for determining the need for work restrictions for health care personnel infected with *bloodborne pathogens.*

   a. **Hepatitis B**
      (1) Administer *hepatitis B vaccine* to personnel who perform tasks involving routine and inadvertent (for example, as with housekeepers) contact with blood, *other body fluids* (including blood-contaminated fluids), and sharp medical instruments or other sharp objects.
      (2) Use both *passive immunization* with *hepatitis B immune globulin* and *active immunization* with hepatitis B vaccine for *postexposure prophylaxis* in susceptible personnel who have had a needlestick, *percutaneous,* or mucous membrane exposure to blood known or suspected to be at high risk for being hepatitis B surface antigen (HbsAg) seropositive.

   b. **Hepatitis C**
      (1) Do not administer *immune globulin* to personnel who have exposure to blood or body fluids positive for antibody to *HCV.*
      (2) Consider implementing policies for postexposure follow-up at baseline and 6 months for health care personnel who have had a percutaneous or mucosal exposure to blood containing antibody to HCV.

CASE REPORTS

The following case reports briefly describe the experiences of four workers who developed latex allergy after occupational exposures.* These cases are not representative of all reactions to latex but are examples of the most serious types of reactions. They illustrate what has occurred in some individuals.

Case No. 1

A laboratory technician developed asthma symptoms after wearing latex gloves while performing blood tests. Initially, the

symptoms occurred only on contact with the gloves; but later, symptoms occurred when the technician was exposed only to latex particles in the air (Seaton et al., 1998).

Case No. 2

A 33-year-old woman sought medical treatment for occupational asthma after 6 months of periodic cough, shortness of breath, chest tightness, and occasional wheezing. She had worked for 7 years as an inspector at a medical supply company, where her job

CASE REPORTS

included inflating latex gloves coated with cornstarch. Her symptoms began within 10 minutes of starting work and worsened later in the day (90 minutes after leaving work). Symptoms disappeared completely while she was on a 12-day vacation, but they returned on her first day back at work.

Case No. 3

A midwife initially suffered hives, nasal congestion, and conjunctivitis. Within a year, she developed asthma, and 2 years later, she went into shock after a routine gynecologic examination during which latex gloves were used. The midwife also suffered respiratory distress in latex-containing environments when she had no direct contact with latex products. She was unable to continue working.

Case No. 4

An intensive care nurse with a history of runny nose, itchy eyes, asthma, eczema, and contact dermatitis experienced four severe allergic reactions to latex. The first reaction began with asthma severe enough to require treatment in an emergency room. The second and third reactions were similar to the first. The fourth and most severe reaction occurred when she put on latex gloves at work. She went into severe shock and was successfully treated in an emergency room.

*U.S. Department of Health and Human Services, CDC, National Institute of Occupational Safety and Health.

CRITICAL THINKING SKILLS REVIEW

1. State why infection control systems were designed.
2. On what are the Universal and Standard Precautions based?
3. What is the most important function of handwashing?
4. State when disposable single-use examination gloves should be worn at your job.
5. State when and why masks and protective eyewear should be worn.
6. State when and why a health care provider should wear a gown or a disposable plastic apron.
7. List 10 procedures that must be followed to prevent infection with sharps or needles.
8. Differentiate between being HIV positive and having AIDS.
9. State the cause of HIV disease.
10. List 10 signs and symptoms of hepatitis.
11. In a health care setting, who must be offered the hepatitis B vaccination?
12. Whose responsibility is it to pay for the hepatitis B vaccine?
13. When should the hepatitis B vaccination be offered to employees?
14. Can employees refuse the vaccination?
15. Is a routine booster dose of hepatitis B vaccine beyond the series of three injections required?
16. What serologic testing must be done on the source individual?
17. When is the exposed employee's blood tested?
18. What information must the employer provide to the health care professional after an exposure incident?
19. What information does the health care professional provide to the employer after an exposure incident?
20. Discuss and differentiate between Standard Precautions and Transmission-Based Precautions.

🖥 INTERNET RESOURCES

Centers for Disease Control and Prevention (CDC)
www.cdc.gov

American Liver Foundation
www.info@liverfoundation.org

OSHA
www.osha.gov

CDC AIDS Clearinghouse
www.cdcnac.org

CDC Hepatitis Branch
www.cdc.gov/ncidod/diseases/hepatitis/hepatitis.htm

The CDC HIV/AIDS Page
www.cdc.gov/diseases/hivqa.html

Harvard AIDS Institute
www.hsph.harvard.edu/Organizations/hai/home_pg/html

HIV InSite
www.hivinsite.ucsf.edu

HIV/AIDS Treatment Information Service
http://sis.nlm.nih.gov/aids/aidstrea.html

Office of AIDS Research
http://sis.nlm.nih.gov/aids/oar.html

World Health Organization
www.who.org

Occupational Safety and Health Administration (OSHA) directive
www.osha-slc.gov/OshDoc/Directive_data/CPL_2-2_44D.html

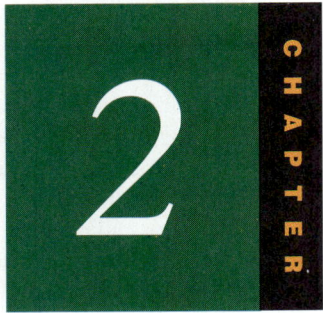

2

Infection Control: Practices of Medical Asepsis and Sterilization

■ Cognitive Objectives

On completion of Chapter 2, the medical assistant student should be able to:

1. Define, spell, and pronounce the terms presented in the vocabulary and throughout the chapter.
2. List the five classifications of microorganisms that are capable of causing a disease process, giving examples of diseases caused by each.
3. List the six factors that are essential for the development of an infectious process, discussing briefly components in each.
4. Differentiate between the types of human reservoirs—overt cases, subclinical cases, and human carriers.
5. Compare direct transmission with indirect transmission of a disease process.
6. List and describe the body's natural defense mechanisms used to control or prevent disease and infection.
7. Briefly discuss the function of the immune system.
8. List and briefly discuss the four critical phases of each immune response.
9. Discuss and compare the various types of immunity.
10. Identify six diseases for which the Centers for Disease Control and Prevention (CDC) has issued guidelines for immunizations to protect health care providers.
11. List the diseases for which there are recommendations for adult immunizations.
12. List the classic signs and symptoms of inflammation and briefly describe the inflammatory process.
13. List five diagnostic tests that may be used to diagnose an infectious process.
14. Differentiate between medical and surgical asepsis; list and describe procedures used to accomplish each and medical situations in which each is used.
15. Differentiate between sanitization, disinfection, and sterilization; describe the procedures used with these methods when working with contaminated instruments, syringes and needles, rubber goods, and other equipment and select the most effective method for controlling microscopic agents.

16. Explain the importance of sterilizing instruments and supplies before using them for medical procedures.
17. List and briefly describe five methods used for sterilizing equipment and two methods used for disinfecting equipment.
18. Describe how items are to be wrapped, positioned, and removed from a sterilizer for sterilization to be effective and how items are to be positioned and removed from a boiler.
19. List three critical factors in steam sterilization.
20. State the recommended exposure times for sterilizing and disinfecting the various types of equipment and supplies that are used in the physician's office.
21. Describe types of and state the reason for using sterilization indicators.
22. Discuss problems encountered in sterilization techniques and causes of insufficient sterilization.
23. Discuss how, where, and how long sterile supplies should be stored.

■ Terminal Performance Objectives

On completion of Chapter 2, the medical assistant student should be able to:

1. Demonstrate how to wash hands, wrists, and forearms, explaining the reasons for the actions taken.
2. Given various items assumed to be contaminated, demonstrate how to sanitize, disinfect, and sterilize each, using the methods discussed in this chapter.
3. Demonstrate how to inspect instruments before they are sterilized and state the reason for the actions taken.
4. Given items to be sterilized, demonstrate how each should be wrapped before placing in the sterilizer.
5. Given packs that have been removed from an autoclave, determine if sterilization has been effective and then store each for use at a later date.
6. Provide instructions and patient education that is within the professional scope of a medical assistant's training and responsibilities as assigned.

The student is to perform these objectives with 100% accuracy 90% of the time (9 out of 10 times).

The consistent use of Universal/Standard Precautions is required by all health care professionals in all health care settings as a method of infection control. It is assumed that these precautions are used in all of the following procedures. Review

Chapter 1 if you have any questions on methods to use because the methods and techniques are not repeated in detail in each procedure presented in this chapter.

Be sure to consult the latest guidelines issued by the Centers for Disease Control and Prevention (CDC) and consult with infection control practitioners when needed to identify specific precautions that pertain to your particular work situation.

VOCABULARY

antiseptic (an'tĭ-sep'tik)—A substance capable of inhibiting the growth or action of microorganisms, without necessarily killing them; generally safe for use on body tissues.

asepsis (a-sep'sis)—The absence of all microorganisms causing disease; absence of contaminated matter. The state of being free from infection or infectious matter.

bactericide (bak-tēr'i-sīd)—A substance capable of destroying bacteria but not spores.

bacteriostatic (bak-te"re-o-stat'ik)—A substance that inhibits the growth of bacteria.

cilia (sil'e-ah)—Small, hairlike processes extending on the outer surfaces of some cells. Cilia beat in a rhythmic way to move the cell or to move mucus or a fluid over the surface.

contaminated, contamination (kon-tam"ĭ-na'shun)—The act of making unclean, soiling, or staining, especially introducing disease germs or infectious material into or on normally sterile objects.

decontaminate—To remove infectious agents from body surfaces or from inanimate surfaces or articles.

disinfectant (dis"in-fek'tant)—A substance capable of destroying pathogens but usually not spores; generally not intended for use on body tissue because it is too strong.

disinfection—A process that destroys most harmful microorganisms but rarely kills spores.

fungicide (fun'jĭ-sīd)—A substance that destroys fungi.

germicide (jer'mĭ-sīd)—A substance that is capable of destroying pathogens.

immunization (im"u-nĭ-za'shun)—The process of rendering a person immune (protected from or not susceptible to a disease) or of becoming immune; often called vaccination or inoculation. A process by which a person is artificially prepared to resist infection by a specific pathogen.

incubation (in"ku-ba'shun) **period**—The interval of time between the invasion of a pathogen into the body and the appearance of the first symptoms of disease.

infection (in-fek'shun)—A condition caused by the multiplication of pathogenic microorganisms that have invaded the body of a susceptible host.

- **acute**—Rapid onset, severe symptoms, and usually subsides within a relatively short time.
- **chronic**—Develops slowly, milder symptoms, and lasts for a long time.
- **latent**—Dormant or concealed; pathogen is ever-present in the host, but symptoms are present only intermittently, often in response to a stimulus. At other times the pathogen is dormant.
- **localized**—Restricted to a certain area.

- **generalized**—Systemic; involving the whole body.

inflammation (in"flah-ma'shun)—A localized protective response of the tissues of the body brought on by destruction or injury of tissues. This response serves to destroy, wall off, or dilute both the agent that caused the injury and the injured tissue. (See also Inflammatory Process in this chapter.)

medical microbiology—The study and identification of pathogens and the development of effective methods for their control or elimination.

necrosis (ne-kro'sis)—The death of a cell or a group of cells because of injury or disease.

normal flora—Microorganisms that normally reside in various body locations such as the vagina, intestine, urethra, upper respiratory tract, and skin. These microorganisms are nonpathogenic and do not cause harm (although they may become pathogenic and cause harm if they are introduced into a body area in which they do not normally reside).

pathogenic (păth"ō-jĕn'ĭk)—Productive of disease. *P. microorganism*—one that produces disease in the body.

reservoir (rez'er-vwar)—The source in which pathogenic microorganisms grow and from which they leave to spread and cause disease.

resistance (re-zis'tans)—The ability of the body to resist disease or infection because of its own defense mechanisms.

sepsis (sep'sis)—A morbid state or condition resulting from the presence of pathogenic microorganisms.

spore (spōr)—A reproductive cell, usually unicellular, produced by plants and some protozoa and possessing thick walls to withstand unfavorable environmental conditions. A spore is also a form assumed by some bacteria. Spore-forming bacteria can cause disease (for example, tetanus, gas gangrene). Bacterial spores are resistant to heat and must undergo a prolonged exposure to extremely high temperatures to be destroyed. This destruction of spores can be accomplished by sterilization techniques.

sterile (ster'il)—Free from all microorganisms and spores.

toxin (tok'sin)—A poisonous substance produced by pathogenic bacteria and some animals and plants. The toxins produced by bacteria include toxic enzymes, exotoxins, and endotoxins. Toxins in the body cause antitoxins to form, which provide a means for establishing immunity to certain diseases.

vaccination (vak"sĭ-na'shun)—The introduction of weakened or dead microorganisms (inoculation) into the body to stimulate the production of antibodies and immunity to a specific disease.

virulence (vir'u-lens)—The degree of ability of a pathogen to produce disease.

BASIC CONCEPTS AND GOALS

Since the early days of civilization, there has been concern with the control of disease and the spread of infection. The history of medicine documents the wealth of knowledge attained by numerous individuals about the anatomy and physiology of the human body, certain diseases, and many therapeutic agents. However, not until the last half of the nineteenth century was a connection between disease and pathogenic microorganisms established through the work of Louis Pasteur and Robert Koch. Among the findings documented, Pasteur discovered important properties of bacteria, and Koch was credited with establishing the germ theory of disease. Koch's theory states that to prove an organism is actually the specific pathogen causing the disease, one must establish a causal relationship between the microbe and the disease.

Microorganisms (microbes) are defined as minute living creatures that are too small to be seen by the naked eye. The classifications or divisions of microscopic life include viruses, rickettsiae, bacteria, fungi, and parasites. Microorganisms in each of these divisions that cause disease are termed **pathogens**. It is important to keep in mind that many members of these microscopic divisions are either beneficial or harmless to humans or animals. The term **medical microbiology** implies the study of pathogens, which involves identification and development of effective methods of control or elimination.

Pathogenic microorganisms are everywhere around us. They are easily spread directly from person to person or indirectly by animate and inanimate vehicles to humans. Disease or infection occurs when pathogens invade a susceptible host. Although antibiotics are available for use in the treatment of many infectious processes, the best means of controlling infection is to prevent the spread of disease-producing microorganisms. It is the responsibility of health professionals to take an active, conscientious role in the process of infection control. Lack of knowledge about how pathogens spread or how to control the process is often the cause of major outbreaks of infection or disease. The **goals of infection control** are to prevent the spread of pathogenic microorganisms, to attain a state of asepsis (absence of pathogens), and to educate the public in the ways that they too can help. **Asepsis**, or aseptic technique, is divided into two categories—medical asepsis and surgical asepsis, and distinguishing between these two methods is important.

The rest of this chapter discusses disease-producing organisms, how they are spread, the body's own defense mechanisms, the immune system, infection control precautions, and medical and surgical asepsis with techniques and sterilization procedures used to prevent transmission of pathogens. Surgical asepsis (aseptic technique) is discussed in greater length in Chapter 6. Universal/Standard Precautions for blood and body substances are presented in Chapter 1.

INFECTIOUS PROCESS AND CAUSATIVE AGENTS

The mere presence of a pathogenic microorganism is not enough to promote infection. For the infectious process to develop, a sequential connection must occur between the following factors (Figure 2-1):

FIGURE 2-1 The chain of the infectious process. To prevent the spread of disease this sequential connection must be broken.

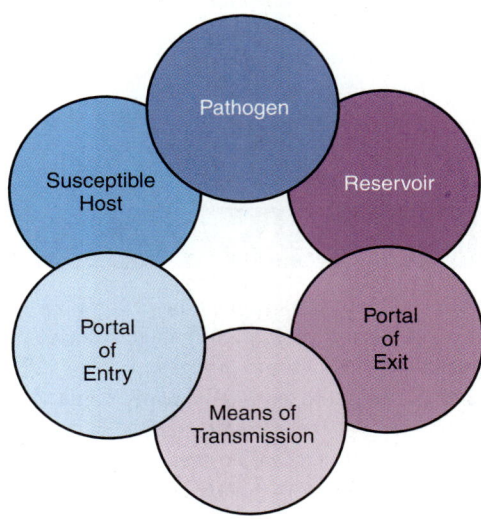

1. A cause or an etiologic (e-tē-o-loj′ ik) agent (pathogen)
2. A source or a reservoir of the etiologic agent
3. A means of escape of the etiologic agent from the reservoir (portals of exit)
4. A means of transmission of the etiologic agent from the reservoir to the new host
5. A means of entry of the etiologic agent into the new susceptible host (portals of entry)
6. A susceptible host

Cause or Etiologic Agent

Infection begins with the invasion of the body by a **pathogen** that is the causative agent of the disease in question. The pathogenic organisms must be present in a sufficiently high concentration and be adequately capable of causing disease. Examples of causative agents or pathogens are viruses, rickettsiae, bacteria, fungi, and parasites.

Viruses.   Viruses (vi′rus) are the smallest pathogens and require susceptible host cells for multiplication and activity. To observe viruses, an electron microscope must be used. A phenomenon that characterizes viral infections as the most insidious is the fact that viruses, as intracellular parasites, can only multiply inside a living cell. Viruses attach themselves to a living cell, inject a compound of protein and nucleic acid, either deoxyribonucleic acid (DNA) or ribonucleic acid (RNA), and take over the normal cellular metabolism. The cell proceeds to make new cells in addition to new viruses, then bursts, dies, and releases numerous viruses that can then invade other cells. Chemotherapy for viral diseases is extremely difficult because the viruses surviving an initial dose of a drug have the ability to change their characteristics so that they rapidly become resistant to the drug.

Viruses are also more resistant to chemical disinfection than bacteria, but they can be destroyed by heat, as is done when sterilizing equipment in an autoclave.

A greater variety of viruses exists than of any other category of microbial agents of disease. Viruses are the causative agents of influenza, poliomyelitis, colds, mumps, measles, rabies, smallpox, and chickenpox, as well as hepatitis A, hepatitis B, herpes simplex I, and herpes simplex II.

Rickettsiae.

Rickettsiae (rik-ĕt′sē-ă) like viruses are obligate intracellular parasites. This means that they can only survive within the host organism. They differ from viruses in that they are visible under a conventional microscope by special staining techniques and are also susceptible to antibiotic suppression of replication.

Rickettsiae are the causative organisms for the various spotted fevers, such as Rocky Mountain spotted fever, and also typhus, Q fever, and trench fever. They are generally tickborne and therefore are not common in sanitary urban areas.

Bacteria.

Bacteria (bak-te′re-ah) can readily multiply outside of living cells. Bacteria are single-celled microorganisms that can be cultivated on artificial media and, with appropriate staining techniques, can be readily visible under a microscope. These characteristics make bacteria much simpler to identify than viruses and rickettsiae. There are many varieties, only some of which cause disease; most are nonpathogenic, and many are useful. Bacteria are classified into the following three groups according to their shape and appearance (morphology) (Figure 2-2):

1. Cocci (kok′si) are spheric bacteria; among the cocci are the following three types:
   a. Staphylococci (stăf″ĭl-o′kŏk′si)—Forming grapelike clusters of cells, these are the most common pus-producing organisms known to humans. They are readily found in pimples, boils, suture abscesses, and osteomyelitis.
   b. Streptococci (strĕp″tō-kŏk′si)—Forming chains of cells, these are the cause of strep throat, rheumatic heart disease (RHD), scarlet fever, and septicemia (infection in the bloodstream).
   c. Diplococci (dip-lō-kŏk′si)—Forming pairs of cells, different types of diplococci are the causative organisms for gonorrhea, pneumonia, and meningitis.
2. Bacilli (bah-sil′i) are rod-shaped bacteria; these organisms cause tuberculosis (TB), typhoid and paratyphoid fever, tetanus (lockjaw), gas gangrene, bacillary dysentery, and diphtheria.
3. Spirilla (spi-ril′ah) are spiral organisms; these organisms cause cholera, syphilis, and relapsing fever.

Fungi.

Fungi (fun′ji) are the lowest form of infectious agents that bridge the gap between free-living and host-dependent parasites.

Fungi are unicellular or multicellular. They can be grown on artificial media and then identified under the microscope. Fungi appear in the form of molds and mushrooms, as well as in microscopic growth. Disease-producing fungi are seen as the causative agent in some infections of the skin, such as athlete's foot and ringworm.

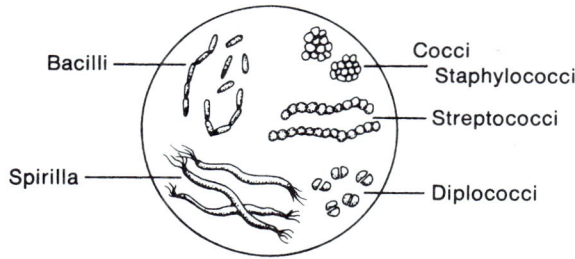

FIGURE 2-2 Classification of bacteria according to their morphology.

The fungus *Candida albicans (Monilia)* is responsible for the disease known as thrush (an infection of the mouth and throat) and also some vaginal infections.

Parasites.

Parasites (par′ah-sīt) are organisms that live in or on another organism from which they gain their nourishment. Parasites include single-celled and multicelled animals, fungi, and bacteria. Viruses are sometimes considered to be parasitic. Examples include the following:

1. Protozoa (pro″to-zo′ah) are single-celled microscopic organisms. Some can be cultivated, fixed, and stained for viewing under a microscope. The most well-known protozoa cause malaria, amoebic dysentery, and *Trichomonas* infections of the vagina.
2. Metazoal (met″ah-zo′al) parasites are multicellular organisms, causing conditions such as pinworms, hookworms, tapeworms, and trichinosis in pork.
3. Ectoparasites (ek″to-par′ah-sīt) can superficially affect the host (for example, lice and scabies mite) or can invade the integument (for example, the larvae of dipterous flies).

Source or Reservoir of Etiologic Agent

Areas where organisms grow and reproduce are called **reservoirs** and are found mainly in human beings and animals. Organisms can also exist in soil, water, and equipment.

Human reservoirs include the following:

- Overt carriers: people who are obviously ill with the disease.
- Subclinical carriers: abortive (undeveloped) and ambulatory (walking) cases of the disease (for example, "walking" pneumonia). Infection goes unnoticed because of lack of symptoms.
- Human carriers: people unaware of their condition who circulate freely in their communities until detected and diagnosed (for example, the Typhoid Marys or people who are in the convalescent stage of an infection).

Animal reservoirs include mainly domestic animals and rodents. Zoonosis (zo″o-no′sis) is the term given to an animal disease that is transmissible to humans. In this case, the infection is usually derived from the animal and is not further transmitted from human to human. An example is rabies.

Means of Escape of Etiologic Agent From Reservoir

Pathogens commonly exit from their reservoir through one or more of the following (*portals of exit*):

- Respiratory tract in secretions from the nose, nasal sinuses, nasopharynx, larynx, trachea, bronchial tree, and lungs
- Intestinal tract through discharge with the feces
- Urinary tract through discharge or in the urine
- Skin or mucous membranes or open lesions or discharges on the surface of the body
- Reproductive tract through discharges
- Blood
- Across the placenta

Means of Transmission of Etiologic Agent From Reservoir to New Host

The means of transmission is the method by which the pathogen is transmitted from the portal of exit in the reservoir to the portal of entry in the new host. After an infecting organism has escaped from its reservoir, it can cause a new infection only if it finds its way to a new susceptible host. Transmission may occur by either of the following:

- *Direct transmission*: The organism passes from one person to another through inhalation, by actual physical contact such as sexual contact or kissing, or by direct contact with an open lesion. The organism goes from one host to another without the aid of intermediate objects. This is also called person-to-person transmission.
- *Indirect transmission*: The organism is capable of survival for a time outside the body and is transferred to the new host by a vehicle, which is either animate or inanimate. Animate vehicles are people who touch contaminated material, do not wash their hands, and then carry the microorganism on their hands to a susceptible host. Other animate vehicles are called vectors and include the various insects that spread infection. Inanimate vehicles, called fomites, are nonliving objects or substances and include water, milk, foods, soil, air, excreta, clothing, bedding, towels, in-struments, syringes and needles, toiletries, or any contaminated article.

Means of Entry of Etiologic Agent Into New Susceptible Host

The infecting organism enters a new host through a part of the body, which is called the portal of entry. The main portals of entry are:

- Respiratory tract—Organisms may be inhaled
- Gastrointestinal tract—Organisms may be ingested
- Skin or mucous membranes—Organisms may be introduced via cuts, abrasions, or open wounds
- Urinary tract—Organisms may be introduced through external body orifices
- Reproductive tract—Organisms may be introduced through external body orifices
- Blood
- Across the placenta

Although avenues of escape or portals of exit correspond to the portals of entry, the pathogen can escape from one site in the reservoir and enter the new host in another site. An example of this is when the pathogen leaves from the respiratory tract in the reservoir (as through sputum or water droplets) and enters the new host through the skin (as through an open wound when a dressing is being changed).

Susceptible Host

For the infectious process to be completed, the pathogenic organism must enter a host whose **resistance** is so low that it cannot fight off the invading organism. Even though a pathogen gains entry to the body, disease or infection may not develop because the body possesses certain defense mechanisms to protect itself. These mechanisms may also help destroy invading pathogens. Such defense mechanisms are called resistance, and if they are great enough, they constitute immunity (ĭ-mū′nĭ-tē).

Table 2-1 outlines the six essential factors of the infectious process for two diseases. All infectious diseases can be outlined in this manner.

TABLE 2–1 Factors of Infectious Process

Disease	Cause/Agent	Reservoir/ Source	Means of Escape From the Reservoir	Means of Transmission From Reservoir to New Host	Means of Entry Into New Host	Susceptible Host
German measles (rubella)	Virus	Humans	Mouth, nasopharynx	Water droplets	Mouth	Humans
Pneumonia	Bacteria	Humans	Mouth, nasopharynx	Droplets; sputum; fomites, such as a pencil (indirect transmission)	Mouth, respiratory mucosa	Humans

Stages of an Infectious Process

The stages of an infectious process generally include the following:

1. The invasion and multiplication of the pathogen in the body
2. The **incubation period,** which may vary from a few days to months or years
3. The **prodromal period,** when the first mild signs and symptoms appear; the person is highly contagious during this period
4. The acute period, when signs and symptoms are at the most severe stage
5. The recovery and convalescent period, when signs and symptoms begin to subside and the body heals itself, returning to a state of health

THE BODY'S DEFENSES AGAINST DISEASE AND INFECTION

The body's resistance level to undesirable microorganisms is influenced by the general health status of the individual and other related circumstances:

- Amount of rest, sufficient or insufficient
- Dietary intake of nutritional foods, adequate or inadequate
- How one copes with stress
- Age of the individual (the young and aged are most susceptible to infection because of the immaturity of the immune system in the young and the decline of this system in the aged)
- Presence of other disease processes in the body
- Condition of the external environment, such as poor living conditions
- Influence of genetic traits (for example, people with diabetes mellitus and sickle cell anemia are more prone to some infections than are other individuals)

Physical and Chemical Barriers

The body has natural defense mechanisms, either physical or chemical, that act as barriers to the invasion of pathogenic organisms.

Skin.   This tissue is the largest barrier against infection. As long as it remains intact, the skin is a physical barrier to a tremendous number of microorganisms. Chemical barriers of the skin include the acid pH of the skin (which inhibits bacterial infection), sweat, and lysozyme (which functions as an antibacterial enzyme in the skin).

Mucous membrane.   This tissue holds in check many microorganisms because of the repelling forces in the secretions that bathe these membranes. The cilia of some mucous membranes serve to keep their surfaces swept clean.

Respiratory tract.   The mucosal lining of this tract is very sensitive and thus readily stimulated by foreign matter. Certain reflexes such as coughing or sneezing help remove foreign matter, including microorganisms. The hairs lining the nostrils, along with the moist membranes, serve as a physical barrier. The cilia lining the bronchi beat upward to carry mucus and small, interfering foreign materials such as dust, bacteria, and soot to the throat. The bending passageway from the mouth to the lungs also serves as a barrier.

Gastrointestinal tract.   Hydrochloric acid in the stomach has an important bactericidal action, destroying many disease-producing agents. Bile in the small intestine is thought to have a germicidal effect.

Blood and lymphoid tissue.   These tissues contain and produce cells and antibodies that can exert a tremendous influence in protecting the body against disease. White blood cells (leukocytes) are particularly active when pathogenic microorganisms invade the body. In the inflammatory process, some leukocytes surround, engulf, and digest the pathogens. This process is known as phagocytosis (fag″o-si-tō′sis), which is basically the ingestion of the pathogen or "cell-eating." Lymphoid tissue produces antibodies, which are protein compounds that help combat infection.

Antigen-Antibody Reaction

Another internal defense mechanism that the body gradually develops against invasion by foreign substances (antigens) is the formation of antibodies. Antibodies are protein substances produced mainly in the lymph nodes, spleen, bone marrow, and lymphoid tissue in response to invasion by an antigen. Different types of antibodies are produced in response to different antigens, with each antibody being effective only against the specific antigen that stimulates its production. The antibodies can either neutralize the antigens, render them harmless, rupture their cell membrane, or prepare the antigen so that they are more susceptible to destruction by phagocytes (cells that ingest and destroy microorganisms, cells, and cell debris).

The antigen-antibody reaction is this reaction of the body to the invasion of antigens. When antibodies are produced in sufficient quantities, the body becomes immune. Because the body is capable of continuing to produce antibodies for weeks to several years, immunity can last for months or years.

Immune System

The immune system is a complex system that defends the body against microorganisms and cancer cells. Its general function is to produce immunity, that is, resistance to disease. The structures of the immune system are not organs. The system is made up of trillions of separate cells and molecules performing many different functions. It includes the white blood cells (especially the neutrophils and lymphocytes), the connective tissue cells or macrophages, and protein molecules or antibodies. Because of recent research, an understanding of this system is increasing significantly. To fully grasp the complexities of the immune system, a thorough knowledge of human biology is required, which is beyond the scope of this book. However, a general view of the immune response is provided in Figure 2-3.

FIGURE 2-3   The four phases of the immune system and how they function. (Courtesy The National Geographic Society.)

CELL WARS

About one trillion strong, our white blood cells constitute a highly specialized army of defenders, the most important of which are depicted here in a typical battle against a formidable enemy.

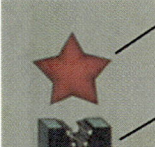

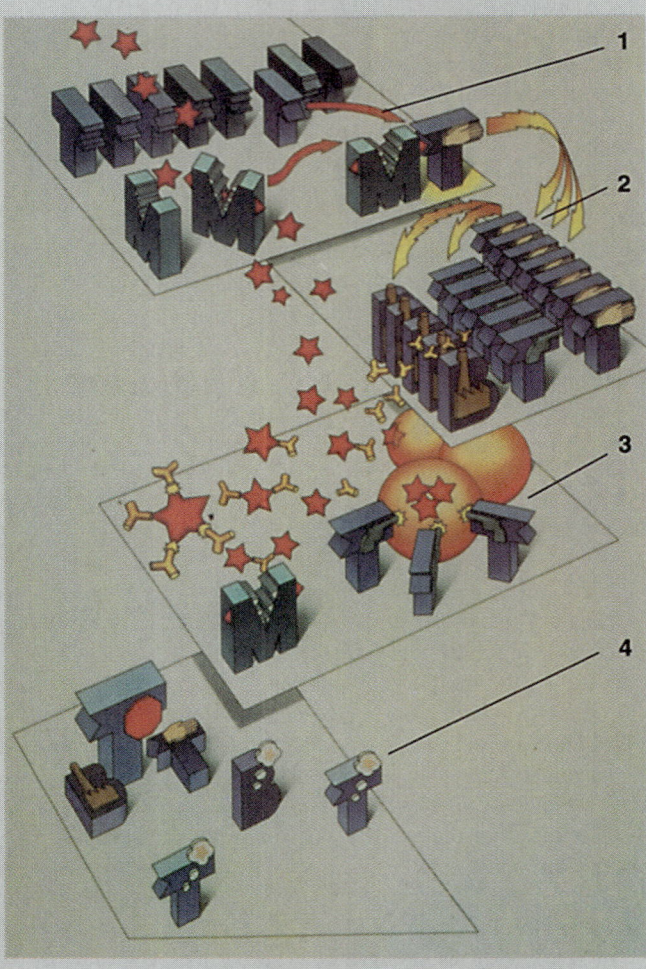

VIRUS
Needing help to spring to life, a virus is little more than a package of genetic information that must commandeer the machinery of a host cell to permit its own replication.

MACROPHAGE
Housekeeper and frontline defender, this cell engulfs and digests debris that washes into the bloodstream. Encountering a foreign organism, it summons helper T cells to the scene.

HELPER T CELL
As a commander in chief of the immune system, it identifies the enemy and rushes to the spleen and lymph nodes, where it stimulates the production of other cells to fight the infection.

KILLER T CELL
Recruited and activated by helper T cells, it specializes in killing cells of the body that have been invaded by foreign organisms, as well as cells that have turned cancerous.

B CELL
Biologic arms factory, it resides in the spleen or the lymph nodes, where it is induced to replicate by helper T cells and then to produce potent chemical weapons called antibodies.

ANTIBODY
Engineered to target a specific invader, the Y-shaped protein molecule is rushed to the infection site, where it either neutralizes the enemy or tags it for attack by other cells or chemicals.

SUPPRESSOR T CELLS
A third type of T cell, it is able to slow down or stop the activities of B cells and other T cells, playing a vital role in calling off the attack after an infection has been conquered.

MEMORY CELL
Generated during an initial infection, this defense cell may circulate in the blood or lymph for years, enabling the body to respond more quickly to subsequent infections.

A miracle of evolution, the human immune system is not controlled by any central organ, such as the brain. Rather it has developed to function as a kind of biologic democracy, wherein the individual members achieve their ends through an information network of awesome scope. Accounting for one percent of the body's 100 trillion cells, these defender white cells arise in the bone marrow. They fall into three groups: the phagocytes, or "cell eaters," of which the stalwart macrophage is one, and two kinds of lymphocytes, called T and B cells. All share one common objective: to identify and destroy all substances, living and inert, that are not part of the human body, that are "not self." These include human cells, which have turned from self to nonself, friend to foe.

There are four critical phases to each immune response: recognition of the enemy, aplification of defenses, attack, and slowdown. Each immune response is a unique local sequence of events, shaped by the nature of the enemies. Chemical toxins and a multitude of inert environmental substances, such as asbestos and smoke particles, are normally attacked only by phagocytes. Organic invaders inlist the full range of immune responses. Besides viruses, these include single-celled bacteria, protozoa, and fungi, as well as a host of multicelled worms called helminths. Many of these enemies have evolved devious methods to escape detection. The viruses that cause influenza and the common cold, for example, constantly mutate, changing their fingerprints. The AIDS virus, most insidious of all, employs a range of strategies, including hiding out in healthy cells. What makes it fatal is its ability to invade and kill helper T cells, thereby short-circuiting the entire immune response.

1. **THE BATTLE BEGINS**
   As viruses begin to invade the body, a few are consumed by macrophages, which seize their antigens and display them on their own surfaces. Among millions of helper T cells circulating the bloodstream, a select few are programmed to "read" that antigen. Binding to the macrophage, the T cell becomes activated.

2. **THE FORCES MULTIPLY**
   Once activated, helper T cells begin to multiply. They then stimulate the multiplication of those few killer T cells and B cells that are sensitive to the invading viruses. As the number of B cells increases, helper T cells signal them to start producing antibodies.

3. **CONQUERING THE INFECTION**
   Meanwhile, some of the viruses have entered cells of the body—the only place they are able to replicate. Killer T cells will sacrifice these cells by chemically puncturing their membranes, letting the contents spill out, thus disrupting the viral replication cycle. Antibodies then neutralize the viruses by binding directly to their surfaces, preventing them from attacking other cells. Additionally, they precipitate chemical reactions that actually destroy infected cells.

4. **CALLING A TRUCE**
   As the infection is contained, suppressor T cells halt the entire range of immune responses, preventing them from spiraling out of control. Memory T and B cells are left in the blood and lymphatic system, ready to move quickly should the same virus once again invade the body.

The four critical phases to each immune response are as follows:

1. *Recognition of the enemy:* When a pathogen enters the body, the immune system must recognize that a foreign agent has invaded the body.
2. *Amplification of defenses:* To be effective, defense mechanisms that fight the recognized pathogen must be produced in large numbers.
3. *Attack:* The T and B cells (the specific cells of the immune system) and the antibodies (produced by the B cells) seek out and destroy infected cells and disable free-floating pathogens.
4. *Slowdown:* After the pathogen has been contained or eliminated, the suppressor T cells halt the entire range of immune responses, preventing them from getting out of control and depleting the system.

A properly functioning immune system is necessary to help prevent or conquer disease once it has invaded the body. Without a normal functioning immune system, the body becomes a victim to serious and potentially life-threatening disease(s).

Immunity.   Immunity, the resistance of the body to pathogenic microorganisms and their toxins occurs as a result of the antigen-antibody reaction. Specific types of immunity follow:

- Active immunity develops when antigens are introduced into the body.
- Passive immunity develops when ready-made antibodies are introduced into the body.
- Natural immunity is an inborn resistance to a disease as a result of antibodies that are normally present in the blood.
- Acquired or induced immunity results from antibodies that are not normally present in the blood.

Active and passive immunity can be either natural or acquired.

Natural immunity.   Natural immunity can be active or passive. *Inherited (active) immunity* is acquired by being a member of a race or species. Some races are more or less susceptible to certain diseases. The longer a race has been exposed to a certain disease, the less susceptible its members become. Humans do not contract many diseases common to lower species of animals, and lower species of animals do not contract most human diseases. *Congenital (passive) immunity* is the immunity possessed at birth; antibodies are passed from the mother through the placenta to the fetus. The duration of this immunity can last from 5 to 6 months.

Acquired immunity.   Acquired immunity can be active or passive. *Natural active immunity* results from being a carrier, recovering from or having a disease, or having an atypical or subclinical case of the disease.

Artificial active immunity is acquired through vaccinations with inactivated (dead) or attenuated (weakened) organisms. Inactivated or dead vaccines include the typhoid, whooping cough, and influenza vaccines, as well as the Salk vaccine for polio. Attenuated vaccines include vaccines for polio (the Sabin vaccine), smallpox, measles (rubeola), mumps, and German measles (rubella). Toxoids are exotoxins that have been modified to reduce the toxicity (for example, diphtheria and tetanus toxoids).

Artificial passive immunity is obtained by injecting various products that are usually prepared commercially to produce a high level of antibodies immediately. These products are used to modify, treat, or prevent disease; they include immune globulin and antitoxins.

Immune globulin, obtained from the blood, is sometimes used for treatment but is more commonly used for the prevention of viral hepatitis and measles. Antitoxins include the following:

- Diphtheria antitoxin, produced by vaccinating horses and then extracting the gamma globulin fraction of the blood, is used for the immediate prevention and treatment of diphtheria.
- Tetanus antitoxin, obtained by extracting the gamma globulin fraction from the blood of people recently vaccinated with the tetanus toxoid, is used for the immediate prevention and treatment of tetanus.
- Immune sera, either bacterial or viral in origin, are obtained from the immune globulin fraction of blood from an artificially immunized animal. The rabies immune sera and the pertussis (whooping cough) immune sera are the most commonly used products.

A summary of immunization recommendations can be found in the *Student Mastery Manual.*

Vaccination records should be kept current. Parents must understand the purposes and possible risk factors when a child is immunized. As of August 1992, federal law states that a parent or guardian must be informed about the recommended vaccines.

Federal law requires that the appropriate Vaccine Information Statement(s) (VISs), which have been developed by the Centers for Disease Control and Prevention (CDC), be given to the patient or parent/guardian before each dose of a vaccine is administered. These statements provide information on the disease and vaccine, including the risks and benefits of the vaccine. The need for the patient or parent/guardian to sign an informed consent form before the vaccine is administered is determined by *state law*. The VISs are *not* to be used as designated informed consent documents. Therefore you must consult *your* state law to determine if there are any specific "informed consent" requirements relating to immunizations (see also Pediatric Examinations in Chapter 5, pp. 249-267, for information on immunizations and the VISs).

In addition to childhood vaccinations, there is a continuing need for adults to receive certain vaccinations. Some vaccine-preventable infections in adults represent a continuing cause of sickness and death, especially among older persons. An increased awareness and education are required of *both* the public and health care providers of the need for adult immunizations. VISs from the CDC are the same for both adults and children (see Health Matters boxes on pp. 252-265). Table 2-2 presents recommendations for adult immunizations.

TABLE 2–2 **California Adult Immunization Recommendations**

Vaccine* or Toxoid†	Indications
Tetanus and diphtheria toxoids (Td)	All adults
Influenza vaccine (Flu)	a. Everyone 65 years of age or older (see comment)
	b. Residents of nursing homes and other long-term care facilities housing persons with chronic medical conditions
	c. Anyone who has a serious long-term health problem with:
	- heart disease - kidney disease
	- lung disease - metabolic disease, such as diabetes
	- asthma - anemia, and other blood disorders
	d. Anyone whose immune system is weakened because of:
	- HIV/AIDS or other diseases that affect the immune system
	- long-term treatment with drugs such as steroids
	- cancer treatment with x-rays or drugs
	e. Anyone 6 months to 18 years of age on long-term aspirin treatment (who could develop Reye syndrome if they contract influenza)
	f. Women who will be in the second or third trimester of pregnancy during the influenza season
	g. Physicians, nurses, family members, or anyone else coming in close contact with people at risk of serious influenza
Pneumococcal vaccine (Pneumo)	a. Everyone age 65 years and over
	b. Adults of any age with significant chronic cardiovascular or pulmonary disorders
	c. Adults of any age with splenic dysfunction, asplenia, Hodgkin's disease, multiple myeloma, cirrhosis, alcoholism, renal failure, cerebrospinal fluid leaks, immunosuppressive conditions
Measles, mumps, rubella vaccines (MMR)	Adults, especially health care personnel born since 1956 who are at risk of exposure to patients with measles or rubella, or who have contact with pregnant patients

*Foreign travel immunizations are not included. Nor are less commonly used vaccines, such as typhoid, rabies, and meningococcal vaccines.

†For all these vaccines and toxoids, (a) delay between doses does not require restarting series or repeating doses.

Schedule	Selected Contraindications	Comments
PRIMARY SERIES: Two doses 4-8 weeks apart, third dose 6-12 months after second **Dose:** 0.5 ml intramuscular (IM) **Booster:** Every 10 years	Neurologic or severe hypersensitivity reaction to prior dose	**WOUND MANAGEMENT:** Patients with three or more previous tetanus toxoid doses: (1) give Td for clean, minor wounds if 10 or more years since last dose; (2) for other wounds, give Td if 5 or more years since last dose. Patients with less than 3 or unknown number of prior tetanus toxoid doses: give Td for clean, minor wounds, and Td plus TIG (Tetanus Immune Globulin) for other wounds.
PRIMARY SERIES: One dose each Fall **Dose:** 0.5 ml IM **Booster:** Each Fall	Anaphylactic allergy to eggs	The age above which influenza immunization is recommended for everyone will likely be lowered from 65 to 50 years, starting by Fall 2000.
PRIMARY SERIES: One dose **Dose:** 0.5 ml IM or subcutaneous (SC) **Booster:** Immunosuppressed or immunodeficient persons: 5 years after first dose. Also, persons aged 65 years and older if first dose given before age 65 and 5 or more years have passed since first dose.		If elective splenectomy or immunosuppressive therapy is planned, give vaccine 2 weeks ahead, if possible.
PRIMARY SERIES: At least one dose on or after first birthday (Two measles-containing vaccine doses, both on or after the first birthday, if in college or in health care profession, with second dose at least 4 weeks after the first.) **Dose:** 0.5 ml SC	a. Immunodeficiency or immunosuppressive therapy b. Anaphylactic allergy to neomycin or gelatin c. Pregnancy d. Recent receipt of immune globulin preparation or blood/blood product (a precaution, but not a contraindication) e. Thrombocytopenia ≤6 weeks after prior dose	MMR is vaccine of choice, even if already immune to 1-2 of its components. Women should avoid pregnancy for 3 months after immunization, but as data show *no* risk to fetus from the vaccine, accidental immunization of a pregnant woman is not an indication for therapeutic abortion.

Continued

TABLE 2-2   **California Adult Immunization Recommendations—cont'd**

Vaccine or Toxoid	Indications
Hepatitis B vaccine (Hep B)	a. Homosexually active men b. Users of illicit injectable drugs c. Household and sexual contacts of hepatitis B virus carriers d. Health care providers frequently exposed to blood or blood-contaminated body fluids e. Clients and staff of institutions for the mentally retarded f. Hemodialysis patients g. Recipients of clotting factor VIII or IX concentrates h. Morticians, emergency medical technicians i. Other persons whose occupation puts them at increased risk of exposure to human blood or other blood-contaminated body fluids j. Sexually active heterosexual persons with multiple sexual partners or recent episode of sexually transmitted disease k. Certain international travelers
Inactivated polio vaccine (IPV)	a. Health care providers and laboratory workers *if* they are in close contact with patients excreting wild poliovirus or who handle specimens from such patients b. Members of community with current disease caused by wild polioviruses c. Travelers to non–polio-free countries
Varicella vaccine (Var)	a. Household contacts of immunocompromised persons b. Health care providers who have contact with immunocompromised, pregnant or other high-risk patients, including premature newborns NOTE: Immunization not necessary if person has reliable history of clinical varicella
Hepatitis vaccine (Hep A)	a. Traveling to or working in developing countries b. Homosexually or bisexually active males c. Patients with chronic liver disease (including HBsAg+ or anti-HCV+ persons if they also have clinical or laboratory evidence of chronic liver disease) d. Users of illegal injecting and noninjecting drugs if local epidemiologic data suggest increased risk e. Persons who receive blood clotting factor concentrates f. Persons who work with hepatitis A infected nonhuman primates or with hepatitis A virus in laboratory settings

In 1998 the CDC released a summary of immunization guidelines for **immunizations to protect health care providers** from vaccine-preventable diseases. Strong recommendations were given for protection against six diseases: hepatitis B, measles, mumps, rubella, influenza, and varicella.

At times people must be vaccinated against particular diseases for travel purposes. A special certificate booklet must be completed verifying the required vaccination(s). These booklets can be obtained from your local U.S. Government Printing Office or from the Superintendent of Documents, U.S. Government Printing Office, Washington, D.C. 20402 (Figure 2-4, pp. 45-46).

Inflammatory Process

The inflammatory process is a nonspecific defense response of the body to an irritating, invasive, or injurious foreign substance. In other words, it is a process by which the body responds to injury. Acute inflammation is stimulated by necrosis and degeneration of tissue (injuries), invading microorganisms (infection), and antigen-antibody reactions (allergies). The in-

Schedule	Selected Contraindications	Comments
PRIMARY SERIES: Three doses. The second dose must be at least 1 month after the first. The third dose must be at least 2 months after the second and at least 4 months after the first. Can start series with one manufacturer's vaccine and finish with another. **Dose:** (Adult): 1.0 ml IM **Booster:** Need unclear. None presently recommended.	Anaphylactic allergy to yeast	a. Persons with serologic markers of prior or continuing hepatitis B infection (carriage) do not need immunization. b. For hemodialysis patients and other immunodeficient or immunosuppressed patients vaccine dosage is doubled or special preparation is used. c. All pregnant women should be sero-screened for HBsAg and, if positive, their infants should be given postexposure prophylaxis starting at birth. d. Postexposure prophylaxis: Consult USPHS (ACIP) recommendations, local health department, or the Immunization Branch.
PRIMARY SERIES: Unimmunized adults: IPV. Two doses at 4–8 week intervals, third dose 6–12 months after second (can be as soon as 2 mo) **Dose:** 0.5 ml SC Partially immunized adults: Complete primary series with IPV schedule shown above; no need to repeat doses if schedule is interrupted. **Booster:** None routinely (see comments)	IPV: a. Pregnancy b. Anaphylactic allergy to neomycin	a. If potential exposure to wild poliovirus is imminent, adults who had only three doses of polio vaccine (IPV or OPV) previously may be given one more dose of IPV. b. OPV no longer routinely available in the United States
PRIMARY SERIES: Two doses 4-8 weeks apart **Dose:** 0.5 ml SC **Booster:** None recommended	a. Immunocompromised b. Anaphylactic reaction to gelatin or neomycin c. Recent receipt of immune globulin or blood product (precaution) d. Pregnancy	If apparent vaccine-caused rash occurs within 26 days after either dose, avoid direct contact with immunocompromised, pregnant, or other high-risk persons for duration of rash.
PRIMARY SERIES: Two doses 6-12 months apart **Dose:** (Adult): 1.0 ml IM **Booster:** None recommended	Anaphylactic allergy to alum (aluminum hydroxide)	a. Can give immune globulin at same time in different extremity. b. Immunization not routinely recommended for food handlers, health care providers, sewage workers, or child-care facility workers.

flammatory process includes dilation of the blood vessels because of increased blood flow; oozing of watery fluids and protein into tissue spaces (exudation) from the dilated blood vessels because of their increased permeability; and infiltration of neutrophils and monocytes (white blood cells) from the blood into the tissue of the injured area to phagocytize (ingest) necrotic tissue and bacteria, if present.

After phagocytosis is complete, the liquefied remains diffuse back into the blood vessels or are carried away by the lymphatic vessels that drain into regional lymph nodes. Here the contents are filtered to prevent the spread of foreign substances or bacteria to other parts of the body. By now the process of repair has started at the original site of inflammation.

Signs and Symptoms.   Classic signs and symptoms of inflammation include both local signs and symptoms, which are a result of the changes seen in the blood vessels and the effect on the surrounding tissues, and systemic signs and symptoms.

Local
    Redness
    Heat or warmth

HEALTH MATTERS

KEEPING YOUR PATIENTS INFORMED ABOUT IMMUNIZATION

THE FLU

Flu, or influenza, is an easily spread virus. Flu shots are for anyone who wants to reduce the risk of catching the disease. They are especially important for people 65 years of age and older, and for those who suffer from chronic health problems like heart or lung disease or diabetes.

Influenza can be prevented with an annual shot taken every fall.

PNEUMOCOCCAL DISEASE

Pneumococcal disease is an infection of the lungs, bloodstream, and/or brain. It kills thousands of older people in the United States each year. Pneumococcal shots are recommended for people 65 and older, and for those with a chronic illness or weak immune system. One vaccination lasts most people a lifetime.

HEPATITIS B

Hepatitis B is caused by a highly infectious virus that attacks the liver. It can lead to liver cancer and death. The virus is found in the blood and other body fluids of infected people.

The hepatitis B vaccine is recommended for sexually active people with multiple sex partners, health care providers, all adolescents, people living among others with the virus, children of immigrants or parents of adopted children from certain countries, Native Americans and Alaskan Natives, people who use street drugs, and international travelers visiting areas where the disease is common.

Three shots are needed to protect against hepatitis B. They are given over a 6-month period.

MEASLES, MUMPS, RUBELLA

Measles, mumps, and rubella are diseases spread by coughing, sneezing, and even talking. Pregnant women who get rubella during the first 3 months of pregnancy put their babies at risk for serious birth defects or even death. Mumps may put pregnant women at risk of spontaneous abortions. One vaccine, the MMR, is available for all these diseases.

Two doses are recommended for adults born after 1956 who cannot prove immunity.

TETANUS/DIPHTHERIA

Tetanus, also called lockjaw, is caused by a germ that enters the body through cuts or wounds. It leads to a severe infection of the nervous system and can be fatal. Diphtheria is spread by bacteria that affects the tonsils, throat, nose, and skin. This disease is easily passed from person to person through coughing, sneezing, or even laughing.

One combination shot, called Td booster, protects against both diseases. It should be taken once every 10 years after age 7.

HEPATITIS A

Hepatitis A, a virus that infects the liver, is usually contracted by eating something prepared under poor sanitary conditions. It can also be spread through sexual contact. The vaccine is recommended for those in direct contact with infected persons, workers and children at day care centers, travelers to developing countries where hepatitis A is common, and men who have sex with men.

Two doses are needed 6 to 12 months apart to ensure long-term protection. Travelers should get the first dose at least 4 weeks prior to departure.

CHICKENPOX

Chickenpox, or varicella, is spread easily through the air from sneezes and coughs or direct contact with infected persons' sores. While chickenpox is a mild disease in children, adults are more likely to develop pneumonia, bacterial infections, and brain inflammation.

People 13 years of age and older who have not had chickenpox can protect themselves by getting 2 doses of the varicella vaccine.

DID YOU KNOW?

- 20,000 Americans die annually from flu-related illnesses.
- Pneumococcal disease leading to pneumonia is to blame for up to 40,000 deaths each year.
- Nearly one-third of adults with hepatitis B don't know how they got infected.
- Adults are 25 times more likely than children to die from chickenpox.

Swelling
Pain or tenderness
Limitation of function in the area
Systemic
　Leukocytosis (increased number of white blood cells in the blood)
　Fever
　Increased pulse rate
　Increased respiration rate

Infection

Signs and Symptoms.   Common signs and symptoms of infection follow. The patient may have only a few of the signs and symptoms listed for each type of infection. At other times, all of the listed signs and symptoms may be present. Common sexually transmitted diseases are discussed in Chapter 11, under Vaginal Smears and Culture Collection and in Table 11-1.

FIGURE 2-4 International certificates of vaccination. Administration of vaccinations necessary for international travel must be documented in this booklet and carried as the person travels. (Courtesy U.S. Department of Health, Education, and Welfare.)

INTERNATIONAL CERTIFICATES OF VACCINATION
AS APPROVED BY
THE WORLD HEALTH ORGANIZATION
(EXCEPT FOR ADDRESS OF VACCINATOR)

CERTIFICATS INTERNATIONAUX DE VACCINATION
APPROUV'ES PAR
L'ORGANISATION MONDIALE DE LA SANT'E
(SAUF L'ADRESSE DU VACCINATEUR)

TRAVELER'S NAME-NOM DU VOYAGEUR

ADDRESS-ADRESSE (Number-Nem'ero)   (Street-Rue)

(City-Ville)

(County-Departement)   (State-Etat)

U.S. DEPARTMENT OF HEALTH, EDUCATION, AND WELFARE
PUBLIC HEALTH SERVICE

PHS-731 (REV.1-74)

INSTRUCTIONS TO TRAVELERS

International Certificate of Vaccination or Revaccination are official statements verifying that proper procedures have been followed to immunize you against a disease which could be a threat to the United States and other countries. The Certificates are second in importance only to your passport in permitting uninterrupted international travel. THEY MUST BE COMPLETE AND ACCURATE IN EVERY DETAIL, or you may be detained at ports of entry.

When your itinerary is complete, you may obtain information on immunizations required or recommended for foreign travel from your local or State Health Department.

How to Complete Your International Certificates of Vaccination

1. Enter your name and address on the cover of the booklet before presenting it to your physician.

2. On the Certificates required for your travel, print your name on the first line; sign your name on the second line; indicate your sex; and indicate your date of birth in the following sequence: day, month, year. Example: 5 June 1980.

3. Vaccination against cholera may be given by any licensed physician in the United States. After the physician completes his part of the Certificate, take it to your local health department to be validated. Yellow fever immunization may be obtained only at a designated Yellow Fever Vaccination Center. The Certificate must be stamped with the official stamp of the Yellow Fever Vaccination Center.

4. It is your responsibility to have the Certificates validated with an "approved stamp." THE CERTIFICATES ARE NOT VALID WITHOUT AN "APPROVED STAMP."

INSTRUCTIONS TO PHYSICIAN

INFORMATION REQUESTED ON EACH CERTIFICATE MUST BE COMPLETE FOR THE CERTIFICATE TO BE VALID.

1. The space for primary vaccination against smallpox is to be used only when a person receives his vaccination for the first time. If unsuccessful, a new Certificate must be used for a repeat primary vaccination.

2. The dates on each Certificate are to be written with the day in arabic numerals, followed by the month in letters and the year in arabic numerals. Example: 1 Jan. 2000.

3. Vaccinations may be given by nurses and medical practitioners. The WRITTEN signature of the physician or other person authorized by him must appear on the Certificate. A signature stamp is not acceptable.

4. If smallpox vaccination is contraindicated on medical grounds, you should provide the patient with a written statement on your letterhead, signed and dated, indicating the nature on the contraindication.

5. Information concerning official immunization requirements for international travel and the location of Yellow Fever Vaccination Centers in your area may be obtained from your local or State Health Department.

DO NOT THROW THIS BOOKLET AWAY. YOU MAY HAVE OCCASION TO USE THE CERTIFICATES FOR FUTURE TRAVEL AND AS A RECORD OF YOUR VACCINATION HISTORY.

Continued

FIGURE 2-4—cont'd   International certificates of vaccination. Administration of vaccinations necessary for international travel must be documented in this booklet and carried as the person travels. (Courtesy U.S. Department of Health, Education, and Welfare.)

PERSONAL HEALTH HISTORY

The information which follows is a record of other immunizations which the traveler has obtained as an additional health protection for international travel. These immunizations are NOT usually required for entrance by any country. Space is also provided for a personal health record in case of illness or accident while traveling abroad.

OTHER IMMUNIZATIONS (Typhus, Typhoid, Plague, Poliomyelitis, Tetanus, etc.)

Date	Vaccine	Dose	Physician's Signature

REMARKS CONCERNING VACCINATIONS-REMARQUES CONCERNANT LES VACCINATIONS

Date	Notes	Physician's signature and address / Signature et adresse du me'decin

This information is to assist any physician called upon to treat an ill traveler.
Cette information est pour aider le me'decin qui peut etre appel'e pour traiter un voyageur malade.

Date	Rh type / Type Rh	Blood group / Groupe sanguin	Name and address of physician / Signature et adresse du me'decin

Name and address of person to notify in case of emergency.
Nom et adresse de la personne a aviser en cas d'urgence.

REMARKS concerning state of health, medical treatments, or known sensitivities:
REMARQUES concernant l'etat de sante, traitements medicaux, ou sensibilites connues:

OPHTHALMIC INFORMATION (Prescription Glasses)

	Sphere	Cylinder	Axis	Prism	Base
(OD) Ocular Dexter					
(OS) Ocular Sinister					

Add _____   Base Curve _____

Other _____

HEALTH **MATTERS**

KEEPING YOUR PATIENTS INFORMED

TEN IMPORTANT FACTS FOR OLDER ADULTS TO KNOW ABOUT VACCINES

1. Each year up to 60,000 adults, many aged 65 or older, die of preventable infectious diseases (influenza, pneumoccocal infection, and hepatitis B).
2. All people 65 years of age or older should receive influenza and pneumococcal vaccines. People who are in a certain high-risk group should receive hepatitis B vaccines.
3. Pneumonia and influenza, together, are the SIXTH LEADING CAUSE OF DEATH in the United States. Most of these deaths occur in people aged 65 or older.
4. Influenza vaccine can prevent up to 70% of hospitalizations and 85% of deaths from influenza-related pneumonia.
5. Because influenza viruses change each year, people should receive the new vaccine annually, usually in the fall. You cannot get influenza from the vaccine.
6. Influenza vaccine WILL NOT protect you from other respiratory infections, such as colds and bronchitis.
7. Pneumococcal pneumonia is the most common type of pneumonia, accounting for up to one third of all types of pneumonias that lead to hospitalization.
8. Pneumococcal vaccine can prevent up to 60% of serious pneumococcal infections, but it WILL NOT protect you from other types of pneumonia.
9. Pneumococcal vaccine is usually a once-in-a-lifetime shot. You cannot get pneumonia from the vaccine.
10. Because most cases of tetanus and diphtheria occur in adults, ALL adults should receive booster shots every 10 years. People who travel outside the United States should be evaluated for other vaccines that may be necessary.

This information was prepared in cooperation with the Centers for Disease Control and Prevention.

Localized infections
    Edema, redness of the area
    Exudate or drainage that is clear, cloudy, serous, purulent, or bloody
    Itching (in some infections)
    Pain
    Redness
    Swelling
    Tenderness
    Warmth
Generalized infections
    Altered mental status
    Confusion
    Congestion
    Convulsions
    Decreased appetite
    Fatigue
    Fever
    Headache
    Hypotension
    Increased pulse rate
    Jaundice (in some infections)
    Joint pain
    Light-headedness
    Malaise
    Muscle aches
    Possible elevation of white blood cell count
    Shock
Respiratory infections
    Abnormal breath sounds
    Chest pain
    Congestion
    Cough
    Elevated white blood cell count
    Fever
    Increased pulse rate
    Positive sputum culture
    Positive throat culture
    Positive x-ray film findings
    Productive cough (sputum)
    Rhinitis
    Shortness of breath
    Sore throat
Genitourinary infections
    Dysuria
    Elevated white blood cell count
    Fever
    Flank or pelvic pain
    Frequency
    Hematuria
    Positive urine culture
    Purulent or foul discharge
    Urgency
Gastrointestinal infections
    Abnormal bowel sounds
    Abdominal cramps
    Anorexia
    Diarrhea
    Distention
    Elevated white blood cell count
    Fever
    Increased pulse rate
    Nausea
    Positive guaiac test
    Vomiting

DIAGNOSTIC DATA

None of the local or systemic signs and symptoms of the inflammatory process are diagnostic in themselves. Many of these signs and symptoms are seen in disease processes other than the infectious process. However, they do provide clues that aid in the diagnosis of a suspected infection. Diagnostic tests in conjunction with an evaluation of the patient's general health status are required to confirm a diagnosis and initiate therapeutic decisions. Examples of diagnostic tests used to obtain data follow. Each of these tests is discussed in detail in its respective chapter.

- Microbiologic tests—bacterial, viral, and fungal cultures and the Gram stain; cultures are commonly obtained from blood, sputum, urine, spinal fluid, aspirates of body fluids, and body discharges at any possible site of infection
- Blood counts
- Urinalysis
- Skin tests
- Radiologic examinations
- Ultrasound examinations
- Gallium scans
- Computed tomography (CT) scans

The techniques for collecting and handling laboratory specimens must be correct to ensure accurate results (see Chapter 11 for the methods of properly handling and collecting specimens.) Inaccurate results lead to a false diagnosis and an inappropriate form of therapy for the patient. Knowledge of the infectious disease process, of the signs and symptoms of an infectious process, and of prevention and control measures are vital to control and prevent all infectious disease processes.

INFECTION CONTROL

To control and prevent the infectious process, the sequential connection between the six factors involved in this process must be broken at the weakest point. Various medical and surgical aseptic practices can break this cycle so that microorganisms cannot spread to and invade a susceptible host (see Figure 2-1).

Medical Asepsis

Medical asepsis refers to the destruction of microorganisms after they leave the body. Techniques used to accomplish this include practices that help reduce the number and transfer of pathogens. Many of these practices are observed in everyday living (for example, washing one's hands after using the bathroom or before handling food; covering one's nose and mouth when sneezing or coughing; and using one's own hair comb, toothbrush, and eating utensils).

Common medical aseptic practices to follow to break the cycle of the infectious process when working with patients include the following:

- Wash your hands before and after handling supplies and equipment and before and after assisting with each patient. The handwashing procedure is discussed in detail in this chapter.
- Handle all specimens as though they contain pathogens.
- Use disposable equipment when available and dispose of it properly, according to office policy. All equipment is considered contaminated after patient use.
- Clean nondisposable equipment before and after patient use.
- Use gloves to protect yourself (see Universal/Standard Precautions in Chapter 1).
- Use clean or sterile equipment and supplies for each patient.
- Avoid contact of used supplies with your uniform to prevent the transfer of pathogens to yourself and other patients.
- Place damp or wet dressings, bandages, and cottonballs in a waterproof bag when discarding them to prevent the possible spread of infection to individuals who handle the garbage.

HEALTH MATTERS

KEEPING YOUR PATIENTS INFORMED

"Infectious diseases are the third-leading cause of death in the United States and the leading cause of death worldwide," states Dr. James Hughes, Director of The National Center for Infectious Diseases at the CDC.

COMMON EVERYDAY PRACTICES FOR EVERYONE TO USE TO PREVENT INFECTIOUS DISEASES

1. Wash your hands frequently, especially in flu and cold seasons.
2. Vaccinate children, adults, and animals according to the immunization recommendations stated by disease control centers.
3. Prepare and store food carefully and according to the directions given. Cook food thoroughly and avoid eating improperly cooked foods.
4. Report any infections that do not get better to a physician.
5. Use antibiotics ONLY as directed. Abuse of antibiotics by many people has given rise to strains of pathogens that are now resistant to antibiotics, making treatment harder and sometimes impossible.
6. Check with your physician or public health centers about possible disease threats in areas of the world when traveling to those places. Keep your vaccination record up-to-date.
7. Avoid high-risk unsafe practices, such as unprotected sex and intravenous drug use and sharing needles.
8. Be cautious around wild or unfamiliar animals.
9. Use insect repellent if in an area that has a lot of insects.
10. Keep yourself informed and help to inform and educate others in ways to prevent and control the spread of infectious diseases.

- Cover any break in your skin as a protective measure against self-infection.
- Discard items that fall on the floor or clean before using because all floors are contaminated.
- Use damp cloths for dusting or cleaning to avoid raising dust, which carries airborne microorganisms.
- If you are unsure whether supplies are clean or sterile, clean or sterilize them before use.

These practices are used during "clean" procedures, which involve parts of the body that are not normally sterile. Specific examples include aseptic procedures used when taking a temperature; obtaining urine, stool, or sputum specimens; obtaining smears or cultures from the throat or vagina; administering oral medications; removing and discarding used supplies; and cleaning a treatment room after use. See Universal/Standard Precautions in Chapter 1.

Handwashing.   To prevent the spread of microorganisms, handwashing is one of the first procedures that all health personnel must learn. **Correct handwashing is the foundation of aseptic technique.** Hands that are not properly cleansed often spread infection because the hands are in constant use when working with or around patients.

This procedure must become an automatic part of your work. Its importance *cannot* be overemphasized, and your conscientiousness *cannot* be overstressed. The time involved to wash the hands, wrists, and forearms well should be 1 to 2 minutes (2 to 4 minutes if they are highly contaminated).

The use of bar soap is being discouraged because of the possibility of cross-contamination between people using it. In addition, a wet bar of soap is a good reservoir for microorganisms. Liquid soap or soap granules are preferred and recommended, especially in areas where many people use the same facilities. When liquid soap is used, the dispenser should be replaced or cleaned and filled with fresh product when empty; liquids should not be added to a partially full dispenser.

Use a plain, nonantimicrobial soap for routine handwashing. Use an antimicrobial agent or waterless antiseptic agent for specific circumstances, such as outbreaks of infectious disease(s).

The following handwashing procedure includes information on using a bar of soap *ONLY* when it is the only form of soap available. Remember, liquid soap is preferred and *MUST* be used when available.

The Centers for Disease Control and Prevention (CDC) recommends the following guidelines:

- Wash your hands for 2 minutes before beginning to work with patients. This provides effective protection.
- Wash your hands for 30 seconds after each patient contact. This ensures minimal spread of infection.
- Wash your hands for 1 minute immediately after handling contaminated equipment, supplies, or organic material.

Also see the section on barrier precautions and handwashing in Chapter 1.

Surgical Asepsis

Surgical asepsis refers to the destruction of all microorganisms and spores, pathogenic as well as nonpathogenic, before they enter the body. The goal of surgical asepsis is to prevent infection or the introduction of microorganisms into the body.

Practices of surgical asepsis are usually referred to as sterile techniques and are used when an area and supplies in that area must be made and kept sterile. These techniques are used in all procedures in which entry into normally sterile body parts occurs (for example, when administering injections and during all surgical procedures). As an additional example, when

---

PROCEDURE 2-1

HANDWASHING

Objective

Understand and demonstrate how to wash your hands, wrists, and forearms, explaining the reasons for the actions taken.

Equipment

Clean paper towels	Soap—liquid preferred
Sink with running water	Orangewood stick or nail brush

PROCEDURE

1. Remove jewelry, except plain wedding band. Remove watch or move it up. Provide complete access to area to be washed.

2. Stand in front of the sink, making sure that your clothing does not touch the sink.

3. Turn water on; adjust it to a lukewarm temperature and a moderate flow to avoid splashing.

RATIONALE

Jewelry may harbor microorganisms.

Sinks are always contaminated.

Warm water makes better suds than cold water; hot water may burn or dry the skin.

PROCEDURE 2-1—cont'd

4. Wet hands and apply soap. When using bar soap, keep the bar in your hands throughout the whole procedure. For liquid soap use approximately 1 teaspoon. Apply enough soap to develop a good lather. If you drop the bar of soap, you must repeat the procedure.

Only the inside of a bar of soap is clean when in use; all other objects are considered contaminated.

5. Wash hands (palm, sides, and back), fingers, knuckles, and between each finger, using a vigorous rubbing and circular motion. If wearing a wedding band, slide it down the finger a bit and scrub skin underneath it. You must wash all areas on the hands. Interlace fingers and scrub between each finger (Figure 2-5).

Friction caused by vigorous rubbing mechanically removes dirt and organisms.

6. During the procedure, keep the hands and forearms at elbow level or below and hands pointed down.

This prevents water from running down to the elbows, which are areas of less contamination than the hands.

7. Rinse hands well under running water.

8. Wash wrists and forearms as high as contamination is likely.

Washing the wrists and forearms after the hands prevents the spread of microorganisms from the hands to these areas.

9. If bar soap was used, rinse it off and drop it on a rack in the dish without touching the dish. Bar soap should ONLY be used when liquid soap or soap granules are not available.

Soap bars are excellent media for the growth of bacteria; therefore they must be rinsed after use. The soap dish is considered contaminated and therefore must not be touched. Bar soap should be kept on racks that allow drainage of water so that the soap can dry.

10. Rinse hands, wrists, and forearms under running water (Figure 2-6).

Running water rinses away the dirt and organisms that have been loosened during the washing process.

11. Clean nails with orangewood stick or nail brush at least once a day when starting work and each time hands are highly contaminated; then rinse well under running water (Figure 2-7).

Microorganisms collect and can remain under the nails unless cleansed away.

12. Repeat steps 3 through 10 when the hands are highly contaminated.

A second washing is necessary when the hands are heavily contaminated to ensure that all the microorganisms have been removed.

13. Thoroughly dry hands, wrists, and forearms with paper towels. Use a dry towel for each hand.

Drying the skin completely prevents chapping.

14. Use another dry paper towel to turn water faucet off (Figure 2-8).

The faucet is contaminated; using a dry paper towel allows the hands to remain clean.

15. Use hand lotion as necessary.

Lotion helps replace the skin's natural oils and prevents chapping. Chapping skin is more difficult to keep clean and more likely to crack. Once the skin is broken, microorganisms can easily enter and cause an infection.

changing dressings on a wound, a sterile field, sterile equipment, and sterile technique are maintained to prevent infection from developing.

Measures used to obtain and provide surgical asepsis include absolute sterilization of all instruments and supplies that come in contact with normally sterile body parts and open wounds, thorough handwashing with a detergent or surgical soap, and wearing sterile gloves during sterile procedures. During surgical procedures, the physician and those directly involved with the procedure also wear a

FIGURE 2-5   Handwashing technique. Interlace the fingers to wash between them. Create a lather with the soap. Keep hands pointed down.

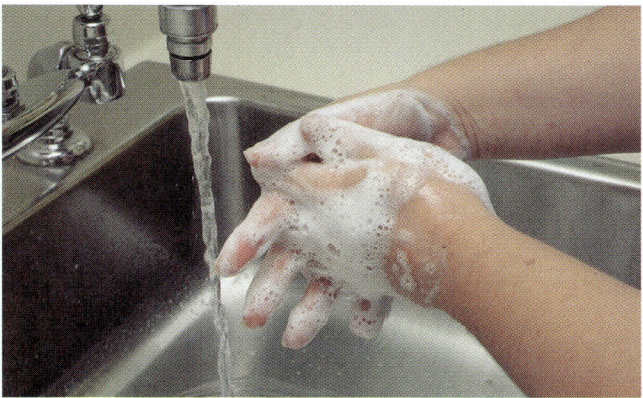

FIGURE 2-8   After drying hands, turn water faucet off, using a dry paper towel.

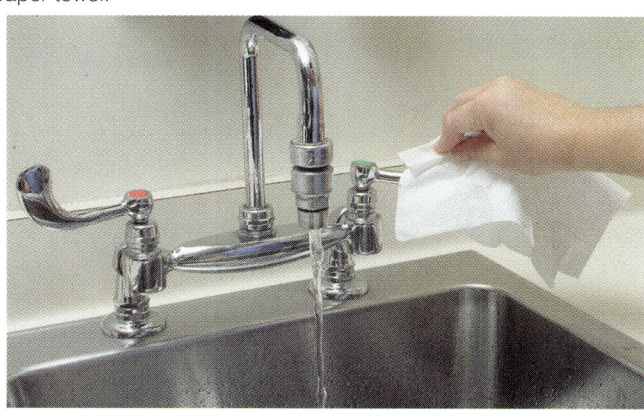

FIGURE 2-6   Rinse hands well, keeping fingers pointed down.

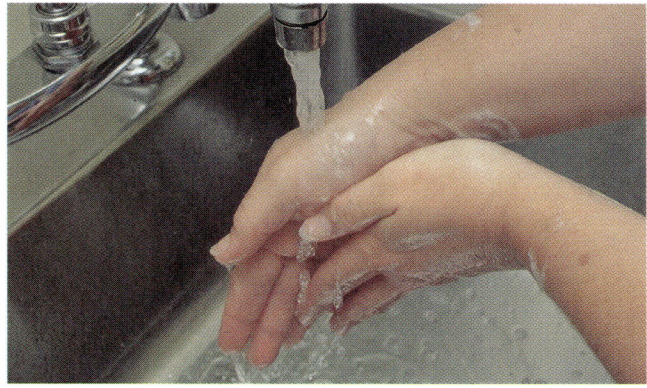

FIGURE 2-7   Use the blunt edge of an orangewood stick to clean under the fingernails.

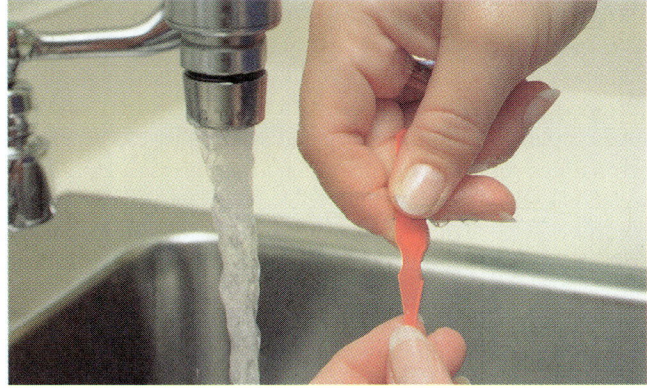

sterile gown, a cap, and a mask to help prevent contamination.

Methods of sterilization and disinfection are discussed in this chapter. The use of other surgical aseptic or sterile techniques and practices is discussed in Chapter 6.

METHODS TO CONTROL MICROSCOPIC AGENTS

Sanitization, disinfection, and sterilization are the three principal methods used for inhibiting the growth of and destroying microscopic life. Each represents a different level of decontamination, and though often used jointly, one must not be confused or substituted for the other.

Sanitization, the first step that must always be done before items can be reliably disinfected or sterilized, is a process of cleansing and scrubbing items with agents such as water and detergents or chemicals. Ultrasonic cleaners are also used (see Figure 2-19).

Disinfection involves methods that destroy "most" infectious microorganisms. However, some resistant and spore-forming bacteria and some viruses, such as the hepatitis B virus, are not adequately destroyed by these methods. Agents used to disinfect items include various types of chemical germicides and boiling water or flowing steam.

Sterilization is a precise scientific term with a single, exact meaning when applied to medical supplies and instruments. Sterilization is defined as the processes or methods that completely destroy all forms of microscopic life, including bacterial spores.

Using specific procedures, sterilization is accomplished by subjecting the object(s) to chemical or physical agents that are capable of killing the microorganisms. It must be emphasized that there are no degrees of sterility—**objects are either sterile or unsterile.**

Sterilization plays a vital role in protecting the health and life of patients who seek treatment in both physicians' offices and hospitals. The use of presterilized disposable equipment has greatly helped reduce the spread of microorganisms and the need for sterilization procedures. Almost all equipment used in a physician's office or clinic is now available in disposable materials. Nonetheless, certain nondisposable items and equipment, such as a stethoscope, are used repeatedly on many patients. Therefore the microorganisms that contaminate nondisposable supplies must be destroyed by appropriate measures.

PROCEDURE 2-2

SANITIZING INSTRUMENTS

PROCEDURE	RATIONALE
1. Bulk rinse the instruments in water containing a blood solvent, a low-sudsing detergent, or any *approved* germicide solution.	*This first step is to clean all debris, oil, blood, and grease off the instruments.*
2. Rinse the instruments in another sink or pan of fresh water.	
3. Scrub each instrument thoroughly with a brush and a warm nonionizing detergent solution (such as Tide or Joy). Keep the instrument under a flow of water or in water when scrubbing with the brush (Figure 2-9). Pay special attention to serrated edges and other areas where blood, oil, or grease may collect.	
4. Using hot water, thoroughly rinse all detergent off the instruments.	*Any detergent residue on an instrument prevents disinfection.*
5. Remove the excess moisture from the instruments by rolling them in a towel.	*Drying instruments helps to prevent rusting.*
6. Check all instruments for working condition and check to see that they are thoroughly cleaned. Never oil instruments, even if they are stiff when using them.	*Oil on an instrument may keep a contaminated area from a sterilizing agent.*
7. Wrap the instruments for sterilization.	
8. When instruments cannot be cleaned immediately after use, soak them in a solution of water and an effective blood solvent. Never soak an instrument in saline.	*Soaking prevents blood or other organic matter from drying or hardening on the instrument (which would be more difficult to remove later). Saline causes corrosion to the instrument.*

Methods used to accomplish sterilization include the following:

- Dry heat
- Moderately heated chemical gas mixtures
- Chemical agents
- Steam under pressure (autoclaves)
- Unsaturated chemical vapor (Chemiclaves)

The first three methods are limited to certain applications and require longer exposure periods to sterilize items; therefore they are not often used. The *autoclave,* the most commonly used sterilizing method, and the *Chemiclave* are considered the most efficient, reliable, and practical answers to meet the sterilizing needs in the physician's office or clinic.

Sterilization

Preparation of materials.   The initial step when sterilizing or disinfecting contaminated items is to remove them from the treatment room to the work area designated for dirty equip-

ment. Take care to avoid contamination to yourself or injury from any sharp instrument and to prevent dulling any sharp blade or scissors while you are handling instruments. When you handle contaminated items or if you have any break in your skin, wear heavy rubber gloves with long cuffs over disposable gloves; a plastic apron or gown; and safety glasses, goggles, or personal glasses with added solid side shields or a chin-length face shield when sanitizing supplies.

After you clean supplies, your hands are contaminated. Wash them as described previously (see also Barrier Precautions in Chapter 1).

Inspection of instruments.   The purpose of checking instruments is to ensure that they are in proper working order and in alignment before they are needed for use in a procedure. Check instruments in a well-lit clean area. Instruments should be dry before you check them.

1. Check that the serrations of each instrument meet evenly.
2. Check that the ratchets close easily and that they do not spring open.

FIGURE 2-9   When scrubbing, wear heavy rubber gloves over disposable gloves.

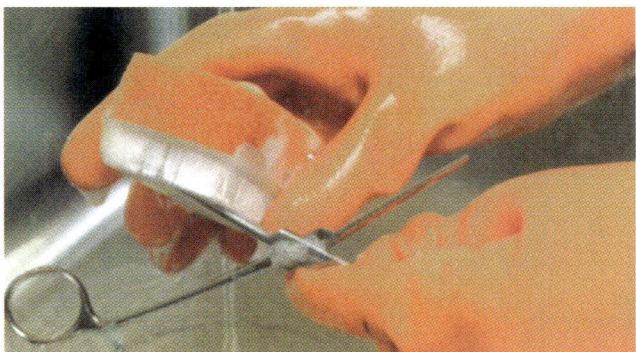

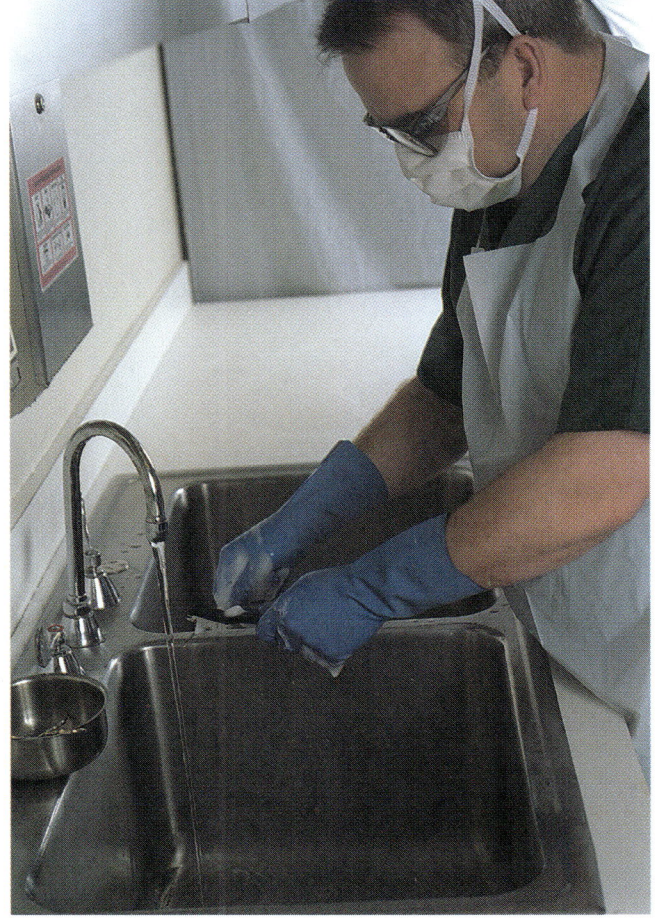

3. Check that the instruments open and close easily.
4. Check that all parts are present (for example, that the screws of a speculum are intact).
5. Coat instruments with a water-soluble lubricant such as instrument milk* to protect from corrosion and to provide lubrication for the hinges.
6. Air-dry for 20 minutes.
7. If imperfections are found, separate out and follow agency policy for dealing with broken equipment.
8. The instruments are now ready to be wrapped for sterilization.

Wrapping instruments and related supplies for sterilization.
The next step before sterilizing items that are to be stored for future use is to wrap them in protective coverings, such as clean muslin or special disposable paper bags. These materials are used because they can be permeated by steam or the chemical vapor from the sterilizer but not by airborne or surface contaminants during handling and storage.

Items that will be used immediately or those that do not have to be sterile when used (for example, supplies used for "clean" procedures) can be sterilized by placing them in the sterilizer tray with muslin or other material designated by the manufacturer under and over them. When you have completed the sterilizing process, remove the items with sterile transfer forceps and then either use or place them in the proper storage area.

Wrap the items that are to be kept sterile for future use. Wrap together materials and instruments that will be used together. Leave hinged instruments such as hemostats open when they are being sterilized for immediate or future use. Sterilize containers with lids on their sides with the lid off; place the lid at the side or bottom of the container, with the inner surface facing outward.

The method for wrapping instruments and other supplies such as dressings is the same. Figure 2-10 explains and illustrates the method to be used for wrapping these items. Study and practice this procedure of preparation. Keep packs small and wrap loosely but firm enough for handling.

Another aid to sterilization has been the introduction of disposable packaging materials, including paper, pouches, and tubing of paper and plastic. They are convenient for sterilizing and storing syringes, tubing, and special purpose items.

ATI Steriline bags are made of a special heavy-duty, wet-strength, surgical grade paper that allows rapid steam penetration during sterilization. They also act as a barrier against airborne bacteria during storage.

Each Steriline bag is printed with a temperature and steam-sensitive indicator consisting of an indicator line that changes color during sterilization to show that an item has been processed through the sterilizer (Figure 2-11, *A*).

ATI pouches and tubing offer a clearly labeled package that can be used either for steam or ethylene oxide (EO) gas sterilization. They offer advantages similar to those of Steriline bags, plus the benefits of content visibility and an easy, peel-open feature. Their use minimizes the risk of damaging expensive items by using the wrong sterilizing method. The steam indicator changes color from blue to grey/black during processing in either a gravity displacement or prevacuum, high-temperature steam sterilizer. The gas indicator changes color from yellow to rust/red during processing in an ethylene oxide gas sterilizer (Figure 2-11, *B*).

*Preplube Solution recommends 1:10. Review and follow the manufacturer's directions.

FIGURE 2-10   Wrapping technique.

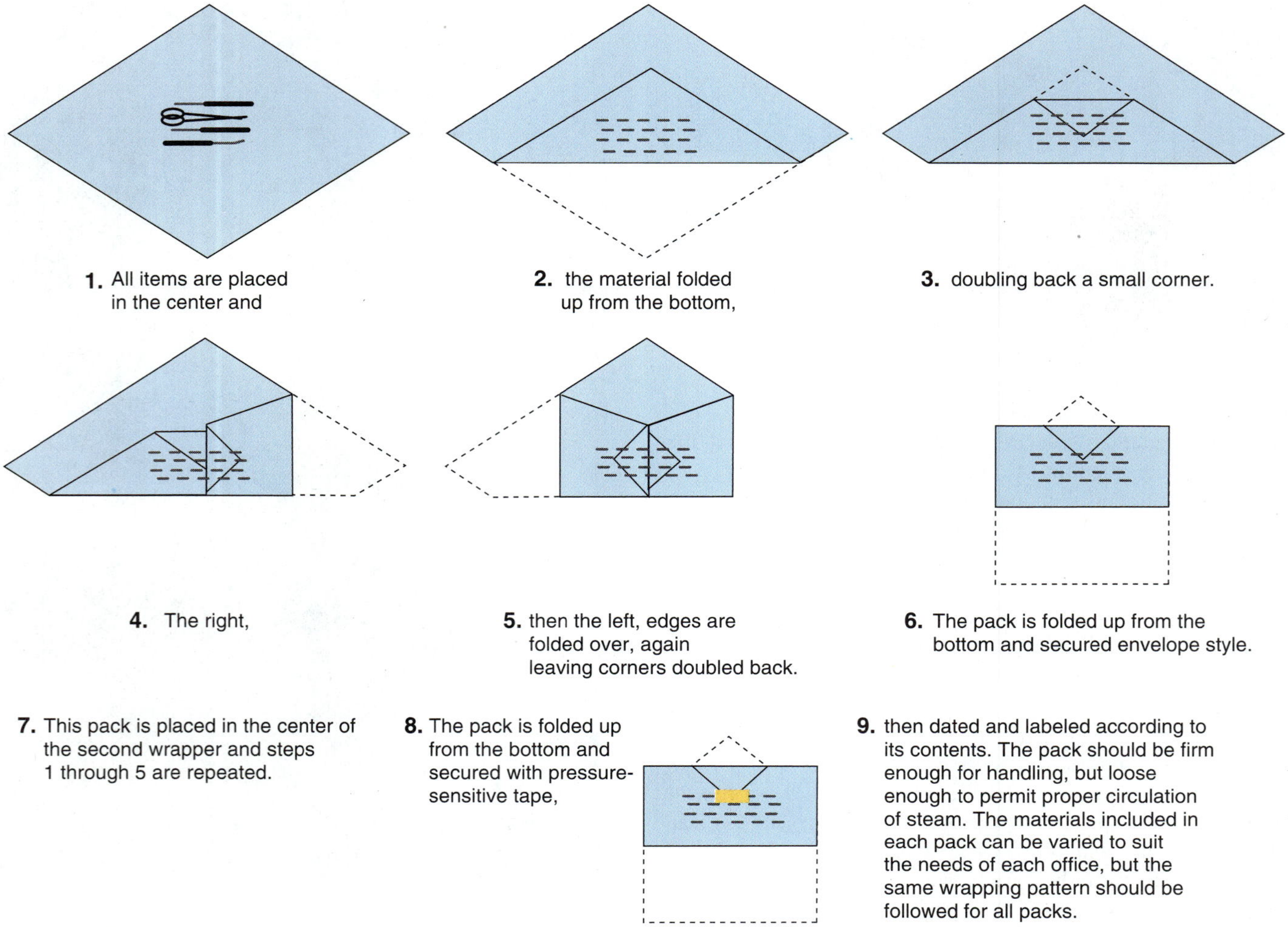

1. All items are placed in the center and

2. the material folded up from the bottom,

3. doubling back a small corner.

4. The right,

5. then the left, edges are folded over, again leaving corners doubled back.

6. The pack is folded up from the bottom and secured envelope style.

7. This pack is placed in the center of the second wrapper and steps 1 through 5 are repeated.

8. The pack is folded up from the bottom and secured with pressure-sensitive tape,

9. then dated and labeled according to its contents. The pack should be firm enough for handling, but loose enough to permit proper circulation of steam. The materials included in each pack can be varied to suit the needs of each office, but the same wrapping pattern should be followed for all packs.

ATI Instrument Protectors are convenient, disposable holders for delicate surgical instruments. They protect instrument tips from being cracked or broken and help prevent the instrument from penetrating the pouch or package in which it is placed. Chemical indicators on each protector verify steam or EO gas processing. To use these holders, first insert the instrument through the slots of the protector until the tip is completely covered by the plastic flap. Open hinged instruments such as scissors, and fold the antilock flap forward between the handles. For added protection and holding ability, tuck the antilock flap into the top slot. Slide the loaded instrument protector into a sterilization pouch, with the instrument facing the film side. Seal the pouch in the normal manner and sterilize (see Figure 2-11).

Wrapping reusable syringes and needles.   Syringes are best wrapped in special disposable paper bags or peel pouches that are available for sterilization (see Figure 2-11).

Autoclave—Steam Sterilization

Any appreciation of infection control must include an understanding of the basic principles and procedures of sterilization.

Although different methods of sterilization are available, steam sterilization still remains one of the most effective, economical, and safe procedures and is considered the method of choice whenever applicable.

The *purpose* of sterilization is to completely destroy all living microorganisms, including spores and viruses that may be present in the item being sterilized. The process must destroy or kill *all* microorganisms, including those that cause infection or disease (pathogens). There is no such thing as an object being "almost sterile" or "partially sterile."

Bacterial Life Cycle.   The reason why sterilization must be an absolute process is based on our knowledge of the bacterium and its life cycle. Bacteria have a very high rate of reproduction and can multiply rapidly into millions within hours. If only a few of these bacteria enter an operative wound from a supposedly sterile item, their multiplication may delay or inhibit recovery. Some may even cause the death of a patient. Bacteria in their vegetative form are easily destroyed by correct sterilization methods, but their spores are far more resistant. Spore forming is a protective mechanism by which the bacteria are able to remain dormant for extended periods, even years. In

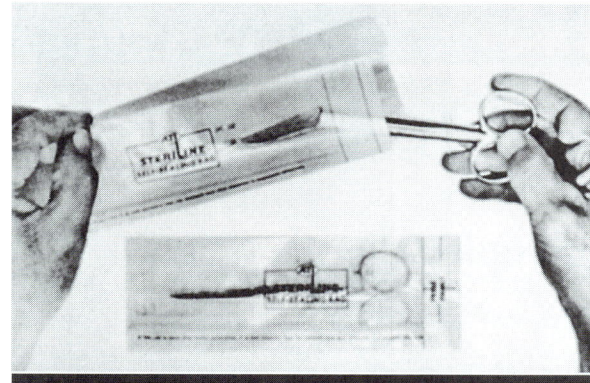

A

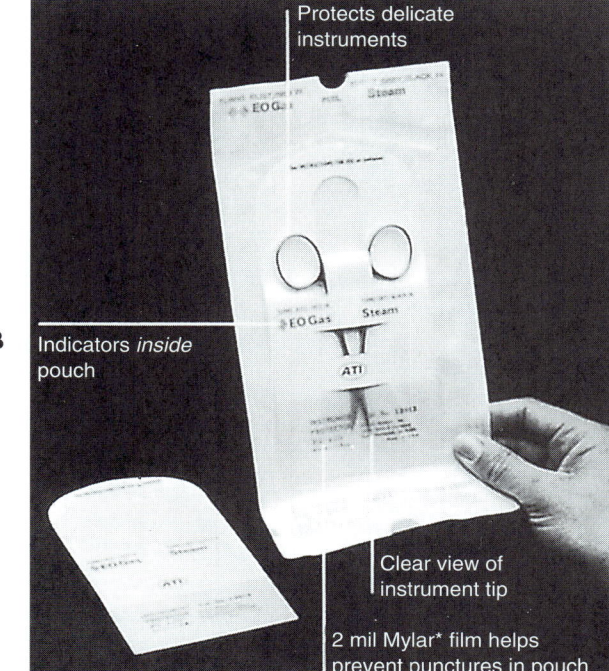

B

Protects delicate instruments

Indicators *inside* pouch

Clear view of instrument tip

2 mil Mylar* film helps prevent punctures in pouch

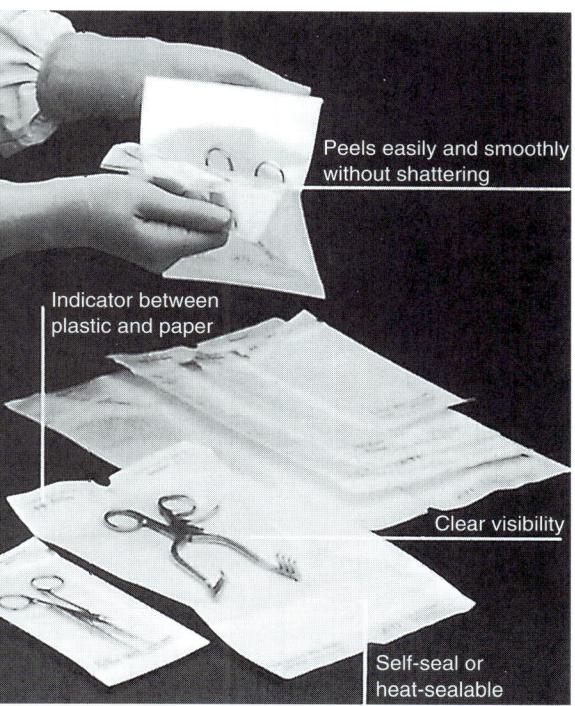

C

Peels easily and smoothly without shattering

Indicator between plastic and paper

Clear visibility

Self-seal or heat-sealable

FIGURE 2-11 **A** through **C,** ATI Instrument Protectors are thick, disposable paper holders designed to protect delicate surgical instruments during sterilization. They hold instruments snugly in place and help prevent the instrument from penetrating the pouch in which they are placed. Each instrument protector has steam and ethylene oxide (EO) gas indicators to verify processing in a sterilizer. (Courtesy ATI, a division of PyMaH Corp, Somerville, NJ.)

this state, they can survive conditions that would quickly kill their active or vegetative form. However, when these spores are again placed in a favorable condition for development, they become active bacteria capable of causing infection and death. Surgically critical microorganisms such as anthrax and *Clostridium* can pose a real threat to the human body if not completely destroyed. Thus sterilization must be absolute and destroy both active bacteria and their spores.

Critical Factors in Steam Sterilization

Heat and moisture.   Because microorganism destruction must be absolute, a knowledge of the factors controlling steam sterilization is essential. The killing power of saturated steam depends on three main factors: *heat, moisture,* and *time*. Heat by itself can readily kill bacteria. This is accomplished by disrupting the cell's life functions through coagulation of cell protein. However, spores are more resistant to dry heat but are readily destroyed by sufficient moist heat. Saturated steam is a gas and is therefore able to circulate by convection. This process allows it to penetrate porous objects in the steam sterilizer.

Time.   At any given temperature, exposure must be for a specific period to completely disrupt and destroy all the microorganisms. Steam sterilization may be adequately accomplished at any temperature above 212° F (100° C), provided the related period of exposure is used. You should always adhere to the required time; otherwise, unsterile supplies may result.

Research recommends a minimum of 12 minutes of direct exposure to saturated steam at 250° F (121° C) for surgical sterilization. In practice, it usually takes longer for direct exposure to take place throughout the pack (see Exposure Times).

When the temperature is increased, the length of time necessary for sterilization decreases. Conversely, if the temperature is lowered, more time is required to ensure sterilization.

PROCEDURE 2-3

WRAPPING REUSABLE SYRINGES AND NEEDLES

Objective
Understand and demonstrate how to wrap reusable syringes and needles for sterilization.

PROCEDURE	RATIONALE
1. Write the size of the syringe and the date on the outside of the bag.	*Size must be indicated for identification. Date must be indicated, because if not used within 21 to 30 days (varies with office or agency preference), it must be rewrapped and resterilized.*
2. Wrap barrel and plunger of the syringe separately in gauze.	
3. Place matching separated syringe barrel and plunger inside the bag (or peel pouch) with the top of both facing the same direction.	
4. Fold the top of the bag and seal securely.	
5. When the needle is to be sterilized with the syringe, place the needle in a disposable paper form.	*The paper form protects the point of the needle, allows steam penetration, provides a means for sterile handling when putting the needle on the syringe tip for use, and also prevents the needle from piercing the bag.*
6. Label the bag with the size of syringe and needle and the date.	
7. Place the needle in the bag with the syringe and plunger; fold the top of the bag and seal.	
8. When the needle is to be sterilized individually, place it in a plastic pouch as described in Figure 2-12, *A* and *B*.	*Consult the latest guidelines issued by the CDC and consult with infection control practitioners as needed to identify specific precautions that pertain to your particular work situation.*

FIGURE 2-12   A and **B,** Needles in packets ready for autoclaving. Some surgical needles are reusable, but the sterilization process is handled by central sterilization supplies in hospitals. Sterilization of needles generally is not handled in offices.

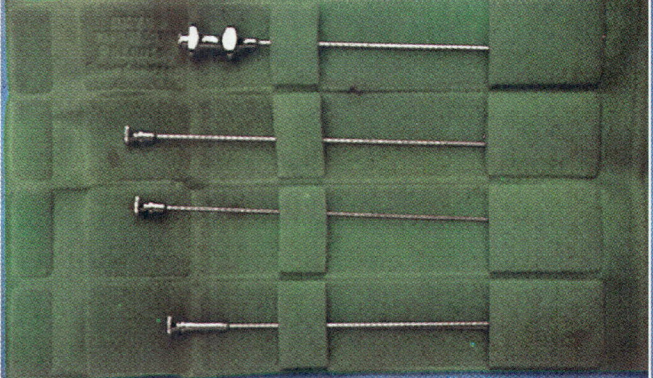
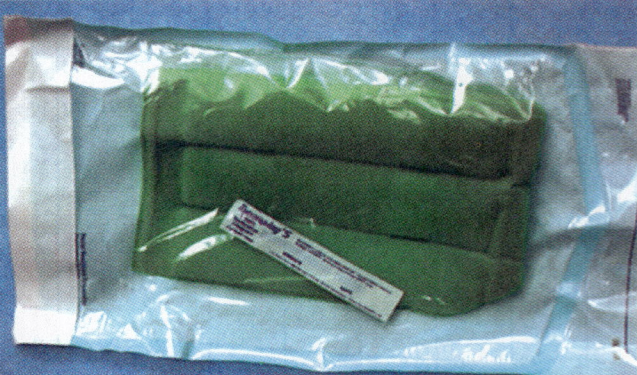

A   B

Temperature and pressure.   Because saturated steam is a gas, it is subject to the physical laws of gases. Although a detailed discussion of the subject is not possible here, two physical relationships between temperature and pressure should be mentioned. First, saturated steam cannot undergo a reduction in temperature without a corresponding lowering of pressure (the opposite is also true). Second, in high-altitude regions, greater steam pressure is necessary to reach the minimum temperature range for sterilization because atmospheric pressure decreases with an elevation in altitude.

Steam quality.   Steam can exist in various physical states, all of which have an effect on sterilizer performance. The three most common forms are:

1. *Saturated steam*: Steam containing pure gaseous water holding as much water as possible for its temperature and pressure. It is the most effective form of steam for sterilization.
2. *Wet steam*: This is usually formed when water from the boiler or condensate from the pipes carrying the steam is injected into the sterilizer. The result is an excess of water that can cause items in the sterilizer to become wet.
3. *Superheated steam*: Steam formed from saturated steam that is further subjected to higher temperatures. The steam becomes "dried out" and lacks sufficient water vapor, resulting in the loss of essential moisture necessary for sterilization.

General Procedures.   Correct sterilization technique is essential for the destruction of microorganisms and their spores. Remember that steam is lighter than air and that air must be eliminated from the sterilizer.

The following is an abbreviated discussion of recommended procedures.

Positioning loads in an autoclave.   Proper positioning of all instruments and materials is extremely important because of the pattern that steam follows as it circulates through the autoclave.

A direction booklet, which must be read carefully, is supplied with every sterilizer. Usually, when the sterilizing cycle begins, steam builds up at the top of the inside chamber and moves downward from the point of admission. Dry, cool air is forced downward and out an exhaust drain at the bottom front part of the chamber. You must place all materials so that steam can flow between the packs and penetrate them. To avoid the formation of air pockets, you must place containers, tubes, cups, and similar items on their sides so that cool air can drain out in a downward direction and be replaced by steam. If they are placed upright, air becomes trapped in the item, which in turn prevents steam from contacting all surfaces, resulting in incomplete sterilization.

Place syringes wrapped in disposable paper bags horizontally (on their sides) in the sterilizer tray so that steam can circulate inside the syringe barrel. Place constriction or test tubes with needles horizontally so that steam can circulate inside the tube. Place linen and dressing packs in a vertical position.

When sterilizing linen packs and hard items in the same load, place the linen packs on top and the hard items on the bottom to prevent water condensation from dripping down on the linen packs. Items should not rest against plastic utensils to allow plastics to retain their shape even though exposed to very high temperatures.

Above all, *do not* overload the sterilizer chamber, regardless of the number of items being sterilized. Place the articles as loosely as possible inside the chamber. Leave a 1- to 3-inch space between all articles and the surrounding walls in the chamber. Correct positioning and spacing of all materials allows

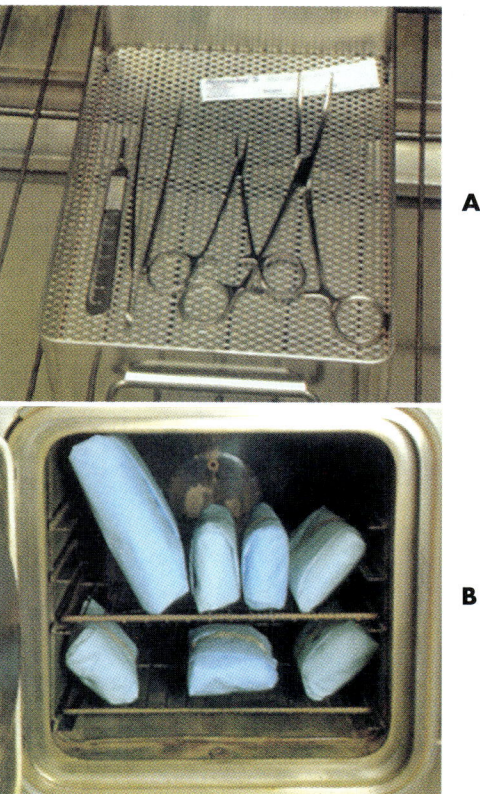

FIGURE 2-13   A, Instruments in autoclave for sterilization must be well spaced and hinged handles left open. **B,** Linen packs spaced correctly in an autoclave.

effective sterilization to occur when the proper *temperature, pressure,* and *time* requirements are also met (Figure 2-13).

NOTE: Do not try to open the door of the sterilizer for any reason once the sterilizing cycle has begun. If you do open the door while the cycle is in progress, the steam under pressure may cause severe injury to you. At that time, it may be impossible to reclose the door because of the pressure remaining inside the sterilizer. If the door is opened before the exhaust phase has been completed, the sterilizing process will be ineffective.

Exposure times.   All loads placed in a sterilizer must be timed carefully after the sterilizer has attained the proper temperature. The length of sterilization time varies with the items and whether a wrapper, paper, or fabric is used. Suppliers of such materials supply correct exposure data to ensure observance of adequate exposure periods.

The *high temperature* attained is the *sterilizing influence* that destroys the microorganisms. The amount of pressure used only makes it possible to develop the high temperature. An accurate thermometer on the autoclave should be used to provide a positive indication that sterilizing conditions have been met in the chamber. Thus the three variables in the sterilizing cycle of an autoclave are *time, temperature,* and *pressure.* Altering any one of these means that you must alter the others.

In the autoclave, when steam is in contact with all surfaces of the items, 30 to 45 minutes and 15 to 17 pounds of pressure

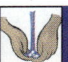

PROCEDURE 2-4

REMOVING LOADS FROM THE STERILIZER

Objective
Understand and demonstrate how to remove equipment from an autoclave after the sterilization cycle is finished.

PROCEDURE	RATIONALE
1. Exhaust steam pressure from the chamber. Read and follow precisely the manufacturer's directions for exhausting steam.	
2. When the pressure has reached 0 and the temperature has decreased to 212° F, open the door of the autoclave slightly (Figure 2-14). Only "crack" open the door.	*Stand back from the door to avoid steam burns to the face and hands. An open sterilizer door allows condensation from outside cool air; this results in wet packs.*
3. Allow the contents to dry for approximately 15 minutes before removing them. Some modern autoclaves automatically provide a sterilization cycle that includes drying, thus eliminating the need for these steps.	*Packs must not be removed wet or damp. If wet or damp packs are touched, they will be contaminated. Also, if a pack is hot and placed on a cool surface, moisture condenses and contaminates the pack.*
4. Regardless of the type of sterilizer you use, all dry, wrapped items and unwrapped items that do not have to remain sterile can then be removed with your clean, dry hands. Do not remove unwrapped metal objects too soon with bare hands.	*Metal retains heat, and you could get burned.*
5. Remove unwrapped items that are to remain sterile for immediate use with sterile transfer forceps; place items to be used later in sterile storage containers.	

at 250° F (121° C) is adequate time to kill all known microorganisms. However, in practice, longer periods are necessary to achieve this exposure. Recommended exposure times for items placed in an autoclave at 250° F (121° C) are as follows.

Wrapped surgical instruments	30 minutes
Wrapped syringes and needles	30 minutes
Wrapped rubber goods (excessive exposure causes heat damage to the rubber)	20 minutes
Wrapped dressings	30 minutes
Wrapped suture materials	30 minutes
Wrapped treatment trays	30 minutes
Unwrapped utensils, glassware, and similar items, when inverted or placed on edge	15 minutes
Unwrapped instruments covered with muslin	20 minutes

Again, you must scrupulously watch methods of wrapping, time of exposure, and temperature because the purpose of autoclaving is to sterilize every article completely. *Each manufacturer's direction booklet must be read and followed carefully to achieve adequate sterilization.*

Care and cleaning of the autoclave. Adherence to the manufacturer's instructions for cleaning and maintenance is es-

sential. Follow the spore check schedule for maintaining the autoclave.

Chemical sterilization indicators. Numerous commercial devices are used to indicate the effectiveness of the sterilization process. Used correctly, these devices, known as chemical sterilization indicators, are adequate assurances that the parameters of the sterilization process are met. These indicators work on the principle that specifically prepared dyes will change color when exposed to the high temperature and saturated steam in the autoclave for a specific time. Individual disposable indicators for which color changes are to be observed after sterilization include the Sterilometer-Plus and Sterilometers (Figure 2-15). Sterilometer-Plus represents one of the most precise, complete chemical indicators available. It consists of two indicator bars covered by a clear plastic overlay. The indicator bars contain a special reactive pigment that changes color from purple to green only in the presence of steam and not in the presence of heat alone (the water molecules in the steam actually are part of the color-change reaction, so the reaction cannot take place without steam present). The clear plastic overlay prevents the indicator areas from coming into contact with items being sterilized.

FIGURE 2-14 When the sterilization cycle is finished, "crack" open the door slightly and allow the contents to dry for 15 minutes before removing them.

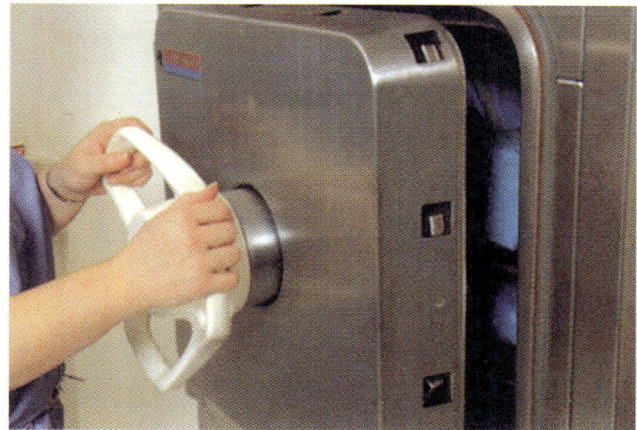

When the indicator is exposed to steam in a sterilizer, the steam begins to work on the indicator inks. The heat energy and water content of the steam react with the purple pigment in the ink and cause it to turn green. The ink contains other chemicals that carefully control the amount of time necessary for the ink to completely change color, so the indicator changes only when the conditions necessary for complete sterilization have been met.

The Sterilometer is a disposable tag that is placed in the center of a pack with the nonindicator end extended outside the wrapper. This feature enables the indicator to be removed without touching the contents of the pack. Sterilization conditions of adequate steam, temperature, and time are ensured if the wide bar at the opposite end has changed completely from white to black. If these color-change standards do not result, the pack must be reprocessed and resterilized.

Also, specific areas or markings on the outside of commercially prepared packages and on special disposable bags that are available for wrapping instruments, syringes, and needles change color if sterilization standards have been met (see Figure 2-15). These preceding indicators are superior to the frequently used *autoclave tape indicators* because the dark diagonal lines that appear on the tape at the end of the sterilization cycle merely indicate that the pack has been exposed to steam and the autoclaving process (Figure 2-16). Many other indicators are available for various types of sterilization processes. Figure 2-17 illustrates the dry heat sterilization indicator on a pressure-sensitive label, which changes from tan to black when exposed for 5 minutes at 340° F. When any sterilization indicator is used, the manufacturer's directions for use must be followed. Sterilization indicators must be stored in a dry place and away from excessive heat.

Evidence of sterility of equipment can *only* be obtained if a culture is taken from the equipment after it has been processed in the sterilizer. This means that the pack would have to be opened, and once opened, it would be contaminated by the air. *Biologic indicators and monitors* in test packs placed in the sterilizer can provide definitive biologic verification that conditions to kill spores were met in the sterilizer. An example of biologic monitors are small strips of specially impregnated paper to which a precise number of live, nonpathogenic resistant spores have been applied. They are designed to validate both the actual sterilizer "kill" function and the operator's wrapping and processing technique. The biologic strips are placed in hard-to-reach parts of the sterilizer, cycled with a normal load of instruments, and then cultured (provided with nutrition and incubation) and tested 24 and 48 hours later. If the spores grow, sterilization has not been achieved. A biologic monitor should be used daily in each sterilizer or according to agency policy to ensure that the sterilization process is effective and safe.

Causes of Insufficient Sterilization.   Failure of the indicators to change colors completely indicates a serious lack of steam penetration into the pack. This is a warning of a sterilizer malfunction or an error in the sterilization technique. *Never neglect this warning.* Causes of sterilization failure are numerous, elusive, and often difficult to locate. The problem may require minute examination of every part of the sterilizer and/or a complete reexamination of preparation, wrapping, and loading techniques. Some of the most common problems are the following:

1. Faulty preparation of materials
2. Improper loading of the sterilizer
3. Faulty sterilizer
4. Air in the sterilizer
5. Wet steam

Regarding technique, sanitize all materials completely beforehand, and wrap and secure them properly as described previously. You must position the load correctly in the sterilizer and not overload the chamber. Timing for adequate exposure times must begin *after* the sterilizer has attained the proper temperature. If all of these conditions have been met satisfactorily and sterilization has not taken place, you must have the equipment checked for a defect and repaired as necessary (Table 2-3).

Storing Sterile Supplies.   Special storage places for each type of supply should be maintained away from areas where contaminated materials are handled. Storage places must be clean, dry, and dustproof. The lowest shelf should be at least 8 inches from the floor. Sterile items wrapped in cloth or special sterilization paper can safely be stored for 21 to 30 days. Wrapped items that are placed in sterile plastic dustcovers can be stored for 6 months, and items wrapped in plastic peel-back packs (special envelopes with one side of transparent plastic and the other side of paper) can be stored for 3 months. When these periods are elapsed, all packs should be reprocessed and resterilized before use. A system should be created for storing supplies (for example, placing loads from the sterilizer or new items on the right side of the shelf and removing them for use from the left side). If supplies are stored in longer, narrower shelves, the oldest supplies are placed in the front and the new in the back. With these systems, the oldest supplies are always stored on the left side or in the front part of the designated shelf so that they will be used first. Once a month a time should be

FIGURE 2-15 A, Sterilometer-Plus sterilization indicators. Color changes from purple to green on the indicator bars, pointing out when the conditions necessary for sterilization have been met. **B,** Sterilometer sterilization indicators. Sterilization conditions are ensured if the wide bar at one end has changed completely from white to black. (Sterilometer-Plus and Sterilometer are registered trademarks of PyMah Corp., Somerville, NJ.)

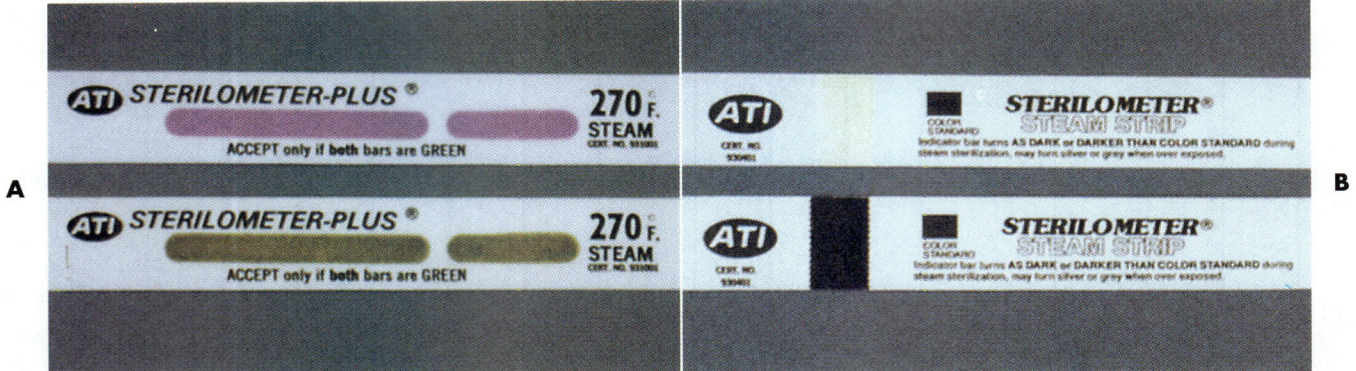

FIGURE 2-16 A, Autoclave indicator tape used to seal and label packages before sterilization. **B,** Dark diagonal lines appear on the tape after the sterilization cycle to indicate that the pack has been exposed to steam and the autoclaving process.

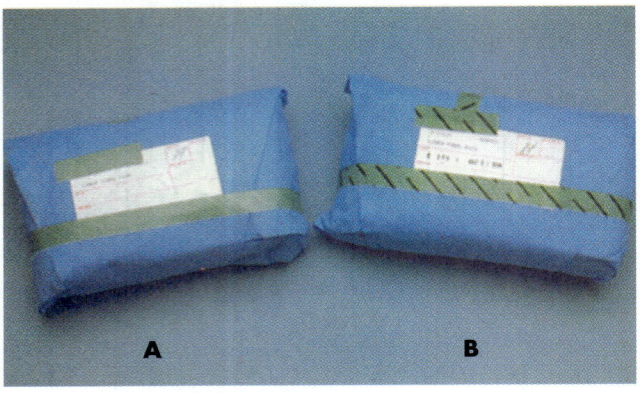

FIGURE 2-17 Dry heat sterilization indicator labels.

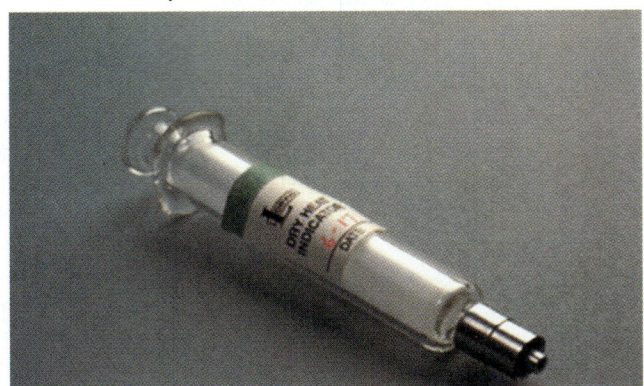

designated to review the examination rooms and all cupboards and shelves to ascertain adequate inventory levels, expired dates, and defective or contaminated packages. Any defective or outdated supplies should be removed and reprocessed for sterilization.

Instruments sterilized unwrapped are to be used immediately and are not to be stored if they are to be sterile when used.

In summary, remember the following points when sterilizing items in an autoclave (steam sterilization). Treat all items as follows:

- Sanitize (clean) properly before sterilization.
- Correctly wrap, seal, and label (for identification) or cover to prevent recontamination; when using cloth or paper wrapper, include a chemical sterilization indicator in and on the pack.
- Position correctly in the sterilizer so steam contacts all surfaces.
- Load only items able to fit easily into the chamber—**do not overload.**

- Expose to saturated steam at 250° F (121° C) for 15 to 30 minutes (varies with the items).
- Allow to dry before removal from the sterilizer.
- Store in specific clean, dry, and dustproof places.
- Check at intervals to determine if the period (date) of sterility has been exhausted.
- Reprocess and resterilize when they are no longer sterile because of wrap damage or date expiration.
- Replace the wrapper and all chemical indicators (inside and outside of the pack) of all items that need to be reprocessed; rewash any fabric items in the package and the wrapper; discard and replace nonwoven wrappers and gauze sponges.

Unsaturated Chemical Vapor Sterilization

A practical, efficient, and reliable method of sterilization, the unsaturated chemical vapor sterilizer (now known as the Harvey Chemiclave, Figure 2-18) depends on pressure, heat, and a specific solution, the Vapo-Steril solution, a formulation of

TABLE 2–3   Problems Encountered in Sterilizing Technique

Probable Causes	Corrections
Damp or wet loads	
Clogged strainer in exhaust line; clogged steam trap	Remove strainer; free openings of lint and sediment daily; use trisodium phosphate solution weekly
Placing warm sterilized packs on cold surfaces	Allow packs to cool before removing from sterilizer or place on surfaces covered with several layers of towels or drapes
Sterilized goods removed too soon from sterilizer after completion of cycle	Allow goods to remain in sterilizer at completion of cycle an additional 15 minutes— door slightly opened ½ inch
Improper loading; tightly loaded packs	Leave space between items; arrange items to present least possible resistance to passage of air and steam through layers of load; position load so water does not collect in utensils; place packs on edge
Pools of water on floor of chamber	Position bottom of sterilizer to lean toward exhaust port so that condensation can drain
Wet steam	Contact manufacturer in charge of maintenance
Deposits on interior	Perform weekly cleaning of sterilizer
Corroded instruments	
Poor cleaning; residual organic debris (for example, blood)	Improve cleaning; do not allow protein to dry on instruments; use correct cleaning solution for each instrument
Improper use of instrument milk or other water-soluble lubricant	Follow procedures for instrument milk or other instrument lubricant used
Moisture—not dried properly	Check sterilizer for drying efficiency; packs should air-dry in sterilizer; store packs in dry area
Exposure to harsh chemicals	Do not expose instruments to harsh chemicals and abrasives such as steel wool and powder cleaner
Metallic deposits resulting from reaction with sterilizer components	Keep sterilizer free of deposits on chamber walls, shelves, and trays

proven effective liquid bactericidal chemicals and minimal water. When it is heated and pressurized to 270° F (132° C) and at least 20 pounds per square inch pressure, all living microorganisms are consistently killed within 20 minutes.

First clean all items to be sterilized. To avoid hand scrubbing of instruments and the possibility of transmitting pathogenic microorganisms among patients and medical personnel, use an ultrasonic cleaning device (Figure 2-19). When the instruments are clean, thoroughly rinse them in cold running water to remove any residue or ultrasonic solution or detergent that would inhibit sterilization or damage the sterilizer and towel dry them before placing them in the sterilizer. Dip small, hard-to-dry items in a shallow tray of Vapo-Steril solution in lieu of drying. Place the items in an instrument tray lined with a Harvey chemically-pure, hard-surface tray liner. If storage of sterile instruments is desired, sterilize them in Harvey Sterilization Indicator bags. These bags permit penetration by the chemical vapor but preclude contamination by airborne bacteria.

The Chemiclave (the unsaturated chemical vapor sterilizer) uses mechanical principles substantially different from those of other systems. The sterilizer is preheated before the initial use and remains at 270° F (132° C) for immediate use. No further

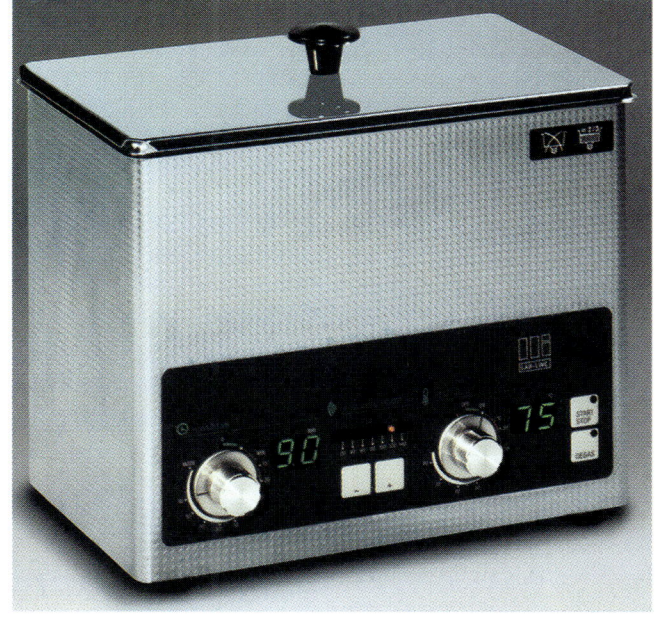

FIGURE 2-18 Harvey Chemiclave EC 6000.

FIGURE 2-19 Ultrasonic cleaner.

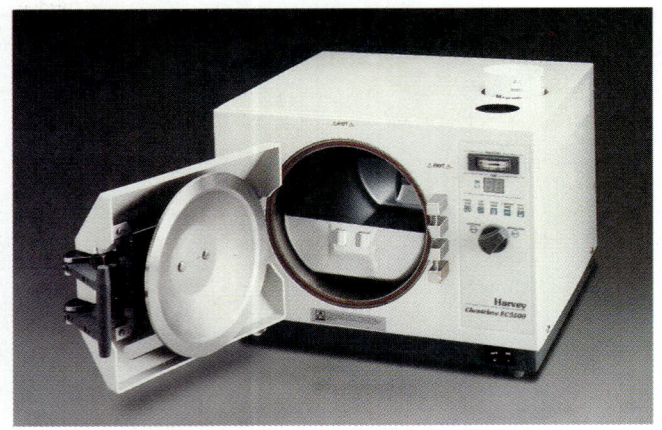

preheating is necessary. Unlike the steam autoclave, in which an unmeasured amount of water is recirculated over the heating element, the unsaturated vapor sterilizer valving system measures a precise amount of solution into the closed, preheated chamber. This solution condenses on the cooler objects in the chamber to begin **bactericidal** activity. As the objects heat, vaporization of the solution occurs, and unsaturated chemical vapor acts to complete the sterilization cycle. Temperature monitoring is unnecessary because this sterilizer provides both audible and visual signaling on completion of the cycle. A thermostatically controlled heating unit maintains the chamber temperature, and a temperature indicator light registers that the heating element is functioning properly. Any failure in the system is immediately evident because the pressure in the chamber will not be attained and, unless all operating criteria are met, the pressure switch will not activate the cycle timer.

Cutting edges, even those of carbon steel, and surgical instruments, handpieces, forceps, and similar items vulnerable to dulling, corroding, rusting, or loss of temper in autoclaves or dry heat units are safely and effectively sterilized in a Chemiclave. Many "soft" items can also be safely sterilized in this unit, and because sterilization is achieved in a water-unsaturated environment, materials such as gauze and cotton are dry and ready for immediate use when the cycle is completed. Only low-grade plastic and rubber items, liquids, agars, and items damaged at 270° F (132° C) *should not* be placed in the Chemiclave. As with all sterilizers, the directions for operation from the manufacturer must be followed explicitly to obtain maximum results.

You must adhere to regulations made by the Environmental Protection Agency (EPA) and the Occupational Safety and Health Administration (OSHA) when using this equipment. In addition, individual states may set additional regulations that you must follow when using this equipment.

Dry Heat Sterilization

To sterilize items with dry heat, a special, combined autoclave–dry heat sterilizer or an individual dry heat sterilizer is necessary. In essence they are like an oven.

Thoroughly clean all items before sterilizing them. Place instruments and glass items such as syringes on the tray or wrap them in aluminum foil. Place sharp items on gauze in racks or wrap them in aluminum foil. Disperse rubber goods and dressings in a container or wrap them in aluminum foil. As for all methods of sterilization, consider both exposure time and temperature. Dry heat sterilizers require longer exposure periods and higher temperatures than do the autoclave (steam under pressure). The exposure time for dry heat is at least 1 hour at 320° F (160° C). If the items being sterilized cannot tolerate this temperature, reduce the temperature and extend the time proportionally. This method is suggested for instruments that corrode easily, sharp cutting instruments, and glass syringes because moist heat dulls the cutting edges and the ground-glass portion of the syringe. Needles, powders, oils, ointments, lensed instruments, dressings, rubber goods, and polyethylene tubing can also be sterilized by this method.

Gas Sterilization

Gas sterilizers that use moderately heated mixtures of ethylene oxide (EO) gas are useful for sterilizing heat and moisture-sensitive items, including rubber and plastic goods, delicate items such as lensed instruments, glass, ophthalmologic surgical instruments, catheters, telescopic instruments (for example, endoscopes, ophthalmoscopes, otoscopes, sigmoidoscopes, and arthroscopes), and anesthesia equipment. Clean, wrap, and position items to be sterilized in the gas chamber using the same steps that were discussed for autoclaving. The temperature in a gas sterilizer is lower (140° F or 50° C); thus the exposure time is extended to suit the temperature, moisture, and gas concentration being used. Time required is 2 to 6 hours, with additional time required for aeration, which can be as long as 5 to 7 days for certain porous materials. Specific instructions for the times and temperatures necessary are supplied by the manufacturer, and you must follow these explicitly. Adhere to EPA and OSHA regulations when this method is used. Physician's offices may contract with outside agencies to process equipment in this manner.

Chemical Sterilization

Many studies have shown that chemical sterilization (cold sterilization) is difficult to accomplish. Therefore this method generally is limited to items that are heat sensitive, such as delicate cutting instruments and nonboilable sutures, or it is used when heat sterilization methods are not available. Chemical solutions are more commonly used for disinfection rather than for sterilization. Nonetheless, a variety of chemical solutions are on the market. Classifications include germicides, bactericides, disinfectants, and antiseptics.

Three chemical solutions that have been recognized as reliable for both sterilization and disinfection procedures are *Cidex, Metricide,* and *glutaraldehyde.* These solutions are capable of destroying bacteria (including spore-forming types) and viruses and are safe to use on instruments, rubber, and plastic goods. Reliable manufacturers always indicate which microorganisms can be expected to be killed by the chemical solution; which items the solution can and cannot be used on; and

PROCEDURE 2-5

PROCEDURE FOR CHEMICAL STERILIZATION

Objective

Demonstrate how to sterilize instruments using a chemical solution; how to remove the instruments from the tray for use.

PROCEDURE

1. Sanitize items as discussed for autoclaving.

2. Pour chemical solution into a designated container with an airtight cover (Figure 2-20). Follow the directions for each chemical accurately.

3. Completely immerse the item into the solution and close the cover.

4. Leave for required time, which varies with the chemical and strength used. Exposure time may be from 20 minutes to 3 hours or more. Items must soak for 1 to 4 hours in Cidex, 1 hour in Metricide, and up to 10 hours in glutaraldehyde.

5. Before using, lift tray out of container and rinse items in pan of sterile distilled water. Wear gloves when handling supplies.

6. Using sterile transfer forceps, remove items from the tray for use.

7. Change the solution in the container every 7 to 14 days or as recommended by the manufacturer.

RATIONALE

Some chemicals must be diluted before use, but if diluted too much, the solution loses its effectiveness.

Correct exposure time is extremely important to ensure sterilization.

Often the solutions used are toxic; therefore items must be thoroughly rinsed before being used on patients.

---

specific directions for use, including the amount of time that the item must soak in the solution.

ULTRASONIC CLEANING AND STERILIZATION PROCEDURES

To avoid cleaning instruments by hand and risking the possibility of contamination, many health care clinics and offices are now using ultrasonic cleaners for sanitizing instruments before they are sterilized. Special instructions are provided by the manufacturer for processing instruments using an ultrasonic cleaner and preparing instruments to be sterilized and stored.

Disinfection Procedures

Chemical disinfection.   Many medical procedures are termed "clean" procedures; therefore they do not require the use of strict aseptic (sterile) technique. Instruments and equipment used in clean procedures are in contact only with the patient's skin or shallow body orifices. Because they do not bypass the body's natural defenses, they can be used safely after being disinfected. Examples of such supplies are thermometers, percussion hammers, laryngeal mirrors, blunt instruments not used on open skin surfaces or on sterile materials (for example,

FIGURE 2-20 Instrument container with cover used for chemical disinfection and sterilization.

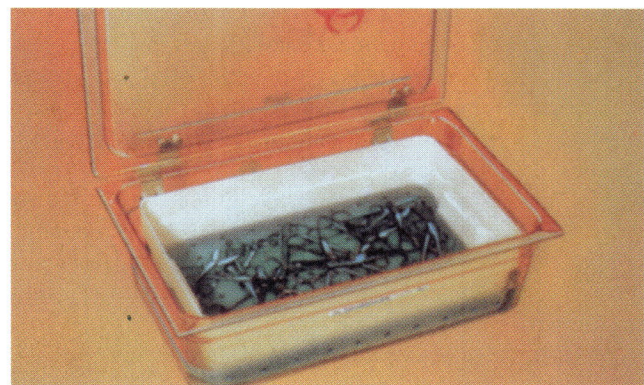

dressings that will touch an open wound), and stainless steel goods such as kidney basins.

When disinfecting such items, thoroughly wash, rinse, and dry as done for sterilization. Then apply a disinfectant or antiseptic solution to the surface of the item or immerse it completely in such a solution (see the procedure for chemical sterilization).

FIGURE 2-21 Disinfecting a stethoscope. Both earpieces and diaphragm should be disinfected after each use.

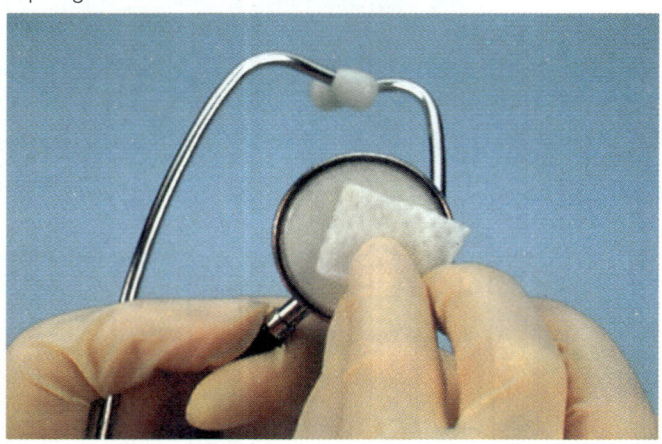

Certain items such as sphygmomanometers, stethoscopes, and ophthalmoscopes may be ruined if washed and immersed in any solution. Disinfect these items only by wiping them off with gauze or cloth moistened with a disinfectant (Figure 2-21). Chemical solutions suggested for use include *Cidex, Solucide, 70% to 90% isopropyl alcohol, Deo-Fect, iodophor solutions, chlorophenyl, and Metricide.*

SUMMARY

When instruments and other equipment are used, the spread of numerous pathogens can be prevented only by the proper sterilization of reusable items or by the use of presterilized disposable items, in addition to meticulous aseptic technique.

Because few procedures more directly affect the continued health of the patient, the physician, and yourself, you must pay conscientious attention to sterilizing all items at all times. Periodically reexamine the techniques used to check their adequacy.

The use of disposable equipment is highly recommended to help control infectious processes and has been found to be most economical in the long run.

CONCLUSION

You have now completed the chapter on infection control. After you have practiced the procedures and are ready to demonstrate your skills and knowledge attained, arrange with your instructor to take a performance test. You will be expected to demonstrate accurately your skill in preparing for and performing all of the procedures outlined in this chapter. In addition, you should be prepared to discuss briefly the infectious process and the methods used for infection control.

REVIEW OF VOCABULARY

Read the following and define the italicized terms.

When *chemically disinfecting* supplies after use, you may use a variety of preparations that are on the market. These are designated as being a *bactericide* or *bacteriostatic, a germicide,* or a *disinfectant.* When making your choice for use, keep in mind that most of these solutions do not destroy *spores* and that the most effective method for decontaminating items is by using the process of *sterilization.* Remember also to keep *contaminated supplies* away from your clean working area.

Sterile or *aseptic technique* is a very important factor in *infection control* and is to be used in numerous medical procedures. A common example of a time when these techniques are used to prevent *infection* from developing is the administration of injections—the syringe and needle used must be sterile, and the patient's skin must be cleansed with an *antiseptic* before the injection is administered.

When a *pathogenic organism* leaves its reservoir, it may invade a new *susceptible host,* and depending on its virulence and the resistance of the new host, it may cause *infection, sepsis,* and even *necrosis* to the tissues involved.

Immunizations (vaccinations) are given to build up resistance to various infectious diseases, such as diphtheria, which has an *incubation period* of 2 to 5 days.

CRITICAL THINKING SKILLS REVIEW

1. State three goals of infection control, and explain how you and the general public can play an active role in this.
2. Differentiate between a local and generalized infection.
3. Differentiate between artificial passive and active immunity.
4. List five diagnostic tests that may be used to help diagnose an infection.

5. Describe the inflammatory process, listing five local and four systemic signs and symptoms of inflammation.
6. You are given three pieces of equipment: one to sanitize, one to disinfect, and the other to sterilize. Explain the differences among these three processes, and list methods used to accomplish each effectively.
7. At your place of employment you have an autoclave, a Chemiclave, a dry heat sterilizer, a gas sterilizer, and chemical solutions. List at least three items that you would sterilize in each of these.

8. If you are busy and cannot clean soiled instruments immediately after use, what should you do?
9. On checking your storage area of sterile supplies, you find a pack that has been there for $1\frac{1}{2}$ months. What should your next action be regarding this pack?
10. When removing a dry pack from the autoclave, you observe that the sterilization indicator has not changed color. What would you do?

PERFORMANCE TEST

In a skills laboratory, a simulation of a joblike environment, the medical assistant student is to demonstrate skill in performing the following procedures without reference to source materials. Time limits for the performance of each procedure are to be assigned by the instructor (see also p. 104).

1. Given soap, perform a medical aseptic handwash.
2. Given reusable syringes and needles and instruments, sanitize these items and then wrap them for sterilization.
3. Given wrapped supplies for sterilization, position these correctly in the chamber of the sterilizer.
4. Given various types of sterilizers and the manufacturer's instructions, sterilize wrapped and unwrapped items, cor-

rectly remove them from the sterilizer on completion of the sterilizing cycle, and determine if sterilization has been effective.
5. Given thermometers, a percussion hammer, and a variety of blunt instruments, correctly disinfect these items using chemicals; disinfect blunt instruments using boiling water.

The student is to perform these activities with 100% accuracy 90% of the time (9 out of 10 times).

The successful completion of each procedure will demonstrate competency levels as required by the American Association of Medical Assistants (AAMA), American Medical Technologists (AMT), and future employers.

🖥 INTERNET RESOURCES

Centers for Disease Control and Prevention (CDC)
www.cdc.gov

National Institutes of Health
www.nih.gov

Health Quality
www.nahq.org

OSHA
www.osha.gov

MedScape
www.medscape.com

Bugs in the News (Information about microbiology in a user-friendly style)
http://falcon.cc.ukans.edu/~jbrown/bugs.html

Health Finder
www.healthfinder.gov

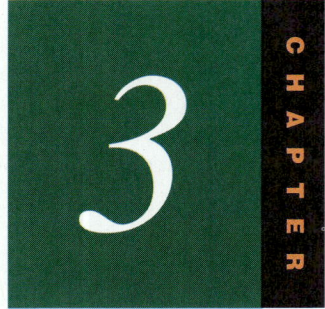

3

CHAPTER

Physical Measurements: Vital Signs, Height, and Weight

■ Cognitive Objectives

On completion of Chapter 3, the medical assistant student should be able to:

1. Define the terms **vital signs, temperature, pulse, apical heartbeat, respiration rate,** and **blood pressure** and list the normal average values for each.
2. Define, spell, and pronounce the listed vocabulary terms that relate to temperature, pulse, respirations, and blood pressure and state verbally or in writing examples of each.
3. List the required equipment for taking a patient's vital signs and the general care for his or her equipment.
4. Recall and state the *general* instructions for taking temperature, pulse rate, respirations, and blood pressure.
5. Describe briefly the methods used to obtain and record a patient's vital signs.
6. When given hourly recordings of patient's temperatures, determine if these sets indicate normal or abnormal variations in daily body temperature.
7. When given the results of 25 patients' vital signs, state which results fall within normal ranges and which do not. State the reasons for the answers given.
8. List five situations in which taking an oral body temperature should be avoided or delayed.
9. For each, list two situations in which to avoid taking rectal and axillary temperatures.
10. Discuss the advantages of tympanic thermometry (infrared radiation temperature measurement).
11. State why the tympanic membrane and surrounding tissue are accurate indicators of true body core temperature.
12. List 10 situations that cause variations in a person's pulse rate.
13. List and locate the seven arteries in the body from which the pulse rate can be obtained with relative ease.
14. Describe what is meant by (a) the rate, rhythm, and volume of the pulse rate and (b) the rate, rhythm, and depth of respirations.
15. List five situations that increase a person's respiratory rate and five that cause this rate to decrease.
16. List five situations that increase a person's blood pressure and five that cause this rate to decrease.
17. List and explain five factors that determine arterial blood pressure.
18. List five methods that may be used to control high blood pressure.
19. List four medical problems that could result if high blood pressure is not treated.
20. State six reasons for measuring a patient's height and weight.

■ Terminal Performance Objectives

On completion of Chapter 3, the medical assistant student should be able to:

1. Demonstrate the correct procedures for obtaining and recording a patient's oral, axillary, rectal, and ear (tympanic) temperature using various types of equipment.
2. Identify and locate pulsations on the seven major arteries used to measure a patient's pulse rate; identify and locate the apical heartbeat.
3. Demonstrate the correct procedure for taking and recording a patient's pulse rate and apical heartbeat.
4. Demonstrate the correct procedure for measuring and recording a patient's respiratory rate.
5. Demonstrate the correct procedure for taking and recording the systolic and diastolic blood pressures on a patient's brachial and popliteal arteries using various types of equipment.
6. Demonstrate the correct procedure for taking and recording a patient's blood pressure using the palpation method.
7. Demonstrate the correct procedure for taking and recording a patient's orthostatic blood pressure.
8. Convert 20 temperature results recorded in Celsius (centigrade) degrees to Fahrenheit degrees.
9. Convert 20 temperature results recorded in Fahrenheit degrees to Celsius (centigrade) degrees.

10. Demonstrate the correct procedures for measuring and recording a patient's weight and height.
11. Convert 20 weight and height results recorded in kilograms and inches to pounds and feet (and inches if applicable).
12. Convert 20 weights recorded in pounds to kilograms.
13. Demonstrate the proper methods for caring for stethoscopes, sphygmomanometers, and thermometers after use.
14. Provide instructions and patient education that is within the professional scope of a medical assistant's training and responsibilities as assigned.

The student is expected to perform these objectives with 100% accuracy. Results obtained for pulse and respiratory rates are acceptable if within two beats or respirations, as determined by

the instructor. Results for blood pressures are acceptable if within 2 to 4 mm Hg, as determined by the instructor.

The consistent use of Universal/Standard Precautions is required by all health care professionals in all health care settings as a method of infection control. It is assumed that these precautions are used in all of the following procedures. Review Chapter 1 if you have any questions on methods to use because the methods or techniques will not be repeated in detail in each procedure presented in this chapter.

Be sure to consult the latest guidelines issued by the Centers for Disease Control and Prevention and consult with infection control practitioners when necessary to identify specific precautions that pertain to your particular work situation.

TEMPERATURE VOCABULARY

constant fever—High fever with a variation not exceeding 1° or 2° Fahrenheit (F) (0.6° or 1.2° Celsius or centigrade [C]) between morning and evening temperatures.

convection—Transfer of heat by the automatic circulation of body fluids.

crisis—Sudden drop of a high temperature to normal or below; generally occurs within 24 hours.

evaporation—Disappearance; loss.

fever—Pyrexia, or elevation of body temperature above normal, 98.6° F (Fahrenheit) or 37° C (centigrade or Celsius) registered orally. Some classify it as:
Low: 99° to 101° F (37.2° to 38.3° C)
Moderate: 101° to 103° F (38.3° to 39.5° C)
High: 103° to 105° F (39.5° to 40.6° C)

intermittent fever—Variations with alternate rises and falls, with the lowest measurement often dropping below 98.6° F (37° C). An intermittent fever reaches the normal line at intervals during the course of an illness (for example, AM: 98° F [36.7° C]; PM: 100° F [37.8° C]; AM: 98.6° F [37° C], PM: 101° F [38.4° C]).

lysis—Gradual decline of a fever.

onset—Beginning of a fever.

oxidation—Combining with oxygen.

radiation—Sending out rays in the form of waves or particles.

remittent fever—Variations in temperature, but always above 98.6° F (37° C); a persistent fever that has a daytime variation of 2° F (1.2° C) or more (for example, PM: 100° F [37.8° C], PM: 103° F [39.5° C]; AM: 99° F [37.2° C], PM: 102.4° F [39.1° C]) (Figure 3-1).

Among the medical assistant's most routine clinical duties are taking and recording the patient's physical measurements, which include vital signs, height, and weight. Therefore the medical assistant must know and understand these measurements and be able to correctly obtain and record the values for each. This chapter discusses these six measurements, along with procedures and related vocabulary.

The medical assistant student should have completed or may currently be studying anatomy and physiology. Therefore detailed explanations of how the body produces vital signs are not included. See also Chapter 18, which is a brief overview of anatomy and physiology.

VITAL SIGNS

Vital signs are measurable, concrete indicators that pertain to and are essential for life. The four vital signs are temperature,

pulse, respirations (TPR), and blood pressure (BP). These signs are routinely measured in each physical examination. Vital signs provide information that helps the physician do the following:

- Determine the patient's condition by comparing the patient's body temperature, pulse, respirations, and blood pressure with normal values
- Determine a diagnosis, the course, and the prognosis of the patient's condition
- Designate the treatment that will be instituted

Temperature

Body temperature, the degree of body heat, is a result of the balance maintained between heat produced and heat lost by the body. This is regulated by a central heat-regulating center located in a portion of the brain, the hypothalamus, that initiates the various mechanisms to increase or decrease heat loss.

FIGURE 3-1 Temperature graph demonstrating the defined terms.

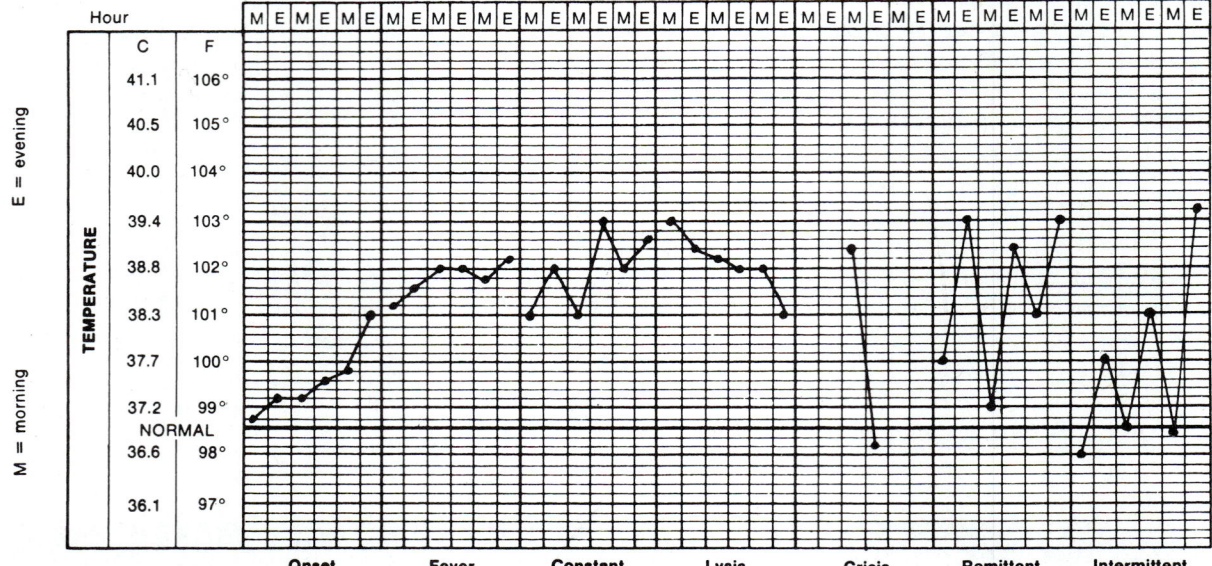

Heat is produced by oxidation of foods in all body cells, especially those in the skeletal muscles and liver. The blood and blood vessels distribute it to other parts of the body. Eighty-five percent of body heat is lost through the skin by **radiation, convection,** and **evaporation** of perspiration. The remainder is lost through the respiratory tract and mouth and through feces and urine.

A variation from the normal range of a patient's temperature may be the first warning of an illness or a change in the patient's condition. As such, it is an important part of the diagnosis and treatment plan for a patient.

Normal temperature readings. Body temperature is measured by a thermometer placed under the tongue, in the rectum, in the axilla, or in the ear (tympanic membrane) because large blood vessels are near the surface at these points. The normal temperature values for these sites based on a statistical average are as follows:

- Oral: 98.6° Fahrenheit (F) or 37° Celsius or centigrade (C)
- Rectal: 99.6° F or 37.6° C
- Axillary: 97.6° F or 36.4° C
- Ear: The thermometer converts the temperature to an oral or rectal equivalent

Accurate rectal temperatures register approximately 1° F or 0.6° C higher than accurate oral temperatures. Accurate axillary temperatures register approximately 1° F or 0.6° C lower than accurate oral temperatures. The ear and then the rectal temperatures are considered the most reliable and accurate readings. The mucous membrane lining of the rectum, with which the thermometer comes into contact, is not exposed to the air, and the conditions do not vary as do those of the mouth or axilla.

The ear (tympanic membrane) and the rectal temperatures are known as the body's **core** temperatures or temperature of deep tissues. Despite external changes in the environment or physical activity the temperature control mechanisms keep the body's core temperature relatively constant. Surface temperatures (oral, axilla, and skin) fluctuate more, depending on blood flow to the skin and the amount of heat lost to the external environment. You will find in clinical practice that a patient's temperature will be within a certain range. No single temperature is normal for all people.

Variations in body temperature. *Normal body temperature* varies from person to person and occurs at different times in each person.

- The daily average oral temperature of a healthy person may vary from 97.6° to 99.6° F (36.4° to 37.3° C).
- The lowest body temperature occurs in the early morning (2 to 6 AM).
- The highest body temperature occurs in the evening (5 to 8 PM).
- In a woman, body temperature may increase *slightly* during the menstrual cycle at the time of ovulation.
- Body temperature is slightly higher during and immediately after eating, exercise, or emotional excitement.
- Body temperature may vary more and is generally higher in an infant or young child than in an adult.

Abnormal temperatures occur when the body's temperature-regulating system is upset by disease or other physical disturbances.

Body temperature *decreases* in some illnesses; if a patient faints, collapses, or hemorrhages; or if the patient is in a fasting state, is dehydrated, or has sustained a central nervous system (CNS) injury. Subnormal temperatures, below 96° F (35.6° C), may occur in cases of collapse and in hypothermia, usually caused from prolonged exposure to cold, for example, as seen in the homeless.

Body temperature *increases* are caused by the following:

- An infectious process
- Following a chill (the muscular activity that occurs in shivering [chills] releases heat and thus increases heat production in the body)
- Activity
- Stress
- Emotions
- Environmental changes
- Age (infants show 1° F higher)
- Reactions to certain drugs
- Amount and type of food eaten (an increase in metabolic rate increases heat production in the body)

Fever usually accompanies infection and many other disease processes. Fever is present when the oral temperature is 100° F (38.8° C) or higher. Temperatures of 104° F (40° C) or higher are common in serious illnesses.

Thermometers.

A thermometer calibrated in Fahrenheit or centigrade (Celsius) degrees is the instrument used to measure body temperature. Various models made of glass or special disposable materials are available. Newer models are electronic or the infrared tympanic thermometers. All good thermometers must pass a rigid inspection for proper calibration according to the standards set by the U.S. National Bureau of Standards.

The often-used **glass thermometers** vary in shape. The rounded, short bulb is used when taking rectal temperatures because it is held better by the rectal muscles and does not traumatize the mucosa. It may also be used when taking an axillary temperature. The slender bulb is considered more effective for oral temperatures. Rounded, short-bulb thermometers are also available for both oral and rectal use. These are usually color coded for easy identification (that is, oral thermometers have a blue identification mark at the end, and rectal thermometers have a red mark). All register the same temperature, although the "normal" temperature arrow is on the 98.6° F (37° C) mark for the oral thermometer and may be on the 99.6° F (37.6° C) mark for the rectal thermometer (Figure 3-2). Various types of disposable thermometers are also available (see Figure 3-2).

Clear plastic, disposable covers called *thermometer sheaths* are available to fit over the stem and bulb of all glass thermometers (Figure 3-3). These can be used when taking the temperature by any method. The rectal sheath is prelubricated for easier insertion. The sheath is placed on the thermometer according to the manufacturer's directions before the thermometer is used and removed before the temperature is read. When the sheath is removed from the thermometer, it turns in on itself, enclosing the area that has been in contact with the pa-

FIGURE 3-2 **A,** Reusable glass thermometers. Slender bulb is best for oral temperatures; rounded bulb is best for rectal temperatures and may also be used for axillary temperatures. **B,** One type of disposable thermometer. The last dot to turn dark indicates the temperature reading.

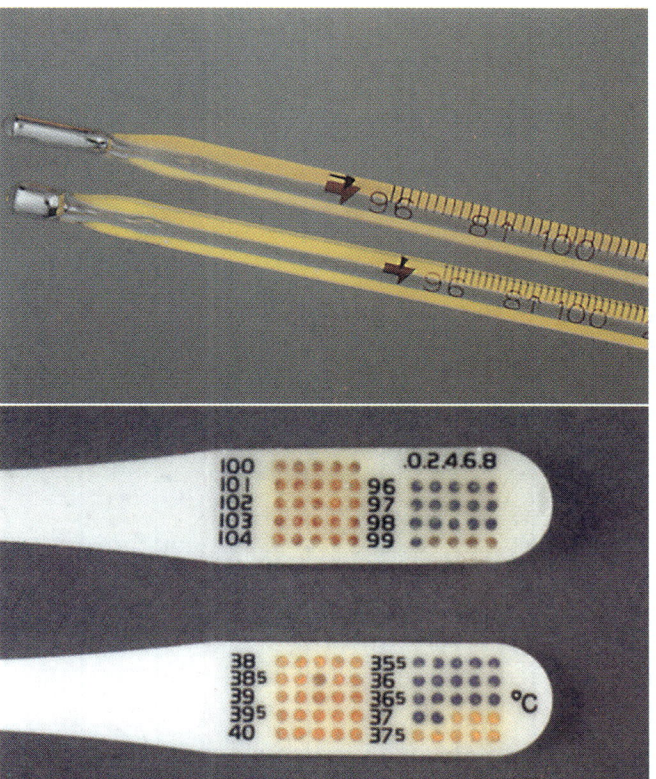

tient's body part, thereby helping to prevent the spread of any infectious agent that is present.

Safe and easy-to-use, battery-operated *electronic thermometers* work rapidly (within 10 to 45 seconds) and are accurately calibrated to within two tenths of a degree. They have disposable covers and interchangeable color-coded probes for both oral and rectal use. The temperature is registered on a dial or on a digital display on the equipment. An example of an electronic thermometer currently used in many medical settings is shown in Figure 3-4.

The newest technology now makes it possible to measure body temperature in the ear in 1 to 2 seconds. This method is referred to as *"infrared tympanic thermometry"* and is thought to be the most accurate method of measuring body temperature. Various models of these thermometers with disposable ear probe covers are available. The thermometer calculates the body temperature, converts it to an oral or rectal equivalent, and displays it on a digital screen (see Figure 3-10, p. 77).

Advantages of the electronic and tympanic thermometers over the glass thermometers are that they are quick and provide protection from infection and the possibility of breakage and mercury spillage. There are some differences between the models available; therefore the manufacturer's directions must be followed for each thermometer.

How to read a glass thermometer.   When reading a thermometer, hold it between your thumb and the index finger of your right hand at the stem (the end away from the bulb.) Rotate the thermometer until you see the center clear (silver) line of mercury toward the bulb. Follow this line up until it ends. Sometimes you can see this line better by changing the direction of the light source. Fahrenheit thermometers are marked off in degrees, with intermediate marks at two tenths of a degree. When the mercury line ends between the two-tenths mark, read the temperature at the next highest two tenths of a degree. Centigrade thermometers are marked off in degrees, with intermediate marks at one tenth of a degree. Centigrade readings can be converted to Fahrenheit readings and Fahrenheit degrees converted to centigrade degrees using the following formulas. Because the metric system is being used more frequently, you should know how to convert Fahrenheit degrees to centigrade degrees. The formula for this is as follows:

$$C° = (F° - 32 \times 5/9)$$

If the Fahrenheit temperature is 98.6°, then:

$$C° = (98.6° - 32) \times 5/9$$
$$C° = 66.6° \times 5/9$$
$$C° = 333/9$$
$$C° = 37°$$

To convert centigrade to Fahrenheit degrees (Table 3-1), the formula is:

$$F° = (C° \times 9/5) + 32$$

Methods and procedures for taking a temperature.   Use the following guidelines to determine which method to use:

1. *Oral* temperature should *never* be taken on the following:
   a.   Children who are not old enough to know how to hold the thermometer in the mouth (4 years old and younger)

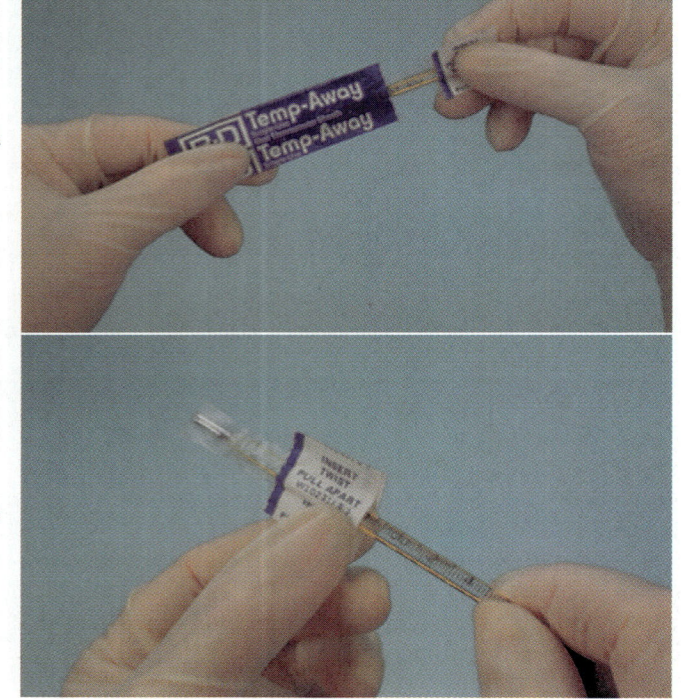

FIGURE 3-3   Disposable thermometer sheath. **A,** Apply the sheath to the thermometer according to the manufacturer's instructions. **B,** Remove the sheath before the temperature is read. Sheath folds back on itself to enclose patient's secretions.

A

B

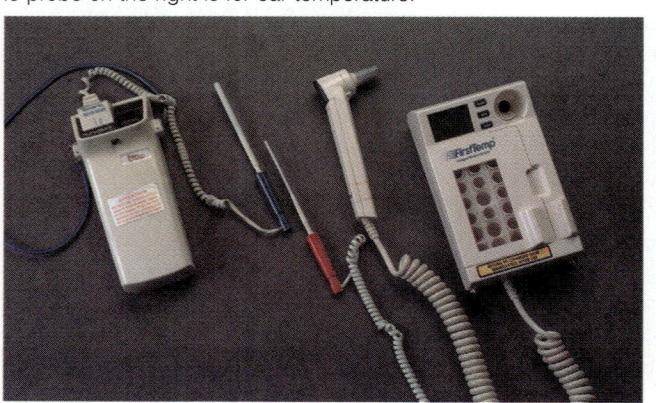

FIGURE 3-4   Some thermometers are electronically operated devices for taking oral, rectal, and ear temperatures safely and accurately. Blue probe is for oral temperature; red is for rectal temperature; the probe on the right is for ear temperature.

TABLE 3–1   **Comparison of Centigrade and Fahrenheit Readings**

°C	°F	°C	°F	°C	°F
34.0	93.2	36.5	97.7	39.0	102.2
34.1	93.4	36.6	97.9	39.1	102.4
34.2	93.6	36.7	98.1	39.2	102.6
34.3	93.7	36.8	98.2	39.3	102.7
34.4	93.9	36.9	98.4	39.4	102.9
34.5	94.1	37.0*	98.6*	39.5	103.1
34.6	94.3	37.1	98.8	39.6	103.3
34.7	94.5	37.2	98.9	39.7	103.5
34.8	94.6	37.3	99.1	39.8	103.6
34.9	94.8	37.4	99.3	39.9	103.8
35.0	95.0	37.5	99.5	40.0	104.0
35.1	95.2	37.6	99.7	40.1	104.2
35.2	95.4	37.7	99.9	40.2	104.4
35.3	95.5	37.8	100.0	40.3	104.5
35.4	95.7	37.9	100.2	40.4	104.7
35.5	95.9	38.0	100.4	40.5	104.9
35.6	96.1	38.1	100.6	40.6	105.1
35.7	96.3	38.2	100.8	40.7	105.3
35.8	96.4	38.3	100.9	40.8	105.4
35.9	96.6	38.4	101.1	40.9	105.6
36.0	96.8	38.5	101.3	41.0	105.8
36.1	97.0	38.6	101.5	41.1	106.0
36.2	97.2	38.7	101.7	41.5	106.7
36.3	97.3	38.8	101.8	42.0	107.6
36.4	97.5	38.9	102.0	42.5	108.5

*Normal oral temperature.

b. Patients with a nasal obstruction, dyspnea, coughing, weakness, a sore mouth, mouth diseases, or oral surgery

c. Patients receiving oxygen

d. Uncooperative, delirious, unconscious, or intoxicated patients

2. **Axillary** temperatures should *never* be taken on the following:

a. Thin patients who cannot make the hollow under the arm airtight

b. Perspiring patients whose axilla cannot be kept dry for the required 10 minutes

3. **Rectal** temperatures should *never* be taken on the following:

a. Rectal surgery patients

b. Children or other patients whose body movements cannot be controlled for the required 3 to 5 minutes (time varies with agency policy)

4. **Tympanic (ear)** temperatures are the easiest and most reliable method. Use this method if a tympanic thermometer is available.

Equipment

- Thermometer
- Oral: Glass thermometers may be stored in a small, covered container with a small pad of cotton in the bottom and labeled "clean oral thermometers" or in individual, clean, labeled envelopes stored in a drawer.
- Rectal: Glass thermometers may be stored in a small, covered container with a small pad of cotton in the bottom and labeled "clean rectal thermometers" or in individual, clean, labeled envelopes stored in a drawer.
- Box of tissues or small cotton squares
- Container for waste
- Containers labeled "soiled oral thermometers" or "soiled rectal thermometers"
- Water-soluble lubricant such as K-Y jelly or Lubafax if taking a rectal temperature
- Disposable, single-use examination gloves if taking a rectal temperature or an infant's temperature

General instructions

1. Handle the thermometer with great care because it is a very delicate instrument.
2. Keep rectal thermometers separate from oral thermometers.
3. Wash your hands before and after handling a thermometer or taking a patient's temperature.
4. Wear disposable, single-use examination gloves when taking a rectal temperature.
5. Read the thermometer with great care to ensure accuracy.
6. Record the reading and indicate if it was other than oral. This notation must be made because of the differences in temperatures when taken in either the axilla or rectum.

Care of glass thermometers after each use

1. Shake mercury down to below 96° F (35.5° C).
2. Wash with soap and cold water, and then rinse with cold running water.
3. Dry the thermometer.
4. Place in a disinfectant solution such as glutaraldehyde (Cidex) or 70% alcohol for 20 minutes; then rinse with *cold* running water and dry with a small piece of cotton before the next use.
5. If the thermometer is not to be reused after being disinfected, dry it and place in a covered container that has cotton in the bottom to protect the bulb. Store in dry containers or individual clean envelopes.

PROCEDURE 3-1

ORAL TEMPERATURE

Objective

Understand and demonstrate the correct procedure for obtaining and recording a patient's oral temperature.

PROCEDURE	RATIONALE
1. Identify and evaluate the patient.	*To avoid a false reading, defer taking for 15 to 20 minutes if the patient has just finished eating, drinking, or smoking. To avoid any accident, do not leave a patient alone unless he or she is absolutely responsible.*
2. Wash your hands. **Use appropriate personal protective equipment (PPE) as indicated by facility.**	
3. Assemble equipment.	
4. Instruct the patient to assume a sitting position and explain the procedure.	*Complete explanations help gain the patient's cooperation and help the patient relax. Provide for the patient's comfort and safety.*
5. Remove clean thermometer from the container.	

Continued

6. If just removing the thermometer from the disinfectant solution, rinse with cold running water and wipe dry from the stem downward to the bulb in a rotating manner with a tissue or cotton square. Discard cotton square.

This removes any disinfectant that may be irritating to the patient. You must use cold water because hot water may cause mercury to expand too much and break the bulb. Wiping in a rotating manner ensures that all sides are wiped.

7. Firmly holding the end of the thermometer, shake it down to 96° F (35.5° C) or lower. Do this by giving the wrist several quick snaps as though cracking a whip. Be careful to avoid contact with nearby objects. *(If you are using a disposable plastic sheath to cover the thermometer, apply it now.)*

Constriction in the mercury reservoir prevents it from going down, unless forced. The mercury must be below 96° F to avoid an error in recording an accurate reading.

8. Place the thermometer well under the patient's tongue into the sublingual pocket.

Temperature reading is produced from heat from superficial blood vessels under the tongue.

9. Instruct the patient to keep lips closed, to breathe through the nose, and not to touch the thermometer with the teeth.

Keeping the mouth closed prevents cooler air from the outside from affecting the temperature reading. Keeping teeth off of the thermometer prevents biting down and possibly breaking it.

10. Leave the thermometer in place for 3 minutes.

11. The pulse and respirations may be taken while the thermometer is registering.

12. Remove the thermometer and wipe it from the stem toward the bulb, using a rotating motion; never place pressure on the mercury bulb end of the thermometer, **or** *remove the disposable plastic sheath if used and dispose of according to agency policy.*

Wiping removes any secretions and makes it easier to read the temperature. Wiping from stem to bulb also prevents contact of microorganisms from the patient's mouth with your fingers.

13. Read the thermometer. Hold it horizontally in your right hand and rotate it slowly until you see the point at which the mercury column stops (Figure 3-5).

14. Record the reading.

15. Shake the mercury down to 96° F (35.5° C) or below and place the thermometer in the container for used oral thermometers or into a container of cool soap solution.

16. If retaking a questionable temperature, check that the thermometer is shaken down to 96° F (35.5° C) or below, **or** use another thermometer **or** use another method, either rectal or axillary. If the temperature is found to be remarkably high or low for no apparent reason, take it again.

17. Wash your hands.

Charting Example

March 2, 20__, 9 am
Oral temp 98.8° F
OR
Temp 98.8° F
J. Sublett, CMA

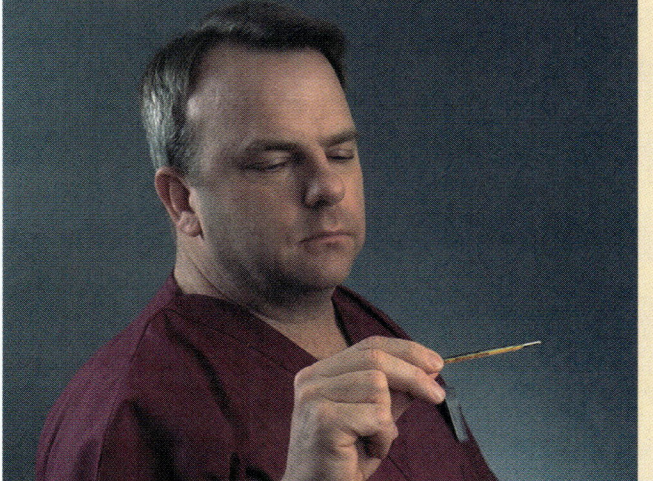

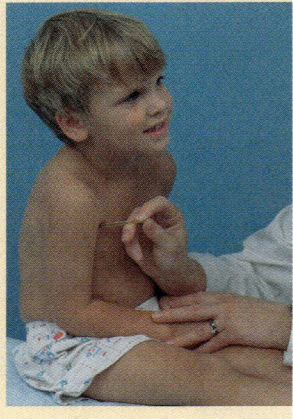

FIGURE 3-6 Placing thermometer for taking an axillary temperature.

FIGURE 3-5 Read the thermometer by holding it horizontally and rotating it slowly until you see the point at which the mercury stops.

PROCEDURE 3-2

AXILLARY TEMPERATURE

Objective

Understand and demonstrate the correct procedure for obtaining and recording a patient's axillary temperature.

PROCEDURE	RATIONALE
1. Perform steps 1 through 7 as for oral temperature technique, using a rounded, short-bulb thermometer.	
2. Blot the axillary region dry with tissue or a cotton square.	*Avoid rubbing because friction increases the blood supply in the area, thus increasing the temperature of the skin.*
3. Place the bulb end of the thermometer in the hollow of the axillary region with the end of the thermometer slanting toward the patient's chest (Figure 3-6).	*Ensures that the thermometer is in direct contact with the skin surface, not touching clothing or exposed to air. Maintains proper position of the thermometer against blood vessels in the axilla.*
4. Have the patient cross the arms over the chest. It may be more comfortable to hold the opposite shoulder.	*This prevents as little air as possible from coming into contact with the thermometer. When the patient is unable to put his or her hand on the opposite shoulder, place it there gently and hold it with your own hand, or hold the patient's arm close to his or her side. When taking a child's axillary temperature, hold the thermometer in place for the entire time.*
5. Leave the thermometer in place for 10 minutes (time may vary according to agency policy).	*This ensures accurate registration of the temperature. A longer time is necessary for the temperature to register than when taking an oral temperature because the axilla is more subject to the influence of air currents.*
6. The pulse and respirations may be taken while the thermometer is registering.	
7. Remove and wipe the thermometer from the stem toward the bulb and read it. Hold a glass thermometer in your right hand to read it.	*Never place pressure on the bulb end of the thermometer.*

Charting Example

January 30, 20___, 11 am
Axillary temp 97.6° F
OR
Temp 97.6° F (A) or (Ax).
M. Kubiak, CMA

8. Record reading.

9. Shake the mercury down to 96° F (35.5° C) or below and place the thermometer in the container for used thermometers.

10. Wash your hands.

PROCEDURE 3-3

RECTAL TEMPERATURE

Objective

Understand and demonstrate the correct prodedure for obtaining and recording a patient's rectal temperature.

PROCEDURE	RATIONALE
1. Perform Steps 1 through 7 as for oral temperature, using a rectal thermometer.	*Never use an oral thermometer for a rectal temperature.*
2. Have the patient turn on the side with the upper leg flexed, if possible.	*Do not expose the patient unnecessarily.*
3. Don disposable, single-use examination gloves.	

4. Apply a water-soluble lubricant to the thermometer. (If you are using a disposable sheath over the thermometer, put it on and then apply the lubricant) (Figure 3-7).

Lubricant allows for easier insertion of the thermometer. Some disposable plastic sheaths are prelubricated.

5. Separate buttocks so that anus is exposed.

6. Gently insert thermometer approximately 1 to 1½ inches into the anal canal and instruct the patient to remain still.

Forceful insertion beyond 1 to 1½ inches may cause damage to the tissues involved. Movement could cause the thermometer to go farther into the rectum and possibly cause tissue damage, or the thermometer could slip out of the rectum. The thermometer could also slip out of the rectum if it is not inserted far enough.

7. Hold thermometer in place for 3 to 5 minutes (time may vary with agency policy.) You may take an adult's pulse and respiration while the thermometer is registering.

Never leave the patient alone when taking a rectal temperature.

8. Remove the thermometer. Remove the sheath covering if used. Wipe the thermometer in a rotating motion going only from the stem toward the bulb to remove any secretions.

Lubricant and any fecal material must be removed from the thermometer to allow for ease in reading the temperature.

9. Wipe the patient's anal area with a tissue to remove any lubricant. Wipe in the direction going toward the back.

Provide for the patient's comfort.

10. Read the temperature accurately. Hold the thermometer horizontally in the right hand and rotate it slowly until you see the point at which the mercury column stops.

Never place pressure on the bulb end of the thermometer. Be certain that all fecal material is removed.

11. Shake the mercury down to below 96° F (35.5° C).

12. Place the thermometer in the container for used rectal thermometers.

13. Remove and dispose of gloves.

14. Wash your hands.

15. Record the reading, noting that a rectal temperature was taken.

16. Assist the patient as needed.

Charting Example

May 19, 20__, 10 am
Rectal temp 99.6° F
OR
Temp 99.6° F Ⓡ
Josh Burns, CMA

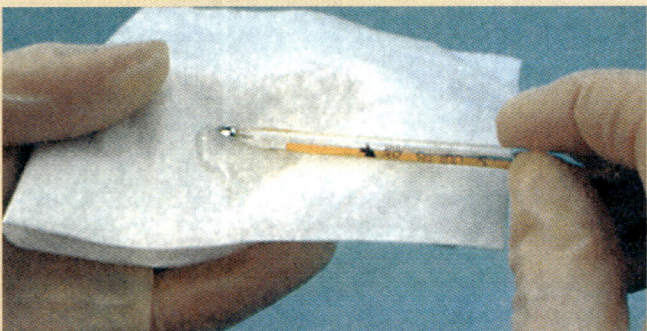

FIGURE 3-7   Lubricating thermometer for taking a rectal temperature. Put some lubricant on a tissue or paper; then put the thermometer into the lubricant so that the first inch of the thermometer is covered with lubricant.

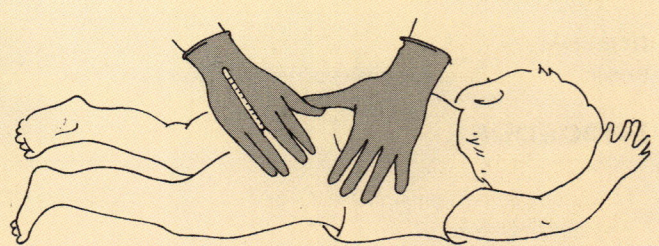

FIGURE 3-8   Position for holding a thermometer and infant while taking the rectal temperature.

Taking an infant's temperature

Objective: Understand and demonstrate the correct method for taking an infant's rectal temperature.

1. Don disposable, single-use examination gloves.
2. Lay the infant on the abdomen on a firm surface.
3. With your left hand, spread the cheeks of the buttocks so that you can see the rectum.
4. With your right hand, insert the lubricated bulb end of the rectal thermometer into the rectum approximately $\frac{1}{2}$ to 1 inch.
5. Place your right hand on the infant's buttocks, hold the buttocks firmly, and pinch the thermometer firmly between your fingers.
6. Place your other hand in the small of the infant's back, with your arm straight, and lean on the infant slightly. This helps hold the infant still (Figure 3-8).
7. Hold the thermometer in place for 3 to 5 minutes (time may vary with agency policy).
8. Remove the thermometer and place it out of reach of the infant.
9. Support the infant. Wipe the anal area to remove excess lubricant.
10. Wipe the thermometer with a tissue, read the temperature registered, and record it promptly.
11. Remove and dispose of gloves.
12. Wash your hands.

Infrared radiation temperature measurement (infrared tympanic thermometry).

All material objects give off electromagnetic waves from their surface. The cooler the object, the less energy these waves carry. The hotter the object, the more energy the waves carry. These waves vary in length, and the longest waves that we can see are red. The energy of the radiation given off from our bodies is lower than these red waves; hence the term **infrared,** meaning below red. Infrared tympanic thermometers are based on the detection of thermal infrared radiation (heat).

Broad scientific research from around the world shows the tympanic membrane (eardrum) and its surrounding tissue to be *the most accurate* indicator of true core body temperature because the eardrum shares blood supply and is near the hypothalamus, the body's thermostat or the temperature control center of the brain (Figure 3-9).

One of the tympanic thermometers available, the handheld Thermoscan (Figure 3-10, *A* and *B*) is like a camera in that it takes a snapshot of infrared heat given off of the eardrum and surrounding tissue and registers it on a sensitive surface. Instead of a lens, a gold-plated wave guide covered by a protective window is used; instead of film, an infrared sensor is used. A shutter is used as it is in a camera. The thermometer then calculates the body temperature, converts it to an oral or rectal equivalent, and displays it on the digital screen—all within 1 second.

Advantages. Tympanic thermometry offers many benefits and advantages over traditional glass mercury, electronic, and digital thermometers (specifically accuracy, safety, speed, comfort, cleanliness, and user convenience). Therefore it is quickly becoming the preferred site for taking body temperature. Different models are available for both professional and home use.

Accuracy. Clinical studies show that the eardrum is an accurate indicator of true core body temperature because it shares blood supply and is near the hypothalamus, the body's "thermostat." The ear canal is a protected cavity, unaffected by environmental factors. Unlike traditional thermometers, tympanic thermometers do not have to be in place for an extended length of time; they are not affected by external factors such as eating, chewing gum, drinking, smoking, and breathing through the mouth—all of which affect oral thermometers; and, as with oral electronic thermometers, they do not depend on where they are placed in the mouth (for example, too far forward in the mouth and away from the sublingual artery). Reading the temperature from a tympanic thermometer is easy because it is displayed as a clear digital readout, thus eliminating the need to visually interpret the mercury column. In addition, the infrared tympanic technique is faster and more accurate than other methods because it measures the patient's temperature as it naturally radiates, not the thermometer's own temperature after extended patient contact. Presence of any form of otitis media (inflammation of the middle ear) does not affect the temperature measurement. Also, cerumen (ear wax) does not affect the tympanic membrane thermometer readings (unless it is on the lens of the thermometer) because cerumen is transparent to infrared energy. Finally, tympanic thermometers can be used when temperatures are difficult or impossible to obtain with conventional contact thermometers.

Safety, cleanliness, and infection control. Infrared tympanic thermometers eliminate potential risks such as bowel perforation, breakage of glass thermometers, and mercury ingestion or contamination. Because they are placed in the ear, which is a dry, nonmucous membrane cavity, tympanic thermometers virtually eliminate the possibility of cross-contamination. The ear canal harbors fewer pathogens than the mouth or rectum. The probe tip is covered with a disposable cover, which is changed for each patient. The disposable probe cover is ejected after use without having to be touched. These thermometers measure temperatures *without* touching the tympanic membrane (that is, there is not membrane contact). The probe tip has been designed to make it impossible to cause damage to the eardrum, regardless of the age of the patient.

Speed. Traditional thermometers may take as long as 5 minutes to display an accurate temperature. In contrast, tympanic thermometers take and display temperatures on an easy-to-read display in 1 second. Because infrared waves travel at the speed of light, readings can be taken almost instantaneously.

Comfort. Tympanic thermometers make temperature taking a fast, painless, noninvasive procedure. Because it is not physically or emotionally threatening, it does not add to the discomfort of any patient, especially a sick child or a nervous or elderly patient. No active cooperation is required; thus it can be used without disturbing a sleeping child or it can be used on an unconscious patient. In terms of ease of access and accuracy of core temperature, the tympanic site is superior to all others.

TYMPANIC MEMBRANE (EAR) TEMPERATURE

Objective

Understand and demonstrate the correct procedure for obtaining and recording a patient's tympanic membrane (ear) temperature.

Equipment

Tympanic thermometer with battery   Disposable probe cover
    (for example, Thermoscan PRO-1
    Instant Thermometer)

NOTE: Accurate measurements depend on correct technique. The following procedure is for the Thermoscan thermometer. Other brands (Ototemp, FirstTemp Genius 3000A) require slightly different techniques. Follow the manufacturer's instructions.

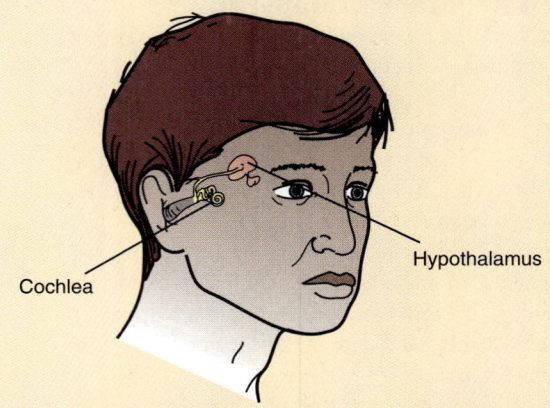

Cochlea

Hypothalamus

FIGURE 3-9   The eardrum is an excellent site to measure body temperature because it is near the hypothalamus, which is the body's temperature control center.

PROCEDURE

1. Wash your hands. **Use appropriate personal protective equipment (PPE) as indicated by facility.**

2. Assemble equipment. Make sure that the sensor lens of the thermometer is clean.

3. Identify and evaluate the patient.

4. Instruct the patient to assume a sitting position and explain the procedure.

5. Apply a disposable cover to the probe tip (Figure 3-11).

6. Select oral or rectal equivalent and press "ON."

7. For adults, gently pull the ear lobe up and back. For children, gently pull the ear lobe down and back.

8. Gently insert the probe tip in the patient's ear until the tip fully "seals off" the ear canal. DO NOT apply pressure (Figure 3-12).

9. Depress and hold the activation button for 1 second.

10. Remove from the ear. Read the temperature and record promptly. The Thermoscan PRO-1 is programmed to display the actual ear temperature, as well as the oral, rectal, or core equivalents (see Figure 3-10, p. 77).

11. Discard the disposable probe cover in the designated waste container.

12. Return the equipment to the designated area.

13. Wash your hands.

14. Attend to the patient as needed.

RATIONALE

Dust or ear wax on the lens obstructs proper functioning of the thermometer, resulting in false-low readings.

Explanations help the patient to relax and cooperate. Also, many people have never heard of taking a temperature in the ear. Provide for the patient's comfort and safety.

Make sure that the thermometer is locked in the mode that you prefer.

This straightens the ear canal to obtain a clear view of the eardrum (See Figure 9-1 on p. 435).

The probe is positioned snugly in the ear canal to get a view of the eardrum and its surrounding tissue, just as a photographic camera is aimed at an object. It does not touch the eardrum.

This allows the unit to measure the infrared heat generated by the eardrum and surrounding tissue. This measurement is then converted into either an oral or rectal equivalent in either Celsius (centigrade) or Fahrenheit degrees. The resulting temperature is displayed in 1 second.

Charting Example

August 1, 20__ 4 pm
Tympanic temp 98.6° F
J. Lee, CMA

FIGURE 3-10 **A,** Thermoscan PRO-1 Instant Thermometer, an infrared tympanic (ear) thermometer designed to display the temperature in less than 1 second. Disposable probe covers are used over the ear probe for each patient. **B,** Thermoscan Instant Thermometer takes a snapshot of the heat given off by the eardrum and surrounding tissue. **C,** Results are displayed on the digital screen.

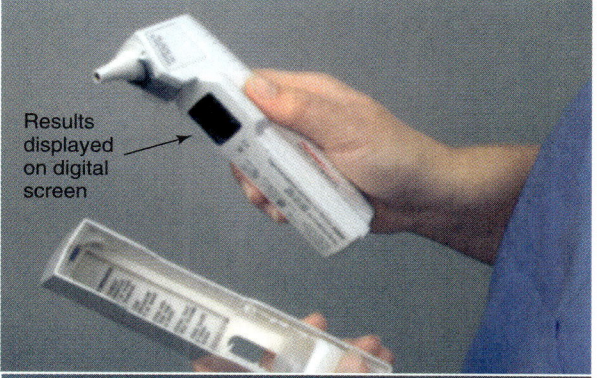

Results displayed on digital screen

A

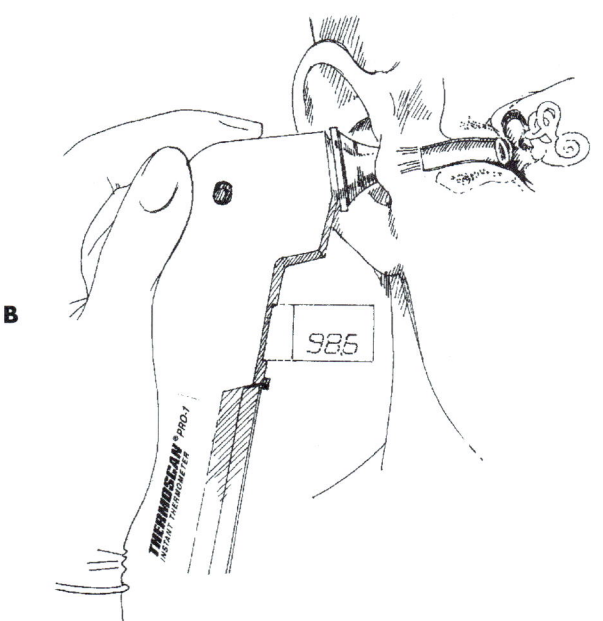

B

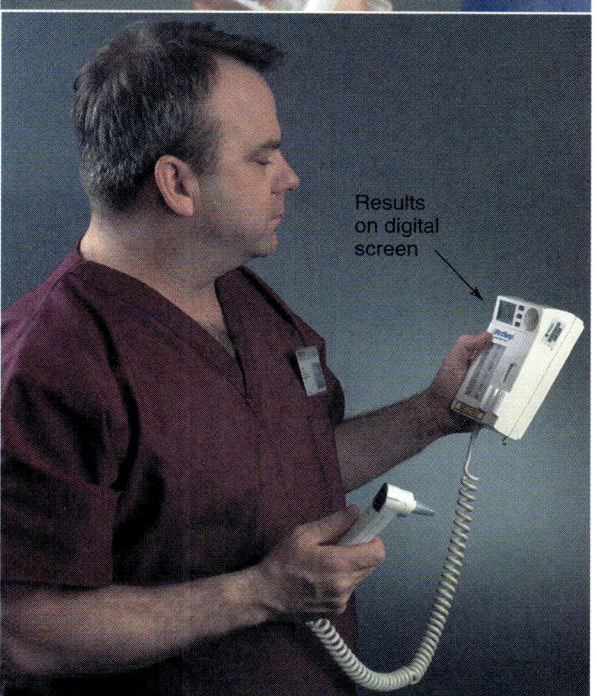

Results on digital screen

C

FIGURE 3-11   Applying disposable cover to the ear probe tip.

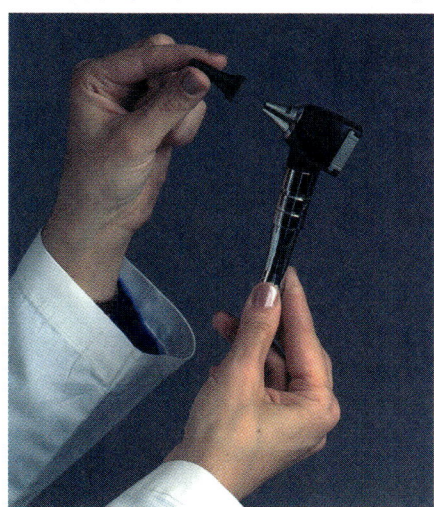

FIGURE 3-12   Gently insert probe tip in the patient's ear until the tip fully "seals off" the ear canal. The probe does not need to touch the ear's tympanic membrane to obtain an accurate temperature reading. The temperature is calculated by detection of the highest level of infrared energy, or heat rays within the ear canal.

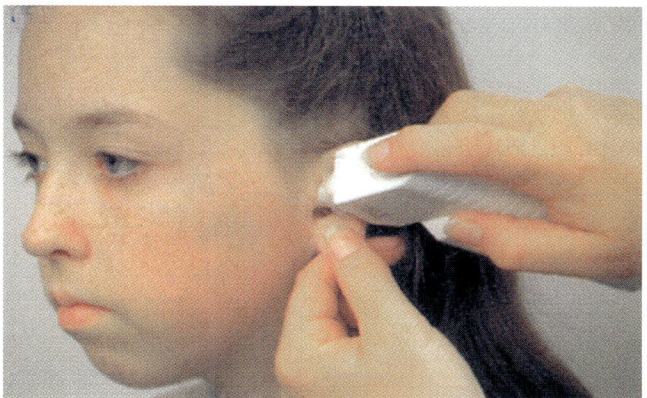

Pulse

The pulse is defined as the beat of the heart as felt through the walls of the arteries. It is produced by the wave of blood that travels along the arteries with each contraction of the left ventricle of the heart.

The pulse can also be described as a throbbing caused by the alternate expansion and recoil of an artery. It is felt best when a superficial artery is pressed against a firm, underlying anatomic structure, such as bone.

Characteristics of the pulse.
When taking a pulse, the four important characteristics to note are the rate, rhythm, and volume of the pulse and the condition of the arterial wall, all of which vary with the size and the elasticity of the artery, the strength of contraction of the heart, and the tissues surrounding the artery.

The **rate** (frequency) of the pulse is the number of pulsations (beats) in a given minute. Normal (average) rates are outlined in the following section. Abnormal rates are those above or below the range of norms, and can be described as bradycardia (slow) or tachycardia (rapid).

The **rhythm** of the pulse pertains to the time interval between each pulse. Normal rhythm is described as regular (that is, intervals between pulsations are of equal length). Abnormal rhythm may be described as irregular, arrhythmic, bigeminal, skipping beats, or intermittent. Skipping an occasional beat occurs in all normal individuals, especially during exercise or after ingesting certain stimulants, such as coffee. Most of these irregularities go unnoticed, but they may concern a patient enough to cause him or her to seek medical advice. When frequent beats are skipped or if the beats are highly irregular, the physician should be alerted because this could be a sign of heart disease. In such cases, it is sometimes useful for one person to take the radial pulse for 1 minute and the other person to take the apical pulse by listening over the heart simultaneously (see p. 83). The findings are recorded and compared. If the apical rate is greater, the difference is referred to as the **pulse deficit**. This could indicate inadequate blood circulation to the arms and legs when the heart contracts.

The pulse deficit is important in the examination of the patient with atrial fibrillation, one of the more common causes of a very irregular pulse. Atrial fibrillation is an irregular heartbeat marked by rapid, inefficient, random contractions of the atria in the heart.

The **volume** (also known as "intensity," "force," "character," or "quality") of the pulse is an indication of the general condition of the heart and the circulatory system. It pertains to the strength of the pulsations and may be described as full, strong, bounding, weak, feeble, thready, febrile, hard, or soft. Volume depends on the force of the heartbeat and the condition of the arterial walls. The pulse may vary in volume in association with irregularities of rhythm. If a pulse varies only in intensity but is otherwise perfectly regular, it is often a manifestation of heart disease.

The **condition of the arterial wall** pertains to the texture of the artery that you feel through the skin surface when palpating the pulse. A normal arterial wall is described as soft and elastic; abnormal conditions include hard, ropy, knotty, and wiry.

Variations in pulse rate.
Individual pulse rates *normally vary* as a result of a person's sex, age, body size, posture, activity level, and health status, as well as functions of the nervous system and the volume and chemical composition of the blood.

In general, the pulse rate is faster in women (70 to 80 beats per minute) than in men (60 to 70 beats per minute) and is usually higher in short people than in tall people. Infants' and children's pulse rates are also more rapid than an adult's. When one is sitting, the rate is more rapid (for example, 70 beats per

PULSE VARIATION VOCABULARY

abdominal pulse—Abdominal aorta pulse.

alternating pulse—Alternating weak and strong pulsations.

arrhythmia (a-rith′mi-a)—Irregularities in pulse or rhythm.

bigeminal pulse (bi-jem′in-al)—Two regular beats followed by a longer pause. It has the same significance as an irregular pulse.

bradycardia (brad-i-kar′di-a)—Slow heart action; extremely slow pulse, generally below 60 beats per minute.

febrile pulse (feb′rile)—A full, bounding pulse at the onset of a fever, becoming feeble and weak when the fever subsides.

formicant pulse (for′mi-kant)—A small, feeble pulse.

intermittent pulse—A pulse in which occasional beats are skipped.

irregular pulse—A pulse with variation in force and frequency; may be caused by an excess of tea, coffee, tobacco, or exercise.

pulse deficit—The apical rate is greater than the radial pulse rate.

pulse pressure—The difference between the systolic and the diastolic blood pressure.

Example: If BP is 120/80,

  120 = systolic pressure

  −80 = diastolic pressure

    40 = pulse pressure

A pulse pressure consistently over 50 points or under 30 points is considered abnormal.

regular pulse—The rhythm of the pulse rate is regular.

slow pulse—A pulse between 40 and 60 beats per minute, often found among the aged and among athletes at rest.

tachycardia (tak″y-kar′di-a)—A pulse of 100 or more beats per minute when the person is at rest; abnormal rapidity of heart action.

thready pulse—A pulse that is very fine and scarcely perceptible, as seen in syncope (fainting).

unequal pulse—A pulse in which some beats are strong and others are weak; pulse in which rates are different in symmetric arteries.

venous pulse—A pulse in a vein, especially one of the large veins near the heart, such as the internal and external jugular. Venous pulse is undulating and scarcely palpable.

minute) than when lying down (for example, 66 beats per minute); the rate increases when standing, walking, or running (for example, 80, 86, and 90 beats per minute, respectively). During sleep or rest, especially in athletes, the pulse rate may be as low as 45 to 50 beats per minute.

The following list indicates some of the common causes of increases or decreases in the pulse.

Increase

- Fear, excitement, or anxiety
- Physical activity or exercise
- Fever
- Certain types of heart disease
- Hyperthyroidism
- Shock
- Pain
- Certain drugs, for example, epinephrine (Adrenalin)
- Many infections
- Hemorrhage

Decrease

- Mental depression
- Certain types of heart disease
- Some chronic illnesses
- Hypothyroidism
- Certain brain injuries that cause increased intracranial pressure
- Certain drugs, such as digitalis
- Hypothermia
- Unrelieved severe pain

Comparing Pulse Rates

Generally Faster

- In women
- In short people
- In infants and children
- When sitting versus lying down
- When standing, walking, or running

Generally Slower

- During rest or sleep
- In well-trained athletes

Normal Pulse Rates (Average Number of Pulsations [Beats] in 1 Minute)

At birth	130 to 160 beats per minute
Infants	110 to 130 beats per minute
Children from 1 to 7 years	80 to 120 beats per minute
Children over 7 years	80 to 90 beats per minute
Adults	60 to 100 beats per minute

Common arteries and body locations for determining pulse rate (Figure 3-13)

- **Apical:** Over the apex of the heart in the fifth intercostal space on the midclavicular line
- **Brachial:** Over the inner aspect at the bend of the elbow
- **Common carotid:** At right and left sides of the neck, at the anterior edge of the sternocleidomastoid muscle
- **Dorsalis pedis:** On the upper surface of the foot between ankle and toes
- **Facial:** Along the lower margin of the mandible
- **Femoral:** The anterior side of the pelvic bone, in the middle of the groin region
- **Popliteal:** At the back of the knee
- **Radial:** Over the inner aspect of the wrist area, on the thumb side; this site is the one most commonly used and accessible in most cases
- **Temporal:** At the temple, on the side of the forehead

Apical pulse.   The apical rate is the rate per minute of the heartbeat as determined by auscultation of the apex of the heart. This is the most accurate pulse site. An apical pulse is taken on all children under 2 years of age, on patients for whom a very accurate rate is needed, and on patients with possible heart problems, regardless of age. It may also be taken when the radial pulse is inaccessible because of a cast or dressing. The *normal range* is 60 to 100 beats per minute; the *average rate* is 80 beats per minute.

To count the apical beat, place the chestpiece of a clean stethoscope over the apex of the heart and count the number of heartbeats for 1 minute.

The apex of the heart is located in the left fifth intercostal space on the midclavicular line (that is, between the fifth and sixth ribs on a line with the midpoint of the left clavicle). This position is usually just below the nipple (see Figure 3-13, *C*).

When recording the results, you must indicate that it was the apical rate that was taken. This can be noted by using the abbreviation "AP." On completion, wipe the earpiece and

---

FIGURE 3-13   **A,** Common arteries for determining pulse rates.

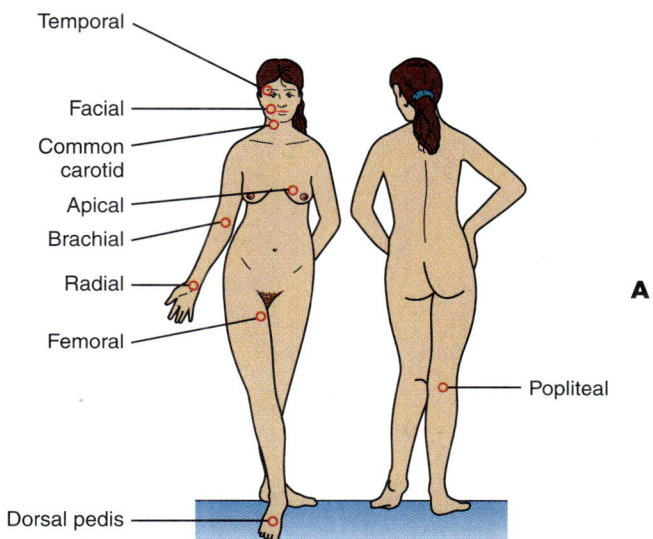

Temporal

Facial

Common carotid

Apical

Brachial

Radial

Femoral

Popliteal

Dorsal pedis

A

FIGURE 3-13—cont'd   **B,** Checking major pulse points head to toe.

CHECKING MAJOR PULSE POINTS HEAD–TO–TOE

As part of your head-to-toe physical examination, you'll need to check for arterial pulses, moving from body region to body region, comparing pulses from side to side to detect any variations. First, you'll palpate the pulses and then, where appropriate, auscultate for abnormal vascular sounds.

Palpation gives you information about pulse rate, rhythm, contour, and amplitude. (See *Tips for palpating pulses.*) A normal pulse in adults ranges from 60 to 80 beats a minute and has a regular rhythm. The pulse's contour should be smooth on both the upstroke and downstroke. The amplitude, or quality, of the pulse is normally easy to palpate. (See *Describing pulse amplitude.*)

The accompanying chart shows major pulse points, explains the proper techniques for palpation and auscultation, and lists abnormal findings and their possible causes.

BRACHIAL PULSE

Technique: Apply firm pressure and palpate just medial to the biceps tendon at the antecubital fossa. The brachial artery can also be palpated higher up on the arm, in the groove between the biceps and triceps muscles.

INTERPRETATION OF ABNORMAL FINDINGS

- *Absent pulse* may indicate occlusion caused by dislodged thrombi (from the left atrium during atrial fibrillation, from the left ventricle following MI, or from diseased or prosthetic valves); embolization caused by intravenous drug abuse, arterial catheterization, arterial blood gas sampling, or indwelling monitoring lines; or closed trauma from a fracture or dislocation.
- *Diminished or absent pulse* may indicate aortic arch syndrome or a proximal atherosclerotic narrowing or occlusion.
- *Exaggerated, widened pulse* may indicate an aneurysm from atherosclerosis, trauma from brachial artery catheterization, or bacterial infection.

TIPS FOR PALPATING PULSES

- When checking each pulse site, make sure you and the patient are in a comfortable position. If you're in an awkward position, this may interfere with your tactile sensitivity.
- Use the distal pads of your index and middle fingers and apply firm pressure. Your fingertips are the most sensitive part of your hand for palpating pulses.
- To help find a pulse in a patient's arm or leg, support and relax any nearby joint with your free hand while palpating with your examining hand.
- If you have difficulty locating a pulse, move your fingers in and around the area, varying the amount of pressure you exert with your fingerpads. Once you've located the pulse, mark the spot with a felt-tip marking pen so the pulse can be found more easily later.
- Make sure you're not confusing the patient's pulse with your own pulsating fingerpads. If this is a problem, palpate your own carotid pulse to determine your heart rate and compare it to the patient's. Usually, the heart rates differ.
- Don't palpate with your thumb because it has strong pulsations that you can easily confuse with the patient's.
- When palpating pulses, don't press too hard; otherwise, you'll block the artery and won't feel a pulse.
- When checking pulse points, keep in mind that an occlusion can affect any artery. The two most common causes of arterial occlusion are embolism (from the heart, aorta, or large arteries) and thrombus formation (from atherosclerosis or trauma). A diminished or absent peripheral pulse may indicate a partial or complete obstruction proximally. Typically, all pulses distal to the occlusion are affected.

POPLITEAL PULSE

Technique: With the patient's knee slightly flexed and his foot resting on the bed, palpate deeply into the popliteal fossa, just lateral to the midline, using both your hands. Or use the same technique with the patient lying prone to better expose the artery.

INTERPRETATION OF ABNORMAL FINDINGS

- *Diminished or absent pulse* (often with a bruit) suggests aortoiliac, popliteal, or femoral occlusive disease, such as atherosclerosis.
- *Exaggerated, widened pulse* may indicate a popliteal aneurysm from atherosclerosis, trauma (blunt or penetrating), previous vascular reconstructive surgery, or bacterial infection.
- *Abrupt absence of all leg pulses* may indicate acute aortic bifurcation occlusion.

POSTERIOR TIBIAL PULSE

Technique: Curve your fingers and palpate behind and slightly below the medial malleolus of the ankle. You may have difficulty palpating this pulse in obese or edematous patients.

INTERPRETATION OF ABNORMAL FINDINGS

- *Diminished or absent pulse* may indicate aortoiliac, femoral, popliteal, or posterior tibial occlusive disease, such as atherosclerosis or Buerger's disease.
- *Abrupt absence of all leg pulses* may indicate acute aortic bifurcation occlusion.

CAROTID PULSE

Technique: Gently place your fingers on the trachea at the level of the cricoid cartilage, rolling your fingers laterally into the groove between the trachea and sternocleidomastoid muscle. Never palpate both sides simultaneously; this can slow the heart rate, cause a drop in blood pressure, or induce cerebral ischemia.

After you palpate each carotid artery, have the patient hold his breath for several heartbeats as you gently place the bell of the stethoscope over the area you palpated. Listen there and at several points along the artery for abnormal vascular sounds, such as bruits (low-pitched blowing sounds caused by turbulent blood flow).

INTERPRETATION OF ABNORMAL FINDINGS

- *Prominent pulsations* may be caused by aortic valve regurgitation or hyperthyroidism.
- *Unilateral pulsation* may indicate a tortuous or kinked carotid artery.
- *Bounding pulse* may be caused by anemia, hyperthyroidism, or aortic valve regurgitation.
- *Diminished pulse* may be caused by aortic valve stenosis, constrictive pericarditis, left ventricular failure from MI, or atherosclerotic narrowing of the carotid artery.
- *Palpable thrill* (a fine rushing vibration) may be caused by atherosclerotic narrowing of the carotid artery, a fistula between the carotid artery and jugular vein, anemia, thyrotoxicosis, or aortic valve stenosis.
- *Systolic bruit* may be caused by atherosclerotic narrowing of the carotid artery or a radiated aortic valve murmur.

DESCRIBING PULSE AMPLITUDE

As you palpate pulse points, you'll need to describe and document the amplitude, or quality, of the pulse at each site. Pulse amplitude gives you information about circulating blood volume, the strength of left ventricular contractions, and blood vessel tone. Make sure you palpate for pulse amplitude during ventricular systole. But remember not to press too hard; otherwise, you'll obliterate the pulse.

Use the following scale to describe pulse amplitude and remember to specify the scale range when documenting your results.

+ 3 = *Bounding.* Easy to palpate; forceful; not easily obliterated by finger pressure.

+ 2 = *Normal.* Easy to palpate; obliterated only by strong finger pressure.

+ 1 = *Weak or thready.* Difficult to palpate; easily obliterated by slight finger pressure.

  0 = *Absent.* Not discernible.

RADIAL PULSE

Technique: Lightly place your fingers in the groove formed along the radial side of the forearm, lateral to the flexor tendon of the wrist.

INTERPRETATION OF ABNORMAL FINDINGS

- *Diminished or absent pulse* may indicate aortic arch syndrome, proximal artherosclerotic narrowing or occlusion, or Buerger's disease.
- *Absent pulse* may indicate occlusion caused by dislodged thrombi (from the left atrium during atrial fibrillation, from the left ventricle following MI, or from diseased or prosthetic valves); embolization caused by intravenous drug abuse, arterial catheterization, arterial blood gas sampling, or indwelling monitoring lines; or closed trauma from a fracture or dislocation.
- *Exaggerated, widened pulse* may indicate an aneurysm from atherosclerosis, trauma from radial artery catheterization, or bacterial infection.

FEMORAL PULSE

Technique: With the patient supine, palpate below the inguinal ligament, halfway between the symphysis pubis and anterior superior iliac spine. For an obese patient, press more firmly (using both hands, one on top of the other, if necessary) and palpate in the crease of the groin halfway between the symphysis pubis and the anterior superior iliac spine.

After palpating each femoral pulse, gently place the bell of the stethoscope over the area you palpated and listen for abnormal vascular sounds.

INTERPRETATION OF ABNORMAL FINDINGS

- *Diminished or absent pulse* (often with a bruit) suggests aortoiliac occlusive disease.
- *Exaggerated, widened pulse* (often with a bruit) may indicate a femoral aneurysm from atherosclerosis, trauma (blunt or penetrating), femoral artery catheterization, previous vascular reconstructive surgery, or bacterial infection.
- *Absent pulse or one that is more diminished than the radial pulse* may indicate coarctation of the aorta.
- *Abrupt absence of all leg pulses* may indicate acute aortic bifurcation occlusion.

PEDAL PULSE

Technique: With the patient supine, gently place your fingers between the great and first toes, and slowly move away from the toes between their extensor tendons until the pulse is palpable. Keep in mind that in some patients, the pedal pulse may be congenitally absent or branch high up in the ankle.

INTERPRETATION OF ABNORMAL FINDINGS

- *Diminished or absent pulse* may indicate aortoiliac, femoral, popliteal, or posterior tibial occlusive disease, such as atherosclerosis or Buerger's disease.
- *Decreased or absent pedal pulses* with normal femoral and popliteal pulses may indicate occlusive disease in the lower popliteal artery or its branches.
- *Abrupt absence of all leg pulses* may indicate acute aortic bifurcation occlusion.
- *Absent pulse* may indicate popliteal artery entrapment.

PROCEDURE 3-5

TAKING A RADIAL PULSE

Objective
Understand and demonstrate the correct procedure for taking and recording a patient's pulse rate.

Equipment
Watch with a sweep second hand
Paper or graphic sheet to record pulse
Pen .

General Instructions
1. Have the patient assume a comfortable position either sitting or lying down, with the arm supported.

2. Do not take a pulse immediately after the patient has been emotionally upset or after exertion, unless so ordered.

3. Never use your thumb to take a pulse because its own pulse is likely to be confused with the one being taken.

4. Always count any unusual pulse for a full minute and repeat if uncertain.

5. When the pulse feels normal and is regular, count the number of pulsations for 30 seconds. Multiply this number by 2 to obtain the pulse rate for 1 minute.

PROCEDURE

1. Identify the patient and explain the procedure.

2. Wash your hands. **Use appropriate personal protective equipment (PPE) as indicated by facility.**

3. Position the patient with the arm supported and at rest.

4. Take a firm hold of the patient's wristbone just over the radial artery, with sufficient pressure to feel the pulsation distinctly. (Pulse rates at other locations previously noted are taken in similar fashion; Figure 3-14.)

5. Count the pulse for 60 seconds. Also see No. 5 under General Instructions.

6. Note the rate, rhythm, volume, and condition of the arterial wall.

7. Write the pulse rate down immediately.

8. Record accurately on the patient's chart.

RATIONALE

Explanations help gain the cooperation and relaxation of the patient.

A firm hold inspires the patient's confidence. Excess pressure prevents the pulse from being felt. Never use your thumb to take a pulse because the pulse in your thumb can be confused with that of the patient.

This gives the total beats per minute and provides adequate time to assess the rate, rhythm, and volume of the pulse. Always report any deviation from normal. If deviations are noted, always count the pulse rate for 1 full minute and repeat if uncertain.

Do not trust it to memory.

Charting Example

July 9, 20 __, 2 pm
Pulse 78
OR
Radial pulse, right arm—78
Regular and strong pulsation
Rae Evans, CMA

diaphragm of the stethoscope with an alcohol sponge and return it to the proper storage area.

Respiration

Respiration is the act of breathing and consists of one inspiration or inhalation (that is, the taking of air containing oxygen into the lungs) and one expiration or exhalation (that is, the expelling of air containing carbon dioxide from the lungs). More technically, respiration is the taking in of oxygen (O_2) and its use in the tissues and the giving off of carbon dioxide (CO_2). For this reason, respiration may be classified as external and internal. External respiration is the interchange of gases that takes place in the lungs between the alveoli and the blood; internal respiration is the interchange of gases that takes place in the tissues between the body cells and blood.

FIGURE 3-13—cont'd **C,** Location for taking an apical pulse.

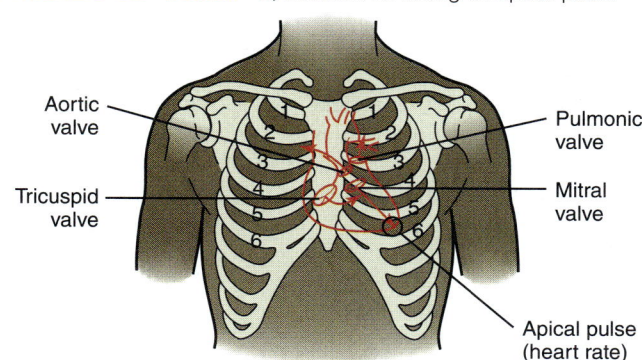

Aortic valve

Pulmonic valve

Tricuspid valve

Mitral valve

Apical pulse (heart rate)

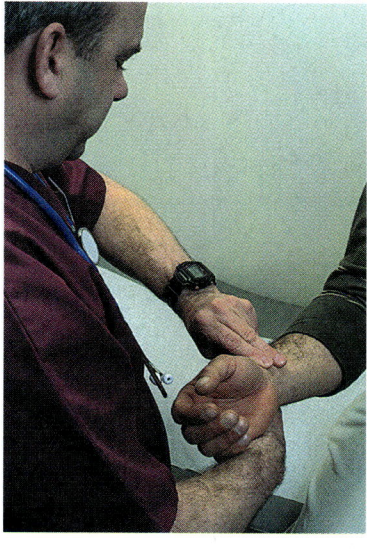

FIGURE 3-14 Taking a patient's pulse. Correct position and technique are very important.

RESPIRATION AND RESPIRATORY RATE VOCABULARY

abdominal respirations—The inspiration and expiration of air by the lungs accomplished primarily by the abdominal muscles and diaphragm.

accelerated respirations—More than 25 respirations per minute, after 15 years of age.

apnea (ap-ne'ah)—Cessation or absence of breathing. May be intermittent (lasting more than 15 seconds) as seen in sleep apnea.

artificial respiration—Artificial methods to restore respiration in cases of suspended breathing.

Biot's respiration—Irregularly alternating periods of apnea and hyperpnea; occurs in meningitis and disorders of the brain.

bradypnea (brad"ip-ne'ah)—The rate of breathing is regular but slower than normal in rate. Less than 12 breaths per minute.

Cheyne-Stokes respiration (chan stoks)—Respirations gradually increasing in rapidity and volume until they reach a climax and then gradually subsiding and ceasing entirely for from 5 to 50 seconds, when they begin again. These are often a sign of impending death. Cheyne-Stokes respirations may be observed in normal persons (especially the aged) during sleep or during visits to higher altitudes.

diaphragmatic respiration—Respirations performed mainly by the diaphragm.

dyspnea (disp-ne'ah)—Labored or difficult breathing.

eupnea (up-ne'ah)—Easy or normal respiration.

forced respiration—Voluntary hyperpnea.

hyperpnea (hy"perp-ne'ah)—Increase in rate and depth of respirations. Respirations may be labored. Occurs normally during exercise and abnormally with pain, fever, hysteria, or any condition in which the supply of oxygen is inadequate, such as cardiac disease or respiratory disease.

hyperventilation—Increase of air in the lungs above the normal amount; abnormally prolonged, rapid, and deep breathing, usually associated with acute anxiety or emotional tensions. Excessive intake of oxygen and blowing off of carbon dioxide occurs. Decreased levels of carbon dioxide in the blood (hypocapnia) result. Immediate treatment consists of rebreathing into a paper bag to replace the carbon dioxide "blow off" while hyperventilating. Also see Chapter 17.

hypoxia (hi-pok'se-ah)—Reduced amounts of oxygen to the body tissues.

labored breathing—Dyspnea or difficult breathing; respiration that involves active participation of accessory inspiratory and expiratory muscles.

orthopnea (or"thop-ne'ah)—Severe dyspnea in which breathing is possible only when the patient sits or stands in an erect position.

rales (rahls)—An abnormal bubbling sound heard on auscultation of the chest; often classified as either moist or crackling and dry.

stertorous (ster'to-rus)—Characterized by a deep snoring sound with each inspiration.

tachypnea (tak"ip-ne'ah)—Rate of breathing is regular but abnormally rapid. More than 20 breaths per minute.

Breathing is controlled spontaneously (autonomically) by the respiratory center in the medulla oblongata in the lower portion of the brainstem. A buildup of carbon dioxide in the blood stimulates respirations to occur automatically.

In the human body a relationship exists among the body temperature, pulse, and respiratory rates. The usual ratio of respiration to pulse is one to four (1:4). Respiration and pulse ordinarily rise proportionally to each degree rise in temperature because of increased metabolism in the tissue cells and the need for more rapid heat dissipation.

Characteristics of respirations. When taking the respiratory rate of a patient, the three important characteristics to note are the rate, rhythm, and depth.

Normal Respiratory Rates

At birth	30 to 60 respirations/minute
Infants	30 to 38 respirations/minute
Children	20 to 26 respirations/minute
Adults	12 to 20 respirations/minute

The **rate** of respirations refers to the number of respirations per minute and is best described as normal, rapid, or slow. In adults, normal resting rates are between 12 and 20 per minute; abnormally slow rates are less than 12 per minute and below and should be considered a serious symptom; above-normal rates at rest are between 24 and 35 per minute; rapid rates are between 36 and 50 per minute. Any rate above 40 should also be considered a serious symptom. Rates of 60 per minute and above are dangerously rapid. Usually rapid respirations are also shallow and are seen with some diseases of the lungs. Deep respirations are characteristically slow, dependent on air exchange, and common in conditions affecting intracranial pressure and in some forms of coma, including diabetic coma.

The **rhythm** may be described as regular or irregular. Regular breathing or respiration is characterized by inhalations and exhalations that are the same in depth and rate, whereas in irregular breathing, the inhalations and exhalations may vary in the amount of air inhaled and exhaled and in the rate of respirations per minute.

The **depth** of respirations depends on the amount of air inhaled and exhaled and is best described as either shallow or deep. In shallow respirations, small amounts of air are inhaled; they are often rapid. In deep respirations, larger amounts of air are inhaled, as in a "deep breath." These breaths are often slower.

Variations in respiratory rate. Certain situations, both in health or in diseased states, cause variations in normal respiratory rates.

Increased respiratory rate

- Excitement
- Nervousness
- Anxiety
- Any strong emotion
- Increased muscular activity, such as running or exercising
- Shortness of breath
- Certain drugs, such as ephedrine, cocaine, and amphetamines
- Diseases of the lungs
- Diseases of the circulatory system
- Fever
- Pain
- Shock
- Hemorrhage
- Gas poisoning
- High altitudes
- Obstructions of the air passages
- An increase in the carbon dioxide levels in arterial blood, which in turn stimulates the respiratory center

Decreased respiratory rate

- Sleep
- Certain drugs, such as morphine and sedatives
- Drug overdose
- Certain diseases of the kidneys, which involve a coma
- Diseases and injuries that cause pressure on the brain tissue (for example, a stroke or skull fracture)
- Decrease of carbon dioxide level in arterial blood (causes the respiratory centers to be depressed, causing decreased respiration rates)

Blood Pressure

Blood pressure (BP) is the pressure of the blood against the walls of the blood vessels. The pressure inside the arteries results from the pumping action of the heart muscle and varies with the contracting and the relaxing phases of the heartbeat cycle. Systole is the phase when the heart contracts, forcing blood through the arteries, and diastole is the phase when the heart relaxes between contractions. Thus when measuring a person's BP, you will take two readings: systolic pressure and diastolic pressure (systole and diastole).

Systolic pressure, measured in millimeters of mercury (mm Hg), represents the force with which blood is pushing against the artery walls when the ventricles of the heart are in a state of contraction. During systole, blood is forced out of the heart into the aorta and pulmonary artery, and the pressure within the arteries is the highest.

Diastolic pressure, also measured in millimeters of mercury, represents the force of the blood in the arterial system when the ventricles of the heart are in a state of relaxation. During diastole, blood flows into the two ventricles of the heart and dilates them, and the pressure within the arteries is at its lowest point.

These measurements provide the physician with valuable information about a patient's cardiovascular system. Systolic pressure provides information about the force of the left ventricular contraction, and diastolic pressure provides information about the resistance of the blood vessels.

Clinically, diastolic pressure is more important than systolic pressure because diastolic pressure indicates the strain or pressure to which the blood vessel walls are constantly subjected. Because diastolic pressure rises or falls with peripheral resistance, it also reflects the condition of the peripheral vessels. For example, if a patient's arteries are sclerosed (hardened), both the peripheral resistance and the diastolic pressure increase.

BP is recorded and discussed as the systolic pressure over the diastolic pressure. A typical BP is expressed as 120/80 (mm Hg) or 120 over 80. The numeric difference between these two readings (in this case, 40 points) is called the **pulse pressure,** which may indicate the tone of the arterial walls. A normal pulse pressure is about 40; if consistently over 50 points or under 30 points, it is considered abnormal. An increase in pulse pressure may be seen in arteriosclerosis, mainly because of an increase in the systolic pressure, or in aortic valve insufficiency, because of both a rise in systolic and a fall in diastolic pressure.

PROCEDURE 3-6

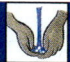

TAKING THE RESPIRATORY RATE

Objective
Understand and demonstrate the correct procedure for measuring and recording a patient's respiratory rate.

Equipment
Watch with a sweep second hand
Paper or graphic sheet to record respiration rate
Pen

General Instructions

1. Have the patient assume a comfortable position.

2. Do not take the respiratory rate immediately after the patient has been emotionally upset or after exertion, unless so ordered.

3. Count any unusual respiratory rate for an additional minute.

4. Regular respirations may be counted for 30 seconds. This number is then multiplied by 2 to obtain the rate per minute.

PROCEDURE

1. Wash your hands. **Use appropriate personal protective equipment (PPE) as indicated by facility.**

2. Do *not* explain procedure to the patient.

3. Place your fingers on the patient's wrist as though counting the pulse.

4. Count each breathing cycle (inhalation and exhalation) as one breath by watching the rise and fall of the chest or upper abdomen.

5. Count for 1 full minute.

6. Record rate on paper immediately.

7. Record on patient's chart. Note (a) any abnormality if present; (b) any pain associated with breathing; and (c) the position the patient assumes, because in some cases it may be significant (for example, when the patient can breathe easier when sitting up or when lying on one side or the other).

RATIONALE

The rate of respirations should be counted and their depth, rate, and rhythm studied without the patient's knowledge. The consciousness of being watched causes an involuntary change in the rate of respiration. A patient can control respirations if he or she wishes to.

When these movements are scarcely perceptible, place the patient's hand gently but firmly on his or her chest, keeping your fingers on the wrist or have the patient lie on his or her back and monitor the rise and fall of the stomach.

Do not trust it to memory.

Charting Example

January 15, 20__, 2 pm
Respirations 22 and regular
L. Quarry, CMA

Factors that determine blood pressure. A number of factors, acting in dynamic equilibrium and united through the central nervous system, determine the arterial BP:

1. *Pumping action of the heart and cardiac output*—How hard the heart pumps the blood, or the force of the heartbeat; how much blood it pumps and how efficiently it does the job
2. *Volume of blood within the blood vessels*—How much blood the heart pumps into the arterial system
3. *Peripheral resistance of blood vessels to the flow of blood*—The size of the lumen, that is, the central core or channel of the arteries, directly influences the resistance to the blood flow. When the lumen is narrow, the BP is higher; with a wider lumen, the BP is lower.
4. *Elasticity of the walls of the main arteries*—The main arteries leading from the heart have walls with strong elastic fibers capable of expanding and absorbing the pulsations

generated by the heart. At each pulsation, the arteries expand and absorb the momentary increase in BP. As the heart relaxes in preparation for another beat, the aortic and pulmonary valves close to prevent blood from flowing back to the ventricles of the heart, and the artery walls spring back, forcing the blood through the body between contractions. In this way the arteries act as dampers on the pulsation and thus provide a steady flow of blood through the blood vessels. This elasticity of the arterial walls lessens with age, and because the arterial wall is less flexible, the BP is higher.

5. *Blood's viscosity, or thickness*—BP increases as the viscosity of blood increases. Polycythemia, an increase in red blood cells, causes this.

How much each factor contributes is not known, but peripheral resistance and cardiac output are thought to have the greatest influence on BP.

BLOOD PRESSURE VOCABULARY

benign hypertension (be-nin)—Hypertension of slow onset that is usually without symptoms.

essential hypertension (idiopathic or primary hypertension)—Hypertension that develops in the absence of kidney disease. **Its cause is unknown.** About 85% to 90% of the cases of hypertension are in this category. Often, high BP runs in families and may be genetically determined.

hypertension (hi′per-ten′shun)—High BP; a condition in which a patient has a higher BP than normal for his or her age (for example, systolic pressure consistently above 160 mm Hg and diastolic pressure above 90 mm Hg). Mild or borderline hypertension is 140/90 to 160/95.

hypotension (hi′po-ten′shun)—A decrease of systolic and diastolic BP to below normal (for example, below 90/50 is considered low BP).

malignant hypertension (mah-lig′nant)—Hypertension that differs from other types in that it is a rapidly developing hypertension and may prove fatal if not treated immediately after symptoms develop, before the blood vessels are damaged. This type occurs most often in persons in their twenties or thirties.

orthostatic BP (or′tho-stat′ik)—BP measured when the patient is changed from a lying position to a sitting or an erect, standing position.

orthostatic hypotension—Hypotension occurring when a patient assumes an erect position from a lying or sitting position. Also called postural hypotension. It is associated with blurred vision, dizziness, and fainting.

postural hypotension—Hypotension occurring on suddenly arising from a recumbent position or when standing still for a long time.

renal hypertension—Hypertension resulting from kidney disease.

secondary hypertension—Hypertension that is traceable to known causes, such as a pheochromocytoma (tumor of the adrenal gland), hardening of the arteries, kidney disease, or obstructions to the kidney blood flow. Approximately 10% to 15% of the cases of hypertension are secondary. Patients with secondary hypertension can often be cured if the underlying cause can be eliminated.

Normal readings and values for blood pressure.

At birth the systolic pressure is about 80 mm Hg. *At age 10* (young people), systolic BP varies normally from 100 to 120 mm Hg, and diastolic pressure varies from 60 to 80 mm Hg. *In adults* the *average* BP is 120/80. The *average ranges* are 90 to 140 mm Hg for systolic pressure and 60 to 90 mm Hg for diastolic pressure. As age increases, the BP gradually increases. *In older people* (around 60 years) the systolic BP normally varies from 140 to about 170 mm Hg, and diastolic varies from 92 to 100 mm Hg because of loss of resilience in the vascular tree and the physiologic changes of aging.

Variations in normal blood pressure.

BP can vary between the sexes (with women usually having a lower pressure than men), between different age groups, and even between individuals of the same age and sex. At birth it is the lowest; it continues to increase with age, usually reaching its peak in advancing age. Variations are also seen at different times of the day and during different activities. BP is higher when a person is standing or sitting than when he or she is lying down. It is normally lowest just before awakening in the morning.

Many other situations produce changes in BP. The following lists indicate some of the common causes of an increase or decrease in a person's pressure.

Increased or elevated
- Exercise
- Stress, anxiety, or excitement
- Conditions in which blood vessels become more rigid and lose some of their elasticity (for example, old age)
- Increased peripheral resistance resulting from vasoconstriction or narrowing of peripheral blood vessels
- Endocrine disorders, such as hyperthyroidism and acromegaly
- Increased weight
- Smoking
- Pain
- Renal disease and diseases of the liver and heart
- Certain drug therapy
- Increased intracranial pressure
- Increased arterial blood volume

NOTE: In the right arm, the pressure is about 3 to 4 mm Hg higher than in the left arm.

Decreased or lowered
- Cardiac failure
- Massive heart attack, that is, myocardial infarction (MI)
- Decreased arterial blood volume (such as in hemorrhage)
- Shock and collapse
- Dehydration
- Drug treatment, for example, antihypertensives (for example, beta-blockers), and diuretics; also drugs used for people going through detoxification
- Disorders of the nervous system, for example, autonomic insufficiency
- Adrenal insufficiency
- Hypothyroidism
- Sleep
- Infections and fevers

- Cancer
- Anemia
- Neurasthenia
- Approaching death

Abnormal readings. Hypertension is commonly referred to as the "silent killer" because patients often exhibit no symptoms. In children around age 10, upper limits of normal are 140/100; systolic pressures greater than 140 mm Hg are generally recognized as being abnormal. The latest guidelines state that adults with a systolic pressure consistently above 140 mm Hg and a diastolic pressure consistently above 90 mm Hg are recognized as being in the first stage of hypertension. If the BP is consistently above this level, it could, if not treated, damage the heart, eyes, kidneys, and even the arteries. It can also be fatal. Diagnosis of hypertension is never based on only one reading. It is based on at least three consecutive daily or weekly pressure readings. Appropriate treatment of hypertension can markedly reduce the untoward effects, such as heart failure, blindness, kidney failure, and stroke.

Hypotension is systolic pressure consistently under 90 with the diastolic pressure in proportion. In the absence of other signs or symptoms, hypotension is generally harmless. An extremely low BP is occasionally a symptom of a serious condition such as shock and may be associated with Addison's disease (underfunctioning of the adrenal glands) and severe iron deficiency anemia (also see terms in the vocabulary).

Prevention, detection, and evaluation of high blood pressure. With a significant increase in hypertensive-related diseases (stroke, heart failure, and end-stage kidney disease), the Joint National Committee (JNC) on Prevention, Detection, Evaluation, and Treatment of High Blood Pressure made important changes in its sixth and most recent report, which was released in November 1997. Major differences in the sixth report are an increased and much stronger emphasis on *prevention,* a new classification system for hypertension, and a more aggressive approach to treatment. *Important to note is that the word "prevention" is used for the first time in the title of the report.*

The JNC on Prevention, Detection, Evaluation, and Treatment of High Blood Pressure has recommended that all adults age 18 and older with *diastolic* BPs of 110 mm Hg or above should be referred promptly to a source of medical care. All persons with BPs of 160/100 to 179/109 mm Hg should have the BP elevation confirmed within 1 month. All persons with a BP between 140/90 and 159/99 mm Hg should be checked every 2 months. All adults with *diastolic* BPs below 90 mm Hg should have their BP checked yearly.

The *purpose* of the BP recheck is to separate persons with initially elevated BP into (1) those whose diastolic BPs have returned to normal and who therefore require only annual BP remeasurement and (2) those with sustained elevation in pressure that warrants treatment or further diagnostic study.

At each repeat visit, the person's BP should be taken two or more times, and the average pressure obtained should be used as the value for the visit. BP measurements should be obtained on at least two occasions before specific therapy is prescribed, unless the initial diastolic BP is greater than 110 mm Hg (Table 3-2).

Patient education begins at the same time the BP is initially measured. Without alarming the patient, the person taking the pressure must carefully communicate the importance of following the recommended action.

Recommendations for evaluation.   The physician often includes the following when evaluating the patient's condition.

1. **History.** The medical history consists of any previous history of high BP or its treatment; the use of all prescribed and over-the-counter drugs, herbal remedies, illicit drugs (some of which may raise BP or interfere with the effectiveness of antihypertensive therapy), birth control pills, or other hormones; cardiac or renal disease, stroke, and other cardiovascular risk factors, including diabetes, cigarette smoking, or dietary habits including intake of caffeine, alcohol, saturated fat, and a high salt intake; lipid abnormalities, or family history of high BP or its complications. A history of weakness, muscle cramps, and polyuria suggests further screening for aldosteronism (electrolyte imbalance caused by an increased secretion of aldosterone from the adrenal gland). A history of headaches, palpitations, or excessive sweating suggests further study for pheochromocytoma (a tumor in the adrenal gland).
2. **Physical evaluation.** In addition to two or more BP measurements taken on both arms (one standing), the pretreatment physical examination includes the items listed below:
   a. Height, weight, and waist circumference
   b. Funduscopic examination of the eyes for hypertensive retinopathy, hemorrhages, exudates, and papilledema; this is especially important in persons with diastolic BPs of 110 mm Hg or higher
   c. Examination of the neck for thyroid enlargement, bruits, and distended veins
   d. Auscultation of the lungs for rales and evidence of bronchospasm
   e. Examination of the heart for increased rate, size, precordial heave, murmurs, arrhythmias, and gallops
   f. Examination of the abdomen for bruits, large kidneys, masses, or dilation of the aorta and abnormal aortic pulsation
   g. Examination of the extremities for edema, peripheral pulses, and neurologic deficits associated with stroke
   h. Neurologic assessment
3. **Basic laboratory tests.** Baseline laboratory tests listed below are obtained before initiating therapy:
   a. Complete blood count
   b. Urinalysis for protein, blood, and glucose (dipstick)
   c. Creatinine and/or blood urea nitrogen
   d. Serum potassium, sodium, creatinine, fasting glucose, total cholesterol, and high-density lipoproteins (HDLs)
   e. Electrocardiogram

TABLE 3-2 Classification of Blood Pressure, Hypertension, and Recommendations for Referral to Treatment

Category[a]	Systolic (mm Hg)		Diastolic (mm Hg)	Follow-up Recommended[d,e]
Optimal[b]	<120	and	<80	—
Normal	<130	and	<85	Recheck in 2 years
High-normal	130-139	or	85-89	Recheck in 1 year[f]
Hypertension[c]				
Stage 1	140-159	or	90-99	Confirm within 2 months[f]
Stage 2	160-179	or	100-109	Evaluate or refer to source of care within 1 month
Stage 3	≥180	or	≥110	Evaluate or refer to source of care immediately or within 1 week depending on clinical situation

From The Sixth Report of the Joint National Committee on Prevention, Detection, Evaluation, and Treatment of High Blood Pressure.

[a]Not taking antihypertensive drugs and not acutely ill. When systolic blood pressures (SBP) and diastolic blood pressures (DBP) fall into different categories, the higher category should be selected to classify the individual's blood pressure status. For example, 160/92 mm Hg should be classified as stage 2 hypertension, and 174/120 mm Hg should be classified as stage 3 hypertension. Isolated systolic hypertension is defined as SBP of 140 mm Hg or greater and DBP below 90 mm Hg and staged appropriately (e.g., 170/82 mm Hg is defined as stage 2 isolated systolic hypertension). In addition to classifying stages of hypertension on the basis of average blood pressure levels, clinicians should specify presence or absence of target organ disease and additional risk factors. This specificity is important for risk classification and treatment.

[b]Optimal blood pressure with respect to cardiovascular risk is below 120/80 mm Hg. However, unusually low readings should be evaluated for clinical significance.

[c]Based on the average of two or more readings taken at each of two or more visits after an initial screening.

[d]If systolic and diastolic categories are different, follow recommendations for shorter time follow-up (e.g., 160/86 mm Hg should be evaluated or referred to source of care within 1 month).

[e]Modify the scheduling of follow-up according to reliable information about past blood pressure measurements, other cardiovascular risk factors, or target organ disease.

[f]Provide advice about lifestyle modifications.

Other tests that may be helpful include a chest x-ray film, blood sugar, low-density lipoprotein (LDL), cholesterol/HDL ratio, serum uric acid and thyroid stimulating hormone (TSH), and microscopic urinalysis. (Ordering automated blood chemistries reduces the cost to the patient.) Clinical judgment or abnormal findings obtained during the routine evaluation may suggest other tests such as an intravenous urogram and urinary catecholamines.

4. **Explanation of findings to the patient and treatment plans.** The patient must be given adequate information to understand the disease and what actions he or she must take, as well as the opportunity to ask questions or discuss points of concern. *It is crucial to high BP control that the patient understand the following:*
   a. The seriousness and lifelong nature of high BP and the possible consequences of not treating it—there is *no* cure; however, hypertension can be controlled
   b. The importance of taking medication as directed to maintain BP control and to call the physician with any trouble—some side effects; BP medications are now available for treating all forms of high BP
   c. The importance of adhering to other methods recommended to control BP. **Lifestyle modifications,** also providing the greatest methods for **prevention,** include weight loss; reduced intake of animal fats and food high in sodium or salt; maintaining adequate intake of dietary calcium, potassium, and magnesium for general health (see Table 18-18, The DASH Diet,

pp. 818-819); not smoking; reduced intake of alcohol (not more than 1½ to 2 drinks per day is the recommendation); and mild-to-moderate exercise programs as prescribed by the physician (commonly 30 to 45 minutes of aerobic activity most days of the week); often the physician recommends some combination of the aforementioned methods for controlling high BP
   d. The **asymptomatic** nature of the disease—how the patient feels may not reflect the level of BP or the need to continue taking medication
   e. The importance of keeping follow-up appointments
   f. That treatment of any form of high BP markedly reduces the risk of stroke, heart attack, heart failure, kidney failure, and blindness

Patients not requiring further study or treatment should be reassured, but the importance of an annual BP measurement must be strongly emphasized.

Risk stratification. The risk of cardiovascular disease in patients with hypertension is determined not only by the level of blood pressure but also by the presence or absence of target organ damage or other risk factors, such as smoking, dyslipidemia, and diabetes, as shown in the box on p. 89. These factors independently modify the risk for subsequent cardiovascular disease, and their presence or absence is determined during the routine evaluation of patients with hypertension (that is, history, physical examination, laboratory tests). Based on this assessment and the level of blood pressure, the patient's

HEALTH MATTERS

KEEPING YOUR PATIENTS INFORMED ABOUT RISK FACTORS FOR HYPERTENSION

MAJOR RISK FACTORS

Smoking

Dyslipidemia (increased blood fats)

Diabetes mellitus

Age older than 60 years

Sex (men and postmenopausal women)

Family history of cardiovascular disease: women under age 65 or men under age 55

TARGET ORGAN DAMAGE/CLINICAL CARDIOVASCULAR DISEASE

Heart diseases

- Left ventricular hypertrophy
- Anginal/prior myocardial infarction
- Prior coronary revascularization
- Heart failure

Stroke or transient ischemic attack

Nephropathy

Peripheral arterial disease

Retinopathy

PREVENTION

Obesity and inactivity also interact with the other risk factors. Preventing hypertension can be greatly influenced by modification of risk factors that we have control over.

HEALTH MATTERS

KEEPING YOUR PATIENTS INFORMED

The National Heart, Lung, and Blood Institute (NHLBI) Information Center offers a toll-free service (1-800-575-WELL) that features messages in Spanish or English about the prevention of high blood pressure and high blood cholesterol. The service allows callers to leave their name and address if they would like to receive additional information on these topics by mail.

LIFESTYLE MODIFICATIONS FOR HYPERTENSION PREVENTION AND MANAGEMENT*

- Lose weight if overweight
- Limit alcohol intake to no more than 1 oz (30 ml) of ethanol (e.g., 24 oz [720 ml] of beer, 10 oz [300 ml] of wine, or 2 oz [60 ml] of

100-proof whiskey) per day or 0.5 oz. (15 ml) of ethanol per day for women and lighter-weight people

- Increase aerobic physical activity (30 to 45 minutes most days of the week)
- Reduce sodium intake to no more than 100 mmol/day (2.4 g of sodium or 6 g of sodium chloride)
- Maintain adequate intake of dietary potassium (approximately 90 mmol/day)
- Maintain adequate intake of dietary calcium and magnesium for general health
- Stop smoking and reduce intake of dietary saturated fat and cholesterol for overall cardiovascular health

*From the Sixth Report of the Joint National Committee on Prevention, Detection, Evaluation, and Treatment of High Blood Pressure, 1998, National Heart Institute (NHI) publication no. 98-4080.

risk group can be determined, as shown on p. 90. This classification puts patients with hypertension into risk groups for therapeutic decisions. The World Health Organization Expert Committee on Hypertension Control recently recommended a similar approach. Obesity and physical inactivity are also predictors of cardiovascular risk and interact with other risk factors, but they are of less significance in the selection of antihypertensive drugs.

Long-term maintenance. Management of high BP must be considered a lifelong endeavor; BP treatment is "considered effective if levels are controlled. Patients must be periodically monitored to ensure control and to make certain that they continue therapy. After control has been

demonstrated and the patient's BP is stable, remeasurement every 3 to 6 months should be adequate for most patients. Physicians order laboratory and baseline tests according to each patient's age, the initial severity of BP, and the target organ damage.

After normal levels are achieved, it may be possible to reduce drug therapy; however, the patient must understand that it is normally impossible to discontinue treatment. BP may be measured at home when appropriate or when frequent monitoring is deemed necessary (see box on p. 90).

Most patients with uncomplicated essential hypertension have few, if any, symptoms related to their hypertension; however, they should be warned about drug therapy that may produce unwanted effects. Every effort should be made to adjust

Risk Groups for Hypertension

Blood Pressure Stages (mm Hg)	Risk Group A (No Risk Factors; No TOD/CCD)	Risk Group B (At Least One Risk Factor, Not Including Diabetes; No TOD/CCD)	Risk Group C (TOD/CCD and/or Diabetes, With or Without Other Risk Factors)
High-normal (130-139/85-89)	Lifestyle modification*	Lifestyle modification	Drug therapy‡
Stage 1 (140-159/90-99)	Lifestyle modification (up to 12 months)	Lifestyle modification† (up to 6 months)	Drug therapy
Stages 2 and 3 (≥160/≥100)	Drug therapy	Drug therapy	Drug therapy

For example, a patient with diabetes and a blood pressure of 142/94 mm Hg plus left ventricular hypertrophy should be classified as having stage 1 hypertension with target organ disease (left ventricular hypertrophy) and with another major risk factor (diabetes). This patient would be categorized as Stage 1, Risk Group C, and recommended for immediate initiation of pharmacologic treatment.

*Lifestyle modification should be adjunctive therapy for all patients recommended for pharmacologic therapy.
†For patients with multiple risk factors, clinicians should consider drugs as initial therapy plus lifestyle modifications.
‡For those with heart failure, renal insufficiency, or diabetes.
TOD/CCD, Target organ disease/clinical cardiovascular disease.

HEALTH MATTERS

KEEPING YOUR PATIENTS INFORMED ABOUT BLOOD PRESSURE MEASURED AT HOME

Often patients are advised to take their blood pressure at home. This allows them to become an active participant in their treatment program.

SELF-MEASUREMENT OF BLOOD PRESSURE

Measurement of blood pressure outside the clinician's office may provide valuable information for the initial evaluation of patients with hypertension and for monitoring the response to treatment. Self-measurement has four general advantages:

1. Distinguishing sustained hypertension from "white-coat hypertension," a condition noted in patients whose blood pressure is consistently elevated in the physician's office or clinic but normal at other times
2. Assessing response to antihypertensive medication
3. Improving patient adherence to treatment
4. Potentially reducing costs

The blood pressure of persons with hypertension tends to be higher when measured in the clinic than outside of the office. There is no universally agreed-on upper limit of normal home blood pressure, but readings of 135/85 mm Hg or greater should be considered elevated.

CHOICE OF MONITORS FOR PERSONAL USE

Although the mercury sphygmomanometer is still the most accurate device for clinical use, it is generally not practical for home use. Therefore either validated electronic devices or aneroid sphygmomanometers that have proven to be accurate according to standard testing are recommended for use, along with appropriately sized cuffs. *Finger monitors are inaccurate.* Periodically, the accuracy of the patient's device should be checked by comparing readings with simultaneously recorded auscultatory readings taken with a mercury device. Independent evaluations of the instruments available to patients are published from time to time.

drugs and their dosages to eliminate or minimize such unpleasant effects and, at the same time, to gain patient acceptance of any that remain. Those responsible for monitoring antihypertensive regimens should also be aware of pharmacologic interactions and adverse effects of antihypertensive agents and should be alert to discover or prevent them.

Numerous reports over the past 20 years show that control of BP can reduce the occurrence of stroke by as much as 40% and the occurrence of heart attacks by 15% in patients with even mild forms of high BP. In patients with severe forms of high BP, treatment can reduce these risks by as much as 70%.

High blood pressure myth. The *major myth* about high BP is that people can feel when their BP is elevated. It is *very rare* that a person can tell when the BP is elevated unless it is very high. Studies have shown that the signs and symptoms that are often associated with hypertension (that is, headache, dizziness, fatigue, shortness of breath, and nosebleeds) are

HEALTH MATTERS

KEEPING YOUR PATIENTS INFORMED

Help your patients learn the answers to the following questions:

- Who can get high blood pressure?
- What are the risk factors for high blood pressure?
- Does age affect blood pressure?
- How does the sex of a person affect blood pressure?

- Does high blood pressure run in families?
- What causes high blood pressure?
- Does diet affect blood pressure?
- What can be done about high blood pressure?
- Who is involved in the treatment of high blood pressure?
- What kind of exercise can help to control blood pressure?
- What *is* high blood pressure?
- What will you do if you are diagnosed with high blood pressure?

FIGURE 3-15   Various types of sphygmomanometers. **A,** Wall mercury sphygmomanometer; **B,** portable sphygmomanometer; **C,** blood pressure cuff sizes (1, 2, 3, 4); **D,** acoustic sphygmomanometer. Wrap cuff around the arm in the usual way. Make sure microphone is over brachial artery. With cuff in place, raise pressure to approximately 30 mm Hg beyond expected systolic pressure. Watch digital countdown as pressure automatically releases. Systolic pressure is displayed first, followed by diastolic pressure as the sphygmomanometer responds to appropriate sounds. When both systolic and diastolic readings are displayed, the touch of a button also lets you read pulse rate. (**A** and **B,** Courtesy Welch-Allyn, Inc., Skaneateles, NY. **C,** From Barkauskas VH: *Health and Physical Assessment,* ed 2, St Louis, 1997, Mosby.)

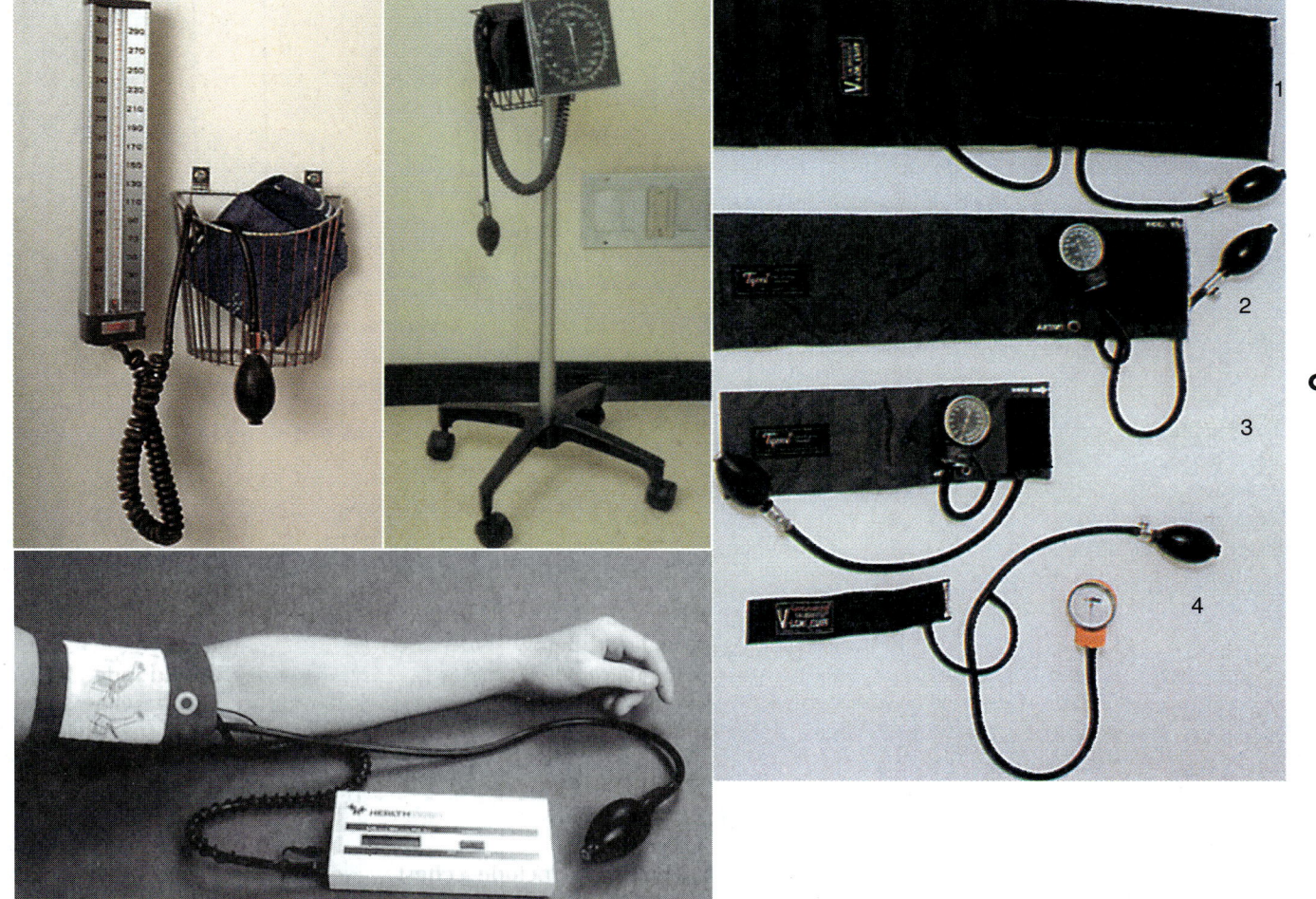

much more common in people with normal BP than they are in patients with hypertension. Therefore it is recommended that everyone has his or her BP measured to determine the reading. If it is within normal ranges, it should be rechecked every 1 to 2 years.

Instruments for measuring blood pressure.
BP is measured with two instruments, a **sphygmomanometer** (sfig″mo-mah-nom′e-ter) and a **stethoscope** (steth′o-skop). Various models of each and combination kits are available (Figure 3-15).

Sphygmomanometers.   Two common types of sphygmomanometers (*sphygmo,* pulse; *manos,* slight; *meter,* to measure) are available for general use: the mercury manometer, which uses a column of mercury to measure the BP, and the aneroid (*a,* not; *neroid,* liquid) manometer, which uses compressed air. Acoustic sphygmomanometers are also available.

Each type has advantages and disadvantages. The mercury manometer offers total reliability because, once calibrated at the factory, accuracy is ensured. However, it can only be used when the column of mercury is in a vertical position, and it is more fragile and larger than the aneroid type. The aneroid manometer, on the other hand, must be adjusted periodically and calibrated against a mercury manometer. However, it is smaller, thus offering more convenience and easier portability. Each manometer has four basic parts (Figure 3-16).

1. **Pressure indicators.** Pressure indicators are the scales used to read the BP. The mercury manometer has a glass tube with numbers on the side to indicate the height of the column of mercury in millimeters. When the cuff is inflated, mercury is forced up into the tube; as the cuff is deflated, the column of mercury falls. At certain points the level of the column of mercury is noted to provide the BP reading. In the aneroid manometer an internal gear rotates in response to inflation and deflation of the cuff, which in turn moves a needle across a calibrated dial to provide the BP reading.

2. **Cuff.** The compression cuff is a rectangular, inflatable rubber bag covered with a nonstretch material. This is wrapped around the patient's arm and secured with Velcro material or with clasps. On older models, the end of the cuff is tucked under one of the turns wrapped around the arm. Various sizes of cuffs are available to ensure a proper fit. Small cuffs are used on children or very thin people; larger cuffs are used on obese people or when taking a pressure reading on the leg (Table 3-3).

3. **Inflation bulb.** This bulb is used to pump air into the cuff through a rubber tube.

4. **Pressure control valve.** A valve on the inflation bulb is regulated with a thumbscrew to allow the air in the cuff to escape at different rates as it is opened and closed.

Stethoscopes.   The second instrument used to measure BP is the *stethoscope,* a basic diagnostic instrument that amplifies sounds produced by the BP, the heart, and other internal body sounds. The key parts of the stethoscope are shown in Figure 3-17.

Measuring blood pressure

Auscultation method.   Auscultation (aws"kul-ta′shun) is the process of listening for sounds representing the pressure inside the arteries. The artery most commonly used is the brachial artery at the antecubital space opposite the elbow. Other locations that may be used are the popliteal artery behind the knee or, less commonly, the pedal artery on the foot.

When measuring BP, you listen for a series of sounds called **Korotkoff sounds.** These sounds are produced by the blood as it flows through the artery. You hear these sounds through the stethoscope placed over the artery as you are deflating the BP cuff. Particular phases of these sounds determine the systolic and the diastolic BP readings (Figure 3-18).

1. **Phase I.** This is the first in a series of faint but clear tapping sounds. These sounds gradually increase in intensity. The first two consecutive sounds represent the systolic pressure.

2. **Phase II.** As the cuff is further deflated, the sounds change to a swishing or murmur. Occasionally these sounds disappear and reappear as the cuff is further deflated by 10 to 40 mm Hg. The period of silence is called the auscultatory gap. This is present especially in patients who have hyper-

TABLE 3–3   Recommended Widths of Compression Cuffs

Age	Width of Inflatable Bladder
Newborn infants	2.5 cm (1 in)
Children (1-4 yr)	6 cm (2.3 in)
Children (4-8 yr)	9 cm (3.5 in)
Adults	13 cm (5.1 in)
Obese adults	20 cm (8 in)

FIGURE 3-16   Four basic parts of a sphygmomanometer.

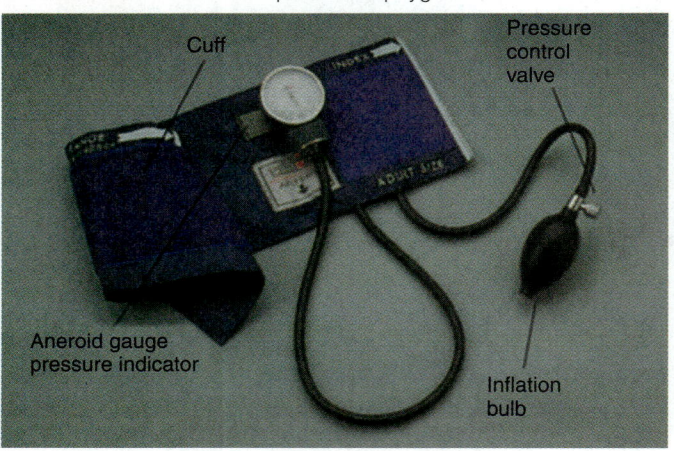

FIGURE 3-17   Key parts of the stethoscope.

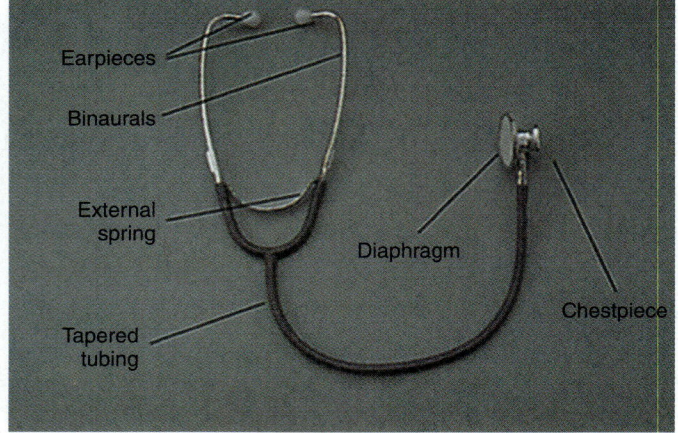

tension (high BP). Failure to notice this gap may cause serious errors in obtaining a BP reading.

3. **Phase III.** The sounds become crisp and loud. The blood is flowing through an increasingly open artery.
4. **Phase IV.** As the cuff is further deflated, the sounds become dull and muffled. This change of sound is the first diastolic sound.

Parts of a Stethoscope

binaurals—Rigid metal tubes that connect the tubing to the earpieces.

chestpiece—Has one, two, or three "heads" consisting of bell-shaped or various diaphragm-type sensors that "pick up" body sounds.

diaphragm—A waferlike sound sensor; its shape and the pressure applied to it determine which sound frequencies, low to high, are picked up.

earpieces—Tips of the stethoscope to be positioned in the examiner's ear.

spring—The external spring that holds the binaural so that the earpiece is firmly positioned in the ear.

tubing—Tapered, flexible rubber or plastic tubing through which sound travels from the chestpiece to the binaurals.

FIGURE 3-18 Phases of Korotkoff sounds that would be recorded as a blood pressure of 120/80/50.

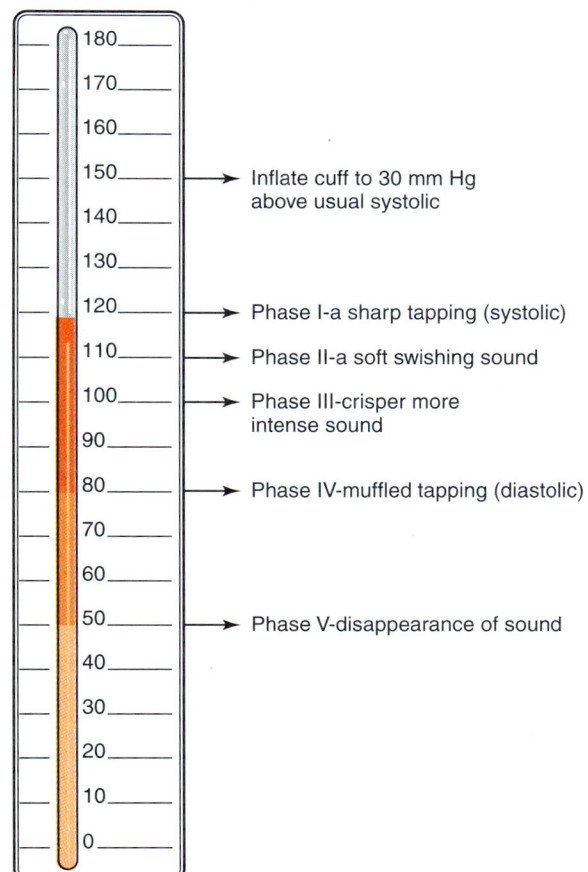

Inflate cuff to 30 mm Hg above usual systolic

Phase I-a sharp tapping (systolic)

Phase II-a soft swishing sound

Phase III-crisper more intense sound

Phase IV-muffled tapping (diastolic)

Phase V-disappearance of sound

5. **Phase V.** This is the point at which all sound disappears. This is the second diastolic sound.

Sometimes two figures are used to record the diastolic pressure. The first one used is the number observed when the sound changes in Phase IV. The second figure used is the number observed at the point when all sound disappears. An example of this type of recording is BP 124/82/0 **or** 124/82-0. If all of the sounds disappeared when the first diastolic sound was heard, the BP would be recorded as 124/82/82 or 124/82-82.

Taking a blood pressure reading on the leg.

1. The procedure is the same as outlined in the box on pp. 94-96, except that the arterial locations differ and the patient should be lying down. A leg pressure may be taken by either of the following methods:
   a. Placing a cuff around the thigh and the bell or diaphragm of the stethoscope over the popliteal artery behind the knee (see Figure 3-13).
   b. Placing the cuff around the calf of the leg and the bell or diaphragm of the stethoscope over the pedal (dorsalis pedis) artery on the foot (see Figure 3-13). *This is not a commonly used procedure.*

These locations can be used when the brachial artery is inaccessible because of a cast or dressing, or when an arteriovenous shunt for hemodialysis is present in the arm.

Palpation method for measuring blood pressure.
This is an alternative method for measuring blood pressure. When the blood pressure is inaudible by stethoscope, you may use this method, but only when the physician directs you to use it because it is generally thought to be inaccurate.

The procedure is similar to the auscultation method, except that you use your fingers rather than a stethoscope.

1. Place your fingers over the patient's brachial artery.
2. Pump cuff to at least 20 to 30 mm Hg after pulsation in the artery has ceased.
3. Release the air valve slowly.
4. Read the *systolic pressure* the moment you feel the first pulsation in the artery.
5. The pulse increases in force and tension and then gradually becomes softer; at this point of change, record the diastolic pressure if you can feel it. (*Some believe that this reading is not accurate because it is difficult to obtain; therefore they do not obtain a diastolic reading for BP taken by the palpation method.*)
6. Chart and indicate that the BP was obtained by palpation on the brachial artery.

Orthostatic blood pressure.
When a patient is receiving antihypertensive drug therapy, dehydrated, or suffering from hemorrhagic shock, the BP may take longer than normal to stabilize when the patient is changed from a lying position to a sitting or standing position. The BP readings taken after this change are known as orthostatic readings.

PROCEDURE 3-7

TAKING BLOOD PRESSURE READING ON THE ARM

Objective

Understand and demonstrate the correct procedure for taking and recording the systolic and diastolic blood pressure on a patient's brachial artery.

Equipment

Sphygmomanometer   Cotton balls or alcohol sponges
Stethoscope   Paper and pencil
70% isopropyl alcohol

General Instructions

1. Before taking the patient's BP, ask if he or she has been or is currently under treatment for high BP. Anyone under treatment should be encouraged to continue, especially if BP is normal at the time of screening, and should be urged to report an elevated BP to the physician. The potential dangers of discontinuing antihypertensive treatment and the desirability of controlling BP must be strongly emphasized.
2. Ensure as much confidentiality as possible during the recording of the BP.
3. Be sure the patient is relaxed and in a comfortable position. Depending on the physician's orders, the patient may be sitting, standing, or lying.
4. If possible, take all subsequent observations with the patient in the same position and using the same arm.
5. Do not leave the cuff inflated any longer than necessary because prolonged pressure affects the accuracy of the readings and is unpleasant for the patient.

6. On all new patients, BP should be taken on both arms. If a discrepancy exists, the arm with the higher pressure is used in future recordings. This discrepancy is to be recorded on the chart.
7. BP is taken routinely on the following patients, the frequency being determined by their condition:
   a. Patients receiving a complete physical examination
   b. Children before entering school
   c. Patients receiving hypertensive drugs
   d. Patients with a history of heart, kidney, or hypertensive disease
   e. New admissions to the hospital
   f. Pregnant patients
   g. Postpartum patients
   h. Preoperative patients
   i. Postoperative patients
   j. Patients in shock or those who are hemorrhaging
   k. *All* patients with neurologic disorders
   l. *All* patients as a preventive health measure
8. Check the sphygmomanometer regularly for loss of mercury and for leaks in the tubing, compression bag, and bulb.
9. Before and after each use of the stethoscope, clean the earpieces and the bell or diaphragm with a cotton ball soaked in alcohol or with an alcohol sponge.
10. Handle these instruments gently; misuse adversely affects their proper functioning.

PROCEDURE

1. Wash hands and obtain equipment. **Use appropriate personal protective equipment (PPE) as indicated by facility.**

2. Identify patient and explain the procedure.

3. Help the patient assume a comfortable position with the arm extended and supported.

4. Place a mercury sphygmomanometer on a level surface, in a position in which the scale can be easily read.

5. Expose the patient's arm well above the elbow.

6. Apply the cuff of the sphygmomanometer over the brachial artery (see Figure 3-13) 1 to 2 inches above the antecubital space, and wrap the remainder of the cuff around the arm so that each turn covers the previous one (Figure 3-19). On older model cuffs, tuck the end under one of the turns; some cuffs have clasps or hooks to fasten, and the newer models with Velcro closures adhere to the last turn on the cuff.

RATIONALE

Explanations help to gain the patient's confidence and relaxation.

The patient may be sitting, standing, or lying down, depending on the physician's orders.

Having a mercury manometer at your eye level enables you to take a more accurate reading.

Clothing should be adjusted to avoid constriction and to prevent rustling of garments.

You should apply the cuff snugly and neatly. The arm may be flexed slightly after the cuff is applied. Use a child's or infant's cuff for small children or for extremely thin patients and use the larger cuff for obese patients to obtain an accurate reading (see Table 3-3 and Figure 3-15, C).

PROCEDURE 3·7—cont'd

7. Locate the strongest pulsation of the brachial artery in the antecubital space by palpating with your fingers at the bend of the elbow (Figure 3-20).

8. Adjust the earpieces of the stethoscope in your ears, place the bell or diaphragm of the stethoscope over the artery pulsation, and hold in place (Figure 3-21).

The bell or diaphragm should always be placed below, not under, the cuff and directly over the strongest pulsation of the brachial artery that is felt.

9. With your dominant hand, close the air valve on the hand bulb by turning the thumbscrew in a clockwise direction. Pump air into the cuff of the manometer rapidly until the level of mercury is about 20 to 30 mm Hg above the palpated or previously measured systolic pressure (the procedure for taking BP by palpation is explained on p. 93).

Blood is cut off when the cuff is inflated. To identify the true systolic pressure, air must be pumped into the cuff rapidly, and then the cuff deflated slowly. Inflating the cuff slowly or sending the mercury to a higher level than necessary is very uncomfortable for the patient. To avoid missing the true systolic reading, pressure can initially be taken by the palpation method, and then 15 to 30 seconds later the pressure reading can be taken by the auscultation method.

10. Turn the thumbscrew counterclockwise to open the air valve slowly. Allow for a slow release of air to the cuff so that the pressure falls only 2 to 3 mm Hg at a time (Figure 3-22).

Rapid deflation of the cuff causes you to miss the exact reading.

11. Listen carefully and read the exact point on the mercury column (or spring gauge if using an aneroid manometer) at which the first distinct sound is heard. Keep this number in mind; this represents the systolic pressure.

This sound is caused by the initial spurt of blood into the collapsed artery as deflation of the cuff occurs. This is Phase I of the Korotkoff sounds.

12. Continue to allow the air to escape, thereby letting the cuff deflate slowly. The sounds get louder and then become like a murmur, then crisp, then dull and soft, and then fade away (Figure 3-23).

This is a continuation of Phases I, II, III and into Phase IV of the Korotkoff sounds.

13. Read the scale when the sound becomes dull or muffled. Keep this number in mind; it represents the diastolic pressure.

The level of mercury at the point where the sound changes from loud to dull or muffled is the diastolic pressure, representing the pressure in the arteries during diastole of the heart. This is Phase IV of the Korotkoff sounds.

14. Continue to deflate the cuff until the sound disappears. This is Phase V of the Korotkoff sounds. Remember this number because many physicians request that both numbers be reported for diastolic readings.

This is Phase V of the Korotkoff sounds.

15. Open the valve completely to release all the air from the cuff.

The blood in the veins in the lower arm is not able to return to the heart if all the air in the cuff is not released.

16. If there is any doubt of an accurate reading, wait 15 seconds, then repeat steps 7 through 15. Do not repeat more than twice on the same arm because the reading will be inaccurate as a result of blood stasis (blood trapped in the arm).

Between readings, the cuff must be completely deflated. Failure to do so produces erroneously high readings.

17. Write the BP down on paper as a mathematical fraction. If your employer doesn't mind, you may inform the patient of the numeric value of the BP.

Do not trust it to memory. Record systolic reading over diastolic reading as a mathematical fraction. (For example, 120/80 or 120/80- 60 (60 indicating where the sounds disappear).

18. Remove the cuff from the patient's arm.

19. See that the patient is comfortable.

Continued

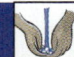
20. Return the equipment to the designated area and prepare it for storage according to the type of apparatus used. Cleanse the earpiece and diaphragm of the stethoscope with an alcohol sponge.

21. Record the BP on the patient's chart.

Charting Example

October 1, 20___, 2 pm
BP 118/86 rt arm
or
118/86-70 rt arm
Ann Banks, CMA

22. Notify the physician if you have obtained a relatively higher or lower reading than previously recorded.

Further evaluation or only periodic measurement may be needed. Because an initial high reading may reflect only a transient increase, which could be caused by anxiety or excitement, the BP should be measured on different days and after the patient has been able to relax for a time.

FIGURE 3-19   Applying the cuff of the sphygmomanometer above the antecubital space of the right arm.

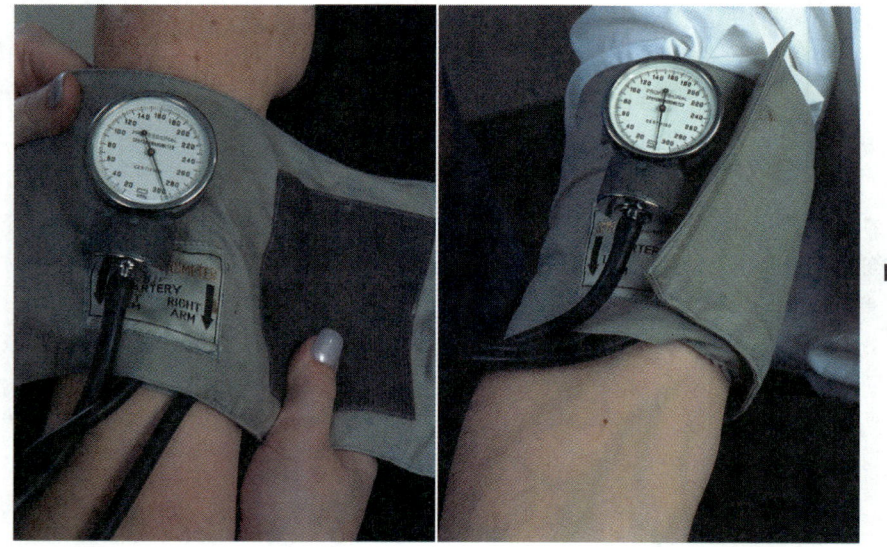

A   B

FIGURE 3-20   Location of strongest pulsation in the antecubital space.

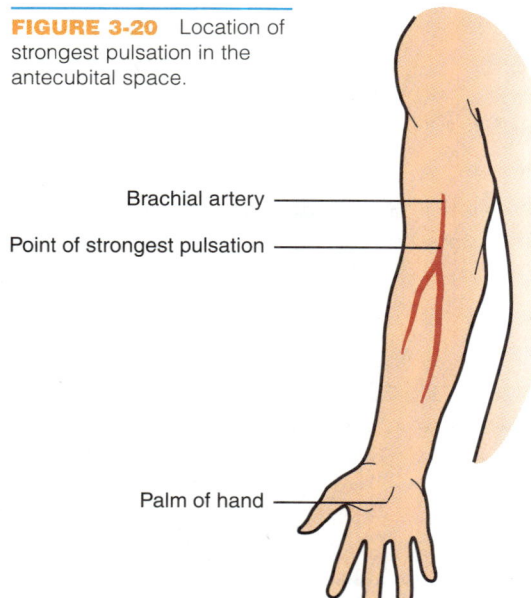

Brachial artery

Point of strongest pulsation

Palm of hand

FIGURE 3-21   Adjusting the stethoscope for taking BP.

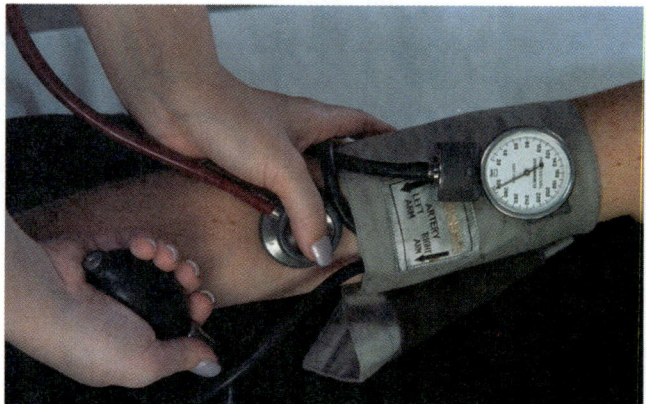

FIGURE 3-22   Technique for taking BP using aneroid sphygmo-manometer.

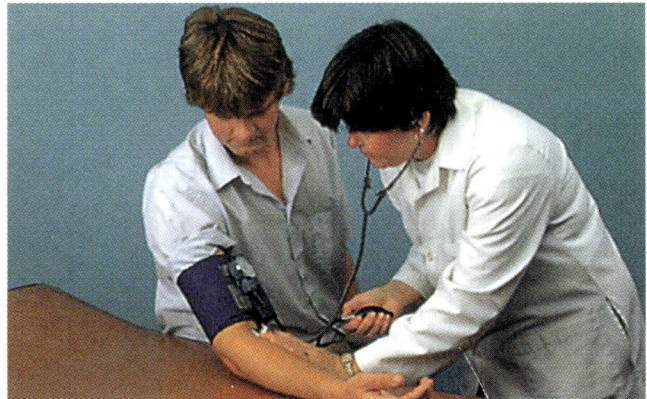

FIGURE 3-23   Mercury column descending as air is released from the cuff.

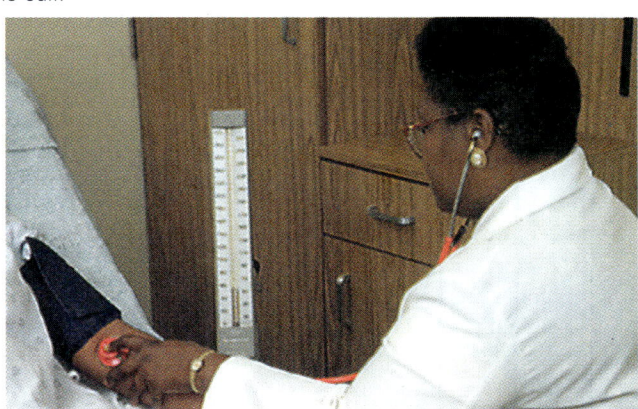

PROCEDURE 3-8
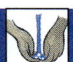

MEASURING ORTHOSTATIC BLOOD PRESSURE

Objective
Understand and demonstrate the correct procedure for taking and recording a patient's orthostatic blood pressure.

Equipment
Sphygmomanometer   Stethoscope

PROCEDURE

1. Identify the patient and explain the procedure.

2. Have the patient assume a recumbent position for 5 minutes, and then take the BP and apical pulse.

3. Instruct the patient to sit up at a 90-degree angle. Take the BP and apical pulse immediately. Ask how the patient feels.

4. Have the patient stand up at the side of the examining table. Take the BP and apical pulse immediately. Question the patient concerning a change in equilibrium.

5. Chart the BPs and apical pulses on the patient's medical record. Indicate which readings were taken when the patient was lying down, sitting, and standing.

6. Report the following to the physician:
  a. Any systolic change greater than 10 mm Hg in lying/sitting or lying/standing positions
  b. Any diastolic change greater than 20 mm Hg in lying/sitting or lying/standing positions
  c. Any apical pulse change greater than 20 beats per minute in a lying/sitting or lying/standing position

RATIONALE

Explanations help gain the patient's confidence and relaxation.

The patient may feel dizzy.

The patient may need to rest between the sitting and standing measurements. Standing pressure may be omitted, depending on the physician's order and/or the patient's condition.

Charting Example

August 22, 20__, 8 am
120/80—lying
110/80—sitting
90/70—standing
T. O'Connell, CMA

PHYSICAL MEASUREMENTS OF HEIGHT AND WEIGHT

The two other important physical or clinical measurements to obtain are the height and weight of the patient. Common practice is to take these measurements as part of a physical examination for the following reasons:

1. Height and weight measurements may provide relevant information for diagnosing, treating, preventing, or evaluating a condition
2. Height and weight are documented to determine a child's growth pattern (see Chapter 5)
3. The patient's weight is used as a guide for determining the dosage to be administered for certain drugs
4. The patient's weight must be known before a magnetic resonance imaging (MRI) examination (see Chapter 14) because the machine used must be adjusted to the patient's weight

Recommended standards have been set for the average weight that individuals should be for their height, but these are only ranges, not absolute standards; differences in body types must be considered.

Being overweight or underweight can cause serious health complications. Common complications of being overweight include hypertension (high BP), heart disease, and diabetes mellitus. Being underweight may indicate malnourishment or metabolic disorders. Either may be the result of psychologic problems.

Many patients are very self-conscious about their weight; therefore the scales should be located in an area that ensures privacy. Also to reduce embarrassment, you may have the patient stand with the back to the numbers on the scale. It is important in this procedure, as in all procedures, that you maintain a neutral facial expression to avoid communicating your impressions to the patient.

Be alert and note any unusual weight gains or losses in established patients and comments regarding changes by new patients, either of which may be an important diagnostic aid.

Some scales are calibrated in kilograms, and others in pounds. To convert a weight, use the following formulas:
To convert kilograms to pounds (kg to lb):

$$1 \text{ kg} = 2.2 \text{ lb}$$

Multiply the number of kilograms by 2.2.
EXAMPLE: If a patient weighs 60 kg, multiply 60 by 2.2:

$$60 \times 2.2 = 132 \text{ lb}$$

To convert pounds to kilograms (lb to kg), divide the number of pounds by 2.2.
EXAMPLE: If a patient weighs 132 lb, divide 132 by 2.2:

$$132 \div 2.2 = 60 \text{ kg}$$

See Table 3-4 for the conversion of pounds to kilograms and Table 3-5 for the average heights and weights for adults.

For convenience, post a conversion chart near the area where you measure weights and heights.

TABLE 3–4   Conversion Table: Pounds to Kilograms*

Pounds	Kilograms	Pounds	Kilograms	Pounds	Kilograms
1	0.45	100	45.36	205	92.99
2.2	1.00	105	47.63	210	95.26
5	2.27	110	49.90	215	97.52
10	4.54	115	52.12	220	99.79
15	6.80	120	54.43	225	102.06
20	9.07	125	56.70	230	104.33
25	11.34	130	58.91	235	106.60
30	13.61	135	61.24	240	108.86
35	15.88	140	63.50	245	111.13
40	18.14	145	65.77	250	113.40
45	20.41	150	68.04	255	115.67
50	22.68	155	70.31	260	117.94
55	24.95	160	72.58	265	120.20
60	27.22	165	74.84	270	122.47
65	29.48	170	77.11	275	124.74
70	31.75	175	79.38	280	127.01
75	34.02	180	81.65	285	129.28
80	36.29	185	83.92	290	131.54
85	38.56	190	86.18	295	133.81
90	40.82	195	88.45	300	136.08
95	43.09	200	90.72		

*To convert:
Pounds to kilograms: multiply number of pounds by 0.45 (0.4536), **or** divide pounds by 2.2.
Kilograms to pounds: multiply number of kilogram by 2.2 (2.204).

TABLE 3–5   **Desirable Weights—Ages 25 to 59—Based on Lowest Mortality**

Men				Woment			
Height (in Shoes With 1-inch Heels)		Small Frame	Medium Frame	Large Frame	Height (in Shoes With 1-inch Heels)		Small Frame	Medium Frame	Large Frame
Feet	Inches	Small Frame	Medium Frame	Large Frame	Feet	Inches	Small Frame	Medium Frame	Large Frame
5	2	128-134	131-141	138-150	4	10	102-111	109-121	118-131
5	3	130-136	133-143	140-153	4	11	103-113	111-123	120-134
5	4	132-138	135-145	142-156	5	0	104-115	113-126	122-137
5	5	134-140	137-148	144-160	5	1	106-118	115-129	125-140
5	6	136-142	139-151	146-164	5	2	108-121	118-132	128-143
5	7	138-145	142-154	149-168	5	3	111-124	121-135	131-147
5	8	140-148	145-157	152-172	5	4	114-127	124-138	134-151
5	9	142-151	148-160	155-176	5	5	117-130	127-141	137-155
5	10	144-154	151-163	158-180	5	6	120-133	130-144	140-159
5	11	146-157	154-166	161-184	5	7	123-136	133-147	143-163
6	0	149-160	157-170	164-188	5	8	126-139	136-150	146-167
6	1	152-164	160-174	168-192	5	9	129-142	139-153	149-170
6	2	155-168	164-178	172-197	5	10	132-145	142-156	152-173
6	3	158-172	167-182	176-202	5	11	135-148	145-159	155-176
6	4	162-176	171-187	181-207	6	0	138-151	148-162	158-179

Courtesy Metropolitan Life Insurance Co., New York, NY.
*Weights in pounds according to frame (in indoor clothing weighing 5 pounds for men and 3 pounds for women).
†For women between ages 18 and 25, subtract 1 pound for each year under 25.

PROCEDURE 3-9

MEASURING HEIGHT AND WEIGHT

Objective
Understand and demonstrate the correct procedures for measuring and recording a patient's height and weight.

Equipment
Weight scale with height measuring bar

PROCEDURE

1. Wash your hands—**Use appropriate personal protective equipment (PPE) as indicated by facility.**

2. Identify the patient and explain the procedure.

3. Place a clean paper towel on the scale foot stand.

4. Balance the scale. Ensure that both weights are on zero and that the balance bar hangs free before the patient steps onto the scale.

5. Have the patient remove shoes and any jacket or heavy outer sweater. In some offices or agencies, the patient may be weighed in a patient gown.

RATIONALE

This is just one form of expected clean technique. Use a clean towel for each patient.

Unbalanced scales result in an inaccurate weight measurement.

The removal of heavy outer clothing provides a more accurate reading.

Continued

PROCEDURE 3-9—cont'd

6. Direct or assist the patient onto the scale. NOTE: You may raise the height bar above the patient's estimated height and have it in position before the patient steps onto the scale to avoid moving and manipulating it later.

7. Ask the patient his or her usual weight and then move the 50-pound weight to the 50-, 100-, 150-, 200-, or 250-pound mark, ensuring that the weight is resting securely in the weight indicator groove (Figure 3-24). Metric scales are marked using 10-kilogram (kg) increments.

Unless the weight is secured correctly in the groove provided, the patient's weight measurement will be off by many pounds.

8. Gradually move the upper weight across the individual pound register until the arm at the right end of the balance bar rests in a position in the center of the metal frame, not touching either edge of this frame.

The weight is read when the balance bar is in the middle.

9. Read the weight accurately to the nearest quarter of a pound or the nearest 0.1 kg. NOTE: Pediatric scales measure weights in pounds and ounces or grams and kilograms.

10. Return the weights to zero.

11. Record the weight on the patient's chart.

When charting, you must indicate if the patient was wearing street clothes or a patient gown.

12. To measure height, either have the patient remain on the scale, standing erect and looking straight ahead, **or** have the patient face away from the scale.

The patient must be standing very straight to obtain the correct height measurement.

13. If the height bar was not raised previously (see Step 6), raise it over the patient's head and extend the hinged arm.

14. Carefully lower the height bar until it touches the top of the patient's head lightly (Figure 3-25).

15. Read the height measurement.

The number (in inches) indicating the patient's height is the last digit or fraction visible at the point where the movable part of the bar enters its stationary holder.

16. Assist the patient off the scale if necessary and return the height bar to the resting position.

17. Record the height accurately in feet and inches. Use accepted abbreviations. Some height bars use the metric scale. The height is then recorded in centimeters (cm).

Charting Example

October 27, 20___, 4 PM
Ht. 5′ 2″
Wt. 112 lb in street clothes, s̄ [without] shoes.
Annie Fox, CMA

FIGURE 3-24 Weighing the patient.

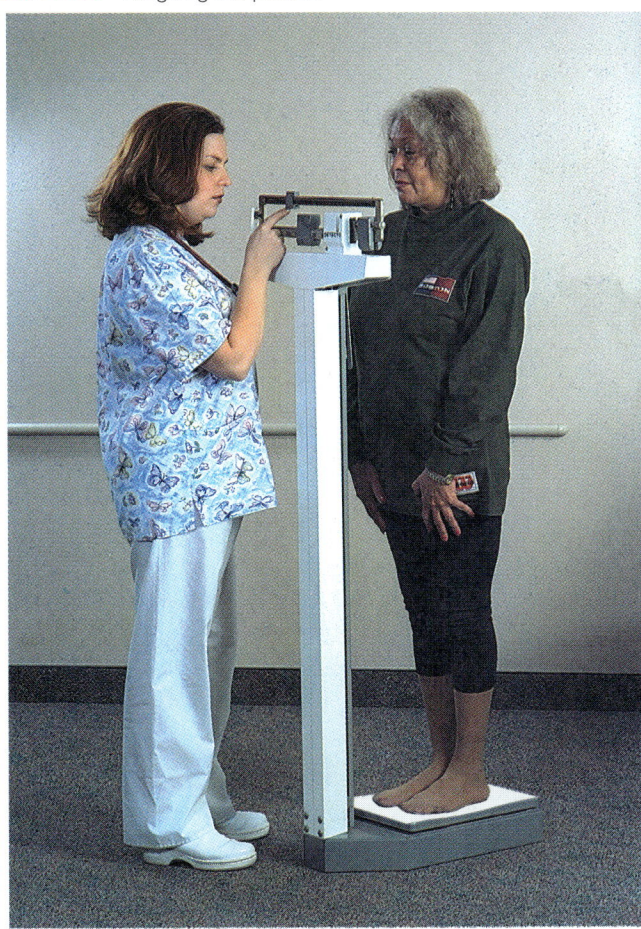

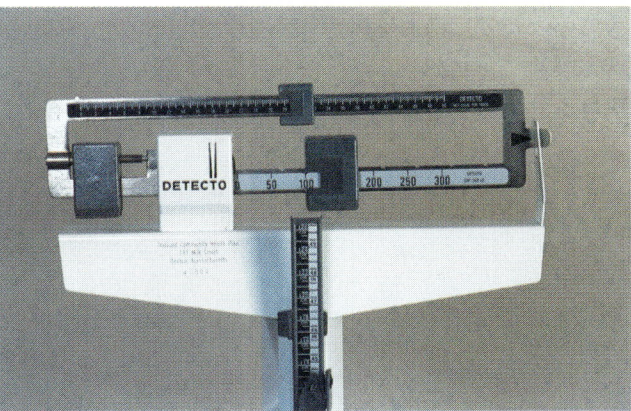

FIGURE 3-25 Measuring the patient's height.

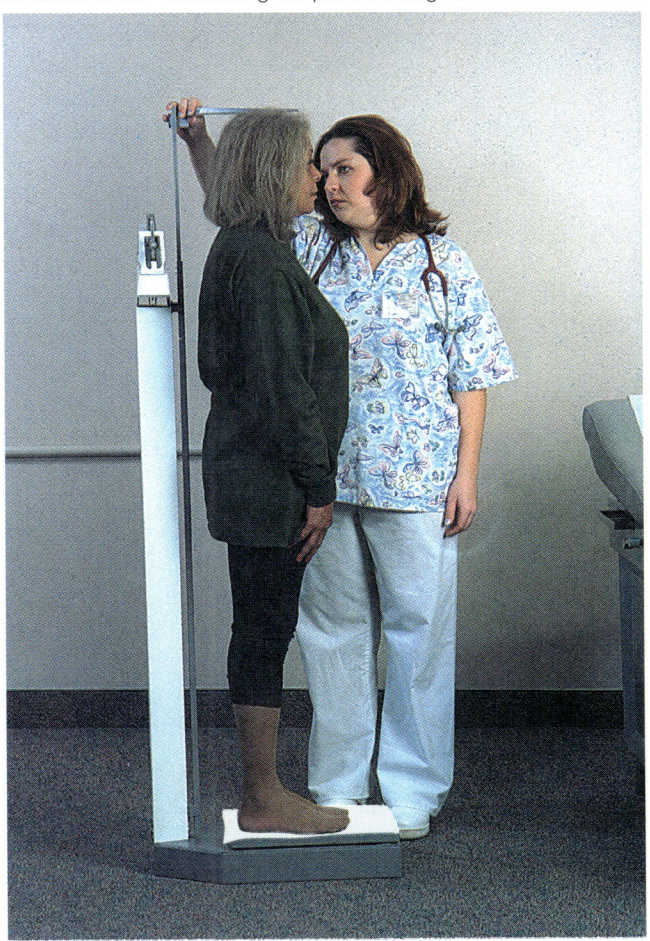

CONCLUSION

You have now completed the chapter on Physical Measurements, the most basic clinical procedures that you may be required to perform. When you have practiced these procedures and feel competent in performing them, arrange with your instructor to take the Performance Test. You will be expected to demonstrate accurately your ability to prepare for and take the vital signs and height and weight measurements on individuals assigned to you by your instructor.

REVIEW OF VOCABULARY

This is a sample of how a physician may write up part of a patient's case history. In the following sentences, words that have been defined for you in the chapter are used. Read this and define the terms in bold.

Physician's Statement of a Patient's Vital Signs

This 40-year-old patient was first seen with the chief complaint of frequent **dyspnea** and **orthopnea** at night. On examination of the chest, **rales** were heard, and **respirations** were **accelerated** to 30 per minute.

- Patient stated that he often **hyperventilated,** especially in stressful situations.
- Patient had a fever of 103° F, which remained **constant** over the first 24 hours after being seen in my office. The **onset** of this **fever** was apparently 2 days before this examination.
- **Bigeminal pulse rate, arrhythmia,** and **pulse deficit** of at least eight beats—**apical pulse rate** was 130; **radial pulse rate** was 122, approximately. Venous pulse in the external jugulars was palpable and also very **irregular.**
- *BP*—**systolic,** 164; **diastolic,** 128.
- **Pulse pressure,** 36. Height, 5′6″; weight, 142 lb.

Family history revealed that this patient's father has **hypertension,** mother has **hypotension,** and sister was diagnosed as having **malignant hypertension** at the age of 29.

For more information on this patient's history, please refer to past notes in the previous chart.

Y. Short, MD

Consultation Letter to Referring Physician

The letter on p. 103 is a sample of a letter received in the physician's office from a consulting physician. After reading this report, you should be able to discuss the contents. A dictionary or other reference source may be used as needed.

CRITICAL THINKING SKILLS REVIEW

1. List three purposes for taking a patient's vital signs.
2. For the following situations, indicate if you would normally see an increase or a decrease in each of the following: temperature, pulse rate, respiratory rate, and BP:
   a. A patient who faints
   b. A patient who has a severe infection in her throat
   c. A patient who is hemorrhaging
   d. A patient who has just jogged for 2 miles
   e. A patient who has a brainstem injury
   f. A patient who becomes extremely excited or upset
   g. A patient who is sleeping
   h. A child as compared with an adult
3. List the normal average readings for the following:
   a. Oral temperature in adults
   b. Axillary temperature in adults
   c. Rectal temperature in adults
   d. Pulse rate in adults
   e. Respiratory rate in adults
   f. BP in adults
4. Convert the following temperatures to centigrade degrees:
   a. 98.6° F
   b. 97.8° F
   c. 100.4° F
   d. 99.6° F
5. Convert the following temperatures to Fahrenheit degrees:
   a. 39.5° C
   b. 36° C
   c. 38.2° C
   d. 37.2° C
6. List four benefits of tympanic thermometry over glass mercury thermometers.
7. Why is the tympanic membrane an accurate indicator of body temperature?
8. List and describe the location of the seven most common arteries where a pulse may be felt.
9. If a patient has an extremely sore mouth, how would you take the temperature?
10. What is meant by the pulse rate? The respiratory rate?

December 15, 200_

Dr. Y. Short
666 South W Street
Anytown, USA

Dear Dr. Short:

Mrs. Alice Price was seen initially on 9/27/01 at your request because of her progressing nocturnal choking sensations during the past year.

It was of interest to learn that I had seen her sometime before 1985 for a respiratory allergy syndrome that was attributed to dust and other inhalants following some testing procedures.

She indicates that she has been living in the same residence for the past 14 years and has had the same pet, a Chihuahua, for the past 12 years. There has been some sputum production without blood with the present illness but no chest pain or peripheral edema. She had retired from her employment as a janitor with the City and County of Anytown 2 years ago.

Past history shows T & A [tonsillectomy and adenoidectomy] age 27, appendectomy and hysterectomy proximate to that date, and a whiplash 3 years ago.

The weight is in the 168-lb range, and she indicates an allergy to pork and fish, which she believes may precipitate her nocturnal dyspneic events. She has had nocturia three times nightly for the past year; she drinks two cups of coffee and tea per day, uses no cigarettes, and her alcohol intake is moderate. Her medications are limited to the Tri-Pro-Hist prescribed by you for her asthma.

The various laboratory data of 9/10/01 were not remarkable, except for liver enzyme elevation, and it was noted the PME equaled 2% on the differential. Chest x-ray film in 1992 was reportedly negative, and no changes were seen on the 9/27/01 repeat film. Physical signs showed height 66 inches, weight 169 lb; the general findings were normal except for BP 160/109.

Vital capacity was 3 liters (90% normal) with mild FEV^1 [full expiration volume 1] delay, and EKG showed an intermediate heart with changes suggesting hypocarbia.

It was my belief that Mrs. Alice Price has the following conditions:
1.   Arterial hypertension, mild
2.   Exogenous obesity, approximately 30 lb
3.   Paroxysmal nocturnal dyspnea, atopic, possibly associated with food and/or inhalants
4.   Hepatic insufficiency, metabolic origin

I advised her of these several entities, prescribed Aldactazide once daily for antihypertensive effect, and suggested that she continue on the antihistamine prescribed by you. When reviewed on 10/3/01, she had had significant diuretic effect, fewer nocturnal events, and BP was 150/92.

I therefore advised her to remain on the Aldactazide daily and supplement the antihistamine with Elixophyllin 0.2 on a prn basis for dyspnea.

She will report back in 1 month, and if there are any unusual circumstances, I shall promptly advise you.
Sincerely yours,

R.G. Lewis, MD

11. What is meant by the rhythm of the pulse rate? The rhythm of the respiratory rate?

12. You have just taken a patient's respiratory rate and found it to be 10 respirations per minute. Would you consider this a normal and adequate rate or a serious symptom of some physiologic change in the body?

13. What action is taking place in the heart during systole? During diastole?

14. Why does BP usually increase in the elderly?

15. If a patient has plaster casts on both arms, where and how would you take the BP?

16. A patient's BP is 130/92. What is the pulse pressure? Is this pulse pressure in the normal range?

17. What medical condition is commonly referred to as the "silent killer"? Explain why.

18. List four conditions that may be prevented if hypertension is treated successfully.

19. List four methods that may be used to control high BP.

20. Convert the following body weights to measurements in pounds:
    a. 52 kg
    b. 68.5 kg
    c. 47 kg
    d. 56 kg

21. Convert the following body weights to measurements in kilograms:
    a. 112 lb
    b. 174 lb
    c. 136 lb
    d. 155 lb

PERFORMANCE TEST

In a skills laboratory, a simulation of a joblike environment, the medical assistant student must demonstrate knowledge and skill in performing the following procedures without reference to source materials. For these activities the student needs a watch with a second hand; ear, rectal and oral thermometers; a stethoscope; a sphygmomanometer; alcohol sponges; containers for used thermometers; a scale with height measuring bar; various individuals to play the role of a patient; and a patient chart. The instructor assigns time limits and the number of patients to be tested for each procedure.

Given an ambulatory patient and the appropriate equipment and supplies, obtain and record the following accurately:

- Oral temperature
- Axillary temperature
- Rectal temperature (a model may be used for this procedure)
- Ear (tympanic membrane) temperature
- Pulse rate
- Respiratory rate
- BP taken on the brachial artery
- BP taken on the popliteal artery
- Apical heartbeat
- Orthostatic BP
- Height and weight

The student is expected to perform these procedures with 100% accuracy.*

The successful completion of each procedure will demonstrate competency levels as required by the AAMA, AMT, and future employers.

Grading

Grading systems are flexible to meet each instructor's preference. The instructor may wish to use a satisfactory/unsatisfactory grading system, a pass/fail system, or a point-value system for each step on the checklist. It is recommended that each procedure be assigned a time limit by the instructor.

Performance Tests, Checklists, and Evaluation Charts for the instructor's use when evaluating the student's performance of a skill are provided in the Instructor's Manual and in the student workbook that accompanies this book.

---

*Results obtained for the pulse rates and the respiratory rates are acceptable if within two beats or respirations, as determined and recorded by the instructor. Results for BP readings are acceptable if within 2 to 4 mm Hg, as determined and recorded by the instructor. The student is expected to become proficient in these procedures before progressing to others in this book.

🖥 INTERNET RESOURCES

American Heart Association
www.americanheart.org

National Institutes of Health, National Heart, Lung and Blood Institute
www.nhibi.nih.gov

North American Association for the Study of Obesity
www.naaso.org

American Heart Association
http://amhrt.org

Medline*plus*
www.nlm.nih.gov.medlineplus

United States National Library of Medicine (information on general health)
www.nlm.nih.gov/medlineplus

Health Finder
www.healthfinder.gov

High Blood Pressure Information for Patients/General Public:
www.nhlbi.nih.gov/nhlbi/cardio/hbp/gp/hbinfgp.htm

Health History and Physical Examination

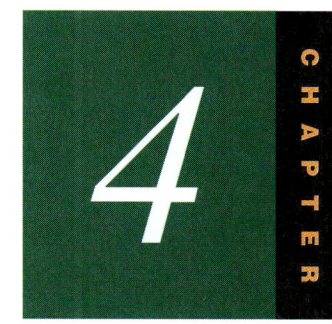

4 CHAPTER

■ Cognitive Objectives

On completion of Chapter 4, the medical assistant student should be able to:

1. Define, spell, and pronounce the vocabulary terms and define the medical abbreviations listed.
2. List the eight major components of a patient's medical history or record and describe the information that is recorded in each.
3. List and define the six parts of the patient's medical history.
4. List eight reasons why information gathered during a history and physical examination is valuable to the physician.
5. List and describe six methods of examination used by the physician when performing a physical examination on a patient, giving an example of when or how each is used.
6. List the essential parts of a physical examination.
7. Differentiate between information obtained in the review of systems and that obtained during the physical examination.
8. Discuss the steps taken by a physician when making a diagnosis.
9. List five forms of treatment.
10. List three reasons for diagnostic studies.
11. Discuss the purpose of the patient's medical record.
12. Discuss the importance of correct documentation and confidentiality of the patient's medical record.
13. State who owns the patient's medical record.
14. State reasons for and demonstrate the technique used to make corrections in a patient's medical record.
15. Discuss options for retaining medical records.
16. Explain the terms *managed health care* and *primary care physician*.
17. State and discuss the goals of managed health care systems.
18. Discuss and explain the patient's rights and responsibilities under a managed health care system.
19. Differentiate between verbal and nonverbal communication.
20. Explain and give an example of effective communication skills between two or more individuals.
21. Discuss the importance of recognizing different forms of communication that may be observed in people from different cultures.
22. Explain the importance of good communication interactions between patients and health care providers.
23. Discuss and explain how cultural influences play a role in health care for both patients and health care providers.
24. Discuss and explain 10 guidelines for relating to patients from different cultures.
25. Discuss and give five examples of guidelines to follow when preparing for and providing patient education. State why it is important for you to develop effective patient teaching skills and how you would develop these skills.
26. Explain and demonstrate how to teach patients to keep records of their symptoms and treatment programs.
27. Discuss and explain 14 guidelines to use when assisting with obtaining a patient's medical history and conducting a patient interview.
28. Explain the purpose and advantages of having an advanced directive and a durable power of attorney for health care. Discuss the legal aspects of advanced directives.
29. List and explain at least 17 of the special provisions and limitations to be discussed when completing a durable power of attorney for health care document.
30. Explain what the problem-oriented medical record is, giving examples of SOAP charting methods used.
31. Identify community and national resources and hotlines for health care information and patient referral.

■ Terminal Performance Objectives

On completion of Chapter 4, the medical assistant student should be able to:

1. Help obtain and record a brief medical history or statement of the patient's chief complaint.
2. Demonstrate cultural sensitivity competencies when relating to patients from different cultures.

3. Provide culturally sensitive care to a diverse society.
4. Demonstrate positive interactive communication skills.
5. Demonstrate patience and good listening skills with patients and co-workers.
6. Develop and demonstrate teaching skills that work effectively with patients of all cultures and with patients who have varied educational levels.
7. Demonstrate the ability to pay close attention to detail.
8. Through continued practice of interacting with patients and co-workers, develop analytical skills that can help in evaluating a situation and developing or changing a well-defined plan of action and care.
9. Develop and review methods used to provide patient education. Have patients perform a demonstration of the skill taught and evaluate the technique used.
10. Listen to the patient attentively and question the patient to clarify, obtain, and confirm information.
11. Demonstrate the ability to obtain information and cooperation from others while projecting confidence and understanding.
12. Communicate information and needs clearly.
13. Create an atmosphere that allows comfortable interactive communication.
14. Provide instructions and patient education that is within the professional scope of a medical assistant's training and responsibilities as assigned.

The student is expected to perform these objectives with 100% accuracy 90% of the time (9 out of 10 times).

The consistent use of Universal/Standard Precautions is required by all health care professionals in all health care settings as a method of infection control. It is assumed that these precautions are used in all of the following procedures. Review Chapter 1 if you have any questions on methods to use because the methods or techniques will not be repeated in detail in each procedure presented in this chapter.

Be sure to consult the latest guidelines issued by the Centers for Disease Control and Prevention and consult with infection control practitioners when necessary to identify specific precautions that pertain to your particular work situation.

VOCABULARY

competence—A state of being capable; possessing the knowledge, skills, and abilities needed to function in a given situation or setting. A person's **"potential ability."**

competency—Competency focuses on a person's **"actual performance"** in a designated situation consistent with standards established by the work setting.

health—The state of mental, physical, and social well-being of an individual; not merely the absence of disease.

negative findings—*No* evidence of disease or body dysfunction.

positive findings—Evidence of disease or body dysfunction.

prodrome—An early symptom indicating the onset of a disease, such as an achy feeling before having the flu.

prognosis—A statement made by the physician indicating the probable or anticipated outcome of the disease process in a patient; usually stated simply as *good, fair, poor,* or *guarded.*

sign—Sometimes called a *physical sign;* any objective evidence (apparent to the observer) representing disease or body dysfunction. Signs may be observed by others or revealed when the physician performs a physical examination; examples include swollen ankles, a distended rigid abdomen, elevated blood pressure, and decreased sensation.

symmetry—Conformity in form, size, and arrangement of parts on opposite sides of the body.

symptom—Sometimes called a *subjective symptom;* any subjective evidence of disease or body dysfunction; a change in the physical or mental state of the body that is perceptible or apparent only to the individual experiencing the change; examples include anorexia, nausea, headache, pain, itching, and dizziness.

syndrome—A combination of symptoms resulting from one cause or commonly occurring together to present a distinct clinical picture; an example is the dumping syndrome, which consists of nausea, weakness, varying degrees of syncope, sweating, palpitation, and sometimes diarrhea and a feeling of warmth. This may occur immediately after eating in patients who have had a partial gastrectomy.

THE MEDICAL RECORD

To provide a basis for decision making and planning for the care of a patient, different kinds of information must be gathered, compiled, and maintained in an orderly and confidential manner. Lack of needed information and confidentiality may jeopardize appropriate patient care. The patient's confidential medical record is a compilation of information concerning the patient, the care provided, the progress, and the results obtained. The medical record is a *confidential legal document belonging to the physician or clinical agency.*

When a physician sees the patient for the first time, identifying information (such as name and address) and all the information necessary for diagnosing the case, prescribing treatment, and planning future care are obtained. Every **diagnostic workup has six major components:** the history, the physical examination, the summary of positive findings, the interpretation of completed diagnostic studies, the examiner's impression based on all the information gathered, and the care plans, including suggested further study.

On subsequent visits the progress or status of the patient's condition is recorded as progress notes. Eventually, when the patient is discharged or the condition has been resolved, the date of discharge and status of the patient at that time are recorded as the discharge summary.

This compilation of information is kept together and called the patient's medical record. These **confidential** records and reports are arranged in a file folder, binder, or other special type of folder, which is generally referred to as the patient's chart or file.

The medical assistant plays an important role in obtaining and maintaining data on patients. This responsibility varies with the preference and specialty of the physician. In some instances the medical assistant is expected to relieve the physician of much of the data collection. In these cases, the medical assistant obtains identifying information from the patient; measures the patient's height, weight, temperature, pulse rate, respiration rate, and blood pressure; and takes the medical history. In other situations, the medical assistant may be required to obtain only the identifying information.

Identifying information includes the patient's name, address, telephone number(s) (home and work), age, date of birth, sex, marital status, occupation, place of employment, and insurance company and policy number. In addition to recording data, the medical assistant is responsible for preparing the examination room for the examination of the patient; preparing the equipment and supplies needed; preparing the patient both physically and mentally; assisting the patient and the physician; collecting specimens as requested; and organizing the results of diagnostic studies (such as laboratory, pathology, and diagnostic imaging reports), operative reports, consultation letters or reports (see also Chapter 10), and consent forms (see Figure 6-16, p. 310) in the patient's record.

Many hospitals have now computerized many parts of their medical records. Physicians have their own secret signature code or password to call up information on their patients. With the appropriate hardware in the office or clinic, physicians can call up certain reports and information about their patients in the hospital to keep them abreast of ongoing care. They can also obtain the discharge summary with a current laboratory summary and recent vital signs for patients leaving the hospital. These reports are then put into the patient's medical record in the office to help the physician provide continuity of care in the clinic or office. Hospital laboratory reports can also be obtained for clinic or office patients.

Federal security and privacy regulations are being phased in to protect the availability, confidentiality, and integrity of these medical records. These regulations are vital because of the increasingly high-tech methods being used for exchanging health care information. Health care providers, health care plans, and clearinghouses must comply with the regulations 2 years after the publication of them in August 1999. Health plans with fewer than 50 members have 3 years to comply with the regulations.

This chapter discusses the components and related information of a patient's medical record, related vocabulary, medical abbreviations, and the problem-oriented medical record. Chapter 5 presents vocabulary, procedures, and techniques used when preparing for and assisting with various types of physical examinations.

Actual medical reports are cited at the end of chapters in the Review of Vocabulary to help the medical assistant student correlate the contents of the chapters with the ways physicians record information about the patient.

The health care system continues to be in a process of change. See the box below and on p. 109 for a discussion on managed care, primary care physicians, and the patient's rights and responsibilities under managed care. Other issues of major importance—communication skills, culturally sensitive health care, patient education and teaching, and the durable power of attorney for health care follow. You must recall and apply *all* of these skills and knowledge when studying the chapters in this book and *always* when working as a medical assistant.

HEALTH MATTERS

KEEPING YOUR PATIENTS INFORMED

PATIENT'S RIGHTS AND RESPONSIBILITIES UNDER MANAGED CARE*
What Is Managed Health Care?

Managed care is a system of medical care that emphasizes primary and preventive care. It guarantees you 24-hour, 7-day-a-week access to a personal physician. All of your medical care will be coordinated through your personal doctor, called a primary care physician, who you select from a list provided by the managed care plan or network. You may hear terms such as health maintenance organization (HMO), independent practice association (IPA), physician hospital organization (PHO), and medical service organization (MSO). These are examples of managed care systems.

What Is a Primary Care Physician?

A primary care physician specializes in caring for your needs as a person or whole family. The primary care physician you select is responsible for coordinating all of your care. Ninety percent of all your medical needs can be taken care of right in the office. For the remaining care, your personal doctor will choose appropriate specialists.

Your primary care physician will also serve as your counselor and advocate in dealing with the health care system. He or she will explain the need of various speciality tests and referrals. This physician will also serve as a "translator" for you in explaining some of the

*This information was reprinted with permission from the National Rural Health Association. For more information, contact the National Rural Health Association, One West Armour Blvd., Suite 301, Kansas City, MO 64111; (816) 756-3140 or access our World Wide Web site at http://NRHArural.org.

Continued

HEALTH MATTERS—cont'd

technical medical terminology and the reasons why the specialists you were referred to are recommending tests. Because your primary care physician knows you as a whole person and is not just looking at the health of a single organ system in the body, he or she may recommend against a test or procedure that you or a specialist think is needed.

Your primary care physician is there for you to talk to. His or her job is to form a partnership with you to keep you healthy. From time to time, there may be a disagreement between you and your physician. If this occurs, discuss it openly with your physician. Most often, this will resolve the matter. On the rare occasion when the two of you cannot resolve the issue, you can change primary care physicians.

What Are the Goals of a Managed Health Care System?

There are seven major goals of a managed care system. They are:

1. To keep you healthy
2. To improve the quality of your care
3. To reduce the cost of your care
4. To educate you so that you can make informed decisions about the type of care you want and need
5. To guarantee you readily accessible health care through a personal physician
6. To treat you in a respectful and compassionate manner
7. To help you become a full partner in your medical care, sharing in the responsibility for your health

These goals are accomplished by:

1. Preventing disease in two ways—through education and regular checkups
2. Treating disease
3. Giving you the information you need to make good decisions about your health care needs
4. Fostering a close, personal relationship with your doctor

What Are Your Rights Under a Managed Health Care System?

You have a right to be informed about how the system works.

You have a right to select any primary care physician. Some plans allow you to do this immediately. Some plans make you wait 30 days.

You have a right to change insurance plans once a year. This is called the open enrollment period.

You have the right to file a complaint about the care you receive to the plan. All plans have grievance procedures and a medical director to review these complaints. If you still think you are not being heard, you have a right to file a grievance with the insurance commissioner of the state where the plan is licensed.

You have the right to obtain health care 24 hours a day.

What Are Your Responsibilities Under a Managed Health Care System?

Ultimately, you are responsible for your own health and well-being. You can keep yourself healthy by doing the following:

1. Eat less fat.
2. Eat less sugar.
3. Exercise.
4. Don't smoke.
5. Don't use illegal drugs.
6. Don't drink to excess.
7. Enjoy sex with only one partner. Protect yourself in all your sexual practices.
8. Avoid violence.
9. Learn how to manage stress and keep a positive mental attitude.
10. Avoid injuries, that is, by wearing seat belts and bicycle helmets.

Your physician can give you the knowledge and the encouragement to keep you healthy and happy, but the decision to do so must come from you.

1. Get regular checkups.
2. Communicate your needs to your physician.
3. Ask questions.
4. Get the information you need to make informed decisions.
5. Call your primary care physician before seeking emergency room care. The exception to this, of course, is if there is a life and death emergency. In that case, call the ambulance first and then call your primary care physician. Examples of this are massive bleeding or if you think you are having a heart attack.
6. Assist your physician in establishing reasonable goals for your health and treatment. Demand quality care, not expensive care. Again, ask questions as to the appropriate use of these things and then decide together with your physician what is best for you.
7. Inform your plan and your legislators if your health care needs are not being served. No matter how good a health care system is, no system is right for everyone. Your input and feedback on how your needs are not being met are an important part of improving the system.

15 Questions to Ask a Managed Health Care Plan

1. What happens if my doctor is not a member of the plan? Can I still go to him or her?
2. If I am already seeing a specialist for a condition, can I continue going to the same specialist?
3. What do I do if I have a medical problem at night or on weekends?
4. What do I do if I am out of the area and I have a medical problem? Is this covered by the plan?
5. Can I use a walk-in or urgent care center?
6. What do I do if I have a life-threatening emergency and cannot get hold of my primary care physician immediately?
7. What do I do if I sincerely disagree with the advice I am getting from my primary care physician? For example, let's say I believe I need specialty care or a procedure and my doctor refuses to let me get it?
8. What happens if there are no specialists of the type I need in the managed care network?

HEALTH M A T T E R S — c o n t ' d

9. What if I need superspecialized care like a heart transplant? Can I choose the center I want or will I have to go to a specific center?

10. What if the doctors in the managed care plan cannot diagnose my condition? Can my primary care physician refer me outside the plan in this case?

11. What if the managed care plan goes bankrupt? Will I still be able to get medical care under the contract or will I have to pay for it myself?

12. Am I allowed to get care outside the plan if I agree to pay for it myself?

13. What do I do if I am unhappy with the specialist I am referred to?

14. What are my options if I choose to join a managed care plan?

15. Can a woman select an obstetrician/gynecologist as a second primary care physician?

Summary

In the managed care system, you are a full partner in promoting your health and well-being. You are responsible for taking care of yourself by living a healthy lifestyle, getting regular checkups, and communicating your needs to your physician. Your physician is responsible for educating you, listening to you, and providing the care you need to be happy and healthy. Your primary care physician also will do this in a way that will allow for efficient use of services so that your financial health can be preserved at the same time as your physical health.

COMMUNICATION SKILLS

Good communication skills are essential both in your professional life and personal life. Communication can be defined as giving and receiving information, verbally or nonverbally, through words, gestures, or writing. Communication is a dynamic, two-way and cyclical process. Effective communication occurs when a person, the sender, sends a message and that message is received and interpreted by the receiver (the listener) with the same meaning that was intended by the sender, *and* the receiver/listener can provide feedback to the sender by verbal or nonverbal means. Feedback indicates that communication has occurred—that is, the receiver of the message has *really listened,* understands or does not understand the message, and can respond. This model of communication can be illustrated as follows.

$$\text{Sender} \rightarrow \text{Message} \rightarrow \text{Receiver}$$
$$\llcorner \text{Feedback} \longleftarrow\lrcorner$$

The sender has intentions that are put into words, actions, or writing and transmits these to the receiver. If communication occurs, the receiver translates the message into meaning and provides a response (feedback) verbally or nonverbally. Feedback lets the sender know that communication has occurred, and the interaction continues until the goal has been achieved or is no longer important. To clarify the message from the sender, you may summarize it in your own words and ask, "Is that what you meant?" This gives the sender the opportunity to confirm or clarify the message or correct any misunderstanding before communication continues.

Communication moves toward a goal, so it is important to establish your goal. This will help you to listen more effectively and focus on what you need to find out from the other person. **Communication competency** is thought of as the ability to accomplish goals through coordinated social interactions. This implies that there is a purpose in communication.

Most commonly, when we think of communication, we think of talking "to" or "with" someone—using words and what they mean to express feelings, thoughts, ideas, requests, opinions, observations, and so on; using words to verbally respond to someone by providing feedback to the sender; or using words to influence one another. *Words* are only a small part of effective communication. **Attitude, tone of voice,** and **body language** affect the words and must complement what is said for the words to be credible and meaningful to the listener.

People respond and express feelings differently. **Observe** their *mannerisms* and *attitude.* **Listen** for the *tone* of the voice/words. Tone is also called vocal cues and includes the *pitch* of the voice—high or low; the *rate*—how fast one speaks; and *inflection* and *volume*—how certain words are stressed or spoken loudly or softly. For example, loud talk could indicate anger, talking softly could mean that the person is nervous or unsure of what he or she is saying, and a high pitch could indicate stress. Speaking fast often indicates anxiety. Also, the quality of a voice, either pleasant or unpleasant, may influence how you listen. If the voice is irritating and whiny, you may not listen with the attentiveness that you would to someone whose voice sounds pleasant or appealing to you. *Pronunciation, articulation,* and *intonation* also play a role in communication, for example: the word "Ooooh" said with pleasant surprise versus "Oh" said with little interest, or the words "Thanks a lot" spoken with sincere gratitude versus "Thanks a lot" spoken sarcastically when told something that is not pleasing to the person.

Body language is nonverbal communication. This is a powerful way of expressing feelings and thoughts. It can involve a variety of facial expressions; eye contact or lack of it; movement and position of hands, shoulders, legs, or torso; and posture. Sometimes learning to interpret what people *don't* say can tell you more than what they *do* say. For example, during a conversation, two people may lean toward each other, demonstrating interest in communicating, and they may have eye contact; or they may lean away from each other when they are not interested or not comfortable being near each other or not wanting to be with each other. Eye contact may or may not be present, but if it is, it will send a different message than eye contact between two people who want to be together. These movements and body positions send out a clear message. Facial expressions and body positions are used to express emotions. Both give **nonverbal feedback** similar to words giving **verbal feedback.** Sometimes nonverbal communication sends a much stronger and even harsher message than verbal communication. Culture also has a greater influence on a person's body language and how others interpret your body language. For example, in some cultures eye-to-eye contact is considered challenging and even hostile; in other cultures it is expected because it conveys friendliness, and if eye contact doesn't occur, some may feel that the person is trying to hide something or is very shy. In some cultures when people speak with each other, they are positioned very close to each other; others need distance between people and will even back up if one comes too close into the other's comfort zone. People react to body language without realizing it or knowing why they do so. Nonverbal communication is an elaborate unwritten code understood by all, yet it may be interpreted differently. Consider how a tendency to make assumptions about another person's behavior can lead to communication problems. Body language can be a building block for more verbal forms of communication. To increase the effectiveness of health care and to communicate more meaningfully with patients, some understanding and appreciation of their culture(s) are needed.

The **quality of the communication** exchange that takes place in health care settings is extremely important for the delivery of good health care. Taking the time to establish good rapport, positive interactions, and good communication skills with patients promotes the well-being of the patient and often leads to greater acceptance and cooperation with examination and treatment regimens. Giving and explaining care to patients, collecting pertinent information from patients, and working well with other members of the health care team depend on the ability of people to communicate.

Because most written medical information and instruction pamphlets are written at the tenth-grade reading level, they cannot be relied on as an effective means of communication for everyone. Some patients may have difficulty reading and understanding printed materials. Others may have difficulty reading but may not readily admit it or may even hide this fact from others. If you have any doubt that patients will understand handwritten or printed materials, focus on whether the patients *understand* the information and necessary skills needed to improve their health. The material (information) given should always be reviewed by asking patients to repeat or demonstrate what they have learned after the information has been provided. Summarize the most important points toward the end of the conversation.

Encourage patients to have open and honest communication and to ask questions about their concerns. This enables health care providers to convey the information and guidance that patients need to improve their overall health and develop healthier lifestyles by making informed decisions. *Remember, good communication is vital. The art of positive and effective communication requires skill and motivation.*

CULTURAL CONSIDERATIONS IN HEALTH ASSESSMENT AND HEALTH CARE

As the population in America becomes more diverse, there is an even greater need to appreciate and understand cultural influences on health behavior and health care. **Culture** is a set of learned values, beliefs, and customs shared by a group that gives standards for behavior and meaning and some predictability to their daily lives. Cultural beliefs, traits, and personal characteristics determine health behaviors, and these can vary and change over time. More than half of all present health problems result from the individual's behavior and lifestyle. Cultural beliefs also determine when people will seek medical care and also from whom and where they will seek it.

Major goals of health care are to care for others and to promote wellness and health while respecting value systems and lifestyles of the people served. To meet these goals, culture-based health attitudes and behaviors must be understood. In addition, a wide diversity of beliefs, behaviors, and ideas about health and illness must be accepted, including many that differ from those held by the health care providers. Knowledge of cultural factors provides a basis for understanding health and illness behaviors, practices, and beliefs. This knowledge also helps physicians when deciding on and providing methods of treatment to meet the needs of the **individual** patient. For some, cultural influences play an important role in developing their habits and beliefs and in accepting standard medical care; for others, **cultural influences** only play a moderate or minor role in their attitudes about health care and compliance with the suggested or prescribed form(s) of treatment. Assumptions should *never* be made about cultural beliefs and behaviors without first receiving confirmation from the patient or the patient's family. Remember that not all members of a cultural group are going to believe and behave in exactly the same way. Do not stereotype people and do not judge other cultures by your own. Someone once said, "One of the problems of being blind is not the blindness but what people think of the blind."

Some of the **first** things that must be done to develop cultural awareness and cultural sensitivity are to recognize that culture diversity *does* exist, to identify and recognize your own cultural values and beliefs and recognize how they influence your attitudes and behaviors, and to respect the uniqueness of people who may or may not be different from yourself.

Major **variables in cultural assessment** of a patient include the person's **values, beliefs,** and **customs.** Values are learned through socialization starting in early childhood and continue to be shaped and reshaped throughout life. Values represent what is important to a person and provide guidance for what is desirable or not desirable. Values form the basis for attitudes, beliefs, and behavior. Beliefs include knowledge, thoughts, ideas, opinions, acceptance, and faith about various aspects of the world. Of special concern in health care is the patient's beliefs about wellness, illness, cause of the illness, type of treatment that is acceptable or unacceptable, expected outcomes, and fears of the illness or condition and treatment. Customs or behaviors that are important to one's health and to health care include dietary practices, communication patterns (verbal and nonverbal behaviors or communications), family relationships, religious beliefs and practices (these may include specific dietary regulations or restrictions, or restrictions on the acceptance of some forms of treatment; for example, some people refuse to have blood transfusions or use medications that contain caffeine or pork products), and health and illness behaviors (these include patient's attitudes toward health and response to illness and symptoms, for example, how much or how little pain that people will tolerate before seeking help or expressing their feelings). Pain is one of the most common complaints in medicine, yet tolerance and reflecting the intensity of pain are often influenced by culture. Some cultures feel that it is unworthy of their maturity to complain and that they must accept pain silently; others find release in complaining profoundly about the smallest to the greatest pain.

It is important to identify major values, beliefs, and customs related to individual health concerns. A person's culture and the influence it has, if any, on the person are not determined by his or her appearance or surname. As we are a more diverse population, it is becoming increasingly important for all patients to have a cultural assessment. More health professionals and specialists in the fields of cultural diversities, sensitivities, and competencies encourage and recommend more culturally sensitive caregiving. They recommend that each patient have a **cultural assessment,** which should include at the very least the following:

1. Place of birth. If the person emigrated to this country, how long has he or she lived here?
2. Ethnic group. How strong is the person's identity with this group? Does he or she live in an ethnic community?
3. Major support systems. Does the person have family, friends, work, school, groups, church, and so on?
4. Religion. How important is religion to the person, what is his or her religion, and how does it, or does it, affect daily living practices?

5. Language(s) spoken. If more than one, which is the primary and which is the secondary language? What are the person's speaking, comprehension, and reading abilities in each language?
6. Description of the person's nonverbal communication style.
7. Food preferences and prohibitions, if any.
8. Economic situation. Is it adequate to meet the person's (and family's, if any) needs?
9. Description of the person's health and illness practices and beliefs.
10. Description of the person's beliefs and customs concerning birth, illness, death, diet and food practices, and medical care.

The subject of cultural diversity and culturally competent and sensitive care encompasses much more than can be presented in this chapter. All medical assistants and health care providers should research, read, and gain a better understanding of these subjects. Some excellent books are available that provide detailed descriptions of the characteristics of different cultural groups, and these can help to guide and shape care that is given. However, these descriptions are generalized and are to be used *only* as guidelines. See the box below regarding guidelines for relating to patients from different cultures.

Often medical assistants are the first contact that patients have with the medical system. Therefore they should acquire and demonstrate an understanding of diverse cultures to reduce the barriers patients come across when accessing medical care.

HEALTH MATTERS

GUIDELINES FOR RELATING TO PATIENTS FROM DIFFERENT CULTURES

1. Assess your personal beliefs surrounding persons from different cultures.
   - Review your personal beliefs and past experiences
   - Set aside any values, biases, ideas, and attitudes that are judgmental and may negatively affect care
2. Assess communication variables from a cultural perspective.
   - Determine the ethnic identity of patient, including generation in America
   - Use the patient as a source of information when possible
   - Assess cultural factors that may affect your relationship with the patient and respond appropriately
3. Plan care based on the communicated needs and cultural background.
   - Learn as much as possible about the patient's cultural customs and beliefs
   - Encourage the patient to reveal cultural interpretation of health, illness, and health care
   - Be sensitive to the uniqueness of each patient

- Identify sources of discrepancy between the patient's and your own conceptions of health and illness
- Communicate at the patient's personal level of functioning
- Evaluate effectiveness of actions and modify the care plan when necessary
4. Modify communication approaches to meet cultural needs.
   - Be attentive to signs of fear, anxiety, and confusion in the patient
   - Respond in a reassuring manner in keeping with the patient's cultural orientation
   - Be aware that in some cultural groups, discussion with others concerning the patient may offend and impede the care process
5. Understand that respect for the patient and communicated needs is central to the therapeutic relationship.
   - Communicate respect by using a kind and attentive approach
   - Learn how listening is communicated in the patient's culture
   - Use appropriate active listening techniques
   - Adopt an attitude of flexibility, respect, and interest to help bridge barriers imposed by culture

HEALTH **MATTERS—cont'd**

6. Communicate in a nonthreatening manner.
   - Conduct the interview in an unhurried manner
   - Follow acceptable social and cultural amenities
   - Ask general questions during the information-gathering stage
   - Be patient with a respondent who gives information that may seem unrelated to the patient's health problem
   - Develop a trusting relationship by listening carefully, allowing time, and giving the patient your full attention
7. Use validating techniques in communication.
   - Be alert for feedback that the patient is not understanding
   - Do not assume meaning is interpreted without distortion
8. Be considerate of reluctance to talk when the subject involves sexual matters.
   - Be aware that in some cultures, sexual matters are not discussed freely with members of the opposite sex
9. Adopt special approaches when the patient speaks a different language.
   - Use a caring tone of voice and facial expression to help alleviate the patient's fears
   - Speak slowly and distinctly, but not loudly
   - Use gestures, pictures, and play acting to help the patient understand
   - Repeat the message in different ways if necessary

- Be alert to words the patient seems to understand and use them frequently
- Keep messages simple and repeat them frequently
- Avoid using medical terms and abbreviations that the patient may not understand
- Use an appropriate language dictionary

10. Use interpreters to improve communication.
    - Ask the interpreter to translate the message, not just the individual words
    - Obtain feedback to confirm understanding
    - Use an interpreter who is culturally sensitive

RECOMMENDED RESOURCES

Books

Geissler E: *Pocket guide to cultural assessment,* St Louis, 1994, Mosby.

Giger J, Davidhizar R: *Transcultural nursing: assessment and intervention,* St Louis, 1991, Mosby.

Leininger M: *Transcultural nursing: concepts, theories, research, and practices,* Columbus, Ohio, 1995, McGraw Hill and Greydon Press.

Minarik PA: *Culture and nursing care: a pocket guide,* San Francisco, 1996, UCSF Nursing Press.

Spector R: *Cultural diversity in health and illness,* East Norwalk, Conn, 1991, Appleton & Lange.

To narrow the gap and reduce barriers between medical care and health care needs of patients, it is important to learn who the patients are—their cultural identity—and how their beliefs about health and illness affect them differently.

Cultural barriers can be overcome with the right combination of good communication and listening skills, creativity, and concern. Learning key points of the cultures of the patients cared for will enhance interactions with patients who maintain a strong identity with their ethnic and cultural heritage. Culturally sensitive health care *will* take into account that patient's values, customs, and beliefs. *Respect the privacy, dignity, and culture of the patient and use skills with these values while always observing the principles of informed consent and confidentiality.*

PATIENT EDUCATION AND PATIENT TEACHING

As a medical assistant, patient teaching will be an important part of your work. Therefore you must have some knowledge of adult patient education principles and strategies. A basic understanding of the adult learner is required for patient teaching. By applying specific knowledge of the teaching and learning process, you will be a more effective educator. Your teaching skills will directly influence the patient's learning. By understanding some basic teaching strategies, you can make the most of whatever time you have to teach patients.

Guidelines for patient teaching can be organized in five groups, described by the acronym TEACH:

T—Tune in to the patient
E—Edit information given to the patient
A—Act on every moment that you have to teach the patient
C—Clarify often
H—Honor the patient as a partner in the teaching process

Tune In

First, listen to the patient. Begin your teaching by finding out what the patient's immediate needs and thoughts are because these must be addressed first. Once the patient's immediate needs and thoughts are attended to, the patient will most often (likely) give his or her full attention to what you are explaining or teaching and will absorb what you feel is important.

Ask questions that permit patients to express themselves when they answer. Avoid questions that would elicit just a "yes" or "no" answer. For example, ask, "Please describe to me what type of pain you are having and show me where you feel it," and not "Are you having sharp pain in the lower leg and knee?" This approach makes patients focus, think about the question, and answer in their own words.

Second, let the information that you teach be directed by the patient's need(s). Most adults like to feel independent and self-directed; however, illness can temporarily interfere with their independence. By involving patients in the teaching process and in identifying goals to work toward, most patients will more likely want to work on and reach those goals because they were also self-directed. Connect the patient's concerns with what must be known for self-care. For example, if the patient wants to get out and around more with minimal difficulties after a knee injury, he or she must be taught and must participate in learning how to use crutches to meet this goal successfully.

Some patients are hesitant to ask questions. Self-direction can still be promoted by offering patients a few topics for discussion and asking them to pick the topics that they feel are most important to them at the time. Even with limited time, you can say, "You will need to know how to use crutches to go up and down stairs at home, which would you like to try first?"

Edit Information

Focus on the most crucial information. Separate it from the "nice to know" information. Remember, the more details you give, the more the patient will forget. For example, the patient must understand the importance of taking high blood pressure medication everyday, even if he or she feels fine, and does not have to understand what the numbers in the blood pressure readings mean, at least right away. More detailed information can be provided at a later time. The patient can recall and retain the most important information when it is given clearly and at the beginning of your teaching period. Divide information into manageable bits, rather than giving an overload. This approach promotes retention of the information or directions.

If the patient understands why it is important to take small steps when using crutches, it is not so imperative that the medical definition of a torn ligament is understood right away. Many patients remember facts that were taught in the first third of the teaching session. Elicit feedback from the patient to see if the most important information can be applied. For example, ask the patient to demonstrate how to climb stairs with crutches, or have the patient demonstrate how to climb stairs with crutches before you explain what a torn ligament is (assuming that the patient wanted to know more about the medical condition).

Be *clear* and *specific* in what you say, making sure that your description is understandable. You can ask the patient to explain the instructions that you just gave to him or her. When giving written instructions, review them with the patient. Make sure that the instructions are clear and to the point, leaving no room for misunderstandings. If you tell the patient to call for an appointment in 2 weeks, do you mean to call in 2 weeks or to make the appointment for 2 weeks from now?

Patient recall and retention can also be improved by grouping related directions, for example, "I will explain and demonstrate how to walk with crutches, then you can practice; then I will explain and demonstrate how to sit down in a chair using crutches, then you can practice; then I will explain and demonstrate how to stand up from a sitting position using crutches, and then you can practice. We will go over each movement and then put them all together."

Act on Teachable Times

Teach at every opportunity. Timing is everything. Adult learners learn better when they need the information or skill to deal with a real-life situation. Illness brings varied changes—pain, anxiety, fatigue, disability, interference with everyday activities, concern for other family members that may be affected by the patient's illness—all of which can be barriers to learning. Illness also brings another change—a need for new information. For example, the patient needs to know how to be more aware of what triggers pain. Teach the patient how to record the time, the type of pain experienced, what he or she was doing at the time the pain started, what relieved the pain, if anything, and how long did relief last. The patient may be ready for new information but may not know what kind is needed. For example, if the patient will be using crutches to walk, he or she may not think of asking how to sit down or get up from a sitting position using the crutches. You can help by giving the information needed for daily activities. Obviously certain times are not suited for patient teaching, for example, if the patient is in a lot of pain, he or she will likely not give his or her full attention to learning how to walk with crutches. After the physician treats the patient's pain and when the pain has been relieved, effective teaching is more likely to occur.

An environment that promotes respect, helpfulness, honesty, and trust is required for effective patient teaching and learning. You must make a conscious effort to create such an environment. Begin by showing that you are interested in the patient as a person. Learning something about the patient's everyday activities can help guide you in determining what type of information is needed, for example, "You can go to work, but could someone drive you to work while you have the leg cast?"

Provide positive feedback whenever possible. Positive feedback acknowledges healthy changes and behaviors and reinforces learning.

Clarify Often

People have different learning styles. Some like to read the information or directions and then ask questions. Others like to have things explained to them, then read the directions, and then ask questions, if they have any. Some patients do not read well, so they do need to have the information explained to them verbally. Ask the patient if he or she prefers to discuss the directions, watch a videotape, read a booklet, or maybe do all three and then ask any questions needed to clarify the information. ***Patient education should be provided verbally and supplemented with educationally appropriate, culturally sensitive written materials.*** Have written materials in different languages when attending to people who read best in a language other than English. When possible, use visual aids to enhance the learning process. Make sure that printed materials have print large enough for patients to read. Some elderly patients may have decreased visual capabilities and may need large print on all materials. You could also suggest that they could use a magnifying glass when reading with or without their regular eyeglasses.

Once again, ask questions that allow patients to express what they have learned or what they need to learn. One way to do this is to present a brief scenario of a situation and ask patients how they would handle things or what they would do. Keep in mind that each patient's concerns are not necessarily every patient's concerns. **All patients must be treated and taught as individuals.** Do not generalize and do not assume anything. Clarify and verify often and seek frequent feedback. This allows patients to explain to you how they would use the information that they have learned. Sometimes you may have to review information and instructions more than once. Remember that the purpose of teaching patients is for them to understand and follow instructions and feel confident with and contribute to the care provided. Be patient with patients. Sometimes patients hesitate to ask questions for fear of being considered stupid, or they might hide their inability to understand the answer if it is given in incomprehensible medical jargon.

If the patient cannot seem to grasp the information and the information is crucial to his or her self-care, you may need to seek the help of the family or friends (with the patient's approval) or seek other referrals that may be helpful, such as the assistance of a medical interpreter for patients who do not understand English well enough to understand and follow the required directions. Always provide information on local *community services, resources,* and *support groups* that are relevant to the patient's needs and concerns.

Honor the Patient as a Partner

The physician cannot properly diagnose a patient's condition if the patient is not honest in describing the symptoms and the medical history. The patient is the expert on what he or she feels and knows. The effectiveness of care and patient teaching depends on attaining understanding and cooperation from the patient. Determine at the time whether the patient is physically, emotionally, and even financially capable of following a prescribed program of treatment. It does little or no good to tell a patient to walk for at least 30 minutes everyday if the patient has severe bunions on both feet that become very painful after walking just 5 to 10 minutes. If a medication is to be taken three times a day after meals, it is important to establish that the patient does eat three regularly spaced meals a day.

Sometimes knowing the patient's background, line of work, and interests can help you to focus on issues that need to be taught. Teaching someone about diet and exercise will be done differently for a person who eats in restaurants everyday than for a person who loves to cook and is physically unable to do a lot of exercise because of an injury or other disability. **Patients are**

the center of the educational process, and ultimately they will make the decision to follow or not to follow the recommended treatment program and teachings. You can provide the best patient education and use various approaches at different times, but the patient will not benefit if he or she is not receptive to learning and following health-promoting ways of doing things. For example, you may teach a patient who is overweight and who has high blood pressure the importance of modifying a high-fat diet and the need for exercise to lose weight; however, this does little good if the patient's attitude is, "Heart disease runs in my family, so I know I'm going to die that way and might as well enjoy what I like when I want it." Even so, you must always strive to motivate patients toward better health, but ultimately the patient has to share responsibility for the process and outcome. *Most* patients who have a better understanding of their medical condition are able to make more informed decisions to improve and maintain their health status. Patients need understandable and culturally relevant information as they try to make choices directed toward positive and sometimes life-changing behaviors for improved health.

It is essential that you share what you know. Communicate knowledge and information by providing quality patient teaching and engaging the patient in the learning process. The teaching-learning process is a joint process that works toward common goals. Remember, "even if you can't change someone's mind, you can introduce new ideas," and maybe, these new ideas will lead to positive health changes, eventually.

Provide information on local community services, resources, and support groups related to the patient's needs and concerns. Examples include the American Heart Association, the American Cancer Society, breast cancer support groups, Arthritis Association and support groups, Diabetic Association and support groups, groups for alcoholics or family members of alcoholics and/or any substance abuse, shelters for victims of abuse and violence, Health Resource Centers on Domestic Violence, Women's Health Resource Centers, food banks, and many others. Also see the box

---

HEALTH MATTERS

KEEPING YOUR PATIENTS INFORMED

HEALTH CARE RESOURCES

The following health care organizations and agencies provide information and material that may help to enhance your patient education goals. Many of these organizations have local and regional agencies that provide community services, and some offer workshops on special topics and patient concerns.

Health on the Net*

Where to search on-line:

- **www.healthfinder.gov**—Government-sponsored gateway to on-line health information. Easy to use and search.
- **igm.nlm.nih.gov**—A project of the National Institutes of Health and the National Library of Medicine. Allows users to search Medline, with its 9 million biomedical journal citations, as well as other health care resources.
- **www.kidshealth.org**—From the Nemours Foundation and its related hospitals, clinics, and centers. Good resource that provides information tailored to young children, teens, and parents.
- **www.ama-assn.org**—The official site of the American Medical Association and its journals. Includes helpful information for consumers.
- **www.hon.ch**—Another good gateway onto Internet health sites, sponsored by the Health on the Net Foundation in Switzerland. It is dedicated to improving medical information on the Internet.

*Source: *St. Petersburg Times.*

HEALTH **M A T T E R S — c o n t ' d**

HOTLINES AND RESOURCES

Aging

National Institute on Aging

1-800-222-2225 (8:30-5 ET)

AIDS

National CDC HIV/AIDS Hotline

1-800-342-2437 (9-5 ET)

General information about HIV/AIDS, referrals

Allergy

American Academy of Allergy and Immunology

1-800-822-2762 (8:30-5 ET)

National Institute of Allergy and Infectious Diseases

301-496-5717 (8:30-5 ET)

Alternative Medicine

Global Navigator's Alternative Medicine Sites

http://www.gnn.com/wic/wics/med.alt.html

The University of Pittsburgh's Alternative Medicine Home Page

http://www.pitt.edu/-cbw/altm.html

Alzheimer's Disease

Alzheimer's Association

1-800-272-3900 (8-5 CT)

Arthritis

Arthritis Foundation

1-800-283-7800 (24-hour recording)

National Institute of Arthritis and Musculoskeletal and Skin Diseases

301-495-4484 (8:30-5 ET)

Breast Cancer

Breast Cancer Information Clearinghouse

http://www.nysernet.org/bcic/

Y-Me National Organization for Breast Cancer Information Support

1-800-221-2141 (9-5 CT)

Presurgery counseling treatment information, peer support, patient literature, and referrals

Cancer

American Cancer Society

http://www.cancer.org/

1-800-ACS-2345 (24-hour recording)

Cancer Information Service of the National Cancer Institute

1-800-4-CANCER

CancerFax (National Cancer Institute)

1-800-624-2511 (24 hours)

Faxes current patient and professional information about causes, diagnoses, and treatment for all forms of cancer

OncoLink

http://www.oncolink.upenn.edu/

Information on most types of cancer provided by the University of Pennsylvania has many links to other useful sites

Child Abuse

National Council on Child Abuse and Family Violence

1-800-222-2000

Chronic Fatigue Syndrome

CFIDS Assoiation

1-800-442-3437 (24-hour recording)

Cosmetic/Reconstructive Surgery

American Society of Plastic and Reconstructive Surgeons

1-800-635-0635 (8:30-4:30 CT)

Dentistry

American Dental Association

http://www.ada.org/index.html

National Institute of Dental Research

301-496-4261 (8:30-5 ET)

Diabetes

American Diabetes Association

1-800-342-2383 (9-5 ET)

National Institute of Diabetes and Digestive and Kidney Diseases

301-496-3583 (8:30-5 ET)

Disease Prevention

Centers for Disease Control and Prevention

http://www.cdc.gov/

404-332-4555 (8-4:30 ET; 24-hour recording)

Information on infections, epidemics, and immunization

Drug/Alcohol Abuse

National Clearinghouse for Alcohol and Drug Information

1-800-729-6686 (8-7 ET)

Information on alcohol, drugs, and tobacco provided by the Center for Substance Abuse Prevention (CSAP), National Institute on Drug Abuse, and National Institute on Alcohol Abuse and Alcoholism

Eating Disorders

Eating Disorders Awareness and Prevention (EDAP)

206-382-3587 (8-5 PT)

National Center for Overcoming Overeating

212-875-0442

Information about binge eating disorder (24-hour recording)

Endometriosis

Endometriosis Association

1-800-992-3636 (24-hour recording)

Continued

HEALTH **MATTERS—cont'd**

Environment and Health

Environment Health Clearinghouse

1-800-643-4794 (9-8 ET)

Scientists from the National Institute of Environmental Health Sciences answer questions related to environment and illness.

Eye Disease

National Eye Institute

301-496-5248 (8:30-5 ET)

American Academy of Ophthalmology's Eyenet

http://www.eyenet.org/

Graphics depicting eye anatomy; information on conditions and treatments

Fibromyalgia

Fibromyalgia Alliance of America

614-457-4222 (10-6 ET; 24-hour recording)

Hearing

National Institute on Deafness and Other Communication Disorders

1-800-241-1044 (voice 8:30-5 ET)

1-800-241-1055 (TDD/TTY/TT)

Heart Disease

American Heart Association

1-800-AHA-USA1 (8:30-4:30 local time)

National Heart, Lung, and Blood Institute

301-251-1222 (8:30-5 ET)

Incontinence

The Simon Foundation for Continence

1-800-237-4666 (24 hours)

Quarterly newsletter and other publications

Infertility

RESOLVE

617-623-0744 (9-4 ET)

Lung Disease

American Lung Association

1-800-LUNG-USA (8-4:30 ET)

Information on respiratory disease

Lyme Disease

Lyme Disease Foundation

1-800-866-LYME (24-hour recording)

Medication

Center for Drug Evaluation and Research

301-594-1012 (8-4:30 ET)

The Food and Drug Administration hotline for information about medicines

Menopause

North American Menopause Society

http://menopause.com

Midlife Women's Network

1-800-886-4354 (8-5 CT)

Mental Health

Depression Awareness

1-800-421-4211 (24-hour recording)

The National Institute of Mental Health's hotline for information about symptoms and treatment of depression

Grief Recovery Helpline

1-800-445-4808 (9-5 PT)

Information on recovering from loss

National Institute of Mental Health

301-443-4513 (8:30-4:30)

Panic Disorder Information Line

1-800-64-PANIC (24-hour recording)

Internet Mental Health Home Page

http://www.mentalhealth.com/p.html

Nutrition and Dietary Health

National Dietetic Association Nutrition Hotline

1-800-366-1655

Information from and referrals to registered dieticians (experts 9-4 CT; recorded messages 8-8 CT)

Osteoporosis

National Osteoporosis Foundation

202-223-2226 (8:30-5:30 ET)

Parenting

National Institute of Child Health and Human Development

301-498-5133 (8-5 ET)

PMS

OMS Access

1-800-222-4767 for information

1-800-558-7046 for referrals to physicians in your area (9-5 CT)

Rare Diseases

National Organization of Rare Diseases

1-800-999-6673 (9-5 ET; 24-hour recording)

Stroke

American Heart Association Stroke Connection

1-800-553-6321 (8:30-5 CT)

Information, referrals, videotapes, and a newsletter

HEALTH MATTERS

KEEPING YOUR PATIENTS INFORMED

TEACHING PATIENTS HOW TO KEEP RECORDS OF SYMPTOMS AND TREATMENT

Recording information on their own symptoms and care can be an effective method in helping patients discover what causes and what relieves a problem, such as chronic headaches, or in aiding patients who must perform special care for themselves everyday, such as diabetics who may have to record blood sugar values and give themselves insulin one or more times a day.

Patients can use preprinted forms or create their own journals to record their information. Recording information on themselves makes patients become more active participants in their care. It also helps the physician and other health care providers understand patients' conditions better.

For patients' own recordings to be of value to them and their physician, they must understand and be taught how to do it correctly. Make sure patients understand the following:

- What should be recorded/documented. For example, a patient who has frequent headaches should record the date and time the headache started, how intense it was, where the pain was located (that is, what side of the head; in the front, top or back of the head; any pain in the eye area), what possibly triggered the headache (for example, bright lights, intense reading, working on the computer), how long the headache lasted, any accompanying signs and symptoms, what was done to help relieve the headache, and how effective were these methods.

- Why this information is important
- How to record the information. If a preprinted form is to be used, review each part of the form with the patient. If a graph or chart is to be used, show the patient how to fill it in with the required information.

Show patients an example of self-recordings. Emphasize how keeping these recordings can help them understand and learn more about their condition and possibly control it better and how they can provide important information for the physician when decisions are made about their care. All this may encourage interest in keeping updated records. Give patients a name and phone number of a contact person to call if they have any questions about their recording(s).

A good self-recording may look like the following:

Headache Diary

2-24-01 3 PM—Mild headache starting. Did deep breathing exercise with no relief. Massaged pressure points on head.

4 PM—Headache worse. Sharp penetrating pain on the right side of the head in the back on top and also in the right eye area.

4:10 PM—Took two Tylenol tablets. This gave some relief. Mild headache continued until bedtime. Possible trigger: working on the computer and reading in a poorly lighted area.

Once you teach patients good recording skills, you may soon be able to show them how this information helped in controlling symptoms and improve their health.

---

on pp. 114 to 117 for many other resources and hotlines that provide valuable and useful information.

HISTORY AND PHYSICAL EXAMINATION

The history and general physical examination are extremely valuable diagnostic tools used by a physician to gather information about the physiologic and sometimes psychologic condition of a patient. Many people now recognize the value of a regular physical examination in preventing disease or treating disease in the early stages. Most medical authorities recommend that everyone have at least one a year.

Information gathered from a history and general or special physical examination can be used by the physician to determine the following:

- The individual's level of health
- The body's level of physiologic functioning
- A tentative diagnosis of a condition or disease
- A confirmed diagnosis of a condition or disease
- The need for additional special examinations or testing
- The type of treatment to be prescribed

- An evaluation of the effectiveness of the prescribed treatment
- Preventive measures to be used

Preventive techniques include **educating patients** about healthful living habits, administering vaccinations to prevent communicable diseases, using screening procedures such as blood pressure checks and Pap smears, and treating conditions in the early stages to avoid more serious diseases.

The order followed by physicians when taking a history and performing a physical examination may vary somewhat, but the end result is the same because the same basic areas are covered. One of two types of forms may be used to record the information obtained: a preprinted outline form (Figure 4-1) or a blank sheet of standard-size paper on which the physician writes out all the information gathered. The preprinted form serves as a reminder so that essential factors will not be overlooked, and it minimizes writing to a narrative record of abnormal findings.

History

The history is a record of the information provided by the patient or family or from the patient's health record. It is the systematic account of past medical and psychosocial occurrences

Text continued on p. 126

FIGURE 4-1 **A,** Preprinted forms used for patient history and physical examination (page 1). (Courtesy Histacount, Thorofare, NJ.)

COMPLETE HISTORY AND PHYSICAL

Name **Age:** **Date: / /**

BP, P, RR, T, WT: Page 1

CHIEF COMPLAINT AND PRESENT ILLNESS:

PAST HISTORY: ANY SERIOUS ILLNESS AS A CHILD? (Answer YES or NO)

______ Mumps
______ Measles
______ Diphtheria
______ Whooping Cough
______ Scarlet or Rheumatic Fever
______ Nephritis
______ Kidney Disease
______ Pneumonia
______ Heart Murmur
______ Mononucleosis
______ Other

ANY OPERATIONS? **DATE** **PLACE**

1.
2.
3.
4.
5.
6.

ANY TRANSFUSIONS? No Yes When

ANY HOSPITALIZATIONS? **DATE** **PLACE**

A

1.
2.
3.
4.
5.
6.
7.

ANY SERIOUS ILLNESS AS AN ADULT? **DATE** **PLACE**

1.
2.
3.
4.
5.

ANY INFECTIOUS DISEASE? **DATE** **PLACE**

1.
2.
3.
4.

ANY SERIOUS ACCIDENTS? **DATE** **PLACE**

1.
2.

ANY STRESS? (WORK, FAMILY, ETC.)

ANY EMOTIONAL OR MENTAL ILLNESS? **DATE** **PLACE**

1.
2.

(0595) H57 HISTACOUNT CORPORATION • 301 GROVE ROAD • THOROFARE, NJ 08086 • 800-645-5220 FORM NO. 3255

FIGURE 4-1—cont'd **A,** Preprinted forms used for patient history and physical examination (page 2).

COMPLETE
HISTORY AND PHYSICAL

Date: / /

Name: _____ Page 2

MEDICINE OR PILLS TAKEN? (List all, even vitamins and aspirin)

Name or Type	Year Begun	Year Stopped	Helped	No Help	Side Effects
			Check Effects		
1.					
2.					
3.					
4.					
5.					
6.					
7.					
8.					
9.					

IMMUNIZATIONS? Answer Yes or No in _____, and place date in (   ).

_____ DPT (Tetanus) (   )   _____ Mumps   (   )   _____ Pneumococcal Vac. (   )

_____ Polio   (   )   _____ Rubella   (   )   _____ Other   (   )

_____ Measles   (   )   _____ "Flu" Vaccine (   )

ANY ALLERGIES TO MEDICINES?   **WHAT EFFECTS?**

1.
2.
3.
4.

ANY ALLERGIES TO FOODS OR OTHER?   **WHAT EFFECTS?**

1.
2.
3.
4.

B

FAMILY HISTORY:

		HEALTH				CAUSE OF DEATH
		Good	Poor	Died	Age	
FATHER						
MOTHER						
BROTHERS 1.						
2.						
3.						
4.						
SISTERS 1.						
2.						
3.						
4.						

DO ANY BLOOD RELATIVES HAVE THE FOLLOWING?

Problem	Relation	Problem	Relation	Problem	Relation
MIGRAINE		EMPHYSEMA		THYROID DISEASE	
EPILEPSY		LUNG DISEASE		OVERWEIGHT	
STROKE		ASTHMA		INFECTIOUS DISEASE	
GLAUCOMA		STOMACH ULCERS		ALLERGIES	
HEARING LOSS		GALLSTONES		ANEMIA	
RHEUMATIC FEVER		KIDNEY DISEASE		GOUT	
HEART MURMUR		NEPHRITIS		BLEEDING TENDENCY	
HEART DISEASE		ARTHRITIS		MENTAL ILLNESS	
HIGH BLOOD PRESS.		DIABETES		OTHER:	
TUBERCULOSIS		CANCER			

Continued

FIGURE 4-1—cont'd **A,** Preprinted forms used for patient history and physical examination (page 3).

Name:	Date:	Page 3.

SOCIAL HISTORY:

OCCUPATION		Position Held	Nature or Description of Work	# Of Years
PREVIOUS	1.			
	2.			
	3.			
PRESENT				

ANY EXPOSURE TO TOXIC OR DANGEROUS MATERIALS?

	No	Yes	When	Name or Type	What Symptoms?	Other People Affected?
INSULATION						
FUMES						
METALS						
CHEMICALS						
PLASTICS						
SOLVENTS						
DYES						
ANIMALS						
OTHER:						

TRAVEL:

U.S.A.
1. (East) _____ When? _____
2. (West) _____ When? _____
3. (South) _____ When? _____
4. (Central) _____ When? _____

FOREIGN
1. _____ When? _____
2. _____ When? _____
3. _____ When? _____
4. _____ When? _____

PETS: CATS _____ DOGS _____ OTHER _____

SINGLE _____   **DIVORCED** _____ When? _____
MARRIED _____ When? _____   **WIDOWED** _____ When? _____

CHILDREN: Boys _____ Girls _____

HABITS	No	Yes	When Started	When Stopped	Amount
SMOKE					PACKS PER DAY _____
COFFEE					CUPS PER DAY _____
ALCOHOL					LIQUOR/DAY _____ BEER/DAY _____ WINE/DAY _____
OTHER DRUGS					

MEALS: REGULAR? YES _____ NO _____ MEALS PER DAY _____ SNACKS PER DAY _____

EMOTIONAL STRESS:
AT WORK _____
FAMILY _____
OTHER _____

EXERCISE:
NONE _____
IRREGULAR _____ TYPE? _____ # OF TIMES/WEEK _____
REGULAR _____ TYPE? _____ # OF TIMES/WEEK _____

SLEEP: REGULAR? YES _____ NO _____ HOURS PER NIGHT _____

Other relevant information that may have bearing on your life and health, in your own words:

FIGURE 4-1—cont'd   **A,** Preprinted forms used for patient history and physical examination (page 4).

MEDICAL ALERT _____

Name _____

REVIEW OF SYSTEMS

Pt. Initials:

PROBLEM	NO	YES	DATE BEGAN	Page 4
Convulsion, Seizure			/ /	
Frequent Headaches			/ /	
Dizzy, Balance Problem			/ /	
Fainting			/ /	
Wear Glasses, Contacts			/ /	
Vision Worse			/ /	
Eye Pain			/ /	
Frequent Earaches			/ /	
Decreased Hearing			/ /	
Sinus Pains			/ /	
Often Stuffy Nose, Sneezing			/ /	
Difficulty Swallowing/Sore			/ /	
High Blood Pressure			/ /	
Chest Pain at Rest			/ /	
Chest Pain Exercising			/ /	
Heart "Races"			/ /	
Heart "Skips Beats"			/ /	
Heart Murmur			/ /	
Short of Breath [At Night			/ /	
Short of Breath [At Rest			/ /	
Short of Breath [Exercising			/ /	
Swelling Feet, Ankles			/ /	
Frequent Cough			/ /	
Coughed Up Blood			/ /	
Bronchitis			/ /	
Pneumonia			/ /	
Pleurisy			/ /	
Asthma Or Wheezing			/ /	
Emphysema			/ /	
Abdominal Pain			/ /	
Frequent Nausea			/ /	
Vomiting Blood			/ /	
Bloody or Black Stools			/ /	
Frequent Diarrhea			/ /	
Frequent Constipation			/ /	
Hepatitis Or Jaundice			/ /	
Cirrhosis Of Liver			/ /	
Pancreatitis			/ /	
Pain On Urination			/ /	
Blood in Urine			/ /	

FIGURE 4-1—cont'd **B,** Patient questionnaire (page 5, side 1).

PATIENT QUESTIONNAIRE

PATIENT'S NAME _____ BIRTH DATE _____ SEX ____ S.M.W.D. ____

ADDRESS _____ TEL. NO. ____

INSURANCE _____ REFERRED BY _____ OCCUPATION _____

INSTRUCTIONS: PUT ☑ IN THOSE BOXES APPLICABLE TO YOU AND IN THE "YES" OR "NO" SPACE. IF LINES ARE PROVIDED WRITE IN YOUR ANSWER.

FAMILY HISTORY

	FATHER	MOTHER	BROTHER 1	2	3	4	SISTER 1	2	3	4	SPOUSE	CHILDREN 1	2	3	4	5	6
AGE (IF LIVING)																	
HEALTH (G) GOOD (B) BAD																	
CANCER																	
TUBERCULOSIS																	
DIABETES																	
HEART TROUBLE																	
HIGH BLOOD PRESSURE																	
STROKE																	
EPILEPSY																	
NERVOUS BREAKDOWN																	
ASTHMA, HIVES, HAY FEVER																	
BLOOD DISEASE																	
AGE (AT DEATH)																	
CAUSE OF DEATH																	

PERSONAL HISTORY

HAVE YOU EVER HAD...	NO	YES	HAVE YOU EVER HAD...	NO	YES	HAVE YOU EVER HAD...	NO	YES
☐ SCARLET FEVER ☐ SCARLATINA			☐ GONORRHEA ☐ SYPHILIS			ANY ☐ BROKEN ☐ CRACKED BONES		
DIPHTHERIA			ANEMIA			RECURRENT DISLOCATIONS		
SMALLPOX			JAUNDICE			☐ CONCUSSION ☐ HEAD INJURY		
PNEUMONIA			EPILEPSY			EVER BEEN KNOCKED UNCONSCIOUS		
PLEURISY			MIGRAINE HEADACHES			☐ FOOD ☐ CHEMICAL ☐ DRUG POISONING		
UNDULANT FEVER			TUBERCULOSIS			EXPLAIN		
☐ RHEUMATIC FEVER ☐ HEART DISEASE			DIABETES					
ST. VITUS DANCE			CANCER					
☐ ARTHRITIS ☐ RHEUMATISM			☐ HIGH ☐ LOW BLOOD PRESSURE			ANY OTHER DISEASE		
ANY ☐ BONE ☐ JOINT DISEASE			NERVOUS BREAKDOWN			EXPLAIN		
☐ NEURITIS ☐ NEURALGIA			☐ HAY FEVER ☐ ASTHMA					
☐ BURSITIS ☐ SCIATICA ☐ LUMBAGO			☐ HIVES ☐ ECZEMA					
☐ POLIO ☐ MENINGITIS			FREQUENT ☐ COLDS ☐ SORE THROAT			WEIGHT: NOW ____ ONE YR. AGO ____		
BRIGHT'S DISEASE			FREQUENT ☐ INFECTIONS ☐ BOILS			MAXIMUM ____ WHEN ____		

ALLERGIES

ARE YOU ALLERGIC TO...	NO	YES	ARE YOU ALLERGIC TO...	NO	YES	ARE YOU ALLERGIC TO...	NO	YES
☐ PENICILLIN ☐ SULFA DRUGS			ANY OTHER DRUGS			ANY FOODS		
☐ ASPIRIN ☐ CODEINE ☐ MORPHINE			EXPLAIN			EXPLAIN		
☐ MYCINS ☐ OTHER ANTIBIOTICS								
☐ TETANUS ☐ ANTITOXIN ☐ SERUMS			ADHESIVE TAPE			☐ NAIL POLISH ☐ OTHER COSMETICS		

SURGERY

HAVE YOU HAD REMOVED...	NO	YES	HAVE YOU HAD REMOVED...	NO	YES	HAVE YOU...	NO	YES
TONSILS			☐ OVARY ☐ OVARIES			HAD HERNIA REPAIRED		
APPENDIX			HEMORRHOIDS			HAD ANY OTHER OPERATIONS		
GALL BLADDER			EVER HAVE A TRANSFUSION			BEEN HOSPITALIZED FOR ANY ILLNESS		
UTERUS			☐ BLOOD ☐ PLASMA			EXPLAIN		

X-RAYS

EVER HAVE X-RAYS OF...	NO	YES	DATE	DISEASE PRESENT
CHEST				
☐ STOMACH ☐ COLON				
GALL BLADDER				
EXTREMITIES				
BACK				
OTHER				

B

FORM NO. 405

HISTACOUNT CORPORATION, 301 GROVE ROAD • THOROFARE, NJ 08086 • 800-342-5274 (0895)

FIGURE 4-1—cont'd   **B,** Patient questionnaire (page 5, side 2).

SYSTEMS

DO YOU NOW HAVE OR HAVE YOU EVER HAD . . .	NO	YES	DO YOU NOW HAVE OR HAVE YOU EVER HAD . . .	NO	YES
ANY ☐ EYE DISEASE ☐ EYE INJURY ☐ IMPAIRED SIGHT			KIDNEY ☐ DISEASE ☐ STONES		
ANY ☐ EAR DISEASE ☐ EAR INJURY ☐ IMPAIRED HEARING			BLADDER DISEASE		
ANY TROUBLE WITH ☐ NOSE ☐ SINUSES ☐ MOUTH ☐ THROAT			BLOOD IN URINE		
FAINTING SPELLS			☐ ALBUMIN ☐ SUGAR ☐ PUS ☐ ETC. IN URINE		
CONVULSIONS			DIFFICULTY IN URINATION		
PARALYSIS			NARROWED URINARY STREAM		
DIZZINESS			ABNORMAL THIRST		
HEADACHES: ☐ FREQUENT ☐ SEVERE			PROSTATE TROUBLE		
ENLARGED GLANDS			☐ STOMACH TROUBLE ☐ ULCER		
THYROID: ☐ OVERACTIVE ☐ UNDERACTIVE ☐ ENLARGED			INDIGESTION		
ENLARGED GOITER			☐ GAS ☐ BELCHING		
SKIN DISEASE			APPENDICITIS		
COUGH: ☐ FREQUENT ☐ CHRONIC			☐ LIVER DISEASE ☐ GALL BLADDER DISEASE		
☐ CHEST PAIN ☐ ANGINA PECTORIS			☐ COLITIS ☐ OTHER BOWEL DISEASE		
SPITTING UP BLOOD			☐ HEMORRHOIDS ☐ RECTAL BLEEDING		
NIGHT SWEATS			BLACK TARRY STOOLS		
SHORTNESS OF BREATH ☐ EXERTION ☐ AT NIGHT			☐ CONSTIPATION ☐ DIARRHEA		
☐ PALPITATION ☐ FLUTTERING HEART			☐ PARASITES ☐ WORMS		
SWELLING OF ☐ HANDS ☐ FEET ☐ ANKLES			☐ ANY CHANGE IN APPETITE ☐ EATING HABITS		
VARICOSE VEINS			☐ ANY CHANGE IN BOWEL ACTION ☐ STOOLS		
EXTREME ☐ TIREDNESS ☐ WEAKNESS			EXPLAIN		

IMMUNIZATION - EKG

HAVE YOU HAD . . .	NO	YES	HAVE YOU HAD . . .	NO	YES
SMALLPOX VACCINATION (WITHIN LAST 7 YEARS)			POLIO SHOTS (WITHIN LAST 2 YEARS)		
TETANUS SHOT (NOT ANTITOXIN)			AN ELECTROCARDIOGRAM WHEN		

HABITS

DO YOU . .	NO	YES	DO YOU USE . . .	NEVER	OCC.	FREQ.	DAILY
EXERCISE ADEQUATELY			LAXATIVES				
HOW?			VITAMINS				
AWAKEN RESTED			SEDATIVES				
SLEEP WELL			TRANQUILIZERS				
AVERAGE 8 HOURS SLEEP (PER NIGHT)			SLEEPING PILLS, ETC.				
HAVE REGULAR BOWEL MOVEMENTS			ASPIRINS, ETC.				
SEX - ENTIRELY SATISFACTORY			CORTISONE				
LIKE YOUR WORK (HOURS PER DAY) ☐ INDOORS ☐ OUTDOORS			ALCOHOLIC BEVERAGES				
WATCH TELEVISION (HOURS PER DAY)			COFFEE (CUPS PER DAY)				
READ (HOURS PER DAY)			TOBACCO: ☐ CIGARETTES (PKS PER DAY)				
HAVE A VACATION (WEEKS PER YEAR)			☐ CIGARS ☐ PIPE ☐ CHEWING TOBACCO				
HAVE YOU EVER BEEN TREATED FOR ALCOHOLISM			☐ SNUFF				
HAVE YOU EVER BEEN TREATED FOR DRUG ABUSE			APPETITE DEPRESSANTS				
RECREATION: DO YOU PARTICIPATE IN SPORTS OR HAVE			THYROID MEDICATION: ☐ NO ☐ YES, IN PAST ☐ NONE NOW NOW ON GR. DAILY				
HOBBIES WHICH GIVE YOU RELAXATION AT			HAVE YOU EVER TAKEN . . .				
LEAST 3 HOURS A WEEK.			☐ INSULIN ☐ TABLETS FOR DIABETES ☐ HORMONE SHOTS ☐ TABLETS ☐ NO				

WOMEN ONLY

MENSTRUAL HISTORY . . .	NO	YES		NO	YES
AGE AT ONSET			ARE YOU REGULAR: ☐ HEAVY ☐ MEDIUM ☐ LIGHT		
USUAL DURATION OF PERIOD DAYS			DO YOU HAVE ☐ TENSION ☐ DEPRESSION BEFORE PERIOD		
CYCLE (START TO START) DAYS			DO YOU HAVE ☐ CRAMPS ☐ PAIN WITH PERIOD		
DATE OF LAST PERIOD			DO YOU HAVE HOT FLASHES		
PREGNANCIES . . .	NO	YES		NO	YES
CHILDREN BORN ALIVE (HOW MANY)			STILL BORN (HOW MANY)		
CESAREAN SECTIONS (HOW MANY)			MISCARRIAGES (HOW MANY)		
PREMATURES (HOW MANY)			ANY COMPLICATIONS		

EMOTIONS

ARE YOU OFTEN . . .	NO	YES	ARE YOU OFTEN . . .	NO	YES
DEPRESSED			JUMPY		
ANXIOUS			JITTERY		
IRRITABLE			IS CONCENTRATION DIFFICULT?		

Continued

FIGURE 4-1—cont'd **B,** Patient physical examination (page 6, side 1).

PHYSICAL EXAM

NAME:

GENERAL: DATE:

		OK	R	L				OK	R	L
HEAD	Bruises				**NEURO**	Mot ⌐Grip			
	Al. Or. × 3					Mot ⌐Leg			
	Mem./Sp.					DTR			
	Facies					Bab, K, B			
EYES	Vision					Cran 2-12			
	Perrla/EOM					Sens.			
	Sclera/Con					Vib/Pos			
	Cornea					Romb/Gait			
	Fundi					RAM			
	Str./Nyst.					FTN/HTT			
	Ton./Other				**BACK**	B & K Crease			
EAR	Canal					Scol.			
	T.M.					Tender			
	Whisper					Spasm			
	Rinne	#1B #2A	WEB. ←→	#1B #2A		SLR/Las.			
						Flex/Ext			
						Rot/LatFlx			
NASAL	Septum				**LYMPH**	Neck			
	Mucosa					Suprclav.			
	Sinuses					Axil			
THROAT	Tongue					Groin			
	Phar/Uv.				**VASC.**	Carotid			
	Teeth					Radial			
	Lips					Fem.			
NECK	Veins					Pop.			
	Thyroid					DP/PT			
	Flex/Ext				**EXTREMITY**	Edema			
	Lat. Rot.					Homan			
LUNG	Tr. Dev/Frem					Varic.			
	Diaph/Perc.					Joints			
	Rales					ROM			
	Rhonchi					Tender			
	Wheezes					Heat/ ⌐Eff.			
COR	Rhyt/Skips					Arm			
	Murmur					Form.			
	Thrill					Meas Thigh			
	Gal/Rub					Calf			
	PMI					Other			
	TORSO –				**DERM.**	Temp/Sweat			
BREASTS	Mass ⌐Hard ■					Moles			
	└Soft ▨					Cyan/Club			
	Tender					Scars			
	Nipples					Other			
	Other				**PELVIC**	Labia			
ABD	Soft/BS					Disch.			
	Megaly					Cervix			
	Tender					Uterus			
	Rebound					Adnexa			
	Bruit					RECTAL –			
	Other					OTHER –			
GU	CVA Tend.								
	Penis								
	Testes								
	Hernia								

H 2 6   (0196)   HISTACOUNT CORPORATION FORM NO. 3256

FIGURE 4-1—cont'd   **B,** Patient physical examination (page 6, side 2). (Courtesy Histacount, Thorofare, NJ.)

CASE NO. _____ PATIENT'S NAME _____ DOB _____

ADDRESS _____ INSURANCE _____ DATE _____

TEL. NO. _____ REFERRED BY _____ OCCUPATION _____ AGE _____ SEX _____ S.M.W.D.

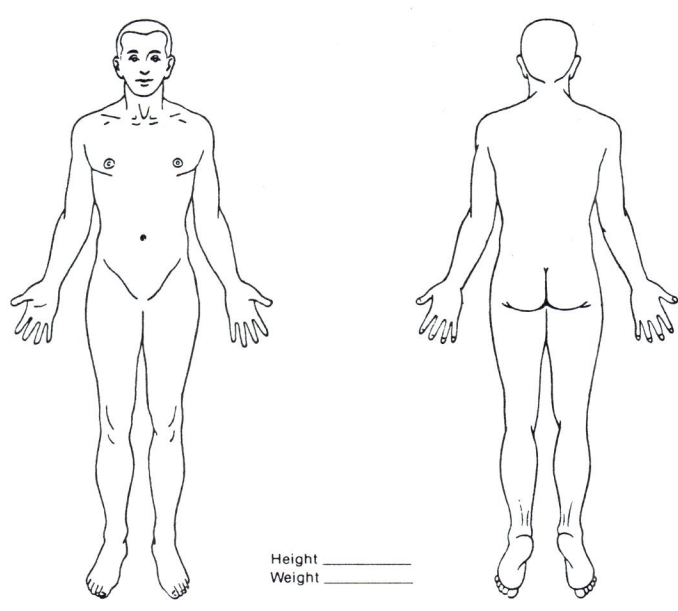

Height _____
Weight _____

Comments: _____

_____

_____

_____

_____

_____

_____

_____

_____

_____

_____

_____

_____

_____

_____

_____

_____

_____

_____

_____

_____

in a patient's life and other factors that may have an effect on the patient's health. It includes a series of questions and answers regarding the patient.

History taking reveals information about the patient's general health status and physical or emotional problem areas, including both current and potential problems that call for preventive care and advice. Focus is also on the patient's behaviors and feelings about the illness.

History is composed of the following (see also Figure 4-1 and Review of Vocabulary on p. 148):

1. **Chief complaint (CC).** The chief complaint is a brief statement made by the patient describing the nature of the illness and duration of symptoms that led the patient to consult the physician. Chief complaint is abbreviated CC.
2. **History of present illness (HPI or PI).** The history of present illness includes the present illness discussed in detail, the health status of the patient until the onset of the present illness, the onset of symptoms, the character and duration of each, and any other pertinent facts or relation to other events, such as shortness of breath after exertion.
3. **Past history (PH).** The past history is a summary of all prior illnesses, allergies, drug sensitivities, childhood diseases, surgical procedures, hospital admissions, and serious injuries and disabilities, including the date of each. For women, the number of pregnancies, live births, and abortions, if any, are also recorded. Past history is abbreviated PH.
4. **Family history (FH).** The family history is the health status and age of immediate relatives; if deceased, the date, age at death, and cause are noted. Diseases among relatives that are thought to have a hereditary or familial tendency or cases in which contact may play a role are also recorded. Examples would be cardiovascular, renal, endocrine, metabolic, mental, or infectious diseases, neoplasms or carcinoma, and allergies.
5. **Social and occupational history.** The social and occupational history (may also be called personal history and patient profile) includes information relating to where the patient has lived, occupation(s), and environment. This includes statements about the patient's lifestyle and habits, any of which may have a bearing on the development of disease, and the patient's general health status and perception of his or her health. These factors may include the following:
   - Use of tobacco, alcohol, drugs, coffee, or tea
   - Diet, sleep, exercise, hobbies, and interests
   - Marital history, children, home life; religious convictions; occupation and employment
   - Sexual orientation(s), problems, and attitudes
   - Causes, levels of, and ways of reacting to stress
   - Defense mechanisms
   - Resources for support and assistance
   - Cultural, educational, and environmental factors that may be related to health status. Cultural preferences or habits and any language barriers should be noted.
   - Violence or abuse, domestic or other. *The need for routine screening, treatment, and documentation of domestic violence is critical.*

6. **Review of systems (ROS).** Review of systems is the last category in the history. The purpose of this systematic review is to reveal subjective symptoms that either the patient forgot to discuss or at the time seemed relatively unimportant to the patient. An analysis of the subjective findings, as related by the patient when questioned by the physician, generally gives a clue to the diagnosis and indicates the nature and extent of the physical examination required.

The following are the major headings in the order in which they appear in the patient's ROS and the items that are usually reviewed by the physician. The physician questions the patient as to the usual or unusual presence, condition, or occurrence of any of these.

The physician asks if there has been or is a history of the following conditions and whether, as well as what, kinds of medications are currently being used for any of the following*:

- General—Chills, fever, sweats, weight gain or loss, fatigue, weakness, nightmares, insomnia, nervousness, loss of memory
- Head—Headaches, trauma, sinus pain, fainting
- Eyes—Vision, pain, burning, eyestrain, redness, photophobia, diplopia, blurred vision, excessive tearing, discharge, any eye diseases, prescription glasses, date of last eye examination
- Ears—Hearing loss, pain, discharge, tinnitus, dizziness, mastoiditis, trauma, noise exposure, vertigo
- Nose—Smell, head colds, discharge, postnasal drip, epistaxis, pain, obstruction, trauma, allergies
- Mouth—Taste; dryness or excessive salivation; condition of lips, tongue, gums, teeth, dentures
- Throat—Redness, sore throat, tonsillitis, hoarseness, laryngitis, voice changes, speech defects, dysphagia
- Neck—Pain, tenderness, swelling, limitation of motion, trauma
- Respiratory—Chest pain, cough, expectoration, hemoptysis, asthma, wheezing, dyspnea, orthopnea, hyperventilation, night sweats, recurrent respiratory tract infections
- Cardiovascular (CV)—Chest pain, hypertension, palpitation, tachycardia, bradycardia, peripheral edema, varicosities, cyanosis, dizziness, syncope
- Gastrointestinal (GI)—Appetite, anorexia, bulimia, abdominal pain, nausea, vomiting, hematemesis, food intolerance, indigestion, dysphagia, diarrhea, constipation, laxatives, color and form of stools, melena, jaundice, distention, flatus, colic, hemorrhoids, rectal pain, presence of blood, pus, or mucus, pruritus ani, hernia or masses
- Genitourinary (GU)—Dysuria, oliguria, polyuria, frequency, hesitancy, nocturia, incontinence, enuresis, urgency, retention, hematuria, pyuria, glycosuria, abnormal

---

*See Appendix A for definitions and pronunciation keys for many of the terms listed.

color or odor, pain, renal colic, stones, pruritus, discharge, sexually transmitted disease(s), sexual habits, potency, prostate disease, testicular masses, history of urinary tract infections

- Female reproductive—Leukorrhea, discharge, itching, pain, dyspareunia, date and results of last Pap smear, breast self-examination routine

  Menses (menstrual periods)—Age at onset, regularity, amount, duration, date of last menstrual period, premenstrual tension, dysmenorrhea, amenorrhea, irregular bleeding, spotting, menopause (age of onset), postmenopausal bleeding, menopausal symptoms

  Obstetric history—Number of pregnancies, live births, and living children; complications during pregnancy and labor; abortions if any

  Birth control—Method if used
- Metabolic—Change in weight and appetite
- Endocrine—Excessive thirst, goiter, hair distribution, falling hair, change in skin texture or color, temperature intolerance, speech, voice, growth changes, sexual vigor and abnormalities, symptoms of diabetes, hormone therapy
- Blood—Bruising or bleeding tendencies, blood disorders
- Skin—Allergies, rash, pruritus, moles, sores or ulcers, color change (redness, jaundice, cyanosis, pallor), infections, dryness, sweating, alopecia, past dermatitis
- Musculoskeletal (MS)—Muscle or joint pain, swelling, stiffness, limitation of movement, spasm, tetany, weakness, numbness, coldness, deformities, atrophy, dislocations, fractures, discoloration, varicosities, cramping, edema, thrombophlebitis
- Neurologic—Headaches, vertigo, fainting, sense of balance, nervousness, sleeping irregularities, tremor, convulsions, loss of consciousness, memory, paralysis, paresthesia, pain
- Psychiatric—Personality type, emotional stability, previous mental illness

Assisting with the patient history or interview.

At times, you may be responsible for obtaining some of the information for the patient history. The interview is often the first step in developing a relationship with the patient, with the patient's well-being established as the mutual concern. A positive relationship opens the door to providing opportunities for *health education* and possibly counseling now or at a later time. You will be collecting data on the various dimensions of the patient's health.

Skillful interviewers direct patients to give information without patients' having to guess what information may be important to give. You cannot assume that patients have the ability or the knowledge to know what you need to know about them. When interacting with others, first impressions are crucial. Research studies have determined that people make their first impression with others within 7 seconds of the interaction, and this is the impression that they will carry away with them. Your gestures, how you sit, and whether you smile or not can make the difference between success or failure in any situation. Nonverbal communication, however subtle, does affect how

and what others think of you—friendly or unfriendly; aggressive, assertive, or passive; trustworthy or untrustworthy; credible or not credible; professional or unprofessional. Being professional does not mean being impersonal. Demonstrating compassion and care is needed when working with patients and to motivate them to do what is needed and when and how to do it. Many patients comment that how medical personnel interact with them is the *most important* component of treatment (Figure 4-2).

To help guide you in this responsibility, keep the following guidelines in mind:

1. Make sure that the environment is as quiet and private as possible. This helps put the patient at ease and also enhances your own concentration.
2. Introduce yourself and explain to the patient what you will be doing and *why* you are doing this interview before the patient sees the physician.
3. Call the patient by name. Express friendliness and concern without losing professional mannerisms or perspective.

   Always use "Mr.," "Ms.," "Miss," "Mrs.," or another appropriate term (for example, Judge, Captain, Reverend, Father, and so on) to address your patient. Some patients prefer to be addressed by their first name or nickname. If this is the case, he or she will most likely tell you. A

FIGURE 4-2 Demonstrating compassion and care is a critical component of the medical interview.

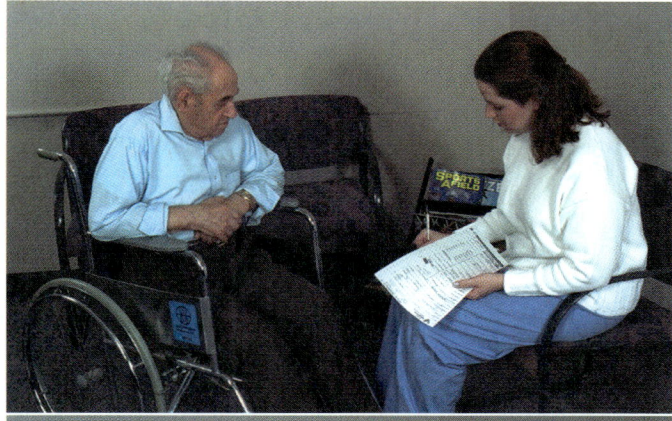
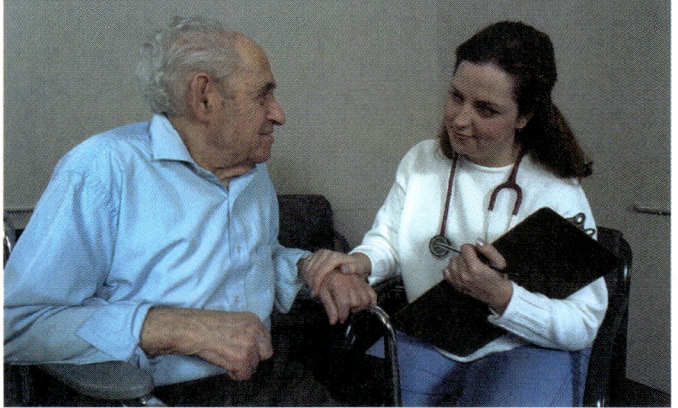

notation could be made on the patient's medical record to this effect to ensure that their preference is used. For example: "Patient prefers to be called Mary rather than Mrs. Jones," or "Rosie rather than Rosemary."

4. Speak slowly, clearly, and distinctly.
5. Listen to the patient attentively.

Make a conscious effort to pay attention and respond to the patient as needed to verify your perceptions. Don't interrupt the patient. Let the patient know that you are listening by using nonverbal signs—for example, nod your head. **Listening well is essential to successfully interacting with patients.** (The ability to listen is a critical thinking skill.)

6. Use eye contact appropriately, observing the patient's body language and facial expressions while doing so. *Do not stare at the patient or at your outline.*

Keep the patient's sociocultural background in mind so that you do not misinterpret his or her nonverbal communication. For example, the patient may look down when you speak to show respect to you and not mean that he or she is anxious or insecure. Direct eye contact means lack of respect in this same culture.

Keep in mind that if you make assumptions about another person's behavior, this could lead to communication problems.

If you are working with patients with an interpreter, including sign language interpreters, introduce the interpreter to the patient and the patient's family if present. Maintain appropriate eye contact with and address questions and information to the patient, *not* the interpreter.

Some deaf patients read lips. In these cases make sure that they can always see your mouth when you ask questions or when speaking with them. Explain to blind patients what you are doing *every* step of the way during your interaction.

7. Treat the patient the way you would want to be treated. Successful interviewing begins with your attitude toward the patient. Think of the interview as a conversation rather than a task of filling out a preprinted form. By doing this, the quality of information that you obtain from the patient will be improved. Avoid interrogation (that is, asking a series of blunt questions). Create an atmosphere of mutual respect and trust by showing genuine interest, concern, and empathy. Be calm. A conversation is a two-way communication. Allow the patient time to complete sentences, even if he or she starts to ramble. You can redirect your questioning as necessary.

Treat each patient as an individual. Good interpersonal skills will complement your technical skills. By being a positive and confident health professional, you can inspire patients to succeed.

8. Encourage the patient to give specific information. This enables both you and the physician to care for the patient's needs. Besides medical information, personal information about the patient, such as stressors at home or work, can help to identify factors that may be affecting the patient's health. A well-documented fact is that stress can lead to a number of physical and emotional problems.

When you need to ask very personal or potentially embarrassing questions, explain why you are doing so. Some facilities will have you ask all patients, "Are you presently or have you ever experienced violence in the home or elsewhere?" and "Are there any cultural or religious practices that the medical provider should know about when providing treatment programs?" For example, in accordance with certain religions, some people do not accept blood transfusions, and others do not eat certain foods. The patient may need to make an appointment with the physician to discuss any special needs if and before they are hospitalized for treatment.

Sometimes you may need to ask the patient if he or she has prepared an **advanced directive (AD) or a durable power of attorney for health care (DPAHC)** outlining health care wishes if he or she is unable to make decisions for himself or herself (see the box on p. 129, which discusses the DPAHC, and Figure 4-3). If the patient has completed these forms, a *copy* should be provided for the physician's office or clinic medical record, and if the person is to be admitted to a hospital, he or she should be directed to take a *copy* to the hospital. The original should be kept with the patient's other important papers or given to the patient's family or agent or attorney. To be *legal*, these forms must be properly *witnessed* and *notarized*. This step must be confirmed before it is put into the patient's medical record.

Often *seniors* are reluctant to bring up certain concerns they may feel are embarrassing or not important, such as depression or sexuality, or to ask too many questions for fear of seeming to waste the physician's or your time. Always encourage patients to ask all the questions they have. Let them know and understand that *all* questions are important. Encourage patients to write their questions down as they think of them and to always bring this list when coming to see the physician.

Take your time when working with seniors. The elderly are very sensitive about being rushed through appointments. Remember, each diverse group brings with it certain health care needs.

9. Use direct and open-ended questions to ask the patient the reason for the visit to the physician and, when applicable, to ask the patient to describe the chief complaint and symptoms or problems that have been experienced. You may start simply by asking, "How are you feeling?" Most patients then focus on their chief complaint. The responses given to these questions help the physician determine the nature and extent of the physical examination required.

When you ask the patient about symptoms, you must collect specific information, but be careful not to influence the patient's answer. You must ask questions that will answer **"what," "where,"** and **"when."** For example, if the patient is complaining of pain (the **"what"**), ask the patient to describe the type of pain experienced. Do not ask, "Is it a sharp or dull pain?" Ask **where** the pain is and have the patient show you where he or she feels the pain. Watch the patient's facial expression and other body language as the

HEALTH MATTERS

KEEPING YOUR PATIENTS INFORMED

Who will make health care decisions for you if you are unable to make them for yourself?

The Patient Self-Determination Act (PSDA) was passed by the U.S. Congress in 1990 and implemented in 1991. This act requires health care providers to inform patients of their rights to make health care decisions and to execute **advance directives (ADs).** ADs outline in advance health care wishes that patients would want should they become physically or mentally unable to make decisions for their own medical care and treatment.

The Durable Power of Attorney for Health Care (DPAHC) is the preferred form of an advance directive because it is flexible and covers the widest scope of possibilities. It also names and gives legal authority to someone (the agent) to make health care decisions when they cannot be made by the patient. This person, the agent, can ensure that the patient's wishes are carried out when the patient is unable to speak for himself or herself. If specific directives are not made, health care decisions for a patient unable to make his or her own decisions are generally left to the patient's family, close friends, and physician(s).

ADs should be reviewed from time to time by the patient to ensure that the directives stated reflect current wishes and that the agent's name, telephone number(s), and address are current. The patient must also check that the agent is still willing to serve in that capacity. Updated signed copies should be given to the physician, close family members, and any other person that may be called on if there is a medical emergency. It is a good idea to put the original copy with other important papers but not in a safe deposit box. Someone close to the patient should know where to locate the document if needed. The patient should also carry a wallet card that will inform any health care provider that an AD has been executed so that the patient's wishes can be followed (see p. 136).

YOUR RIGHT TO MAKE DECISIONS ABOUT MEDICAL TREATMENT*
Who Decides About My Treatment?

Your doctors will give you information and advice about treatment. You have the right to choose. You can say "Yes" to treatments you want. You can say "No" to any treatment you don't want—even if the treatment might keep you alive longer.

How Do I Know What I Want?

Your doctor must tell you about your medical condition and about what different treatments can do for you. Many treatments have "side effects." Your doctor must offer you information about serious problems that medical treatment is likely to cause you.

Often, more than one treatment might help you—and people have different ideas about which is best. Your doctor can tell you which treatments are available to you, but your doctor can't choose for you. That choice depends on what is important to you.

What If I'm Too Sick to Decide?

If you can't make treatment decisions, your doctor will ask your closest available relative or friend to help decide what is best for you. Most of the time, that works, but sometimes everyone doesn't agree about what to do. That's why it is helpful if you say in advance what you want to happen if you can't speak for yourself. There are several kinds of "advance directives" that you can use to say *what* you want and *who* you want to speak for you.

One kind of advance directive under California law lets you name someone to make health care decisions when you can't. This form is called a **Durable Power of Attorney for Health Care.**

Who Can Fill out This Form?

You can if you are 18 years or older and of sound mind. You do not need a lawyer to fill it out.

Who Can I Name to Make Medical Treatment Decisions When I'm Unable to Do So?

You can choose an adult relative or friend you trust as your "agent" to speak for you when you're too sick to make your own decisions.

How Does This Person Know What I Would Want?

After you choose someone, talk to that person about what you want. You can also write down in the *Durable Power of Attorney for Health Care* when you would or wouldn't want medical treatment. Talk to your doctor about what you want and give your doctor a copy of the form. Give another copy to the person named as your agent. Also, take a **copy** with you when you go into a hospital or other treatment facility.

Sometimes treatment decisions are hard to make, and it truly helps your family and your doctors if they know what you want. The *Durable Power of Attorney for Health Care* also gives them legal protection when they follow your wishes.

What If I Don't Have Anybody to Make Decisions for Me?

You can use another kind of advance directive to write down your wishes about treatment. This is often called a **"living will"** because it takes effect while you are still alive but have become unable to speak for yourself. The California Natural Death Act lets you sign a living will called a *Declaration*. Anyone 18 years or older and of sound mind can sign one.

When you sign a *Declaration,* it tells your doctors that you don't want any treatment that would only prolong your dying. All life-sustaining treatment would be stopped if you were terminally ill and your death was expected soon or if you were permanently unconscious. You would still receive treatment to keep you comfortable, however.

The doctors must follow your wishes about limiting treatment or turn your care over to another doctor who will. Your doctors are also legally protected when they follow your wishes.

*From the California Department of Health Services.

HEALTH MATTERS—cont'd

Are There Other Living Wills I Can Use?

Instead of using the *Declaration* in the Natural Death Act, you can use any of the available living will forms. You can use a *Durable Power of Attorney for Health Care* form without naming an agent. Or you can just write down your wishes on a piece of paper. Your doctor and family can use what you write in deciding about your treatment. However, living wills that don't meet the requirements of the Natural Death Act don't give as much legal protection for your doctors if a disagreement arises about following your wishes.

What If I Change My Mind?

You can change or revoke any of these documents at any time as long as you can communicate your wishes.

Do I Have to Fill out One of These Forms?

No, you don't have to fill out any of these forms if you don't want to. You can just talk with your doctors and ask them to write down what you've said in your medical chart. You can talk with your family, but people will be more clear about your treatment wishes if you write them down. Also, your wishes are more likely to be followed if you write them down. (See the forms following.)

Will I Still Be Treated If I Don't Fill out These Forms?

Absolutely. You will still get medical treatment. We just want you to know that if you become too sick to make decisions, someone else will have to make them for you. Remember that:

- A *Durable Power of Attorney for Health Care* lets you name someone to make treatment decisions for you. That person can make most medical decisions—not just those about life-sustaining treatment—when you can't speak for yourself. Besides naming an agent, you can also use the form to say when you would and wouldn't want particular kinds of treatment.
- If you don't have someone you want to name to make decisions when you can't, you can sign a **Natural Death Act Declaration.** This *Declaration* says you do not want life-prolonging treatment if you are terminally ill or permanently unconscious.

How Can I Get More Information About Advance Directives?

Ask your doctor, nurse, medical assistant, or social worker to get more information for you.

It is your responsibility to supply a **copy** of your advance directive to the hospital so that it can be kept with your records. If you have any questions about any of these forms, please talk to your doctor, your nurse, your medical assistant, or your social services representative.

---

pain area is pointed out. Ask **when** the pain first occurred and if there are any special times that it occurs; ask whether anything seems to bring on the pain, and how long it lasts. If the patient can't remember when the pain first started, try to pinpoint the time by asking questions such as, "Did you have pain on the July 4th holiday?" or similar questions. Be aware that some patients may prefer to use another word rather than pain (for example, a pediatric patient may associate better with the word "hurt"). (See also Vocabulary Used to Describe Pain on pp. 143-144).

10. Listen carefully to the patient and pay attention to the sound and tone of his or her voice. The patient may be anxious or upset, or maybe the pain is so intense that the patient is about to cry. Listen for offhand comments, such as, "I probably have this pain because I'm under so much stress. I really shouldn't be here at all." You must reassure the patient that the right decision was made by coming to see the doctor and encourage the patient to discuss any problems with the physician. Alert the physician to these types of comments. The physician can then ask the patient what is really bothering him or her. It may be that the patient does not wish to disclose an intimate problem to you but may be more willing to discuss it if the physician appears to be receptive and willing to inquire and listen.

11. When asking patients about the medications that they are taking, always ask if they are using nicotine gum or patches, which are smoking cessation methods. Both of these can interact with other medications. These methods are very common, and many people do not think of them as medications. Also ask patients about their use of alternative/complementary/integrative therapies, including herbal medicines. Again, many people do not think of herbal remedies as medication, but they are and could contain chemicals that if taken with other drugs could cause undesirable side effects. Research on the effects of herbal medicine is limited, so information on side effects or herbal drug interactions is not as available as for drugs that are regulated by government quality assurance standards.

Be aware that diuretic medications are often referred to by patients as their "water pill."

Ask patients to keep a diary of all the medications and therapies that they use and to bring this information for review each time they have a doctor's appointment.

Text continued on p. 136

Optional Statement of Desires, Special Provisions, and Limitations for Durable Power of Attorney for Health Care

If I develop any incurable, progressive, or degenerative disease stated to be terminal with respect to outcome (not with respect to time) and no cure is available and treatment only prolongs dying, I request that my physician follow my guide regarding life support and life-sustaining intervention listed below. If my desires are not known and life-sustaining or life support procedures are used in an emergency situation, I request that my desires be respected and followed once they are known to my professional care team. I do not want to be kept alive in a vegetative state.

	I want	I do not want	I want tried, but stopped if I do not improve	I am undecided
Pacemaker Any device that substitutes for the normal heartbeat.	❏	❏	❏	❏
Peritoneal Dialysis or Kidney Dialysis Alternative means of filtering poisons from the body when the kidneys fail.	❏	❏	❏	❏
Respirator A breathing machine attached to a tube inserted into the lungs through the nose or mouth.	❏	❏	❏	❏
Cardiopulmonary Resuscitation (CPR) Intervention given by person, machine, or drugs when the heart and/or lungs stop working.	❏	❏	❏	❏
Feeding Tube for Food or Fluids A tube placed into the stomach or bowel to give fluid and/or nutrition.	❏	❏	❏	❏
Hypodermoclysis for Nutrition or Fluid Placing fluid under the skin outside a vein with a needle; the body will absorb this fluid.	❏	❏	❏	❏
Intravenous (IV) Tubes for feeding and hydration.	❏	❏	❏	❏
Antibiotics To treat pneumonia or any other infection.	❏	❏	❏	❏
Cancer Therapy or Radiation X-ray treatments for tumors or cancers.	❏	❏	❏	❏
Chemotherapy Cancer medicine given by mouth or intravenously.	❏	❏	❏	❏
Transfusion Blood or blood products given into a vein.	❏	❏	❏	❏
Medical Treatment, Diagnostic Procedures, and Tests Further tests and procedures to monitor failing condition.	❏	❏	❏	❏
Surgery An operation only if it provides for my comfort and dignity.	❏	❏	❏	❏
Paramedic	❏	❏	❏	❏
Uniform Gift Act, organ transplant Donation of body parts; please specify:	❏	❏	❏	❏
Autopsy Complete autopsy or selective autopsy to confirm my diagnosis.	❏	❏	❏	❏
Research Consent	❏	❏	❏	❏

Other Concerns or Corrections:

_____
_____
_____

I wish:
1. Caring and supportive nursing and medical care to relieve pain and suffering including narcotics to relieve pain even if respiration is depressed.
2. Food and fluids to be offered as long as I am conscious to take them by mouth and then moist sponges to moisten my lips to relieve the sensation of dehydration.

Signature: _____ Date: _____
Name (print): _____

To be included in my Durable Power of Attorney for Health Care.

Mills-Peninsula Wellness Center, 100 S. San Mateo Drive, San Mateo, CA 94401, 1-800-654-9966

FIGURE 4-3   **A,** CMA Durable Power of Attorney for Health Care.

California Medical Association
DURABLE POWER OF ATTORNEY FOR HEALTH CARE DECISIONS
(California Probate Code Sections 4600-4753)

A

WARNING TO PERSON EXECUTING THIS DOCUMENT

This is an important legal document. Before executing this document, you should know these important facts:

This document gives the person you designate as your agent (the attorney-in-fact) the power to make health care decisions for you. Your agent must act consistently with your desires as stated in this document or otherwise made known.

Except as you otherwise specify in this document, this document gives your agent power to consent to your doctor not giving treatment or stopping treatment necessary to keep you alive.

Notwithstanding this document, you have the right to make medical and other health care decisions for yourself so long as you can give informed consent with respect to the particular decision. In addition, no treatment may be given to you over your objection, and health care necessary to keep you alive may not be stopped or withheld if you object at the time.

This document gives your agent authority to consent, to refuse to consent, or to withdraw consent to any care, treatment, service, or procedure to maintain, diagnose, or treat a physical or mental condition. This power is subject to any statement of your desires and any limitations that you include in this document. You may

state in this document any types of treatment that you do not desire. In addition, a court can take away the power of your agent to make health care decisions for you if your agent (1) authorizes anything that is illegal, (2) acts contrary to your known desires or (3) where your desires are not known, does anything that is clearly contrary to your best interests.

This power will exist for an indefinite period of time unless you limit its duration in this document.

You have the right to revoke the authority of your agent by notifying your agent or your treating doctor, hospital, or other health care provider orally or in writing of the revocation.

Your agent has the right to examine your medical records and to consent to their disclosure unless you limit this right in this document.

Unless you otherwise specify in this document, this document gives your agent the power after you die to (1) authorize an autopsy, (2) donate your body or parts thereof for transplant or therapeutic or educational or scientific purposes, and (3) direct the disposition of your remains.

If there is anything in this document that you do not understand, you should ask a lawyer to explain it to you.

1. CREATION OF DURABLE POWER OF ATTORNEY FOR HEALTH CARE

By this document I intend to create a durable power of attorney by appointing the person designated below to make health care decisions for me as allowed by Sections 4600 to 4753, inclusive, of the California Probate Code. This power of attorney shall not be affected by my subsequent incapacity. I hereby revoke any prior durable power of attorney for health care. I am a California resident who is at least 18 years old, of sound mind, and acting of my own free will.

2. APPOINTMENT OF HEALTH CARE AGENT

(Fill in below the name, address and telephone number of the person you wish to make health care decisions for you if you become incapacitated. You should make sure that this person agrees to accept this responsibility. The following may not serve as your agent: (1) your treating health care provider; (2) an operator of a community care facility or residential care facility for the elderly; or (3) an employee of your treating health care provider, a community care facility, or a residential care facility for the elderly, unless that employee is related to you by blood, marriage or adoption, or unless you are also an employee of the same treating provider or facility. If you are a conservatee under the Lanterman-Petris-Short Act (the law governing involuntary commitment to a mental health facility) and you wish to appoint your conservator as your agent, you must consult a lawyer, who must sign and attach a special declaration for this document to be valid.)

I, _____ , hereby appoint:
        (insert your name)

Name _____

Address _____

Work Telephone (_____) _____   Home Telephone (_____) _____

as my agent (attorney-in-fact) to make health care decisions for me as authorized in this document. I understand that this power of attorney will be effective for an indefinite period of time unless I revoke it or limit its duration below.

(Optional) This power of attorney shall expire on the following date: _____ .

© California Medical Association 1996 (revised)

3. AUTHORITY OF AGENT

If I become incapable of giving informed consent to health care decisions, I grant my agent full power and authority to make those decisions for me, subject to any statements of desires or limitations set forth below. Unless I have limited my agent's authority in this document, that authority shall include the right to consent, refuse consent, or withdraw consent to any medical care, treatment, service, or procedure; to receive and to consent to the release of medical information; to authorize an autopsy to determine the cause of my death; to make a gift of all or part of my body; and to direct the disposition of my remains, subject to any instructions I have given in a written contract for funeral services, my will or by some other method. I understand that, by law, my agent may <u>not</u> consent to any of the following: commitment to a mental health treatment facility, convulsive treatment, psychosurgery, sterilization or abortion.

4. MEDICAL TREATMENT DESIRES AND LIMITATIONS (OPTIONAL)

(Your agent must make health care decisions that are consistent with your known desires. You may, but are not required to, state your desires about the kinds of medical care you do or do not want to receive, including your desires concerning life support if you are seriously ill. If you do not want your agent to have the authority to make certain decisions, you must write a statement to that effect in the space provided below; otherwise, your agent will have the broad powers to make health care decisions for you that are outlined in paragraph 3 above. In either case, <u>it is important that you discuss your health care desires with the person you appoint as your agent and with your doctor(s).</u>

(Following is a general statement about withholding and removal of life-sustaining treatment. If the statement accurately reflects your desires, you may initial it. If you wish to add to it or to write your own statement instead, you may do so in the space provided.)

I do **not** want efforts made to prolong my life and I do **not** want life-sustaining treatment to be provided or continued: (1) if I am in an irreversible coma or persistent vegetative state; or (2) if I am terminally ill and the use of life-sustaining procedures would serve only to artificially delay the moment of my death; or (3) under any other circumstances where the burdens of the treatment outweigh the expected benefits. In making decisions about life-sustaining treatment under provision (3) above, I want my agent to consider the relief of suffering and the quality of my life, as well as the extent of the possible prolongation of my life.

If this statement reflects your desires, initial here: _____

Other or additional statements of medical treatment desires and limitations: _____

_____

_____

_____

(You may attach additional pages if you need more space to complete your statements. Each additional page must be dated and signed at the same time you date and sign this document.)

5. APPOINTMENT OF ALTERNATE AGENTS (OPTIONAL)

(You may appoint alternate agents to make health care decisions for you in case the person you appointed in Paragraph 2 is unable or unwilling to do so.)

If the person named as my agent in Paragraph 2 is not available or willing to make health care decisions for me as authorized in this document, I appoint the following persons to do so, listed in the order they should be asked:

First Alternate Agent: Name _____

Address _____

Work Telephone (_____) _____   Home Telephone (_____) _____

Second Alternate Agent: Name _____

Address _____

Work Telephone (_____) _____   Home Telephone (_____) _____

6. USE OF COPIES

I hereby authorize that photocopies of this document can be relied upon by my agent and others as though they were originals.

Continued

FIGURE 4-3—cont'd   A, CMA Durable Power of Attorney for Health Care.

DATE AND SIGNATURE OF PRINCIPAL
(You must date and sign this power of attorney)

I sign my name to this Durable Power of Attorney for Health Care at _____, _____

(City)   *(State)*

on _____ . _____

(Date)   *(Signature of Principal)*

STATEMENT OF WITNESSES

(This power of attorney will not be valid for making health care decisions unless it is either (1) signed by two qualified adult witnesses who are present when you sign or acknowledge your signature <u>or</u> (2) acknowledged before a notary public in California. If you elect to use witnesses rather than a notary public, the law provides that none of the following may be used as witnesses: (1) the persons you have appointed as your agent and alternate agents; (2) your health care provider or an employee of your health care provider; or (3) an operator or employee of an operator of a community care facility or residential care facility for the elderly. Additionally, at least one of the witnesses cannot be related to you by blood, marriage or adoption, or be named in your will.

(SPECIAL RULES FOR SKILLED NURSING FACILITY RESIDENTS: If you are a patient in a skilled nursing facility, you <u>must</u> have a patient advocate or ombudsman sign both the statement of witnesses below <u>and</u> the declaration on the following page. You must also have a second qualified witness sign below <u>or</u> have this document acknowledged before a notary public.)

I declare under penalty of perjury under the laws of California that the person who signed or acknowledged this document is personally known to me to be the principal, or that the identity of the principal was proved to me by convincing evidence;* that the principal signed or acknowledged this durable power of attorney in my presence, that the principal appears to be of sound mind and under no duress, fraud, or undue influence; that I am not the person appointed as attorney in fact by this document, and that I am not the principal's health care provider, an employee of the principal's health care provider, the operator of a community care facility or a residential care facility for the elderly, nor an employee of an operator of a community care facility or residential care facility for the elderly.

First Witness: Signature _____

Print name _____

Date _____

Residence Address _____

Second Witness: Signature _____

Print name _____

Date _____

Residence Address _____

(AT LEAST ONE OF THE ABOVE WITNESSES MUST ALSO SIGN THE FOLLOWING DECLARATION)

I further declare under penalty of perjury under the laws of California that I am not related to the principal by blood, marriage, or adoption, and, to the best of my knowledge I am not entitled to any part of the estate of the principal upon the death of the principal under a will now existing or by operation of law.

Signature: _____

---

*The law allows one or more of the following forms of identification as convincing evidence of identity: a California driver's license or identification card or U.S. passport that is current or has been issued within five years, or any of the following if the document is current or has been issued within five years, contains a photograph and description of the person named on it, is signed by the person, and bears a serial or other identifying number: a foreign passport that has been stamped by the U.S. Immigration and Naturalization Service; a driver's license issued by another state or by an authorized Canadian or Mexican agency; or an identification card issued by another state or by any branch of the U.S. armed forces. If the principal is a patient in a skilled nursing facility, a patient advocate or ombudsman may rely on the representations of family members or the administrator or staff of the facility as convincing evidence of identity if the patient advocate or ombudsman believes that the representations provide a reasonable basis for determining the identity of the principal.

FIGURE 4-3—cont'd. **A,** CMA Durable Power of Attorney for Health Care.

SPECIAL REQUIREMENT: STATEMENT OF PATIENT ADVOCATE OR OMBUDSMAN

(If you are a patient in a skilled nursing facility, a patient advocate or ombudsman must sign the Statement of Witnesses above __and__ must also sign the following declaration.)

I further declare under penalty of perjury under the laws of California that I am a patient advocate or ombudsman as designated by the State Department of Aging and am serving as a witness as required by subdivision (e) of Probate Code Section 4701.

Signature: _____   Address: _____

Print Name: _____   _____

Date: _____   _____

CERTIFICATE OF ACKNOWLEDGMENT OF NOTARY PUBLIC

(Acknowledgment before a notary public is __not__ required if you have elected to have two qualified witnesses sign above. If you are a patient in a skilled nursing facility, you __must__ have a patient advocate or ombudsman sign the Statement of Witnesses on page 3 __and__ the Statement of Patient Advocate or Ombudsman above)

State of California   )
)ss
County of _____   )

On this _____ day of _____, in the year _____,

before me, _____,
                              (here insert name and title of the officer)

personally appeared _____
                                   (here insert name of principal)

personally known to me (or proved to me on the basis of satisfactory evidence) to be the person(s) whose name(s) is/are subscribed to this instrument and acknowledged to me that he/she/they executed the same in his/her/their authorized capacity(ies), and that by his/her/their signature(s) on the instrument the person(s), or the entity upon behalf of which the person(s) acted, executed the instrument.

WITNESS my hand and official seal.

_____
        (Signature of Notary Public)

                                                                        NOTARY SEAL

COPIES

YOUR AGENT MAY NEED THIS DOCUMENT IMMEDIATELY IN CASE OF AN EMERGENCY. YOU SHOULD KEEP THE COMPLETED ORIGINAL AND GIVE PHOTOCOPIES OF THE COMPLETED ORIGINAL TO (1) YOUR AGENT AND ALTERNATE AGENTS, (2) YOUR PERSONAL PHYSICIAN, AND (3) MEMBERS OF YOUR FAMILY AND ANY OTHER PERSONS WHO MIGHT BE CALLED IN THE EVENT OF A MEDICAL EMERGENCY. THE LAW PERMITS THAT PHOTOCOPIES OF THE COMPLETED DOCUMENT CAN BE RELIED UPON AS THOUGH THEY WERE ORIGINALS.

Additional forms can be purchased from: CMA Publications, P.O. Box 7690, San Francisco, CA 94120-7690 • (415) 882-5175

FIGURE 4-3 **B,** Durable Power of Attorney for Health Care wallet identification card. (**A** and **B,** Courtesy and Copyright California Medical Association 1998. Published with permission of and by arrangement with the California Medical Association. Copies of this form, as well as an accompanying brochure and wallet card, may be obtained from CMA Publications at 800-822-1-CMA.)

DURABLE POWER OF ATTORNEY FOR HEALTH CARE WALLET IDENTIFICATION CARD

The attached wallet card is provided for the purpose of alerting emergency medical personnel to the existence of a Durable Power of Attorney for Health Care (DPAHC) in the event that you require medical treatment and are unable to verbally inform health care providers that an agent has been appointed to act in your behalf. It is recommended that you complete the card by filling in the indicated names and telephone numbers and carry it with you at all times.

Instructions:

B

1. On the **front** of the card, print your full name in the space labeled "principal's name."

2. On the **back** of the card, print the names and telephone numbers of the persons you have appointed as your **health care agent** and (first) **alternate agent** in the spaces provided. (Make sure the names and telephone numbers are the same as those listed in your DPAHC form.) Space is also provided on the card to write in the name and telephone number(s) of a third person who has a copy of your DPAHC form. This may be the person you have named as your "second alternate agent" or, if you have not designated a second alternate agent, any other person to whom you have given a copy of your completed form.

3. Carefully tear off the card along the perforated line and place it in a conspicuous place in your wallet or billfold. Be sure to update the information on the card if there is a change in the telephone number(s) of any of the people you have listed on it, or if you subsequently complete a new DPAHC form in which different individuals are designated to act as your agent and/or alternate agent(s).

IMPORTANT NOTICE TO EMERGENCY MEDICAL PERSONNEL

I, _____,
(principal's name)
have executed a DURABLE POWER OF ATTORNEY FOR HEALTH CARE pursuant to California Probate Code §§4600-4753 (or §§4770 et. seq.). If I am unable to make my own health care decisions, my designated agent has the legal authority to make those decisions on my behalf, including decisions concerning life-sustaining treatment. In such an event, one of the persons listed on the reverse of this card who has a copy of my Durable Power of Attorney should be contracted immediately, in the order listed.
(See Reverse)

1. Agent's Name: _____
   Work: (_____) _____
   Home: (_____) _____
2. Alternate Agent: _____
   Work: (_____) _____
   Home: (_____) _____
3. Other: _____
   Work: (_____) _____
   Home: (_____) _____

(See Reverse)

12. Accept what the patient states. Often saying "um-hm" or giving a nod will encourage the patient to go on.
13. Summarize the information that you have gathered. Ask the patient if there is anything else that he or she would like to add or if there is anything that you may have left out.
14. Be willing and prepared to answer questions that the patient may have. Respond with interest. If you cannot answer the question, refer it to the physician. Explain that the physician will discuss the answer to the patient's question(s).

Physical Examination

After the history is completed, the physician proceeds with the physical examination, often referred to as a physical or a PE. This differs from the history in that it involves a thorough examination of the patient from head to toe for anatomic and physiologic functioning.

The key to a physical examination is systematic thoroughness. Generally a physician formulates a logical, methodic approach by examining each body system or part, beginning with the head and working down. The information obtained in the history or the chief complaint as stated by the patient helps determine the extent of the examination to be performed. Some-times either a limited or a specific examination of one body part or system may be indicated.

The physician uses various methods of physical examination to learn about the patient's condition. The standard methods follow (Figure 4-4).

Methods of Physical Examination

Inspection. Inspection is the visual observation of the body as a whole and of its individual parts. The physician observes the patient's general appearance, the color of the skin, and the size and shape of the body as a whole and of the individual parts. The physician also notes any rashes, scars, trauma, deformities, swelling, injuries, nervousness, and any sounds coming from the patient, such as a sigh, cough, wheezing, and so on.

In the detailed examination, the physician uses the otoscope to look into the ears and the ophthalmoscope to inspect the eyes. A tongue blade is helpful when inspecting the mouth and throat.

Palpation. Palpation is performed by applying the tips of the fingers, the whole hand, or both hands to the body part. Pressure may be slight or forcible, continuous or intermittent. The physician feels, touches, and sometimes manipulates the external sur-

FIGURE 4-4   Methods of physical examinations. **A,** Inspection. **B,** Palpation. **C,** Percussion. **D,** Auscultation.

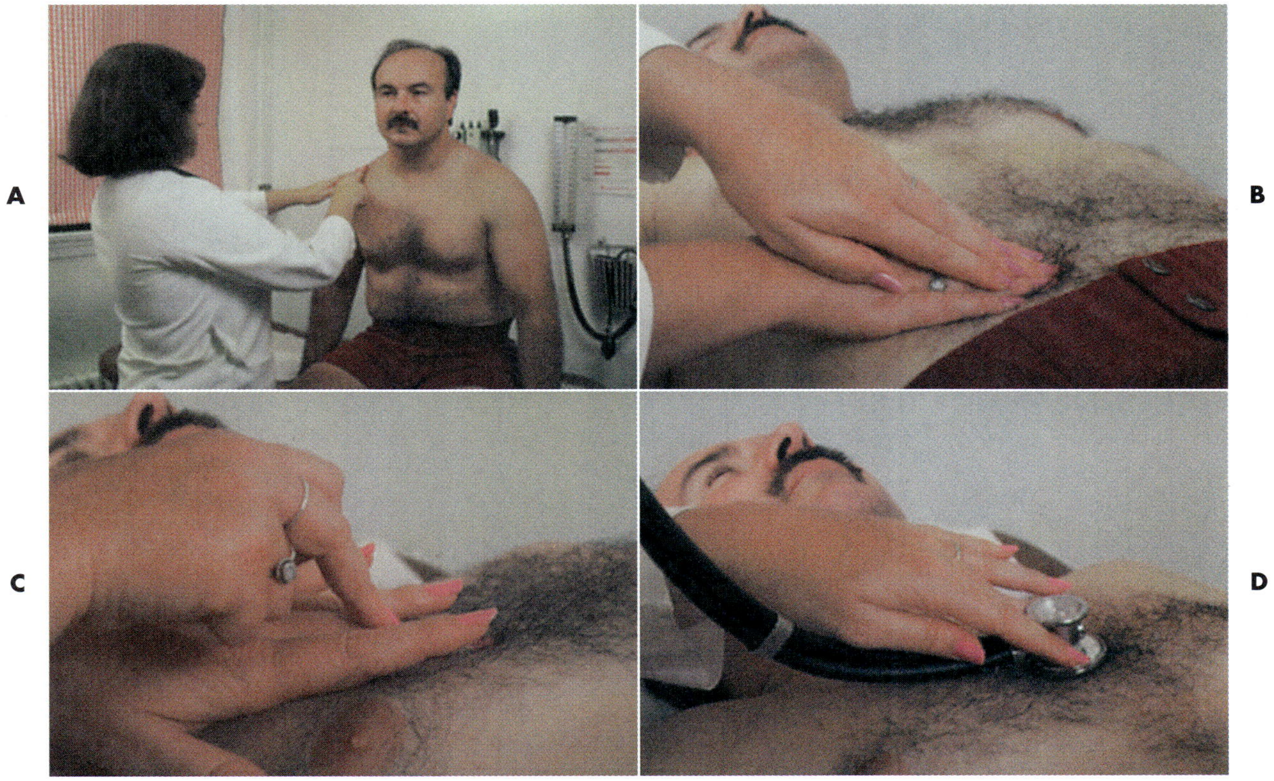

face of the various parts of the body to determine the physical characteristics of tissues or organs and also to note if pain or tenderness is present.

Also involved are the physician's senses of temperature, vibration, position, and kinesthesia (the sense used to perceive movement, position, and weight) as the examination is in progress. Some of the organs and parts of the body examined by this method are the breast, chest, abdomen, liver, kidney, bladder, and lymph nodes. In conjunction with external palpation, internal palpation may be done on the uterus, ovaries, rectum, and prostate. Palpation is used to determine the size, position, and location of pelvic and abdominal organs and if any abnormalities or masses are present.

Percussion.   In medical diagnosis, percussion is done by tapping the body lightly but sharply with the fingers. The physician places one or two fingers of one hand on the part of the body to be examined and then strikes those fingers with the index or middle finger of the other hand.

The purpose of percussion is to determine the density, size, and position of the underlying organs and also to determine the presence of pus or fluid in a cavity. The differing densities of the various parts of the body give off different sounds when struck by the examiner's fingers. The more hollow the part struck, the more drumlike the sound. The sounds that are emitted help the physician make a diagnosis. A solid mass in a hollow organ can be noted because of a change from the normal

density. Also, the borders of certain organs such as the heart can be mapped out by comparing the density in the organ with surrounding tissues. Percussion is most commonly used on the chest and back for examination of the heart and lungs but may also be done on the abdomen, bladder, or bones.

A physician may also use an instrument, the percussion hammer, to check a patient's reflexes by striking the tendon just below the knee and also at the elbow or ankle. Failure of the desired reflex gives the physician more information for a diagnosis.

Auscultation.   Auscultation is the process of listening to sounds produced in some of the body cavities as the organs perform their functions. A stethoscope is usually used, but it can also be done by placing an ear directly over a bare or thinly covered body surface. It is used chiefly on the chest to listen to the heart and lungs and also on the abdomen to diagnose an abdominal aneurysm or listen to fetal heart sounds or peristaltic waves. Listening to the sounds produced in these body cavities helps determine the physical condition of the organs.

Mensuration.   Mensuration is the process of measuring. Clinical measurements include weight, height, temperature, pulse rate, respirations, and blood pressure. Head circumference is also measured in young children. When recorded and compared with previous measurements, these are extremely important guides for some diagnoses. The chest may also be measured to ascertain the amount of expansion and retraction on each side that accompanies inspiration and expiration. This is important when diagnosing or treating chest conditions such as emphysema, in which there is often a loss of elasticity of the lungs. Circumference of the extremities may be measured, especially when determining neuromuscular problems.

Smell. Smell is a less commonly used method, but it is still a relevant method for detecting a disease process. Odors from the breath, sputum, urine, feces, vomitus, or pus can provide valuable information to help the physician make a diagnosis.

Essentials of a thorough physical examination.
The physician observes, tests, and measures each of the following for normal or abnormal structure and function and records his or her findings. *See Appendix A, Part 2, on pp. 833-835, for vocabulary used in recording physical findings.*

- General inspection—General appearance, nutritional status, apparent age, color, sex, height, weight, attitude, communication
- Vital signs—Temperature, pulse rate, respirations, blood pressure
- Skin—Color, texture, turgor, warmth, hair distribution, pigmentation, rashes, scars, lesions, moles, warts
- Head—Position, proportion to rest of body, distribution of hair, masses, evidence of trauma
- Face—Symmetry, size, appearance, facial expression, tenderness
- Eyes—Visual fields, visual acuity, eyeball movement, conjunctiva, sclera, cornea, iris, pupils, eyelids, ptosis, tearing, discharges
- Ears—Hearing, ear canals, tympanic membranes, cerumen, discharge
- Nose—Size, shape, color, deformity, septum, airways, mucosa, discharge, bleeding
- Mouth—Breath, lips, gums, teeth, tongue, mucosa
- Throat—Tonsils, pharynx, larynx
- Neck—Suppleness, thyroid gland, lymph nodes, vessels, carotid pulses, position of trachea, tenderness, stiffness, masses
- Breasts—Size, contour, symmetry, nipples, masses, discharge, tenderness
- Chest—Shape, symmetry, expansion, lesions
- Lungs—Rate and quality of respirations, breath sounds, cough, sputum, friction rubs, resonance, fremitus
- Heart—Rate, rhythm, point of maximum impulse (PMI), sounds, murmurs, dullness, thrills, gallop
- Arteries—Pulses, vessel walls, bruits
- Veins—Pulsation, dilation, filling
- Lymph nodes—Enlargement
- Abdomen—Contour; appearance; liver, kidneys, and spleen (LKS); bladder; scars, peristalsis; tenderness; rigidity; spasm; masses; fluid; hernia
- Female genitalia—External appearance, Bartholin's and Skene's glands, discharge, masses; vaginal—bimanual examination of uterus and adnexa, tenderness, masses, Pap smear if required
- Male genitalia—Penis, scrotum, scars, lesions, discharge, tenderness, masses, atrophy, enlargement
- Rectum—Sphincter tone, prostate gland, seminal vesicles, fissure, fistula, hemorrhoids, masses, discharge, feces
- Back and spine—Posture, curvature, balance, mobility, gait, tenderness, masses, costovertebral tenderness
- Extremities—Proportion to trunk, range of motion, color, pulses, edema, swelling, deformity, tenderness, ulcers, varicosities
- Fingernails—Contour, color
- Neurologic status—Consciousness; cranial nerves; reflexes; coordination; gait; balance; muscle tone and strength; tactile, pain (deep and superficial), and discriminatory sensations
- Mental status—Orientation to time, place, and person; appearance, behavior; mood and thought content

Other tests that a physician may have performed as part of the physical examination include a routine urinalysis (UA), a complete blood count (CBC), a chest x-ray film, and electrocardiogram (ECG or EKG). A physical examination varies according to the needs or complaints of a patient. Often a patient may have a complaint or situation that can be handled in a few minutes or one that requires a special type of examination, such as a sigmoidoscopy. Other patients may require a complete physical examination. In this case, all of the preceding information is obtained.

Special examinations.
Certain types of examinations are more specific and restricted. These are local or special examinations, which are confined to specific parts and organs or special functions of the body. They are extensive and detailed and performed to establish complete information of a complex nature. Often they are done to examine the interior of body cavities and passages. Some of the local or special examinations are vaginal and obstetric examinations, proctoscopy, sigmoidoscopy, cystoscopy, bronchoscopy, and skin tests. Other specialized examinations include ultrasound, roentgenologic, neurologic, ophthalmologic, and cardiac studies.

SUMMARY OF POSITIVE FINDINGS

On the basis of the subjective findings related by the patient and the objective findings found by the physician during the physical examination, the physician sometimes briefly summarizes all of the positive findings of the case.

DIAGNOSTIC DATA

Diagnostic studies are performed for the following reasons:

- To determine (diagnose) the condition from which the patient is suffering so that treatment may be started if feasible.
- To discover disease in its early stage before the patient has any signs or symptoms. This is called **screening.** Screening often makes it possible to cure or delay the progression

of a disease, such as cancer or hypertension, because treatment can be started in the early stages.

- To evaluate past or ongoing treatment received by the patient.

As the field of medical science continues to expand, newer, more accurate, and more sophisticated techniques are made available to help physicians diagnose disease processes. Diagnostic procedures and studies include but are not limited to physical examinations, surgical intervention, and laboratory studies. Laboratory data may include a set of routine laboratory examinations that were performed at the time of the patient's physical examination, with the results recorded if the tests have been completed. Other procedures used in diagnosing and treating disease processes may involve the specialized areas of radiology (roentgenology), nuclear medicine, special skin tests, physical medicine, physiotherapy, and electrocardiography. These areas of health care and treatment are discussed further in later chapters. (Also see Summary of Studies Used for Diagnosing Conditions Affecting Body Organs and Systems in the *Student Mastery Manual.*)

IMPRESSION

Once all of this information has been gathered, the physician gives an impression of the patient's condition that may include any or all of the following:

- **Diagnosis**
  Primary diagnosis—A statement that indicates the cause of the patient's current, most important problem or condition
  Secondary diagnosis—A statement that indicates a problem or condition that is less important or urgent than the patient's primary diagnosis
- **Tentative or provisional diagnosis**—A probable diagnosis that reflects the physician's impression of the patient's condition, but it is made before any further tests have been completed and a final diagnosis has been reached
- **Differential diagnosis**—A possible diagnosis that is based on comparison of the signs and symptoms of two or more similar diseases to determine, by a process of elimination, the disease from which the patient is suffering
- **Rule out (R/O)**—A statement that indicates the conditions that the physician believes might be causing the patient's problem. Each condition is investigated thoroughly and ruled out as a diagnosis, if and when negative testing results are obtained. Again, by a process of elimination, a diagnosis may be reached. (Currently the term *rule out* is being replaced by the term *possible diagnosis,* which some believe to be a better description of the process.)
- **Problem list**—This is used in the most recent system of recording called the problem-oriented system (POS). A problem is any situation, disease, or condition for which the patient needs help or any question that requires a solution. In the problem list, each problem drawn from the database is numbered, dated, and listed in order of occurrence. (Database refers to all of the preceding parts of the

medical record as discussed.) Problems may be stated in terms of the following:
  Diagnosis
  Symptom of physical findings
  Physiologic findings
  Abnormal laboratory results
  Social or personal problems
  Environmental problems
  Behavioral factors
  Patient education
- Additional explanations of the POS and the problem-oriented record are discussed at the end of this chapter
- **Prognosis**—A statement of the probable or anticipated outcome of the patient's condition

CARE PLANS AND SUGGESTED FURTHER STUDY

The next part of the medical record details the physician's specific plans, which may include one or a combination of the following forms of treatment: drug therapy, physical therapy, diet therapy, surgery, and psychotherapy. Treatments prescribed and medications ordered are entered on the record in detail. If hospitalization is required, this is noted. Patient education should be included for all of these treatments.

Suggested further studies list the laboratory tests, x-ray film studies, or any other special tests that the physician deems necessary for the treatment and care of the patient. Instructions for follow-up visits are stated. A statement is made that the patient has been referred to another physician for consultation or treatment when this is advisable.

After special tests or consultations are completed, a report is made, which is then incorporated into the patient's medical record.

Consent Forms

See Chapter 6, p. 309, and Figure 6-16, p. 310.

REPORTS FROM DIAGNOSTIC STUDIES, TREATMENT PLANS, AND CONSULTATION SERVICES

The results of all diagnostic studies are provided on a variety of forms specific to the agency. Many reports are computer generated, and some can be accessed by the physician using the computer code that he or she has established with the facility performing the test(s). Surgical reports are dictated by the physician after surgery. After these reports are typed, copies are sent for the patient's hospital chart and the patient's medical record in the physician office or clinic.

When patients are referred to a consulting physician for a review and second opinion or for special procedures or examinations, the consulting physician then sends a report of the examination or test results and findings to the referring physician as a matter of professional courtesy. Sometimes this report is outlined in a letter; other reports are recorded using a special format or specific forms. Reports with information discussing the patient's care and treatment from outside sources must be filed in the appropriate section of the patient's office or clinic medical record. The medical assistant must develop a system for ensuring that *laboratory tests, pathology reports, x-ray films, consultations,* or *surgical reports* from outside sources are received for the physician to review and then filed in the patient's medical record.

Samples of medical reports are provided at the end of all chapters showing a variety of ways for recording the findings and results of medical procedures and examinations.

Remember that one of the patient's rights is that ALL such information and discussions are privileged and confidential information and must be treated accordingly. The patient's medical record is a legal confidential file. Information in all medical records is to be viewed only when dealing with the medical care of the patient, when used for medical training and learning experiences, when the record is needed for legal cases, and also for obtaining general patient information and information on insurance carriers for billing purposes.

PROGRESS NOTES

After each future visit, the physician's observations, the status of the patient's condition, and the patient's own report, if it is relevant, are added to the medical record. Any change in treatment or medication is recorded. This is called the progress report or progress note, and each entry must be dated and signed. In a hospital, other health care providers (for example, physical therapists) write progress notes.

DISCHARGE SUMMARY

If the patient is discharged, the date and final statement about the patient's health and condition at that time are recorded on the medical record. These may be written at the end of the progress notes or on a separate form.

If the patient dies, a statement describing the cause of death is recorded, and the history is marked *"deceased."*

Hospital discharge summaries contain more detailed information, including:

- Admission date, discharge date
- Admitting diagnosis, final diagnosis
- Summary of the history—sex, age, chief complaint, brief history of present illness, pertinent past history
- Pertinent physical findings
- Pertinent laboratory and x-ray film findings
- Treatment (for example, surgery, drugs, x-ray films, and diet)
- Hospital course (uneventful or list of any complications)
- Condition on discharge
- Prognosis (good, fair, poor, guarded)
- Recommendations on discharge (for example, special orders, follow-up care, and medications)
- Date, hour, and physician's signature

A copy of the patient's hospital discharge summary should be obtained from the hospital for the patient's permanent office record. The summary is helpful to the physician for providing continuity of care to the patient on return visits to the office or clinic. It is also used for research, statistical, insurance, billing, and legal purposes.

PROBLEM-ORIENTED MEDICAL RECORD

Over the years, the problem-oriented medical record (POMR) has gained great momentum and support from health care providers in a variety of settings. Pioneered by Lawrence L. Weed, MD, of the University of Vermont College of Medicine, the POMR provides a systematic way of recording data pertinent to patient care. Its purpose is to obtain and record in an organized manner all the facts needed to accurately diagnose, treat, and provide complete follow-up care for a patient's condition, disease, or situation. It consists of the following four basic parts.

1. Database
2. Problem list
3. Plans
4. Progress notes

The **database** provides the essential data necessary to identify and solve the problem(s). It consists of the patient's medical history, the physical examination, and known laboratory data, all of which were described previously.

The **problem list** results from the information obtained in the database. All the problems identified are titled, numbered, and dated in order of occurrence. This information is usually placed on the front page of the patient's chart to provide a quick diagnostic profile of the patient. The problems may be stated in various terms as outlined in the following paragraphs.

At subsequent visits any new problems are noted as they arise, dated, and numbered consecutively. As problems are resolved, the fact is noted with the date of occurrence. The number of a resolved problem is not used again for another problem.

The problem list can be adapted in various ways to accommodate short-term or temporary problems that are seen frequently in the physician's office or clinic. One recommendation is the use of two problem lists: one for short-term or temporary problems, the other for long-term or permanent problems. When a short-term problem persists beyond a reasonable time or when it recurs frequently, it is removed from the short-term list and added to the long-term or permanent list.

Another recommendation is to use only one problem list but not to record quickly resolved temporary problems on it. Temporary problems are simply indicated as such in the progress notes and are not numbered.

Plans state what will be done to start to solve the problem(s). They are made for each titled and numbered problem. A plan for a problem may be classified as follows:

- *Diagnostic,* that is, evaluative studies such as laboratory tests and x-ray films, consultations requested, and interviews with the patient's family, all of which help acquire additional information.

- *Therapeutic,* that is, medical, surgical, diet, psychologic, or physical treatment used to meet the goals of the physician when providing health care.
- *Educative,* that is, what the patient is told about the therapy and condition, what instructional material, if any, the patient received, and what the patient is expected to do as a partner in the care and treatment plan.

The **progress notes** are added to the record as the plan(s) are carried out. Each progress note is dated, titled, and numbered according to the corresponding problem number. Each problem is evaluated for current status, with a notation of new findings or thoughts, changes in treatment plans, and resolution of the problem.

Each progress note should contain four parts and should be recorded according to the following format (SOAP):

Number and title of the problem

S *Subjective findings*—Statements made by the patient, how the patient feels, other information from the patient's family.

O *Objective findings*—What the examiner observes or measures; specific things done for or to the patient; results of laboratory, x-ray film, and other diagnostic reports.

A *Assessment*—Evaluation and interpretation of the patient's status (S plus O). Assessment may be what the examiner thinks is happening, reasons for changing management of the problem, or significance of the findings; it may be expressed as an impression or as a diagnosis.

P *Plan*—Diagnostic, therapeutic, and/or educative methods that will be used.

After the database has been completed and evaluated, the POMR may appear as follows:

Problem list

Nov. 4, 20__
　　Problem No. 1: Hypertension, essential arterial
　　Problem No. 2: Obesity, exogenous
　　Problem No. 3: Upper abdominal pain—Resolved 11/7/__

Plan

Nov. 4, 20__
　　Problem No. 1: Aldactazide 50 mg, 1 tab bid; recheck patient in 1 week
　　Problem No. 2: 1200-calorie diet; multivitamin ×1 daily; suggested to patient to join a weight-reducing group
　　Problem No. 3: UGI series; oral cholecystogram

Progress notes

Nov. 4, 20__
　　Problem No. 1: Hypertension, essential arterial
　　　　S—patient states that fatigue and headaches decreasing somewhat
　　　　O—BP ↓ 20 points to 160/84

　　　　A—positive effects from the medication
　　　　P—continue medication for 2 weeks; then to be checked
　　Problem No. 2: Obesity
　　　　S—patient has joined a weight-reducing group but states that she hates dieting
　　　　O—wt down 4 lb to 176 lb
　　　　A—dieting effective
　　　　P—continue 1200-calorie diet and multivitamin ×1 daily
　　Problem No. 3: Upper abdominal pain
　　　　S—patient states that the abdominal pain is less severe but persists
　　　　O—UGI and GB series negative; no abdominal distention
　　　　A—deferred until all results complete
　　　　P—abdominal ultrasound
Nov. 11, 20__
　　Problem No. 1: Hypertension
　　　　S—patient states that headaches have stopped, but she still remains fatigued
　　　　O—BP 140/84
　　　　A—medication effective
　　　　P—reduce Aldactazide to 1 tab daily
　　Problem No. 2: Obesity
　　　　S—patient states is now adjusting to the diet much better
　　　　O—wt ↓ 2 lb to 174
　　　　A—weight loss will benefit problem No. 1
　　　　P—continue 1200-calorie diet
　　Problem No. 3: Upper abdominal pain
　　　　S—patient states pain has subsided 11/7/__
　　　　O—x-ray results and ultrasound reports negative
　　　　A—temporary condition, resolved 11/7/__
　　　　P—patient to report if pain recurs and advised that x-ray film studies and ultrasound were negative

As you can see, the POMR is an orderly method of providing a chronologic profile of a patient that helps the physician and other health care providers conduct total patient care. This system provides a quick current reference of the patient's medical record, including problem management. It greatly reduces the possibility of an oversight, especially for patients receiving long-term care or those with multiple problems.

RECORDS MANAGEMENT

Records and Documentation

The medical record is the most important tangible element in legal medicine. The patient's record provides the information necessary to determine if medical services were given in accordance with the standards of care recognized by law, and it should include the patient's acceptance or refusal of medical advice. The record should clearly indicate the patient's failure to comply with treatment plans or keep necessary appointments for follow-up care and the physician's attempts to inform the patient of the necessity of care.

The physician and any other personnel responsible for making contributions to the patient's record should be careful to avoid unprofessional comments such as slang or colloquial terms; criticisms of patient's lifestyle, previous physicians, or medical care; or terms such as *error, mistake,* and *inadvertently.*

Although the *medical record* is considered the *property of the physician* or the physician's place of employment because he or she acquired, compiled, and interpreted the information, other persons have legal access to it. Patients or their attorneys may acquire copies for review. If a lawsuit is filed, the patient's records become available to the legal representatives of the plaintiff and defendant and to the court. They are also available to federal or state agencies responsible for payment of the medical care or private (health, life, or disability) insurance companies with the written consent of the patient.

It is in the patient's and the physician's best interests if the records are accurate, complete, and legible. If these three criteria are met, the physician has an important tool in the prevention of or defense against professional liability claims.

Confidentiality.   Properly maintaining and storing patients' medical records ensure the confidentiality of the information contained in them. You should think of the record as the person and provide the same privacy for the record as you would provide for the patient. This creates an atmosphere in which the patient can feel confident in being totally frank with the physician.

Permanent protection.   A medical record is a permanent proof of care and is credible, regardless of the time elapsed since an entry was made. Because a lawsuit may be filed years after an event, the record is considered more reliable than the physician's memory. For the record to provide protection, it must be carefully prepared and maintained.

Entries
Unalterable entries.   The entries in a medical record are unalterable. In other words, notes written in a patient's medical record *cannot* be changed or removed. Should an error be recognized, a specific technique should be used to correct it. If records are handwritten, all notations should be made in a neat and legible manner in blue or black ink.

Authorized personnel.   Because of the importance of the medical record, office policy should be established that indicates which personnel are authorized to make entries in a patient's record. As a professional medical assistant, you will undoubtedly be responsible for medical records, including entry making. You must always keep in mind the importance of the medical record for patient care and for legal purposes.

Entries to be avoided.   A thoughtless comment in a patient's chart could give the impression that the physician is uninterested in the care or prejudiced in his or her opinion of the patient. This impression can influence the credibility of the physician and the quality of care provided. Humorous or sarcastic remarks should never be written in a patient's record. Physicians and assistants should also take care not to attempt to describe another physician's findings or treatments. Information provided by the patient can be enclosed in quotation marks to indicate the source. If more information is required, the patient can sign a records release so that the other physician's records can be acquired.

Corrections
Reasons for corrections.   Occasionally it is necessary to make a correction in the progress notes of a patient's record. This occurs when incorrect data are recorded in the patient's record or when an entry is made in the wrong chart. For example, as you record a patient's weight as 103 pounds, you note that it was recorded as 156 pounds on a previous visit. One of the notations must be incorrect. The fact should be rechecked, and the entry corrected. If you have several charts in your hands at one time, you could inadvertently make an entry intended for the chart of one patient in the progress notes of another. Again, a correction is in order.

Correction technique.   Any information noted in the chart, whether factual or not, becomes part of the permanent record. You must *never* attempt to obliterate a chart entry. If an error in charting is discovered, you should correct is as follows:

1. Strike a single line through the error.
2. Date and initial the strikeout.
3. If the data are incorrect, enter the correct information directly below the strikeout. Date and initial the entry.
4. If the entry is made in the wrong chart, follow Step 1 and note "Recorded in chart by error. Information transferred to chart of John C. Adams."
5. Date and sign the strikeout and explanation.

Step four is vital for legal purposes because the information can be verified, and moving the information from one file to another is not considered a breach of confidentiality.

Always identify the reason for the correction, for example:

~~4/24/01   3pm BP 186/84~~   4/24/01   J. Wright CMA
4/24/01—3:05 PM Mistaken entry above. BP 136/84
    J. Wright, CMA

Statistical information.   Physicians may wish to gather and evaluate data on the effectiveness of a treatment plan or follow the course of several patients with the same diagnosis. Medical records can provide this information, which can be abstracted and maintained in a separate file. The increasing use of computers to store records and abstract data is a great help with statistical information. However, this information, whether abstracted by you or a computer, is still confidential and must be protected.

Retention of Medical Records
Period of retention.   Debates are ongoing concerning the amount of time that records should be retained after certain events such as treatment of a minor, closure of a case, death of a patient, retirement of the physician, and death of the physi-

cian. Opinions vary from one state to another and according to whether they belong to an attorney, a medical association, or a management consultant.

When care involves a minor, the record should always be kept at least until the child becomes an adult and thereafter until the local statute of limitations runs out.

Closure of a case (for example, the care of a specialist) may warrant destroying a chart after a given period. Most agree that the chart should be retained for at least 10 years.

If the death of a patient is uncomplicated, some suggest that the chart be retained through the statute of limitations and then destroyed.

If a physician retires, the charts of deceased patients may be destroyed after a specified time following the death. After appropriate notification, the records of living patients may be transferred to the physician who continues the practice or to a physician of the patient's choice on receipt of a written authorization.

When a physician dies, the patient's records are put under the care of a custodian of records, often the physician's spouse or a former employee who is willing to perform the duties involved. The disposition of the record is similar to that done for a physician's retirement.

General advice.   Because of the increasing frequency of professional liability suits and the variations in statutes, many authorities are beginning to agree that the only safe option is to retain medical records forever. If the physician retires or dies, records that are requested should be forwarded and the others retained by the physician or his or her heir.

Storage sites.   Inactive records may be stored in specifically designed file-storage boxes in a storage area on the office premises, with a professional storage company, or on microfilm. For an ongoing practice, storing the records on the premises is ideal because inactive records may be needed from time to time. Professional storage facilities are appropriate if the physician has retired or dies. Microfilm is an ideal option from the perspective of saving space, but it is relatively expensive.

SPECIAL VOCABULARY

Vocabulary Used to Describe Pain

In performing the complete history and physical examination, the examiner must deal with a variety of terms relating to pain. The following are some of these particular terms, along with an explanation of each.

Pain is a very **subjective symptom**, usually having both a physical and a mental component. The experience and related feelings vary greatly among people. How a person expresses, does not express, or tolerates pain is also subjective. Some people don't express pain, but that doesn't mean they are not experiencing it; often they adapt to it. Adaptation can be dangerous because pain may be a warning signal, and becoming used to it and ignoring it can result in damage to the body. On the other hand, people who have pain for long periods often have a

decreased tolerance to pain. All pain is real and must be acknowledged. Recognition and proper management of pain are important in total patient care. (See the box on p. 144.)

PAIN VOCABULARY

colicky—Acute intermittent abdominal pain usually caused by spasmodic contractions.

excruciating—Torturing, extreme pain, often intractable.

exquisite—Immense pain to which an individual is extremely sensitive.

guarding—A reflex usually related to abdominal pain; the action of tensing muscles, drawing up knees, and/or placing a hand over a part to prevent examination or protect against increasing pain.

intractable—Unmanageable; not controllable with conventional means such as rest, heat, or medication.

radiating—Diverting from a common central point (for example, gallbladder pain begins in the right upper quadrant of the abdomen, and it is diverted from that central point to the right flank and right scapular area).

rebound tenderness—A sensation of pain felt when pressure applied on a body part is released.

stabbing—Deep, sharp, intermittent pain.

threshold—The level that must be exceeded for an effect to be produced; the level of pain that an individual can tolerate without external intervention. Threshold is unique to each individual, and the overall physiopsychologic makeup of an individual must be considered when evaluating pain.

transient—Fleeting, brief, passing, coming and going.

types of pain
- Superficial or cutaneous
- Deep pain—From muscles, tendons, joints
- Visceral pain—From the viscera (any large interior organ in any great body cavity, especially in the abdomen)

Vocabulary Used When Recording Physical Findings

The following vocabulary lists *some* of the terms that the examiner may use when recording the **objective** findings of the physical examination of a patient. Each term is presented under the body part or system for which it is used when describing the findings of the physical examination. If you have completed studies in medical terminology, these terms should be familiar; if not, by referring to Appendix A, you should be able to define, pronounce, and become familiar with each term.

Skin

Abrasion	Laceration
Avulsion	Petechiae
Contusion	Purpura
Cyanosis	Turgor
Ecchymosis	Ulcer
Erythema	Urticaria
Jaundice	

HEALTH **MATTERS**

PAIN ASSESSMENT: THE FIFTH VITAL SIGN

Assembly Bill 791 (Thomson) was signed into law by Governor Gray Davis on September 15, 1999, and became effective January 1, 2000. Section 1254.7 was added to the Health and Safety Code (HSC) as part of this bill. HSC 1254.7 reads:

(a) It is the intent of the Legislature that pain be assessed and treated promptly, effectively, and for as long as pain persists.

(b) Every health facility licensed pursuant to this chapter shall, as a condition of licensure, include pain as an item to be assessed at the same time as vital signs are taken. The health facility shall insure that pain assessment is performed in a consistent manner that is appropriate to the patient. The pain assessment shall be noted in the patient's chart in a manner consistent with other vital signs.

This legislative mandate is consistent with state and federal concerns regarding appropriate pain management for all persons. The Veterans Administration has adopted similar policies, referring to pain as the fifth vital sign.

In 1994, the BRN adopted a pain management policy for RN practice and pain management curriculum guidelines for nursing programs. Both of these documents include a standard of care for California RNs of assessing pain and evaluating response to pain management interventions using a standard pain management scale based on patient self-report. This new law places a similar requirement on licensed health care facilities. Nursing programs need to integrate pain as the fifth vital sign into their curricula and health facilities need to educate staff regarding pain management.

It is now required that all health care staff record pain assessment each time that vital signs are recorded for each patient. If the institution is using the zero-to-ten pain assessment scale, a recording of "pain 2/10" fulfills the requirements of this law. The Board reminds RNs that pain assessment is based on patient self-report and that patients can be asleep and still experience significant pain; appropriate charting would be to write "asleep" for the pain rating. Registered nurses will continue to be required to monitor all five vital signs and take appropriate action based on deviations from normal. In other words, a competent RN intervenes when the patient's pain is not being managed according to the agreed-upon comfort level.

Registered nurses should remember that *prn* means "in the nurse's judgment." In regards to pain medications that are ordered prn, RNs can choose to give the medication routinely, around the clock. In many acute pain situations, such as postoperative or post-trauma, medications ordered q 4h prn (every 4 hours as needed), for example, should be given (or at least offered) q 4h (every 4 hours) routinely for the first 24 to 48 hours to keep ahead of the patient's pain. Research shows that when a patient's acute pain is managed around the clock and the pain level is kept from becoming severe, the total amount of opioid needed is reduced. (See Fig. 5-44, *C*, p. 233.)

From: The BRN Report, California Board of Registered Nursing, Sacramento, CA.

Eyes
Acuity	Nystagmus
Adnexa	Papilledema
Arcus senilis	Ptosis
Fundus of the eye	

Ears
Cerumen	Tympanic membranes

Nose
Nares	Nasal septal defect

Neck
Carotid pulse	Supple
Range of motion	

Cardiovascular system (CVS)
Bruit	Ischemia
Congestion	Murmur
Ecchymosis	Petechiae
Engorgement	Purpura
Erythema	Resuscitation
Gallop	Rub
Infarction	Thrill

Respiratory system
Fremitus	Rhonchi
Friction rub	Sputum
Rales	Stridor
Resonance	

Abdomen
Ascites	Hernia
Contour	Protuberant
Distention	Rigidity
Flaccid	Scaphoid

Gastrointestinal (GI) system
Caries	Fistula
Distention	Hemorrhoid
Fissure	Peristalsis

Reproductive system
Adnexa	Introitus
Atrophy	Involution
Gravida	Para

Genitourinary (GU) system
Discharge	Introitus

Musculoskeletal (MS) system—neurologic and extremities examination
Claudication	Lordosis
Clubbing	Passive congestion
Crepitation	Protuberance
Edema	Rigidity

Exostosis
Flaccid
Gait
Kyphosis

Scoliosis
Supple
Ulcer
Varicosity

General

Cachexia
Dehydration
Diaphoresis
Emaciation

Fingerbreadth
Lethargic
Patulous *or* distended
Tenderness

MEDICAL ABBREVIATIONS

In a patient's medical case history, physical examination report, and notes on the chart, you will encounter a variety of abbreviations. The following list includes some of the more common abbreviations. They are grouped together according to general usage. Pay special attention to when capital letters are and are not used. Prescription abbreviations are given in Chapter 7, and others are given in the appropriate chapters.*

Body systems

HEENT—head, eyes, ears, nose, and throat
ENT—ear, nose, and throat
CR—cardiorespiratory
CVS—cardiovascular system
GI—gastrointestinal
GU—genitourinary
CNS—central nervous system
MS—musculoskeletal
NS—nervous system
NM—neuromuscular

Patient's history

CC—chief complaint
PI *or* HPI—present illness *or* history of present illness
PH—past history
LMD—local medical doctor
UCHD *or* UCD—usual childhood diseases
FH—family history
a & w *or* A & W—alive and well
ROS—review of systems
PTA—prior to admission
c/o—complains of

Physical examination (PE)

wd—well-developed
wn—well-nourished
IPPA—inspection, percussion, palpation, and auscultation
P & A—percussion and auscultation
BP—blood pressure
TPR—temperature, pulse, and respirations
WNL—within normal limits
wt—weight
ht—height

Diagnosis

Diag *or* Dx—diagnosis
R/O—rule out
POS—problem-oriented system

Ears

TM—tympanic membrane(s)

Eyes

REM—rapid eye movement
L & A—light and accommodation
PERLA—pupils equal and reacting to light and accommodation
EOM—extraocular movement
RRE—round, regular, and equal
OS—left eye
OD—right eye
OU—both eyes

Chest (heart and lungs)

P & A—percussion and auscultation
PND—paroxysmal nocturnal dyspnea
SOB—shortness of breath
PMI—point of maximal intensity (or impulse)
MCL—midclavicular line
ICS—intercostal space
NSR—normal sinus rhythm
RSR—regular sinus rhythm
RRR—regular rate and rhythm
ASCVD—arteriosclerotic cardiovascular disease
cva—costovertebral angle
ASHD—arteriosclerotic heart disease
MI—myocardial infarction
EKG *or* ECG—electrocardiogram
AV—arteriovenous, atrioventricular
CHF—congestive heart failure
RHD—rheumatic heart disease
URI—upper respiratory infection
CPR—cardiopulmonary resuscitation
PVC—premature ventricular contraction
COPD—chronic obstructive pulmonary disease
CHD—coronary heart disease

Abdomen and GI

LKS—liver, kidney, spleen *or* LKKS—liver, kidneys, and spleen
GB—gallbladder
BM—bowel movement
DRE—digital rectal examination

Female reproductive system

BUS—Bartholin, urethral, and Skene glands
LMP—last menstrual period
OB—obstetrics
PID—pelvic inflammatory disease
GYN—gynecology
EDC—expected date of confinement
FHT—fetal heart tones
FHR—fetal heart rate
L & D—labor and delivery
PP—postpartum
IUD—intrauterine device

*According to the style of the American Medical Association, medical and pharmaceutical abbreviations are to be written *without* the use of periods (for example, rather than writing *a.c.,* as was done in the past, you will now write *ac*).

SAB—spontaneous abortion (miscarriage)
TAB—therapeutic abortion

Musculoskeletal system

EMG—electromyogram
MS—multiple sclerosis
LOM—loss of movement or motion
cva—costovertebral angle
DTR—deep tendon reflexes
L1, L2, etc.—first lumbar vertebra, second lumbar vertebra, etc.
T1, T2, etc.—first thoracic vertebra, second thoracic vertebra, etc.
RUE—right upper extremity
LUE—left upper extremity
RLE—right lower extremity
LLE—left lower extremity
DJD—degenerative joint disease
ROM—range of motion
A/P—anterior/posterior
NSAID—nonsteroidal antiinflammatory drug(s)

Central nervous system (CNS)

CSF—cerebrospinal fluid
CVA—cerebrovascular accident
EEG—electroencephalogram
DTR—deep tendon reflexes

Laboratory

HIV—human immunodeficiency virus
HAV—hepatitis A virus
HBV—hepatitis B virus
HCV—hepatitis C virus
HDV—hepatitis D virus
HEV—hepatitis E virus
HSV—herpes simplex virus
HPV—human papilloma virus
CBC—complete blood count
UA—urinalysis
O_2—oxygen
CO_2—carbon dioxide
CSF—cerebrospinal fluid
SMA—sequential multiple analysis
HGB *or* HG *or* Hb *or* Hgb—hemoglobin
Hct—hematocrit
WBC—white blood (cell) count
RBC—red blood (cell) count
Diff—differential (blood count)
Protime *or* PT—prothrombin time
PTT—partial thromboplastin time
pH—hydrogen ion concentration, referring to the degree of acidity or alkalinity of a solution
BUN—blood urea nitrogen
Sedrate—sedimentation rate
ESR—erythrocyte sedimentation rate
Rh—Rhesus blood factor
PKU—phenylketonuria
FBS—fasting blood sugar
GTT—glucose tolerance test

PBI—protein-bound iodine
PCV—packed cell volume
RF—rheumatoid factor
RhA—rheumatoid arthritis
STS—serologic test for syphilis
VDRL—Venereal Disease Research Laboratory (blood test for syphilis)
RPR—rapid plasma reagin
PSA—prostate-specific antigen
C & S—culture and sensitivity
CPK—creatine phosphokinase
LDH—lactate dehydrogenase
SGOT—serum glutamic oxaloacetic transaminase (now known as AST)
AFB—acid-fast bacillus
O & P—ova and parasites
Chol—cholesterol
HDL—high-density lipoprotein
LDL—low-density lipoprotein
HGH—human growth hormone
EMIT—enzyme immunoassay for drug screening
staph—*Staphylococcus*
strep—*Streptococcus*
2 hr pc—2 hours post cibum (2 hours after a meal)
2 hr pp—2 hours postprandial (2 hours after a meal)
T_3, T_4—thyroid tests
TSH—thyroid stimulating hormone

X-ray film studies

A-P and Lat—anterior-posterior and lateral
IVP—intravenous pyelogram
GBS—gallbladder series
CT—computed tomography
MRI—magnetic resonance imaging
BE—barium enema
KUB—kidneys, ureter, bladder
UGI—upper gastrointestinal series

Surgical terms

T & A—tonsillectomy and adenoidectomy
D & C—dilation and curettage
I & D—incision and drainage
TUR—transurethral resection
TURP—transurethral resection of the prostate

Hospital departments

ICU—intensive care unit
CCU—coronary care unit
ER *or* ED—emergency room *or* emergency department
OR—operating room
RR *or* PAR—recovery room *or* postanesthetic room
Lab—laboratory
Path—pathology
SNF—skilled nursing facility
OPD—outpatient department
Peds—pediatrics
OB-GYN—obstetrics and gynecology
RT—respiratory therapy

PT—physical therapy
OT—occupational therapy

General

Pt *or* pt—patient
c/o—complaining of
Hx—history
ADL—activities of daily living
Ca *or* CA—cancer or carcinoma
d/c *or* D/C—discontinue
DOA—dead on arrival
OD—overdose
cm—centimeter
lb—pound
kg or kilos—kilograms
ac—before meals
pc—after meals
stat—immediately
prn—whenever necessary
ad lib—as desired
ASAP—as soon as possible
BR—bed rest
BP—blood pressure
I & O—intake and output
IM—intramuscular
IV—intravenous
sc or SubQ—subcutaneous
LP—lumbar puncture
NPO—nothing by mouth
D/W—dextrose in water
S/W—saline in water
NS—normal saline
DOB—date of birth
FUO—fever of unknown (or undetermined) origin
CDC—Centers for Disease Control and Prevention
DPT—diphtheria, pertussis, tetanus (immunizations)
Td—tetanus and diphtheria
Dx—diagnosis
Rx—prescription; also often used for "treatment"
STD—sexually transmitted disease (the newer term replacing VD for venereal disease)
TB—tuberculosis
LLQ—left lower quadrant (of the abdomen)

LUQ—left upper quadrant (of the abdomen)
RLQ—right lower quadrant (of the abdomen)
RUQ—right upper quadrant (of the abdomen)
WF, BF—white female, black female
WM, BM—white male, black male
y/o—years old
GC—gonococcus or gonorrhea
K—potassium
LE—lupus erythematosus
SLE—systemic lupus erythematosus
STG—short-term goals
LTG—long-term goals
w/—with
w/o—without
h—hour
NYD—not yet diagnosed
PM—postmortem
O_2—oxygen
CO_2—carbon dioxide
TLC—tender loving care

Symbols

>—greater than
<—less than
♂—male
♀—female
↑—above, increase
↓—below, decrease
×—times (multiply by)
%—percentage
#—number *or* pound
=—equals
+—plus *or* positive
−—minus *or* negative
$\bar{o}$—none
$\bar{c}$—with
$\bar{s}$—without
$\bar{a}$—before
$\bar{p}$—after
×/d—times per day

Additional abbreviations frequently used for medications are given in Chapter 7.

CONCLUSION

You have now completed the chapter on health history and physical examinations. You will be expected to discuss the parts of a patient's health history and its importance, together with other components that make up a medical record. In addition, you should be able to describe the methods used by a physician when performing a physical examination. When you are familiar with the contents of this chapter, arrange with your instructor to take a performance test.

REVIEW OF VOCABULARY

The following are samples of a patient's medical history and physical examination and samples of SOAP charting. A consultation letter and a hospital discharge summary as dictated by a physician are also included. *These are to help familiarize you with the format and contents of medical reports.* Read these and be prepared to discuss the contents and define all the medical terms that are used. You should recognize some of the terms; others are new, and you may have to refer to Appendix A or to a medical dictionary for the definitions.

History and Physical Examination
PATIENT: Patrick Nelson
PHYSICIAN: S. Kennedy, MD
DATE: November 12, 20__
CHIEF COMPLAINT: None
HISTORICAL DATA: This 27-year-old white male enters for a physical evaluation. Actually he has no complaints but thinks that it is wise to have a general physical evaluation.
PAST MEDICAL HISTORY: The patient states that he had the usual childhood diseases. He had the flu in 1984, moderately severe. The patient received all of his immunizations.
Operations: Tonsillectomy as a child.
Injuries: Broken bones and unconsciousness, none.
PERSONAL HISTORY: The patient is single and works with his father.
FAMILY HISTORY: His father and mother are both living, of middle age, and well. He has an older sister and a younger brother, both in good health.
HABITS: The patient smokes a package to a package and a half of cigarettes per day. Alcoholic intake, about 4 oz per week.
MEDICATIONS: None.
SYSTEM REVIEW
Head and neck
　　Eyes: The patient is myopic and wears glasses all the time. He denies headaches or visual disturbances.
　　Ears, nose, and throat: Not remarkable.
Cardiorespiratory: The patient denies all symptoms in this system, except for being soft. He states that he gets no regular exercise and when he does sudden exercise, he becomes short of breath.
Gastrointestinal: His appetite is excellent. His weight is stable at approximately 160 pounds. Digestion is good. Bowels are regular with use of laxatives. He states that he had some minor hemorrhoid problems in the past.
Genitourinary: The patient denies nocturia. He urinates several times daily without difficulty. There is no history of kidney stones, bladder infections, or bleeding.
Neuromuscular osseous: The patient recently had a backache from which he has made a satisfactory recovery. Orthopedic consultation at that time was negative.
PHYSICAL EXAMINATION
Height: 72 inches.
Weight: 167 pounds.
Blood pressure: 144/80.

Temperature: 98.6° F
Pulse rate: 76 and regular.
Respirations: 16 per minute.
The general impression is that of a well-developed, well-nourished white male, who appears to be in no acute distress. He is slightly obese, pleasant, and cooperative.
Head and neck
Eyes: Patient has a positive cover test, with a latent exophoria. He is highly myopic. Funduscopic examination is otherwise not remarkable.
Ear, nose, and throat: Normal. The neck is supple. The trachea is in the midline. The thyroid is not palpable. The neck veins are collapsed.
Chest: Clear to percussion and auscultation. There is good diaphragmatic descent bilaterally. Breath tones are normal. No adventitious sounds are heard.
Heart: The left border of cardiac tonus is 6 cm from the mid-sternal line, with the point of maximum impulse at the fourth intercostal space. The rhythm is regular. No murmurs or adventitious sounds are heard.
Abdomen: Slightly rotund. The liver, spleen, and kidneys are not palpable. There are no masses or tenderness.
Genitalia: There is a normal male escutcheon. The penis is circumcised. Testes are in the scrotum. The inguinal rings are intact.
Rectal: Examination discloses good sphincter tone. The prostate is small, smooth, and symmetric. The ampulla is filled with soft, brown stool.
Extremities: There is no evidence of edema, cyanosis, or jaundice. Peripheral pulses are adequate. Most notable is the finding of several small glomus tumors on the fingers. Some of these are painful; others are not.
Neurologic: Intact.
Skin: Negative.
Lymphatics: Negative.
IMPRESSIONS
　1.　Normal, healthy male.
　2.　Glomus tumors.
　3.　Latent exophoria.
RECOMMENDATIONS
　1.　Routine urine and CBC.
　2.　Chest x-ray film.
　3.　Lose 10 pounds of weight.
　4.　Return as needed.

S. Kennedy, MD

Discharge Summary
HISTORY: The patient is a 36-year-old male, juvenile-onset diabetic, with multiple problems involving the gastrointestinal, genitourinary, and musculoskeletal systems.
PROBLEM NO. 1: Diabetes mellitus: onset at age 15 years, with two episodes of diabetic ketoacidosis at ages 15 and 20, with multiple admissions for hypoglycemic and hyperglycemic

symptoms. The patient states he has taken 55 units of Lente in the morning and 15 units of Lente in the evening for 20 years, with slight increases in these periodically, covering himself with regular, 15 units in the AM and 10 units in the PM. The patient is presently on 45 units of Lente and 15 units of regular in the morning, and 15 Lente and 10 regular in the PM, with urines running negative to 2+, with no ketones. The patient states he has not changed his dose or altered his eating habits or skipped a dose in the past 48 hours.

Twelve hours before admission, the patient noted the onset of mild nausea and vomiting, with abdominal distention, bloating, and intermittent diarrhea (brown). The patient denies bright red blood per rectum or per mouth, or melena. He denies loss of consciousness or lethargy, fever, chills, night sweats, cough, dysuria, pyuria, but does admit to polydipsia on a chronic basis. Complications from the diabetes include retinopathy, which was first noted in 1996 and treated with lasers; he denies any renal or neurologic complications (impotence, bladder, bowel). The patient has also had numerous abscesses in the perianal area and urinary tract infections, including pyelonephritis times one.

PROBLEM NO. 2: Gastrointestinal complaints: The patient has a greater than 15-year history of peptic ulcer disease, with a history of hematemesis and melena in 1994, for which he had an upper GI series that showed a suggestion of a swollen duodenal bulb and an endoscopy that read out as a normal examination. The patient also had acid studies done, which showed a basal secretion of 7.86 mEq per hour, going to a post-Histalog stimulation level of 35.7 mEq per hour. The findings were consistent with an ulcerogenic picture. It was elected not to do surgery at that time because of the lack of anything treatable. The patient was noted to have decreased gastric emptying, which was thought to be caused by an inadvertent vagotomy during his hiatal hernia repair in 1995.

The patient presently complains of epigastric pain, worse on lying, with heartburn, relieved by eating and taking antacids. The patient gives a history of melena for 3 days and hematemesis, two episodes in the past 2 months, without recurrence. The patient also takes aspirin for back pain. The patient has a past history of hepatitis A, treated in 1990, without recurrence.

PROBLEM NO. 3: Back pain, chronic: In 1995 the patient suffered trauma to his back, secondary to lifting a heavy object, which resulted in marked decrease in the strength in his lower extremities. The patient was evaluated at that time with an electromyogram (EMG), which was normal, and a myelogram, which showed protrusion of the nucleus pulposus in the L4-5 area. The patient was taken to surgery, where partial hemilaminectomy was done in December 1995. The patient states that he has had no cessation or relief of his back pain secondary to the operation. The patient denies any paresthesia, weakness, or asymmetry in motor sensory involvement in his lower extremities.

PROBLEM NO. 4: Chest pain, hypertension: The patient has a history of cardiac "attacks" in 1994 and 1995 times two and in 1996, requiring hospitalization. The patient was told each time that there was no heart damage. The patient describes the pain as substernal, radiating to the neck and back, without associated shortness of breath, palpitations, diaphoresis, but does state that it is precipitated by exercise on occasion or emotional stress. The patient has never had any EKG changes consistent with ischemia and/or infarct. The patient's history of high blood pressure runs in the 140/90 range and has been treated for 1½ years in the past, but he has presently been off medications. The patient states that episodes of chest pain come approximately one to two times per month and only last for seconds. The patient has been treated in the past with nitroglycerin in 1996 but no longer takes the medication.

PROBLEM NO. 5: Kidney problems: At the age of 10 years, the patient had pyelonephritis and subsequent recurrent urinary tract infections, which may or may not have included flank pain, fever, and chills. The patient has been treated in the past with antibiotics for his urinary tract infections, the most recent being 7 years ago. The patient has a past history of renal stones in 1996, left-sided, with a normal intravenous pyelogram. The patient was evaluated for calcium, phosphate, and oxalate in his urine, which were all within the normal range. The patient's creatinine level in the past has run around 1, with a BUN around 18 in 1996.

PAST MEDICAL HISTORY: Allergies: None. Illness: As above. Surgery: Note above. Habits: 25 years of smoking a pack a day; no alcohol. Medications: Note history of present illness.

SOCIAL HISTORY: The patient lives in Anytown, California, works as a chef, and presently is living with a girlfriend. The patient has been married three times and has one child, who is 14 years old, by his first wife.

FAMILY HISTORY: The family history is positive for diabetes in a maternal uncle and maternal great-grandmother. There is no history of myocardial infarction, high blood pressure, cerebrovascular accident, tuberculosis, rheumatic heart disease, endocrinopathies, or cancer.

REVIEW OF SYSTEMS: This is significant for head, eyes, ears, nose, and throat. He did have a headache in 1996, which was evaluated with an EEG and skull films, all of which were within normal limits; presently without complaint of headache. Lungs: He has been without pneumonia; negative PPD within the last year and half. Neurologic: The patient has a questionable history of psychiatric disease in the past with "rage attacks." The patient has not been evaluated further.

PHYSICAL EXAMINATION: Blood pressure was 140/96 lying, with a pulse rate of 92, going to 140/100 standing up, with a pulse rate of 116. Respirations were 20, temperature was 37° C. Generally, a well-developed male, appearing in no acute distress.

Skin: The skin had a midline abdominal scar and an abscess scar on the left medial buttock area. There were ingrown hairs on his anterior and posterior thoracic walls. There was no diaphoresis.

Head, eyes, ears, nose, and throat: Atraumatic; extraocular movements were positive; pupils were equal, round, and reactive to light, without nystagmus. The fundi were remarkable for increased tortuosity of his vessels, with hemorrhages and exudates present in both retinae; his discs were flat. Tympanic membranes showed old scarring, but normal light reflexes. Oropharynx was clear and edentulous.

Neck: Supple, without increase, decrease, or asymmetric thyroid enlargement; there were no bruits.

Node: No cervical, supraclavicular, axillary, or epitrochlear nodes. He did have positive occipital and inguinal nodes, old.

Lungs: Decreased respiratory movements; there was a slight increase in his AP diameter; positive end-inspiratory wheezing, with inspiration/expiration ratio of 1:1.2. The patient was without rales; he did have scattered rhonchi. No increased or decreased vocal or tactile fremitus was noted.

Cardiovascular examination: The cardiovascular examination showed a point of maximal impulse in the fifth intercostal space, midclavicular line; no heave, thrill, or thrust; no S-3, S-4, or murmur. Pulses were +2 and equal throughout, without bruits. The carotids were good and up bilaterally, without bruits.

Abdomen: The liver was 12 cm by percussion; no spleen, kidney, or bladder palpable; bowel sounds were active, without distention.

Rectal examination: The rectal examination was guaiac-negative; prostate was symmetrically enlarged, without nodularity or mass.

Extremities: There was full range of motion, without cyanosis, clubbing, or edema.

Neurologic examination: Oriented times three. Abstract thought and short- and long-term memory were intact. There was no sensory, motor, or cerebellar abnormality in his lower or upper extremities. Cranial nerves II through XII were within normal limits. His reflexes were +1 and equal throughout, except for absent ankle jerks, with down-going toes. Negative straight-leg raising. No root, grasp, or suck reflexes were noted.

LABORATORY DATA: He had a pH of 7.38, Po_2 of 67, and a Pco_2 on room air, with a bicarbonate of 24. His glucose was 855. His urinalysis showed +4 glucose, negative ketones. Chest x-ray film was without cardiopulmonary disease, and there was no air under the diaphragm. KUB showed no abnormalities. Sodium was 122, potassium 3.6, bicarbonate 28; BUN was 21, and creatinine level was 1.6. His EKG showed normal sinus rhythm, without acute changes.

HOSPITAL COURSE: The patient's hospital course was one of treatment with intravenous insulin and normal saline to correct the abnormalities noted from the hyperosmolar effect of the increased glucose load intravascularly. The patient responded well to rehydration and to IV insulin, receiving 10 units of IV insulin over a 4- to 6-hour period, with a blood glucose drop from 855 to 328. The patient at no time showed any evidence of ketoacidosis, with urines running in the 3 to 4+ range, with negative ketones, and bicarbonate staying in the 28 to 30 range. By morning, the glucose was 106, with negative-negative urine and a bicarbonate of 30. The patient was treated as an outpatient and started on a normal regimen, with 45 units of Lente and 15 units of regular in the morning, and 15 units of Lente and 10 units of regular in the evening. The patient responded well to therapy and is being discharged today for follow-up in my clinic.

The patient continued to be guaiac-negative in the hospital for the 2 days. The patient's epigastric complaints will be followed on an outpatient basis and worked up accordingly.

CHEST PAINS: The patient did have one episode of chest pain while in the hospital, with EKG during chest pain showing no abnormalities. The pain lasted for seconds and went away without medication.

The patient is being discharged with the following medications: Lente and regular insulin—45 units of Lente and 15 units of regular in the AM, and 15 units of Lente and 5 units of regular in the PM. Tylenol and codeine, one po q4h prn for low back pain.

Discharge Diagnosis

Diabetes, out of control, secondary to noncompliance
Epigastric pain
Low back pain
Chest pain

N.J. Hopew, MD

October 1, 20__

W.F. Mayhan, MD
124 Medical Drive
San Francisco, CA 94119

Dear Doctor Mayhan:

Ms. Catherine Holmes was seen for neurologic evaluation on September 28, 20__.

She is a 21-year-old, white, right-handed, single supermarket checker who complains of headaches.

The patient stated that on the evening of September 27, 20__, she fell and struck the back of her head against an upholstered arm of a couch. She was not rendered unconscious but did have a headache afterwards. Nevertheless, the remainder of the evening passed uneventfully, and she went to bed. The following morning she woke up and went to work. However, at approximately 10 o'clock she had the onset of a relatively severe headache with a feeling that her ears were popping and her eyes were glassy. In addition, she felt very tired. She complained of some nausea but did not vomit. She took aspirin, which has given her some degree of relief.

At the time of her examination, the patient was continuing to complain of a mild headache, but one that was not severe. She did feel extremely tired and wanted to rest at home. Approximately 1 year ago the patient had a concussion; however, she was not hospitalized and suffered no long-term adverse effects. She denies any history of other neurologic or general medical problems. She did have eye surgery a number of years ago for an extraocular muscle imbalance. She denied any history of surgery, fractures, or allergies. She smokes approximately a package of cigarettes per day and occasionally partakes of wine. Currently she is taking birth control medication, but no other agents.

Family history reveals her father to be suffering from hypertension. Her mother died approximately a year ago at the age of 46 from a cerebral hemorrhage, which, from her description, may have been a ruptured aneurysm. While speaking of her mother, the patient did become quite tearful.

EXAMINATION: The examination revealed a well-developed, well-nourished, white female. She was in no acute distress. She was alert, oriented, and cooperative.

Cranial nerve examination was normal. Deep tendon reflexes were active and symmetric. Plantar responses were downgoing.

Motor testing showed no upper extremity drift. No other evidence of gross or focal motor weakness was noted.

Sensory testing was intact to pinprick, as well as vibratory, sensation. Romberg test was negative.

Cerebellar testing showed no incoordination or decomposition of movements.

The patient's gait was normal for all modalities, including heel, toe, and tandem. No cranial or carotid bruits were heard. There was a full range of motion to her head and neck. Blood pressure was 100/60, right arm, sitting.

IMPRESSION: Status 1 day after head injury.

DISCUSSION: This patient's neurologic examination is unremarkable. She does complain of a residual headache that is the result of the blow she received to her head the evening before this examination. Currently she is feeling better with very minimal symptomatic treatment, and it is quite possible that this will resolve without any further aggressive management. I have given her a prescription for Darvocet-N 50 mg in the event her headache recurs or becomes more severe. In addition, I have indicated to her that if further difficulties arise, she should again contact us.

Thank you for giving me the opportunity to meet this very nice patient.

With best personal regards,

E. Schroeder, MD

SOAP Charting Examples

PROGRESS NOTES

DATE: 10/21/00

BP 139/81 Heart Rate: 85 wt: 185

DOB: 12/24/51

Problem: PE

S: Patient is applying to be a part-time employee at Derol Home Care. She is currently working as a NA at Lake Shore where she has been for 18 years. She would like to get some additional employment. She is generally feeling well although concerned about her weight. Main medical problems: asthma which is controlled with terbutaline 1 bid, Theo-Dur 200 mg 1½ tabs bid, Vanceril 2 puffs qd and may advance to 5-10 x/d if having asthma exacerbation, Albuterol nebulizer (not using this any longer), Serevent inhaler 2 puffs q12h, and Accolate 20 mg 1 bid. Patient also dealing with her eczema for which she uses triamcinolone 0.1% or hydrocortisone cream 1% if under good control. No longer taking Modicon. Using condoms intermittently. LMP: 10/6

O: See PE form

A: • Chronic asthma, under maximal treatment and doing quite well
    • Chronic eczema, doing fairly well with meds as above
    • Past motor vehicle accident with fracture of femur and humerus
    • Past bilateral ptosis
    • Intermittent depression, well at this time
    • Degenerative joint disease

P: Dx: PPD. CBC, metabolic panel, liver panel, TSH. UA is negative.
    EKG next visit as there was no nurse available for this today. Patient will phone with PPD results in 2 days, at which time I will complete her form for future employer.

PROGRESS NOTES

DATE: 4/3/01

BP: 110/70 HR: 72 wt: 125½

Problem: R shoulder pain

S: 48 y/o F, business analyst for PG Company, fell while on a cruise on the wet stairs. She injured her right shoulder on 2/15/01. Pt has had pain in the shoulder since that time. She also has reduced ROM. She does not think that there is a fracture but is worried because it has not improved.

O: ROM of R shoulder is somewhat reduced particularly in abduction. There is no tenderness over the acromion or the bicipital groove. She has limited ability on internal rotation. Standing: shoulders at unequal height.

A: 1. R shoulder injury, 2/15/99

P: Dx: X-ray of R shoulder
    Rx: May use ibuprofen for pain relief.

DATE: 8/12/01

Problem: Patient comes in complaining of pain in her neck.

S: She has been seeing a chiropractor, off plan, but she now has an insurance that does cover chiropractor care. She is on a computer all the time. She states that the adjustments to her neck and first rib help, but they don't seem to hold.

P: I gave her a slip to get a C-spine series and also a mammogram, which is overdue. I also gave her a slip to go to PT, although she wants to go to someplace downtown if at all possible. If that doesn't give her any improvement, she will consider chiropractic referral within her network.

CRITICAL THINKING SKILLS REVIEW

1. Information gathered on a history and physical examination is used for various purposes. List four of these purposes.
2. List and define the six parts of a patient's history.
3. The following information has been obtained from the physician's notes. For each statement, indicate where on the patient's record this information is recorded. Choose your answers from the following headings: chief complaint, history of present illness, past history, family history, social or occupational history, review of systems, physical examination, and impression.
   a. The patient is a 25-year-old white, obese female who was in good health until approximately 10 PM last evening.
   b. There is no history of past operations.
   c. Neck: Thyroid is not enlarged.
   d. Head: There is no history of headaches, sinus pain, or trauma.
   e. The arteries are full, soft, and readily compressible.
   f. "I have a lump in my left breast."
   g. Patient had measles and chickenpox when she was a child.
   h. R/O diabetes.
   i. Muscle tone is decreased in all four extremities.
   j. Patient's father has a history of hypertension for 5 years.
   k. GU system: There is no history of dysuria, hematuria, frequency, or nocturia.
   l. The patient denies the use of alcohol, tobacco, and drugs of any kind.
4. Define the following methods of examination, and state one body part or system that is examined in each method.
   a. Inspection
   b. Percussion
   c. Palpation
   d. Auscultation
   e. Mensuration
5. Describe the difference between the ROS and the PE.
6. List five forms of treatment that may be used for the care of a patient.
7. List three reasons why diagnostic studies are important for patient care.
8. State the purpose of the problem-oriented medical record.
9. List and explain the four parts of the problem-oriented medical record.

PERFORMANCE TEST

In a skills laboratory, a simulation of a joblike environment, the medical assistant student is to demonstrate knowledge and skill in obtaining identifying information and the medical history from a patient. The student may use a preprinted history form or make a list of questions that should be asked of the patient from the information presented in this chapter. For these activities the student needs a person to play the role of the patient and the necessary supplies. Time limits for the performance of this procedure are to be assigned by the instructor. (See also Grading on p. 104 in Chapter 3.)

The student is to perform these procedures with 100% accuracy 90% of the time (9 out of 10 times.)

The successful completion of each procedure will demonstrate competency levels as required by the AAMA, AMT, and future employers.

 ## INTERNET RESOURCES

National Association for Healthcare Quality
www.nahq.org

Healthfinder
(Maintained by the U.S. Department of Health and Human Services, this site provides basic self-care information and government health news.)
www.healthfinder.gov

Mayo Clinic Health Oasis
www.mayohealth.org

MedScape
www.medscape.com

CBS HealthWatch
www.cbshealthwatch.medscape.com

RealAge (news and health assessment tools)
www.realage.com

United States National Library of Medicine (information on general health)
www.nlm.nih.gov/medlineplus

MedicAlert
www.medicalert.org

The Alternative Medicine Homepage
www.pitt.edu/~cbw/altm.html

Choice in Dying
www.choices.org

The National Council on the Aging
www.ncoa.org

American Society on Aging
www.asaging.org

Cross cultural information affecting treatment and management for clinicians
http://healthlinks.washington.edu/clinical/ethnomed

Cultural competency training resources
www.yale.edu/implicit/raced/race1.html

Wellness Web Patient's Network
http://wellweb.com

Health Resources for Women of Color: Information from HHS Agencies and Programs (National Women's Health Information Center)
www.4women.gov/nwhic/minority.htm

Columbia University's Health Education Site
www.goaskalice.columbia.edu/Cat2.html

The National Institute of Diabetes and Digestive and Kidney Disease of The National Institute of Health
www.niddk.nih.gov/health/diabetes/dylb/home/htm

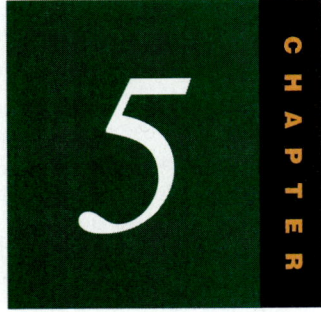

5

CHAPTER

Preparing for and Assisting With Routine and Special Physical Examinations

■ Cognitive Objectives

On completion of Chapter 5, the medical assistant student should be able to:

1. Define, spell, and pronounce the vocabulary terms.
2. State in summary form the medical assistant's responsibilities when assisting the physician during the examination of a patient.
3. List, identify, and state the function of each instrument commonly used during a complete physical examination, including rectal and vaginal examinations, a proctosigmoidoscopy, a neurologic examination, an ear examination, and an eye examination.
4. State two purposes for positioning a patient and three purposes for gowning and draping a patient for physical examinations.
5. State the purpose of and discuss the following special examinations: neurologic, ear, eye, gynecologic, obstetric, 6-weeks-postpartum visit, breast self-examination, and pediatric.
6. Discuss the special instructions that must be given to the patient before a Papanicolaou (Pap) smear is taken.
7. Discuss the Bethesda system that is used to report the results of a Pap smear.
8. List the information that should be included on a laboratory requisition when sending a specimen for a cytologic examination.
9. Identify and discuss regular clinical preventive services that are recommended by most U.S. medical authorities for normal-risk adults.
10. Explain the importance of breast and testicular self-examinations. Explain how these examinations should be performed.
11. Explain and compare the different methods of birth control available. Discuss the effectiveness of each method.
12. Explain which examinations are performed in a gynecologic examination. Discuss the purpose of each examination.
13. Explain what is done in a sigmoidoscopy. State three complications (however rare) that may occur following the examination.
14. Explain and discuss the special preparation required for a sigmoidoscopy and the consent form the patient must sign before the physician performs the examination.
15. Discuss the American Cancer Society's guidelines for examinations for the early detection of cancer in people without symptoms.
16. List and explain seven warning signals of cancer.
17. Differentiate between cancer that is localized and cancer that has metastasized.
18. Briefly discuss major cancer sites with reference to:
    a. Risk factors
    b. Risk reduction
    c. Examinations used for early detection
    d. Warning signs
    e. Treatment
    f. Special information listed
19. State the purpose for the Snellen Big E eye chart and when it is used.
20. Discuss the special instructions that must be given to a pregnant woman before she is tested for gestational diabetes.
21. Differentiate between an alpha-fetoprotein blood test, an amniocentesis, and a chorionic villi sampling test. State the purpose(s) of each test.
22. State the two broad classifications of pediatric patient physician office visits. State the purpose of each type of visit.
23. Discuss the guidelines for health supervision for a child's care.
24. Discuss general points that should be considered for a physical examination and office visit of a pediatric patient.
25. Discuss the reasons why keeping growth charts for infants and children is important. List the measurements that are recorded on these charts.

26. Discuss the disease *phenylketonuria (PKU)* and the recommended treatment. List the tests performed to diagnose this condition and state when each is usually performed.

27. Discuss the recommended schedule for an immunization program for an infant and child.

28. List six common immunizations given to children. State how each is administered.

29. Explain the purpose of giving the parent or legal representative of a child the Centers for Disease Control and Prevention (CDC) Vaccine Information Statements before a child can be vaccinated.

30. Explain how lead may enter the body. Discuss why lead poisoning is of special concern especially for children.

31. Identify five common sources of lead exposure for a child.

32. Discuss blood level screening for children and the importance of this procedure.

33. Discuss six methods that can be used to prevent lead poisoning.

34. Explain what is occurring in the breathing passageways of a person with asthma.

35. State what age group can be affected by asthma.

36. State four common signs and symptoms of asthma and recognize 10 early warning signs that can occur before breathing becomes difficult.

37. Discuss eight "triggers" that can lead to an asthma attack.

38. Summarize how a diagnosis of asthma is determined, along with some of the essential patient education and common treatment plans.

39. Explain the significance of peak flow values, comparing the three zones of values.

40. Discuss the purpose of pulse oximetry, indicating some common uses.

41. State five factors that can affect the accuracy of a pulse oximeter.

42. Explain the purposes for pulmonary function tests.

43. Discuss at least three causes of chronic obstructive pulmonary disease (COPD).

44. Explain nine common spirometry measurements.

45. Identify five reasons why a spirometry test should be delayed and done at a later time.

46. Explain to a patient how a spirometry test will be performed. Review the reasons for the test and any special instructions.

■ Terminal Performance Objectives

On completion of Chapter 5, the medical assistant student should be able to:

1. Prepare a patient for a physical examination by providing clear, simple instructions and explanations that are easy to understand.

2. Position and drape a patient in the positions outlined in this chapter.

3. Select, identify, and prepare equipment and supplies required for:
   a. A complete physical examination, which is to include a rectal examination and a pelvic examination with Pap smear.
   b. A proctosigmoidoscopy.

4. Demonstrate correct assisting techniques during physical examinations.

5. Assist the patient before, during, and after the examination.

6. Record the procedures and results (when applicable) of physical examinations.

7. Perform a breast self-examination if female. Explain this method of examination to a female patient.

8. Perform a testicular self-examination if male. Explain this method of examination to a male patient.

9. Measure a preschooler's and an adult's distance visual acuity using the Snellen eye charts.

10. Measure a patient's near visual acuity.

11. Measure color vision in a patient.

12. Assist a parent or caregiver in completing an initial health history form for a pediatric patient.

13. Demonstrate how to carry an infant in the cradle, upright, and football positions.

14. Take the following measurements on a child and record the results in the medical record and on the growth chart:
   a. Length or stature
   b. Weight
   c. Head circumference
   d. Chest circumference
   e. Vital signs

15. Demonstrate the method used to obtain a urine specimen from a child that is not toilet trained.

16. Obtain a blood specimen from an infant for a screening test for phenylketonuria (PKU).

17. Demonstrate the procedures used for performing a urine test to screen an infant for PKU.

18. Locate the sites and demonstrate the procedure used to give an intramuscular injection to a child.

19. Record the required information on a child's medical record after a vaccination has been administered.

20. Demonstrate and explain how to measure peak expiratory flow rates; record and discuss the results.

21. Demonstrate how to measure arterial blood oxygen saturation using a pulse oximeter and record the results.

22. Prepare a patient for a spirometry test. Demonstrate a correct method used to perform a single breath spirometry test.

23. Provide instructions and patient education that is within the professional scope of a medical assistant's training and responsibilities as assigned.

The student is to perform these skills with 100% accuracy 90% of the time (9 out of 10 times).

VOCABULARY

ACS—American Cancer Society

bimanual (bi-man'u-al)—With both hands, as in bimanual palpation.

bronchoscopy (bron-kos'kō-pĭ)—Internal inspection of the tracheobronchial tree with the use of a bronchoscope; used for diagnostic or treatment purposes. For diagnosis, the physician inspects the interior of the bronchi and may obtain a sample of secretions or a biopsy of tissue; for treatment, foreign bodies or mucous plugs that may be causing an obstruction to the air passages can be located and removed.

cystoscopy (sis-tos'ko-pĭ)—Internal examination of the bladder with a cystoscope. Samples of urine for diagnostic purposes can be obtained by passing a catheter through the cystoscope into the bladder or beyond, up into the ureters and kidneys. Also, radiopaque dyes may be injected through the cystoscope into the bladder or up into the ureters when taking x-ray films of the urinary tract.

digital (dij'it-al)—The use of a finger to insert into a body cavity such as the rectum for palpating the tissue.

endoscopy (en-dos'ko-pĭ)—Visual examination of internal cavities of the body with an endoscope (for example, a proctoscope, bronchoscope, cystoscope, gastroscope, and laryngoscope). (See Figure 5-1.)

gastroscopy (gas'tros'ko-pĭ)—Internal inspection of the stomach with a gastroscope.

oral examination—Examination pertaining to the mouth.

Papanicolaou (Pap) smear or test (pap"ah-nik"o-la'oo)—A smear examined microscopically to detect cancer cells from body excretions (urine and feces), secretions (vaginal fluids, sputum, or prostatic fluid), or tissue scrapings (as obtained from the stomach or uterus); most commonly done on a cervical scraping to detect abnormal or cancerous cells in the mucus of the uterus and cervix.

pelvic examination—Examination of the external and internal female reproductive organs.

prodrome—An early symptom indicating the onset of a disease (for example, an achy feeling before having the flu).

roentgenologic (rent-gĕn-ōl'oj-ic)—Pertaining to an examination with the use of x-ray film (radiographs).

sign (physical sign)—Any objective evidence (apparent to the observer) of disease or body dysfunction. Signs may be observed by others or revealed when a physician performs a physical examination (for example, swollen ankles, a distended rigid abdomen, elevated blood pressure, or decreased sensation). Signs often accompany symptoms, for example, a rash is often seen when a patient complains of itchiness.

symptom—Any subjective evidence of disease or body dysfunction; a change in the physical or mental state of the body that is perceptible or apparent only to the individual (for example, anorexia, nausea, headache, pain, or itching).

syndrome—A combination of symptoms having one cause or commonly occurring together to present a distinct clinical picture; an example is the dumping syndrome, which consists of nausea, weakness, varying degrees of syncope, sweating, palpitation, and sometimes diarrhea and a feeling of warmth. This may occur immediately after eating in patients who have had a partial gastrectomy.

subjective symptom—Symptom of internal origin that is apparent or perceptible only to the patient (for example, pain or dizziness [vertigo]).

symmetry (sim'et-ri)—Conformity in form, size, and arrangement of parts on opposite sides of the body.

INSTRUMENTS USED FOR PHYSICAL EXAMINATIONS (FIGURE 5-1)

anoscope (an'no-skōp)—A speculum or endoscope inserted into the anal canal for direct visual examination.

applicator—A slender rod of wood with a pledget of cotton on one end used to apply medicine or to take a culture from the body.

biopsy (bi'op-se) **forceps**—Two-pronged instruments of varying sizes and shapes used to remove tissue from the body for examination.

bronchoscope (brong'ko-skōp)—An endoscope designed specifically for passage through the trachea to allow visual examination of the interior of the tracheobronchial tree.

cystoscope (sist'o-skōp)—A hollow metal tube instrument (endoscope) designed specifically for passing through the urethra into the urinary bladder to permit internal inspection. The bladder interior is illuminated by an electric bulb at the end of the cystoscope. Special lenses and mirrors allow the bladder mucosa to be examined for calculi (stones), inflammation, or tumors.

endoscope (en'do-skōp)—A specially designed instrument made of metal or rubber (rigid or flexible) that is used for direct visual examination of hollow organs or body cavities. All endoscopes have similar working elements, even though the design varies according to its specific use. The viewing part (scope) is a hollow tube fitted with a lens system that allows viewing in a variety of directions. Each endoscope has a light source, power cord, and power source; examples include bronchoscope, cystoscope, proctoscope, and sigmoidoscope.

insufflator (in'suf'fla-tor)—An instrument, device, or bag used for blowing air, powder, or gas into a cavity.

laryngeal (lar-in'je-al) **mirror**—An instrument used to view the pharynx and larynx, consisting of a small, rounded mirror attached to the end of a slender (metal or chrome plate) handle.

laryngoscope (lar-in'go-skōp)—An endoscope used to examine the larynx. It is equipped with mirrors and a light for illumination of the larynx.

nasal speculum (na'zl spĕk'u-lŭm)—A short, funnel-like instrument used to examine the nasal cavity.

FIGURE 5-1 Instruments used for physical examinations. **A,** Laryngoscope; **B,** Sonnenschein nasal speculum; **C,** tuning forks; **D,** otoscope; **E,** Boucheron and Toynbee ear specula to be used with an otoscope; **F,** Miltex fiberglass tape measure; **G,** Tischler cervical biopsy punch forceps. (**B, C,** and **E** through **G** courtesy Miltex Instrument Co., Division of Miltenberg, Inc., Lake Success, NY.)

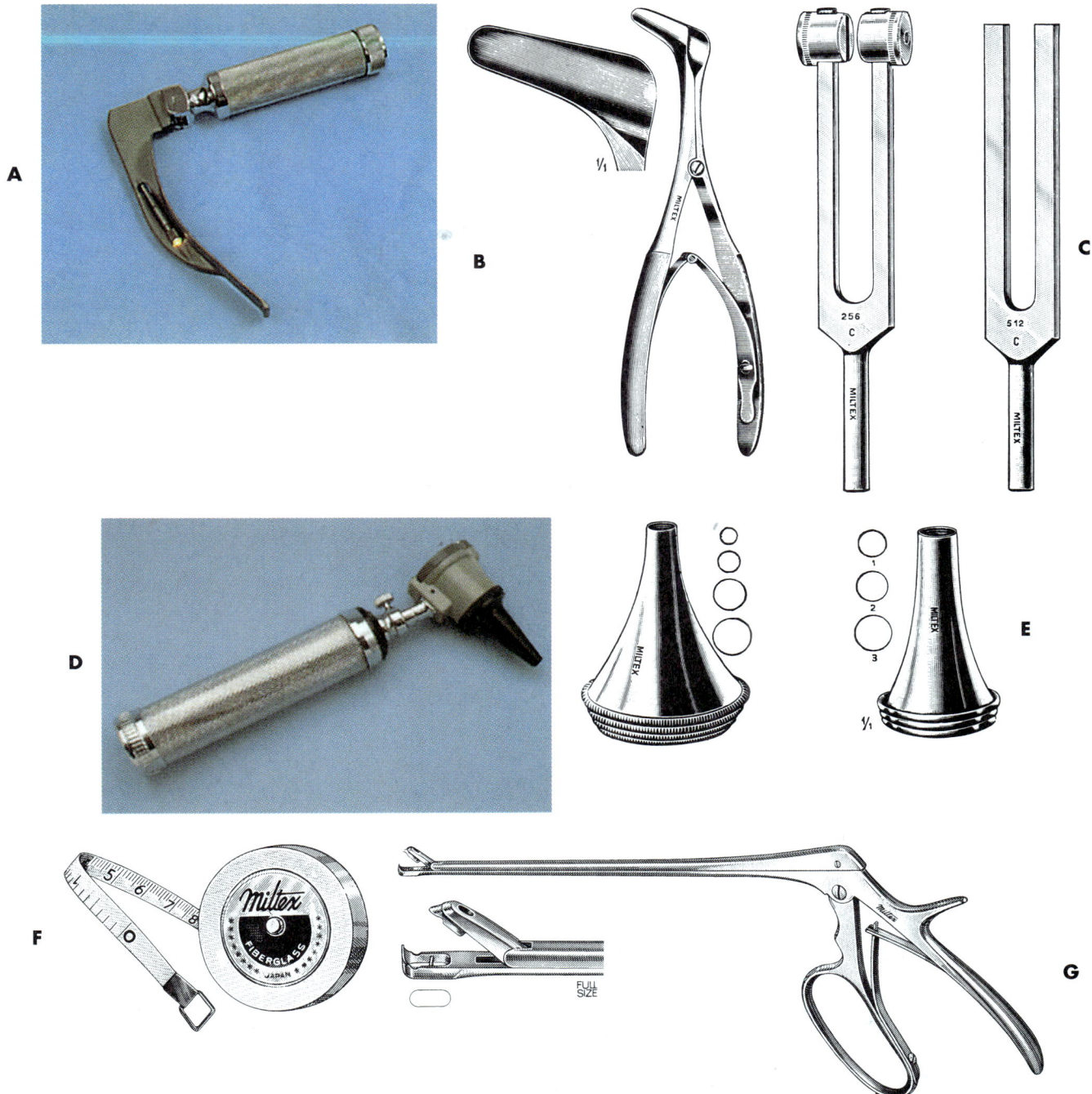

FIGURE 5-1—cont'd   Instruments used for physical examinations. **H,** Frankel head band and mirror set; **I,** Wartenberg neurologic pinwheel; **J,** laryngeal mirror; **K,** insufflator; **L,** percussion hammer; **M,** Graves vaginal speculum; **N,** ophthalmoscope. (**H** through **J, L,** and **M** courtesy Miltex Instrument Co., Division of Miltenberg, Inc., Lake Success, NY.)

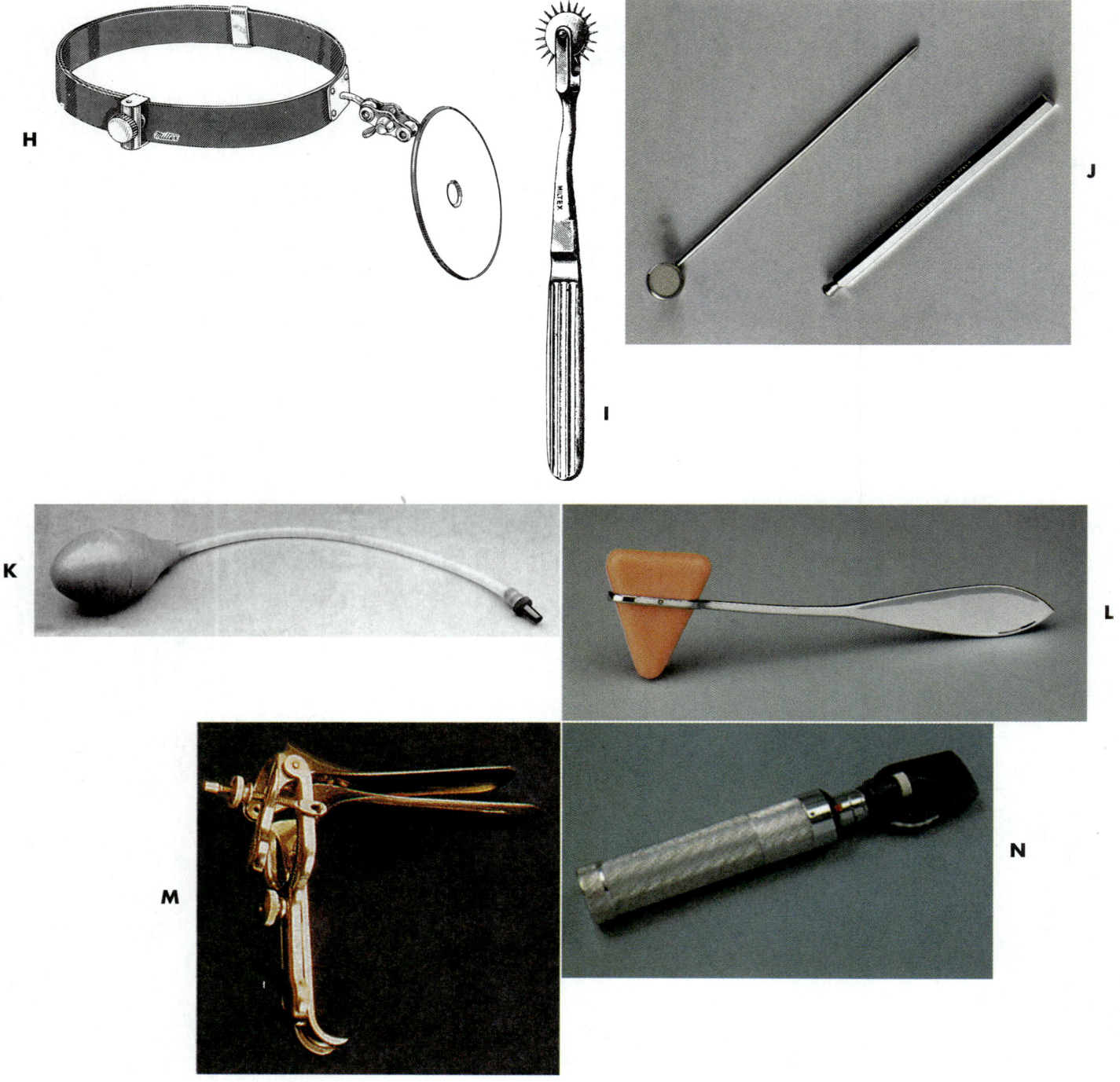

FIGURE 5-1—cont'd   Instruments used for physical examinations. **O,** Kelly proctoscope; **P,** Hirschman anoscope; **Q,** Schiotz tonometer with three weight (7.5, 10, and 15 g). **R,** Yeoman biopsy forceps; **S,** 60-cm fiberoptic flexible sigmoidoscope; **T,** metal 25- to 30-cm sigmoidoscope. (**O** through **R** courtesy Miltex Instrument Co., Division of Miltenberg, Inc., Lake Success, NY.)

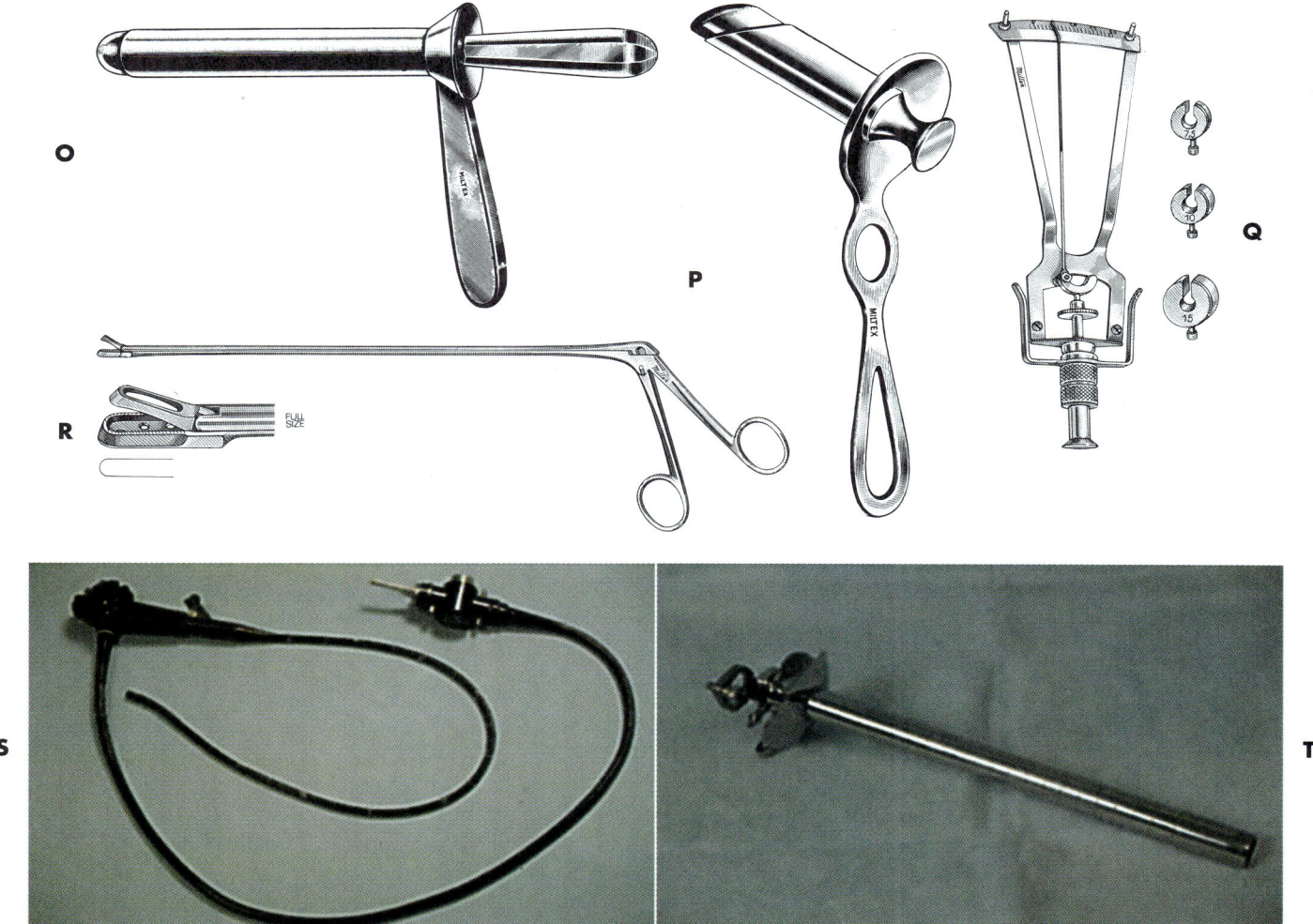

ophthalmoscope (ŏf'thăl'mō-skōp)—An instrument used for examining the interior parts of the eye. It contains a perforated mirror and lens. When the ophthalmoscope is turned on and brought close to the eye, it sends a narrow, bright beam of light through the lens of the eye. By looking through the lens of the instrument, the physician is then able to examine the interior parts of the eye, including the lens, anterior chamber, retinal structures, and blood vessels, to detect any possible disorders. Many ophthalmoscopes come with an interchangeable otoscope, throat illuminator head, or nasal illuminator head.

otoscope (o'tō-skōp)—An instrument used to examine the external ear canal and eardrum.

percussion (pur-kush'un) **hammer**—A small hammer with a triangular-shaped rubber head used for percussion.

proctoscope (prŏk'to-skōp)—A specially designed tubular endoscope that is passed through the anus to permit internal inspection of the lower part of the large intestine.

sigmoidoscope (sĭg-moy'dō-skōp)—A tubular endoscope used to examine the interior of the sigmoid colon.

speculum (spĕk'ū-lŭm)—An instrument used for distending or opening a body cavity or orifice to allow visual inspection; a bivalve speculum is one having two parts or valves.

Sims' vaginal speculum—A form of bivalve speculum used in the examination of the vagina and cervix. Vaginal specula come in three sizes: small, medium, and large. They are made of metal or disposable plastic.

stethoscope—An instrument used in auscultation to amplify the sounds produced by the lungs, heart, intestines and other internal organs; also used when taking a blood pressure reading (see p. 92).

tongue blade—A flat, thin, smooth piece of wood or metal with rounded ends approximately 6 inches long; also called a tongue depressor. It is used for pressing tissue down to permit a better view when examining the mouth and throat. In addition, it may be used for application of ointments to the skin.

tonometer (to-nom'e-ter)—An instrument used to measure tension or pressure, especially intraocular pressure.

tuning fork—A steel, two-pronged, forklike instrument used for testing hearing; the prongs give off a musical note when struck.

The consistent use of Universal/Standard Precautions is required by all health care professionals in all health care settings as a method of infection control. It is assumed that these precautions are used in all of the following procedures. Review Chapter 1 if you have any questions on methods to use because the methods or techniques are not repeated in detail in each procedure presented in this chapter.

Be sure to consult the latest guidelines issued by the Centers for Disease Control and Prevention (CDC) and consult with infection control practitioners when necessary to identify specific precautions that pertain to your particular work situation.

PREPARING FOR AND ASSISTING WITH PHYSICAL EXAMINATIONS

The physical examination is done in an examination or treatment room, whereas the history is commonly obtained from the patient in the physician's private office.

This chapter covers gowning, positioning, and draping the patient for an examination and preparing for and assisting with the common examinations performed by a physician—*one* method of conducting examinations and *one* group of instruments and equipment are included for each. The physician(s) or agency for whom you work may use other methods and equipment; you must be able and willing to adapt to individual needs as required.

General instructions to be followed and responsibilities to be assumed by medical assistants when assisting with every procedure and examination are listed in the next section. Keep them in mind as you prepare for all examinations because they are not repeated in each individual procedure.

Often, during any of the examinations that are outlined in this chapter, various types of specimens may be obtained. Detailed information for collecting and labeling specimens is covered in Chapter 11.

Cleansing and sterilization techniques for the care of used, nondisposable equipment are discussed in Chapter 2. Refer to these chapters for more specific information.

GENERAL INSTRUCTIONS AND RESPONSIBILITIES FOR THE MEDICAL ASSISTANT

1. Always wash your hands thoroughly before setting up the required equipment for an examination and assisting the physician.
2. Prepare the patient, the examination room, and the equipment and instruments required by the physician for the examination according to office or agency policy.
3. Make certain that electrical and battery-operated equipment and all lights are in working condition.
4. Place the equipment for the examination so that it is conveniently located for the physician's use.
5. Make sure that the examination room is comfortably warm, well aired, and spotlessly clean.
6. Cover the examination table with a clean cover, either a cotton or muslin sheet, crepe paper, or a covered rubber sheet on the lower part of the table. A towel may be placed over a pillow at the end of the table.
7. Always have the patient empty his or her bladder before an examination begins. If a urine specimen is needed, collect it at this time.
8. Assist the patient as required. Have a sturdy step stool for the patient to use when getting on and off the examining table. Offer support; guard against falling. **Never leave a confused patient or a child alone on the examining table because of the danger of falling.**
9. Assist the physician as required. You must learn the physician's methods and preferences for each examination.
10. *Never* expose the patient unnecessarily. Only those parts of the body being examined are to be exposed.
11. A female assistant should remain in the room if the patient is female and the physician is male, especially for a gynecologic examination (pelvic examination, Pap smear, and breast examination). Your presence may not only help the anxious patient to feel more relaxed, but it also protects the physician from unwarranted lawsuits. No false allegations can be made if you witness the entire examination.
12. Observe the patient for various types of reactions. A change in facial expression may indicate that the patient is apprehensive or experiencing pain. Note any unusual weakness, change in breathing pattern, change in skin color, or fainting. Your observations may provide the physician with important information that will help make a diagnosis and provide treatment for the patient.
13. **Inform the patient of any special instructions.** When the physician has completed the examination, inform the patient that he or she is free to leave after getting dressed or, if required, to check at the front desk to schedule a future appointment or a laboratory or x-ray examination. Often the physician requests that certain tests be run or specimens be gathered. Some offices and agencies have a printed sheet on which the physician can check each test that is to be performed on the patient. The medical assistant makes the proper arrangements, notifies the technologist, or collects the specimens requested before the patient leaves. Provide any special instructions that are required for the test(s), for example, nothing by mouth for 12 hours before the test. If the patient is to go to an outside laboratory or other facility, give the patient, **in writing,** the name, address, and telephone number of the facility. Let the patient know if and how the results will be reported to him or her. You *must* also make sure that the patient fully understands the directions given by you or the physician. Ask the patient if he or she understands the directions. *Never assume anything.*
14. Handle specimens obtained according to office or agency policy.

15. On completion of the examination, carry out your responsibilities for the disposal, cleansing, disinfecting, or sterilizing of the used equipment and the treatment room to prevent the spread of microorganisms.

16. **GUIDE FOR CHARTING.** Record findings from the examination accurately and completely. Use correct medical abbreviations, when applicable, in recording all information. Most physicians record all the necessary information on the patient's chart; thus this is commonly not one of the medical assistant's responsibilities. The policy regarding this varies and is established by the physician or agency for whom you work. If it is your responsibility, the following items are usually to be included:

    a. Date, time, and type of examination and the findings or results, when applicable

    b. Name of the examiner

    c. If specimens were obtained, the type, how they were handled, and the test(s) to be performed

    d. Any pertinent observations that you have made to describe the patient's general condition; be specific in the type of information you record (for example, "patient complained of slight nausea and a transient pain in the right lower abdominal quadrant")

    e. Future directions given to the patient. Be *very* specific. State exactly what special education or directions were given.

    f. Your signature

17. **PATIENT EDUCATION.** Always provide patient education orally and have available **educationally appropriate** and **culturally sensitive** printed materials to give to a patient. Printed materials can also be left in the waiting room so that patients can become more informed while they are waiting to see the physician. A notation should be posted, such as, "Feel free to take a copy of these materials with you." Many people will pick up copies of *free* material wherever they are. This is a positive way to encourage patient education.

A major emphasis in health care today is focused on *prevention*, and a major part of prevention is *patient education*. Research studies provide strong evidence that a variety of clinical preventive services can help in preventing some of the leading causes of death and disability in the United States today. The Surgeon General, the Agency for Health Care Policy and Research (AHCPR) and the Office of Disease Prevention and Health Promotion (ODPHP) urge practitioners, health care plans, and consumers to work together to make prevention—screening, immunizations and counseling for *health behavior change*—a part of *every* health care visit, in *every* clinical setting.

To have positive health behavior change, we need knowledge (information); therefore patient education at every opportune time must be practiced and promoted. With knowledge, attitudes are developed (and quite possibly, a positive change in attitude). Following this comes behavior—quite possibly an improved health behavior, which often develops slowly. Change takes time, support, and encouragement, and it needs a goal or a reason for the change. Understanding is a significant part of change. People need to understand what the change is, why it may be advised, and the possible outcomes if it does or does not occur. Motivation is also important to bring about change. People need reasons to change and the will to change; it is their attitudes that will aid or discourage the change(s). Health care providers at various levels can influence and even guide consumers' health behaviors and changes. We need to focus more on patient education and to take the time to communicate, listen, motivate, encourage, support, and participate in positive health behavior change(s). These actions are all part of patient education.

Scientific and health care research shows that prevention and behavior change can help people stay healthier and live a longer and healthier life. By improving the delivery of clinical preventive care, we have the potential to make significant improvements in our own health and the health of others, as well as improvements in the quality of health care that is provided to consumers. A variety of programs have begun to engage and practice prevention policies and methods. One such program is the "Put Prevention into Practice." This is a national, research-based public-private program that is assisting others in increasing the appropriate use of clinical preventive services. They and many other health-related agencies provide materials to assist health providers and consumers in promoting a *team* approach to the delivery of preventive services. Some materials are geared toward tracking and prompting preventive services, and some are made to remind practitioners, health care providers, and patients when preventive care is recommended (Table 5-1). These and similar tools can be used to stimulate discussions between patients and the health care team about preventive care. Personal health guides can be used as teaching tools and as a way of **encouraging patients to be** *active* **participants** in their own health and preventive care. A personal prevention record can be used to keep track of the preventive care received or that will be needed in the future.

GOWNING, POSITIONING, AND DRAPING THE PATIENT FOR PHYSICAL EXAMINATIONS

A physical examination is facilitated by the use of an examining table and proper gowning, positioning, and draping of the patient. **The purposes of positioning a patient are:**

- To allow better visibility and accessibility for the physician during the examination of the patient.
- To provide support for the patient when being examined.

The purposes of gowning and draping the patient are:

- To avoid unnecessary exposure of the patient's body during an examination, thereby protecting the patient's modesty.
- To contribute to the patient's feeling of being cared for, which helps the patient relax.
- To provide some comfort and warmth and to avoid chilling.

TABLE 5–1   Clinical Preventive Services for Normal-Risk Adults

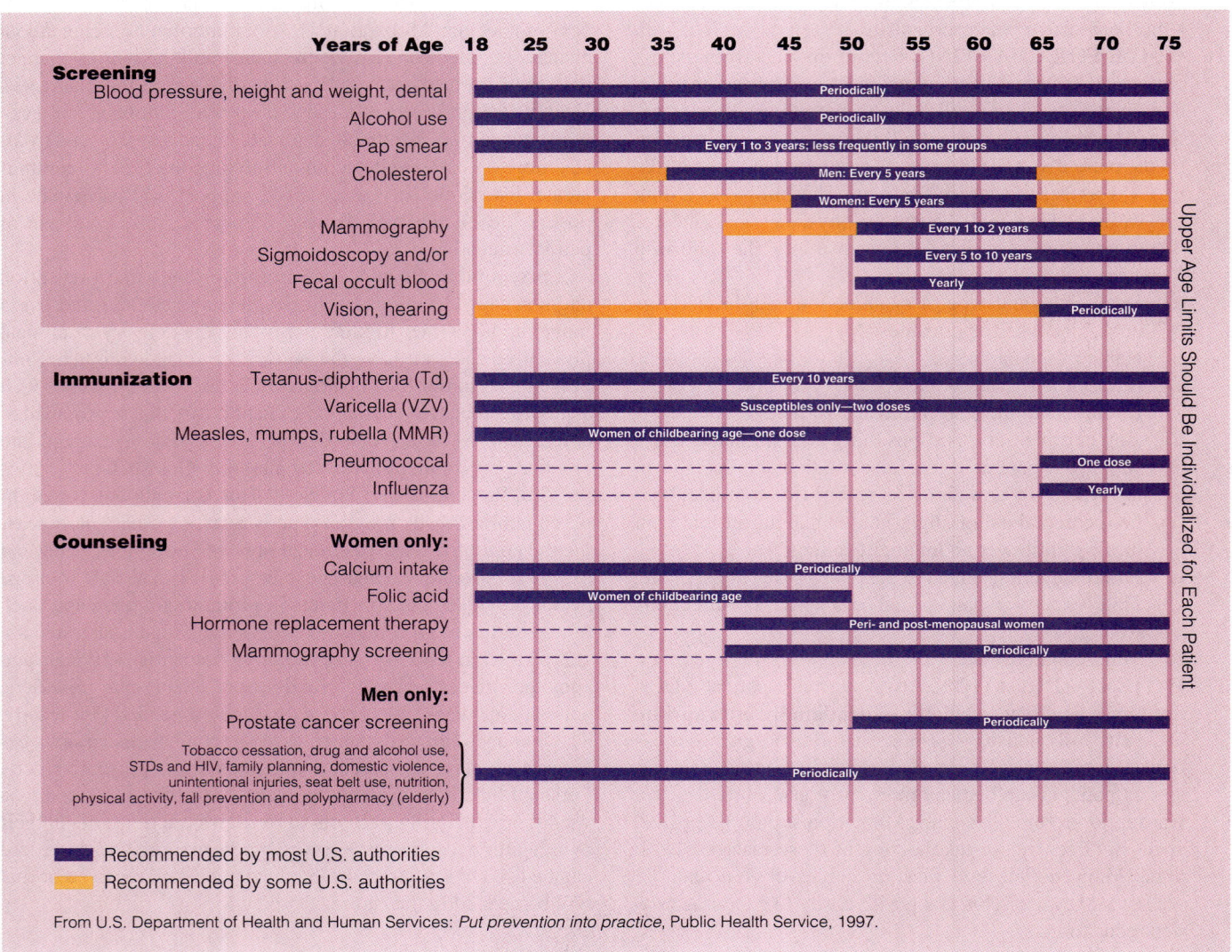

Years of Age	18	25	30	35	40	45	50	55	60	65	70	75
Screening												
Blood pressure, height and weight, dental	Periodically											
Alcohol use	Periodically											
Pap smear	Every 1 to 3 years; less frequently in some groups											
Cholesterol				Men: Every 5 years								
				Women: Every 5 years								
Mammography						Every 1 to 2 years						
Sigmoidoscopy and/or							Every 5 to 10 years					
Fecal occult blood							Yearly					
Vision, hearing										Periodically		
Immunization												
Tetanus-diphtheria (Td)	Every 10 years											
Varicella (VZV)	Susceptibles only—two doses											
Measles, mumps, rubella (MMR)	Women of childbearing age—one dose											
Pneumococcal										One dose		
Influenza										Yearly		
Counseling	**Women only:**											
Calcium intake	Periodically											
Folic acid	Women of childbearing age											
Hormone replacement therapy						Peri- and post-menopausal women						
Mammography screening						Periodically						
Men only:												
Prostate cancer screening							Periodically					
Tobacco cessation, drug and alcohol use, STDs and HIV, family planning, domestic violence, unintentional injuries, seat belt use, nutrition, physical activity, fall prevention and polypharmacy (elderly)	Periodically											

Upper Age Limits Should Be Individualized for Each Patient

█ Recommended by most U.S. authorities
█ Recommended by some U.S. authorities

From U.S. Department of Health and Human Services: *Put prevention into practice*, Public Health Service, 1997.

The **principle of gowning and draping** is that only the part of the body that is being examined should be exposed, other than the head, arms, and sometimes the legs, and only when the physician is about to begin the examination.

Different positions are used for various types of examinations. In all positions the patient must be well supported because most positions are uncomfortable and difficult to maintain for any length of time. The position chosen depends on the type of examination or procedure to be performed and on the patient's age, sex, and physical and emotional condition. The various positions used most commonly in a general or special physical examination are presented, along with the instructions for gowning, positioning, and draping the patient.

Supine Position

The patient lies flat on the back, with arms placed at the side and head elevated slightly on a pillow. This position is used for examinations of the abdomen and breasts, for some surgical and x-ray film procedures, and on occasion for examination of the chest (Figure 5-2).

Prone Position

The patient lies flat on the abdomen, with arms flexed under the head, which is turned to one side. This position may be used in examinations of the back in musculoskeletal and neurologic examinations and for some surgical procedures (Figure 5-3).

Fowler's Position

The patient is sitting up. This position is used for examining the head, ears, eyes, nose, throat, neck, chest, and breasts (Figure 5-4).

Semi-Fowler's position.   The patient is lying in a supine position, with the head of the table or bed raised 18 to

FIGURE 5-2   Supine position.

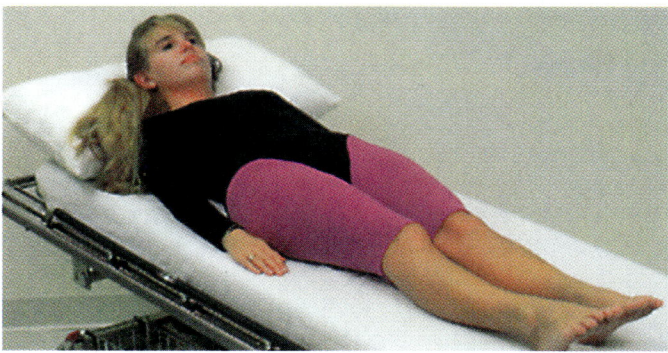

FIGURE 5-3   Prone position.

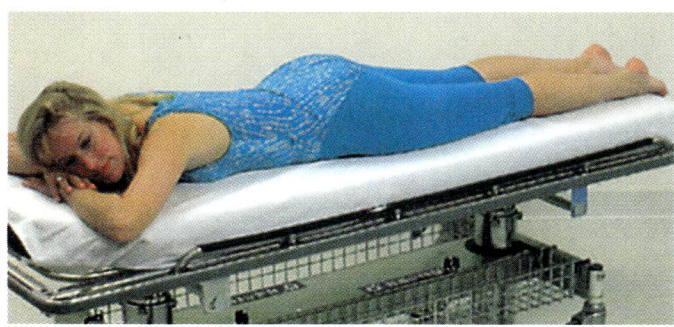

FIGURE 5-4   Fowler's (sitting) position.

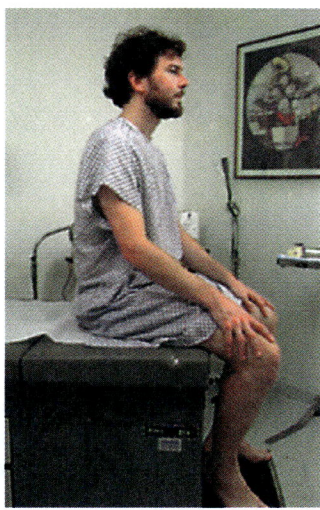

FIGURE 5-5   Semi-Fowler's position.

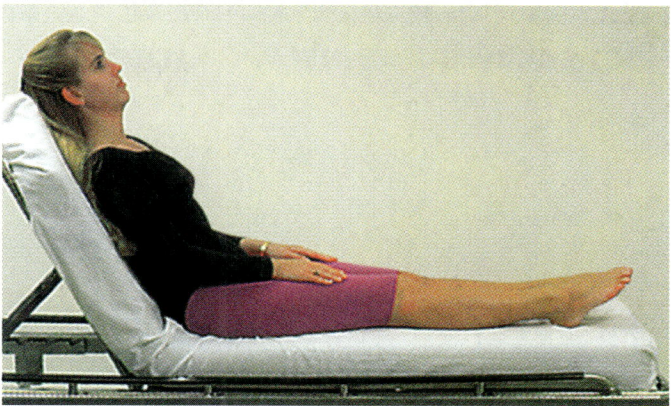

FIGURE 5-6   Standing position.

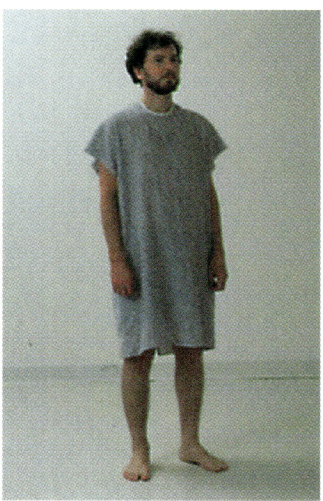

20 inches above the level of the feet. This may be used rather than the supine or Fowler's position when required for the comfort and physical condition of the patient (for example, for a patient with dyspnea [Figure 5-5]).

Erect or Standing Position

The patient stands erect with arms at the sides and feet facing forward. This position is used for part of a neurologic and mus-culoskeletal examination and also during some x-ray film procedures (Figure 5-6).

The following instructions apply to positioning and draping the patient in the supine, prone, Fowler's and semi-Fowler's positions.

1. Provide the patient with a gown. Depending on the examination to be performed, the patient should be instructed to disrobe completely; at times the patient may leave underpants on. If the chest is to be examined, it is advisable to instruct the patient to put the gown on with the opening in the front because this provides for comfort and easier accessibility to this region during the examination.
2. Instruct and assist the patient in assuming the correct position as required.
3. Place a drape sheet over the midtrunk and legs.
4. When the examination begins, the drape sheet may be folded back to expose the area on the body that is being examined.

Text continued on p. 175

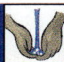

DORSAL-RECUMBENT AND LITHOTOMY POSITIONS

Objective
Understand the reasons for and demonstrate the correct procedure for assisting the patient to assume the dorsal-recumbent and the lithotomy positions.

Equipment
Examination table
Patient gown, either cotton or disposable paper
Paper or sheet to cover the table
Small towel, cloth or paper
Small pillow
Drape sheet
Stirrups on the examining table for the lithotomy position

In the lithotomy position the patient's feet normally are placed in stirrups that are raised approximately 12 inches from table level, although the stirrups on some examining tables cannot be elevated. These positions are used almost exclusively for pelvic, bladder, and rectal examinations (Figures 5-7 and 5-8).

- The patient lies on the back with the legs separated and flexed.
- The feet are supported in stirrups, or the soles of the feet are flat on the table.
- The buttocks are brought to the edge of the examining table.
- The arms are placed either at the side or crossed over the chest or under the head.

PROCEDURE

1. Place clean paper or sheet on the examination table.

2. Identify the patient and explain the procedure.

3. Have the patient disrobe and put on the patient gown.

4. Have the patient lie down on the table; place a small pillow under the head.

5. Cover the patient with a drape sheet, placing it in a rectangular arrangement. One point of the sheet faces the patient's neck and covers the chest; the opposite corner is placed between the legs or feet. The other corners extend over the sides of the patient.

6. Have the patient move buttocks down to the extreme edge of the table with knees flexed and the feet firmly on the table or at table level in stirrups.

RATIONALE

The medical assistant must explain what is required and why it is necessary, to gain full cooperation from the patient. Clear explanations also help reassure the patient.

For a pelvic examination the patient should disrobe from the waist down. For a pelvic and breast examination, the patient should disrobe completely and put the gown on with the opening in the front.

Help make the patient as comfortable as possible.

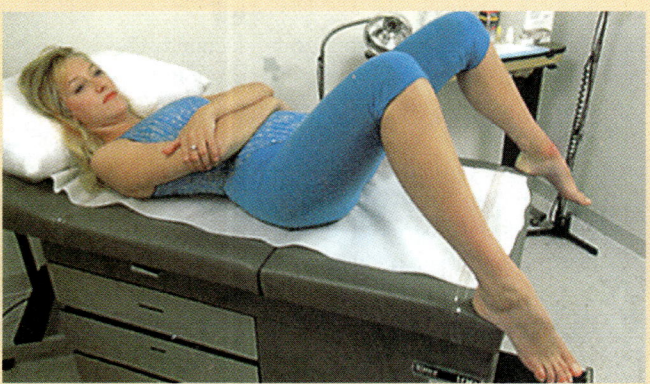

FIGURE 5-7   Dorsal-recumbent position.

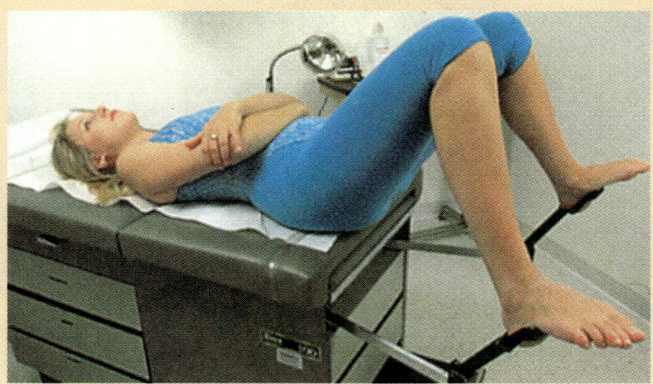

FIGURE 5-8   Lithotomy position.

PROCEDURE 5-1

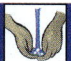

DORSAL-RECUMBENT AND LITHOTOMY POSITIONS—cont'd

7. Place a small towel under the buttocks.

This catches discharge that may be excreted from the patient's body.

8. Have the patient cross arms under the head or over the chest or place along the sides of the body.

9. Take the lateral corners of the sheet and wrap them around the feet in a spiral fashion.

10. When the examination begins, the corner of the sheet that covers the perineum is pulled back and upward toward the abdomen to expose the perineal area. Place this part of the sheet neatly over the patient's abdomen.

Avoid letting the sheet fall over the perineum because this would obstruct the physician's examination.

11. If you are to position the patient in the **lithotomy position,** the same procedure is followed, except that the patient's legs are elevated in the stirrups. In this position the lateral corners of the sheet are wrapped around the legs and feet that are supported in the stirrups. The stirrups are generally raised at least 1 foot above the table level and positioned to the sides of the table.

The knees are placed sufficiently apart to expose the perineum.

PROCEDURE 5-2

JACKKNIFE OR PROCTOLOGIC POSITION

Objective

Understand the reasons for and demonstrate the correct procedure for assisting the patient to assume the jackknife or proctologic position.

Equipment

Examination table
Patient gown, either cotton or disposable paper
Paper or sheet to cover the table
Small towel, cloth or paper
Small pillow
Drape sheet; two drape sheets are needed for the jackknife
    position

General Instructions

The patient lies on the abdomen with both the head and legs lowered so that the buttocks are elevated. Arms are placed along the side of the head.

This position is used for rectal examinations and occasionally for surgery. A special examining table that can be adjusted to facilitate this position is required.

PROCEDURE

RATIONALE

1. Place clean paper or sheet on table and a small towel over the area of the table where it will be split.

The towel helps soak up any discharge that may be excreted from the patient during the examination and can be removed or folded over before the patient gets up.

2. Identify the patient and explain the procedure.

This helps to put the patient at ease and cooperate.

3. Have the patient disrobe completely and put on a patient gown with the opening in the back.

If only a rectal examination is to be done, a female patient does not have to remove her bra.

Continued

PROCEDURE 5-2

JACKKNIFE OR PROCTOLOGIC POSITION—cont'd

4. Have the patient lie on the table and roll over onto the abdomen.

5. The table is split so that the patient's head and legs are lowered, and the buttocks are elevated. Arms may be placed under the head or stretched out in front of the head.

   The patient's legs are braced against the lowered part of the table. Good support is required because this position is difficult to maintain.

6. Place a small pillow under the patient's head.

   Make the patient as comfortable as possible.

7. Cover the patient's body with one sheet and put another sheet over the legs.

   Do not bind the legs together because commonly it is necessary for them to be separated for proper examination.

8. When the examination begins, the lower part of the sheet covering the patient's body is drawn back and folded over the lumbar region.

   This exposes only the rectal region, which is being examined, and maintains the patient's modesty as well as can be expected.

PROCEDURE 5-3

KNEE-CHEST POSITION

Objective
Understand the reasons for and demonstrate the proper procedure for assisting a patient to assume the knee-chest position.

Equipment
    Examination table
    Patient gown, either cotton or disposable paper
    Paper or sheet to cover the table
    Small towel, cloth or paper
    Small pillow
    Two drape sheets

General Instructions
The patient rests on the knees and chest, with the head turned to one side. Arms may be placed under the head to partially help support the patient. Buttocks extend up in the air, and the back is straight.

    This position is used for the rectal examination and sometimes for vaginal and prostatic examinations (Figure 5-9).

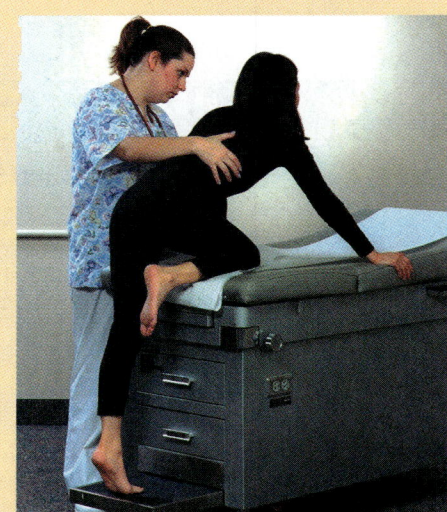

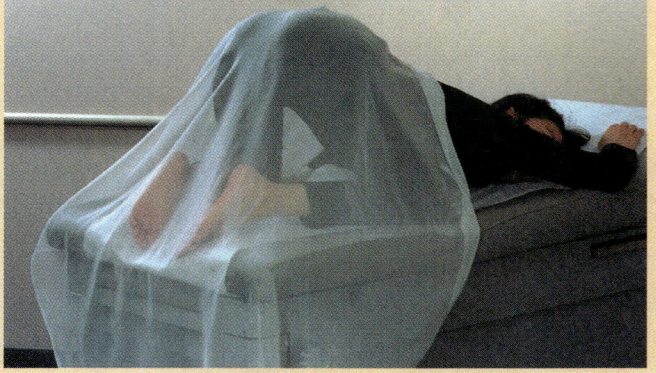

FIGURE 5-9 Knee-chest position.

PROCEDURE 5-3

KNEE-CHEST POSITION—cont'd

PROCEDURE	RATIONALE
1. Place clean paper or sheet on the table.	
2. Identify the patient and explain the procedure.	This helps reassure the patient and helps the patient understand what to expect and the reason for assuming this position.
3. Have the patient disrobe and put on the patient gown. The opening of the gown should be in the back.	
4. Have the patient kneel on the table, keeping the buttocks elevated and back straight.	The patient is resting on the chest in this position.
5. Have the patient turn the head to one side. A small pillow may be placed under the chest for support and comfort.	
6. The arms should be flexed at the elbow and extended, placing them under or near the side of the head.	This helps support the patient.
7. Cover the patient's body with a drape sheet and place a smaller drape sheet over the legs.	The patient should be fully draped.
8. When the examination begins, the drape sheet is pulled back and folded over the top of the buttocks.	This exposes only the rectal and vaginal areas, which are to be examined.

PROCEDURE 5-4

SIMS OR LEFT LATERAL POSITION

Objective

Understand the reasons for and demonstrate the proper procedure for assisting the patient to assume the Sims or left lateral position.

Equipment

    Examination table
    Patient gown, either cotton or disposable paper
    Paper or sheet to cover the table
    Small towel, cloth or paper
    Small pillow
    Drape sheet

General Instructions

The patient lies on the left side and chest, with the left leg slightly flexed and the right leg sharply flexed on the abdomen.
The left arm is drawn behind the body with the body inclining forward.
The right arm is positioned forward according to the patient's comfort.
The buttocks are brought up to the long edge of the table.

This position is commonly used for rectal examinations and when giving enemas. The vagina and abdomen can also be examined in this position, and it may be used for older women when the lithotomy position is too difficult to maintain (Figure 5-10).

PROCEDURE	RATIONALE
1. Place clean paper or sheet over table.	
2. Identify the patient and explain the procedure.	This provides the patient with some understanding of why this position is to be assumed, thus enabling the patient to cooperate.
3. Have the patient disrobe completely and put on the patient gown. The opening of the patient gown should be in the back.	

Continued

PROCEDURE 5-4

SIMS OR LEFT LATERAL POSITION—cont'd

4. Instruct the patient to lie down on the table and then to roll over onto the left side and chest, moving the buttocks up to the long edge of the table. You may help the patient assume this position properly by placing your hand along the long side of the table, so that the patient's buttocks touch your hand when they are over to the side far enough.

5. The left arm is drawn behind the body with the body inclining forward. The right arm is positioned in front of the body, where it provides support and is most comfortable for the patient.

6. Place a small pillow under the patient's head. One may also be placed under or near the chest.

7. Instruct the patient to flex the right leg sharply over the abdomen and to flex the left leg slightly.

8. Place a small towel under the buttocks.

9. Cover the patient with the drape sheet.

10. When the examination begins, fold back the drape sheet so that only the anal and vaginal areas are exposed.

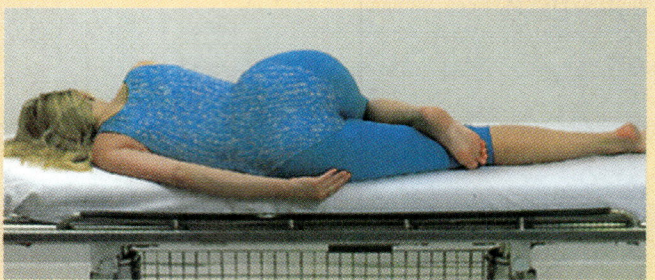

FIGURE 5-10   Sims or left lateral position.

Provides comfort and support for the patient.

This position provides good access to the anal canal, rectum, and sigmoid colon.

The towel catches discharge and can be removed before the patient gets up.

PROCEDURE 5-5

TRENDELENBURG POSITION

Objective
Understand the reasons for and demonstrate the proper procedure for assisting the patient to assume the Trendelenburg position.

Equipment
Examination table
Patient gown, either cotton or disposable paper
Paper or sheet to cover the table
Small towel, cloth or paper
Small pillow
Two drape sheets
A binder to support the patient on the table

General Instructions
In the Trendelenburg (trĕn-dĕl'ĕn-burg) position, the patient lies on the back with the head lower than the rest of the body. The body is elevated at an angle of about 45 degrees, and the knees are flexed over the lower section of the examining table, which is lowered. The patient should be well supported to prevent slipping.

This position is not used routinely for an office examination, but often it is used in the operating and x-ray rooms. It displaces the intestines into the upper abdomen.

An alternate form of the Trendelenburg position is one in which the patient's body is placed on an incline with the feet elevated at an angle of 45 degrees and the head lowered. This position is used to prevent shock or when the patient is in a state of shock or has low blood pressure. It is also used for some abdominal surgery. Some physicians have the patient positioned in the Sims position, along with this form of the Trendelenburg position, for rectal examinations (Figure 5-11).

PROCEDURE 5-5

TRENDELENBURG POSITION—cont'd

PROCEDURE

1. Place clean paper or sheet on the examining or x-ray table.

2. Identify the patient and explain the procedure.

3. Have the patient disrobe and put on the patient gown. The opening of the gown should be in the front.

4. Assist the patient onto the table and instruct the patient to assume a supine position. Place a small pillow under the head.

5. Instruct the patient to cross arms over the chest region or place alongside the body.

6. Cover the patient from the shoulders to the feet with a drape sheet.

7. Support the patient with a binder to prevent slipping. This is placed over the abdominal region and secured to both sides of the table.

8. Adjust the examining table. The body is on an inclined plane with the head slightly lowered. In the operating room the knees will be flexed over the lower end of the table. In the x-ray room, the table is raised so that the head is lowered and the feet are elevated. Feet and legs are straight.

RATIONALE

This enables the patient to understand the need for this position and what to expect. Your caring attitude will also help reassure the patient.

Make the patient as comfortable as possible.

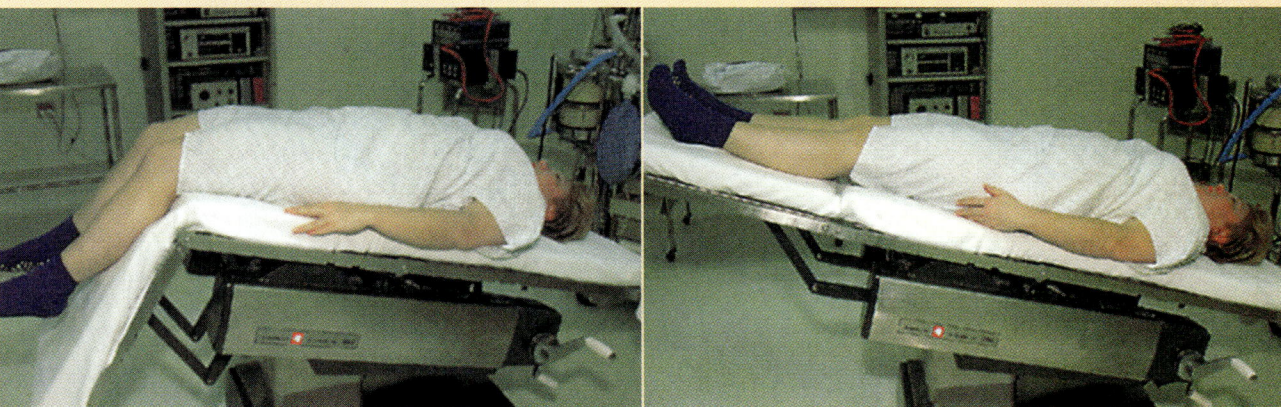

FIGURE 5-11   **A** and **B,** Trendelenburg positions.

PROCEDURE 5-6

COMPLETE PHYSICAL EXAMINATION

Objective
Understand and demonstrate the proper procedure for preparing the patient for a physical examination and assisting the physician. Inform the patient of any special instructions and record the procedure on the patient's chart.

Equipment
The exact amount and type of equipment to be assembled for a physical examination depends on the following:

Purpose of the examination
Type and extent of the examination
Preferences of the physician
Condition of the patient

In some physician's offices and agencies, the equipment required for examination is kept on a special tray ready for use and in a central location. In others it may be necessary for you to assemble all the equipment that will be needed.

Although there are differences among physicians and agencies, the following list includes items that are commonly used and should be available, ready for use (Figure 5-12).

Examination table covered with a clean sheet
Patient gown, either cloth or paper
Draping material, drape sheet, small towel
Watch with a sweep second hand
Stethoscope
Thermometer
Sphygmomanometer
Scale with height measure rod
Tape measure
Tuning fork

Percussion or reflex hammer
Tongue blades
Laryngeal mirror
Head mirror
Flashlight and/or gooseneck lamp
Otoscope
Ophthalmoscope
Nasal speculum
Safety pin
Footsense 5.07 monofilament (to test a diabetic's feet)
Tissues
Cotton balls
Alcohol or prepackaged alcohol swabs
Urine specimen bottle
Laboratory request form
X-ray film request form
Emesis basin or waste container used for soiled equipment and/or waste

Additional equipment is required for a visual acuity test, vaginal examination, and rectal examination. This varies with the purpose of the examination, the condition of the patient, and the physician's preference.

Visual Acuity Test
Snellen eye chart is used most often to measure distance visual acuity.

Vaginal Examination
Vaginal speculum
Disposable, single-use examination gloves
Water-soluble lubricant, such as K-Y jelly
Uterine sponge or uterine dressing forceps

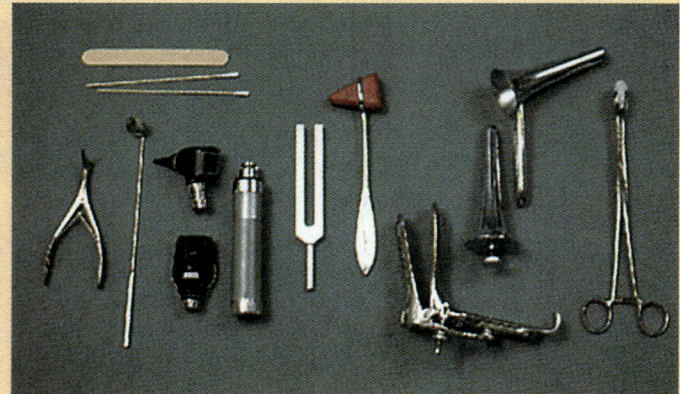

FIGURE 5-12 Instruments and supplies commonly used for a physical examination. *Left to right,* Nasal speculum, laryngeal mirror, otoscope *(top)* and ophthalmoscope *(bottom)* attachments with battery-operated handle, tuning fork, percussion hammer, vaginal speculum, anoscope, and sponge stick (forceps) with sponge; *top left corner,* tongue blade, cotton-tipped applicators.

PROCEDURE 5-6

COMPLETE PHYSICAL EXAMINATION—cont'd

Sponges

Two glass slides for smears *or* one glass slide and one sterile culture tube with applicator

Cotton-tipped applicators or wooden cervical spatulas and/or brush, for example, Cytobrush or Cervex-brush

Fixative spray or cytology jar with solution

Plastic container for slides if using the fixative spray

Laboratory request form

Rectal examination

Rectal glove or sterile rubber gloves or rubber finger cot

Lubricant, such as K-Y jelly

Rectal speculum, proctoscope, or anoscope (depending on the extent of the examination)

Tissues

Sponge forceps

Sponges

Cotton-tipped applicators

PROCEDURE

1. **Wash your hands. Use appropriate personal protective equipment (PPE) as indicated by facility.**

2. Assemble and prepare the necessary equipment for the physician. Equipment is to be arranged on a table or tray covered with a clean towel.

3. Identify the patient and explain the procedure.

4. Have the patient void to empty the bladder. Instruct the patient on how to collect a urine specimen if one is required (see Chapter 11, pp. 480-482).

5. Take the following physical measurements and record accurately:

   TPR
   BP
   Height
   Weight
   This varies with your job requirements. At times the physician may wish to do these tests rather than have you do them. Height and weight should be taken after the patient removes shoes and heavy outer clothing.

6. Instruct the patient to disrobe completely and put on a patient gown with the opening in the front.

7. Have the patient sit on the edge of the examining table with a towel under the buttocks. Place a drape sheet over the patient's lap.

8. Call the doctor when the patient is ready and when you have completed all the necessary recordings and assembled the equipment. Give the patient's chart to the physician before the examination begins. A female assistant should remain in the room if the patient is female and the physician is male and/or if the physician requires your assistance when performing the examination (see p. 160, No. 11).

RATIONALE

An explanation helps the patient to understand the procedure (that is, what will occur, how it may feel, and how she or he can help in the examination). It also helps to reassure the patient.

When the bladder is full, it is difficult for the physician to palpate the abdomen adequately. It is also very uncomfortable for the patient to have a full bladder while being examined.

Gown donned with opening in the front permits access to the chest for examination while the shoulders and back are still covered.

Continued

PROCEDURE 5-6

COMPLETE PHYSICAL EXAMINATION—cont'd

9. Assist the physician as required. Depending on the physician's preference, you may have to be ready to hand the instruments as needed. The physician proceeds with the examination from head to toe, examining the body systems and parts as described previously under the physical examination in Chapter 4.

10. While the patient is in a sitting position, the physician examines the head, ears, eyes, nose, mouth, and throat; the neck and axillae; the chest, breasts, and heart; and the neuromuscular reflexes and sensations, such as the pinprick, as well as general observation of skin and body symmetry. Diabetics especially need to have their feet examined and tested for loss of protective sensation (LOPS) at least once but preferably 3 or 4 times a year. LOPS is the degree of sensory loss that allows skin injury to occur without it being felt by the person as painful. (See also Chapter 17 for more information on diabetes).

Equipment

Tuning fork	Head mirror
Otoscope	Laryngeal mirror
Ophthalmoscope	Stethoscope
Nasal speculum	Safety pin
Tongue blade	Percussion hammer
Flashlight	Footsense 5.07 monofilament to test a diabetic's feet

Nearly half of all diabetic patients suffer from diabetic neuropathy. This complication suppresses the warning signals of pain that help others to avoid injury or alert them to a problem if pain is present. LOPS resulting from neuropathy is a major factor in the cause of foot injury, which often leads to ulceration, infection, and, potentially, amputation. Complications from diabetes are the cause for approximately 50% of all nontraumatic amputations in the United States today. (See the box, Foot Care Guidelines for Patients With Diabetes).

11. If handing used equipment or specimens, don gloves. When handing or accepting a tongue blade from the physician, hold it in the center. Without touching the end used, discard in the emesis basin or waste container.

By handling the tongue blade in this way, you avoid contamination to the patient and also to yourself.

12. Warm the laryngeal mirror by placing the mirrored end under warm running water or in a glass of warm water. Be sure to dry it before it is used.

It must be warmed to prevent fogging.

13. After Step 10 is completed, the patient is to assume a supine position. Help the patient attain this position if necessary. Give reassurance and support as needed.

Often just placing your hand on the patient's shoulder or arm gives the patient a feeling of support and of being cared for.

14. Place the drape sheet to cover the patient from shoulders to feet. Move it down when the physician is ready to examine the breasts and abdomen. When the physician examines the breasts, fold the sheet down to the patient's waist and open the patient's gown. When the patient is in this position, the physician palpates breasts, liver, spleen, and other abdominal organs. The groin is checked for a possible hernia.

When the abdomen is being examined, the patient's gown can be used to cover the breasts; fold the drape sheet down to the pubic hair line. The physician may use a stethoscope to listen to abdominal sounds as part of the examination of the abdomen.

PROCEDURE 5-6

COMPLETE PHYSICAL EXAMINATION—cont'd

15. For a vaginal and rectal examination, help the patient assume the correct position. Assist the physician as required. Positions and procedures for these examinations are discussed next. Vaginal and rectal examinations are included in the complete physical examination of a female patient. For the male patient, the physician examines the genitals, rectum, and prostate gland.

16. Observe the patient for any unusual reactions, such as a feeling of weakness or pain, facial grimace, or change in color.

17. When the examination has been completed, the patient may sit up. It may be advisable to allow the patient to remain in the supine position for a few minutes before getting up.

18. Ask if patient has any questions.

Often a patient may have questions but does not feel free to ask or may feel that there isn't time to do so.

19. Inform the patient of any special instructions. See p. 160, No. 13.

Patients are often left in the room after the examination, not knowing if they are to talk further to the physician or are free to leave. Do not let this happen.

20. If necessary, help the patient dress; otherwise, leave the room so that the patient may have some privacy.

21. On returning to the examining room, assemble all used equipment and supplies to be disposed of properly. Remove all linens and place in the soiled laundry. Place disposable equipment in a covered waste container. Take instruments to your cleanup area. You may rinse some instruments with cool water or wash or soak them in soap and water until you are ready to prepare them for sterilization or disinfection (see Chapter 2). For others (for example, the tuning fork), you may wipe off and replace them in the usual storage area.

22. Resupply clean equipment as needed.

23. Clean the examination table and put on a fresh cover.

24. If smears or cultures were obtained, send them to the laboratory or place them in a refrigerator or a cool dark place until you can transfer them to the laboratory. Make sure that specimens are properly labeled and that you have completely filled out the appropriate laboratory request form.

25. Remove gloves if worn. **Wash your hands.**

26. Do any recording required of you completely and accurately (see No. 16, p. 161). Use accepted medical abbreviations when recording.

Charting Example

January 27, 20__, 1 PM
Complete physical examination done by Dr. Short. Patient referred to lab for a CBC (complete blood count) and UA (urinalysis) and to the x-ray department for a chest x-ray film. Patient to return in 1 week to discuss the results of these tests with the doctor.
Ann O'Reilly, CMA

HEALTH **MATTERS**

FOOT CARE GUIDELINES FOR PATIENTS WITH DIABETES

GENERAL CARE AND HYGIENE

Never go barefoot either indoors or outdoors. Your feet may be numb and you will not feel an injury as it occurs.

Inspect your feet daily. Use a mirror and pay particular attention to soles and between toes. Check for dryness, redness, tenderness, and localized areas that rub (hot spots). Dry, cracked skin breaks down more quickly than moisturized skin. Ask a family member for help if necessary.

Wash your feet daily. Test the water first with your forearm or elbow to be sure it is not too hot. Keep toes clean and free of debris between them.

For dry feet, use a very thin coat of lubricating cream or oil. Apply after bathing and drying the feet. Do not put oil or cream between toes as this may cause too much moisture and cause the skin to breakdown. Never use antiseptic solutions or astringents on your feet; this may be too drying for skin.

If feet are cold at night, wear loose socks to bed. If feet are hot, do not ice down. Avoid exposing your feet to extremes in temperature.

- Check temperature of bath water with forearm or elbow before bathing.
- Do not apply hot water bottles or heating pads.
- Do soak feet in hot water.
- Never walk on hot sand or pavement.
- Protect your feet against sunburn with sunscreen.
- Beware of car heaters on long trips.
- Cut nails straight across. Do not cut deep down the sides or corners. If vision is impaired, a family member or friend should be instructed on how to help.
- Never cut corns or calluses yourself.
- Do not use commercial corn or callus removers, foot pads, or arch supports.
- Do not use adhesive tape on your feet.
- Do not use garters or elastic to hold up stockings. These may be too tight and a source of rubbing, which could cause an ulcer.
- Do not use panty girdles that are too tight around the legs. Girdles may be too tight and cause swelling of the lower legs.

PHYSICIAN COMMUNICATION

Be sure to see your doctor 3 to 4 times every year. Be sure your doctor knows that you have diabetes. See your doctor or podiatrist promptly if you develop a blister, puncture, or sore on your foot or if a callus or corn appears. Always remove your shoes and socks when you visit your doctor. Remind your doctor to check your feet if necessary.

FOOTWEAR
Shoes

Buy only comfortable, well-fitting shoes. Have the clerk fit them for you. Walk around in them and be sure that they are comfortable immediately. People whose feet are numb tend to wear shoes that are too small, causing rub spots.

Buy new shoes late in the day. Feet enlarge slightly during the day, and shoes that fit in the morning may be too tight by noon.

Choose shoes with soft leather uppers that can mold to the shape of your feet. Shoes should be wide enough across the toes. Modern walking or running shoes may be beneficial.

Never buy shoes with open toes or heels. Inspect the inside of shoes daily for foreign objects, nail points, torn linings, and rough areas. These could be sources of pressure and skin breakdown.

Have your doctor or podiatrist inspect new shoes to be sure of proper fit and construction.

Never wear new shoes more than 2 hours at a time. If they are tight in an area, wearing them for short periods will reduce the risk of skin breakdown. Slowly increase wearing time over several days. Don't wear any shoes for more than 5 hours at a time. You should have one pair for morning, one for the afternoon, and one for evening around the house.

Never wear or buy sandals, particularly those with thongs between toes.

Always inspect the inside of your shoes carefully before putting them on and after taking them off.

Hosiery

Never wear socks or stockings with seams. Seams can cause areas of pressure and rubs, which cause skin breakdown.

Check with your physician or podiatrist for socks or stockings made specifically for people with diabetes. Some synthetics can be a source of dryness, and diabetic feet tend to be dry.

Wear only clean socks and change them daily.

Inspect socks or stockings carefully before and, particularly, after wearing them.

If you have any questions or your skin begins to break down, contact your physician immediately.

These guidelines are in the public domain and may be photocopied for distribution to patients.

PHYSICAL EXAMINATIONS

GYNECOLOGIC EXAMINATION

Gynecology is the branch of medicine that deals with maintaining the health of the female reproductive tract and the diseases and conditions that affect it. The medical specialist in this branch of medicine is called a **gynecologist.**

A **gynecologic examination** may be included as part of a complete physical examination of a female as discussed in the previous procedure or it may be performed as a separate examination. When performed by itself, a gynecologic examination generally includes the following:

- A breast examination performed by the physician and instructions to the patient on how to perform a breast self-examination (BSE) (Figure 5-13)
- A pelvic examination
- A Pap smear
- Individual cultures and smears for suspected vaginal infections (for example, trichomoniasis vaginitis, candidiasis, gonorrhea, chlamydia, herpes simplex virus (HSV), and human papilloma virus [HPV, or genital warts]). These infections and the cultures and smears that are used to diagnose them are discussed in Chapter 11 (also see Table 11-1).
- Rectal-vaginal examination
- A discussion of birth-control methods (when needed). (See the accompanying box.)

Breast Self-Examination (BSE)

Generally the physician examines the patient's breasts at each physical examination. Between examinations, women should examine their own breasts to detect any abnormality, which can be brought to the physician's attention immediately. The following information is supplied to the public for their general information by the American Cancer Society.

Reasons for monthly BSE.   Most breast cancers are first discovered by women themselves. Because breast cancers found early and treated promptly have excellent chances for cure, learning how to examine your breasts properly can help save your life. Use the sample six-step BSE procedure shown in Figure 5-13.

Best time to perform BSE.   Follow the same procedure once a month about a week after your period, when breasts are usually not tender or swollen. After menopause, check breasts on the first day of each month. After hysterectomy, check with your doctor or clinic for an appropriate time of the month. A monthly BSE coupled with an annual physical examination reassures you that nothing is wrong.

What to do if you find a lump or thickening.   If a lump or dimple or discharge is discovered during BSE, it is important to see your doctor as soon as possible. Don't be frightened. Most breast lumps or changes are not cancer, but only your doctor can make the diagnosis.

The medical assistant should see that the office or clinic has literature for women on this subject. (See also Mammography in Chapter 14.)

Pelvic Examination and a Pap Smear

Pelvic (vaginal) examinations and Papanicolaou (Pap) smears are essential for the adult female. Most general practitioners and internists, as well as gynecologists and obstetricians, perform them routinely. These examinations, done for diagnostic purposes of the female reproductive system, include inspection of the vulva, vagina, and cervix for any abnormalities and a bimanual palpation of the uterus, fallopian tubes, and ovaries. The physician notes the size, shape, position, and consistency of the uterus and whether any masses are present in the uterus, fallopian tubes, or ovaries. Developed by Dr. George Papanicolaou in the 1940s, the **purpose** of the Pap smear, used as a **screening test,** is to detect precancerous conditions or any unusual cell growth and to detect cancer of the cervix. The value of the test is that it can detect potential problems early so that they can be treated. It is recommended that all women have a pelvic examination every 3 years and that all women who are age 18 or who have been sexually active before age 18 have an annual Pap smear and pelvic examination. After three or more consecutive normal examinations, the Pap test may be performed less frequently at the discretion of the woman's physician.

More frequent testing may be recommended for women who have had abnormal results in the past, those with sexually transmitted diseases, and those with a family history of cervical cancer.

Special instructions must be given to the patient before they have a Pap smear taken. The medical assistant is often responsible for providing the patient with the following information.

1. Do not douche or put any vaginal medications, creams, foams, lubricants, or contraceptive products such as spermicides in the vagina for 24 hours (some suggest 48 to 72 hours) before having a Pap smear taken. These products interfere with the specimen obtained and make the test invalid.
2. Abstain from sexual intercourse for 1 to 2 days before the test.
3. Try to schedule the Pap smear so that it takes place between the twelfth and sixteenth days of the menstrual cycle. A Pap smear must not be taken during the patient's menstrual period because the red blood cells interfere with obtaining accurate findings.

The federal government and several states have passed legislation to regulate the laboratories that evaluate Pap smears. These relatively new laws establish training requirements and proficiency testing for technologists and place a limit on the number of slides that they can review in 1 day. The smear should be examined in a certified laboratory by a pathologist or qualified technologist who reports the findings according to The Bethesda System (TBS) that was developed

Text continued on p. 182

FIGURE 5-13 Breast self-examination: a new approach. (Courtesy American Cancer Society, San Francisco, Calif.)

Breast Self-Examination:
A NEW APPROACH

All women over 20 should practice monthly breast self-examination (BSE). Regular and complete BSE can help you find changes in your breasts that occur between clinical breast examinations (by a health professional) and mammograms.

Women should examine their breasts when they are least tender, usually seven days after the start of the menstrual period. Women who have entered menopause, are pregnant or breast feeding, and women who have silicone implants, should continue to examine their breasts once a month. Breast feeding mothers should examine their breasts when all milk has been expressed.

If a woman discovers a lump or detects any changes, she should seek medical attention. Most women will not develop breast cancer and most breast changes are *not* cancerous.

Remember the seven P's for a complete BSE:

1 Positions
2 Perimeter
3 Palpation
4 Pressure
5 Pattern
6 Practice with Feedback
7 Plan of Action

1 Positions
Visual Inspection: Standing

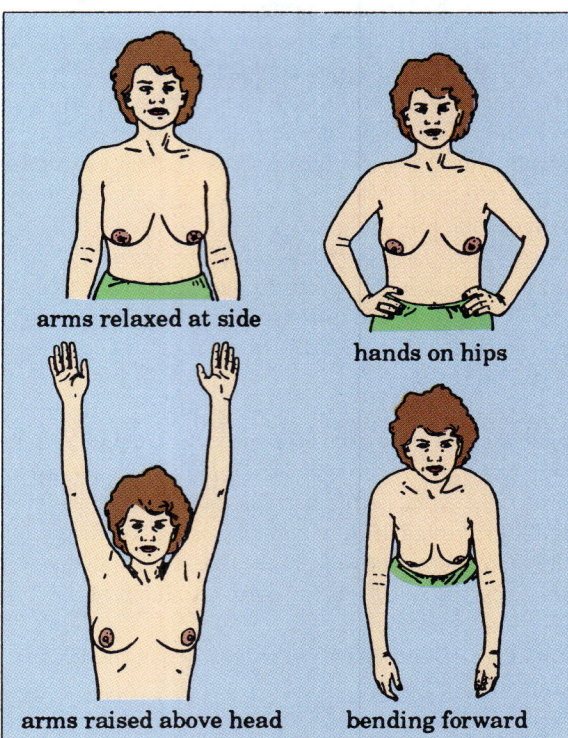

arms relaxed at side

hands on hips

arms raised above head

bending forward

In each position, look for changes in contour and shape of the breasts, color and texture of the skin and nipple, and evidence of discharge from the nipples.

Palpation: Side-lying & Flat

Use your left hand to palpate the right breast, while holding your right arm at a right angle to the rib cage, with the elbow bent. Repeat the procedure on the other side. The side-lying position allows a woman, especially one with large breasts, to most effectively examine the outer half of the breast. A woman with small breasts may need only the flat position.

Side-lying Position:

Lie on the opposite side of the breast to be examined. Rotate the shoulder (on the same side as the breast to be examined) back to the flat surface.

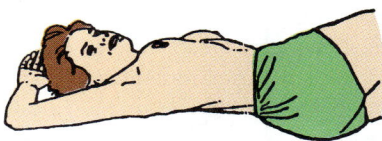

FIGURE 5-13—cont'd   Breast self-examination: a new approach. (Courtesy American Cancer Society, San Francisco, Calif.)

Flat Position:

Lie flat on your back with a pillow or folded towel under the shoulder of the breast to be examined.

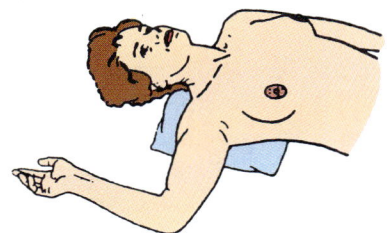

2 Perimeter

The examination area is bounded by a line which extends down from the middle of the armpit to just beneath the breast, continues across along the underside of the breast to the middle of the breast bone, then moves up to and along the collar bone and back to the middle of the armpit. Most breast cancers occur in the upper outer area of the breast (shaded area below).

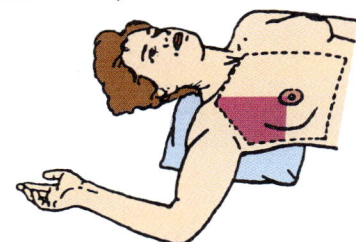

3 Palpation With Pads of the Fingers

Use the pads of three or four fingers to examine every inch of your breast tissue. Move your fingers in circles about the size of a dime.

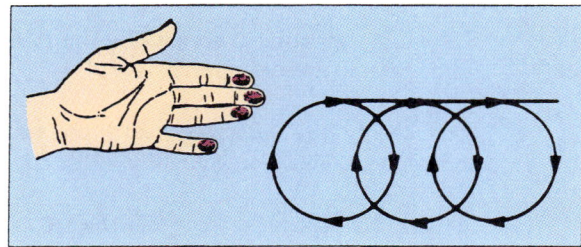

Do not lift your fingers from your breast between palpations. You can use powder or lotion to help your fingers glide from one spot to the next.

4 Pressure

Use varying levels of pressure for *each palpation*, from light to deep, to examine the full thickness of your breast tissue. Using pressure will not injure the breast.

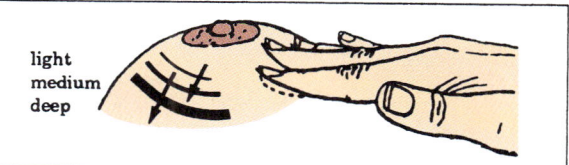

5 Pattern of Search

Use one of the following search patterns to examine all of your breast tissue. Palpate carefully beneath the nipple. Any incision should also be carefully examined from end to end. Women who have had any breast surgery should still examine the entire area and the incision.

Vertical Strip:

Start in the armpit, proceed downward to the lower boundary. Move a finger's width toward the middle and continue palpating upward until you reach the collarbone. Repeat this until you have covered all breast tissue. Make at least six strips before the nipple and four strips after the nipple. You may need between 10 and 16 strips.

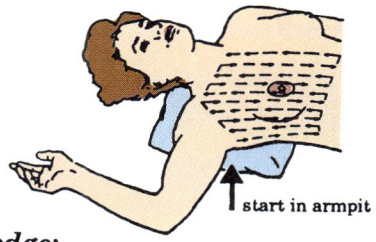

Wedge:

Imagine your breast divided like the spokes of a wheel. Examine each separate segment, moving from the outside boundary toward the nipple. Slide fingers back to the boundary, move over a finger's width and repeat this procedure until you have covered all breast tissue. You may need between 10 and 16 segments.

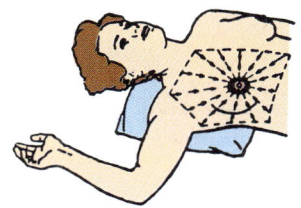

Continued

FIGURE 5-13—cont'd   Breast self-examination: a new approach. (Courtesy American Cancer Society, San Francisco, Calif.)

Circle:

Imagine your breast as the face of a clock. Start at 12 o'clock and palpate along the boundary of each circle until you return to your starting point. Then move down a finger's width and continue palpating in ever smaller circles until you reach the nipple. Depending on the size of your breast, you may need eight to ten circles.

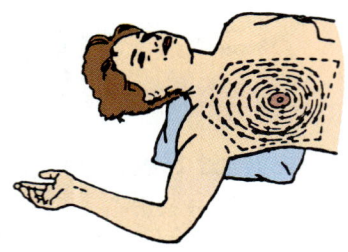

Nipple Discharge:

Squeeze your nipples to check for discharge. Many women have a normal discharge.

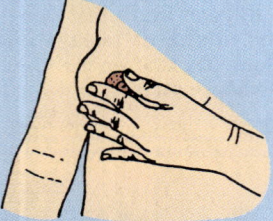

Axillary Examination:

Examine the breast tissue that extends into your armpit while your arm is relaxed at your side.

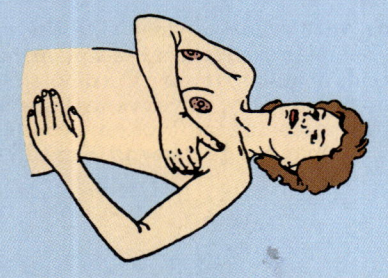

6 Practice With Feedback

It is important that you perform BSE while your instructor watches to be sure you are doing it correctly. Practice your skills under supervision until you feel comfortable and confident.

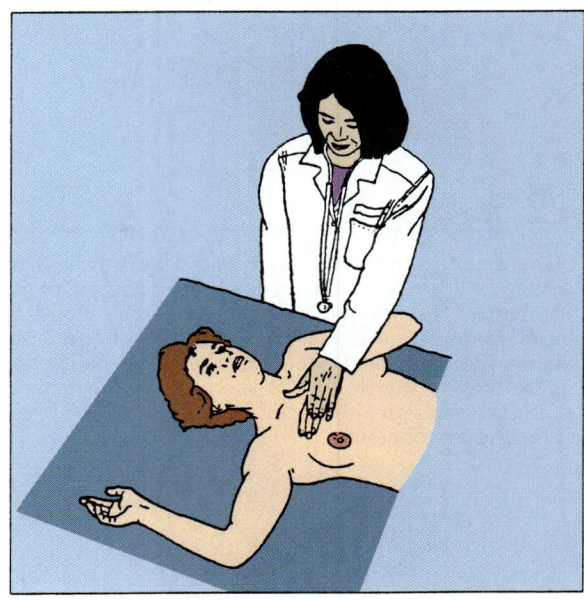

7 Plan of Action

Every woman should have a personal breast health plan of action:

✔ Discuss the American Cancer Society's breast cancer detection guidelines with your health care professional.

✔ Schedule your clinical breast examination and mammogram as appropriate.

✔ Do monthly BSE. Ask your health professional for feedback on your BSE skills.

✔ Report any changes to your health care professional.

HEALTH **MATTERS**

METHODS OF BIRTH CONTROL

BIRTH CONTROL IS YOUR RESPONSIBILITY

Sex is one of life's most pleasurable experiences. However, with pleasure, there is responsibility: sexual intercourse between a male and a female carries with it the risk of pregnancy. For many, especially teenagers, pregnancy would not be a welcome event. Any couple who decides to have sexual intercourse needs to use some form of birth-control method to reduce risk of an unwanted pregnancy. The following are options for birth control.

TYPES OF BIRTH CONTROL
Abstinence (Not Having Sex)

When it comes to preventing pregnancy, abstinence is the only method of birth control that is totally safe and 100% effective. Abstinence means having no intercourse, so there is no chance of pregnancy and a reduced chance of contracting a sexually transmitted disease (STD). The advantage is that no birth-control devices are necessary; however, this method can sometimes cause stress. If someone pressures you for sex, remember that it's *your* body—you can always say no.

Sterilization

Sterilization is a surgical procedure that makes you unable to reproduce. It is available for both men and women.

- **Vasectomy:** Vasectomy is the most common type of male sterilization. It is a simple, 20-minute procedure done in a doctor's office. The tubes that take the man's sperm to the penis are cut and closed. A vasectomy should have no effect on a man's sexual desire, erections, ejaculations, or sexual performance. Vasectomies are safe and, in most cases, 100% effective. A vasectomy should be considered permanent, although in some cases it can be reversed. Because a vasectomy is minor surgery, there is a slight risk of complications.

- **Tubal ligation:** Tubal ligation is the most common type of female sterilization. In this procedure, the fallopian tubes are cut, sealed off, or clamped. This prevents the egg from moving to where it can be fertilized by sperm. Tubal ligation can be done as an outpatient procedure. The surgery is usually performed using a small, lighted instrument, which is inserted through a tiny incision in the abdominal wall. After tubal ligation, there is almost no chance of pregnancy. Tubal ligation should be considered permanent. However, in some cases, it can be reversed with surgery to connect the fallopian tubes. Risks of tubal ligation include bleeding, infection, and other complications.

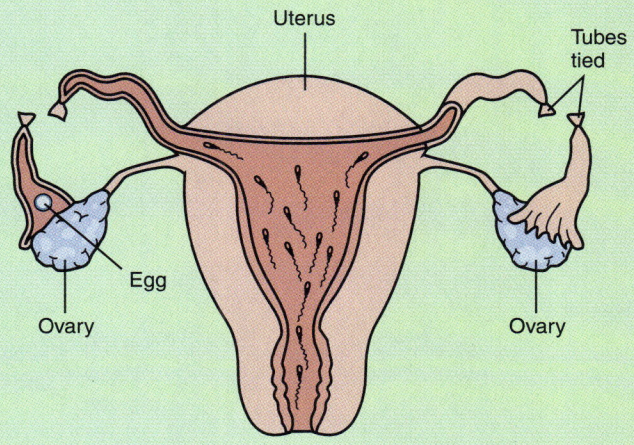

Diaphragms

A diaphragm is a round, flexible rubber disc that covers the opening of a woman's uterus. Before having sex, the woman spreads spermicide on the diaphragm and inserts it into her vagina. The diaphragm must be left in place at least 6 hours after intercourse. This prevents sperm from entering and fertilizing the egg. The diaphragm is fitted by a doctor and is reusable. Some people are allergic to the spermicides, but for many, it works well and is 82% to 94% effective. Oil-based lubricants should not be used with the diaphragm. It may offer some protection against STDs when used with spermicide.

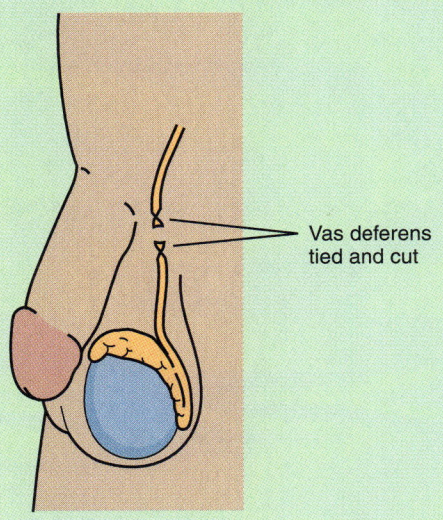

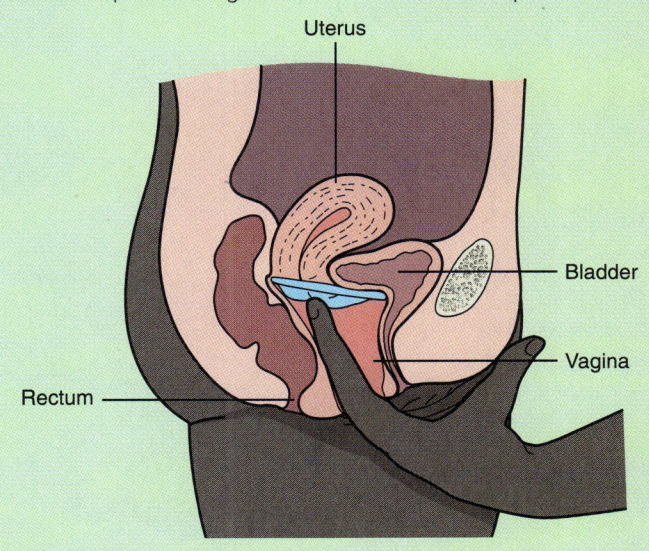

Continued

Cervical Caps

A cervical cap is a small, latex, thimble-shaped cup used with a spermicide to block sperm from reaching the uterus. It fits over the cervix and is 82% to 91% effective. It can be put in place several hours before intercourse so it does not interrupt foreplay, and it may offer some protection against STDs when used with a spermicide. To avoid toxic shock syndrome, the cap should not be left in place for more than 24 hours. It must be fitted by a doctor but is reusable and available with a prescription. As with the diaphragm, oil-based lubricants should not be used with the cervical cap. Some women may be allergic to the spermicides used with the cervical cap.

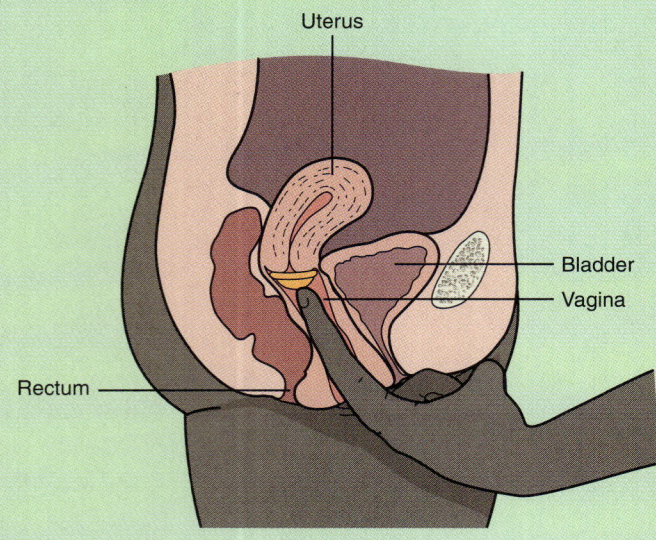

Female Condom

The female condom is a polyurethane sheath with a flexible ring at each end. The smaller ring fits over the cervix and acts as an insertion guide and anchor during use. The larger ring lies outside the vagina, covering the genitals. The female condom can be inserted into the vagina up to 8 hours before intercourse and is 79% to 95% effective. It is available without a prescription. Because the female condom is made of polyurethane, oil-based products may be used for lubrication. The female condom should not be used with the male

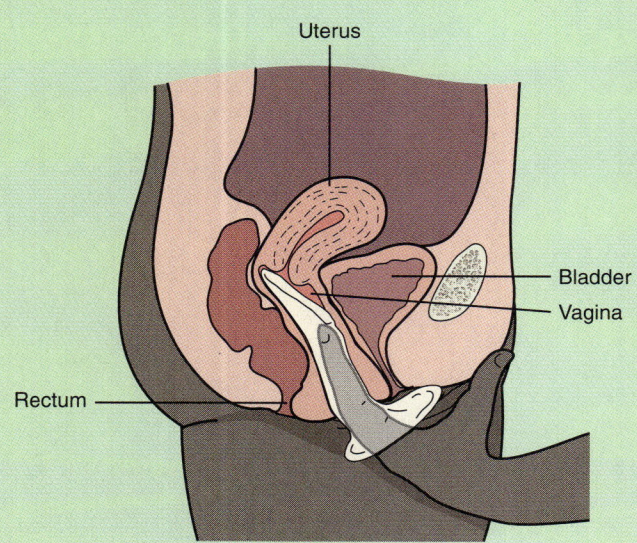

condom. For women who are unsuccessful in convincing their male partner to wear a condom, the female condom may provide the best protection against STDs, including HIV/AIDS.

Vaginal Spermicides

Spermicides are chemicals that are put into a woman's vagina before sexual intercourse. These chemicals kill sperm before they can enter the uterus and fertilize the egg. Spermicides are available as creams, films, foams, gels, jellies, suppositories, or tablets. They may come in tubes with plastic applicators. Spermicides must be reapplied each time there is intercourse. They are somewhat messy. A few people have allergic reactions to spermicides, but they are 79% to 94% effective. Spermicides can be bought at a drugstore without a prescription.

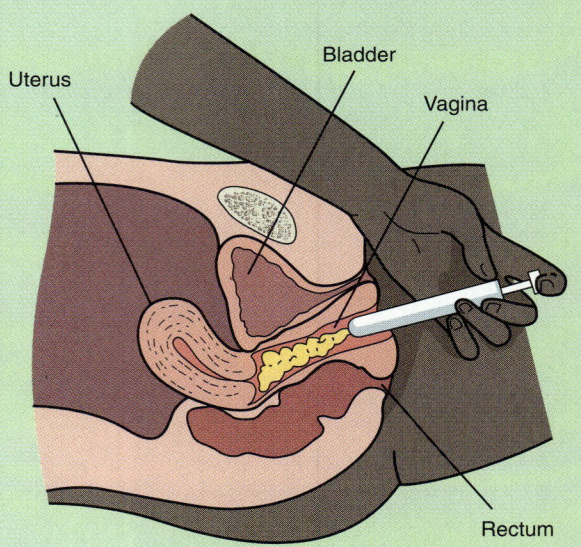

Intrauterine Devices (IUDs)

An IUD is a small piece of flexible plastic that is placed in a woman's uterus by a doctor. An IUD is about 98% to 99% effective, but most doctors no longer recommend an IUD unless a woman has already been using one without complications. Some minor, short-term effects of IUD use include cramping, dizziness, bleeding between periods, and backache. They are not recommended for women under 25 years old and do not provide protection against STDs.

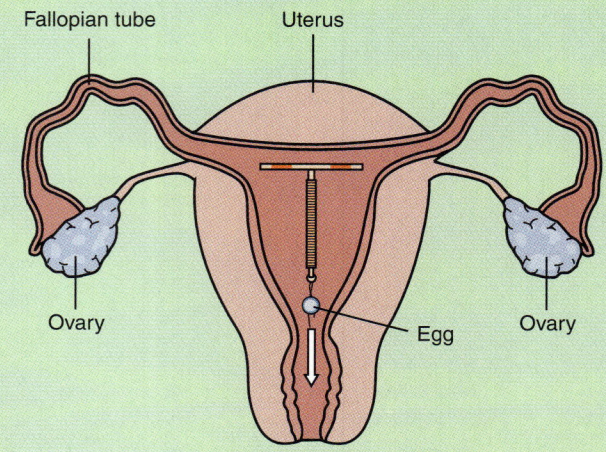

HEALTH **MATTERS—cont'd**

Hormonal Birth Control

Birth-control pills help prevent pregnancy with synthetic versions of female hormones. They work either by stopping the release of eggs from the ovaries or by making the uterus reject a fertilized egg. The pills come in different types, brands, and strengths and are taken for 21 or 28 days each menstrual cycle. Pills require a doctor's prescription and must be taken on a strict schedule. They are 97% to 99% effective but can cause weight gain, tender breasts, spotting, nausea, headache, bowel irregularities, high blood pressure, and abnormal blood clotting. Pills do not provide protection against STDs.

Depo-Provera, an injectable form of contraception, protects against pregnancy for a full 3 months. The active ingredient is a chemical similar to the natural hormone progesterone, which is produced by the ovaries during the second half of the menstrual cycle. Although Depo-Provera offers benefits (convenient, long-lasting, private, reversible), there are risks and side effects that a woman should discuss with a health care provider before deciding on this method. It offers no protection against STDs.

Norplant is another hormonal method. In this method, small, thin, flexible capsules are implanted beneath the skin of the underside of a woman's upper arm. The capsules automatically release a hormone over a period of 5 years. Unlike the pill, implants provide a steady, regular supply of hormone. If pregnancy is desired, the implants can be removed by a physician at any time. The implant is highly effective and needs no daily monitoring. However, it is one of the most expensive methods of birth control and offers no protection against STDs.

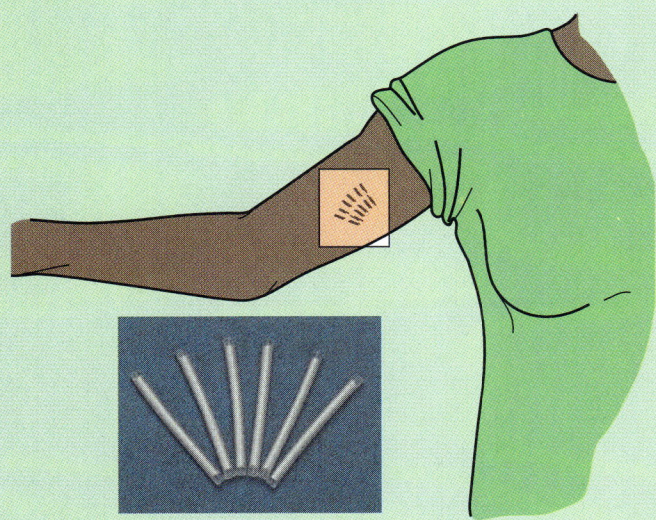

Male Condoms

Condoms are the most widely used male birth-control method. They are also known as "rubbers." A condom is a thin, latex or polyurethane sheath that looks like a balloon. It is placed over a man's erect penis before sex and prevents the sperm from entering the vagina. Latex or polyurethane condoms may also help protect either partner against STDs, including HIV/AIDS, especially if used with a spermicide. They are available without a prescription in drug-

stores. Condoms are fairly effective—88% to 97% when used properly. However, there is a risk of the condom breaking or slipping off during intercourse. Many use condoms during anal sex (inserting the penis into the rectum instead of the vagina); however, anal sex can be dangerous. Aside from tearing the delicate tissues of the anus and rectum, anal sex puts you at greater risk of getting an STD, including HIV/AIDS, even when using a condom.

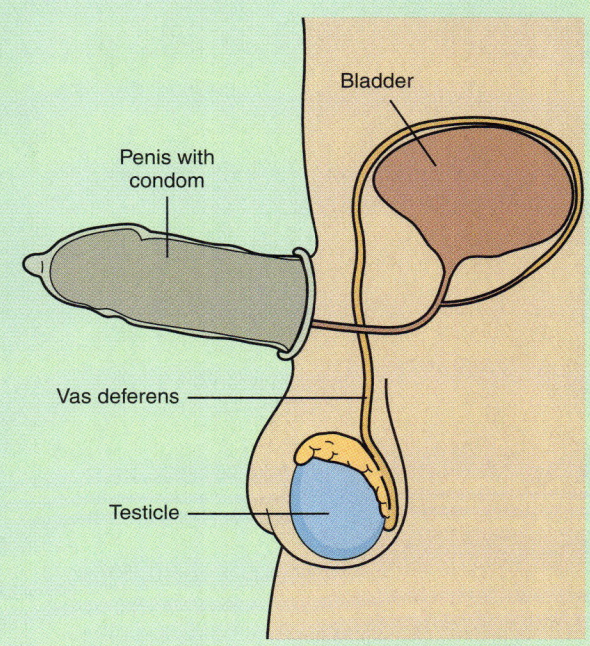

Natural Family Planning

Natural family planning (NFP) methods use no devices or chemicals. A couple observes, records, and interprets signs of fertility in the woman's body. Pregnancy is avoided by not having sex on those few days. NFP methods can be effective birth-control methods for couples who properly and consistently use them. NFP methods are much better techniques than the "rhythm method," which tries to estimate the menstrual period. Both partners should be trained by an expert. NFP methods include:

- **Basal body temperature (BBT):** BBT is a person's lowest body temperature, which is usually in the morning. After waking up, a woman takes her temperature and records it. During the time an egg is being released (ovulation), the BBT rises. To avoid pregnancy, the couple does not have sex for about 2 weeks while the BBT is elevated.
- **Cervical mucus method (CMM):** With CMM, the woman feels for the daily changes in the cervical mucus in her vagina. During a fertile phase (about 6 days), the mucus will be wet, even slippery. After the fertile phase has passed, the mucus will thicken and dry up. To avoid pregnancy, the couple does not have sex on those days when cervical mucus is present.
- **Sympto-Thermal Method (STM):** STM uses both the BBT and CMM to estimate when a woman is fertile. Other signs of

Continued

HEALTH MATTERS—cont'd

fertility like abdominal cramps, bleeding, sensitive breasts, nausea, headaches, and increased sexual desire are also noted. For couples who are motivated and properly instructed, STM is the most reliable form of natural family planning.

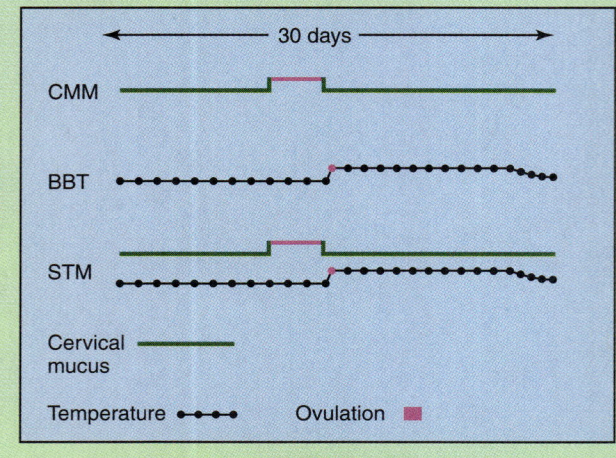

FERTILITY

BIRTH-CONTROL "METHODS" THAT DON'T WORK

Withdrawal

Withdrawal is when a man interrupts sexual intercourse by taking his penis out of the woman's vagina before he ejaculates. Because most males do not have the self-control to time their ejaculation, withdrawal is a very unreliable method of birth control. A further risk is that sperm may escape from the penis long before ejaculation and cause pregnancy. STDs are also a risk. In addition, withdrawal interferes with sexual pleasure.

Douching

Douching is a procedure in which a cleansing solution in warm water is used to wash the vagina. Douching after intercourse does not prevent pregnancy because sperm can reach an egg in less than 90 seconds. Douching does not prevent STDs.

Makeshift Condoms

Some people think that using plastic wrap or plastic bags will work just as well as a condom. Makeshift condoms slip, break, or tear and do not prevent pregnancy or STDs, including HIV/AIDS.

Standing Up

Some couples believe sperm cannot travel upward and that standing up during sex prevents pregnancy. However, the truth is that sperm travel upward very well. Having sex while standing up does not prevent pregnancy.

TEST QUESTIONS

Take this exam before and after reading the text.

T F   1. There is no such thing as a female condom.
T F   2. Douching does not work as a method of birth control.
T F   3. Male or female sterilization should be thought of as a permanent form of birth control.
T F   4. Birth-control pills contain hormones.
T F   5. Most doctors no longer recommend the use of an IUD.
T F   6. Diaphragms should not be used with spermicides.
T F   7. Latex condoms are a good method of birth control and can help prevent the spread of sexually transmitted diseases.
T F   8. A female condom can be left in the vagina up to 24 hours.
T F   9. Withdrawal is a very unreliable method of birth control.
T F   10. Cervical caps are thimble shaped and fit over the cervix.

Answers

(1) F (2) T (3) T (4) T (5) T (6) F
(7) T (8) F (9) T (10) T

Courtesy of Health EDCO, A Division of WRS Group, Inc., Waco, Texas. Phone: (800) 299-3366, ext. 295. Website: http://www.healthedco.com

---

in 1988 and modified in 1991 by the National Cancer Institute. This system includes an evaluation and report on the following:

1. **Adequacy of the specimen:**
   - Satisfactory for evaluation
   - Satisfactory for evaluation but limited by (disease specified)
   - Unsatisfactory for evaluation (reason specified)
2. **General categorization (this is optional)**
   - Within normal limits (WNL)
   - Benign cellular changes (see descriptive diagnosis)
   - Epithelial cell abnormality (see descriptive diagnosis)
3. **Descriptive diagnosis**
   - *Benign cellular changes*

- Infection: *Trichomonas,* fungal organisms, coccobacilli, cellular changes associated with herpes simplex virus
- Reactive cellular changes associated with inflammation, atrophy, radiation therapy, the presence of an intrauterine device in the patient's uterus, and other nonspecific causes
  - *Epithelial cell abnormalities*
- Squamous cell: atypical, low-grade and high-grade squamous intraepithelial lesions, and squamous cell carcinoma
- Glandular cell: endometrial cells (benign), atypical glandular cells, endocervical adenocarcinoma, endometrial adenocarcinoma, extrauterine adenocarcinoma, and adenocarcinoma
  - *Other malignant neoplasms*

Abnormal findings indicate the need for further diagnostic studies. Often a physician first performs a colposcopy. In this examination an instrument called a colposcope magnifies and focuses an intense light on the cervix, allowing the physician to observe the cervical anatomy in greater detail. If the colposcopy reveals an inflammatory process, a vaginal cream may be all that is needed for treatment. If the colposcopy reveals areas of abnormal tissues, the physician may use one or more diagnostic and therapeutic procedures, including a biopsy, cryosurgery, endocervical curettage, or possibly a cone biopsy using either traditional surgery, laser surgery, or more extensive surgery (also see Table 5-3).

New uses for the Pap smear.   Technologic advances combined with the traditional techniques and better sampling and interpretation guidelines are making the Pap smear more effective than ever in detecting early disease. The PAPNET, a computerized method for analyzing Pap smears, is being used to retest Pap smears that have been interpreted by technologists. The PAPNET computer duplicates the process that the human eye and mind use to identify abnormal cells. It scans each slide and selects the 128 most unusual cells. Pathologists then examine the suspicious cells and decide if anything is amiss. This is a more expensive examination, but it is hoped that this method will eventually replace many of the examinations now done by hand.

Another test, the *ViraPap,* was approved by the Food and Drug Administration (FDA) in 1989. It is used to screen for the presence of HPV or genital warts in Pap smear samples. HPV is linked to the incidence of cervical cancer, and this test could detect the disease before cancer develops.

PROCEDURE 5-7

PELVIC EXAMINATION AND PAP SMEAR

Objective
Understand and demonstrate the proper procedure for assisting the patient and physician during a pelvic examination and Pap smear. Inform the patient of any special instructions and record the procedure on the patient's chart.

Equipment (Figure 5-14)
Examination table (stirrups if available) covered with a clean sheet or paper

Patient gown
Drape sheet
Small towel
Small pillow
Gooseneck lamp
Vaginal speculum (metal or disposable plastic)
Water-soluble lubricant, such as K-Y jelly
Disposable, single-use examination gloves
Uterine sponge or uterine dressing forceps

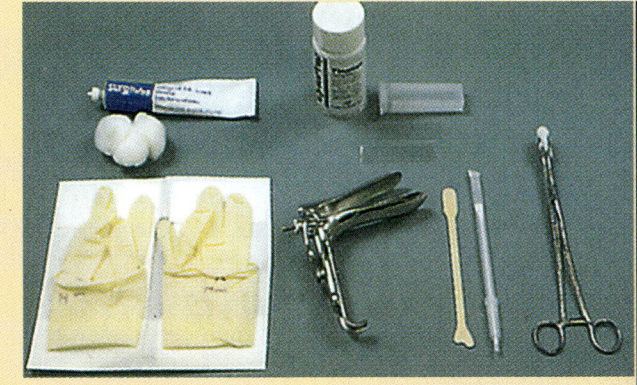
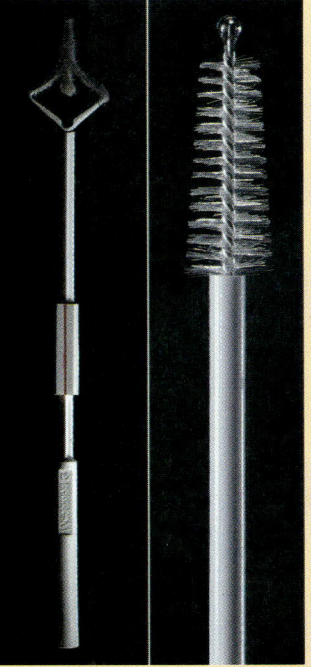

FIGURE 5-14   A, Equipment for pelvic examination and Pap smear. **B,** *Left to right,* Cervex-brush and Cytobrush used for obtaining a Pap smear.

Continued

PROCEDURE 5-7

PELVIC EXAMINATION AND PAP SMEAR—cont'd

Sponges or cotton balls

Two glass slides for smears or one glass slide and one sterile culture tube with applicator

One or two cotton-tipped applicators or wooden cervical spatulas and a cervical brush device (varies with physician preference)

Usually the cotton-tipped applicator/swab is used only for patients who have had a hysterectomy. Brushes are now being used with or instead of the spatula to improve the quality of cells obtained. The cylindric brush (for example, the Cytobrush Plus) collects only endocervical cells. The paintbrush-type brush (for example, the

Cervex-brush) or the Accellon Combi cervical biosampler brush are used to collect *both* ectocervical and endocervical cells at the same time. When these last two types of brushes are used, only one slide is used for the smear. This smear would contain cells from both the ectocervical and endocervical areas (Figure 5-14, *B*).

Fixative spray such as Cyto-Fix or Spray-Cyte *or* cytology jar with solution (for example, 95% isopropyl alcohol solution is preferred, although formalin 10% may be used)

Plastic container for slides when using the fixative spray

Tissues

Laboratory request form (see Chapter 11, Figure 11-12, p. 499)

PROCEDURE

1. Wash your hands. Use appropriate personal protective equipment (PPE) as indicated by facility.

2. Assemble and prepare the necessary instruments and equipment. Prepare the room. Make sure the lamp is working and that there is a clean paper or sheet on the table.

3. Identify the patient. Explain the procedure, and reassure the patient.

4. Have the patient empty her bladder. Explain to the patient how to collect a specimen if a urinalysis is to be done.

5. You may be required to take the patient's pulse rate and blood pressure.

6. Provide a patient gown and have the patient remove all clothing from the waist down. Shoes may be left on if the heels fit into the stirrups.

7. Position the patient on the table in a dorsal-recumbent or lithotomy position and drape as explained previously.
   a. Place the stirrups far enough out so the knees are apart.
   b. Avoid exposing the patient unnecessarily.
   c. Make sure there is a small towel under the buttocks.

8. Call the physician. NOTE: You may call the physician into the room and then have the patient assume the required position. Remain in the room (refer to No. 11, p. 160).

9. Assist the physician as required.
   a. Lower the foot of the examining table (if it is a table that splits) or push the footpiece in on newer-model tables.
   b. Pull back the drape sheet, exposing only the perineal region.

RATIONALE

An explanation helps the patient understand the need for the examination and what to expect (that is, what will occur and how it may feel).

This is usually done if the woman is taking birth-control pills and often routinely in many offices as a screening process for high blood pressure.

This varies with the physician's preference and the patient's condition. The Sims position may also be used for a vaginal examination of an elderly woman.

PROCEDURE 5-7

PELVIC EXAMINATION AND PAP SMEAR—cont'd

If you do not have to assist the physician with the instruments and materials, give your attention to the patient. You may stand by the patient on one side and offer support and reassurance. Often, support can be given just by having your hand placed gently on the patient's arm or shoulder.

10. Be prepared to hand the physician the various instruments and materials that may be needed. Some physicians request that you put some water-soluble lubricant such as K-Y jelly out on a gauze sponge; others squeeze it out when they are ready to lubricate the disposable, single-use examination gloves and vaginal speculum. Direct the light on the area being examined. The vaginal speculum may be warmed by running warm water over it. Alternatives used in some offices and agencies are to keep the instruments on a heating pad or in a warming pan. Other agencies use plastic, disposable specula; it is not necessary to warm them.

11. If a smear is to be obtained, mark the patient's name on the slides and the cytology jar *or* on the container where they will be placed after using a fixative spray. Label the slides No. 1 and No. 2. Attach paper clips to the ends of the slides.

Attaching paper clips to the ends of the slides prevents them from sticking together if they are to be placed in a cytology jar with the isopropyl alcohol or formalin solution.

12. You may instruct the patient to breathe deeply through the mouth.

This helps relax muscles.

13. The *physician* begins the examination. If a Pap smear is to be obtained, the physician:
   a. Inserts a dry speculum into the vagina (Figure 5-15).
   b. Opens the speculum so that he or she can see the cervix clearly.
   c. Inserts a cotton-tipped applicator or wooden vaginal spatula and draws it across the cervix to obtain a specimen, which is then smeared evenly and moderately thinly across the No. 1 glass slide (Figure 5-16). This is the ectocervical specimen.
   d. Inserts another applicator or spatula and draws it across the posterior fornices or pools of the vaginal canal to obtain a second specimen, which is then smeared evenly and moderately across the No. 2 glass slide. If the material is spread too thickly, it is difficult for the laboratory worker to visualize individual cells.

NOTE: If a smear is not to be obtained, the speculum is lubricated for easier insertion into the vagina. Steps (c) through (e) would then be omitted.

NOTE: Often an endocervical smear is more desirable than one obtained from the posterior vaginal pool. In this case, the physician inserts an applicator or brush into the cervical os, rotating it completely around the os until the cotton is saturated. A smear is then prepared with this specimen (Figure 5-17).

Continued

PROCEDURE 5-7

PELVIC EXAMINATION AND PAP SMEAR—cont'd

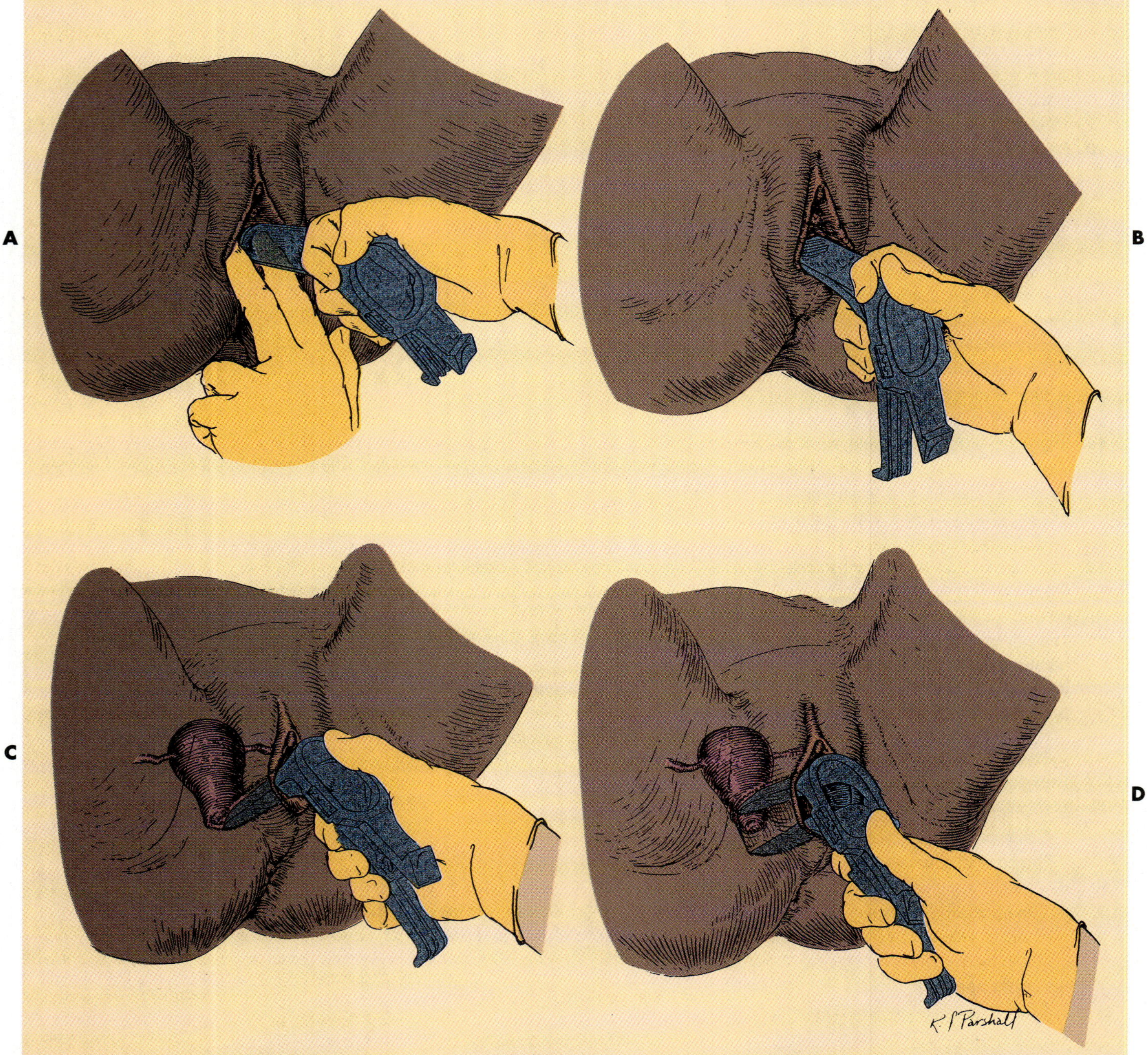

A

B

C

D

FIGURE 5-15   Procedure for vaginal examination. **A,** Opening of the introitus; **B,** oblique insertion of the speculum; **C,** final insertion of the speculum; and **D,** opening of the speculum blades. (From Malasanos L et al: *Health assessment,* ed 4, St Louis, 1990, Mosby.)

PROCEDURE 5-7

PELVIC EXAMINATION AND PAP SMEAR—cont'd

   e. Places these two slides immediately (within 4 seconds to prevent drying and death of cells) into the cytology jar with solution or sprays them thoroughly with the cytologic fixative spray and places them in the designated container after the fixative has dried thoroughly (drying takes about 5 to 10 minutes). NOTE: **The medical assistant may** be required to hold the slide while the physician smears the specimen on the slide and then to spray the slide with the cytologic fixative spray. Don disposable, single-use examination gloves if you will be handling the slides. (See also Chapter 1 and the CDC guidelines for handling specimens.) When spraying the slides, hold the nozzle of the can at least 5 to 6 inches away from the slide and spray lightly from left to right and then from right to left (Figure 5-18). Allow the slides to dry thoroughly before placing them in the designated container for transport to an outside laboratory (Figure 5-19).

   NOTE: Send these slides with a properly labeled cytology laboratory request form to the laboratory for cytologic examination. Enter the following on the request form:

- Date
- Physician's name and address
- Patient's name and age
- Source of specimen
- Test(s) requested

Also enter all of the following that apply:

- Date of last menstrual period (LMP)
- Hormone treatment (which includes birth-control pills)
- Postmenopausal
- Postpartum
- Pregnant
- Previous surgery
- Radiation therapy
- Previous normal results
- Previous abnormal results and date
- Any present or past history of sexually transmitted disease(s)

NOTE: Rather than making two smears, many agencies and physicians obtain one endocervical smear for cytology studies and one culture for gonorrhea screening. This is done more commonly now because often an infection is present without any signs or symptoms. This screening process has been very beneficial in enabling early treatment when an asymptomatic infection is present. *Other* specimens may be obtained at this time for any suspected vaginal infection(s).

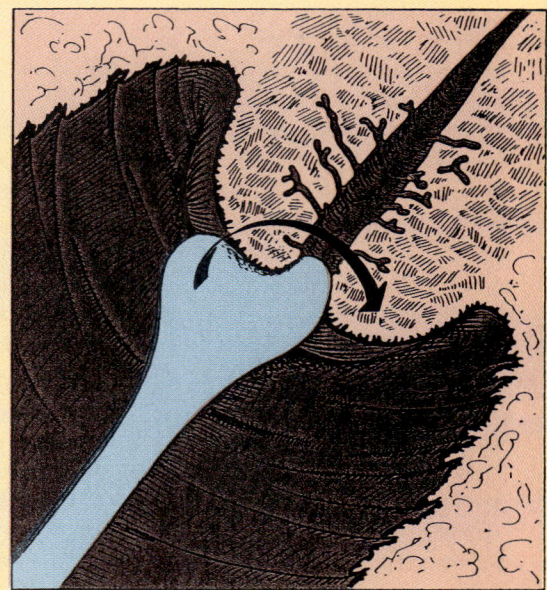

FIGURE 5-16   Cervical smear. (From Malasanos L et al: *Health assessment,* ed 4, St Louis, 1990, Mosby.)

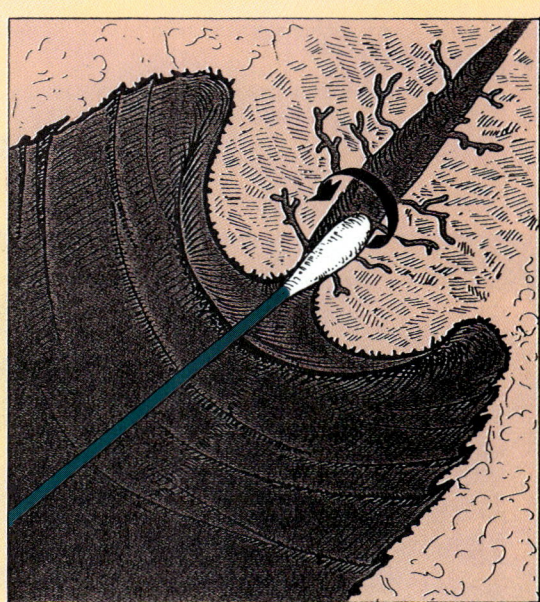

FIGURE 5-17   Endocervical smear. (From Malasanos L et al: *Health assessment,* ed 4, St Louis, 1990, Mosby.)

Continued

PROCEDURE 5-7

PELVIC EXAMINATION AND PAP SMEAR—cont'd

f. Removes the speculum and places it in an area designated for used equipment.

g. Applies water-soluble lubricant to the gloved index finger of the dominant hand.

h. **The bimanual pelvic examination.** The physician inserts the gloved, lubricated finger into the vagina to palpate the Skene and Bartholin glands and the perineum. Then the physician inserts the index and middle fingers to palpate internally for any abnormalities, such as displacement or growths of the uterus, cervix, ovaries, and fallopian tubes. The physician places the other hand on the patient's abdomen and applies pressure so that the movable abdominal organs may be felt more easily during bimanual examination (Figure 5-20). A culture would be obtained if any abnormal discharge is present.

i. **The rectal-vaginal examination.** Most physicians perform this examination while the patient is in this position. The physician inserts the gloved index finger into the vagina and the middle finger into the rectum for the rectal-vaginal examination. After this is completed, the physician would complete a rectal examination.

The rectal-vaginal examination is performed to evaluate the posterior portion of the uterus and other pelvic organs and structures; to confirm the position of the uterus (normal or otherwise); and to palpate the rectovaginal septum along the anterior wall for thickness, tone, and nodules.

14. When the physician has completed the examination, wipe off the excess lubricant or discharge from the patient's perineal region. You may use tissues or the small towel that was placed under the patient's buttocks.

15. Remove small towel from under the patient's buttocks.

16. Raise or pull out the foot of the examining table.

This varies with the type of examining table used.

17. Help the patient remove her feet from the stirrups and place her legs down on the table.

If you are helping the patient lower her legs, lift and move both legs together to avoid any undue strain to the pelvic area.

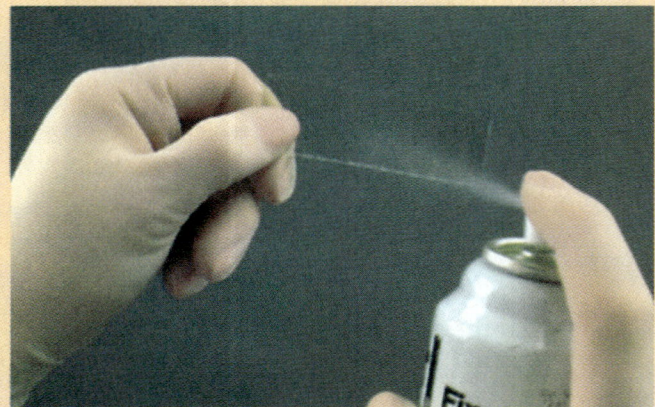

FIGURE 5-18 Spraying smear with a cytologic fixative spray.

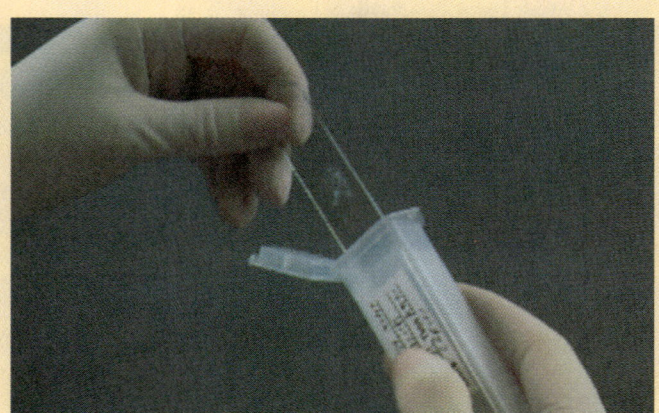

FIGURE 5-19 Placing slides in container for transport to laboratory.

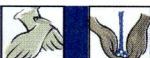

PROCEDURE 5-7

PELVIC EXAMINATION AND PAP SMEAR—cont'd

18. The patient may now slide up toward the head of the table and then sit up. Often it is desirable or advisable to allow the patient to rest for a few minutes before getting up.

19. Remove drape sheet.

20. If necessary, help the patient get up and get dressed. Provide extra tissue and a sanitary pad and belt if required.

Always provide for the patient's safety, comfort, and well-being.

21. Inform the patient of any special instructions, if she is free to leave after she is dressed, or if the physician wishes to speak to her further. Ask the patient if she has any questions (see No. 13, p. 160). Provide accurate and complete information or refer the patient's questions to the physician if you cannot answer them. Inform the patient that usually she *will not* be notified unless further evaluation is required. Provide printed information on birth-control methods if needed.

Part of patient care includes patient education and providing information and answers as necessary.

22. Leave the patient to dress in privacy if your assistance is not required.

23. Don gloves and return to the examining room to assemble all used equipment and supplies to be disposed of properly.

Remove any linens and place them in the soiled laundry. Place disposable equipment in a covered waste container.

Take instruments to your cleanup area. Rinse the instruments with cool water. They can be soaked in soap and water until you are ready to prepare them for sterilization (see Chapter 2).

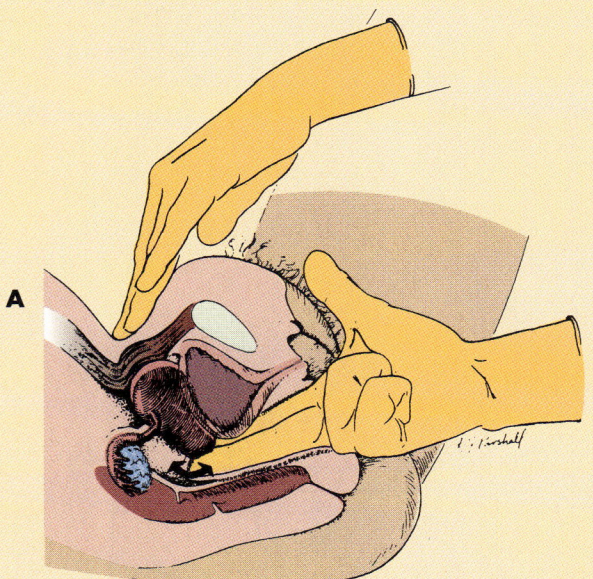
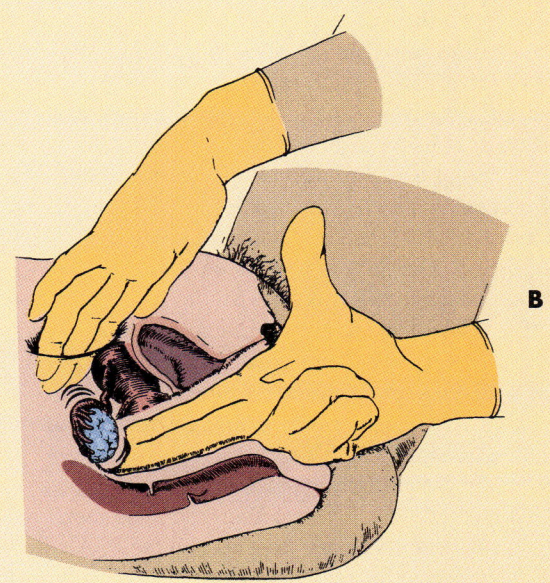

FIGURE 5-20   A, Bimanual palpation of the uterus; **B,** bimanual palpation of the adnexa. (From Malasanos L et al: *Health assessment,* ed 4, St Louis, 1990, Mosby.)

Continued

PROCEDURE 5-7

PELVIC EXAMINATION AND PAP SMEAR—cont'd

24. Resupply clean equipment as needed.

25. Clean the examination table and put on a fresh cover.

26. If smears or cultures were taken, send them to the laboratory with request form; or place in a cool, dark place until you can transfer them to the laboratory. It is important that all the required information appears on the cytology laboratory request, including notation of cervical and vaginal smears (see NOTE to No. 13[e] of this procedure).

27. Remove gloves.

28. Wash your hands.

29. Do any recording required of you completely and accurately (see No. 16, p. 161).

Charting Example

January 27, 20__, 2 PM
    Pelvic exam done by Dr. Short. Pap smear sent to laboratory for cytology studies. Patient had no specific complaints and left office in good spirits.
    Sandi Wilcox, CMA

RECTAL EXAMINATION

The rectal examination is used to detect polyps, early cancer, lesions, inflammatory conditions, and hemorrhoids. In addition, examination of the rectum can show how far the uterus is displaced and if there are any masses in the rectum or pelvic region in a woman and can show the size, any enlargement, and texture of the prostate gland in a man.

The prostate is a gland just below the bladder in the male genital tract. It has the second highest incidence of cancer in men 55 years of age and older. Recommendations for prostate cancer screening for men over age 50 include a digital rectal examination (DRE) and a blood test—the prostate-specific antigen (PSA). The PSA is a very sensitive test used to screen for prostate disease, but it is not specific for cancer. Some elevated PSA test results are discovered that are not related to cancer, and some cancer patients have normal PSAs. However, the DRE and PSA test together are an excellent screen for prostate cancer. One without the other is thought to be inadequate by many physicians.

For the most accurate results, the PSA blood test *must* be done *before* the DRE. When making appointments, it is very important to check with male patients that the PSA will be done *before* they come in for the physical examination of the prostate. The American Cancer Society recommends that after age 40 an annual health checkup for everyone include a DRE. A more extensive examination of the interior surfaces of the rectum is done by a proctoscopy.

TESTICULAR SELF-EXAMINATION (TSE)

Generally the physician will examine a male's testes at each physical examination. Between examinations, men should examine their own testes to detect any abnormality, which can be brought to the physician's attention immediately. The following information is supplied to the public for their general information by the National Cancer Institute. The medical assistant should see that the office or clinic has literature on this subject for patients.

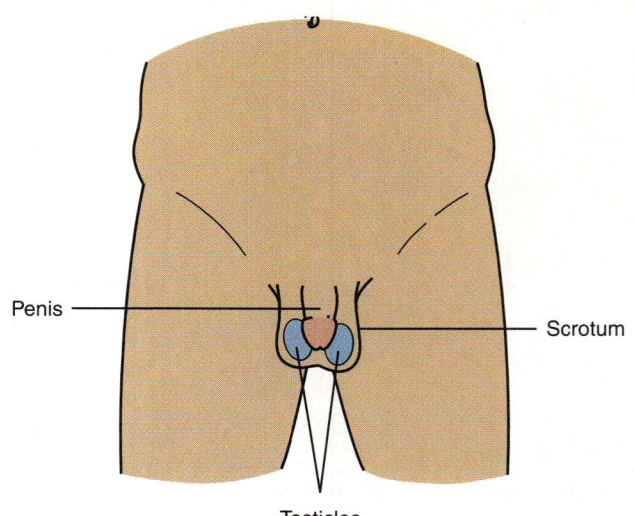

Text continued on p. 194

PROCEDURE 5-8

RECTAL EXAMINATION

Objective

Understand and demonstrate the correct procedures for assisting the patient and the physician during a rectal examination; provide the patient with any special instructions and record the procedure on the patient's chart.

Equipment (Figure 5-21)

Examination table
Sheet or paper to cover the table
Patient gown
Drape sheet
Small pillow
Small towel
Tissues
Disposable, single-use examination gloves
Water-soluble lubricant, for example, K-Y jelly
Sponge forceps
Sponges
Rectal speculum and/or anoscope
Cotton-tipped applicators
Culturette if a culture is obtained

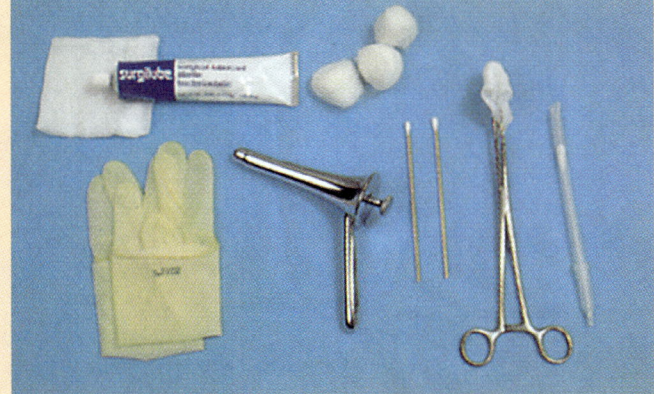

FIGURE 5-21   Equipment for rectal examination including a Culturette (on the far right) to obtain a culture.

PROCEDURE

RATIONALE

1. **Wash your hands. Use appropriate personal protective equipment (PPE) as indicated by facility.**

2. Identify the patient and explain the procedure.

   An explanation helps the patient understand the need for the examination and provides some reassurance.

3. Have the patient empty the bladder. Explain to the patient how to collect a specimen if a urinalysis is to be done (see Chapter 11).

4. Provide a patient gown; have the patient remove all clothing from the waist down and put the gown on with the opening in the back.

5. Assemble the necessary instruments and equipment.

   This varies somewhat, depending on the extent of the examination to be done and the physician's preference. Often only the glove and lubricant are necessary.

6. Position the patient on the examination table in a Sims, jack-knife, or knee-chest position.

   This varies according to the physician's preference.

7. Drape the patient. Refer to pp. 165 to 168 for positioning and draping techniques.

8. Call the physician.

   NOTE: You may call the physician and then position the patient. By doing this, you prevent the patient from having to be in an uncomfortable position for an excessive time.

9. When the examination is ready to begin, pull the drape sheet back, exposing only the rectal area.

   Avoid exposing the patient unnecessarily.

Continued

PROCEDURE 5-8

RECTAL EXAMINATION—cont'd

10. Assist the physician as required. A female assistant should remain in the room if the patient is female and the physician is male, even if she does not have to assist during the examination (see. No. 11, p. 160).

11. Be prepared to hand the physician the various instruments and equipment. Some physicians request that you put some water-soluble K-Y jelly out on a piece of gauze; others get it themselves to lubricate the gloved finger and anoscope if used. If a light is used, direct it on the part to be examined (the rectal region).

12. If you do not have to assist the physician, give your attention to the patient. Provide support and observe for any unusual reactions, such as a feeling of weakness, a change in skin color, or facial grimace, which may be an indication of pain.

13. The **physician** begins the digital rectal examination by inserting a gloved, lubricated finger into the rectum, then palpating the rectum internally to determine if there are any hemorrhoids, polyps or other observations, growths, or enlargements. This is done gently because it is often painful for the patient. In men, the physician will palpate the posterior surface of the prostate gland. The size, contour, consistency, and mobility of the prostate are noted. If the anoscope is used, it is lubricated; then the physician inserts it into the anal canal gently and removes the obturator. If any bleeding or discharge results, the physician may insert the sponge forceps and sponge through the anoscope to swab the area dry. This allows better viewing of the internal surfaces. A good light is needed so that the physician can view the internal lining of the anal canal. If a culture is to be taken, the physician puts a cotton-tipped applicator through the anoscope and swabs the area. The cotton-tipped applicator is then placed in a sterile culture tube, often one that has a special broth solution in it, so that the culture does not dry out.

14. When the physician has completed the examination, wipe the patient's anal region for any excess lubricant or discharge. You may use tissues, or the small towel under the patient's buttocks, which is then removed.

15. Help the patient, if required, assume a supine position. Often it is desirable to allow the patient to remain lying down for a few minutes.

16. Remove the drape sheet.

17. If required, assist the patient to a standing position and in getting dressed. Provide extra tissues to the patient, if required, for additional cleansing of the anal region.

Always provide for the comfort and welfare of the patient at the conclusion of an examination.

RECTAL EXAMINATION—cont'd

18. Tell the patient of any special instructions, if the patient is free to leave after getting dressed, or if the physician wishes to speak further to the patient in the office. Inquire if the patient has any questions. (see No. 13, p. 160). Instruct the patient to notify the physician if there is a large amount of bleeding after the examination. Always provide complete and accurate information. Refer the patient's questions to the physician if you cannot answer them completely and accurately. Never leave a patient in the examining room wondering if the office visit and examination are completed.

19. If your assistance is not required, leave the patient to dress in private.

20. On returning to the examining room, assemble all used equipment and supplies to be disposed of properly. Don disposable gloves and remove any linens and place in soiled laundry. Place disposable equipment in a covered waste container. Take instruments to your cleanup area; rinse with cool water. These may be soaked in soap and water until you are ready to prepare them for sterilization (see Chapter 2). Follow Universal/Standard Precautions for cleanup activities (see Chapter 1).

21. Resupply clean equipment as needed.

22. Clean the examination table and put on a fresh cover.

23. If smears or cultures were obtained, send them to the laboratory or place them in a refrigerator or a cool, dark place until you can transfer them to the laboratory. See Chapter 11 for the technique for obtaining a stool specimen. Make sure that specimens are properly labeled and that you have completely filled out the appropriate laboratory request form. Proper care and labeling of specimens is essential.

24. Wash your hands.

25. Do any recording required of you completely and accurately (see No. 16, p. 161).

Charting Example

January 27, 20__, 3 PM
Rectal exam done by Dr. Short. No specimens were obtained. Patient complained of a sharp, continuous pain in the anal region when leaving the office and will call the doctor if it continues.
Betty Fox, CMA

The Testicles

The testicles (also called testes or gonads) are the male sex glands. They are located behind the penis in a pouch of skin called the scrotum. The testicles produce and store sperm, and they are also the body's main source of male hormones. These hormones control the development of the reproductive organs and other male characteristics, such as body and facial hair, low voice, and wide shoulders.

Testicular Cancer

Cancer that develops in a testicle is called testicular cancer. When testicular cancer spreads, the cancer cells are carried by blood or by lymph, an almost colorless fluid produced by tissues all over the body. The fluid passes through lymph nodes, which filter out bacteria and other abnormal substances, such as cancer cells. Surgeons often remove the lymph nodes deep in the abdomen to determine whether testicular cancer cells have spread.

Symptoms.   Testicular cancer is one of the most common cancers in young men between the ages of 15 and 34. However, this disease also occurs in other age groups, so all men should be aware of its symptoms.

Most testicular cancers are found by men themselves, either by accident or when doing a testicular self-examination (TSE). The testicles are smooth, oval, and rather firm. Men who examine themselves regularly become familiar with the way their testicles normally feel. Any changes in the way they feel from month to month should be reported to a doctor.

Testicular cancer can cause a number of symptoms. Warning signs that men should watch for include the following:

- Lump in either testicle
- Any enlargement of a testicle
- Feeling of heaviness in the scrotum
- Dull ache in the lower abdomen or the groin
- Sudden collection of fluid in the scrotum
- Pain or discomfort in a testicle or in the scrotum
- Enlargement or tenderness of the breasts

These symptoms are not sure signs of cancer. They can also be caused by other conditions. However, it is important to see a doctor if any of these symptoms lasts as long as 2 weeks. Any illness should be diagnosed and treated as soon as possible. **Early diagnosis** of testicular cancer is *especially important* because the sooner cancer is found and treated, the better a man's chance for complete recovery.

Diagnosis.   When a man's symptoms suggest that he might have cancer in a testicle, the doctor will obtain a personal and family medical history and perform a complete physical examination. In addition to checking general signs of health (temperature, pulse rate, blood pressure, and so on), the doctor will carefully examine the scrotum. Also, the patient will usually have a chest x-ray film and blood and urine tests done. If the physical examination and laboratory tests do not show an infection or another disorder, the doctor is likely to suspect cancer because most tumors in the testicles are cancerous.

The only sure way to know whether cancer is present is for a pathologist to examine a sample of tissue under a microscope. To obtain the tissue, the affected testicle is removed through the groin. This operation is called inguinal orchiectomy. The surgeon does not cut through the scrotum and does not remove just a part of the testicle because if the problem is cancer, cutting through the outer layer of the testicle might cause local spread of the disease.

The most **common types** of testicular cancer are seminoma and nonseminoma.

- Seminomas make up about 40% of all cases.
- Nonseminomas are actually a group of cancers. They include choriocarcinoma, embryonal carcinoma, teratoma, and yolk sac tumors.

Each of these two major types of testicular cancer grows and spreads differently; therefore they are treated differently.

Treatment.   Testicular cancer is almost always curable if it is found early. This disease responds well to treatment, even if it has spread to other parts of the body.

How to Do Testicular Self-Examination

Men can improve their chance of finding a tumor by performing a testicular self-examination (TSE) once a month.

TSE should be performed after a warm bath or shower. The heat relaxes the scrotum, making it easier to find anything unusual. The procedure itself is simple and takes only a few minutes:

- Stand in front of a mirror. Look for any swelling on the skin of the scrotum.
- Examine each testicle with both hands. The index and middle fingers should be placed under the testicle while the thumbs are placed on the top. Gently roll the testicles between the thumbs and fingers. It is normal for one testicle to be larger than the other.

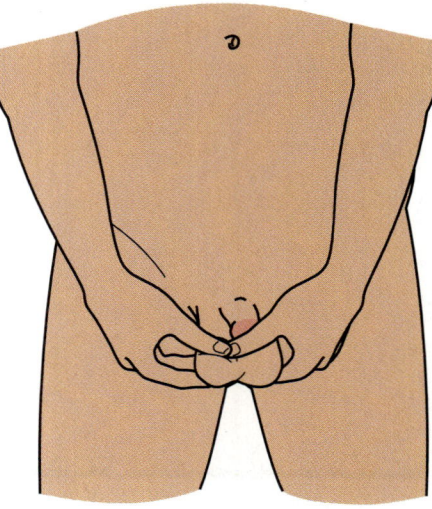

- Find the epididymis (the soft, tubelike structure at the back of the testicle that collects and carries the sperm). Do not mistake the epididymis for an abnormal lump.

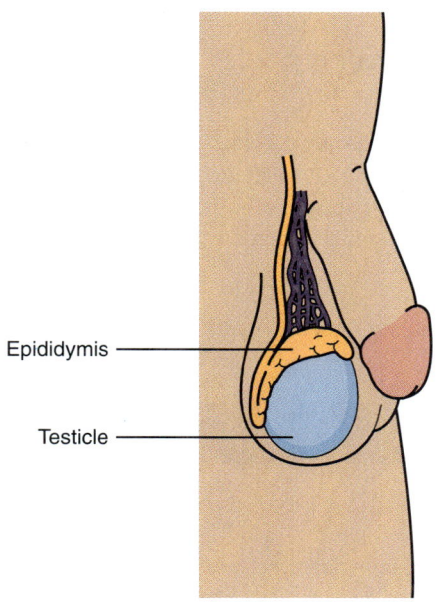

Epididymis

Testicle

If you find a lump, contact your doctor right away. Most lumps are found on the sides of the testicles, but some appear on the front. Remember that testicular cancer is highly curable, especially when treated promptly.

TSE performed regularly is an important health habit, but it cannot substitute for a physician's examination. Your doctor should check your testicles when you have a physical examination. You also can ask your doctor to teach you how to perform a TSE.

ENDOSCOPIC EXAMINATIONS: PROCTOSCOPY AND SIGMOIDOSCOPY

The **purpose** of a proctoscopy (prŏk-tŏs′ kō-pi) and sigmoidoscopy (sig″moi-dos′ ko-pi) is to examine the rectum and lower sigmoid colon for possible lesions, tumors, ulcers, polyps, inflammatory conditions, strictures, varicosities, and hemorrhages. Carcinoma may appear as a nodular, often cauliflower-like growth with superficial ulceration. Polyps are recognized easily by their pedicle. In doubtful cases, a biopsy of the growth is done.

If found early and treated properly, 75% to 80% of all cases of cancer of the rectum and lower bowel can be cured. Most cases occur in men and women at equal rates, between 55 to 75 years of age. Bowel cancers tend to grow slowly and are possible to detect at the most curable stage, before symptoms appear. Anyone with a personal or family history of rectal or colon cancer, of polyps in the rectum or colon, or of ulcerative colitis should be examined carefully. If cancer is found, surgery, sometimes combined with radiation therapy, is the most effective method of treatment. Recently chemotherapy has shown to be beneficial when given to patients after surgery in certain early colon cancer cases.

FIGURE 5-22   Examinations of the rectum and colon. *1,* Anus; *2,* rectum; *3,* limit of digital-rectal examination; *4,* colon; *5,* limit of rigid proctoscope examination; *6,* limit of flexible sigmoidoscope (35 cm) examination; *7,* limit of flexible sigmoidoscope (60 cm) examination; *8,* limit of stool blood test.

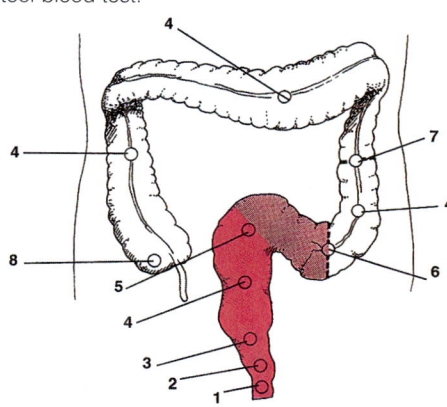

The American Cancer Society recommends that individuals have all of the following (Figure 5-22):

- Annual digital rectal examination after age 40
- Annual stool test for occult (hidden) blood after age 50 (see Chapter 11)
- Proctosigmoidoscopy examination every 5 years after age 50 **or** a colonoscopy every 10 years at age 50 and over

These guidelines apply only to people without symptoms. If a person has a change in bowel habits or has rectal bleeding, they should see a physician immediately.

Many physicians also recommend that a sigmoidoscopy be included as part of the annual physical examination for men over age 40 because of the relatively high incidence of cancer of the rectum and sigmoid colon in this age group.

A proctosigmoidoscopy takes approximately 10 to 15 minutes and requires **special preparation** of the patient beforehand.

Check with your physician or agency for specific instructions. Provide the patient with **printed instructions**. It is the medical assistant's responsibility to check that the patient is prepared before the examination begins. Generally the preparation includes a laxative the evening before (type and amount as prescribed by the physician), only liquids for breakfast, and tap water or saline enemas until the return is clear, usually 1 hour before the examination. NOTE: Enemas are usually avoided for patients who have colitis, bleeding from the rectum, or Crohn's disease.

Another preparation is for the patient to have nothing by mouth except *clear liquids* (for example, Jell-O, apple juice, 7-Up, ginger ale, beef or chicken bouillon) after 5 PM the night before and until the procedure is completed. Two hours before the procedure the patient is to give himself or herself a Fleet enema, hold the enema for 5 to 10 minutes, and then evacuate; then give himself or herself a second enema, hold the enema for 5 to 10 minutes, and then evacuate. The Fleet enema kit can be purchased at a pharmacy without a prescription.

An alternative preparation is the *GoLYTELY prep,* a commonly used prescription drug (cathartic or purgative) used to promote defecation and bowel evacuation. GoLYTELY is supplied in powder form in a plastic 1-gallon (4-L) container. Water is to be mixed with the powder as directed. Many suggest that the mixture tastes better if it is premixed and refrigerated for a few hours before being ingested. No solid foods are to be eaten 3 to 4 hours before drinking the GoLYTELY mixture. Clear fluids are allowed until the patient starts to drink the mixture at intervals as directed.

Depending on the physician's orders and the time of the examination, the patient may drink the GoLYTELY the night before or 2 hours before the examination begins. The patient must have clear liquid bowel movements at least 1 hour before the examination begins.

The *Colyte prep* is very similar to the GoLYTELY prep described in the preceding paragraphs, but it has the advantage of being supplied in a pineapple flavor, which is appealing to some patients.

CANCER FACTS

How Cancer Works*
Normally the cells that make up the body reproduce in an orderly manner so that worn-out tissues are replaced, injuries are repaired, and growth of the body proceeds.

Text continued on p. 200

---

*Courtesy American Cancer Society, San Francisco, Calif.

PROCEDURE 5-9

PROCTOSCOPY AND SIGMOIDOSCOPY

Objective
Understand and demonstrate the proper procedure for assisting the patient and the physician during proctoscopy and sigmoidoscopy examinations; provide the patient with any special instructions, and record the procedure on the patient's chart.

Equipment
Examination table covered with a clean sheet
Patient gown
Drape towel
Drape sheet
Small towel
Small pillow
Place and assemble the following equipment from the contents of the rectal diagnostic set on a clean drape towel (Figure 5-23):

    Sigmoidoscope with obturator (depending on the physician's request, either a 30- to 65-cm, flexible fiberoptic sigmoidoscope or a rigid, 30-cm sigmoidoscope; with the flexible fiberoptic sigmoidoscope the physician can view a greater portion of the intestinal tract)
    A rigid 15-cm proctoscope with obturator (depending on the physician's request)
    Transilluminators (light source)
    Rheostat
    Extension cord
    Insufflator with bulb attachment
    Suction tip for suction machine
    Biopsy forceps (sterile)
    Metal sponge holder or 12-inch long sponge sticks

When the above have been assembled, add:
    Disposable, single-use examination gloves
    Doctor's fluid-resistant gown
    Rectal dressing forceps
    Cotton-ball sponges
    4 × 4 inch gauze
    Tissues
    Water-soluble lubricant (such as K-Y jelly)
    Specimen bottle with preservative if biopsy is to be taken
    Laboratory request form
    Kidney basin
    Suction machine

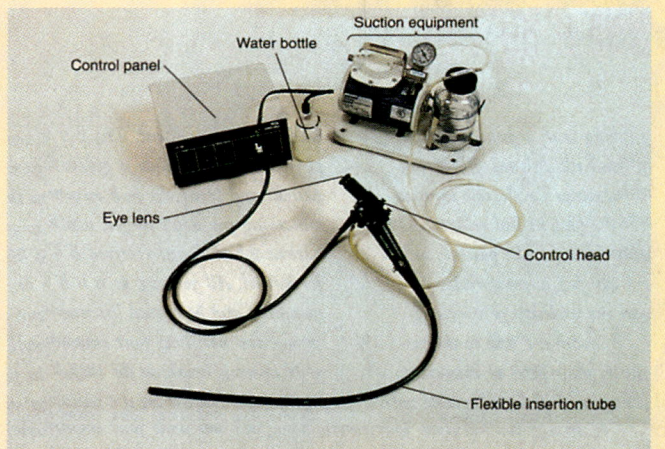

FIGURE 5-23 Equipment for sigmoidoscopy.

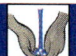

PROCTOSCOPY AND SIGMOIDOSCOPY—cont'd

PROCEDURE	RATIONALE

1. Wash your hands. Use appropriate personal protective equipment (PPE) as indicated by facility.

2. Assemble and prepare the necessary equipment and supplies on a clean drape towel. Disposable scopes may be used instead of the metal ones.

3. Test the suction apparatus and the light on the scopes.

Make sure they are working properly.

4. Identify the patient and explain the procedure carefully. Have the patient read and sign the consent form for the procedure (Figure 5-24). Answer any questions that the patient may have before the procedure begins.

This helps the patient understand the need for the examination and what to expect (that is, what will occur and how it may feel). It also enables the patient to cooperate more readily and to feel somewhat reassured.

5. Have the patient empty the bladder. Explain to the patient how to collect a specimen if a urinalysis is to be done. (Refer to Chapter 11 for specimen collection procedure.)

6. Have the patient remove all clothing from the waist down and put on the patient gown.

7. Position the patient.
   a. Knee-chest position: Many examining rooms have a special proctoscopic table that is tilted in a way that supports the patient in the knee-chest position (see Figure 5-9). Draping remains the same.

This is often preferred because it allows the abdominal contents to fall away from the pelvis, making it easier and less painful for the patient to be examined. NOTE: This is an uncomfortable position and usually cannot be tolerated for a long period.

CONSENT FOR FLEXIBLE SIGMOIDOSCOPY

It is possible to visualize the inside of the rectum and part of the colon with a flexible fiberoptic tube (flexible sigmoidoscopy). This examination is very helpful in evaluating patients with lower abdominal pain, abnormal bowel habits, or rectal bleeding. In addition, since most tumors (benign and malignant) of the colon occur within the reach of this instrument, it is a good screening test.

After preparation of the bowel with enemas, the sigmoidoscope is inserted directly into the rectum and advanced gradually in the colon. To facilitate this process, your colon may be distended with air injected through the sigmoidoscope. Some bloating or cramping may be felt during this process. If necessary, small samples of tissue may be removed for microscopic examination (biopsy) during the procedure. There is no discomfort associated with this.

The examination requires 5 to 15 minutes. You may have mild bloating afterward but there usually are no other side effects. Complications are very, very rare (less than one in 10,000) but include perforation of the bowel and bleeding. This could require surgery.

Complications may result from almost any medical procedure. It is good medical practice to inform patients about any procedure or test they are to have done. Consequently, you are asked to read this statement and sign it indicating that you understand the nature and indications for the procedure.

Date _____ Signature _____

Witness _____

FIGURE 5-24 Consent form to be signed by the patient before a sigmoidoscopy. Note that the patient is signing that he or she understands the nature and indications for the procedure.

Continued

PROCEDURE 5-9

PROCTOSCOPY AND SIGMOIDOSCOPY—cont'd

b. Sims or left lateral position: Position of the patient may vary with the physician's preference (see Figure 5-10).

This may be more comfortable for the patient, depending on age, weight, and condition.

8. Drape the patient completely. Refer to draping procedures on pp. 167-168.

9. Call the physician into the room.

NOTE: You may call the physician into the room and then position the patient, as this would avoid the necessity of having the patient in an uncomfortable position for an excessive amount of time.

10. When the physician is ready to begin the examination, pull the drape sheet back to expose only the anal area.

Avoid exposing the patient unnecessarily.

11. Assist the physician as required. Be prepared to hand the physician the various instruments and equipment. A female assistant should always remain in the room if the patient is female and the physician is male (see No. 11, p. 160). If you do not have to assist the physician, give your full attention to the patient. Provide support and reassurance. Observe the patient for any unusual reactions.

12. The physician begins the examination.

a. Put a generous amount of water-soluble lubricant on a 4 × 4 inch gauze square and place on the towel with the equipment. Use this for lubricating the instruments and the physician's gloved finger when the examination begins.

Method of examination: The physician first does a manual rectal examination. A liberal amount of lubricant is applied to the gloved index finger for easier insertion into the anal canal.

b. Warm the metal scopes by placing them in warm water or by rubbing them with your hand. Avoid additional discomfort for the patient that a cold instrument would cause.

This varies with office or agency preference. Disposable scopes do not need to be warmed.

c. Hand the physician the scope. Attach the inflation bulb to the scope.

The physician or you then lubricates the distal end of the scope with the obturator in place.

d. To help the patient relax the anal sphincter for easier insertion of the scope, instruct the patient to bear down slightly, as though having a bowel movement, at the same time the physician inserts the scope. Also, instruct the patient to take deep breaths through the mouth because this also helps relax the anus and rectum.

If right-handed, the physician separates the buttocks with the left hand and then slowly and gently inserts the scope about 3 to 4 cm. Force is never used when inserting the scope because it could cause injury to the bowel. The obturator is removed and can be placed in the kidney basin.

e. Attach the light source to the scope and adjust the light to the proper intensity. NOTE: You may turn off the lights in the room when the physician begins the visual examination through the scope. This allows for better inspection.

The physician visually inspects the bowel thoroughly as he or she advances the scope to its full length.

f. Observe the patient throughout the procedure for fatigue, weakness, or fainting.

Next, the physician pumps the inflator bulb attachment slowly to inject a small amount of air into the bowel. Although this is quite painful for the patient, it is necessary for proper inspection of the bowel. NOTE: This step is omitted in cases of ulcerative colitis or diverticulitis because of fragility of the bowel.

g. Turn on the suction machine if it is to be used.

h. You may hand the biopsy forceps to the physician. A biopsy forceps is placed through the scope if a biopsy is required.

When there is bleeding or loose discharge in the bowel, the physician may place a long, metal sponge holder with a sponge through the scope to swab the area clean, or the suction tip may be used.

PROCEDURE 5-9

PROCTOSCOPY AND SIGMOIDOSCOPY—cont'd

i.   Have ready a labeled specimen jar.

When a specimen is obtained, it should be placed immediately into the labeled specimen jar.

j.   Continue to offer reassurance and support to the patient. Often, just placing your hand on the patient's shoulder, arm, or hand gives the patient a feeling of being cared for as an individual.

On completing the examination, the physician removes the scope slowly, which may then be placed in the kidney basin.

13.   At the completion of the examination, take tissues and wipe the anal area for any lubricant or body discharge.

Provide for the patient's comfort.

14.   Help the patient assume a supine position. Often, it is desirable to allow the patient to rest for a few minutes before getting up because he or she may feel faint.

15.   Remove the drape sheet.

16.   When required, help the patient get up and get dressed. Provide the patient with extra tissues to cleanse the anal region more completely.

Always provide for the safety and comfort of the patient.

17.   Inform the patient of any special instructions. Inquire if the patient has any questions (see No. 13, p. 160). Provide complete and accurate information. Never leave a patient alone in a room after an examination without an understanding of what is to be done after getting dressed. Complications are rare, but the patient must be made aware of the following as early signs of possible complications and be instructed to call the physician if any occur:

- Severe abdominal pain
- Rectal bleeding of more than a cup; NOTE: Rectal bleeding may occur up to several days after a biopsy.
- Fever and chills

   Provide the patient with a printed form that has a short summary of recommended cancer-related checkups for the asymptomatic person (see Table 5-3). Explain this form to the patient when you give it to him or her.

18.   If your assistance is not required, leave the patient to dress in privacy.

19.   If specimens were obtained, send them to the laboratory. Be sure that all specimens are properly labeled and sent to the laboratory with the correct requisition form.

20.   Don disposable, single-use examination gloves and return to the examining room to assemble all used equipment and supplies. Remove linens and place in soiled laundry. Take the instruments to your cleanup area. Following Universal/Standard Precautions (see Chapter 1), rinse thoroughly with running water. You may then soak the instruments in soap and water until you are ready to prepare them for sterilization (see Chapter 2).

Continued

PROCEDURE 5-9

PROCTOSCOPY AND SIGMOIDOSCOPY—cont'd

NOTE: Do not soak the light attachment for the scope; cleanse it thoroughly with an alcohol sponge. Disposable equipment should be removed and placed in a covered waste container.

21. Wash the examination table with a disinfection solution and cover with a clean sheet or paper.

This prepares the examination room for the next patient.

22. Resupply clean equipment as needed.

23. Wash your hands.

24. Do any recording required of you completely and accurately (see No. 16, p. 161).

Charting Example

January 29, 20__, 1:15 PM
Sigmoidoscopy done by Dr. Short. Tissue biopsy sent with requisition to laboratory.
Gary Greaves, CMA

TABLE 5-2   **Five Most Common Cancer Sites by Age and Sex, 1995**

Age:	0-19	20-34	35-44	45-54	55-64	65-74	75+
Rank				**Males**			
1	Leukemia	Testis	Kaposi's sarcoma	Lung	Prostate	Prostate	Prostate
2	Brain	Kaposi's sarcoma	Non-Hodgkin's lymphoma	Prostate	Lung	Lung	Lung
3	Non-Hodgkin's lymphoma	Non-Hodgkin's lymphoma	Melanoma	Colorectal	Colorectal	Colorectal	Colorectal
4	Soft tissue	Melanoma	Testis	Non-Hodgkin's lymphoma	Bladder	Bladder	Bladder
5	Testis	Hodgkin's disease	Colorectal	Melanoma	Oral	Non-Hodgkin's lymphoma	Non-Hodgkin's lymphoma
Rank				**Females**			
1	Leukemia	Breast	Breast	Breast	Breast	Breast	Breast
2	Brain	Thyroid	Cervix	Lung	Lung	Lung	Colorectal
3	Hodgkin's disease	Melanoma	Melanoma	Uterus	Colorectal	Colorectal	Lung
4	Kidney	Cervix	Thyroid	Colorectal	Uterus	Uterus	Uterus
5	Thyroid	Ovary	Ovary	Ovary	Ovary	Ovary	Non-Hodgkin's lymphoma

Courtesy American Cancer Society, San Francisco, Calif.

Occasionally certain cells undergo an abnormal change and thus begin a process of uncontrolled growth and spread. These cells may grow into masses of tissue called tumors. Some tumors are benign, and others are malignant (cancerous).

The danger of cancer is that it invades and destroys normal tissue. In the beginning, cancer cells usually remain at their original site, and the cancer is said to be localized. Later, cancer cells may metastasize (that is, they invade distant or neigh-

TABLE 5–3   **Summary of American Cancer Society Recommendations for the Early Detection of Cancer in Asymptomatic People**

Cancer Site	Test or Procedure	Sex	Age	Frequency
Breast	Breast self-examination (BSE)	F	20 and over	Every month
	Clinical breast examination (CBE)	F	20-40	Every 3 years
			Over 40	Every year
	Mammography*	F	40 and over	Every year
Cervix uteri	Pap test†	F	Women who are or who have been sexually active or have reached age 18	Every year; may be less frequent after three or more consecutive satisfactory normal annual examinations
	Pelvic examination	F	18-40	Every 1-3 years
			Over 40	Every year
Colorectal	Stool blood test	M and F	50 and over	Yearly
	and			
	flexible sigmoidoscopy	M and F	50 and over	Every 5 years
	or			
	total colon examination with double-contrast barium enema	M and F	50 and over	Every 5-10 years
	or			
	colonoscopy		50 and over	Every 10 years
Prostate	Digital rectal examination (DRE)‡	M and F	50 and over	Every year
	Prostate Specific Antigen (PSA)	M	50 and over	Every year
Other	Health counseling and	M and F	Over 20	Every 3 years
	cancer checkup§	M and F	Over 40	Every year

*Screening mammography should begin by age 40.

†*Endometrium:* Women at high risk for cancer of the uterus should have a sample of endometrial tissue examined when menopause begins. History of infertility, obesity, failure to ovulate, abnormal uterine bleeding, or unopposed estrogen or tamoxifen therapy.

‡Annual digital rectal examination and prostate-specific antigen should be performed on men age 50 and older. If either is abnormal, further evaluation should be considered.

§To include examination of cancers of the thyroid, testicles, ovaries, lymph nodes, oral region, and skin.

Nutrition guidelines
1. Maintain a desirable body weight.
2. Cut down on total fat intake.
3. Include a variety of both vegetables and fruits in the daily diet.
4. Eat more high-fiber foods, such as whole grain cereals, legumes, vegetables and fruits.
5. Limit consumption of alcoholic beverages, if you drink at all.
6. Limit consumption of salt cured, smoked, and nitrate-preserved foods.
7. Eat a varied diet.

Courtesy American Cancer Society, San Francisco, Calif.

Cancer's seven warning signals
1. Change in bowel or bladder habits
2. A sore that does not heal
3. Unusual bleeding or discharge
4. Thickening or lump in breast or elsewhere
5. Indigestion or difficulty in swallowing
6. Obvious change in wart or mole
7. Nagging cough or hoarseness

If you have a warning signal, see your doctor.

boring organs or tissues). This occurs either by direct extension of growth or by cells becoming detached and carried through the lymph or blood systems to other parts of the body.

Metastasis may be regional—confined to one region of the body—when cells are trapped by lymph nodes. If left untreated, however, the cancer is likely to spread throughout the body. That condition is known as advanced cancer and usually results in death. Because cancer becomes more serious with each stage, it is important to detect it as early as possible. Aids to early detection include the seven warning signals and the cancer risk factors (Tables 5-2 to 5-4).

Cancer risk varies considerably by age, with fewer than 1% of all cancers occurring before the age of 15 and 58% occurring after the age of 65. In fact, 50% of all cancers occur between the ages of 55 to 74, and more cancers occur after age 85 than between birth and age 35.

Text continued on p. 206

TABLE 5–4 Major Cancer Sites

	Cancer Risk Factors	Risk Reduction	Early Detection (Asymptomatic Persons)
Bladder (urinary)	Tobacco use; aniline dye used in textile and rubber industries; personal history of bladder cancer.	Avoid use of tobacco products; use workplace safety precautions if working in high-risk industry.	Health-related checkups may identify early signs and symptoms.
Brain	Increasing among older persons; second leading cause of death in children.	None known.	Health-related checkups may identify early signs and symptoms.
Breast	Age; family history in mother or sisters; precancerous condition on breast biopsy; first child born after age 30; obesity; obesity in postmenopausal women never having had children; cancer genes have been identified.	Follow ACS's nutrition guidelines; maintain normal weight; exercise 3 times per week.	Mammography; breast self-examinations; annual clinical breast examinations.
Cervix uteri	Papilloma virus infections; early age at first intercourse; multiple sexual partners; smoking; low-socioeconomic status; poor compliance to screening programs or never having had screening.	Safe sex; avoid use of tobacco products.	Pap smear and pelvic examination.
Colorectal cancer	Personal or family history of colorectal cancer, colorectal polyps; diets high in fat and low in fiber; inflammatory bowel disease.	Removal of polyps; follow the ACS's nutrition guidelines for diets high in fiber and low in fats; recent studies suggest drugs like aspirin may reduce risk.	Flexible sigmoidoscopy; digital rectal examination; stool blood test or total colon examinations.
Endometrium (uterine cancer)	Some forms of infertility; obesity; use of unopposed postmenopausal estrogens; diabetes.	When considering estrogen replacement therapy, benefits and risks must be considered by woman and her physician.	Pelvic examination; endometrial tissue sampling at menopause if high risk.
Hodgkin's disease	Viral causes have been suggested but not proven.	None known.	Health-related checkups may identify early signs and symptoms.
Lymphoma (non-Hodgkin's)	AIDS in some cases; transplantation and immunosuppression therapy; viral causes have been suggested in some types; increased risk is associated with certain genetic diseases.	None known.	Health-related checkups may identify early signs and symptoms.

ACS, American Cancer Society.

TABLE 5–4   **Major Cancer Sites—cont'd**

Warning Signs	Treatment	Special Information
Blood in urine.	In situ stage—surgery and possible instillation of drugs. Later stages—surgery at times with radiation therapy or chemotherapy. Metastatic disease—radiation therapy and chemotherapy.	Modifications of surgical techniques to preserve bladder continence are under study.
Headaches, convulsions, personality changes, visual problems, unexplained vomiting.	In adults—surgery, possibly chemotherapy or radiation therapy. In children—surgery, chemotherapy, and radiation therapy.	Metastases to brain occur with many other cancers. Symptoms may be reduced by using cortisone-like drugs and radiation therapy.
Breast lump or a thickening, bleeding from nipple, skin irritation, retraction.	Early stage—mastectomy or local removal with radiation therapy. Adjuvant therapy—hormones and/or combination chemotherapy. Later stage—combination chemotherapy or hormones and radiation therapy for selected clinical problems.	Bone-marrow transplantation is being tested in women with advanced disease. Breast reconstruction after mastectomy has had good cosmetic results. ACS has special Reach to Recovery programs to help women.
Abnormal vaginal bleeding.	Precursor lesions—cryotherapy (kills cells by cold), electrocoagulation (kills cells by heat from an electrical current), surgery. Localized—surgery or radiation therapy. Invasive—surgery or radiation therapy. Metastatic—chemotherapy and radiation therapy.	The use of the Pap test has greatly reduced the death rate from cervical cancer. The Pap test must be made available to women who have never had the test or who have had infrequent screening. Mature and underserved women may not have the test available. Such women should be prime targets for screening programs.
Rectal bleeding, change in bowel habits, blood in the stools.	Surgery at times combined with radiation therapy or chemotherapy. Chemotherapy in advanced cases is under study.	Colostomy is seldom necessary now for colon cancer and is infrequently needed for rectal cancer patients. New helpful adjuvant treatments have been reported recently.
Vaginal bleeding after menopause.	For uterine hyperplasia, progestins may be used. Surgery sometimes with radiation therapy. Advanced metastases—progestins/chemotherapy.	The cure rate for endometrial cancer is high because tumors tend to be well differentiated and localized.
Night sweats, itching, unexplained fever, lymph node enlargement.	Early stages—radiation therapy sometimes with chemotherapy. Advanced stages—combination chemotherapy.	There has been dramatic improvement in the outcome of this cancer. Most patients are cured.
Lymph node enlargement, fever.	Usually disseminated at time of diagnosis; chemotherapy is used. At times, autologous bone marrow transplantation may be used.	Surgery may be useful when lymphoma is found in the gastrointestinal tract and to remove the spleen when it is overactive.

Continued

TABLE 5–4   **Major Cancer Sites—cont'd**

	Cancer Risk Factors	Risk Reduction	Early Detection (Asymptomatic Persons)
Leukemia	Persons with genetic abnormalities such as Down syndrome; ionizing radiation; exposure to certain chemicals, cytotoxic drugs; certain forms are related to retrovirus, HTLV-1.	Reduce exposure to radiation and hazardous chemicals.	Health-related checkups may identify early signs and symptoms.
Lung	Tobacco use; voluntary and involuntary smoking; occupational exposure to hazardous substances such as asbestos.	Avoid tobacco products in all forms; stop smoking; avoid second-hand smoke; follow workplace safety practices.	Chest x-ray studies for high-risk persons only.
Melanoma (skin)	Fair skin; sun exposure; severe sunburn in childhood; familial conditions such as dysplastic nevus syndrome; large congenital moles.	Protect against sun exposure, especially in childhood; use protective clothing and sunscreens with SPF 15 or greater when exposed to the sun.	Annual skin examinations by an experienced physician; monthly self-examinations.
Oral	Tobacco use; excessive use of alcohol; poor dentition.	Avoid tobacco products in all forms and, if you must drink alcohol, do so in moderation.	Regular oral examinations.
Ovary	Increases with age; possible dietary factors; older women who have never had children are at risk; history of breast, endometrial, or colon cancer; family history; genes have been identified.	Following ACS's nutrition guidelines may be helpful. Prophylactic ovarian removal.	Health-related checkups may identify early signs and symptoms.
Pancreas	Increases after age 50 with most cases between ages 65 and 79; more common in smokers; occurs more often in African Americans; may be associated with pancreatitis, diabetes, and diet.	Following ACS's nutrition guidelines may be helpful.	Health-related checkups may identify early signs and symptoms.
Prostate	Age is the most important risk factor; 80% of all prostate cancer occurs in men over age 65; dietary fat may play a role; high in African Americans.	Although not certain, prudent action would be to follow ACS's nutrition guidelines.	Digital rectal examination; prostate-specific antigen (PSA) test.
Stomach	Occurs in those 50 to 70 years old; pernicious anemia; certain types of gastritis; possible gastric ulcers; dietary factors.	Avoid food high in nitrates; consume foods with selenium, beta-carotene, and vitamin E.	Health-related checkups may identify early signs and symptoms.
Testis	Undescended testis.	None known.	Testicular self-examination in young men has been suggested.

HTLV-1, Human T-cell lymphotropic virus.

TABLE 5–4   Major Cancer Sites—cont'd

Warning Signs	Treatment	Special Information
Fatigue, pallor, repeated infection, easy bruising, nose bleeds.	Combination chemotherapy; bone marrow transplantation may be used in some cases.	There has been dramatic improvement in the outcome of acute childhood leukemia. The majority of children are cured and live into adulthood leading normal lives.
Nagging cough, coughing up blood, unresolved pneumonia.	Surgery, radiation therapy, and chemotherapy depending on type. In small-cell lung cancer, chemotherapy alone or combined with radiation therapy may be the first choice.	Lung cancer rates in men have begun to decrease, but the rates in women continue to increase as a result of smoking.
A change in a mole or a sore that does not heal.	Early stage—surgery. Advanced stages—surgery, radiation therapy, chemotherapy, immunotherapy.	Melanoma is increasing because of environmental and lifestyle changes. For early detection, follow ABCD rule: A—asymmetry of mole (one side does not match the other); B—Border irregularity (edges are irregular); C—color (is not uniform); D—diameter (the size is greater than 6 mm).
Sore in mouth that does not heal; color change in an area of the mouth.	Radiation therapy and surgery; chemotherapy is being studied.	This cancer is significantly affected by alcohol and tobacco use.
Often "silent"; abdominal symptoms, pain.	Surgery, radiation therapy, and chemotherapy.	Health-related checkups may identify early signs and symptoms.
Vague abdominal symptoms, pain.	Surgery, radiation therapy, and chemotherapy may be used. Disease is often advanced at the time of diagnosis.	Two percent of pancreatic cancers occur in the insulin-producing cells. Thirty percent of these patients live 3 years or more after diagnosis.
Difficulty passing urine; blood in urine. These symptoms can be due to benign (noncancer) conditions.	Early stage—surgery or radiation therapy. Advanced stages—radiation therapy, hormone treatments, or anticancer drugs. Radiation therapy can ease painful areas in the bones.	New operations that save nerves and blood supply can preserve potency. New hormonal treatments are being tested.
Indigestion.	Surgery; combination chemotherapy may be helpful.	Decreasing worldwide but a prevalent cancer in Japan, Chile, Iceland, and other countries.
Testicular mass or enlargement.	Early stage—surgery at times with radiation therapy. Advanced stages—chemotherapy.	Survival rates for this cancer have seen a dramatic improvement as a result of therapy. Many patients are cured of this disease.

Cancers occurring before the age of 20 are typically nonepithelial in origin, with the most common types being leukemias, tumors of the brain and nervous system, and lymphomas. Five-year survival rates for childhood cancers vary considerably, depending on the type of cancer, but in general survival is excellent.

Within California, cancer patterns in young adult men differ somewhat from patterns in other geographic areas in that the most common cancer among men between ages 20 and 44 is Kaposi's sarcoma. Melanoma is an important cancer among young adults of both sexes. Breast cancer is the most common cancer among all ages of adult women. After age 45, lung cancer is among the top three cancers for both men and women. Cancer patterns change relatively little after age 65, with the four most common cancers remaining the same within each sex group.

OTHER SPECIAL EXAMINATIONS

Numerous other special or more specific examinations may be performed to gain pertinent information about a body part or system.

NEUROLOGIC EXAMINATION

The neurologic examination tests for adequate functioning of the cranial nerves, the motor or sensory systems, and the superficial and deep tendon reflexes.

Equipment and supplies

- Pins and cotton to test the senses of touch, sensation, and pain on the external surfaces of the body (Figure 5-25)
- Tuning fork to test hearing
- Ophthalmoscope to examine the interior of the eye

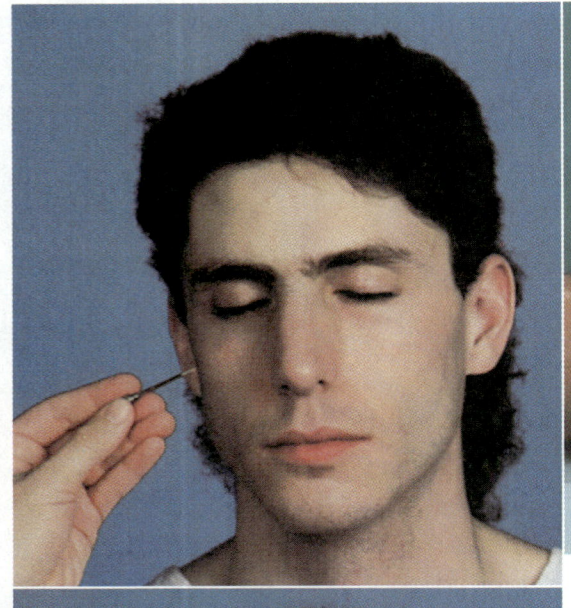

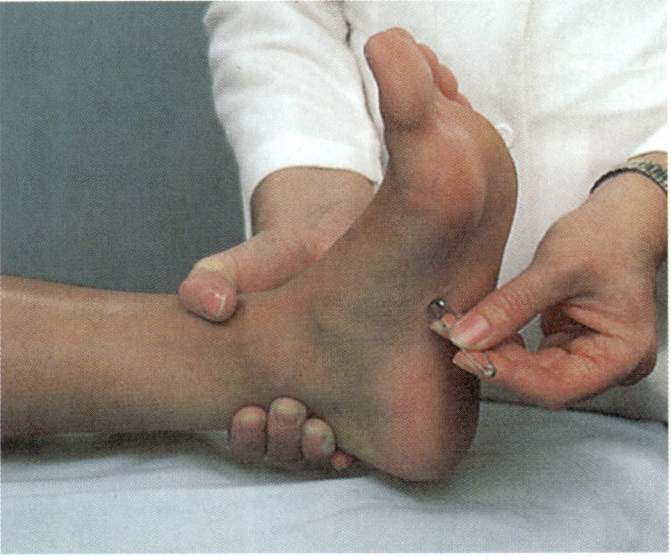

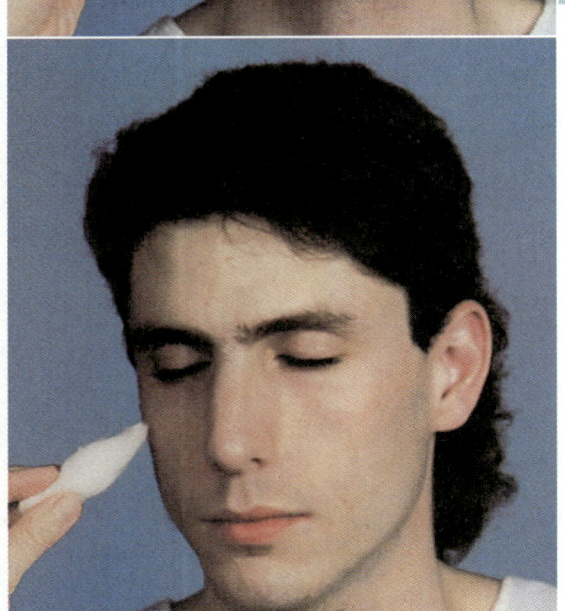

FIGURE 5-25   **A,** Evaluation for sensation and superficial pain using the sharp point of a safety pin. **B,** Alternate use of the dull end of the pin for evaluation of sensation and pain. **C,** Test of light touch sensation using cotton applied to stimulate the sensory nerve endings.

- Flashlight to test pupil reactions and equality
- Tongue depressor to test the gag and corneal reflexes, as well as pharyngeal sensation
- Percussion hammer to test superficial and deep tendon reflexes (Figure 5-26)
- Test tubes with hot and cold water to test the skin for heat and cold sensation
- Bottles of sweet, bitter, salty, and sour solutions to test the sense of taste
- Bottles of substances that have common familiar odors to test the sense of smell

The physician also observes the patient's level of consciousness, behavior, and the higher functions of speech and writing. Coordination, balance, gait, muscle tone, and strength are noted for adequate functioning of the motor system. The sense of touch, pain (deep and superficial), temperature, and discriminatory sensations are noted in the examination of the sensory system.

HEARING EXAMINATION

To detect impaired hearing, the physician uses an otoscope to inspect the external ear canal and eardrum (Figure 5-27) and a tuning fork to test for hearing acuity.

Using the **otoscope**, the physician examines the ear canal for the presence of cerumen (ear wax), redness, swelling, le-sions, discharge, or foreign bodies. Then he or she inspects the color, contour, and landmarks of the eardrum.

The **tuning fork** is used to determine the distance at which the patient can hear a certain sound (**air conduction test**) and for **bone conduction tests.** In **Weber's** bone conduction test, the vibrating end of the tuning fork is placed on the patient's skull or forehead. This test is valuable in distinguishing between perceptive and transmission deafness (Figure 5-28).

The **Rinne** test checks for both bone conduction and air conduction. The base of the vibrating tuning fork is placed on the mastoid bone (behind the earlobe). The examiner times the interval until the patient no longer hears any sound, then quickly places the still vibrating tines of the tuning fork approximately $\frac{1}{2}$ to 1 inch from the ear canal and continues to count the time until the patient no longer hears any sound by air conduction. The patient who does not have any hearing loss will hear the sound by air conduction twice as long as by bone conduction. For example, if the patient's hearing is normal, he or she may hear a sound for 15 seconds when the handle of the tuning fork is placed on the mastoid bone and hears a sound for an additional 30 seconds when the tines are placed $\frac{1}{2}$ to 1 inch from the ear.

A more accurate test to gauge and record the hearing sense is done with the use of an audiometer, a delicate instrument consisting of complex parts. For audiometry the patient is placed in a soundproof room and puts on earphones. Timing circuits, sound wave generators, and other complex pieces of

FIGURE 5-26   Elicitation of the patella reflex. A tap with the percussion hammer is applied directly inferior to the patella: **A,** with the patient sitting and legs hanging over the examining table; **B,** with the patient in a supine position. The normal response is the leg kicking out or extension of the leg.

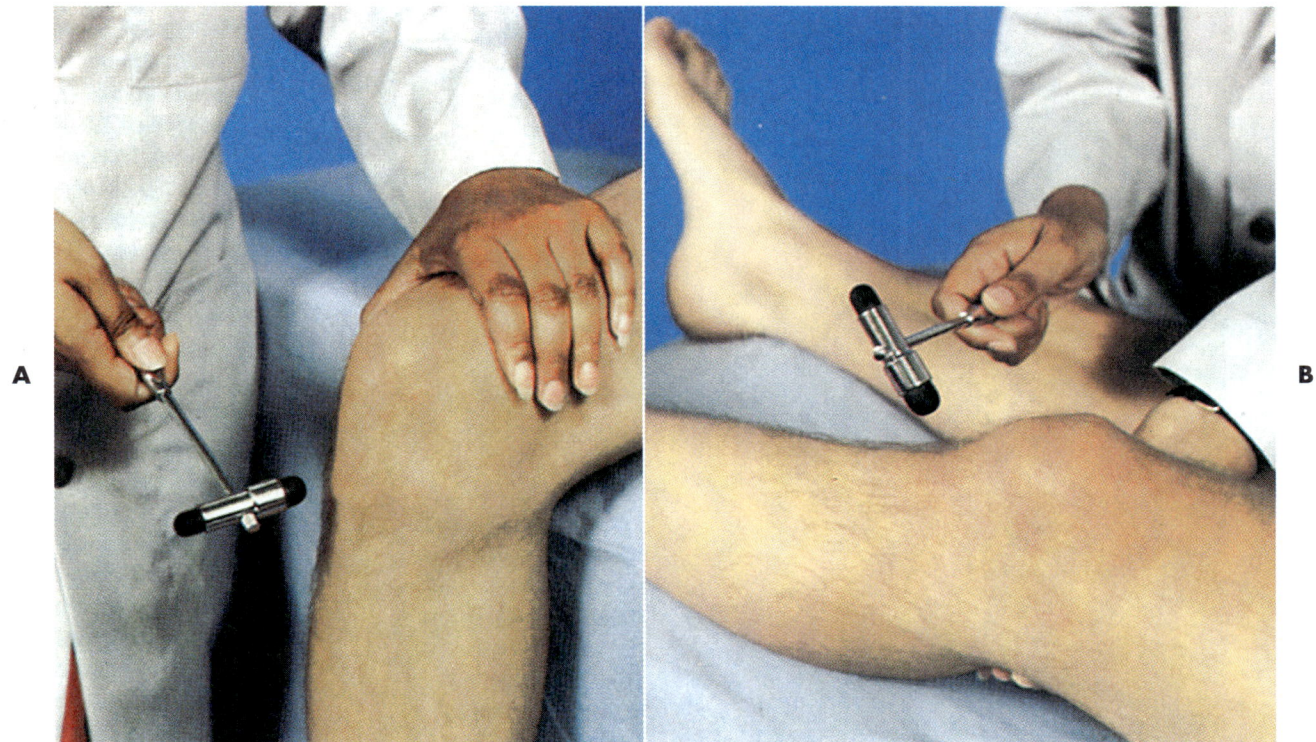

FIGURE 5-27 The patient's head is tipped toward the opposite shoulder for examination of the ear with an otoscope.

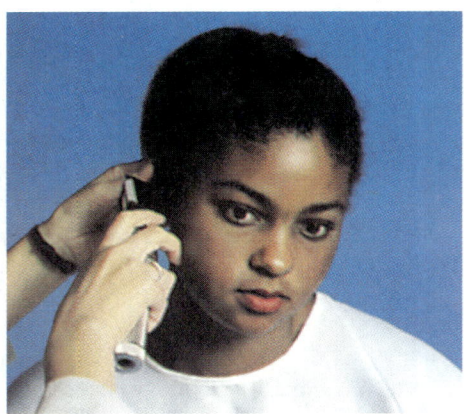

FIGURE 5-28 Hearing examination. **A,** Weber's bone conduction test. **B,** Rinne bone conduction test. **C,** Rinne air conduction test.

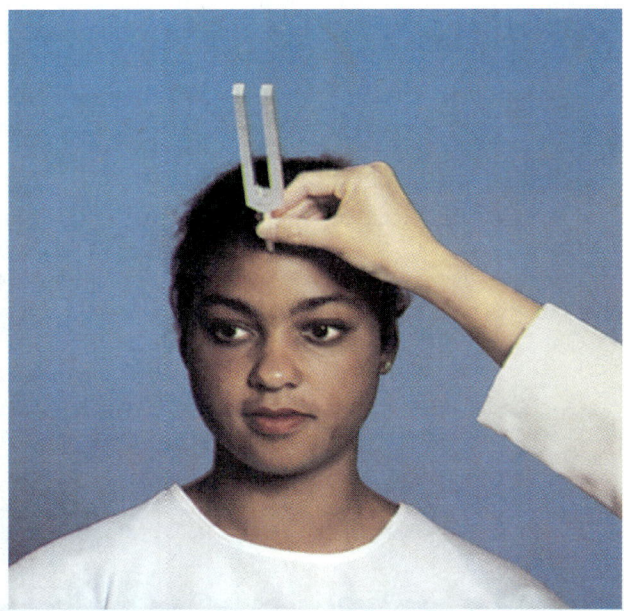

A

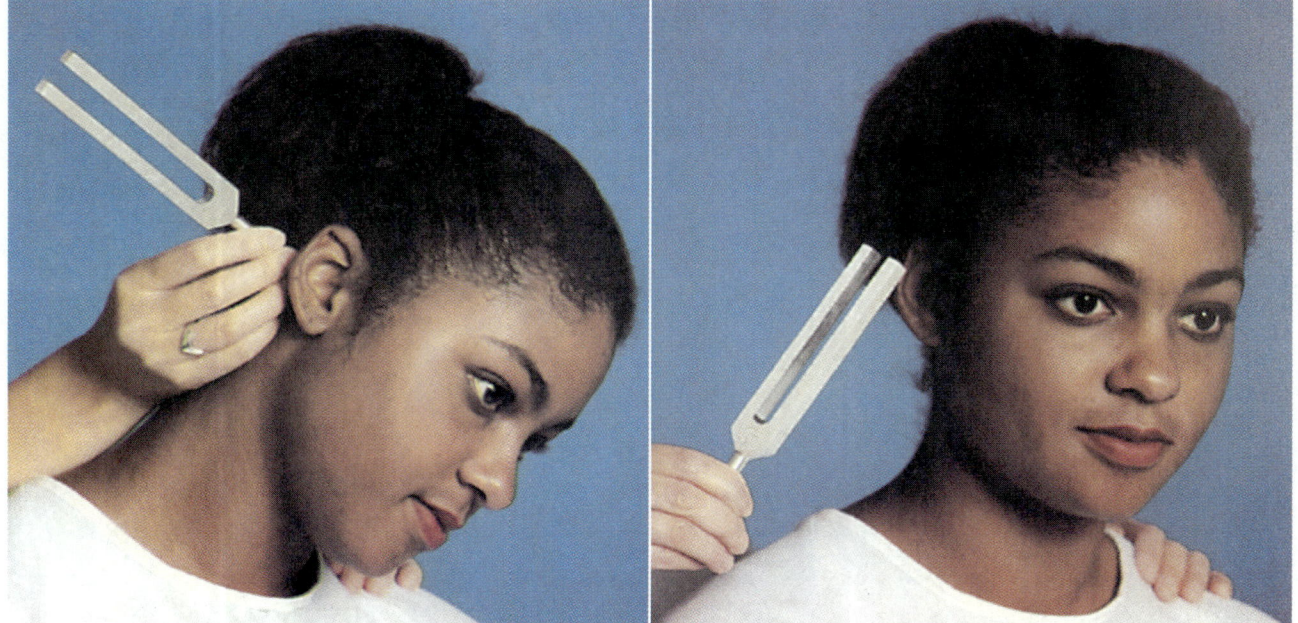

B

C

equipment are used to measure the patient's acuity of hearing for the various frequencies of sound waves. Each ear is assessed separately. Results are plotted on a graph called an audiogram, and these results can indicate if the patient has a hearing loss. If there is a loss of hearing, audiometry can indicate whether it is caused by a problem in the outer, middle, or inner ear or by a problem with the acoustic nerve. No special preparation of the patient is required for this test. Physicians, audiometric technicians, or other specially trained individuals perform this test (Figure 5-29). Also see the box below.

FIGURE 5-29   Audiometer is used to measure the patient's acuity of hearing bilaterally. Patient dons earphones and responds to various frequencies of sound waves by hand signaling.

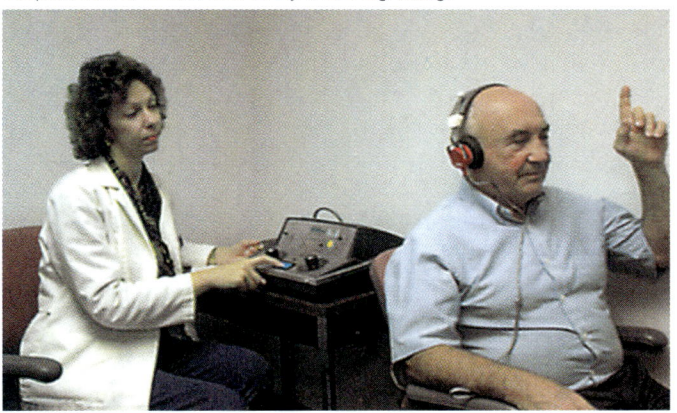

EYE EXAMINATION

External Eye Examinations

Distance visual acuity.   Visual acuity means acuteness or clarity of vision. Visual acuity may be measured on patients having complete physical examinations; but more specifically, it is measured because patients have a specific visual complaint, because of employment requirements, or to meet requirements of the Department of Motor Vehicles for obtaining specific types of drivers' licenses, such as a chauffeur's or truck driver's license. The visual acuity test is also performed in schools and on preschool-age children as a means of vision screening.

Imperfect refractive powers of the eye include conditions known as **myopia** (nearsightedness), **hyperopia** (farsightedness), and **astigmatism** (another refractive error of the eye resulting from irregularities in the curvature of the cornea and/or surfaces of the lens of the eye).

Myopia occurs when the lens of the eye is too thick or the eyeball is too long. Correction is made by using a concave lens to help the light rays come to a focus on the retina. Within the last 10 years, technologic advances have ushered in a new era for treatment of myopia using a surgical procedure called radial keratotomy (RK). This surgery is of special interest to people who do not want to depend on glasses or contact lenses for corrected vision.

Recently two surgical procedures using the excimer laser have been preferred over RK because they are thought to be

---

HEALTH MATTERS

KEEPING YOUR PATIENTS INFORMED

Hearing loss, whether acquired or congenital, is the most common disability in the United States. It is estimated that one in every five Americans experiences some degree of hearing loss. The two major types of hearing loss are nerve loss and conductive hearing loss. **Nerve loss (sensorineural hearing loss),** the most common type, is caused by a defect in the inner ear or auditory nerve. This type of hearing loss is the one most commonly associated with aging. As we age, a natural deterioration of nerve cells can occur. The term **presbycusis** (which means elder's ear) is used to describe hearing sensitivity and nerve loss in the higher sound frequencies associated with aging. Nerve loss is also related to long-term exposure to loud noise, hereditary factors, and diminished blood supply to the inner ear. High cholesterol and tobacco use are related to decreasing the blood supply to the inner ear. Direct trauma can also be the cause of nerve damage. Presbycusis can usually be improved with the use of a hearing aid.

In **conductive hearing loss,** transmission of sound to the inner ear is partially or totally limited. This can be due to disease or injury, such as thickening or perforation of the eardrum, or a disease or

functional change in the middle ear that affects one or more of the ossicles. Chronic ear infections, fluid behind the eardrum, and trauma can also cause conductive hearing loss. Surgery can help some types of conductive hearing loss.

People often do not notice that their hearing has changed until someone else notices that they can't hear as well as they did before, they are talking much louder than usual, or they frequently misunderstand what someone has said to them. Others may notice that they cannot hear background noises, they constantly hear a noise or ringing (tinnitus) in their ears, and they may complain of not understanding what is being said, especially in noisy environments.

Despite whether they notice that their hearing has changed, older adults should have their hearing tested every year or every 2 years.

RESOURCES

- Self Help for Hard of Hearing People (SHHH)
  301-657-2249 (TTY), 301-657-2248 (voice)
  on-line: http://www.shhh.org.
- National Institute on Deafness and Other Communication Disorders
  http://www.nih.gov/nidcd/

safer, more precise, and longer lasting. These laser surgical procedures are photorefractive keratectomy (PRK) and laser-assisted in situ keratomileusis (LASIK). Both procedures can also be used to correct an astigmatism. PRK and LASIK can be performed in an ophthalmologist's office or clinic with the use of anesthetic eyedrops and 30 to 90 seconds of actual laser time. Vision correction in up to 98% of the patients will reach at least 20/40, and about 80% of the patients will reach 20/20 vision.

Hyperopia occurs when the lens of the eye is too thin or the eyeball is too short, causing rays of light entering the eye to come into focus behind the retina. With hyperopia a person finds it difficult to view objects at an average reading distance. Correction is made by using a convex lens to help light rays focus on the retina. As people age, another type of farsightedness, called **presbyopia,** often develops. This condition results from a loss of elasticity of the lens of the eye.

In an **astigmatism,** light rays cannot be focused clearly in a point on the retina because of an uneven curvature of the cornea or lens. Vision is blurred, thereby causing discomfort. Correction is made by using contact lenses or eyeglasses ground to neutralize the defect.

These conditions can be detected by using the **Snellen eye chart** to measure distance visual acuity. The *Snellen eye chart* (Figure 5-30) consists of block letters arranged in rows in gradually decreasing sizes. Another chart used for preschoolers, individuals unable to speak English, slow learners, and those unable to read is the **E chart,** which consists of the letter "E"

arranged in different directions in decreasing sizes. Charts with pictures of common objects such as a house and truck are available to use when testing preschoolers, although some children are unable to identify the objects because of lack of knowledge rather than a defect in visual acuity (see Figure 5-30, *C*).

On the *Snellen* chart there are two standardized numbers on the side of each row of letters; these numbers, shown one on top of the other, indicate the degree of visual acuity measured from a distance of 20 feet, the standard testing distance. The top number is 20, indicating the number of feet between the chart and the person taking the test; the bottom number indicates the distance in feet from which the normal eye can read the row of letters. The large letter on the top of the chart can be read by the normal eye at a distance of 200 feet. This is indicated as 20/200. In each of the succeeding rows, from top to bottom, the size of the letters decreases to the point at which the normal eye can read the row of letters at distances of 100, 70, 50, 40, 30, 25, 20, 15, 13, and 10 feet. The row marked 20/20 indicates normal visual acuity and is expressed as 20/20 vision. A measurement of visual acuity of less than 20/20 vision indicates a refractive error or some other eye disorder (for example, when the letters on the row marked 20/50 are read, the person is said to have 20/50 vision, which means that the person can read at only 20 feet what the normal eye can read at 50 feet). The larger the bottom number of the row that can be read, the poorer the vision. A reading of 20/15 indicates above-average distance vision (see Figure 5-30, *A* and *B*).

FIGURE 5-30   A, Snellen eye chart consisting of varied letters arranged in rows of gradually decreasing sizes; **B,** Snellen Big E eye chart consisting of the letter "E" arranged in different directions in decreasing sizes. These charts are used to measure distance visual acuity; **C,** objects chart for testing preschoolers.

A   **B**   **C**

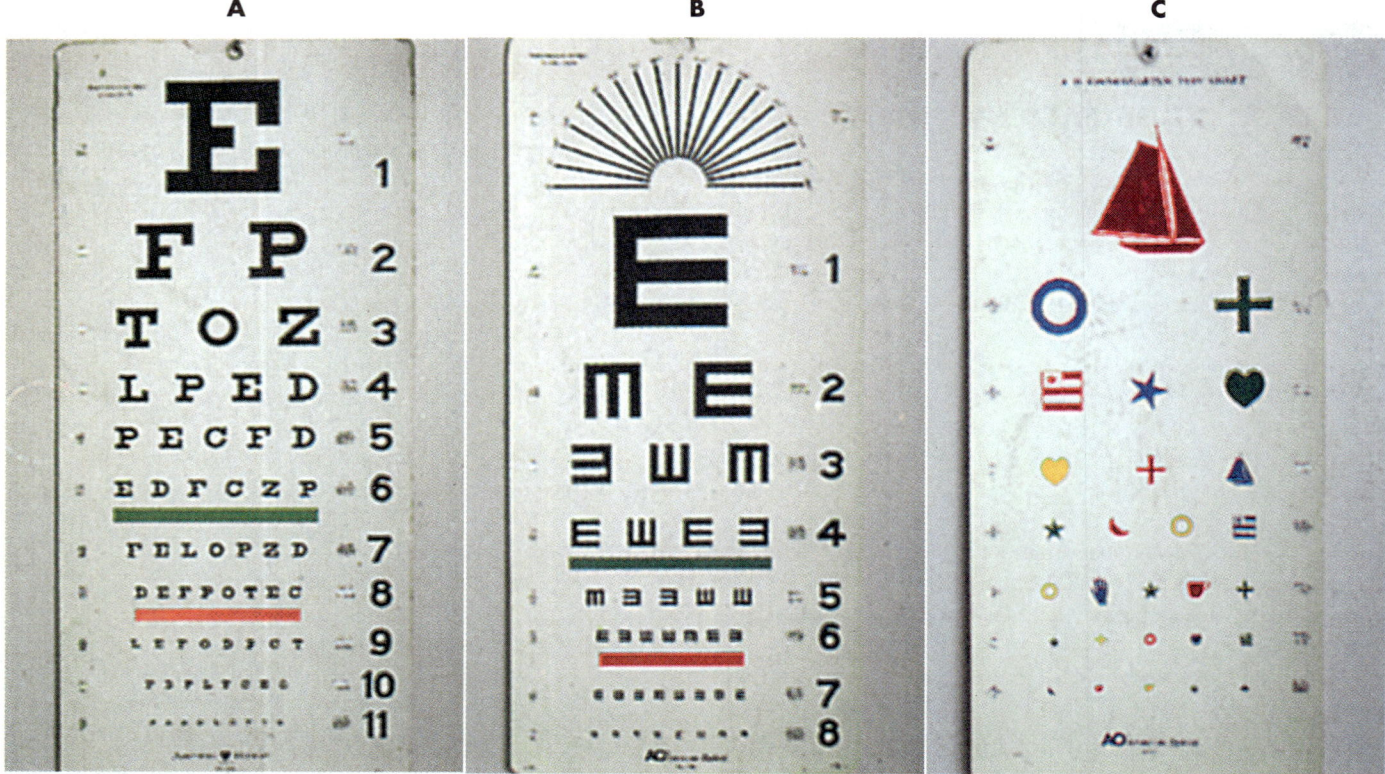

This test is to be given in a well-lit room, with the person taking the test standing or sitting 20 feet away from the chart and the chart placed at eye level to the person. Each eye is to be tested separately, with and without glasses or contact lenses. **Many physicians prefer that patients who wear glasses regularly keep the glasses or contact lenses on during the test. In this case, it *must* be charted that the patient wore glasses or contact lenses during the test.**

However, reading glasses should not be worn during the test because they tend to blur distant vision. The results must be recorded indicating the reading for each eye without and with glasses or contact lenses. Usually, each eye is tested separately because the stronger eye usually compensates for the weaker eye. Patients who are unable to see even the largest numbers on the Snellen chart (top line 20/200) are given additional tests to determine if they can see enough to count fingers (this is recorded as CF), perceive hand movements (HM), perceive light (LP), or perceive light with projection (LPcP). NLP is used to record "no light projection." An ophthalmologist considers patients to be blind when they cannot even perceive light. **Legal blindness** is defined as vision of 20/200 or less in both eyes when wearing correction glasses.

For office space that does not have a 20-foot hallway or space, charts are available that can be used at a distance of 10 feet; or the patient can stand or sit 10 feet away from the standard Snellen chart, and the results recorded would indicate that the test was performed at a distance of 10 feet (for example, if the patient's distance visual acuity was measured using the standard eye chart at a distance of 10 feet, the results would be recorded as "20/20 at 10 feet"). The physician then converts the results. This test is not as reliable as the test recorded at 20 feet because at a distance of 10 feet the eye has to focus, whereas at a distance of 20 feet the eye does not have to focus.

Electric vision testing devices. *Electric testing devices* such as the Titmus II Vision Tester, which is the product of advances in computer-designed optics (Figure 5-31), are also on the market. This one compact instrument, using eight test slides, can screen patients of *all* ages (preschool through adults) for all common vision problems—problems that the standard wall chart misses. *The Titmus II Vision Tester measures acuity (both far and near), hyperopia, binocularity, muscle balance, color perception, depth perception, and, with the optional equipment, peripheral vision and intermediate vision, all within 5 minutes.* The standard wall chart measures only distance vision. The fiber-optic perimeter system determines if peripheral vision is adequate, a basic requirement for employees who operate machinery and mobile equipment. The intermediate distance feature tests the intermediate distance (20 to 40 inches), viewing capabilities important to machine workers and to the increasing number of video display terminal operators. Because of its extremely compact and lightweight design, the Titmus II Vision Tester can be used virtually anywhere. It is especially convenient when performing vision screening tests on large groups or in small areas where space is less than 20 feet. Only 5 square feet of space is required for using this instrument. Patients of all ages and statures can be easily screened

because of the unit's balanced height adjustment. The face mask of the unit eliminates outside light and is designed to accommodate all sizes and types of eyeglasses. A training manual complete with an instructional cassette supplied as standard equipment provides correct testing techniques that are easy to learn. The Titmus II Vision Tester is a complete system for all vision screening in each individual office situation (see Figure 5-31).

Measuring distance visual acuity in preschoolers.   For testing distance visual acuity in preschoolers *(and also for testing non–English-speaking or illiterate people),* the **Snellen Big E eye chart** can be used (see Figure 5-30, *B*). This chart uses the capital letter "E" pointing in four directions. This test is very similar to the preceding procedure using the Snellen eye chart. Children and others "read" the chart by showing the direction of the letter E or use a large duplicate E to match the E that you are pointing to on the chart. Before beginning the test, use a practice E card and have the child practice identifying which direction the "legs of the E" are pointing (Figure 5-32, *A*). Teach the child how to use the eye cover to cover one eye while the other eye is being tested (Figure 5-32, *B*). Instruct the child to keep both eyes open during the test. Position the child comfortably, either standing or sitting, 20 feet away from the chart.

If the child wears glasses, test only with the glasses on. First test both eyes together; then the right eye, and then the left eye. Begin with the 40- or 30-foot line and proceed. If the child is thought to have very poor vision, begin the test using the 200-foot line and proceed until three out of four or four out of six symbols cannot be read. Use a pointer to point to one symbol at a time. Observe the child's eyes during the test and record any evidence of excessive blinking, tearing, squinting, or redness and any head tilting or thrusting the head forward. Record the results of the test accurately.

FIGURE 5-31   Titmus II Vision Tester. (Courtesy Titmus Optical, Inc., Petersburg, Va.)

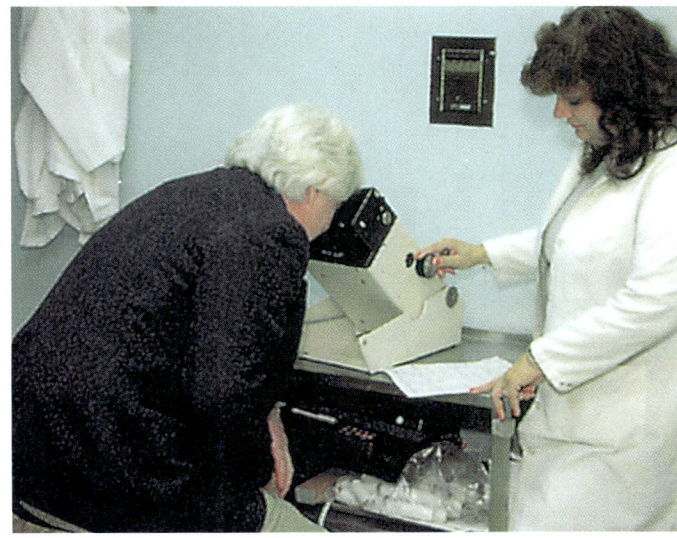

FIGURE 5-32 **A,** Have a child point to the direction in which "the legs of the E" are pointing; **B,** teach a child how to cover one eye with an eye cover/occluder while the other eye is being tested.

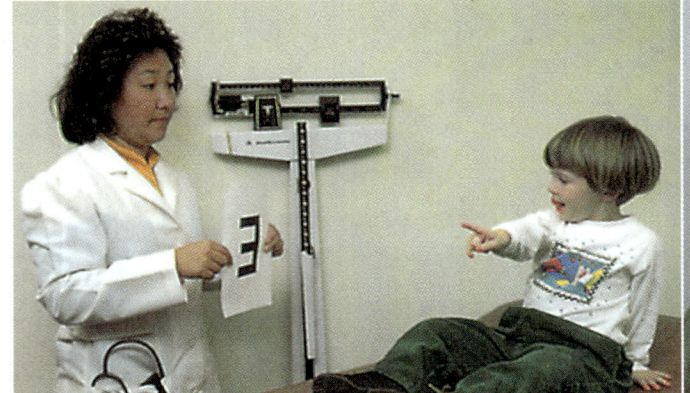
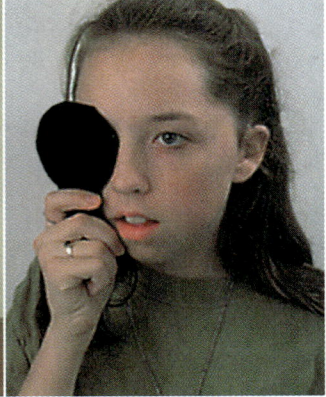

A   B

HEALTH MATTERS

KEEPING YOUR PATIENTS INFORMED

All children should have their eyes and vision checked by age 3. Screening evaluations are very important because they may detect problems in an early stage and at a young age. The earlier the diagnosis of a problem is made, the earlier treatment can be started. This detection gives the child a greater chance of the problem being successfully treated.

SIGNS AND SYMPTOMS OF SOME VISION PROBLEMS IN CHILDREN

- Eyes are misaligned
- Head is frequently tilted to one side
- Tendency to close or cover one eye
- Drooping eyelid(s)
- Frequent squinting
- Much sensitivity to light
- Pupil(s) of the eye(s) is/are white or discolored
- Eyes are red or watery/teary
- Excessive tearing of the eyes
- Difficulty with tasks that require depth perception
- Sitting very close to the TV or holding objects close to the eyes
- Frequent complaints of headaches

PROCEDURE 5-10

MEASURING DISTANCE VISUAL ACUITY (SNELLEN CHART)

Objective
Understand and demonstrate the proper procedure for measuring a patient's distance visual acuity and record the results on the patient's chart.

Equipment
Snellen eye chart (see Figure 5-30, *A* and *B*)
Opaque card or eye cover or occluder
Pen
Paper

PROCEDURE

1. **Wash your hands. Use appropriate personal protective equipment (PPE) as indicated by facility.**

2. Prepare the room; determine location of 20 feet from where the chart will be posted to where the patient will be positioned. When this test is used frequently, this distance can be permanently marked to save time.

3. Assemble the supplies and equipment.

RATIONALE

PROCEDURE 5-10

MEASURING DISTANCE VISUAL ACUITY (SNELLEN CHART)—cont'd

4. Identify the patient and explain the procedure. Do not allow time for the patient to study and memorize the chart before the examination begins.

Explanations help the patient to feel comfortable and more relaxed, in addition to gaining the patient's confidence as you proceed with the examination.

5. Position the patient comfortably, either standing or sitting, 20 feet from the location of the chart.

Twenty feet is the standard testing distance.

6. Position the center of the Snellen eye chart at eye level to the patient.

To position the chart correctly, the patient must first be positioned.

7. Provide the patient with the opaque card or eye cover or occluder. Instruct the patient to cover the left eye with the card, keep the left eye open at all times, and not to put pressure on the eye with the card or occluder.

The right eye (OD) is traditionally tested first. The hand or fingers are not to be used to cover the eye not being tested. The covered eye is to be kept open because closing one eye often causes the other to squint inadvertently.

8. Instruct the patient to use the right eye and to verbally identify the letters as you point to each row. Start at row 20/70 (or a row several rows above the 20/20 row) (Figure 5-33). The patient is to read as many letters as possible in the rows as you point to them.

Starting with row 20/70, which has larger letters than those on row 20/20, allows the patient to gain confidence in identifying the letters.

9. As the patient identifies the letters in the first row that you point to, proceed down the chart until the patient has identified as many rows of letters as possible. Proceed until three out of four symbols, three out of five symbols, or four out of six symbols cannot be read. If the patient is unable to identify row 20/70, proceed up the chart, having the patient identify the rows of letters until the smallest row of letters is identified.

To obtain the correct visual acuity measurement, the patient is to identify the smallest letters possible.

10. Provide instructions to the patient during the test, such as what line to read and not to squint. Observe the patient for any unusual reactions, such as tearing of the eyes, blinking, squinting, or leaning forward to read the chart.

These reactions may indicate the patient is experiencing difficulty with the test and must be recorded.

11. Continue testing until the smallest line of letters that the patient can read is reached or until a letter is misread.

12. Record the results of visual acuity of the right eye on a piece of paper. It is important to write the result down when it is determined to avoid errors when charting the results on the patient's record. When testing the covered eye, allow time for the eye to adjust to the room's lighting before starting the test.

13. Instruct the patient to cover the right eye with the opaque card or eye cover and keep the eye open (see Figure 5-32, *B*).

14. Measure the visual acuity of the left eye (OS), using the method described in steps 8 through 12.

15. Give further instructions to the patient as required.

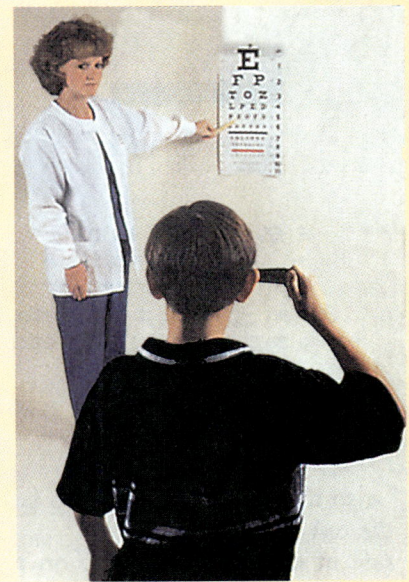

FIGURE 5-33   Using the Snellen chart for distance visual acuity testing.

PROCEDURE 5-10

MEASURING DISTANCE VISUAL ACUITY (SNELLEN CHART)—cont'd

16. Replace equipment and leave the room neat and clean.

17. Record the results for each eye on the patient's chart, using proper medical abbreviations. When one or two letters are missed or misread in a row, the results are recorded with a minus sign. The number of letters missed or misread is recorded next to the bottom number (for example, if the patient identified the rows of letters down to row 20/25 and could not read two letters in this row, you would record this result as 20/25−2, that is, 20/25 *minus* 2). Record as s̄ correction (without correction) when the patient isn't wearing glasses or contact lenses, and c̄ correction (with correction) when the patient is wearing glasses or contact lenses.

Charting Example

| October 31, 20__, 5 PM |
| Snellen chart eye test given. Results without glasses: |
| OD 20/20 s̄ correction |
| OS 20/14 − 2 s̄ correction |
| H. McMullen CMA |

Measuring near visual acuity. The tests for near vision are used to determine if the patient can read average-sized type at a normal reading distance of 14 inches. A sample of newspaper printing or a specially designed chart such as the Rosenbaum or Jaeger charts can be used. The Rosenbaum chart consists of a series of numbers, *E*'s positioned in different ways, *X*'s, and *O*'s, all in varying sizes. Each eye should be tested separately, traditionally beginning with the right eye. The eye not being tested should be kept covered with an eye occluder or an opaque card. If the patient wears reading glasses, they should be worn during the test. This must be recorded along with the results. In a well-lit area, have the patient assume a comfortable position, hold the chart 14 inches away from the eye, and read the smallest line possible. The test results are recorded as either distant equivalents such as 20/25 or 20/30 or Jaeger equivalents such as J-1 or J-2. Both of these measurements are given on the chart. J-2 indicates normal near visual acuity. If you give the patient a newspaper to read for this test, he or she should be able to read it without difficulty when it is held at least 14 inches away from the eyes (Figure 5-34, *A* and *B*). State the distance tested when recording the results.

Visual fields. The patient is asked to look directly at a central point; then the extent of peripheral and side vision is spot checked with an instrument called a perimeter. A target screen method may also be used. The patient is asked to focus on a small target that is moved to different points on a screen. The patient has a visual field defect in the areas where the target cannot be seen.

Color vision. Color vision should be tested when a defect is suspected or when employment requires a person to be able to differentiate colors, such as is required in certain vehicle operation and industrial jobs. Deficiency in color perception is inherited in approximately 7% of men and 0.5% of women. Visual acuity is normal, but perceptions of color are depressed to varying degrees. Diseases of the optic nerve and the fovea centralis (an area at the center of the retina of the eye where cone cells are concentrated and there are no rod cells), some nutritional disturbances, and ingestion of toxic drugs can all interfere with color vision. Testing color vision should include testing with color plates. The plates have numbers outlined in one color surrounded by confusion colors that are similar in color or intensity. The tests vary in degree of difficulty. The patient is asked to identify colored numbers on various color plates from a standardized distance, usually 75 cm (30 inches). The color-deficient person is unable to see the numbers on color plates, numbers that are easily recognizable to the person with normal color vision.

Commonly used color plates for color vision screening are the Ishihara plates. This series provides quick and easy assessment of total color blindness or a red-green deficiency, both of congenital origin. The red-green deficiency is the most common deficiency seen. The Ishihara book contains 24 test plates. The first 17 plates consist of primary colored dots arranged to form different numbers against a background of dots in contrasting colors. The patient is asked to identify the number on each of these plates within 3 seconds. The first plate is designed to be read correctly by everyone so that it can be used to explain the method of the test to the patient. Plates 18 through 24 are used for patients who cannot read numbers such as non–English-speaking or illiterate patients and preschoolers. The patient is asked to trace with a brush winding colored lines between two *X*'s. Each tracing should be completed within 10 seconds. The plates should be held 75 cm (30 inches) away from and at right angles to the patient's line of vision (Figure 5-35).

It is not necessary to use the whole series of plates for every screening. Omit plates 16 and 17 if you are testing primarily to determine a color defect versus normal color appreciation. The test may also be simplified to an examination of only six plates. For this you would use the following:

- Plate No. 1
- One of plates Nos. 2, 3
- One of Nos. 4, 5, 6, 7
- One of Nos. 8, 9
- One of Nos. 10, 11, 12, 13
- One of Nos. 14, 15

FIGURE 5-34   **A,** Rosenbaum chart for testing near vision. **B,** Patient's near vision being tested with the Rosenbaum chart. (From Seidel H et al: *Mosby's guide to physical examinations,* ed 2, St Louis, 1991, Mosby.)

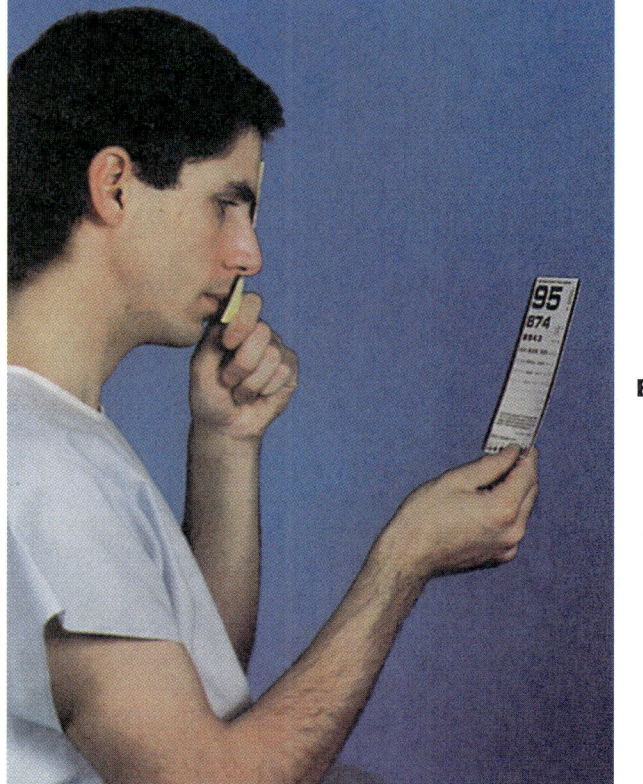

ROSENBAUM POCKET VISION SCREENER

		Point	Jaeger	distance equivalent
95				$\frac{20}{800}$
874				$\frac{20}{400}$
2843		26	16	$\frac{20}{200}$
638 E Ш Ǝ X O O		14	10	$\frac{20}{100}$
8745 Ǝ m Ш O X O		10	7	$\frac{20}{70}$
63925 m E Ǝ X O X		8	5	$\frac{20}{50}$
428365 Ш E m O X O		6	3	$\frac{20}{40}$
374258 Ǝ m Ш X X O		5	2	$\frac{20}{30}$
937826 Ш m E X O O		4	1	$\frac{20}{25}$
428739 E Ш m O O X		3	1+	$\frac{20}{20}$

A

Card is held in good light 14 inches from eye. Record vision for each eye separately with and without glasses. Presbyopic patients should read through bifocal segment. Check myopes with glasses only.

DESIGN COURTESY J. G. ROSENBAUM, M.D.

PUPIL GAUGE (mm.)

2 3 4 5 6 7 8 9

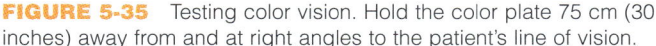

FIGURE 5-35   Testing color vision. Hold the color plate 75 cm (30 inches) away from and at right angles to the patient's line of vision.

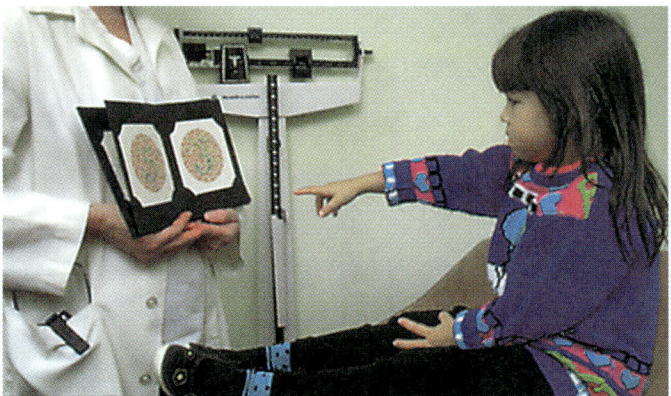

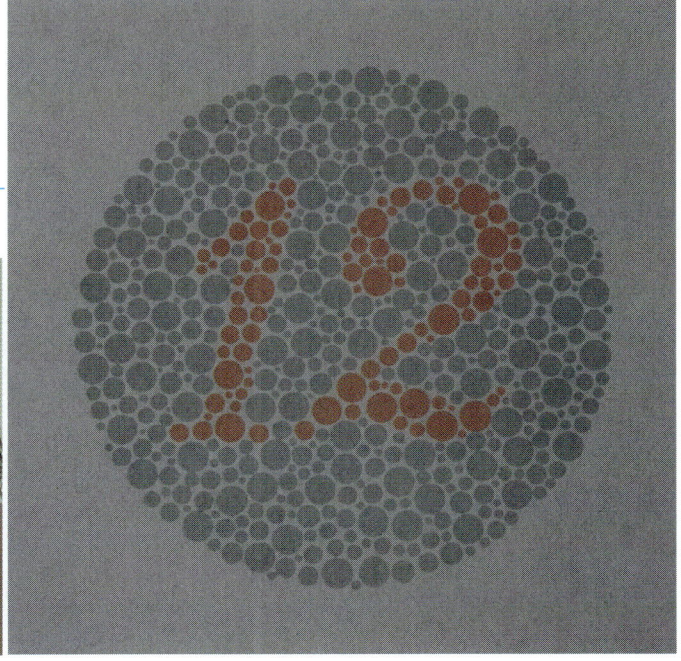

Explanation of the plates and how the test is interpreted is provided with the plates. An assessment of the results obtained from the reading of plates 1 to 15 determines if color vision is normal or defective. Color vision is regarded as normal if 13 or more plates are read normally. **Color vision** is regarded as **deficient** if nine or less plates are read normally. It is rare to find a person whose recording of normal answers is between 14 and 16 plates. For the shorter version of the test when only six plates are used, a normal recording of all plates indicates normal color vision. *The test is to be given in a room well lit by natural daylight.* Unnatural light can lead to inaccurate results because it may cause a change in the appearance of the shades of color. When not in use, the book of test plates should be kept closed to help prevent fading of the colors on the plates.

Refraction.   A physician instills atropine drops (or any mydriatic, a drug used to dilate the eyes) into the eye. With the use of these drops, the lens of the eye is unable to accommodate, thus allowing the physician to determine eye function when the lens is at rest.

Internal Eye Examinations
Ophthalmoscopic examination.
With the use of the ophthalmoscope, the physician examines the anterior chamber, the lens, the vitreous body, and the retina of the eye. When using the ophthalmoscope, the physician may want the room darkened because this causes the pupils to dilate and thus aids the examination. Visualization of the retina with the ophthalmoscope is known as a funduscopic examination (Figure 5-36).

Tonometry.   After instillation of a local anesthetic into the eye, a tonometer is gently rested on the eyeball, or other special equipment is used to touch the eyeball to measure the tension of the eyeball and intraocular pressure. This method is referred to as **applanation tonometry** and is the most accurate method. **"Puff" tonometry** is a type of noncontact tonometry (NCT). This method does not require an anesthetic. Puff tonometry uses a special piece of equipment to determine intraocular pressure.

Tonometry is an important test to determine the presence of an eye condition termed **glaucoma,** in which the pressure within the eyeball is increased.

Most glaucoma is a chronic condition in which the fluid pressure in the eye is abnormally high. If left untreated, the buildup of this pressure damages the sensitive visual structures

FIGURE 5-36   A, Physician using the ophthalmoscope to examine the lens and vitreous body of the eye from a distance of about 12 inches. **B,** Physician using the ophthalmoscope to examine the retina of the eye. Physician uses the right hand and right eye to examine the patient's right eye.

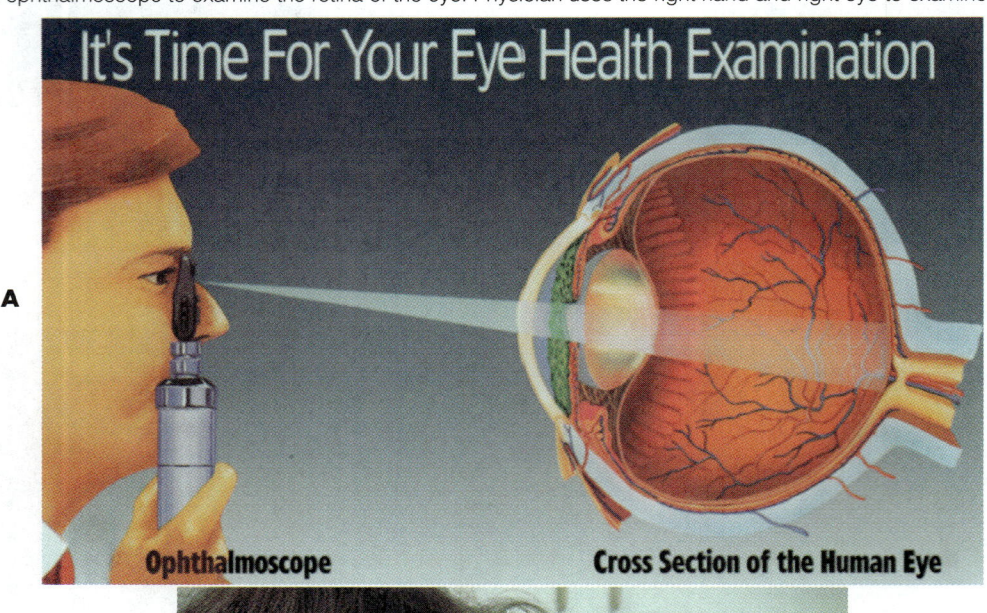

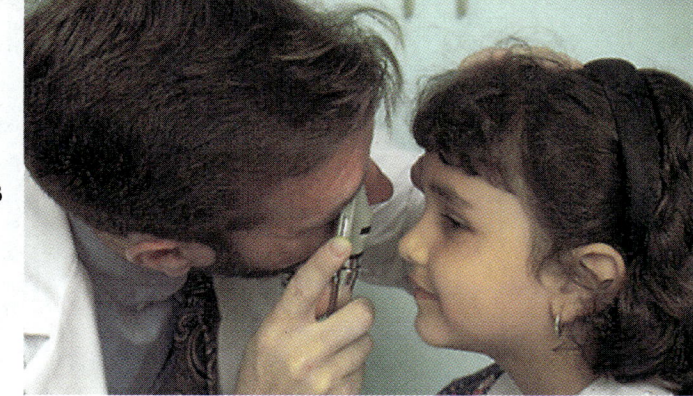

in the back of the eye and results in a gradual loss of vision. Left untreated, glaucoma can cause total blindness. It is the second most common cause of new blindness in the United States.

Special eyedrops are the most common form of treatment for glaucoma. Other treatment choices include ointments and pills. However, when none of these treatments work, traditional ocular surgery or a new infrared laser surgery using a highly concentrated beam of light is necessary to relieve the pressure. When applied, one type of laser will create an opening that allows fluid to drain, thereby reducing the pressure in the eyeball. Another type of laser is used to stretch the tiny holes through which eye fluid drains, thereby again reducing the pressure in the eyeball. **Because glaucoma seldom causes symptoms until it is very advanced, ophthalmologists recommend that every adult over the age of 40 get regular eye pressure checks. Normal tonometry reading is 11 to 22 mm Hg. A reading of 24 to 32 mm Hg suggests glaucoma.**

OBSTETRIC EXAMINATIONS AND RECORD

Obstetrics is the branch of medicine that deals with the care of the mother and fetus during pregnancy, labor, and delivery, and the immediate postpartum period, which is called the puerperium. Pregnancy lasts approximately **280 days** or **40 weeks** from the day of fertilization. The puerperium lasts about 6 weeks after delivery. During that time the mother's body, which has undergone many anatomic and physiologic changes during pregnancy, returns to a normal prepregnancy state, and the mother adjusts to the new responsibilities of motherhood. When a woman suspects that she may be pregnant after missing her regular menstrual period, she may call the physician's office or clinic for an appointment to be tested for pregnancy. To test for pregnancy, most laboratories now do a blood test, called the **human chorionic gonadotropin (HCG) beta subunit test,** commonly referred to as the **serum pregnancy test.** This test can be done 10 to 14 days after the woman thinks she may have conceived. Other laboratories prefer to do the blood test 6 weeks after the date of the first day of the woman's last menstrual period, or 1 to 2 weeks after the first missed menstrual period. The results of this test are reported as either + (positive) or − (negative). Results of 100 mIU/ml of HCG per milliliter or greater are positive. In special circumstances an HCG quantitative serum pregnancy test or a radioimmunoassay (RIA) test may be ordered to rule out the possibility of an ectopic pregnancy or a spontaneous abortion (SAB). The results of this test are reported as a number. Any number less than 5 mIU/ml HCG indicates a negative result (Figure 5-37). In the medical office, urine pregnancy tests are often used because they provide immediate results and are easy to perform (see Chapter 12, p. 558, and Figure 12-14).

FIGURE 5-37   Laboratory request form to order a pregnancy test.

CODE	TEST	NORMAL	RESULTS
3150	T₃ AND T₄ COMBINATION (includes free thyroxine index)		
3151	T₃ UPTAKE	30-40%	%
3153	T₄	4.5-11.5 ug%	ug%
	FREE THYROXINE INDEX	0.5-1.7	
3163	FERRITIN	25-125 ng/ml	ng/ml
3579	HBₛAG	NEG.	
3165	SERUM PREGNANCY		
6268	SERUM ESTRIOL		
3384	TSH	0.8-5.0 mIu/ml	
3167	HCG QUANT		

RIA   GL 4063 | ST | BD

DRAWN BY   REMARKS

ROUTINE REQUEST   DRAWN AT: TIME   DATE

IF REQUEST IS OTHER THAN ROUTINE, PLACE STICKER WITH APPROPRIATE INSTRUCTIONS IN THIS SPACE

DATE   VERIFYING NURSE   DIAGNOSIS

LAST NAME   FIRST NAME
ADDRESS
BIRTHDATE   AGE   SEX   CLASS
PHYSICIAN   ROOM NO.   HOSP. NO.
DATE   PHONE

RIA — PLEASE PRINT — PRESS HARD

TIME IN   TECHNOLOGIST   TIME TELEPHONED OR TELETYPED   TIME OUT

MEDICAL RECORD

After pregnancy has been confirmed, monitoring both the physical well-being of mother and fetus and the progress of the pregnancy is highly recommended and considered vital by some. Prevention of health problems or early detection, diagnosis, and treatment of health problems is accomplished by close supervision of the mother throughout the entire pregnancy. The mother should be seen by the physician at regular intervals. After the initial visit, the expectant mother should see the physician once a month for the first 6 months, every 2 weeks during the seventh and eighth months, and then once a week until the baby is born. For patients with medical problems such as diabetes, these prenatal visits are often scheduled every week throughout the pregnancy.

Six weeks after the baby is born, the mother should return to the office or clinic for a postpartum physical examination to have her general physical condition evaluated.

Health Care During Pregnancy

To provide the best care and supervision of the expectant mother during her pregnancy, the physician must know the patient as an individual and as a member of her family. On the basis of her health status, the physician can determine what, how much, and when care is required. The initial assessment is made on the basis of the mother's medical history and the results of a physical examination. The data gathered initiate the **prenatal or antepartum record** (Figure 5-38, *A* to *C*). This record contains much of the same information as the health history and physical examination discussed in Chapter 4. The data collected are also essential in identifying high-risk patients. Follow-up visits and examinations are conducted to monitor the progress of the pregnancy.

Patient history.   This history includes the patient's past medical history and also an obstetric history if this is not the first pregnancy; the family history, which also includes information on the father's health and family history; the social and occupational history; the review of systems, including the history of the patient's menstrual cycles—the age at onset, regularity, amount, duration, and the date of the last menstrual period (LMP) (see p. 222 and Figure 5-38). Particular attention is given to habits, and conditions, or diseases that could influence the health of the mother and fetus during the pregnancy. The physician plans to watch and give more care during and after the pregnancy if the patient has a present or past history of one or more of the following:

- Age under 17 or over 35 years
- Problematic pregnancies, which may include repeated spontaneous abortions, premature deliveries, stillbirths, eclampsia, or toxemia
- Previous cesarean section(s)
- An infectious disease such as a sexually transmitted disease or a urinary tract infection
- Medical conditions such as kidney, cardiovascular, or respiratory diseases; hypertension; obesity; and nutritional deficiencies
- Metabolic disorder such as hyperthyroidism or diabetes
- Family history of genetic diseases

- Rh-negative blood when the father has Rh-positive blood
- Use of alcohol, tobacco, or drugs (which includes herbal and all other over-the-counter, prescription, or street drugs)

In addition, with domestic violence seen as "epidemic," the Surgeon General of the United States is asking all health care providers to take an active role in addressing this public health concern. Assessment for abuse during pregnancy must be standard care for all pregnant women.

Personal history of the present pregnancy. The personal history of the pregnancy includes the date of the first day of the LMP, symptoms of pregnancy, warning signs, and the expected date of confinement (EDC).

The patient is asked to explain what, if any, **early symptoms of pregnancy** she has experienced. These symptoms may include fatigue, nausea and vomiting (morning sickness), frequent urination, and breast changes, such as a tingling sensation in the breasts, tenderness, enlargement of the nipples, and darkening of the areolae.

The patient is also asked if she has experienced any **warning signs.** The physician must explain what these warning signs are and stress that the patient must notify the physician if and when any of the following appear:

- Sudden increase in vaginal discharge
- Bleeding from the vagina—especially if it is heavy or coupled with abdominal or back pain because bleeding and cramping early in pregnancy may signal a miscarriage
- Sudden continuous or intermittent abdominal pain or cramping
- Continuous or severe nausea and vomiting
- Blurred vision or seeing spots before her eyes
- Chills and/or fever
- Severe pain in the lower abdomen, often beginning on one side, during early pregnancy—a classic indication of an ectopic pregnancy

Later in the pregnancy, **additional warning signs** to watch for and report include the following:

- Pelvic pressure
- Sudden gush of water from the vagina with subsequent leakage, indicating that the amniotic sac has ruptured
- Fainting spells or loss of consciousness
- Swelling or puffiness of the hands or face and/or marked swelling of the ankles and feet
- Rapid weight gain in a short period
- Pain or a burning sensation on urination
- Painless contractions
- Low, dull backache
- Rashes or lesions

By using **Nägele's rule** and the date of the first day of the LMP, you or the physician may determine the EDC. This is done by adding 7 days to the date of the first day of the LMP, subtracting 3 months, and adding 1 year.

FIGURE 5-38   **A** to **C,** Prenatal records.

OBSTETRICS AND GYNECOLOGY CLINIC

PROBLEM LIST	ONSET	COMMENTS	PLAN
1.			
2.			
3.			
4.			
5.			
6.			
7.			

A

DATING SHEET

LNMP _____ ⟶ EDC _____ LMP _____ ⟶ EDC _____

FIRST SYMPTOMS OF PREGNANCY (date) _____

(+)   PREGNANCY TEST   a. URINE (date) _____ at _____ wks

b. SERUM (date) _____ at _____ wks

FIRST EXAM (date) _____ SIZE _____ at _____ wks GA

QUICKENING (date) _____ at _____ wks GA

20 WK STETH FHT (date) _____ at _____ wks GA

Utx at umbilicus? _____

SIZE = DATES?

SONO #1 (date) _____ (findings) _____ ⟶ SONO EDC

SONO #2 (date) _____ (findings) _____ ⟶ SONO EDC

BEST ESTIMATE OF EDC

Continued

FIGURE 5-38—cont'd **A** to **C**, Prenatal records.

ANTEPARTUM RECORD

LAST NAME	FIRST NAME

☐ IDENTIFIED HIGH RISK

PEDIATRICIAN

ADDRESS

BIRTHDATE	AGE	SEX	CLASS

PHYSICIAN

DATE	PHONE

PATIENT (LAST NAME - FIRST NAME)	MAIDEN NAME	REFERRED BY

PATIENT'S ADDRESS (STREET, CITY, STATE, ZIP CODE)	HOME PHONE	BUSINESS PHONE

AGE	BIRTHDATE	BIRTHPLACE	RELIGION	HEIGHT FT. IN.	AVER. WT. LB.	OCCUPATION	MAY WORK UNTIL (DATE)

MARRIED ☐ YES ☐ NO	FATHER'S NAME	AGE	HEIGHT	WEIGHT LB.	BLOOD TYPE	OCCUPATION	

FATHER'S HEALTH HISTORY	FATHER'S FAMILY HISTORY

HISTORY

CTA ONSET DATE	INTERVAL (DAYS)	DURATION (DAYS)	AMOUNT	DYSMENORRHEA	LMP	EDC

PRESENT PREGNANCY HISTORY

	QUICKENING DATE	MOTHER TO NURSE? ☐ YES ☐ NO	ANESTHETIC

PREVIOUS PREGNANCIES – PARITY

YEAR	DURATION	LABOR	ANESTHESIA	SEX	WEIGHT	RHOGAM	*PREMATURITY	*FETAL LOSS

*RECORD REASON

FAMILY

DIABETES	HYPERTENSION	TWINS	CONGENITAL DEFECTS

PERSONAL

RH. FEV.	DIABETES	HEPATITIS	RUBELLA	ANEMIA	CARDIAC	THYROID	ALLERGIES

DRUGS	TRANSFUSIONS	URINARY TRACT	CONVULSIONS	PHLEBITIS	VARICOSITIES

SERIOUS ILLNESS, SURGERY, HOSPITALIZED:

INITIAL PHYSICAL EXAMINATION

BLOOD PRES.	PULSE	ENT	TEETH	HEART	LUNGS	EXTREMITIES

ABDOMEN	BREASTS

PELVIMETRY	PELVIC
D.C.	OUTLET
BIS	VAGINA
SPINES	CERVIX
S.S. LIG.	CORPUS
ARCH.	ADNEXA
SACRAL HOLLOW	RECTUM
FORE PELVIS	
DATE	SIGNATURE

INITIAL LABORATORY WORK

PCV.	HGB.	SEROLOGY	BLOOD TYPE	RH.	ALBUMIN	SUGAR	ATYPICAL ANTIBODIES	Rh TITRE	CYTOLOGY

COPY TO HOSPITAL IN APPROXIMATELY 30 WEEKS   PHYSICIAN

B

FIGURE 5-38—cont'd **A** to **C,** Prenatal records.

ANTEPARTUM RECORD (CONTINUATION)

LAST NAME			FIRST NAME	
ADDRESS				
BIRTHDATE		AGE	SEX	CLASS
PHYSICIAN				
DATE			PHONE	

NAME

SUBSEQUENT VISITS

DATE	WEIGHT	BLOOD PRESSURE	HEIGHT OF FUNDUS	POSITION AND PRESENTATION	FETAL HEART	URINE			SYMPTOMS						INITIALS
						ALBUMIN	SUGAR	HEMOGLOBIN	HEADACHE	DIZZINESS	EDEMA	NAUSEA AND VOMITING	BLEEDING		

DATE	PROGRESS NOTES	TEST	DATE	FINDINGS
		Rh TITRE		
		AMNIO-CENTESIS		
		ULTRA-SONOGRAM		
		X-RAY		
		OTHER		

QUICKENING DATE	MOTHER TO NURSE? ☐ YES ☐ NO	ANESTHETIC	PEDIATRICIAN

SEND COPY TO HOSPITAL AT APPROXIMATELY 38 WEEKS.

_____ M.D.
SIGNATURE

PHYSICIAN

C

EXAMPLE:

$$EDC = \text{date of first day of LMP}$$
$$+7 \text{ days} -3 \text{ months} +1 \text{ year}$$
$$EDC = \text{April 4, 20}\_\_\_ \text{ plus 7 days}$$
$$= \text{April 11, 20}\_\_\_$$
$$-(\text{minus}) \text{ 3 months}$$
$$= \text{January 11, 20}\_\_\_$$
$$+(\text{plus}) \text{ 1 year}$$
$$= \text{January 11 of the following year}$$

Thus the baby will be delivered on approximately January 11 of the following year, or more commonly within 1 week before or 1 week after the EDC (Table 5-5).

Initial prenatal physical examination and diagnostic tests.

The initial prenatal examination includes a physical examination as described on pp. 170-173. Among other findings, the patient's **blood pressure** and **weight** are recorded *at this* and *all subsequent* visits. By keeping a continuous record of the blood pressure and weight, the physician can determine any excessive elevation of the BP or a sudden and rapid weight gain from one visit to the next. Such elevations may be early warning signs of a serious problem, such as preeclampsia, and require further follow-up. Weight measurements are also helpful in determining the stages of fetal growth. The American College of Obstetrics and Gynecology recommends a **weight gain of 22 to 26 lb** during pregnancy. Just as important as total weight gain is the rate of the gain. The mother's weight should increase only slightly in the first 3 months—about 1 lb per month. Then she should begin a steady rate of gain of $\frac{1}{2}$ to 1 lb per week until the birth of the baby. It is critical that the added weight gain be from increased consumption of the necessary food groups, not simply overloading on calories.

Of particular importance during the physical examination are the **breast, abdomen,** and **pelvic examinations.** In addition to the routine examinations of these areas of the body, the breasts are observed for any breast changes that accompany pregnancy as described previously. During the abdominal examination the initial measurement of the height of the fundus of the uterus is recorded. This is the distance in centimeters between the superior aspect of the symphysis pubis and the top of the fundus of the uterus (Figure 5-39). This provides a baseline for future measurements. During the pelvic examination a **Pap smear** and a **culture for gonorrhea and chlamydia** are usually taken. By feeling the uterus, the physician can learn about its position, shape, and size and how long the patient has been pregnant. An estimation of pelvic measurements is also made to determine a difficult delivery in cases of cephalopelvic disproportions. The **vaginal examination** is done to check the birth canal for any abnormalities and obtain further pelvic measurements.

Samples of urine and blood are collected for the following tests. (At times the patient may be sent to an outside laboratory to have these specimens collected.) On the first visit a **complete urinalysis** is performed; then on subsequent visits the urine is checked for **albumin and sugar.** The presence of albumin in the urine can be an early warning sign of toxemia. The presence of sugar in the urine can be a warning sign of a prediabetic state or diabetes. Both of these conditions require careful medical supervision and treatment. **Blood tests** to be performed include a *complete blood count* to assess the general health status of the expectant mother. Of special importance are the *hemoglobin* and *hematocrit* results, which determine if the mother is anemic. If anemia is present, special treatment is given, and further hemoglobin and hematocrit evaluations are done. **Other blood tests** include the *Rh factor* and *blood typing of the ABO blood groups,* a *Venereal Disease Research Laboratory (VDRL)* or a *rapid plasma reagin (RPR)* test for syphilis, and a *rubella titer* to determine if the patient has immunity to rubella (German measles) (see also Chapters 12 and 13 for urine and blood tests).

A blood test that *screens for hepatitis B* is also performed. This is a blood serum test that checks for the presence of the hepatitis B surface antigen (HBsAG). If the results are positive, a liver function test may then be performed. Also, *HIV screening* **should be offered** (see Chapter 1 for more information on HIV, AIDS, and hepatitis).

Some physicians may order a **Mantoux test** to screen the patient for tuberculosis (see also Chapter 8). The physician usually only orders a chest x-ray film to screen for tuberculosis if the patient has had a positive tine or Mantoux test in the past, when the mother has been exposed to tuberculosis, or if other family members have tuberculosis.

After the examination has been completed, the physician discusses with the patient **general health care during pregnancy;** care of the teeth; proper diet; the need for rest and relaxation; types of exercise and work that can be continued; weight gain; the use of tobacco, alcohol, and drugs; and the need for follow-up prenatal visits. Pamphlets containing similar information may be given to the patient to use as a reference. Many obstetric offices also have videotapes on pregnancy used for teaching the patient.

Follow-up prenatal visits.

The **antepartum record** also includes essential data obtained during the follow-up prenatal visits (see Figure 5-38). Data measured and recorded include the patient's weight, blood pressure, height of the uterine fundus, position and presentation of the fetus, the fetal heart rate after the fourth month (Figure 5-40), urine tests for albumin and sugar, blood tests for hemoglobin and hematocrit levels or a complete blood count if deemed necessary, any symptoms or early warning signs experienced by the patient, and any concerns or questions that the patient may have.

Another recommendation is that all pregnant women be tested for **gestational diabetes mellitus (GDM)** between weeks 24 and 28 of pregnancy. The test used to determine this is a 1-hour or a 3-hour glucose tolerance test. The patient must be provided with written instructions for preparation of this test. **Special instructions** include eating adequate amounts of carbohydrates (at least 150 to 200 g/day) for at least 3 days before the test and then fasting for 12 hours before the test. During the test, fasting blood and urine specimens are obtained; then the patient is given a glucose solution to drink. After the patient has ingested all of the glucose solution, urine and blood specimens are obtained at 30 minutes and then at hourly periods.

TABLE 5-5 Pregnancy Table for Expected Date of Delivery

Find the date of the last menstrual period in the top line (lightface type) of the pair of lines. The dark number (boldface type) in the line below will be the expected day of delivery.

	1	2	3	4	5	6	7	8	9	10	11	12	13	14	15	16	17	18	19	20	21	22	23	24	25	26	27	28	29	30	31	
Jan.	1	2	3	4	5	6	7	8	9	10	11	12	13	14	15	16	17	18	19	20	21	22	23	24	25	26	27	28	29	30	31	
Oct.	**8**	**9**	**10**	**11**	**12**	**13**	**14**	**15**	**16**	**17**	**18**	**19**	**20**	**21**	**22**	**23**	**24**	**25**	**26**	**27**	**28**	**29**	**30**	**31**	**(1**	**2**	**3**	**4**	**5**	**6**	**7**	**Nov.**
Feb.	1	2	3	4	5	6	7	8	9	10	11	12	13	14	15	16	17	18	19	20	21	22	23	24	25	26	27	28				
Nov.	**8**	**9**	**10**	**11**	**12**	**13**	**14**	**15**	**16**	**17**	**18**	**19**	**20**	**21**	**22**	**23**	**24**	**25**	**26**	**27**	**28**	**29**	**30**	**(1**	**2**	**3**	**4**	**5**				**Dec.**
Mar.	1	2	3	4	5	6	7	8	9	10	11	12	13	14	15	16	17	18	19	20	21	22	23	24	25	26	27	28	29	30	31	
Dec.	**6**	**7**	**8**	**9**	**10**	**11**	**12**	**13**	**14**	**15**	**16**	**17**	**18**	**19**	**20**	**21**	**22**	**23**	**24**	**25**	**26**	**27**	**28**	**29**	**30**	**31**	**(1**	**2**	**3**	**4**	**5**	**Jan.**
April	1	2	3	4	5	6	7	8	9	10	11	12	13	14	15	16	17	18	19	20	21	22	23	24	25	26	27	28	29	30		
Jan.	**6**	**7**	**8**	**9**	**10**	**11**	**12**	**13**	**14**	**15**	**16**	**17**	**18**	**19**	**20**	**21**	**22**	**23**	**24**	**25**	**26**	**27**	**28**	**29**	**30**	**31**	**(1**	**2**	**3**	**4**		**Feb.**
May	1	2	3	4	5	6	7	8	9	10	11	12	13	14	15	16	17	18	19	20	21	22	23	24	25	26	27	28	29	30	31	
Feb.	**5**	**6**	**7**	**8**	**9**	**10**	**11**	**12**	**13**	**14**	**15**	**16**	**17**	**18**	**19**	**20**	**21**	**22**	**23**	**24**	**25**	**26**	**27**	**28**	**(1**	**2**	**3**	**4**	**5**	**6**	**7**	**Mar.**
June	1	2	3	4	5	6	7	8	9	10	11	12	13	14	15	16	17	18	19	20	21	22	23	24	25	26	27	28	29	30		
Mar.	**8**	**9**	**10**	**11**	**12**	**13**	**14**	**15**	**16**	**17**	**18**	**19**	**20**	**21**	**22**	**23**	**24**	**25**	**26**	**27**	**28**	**29**	**30**	**31**	**(1**	**2**	**3**	**4**	**5**	**6**		**April**
July	1	2	3	4	5	6	7	8	9	10	11	12	13	14	15	16	17	18	19	20	21	22	23	24	25	26	27	28	29	30	31	
April	**7**	**8**	**9**	**10**	**11**	**12**	**13**	**14**	**15**	**16**	**17**	**18**	**19**	**20**	**21**	**22**	**23**	**24**	**25**	**26**	**27**	**28**	**29**	**30**	**(1**	**2**	**3**	**4**	**5**	**6**	**7**	**May**
Aug.	1	2	3	4	5	6	7	8	9	10	11	12	13	14	15	16	17	18	19	20	21	22	23	24	25	26	27	28	29	30	31	
May	**8**	**9**	**10**	**11**	**12**	**13**	**14**	**15**	**16**	**17**	**18**	**19**	**20**	**21**	**22**	**23**	**24**	**25**	**26**	**27**	**28**	**29**	**30**	**31**	**(1**	**2**	**3**	**4**	**5**	**6**	**7**	**June**
Sept.	1	2	3	4	5	6	7	8	9	10	11	12	13	14	15	16	17	18	19	20	21	22	23	24	25	26	27	28	29	30		
June	**8**	**9**	**10**	**11**	**12**	**13**	**14**	**15**	**16**	**17**	**18**	**19**	**20**	**21**	**22**	**23**	**24**	**25**	**26**	**27**	**28**	**29**	**30**	**(1**	**2**	**3**	**4**	**5**	**6**	**7**		**July**
Oct.	1	2	3	4	5	6	7	8	9	10	11	12	13	14	15	16	17	18	19	20	21	22	23	24	25	26	27	28	29	30	31	
July	**8**	**9**	**10**	**11**	**12**	**13**	**14**	**15**	**16**	**17**	**18**	**19**	**20**	**21**	**22**	**23**	**24**	**25**	**26**	**27**	**28**	**29**	**30**	**31**	**(1**	**2**	**3**	**4**	**5**	**6**	**7**	**Aug.**
Nov.	1	2	3	4	5	6	7	8	9	10	11	12	13	14	15	16	17	18	19	20	21	22	23	24	25	26	27	28	29	30		
Aug.	**8**	**9**	**10**	**11**	**12**	**13**	**14**	**15**	**16**	**17**	**18**	**19**	**20**	**21**	**22**	**23**	**24**	**25**	**26**	**27**	**28**	**29**	**30**	**31**	**(1**	**2**	**3**	**4**	**5**	**6**		**Sept.**
Dec.	1	2	3	4	5	6	7	8	9	10	11	12	13	14	15	16	17	18	19	20	21	22	23	24	25	26	27	28	29	30	31	
Sept.	**7**	**8**	**9**	**10**	**11**	**12**	**13**	**14**	**15**	**16**	**17**	**18**	**19**	**20**	**21**	**22**	**23**	**24**	**25**	**26**	**27**	**28**	**29**	**30**	**(1**	**2**	**3**	**4**	**5**	**6**	**7**	**Oct.**

FIGURE 5-39   Measuring the height of the uterine fundus.

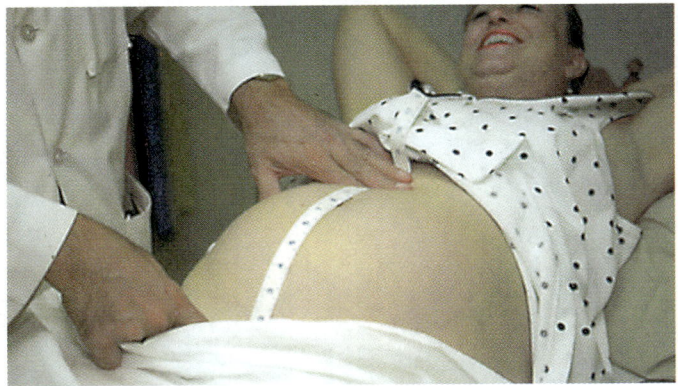

FIGURE 5-40   Listening to the fetal heart rate.

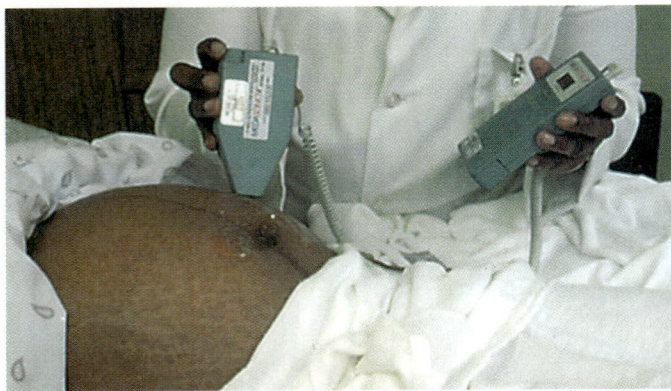

A patient has gestational diabetes when she has any two of the following:

- A fasting plasma glucose of *more than* 105 mg/dl
- A 1-hour glucose level of *more than* 190 mg/dl
- A 2-hour glucose level of *more than* 165 mg/dl
- A 3-hour glucose level of *more than* 145 mg/dl

If the patient is found to have gestational diabetes, she would then receive diabetic education concerning her diet, activity, general health care, and medications. Treatment usually consists of insulin injections, a high-protein diet, and adequate intake of calcium and iron. Usually after the baby is born, the mother's system returns to normal, and she no longer needs the insulin.

A **vaginal examination** is done only periodically and usually 2 to 3 weeks before the EDC. All this information aids the physician in determining and evaluating the progress of the pregnancy and in planning good patient care.

All visits should also include **educating the mother** in healthful living habits and various aspects of her pregnancy because education is an integral part of antepartum care. The follow-up visits present the perfect opportunity to reinforce healthful living habits to the mother, explain the physical and

emotional changes that she is experiencing, and provide explanations about the growth pattern of the fetus. Information on the Lamaze method of childbirth may be given later in the pregnancy. You may be responsible for scheduling the Lamaze childbirth classes, as well as classes on the fundamentals of newborn care for the mother and father.

Other topics to be discussed and reviewed include exercise, rest, diet, sexual intercourse, partner support, labor (the signs of labor, how long it will last, anesthetics), delivery of the baby, postpartum care, and, possibly, family planning.

Other prenatal tests.   In California and a few other states, it is now a state law that the **alpha-fetoprotein (AFP)** blood test be offered to the mother between 15 and 20 weeks of pregnancy. The best time for the blood test to be done is in weeks 16 to 17. The mother is at liberty to accept or deny this test. AFP is produced in the fetus's liver and gastrointestinal tract and is normally found in the mother's blood. The AFP test is nondefinitive and is used *only* as a screening test. It may be used to help rule out conditions such as neural tube defects, abdominal wall defects, chromosome problems, Down syndrome, fetal demise, and also twins. If the results of this test are positive, *further testing is required.* First an ultrasound examination is performed to check for the exact gestational time because AFP levels vary at different times during pregnancy. This procedure may be followed by a repeat serum test and/or amniocentesis and possibly another ultrasound examination. **Counseling and patient education are vital during all of this testing.**

Recent research studies found a correlation between high levels of AFP in a mother's blood and late miscarriage, usually in the third trimester. This is an important development in terms of defining high-risk pregnancies, which is a serious problem in obstetrics. The AFP test is different from other prenatal tests available for early diagnosis of genetic and biochemical disorders in a fetus, for example, **chorionic villi sampling (CVS) and amniocentesis.** The latter tests are currently recommended only for certain pregnant women:

- Women age 35 years or older
- Women who have previously borne a child with chromosomal abnormalities
- Women who are likely to bear a child with other genetic abnormalities because they are known carriers of a detectable genetic disorder, including sickle cell anemia, Tay-Sachs disease, and thalassemia

The primary advantage of **CVS** over amniocentesis is earlier prenatal diagnosis of disorders. This procedure is performed between the eighth to the tenth week of pregnancy. A small amount of tissue surrounding the fetus, the chorionic villi, is suctioned out for laboratory analysis. Results are reported in less than a week. Some controversy still exists over CVS because of isolated cases of fetal damage or the potential for such damage and the increased risk of spontaneous abortion after this test is performed—especially in women who have a history of spontaneous abortion, who have spotting or

FIGURE 5-41   **A,** Chorionic villi sampling. **B,** Amniocentesis.

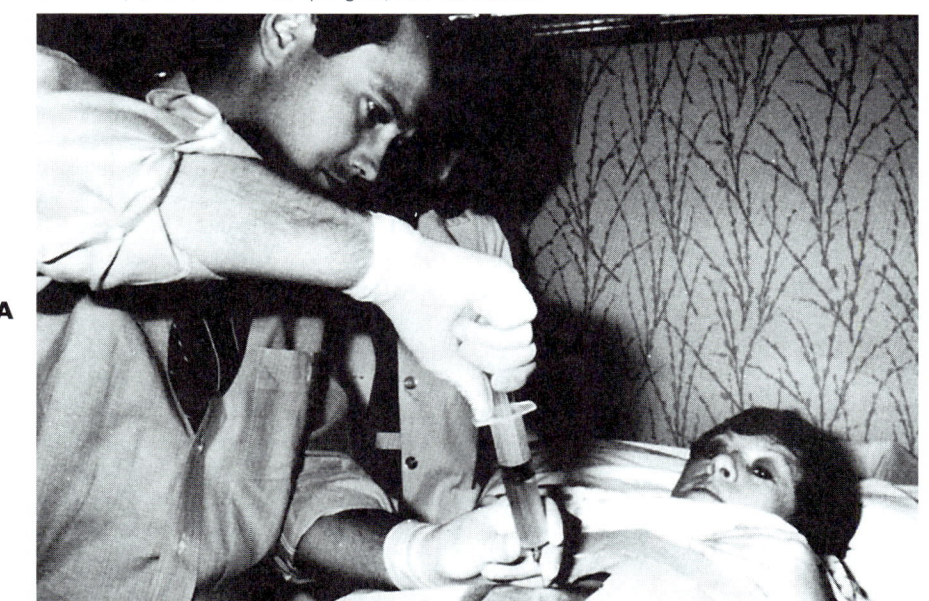

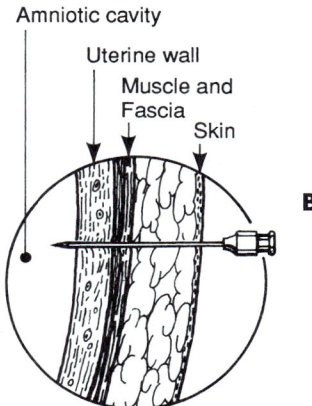

bleeding during pregnancy, or whose placenta is located on either side of the uterus or in the area of the uterus farthest from the cervix.

Amniocentesis is performed around the fourteenth to the sixteenth week of pregnancy. For this procedure a local anesthetic is given to the woman's abdominal region, and the position of the fetus and placenta is determined by ultrasound scanning techniques. The physician inserts a long, thin needle through the woman's abdominal wall, through the uterine wall, and into the amniotic sac to a location where there is the least chance of touching the fetus or placenta with the needle. A small amount of amniotic fluid (20 to 25 ml) is withdrawn from the amniotic sac and sent to the laboratory for analysis. The fluid contains cells that are shed from the fetus. These cells will be grown in a tissue culture and then examined for genetic and chromosomal abnormalities. Results are reported in 2 to 3 weeks (Figure 5-41, *A* and *B*).

Another prenatal screening test, **ultrasound,** uses high-frequency sound waves to produce an image of the fetus on a video screen and on a photographic picture. Ultrasound may be used to confirm the presence of twins, to check fetal age, and to identify defects in the structure of the fetus. (See also Diagnostic Ultrasound on p. 647 and Figure 14-10.)

Counseling and patient education are vital before, during, and after any of these tests.

Six weeks' postpartum visit.   Six weeks after a vaginal delivery, the patient is advised to return to the physician's office for a visit so that her general condition can be evaluated. If the patient had a cesarean section, she should return for a checkup 2 weeks after delivery and then 4 to 6 weeks postpartum. Procedures that are performed at this visit include the following:

- Vital signs (temperature, pulse, and respirations [TPR] and blood pressure [BP])—Any unusual elevation must be noted because it could indicate potential problems.
- Weight—The patient's weight loss after delivery is noted. Nutritional counseling may be necessary if the mother is having difficulty losing the weight that she gained during pregnancy.
- Breast examination—The breasts are checked for any unusual lumps or masses. Any tenderness should be noted. The nipples are examined for cracks, soreness, and redness in mothers who are breastfeeding.
- Abdominal and pelvic examination—The physician determines if the uterus has returned to its normal size and state, if the cervix has healed, and if the abdominal wall and pelvic floor have regained muscle tone. The vagina is checked for any abnormal discharge. Some physicians do a Pap smear at this time; others wait until 3 months after delivery before doing a Pap smear.
- Rectal examination—The physician examines for the presence of hemorrhoids.
- Blood tests—Hemoglobin and hematocrit levels are done to screen for anemia, which may have resulted from blood loss during delivery.

The physician also discusses breastfeeding, any problems the patient may be having with it (if doing so), sexuality, birth control (see Table 5-1), diet, exercise, and any other concerns that the patient may have. It is an opportune time for **patient education** and to reinforce healthful living habits.

Medical Assistant's Responsibilities

In addition to the general instructions and responsibilities for the medical assistant listed on pp. 160 and 161 and the procedures for assisting with a physical examination as outlined on pp. 170 to 173, the medical assistant's responsibilities include the following:

- Acquire some of the information to be recorded on the antepartum record (see Figure 5-38). The amount of information collected by the medical assistant varies according to the physician's preference. Some physicians may obtain all of the history and have the medical assistant obtain only the vital signs and height and weight measurements.
- Assemble **additional equipment** that is required for prenatal examinations. This would include:
  Flexible centimeter tape measure used to measure the height of the fundus of the uterus.
  Pelvimeter used for taking pelvic measurements.
  Fetoscope or Doppler fetal pulse detector and an ultrasound coupling agent used to listen to the fetal heart tones.
- Develop a good rapport with the patient so that she feels comfortable and confident enough to ask questions of you and the physician; help the patient to relax and gain confidence in your abilities and functions.
- Schedule the follow-up prenatal visits.
- Make certain that the patient understands all of the instructions that were given to her.
- Reinforce the need for healthful living habits.
- **Take part in patient education as discussed previously.**
- Remind the patient to call the physician immediately if she experiences any of the early warning signs of problems during the pregnancy.
- Remind the patient to call the office with any questions she may have about the pregnancy and her care.

PEDIATRIC EXAMINATIONS

Pediatrics is the branch of medicine that deals with the care and development of neonates (the first 28 days of life), infants, children, and adolescents and with the diseases and treatments affecting them. The physician specialist in pediatrics is called a **pediatrician.**

The **two** broad classifications of pediatric-patient physician office visits are the **well-child visit** and the **sick-child visit.** To accommodate working parents, pediatric practices often have extended office hours. It is not unusual for a pediatrician's office to be open on evenings as late as 9 PM and at least part of the day on Saturday. During both types of visits, health teaching and anticipatory guidance can and should be provided. Family interrelationships can be observed, and progress of any chronic problem(s) can be assessed. Parents (and patients) are often ready and motivated to learn when they are seeking help for a medical problem. *All information given, observed, or obtained should be recorded on the patient's chart.* In this way, proper treatment and referrals can be made.

During both the well-child and the sick-child visit, the medical assistant may perform or assist with many of the procedures already discussed in this chapter or in other chapters (for example, measuring and recording TPR and BP, assisting with different types of examinations, and measuring distance

visual acuity). Procedures and techniques that are specifically related to the pediatric patient are presented here.

Well-Child Visits

A schedule of well-child visits should be planned for each child to assess growth and development (that is, physical, mental, and emotional maturation), provide immunizations, detect deviations, and provide health teaching and anticipatory guidance. Assessing the child's growth and development is best accomplished by monitoring and comparing each child's growth and development with that of other children within the same age group using established norms and expectations (Figure 5-42; also see Figure 5-45). Guidelines for health supervision for a child's care are outlined in Table 5-6. Table 5-7 contains general trends in physical growth during childhood. The guidelines in Table 5-6 are for children who have no apparent health problem and who are growing and developing satisfactorily. When any variation from the normal standards are detected, additional visits and care may become necessary. (See Table 5-8 for more current recommendations for immunizations and the Summary of Pediatric Immunization Recommendations in the *Student Mastery Manual* for expanded information on the most current immunization recommendations.) In addition, in December 1992 the American Medical Association (AMA) established new Guidelines for Adolescent Preventive Services (GAPS), which call for physicians to make preventive services a greater part of their clinical practice. The main issues of the new recommendations of the GAPS plan suggest that all adolescents ages 11 to 21 years "should have an annual preventive services visit that addresses both the biomedical and psychosocial aspects of health." A physical examination and health guidance for the patients and their adult caregivers or parents should be provided in three of these visits—one each during early, middle, and late adolescence. Annually, physicians should screen and ask adolescents about each of the following:

- Eating and other emotional disorders
- High blood pressure and other heart disease risks, such as obesity, sedentary lifestyle, diabetes, stress, family history of heart attacks, high blood cholesterol
- Alcohol, tobacco, or drug use or abuse
- Sexual behavior that could lead to sexually transmitted diseases (STDs) or unwanted pregnancy

The specialists who developed the guidelines for health supervision emphasize the great importance of **continuity of care.** Prenatal visits, as discussed earlier under Obstetric Examinations in this chapter, for anticipatory guidance are strongly recommended. Health supervision for the newborn should begin in the hospital at the time of birth. The medical assistant should emphasize to the parent(s) or caregiver(s) the need for well-child visits. When the parent(s) or caregiver(s) do not follow the recommendations for physician visits, follow-up should be provided. This can be accomplished by mailing special reminders to the parents or caregivers or by a phone call suggesting a date and time for the visit. A brief explanation of what the visit will include should also be provided so that the

FIGURE 5-42   Guideposts in motor development, emphasizing the average child. (From Cole G: *Basic nursing skills and concepts,* St Louis, 1991, Mosby.)

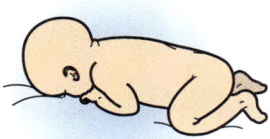

Birth
Keeps his legs tucked up under him and bears his weight
on his knees, abdomen, chest, and head.

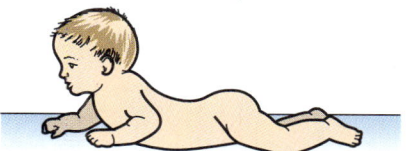

2-3 months
Extends his legs and lifts his chest and
head to look around.

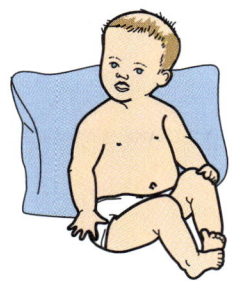

5-6 months
Can sit up with support, hold his head up,
and is alert to surroundings.

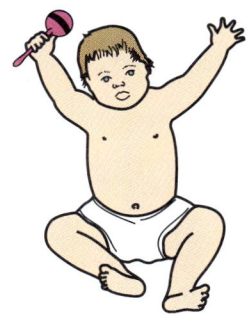

6½-7½ months
Sits up alone and steadily without support.
Legs are bowed to help balance.

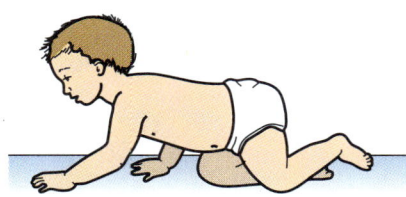

8-9 months
Creeping; the trunk is carried free from floor. With practice,
rhythm appears and only one limb moves at a time.

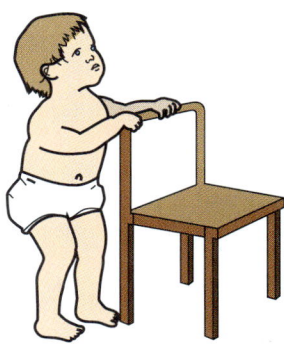

9-11 months
Pulls himself up and stands holding onto furniture.
Feet far apart, head and upper trunk carried forward.

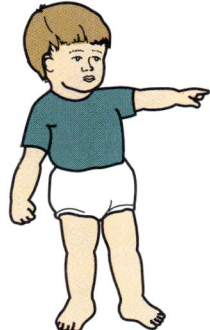

11-12 months
Stands alone, can walk with help.

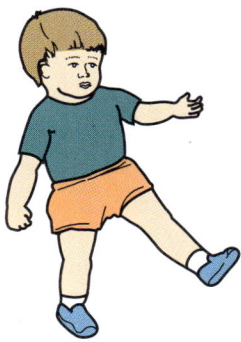

12-14 months
Walks alone on wide base with legs far apart.

TABLE 5–6   Guidelines for Health Supervision

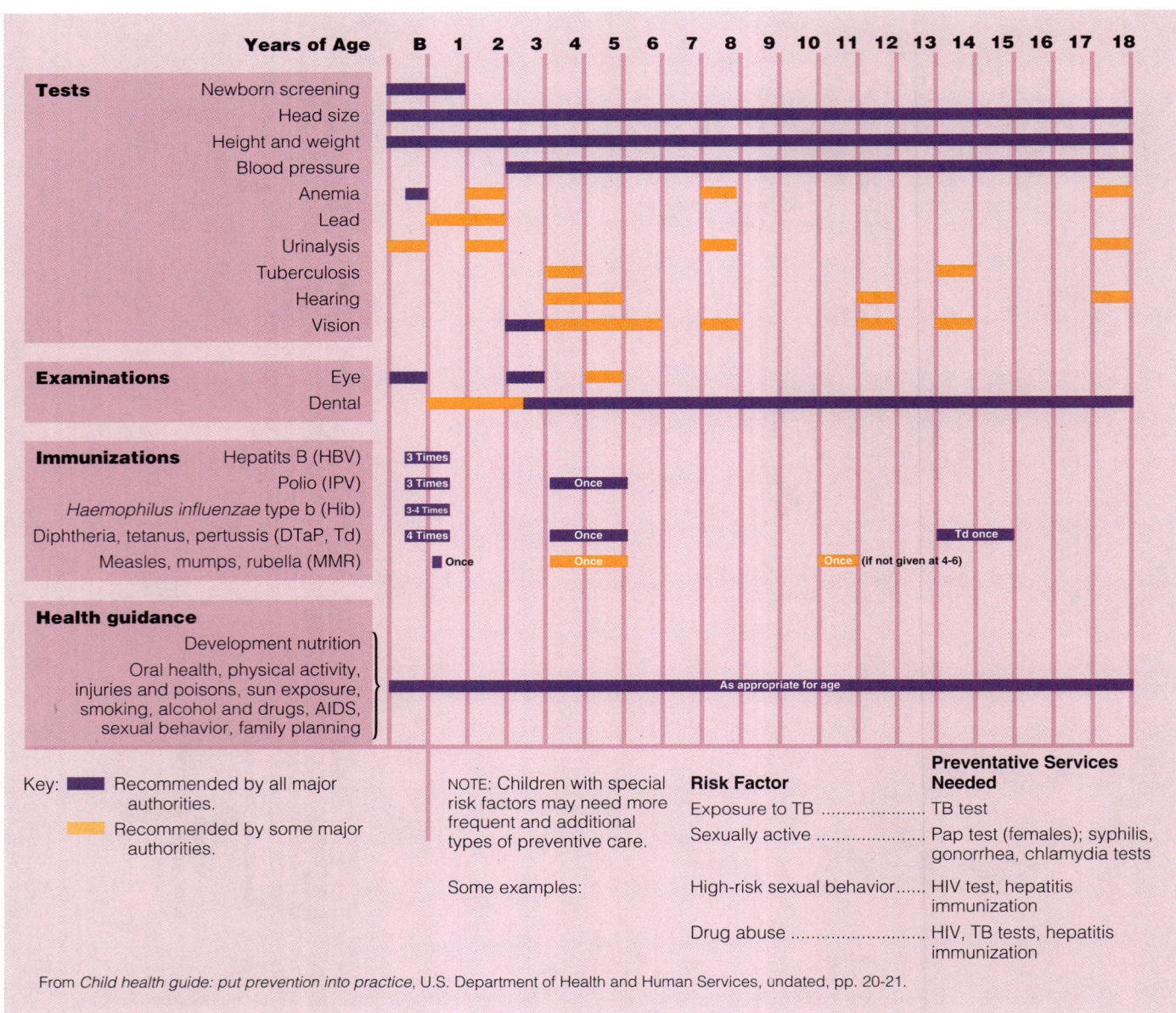

parent or caregiver understands the need for completing the recommended schedule of visits.

A sample of a health history that the parent may fill out before the physician examines the child is shown in Figure 5-43. The medical assistant may have to explain parts of this form to the parent or help the parent to complete the form.

Today's well-child checkups are designed to prevent, detect, and stop health problems early. By monitoring a child's growth and such things as dietary habits through routine visits, situations such as a tendency toward obesity and heart disease can be detected early, and steps can be taken to avoid these conditions. The checkups cover routine health tests, immunizations, behavioral problems, and diet and exer-

cise programs. Home safety is a topic that should be discussed at every checkup because most parents do not realize that accidents, not disease, are the number-one cause of death among children. By the time the child is 2 years old, some doctors start making recommendations for a low-fat diet. Because of today's busy lifestyles, the physician must also help the families come up with a plan that includes the right foods and plenty of exercise (rather than the frequent use of fast-food items that commonly are high in fat and salt). **Cultural, ethnic,** and **socioeconomic factors** should be included in the plan of action for review and follow-up care because they may influence the assessment of growth and development of the child.

TABLE 5–7 **General Trends in Physical Growth During Childhood**

Age	Weight*	Height*
Infants		
Birth-6 months	Weekly gain: 140-200 g (5-7 oz)	Monthly gain: 2.5 cm (1 inch)
	Birth weight doubles by end of first 6 months†	
6-12 months	Weekly gain: 85-140 g (3-5 oz)	Monthly gain: 1.25 cm (0.5 inch)
	Birth weight triples by end of first year	Birth length increases by approximately 50% by end of first year
Toddlers	Birth weight quadruples by age 2½ years	Height at 2 years is approximately 50% of eventual adult height
	Yearly gain: 2-3 kg (4.4-6.6 lb)	Gain during second year: about 12 cm (4.8 inches)
		Gain during third year: about 6-8 cm (2.4-3.2 inches)
Preschoolers	Yearly gain: 2-3 kg (4.4-6.6 lb)	Birth length doubles by 4 years of age
	Yearly gain: 6-8 cm (2.4-3.2 inches)	
School-age children	Yearly gain: 2-3 kg (4.4-6.6 lb)	Yearly gain after 6 years: 5 cm
(2 inches)		Birth length triples by about 13 years of age
Pubertal growth spurt		
Females—between	Weight gain: 7-25 kg (15-55 lb)	Height gain: 5-25 cm (2-10 inches);
10 and 14 years	Mean: 17.5 kg (38.1 lb)	95% of mature height achieved by onset of menarche or skeletal age of 13 years
		Mean: 20.5 cm (8.2 inches)
Males—between	Weight gain: 7-30 kg (15-65 lb)	Height gain: 10-30 cm (4-12 inches); approximately 95% of mature
12 and 16 years	Mean 23.7 kg (52.1 lb)	height achieved by skeletal age of 15 years
		Mean: 27.5 cm (11 inches)

Reproduced from Wong: *Essentials of pediatric nursing,* ed 4, St. Louis, 1993, Mosby.

*Yearly height and weight gains for each age group represent averaged estimates from a variety of sources.

†A study has shown the mean doubling time for birth weight to be 4.7 months and mean tripling time to be 14.7 months (Jung E, Czaijka-Narins DM: Birth weight doubling and tripling times: an updated look at the effects of birth weight, sex, race, and type of feeding, *Am J Clin Nutr* 42:182-189, 1985).

General points for pediatric visits. Any physical examination is approached on the basis of the child's age, development, level of wellness or illness, and past experience with the health care system. The examiner and attendants take into consideration physical, mental, and emotional developmental milestones to reduce or eliminate anxiety that many children experience during a physical examination. The examiners should begin to observe from the time the child and parent or caregiver enter the physician's office. Everyone involved in the process must work together to make the visit and examination a positive experience for the child, the parent or caregiver, and the medical personnel. It is very important that a feeling of trust and confidence be developed among the child, the parent, and the health care workers. A special rapport should be established to solicit cooperation between the child and medical personnel. Interacting with children requires special skills and practice. Knowledge of normal growth and development patterns and how to approach children of different ages is particularly helpful. (You should refer to a pediatric textbook and other books and pamphlets to review the stages and changes for growing and developing children because this text does not describe growth and development in detail.) Also important to note is that it is quite normal for a sick child to regress to an earlier stage of expected behavior.

Explanations are of the utmost importance. *Always explain a procedure to children who are capable of understanding and to the parent.* Both need reassurance. Be honest when you are describing a procedure. If the procedure will hurt, *never* tell children that it will not hurt. Tell them that it will hurt but just for a short time; then offer praise after the procedure, telling them how brave they were, because this will help them feel a little better and accept what has occurred in a more positive way. Children between the ages of 2 and 3 have short attention spans. They often respond well if you make the procedure a game or get them to assist you. You may let them listen to your heartbeat with the stethoscope and then to their own heartbeat before you attempt to take their apical heart rate or blood pressure (Figure 5-44, *A* and *B*). Compliment children during and after the procedure, and ask them questions (for example, "What is your favorite game?"). Be friendly, and talk to children during a procedure. You can also use actions to demonstrate what you want to convey to children. Use hand gestures or point to the item while you are talking. Be sensitive to children and note their psychologic attitude (for example, whether they are happy, sad, depressed, anxious, irritable, or withdrawn). When asking children to describe how they feel, that is, whether they are happy or how much pain (hurt) they feel, you may want to use the **Wong-Baker Faces Pain Rating Scale** (Figure 5-44, *C*) and let them identify their feelings from the diagrams.

Infants under 2 years of age have not yet associated pain and discomfort with the physician's office; thus they are often very agreeable to being weighed and measured or to other procedures, although some may cry when being undressed. In this

Text continued on p. 232

FIGURE 5-43   Pediatric patient history.

PEDIATRIC PATIENT HISTORY

Name: _____ Birthdate: _____ Age: _____

    last   first

Phone number: home (H) _____ work (W) _____

Informant: (indicate relationship to child) _____

Previous pediatrician _____ Location _____

_____

Present concerns (if "none", please state):

Past medical history

Birth history: Birthplace (indicate hospital) _____

HISTORY OF PREGNANCY

1. Illness	No	Yes
2. Drugs/medicine	No	Yes
3. Prematurity	No	Yes
4. Hospitalized	No	Yes
5. Bleeding	No	Yes
6. Smoking	No	Yes
7. Drinking	No	Yes
8. Other	_____	

Comments on "Yes" responses

LABOR AND DELIVERY

9. Caesarean section	No	Yes
10. Prolonged	No	Yes
11. Complications	No	Yes

Newborn History birth weight _____

12. Prolonged stay	No	Yes
13. Yellow jaundice	No	Yes
14. Other		

CHILD'S HISTORY (AS APPLICABLE)

1. Allergies to

a. medications	No	Yes
b. others	No	Yes

2. Childhood illnesses

a. ear infections	No	Yes
b. chickenpox	No	Yes
c. strep throat	No	Yes
d. other	No	Yes

3. Dental problems	No	Yes
4. Injuries/poisonings	No	Yes
5. Emergency room visits	No	Yes
6. Vaccination reactions	No	Yes
7. Hospitalizations	No	Yes
8. Surgeries	No	Yes
9. Blood transfusions	No	Yes
10. Current medications	No	Yes

Comments on "Yes" responses:

FIGURE 5-43—cont'd   Pediatric patient history.

GROWTH AND DEVELOPMENT (AS APPLICABLE)

Nutrition

			Bowel/bladder habits		
Breastfed	No	Yes	Bedwetting	No	Yes
if yes, how long? _____			Constipation/soiling	No	Yes
problems with?	No	Yes	Diarrhea	No	Yes
feeding	No	Yes	Toilet-trained	No	Yes
weight	No	Yes			
anemia	No	Yes	**Behavioral problems**		
other _____			At home	No	Yes
Sleeping difficulties	No	Yes	At school	No	Yes
			With peers	No	Yes

Development

Do you have specific concerns about your child's physical, language, or social development?   No   Yes

Comments on "Yes" responses:

Education (if applicable):

Name and location of child's day care or school:

Grade level:

Is your child's performance thought to be satisfactory?:

Family history

Any immediate family members who have a special medical problem or who
are on special medications?   No   Yes _____

Any immediate family members who have died of medical reasons under the
age of 50?   No   Yes _____

Any immediate family members with the following conditions?

Allergies (asthma, eczema)	No	Yes
High cholesterol, triglycerides	No	Yes
Tuberculosis or positive skin test	No	Yes
Anemia, blood disorder or bleeding	No	Yes
Diabetes	No	Yes
Visual or hearing problems	No	Yes
Speech or learning problems	No	Yes
High blood pressure	No	Yes
Heart disease	No	Yes
Cancer	No	Yes
Seizure disorder (fits)	No	Yes
Alcoholism/drug dependency	No	Yes
Birth defects	No	Yes
Mental disorder	No	Yes
Liver or liver problems	No	Yes
Sudden infant death (crib death)	No	Yes

Continued

FIGURE 5-43—cont'd Pediatric patient history.

Family environment

Are there any special circumstances that could potentially have an impact on the health of your child?   No   Yes

Family Unit

Persons living at home (indicate age and relation to patient)

Usual language(s) spoken at home:
Usual caretaker(s) of child:

Family resources

Occupation of family members

Father	Place of work	WK No.
Mother	Place of work	WK No.
	Place of work	WK No.
	Place of work	WK No.

Family pedigree (to be completed by physician):

Signature_____   Reviewed by_____M.D.
                                                    Date_____
        (relationship to child)

Additional comments:

case, have the parent undress the child. Often these children do not cry before an immunization and can be comforted quickly after the injection by you, the parent, or a toy.

Toddlers and preschool-age children may be more disagreeable and reluctant to be examined and treated. By this age, children have learned to associate pain with visits to the physician and may be fearful of all equipment that they see, even the scale or thermometer. They can associate past pain with this visit. Here you may let the child hold the thermometer before you use it. Often when children become familiar with an instrument, they are more apt to let you use it on them. This age group often reacts to a situation or injury by crying and kicking in anticipation of the effects.

School-age children often approach the examination room with apprehension. Many 10- to 12-year-olds prefer to see the physician without their parent present in the examination room. Check with the physician as to how he or she prefers to handle these situations.

Text continued on p. 242

FIGURE 5-44 **A,** Make a game of the procedure; **B,** let the child listen to his or her own heartbeat; **C,** Wong-Baker Faces Pain Rating Scale. (From Wong D, Whaley L: *Clinical manual of pediatric nursing,* ed 4, St Louis, 1993, Mosby.)

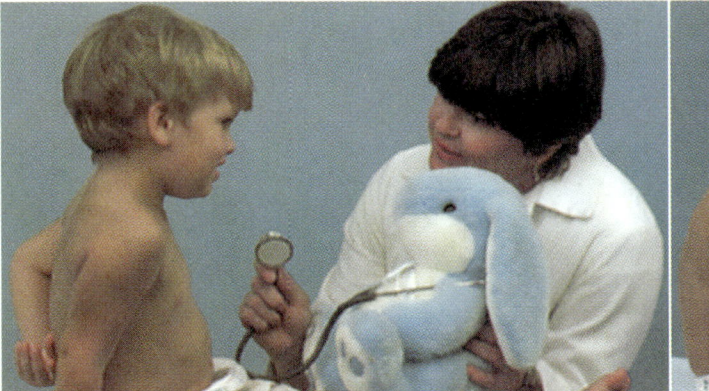

A

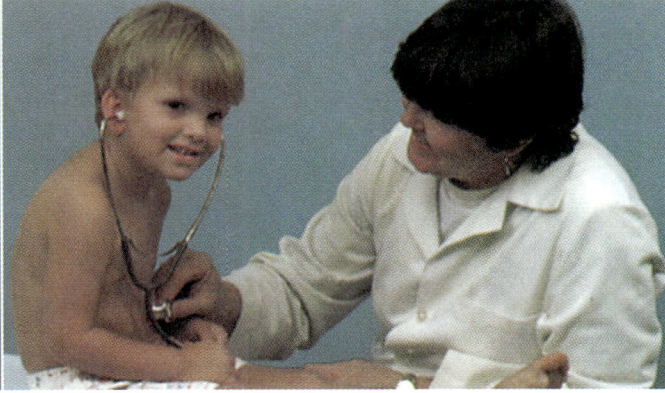

B

Pain scale	Instructions	Comments
Faces Scale* (Wong and Baker, 1988)	Explain to child that each face is for a person who feels happy because there is no pain (hurt) or sad because there is some or a lot of pain. Face 0 is very happy because there is no hurt. Face 1 hurts just a little bit. Face 2 hurts a little more. Face 3 hurts even more. Face 4 hurts a whole lot, but Face 5 hurts as much as you can imagine, although you don't have to be crying to feel this bad. Ask child to choose face that best describes how the pain feels.	Can be used with children as young as 3 years.

| 0 | 1 | 2 | 3 | 4 | 5 |

Pain scale	Instructions	Comments
Poker Chip (Hester, 1979, 1989)	Use four red plastic (poker) chips. Explain to child that these are "pieces of hurt." One piece is a "little bit of hurt," and four pieces is the "most hurt." Ask child to choose number of pieces that describes the pain. If child replies "no pain," record a 0.	Recommended for children as young as 4½ years.
Color Tool (Eland, 1985)	Ask child to identify things that have hurt in the past and what has hurt the worst. Give child 8 crayons or markers (yellow, orange, red, green, blue, purple, brown, and black) in a random order. Ask child which color is like the worst pain experienced. Place that crayon or marker aside and ask child to identify crayon that is like a hurt not quite as bad as the worst hurt. Place that crayon aside and ask which other crayon is like something that hurts just a little. Place that crayon with the others and ask child which crayon is like no hurt at all. Show four crayon choices to child in order from worst hurt color to no hurt color. Ask child to show on body outline where it hurts using crayon of color that most nearly is like the pain feeling. When colors are ranked, assign them a numeric value of 0 to 3.	Recommended for children as young as 4 years provided children know their colors and are not color blind.
Oucher† (Beyer, 1988)	Consists of six photographs of child's face representing "no hurt" to "biggest hurt you could ever have." Child chooses face that most nearly describes the pain. Also includes a vertical scale with numbers from 0 to 100. Child chooses number that best describes the pain.	Photographic scale may be appropriate for children as young as 3 years; use numeric scale for children who can count to 100 by ones.
Numeric Scale	Explain to child that at one end of the line is a 0, which means that a person feels no pain (hurt). At the other end is a 10, which means the person feels the worst pain imaginable. The numbers 1 to 9 are for a very little pain to a whole lot of pain. Ask child to choose the number that best describes how the pain feels.	May be appropriate for children as young as 5 years, although children who cannot count may have difficulty with scale.

No pain   Worst pain

| 0 | 1 | 2 | 3 | 4 | 5 | 6 | 7 | 8 | 9 | 10 |

Pain scale	Instructions	Comments
Simple Descriptive Scale	Explain to child that at one end of line is *no pain* because person feels no hurt. At the other end is *worst pain* because person feels the worst pain imaginable. The words in between are *mild* for just a little pain, *moderate* for a little more, *quite a lot* for even more, and *very bad* for a whole lot of pain. Ask child to choose word that best describes how the pain feels.	May be appropriate for children as young as 5 years, although words may need explanation.

No pain	Mild	Moderate	Quite a lot	Very bad	Worst pain
0	1	2	3	4	5

C

Use any opportunity that arises to **inform** and **teach** the patient and parent about health and prevention of illness or about the form of treatment that the patient will be receiving. Tell them to write all of their questions down so that they remember to ask the physician. This suggestion also is a form of reassurance; you are letting them know that you are interested in them and in their treatment. You may also refer parents to classes on child development that are offered in your community, so it is wise to keep a list of these classes readily available. Let the parent be as involved with caring for the child as is possible during the visit (for example, the mother may hold the baby or child on her lap while the physician is doing part of the examination, or the mother may help in restraining the child during a procedure or part of the examination). Ask the parent if the child knows why she or he is seeing the physician. The child deserves to be told the truth. When the parent and child are ready to leave the office, always check to see if either one still has questions. Reconfirm the information that the parent and patient have received, check if they both understand it, check if the physician provided explanations to their satisfaction, and set up the next appointment if one is needed.

When scheduling appointments, avoid having a lot of children in the reception room at the same time. When possible, schedule well-child visits at certain hours of the day and sick-child visits at other times. In this way you can avoid exposing well children to sick children who may have an infectious disease that could be readily transmitted.

Growth patterns.   Assessing growth and development of a child requires measuring and comparing the child's growth and development with that of other children within the same age group. **Length,** or **stature,** and **weight** should be measured and plotted on a standardized chart (Figure 5-45) at least five times during the first year of life and then yearly through adolescence at each physical examination. Length and weight should be obtained on a newborn to use as a baseline. The average length for a newborn is 18 to 20 inches. The average weight of a newborn ranges from 7 to 7½ lb. Male infants on average are usually longer and heavier than female infants.

The **growth charts** show the growth pattern of the child over time. They can give the physician an indication as to whether the child is maintaining his or her own growth pattern as compared with the accepted ranges. Any child who is plotted on the chart and is found to be in the 5th percentile or lower or in the 95th percentile or higher requires careful evaluation. The most common causes of a child's growth deviation from the accepted norm on the chart are related to the genetic influences of both parents and grandparents and to nourishment (see Table 5-7).

Another measurement that is routinely measured and plotted on the chart is the **head circumference.** When comparing the head circumference with the **chest circumference,** height, and weight, the physician can determine if the head is growing normally or if a pathologic condition may exist. Head circumference is usually measured in children under 36 months of age or in any child whose head size appears abnormal. At birth the infant's head circumference exceeds the chest circumference by 1 inch (2 to 3 cm). At age 1 to 2 years, the head circumference equals the chest circumference, and during childhood, the chest circumference will exceed the head circumference by about 2 to 3 inches (5 to 7 cm).

Recording growth patterns.   The medical assistant may be responsible for taking these measurements and plotting the results on the growth charts (see Figure 5-45).

1. To record the results on the growth charts, follow the following procedure:
    a. In the vertical column, locate the length or stature or weight of the child. (Record recumbent length on 0- to 36-month chart and stature on 2- to 18-year chart.)
    b. In the horizontal column, locate the child's age.
    c. Using imaginary lines extending from these values, locate the point at which the two lines would cross on the graph.
    d. Place an "X" at this location on the chart.
2. To determine the percentile in which the child is compared with that of other children, proceed as follows:
    a. From the marked "X," follow the percentile line or the area between the two percentile lines upward to the right side of the chart.
    b. Read the percentile value located on the right side of the chart.

Vital signs

Temperature.   Many now recommend that the temperature be taken by the axilla method in children up to the age of 5 to 6 years and then orally. In the past, for most children under the age of 5, the temperature was taken rectally. The rectal method is used less often now because of the possibility of causing trauma to the rectal area and because of cultural complaints from parents about penetrating the child's body with a thermometer. If the accuracy of the axilla or oral temperature is in doubt, the rectal method should be used. Also, when the child is very sick or septic, a rectal temperature is still the method of choice. In many facilities the use of tympanic thermometry is becoming more common. See Chapter 3 regarding procedures for all of the methods listed.

Pulse rate.   The pulse rate in children is usually obtained apically or radially. An apical pulse rate should be taken in children under 2 years of age. In a child the pulse rate should be counted for a full minute because often there are some normal irregularities. See Chapter 3 for the procedure for taking a pulse rate.

Respiration rate.   Count the respiration rate for a full minute. Note the rate, rhythm, and any retractions. See Chapter 3 for the procedure for taking the respiratory rate.

Blood pressure.   Take the blood pressure before the child becomes excited. Blood pressure in a child can be measured by either the auscultation or the palpation method. The size of the

Text continued on p. 243

FIGURE 5-45   Growth charts.

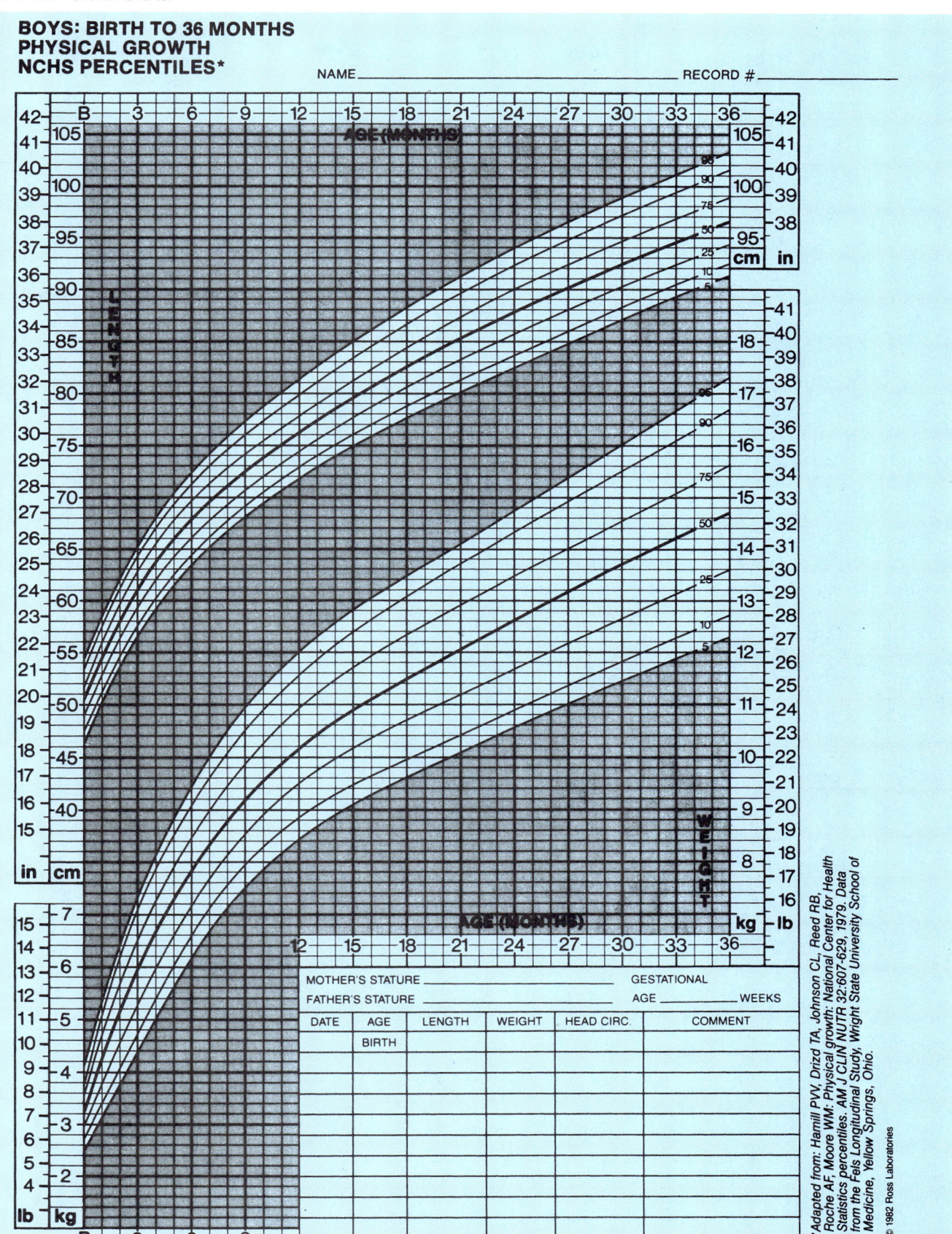

FIGURE 5-45—cont'd Growth charts.

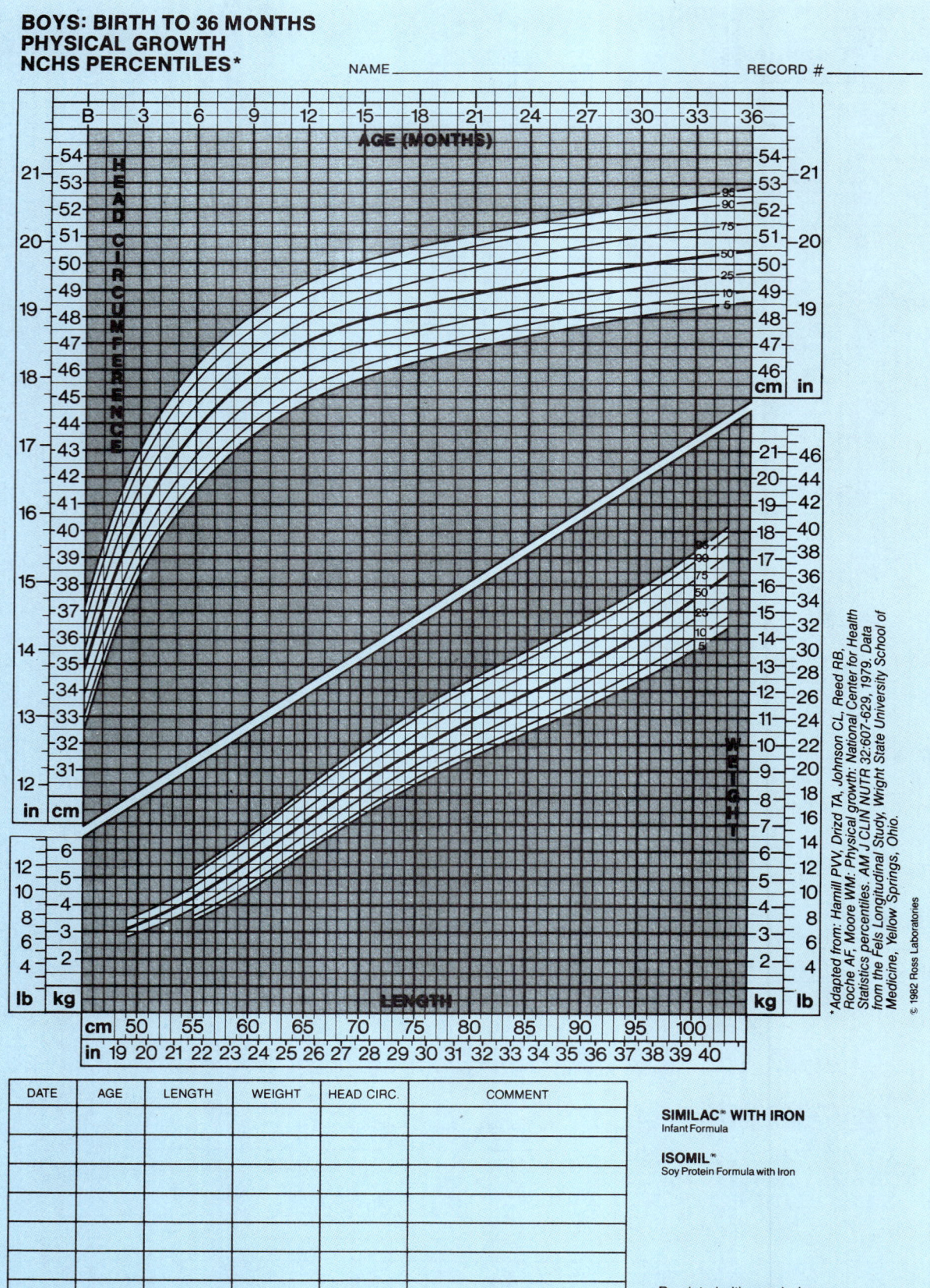

BOYS: BIRTH TO 36 MONTHS
PHYSICAL GROWTH
NCHS PERCENTILES*

NAME _____ RECORD # _____

*Adapted from: Hamill PVV, Drizd TA, Johnson CL, Reed RB, Roche AF, Moore WM: Physical growth: National Center for Health Statistics percentiles. AM J CLIN NUTR 32:607-629, 1979. Data from the Fels Longitudinal Study, Wright State University School of Medicine, Yellow Springs, Ohio.

© 1982 Ross Laboratories

DATE	AGE	LENGTH	WEIGHT	HEAD CIRC.	COMMENT

SIMILAC® WITH IRON
Infant Formula

ISOMIL®
Soy Protein Formula with Iron

Reprinted with permission of Ross Laboratories

FIGURE 5-45—cont'd Growth charts.

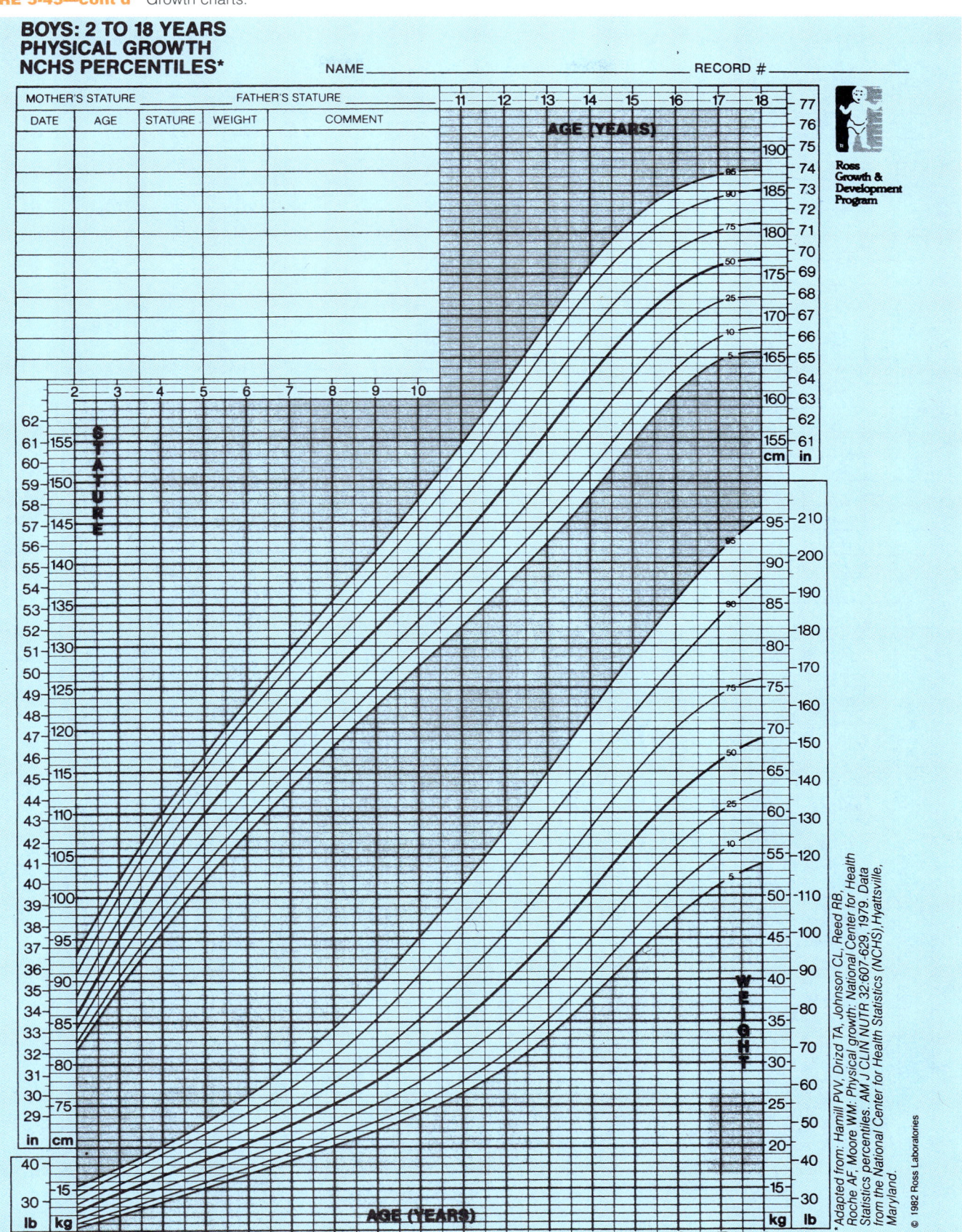

FIGURE 5-45—cont'd   Growth charts.

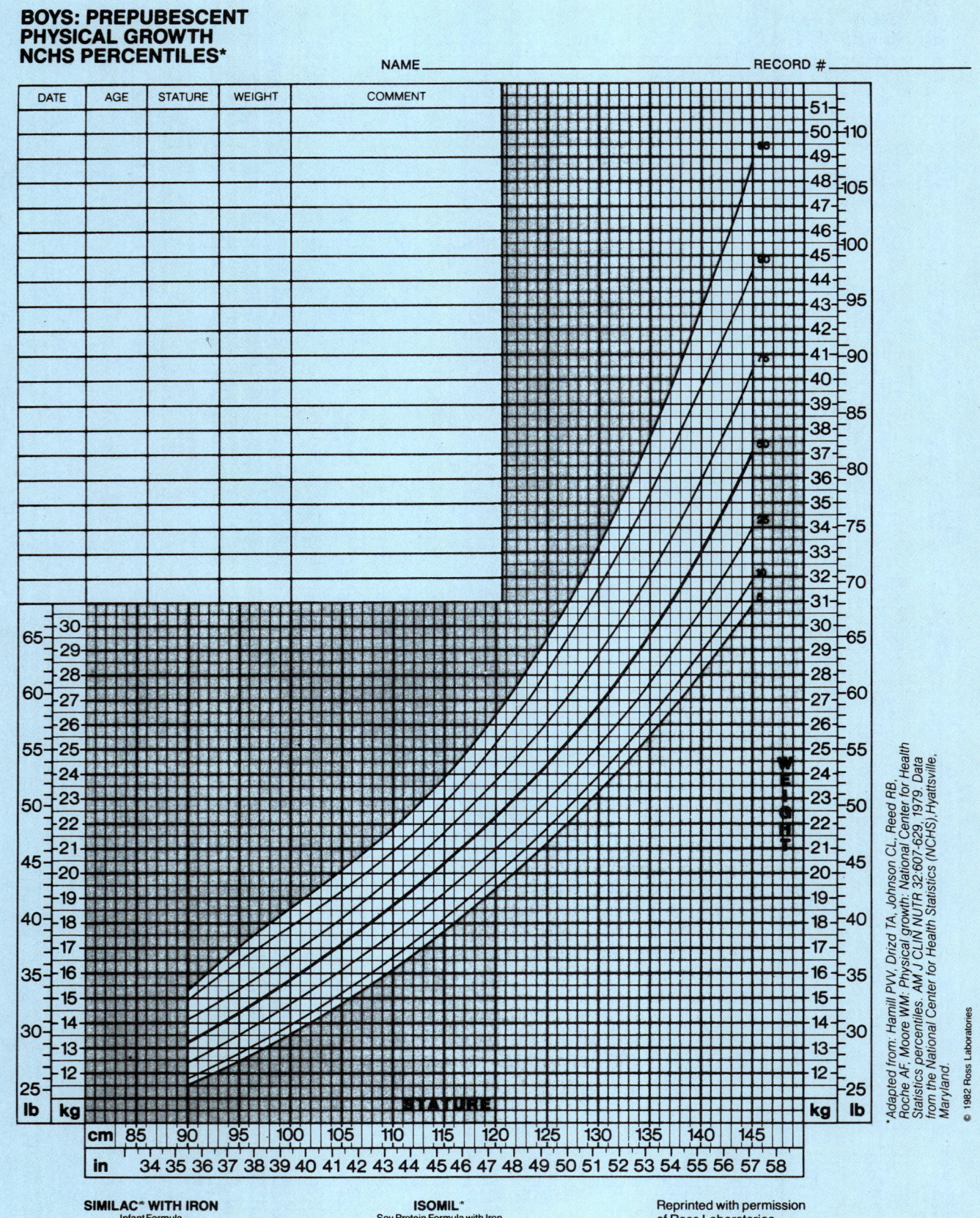

SIMILAC® WITH IRON
Infant Formula

ISOMIL®
Soy Protein Formula with Iron

Reprinted with permission
of Ross Laboratories

FIGURE 5-45—cont'd   Growth charts.

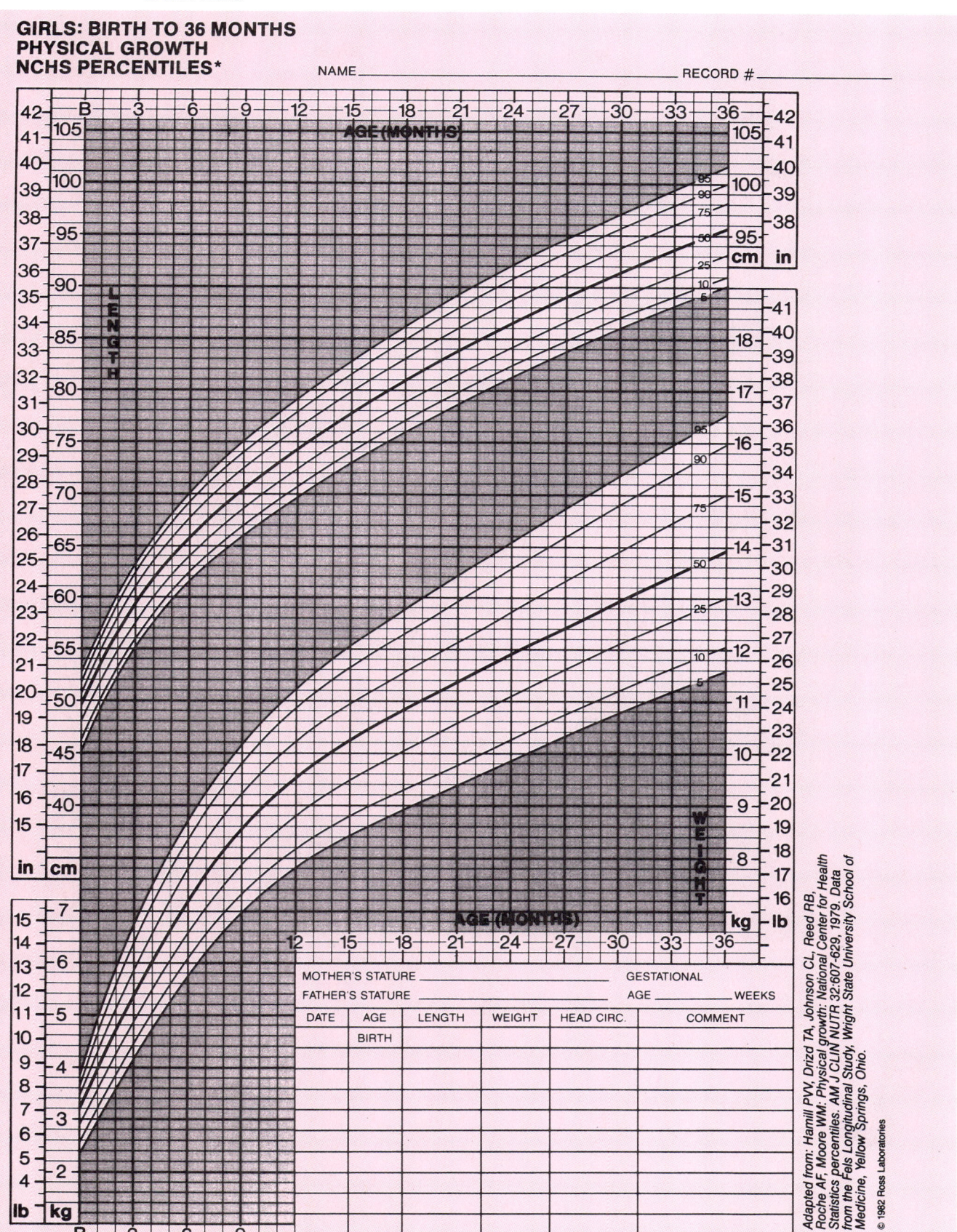

FIGURE 5-45—cont'd Growth charts.

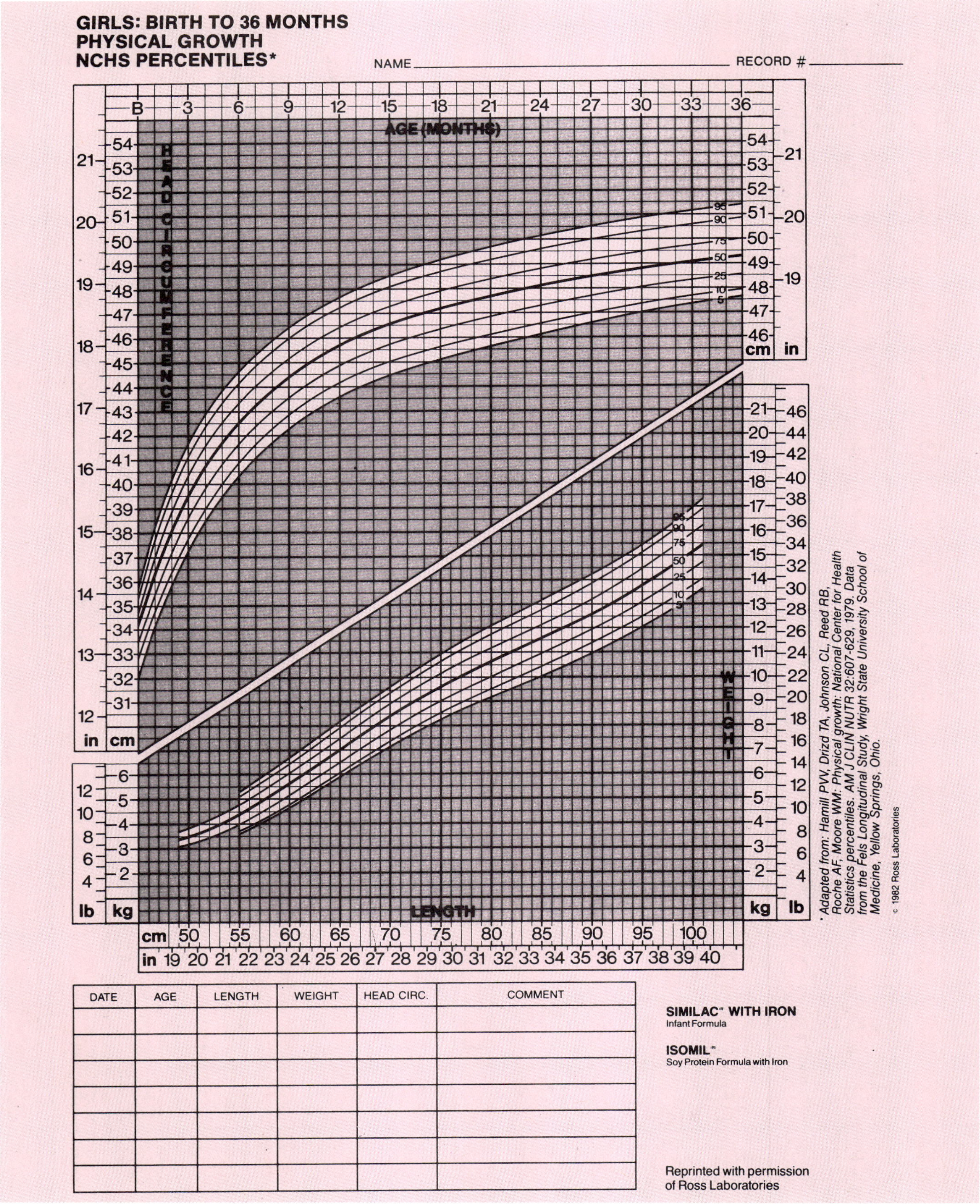

GIRLS: BIRTH TO 36 MONTHS
PHYSICAL GROWTH
NCHS PERCENTILES*
NAME
RECORD #
AGE (MONTHS)
HEAD CIRCUMFERENCE
WEIGHT
LENGTH
DATE
AGE
LENGTH
WEIGHT
HEAD CIRC.
COMMENT
SIMILAC® WITH IRON
Infant Formula
ISOMIL®
Soy Protein Formula with Iron
Reprinted with permission of Ross Laboratories
*Adapted from: Hamill PVV, Drizd TA, Johnson CL, Reed RB, Roche AF, Moore WM: Physical growth: National Center for Health Statistics percentiles. AM J CLIN NUTR 32:607-629, 1979. Data from the Fels Longitudinal Study, Wright State University School of Medicine, Yellow Springs, Ohio.
© 1982 Ross Laboratories

FIGURE 5-45—cont'd Growth charts.

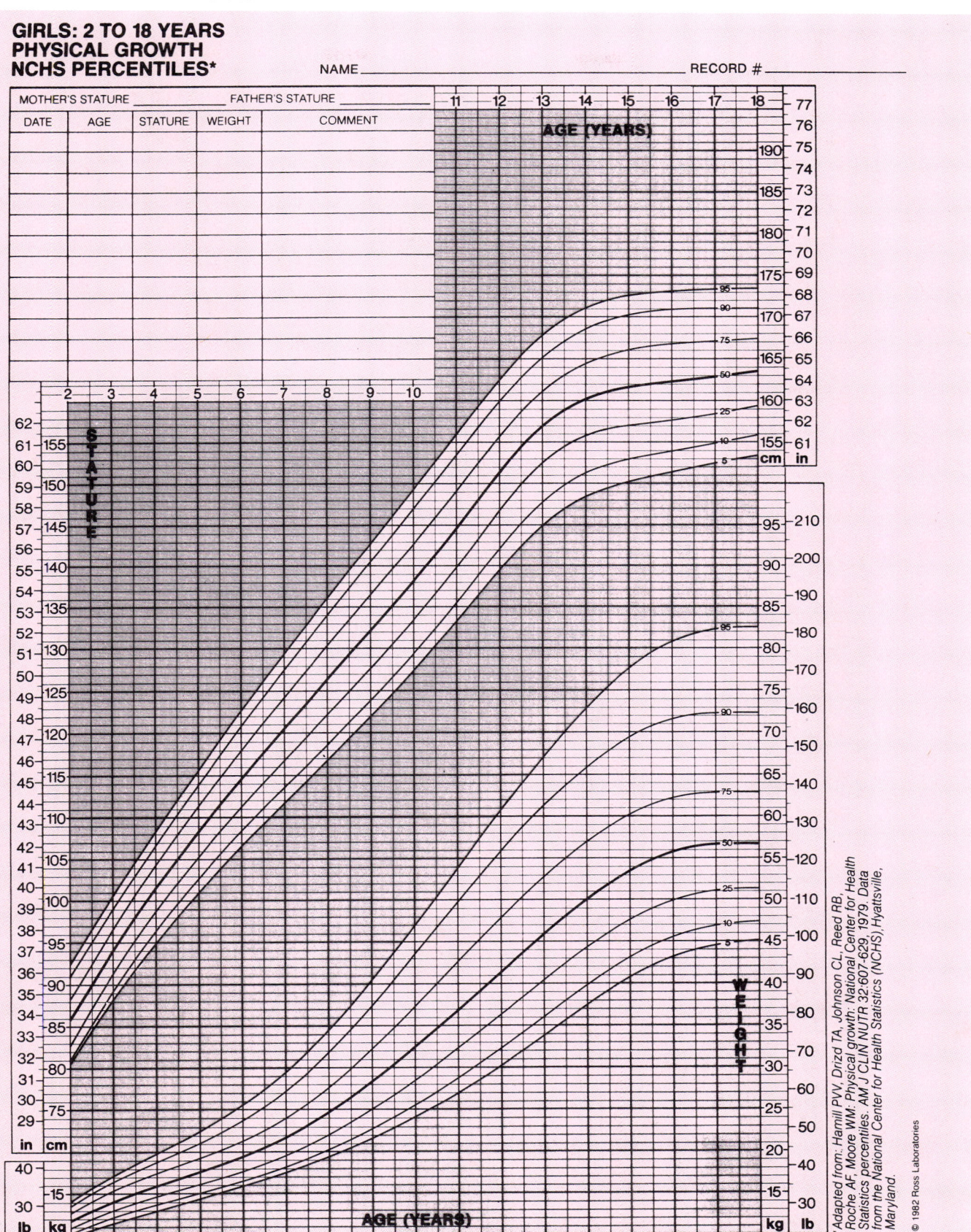

Continued

FIGURE 5-45—cont'd Growth charts.

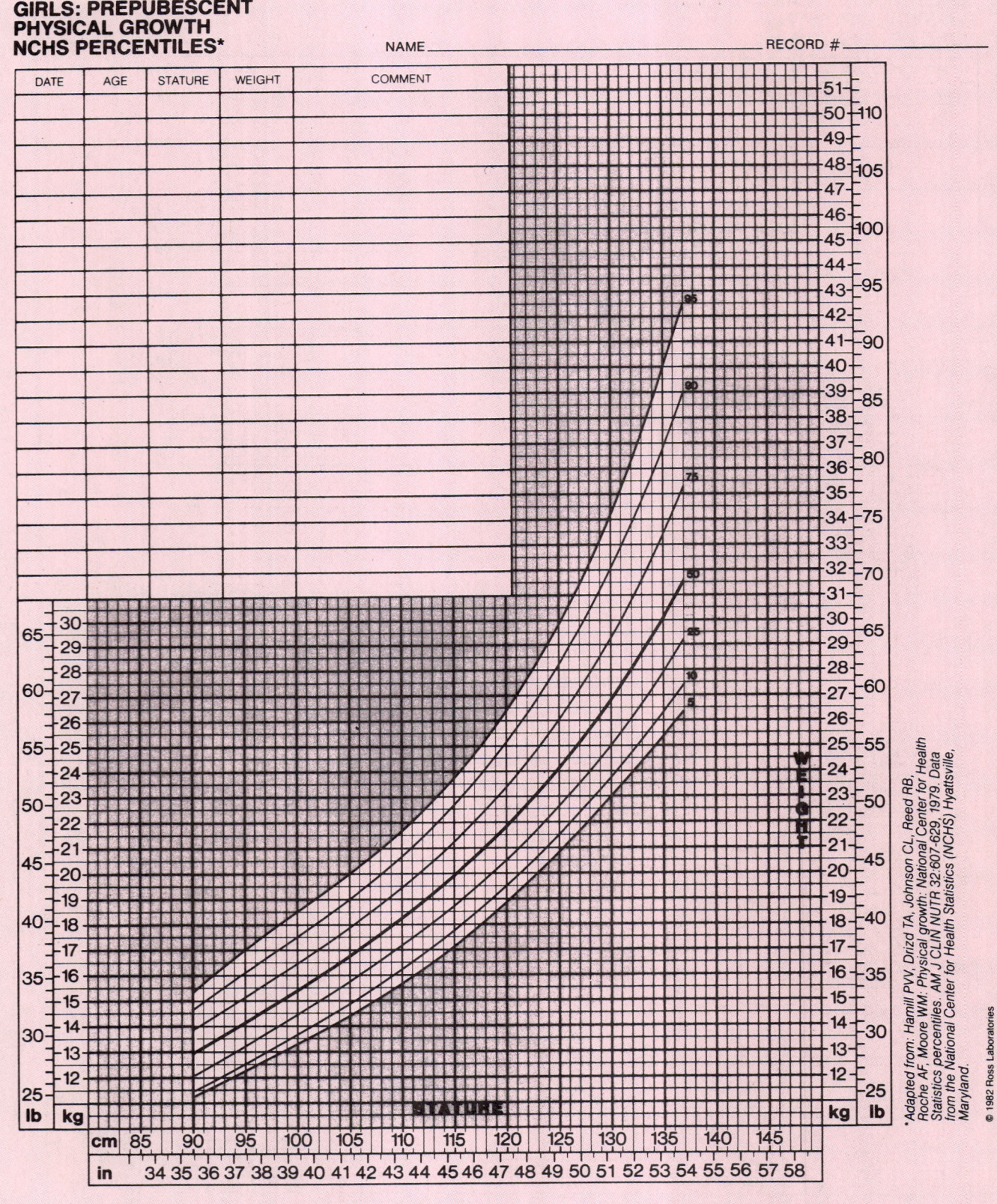

cuff is important for both of these methods. See Chapter 3 for the procedures for taking a blood pressure and the recommended size of cuff to use. In many facilities, automatic blood pressure monitors are used. One such monitor is the Dinamap adult/pediatric monitor. The machine is set according to the manufacturer's directions, the cuff is placed on the patient's arm, the machine is turned on, and the results are displayed on the monitor within seconds.

Blood pressure should be measured once a year in children 3 years of age through adolescence, in children with a tendency toward hypertension, and in high-risk infants.

Techniques for carrying an infant.

When lifting or carrying an infant, you must ensure his or her safety and comfort. You must always provide support for the infant's head and neck because the muscles in these areas are not as strong at this age as they will be in the future years. Three basic carrying and lifting techniques follow.

Cradle position.   When you carry the infant in the cradle position, you support the head, buttocks, and back adequately by your arms (Figure 5-46).

- Slide your right arm under the infant's head and back and gently grasp the infant's upper arm with your hand.
- Slide your left arm up and under the infant's buttocks. Let your hand provide support for the infant's back.
- The infant is cradled in your arms with his or her body resting against your chest.

Upright position.   With fingers spread apart, put your left hand against the infant's head and neck. Always support the head and neck until the infant can do so for himself or herself (Figure 5-47).

- Put your right forearm under the infant's buttocks. This supports the weight of the infant.
- Allow the infant to rest against your chest with the cheek on your shoulder. The infant's head should not come in contact with your face.

Football position.   In the football position you support the infant's head with your hand and the neck and back with your forearm, and you maintain a firm hold by supporting the infant's buttocks between your hip and elbow (Figure 5-48).

FIGURE 5-46   Cradle position.

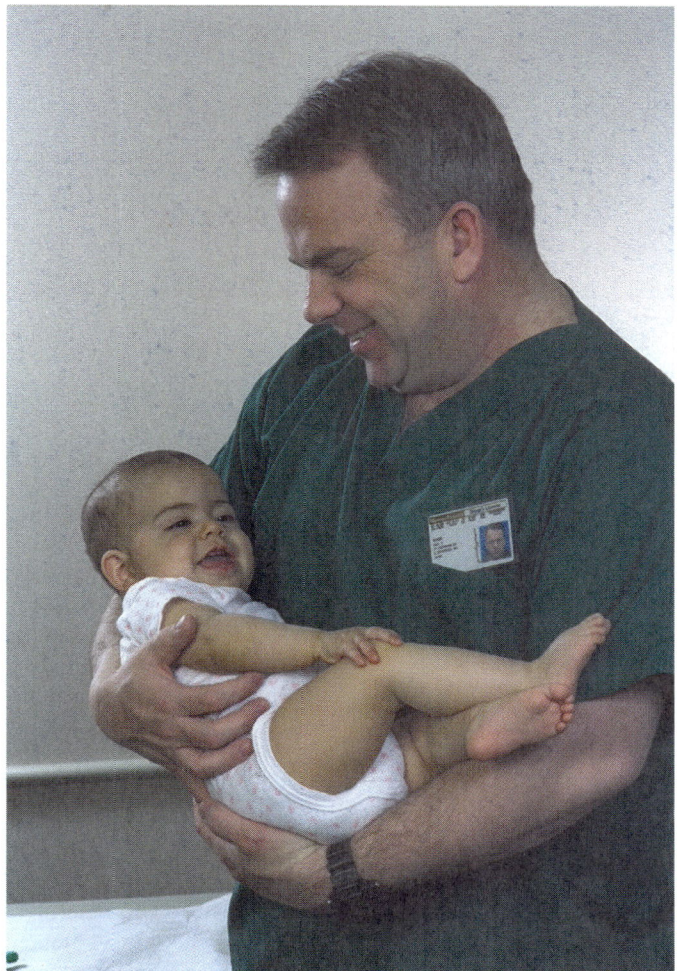

FIGURE 5-47   Upright position.

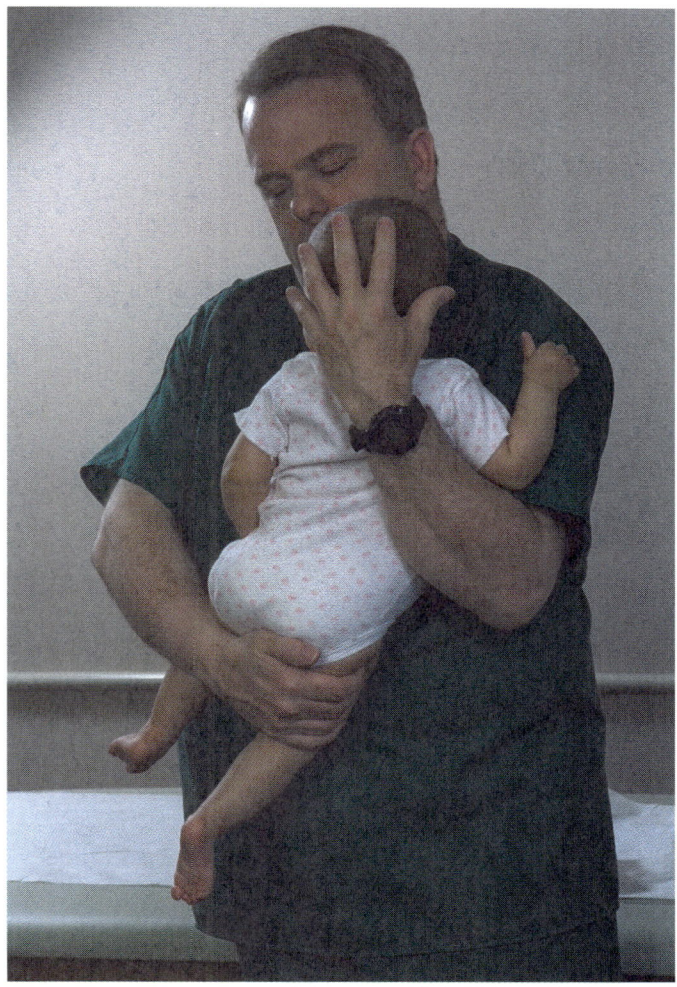

FIGURE 5-48 Football position.

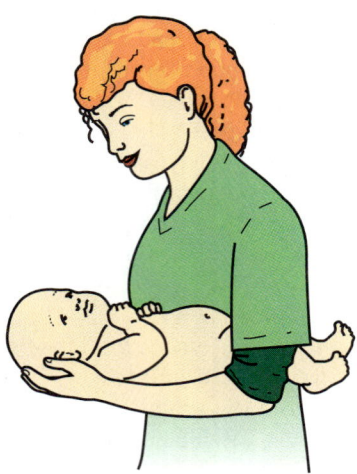

- With fingers spread, place your left hand under the infant's head and neck.
- The infant's back rests on your forearm.
- Maintain security by gently pressing the infant's buttocks between your hip and elbow.

This position is very useful when you need your other hand free for another activity.

Measuring the weight of an infant.

An infant must be weighed accurately because the weight reflects the status of the infant and is used for determining nutritional needs and medication dosages when administered. A **baby scale or pediatric scale** is used for children up to 14 months of age. This is a basket-type scale (Figure 5-49). When the child can stand alone, a regular scale is used (see Chapter 3), or the parent may hold the child on a regular scale, in which case the parent's weight is subtracted from the total weight of parent and child together. The procedure for using a pediatric scale follows.

1. **Wash your hands. Use appropriate personal protective equipment (PPE) as indicated by facility.**
2. Identify the infant.
3. Explain the procedure to the parent or caregiver.
4. Place a clean, impervious paper on the scale basket. Do not use linen to drape the scale because fluids such as urine may seep through the material and contaminate the scale. The paper drape on the scale *must* be changed between each infant. The use of a drape on the scale makes the surface warmer for the infant and also prevents the indirect spread of infection.
5. Ensure that the scale is balanced after the drape has been placed on it.
6. Undress the infant *or* have the parent undress the infant.
7. Gently place the infant in the basket of the scale, face facing up.
8. Place your hand over the infant to protect him or her from falling. Do not touch the infant (see Figure 5-49).

FIGURE 5-49 **A,** Weighing an infant lying on a scale; **B,** weighing an infant sitting on a scale.

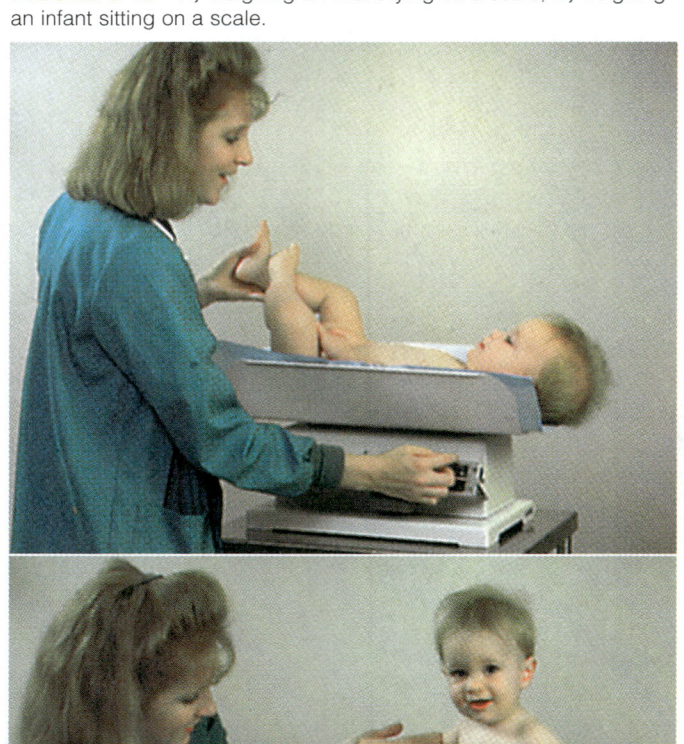

9. Adjust the weight on the scale. Adjust the pound weight and then the ounce weight. Read the results in pounds and ounces.
10. Return the weights to zero.
11. Remove the infant from the scale. You may have the parent hold the infant while you record the weight or you may proceed to measure the infant.
12. Record the infant's weight in the chart. Give the time, date, and infant's age. Sign your name.
13. Remove and discard the drape.

NOTE: Weigh older children in their underwear (no shoes) standing on an upright scale (see the weighing procedure in Chapter 3). When recording the weight, indicate what the child was wearing when weighed.

The procedure for weighing an adolescent is the same as the procedure for weighing an adult (see Chapter 3).

Measuring the length of an infant.

To determine the length of a child up to 24 to 36 months old, the recumbent length is measured (Figure 5-50). This is the measurement from

FIGURE 5-50   Measuring the length of an infant.

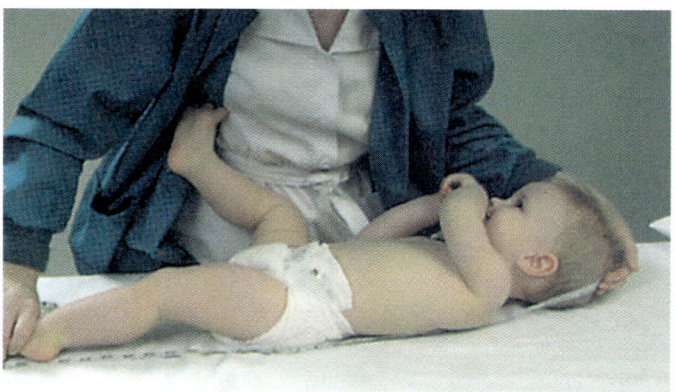

FIGURE 5-51   Measuring the head circumference of an infant.

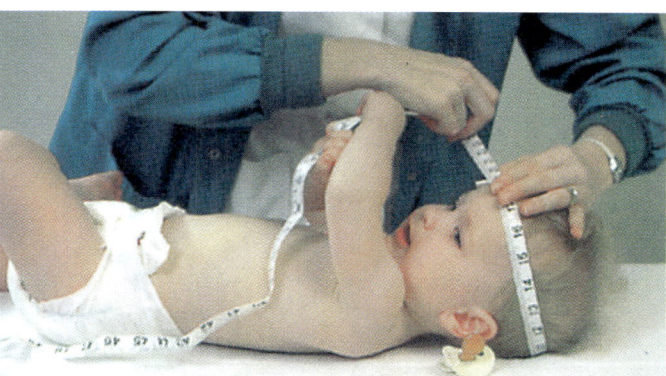

the top of the head to the heels of the feet when the child is lying flat and straight with toes pointing upward. Older children can be measured in a standing position on a scale with a height bar, as described in Chapter 3, or by having the child stand erect with back to the wall (with shoes removed) against a measuring scale. Standing height is also called stature. Note this on the growth charts in Figure 5-45. The procedure for measuring length follows.

1. **Wash your hands. Use appropriate personal protective equipment (PPE) as indicated by facility.**
2. Identify the infant.
3. Explain the procedure to the parent or caregiver. You may wish to ask the parent for help in supporting the infant while you take the measurement.
4. Have a clean disposable drape on the examining table.
5. Place the infant on the back of the disposable drape.
6. Place the vertex (top) of the head at the beginning of the measuring tape.
7. Grasp the knees and gently push them toward the table so that the infant's legs are fully extended. While you are extending the infant's legs, the parent can be holding and supporting the infant's head in position.
8. Take the measurements from the top of the infant's head to the heels of the feet with the toes pointing upward.
9. If you are doing this procedure alone, position the infant's head and draw a pencil mark on the disposable drape at the tip of the head. Then grasp and straighten the knees and draw another pencil mark on the disposable drape where the heels of the feet are. Remove the infant from the table and ensure his or her safety. With a tape measure, measure the distance between the head and feet marks to obtain the length of the infant.
10. Record the measurement on the infant's chart. If required, record the measurement on the infant's growth chart. Give the date, time, and infant's age and sign your name to the record.

Measuring head circumference.   To measure the infant's head circumference, place the infant in a supine position or have the parent hold him or her. Place a measuring tape

around the greatest circumference of the head (that is, from slightly above the eyebrows and top point of the earlobes to the occipital prominence of the skull in the back of the head) (Figure 5-51).

Measuring chest circumference.   Place the infant in a supine position. Place a measuring tape around the chest and across the nipple line. Ideally, take a measurement during inspiration and a measurement during expiration. Take the average of these two measurements as the chest circumference.

Obtaining a urine specimen from a child who is not toilet trained.   A plastic disposable urine collector can be affixed to the perineal area of an infant to obtain a urine specimen. **Wearing gloves,** clean the perineal area of the infant with soap and water or other cleansing agent. Dry the skin thoroughly. Peel off the gummed backing on the urine collector; spread the infant's legs apart and place the adhesive portion of the bag firmly against the infant's perineal region (Figure 5-52, *A* and *B*). The adhesive adheres to the skin. To aid the flow of urine by gravity, you can place the infant in a sitting position. Check the bag frequently until the desired amount of urine is obtained. When the desired amount of urine is voided, remove the bag. Hold it against the child's skin at the bottom and gently peel the adhesive from the skin from top to bottom. Transfer the urine to a specimen bottle. The specimen is now ready to be tested in the office, or you should prepare it to be sent to the laboratory for testing (see Chapter 11).

Sick-Child Visits

Any sign or symptom of illness or disease should be evaluated by the physician to ensure proper and adequate diagnosis and treatment. Follow-up visits or phone calls to note the patient's progress are also very important.

Today it is possible for children to be treated in the physician's office for illnesses that once required hospitalization. For example, children suffering from a variety of childhood infections can receive injectable antibiotics in the office. Also, many outpatient treatments for children with asthma or those who need potent antibiotics are available, and some of these can even be administered at home. The physician discusses the

FIGURE 5-52 Obtaining a urine specimen from a child who is not toilet trained. **A,** Female; **B,** Male. (Boy sketch from Sorrentino S: *Mosby's textbook for nursing assistants,* ed 3, St Louis, 1992, Mosby).

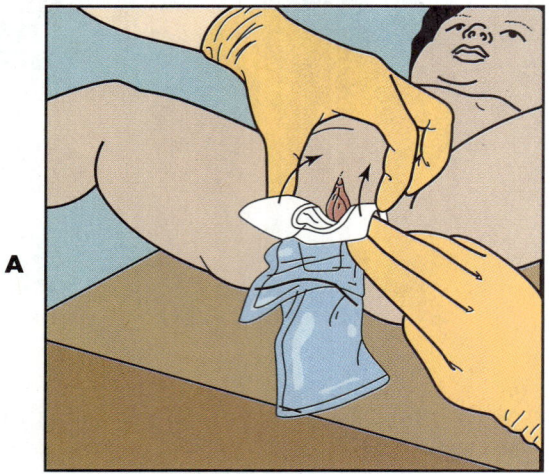

Female

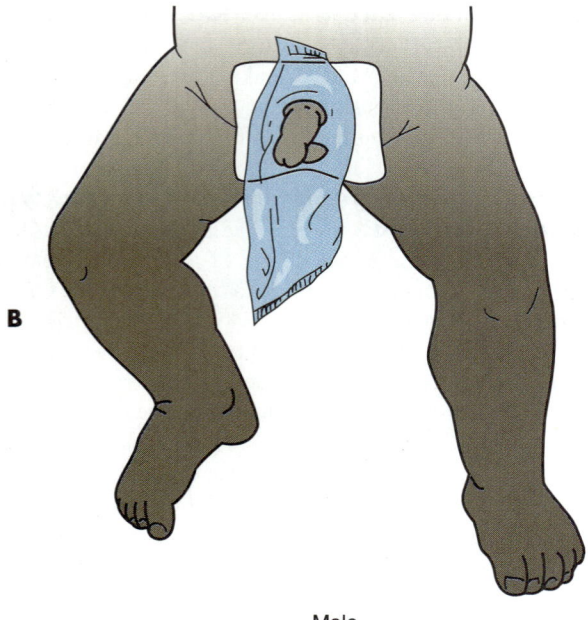

Male

diagnosis, treatment, and home care for the specific illness with the parent and the patient, if he or she is old enough to understand. Both parent and patient must understand medication directions and any other instructions. The need for specific follow-up visits must be reemphasized and understood by the parent and patient.

Phenylketonuria.
Phenylketonuria (PKU) is an **inherited disease** that must be diagnosed early to avoid serious brain damage and mental retardation. Although it is not a common condition, it is thought to affect 1 in every 10,000 births. This disease is characterized by a deficiency of the liver enzyme, phenylalanine hydroxylase, which is essential for converting phenylalanine to tyrosine. Phenylalanine is an essential amino

acid that is necessary for growth. Any excess of phenylalanine in the body should be converted to tyrosine. However, a newborn with PKU is unable to convert any excess. Phenylalanine and its metabolites then accumulate in the body and can lead to severe developmental delays and other neurologic problems. Eventually the phenylalanine spills over into the urine. If the condition is not treated, severe mental retardation and brain damage can result. Dietary control is used to help regulate the amount of phenylalanine present in the body. This therapy must begin early because if the amount of phenylalanine is not restricted, mental retardation progresses.

Blood and **urine tests** are available to diagnose PKU. The most common blood test is the Guthrie test. The Guthrie blood test is required in all states in an effort to screen newborns for PKU. This test is normally done before the newborn is discharged from the hospital. If it is not done in the hospital, arrangements should be made to have it done as soon as possible after discharge. Proper timing for this test is important. The newborn must have ingested an ample amount of phenylalanine, which is a constituent of both human and cow's milk. Therefore it is recommended that this test not be performed before the infant has had breastfeedings or formula for 2 to 3 days. See the procedure on pp. 247-248.

A urine test (the diaper test) is usually done 6 weeks after birth and commonly at the infant's first checkup. If the first test was negative, this follow-up test is usually done to ensure that the first test was not a false negative as a result of inadequate ingestion of milk. It is also done to ensure identification of all those with the deficiency so that special dietary protocols can be started. When the urine PKU test is positive, a blood phenylalanine test should be performed to confirm the findings.

The following should be done before any of the tests are performed:

- Explain to the parent(s) the purpose of the test and the procedure.
- Assess the infant's eating patterns. The test must be done 2 to 3 days after milk feedings. Inadequate amounts of ingested protein before the test can cause false-negative results.
- Check the infant's age. Urine tests are recommended for infants who are at least 6 weeks old.
- Complete the information section on the test card.

Diaper test. This urine test to screen for PKU is *not* to be used until the infant is at least 6 weeks old. The diaper test is often performed at the infant's first checkup after discharge from the hospital.

Drop 10% ferric chloride on a diaper that contains fresh urine. A green spot on the diaper is considered a positive result. This test indicates the *possibility* of PKU.

Positive test results. When all tests are positive, the infant is given a formula low in phenylalanine, such as Lofenalac. Because phenylalanine is necessary for growth, it must be included in the diet. Severe neurologic impairment can be prevented if the patient remains on a diet low in phenylalanine. There is disagreement as to how long this special diet must

PROCEDURE 5-11

GUTHRIE BLOOD TEST TO SCREEN FOR PKU

Objective

Understand and demonstrate the proper procedure for obtaining samples of an infant's blood and prepare it to send to the laboratory to be tested for PKU by the Guthrie method. Record the procedure on the patient's chart.

Equipment

PKU Guthrie test card (filter paper) (Figure 5-53)

Mailing envelope for the test card

Sterile lancet

Alcohol sponge

Cotton balls

Disposable, single-use examination gloves

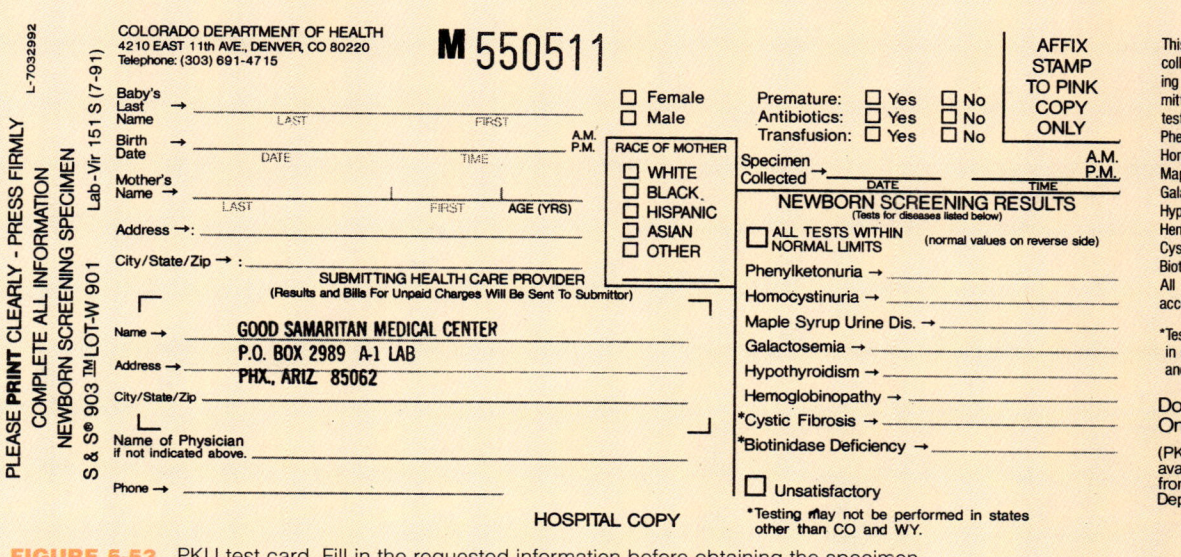

FIGURE 5-53   PKU test card. Fill in the requested information before obtaining the specimen.

PROCEDURE

RATIONALE

1. **Wash your hands**, assemble equipment, and don disposable, single-use examination gloves. **Use appropriate personal protective equipment (PPE) as indicated by facility.**

2. Place the infant prone on a flat surface. Make the heel accessible.

   This position lessens the opportunity for the infant to kick at you.

3. Grasp the infant's heel and cleanse with the alcohol sponge. Allow the alcohol to dry.

4. Grasp the infant's heel. With the sterile lancet, puncture the side of the heel at a right angle (Figure 5-54). The puncture should be at right angles to the lines on the skin and approximately 2 to 3 mm deep.

5. Wipe away the first drop of blood.

   The first drop of blood may be diluted with tissue fluid.

6. Collect the next drops of blood in the circles on the special test filter paper (Figure 5-55). Press the filter paper against the infant's heel and exert enough gentle pressure to obtain an adequate sample.

Continued

PROCEDURE 5-11

GUTHRIE BLOOD TEST TO SCREEN FOR PKU—cont'd

7. Fill each of the circles on the test card with blood. The blood must soak through the filter paper from one side to the other.

An adequate sample is required for testing. The test would have to be repeated if the blood sample was not adequate.

8. Apply pressure with a cotton ball to the puncture site.

This aids in controlling bleeding from the puncture site.

9. Observe the infant after collecting the specimen.

Ensure that clotting takes place and bleeding is prevented.

10. Remove your gloves and **wash your hands.**

11. Allow the test card to dry on a nonabsorbent surface. Do not stack cards on top of one another. Drying takes approximately 2 hours.

A wet specimen cannot be sent in the protective envelope. This would cause contamination plus invalidate the test.

12. Record the procedure in the patient's chart.
    Record on the laboratory slip the infant's date and time of birth and the number of days taking milk, in addition to the usual identifying information requested.

13. Place the dry test card in the protective envelope supplied with the test card and send it to the laboratory within 48 hours for testing.

Charting Example

October 10, 20__, 2 PM
Rt heel puncture for PKU testing. Specimen on filter paper sent to laboratory at 4 PM. Small amount of bleeding after heel puncture. Mother instructed about the test and gave permission. She expressed interest in the results.
J.A. Lee, CMA

The laboratory should receive the test within 48 hours to ensure accurate testing.

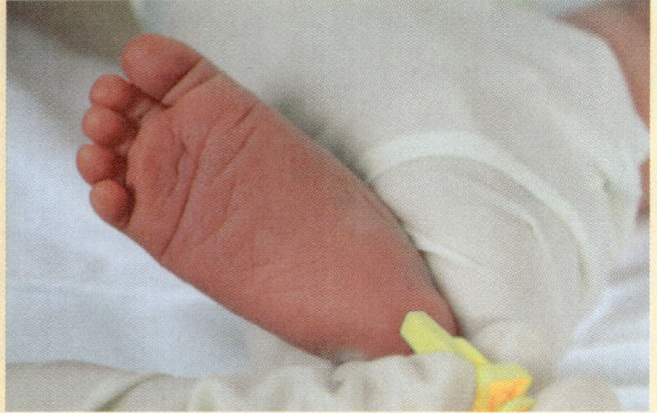

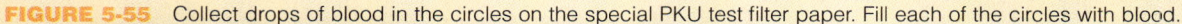

FIGURE 5-54   Grasp the infant's heel. Using a sterile lancet puncture the side of the heel at a right angle to obtain a blood sample.

FIGURE 5-55   Collect drops of blood in the circles on the special PKU test filter paper. Fill each of the circles with blood.

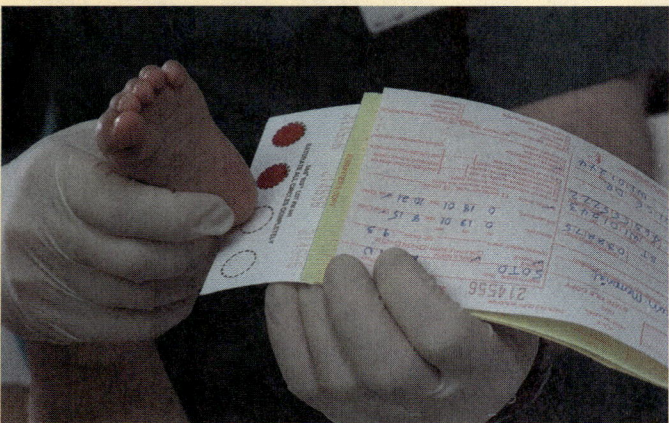 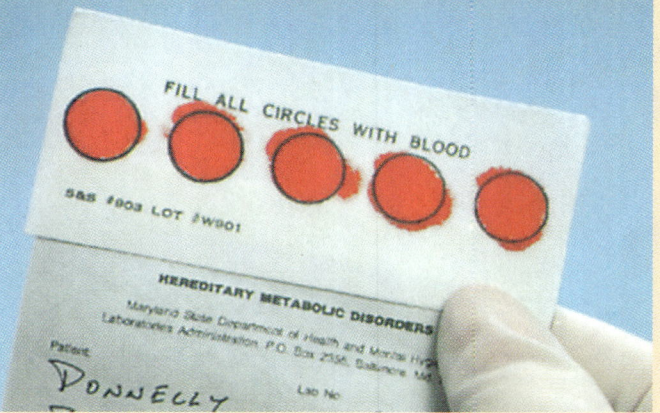

be followed. Some believe that it should be maintained for life; others suggest that it should continue through the sixth year of life when maximum brain development occurs. Therefore close supervision and long-term follow-up, especially nutritional counseling, is very important. Explanation, counseling, and support must be given to the parents of the infant. The dietary treatment is monitored by urine and blood testing.

A woman who has PKU and wants to become pregnant should be instructed to begin a low-phenylalanine diet before conception and continue it throughout the pregnancy (assuming that she has not been following this type of diet for some time). If the woman continues on a general diet, the risk of having a mentally retarded infant is very high.

Intramuscular, subcutaneous, and intradermal injections.

The techniques for administering injections to a child are the same as those used for an adult (see Chapter 7 and Figure 5-56). The child may need to be restrained before the injection is given. Another person should help you with this. Even the parent can hold and restrain the child while you are administering the medication. Tell the child that the medicine will help him or her to feel better and that it will hurt a little bit but only for a very short time. Praise the child after the injection is given, telling the child how brave he or she was. You or the parent can give an infant a hug. Give the child something to play with after the injection is given. This helps to distract the child and allows him or her to associate something pleasant with the experience other than discomfort. You can also place

FIGURE 5-56   Intramuscular injection sites in children. **A,** Vastus lateralis; **B,** ventrogluteal. (From Wong D, Whaley L: *Clinical manual of pediatric nursing,* ed 4, St. Louis, 1993, Mosby, pp. 226 and 227.)

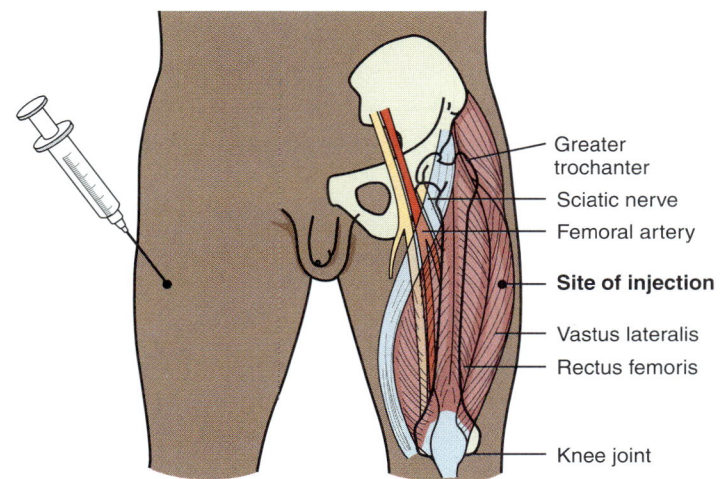

LOCATION
Palpate to find greater trochanter and knee joints; divide vertica distance between these two landmarks into quadrants; inject into middle of upper quadrant.

NEEDLE INSERTION AND SIZE
Insert needle at 45° angle toward knee in infants and in young children or needle perpendicular to thigh or slightly angled toward anterior thigh.
22 to 25 gauge, ⅝ to 1 inch

ADVANTAGES
Large, well-developed muscle that can tolerate larger quantitie of fluid (0.5 ml [infant] to 2.0 ml [child])
No important nerves or blood vessels in this location
Easily accessible if child is supine, side-lying, or sitting

DISADVANTAGES
Thrombosis of femoral artery from injection in midthigh area
Sciatic nerve damage from long needle injected posteriorly an medially into small extremity

A

LOCATION
Palpate to locate greater trochanter, anterior superior iliac tubercle (found by flexing thigh at hip and measuring up to 1 to 2 cm above crease formed in groin), and posterior iliac crest; place palm of hand over greater trochanter, index finge over anterior superior iliac tubercle, and middle finger along crest of ilium posteriorly as far as possible; inject into center of V formed by fingers.

NEEDLE INSERTION AND SIZE
Insert needle perpendicular to site but angled slightly toward iliac crest.
22 to 25 gauge, ½ to 1 inch

ADVANTAGES
Free of important nerves and vascular structures
Easily identified by prominent bony landmarks
Thinner layer of subcutaneous tissue than in dorsogluteal site, thus less chance of depositing drug subcutaneously rather than intramuscularly
Can accommodate larger quantities of fluid (0.5 ml [infant] to 2.0 ml [child])
Easily accessible if child is supine, prone, or side-lying
Less painful than vastus lateralis

DISADVANTAGES
Health professionals' unfamiliarity with site

B

FIGURE 5-56—cont'd   Intramuscular injection sites in children. **C,** Dorsogluteal; **D,** deltoid. (From Wong D, Whaley L: *Clinical manual of pediatric nursing,* ed 4, St. Louis, 1993, Mosby, pp. 226 and 227.)

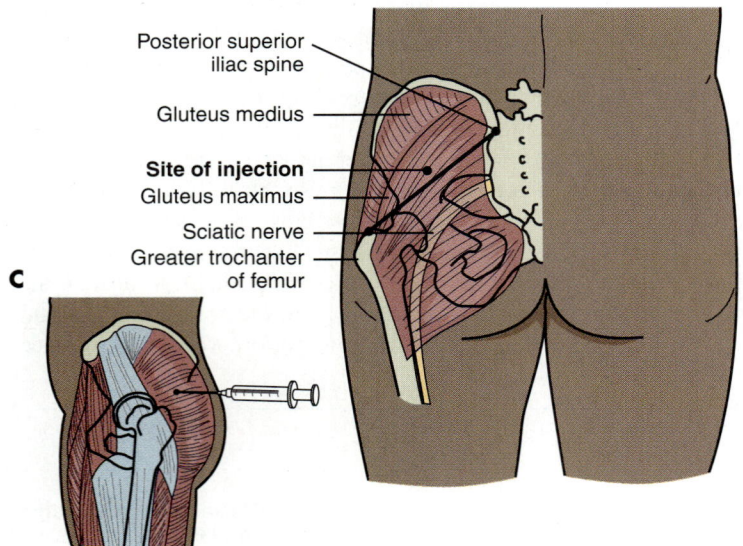

Posterior superior
iliac spine

Gluteus medius

Site of injection

Gluteus maximus

Sciatic nerve

Greater trochanter
of femur

C

LOCATION
Locate greater trochanter and posterior superior iliac spine; draw imaginary line between these two points and inject lateral and superior to line into gluteus muscle.

NEEDLE INSERTION AND SIZE
Insert needle perpendicular to surface on which child is lying when prone.
20 to 25 gauge, ½ to 1½ inches

ADVANTAGES
In older child large muscle mass; well-developed muscle can tolerate greater volume of fluid up to 2.0 ml
Child does not see needle and syringe
Easily accessible if child is prone or side-lying

DISADVANTAGES
Contraindicated in children who have not been walking for at least 1 year
Danger of injury to sciatic nerve
Thick, subcutaneous fat, predisposing to deposition of drug subcutaneously rather than intramuscularly
Inaccessible if child is supine
Exposure of site may cause embarrassment in older child

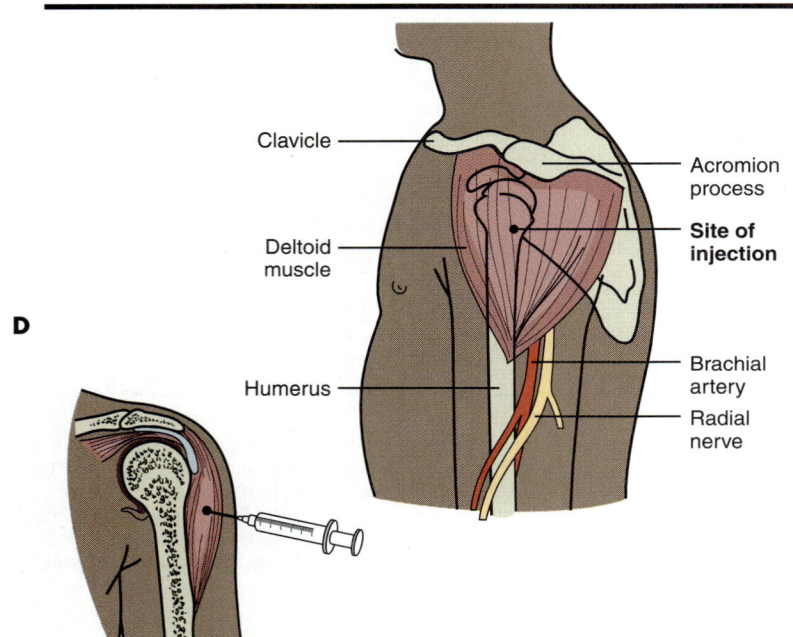

Clavicle

Acromion
process

Deltoid
muscle

Site of injection

D

Humerus

Brachial
artery

Radial
nerve

LOCATION
Locate acromion process; inject only into upper third of muscle that begins about 2 finger-breadths below acromion.

NEEDLE INSERTION AND SIZE
Insert needle perpendicular to site but angled slightly toward shoulder.
22 to 25 gauge, ½ to 1 inch

ADVANTAGES
Faster absorption rates than gluteal sites
Easily accessible with minimal removal of clothing

DISADVANTAGES
Small muscle mass; only limited amounts of drug can be injected (0.5 to 1.0 ml)
Small margins of safety with possible damage to radial nerve
Pain with repeated injections

an adhesive strip with a happy face decoration over the puncture mark. This can be comforting to the child and provides a distraction.

Immunizations.
Immunization is the process of rendering a person immune (protected from or not susceptible to a disease) or of becoming immune. It is often called vaccination or inoculation. Immunization is a process by which a person is artificially prepared to resist infection by a specific pathogen. Immunity, the antigen-antibody reaction, and the different types of immunity are discussed in Chapter 2.

Several vaccines are available for routine use to protect children from many communicable diseases. They should be administered according to a standardized schedule during well-child visits. Common vaccines available include the following:

- Diphtheria and tetanus toxoid combined with pertussis vaccine (DTP) or diphtheria and tetanus toxoid and acellular pertussis (DTaP). This is given intramuscularly.
- Diphtheria-tetanus toxoid (Td or DT). This is given intramuscularly.

- Inactivated poliovirus vaccine (IPV). This is given subcutaneously.
- Trivalent oral polio vaccine (OPV). This is given by mouth. **This vaccine is no longer recommended except in limited circumstances.** See also the Vaccine Information Statement on p. 262.
- Measles (rubeola), mumps (parotitis), and rubella (German measles) (MMR). This is given subcutaneously.
- *Haemophilus* b polysaccharide vaccine (HBPV) (also called *Haemophilus influenzae* type b [Hib] vaccine). This is given intramuscularly.
- Hepatitis B vaccine (in late 1992 specialists started to recommend hepatitis B vaccine for all children under 6 years of age). See Table 5-8 for current recommendations. This is given intramuscularly.
- Varicella vaccine (chickenpox). This is given subcutaneously.

Anatomic sites preferred for the aforementioned routes of administration are as follows:

- Adult—deltoid muscle
- Infant—anterolateral thigh (vastus lateralis) muscle
- Child—anterolateral thigh muscle, deltoid muscle

DO NOT use the buttocks (gluteus maximus muscle) for vaccines. Research studies have shown that vaccines *are not* absorbed as well through the tissues in the buttocks.

Vaccine administration.
Local injection-site reactions to immunization can cause significant discomfort and soreness in vaccine recipients. Local reactions are often caused by inadvertent subcutaneous delivery of vaccines intended for intramuscular (IM) administration. Local reactions include irritation, pain, redness, swelling, and can cause decreased use of the affected extremity for a short time (e.g., small children may limp or avoid walking temporarily). Studies found less swelling, redness, and tenderness at injection sites in infants when a longer (25 mm [1 inch]) needle was used.

Health care providers can easily avoid depositing the vaccine in the subcutaneous tissue by using the correct length needle. A 1-inch, 22- to 25-gauge needle is the preferred length and gauge for all IM immunizations—including influenza—for most vaccine recipients. A $\frac{7}{8}$-inch, 22- to 25-gauge needle is the preferred length and gauge for IM injections in infants younger than 4 months. A longer needle ($1\frac{1}{2}$-inch) may be needed to reach the muscle in very large adolescents and adults. A $\frac{5}{8}$-inch needle is not long enough to adequately deliver IM vaccines. *A $\frac{5}{8}$-inch needle should only be used for vaccines delivered subcutaneously.* Correct delivery of vaccine assures optimum immune response and assists in reducing the occurrence of local immunization reactions.

Medical assistants should be familiar with the different types of vaccinations given, the use of each, the contraindications, the possible side effects, the dosage, the route of administration, and the methods of storage and handling. Package inserts provided with each vaccine contain valuable information. Drug reference books can also be used for obtaining the necessary information. Also see Table 5-8, the box on Vaccine Information Statements, and the Summary of Pediatric Immunization Recommendations in the *Student Mastery Manual*.

Before a child receives a vaccination, information must be provided to the parent/legal representative. Forms containing information for each immunization must be given to the parent so that he or she understands the importance of the immunization and the possible side effects.

Screening questions should also be asked (Figure 5-57). **The National Childhood Vaccine Injury Act requires all health care providers in the United States who administer the previously listed vaccines,** *before* **the administration of** *each dose* **of the vaccine, to provide a copy of the relevant Vaccine Information Statement (VIS) produced by the Centers for Disease Control and Prevention (CDC) to the parent or legal representative of the child to be vaccinated and to any adult who is to receive the vaccine** (see Health Matters box, pp. 253 to 264). (In 1994 an amendment to the act deleted the language that allowed providers the flexibility to develop their own materials.) These materials must be supplemented with visual presentations or oral explanations in appropriate cases.

It is also recommended that health care providers give parents copies of all vaccine information materials *before* the first visit for immunization. Some hospitals provide these materials when the baby is born, and others give them at the first well-baby visit. A notation must be made in each patient's permanent medical record at the time vaccine information materials

FIGURE 5-57   Screening questions before vaccines administered.

SCREENING QUESTIONS

If parent answers "no" to all these questions, immunize the child.

If parent answers "yes" to any question, refer to "Guide to Contraindications to Childhood Vaccines."

1. Is your child sick today or does he/she have a high fever?
2. Is your child, or anyone else at home, taking steroids (such as cortisone or prednisone) or cancer treatment now, or have they taken them within the past 3 months?
3. Does your child, or anyone else in your home, have cancer, leukemia, HIV/AIDS or some other immune system problem?
4. Has your child ever had a reaction to a vaccine which was so bad that your had to take him/her to the doctor or hospital?
5. Has your child ever had convulsions or seizures?* Does your child have any other problems affecting his/her brain or nerves?
6. Does your child have an allergy to any of the following things which is so severe that it needs medical treatment: Eggs, neomycin, streptomycin, thimerosal, gelatin, yeast?
7. Has your child had a blood transfusion or a gamma globulin shot in the past year?
8. Is your child currently taking aspirin? (Except in rare cases, children should not be given aspirin, especially after varicella vaccine.)
9. (For adolescent girls) Could you be pregnant?

Text continued on p. 265

TABLE 5–8 Recommended Childhood Immunization Schedule

Vaccines[1] are listed under routinely recommended ages. ⬛ Bars ⬛ indicate range of recommended ages for immunization. Any dose not given at the recommended age should be given as a "catch-up" immunization at the subsequent visit when indicated and feasible.

⬮ Ovals ⬮ indicate vaccines to be given if previously recommended doses were missed or given earlier than the recommended minimum age.

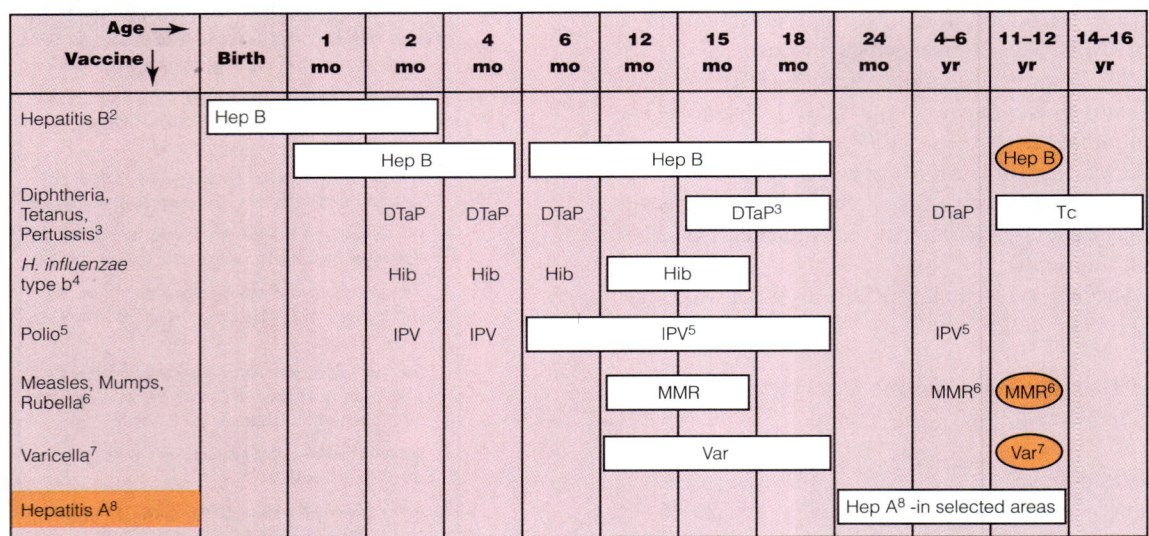

Age → Vaccine ↓	Birth	1 mo	2 mo	4 mo	6 mo	12 mo	15 mo	18 mo	24 mo	4–6 yr	11–12 yr	14–16 yr
Hepatitis B[2]	Hep B											
		Hep B			Hep B						Hep B	
Diphtheria, Tetanus, Pertussis[3]		DTaP	DTaP	DTaP		DTaP[3]				DTaP	Tc	
H. influenzae type b[4]		Hib	Hib	Hib	Hib							
Polio[5]		IPV	IPV	IPV[5]						IPV[5]		
Measles, Mumps, Rubella[6]					MMR					MMR[6]	MMR[6]	
Varicella[7]					Var						Var[7]	
Hepatitis A[8]									Hep A[8] -in selected areas			

Approved by the Advisory Committee on Immunization Practices (ACIP), the American Academy of Pediatrics (AAP), and the American Academy of Family Physicians (AAFP).

NOTE: On October 22, 1999, the Advisory Committee on Immunization Practices (ACIP) recommended that Rotashield (RRV-TV), the only U.S.-licensed rotavirus vaccine, no longer be used in the United States (*MMWR*, Volume 48, Number 43, Nov. 5,1999). Parents should be reassured that their children who received rotavirus vaccine before July 1999 are not at increased risk for intussusception now.

[1]This schedule indicates the recommended ages for routine administration of currently licensed childhood vaccines as of November 1, 1999. Additional vaccines may be licensed and recommended during the year. Licensed combination vaccines may be used whenever any components of the combination are indicated and its other components are not contraindicated. Providers should consult the manufacturers' package inserts for detailed recommendations.

[2]**Infants born to HBsAg-negative mothers** should receive the first dose of hepatitis B (Hep B) vaccine by age 2 months. The second dose should be administered at least 1 month after the first dose. The third dose should be administered at least 4 months after the first dose and at least 2 months after the second dose, but not before 6 months of age.
Infants born to HBsAg-positive mothers should receive hepatitis B and 0.5 ml hepatitis B immunoglobulin (HBIG) within 12 hours of birth at separate sites. The second dose is recommended at 1 month of age and the third dose at age 6 months of age. **Infants born to mothers whose HBsAg status is unknown** should receive hepatitis B vaccine within 12 hours of birth. Maternal blood should be drawn at the time of delivery to determine the mother's HBsAg status; if the HBsAg test is positive, the infant should receive HBIG as soon as possible (no later than 1 week of age). **All children and adolescents (through 18 years of age)** who have not been immunized against hepatitis B may begin the series during any visit. Special efforts should be made to immunize children who were born in or whose parents were born in areas of the world with moderate or high endemicity of hepatitis B virus infection.

[3]The fourth dose of DTaP (diphtheria and tetanus toxoids and acellular pertussis vaccine) may be administered as early as 12 months of age, provided 6 months have elapsed since the third dose and the child is unlikely to return at age 15-18 months. Td (Tetanus and diphtheria toxoids) is recommended at 11-12 years of age if at least 5 years have elapsed since the last dose of DTP, DTaP, or DT. Subsequent routine Td boosters are recommended every 10 years.

[4]Three *Haemophilus influenzae* type b (Hib) conjugate vaccines are licensed for infant use. If PRP-OMP (PedvaxHIB or ComVax [Merck]) is administered at 2 and 4 months of age, a dose at age 6 months is not required. Because clinical studies in infants have demonstrated that using some combination products may induce a lower immune response to the Hib vaccine component, DTaP/Hib combination products should not be used for primary immunization in infants at 2, 4, or 6 months of age, unless FDA-approved for these ages.

[5]To eliminate the risk for vaccine-associated paralytic polio (VAPP), an IPV (inactivated poliovirus vaccine) schedule is now recommended for routine childhood polio vaccination in the United States. All children should receive four doses of IPV at 2 months, 4 months, 6-18 months, and 4-6 years. Oral poliovirus vaccine (OPV) (if available) may be used **only** for the following special circumstances:
1. Mass vaccination campaigns to control outbreaks of paralytic polio.
2. Unvaccinated children who will be traveling in less than 4 weeks to areas where polio is endemic or epidemic.
3. Children of parents who do not accept the recommended number of vaccine injections. These children may receive OPV only for the third or fourth dose or both; in this situation, health care providers should administer OPV only after discussing the risk for VAPP with parents or caregivers.
4. During the transition to an all-IPV schedule, recommendations for the use of remaining OPV supplies in physicians' offices and clinics have been issued by the American Academy of Pediatrics (see *Pediatrics*, December 1999).

[6]The second dose of measles, mumps, and rubella (MMR) vaccine is recommended routinely at 4-6 years of age but may be administered during any visit, provided at least 4 weeks have elapsed since receipt of the first dose and that both doses are administered beginning at or after 12 months of age. Those who have not previously received the second dose should complete the schedule by the 11- 12-year-old visit.

[7]Varicella (Var) vaccine is recommended at any visit on or after the first birthday for susceptible children, that is, those who lack a reliable history of chickenpox (as judged by a health care provider) and who have not been immunized. Susceptible persons 13 years of age or older should receive two doses, given at least 4 weeks apart.

[8]Hepatitis A (Hep A) is shaded to indicate its recommended use in selected states and/or regions; consult your local public health authority. (Also see *MMWR*, Oct. 1, 1999/48 (RR12):1-37.)

HEALTH MATTERS

USE OF THE VACCINE INFORMATION STATEMENTS (VISs)

Must I use the VISs?

YES! *All the U.S. health care providers* must use them if they administer any of the following vaccines or toxoids, alone or in combination:

Diphtheria	Measles
Tetanus	Mumps
Pertussis	Rubella
Hepatitis B	Varicella
Haemophilus influenzae type b (Hib)	
Polio (either live or inactivated)	

The relevant VIS must be given *before* administration of *every dose* of the vaccine. This is required under the National Childhood Vaccine Injury Act.*

In addition to the VISs, providers should give visual and oral explanations to people who might not otherwise understand.

May I change the VIS or make up my own?

No. Federal law requires that the VISs produced by the Centers for Disease Control and Prevention (CDC) be used. You may add the name, address, and so on of your practice, but substantive changes are not acceptable.

To whom do I give the VIS?

Federal law says a VIS must go to:

1. Any adult receiving one of the vaccines, or
2. The parent or legal representative of any child receiving one of the covered vaccines.

"Legal representative" is defined as a person who is qualified to consent to immunization of a minor under state law.

*42 U.S.C. §300aa-26.

May I give VISs at other times, too?

Yes. In addition to the required use, it is a good idea to give parents copies of all VISs before the first visit for immunization.

How should we record that we have given the VIS?

Health care providers must note in each patient's permanent medical record at the time a VIS is given: **which** specific VIS was given (for example, polio), the **date of publication** of the VIS (on the back, bottom right), and the **date the VIS was provided.**

Federal law also requires that all health care providers record in the patient's permanent medical record (or a permanent office log):

- The **name, address**, and **title of the person** who administered the vaccine
- The **date of administration**
- The vaccine **manufacturer**
- The **lot number** of the vaccine used†

Know your state requirements

Health care providers should consult their legal counsel to determine additional state requirements pertaining to immunization. The federal requirement to provide the VISs is in addition to any applicable state law and no state law can negate that requirement.

How can I get copies of the VISs?

Single camera-ready copies of the VISs are available from state health departments. The VISs are also available on the Internet at **www.cdc.gov/nip/publications/vis/.** More detailed instructions regarding the use of the VISs can also be found on the National Immunization Program (NIP) Website.

†42 U.S.C. §300aa-25.

VACCINE INFORMATION STATEMENTS

I. HEPATITIS A VACCINE: WHAT YOU NEED TO KNOW (VIS published 8/25/98)

1. What is hepatitis A?

Hepatitis A is a serious liver disease caused by the hepatitis A virus (HAV). HAV is found in the stool of persons with hepatitis A. It is usually spread by close personal contact and sometimes by eating food or drinking water containing HAV.

Hepatitis A can cause:

- Mild flulike illness
- Jaundice (yellow skin or eyes)
- Severe stomach pains and diarrhea

People with hepatitis A infection often have to be hospitalized. In rare cases, hepatitis A causes death.

A person who has hepatitis A can easily pass the disease to others within the same household.

Hepatitis A vaccine can prevent hepatitis A.

2. Who should get hepatitis A vaccine and when?

- Persons 2 years of age and older traveling or working in countries with high rates of hepatitis A, such as those located in Central or South America, the Caribbean, Mexico, Asia (except Japan), Africa, and southern or eastern Europe. *The vaccine series should be started at least 1 month before traveling.*
- Persons who live in communities that have prolonged outbreaks of hepatitis A
- Persons who live in communities with high rates of hepatitis A: for example, American Indian, Alaska Native, and Pacific Islander communities and some religious communities

Continued

VACCINE INFORMATION STATEMENTS—cont'd

- Men who have sex with men
- Persons who use street drugs
- Persons with chronic liver disease
- Persons who receive clotting factor concentrates

Two doses of the vaccine, given at least 6 months apart, are needed for lasting protection.

Hepatitis A vaccine may be given at the same time as other vaccines.

3. Some people should not get hepatitis A vaccine or should wait.

People who have ever had a *serious* allergic reaction to a previous dose of hepatitis A vaccine should not get another dose.

People who are mildly ill at the time the shot is scheduled should get hepatitis A vaccine. People with moderate or severe illnesses should usually wait until they recover. Your doctor or nurse can advise you.

The safety of hepatitis A vaccine for pregnant women is not yet known. But any risk to either the pregnant woman or the fetus is thought to be very low.

Ask your doctor or nurse for details.

4. What are the risks from hepatitis A vaccine?

A vaccine, like any medicine, is capable of causing serious problems, such as severe allergic reactions. The risk of hepatitis A vaccine causing serious harm, or death, is extremely small.

Getting hepatitis A vaccine is much safer than getting the disease.

Mild problems

- Soreness where the shot was given (about 1 out of 2 adults, and up to 1 out of 5 children)
- Headache (about 1 out of 6 adults and 1 out of 20 children)
- Loss of appetite (about 1 out of 12 children)
- Tiredness (about 1 out of 14 adults)

If these problems occur, they usually come 3 to 5 days after vaccination and last for 1 or 2 days.

Severe problems

- Serious allergic reaction, within a few minutes to a few hours of the shot (very rare)

5. What if there is a moderate or severe reaction?
What should I look for?

Any unusual condition, such as a high fever or behavioral changes. Signs of a serious allergic reaction can include difficulty breathing, hoarseness or wheezing, hives, paleness, weakness, a fast heartbeat, or dizziness.

What should I do?

- Call a doctor, or get the person to a doctor right away.
- Tell your doctor what happened, the date and time it happened, and when the vaccination was given.
- Ask your doctor, nurse, or health department to file a Vaccine Adverse Event Reporting System (VAERS) form, or call VAERS yourself at **1-800-822-7967**.

6. How can I learn more?

- Ask your doctor or nurse. They can give you the vaccine package insert or suggest other sources of information.
- Call your local or state health department.
- Contact the Centers for Disease Control and Prevention (CDC):
  - Call **1-800-232-2522** (English)
  - Call **1-800-232-0233** (Español)
  - Visit the National Immunization Program's website at **http://www.cdc.gov/nip,** or CDC's hepatitis website at **http://www.cdc.gov/ncidod/diseases/hepatitis/ hepatitis.htm.**

Immune Globulin (IG)

Immune globulin can provide *temporary* immunity to hepatitis A.

Who should get IG?

- Persons who have been exposed to HAV and can get IG within 2 weeks of that exposure
- Travelers to areas with high rates of hepatitis A, if they do not receive hepatitis A vaccine

When should IG be given?

It can be given before exposure to HAV or within 2 weeks after exposure.

Benefits

IG protects against HAV for 3 to 5 months, depending on dosage.

Risks

Rare: swelling, hives, or allergic reaction.

From the U.S. Department of Health and Human Services, Centers for Disease Control and Prevention National Immunization Program, Hepatitis A (8/25/98) Vaccine Information Statement.

II. HEPATITIS B VACCINE: WHAT YOU NEED TO KNOW (VIS published 8/23/00)

1. Why get vaccinated?

Hepatitis B is a serious disease. The hepatitis B virus can cause short-term (acute) illness that leads to:

- Loss of appetite
- Tiredness
- Pain in muscles, joints, and stomach
- Diarrhea and vomiting
- Jaundice (yellow skin or eyes)

HEALTH **MATTERS—cont'd**

It can also cause long-term (chronic) illness that leads to:

- Liver damage (cirrhosis)
- Liver cancer
- Death

About 1.25 million people in the United States have chronic hepatitis B virus infection.

Each year it is estimated that:

- 200,000 people, mostly young adults, get infected with hepatitis B virus
- More than 11,000 people have to stay in the hospital because of hepatitis B
- 4000 to 5000 people die from chronic hepatitis B

Hepatitis B vaccine can prevent hepatitis B. It is the first anticancer vaccine because it can prevent a form of liver cancer.

2. How is hepatitis B virus spread?

Hepatitis B virus is spread through contact with the blood and body fluids of an infected person. A person can get infected in several ways, such as:

- During birth when the virus passes from an infected mother to her baby
- By having sex with an infected person
- By injecting illegal drugs
- By being stuck with a used needle on the job
- By sharing personal items, such as a razor or toothbrush, with an infected person

People can get hepatitis B virus infection without knowing how they got it. About one third of hepatitis B cases in the United States have an unknown source.

3. Who should get hepatitis B vaccine and when?

- Everyone 18 years of age and younger
- Adults over age 18 who are at risk

Adults at risk for hepatitis B virus infection include people who have more than one sex partner, men who have sex with other men, injection drug users, health care workers, and others who might be exposed to infected blood or body fluids.

If you are not sure whether you are at risk, ask your doctor or nurse.

People should get three doses of hepatitis B vaccine according to the following schedule. *If you miss a dose or get behind schedule, get the next dose as soon as you can. There is no need to start over.*

Adolescents 11 to 15 years of age may need only two doses of hepatitis B vaccine, separated by 4 to 6 months. Ask your health care provider for details.

Hepatitis B Vaccination Schedule

	WHO?		
	Infant whose mother is infected with hepatitis B virus	**Infant whose mother is *not* infected with hepatitis B virus**	**Older child, adolescent, or adult**
WHEN?			
First dose	Within 12 hours of birth	Birth-2 months of age	Any time
Second dose*	1-2 months of age	1-4 months of age (at least 1 month after first dose)	1-2 months after first dose
Third dose†	6 months of age	6-18 months of age	4-6 months after first dose

*The second dose must be given at least 1 month after the first dose.

†The third dose must be given at least 2 months after the second dose and at least 4 months after the first. The third dose should *not* be given to infants younger than 6 months of age.

Hepatitis B vaccine may be given at the same time as other vaccines.

4. Some people should not get hepatitis B vaccine or should wait.

People should not get hepatitis B vaccine if they have ever had a life-threatening allergic reaction to **baker's yeast** (the kind used for making bread) or to a **previous dose of hepatitis vaccine.**

People who are moderately or severely ill at the time the shot is scheduled should usually wait until they recover before getting hepatitis B vaccine.

Ask your doctor or nurse for more information.

5. What are the risks from hepatitis B vaccine?

A vaccine, like any medicine, is capable of causing serious problems, such as severe allergic reactions. The risk of hepatitis B vaccine causing serious harm, or death, is extremely small.

Getting hepatitis B vaccine is much safer than getting hepatitis B disease.

Most people who get hepatitis B vaccine do not have any problems with it.

Mild problems

- Soreness where the shot was given, lasting a day or two (up to 1 out of 11 children and adolescents, and about 1 out of 4 adults)
- Mild to moderate fever (up to 1 out of 14 children and adolescents and 1 out of 100 adults)

Severe problems

- Serious allergic reaction (very rare)

Continued

HEALTH MATTERS—cont'd

VACCINE INFORMATION STATEMENTS—cont'd

6. What if there is a moderate or severe reaction?
What should I look for?

Any unusual condition, such as a serious allergic reaction, high fever, or behavioral changes. Signs of a serious allergic reaction can include difficulty breathing, hoarseness or wheezing, hives, paleness, weakness, a fast heartbeat, or dizziness. If such a reaction were to occur, it would be within a few minutes to a few hours after the shot.

What should I do?

- Call a doctor, or get the person to a doctor right away.
- Tell your doctor what happened, the date and time it happened, and when the vaccination was given.
- Ask your doctor, nurse, or health department to file a Vaccine Adverse Event Reporting System (VAERS) form, or call VAERS yourself at **1-800-822-7967**.

7. The National Vaccine Injury Compensation Program

In the rare event that you or your child has a serious reaction to a vaccine, a federal program has been created to help you pay for the care of those who have been harmed.

For details about the National Vaccine Injury Compensation Program, call **1-800-338-2382** or visit the program's website at **http://www.hrsa.dhhs.gov/bhpr/vicp.**

8. How can I learn more?

- Ask your doctor or nurse. They can give you the vaccine package insert or suggest other sources of information.
- Call your local or state health department's immunization program.
- Contact the Centers for Disease Control and Prevention (CDC):
  - Call **1-800-232-2522 or 1-888-443-7232** (English)
  - Call **1-800-232-0233** (Español)
  - Visit the National Immunization Program's website at **http://www.cdc.gov/nip** or CDC's Hepatitis Branch website at **http://www.cdc.gov/ncidod/diseases/hepatitis/**

From the U.S. Department of Health and Human Services, Centers for Disease Control and Prevention National Immunization Program, Hepatitis B (8/23/00) Vaccine Information Statement.

III. MEASLES, MUMPS, AND RUBELLA VACCINES: WHAT YOU NEED TO KNOW (VIS published 12/16/98)

1. Why get vaccinated?

Measles, mumps, and rubella are serious diseases.

Measles
- Measles virus causes rash, cough, runny nose, eye irritation, and fever.
- It can lead to ear infection, pneumonia, seizures (jerking and staring), brain damage, and death.

Mumps
- Mumps virus causes fever, headache, and swollen glands.
- It can lead to deafness, meningitis (infection of the brain and spinal cord covering), painful swelling of the testicles or ovaries, and, rarely, death.

Rubella (German measles)
- Rubella virus causes rash, mild fever, and arthritis (mostly in women).
- If a woman gets rubella while she is pregnant, she could have a miscarriage or her baby could be born with serious birth defects.

You or your child could catch these diseases by being around someone who has them. They spread from person to person through the air.

Measles, mumps, and rubella (MMR) vaccine can prevent these diseases.

Most children who get their MMR shots will not get these diseases. Many more children would get them if we stopped vaccinating.

2. Who should get MMR vaccine and when?

Children should get *two doses* of MMR vaccine:

- The first at **12 to 15 months of age**
- and the second at **4 to 6 years of age**

These are the recommended ages. But children can get the second dose at any age, as long as it is at least 28 days after the first dose.

Some **adults** should also get MMR vaccine. Generally, anyone 18 years of age or older, who was born after 1956, should get at least one dose of MMR vaccine, unless they can show that they have had either the vaccines or the diseases.

Ask your doctor or nurse for more information.

MMR vaccine may be given at the same time as other vaccines.

3. Some people should not get MMR vaccine or should wait.

- People should not get MMR vaccine who have ever had a life-threatening allergic reaction to **gelatin,** the antibiotic **neomycin,** or a **previous dose of MMR vaccine.**
- People who are moderately or severely ill at the time the shot is scheduled should usually wait until they recover before getting MMR vaccine.
- Pregnant women should wait to get MMR vaccine until after they have given birth. Women should not get pregnant for 3 months after getting MMR vaccine.
- Some people should check with their doctor about whether they should get MMR vaccine, including anyone who:
  - Has HIV/AIDS, or another disease that affects the immune system

- Is being treated with drugs that affect the immune system, such as steroids, for 2 weeks or longer
- Has any kind of cancer
- Is taking cancer treatment with x-rays or drugs
- Has ever had a low platelet count (a blood disorder)
- People who recently had a transfusion or were given other blood products should ask their doctor when they may get MMR vaccine.

Ask your doctor or nurse for more information.

4. What are the risks from MMR vaccine?

A vaccine, like any medicine, is capable of causing serious problems such as severe allergic reactions. The risk of MMR vaccine causing serious harm, or death, is extremely small.

Getting MMR vaccine is much safer than getting any of these three diseases.

Most people who get MMR vaccine do not have any problem with it.

Mild problems

- Fever (up to 1 person out of 6)
- Mild rash (about 1 person out of 20)
- Swelling of glands in the cheeks or neck (rare)

If these problems occur, it is usually within 7 to 12 days after the shot. They occur less often after the second dose.

Moderate problems

- Seizure (jerking or staring) caused by fever (about 1 out of 3000 doses)
- Temporary pain and stiffness in the joints, mostly in teenage or adult women (up to 1 out of 4)
- Temporary low platelet count, which can cause a bleeding disorder (about 1 out of 30,000 doses)

Severe problems (very rare)

- Serious allergic reaction (less that 1 out of a million doses)
- Several other severe problems have been known to occur after a child gets MMR vaccine. But this happens so rarely, experts cannot be sure whether they are caused by the vaccine or not. These include:
    - Deafness
- Long-term seizures, coma, or lowered consciousness
- Permanent brain damage

5. What if there is a moderate or severe reaction?
What should I look for?

Any unusual conditions, such as a serious allergic reaction, high fever, or behavioral changes. Signs of a serious allergic reaction include difficulty breathing, hoarseness or wheezing, hives, paleness, weakness, a fast heartbeat, or dizziness within a few minutes to a few hours after the shot. A high fever or seizure, if it occurs, would happen 1 or 2 weeks after the shot.

What should I do?

- Call a doctor, or get the person to a doctor right away.
- Tell your doctor what happened, the date and time it happened, and when the vaccination was given.
- Ask your doctor, nurse, or health department to file a Vaccine Adverse Event Reporting System (VAERS) form, or call VAERS yourself at **1-800-822-7967**.

6. The National Vaccine Injury Compensation Program

In the rare event that you or your child has a serious reaction to a vaccine, a federal program has been created to help you pay for the care of those who have been harmed.

For details about the National Vaccine Injury Compensation Program, call **1-800-338-2382** or visit the program's website at **http://www.hrsa.dhhs.gov/bhpr/vicp**

7. How can I learn more?

- Ask your doctor or nurse. They can give you the vaccine package insert or suggest other sources of information.
- Call your local or state health department's immunization program.
- Contact the Centers for Disease Control and Prevention (CDC):
    - Call **1-800-232-2522** (English)
    - Call **1-800-232-0233** (Español)
    - Visit the National Immunization Program's website at **http://www.cdc.gov/nip**

From the U.S. Department of Health and Human Services, Centers for Disease Control and Prevention National Immunization Program, MMR (12/16/98) Vaccine Information Statement.

IV. CHICKENPOX VACCINE: WHAT YOU NEED TO KNOW (VIS published 12/16/98)
1. Why get vaccinated?

Chickenpox (also called varicella) is a common childhood disease. It is usually mild, but it can be serious, especially in young infants and adults.

- The chickenpox virus can be spread from person to person through the air or by contact with fluid from chickenpox blisters.
- It causes a rash, itching, fever, and tiredness.
- It can lead to severe skin infection, scars, pneumonia, brain damage, or death.
- A person who has had chickenpox can get a painful rash called shingles years later.
- About 12,000 people are hospitalized for chickenpox each year in the United States.
- About 100 people die each year in the United States as a result of chickenpox.

VACCINE INFORMATION STATEMENTS—cont'd

Chickenpox vaccine can prevent chickenpox.

Most people who get chickenpox vaccine will not get chickenpox. But if someone who has been vaccinated *does* get chickenpox, it is usually very mild. They will have fewer spots, are less likely to have a fever, and will recover faster.

2. Who should get chickenpox vaccine and when?

Children should get one dose of chickenpox vaccine between 12 and 18 months of age, or at any age after that if they have never had chickenpox.

People who do not get the vaccine until 13 years of age or older should get **two doses,** 4 to 8 weeks apart.

Ask your doctor or nurse for details.

Chickenpox vaccine may be given at the same time as other vaccines.

3. Some people should not get chickenpox vaccine or should wait.

- People should not get chickenpox vaccine if they have ever had a life-threatening allergic reaction to **gelatin,** the antibiotic **neomycin,** or (for those needing a second dose) a **previous dose of chickenpox vaccine.**
- People who are moderately or severely ill at the time the shot is scheduled should usually wait until they recover before getting chickenpox vaccine.
- Pregnant women should wait to get chickenpox vaccine until after they have given birth. Women should not get pregnant for 1 month after getting chickenpox vaccine.
- Some people should check with their doctor about whether they should get chickenpox vaccine, including anyone who:
  - Has HIV/AIDS or another disease that affects the immune system
  - Is being treated with drugs that affect the immune system, such as steroids, for 2 weeks or longer
  - Has any kind of cancer
  - Is taking cancer treatment with x-rays or drugs
- People who recently had a transfusion or were given other blood products should ask their doctor when they may get chickenpox vaccine.

Ask your doctor or nurse for more information.

4. What are the risks from chickenpox vaccine?

A vaccine, like any medicine, is capable of causing serious problems, such as severe allergic reactions. The risk of chickenpox vaccine causing serious harm, or death, is extremely small.

Getting chickenpox vaccine is much safer than getting chickenpox disease.

Most people who get chickenpox vaccine do not have any problems with it.

Mild problems

- Soreness or swelling where the shot was given (about 1 out of 5 children and up to 1 out of 3 adolescents and adults)
- Fever (1 person out of 10, or less)

- Mild rash, up to a month after vaccination (1 person out of 20, or less). It is possible for these people to infect other members of their household, but this is *extremely* rare.

Moderate problems

- Seizure (jerking or staring) caused by fever (less than 1 person out of 1000)

Severe problems

- Pneumonia (very rare)

Other serious problems, including severe brain reactions and low blood count, have been reported after chickenpox vaccination. These happen so rarely experts cannot tell whether they are caused by the vaccine or not. If they are, it is extremely rare.

5. What if there is a moderate or severe reaction?
What should I look for?

Any unusual condition, such as a serious allergic reaction, high fever, or behavioral changes. Signs of a serious allergic reaction can include difficulty breathing, hoarseness or wheezing, hives, paleness, weakness, a fast heartbeat, or dizziness within a few minutes to a few hours after the shot. A high fever or seizure, if it occurs, would happen 1 to 6 weeks after the shot.

What should I do?

- Call a doctor, or get the person to a doctor right away.
- Tell your doctor what happened, the date and time it happened, and when the vaccination was given.
- Ask your doctor, nurse, or health department to file a Vaccine Adverse Event Reporting System (VAERS) form, or call VAERS yourself at **1-800-822-7967**.

6. The National Vaccine Injury Compensation Program

In the rare event that you or your child has a serious reaction to a vaccine, a federal program has been created to help you pay for the care of those who have been harmed.

For details about the National Vaccine Injury Compensation Program, call **1-800-338-2382** or visit the program's website at **http://www.hrsa.dhhs.gov/bhpr/vicp**

7. How can I learn more?

- Ask your doctor or nurse. They can give you the vaccine package insert or suggest other sources of information.
- Call your local or state health department's immunization program.
- Contact the Centers for Disease Control and Prevention (CDC):
  - Call **1-800-232-2522** (English)
  - Call **1-800-232-0233** (Español)
  - Visit the National Immunization Program's website at **http://www.cdc.gov/nip**

From the U.S. Department of Health and Human Services, Centers for Disease Control and Prevention National Immunization Program, Varicella (12/16/98) Vaccine Information Statement.

V. DIPHTHERIA, TETANUS, AND PERTUSSIS VACCINES: WHAT YOU NEED TO KNOW (VIS published 8/15/97)

1. Why get vaccinated?

Diphtheria, pertussis, and tetanus are serious diseases.

Diphtheria

- Diphtheria causes a thick covering in the back of the throat.
- It can lead to breathing problems, paralysis, heart failure, and even death.

Tetanus (lockjaw)

- Tetanus causes painful tightening of the muscles, usually all over the body.
- It can lead to "locking" of the jaw so the person cannot open his or her mouth or swallow. Tetanus can lead to death.

Pertussis (whooping cough)

- Pertussis causes coughing spells so bad that it is hard for infants to eat, drink, or breathe. These can last for weeks.
- It can lead to pneumonia, seizures (jerking and staring spells), brain damage, and death.

Diphtheria, tetanus, and pertussis vaccines prevent these diseases. Most children who get all their shots will be protected during childhood. Many more children would get these diseases if we stopped vaccinating.

2. Diphtheria, Tetanus, and Pertussis Vaccines

DTP vaccine

- Protects against diphtheria, tetanus, and pertussis
- Used for many years

DTaP

- Protects against diphtheria, tetanus, and pertussis
- Newer than DTP

The Centers for Disease Control and Prevention (CDC) recommends DTaP over DTP. This is because DTaP is less likely to cause reactions than DTP.

Related vaccines

- Combinations: To reduce the number of shots a child must get, DTP or DTaP may be available in combination with other vaccines.
- DT protects against diphtheria and tetanus, but *not* pertussis. It only is recommended for children who should not get *pertussis* vaccine

3. What are the risks from these vaccines?

- As with any medicine, vaccines carry a small risk of serious harm, such as a severe allergic reaction or even death.

- If there are reactions, they usually start within 3 days and don't last long.
- Most people have no serious reactions from these vaccines.

Mild reactions (common)

- Sore arm or leg
- Fever
- Fussy
- Less appetite
- Tired
- Vomiting

Mild reactions are much less likely after DTaP than after DTP.

Moderate to serious reactions (uncommon)

Moderate to serious reactions have been uncommon with DTP vaccine:

- Nonstop crying (3 hours or more)—100 of every 10,000 doses
- Fever of 105° F or higher—30 of every 10,000 doses
- Seizure (jerking or staring)—6 of every 10,000 doses
- Child becomes limp, pale, less alert—6 of every 10,000 doses

With DTaP vaccine, these reactions are much less likely to happen.

Severe reactions (very rare)

There are two kinds of serious reactions:

- Severe allergic reaction (breathing difficulty, shock)
- Severe brain reaction (long seizure, coma, or lowered consciousness)

Is there lasting damage?

- Experts disagree on whether pertussis vaccines cause lasting brain damage.
- If they do, it is very rare.

*Most experts believe serious reactions will be **more rare** after DTaP than after DTP.*

4. When should my child get vaccinated?

Most children should get a dose at these ages: 2 months; 4 months; 6 months; 12 to 18 months; and 4 to 6 years.

At 11 to 12 years of age and every 10 years after that, you should get a booster to prevent diphtheria and tetanus.

5. What can be done to reduce possible fever and pain after this vaccine?

Give your child an **aspirin-free** pain reliever for 24 hours after the shot.

Continued

VACCINE INFORMATION STATEMENTS—cont'd

This is important if your child has had a seizure or has a parent, brother, or sister who has had a seizure.

6. Some children should not get these vaccines or should wait.

Tell your doctor or nurse if your child:

- Ever had a moderate or serious reaction after getting vaccinated
- Ever had a seizure
- Has a parent, brother, or sister who has had a seizure
- Has a brain problem that is getting worse
- Now has a moderate or severe illness

Your doctor or nurse has information on what to do in this case (for example, give one of these vaccines, wait, give medicine to prevent fever).

7. What if there is a moderate to severe reaction?
What should I look for?
- Any unusual conditions, such as those in item 3

What should I do?
- Call a doctor, or get the person to a doctor right away.
- Tell your doctor what happened, the date and time it happened, and when the vaccination was given.

- Ask your doctor, nurse, or health department to file a Vaccine Adverse Event Reporting System (VAERS) form, or call VAERS yourself at **1-800-822-7967**.

8. The National Vaccine Injury Compensation Program
The National Vaccine Injury Compensation Program is a federal program that helps pay for the care of those seriously injured by vaccines.

For details call **1-800-338-2382** or visit the program's website at **http://www.hrsa.dhhs.gov/bhpr/vicp/new.htm**

9. How can I learn more?
- Ask your doctor or nurse. They can give you the vaccine package insert or suggest other sources of information.
- Call your local or state health department's immunization program. They can give you the *Parents Guide to Childhood Immunization* or other information.
- Contact the Centers for Disease Control and Prevention (CDC):
  - Call **1-800-232-2522** (English)
  - Call **1-800-232-0233** (Spanish)
  - Visit the CDC website at **http://www.cdc.gov/nip**

From the U.S. Department of Health and Human Services, Centers for Disease Control and Prevention National Immunization Program, DTP/DTaP/DT (8/15/97) Vaccine Information Statement.

VI. TETANUS AND DIPHTHERIA VACCINE (TD): WHAT YOU NEED TO KNOW (VIS published 6/10/94)
About the Diseases
Tetanus (lockjaw) and diphtheria are serious diseases. Tetanus is caused by a germ that enters the body through a cut or wound. Diphtheria spreads when germs pass from an infected person to the nose or throat of others.

Tetanus causes:
- Serious, painful spasms of all muscles

It can lead to:
- "Locking" of the jaw so the patient cannot open his or her mouth or swallow

Diphtheria causes:
- A thick coating in the nose, throat, or airway

It can lead to:
- Breathing problems
- Heart failure
- Paralysis
- Death

About the Vaccines
Benefits of the vaccines
Vaccination is the best way to protect against tetanus and diphtheria. Because of vaccination, there are many fewer cases of these diseases. Cases are rare in children because most get DTP (diphtheria, tetanus, and pertussis), DTaP (diphtheria, tetanus, and acellular pertussis), or DT (diphtheria and tetanus) vaccines. There would be many more cases if we stopped vaccinating people.

When should you get Td vaccine?
Td is made for people 7 years of age and older.

People who have not gotten at least three doses of any tetanus and diphtheria vaccine (DTP, DtaP, or DT) during their lifetime should do so using Td. After a person gets the third dose, a Td dose is needed **every 10 years all through life.**

Other vaccines may be given at the same time as Td.

Tell your doctor or nurse if the person getting the vaccine:

- Ever had a serious allergic reaction or other problem with Td, or any other tetanus and diphtheria vaccine (DTP, DTaP, or DT)
- Now has a moderate or severe illness
- Is pregnant

If you are not sure, ask your doctor or nurse.

What are the risks from Td vaccine?
As with any medicine, there are very small risks that serious problems, even death, could occur after getting a vaccine.

The risks from the vaccine are *much smaller* than the risks from the diseases if people stopped using vaccine.

Almost all people who get Td have no problems from it.

Mild problems

If these problems occur, they usually start within hours to a day or two after vaccination. They may last 1 to 2 days:

- Soreness, redness, or swelling where the shot was given

These problems can be worse in adults who get Td vaccine very often.

Acetaminophen or ibuprofen (nonaspirin) may be used to reduce soreness.

Severe problems

These problems happen *very rarely*:

- Serious allergic reaction
- Deep, aching pain and muscle wasting in upper arm(s). This starts 2 days to 4 weeks after the shot and may last many months.

What to do if there is a serious reaction

- Call a doctor, or get the person to a doctor right away.
- Write down what happened and the date and time it happened
- Ask your doctor, nurse, or health department to file a Vaccine Adverse Event Reporting System (VAERS) form, or call VAERS yourself at **1-800-822-7967**.

The National Vaccine Injury Compensation Program is a federal program that gives compensation (payment) for persons thought to be injured by vaccines. For details call:

1-800-338-2382

If you want to learn more, ask your doctor or nurse. She or he can give you the vaccine package insert or suggest other sources of information.

From the U.S. Department of Health and Human Services, Centers for Disease Control and Prevention National Immunization Program, Td (6/10/94) Vaccine Information Statement.

VII. POLIO VACCINE: WHAT YOU NEED TO KNOW (VIS published 1/1/2000)

1. What is polio?

Polio is a disease caused by a virus. It enters a child's (or adult's) body through the mouth. Sometimes it does not cause serious illness. But sometimes it causes *paralysis* (can't move arm or leg). It can kill people who get it, usually by paralyzing the muscles that help them breathe.

Polio used to be very common in the United States. It paralyzed and killed thousands of people a year before we had a vaccine for it.

2. Why get vaccinated?

Inactivated polio vaccine (IPV) can prevent polio.

History:

A 1916 polio epidemic in the United States killed 6000 people and paralyzed 27,000 more. In the early 1950s there were more than 20,000 cases of polio each year. Polio vaccination was begun in 1955. By 1960 the number of cases had dropped to about 3000, and by 1979 there were only about 10. The success of polio vaccination in the United States and other countries has sparked a worldwide effort to eliminate polio.

Today:

No wild polio has been reported in the United States for over 20 years, but the disease is still common in some parts of the world. It would only take one case of polio from another country to bring the disease back if we were not protected by vaccine. If the effort to eliminate the disease from the world is successful, some day we won't need polio vaccine. Until then, we need to keep getting our children vaccinated.

3. Who should get polio vaccine and when?

IPV is a shot, given in the leg or arm, depending on age. Polio vaccine may be given at the same time as other vaccines.

Children

Most people should get polio vaccine when they are children. Children get four doses of IPV, at these ages:

- A dose at 2 months
- A dose at 4 months
- A dose at 6 to 18 months
- A booster dose at 4 to 6 years

Adults

Most adults do not need polio vaccine because they were already vaccinated as children. But three groups of adults are at higher risk and *should* consider polio vaccination:

- People traveling to areas of the world where polio is common
- Laboratory workers who might handle polio virus
- Health care workers treating patients who could have polio

Adults in these three groups who **have never been vaccinated against polio** should get three doses of IPV:

- The first dose at any time
- The second dose 1 to 2 months later
- The third dose 6 to 12 months after the second

Adults in these three groups who **have had one or two doses** of polio vaccine in the past should get the remaining one or two doses. It doesn't matter how long it has been since the earlier dose(s).

Adults in these three groups who **have had three or more doses** of polio vaccine (either IPV or OPV) in the past may get a booster dose of IPV.

Ask your health care provider for more information.

Continued

HEALTH MATTERS—cont'd

VACCINE INFORMATION STATEMENTS—cont'd

Oral polio vaccine: no longer recommended

There are two types of polio vaccine: **IPV,** which is the shot recommended in the United States today, and a live, oral polio vaccine **(OPV),** which is drops that are swallowed.

Until recently OPV was recommended for most children in the United States. OPV helped us rid the country of polio, and it is still used in many parts of the world.

Both vaccines give immunity to polio, but OPV is better at keeping the disease from spreading to other people. However, for a few people (about 1 in 2.4 million), OPV actually causes polio. Because the risk of getting polio in this country is now extremely low, experts believe that using oral vaccine is no longer worth the slight risk, except in limited circumstances, which your doctor can describe. The polio shot (IPV) does not cause polio. **If you or your child will be getting OPV, ask for a copy of the OPV supplemental Vaccine Information Statement.**

4. Some people should not get IPV or should wait.

These people should not get IPV:

- Anyone who has ever had a life-threatening allergic reaction to the antibiotics **neomycin, streptomycin,** or **polymyxin B** should not get the polio shot.
- Anyone who has a severe allergic reaction to a polio shot should not get another one.

These people should wait:

- Anyone who is moderately or severely ill at the time the shot is scheduled should usually wait until they recover before getting polio vaccine. People with minor illnesses, such as a cold, *may* be vaccinated.

Ask your health care provider for more information.

5. What are the risks from IPV?

Some people who get IPV get a sore spot where the shot was given. The vaccine used today has never been known to cause any serious problems, and most people don't have any problems at all with it.

However, a vaccine, like any medicine, could cause serious problems, such as a severe allergic reaction. *The risk of a polio shot causing serious harm, or death, is extremely small.*

6. What if there is a serious reaction?

What should I look for?

Look for any unusual condition, such as a serious allergic reaction, high fever, or unusual behavior.

If a serious allergic reaction occurred, it would happen within a few minutes to a few hours after the shot. Signs of a serious allergic reaction can include difficulty breathing, weakness, hoarseness or wheezing, a fast heartbeat, hives, dizziness, paleness, or swelling of the throat.

What should I do?

- Call a doctor, or get the person to a doctor right away.
- Tell your doctor what happened, the date and time it happened, and when the vaccination was given.
- Ask your doctor, nurse, or health department to file a Vaccine Adverse Event Reporting System (VAERS) form, or call VAERS yourself at **1-800-822-7967**.

Reporting reactions helps experts learn about possible problems with vaccines.

7. The National Vaccine Injury Compensation Program

In the rare event that you or your child has a serious reaction to a vaccine, a federal program has been created to help you pay for the care of those who have been harmed.

For details about the National Vaccine Injury Compensation Program, call **1-800-338-2382** or visit the program's website at **http://www.hrsa.gov/bhpr/vicp.**

8. How can I learn more?

- Ask your doctor or nurse. They can give you the vaccine package insert or suggest other sources of information.
- Call your local or state health department's immunization program.
- Contact the Centers for Disease Control and Prevention (CDC):
    - Call **1-800-232-2522** (English)
    - Call **1-800-232-0233** (Español)
    - Visit the National Immunization Program's website at **http://www.cdc.gov/nip.**

From the U.S. Department of Health and Human Services, Centers for Disease Control and Prevention National Immunization Program, Polio (1/1/2000) Vaccine Information Statement.

VIII. *HAEMOPHILUS INFLUENZAE* TYPE B (Hib) VACCINE: WHAT YOU NEED TO KNOW (VIS published 12/16/98)

1. What is Hib disease?

Haemophilus influenzae **type b (Hib) disease is a serious disease caused by a bacterium.** It usually strikes children under 5 years old.

Your child can get Hib disease by being around other children or adults who may have the bacteria and not know it. The germs spread from person to person. If the germs stay in the child's nose and throat, the child probably will not get sick. But sometimes the germs spread into the lungs or the bloodstream, and then Hib can cause serious problems.

Before Hib vaccine, Hib disease was the leading cause of bacterial meningitis among children under 5 years old in the United States. Meningitis is an infection of the brain and spinal cord coverings, which can lead to lasting brain damage and deafness. Hib disease can also cause:

HEALTH M A T T E R S — c o n t ' d

- Pneumonia
- Severe swelling in the throat, making it hard to breathe
- Infections of the blood, joints, bones, and covering of the heart
- Death

Before Hib vaccine, about 20,000 children in the United States under 5 years old got severe Hib disease each year, and nearly 1000 people died.

Hib vaccine can prevent Hib disease. Many more children would get Hib disease if we stopped vaccinating.

2. Who should get Hib vaccine and when?
Children should get Hib vaccine at:

- 2 months of age
- 4 months of age
- 6 months of age*
- 12 to 15 months of age

If you miss a dose or get behind schedule, get the next dose as soon as you can. There is no need to start over.

Hib vaccine may be given at the same time as other vaccines.

Older children and adults
Children over 5 years old usually do not need Hib vaccine, but some older children or adults with special health conditions should get it. These conditions include sickle cell disease, HIV/AIDS, removal of the spleen, bone marrow transplant, or cancer treatment with drugs. Ask your doctor or nurse for details.

3. Some people should not get Hib vaccine or should wait.
- People who have ever had a life-threatening allergic reaction to a previous dose of Hib vaccine should not get another dose.
- Children less than 6 weeks of age should not get Hib vaccine.
- People who are moderately or severely ill at the time the shot is scheduled should usually wait until they recover before getting Hib vaccine.

Ask your doctor or nurse for more information.

4. What are the risks from Hib vaccine?
A vaccine, like any medicine, is capable of causing serious problems, such as severe allergic reactions. The risk of Hib vaccine causing serious harm or death is extremely small.

Most people who get Hib vaccine do not have any problems with it.

*Depending on what brand of Hib vaccine is used, your child might not need the dose at 6 months of age. Your doctor or nurse will tell you if this dose is needed.

Mild problems
- Redness, warmth, or swelling where the shot was given (up to one fourth of children)
- Fever over 101° F (up to 1 out of 20 children)

If these problems happen, they usually start within a day of vaccination. They may last 2 to 3 days.

5. What if there is a moderate or severe reaction?
What should I look for?
Any unusual condition, such as a serious allergic reaction, high fever or behavior changes. Signs of a serious allergic reaction can include difficulty breathing, hoarseness or wheezing, hives, paleness, weakness, a fast heartbeat, or dizziness within a few minutes to a few hours after the shot.

What should I do?
- Call a doctor, or get the person to a doctor right away.
- Tell your doctor what happened, the date and time it happened, and when the vaccination was given.
- Ask your doctor, nurse, or health department to file a Vaccine Adverse Event Reporting System (VAERS) form, or call VAERS yourself at **1-800-822-7967**.

6. The National Vaccine Injury Compensation Program
In the rare event that you or your child has a serious reaction to a vaccine, a federal program has been created to help you pay for the care of those who have been harmed.

For details about the National Vaccine Injury Compensation Program, call **1-800-338-2382** or visit the program's website at **http://www.hrsa.dhhs.gov/bhpr/vicp.**

7. How can I learn more?
- Ask your doctor or nurse. They can give you the vaccine package insert or suggest other sources of information.
- Call your local or state health department's immunization program.
- Contact the Centers for Disease Control and Prevention (CDC):
  - Call **1-800-232-2522** (English)
  - Call **1-800-232-0233** (Español)
  - Visit the National Immunization Program's website at **http://www.cdc.gov/nip**

From the U.S. Department of Health and Human Services, Centers for Disease Control and Prevention National Immunization Program, Hib (12/16/98) Vaccine Information Statement.

Continued

HEALTH MATTERS—cont'd

VACCINE INFORMATION STATEMENTS—cont'd

IX. LYME DISEASE VACCINE: WHAT YOU NEED TO KNOW (VIS published 11/1/99)

1. What is Lyme disease?

Lyme disease is caused by infection with a bacterium. People get Lyme disease by being bitten by an infected tick.

You cannot get Lyme disease from another person or from an infected animal.

A common sign of Lyme disease is a round, red, expanding rash 2 inches or more in diameter, which appears between 3 days and a month after the tick bite. People with Lyme disease might get chills and fever, headaches, or muscle and joint pain and often feel tired.

If Lyme disease isn't treated properly, other signs can appear weeks or months after the tick bite. These include:

- Arthritis (pain and swelling in the joints, especially the knees)
- Numbness or paralysis (often in the face muscles)
- Problems with the heart rhythm
- Problems with memory or concentration

Very few, if any, people die from Lyme disease. About 12,000 to 15,000 cases of Lyme disease are reported each year in the United States, mainly in the Northeast and North Central parts of the country and in parts of California.

Lyme disease vaccine can help prevent Lyme disease.

2. Who should get Lyme disease vaccine and when?

Lyme disease vaccine may be given to people between 15 and 70 years of age. The vaccine should be considered for people in this age range who live in areas where Lyme disease is a problem and who work or spend leisure time in wooded, brushy, or overgrown areas where ticks live. People who travel to areas where Lyme disease is common may consider the vaccine if they plan to spend time in wooded or overgrown areas.

The vaccine is not recommended for people with little or no exposure to wooded or overgrown areas that are infested by Lyme disease–bearing ticks.

The Lyme disease vaccine is given as an injection. **Three doses are recommended:**

- The first dose may be given at any time but ideally should be given in January, February, or March.
- The second dose should be given 1 month after the first.
- The third dose should be given 12 months after the first.

It is not known yet how long protection lasts, but no schedule for booster doses has been determined at this time.

3. Some people should not get Lyme disease vaccine.

- Children younger than 15 years of age should not get Lyme disease vaccine.
- Pregnant women should not get Lyme disease vaccine.
- Anyone with arthritis caused by a previous case of Lyme disease, which has not responded to antibiotic treatment, should not get Lyme disease vaccine. (Others who have had Lyme disease may get the vaccine.)
- Anyone who has had an allergic reaction to a previous dose of Lyme disease vaccine should not get another dose.
- People with immune system problems should check with their doctor before getting Lyme disease vaccine.

4. What are the risks from Lyme disease vaccine?

A vaccine, like any medicine, is capable of causing serious problems, such as severe allergic reactions. The risk of a vaccine causing serious harm, or death, is extremely small.

In clinical trials, Lyme disease vaccine has been associated only with mild problems, such as soreness where the shot is given.

Most people who get Lyme disease vaccine do not have any problems with it.

Mild problems

- Soreness where the shot was given (about 1 person out of 4)
- Redness or swelling where the shot was given (less than 1 person out of 50)
- Muscle aches, joint pain, fever, chills (about 1 person out of 15 or less)

5. What if there is a moderate or severe reaction?
What should I look for?

Any unusual condition, such as a high fever or discomfort. Signs of a serious allergic reaction can include difficulty breathing, hoarseness or wheezing, hives, paleness, weakness, a fast heartbeat, or dizziness, occurring within a few minutes to a few hours after the vaccination. A high fever, should it occur, would be within a week after the vaccination.

What should I do?

- Call a doctor, or get the person to a doctor right away.
- Tell your doctor what happened, the date and time it happened, and when the vaccination was given.
- Ask your doctor, nurse, or health department to file a Vaccine Adverse Event Reporting System (VAERS) form, or call VAERS yourself at **1-800-822-7967**.

6. How can I learn more?

- Ask your doctor or nurse. They can give you the vaccine package insert or suggest other sources of information.
- Call your local or state health department's immunization program.
- Contact the Centers for Disease Control and Prevention (CDC):
  - Call **1-800-232-2522** (English); **1-800-232-0233** (Español)
  - Visit the National Immunization Program's website at **http://www.cdc.gov/nip**

From the U.S. Department of Health and Human Services, Centers for Disease Control and Prevention National Immunization Program, Lyme Disease (11/1/99) Vaccine Information Statement.

HEALTH MATTERS

AFTER THE SHOTS . . .

WHAT TO DO IF YOUR CHILD HAS DISCOMFORT

Your child may need extra love and care after getting immunized. Many of the shots that protect children from serious diseases can also cause discomfort for awhile. Here are answers to questions many parents have about the fussiness, fever, and pain their children may experience after they have been immunized. If you don't find the answers to your questions, call the clinic!

My clinic phone number: _____

My child has been fussy since being immunized. What should I do?

After immunization, children may be fussy because of pain or fever. You may want to give your child acetaminophen, a medicine that helps to reduce pain and fever. Some examples of acetaminophen are Tylenol, Panadol, and Tempra. DO NOT GIVE ASPIRIN (see the list below). If the fussiness lasts for more than 24 hours, you should call the clinic.

My child's arm (or leg) is swollen, hot, and red. What should I do?

- A clean, cool washcloth may be applied over the sore area as needed for comfort.
- If there is increasing redness or tenderness after 24 hours, call the clinic.
- For pain, give acetaminophen (see the table below). DO NOT GIVE ASPIRIN.

I think my child has a fever. What should I do?

Check your child's temperature to find out if there is a fever. The most accurate way to do this is by taking a rectal temperature. (Be sure to use a lubricant, such as petroleum jelly, when doing so.) If your child's fever is 105° F or higher by rectum, you need to call the clinic.

If you take the temperature by mouth (for an older child) or under the arm, these temperatures are generally lower and may be less accurate. Call your clinic if you are concerned about these temperatures.

Here are some things you can do to reduce fever:

- Give your child plenty to drink.
- Clothe your child lightly. Do *not* cover or wrap your child tightly!
- Give your child acetaminophen. DO NOT GIVE ASPIRIN.
- Sponge your child in a few inches of lukewarm (not cold) bath water.

My child seems really sick. Should I call the doctor?

If you are worried AT ALL about how your child looks or feels, please call the clinic!

Call the clinic if you answer "yes" to any of the following questions:

- Does your child have a rectal temperature of 105∞ F or higher? (Remember, a temperature taken under the arm or by mouth usually registers lower than a rectal temperature. You should call the clinic if you are concerned about these temperatures.)
- Is your child pale or limp?
- Has your child been crying for over 3 hours and just won't quit?
- Does your child have a strange cry that isn't normal (a high-pitched cry)?
- Is your child's body shaking, twitching, or jerking?

Adapted from the state of California, Immunization Branch by the Immunization Action Coalition, St. Paul, Minnesota.

HOW MUCH FEVER-REDUCING MEDICINE (ACETAMINOPHEN) SHOULD I GIVE MY CHILD?*

Dose of acetaminophen to be given every 4-6 hours, by age or by weight				
1-3 months 6-11 lbs.	4-11 months 12-17 lbs.	12-23 months 18-23 lbs.	2-3 years 24-35 lbs.	4-5 years 36-47 lbs.
½ dropperful	1 dropperful	1½ droppersful	1 teaspoon of syrup	1½ teaspoon of syrup
	or ½ teaspoon of syrup	or ¾ teaspoon of syrup	or 2 chewable (80mg) tablets	or 3 chewable (80mg) tablets

*Acetaminophen may be given before immunization and every 4 hours for 24 hours to minimize minor discomfort or fever. This is especially recommended for children with a family history of seizures or a personal history of seizures not related to a prior DTP/DTaP vaccine dose.

---

are provided, indicating the edition (date of publication) of the materials and the date these materials were provided.

A VIS *must* be given out with *every* vaccination, including each dose of a multidose series, because the statement might have been updated between visits or the health status of the child could have changed.

Signature of the patient, parent, or legal representative acknowledging receipt of the VISs is **not** required; however, you should consult your state law to determine if any specific "informed consent" requirements relate to immunization. **The VIS forms cover both the benefits and the risks associated with**

the vaccination so that they provide enough facts to adequately inform anyone reading them. If patients are unable to read the VISs, it is the provider's responsibility to ensure that they receive the information, by either reading or paraphrasing the VISs to the patients and then confirming that they understand. VISs are now available in 15 languages—Armenian, Cambodian, Chinese, English, Farsi, Japanese, Laotian, Hmong, Portuguese, Russian, Romanian, Samoan, Spanish, Tagalog, and Vietnamese.

The patients or their representatives should take home copies of the VISs because these include information that may be needed later, for example, the recommended schedule for vaccines, information concerning what to look for and do after the vaccination, and what to do if a serious reaction occurs. A form regarding reactions to vaccinations (see the box "After the Shots . . .") should be provided for the parent.

Once an infant or child is immunized, an immunization card should be given to the parents for their permanent home records. This record may also be needed for school or travel purposes (Figure 5-58).

The National Childhood Vaccine Injury Act of 1988 requires the following information to be recorded in the child's permanent medical record for all childhood-mandated vaccinations (Figure 5-59):

1. Type, manufacturer, and lot number of the vaccine
2. Date of administration
3. Name, address, and title of the person administering the vaccine; the address should be the address where the medical record is kept

Other information that is suggested to be recorded includes the following:

1. Site and route of administration
2. Expiration date of the vaccine

Adult immunization.
According to the CDC, vaccine-preventable infections of adults are now about 100 times more likely to kill an American adult than a child. Their major impact is among people of age 65 or older and those with chronic health conditions, such as heart disease, lung disease, diabetes, cancer, or immunodeficiency. For these people, the flu *can* lead to pneumonia and even death. Many of these cases could be prevented by annual flu vaccinations and much greater public education. Health care providers must take advantage of every opportunity possible to inform and educate more adults about the availability and advantage of immunizations for adults. Review Table 2-2, pp. 40-41, for more information on immunizations recommended for adults.

Reporting vaccine-preventable diseases.
Public health officials depend on the prompt reporting of vaccine-preventable diseases to local or state health departments by health care providers to effectively monitor the occurrence of such diseases for prevention and control efforts.

Nearly all vaccine-preventable diseases in the United States are notifiable; individual cases should be reported to local or state health departments. State health departments report these diseases each week to the CDC. All these organizations use the surveillance data to determine whether outbreaks or other unusual events are occurring and to evaluate prevention and control strategies. In addition, the CDC uses these data to evaluate the impact of national policies, practices, and strategies for vaccine programs.

In late 1998 the CDC declared the childhood vaccination program for *Haemophilus influenzae* type b (Hib) a success. Since the introduction of this vaccine in 1988, cases of the disease have dropped 99%. In 1997 fewer than 300 invasive cases were reported, compared with more than 20,000 cases annually in the early 1980s before the vaccine was available. This result is an example of what typically happens when vaccines are effective. The key to a successful vaccination program depends on health care professionals who keep people informed about a child's vaccination schedule.

Hib is a life-threatening disease, especially to children under the age of 1 year, who are particularly at risk for invasive Hib disease. This form of the disease can cause bacterial meningitis.

LEAD POISONING

Childhood lead poisoning is a serious, preventable environmental health problem. Lead enters the body either by inhalation or ingestion. Also, if a woman is exposed to lead during pregnancy, it can cross the placental barrier and pass over to the fetus. Lead is harmful to the developing brain and nervous system of a fetus and young child. Lead can build up in the body over many years and can cause damage to the brain and nervous system, red blood cells, and kidneys. Lead exposure has been associated with reproductive disorders, anemia, and hypertension, and it is especially harmful to children and pregnant women. Serious learning disabilities and neurologic disorders can result from lead poisoning. These problems may or may not be reversible. Severe irreversible effects of lead poisoning could lead to convulsions, mental retardation, paralysis, blindness, and ultimately coma and death.

Common sources of lead exposure include the following:

1. Deteriorating lead-based paint inside and outside of older homes and buildings. Lead levels in paint were reduced in 1950 and again in 1978. Paint sold today has very little lead. Children get lead into their bodies by chewing on lead-painted surfaces and also by eating paint that is peeling or chipping.
2. Lead-contaminated soil, dust, and water. Lead-based paint on the inside or outside of older homes can wear down and mix in with surrounding household and outside dust and dirt. This dust and dirt can get on toys, on a child's fingers, and into the child's mouth. Water contaminated from lead in soldered joints of old pipes is another source. A major source of lead poisoning in infants is seen when lead-contaminated water is used to prepare baby formula.
3. Lead-containing materials used in some occupations or hobbies, such as in a battery manufacturing factory or in a radiator or automotive repair shop, and in hobbies, such as making stained glass items or when soldering. The use of unleaded gasoline has significantly reduced the amount of lead in the air caused by the use of gasoline-operated vehicles. However, lead from gas is also found in dirt and yards near busy roads. Air can become contaminated from fumes from industries such as lead smelters.

Text continued on p. 270

FIGURE 5-58 Immunization record for patient's home record.

VACCINE		DATE GIVEN	DOCTOR OFFICE OR CLINIC	DATE NEXT DOSE DUE
VARICELLA (chickenpox) ☐ Had disease				
HEPATITIS A	1			
	2			
PNEUMOCOCCAL Conjugate	1			
	2			
	3			
	4			

TB SKIN TESTS Pruebas de la Tuberculosis	Type*	Date given	Given by	Date read	Read by	mm indur	Impression
	☐ PPD-Mantoux ☐ Other ____	/ /		/ /			☐ Pos ☐ Neg
	☐ PPD-Mantoux ☐ Other ____	/ /		/ /			☐ Pos ☐ Neg

* If required for school entry, must be Mantoux unless exception granted by local health department.

CHEST X-RAY (Necessary if skin test positive.)	Film date: ____/____/____ Impression: ☐ normal ☐ abnormal Person is free of communicable tuberculosis: ☐ yes ☐ no Signature/Agency: ________________

Parents: Your child must meet California's immunization requirements to be enrolled in school. Keep this Record as proof of immunization. **Padres:** Su niño debe cumplir con los requisitos de vacunas para asistir a la escuela. Mantenga este Comprobante: lo necesitará.

IMMUNIZATION RECORD

Comprobante de Inmunización

THE GREAT SEAL OF THE STATE OF CALIFORNIA

EUREKA

Name
nombre ____________________

Birthdate
fecha de nacimiento ____________________

Allergies
alergias ____________________

Vaccine Reactions
reacciones a cualquier vacuna ____________________

RETAIN THIS DOCUMENT — *CONSERVE ESTE DOCUMENTO*

FIGURE 5-58—cont'd Immunization record for patient's home record.

	VACCINE *vacuna*	DATE GIVEN *fecha de vacunación*	DOCTOR OFFICE OR CLINIC *médico o clinica*		DATE NEXT DOSE DUE *próxima vacuna*
Name			**Sex** **Birthdate**		
	POLIO 1		☐ IPV ☐ OPV		
	2		☐ IPV ☐ OPV		
	3		☐ IPV ☐ OPV		
	4		☐ IPV ☐ OPV		
	DTaP Td DT 1		☐ DTaP ☐ DT/Td		
	2		☐ DTaP ☐ DT/Td		
	3		☐ DTaP ☐ DT/Td		
	4		☐ DTaP ☐ DT/Td		
	5		☐ DTaP ☐ DT/Td		
			☐ Td		
	HIB 1				
	2				
	3				
	4				
	MMR 1				
	2				
	HEPATITIS B 1				
	2				
	3				

PROVIDERS: If using combination vaccines, remember to record dose in all appropriate spaces.

DTaP= diphtheria, tetanus, pertussis (whooping cough) *difteria, tétano y tos ferina*
MMR = measles, mumps, rubella *sarampión, paperas y sarampión aleman*   IPV = inactivated polio
HIB = Hib meningitis (Haemophilus influenzae type B) *meningitis Hib*   OPV = oral polio

PM 298 (3/00) IMM-75

FIGURE 5-59   Child immunization record for the medical record.

CHILD IMMUNIZATION FLOW SHEET

PUT PREVENTION INTO PRACTICE

Disease(s)	Vaccine Type	Vaccine Name	Recommended Age	Date Given	Age Given	Manufacturer	Lot Number	Site	Signature of Person Giving Vaccine	Handout Pub. Date	Signature of Parent or Guardian in Response to Informed Consent Statement	Informed Consent Statement
Diphtheria Tetanus Pertussis	DTaP or DTP		2 mos.									"I have been given a copy of, and have read or have had explained to me, information about each of the diseases and the vaccines listed at left. I have had a chance to ask questions, and they were answered to my satisfaction. I believe I understand the benefits and risks of each vaccine and ask that they be given to the minor named above (for whom I am authorized to make this request)."
	DTaP or DTP		4 mos.									
	DTaP or DTP		6 mos.									
	DTaP or DTP		15-18 mos.									
	DTaP or DTP		4-6 yrs.									
	Td		11-16 yrs.									
Haemophilus influenzae type b	Hib #1		2 mos.									
	Hib #2		4 mos.									
	Hib #3		6 mos.									
	Hib #4		12-15 mos.									
--- OR --- Combined vaccine DTP/Hib	DTP/Hib #1		2 mos.									
	DTP/Hib #2		4 mos.									
	DTP/Hib #3		6 mos.									
	DTP/Hib #4		12-15 mos.									
Polio Choose one: • IPVx2 and OPVx2 • IPVx4 • OPVx4	IPV		2 mos.									
	IPV		4 mos.									
	IPV or OPV*		6-18 mos. (if OPVx4), otherwise 12-18 mos.									
	IPV or OPV		4-6 yrs.									
Measles Mumps Rubella	MMR #1		12-15 mos.									
	MMR #2		4-6 yrs. *OR* 11-12 yrs.									
Hepatitis B	HBV #1		Birth-2 mos.									
	HBV #2		1-4 mos.									
	HBV #3		6-18 mos.									
Varicella	VZV #1		1-12 yrs. *OR* ≥13 yrs.									
	VZV #2		2nd dose only if ≥13 yrs.									

*Year 2000—OPV is no longer recommended or available.

FIGURE 5-60   Childhood lead poisoning evaluation questionnaire.

CHILDHOOD LEAD POISONING EVALUATION QUESTIONNAIRE

Name: _____

DOB: _____

Medical #: _____

Note: These questions may not be adequate to assess risk for all children, and are not a substitute for blood lead testing. All children should be tested at about 12 months, and again at 24 months, if feasible.

	Date __/__/__		Date __/__/__		Date __/__/__		Date __/__/__	
1 Does your child live in or regularly visit a house or other location built before 1960 with peeling or chipping paint? (This can include a day care center, preschool, barn, home of babysitter, relative, friend, etc.)	YES ☐	NO ☐	YES ☐	NO ☐	YES ☐	NO ☐	YES ☐	NO ☐
2 Does your child live in or regularly visit a house built before 1960 with recent or ongoing renovation or remodeling?	YES ☐	NO ☐	YES ☐	NO ☐	YES ☐	NO ☐	YES ☐	NO ☐
3 Does your child have a parent, brother, sister, housemate or playmate who is being treated or followed for lead poisoning? (For example, blood lead >10 µg/dL. This is a unit of measure to determine blood lead levels.)	YES ☐	NO ☐	YES ☐	NO ☐	YES ☐	NO ☐	YES ☐	NO ☐
4 Does your child live with someone whose job or hobby involves exposure to lead? (For example, painting, soldering, automobile battery manufacturing or recycling, vehicle radiator repair.)	YES ☐	NO ☐	YES ☐	NO ☐	YES ☐	NO ☐	YES ☐	NO ☐
5 Does your child live near an active lead smelter or battery recycling plant or other industry likely to release lead?	YES ☐	NO ☐	YES ☐	NO ☐	YES ☐	NO ☐	YES ☐	NO ☐

4. Lead in some pottery, china, pewter, and cookware, especially in the paint or glaze that was used to decorate these items. Eating food prepared or stored in these products can be a source for lead poisoning.

5. Lead found in some traditional or folk home remedies and medications from other countries, such as Azarcon, Greta, and Coral (Mexican); Pay-loo-ah (Hmong); Bokoor and Ceruse (Arabic-Middle East); and Kandu, Bala goli and Ghasard (Asian-Indian). Some cosmetics from other countries may contain lead, for example, Kohl and Alkohl (Arabic-Middle East) and Surma (Asian-Indian, Armenian).

Blood Lead Level Screening for Children

The goal of screening children for blood lead levels (BLLs) is to identify children who need individual interventions to reduce their blood lead level. Children who live in older homes, those who are exposed to lead taken home from an adults' workplace usually in the form of lead dust on clothing, and those exposed to other sources as noted in Figure 5-60 are at the greatest risk for lead poisoning. Children are more likely than adults to be exposed to lead because they have more hand-to-mouth activity than adults and they absorb it more readily than adults. Most children who have lead poisoning do not act or look sick (at first). Screening is done on either a venous or capillary (finger-stick) blood specimen. The CDC suggests that health care providers follow local health department recommendations on screening and in the absence of recommendations, screen all children at ages 1 and 2 years and children 36 to 72 months of age who have not been previously screened. Some facilities include a BLL screening as part of a well-child health assessment. Other facilities use a routine questionnaire (see Figure 5-60) to help identify children who should receive this blood test. If there are any positive answers on the questionnaire, a blood test would then be recommended. BLL testing should also be performed when children have unexplained symptoms or signs that are consistent with lead poisoning. **In children with lead poisoning, you may see developmental delay, attention deficit disorder, hyperactivity, other behavioral problems, hearing loss, seizures and other neurologic symptoms, and anemia.**

Lead Poisoning Prevention Methods

Health care providers should give information, guidance, routine screening, family lead education, diagnostic and follow-up testing for those with elevated BLLs, clinical management as needed, and follow-up care in collaboration with public health agencies.

Family education.   The causes and consequence of elevated BLLs must be explained to the family, for example, the need for follow-up testing and treatment, the need to control lead hazards in the child's surroundings, the potential for future learning disabilities, and the availability of early intervention services. Videos, printed materials, referral services such as parent-support groups, and, if needed, referrals for housing services and social service agencies may be provided. See the box below and on page 272, screening for blood lead levels and steps to prevent lead poisoning in your child.

ASTHMA

Asthma is a **chronic inflammatory lung disease** characterized by recurrent breathing problems. An estimated 12 million Americans of all ages have asthma. A person may have childhood asthma, then it goes away, and then it may come back 30 years later for no apparent reason. Others may have it as a child, and then it goes away forever; whereas others develop it as an adult. In the past 20 years a 20% to 30% increase in asthma has occurred *worldwide*. Many theories are held as to why asthma has developed in such massive numbers, such as people being exposed to more pollution, the immune system of some not maturing the way it should, people having too many infections, and many other unknown reasons.

In asthma the lining of the bronchial tubes become inflamed, the lining swells, and the breathing passageways narrow. Increased sensitivity in the airways leads to bronchospasm, and this condition can cause further narrowing in the bronchi, leading to varying degrees of obstructed airflow and difficult breathing. In some people, the airway is further obstructed by an excessive production of mucus from the mucous glands in the bronchi.

Signs and Symptoms

Common signs and symptoms of asthma include coughing, wheezing, shortness of breath, and a feeling of tightness in the chest. These symptoms can vary at different times and can range from mild, to moderate, to severe and can even be life threatening. Some people are affected only occasionally or even seasonally, whereas other people have a more chronic form and may have symptoms daily. Some people have asthma attacks when symptoms seem to come on very suddenly. An asthma attack can be mild or severe and lasts for varying

HEALTH MATTERS

KEEPING YOUR PATIENTS INFORMED

BLOOD LEAD LEVELS: WHAT DO THEY MEAN?

The blood test gives an idea of how much lead your child has been exposed to over the last month or so. The meaning of the blood lead test results are explained below, with levels given in micrograms of lead per deciliter of blood (μg/dl).

Below 10 μg/dl

This is a *normal* blood lead level.

- If you live in an older home with peeling paint, your child(ren) under age 6 may need to be tested again within the next year.

10 to 14 μg/dl

This level is *slightly above* the level that is considered normal.

- Your child may need to be tested again in 3 to 6 months. Talk with your doctor.
- Look for lead hazards around your home—we'll send you information that will help you.

15 to 19 μg/dl

This level means your child has a *mild* exposure to lead.

- Your child needs another blood test in 3 months. Talk with your doctor.
- We will provide information and a home visit to help you look for hazards around your home.
- If your child has a second blood lead test result in this range, we will test your home for lead.

20 to 44 μg/dl

This level means your child has a *moderate* to *high* exposure to lead.

- Immediately make a medical appointment for a confirming blood lead test and lead poisoning checkup.
- Lead hazards must be found and reduced. We will provide information and test your home for lead.
- Follow your doctor's recommendations for retesting and keep all medical appointments.

Above 44 μg/dl
Lead poisoning at this level is serious.

- Your child needs a full medical checkup and treatment **NOW**!
- Your child may need to be in the hospital for specialized treatment. Your doctor will advise you.
- Lead hazards must be found and removed. Your child needs a lead-safe home to get well. The Lead Program will test your home and provide recommendations for decreasing exposure to lead.
- Follow your doctor's recommendations for retesting and keep all medical appointments.

A blood lead level over 70 μg/dl requires immediate medical attention!

The most common source of lead poisoning in children is dust that comes from peeling paint in older homes. You can help prevent lead poisoning by washing children's hands often, wet cleaning floors and window sills every week, and feeding children good meals with lots of iron and calcium.

For more information, contact the San Francisco Childhood Lead Prevention Program at 415-554-8930.

amounts of time. It is important for the person to recognize early warning signs so that precautions can be used to lessen the severity of an attack or episode.

Triggers of Asthma

A variety of known triggers can set off an asthma attack. These include the following:

- Allergens, such as house dust, pollen, cats, feathers (as in feather pillows), foods, mold
- Irritants in the air, such as tobacco smoke, strong odors (for example, cologne), exhaust fumes, frying foods, and air pollution
- Respiratory infections—colds, flu, sore throats
- Emotional stress (Asthma is *not* of psychologic origin. Stress will not cause an asthma attack *unless* one already has hyperactive airways. Asthma begins in the lungs, not in the head.)
- Too much physical exertion or strenuous exercise
- Breathing cold air, windy weather, or sudden changes in the weather
- Sensitivity to some drugs (such as aspirin), some food additives (such as those sometimes found in dried fruits), some processed foods, wine, and beer
- Some 200 chemicals used in industry (These have been shown to cause occupational asthma.)

Diagnosis

To distinguish asthma from other conditions, a physical examination relies on a combination of factors, which include the following:

- A *detailed* medical history including the pattern of symptoms and what seems to trigger them
- A thorough physical examination

- Pulmonary function tests such as spirometry (see pp. 276 and 281-284), which measures the amount of air inhaled and exhaled. These tests can show obstruction in the airways.
- Peak flow monitoring (another measure of lung function; see pp. 273-274)
- Chest x-rays. The results are usually normal in a person who has asthma.
- Sometimes blood tests and allergy tests
- The patient's response to asthma medications

Management

Because asthma is a chronic condition, close monitoring by the person or parent of the child and the physician is advised. This involves keeping track of early warning signs for a few weeks, using a peak flow meter to measure the peak expiratory flow rates, preventing attacks or episodes by discovering and avoiding substances that trigger an asthma attack, and controlling an asthmatic attack once it starts.

Common early warning signs, which can occur before breathing becomes difficult, include the following:

- Coughing
- Sneezing
- Breathing changes
- Runny, stuffy nose
- Throat itchiness
- Headache
- Fatigue
- Moodiness
- Sleeping difficulties
- Trouble breathing at night

Patient education is an extremely important part of total patient care and is an *essential* part of asthma management. Classes are often available for patients to attend. If asthma education classes are not available, patient education must be initiated and completed in the physician's office or clinic. It is important for the patient and parent or caregiver to understand the different types of asthma, what is happening in the breathing passageways, the signs and symptoms of an impending attack, how to monitor breathing with a peak flow meter, how to identify triggers of attacks, and how to use an inhaler with the medication(s). They should also be aware of their personal action plan, including the use of antiinflammatory or bronchodilator medications; how to work with the physician; and whether any support groups are available. With education a person can often predict when an attack will happen and stop it before it becomes severe. There is no cure for asthma, but major medical advances have made it possible to reduce the severity and frequency of the symptoms and to enable people to be better prepared when they do occur. By understanding their condition, patients have more personal control on managing it and leading a more normal life.

Treatment programs must be individualized for each person's needs. Monitoring asthma and working with the physician on an ongoing basis are crucial for individuals to ensure that their treatment program is the best for them.

It is also important for the patient to receive the following instructions:

Call the physician *immediately* if any of the following conditions occur:
- Severe wheezing
- Labored breathing
- Unable to speak or sleep
- Lips are turning bluish in color
- Chest or neck pain develop
- Vomiting the medications taken
- Wheezing that *has not* improved *after* the *second dose* of asthma mediations

Call the physician *within 24 hours* if any of the following conditions occur:
- The presence of a yellow nasal discharge or congested sinuses
- Vomiting or stomach pain thought to be caused by the asthma medications
- Wheezing still present after 5 days
- Hospitalization within the past year for asthma
- Questions and concerns about the treatment and their condition

Peak Expiratory Flow Rate and Treatment Plan

Changes in the airways and airflow of people with asthma often occur gradually, and often signs and symptoms of a worsening condition are not detected by them until they experience up to a 25% or greater decrease in lung function. By using a small, easy-to-use handheld instrument, the peak flow meter, people can measure lung function by determining their peak expiratory flow rate (PEFR). The PEFR measures how fast air can be forcefully exhaled after taking in a deep breath. It is measured in liters per minute (L/min). The daily results ob-

tained when using the peak flow meter can provide early warning signs of airway changes and obstruction within hours or up to a day or two before an asthmatic attack. By identifying these changes, people can take steps to prevent an impending attack.

The **results** obtained when using a peak flow meter provide both patient and physician with information needed to make decisions for a treatment plan. The peak flow number is used to decide when to add or stop medication(s) or when to seek emergency care, to determine what environmental control measures are needed, to perform personal assessments, and also to determine the effectiveness of asthma medications. The physician can determine peak flow values that are normal for a patient and the steps to take when values drop. Many specialists use **the three-zone system for peak flow values** when making decisions for treatment. This system is based on the patient's *"personal best* peak flow rate." The personal best number is the highest of three peak flow readings attained when the person's asthma is under control. Asthma is under control when there are no asthma symptoms, including nighttime symptoms, and the person can maintain a normal level of activity. Peak flow values are usually highest in the midday and early evenings, so these are the values to use to determine the personal best value. The three zones are determined from this number, and the zones indicate how well a person is breathing. The zone system is compared with the colors of a traffic light, as follows:

Green zone: This zone ranges from 80% to 100% of the patient's *personal best*. Green indicates ALL CLEAR and good lung function. Regular activities and the routine treatment plan for maintaining asthma control should be followed.

Yellow zone: This zone ranges from 50% to 80% of the patient's *personal best*. Yellow indicates CAUTION. More aggressive treatment may be needed. This could include a temporary increase in the prescribed medications.

Red zone: This zone is 50% or less of the patient's *personal best*. Red signals a MEDICAL ALERT. **Immediate treatment** with a bronchodilator is needed. The physician must be contacted or emergency care sought if the peak flow numbers do not immediately return and stay in the yellow or green zones.

For example, if a patient's personal best value is 500 L/min, then the green zone would be from 400 to 500, the yellow zone would be from 250 to 400, and the red zone would be anything below 250 L/min.

Colored tape or lines could be put on the peak flow meter to indicate the different zones. This color system helps people to understand their peak flow readings and how they relate to managing their asthma. The peak flow percentages mentioned previously are to be used only as guidelines. Each person has to establish his or her own peak flow zones with the physician. Each person should keep a record of his or her peak flow values, asthma symptoms, use of inhaled medications, activity level, and nighttime awakenings resulting from asthma. By doing this, changes in lung function can be monitored, and the appropriate treatment can be followed. The severity of the asthma, the season, and the pattern of symptoms determine how often peak flow values must be measured. Graphs or charts for recording the peak flow values often come with the meter when purchased and can be photocopied for regular use. Graphs provide a quick reference when reviewing lung function for any period. *Care for asthma requires good communication, education, and a partnership between the person and the physician.* A **written action plan** should be developed to guide the overall treatment and to specify treatment when acute symptoms develop. Which medications to take, when to call the physician, and when to go to an emergency room must all be outlined in this plan (Figure 5-61, *A*). Asthma is considered an inflammatory disease and not simply abnormal airway constriction; therefore treatment is aimed at reducing the airway inflammation in the long run, as well as dilating the airways when they do constrict. One of the main treatment goals is long-term suppression of the airway inflammation that triggers asthma attacks so that the person can maintain a normal, active lifestyle.

For almost everyone except those with the mildest asthma, regular daily inhalations of an **antiinflammatory drug** (for example, corticosteroids) or regular use of oral medications (for example, zafirlukast [Accolate] or zileuton [Zyflo]) are used to reduce and prevent the inflammation that narrows the bronchial tubes (airways). The other commonly inhaled asthma drugs, **bronchodilators,** do not prevent inflammation but open the airways during an asthma attack.

Suggestions to reduce exposure to asthma triggers include not having pets; encasing pillows and mattresses in dustproof coverings and washing them—in addition to bed linens—twice a week; and removing carpeting, especially from the bedroom. Dehumidifying bathrooms and basements can help to eliminate mold. Also, installing an air purifier can be helpful.

Children with asthma often are sedentary and gain weight because they are afraid of suffering from an asthma attack while exercising. Exercise physiologists have designed **fitness programs** to help children control their asthma and weight through exercise, good diet, and improved motivation. Studies have shown that regular exercise can help in managing asthma.

How to use a peak flow meter.
The following instructions must be given to the person with asthma. Verify that the person understands the directions by having him or her demonstrate how to use the meter and record the peak flow values (see Figure 5-61).

1. Place the indicator at the bottom of the numbered scale on the peak flow meter.
2. Stand up.
3. Inhale as deeply as you can.
4. Place the meter in the mouth and close the lips around the mouthpiece. Do not put the tongue in the hole of the mouthpiece.
5. Blow out as hard and as fast as possible. You must put forth a good effort to blow hard and fast to have reliable and consistent results.
6. Read and record the number that the indicator has moved up to.

7. Repeat steps 1 through 6 two more times.
8. Record the highest of the three numbers obtained and record it on your graph or chart, noting the date and time.
9. Follow the manufacturer's directions for cleaning the meter. This helps to ensure accuracy of the meter.

Also see Review of Vocabulary section at the end of this chapter for a sample Pulmonary Preventative Care Record.

TESTS TO MEASURE THE ADEQUACY OF VENTILATION AND OXYGENATION

Tests used to assess the adequacy of ventilation and oxygenation are **oximetry, pulmonary function tests,** and **peak expiratory flow rates.** Blood work includes a **complete blood count (CBC)** and **arterial blood gas (ABG).**

Most body cells acquire their energy from chemical reactions involving oxygen and the elimination of carbon dioxide. The exchange of these gases occurs between the blood and the environmental air. The transport system for these gases consists of the lungs and the cardiovascular system. When we breathe air into our lungs (inhalation), it passes through passageways, ending in the alveoli or air sacs of the lungs. From the alveoli, oxygen passes into the surrounding capillary beds. Eventually the blood in these vessels with a fresh supply of oxygen (oxygenated blood) flows back to the left side of the heart through the pulmonary veins. As the heart continues beating, this blood goes from the left atrium into the left ventricle and then out through the aorta to a network of blood vessels throughout the body. At all body sites, oxygen passes over through the blood vessel walls to the body cells and tissues to provide energy and allow proper functioning. In turn, the waste gas, carbon dioxide, leaves the cells and goes back into the blood. This blood, now lower in oxygen content (deoxygenated blood), passes through many vessels that eventually take the blood to the superior and inferior venae cava and back to the right atrium on the heart. The blood flows from the right atrium down to the right ventricle and then out through the pulmonary arteries to the lungs. After passing through the various vessels, the blood reaches the tiny capillaries surrounding the air sacs, and when we breathe out (exhale), the carbon dioxide in the blood goes through the air sacs and out through the breathing passages (bronchi). The three steps involved in the process of oxygenation are **ventilation** (the process of moving gases into and out of the lungs), **perfusion** (moving blood to and from the alveolar-capillary membrane to allow gases to exchange), and **diffusion** (the movement of molecules from an area of higher concentration to an area of lower concentration). Diffusion of respiratory gases occurs at the alveolar-capillary membrane in the lungs. Oxygen diffuses across the alveolar-capillary membrane into arterial blood. The blood's capability to carry oxygen is affected by the following:

1. The amount of oxygen dissolved in the plasma. Normally, this is only about 3%.
2. The amount of hemoglobin. Hemoglobin is a complex iron-protein compound in the red blood cells. It is the hemoglobin in the blood that carries oxygen to the cells from

FIGURE 5-61   **A,** Action plan for controlling asthma. **B,** Peak flow meters. **C,** Using peak flow meter to determine peak flow values.

PEAK FLOW ACTION PLAN

Tracking Peak Flow Rates.
Your peak flow meter tells you if you are having an asthma attack or "flare-up." By reading the peak flow number, you can tell how severe an attack is. Because your airway passages narrow even before symptoms of an attack begin, your peak flow meter works as an "early warning device" for asthma attacks.

Having a plan of action before an asthma flare-up is important. Be prepared! Always carry a bronchodilator inhaler with you. Keep emergency phone numbers handy. Have a plan for getting to the emergency department quickly in the event of a medical alert asthma episode.

Your baseline (or best peak flow) value is: _200-210 (pts personal best)_

Measure your peak flow every day, or when you are feeling symptoms, and compare them to the numbers on this page.

☺   **Your Green Zone is:** _160-210_ **ALL CLEAR**
Continue with current medications and dosages.

☹   **Your Yellow Zone is:** _105-160_ **WARNING**
Action to take:
Bronchodilator _Albuterol X2 puffs up to 4-6 times a day_
Anti-Inflammatory Agent _Vanceril dose may need to go up per MD_
Prednisone: No or Yes _May require if no improvement_
Other _____

☹   **Your Red Zone is:** _less than 100-105_ **MEDICAL ALERT**
Action to take: **CALL YOUR DOCTOR OR GO TO ER**
Bronchodilator _____
Anti-Inflammatory Agent _____
Prednisone: No or Yes _____
Other _____

If there is no improvement after 20-30 minutes, call 911 or go to a local emergency room.

A

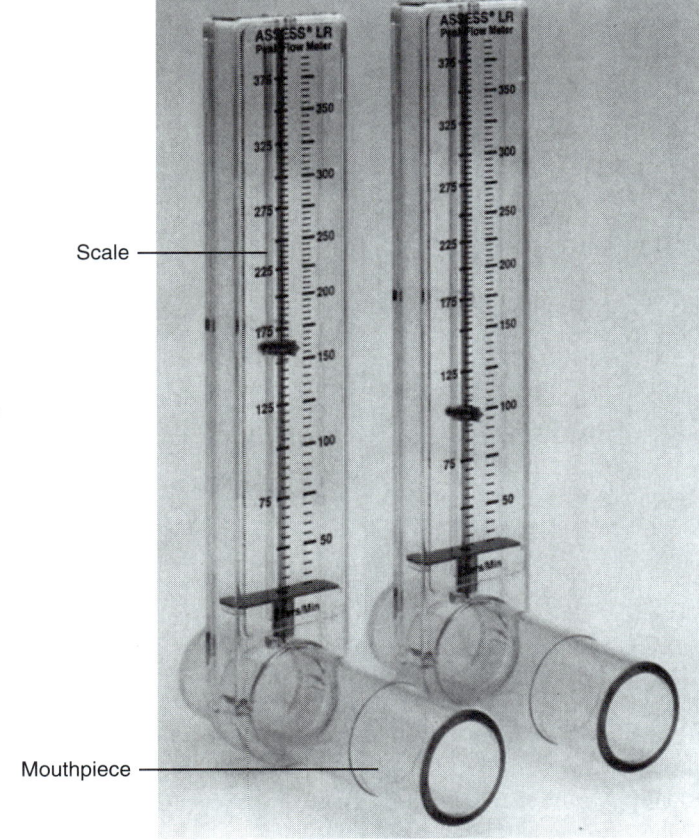

B

Scale

Mouthpiece

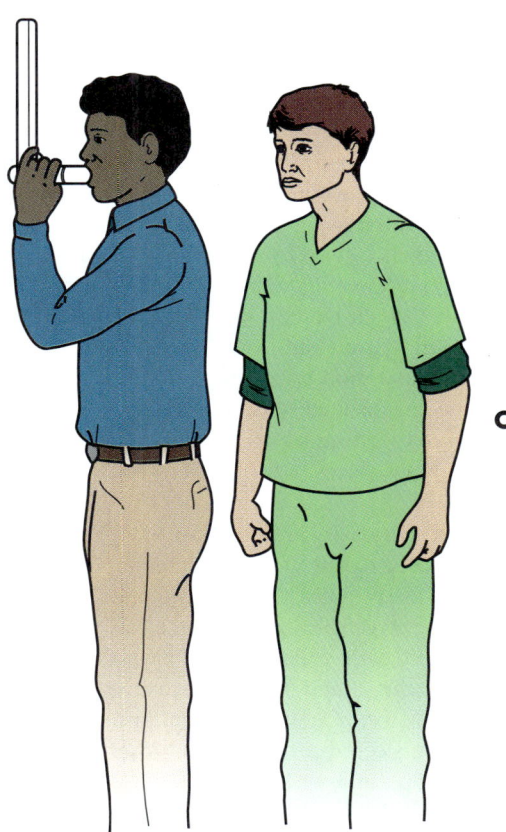

C

the lungs and carbon dioxide away from the cells to the lungs. In arterial blood, hemoglobin is about 97% saturated with oxygen. This gives the blood a bright red color. In venous blood the hemoglobin is only about 20% to 70% saturated with oxygen. Venous blood is a darker red color as a result of the lower oxygen content.

3. The tendency of oxygen is to bind with hemoglobin, forming oxyhemoglobin. The formation of oxyhemoglobin can be easily reversed. When it does reverse, it allows hemoglobin and oxygen to dissociate so that now the oxygen is free to enter the tissues.

Pulse Oximetry

Pulse oximetry is a rapid, noninvasive, and simple method used to determine a patient's arterial blood oxygen saturation (SaO_2). This is the ratio of oxygenated hemoglobin to the total amount of hemoglobin or the percent to which hemoglobin is filled with oxygen. The result is read as a percentage. For example, a saturation of 96% means that 96% of the total amount of hemoglobin in the body is filled with oxygen. A range of 95% to 100% is considered normal. An amount below 90% could quickly lead to serious complications.

To **measure arterial saturation,** a pulse oximeter may be used that has a self-contained finger clip sensor for interpreting the SaO_2 (Figure 5-62, *A* and *B*). Handheld oximeters and larger ones contain a clip sensor probe that is connected to a main unit containing a microprocessor, which interprets the results (Figure 5-63). For adults the sensor can be attached to a finger, ear, forehead, or toe (Figure 5-64, *A* and *B*). For infants the sensor can be attached to the foot (Figure 5-65). The pulse oximeter shines red and infrared light through the tissue and detects the fluctuating signals caused by arterial blood pulses. The ratio of the fluctuation of the red and infrared light signals received determines the oxygen saturation content. This number is displayed as a digital readout. Most units also display the pulse rate. Oxygen saturation levels measured with pulse oximeters are noted as SpO_2 instead of SaO_2. This differentiates the readings from an oxygen saturated level obtained by arterial blood gas (ABG) analysis.

Uses.   Oximetry was first used in the operating room and then in emergency rooms, intensive care units, and medical-surgical units in the hospital. Now it is applied in outpatient settings, in field emergencies, and in home care. Pulse oximetry is commonly used with patients who have pneumonia, chronic bronchitis, asthma, emphysema, congestive heart failure, or a pulmonary embolism. Continuous monitoring may be employed when assessing sleep disorders, during exercise tolerance testing (Figure 5-66), and when evaluating a patient's progress in pulmonary rehabilitation programs. It is also used during diagnostic imaging studies when sedative drugs have been given because the drugs could cause respiratory depression.

Factors that can affect accuracy.   Pulse oximeters are generally reliable; however, a few factors can still affect accuracy. These include the following:

1. **Movement.** If the patient moves or the sensor moves, the ability of the light to travel through the vascular bed is affected. Also, any tremor, such as seen in patients with Parkinson's disease, seizure activity, shivering, or vibrations caused by air or ground transportation also affect the readings. Placing the sensor on the ear may help to avoid these problems.

2. **Excessive or flickering light in the area.** Direct sunlight on the sensor or light from an overhead examination light can give false readings. To fix these problems, either move the patient or the light source or cover the sensor with a washcloth.

3. **Weak pulse rate, cold fingers or toes, hypothermia, or hypotension.** If the oximeter measures the pulse rate, check the pulse rate displayed on the oximeter with the patient's pulse rate that you palpate. If these two rates do not match, the oximeter is probably not picking up reliable SpO_2 readings. Warming the finger or toe or moving the sensor to the ear may help.

4. **Fingernail polish.** Whether this factor causes unreliable readings is debated; however, generally the darker the polish, the more likely the reading will be inaccurate. Green, blue, and black polishes seem to cause the most problems. If you cannot put the sensor on a finger without polish, put it on the toe or ear. If that is not possible, place the sensor sideways on the finger rather than over the nailbed. You may need to tape the sensor in this position so that it does not move. *Artificial nails* also interfere with accurate readings.

5. **Mechanical problems.** Periodically compare the pulse reading from the monitor or sensor with the patient's actual pulse rate. If the sensor is battery operated, check the batteries. Check the position of the sensor because it must be in the correct position to give accurate readings. Refer to the manufacturer's direction booklet. Also, put the sensor on your own finger and compare the pulse readout with your own pulse rate. If you do not obtain a normal reading, use a different oximeter.

Pulmonary Function Tests

Pulmonary function tests are used to assess respiratory health and respiratory function; to diagnose the presence, the degree of, and the progression of respiratory disease (although the same functional abnormality may occur in different diseases); and to study the effects of treatment. These tests measure the ability of the lungs to exchange oxygen and carbon dioxide efficiently. Basic ventilation studies are performed with a **spirometer,** an instrument that measures and records the volume of inhaled and exhaled air. Spirometers were computerized in the mid-1980s so the instrument can gather and analyze detailed volumetric information. This information is recorded on a chart called a **spirogram.** Spirometry readings are expressed in volumes and capacities, and these in turn are expressed as a percentage of the normal.

In some occupations, particularly in industrial settings, spirometry testing can be an important part of an annual em-

FIGURE 5-62 **A,** Pulse oximeter finger clip sensor that is self-contained for interpreting arterial blood oxygen saturation. **B,** Finger pulse oximeter applied. (Courtesy Nonin Medical, Inc., Plymouth, Minn.)

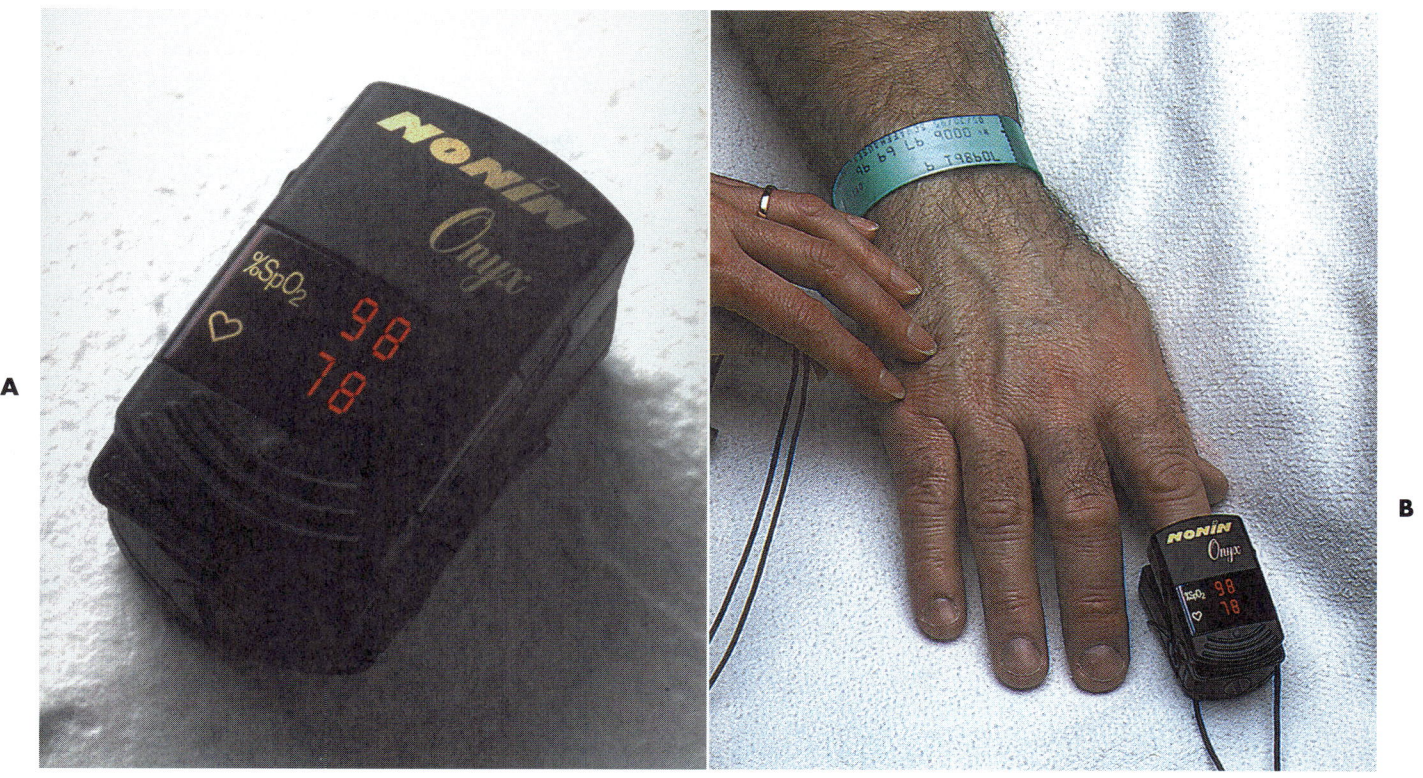

A

B

FIGURE 5-63; **A** and **B,** Handheld pulse oximeter with sensor attached to patient's finger. (Courtesy Nonin Medical Inc., Plymouth, Minn.)

A

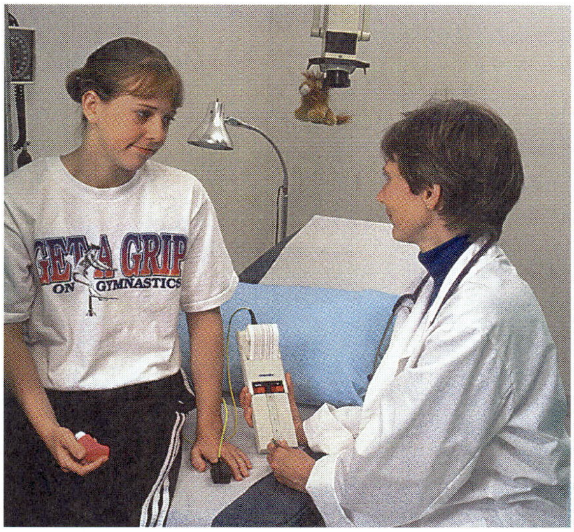

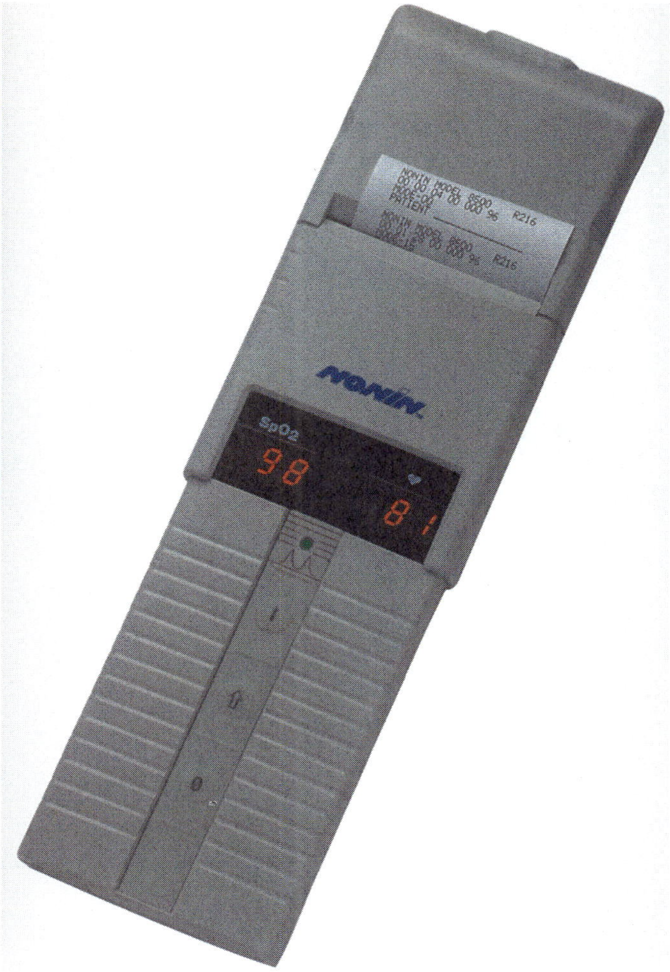

B

FIGURE 5-64   Sensor for the oximeter attached to earlobe **(A),** and forehead **(B).** (Courtesy Nonin Medical Inc., Plymouth, Minn.)

A

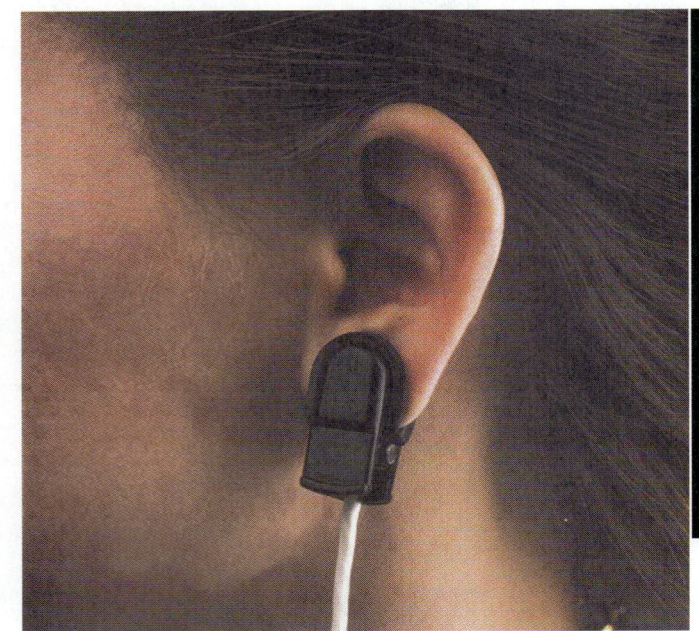

B

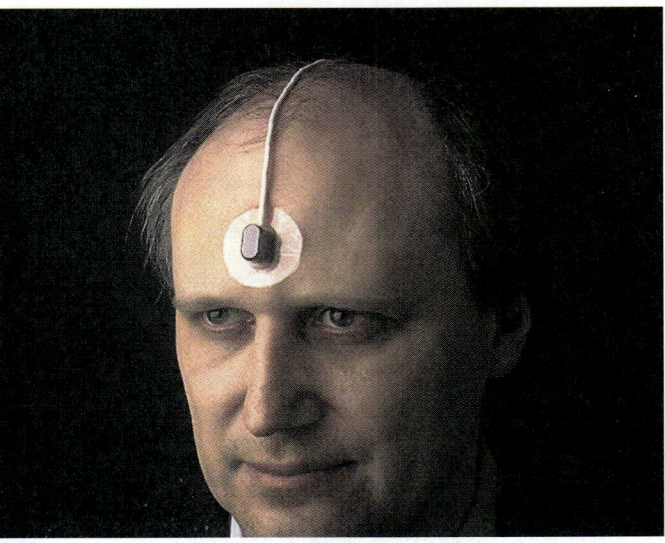

FIGURE 5-65   Oximeter sensor attached to infant's foot. (Courtesy Nonin Medical Inc., Plymouth, Minn.)

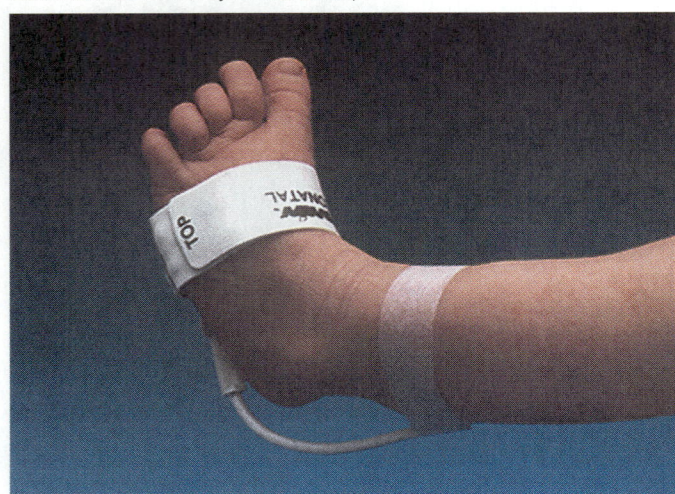

FIGURE 5-66   Continuous fingertip oximetry monitoring during exercise tolerance test. (Courtesy Nonin Medical Inc., Plymouth, Minn.)

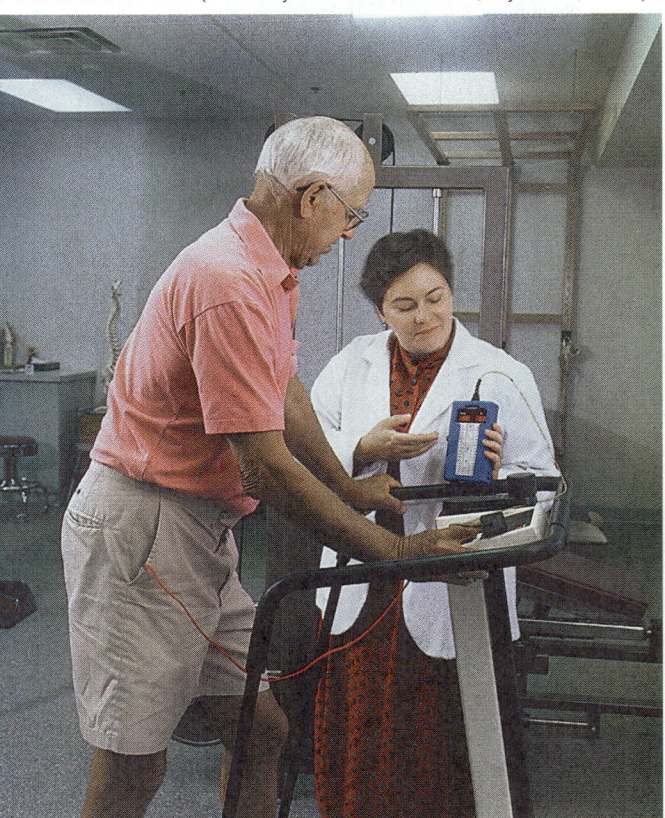

ployee physical examination. Spirometry is an effective way of detecting respiratory disease years *before* symptoms such as shortness of breath occur. Early detection of disease can often lead to successful treatment. Lung disease is the third most common cause of work-related total disability. The most common cause of chronic lung disease is chronic obstructive pulmonary disease (COPD), a preventable, but irreversible, progressive respiratory disorder that is a combination of wheezing, asthma, bronchitis, and emphysema. (COPD is also called chronic obstructive lung disease.) COPD develops slowly over many years and is often in advanced stages before symptoms develop.

COPD is characterized by decreasing inspiratory and expiratory capacities of the lungs. When symptoms develop, they include dyspnea with physical exertion, difficulty in inhaling and exhaling deeply, and sometimes a chronic cough. The use of spirometry can help in detecting COPD many years before abnormalities or symptoms are evident. Spirometry can detect COPD, but it cannot determine the cause. Over 90% of COPD cases are thought to be caused by smoking. Other contributing factors include occupational exposure to inhaled dusts and chemicals, air pollution, and some childhood respiratory illnesses.

Research has shown that over 200 chemicals and dusts are known to cause lung disease. The Occupational Safety and Health Administration (OSHA) requires that annual spirometry testing be performed on employees exposed to many of these agents. Environmental control and elimination of dangerous chemicals and dusts in the workplace are given top priority, but their achievement is not always possible. Regular spirometry testing can help to determine if employees are slowly developing airway changes and airway obstruction. The first test done establishes a baseline of lung volumes and capacities. This test is then compared with future tests to provide visible evidence of lung volume and capacity changes when present. To prevent future disability and increased lung damage, employees with lung and breathing changes should be removed from any occupational-related risks, and those who smoke should be encouraged to quit. Many are also advised to have follow-up spirometry tests every 3 to 5 years.

Common spirometry measurements or calculations include the following (Figure 5-67):

1. **Tidal volume (TV or V_T):** Volume of air inhaled or exhaled during normal breathing.
2. **Minute volume:** Volume of air inhaled and exhaled in 1 minute of normal breathing.
3. **Inspiratory reserve volume (IRV):** Maximal volume of air that can be inspired *after* a normal respiration.

PROCEDURE 5-12

PROCEDURE FOR PULSE OXIMETRY

Objective
Understand and demonstrate for the proper procedure for using a pulse oximeter to determine a patient's pulse oximetry and to record the procedure on the patient's chart.

Equipment
Pulse oximeter and probe or sensor

PROCEDURE

1. Wash your hands.

2. Assemble and prepare the equipment. Review the instructions for use if necessary. Different name brands may have variations in how they work.

3. Identify the patient and explain the procedure.

4. Have the patient sit in a comfortable position with the arm well supported on a table or on the examining table.

5. Clip the monitoring probe or sensor to the patient's index, middle, or ring finger. Center the finger. Make sure that the sensor is on securely and that the emitting and receiving sensors are aligned directly opposite each other (see Figure 5-62, *B*). Once activated, a beam of light passes through the tissue.

6. Allow the system to stabilize. Most oximeters go through an initialization sequence.

7. Read the pulse rate and the arterial blood oxygen saturation on the digital display.

8. Remove the sensor or probe from the patient's finger.

9. Wash your hands.

10. Record the results on the patient's chart.

Charting Example

June 26, 20__, 2 PM
Index finger pulse oximetry results: Pulse: 78
SpO_2: 96
J.A. Lee, CMA

HEALTH MATTERS

KEEPING YOUR PATIENTS INFORMED

QUITTING SMOKING

Your doctor has told you to quit smoking. You want to, but you're not sure of the best way. Perhaps you've tried before, or you're afraid that you will gain weight.

What is the best way to quit?

There are many ways to quit smoking, but you need only one thing— *the desire to quit.* Once you have that all-important ingredient, you will succeed.

You can quit "cold turkey," or you can set a quit date and taper off gradually over a 2-week period. Some people find it helpful to have support from others who are quitting at the same time. Your local chapter of the American Lung Association, the American Cancer Society, or the American Heart Association or a hospital in your community can help you locate a smoking-cessation class. Or, you can use the "buddy system"—make a pact with a friend who wants to quit and provide support for each other.

Many people find chewing nicotine gum or using a nicotine patch helpful for the first few weeks. Talk to your doctor about prescribing one of these for you.

Adopt as many techniques as you think will work for you and use them all.

What about withdrawal symptoms?

Keep in mind that most smokers actually have a double addiction: physical and psychologic. You will need to deal with both aspects.

Physical withdrawal can be a problem for heavy smokers (more than one pack a day). The symptoms vary from one person to another, but common complaints are headaches, constipation, irritability, nervousness, trouble concentrating, and insomnia. You may even cough more for the first week after quitting as your cilia become active again. This is actually a sign that your body is healing itself.

You can do several things to ease the withdrawal symptoms. Although you may fear that you'll be craving a cigarette all the time, each urge actually lasts only 2 or 3 minutes. When it hits, do a minute or two of deep-breathing exercises to calm the urge; close your eyes, take a deep breath, and slowly let it out. If you still feel a craving, change your activity—walk around or do something that requires both hands or do something that you especially enjoy.

Drink lots of water to help flush the toxins from your body. Eat a healthy, well-balanced diet. Many authorities say that eating less meat and more fresh vegetables and fruits helps reduce withdrawal symptoms. To combat aftermeal cravings, leave the table immediately and brush your teeth. Sugarless gum or hard candy; a toothpick; or unsalted, shelled sunflower seeds satisfy the oral craving without adding calories.

Daily exercise (unless your doctor advises not to) will help relax you and hasten recovery from the effects of nicotine.

Try to avoid situations that you associate with smoking, such as a morning cup of coffee or a before-dinner drink. You may need to modify your habits for a while until the withdrawal period is over. This also means avoiding spending much time around other smokers.

Write down all your reasons for quitting smoking to remind yourself whenever you feel discouraged or are tempted to smoke. Keep the list handy and look at it often. Feel proud of yourself for quitting.

Won't I gain weight?

According to recent studies, only about one third of ex-smokers gain some weight; one third lose weight, and one third stay the same. The key to not gaining weight is not to eat every time you crave a smoke. As long as you maintain a well-balanced diet, don't snack between meals, and exercise, you shouldn't experience any weight problems.

What if I fail?

Many people who have successfully quit smoking failed the first time they tried. Often they describe these "failures" as valuable learning experiences that helped them succeed the next time. Whatever you do, don't give up. More than 36 million Americans have already quit. You can, too.

From *Patient teaching guides for health promotion,* St. Louis, 1997, Mosby, p. 15.

---

4. **Expiratory reserve volume (ERV):** Maximal volume of air that can be expired forcefully after a normal expiration.
5. **Residual volume (RV):** The amount of gas left in the lungs after exhaling all that is physically possible.
6. **Forced expiratory volume (FEV) or the FEV in 1 second (FEV$_1$):** Amount of air forcibly exhaled in the first second after a maximal inspiration.

7. **Vital capacity (VC):** Maximum amount of air that can be exhaled. It is usually measured after forced exhalation and then called forced vital capacity (FVC).
8. **Total lung capacity (TLC):** Sum of the vital capacity and the residual volume.
9. **Functional residual capacity (FRC):** Sum of the expiratory reserve volume and the residual volume.

FIGURE 5-67   Components of lung capacity commonly measured in pulmonary function tests.

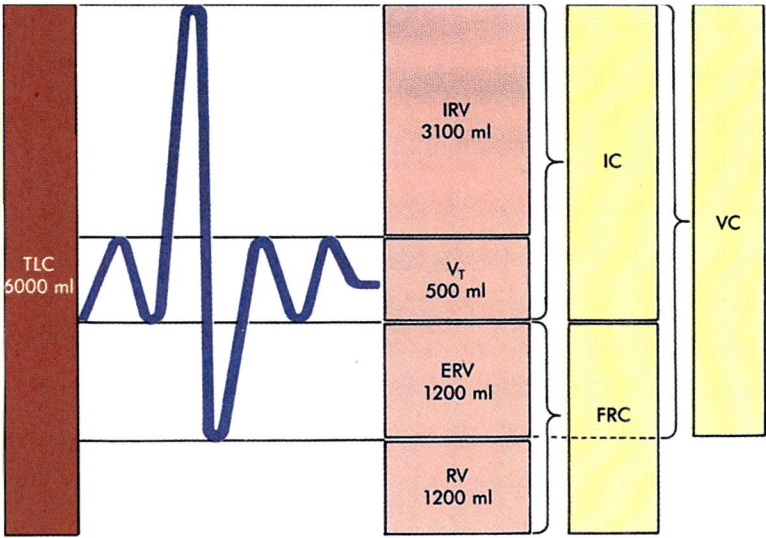

TLC = Total lung capacity

IRV = Inspiratory reserve volume
V_T = Tidal volume
ERV = Expiratory reserve volume
RV = Residual volume

IC = Inspiratory capacity
FRC = Functional residual capacity
VC = Vital capacity

PROCEDURE 5-13

SINGLE BREATH SPIROMETRY TEST (FVC MANEUVER) (FIGURE 5-68)

Objective

Understand and demonstrate the correct procedure for having a patient take a single breath spirometry test and record the procedure on the patient's chart.

Equipment

    Spirometer with hose/connecting tube
    Disposable mouthpiece
    Nose clips
    Disposable, single-use examination gloves

PROCEDURE

RATIONALE

1. **Wash your hands. Use appropriate personal protective equipment (PPE) as indicated by facility.**

2. Prepare equipment for use. Check that the unit is plugged in and turned "ON," ready for use. Insert the disposable mouthpiece into the hose/connecting tube adapter. Read the manufacturer's instructions provided with the machine because different ones may have special instructions.

3. Identify the patient.

4. **Prepare the patient for the test.**
   a.   Explain the purpose of the test. The test will measure and evaluate lung function and air capacity of the lung.

An explanation helps the patient understand the need for the test and provides some reassurance.

PROCEDURE 5-13

SINGLE BREATH SPIROMETRY TEST (FVC MANEUVER)—cont'd

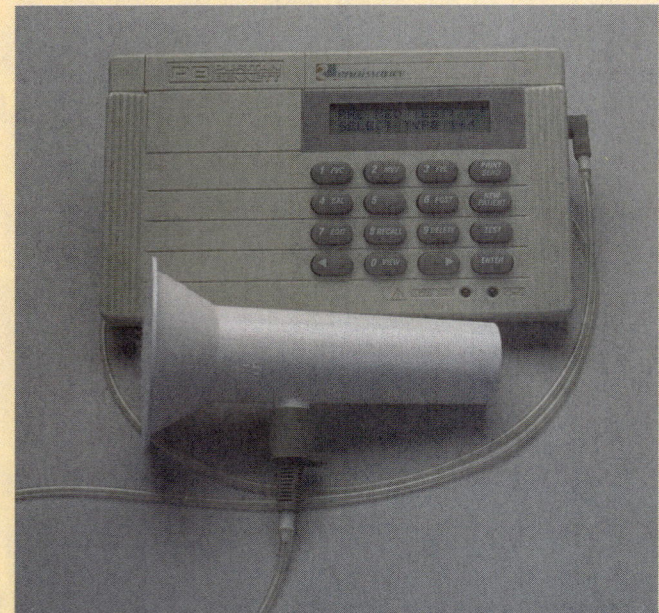

A

B

C

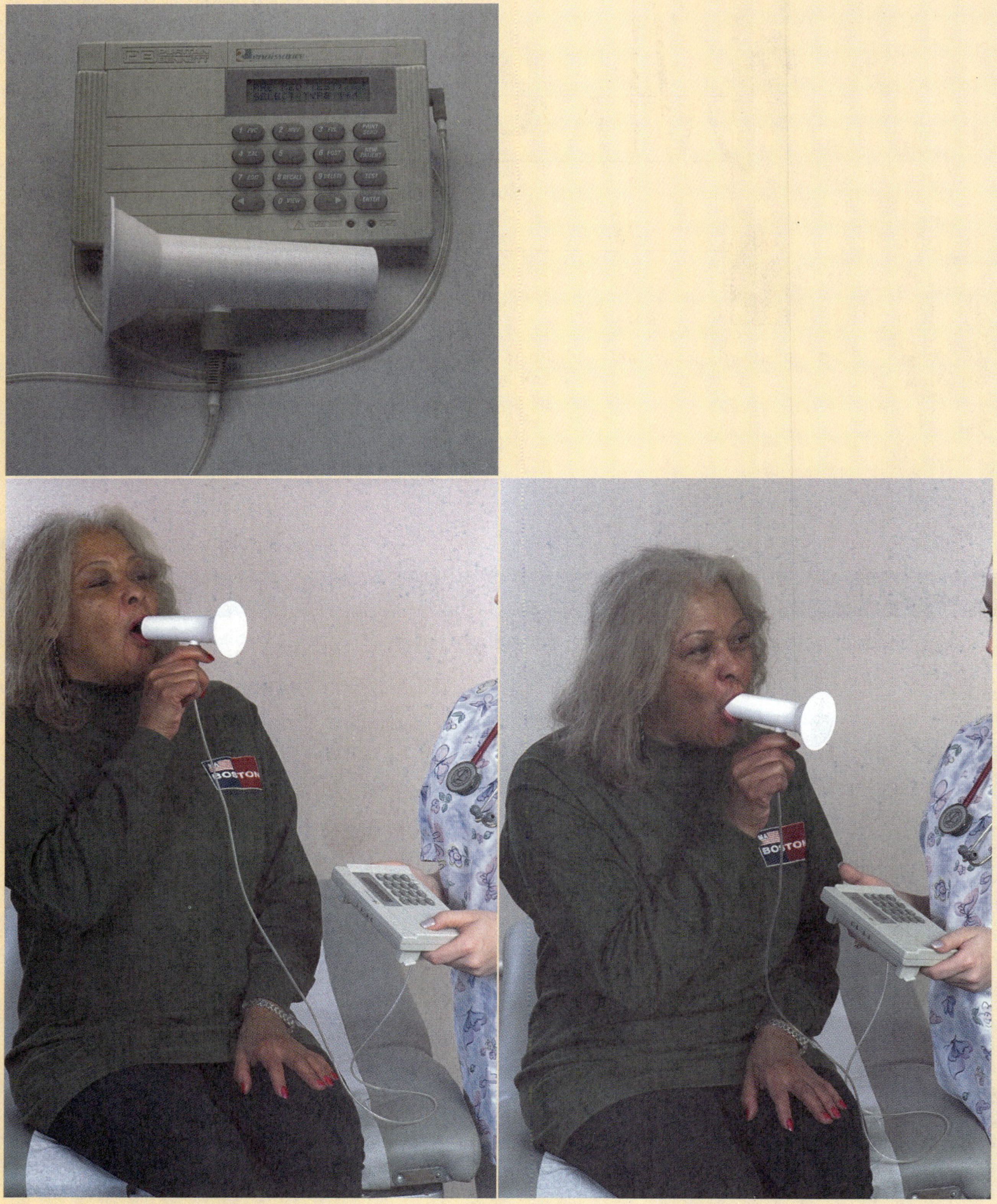

FIGURE 5-68   Spirometry testing can help screen for lung diseases. **A,** Spirometer; **B,** and **C,** person taking single breath test.

PROCEDURE 5-13

SINGLE BREATH SPIROMETRY TEST (FVC MANEUVER)—cont'd

b. Determine if there are any reasons why the test should not be done at this time.

Different conditions can influence test results. The test must be delayed if the patient (1) has eaten a heavy meal, smoked a cigarette, or taken a bronchodilator within the last hour; (2) has had a viral infection or other acute illness within the last 2 or 3 weeks, especially if the test is being done for occupational screening and will be compared with other tests over time; or (3) has had a serious illness, such as recent myocardial infarction, pulmonary emboli, and so on.

c. Obtain the patient's height and weight.

Results of spirometry are often compared with predicted or reference values. To do this correctly, height, age, and sometimes weight are needed.

d. Position the patient either sitting or standing. Have the patient do what is most comfortable.

There is no difference in results between sitting or standing.

   (1) Elderly patients and patients with high blood pressure should sit.

   (2) Very obese patients should stand for proper results.

Sitting offers support and may be safer because dizziness could occur with forced expirations.

e. Loosen tight clothing such as neckties, belts, and bras.

Tight clothing may restrict fast and hard breathing that is required.

f. Remove dentures if they are loose or fit poorly.

Loose or poorly fitting dentures may interfere with the test.

g. *Explain the procedure.*

Explanations help gain the patient's cooperation and provide some reassurance.

   (1) Show the mouthpiece and nose clips to the patient.

   (2) Explain how the mouthpiece fits into the mouth and that the lips must be sealed tightly and the tongue must not stick into the mouthpiece.

The patient's cooperation is critical to ensure accurate results.

   (3) Show the patient the proper neck and chin position. The chin should be slightly elevated and the neck slightly extended.

   (4) Put nose clips on nostrils.

Nose clips will prevent breathing through the nose during the test.

   (5) Give specific instructions in simple terms. For example, "I want you to take a deep breath in, put the mouthpiece in your mouth, seal your lips, and then blow out as hard as possible."

5. **Instruct the patient to:**

   a. Take the deepest breath possible and hold it.

   b. Put the disposable mouthpiece in the mouth and seal the lips firmly around it.

There must be a tight seal around the mouthpiece so that the air does not escape.

   c. Keep the tongue away from the opening in the mouthpiece.

The tongue must not block the opening in the mouthpiece.

   d. Exhale/breathe as hard, as quickly, and as completely as you can. Coach the patient by saying, "Blow harder, harder, faster, faster, faster, go, go, more, more." The patient should blow out for at least 6 seconds, up to a maximum of 15 to 20 seconds.

For an acceptable test, the start of the test must be quick and forceful. It is important to pay attention to the expiratory time to obtain acceptable results.

6. Do *three* separate successive tests. For a test to be acceptable, the patient must not cough. If the patient does cough, start the test again.

   a. Between each test, instruct the patient to remove the mouthpiece from the mouth and hold it away from the face.

   b. Then start the test again repeating the instructions in step 5.

PROCEDURE 5-13

SINGLE BREATH SPIROMETRY TEST (FVC MANEUVER)—cont'd

    c. Try up to eight times to achieve an acceptable test. Stop after this amount because the patient most likely cannot perform adequately for the test.

    d. Record that the patient coughed with each test and that is all that could be obtained.   *This explains why the test does not show adequate results.*

7. After the last test, wearing gloves remove the disposable mouthpiece from the hose and discard it in the biohazard waste container.

8. Attend to the patient's safety and comfort. Check to ensure that the patient does not feel dizzy or have any discomfort or pain. Tell the patient when the physician will discuss the results with him or her and if a future appointment is required.

9. Clean the equipment after use according to the manufacturer's directions. Wear disposable gloves when handling and cleaning used equipment.

10. Wash your hands.

11. Do any recording required of you completely and accurately.

Charting Example

February 6, 20__, 1 PM
Three spirometry tests performed. Patient appeared to tolerate the tests well and had no complaints.
Shannon Leigh, CMA

CONCLUSION

You have now completed the chapter on preparing for and assisting with routine and special physical examinations. After you have practiced the procedures and are ready to demonstrate your skills and knowledge attained, arrange with your instructor to take a performance test. You will be expected to accurately demonstrate your ability in preparing for and assisting with procedures and examinations discussed in this chapter, to measure a patient's distance and near visual acuity, and to perform other examinations discussed in the chapter. In addition, when questioned by your instructor, you will be expected to identify by name the equipment and instruments used for each examination, and explain why each procedure is performed.

REVIEW OF VOCABULARY

The following are samples of a patient's admission note and a hospital discharge note as dictated by a physician. These are to help familiarize you with the format and contents of medical reports. Read these and be prepared to discuss the contents and define all the medical terms that are used. You should recognize some of the terms; others are new, and you may have to refer to Appendix A or a medical dictionary for the definitions.

Admission Note

Medical Center
PHYSICIAN'S REPORT

PATIENT: [X] ADMISSION NOTE
  McFerrin, Sandra   [ ] CONSULTATION
PHYSICIAN:
  Robert Scott, MD   [ ] DISCHARGE SUMMARY
                   9/13/__ Admitted
                   _____ Discharged

CHIEF COMPLAINT: Abdominal pain.

PRESENT ILLNESS: The patient is a 19-year-old woman who, for the first 5 days, has had progressively severe abdominal pain. There has been no nausea until the day of admission, when she became nauseated driving over to the hospital. There has been no vomiting, chills, or fever. The patient has not been bothered by constipation or diarrhea. She had a normal bowel movement the day before admission. The patient's menstrual period started the day before admission, and the previous one approximately a month ago was normal.

The patient was seen in my office the day before admission, and epigastric tenderness was noted. Donnatal and Maalox were prescribed, but this afforded little if any relief. The pain became more acute, more severe, and awoke the patient from sleep and prompted her present admission.

PAST HISTORY: The patient's past health has been quite good, except for an automobile accident approximately a year and a half ago in which her pelvis and bladder were fractured and lacerated, respectively. No sequelae followed. Approximately 7 to 8 years ago, patient was treated prophylactically with INH for a year for exposure to tuberculosis.

FAMILY HISTORY: There is no family history of diabetes, cancer, or premature cardiac disease. The patient's sister had pulmonary tuberculosis when the patient was young, and the patient received a year's course of prophylactic INH. The patient's skin test was positive.

REVIEW OF SYSTEMS: There are no symptoms of respiratory, cardiac, or genitourinary disease.

PHYSICAL EXAMINATION: Blood pressure 130/80, pulse 90, temperature 36.6° C.

General appearance: The patient is a young, well-developed woman who is lying in bed crying because of abdominal pain. *Skin:* No rash. *Eyes:* Sclera clear. The pupils are round, regular, and equal. *ENT:* The tongue and mucous membrane are somewhat dry. *Neck:* Supple. *Breasts:* Clear. *Heart:* Normal sinus rhythm, no murmurs. *Lungs:* Clear. *Abdomen:* Flat, the bowel sounds are hypoactive. There is marked epigastric and left upper quadrant tenderness. There is no guarding or rigidity. There is no rebound tenderness. There is no adnexal tenderness. Rectal examination negative. Extremities negative.

IMPRESSION: Acute abdominal pain, etiology to be determined.

RS: vy
D: 9/13/___
T: 9/13/_____

Robert Scott, MD

Discharge Note

PATIENT: Marion Dale
PHYSICIAN: Scott Douglas, MD
DATE: April 15, 20___

The patient is a 45-year-old, premenopausal white woman presenting a history of a recent dark vaginal discharge with a negative Pap test in April of last year, but a recent Pap test showed dyskeratotic cells and atypical class III cells. Biopsy the next month was positive for epidermoid carcinoma with lymphatic permeating present.

Pelvic examination revealed a lacerated eroded cervical canal, and, under anesthesia, pelvic examination showed uterine enlargement to approximately twice the normal size with a freely mobile uterus; however, no evidence of parametrial induration or other pelvic pathology was present.

Following endometrial curettage, a tandem and colpostat radium-containing applicator were inserted, with the applicator carrying a total of 90 mg homogenous distribution in a circular e.5 cm colpostat, 20 mg radium in the base, and 20 mg in the tip of the tandem with $\frac{1}{2}$ mm platinum intrinsic filtration and 1.5 mm Monel extrinsic filtration, representing total equivalent of 1 mm platinum filtration.

The applicator was inserted to be removed after 72 hours for a total dosage of 6480 mg hours. Following the course of radium, a complete pelvic cycle with external irradiation is recommended. Intravenous pyelogram showed no obstructive nephropathy or ureteral constriction or displacement. Portable AP and lateral views of the pelvis confirming the position of the applicator in situ are to be obtained. Three rolls of iodoform packing in the vaginal canal firmly secured the applicator in contact with the cervical lips, and a loose ligature affixed the colpostat to the anterior cervical lip during the surgical procedure.

Scott Douglas, MD

The following are samples of how information may be charted during and after a patient's visit and examination in the medical office or clinic. Read these and be prepared to define and explain all of the medical terms that are used. A medical dictionary, other reference books, and information given in other chapters of this book may be used as references for obtaining definitions or explanations of the contents of these reports.

Pulmonary Preventive Care Record

Client's name: _____
Date of birth: _____12/24/51_____
Physician: _____

March 11, 20__

Ms. Diane is a long-time asthmatic referred for education by S. Dyer, FNP, of Dr. Jason's office. She presents with decreased breath sounds bilaterally. Expiratory wheezes noted with forced exhalation, room air O_2 sat = 96% HR 89. Simple spirometry performed results indicating borderline obstruction/severe restriction, forced expiration volume, <1 liter. Patient gave three good efforts during test. Had patient perform peak flow with best results only 150L/min! Predicted value is 430 L/min putting her around 35% of predicted. Currently on approximately six respiratory medications, which include terbutaline, Theo-Dur, albuterol, Vanceril, Serevent, and Accolate. Patient

Pulmonary Preventive Care Record

Client's name: _____
Date of birth: _____
Initial visit: _____ 3/11/00 _____
Referring physician: _____
Follow-up date: _____ 3/25/00 _____
Instruction given to: [X] Client   [ ] Parent
        [ ] Other (specify) _____

PROGRESS NOTES

Date
1/16/02

Teaching Session	Date	Initials	Client Teaching Outcome	Date	Initials
Anatomy and normal function of the respiratory system	3/11/00	Visuals used JL	Understands and explains basic anatomy and normal function of the respiratory system.	3/25/00	JL
Changes to the lungs during an asthma attack	3/11/00	Visuals used JL	Understands and explains changes occurring during an asthma attack. What happens to them personally.	3/25/00	JL
Identify asthma triggers and avoidance	3/11/00	JL	Identifies personal triggers and ways to avoid them.	3/25/00	JL
Medications: purpose, dose, and adverse affects	3/11/00	JL	Understands asthma medications, indications. Importance of adhering to schedule. Aware of adverse effects.	3/25/00	JL
Instruction of MDI with spacer device	3/11/00	JL	Exhibits proper technique of MDI w/ spacer device. Understands reason for use.	3/25/00	JL
Peak flow instructions and tracking	3/11/00	JL	Understands purpose of PF monitoring + tracking results. Exhibits proper technique.	3/25/00	JL
Pursed lip breathing technique	3/11/00	JL	Understands and demonstrates proper pursed lip breathing.	3/25/00	JL
EDUCATIONAL MATERIALS (TITLES)	3/11/00	JL	**PEAK FLOW RESULTS:** 3/11/00: 150 L/min 3/25/00: 210 L/min	3/25/00	JL
Asthma Taking Control for a Healthier Life	3/11/00	JL	**OXYGEN SATURATION:** 3/11/00: 99% room air SPIROMETRY PRE-POST BRONCHODILATOR (Results attached)	3/25/00 3/9/00 3/25/00	JL JL
			DEVICES DISTRIBUTED: Peak flow meter/Personal best Spacer device/Aerochamber	3/11/00 3/11/00	JL JL
Signature		**Initials**	**Signature**		**Initials**
Joan Larson, RRT		JL	Joan Larson, RRT		JL

states using Serevent × 2 bid but Vanceril × 2 currently tid. Also using albuterol × 2 bid and prn. Patient states she is unable to exert herself without becoming short of breath after 2 min on the treadmill. At rest did not appear in resp. distress but did continually rub her nose and eyes, as well as having a nasal discharge along with periodic cough throughout the visit. Patient complains of having a "jittery feeling" in the morning after taking her morning inhalers, which include Serevent, Vanceril, and albuterol. Encouraged her not to take the albuterol right after the Serevent but to wait a few hours. Other medications may also be contributors to that feeling. Taught patient to use spacer device with inhalers because she admitted she wasn't already doing so. She may have been undermedicating herself up to this point secondary to technique. Also asked pt to monitor and document daily peak flow readings. Will contact S. Dyer, FNP, at Dr. Jason's office to confer about current status and follow-up.

Joan Larson, RRT

Addendum 3-12-00 at 10:10 am
Spoke via phone to S. Dyer, FNP, and will send test results to office ASAP—Joan Larson, RRT

March 25, 2000
Returned for follow-up session. Found her feeling better. Upon auscultation breath sounds were decreased but clear of wheezing. Room air oximeter was 97% with HR 95.
Patient kept record of peak flow results for last 2 weeks. Personal best = 200-210
Based on that number—zones and Peak Flow Action Plan developed. Patient had been told to increase Vanceril dose since last visit. Seems to have improved her status. Pre-post albuterol spirometry show improvement since previous visit with some response to the albuterol in some flows.

PROGRESS NOTES

BP: 120/70   HR: 80   WT: 117   LMP: 10/2/01
Pt comes in for a Pap smear.
S: Pt states that she has not had a period since Oct., was using the Progest cream but stopped as she hadn't had a period for 6 weeks, and is now starting to get hot flashes.
O: Breasts: no masses felt. BUS neg. Vulva and vagina: very atrophic and very painful on doing the exam. Cervix: short within the vagina. Corpus anterior. Adnexa neg.
A: Atrophic vaginitis; otherwise, probably menopausal.
P: I told her to continue the Progest cream qd as I think that would help her symptoms. I asked her to call me a week before her exam next year so that she could get some estrogen cream to use a week prior to the exam. This would make the exam more comfortable. She had a mammogram today. I'll see her back prn.

Shoulder pain.
S: Pt was seen in Aug. w/ pain in her neck and shoulder. She had gone to a chiropractor and she had tried to go to PT,

but it's still not really all that much better. She's considering acupuncture.
P: I asked her to try to deal w/ the acupuncture if it's covered through her insurance. If not, I would probably send her to an orthopedist if it does not get better.

Cytology Reports

The following Pap smear reports were received in a physician's office. After reading these, you should be able to discuss the contents of these reports with your instructor. Reference sources may be used to obtain definitions of terms with which you are not familiar.

PATIENT NO. 1

01/21/02
Sex/DOB/Age: F   10/09/73   27
Med Rec #:

FINAL DIAGNOSIS
Cervical/vaginal smear—atypical cells identified consistent with low-grade squamous intraepithelial lesion (encompasses HPV/CIN I).*
(Med Class: Squamous intraepithelial lesion)

CYTOLOGY CLINICAL HISTORY

Specimen taken on:	01/15/02
Specimen received date:	01/16/02
Number of slides:	1
Last menstrual period:	1/2/02
Other information:	No hormones

TISSUES: Cervix uteri
MICROSCOPIC-CYTOLOGY: Smear adequate for cytologic evaluation.
Original report read and signed _____ 01/22/02
John Brown, MD

PATIENT NO. 2

01/21/02
Sex/DOB/Age: F   10/10/82   19
Med Rec #:

FINAL DIAGNOSIS
Cervical/vaginal smear—atypical squamous cells of uncertain significance identified.
Comment: suggest further evaluation
(Med Class: atypia)

CYTOLOGY CLINICAL HISTORY

Specimen taken on:	01/14/01
Specimen received date:	01/15/01
Number of slides:	1
Last menstrual period:	1/5/01
Other information:	Prev: WNL*

---

*HPV: Human papilloma virus
CIN: Cervical intraepithelial neoplasia
CIN I: Cervical intraepithelial neoplasia; mild dysplasia
WNL: Within normal limits

TISSUES: Cervix uteri
MICROSCOPIC-CYTOLOGY: Smear adequate for cytologic
evaluation.
Original report read and signed _____ 01/22/02
Jack Black, MD

PATIENT NO. 3

01/21/02
Sex/DOB/Age: F   09/17/63   39
Med Rec #:

FINAL DIAGNOSIS

Cervical/vaginal smear—atypical cells identified consistent
with high grade squamous intraepithelial lesion (encompasses CIN II-III).*

_____

*CIN II: Cervical intraepithelial neoplasia; moderate dysplasia
CIN III: Cervical intraepithelial neoplasia; severe dysplasia

Comments: suggest biopsy to confirm diagnosis
This confirms a phone report to the physician's office.
(Med Class: Squamous intraepithelial lesion)

CYTOLOGY CLINICAL HISTORY
Specimen taken on: 01/15/02
Specimen received date: 01/16/02
Number of slides: 1
Last menstrual period: 12/30/01
Other information: Prev: taken elsewhere

TISSUES: Cervico-Vaginal
MICROSCOPIC-CYTOLOGY: Smear adequate for cytologic
evaluation.
Original report read and signed _____ 01/22/02
Jack Black, MD

CRITICAL THINKING SKILLS REVIEW

1. Explain and summarize the medical assistant's general responsibilities when assisting the physician with a complete
   physical examination.
2. Identify what body part or system is examined with the following instruments:
   a. Otoscope
   b. Laryngeal mirror
   c. Ophthalmoscope
   d. Anoscope
   e. Tuning fork
   f. Bronchoscope
   g. Cystoscope
   h. Percussion hammer
   i. Stethoscope
3. Explain the position that the patient is placed in for:
   a. A vaginal or pelvic exam
   b. A rectal examination and proctosigmoidoscopy
   c. A chest examination
   d. An examination of the ears and eyes
4. Explain the purpose(s) and state the common instruments
   required for the following examinations:
   a. General physical examination
   b. Vaginal examination
   c. Pap smear or test
   d. Rectal examination
   e. Proctosigmoidoscopy
5. If a physician suspects a growth in the sigmoid colon that
   is considered doubtful as to being benign or malignant,
   what procedure does he or she usually perform?
6. You have a 50-year-old obese patient who cannot tolerate
   the jackknife position for a sigmoidoscopy. Name and
   explain an alternate position that may be used for this
   examination.
7. Explain why it is important for a female assistant to remain
   in the room when a female patient is being examined by a
   male physician.
8. Identify some of the common unusual reactions for which
   you observe a patient during an examination.
9. Explain why it is important that you check battery-
   operated and electrical equipment before an examination.
10. List and identify the instruments and equipment that are
    used for a neurologic examination.
11. Explain what a Snellen chart is and how it is used.
12. When increased pressure is present in the eyeball, what
    common condition is suspected?
13. Albumin in the urine during a pregnancy is thought to be a
    serious sign of what condition?
14. List seven warning signals of cancer.
15. Explain how a woman can perform a breast self-examina-
    tion.
16. Explain why every woman should examine her breasts
    monthly.
17. When is the best time of the month for a woman to exam-
    ine her breasts for any unusual lump or thickening?
18. List two types of pediatric visits.
19. Explain why blood lead level screening is needed for children.
20. Explain what is occurring in the respiratory system in
    asthma. State four common signs and symptoms of asthma.
21. Explain why using a peak flow meter is an important part
    of a treatment program for people who have asthma.
22. Explain what pulse oximetry determines.
23. Explain why pulmonary function tests are used.

PERFORMANCE TEST

In a skills laboratory, a simulation of a joblike environment, the medical assistant student is to demonstrate knowledge and skill in performing the following procedures without reference to source materials. For these activities, the student needs a person to play the role of a patient and the necessary equipment and supplies. Time limits for the performance of each procedure are to be assigned by the instructor (see also p. 104).

1. Given an ambulatory patient, the student is to position and drape the patient in the following positions and state when each is used:
   a. Dorsal-recumbent
   b. Lithotomy
   c. Sims
   d. Knee-chest
   e. Supine
   f. Prone
   g. Trendelenburg
2. Given an ambulatory patient, the student is to prepare for and assist with the following:
   a. A complete physical examination that is to include a vaginal and rectal examination
   b. A proctosigmoidoscopy, including a description of the patient preparation that is to be completed before the examination
   c. A pelvic examination and a Papanicolaou smear
   d. An obstetric examination
   e. Pediatric examinations
3. Given an ambulatory patient, the student is to prepare for and measure:

   a. Distance visual acuity using the Snellen eye chart
   b. Near visual acuity
   c. Color vision
4. Demonstrate how to carry an infant in the cradle, upright, and football positions.
5. Demonstrate how to obtain the following measurements on an infant:
   a. Length/height
   b. Weight
   c. Head circumference
   d. Chest circumference
6. Demonstrate the procedure used for performing a urine test to screen an infant for phenylketonuria.
7. Demonstrate the method used to obtain a blood specimen from an infant to perform a test to screen for phenylketonuria.
8. Given an ambulatory patient, the student is to instruct and assist the patient with the performance of a breast self-examination (females) or a testicular self-examination (males).
9. Given an ambulatory patient, the student is to:
   a. Give the patient instructions for using a peak flowmeter.
   b. Determine the patient's arterial blood oxygen saturation using a pulse oximeter.
   c. Perform a spirometry test.

The student is expected to perform these procedures with 100% accuracy 90% of the time (9 out of 10 times).

The successful completion of each procedure will demonstrate competency levels as required by the AAMA, AMT, and future employers.

🖥 INTERNET RESOURCES

American Cancer Society
www.cancer.org

National Cancer Institute
www.nci.nih.gov

Men's Health
www.healthfinder.gov

National Association for Healthcare Quality
www.nahq.org

The World Foundation for Medical Studies in Female Health
www.wffh.org

National Cancer Institute's Cancer Net Web Site
(information about colorectal cancer screening, prevention, and treatment, including how to participate in clinical trials)
http://cancernet.nci.nih.gov

Female Health
www.wwfh.org

Women's Health
www.healthfinder.gov/justforyou/women/default.htm

American Association for Respiratory Care
www.AARC.org

National Association for Women's Health
www.nawh.org

Arthritis Foundation
www.arthritis.org

American Diabetes Association
www.diabetes.org

Smoking Cessation
www.cdc.gov/nccdphp/osh/quittip.htm

The National Institute of Diabetes and Digestive and Kidney Diseases of The National Institute of Health
www.niddk.nih.gov/health/diabetes/dylb/home/htm

Ask-the-Doctor (by pediatrician, Alan Greene, M.D.)
www.DrGreene.com

Planned Parenthood
www.ppfa.org/ppfa

American College of Obstetricians and Gynecologists
www.acog.org

Internet Resources for Special Children
www.irsc.org

Allergy and Asthma Network/Mothers of Asthmatics, Inc.
www.aanma.org

Global Initiative for Asthma
www.ginasthma.com

JAMA's Asthma Information Center
www.ama-assn.org/special/asthma

TransWeb
www.transweb.org

National Asthma Education and Prevention Program
www.nhlbi.nih.gov/about/naepp/index.htm

National Action Plan on Breast Cancer
www.napbc.org

Susan G. Komen Breast Cancer Foundation
http://komen.org

Susan Love, M.D. (breast cancer)
www.susanlovemd.com

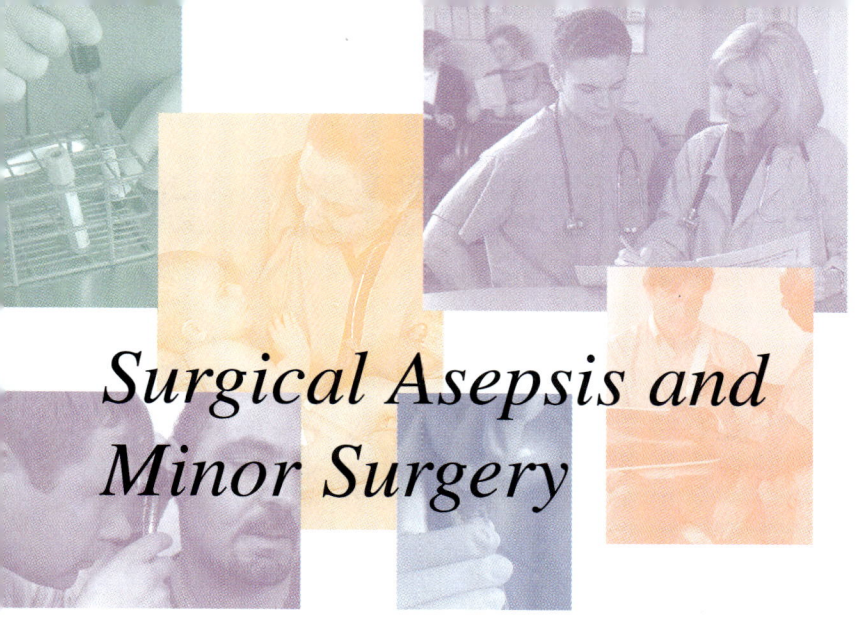

Surgical Asepsis and Minor Surgery

CHAPTER 6

Cognitive Objectives

On completion of Chapter 6, the medical assistant student should be able to:

1. Define, spell, and pronounce the vocabulary terms.
2. State at least 15 principles and practices of surgical aseptic technique.
3. Describe how to handle sterile supplies to avoid contamination—that is, how to open sterile peel-down and envelope-wrapped packages, how to pour sterile solutions into sterile containers, and how to don sterile gloves.
4. List at least six minor surgical procedures that may be performed in a physician's office and list three responsibilities of the medical assistant during each procedure.
5. List and differentiate between three types of local anesthesia.
6. State the information that must be obtained from a patient before administering a local anesthetic and explain why this is important.
7. State the purpose of suture materials, differentiate between absorbable and nonabsorbable suture material, give an example of each, and state when each may be used.
8. Given the numeric sizes of suture material, identify which is the thickest, and arrange in order down to the thinnest; state a procedure in which each size may be used.
9. Discuss and differentiate between the types of suture needles available.
10. Discuss the meaning and purpose of an "informed consent."
11. Discuss the preparation of the patient for minor surgery.
12. List the equipment and supplies that are (a) basic to all minor surgical procedures, (b) required for preparing the patient's skin, (c) required for the administration of a local anesthetic, and (d) required for the minor surgical procedures as outlined in this chapter.
13. Differentiate between an open wound and a closed wound. Give one example of a closed wound and five examples of open wounds.
14. Describe briefly the healing process of wounds.
15. List two goals of wound care.
16. Differentiate between dressings and bandages and know the types and purposes of each. List eight purposes of dressings and four purposes of bandages.
17. Explain the criteria for acceptable bandaging techniques.
18. Describe the five basic turns used to apply roller bandages and explain when each is most appropriately used.
19. State the purposes of casts. Discuss instructions for the patient on the care of a cast.

Terminal Performance Objectives

On completion of Chapter 6, the medical assistant student should be able to:

1. Open and handle sterile supplies and equipment in a manner that prevents contamination.
2. Don sterile gloves in a manner that prevents contamination.
3. Prepare the patient physically and mentally for a minor surgical procedure.
4. Select, assemble, and prepare sterile and nonsterile supplies and equipment needed for a minor surgical procedure using aseptic technique.
5. Assist the patient and the physician during a minor surgical procedure.
6. Prepare the patient's skin for a minor surgical procedure.
7. Remove sutures as directed by the physician.
8. Assist the physician with the application of a cast.
9. Change the patient's dressing and obtain a wound culture.
10. Identify by name and explain the use and care of the instruments and supplies used in minor surgical procedures.
11. Apply roller, triangular, and Tubegauz bandages.
12. Provide instructions and patient education that is within the professional scope of a medical assistant's training and responsibilities as assigned.

The student is to perform these objectives with 100% accuracy 90% of the time (9 out of 10 times).

VOCABULARY

abscess (ab"ses)—A cavity containing pus and surrounded by inflamed tissue. An abscess is usually caused by specific microorganisms (characteristically staphylococci) that invade tissues often by way of small breaks or wounds in the skin. Healing usually occurs when an abscess drains or is incised.

anesthesia (an"es-the'ze-ah)—The loss of sensation or feeling.

asepsis (a-sep'sis)—The state of being free from infection or infectious matter. The absence of all microorganisms causing disease; absence of contaminated matter.

biopsy (bi'op-se)—Removal of tissue from the body for examination.

incisional biopsy—Incision into and removal of part of a lesion.

excisional biopsy—Removal of an entire small lesion.

aspiration/needle biopsy—Removal of matter from an internal organ by means of a hollow needle inserted through the body wall and into the affected tissue.

fine-needle aspiration (FNA) biopsy—Insertion of a thin needle into a lump from which a cell specimen is taken and evaluated for cancer. FNA has been used to diagnose lesions and lumps of the breast, thyroid, lymph nodes, soft tissue, prostate, abdomen, lung, salivary glands, liver, and brain.

punch biopsy—Biopsy in which tissue is obtained by a punch (a type of instrument).

cautery (kaw'ter-e)—An instrument using electric current to cut or destroy tissue, causing hemostasis.

cyst (sist)—A closed capsule or sac containing fluid or a semisolid substance.

sebaceous (se-ba'shus) **cyst**—A benign cyst of a sebaceous gland containing the fatty secretion of the gland; also called a wen. They are most common on the back, scrotum, and scalp.

don—To put an article on, such as gloves or a gown.

ligate (li'gat)—To apply a ligature; to tie off and close.

ligature (lig'ah-tur)—A suture; any material, such as thread or wire, used to tie off blood vessels to prevent bleeding or to constrict tissues.

Mayo (ma'o) **stand**—A stand with a flat metal tray used to hold sterile supplies during an aseptic procedure.

postoperative (post-op'er-ah-tiv)—Pertaining to the time following surgery.

preoperative (pre-op'er-ah-tiv)—Pertaining to the time preceding surgery.

sterile (ster'il)—Free from all living microorganisms. *Also see* asepsis.

sterile field—A work area prepared with sterile drapes (coverings) to hold sterile supplies during a sterile procedure.

sterile setup—Specific sterile supplies used in a specific sterile procedure.

suture (soo'cher)—Various types and sizes of absorbable and nonabsorbable materials used to close a wound with stitches.

transfer forceps—A type of instrument (forceps) that is kept in a chemical disinfectant or germicide and used for transferring or handling sterile supplies and equipment.

The consistent use of Universal/Standard Precautions is required by all health care professionals in all health care settings as a method of infection control. It is assumed that these precautions are used in all of the following procedures. Review Chapter 1 if you have any questions on methods to use because methods or techniques are not repeated in detail in each procedure presented in this chapter.

Be sure to consult the latest guidelines issued by the Centers for Disease Control and Prevention and consult with infection control practitioners when necessary to identify specific precautions that pertain to your particular work situation.

This unit discusses the common practices of, and some procedures requiring, surgical asepsis (sterile technique). To control the sources and spread of infection when performing and assisting with certain medical procedures, knowledge of and adherence to the correct performance of aseptic practices are essential.

It is helpful to review Chapter 2, which discussed concepts of infection control, medical and surgical asepsis, practices of medical asepsis, and the disinfection and sterilization of supplies.

BACKGROUND OF STERILE TECHNIQUE

Sterile techniques used today have gradually evolved since the turn of the century. The history of medicine shows evidence of some understanding of asepsis as early as the time of Hippocrates, the father of medicine, in 460 BC. It was Hippocrates who started to use boiled water when irrigating wounds; later Galen (AD 131-210) boiled instruments before using them when caring for wounds. Throughout the centuries up to the present, numerous individuals, too many to mention here, played vital roles in describing diseases and their causes, theories for contagious diseases, the spread of infection by improperly washed hands, the role of bacteria in causing disease, the inhibition of the growth of microorganisms by heat, and the germ theory for the causes of disease.

Joseph Lister (1827-1912) introduced the use of chemicals to destroy microorganisms in the infected wounds (antisepsis) and later procedures to exclude bacteria from surgical fields (asepsis). Surgery as we know it today was essentially Lister's gift to humanity.

In the late nineteenth century, the concept of vaccinations against disease was introduced. Edward Jenner discovered the value of vaccination against smallpox, and this discovery led to further advances, such as Louis Pasteur's principle of inoculation by means of vaccines against viral and bacterial diseases.

Sterilization of items by boiling began around 1880, and the principles and practices of autoclaving (steam under pressure) began around 1886. Rubber gloves were first used to protect the hands from harsh antiseptics. Eventually they were accepted and used as a protective measure to prevent contamination to the patient. Thus sterile technique or aseptic practices, as we know them, evolved.

PRINCIPLES AND PRACTICES OF SURGICAL ASEPSIS

Surgical asepsis, more commonly called **sterile technique** or **aseptic technique,** is the practice used when an area and supplies in that area are to be made and kept sterile. The **goal of surgical asepsis** is to prevent infection or the introduction of microorganisms into the body. These techniques are used in all procedures in which entry is made into normally sterile body parts, such as when administering an injection, when making a surgical incision, or when caring for any break in the skin such as open wounds or skin ulcers. Strict sterile or surgical aseptic technique is required at all times in such procedures because body tissues can easily become infected. Breaks in technique may lead to infections that the body cannot combat. Even mild infections delay recovery and are costly—*mentally, physically,* and *financially*—to the patient. The medical assistant and the physician are responsible for adhering to the following principles and practices at all times when assisting with or performing a sterile procedure:

1. Sterilize all supplies used for sterile procedures either previously or at the time for immediate use.
2. When in doubt about the sterility of anything, consider it nonsterile.
3. When putting sterile gloves on, do not touch the outside of the gloves with bare hands.
4. People who are wearing sterile gloves must touch only sterile articles; people who are not gloved must touch only nonsterile articles, except when using sterile transfer forceps to move sterile items.
5. During a sterile procedure, if a glove is punctured by a needle or an instrument, remove the damaged glove, wash your hands, and put on a new glove as promptly as patient safety permits. Remove the needle or instrument from the sterile field.
6. The outer wrappings and the edges of packs that contain sterile items are not sterile and thus are handled and opened by the person who is not wearing sterile gloves.
7. Open sterile packages with the edges of the wrapper directed away from your body to avoid touching your uniform or reaching over a sterile field.
8. Touch only the outside of a sterile wrapper.
9. Once a sterile pack has been opened, use it; if it is not used, replace any fabric items, sponges, and dressing materials and rewrap and resterilize the pack.
10. Avoid sneezing, coughing, or talking directly over a sterile field or object.
11. Do not reach across or above a sterile field or wound. Your clothes and skin are not sterile. If you touch the sterile field or drop debris onto it or into the wound, contamination results. Movements around the area should be kept to a minimum.
12. Avoid spilling solutions on a sterile setup. Any moisture that soaks through a sterile area to a nonsterile one produces a means of transporting bacteria to a sterile area. Thus the wet areas are considered contaminated and must either be covered with sterile towels or drapes until the top surface is dry or be removed and redraped.
13. Hold sterile objects and gloved hands above waist level or level to the sterile field. Anything below this level is considered unsterile. Keeping objects or hands in sight helps avoid contamination.
14. Because skin cannot be sterilized, any object that touches it is considered contaminated.
15. Have a special receptacle or plastic bag to receive contaminated materials.
16. A sterile field should be away from drafts, fans, and windows. Microorganisms can be carried in air currents to the patient or the sterile field.
17. Store sterile packages in dry areas. If they become wet, they must be repacked and resterilized or discarded.
18. Hands are the greatest source of contamination; therefore wash frequently, using correct technique.
19. Be constantly aware of the need for very clean surroundings.

In summary, remember these five basic rules:

- Know what is sterile.
- Know what is not sterile.
- Keep sterile items separate from nonsterile items.
- Prevent contamination.
- Remedy a contaminated situation immediately.

HANDLING STERILE SUPPLIES

Opening Sterile Packages

Many commercially prepared sterile packages have instructions for opening printed on them. Read these directions carefully before opening the package to avoid contamination of the contents. To open peel-down packages, such as those in which syringes and dressing materials are supplied, use the accompanying procedure.

You now have a **sterile field** that can be used as a sterile work area. Additional sterile items that may be needed for the procedure may be added to this sterile field. To organize the items contained in the package you just opened, use individually wrapped sterilized hemostats or **don** sterile gloves (see Figure 6-5). Small packages can be held in the hand and unwrapped in the same fashion. Have someone who is wearing sterile gloves take the item from the opened wrap, or remove it with sterile transfer forceps, or carefully place the item on a sterile field, avoiding contamination to the item and field. Be sure that the wrapper corners do not touch the sterile field.

Treat the edges of a sterile field on a flat surface as if they were contaminated. Some recommend that the outside 1-inch border of the field be considered contaminated. Parts of the wrap that fall over the side of the surface are considered contaminated (see Figure 6-5, *G*).

Text continued on p. 298

PROCEDURE 6-1

OPENING PEEL-DOWN PACKAGES

Objective

Understand and demonstrate the correct procedure for opening a peel-down package to obtain the sterile contents without contamination.

PROCEDURE

RATIONALE

1. **Wash your hands. Use appropriate personal protective equipment (PPE) as dictated by facility.**

2. Using both hands, grasp both sides of the extended edges provided.

3. Pull evenly along the sealed edges (Figure 6-1, *A*).

   Pull evenly in a downward motion to avoid tearing.

4. Do not touch the inside of the wrapper; place on a flat surface.
   or
   Using sterile forceps, remove the contents from the wrapper and transfer to a sterile field or use immediately in a sterile procedure such as a dressing change (Figure 6-1, *B*).
   or
   Holding the bottom of the package with the edges folded back, allow a person wearing sterile gloves to take the contents.
   or
   If the item is a syringe to be used by you, grasp the plunger end of the syringe with one hand while holding onto the package with your other hand.

   The inside of the wrapper is sterile and can be used as a sterile field until using the contents.

   Keep your fingers away from the contents to avoid contamination.

   The bottom part of the plunger does not have to remain sterile because this is how you take hold of the syringe to remove it from the sterile package, provided you are going to use it immediately and not place it on a sterile field.

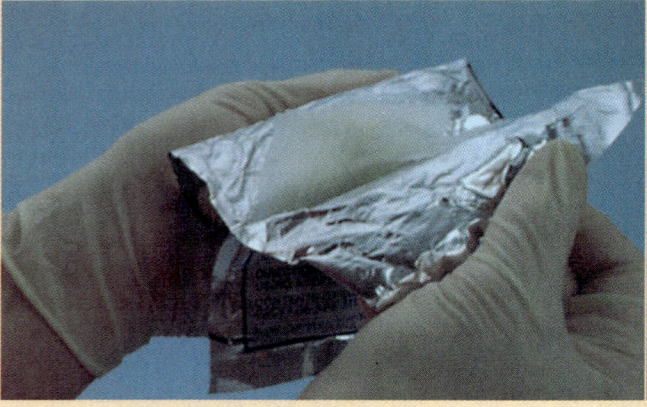
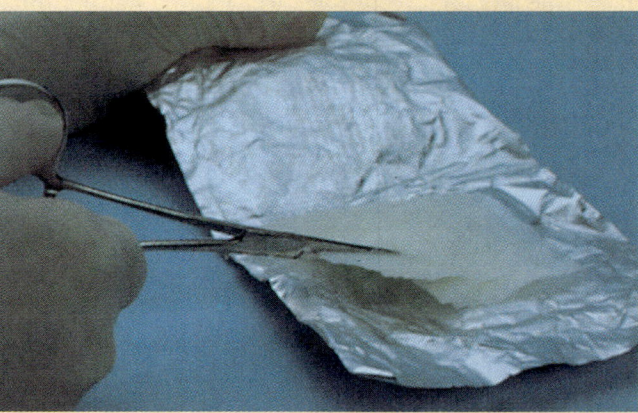

FIGURE 6-1   A, Technique for opening peel-down package with sterile contents. **B,** Technique for removing a sterile dressing from package.

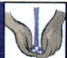

OPENING AN ENVELOPE WRAP

Objective

Understand and demonstrate the correct procedure for opening an envelope wrap package containing sterile supplies.

PROCEDURE

1. **Wash your hands. Use appropriate personal protective equipment (PPE) as dictated by facility.**

2. Place package on a flat surface so that the folded edges are on top.

3. Remove tape or string fastener and discard in waste container. At this time you should also check the date and sterilization indicator.

4. Pull out the corner that is tucked under, if present, and unfold this top flap away from you (Figure 6-2). Avoid touching the pack with your uniform or person.

5. Using both hands, grasp the second layer of folded corners and open these flaps to the sides of the package (Figure 6-3), or open first one side and then the other. The contents of the package are still covered with the last layer of the wrapper.

6. Without reaching over any of the uncovered area, grasp the last fold or fourth corner and open toward your body (Figure 6-4). Lift this corner up and toward you, dropping it on the surface holding the package. Do not touch the inside of the package or the contents with bare hands.

RATIONALE

Check to make sure that the contents are safe for use.

Unfolding away from you avoids the necessity of reaching over the sterile field later and causing contamination.

Touching would contaminate everything.

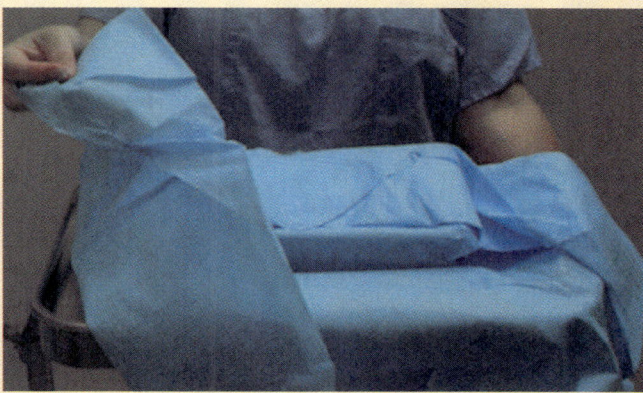

FIGURE 6-3   Open second layer of flaps to each side.

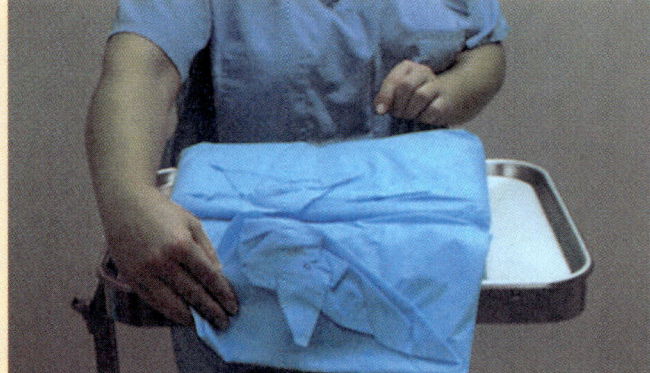

FIGURE 6-2   Unfold top flap away from you.

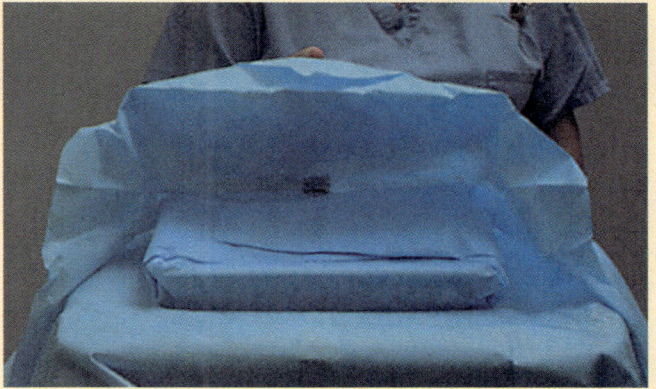

FIGURE 6-4   Open last flap toward your body.

FIGURE 6-5   **A,** Using sterile gloves, arrange sterile supplies on sterile field for use. **B,** Remove sterile forceps from pack to use as sterile transfer forceps. **C,** Use sterile forceps to arrange sterile supplies on sterile field. **D,** Carefully place unwrapped sterile bowl onto sterile field. **E,** Open pack and drop sterile suture pack onto sterile field.

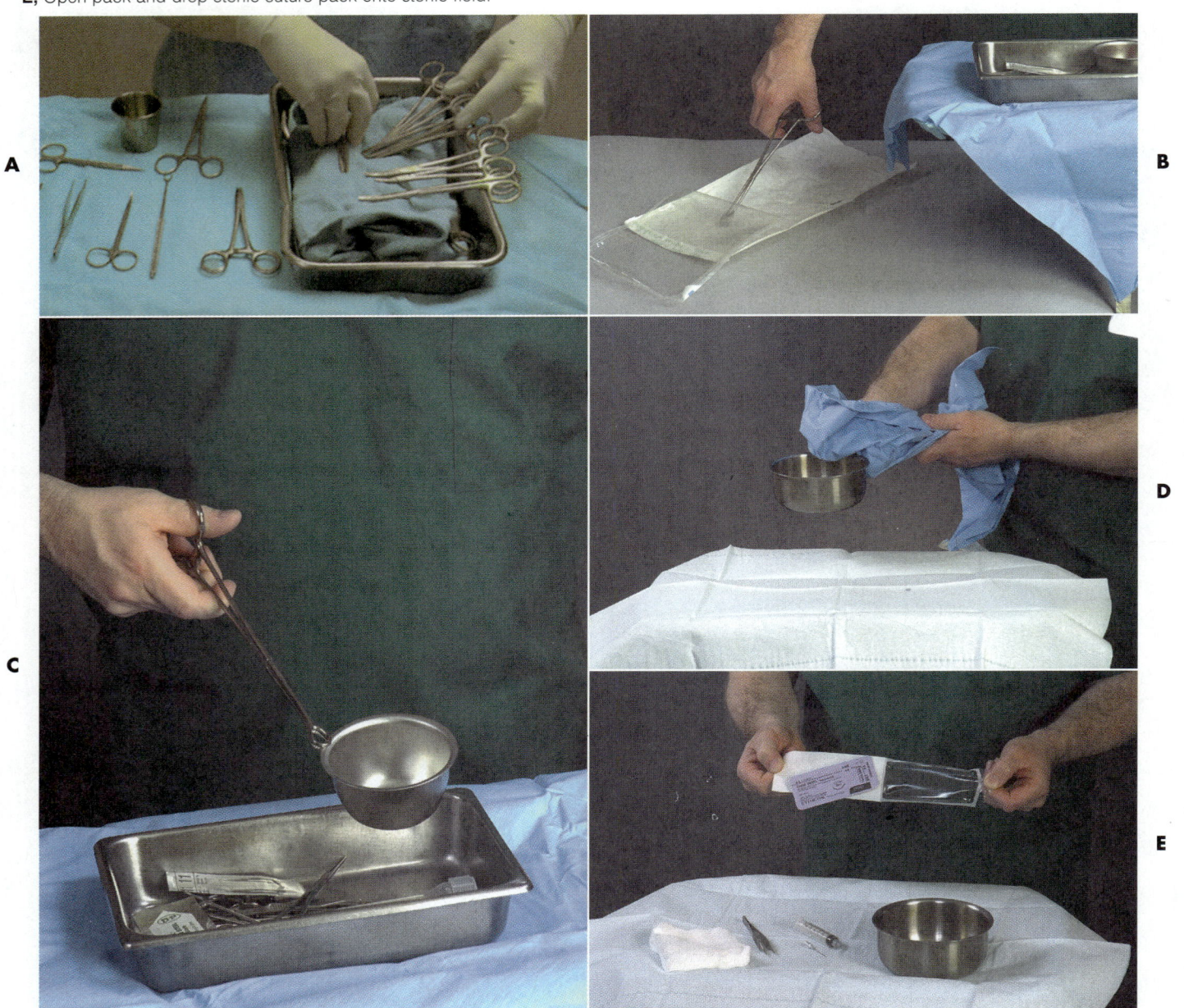

FIGURE 6-5—cont'd **F,** Place sterile instrument from opened sterile pack onto sterile fields. **G,** Sterile fields indicated by red border tape.

F

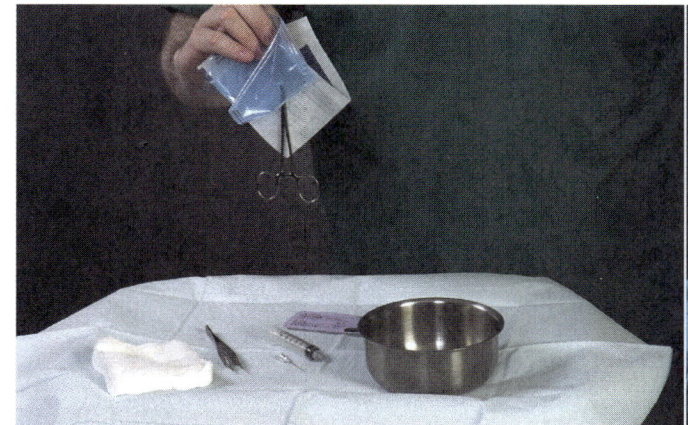

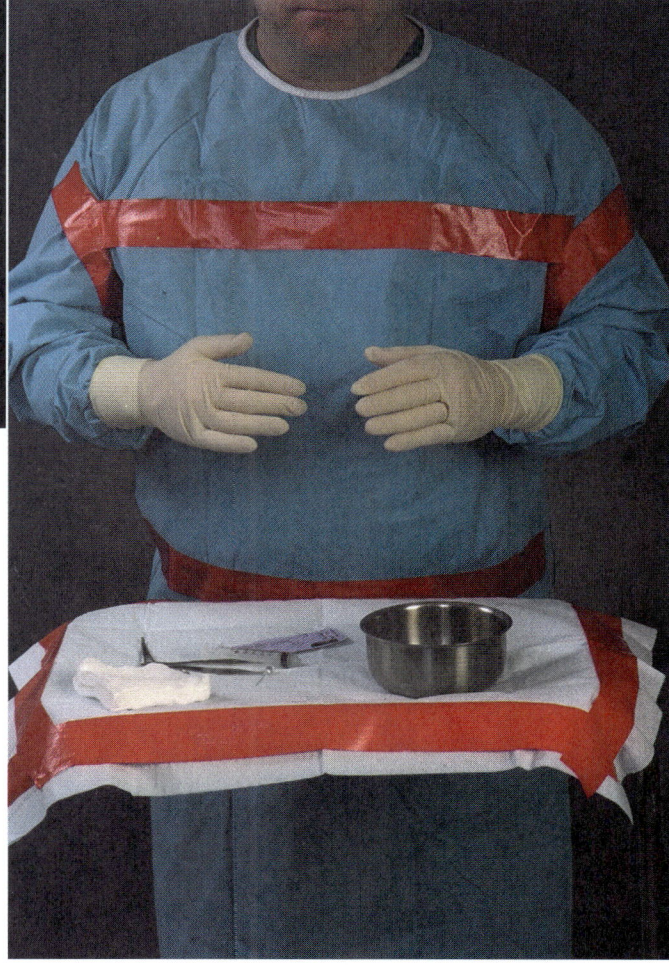

G

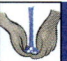

PROCEDURE 6-3

POURING STERILE SOLUTIONS

Objective

Understand and demonstrate the correct methods for checking the name of a sterile solution, then pouring it into a container; pouring it on a sponge.

PROCEDURE

1. **Wash your hands. Use appropriate personal protective equipment (PPE) as dictated by facility.**

2. Obtain the solution and check the label.

3. Obtain sterile container to be used for the solution and unwrap. Follow procedure for unwrapping as described previously.
   NOTE: When using prepackaged sterile trays, a container for the solution may be included in the pack.

RATIONALE

Solutions are drugs. All drug labels must be checked three times before using or administering:
- *When removing from storage area*
- *Before pouring*
- *When replacing container in the storage area*

Continued

POURING STERILE SOLUTIONS—cont'd

4. Remove bottle cap; place on a level surface with the top of the cap resting on the surface or hold it in your hand with the top facing downward.

5. Check the label again. Hold the bottle with the label in the palm of your hand about 6 inches above the container (or less, when pouring very small amounts of solution) and pour the solution (Figure 6-6). Pour a small amount of solution into a waste container to cleanse the side of the bottle and then pour from the same area.

6. When pouring a solution on a sponge, pick up the sponge with forceps and pour the solution over the sponge. The excess solution will drip into the basin or discard container (Figure 6-7).

7. Pick the cap up by the sides and replace it on the bottle securely.

8. Check the label of the bottle and replace it in the correct storage area.

The inner part of the cap is considered sterile. If you place the cap with top facing up, you have contaminated the inner surface, which then cannot be replaced on the container until it has been resterilized.

Holding the bottle this way prevents damage to the label if the solution runs or spills; you also avoid undue splashing.

Do not contaminate the inside of the cap because it is considered sterile and must cover the sterile solution in the bottle.

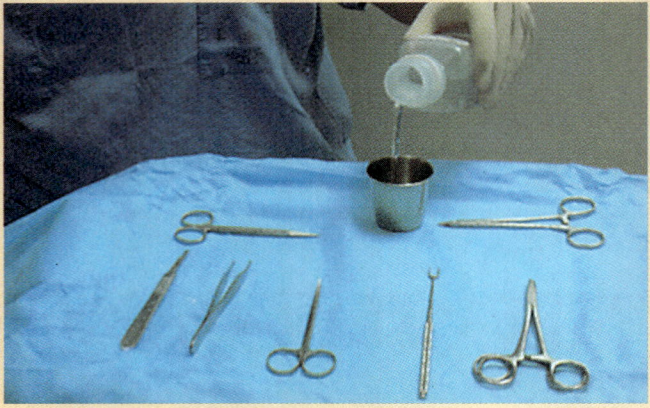

FIGURE 6-6   Pouring solution into container on sterile field. Hold top of container in your hand with top facing downward.

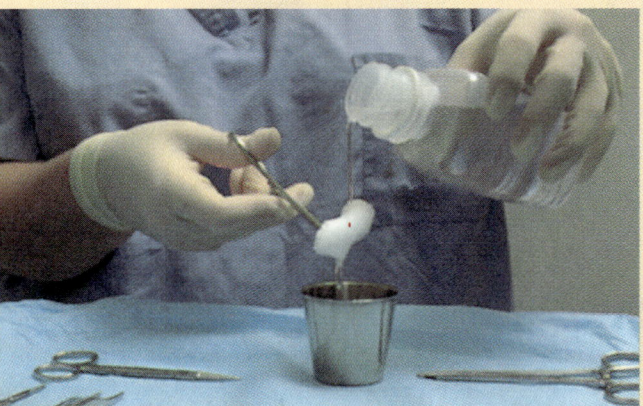

FIGURE 6-7   Pouring solution onto sterile sponge.

Pouring Sterile Solutions

When required to pour a sterile solution, you must use aseptic technique to avoid contaminating the solution.

Donning and Removing Sterile Gloves

Sterile gloves are worn to protect the patient from infection caused by microorganisms that may be on your hands and to provide a means of safely handling sterile supplies and equipment without contaminating these items. Gloves are also worn to protect the health care worker from possible contamination or infection (see also Chapter 1).

MINOR SURGERY

Minor surgery is sometimes performed in the physician's office, although often even these procedures are done in the emergency room or outpatient department of a hospital or in a clinic or freestanding center that is not associated with a hospital.

Minor surgical procedures include those that can be done with or without the use of a local anesthetic, such as the suturing of a laceration; the incision and drainage of an abscess or cyst; incision and removal of foreign bodies in subcutaneous tissues; removal of small growths, such as warts, moles, and skin tags; various types of biopsies; cauterization of tissue

Text continued on p. 302

PROCEDURE 6-4

DONNING AND REMOVING STERILE GLOVES

PROCEDURE	RATIONALE

1. **Wash your hands. Use appropriate personal protective equipment (PPE) as dictated by facility.**

2. Place wrapped gloves on a clean, dry, flat surface with the cuff end toward you.

3. Open the outside and inside wrapper by handling only the outside of the packages.

The inside part of the wrappers is sterile.

4. Using your left hand, pick up the right-hand glove by grasping the folded edge of the cuff and lift up and away from the wrapper (Figure 6-8). The folded edge of the cuff will be against your skin and is contaminated as soon as you touch it. *Do not* touch the outside of the glove with your ungloved hand.

5. Pulling on the edge of the cuff, pull the right glove on. Keep your fingers away from the rest of the glove.

6. Place fingers of the right gloved hand under the cuff of the left-hand glove (Figure 6-9). Be sure that your gloved fingers do not touch your skin.

The area inside the folded cuff is considered sterile.

7. Lift the glove up and away from the wrapper and pull it onto your left hand. Be sure that the left thumb does not stray up and touch the right glove. Keep the right gloved fingers under the cuff and straight; keep the right gloved thumb back.

Avoid touching skin.

8. Continue pulling the left glove up over your wrist (Figure 6-10).

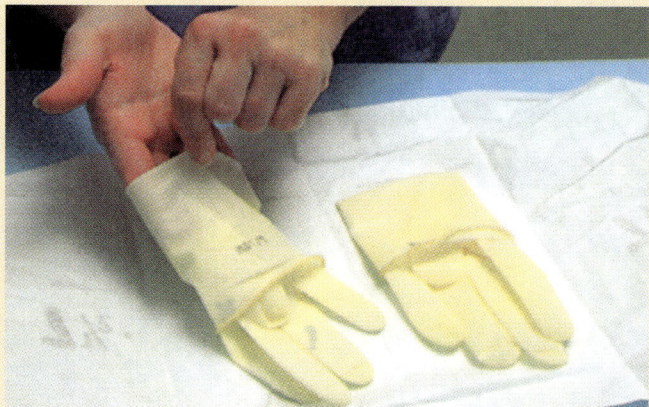

FIGURE 6-8 Technique for donning first sterile glove. Grasp folded edge of cuff, lift up and away from wrapper, and pull onto right hand.

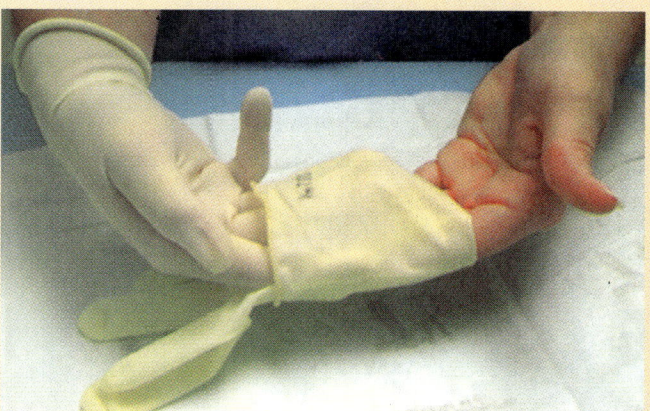

FIGURE 6-9 Technique for donning second sterile glove. Place fingers of gloved hand under cuff of other glove and pull onto left hand.

Continued

PROCEDURE 6-4

DONNING AND REMOVING STERILE GLOVES—cont'd

9. With the gloved left hand, place fingers under the cuff of the right glove and pull the cuff up over your right wrist.

The area inside the folded cuff is considered sterile.

10. Adjust the fingers of the gloves as necessary. If, when putting on either glove, the fingers get into the wrong space, you must proceed with the rest of the gloving procedure and then adjust the gloves with gloved hands.

11. If either glove tears during the procedure, remove and discard. Begin the procedure again with a new pair of gloves.

12. **TO REMOVE GLOVES:**
    a. Grasp the cuff of the right-hand glove with your left hand (Figure 6-11, *A*).
    b. Pull the glove down over the hand (Figure 6-11, *B*).
    c. Discard in appropriate place.
    d. Repeat, using the right hand to remove left glove. Grasp the inside and top of the left-hand glove with your right hand, pull the glove down over the hand, and discard. Reusable gloves must be washed and resterilized; disposable gloves are discarded in the appropriate waste container. Do not touch the outside of the glove (Figure 6-11, *D*).
    e. **Wash your hands thoroughly.**

NOTE: *An alternative method is as follows:*

    a. Grasp the outside of the right hand glove 1 to 2 inches from the top.
    b. Pull the glove down over the hand and off and hold it in your left gloved hand (Figure 6-11, *B*).
    c. Grasp the inside near the top of the left-hand glove with fingers of your right hand and pull the glove down and off your hand. As you pull this glove off, it turns inside out and also encloses the first glove that you are holding in your left hand (Figure 6-11, *C*).
    d. Discard both gloves in the appropriate place or container.
    e. **Wash your hands thoroughly.**

Glove touches glove. You do not touch your skin, thus avoiding contamination of your skin.
The glove turns inside out as it comes off.
The glove is considered contaminated after use.
Skin touches skin. The outside of the glove is considered contaminated.

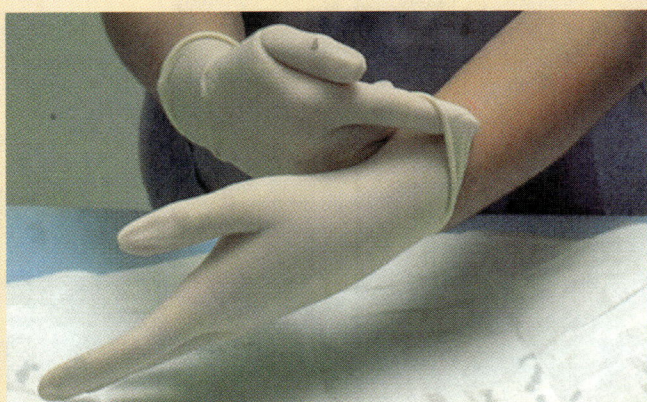

FIGURE 6-10 Technique for donning sterile glove. Adjust cuffs on gloves, avoiding contamination.

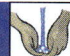

PROCEDURE 6-4

DONNING AND REMOVING STERILE GLOVES—cont'd

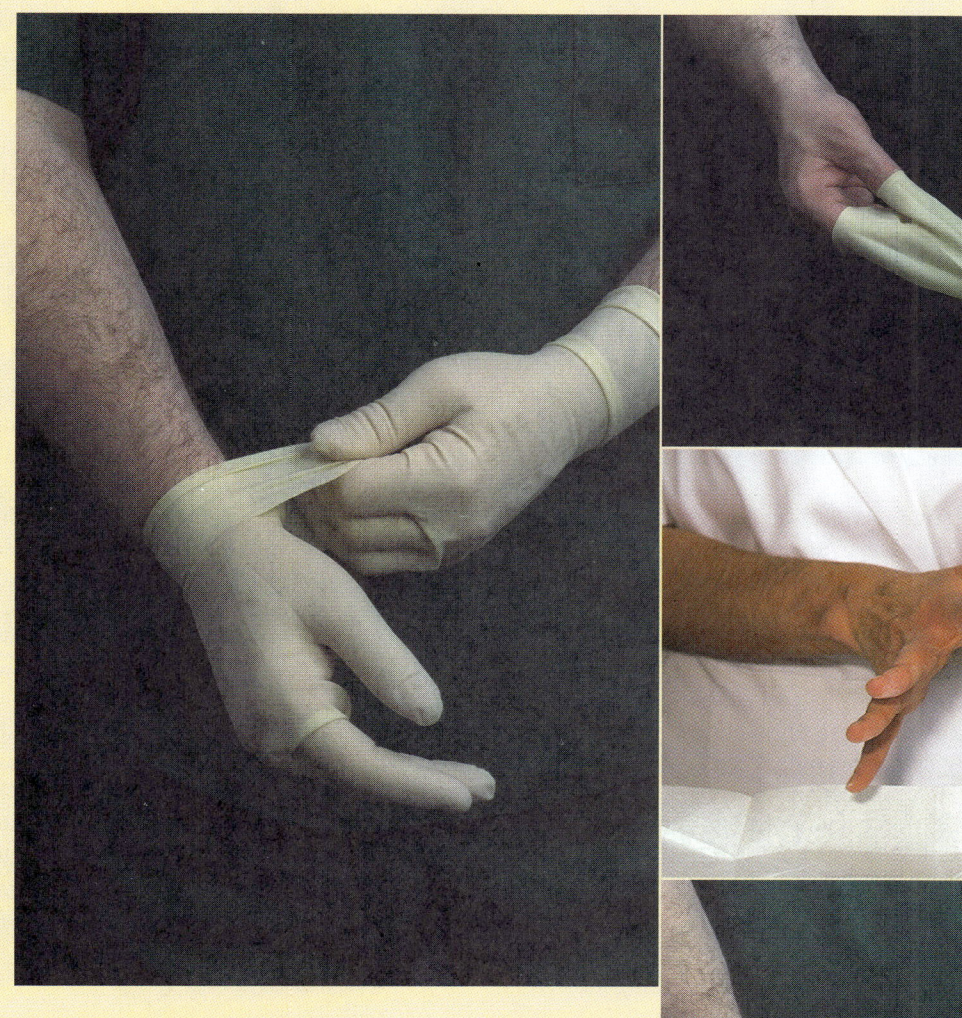

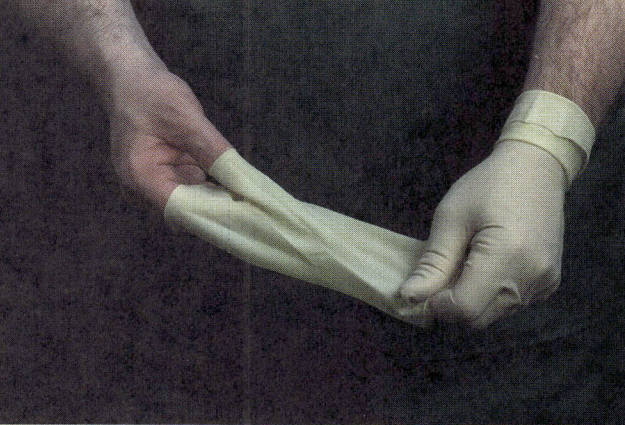

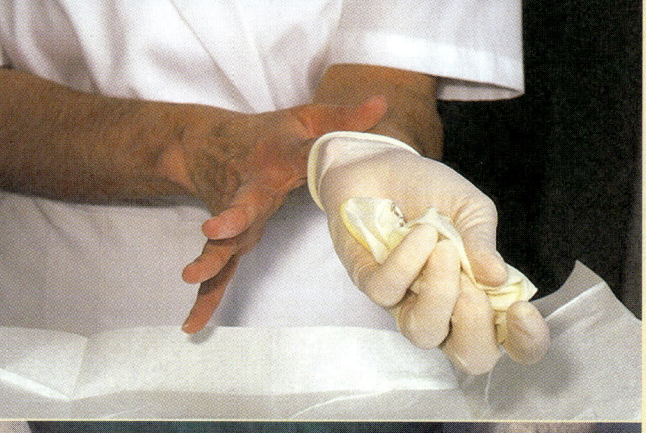

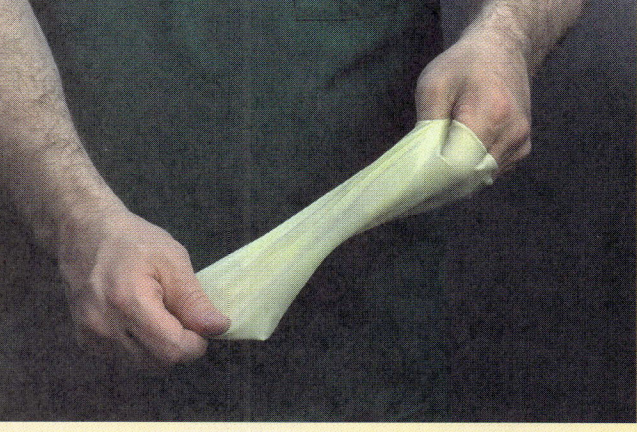

FIGURE 6-11 Techniques for removing sterile gloves. **A,** Grasp *outside* or cuff of right glove near top; **B,** pull glove down and off of right hand; **C,** grasp *inside* top of left glove; **D,** pull glove down and off. Do not touch outside part of gloves because they are considered contaminated.

(such as cauterization of the uterine cervix or of a wart, mole, or skin tag); and insertion of an intrauterine device (IUD). After minor surgery performed in the office or at the hospital, the patient may come to the physician's office for dressing changes and for the removal of sutures as part of the postoperative care. The wound is also inspected at that time to determine the amount of healing that has occurred and to ensure the absence of a developing infectious process.

As the physician's assistant, you may be called on to assist with the surgical procedures or to change a dressing for a patient. Assisting in any surgical procedure is a highly responsible job, and you must always use strict surgical aseptic technique. The nature of the surgery or postoperative care governs the duties and responsibilities of the medical assistant.

Anesthesia

For minor surgery and extremely painful treatments, some type of local anesthetic is usually required. **Local anesthesia** refers to the absence of feeling or sensation and pain in a limited area of the body without the loss of consciousness. The extent and severity of the procedure determine the type and amount of anesthetic used, which can be administered by injection or topical application. Local anesthetics produce their effects in 5 to 15 minutes. These effects may last from 1 to 3 hours, depending on the type and dose administered.

Types of local anesthesia

- **Infiltration**—The anesthetic solution is injected under the skin to anesthetize the nerve endings and nerve fibers at the site of the procedure. The sensory nerves become insensitive and remain so for several hours, depending on the amount of drug administered. (Rules for the administration of medications and injections described in Chapter 7 apply here.) Examples of infiltration anesthetics include procaine (Novocain) 1% to 2% and lidocaine (Xylocaine) 1% to 2%.

- **Nerve block or block anesthesia**—The anesthetic solution is injected into or adjacent to accessible main nerves, thus desensitizing all the adjacent tissue. Examples of nerve block anesthesia include procaine (Novocain) 1% to 2% and lidocaine (Xylocaine) 1% to 2%.

- **Topical or surface anesthesia**—The anesthetic solution is painted or sprayed directly onto the skin or mucous membrane involved to deaden sensation and relieve pain. Examples of topical anesthetics include lidocaine 4% and 5% and 10% cocaine solutions for accessible mucous membranes of oral and nasal cavities and ethyl chloride spray for external topical use, because it is too harsh for use on mucous membranes. A topical refrigerant anesthetic such as Fluor-ethyl aerosol spray is used as a surface coolant and anesthetic. Before a topical anesthetic is applied, the patient's skin must be washed and dried well.

Allergic reactions.   Before the administration of a local anesthetic, you must ask every patient if he or she is allergic to any drug, if he or she has any cardiac or respiratory problems, and if he or she has had any type of anesthetic before. This information is most important because some local anesthetics can cause anaphylactic shock or violent allergic reactions. Often skin tests are made beforehand when deemed necessary. An **emergency tray** with sterile syringes and needles, sterile alcohol sponges, and ampules of a stimulant such as epinephrine (Adrenalin) must be kept in reach when an anesthetic is to be administered, in case an emergency does arise. (See also discussion in Chapter 7 on emergency tray, p. 363).

Suture Materials and Needles

The purpose of sutures is to hold the edges of a wound together until healing occurs. When suture materials are necessary for a procedure, they can be added to your sterile field. Those most commonly used are the sterile prepackaged sutures with or without an attached suture needle (Figure 6-12). The label on these packages indicates the type, length, and size of the suture and the type and size of the needle enclosed. Sutures are prepared from materials that are either absorbable or nonabsorbable. **Absorbable sutures** do not have to be removed when used because they are absorbed or digested by the body fluids and tissues during and after the healing process, usually 5 to 20 days after insertion, varying with the type used. An example of absorbable suture material is surgical gut (catgut), which is made from the submucosa of sheep intestines. Absorbable suture material is generally used in surgical procedures involving the suturing of internal organs and subcutaneous tissue and when ligating vessels.

Nonabsorbable sutures used on outer skin surfaces are removed after the wound has healed because body fluids and cells do not absorb or digest them (for example, cotton, silk, nylon, and stainless steel and metal clips or staples). When used internally, they are not removed and remain as foreign bodies; usually they become encysted and cause no trouble. The most commonly used nonabsorbable suture material is black surgical silk. The silk is dyed black so that it can readily be seen in the tissue in which it is used. The size, or gauge, of most sutures is labeled in terms of 0s (for example, 0, which is the thickest, followed by 00, 000, each decreasing in size up to 10-0, which is the thinnest). Sizes 2-0 up to 6-0 are used most often; 4-0 black silk may be used to suture a laceration on the arm; and 5-0 and

---

FIGURE 6-12 Prepackaged sterile suture materials. Cover of package indicates type, length, and size of suture material. Curved line under the suture label represents type and size of needle included.

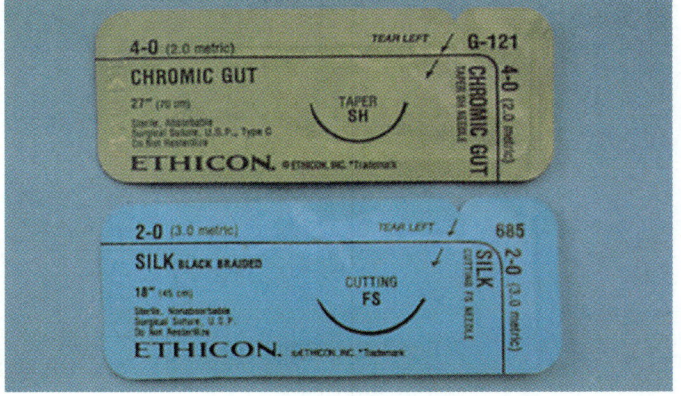

6-0 are commonly used for repairing delicate tissues such as in the face and neck. The finer the suture, the less scar formation; therefore fine sutures are most desirable when cosmetic results are important. 10-0 silk, which is extremely fine, is used for ophthalmologic and vascular procedures. A few types of sutures are designated as 1, 2, 3, 4, and 5 (the thickest); others are designated simply as fine, medium, and coarse. The size and type of the suture used is determined by the area and the purpose, as well as the physician's preference. Thicker sutures are used when closing large wounds; medium ones are used on lacerations; and very fine sutures are used on more delicate tissues, such as the eye or facial tissues.

Sutures must remain in place until the incision or break in the tissue has healed. The physician decides when to remove sutures. Generally, sutures in the skin on the neck or head are removed in 3 to 5 days; sutures in the skin of the hand, arms, legs, and other areas are removed in 7 to 10 days.

Suture needles are either straight or curved and have either a sharp, cutting point or a round, noncutting point. They are supplied in individual packages or in packages with suture materials (see Figure 6-12). Some needles have an eye through which the suture material is threaded. Other needles come attached to the suture material as one unit. These are called **swaged needles** (Figure 6-13). Packages are labeled with the type and size of the needle and the type, size, and length of the suture material.

Sharp cutting needles are used on stable tissues, such as the skin, where the sharp point is useful in getting the needle through the tissue. Round, noncutting needles are used on less firm tissues, such as subcutaneous tissues and on the internal organs of body cavities. Curved needles are held in a needle holder (see Figure 6-13, *B*) when used to be able to get in and out of the tissue, as when suturing small skin incisions. Straight needles are used by hand as they are pushed through adjoining tissues, as when suturing large skin incisions. The size and type of suture needle chosen is determined by the area and the purpose for which it will be used.

An *alternative* to sutures for holding the edges of tissue together is the use of **adhesive skin closures.** These are sterile nonallergic tapes that are supplied in a variety of lengths and

FIGURE 6-13   Types of suture needles: **A,** Straight; **B,** swaged needle positioned for use in needle holder; **C,** curved with sharp point; **D,** swaged. (**A, C,** and **D** courtesy Miltex Instrument Co, Lake Success, NY.)

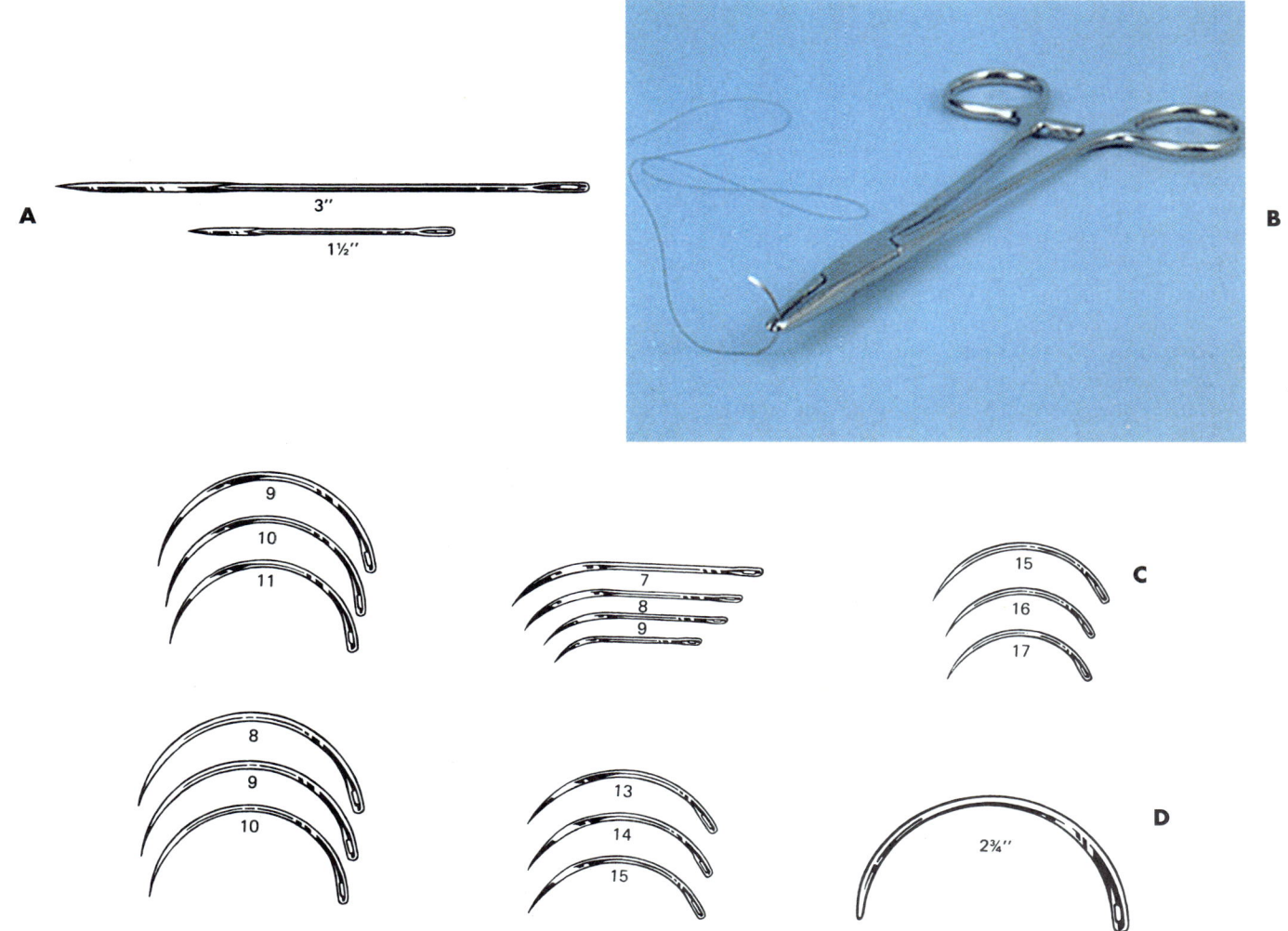

widths. An example of a commercial adhesive skin closure is the Steri-Strip. The edges of the tissue are held together, and the Steri-Strips are applied transversely across this area and left in place until the wound has healed.

The medical assistant may be responsible for setting up the supplies needed by the physician for suturing tissue. The physician chooses the size and type of suture material and needle that will be used. Materials required for suturing tissue are given on p. 318.

Instruments Used for Minor Surgery

Surgical instruments are tools or devices designed to perform a specific function, such as cutting, grasping, retracting, or suturing (Figure 6-14). They are usually made of steel and are treated so that they are durable, rust resistant, heat resistant, and stainproof. Proper care of all surgical instruments is essential. You must see that they are used correctly, handled carefully, inspected for any defects, and sterilized and stored correctly. As a medical assistant, you should be able to identify a variety of surgical instruments; know how they are used, sterilized, and stored; and be able to select the correct instruments for a variety of minor surgical procedures that may be performed in the physician's office or clinic. Some of the more common surgical instruments are discussed. Figure 6-14 illustrates many of these instruments. Additional figures in this chapter illustrate tray setups for specific procedures with some of these instruments.

Scalpels (see Figure 6-14).
Scalpels (skal´pel) are used to make incisions into tissue. They are small surgical knives that usually have a convex (rounded, somewhat elevated) edge. Scalpel *blades* are supplied in various sizes and shapes that are designed for making different types of incisions in various tissues. Scalpels are now disposable, and some are supplied with a disposable handle. The No. 3 and No. 7 *handles* are the most commonly used, the No. 7 handle being thinner.

Scissors (see Figure 6-14).
Surgical scissors *are used to **cut** or **dissect** tissues and to cut sutures.* Others *are used to cut bandages* when they are to be removed. These instruments consist of two opposing cutting blades, which may be *straight or curved.* The tips on the blades vary. On some scissors both tips are *sharp,* whereas on others both tips are *blunt;* others have one sharp tip and one blunt tip. **Bandage scissors** have one blunt tip and one tip that has a flat blunt probe. These are *used* to remove bandages and dressings without puncturing the tissues. **Suture scissors,** *used* to remove sutures, have one blunt tip and a hook on the second tip. When removing sutures, the hook goes under the suture. The blunt tip prevents puncture to the tissue. **Short, straight Iris scissors** with two sharp tips are also *used* to remove sutures. Common **dissecting scissors** are the straight or curved Mayo scissors; the short, curved Metzenbaum scissors, which are *used* on superficial, delicate tissue; and the long, blunt, curved Metzenbaum, which are *used* on deep, delicate tissue. The tips of dissecting scissors are blunt so that tissue is not inadvertently punctured. **Operating scissors** have straight blades and may have any of the combination types of blades (*sharp/sharp,*

blunt/blunt, or *sharp/blunt*). The type of scissors used in a procedure varies, depending on its intended function and the physician's preference.

Forceps (see Figure 6-14).
Forceps are instruments of varied sizes and shapes *used for* **grasping, compressing,** or **holding** *tissue or objects.* They are two-pronged instruments with either a spring handle or a ring handle with a ratchet closure. The ratchet is a toothed clasp that allows different degrees of tightness to be applied to the tissue or object on which the instrument is used. The inner surfaces of some forceps have sawlike teeth that are called serrations (Figure 6-15). **Serrations** prevent tissue from slipping out of the forceps jaw. The tips may be either *straight* or *curved* and *plain tipped* or *toothed tipped.* **Plain-tipped forceps** are *used* to pick up tissue, dressings, or other sterile objects.

Plain-tipped forceps include standard thumb forceps, plain splinter forceps (these have sharp points), Adson dressing forceps, and the Halsted mosquito, Kelly, and Rochester-Pean hemostatic forceps.

A **toothed-tipped forceps** is especially useful for grasping tissue. The teeth prevent the tissue from slipping out of the grasp of the instrument. **Forceps** with a **toothed tip** include standard tissue forceps, Allis tissue forceps, and Ochsner-Kocher hemostatic forceps.

Examples of **forceps** with a **spring handle** are the thumb, tissue, splinter, and dressing forceps. Examples of forceps with a **ring handle** and **ratchet closure** are Allis tissue forceps, Foerster sponge forceps, Backhaus towel clamps, and straight or curved hemostatic forceps or hemostats. Hemostats include Halsted mosquito hemostatic forceps, Kelly hemostatic forceps, Rochester-Pean hemostatic forceps, and Ochsner-Kocher hemostatic forceps.

Sponge forceps are *used* for holding sponges and have serrated ringlike tips. **Towel clamps** have two sharp points and are *used* to hold the edges of sterile drapes or towels together. **Hemostats** are *used* to compress, hold, or grasp a blood vessel. They are also used by some people to apply or remove a dressing.

A **uterine** or **cervical tenaculum** is a clamp or forceps with long handles and short hooks used to hold or grasp the cervix.

Needle Holders (see Figure 6-14).
Needle holders have a ring handle, a ratchet closure, and serrated tips. Some needle holders have a groove in the middle of the serrations (see Figure 6-15). These instruments are designed to hold a curved needle used for suturing tissues.

Retractors (see Figure 6-14).
Retractors are instruments *used* to hold back the edges of tissues or organs to maintain exposure of the operative area. Examples include a double-ended Richardson retractor and a Volkmann rake retractor.

Probes (see Figure 6-14).
Probes are slender, long instruments *used* for exploring wounds or body cavities or passages. The end of a probe may be straight or curved. The body area being explored determines the type of probe to be used.

Sounds (see Figure 6-14).   A **sound** is an instrument used to find the opening of a cavity or canal, to determine the depth of a cavity such as the uterus, or to check if a canal is open.

Biopsy Instruments (see Figure 6-14).   **Biopsy instruments** are *used* to obtain a small piece of tissue from the body for examination. Biopsy forceps are available in various sizes and shapes. Three common ones seen in offices or clinics are the rectal biopsy punch, the cervical biopsy forceps, and a 6-mm biopsy punch used to obtain a small sample of skin.

Instrument care.   Keep in mind the following points for the care of instruments:

1. Use the instrument *only* for the intended purpose and in the correct manner. "Handle with care."
2. Rinse or soak and then sanitize and sterilize instruments, as described in Chapter 2, as soon as possible after use.
3. Inspect each instrument for proper working condition and for any defect.
4. Never toss instruments around or pile them on top of each other; damage could result.

Text continued on p. 309

FIGURE 6-14   **A,** Surgical blades (scalpels) and instruments used for minor surgery. (**A** Courtesy Miltex Instrument Co, Lake Success, NY.)

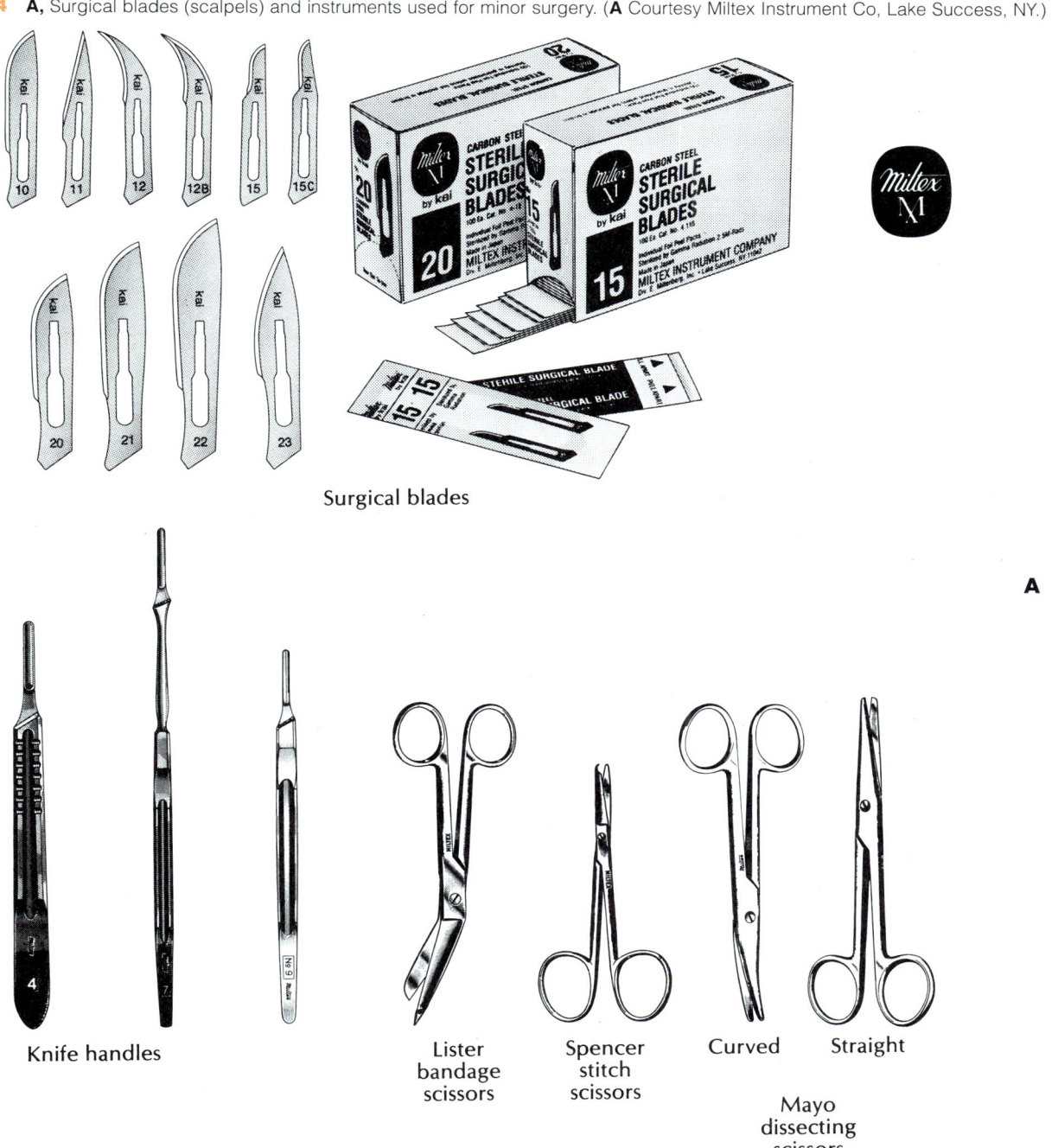

Surgical blades

Knife handles   Lister bandage scissors   Spencer stitch scissors   Curved   Straight

Mayo dissecting scissors

A

Continued

FIGURE 6-14—cont'd   **A,** Surgical blades (scalpels) and instruments used for minor surgery. (**A** Courtesy Miltex Instrument Co, Lake Success, NY.)

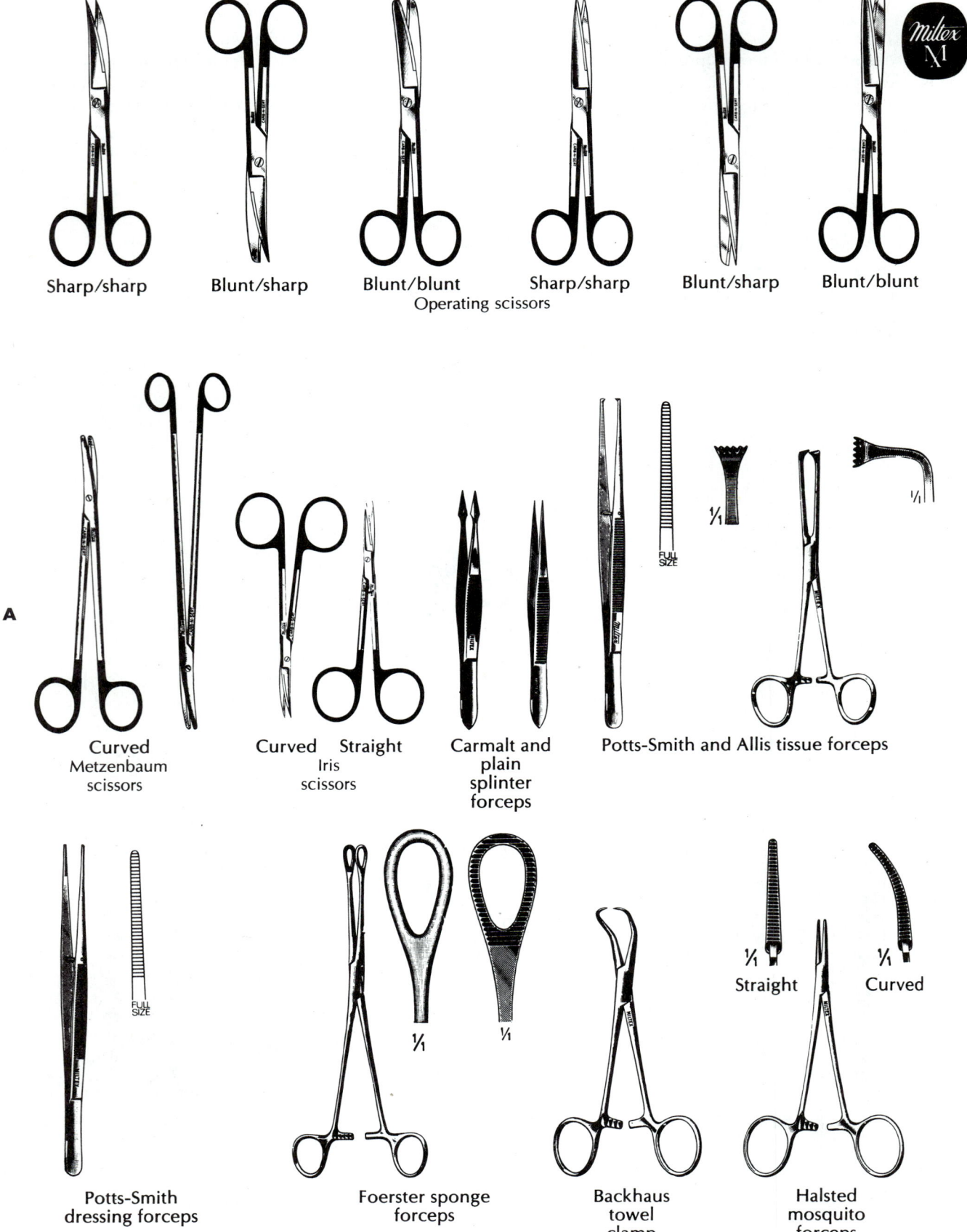

Sharp/sharp   Blunt/sharp   Blunt/blunt   Sharp/sharp   Blunt/sharp   Blunt/blunt

Operating scissors

Curved Metzenbaum scissors

Curved   Straight
Iris scissors

Carmalt and plain splinter forceps

Potts-Smith and Allis tissue forceps

Potts-Smith dressing forceps

Foerster sponge forceps

Backhaus towel clamp

Halsted mosquito forceps

Straight   Curved

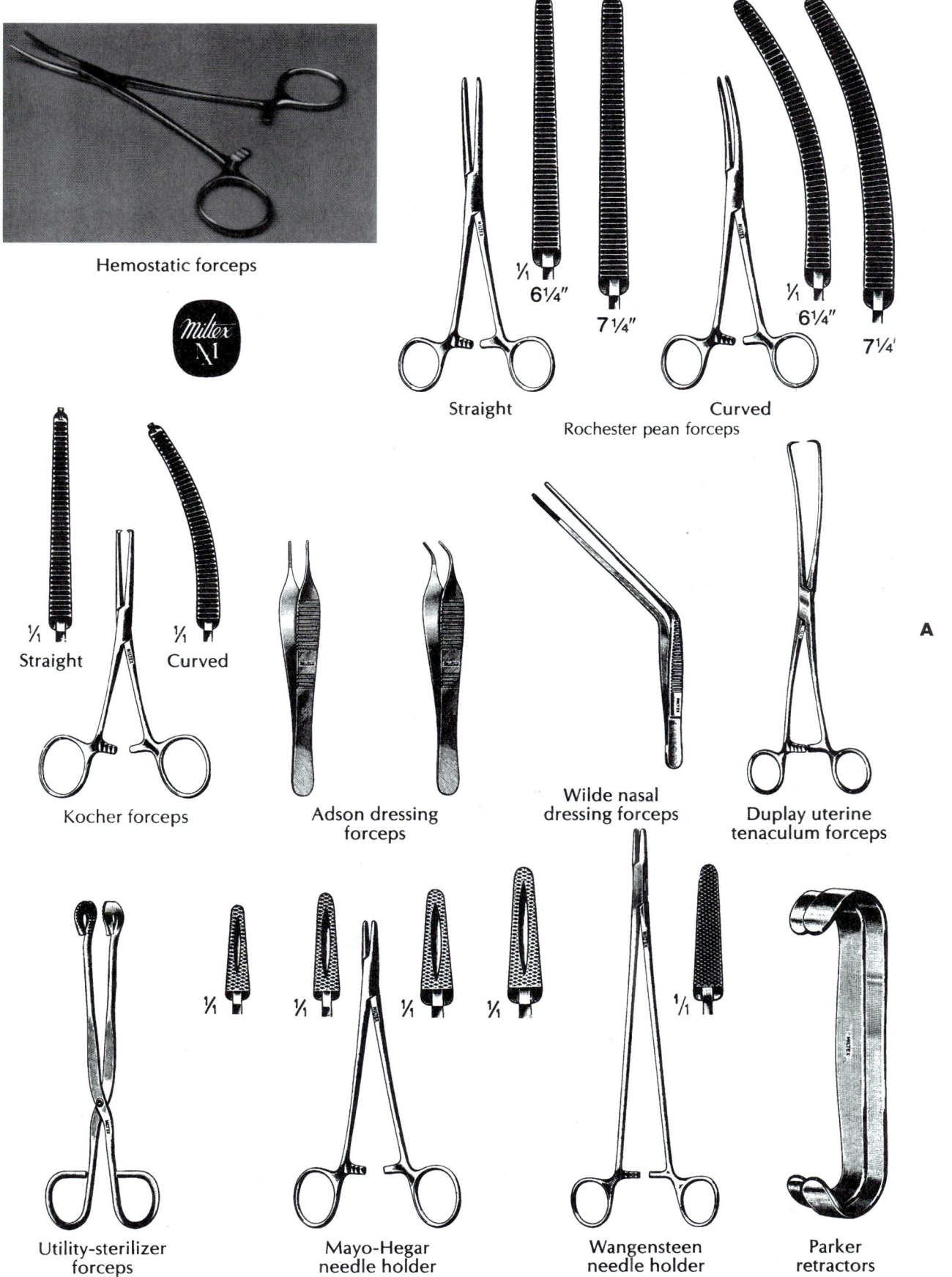

Hemostatic forceps

¹/₁
6¼″
7¼″
Straight

¹/₁
6¼″
7¼′
Curved

Rochester pean forceps

A

¹/₁
Straight

¹/₁
Curved

Kocher forceps

Adson dressing
forceps

Wilde nasal
dressing forceps

Duplay uterine
tenaculum forceps

¹/₁

¹/₁   ¹/₁   ¹/₁   ¹/₁   ¹/₁

Utility-sterilizer
forceps

Mayo-Hegar
needle holder

Wangensteen
needle holder

Parker
retractors

Continued

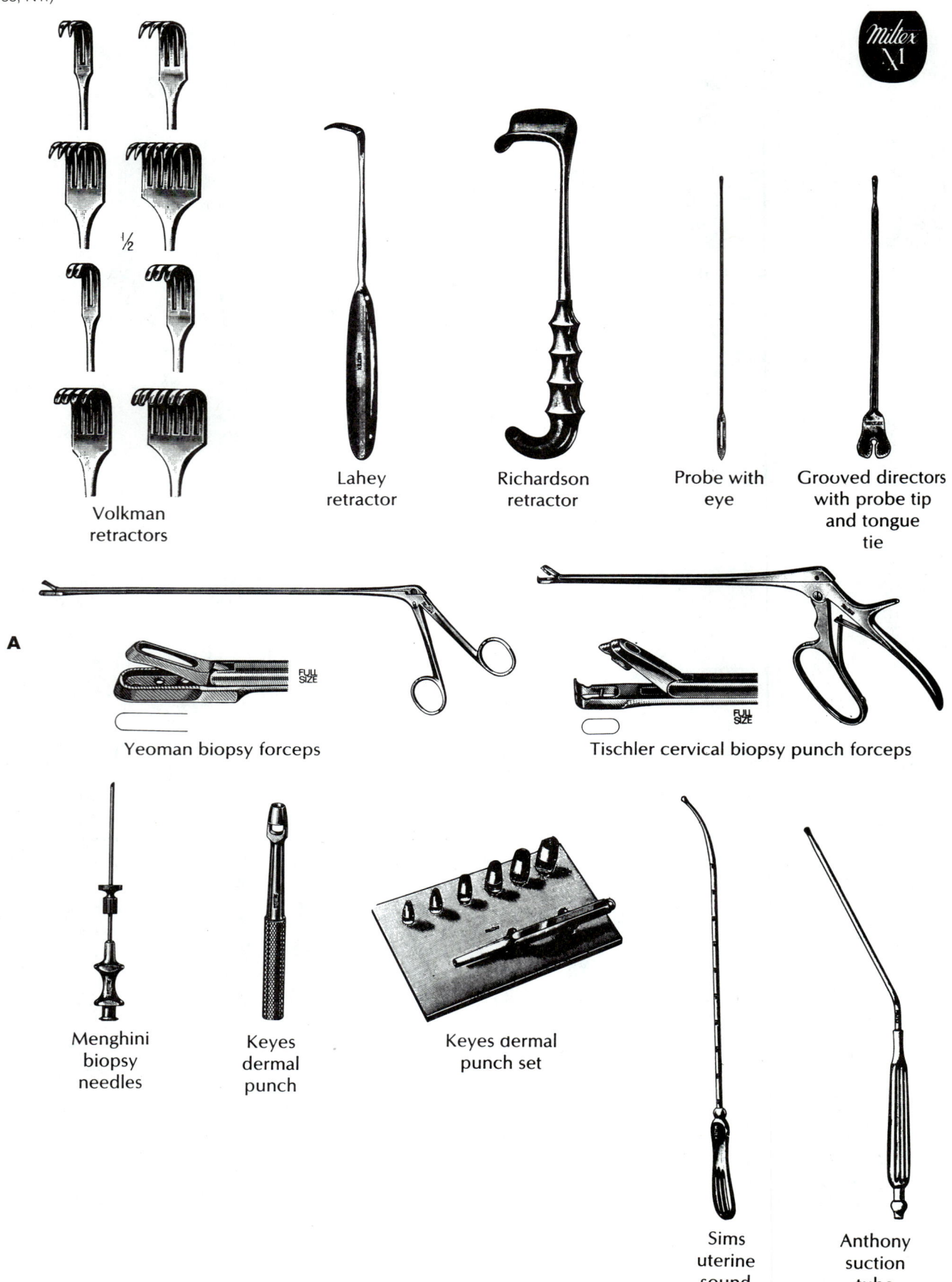

Volkman retractors

½

Lahey retractor

Richardson retractor

Probe with eye

Grooved directors with probe tip and tongue tie

A

Yeoman biopsy forceps

Tischler cervical biopsy punch forceps

Menghini biopsy needles

Keyes dermal punch

Keyes dermal punch set

Sims uterine sound

Anthony suction tube

FIGURE 6-14   **B,** Cryosurgery unit and probe.

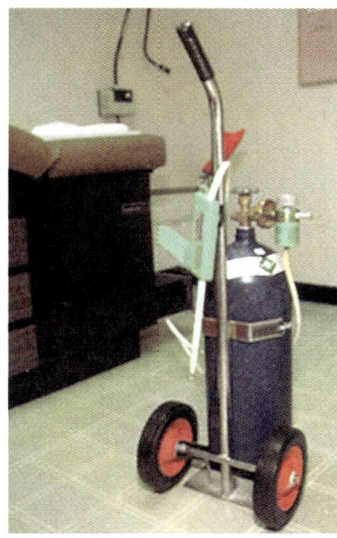

B

FIGURE 6-15   *Left,* Serrated tip on forceps; *right,* serrated tip with groove in the middle, as seen on some needle holders.

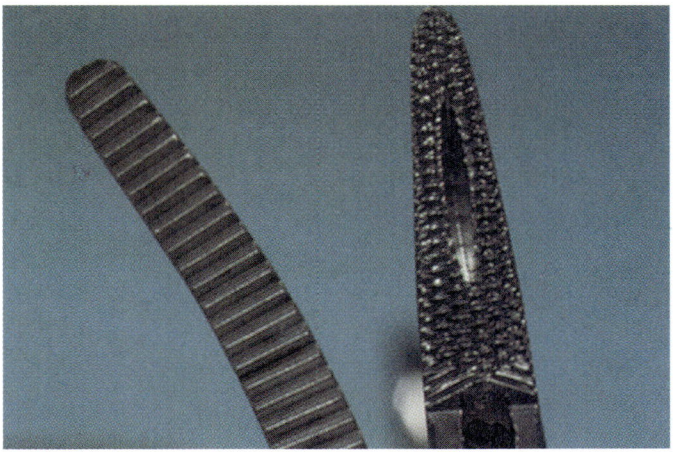

5. Keep sharp and lensed instruments separate from other instruments to prevent damage.
6. Keep ratchet handles open when not in use. This prolongs the usefulness of the instrument.

Preparing the Patient for Minor Surgery

When a patient is to have minor or major surgery or other major forms of therapy, the physician must explain the nature, benefits, and risks of the procedure and the alternatives available, as well as the probable outcome if the procedure is not performed. These details allow the patient to give an **informed consent** for the procedure. Informed consent is a *right,* not merely a privilege. By law, the patient's consent is required for these types of treatment. A consent form (Figure 6-16) giving the physician permission to perform the procedure must be signed by the patient before the procedure is started. Consent forms are usually specific to each facility. The patient *must understand* what he or she is signing. If this is not done, numerous legal complications may result. The consent form documents that the patient understands the services that will be provided by the physician. To safeguard against errors, the consent form *should* also provide details that can be used to verify the operative site, such as a biopsy of the *left* breast.

Although the explanation is the physician's responsibility, often the medical assistant must briefly explain the procedure once again on the day of the surgery while preparing the patient and be ready to answer numerous questions that the patient may have. Remember, any surgical procedure is an invasion into body parts; although the surgical procedure may be minor, it often does not appear minor to the patient. Many patients are anxious, nervous, or concerned about what is going to happen. You can and must help the patient relax and allay any fears or apprehensions. Prepare supplies and equipment required for the procedure in advance. Have everything ready when the patient arrives. Make sure that the room is spotlessly clean, well lit, and at a comfortable temperature. Do not have instruments exposed for the patient's view because seeing them may make some patients more apprehensive.

When the patient arrives in the office, greet and usher him or her into the treatment room. Have the consent form ready to sign. Provide a patient gown and give directions for the removal of clothing. Attend to the patient's needs for comfort *and* communication and give emotional support and reassurance. Once again, a simple explanation of the procedure may be needed. Be willing to answer any questions that the patient may have. Always maintain a calm and confident manner as you are preparing the patient. This in itself can help to reassure and relax the patient.

The best of care can be enhanced by evaluating every patient and situation individually. In this way you can provide the most suitable environment for each individual. Also, when deemed necessary, ascertain that the patient has arranged to have someone accompany her or him to the office or clinic and provide transportation home.

Assisting With Minor Surgery

Careful preparation and adherence to aseptic technique are required when preparing for office or clinic surgery. The responsibilities of the medical assistant during minor surgery include preparing the room and supplies; preparing the patient, both physically and mentally; and assisting the physician as needed. An efficient assistant can make the procedure easier for the patient and the physician by giving attention to both. Similar preparatory steps and equipment are used in most minor surgical procedures, although they may vary according to the physician's preferences. A general procedure for assisting with minor surgery is presented, followed by sample lists of materials needed for the most common surgical procedures performed in a physician's office or clinic.

Text continued on p. 317

FIGURE 6-16   Sample consent form required for surgical procedures and other medical procedures.

AUTHORIZATION AND CONSENT TO SURGERY OR SPECIAL DIAGNOSTIC OR THERAPEUTIC PROCEDURES

To: _____

Name of Patient

This Medical Center maintains personnel and facilities to assist your Surgeon and Physician in performing various surgical procedures and other diagnostic and therapeutic procedures.

This form is meant to insure those of us responsible for your care that you have been informed about the nature of the operation or procedure(s).

1. Your attending physician(s) is/are: _____

_____

_____

2. You have been scheduled for the following operation or procedure(s): _____

_____

_____

3. _____ will be responsible for conducting this/these operation or procedure(s). He/she may be assisted by interns and residents. He/she may also be assisted by anesthesiologists, pathologists, and radiologists from the medical staff of the Medical Center. These persons are in attendance for the purpose of performing specialized medical services, such as anesthesia, pathology, or radiology. Except for interns and residents, none of the foregoing is an agent or employee of the Medical Center or your attending physician because they are independent contractors who have agreed to provide services to you.

4. You have been informed of the purpose, the nature, and risks of this/these operation or procedure(s), of their expected benefits or effects and of available alternative methods of treatment and their risks and benefits by your physician(s) and surgeon(s).

5. You have the right to authorize or refuse any proposed operation or procedure any time before it is performed. Should an emergency occur, additional procedures may be carried out as considered to be necessary by your physician or surgeon.

6. The pathologist is hereby authorized to use his/her discretion in disposing of any member, organ, or other tissue removed from your person during the operation or procedure(s).

YOUR signature is your acknowledgment:

7. a. That you have read, understood, and agreed to the above.

   b. That your physician(s) has/have explained the proposed operation or procedure(s) to your satisfaction, including providing you with all of the information described above.

   c. That you authorize and consent to the performance of the operation or procedure(s).

Date: _____   _____

Time: _____   Patient/Parent/Guardian/Conservator

_____   _____

           Witness   (If signed by other than Patient, indicate relationship)

HEALTH MATTERS

KEEPING YOUR PATIENTS INFORMED

The following information may be printed as an informational sheet that is given to a patient before the procedure is performed.

WOMAN'S CLINIC
Laparoscopy

Your doctor has recommended a procedure called laparoscopy. This procedure is usually a same-day surgery procedure. This means that a light general anesthesia is administered. You can return home the same day after you have recovered and may be able to resume your routine activities in a few days. Strenuous work or sports should be avoided for about a week.

A laparoscope is a long, slender telescope with a light that the physician uses to view the abdomen and possibly diagnose injury or disease of the abdominal organs. It is very valuable in determining causes of infertility, including endometriosis, scar tissue, tubal quality, abdominal masses, ovarian enlargement, fibroids, and infections. This is also a means of performing permanent sterilization (tubal ligation).

After the anesthesia has taken effect, the doctor will make a small incision below the naval. A needle is inserted, and the abdomen is filled with carbon dioxide, which separates the organs for a clear view through the laparoscope. At the end of the procedure the laparoscope is removed, and this gas is released through the incision. The incision is closed with a suture and covered with a Band-Aid. You will recover in the Same-Day Surgical Unit, where a nurse will check your blood pressure and monitor your recovery until you are ready to go home. Someone must come to the hospital to take you home.

After laparoscopy, some discomfort may be noticed. Occasionally, abdominal or shoulder pain results from the gas, which normally is absorbed within 24 hours. Pain can also occur in the neck and throat. A slight discomfort may be felt at the site of the incision. Sometimes patients do experience immediate postoperative nausea or chest discomfort.

You will be given a follow-up appointment in the clinic to go over the results following the procedure and to check the incision in 2 weeks. If you experience severe abdominal pain, unexplained fever, redness, swelling, drainage from the incision, or any other severe symptoms, you must report these to your physician.

HEALTH MATTERS

KEEPING YOUR PATIENTS INFORMED

When patients are going to have surgery, preoperative information will be given or mailed to them. It is vital that they understand all directions to enable the best of care. After outpatient minor surgery, written postoperative instructions will be provided to the patient. The following are examples of preoperative information and postoperative directions that may be given to the patient. Read these to become familiar with the types of directions that are provided as part of total patient care and education.

MEDICAL CENTER

Welcome and thank you for selecting the Medical Center for your health care needs!

You are scheduled to have surgery at the Medical Center located at 123 Elm Street on _____ at

_____.

The following is some information that we hope will clarify the presurgical preparation process for you. Your physician will schedule your surgery under one of two types of anesthesia:

Type of anesthesia	Required number of hours, nothing to eat or drink before surgery (*DO NOT* drink even water or coffee)	Time to arrive to the hospital
Monitored care/local standby, regional, or general anesthesia	*8 hours before surgery*. Nothing to eat or drink after midnight the night before and nothing to eat or drink on the morning of the surgery.	1½ hours before scheduled surgery. Register on the first floor and report to the third floor
Local anesthesia	May eat lightly unless physician states otherwise. ***No*** milk products	1 hour before scheduled surgery

We require preregistration between 24 hours and 96 hours before surgery. This is done in the Registration area, ground floor, between the hours of 8 AM and 5 PM. No appointment is necessary. Please bring with you any insurance card(s) that you may have. Please register first at admitting and then please go to the nurse's station located around the corner from admitting.

OR

The nurse will call you to schedule a time to register.

At the time of preregistration, you will meet our Surgical Nurse Facilitator, who will review your health history, give you instructions for the day of surgery, and answer any questions that you may have. If you need any laboratory, x-ray, or EKG studies, these can be completed at this time.

Continued

Reminders:

- Do not take any aspirin for 1 week before surgery ____(date)____ _____. You may take Tylenol or Advil for pain before surgery.
- If you take medication(s) on a daily basis, please bring them with you on the day you preregister.
- If you are scheduled to see an internist or family doctor to have a physical examination, please let him or her know that your surgery will be done at the MEDICAL CENTER so that he or she may direct any reports or laboratory results to the MEDICAL CENTER.
- If you have a monitored care/local standby, regional, or general anesthetic, you are required to have someone accompany you home. Please be prepared to let the Surgical Nurse Facilitator know who will be taking you home.
- After surgery you may purchase any medication(s) that your physician prescribes for you at the Medical Center or the pharmacy of your choice.
- Parking at a nominal fee is available at the MEDICAL CENTER (Valet Parking) or at the Elm Street garage (self-park).

Please call if you have any questions or concerns.

Phone numbers:

Registration	123-4567
Ambulatory Surgery Unit	123-4578
Surgical Nurse Facilitator	123-4589
Ambulatory Surgery Unit Fax	123-0051
Admitting Fax	123-0052

POSTOPERATIVE INSTRUCTIONS: BREAST BIOPSY

1. You can expect some pain and swelling in the area of your incision. This is normal and will go away with time. You may also note a firm ridge under the incision in the next few weeks. This is called a *healing ridge* and is a sign that the wound is healing properly. This too will resolve in the next few months.
2. You may note some bruising form around your incision. This is a common occurrence and should resolve in time.
3. It is advised that you wear your bra for support for the first 2 to 4 weeks.
4. An ice pack over the wound helps cut down on pain and swelling and will assist your postoperative recovery.
5. You may remove the outer gauze dressing on the second day after surgery and resume showering or bathing. There may be tapes on the skin crossing the actual incision. These are called *Steri-strips* and need to be left in place to support the wound. There are no sutures to remove because they are internal and will be absorbed by your body.
6. You should avoid aggressive physical sports or exercise for the next 3 to 4 weeks because the wound is healing. Walking is a good temporary replacement to your usual routine.
7. You must make an appointment to see your surgeon in the next 7 to 10 days. Please call 112-3344 to schedule the appointment.
8. **IF YOU HAVE ANY PROBLEMS OR QUESTIONS, DO NOT HESITATE TO CALL US AT 112-3344.**
9. Please call our office for your biopsy results if you have not heard from us by 4 PM on the third day after your surgery.
10. Pain medicine has been prescribed to relieve your discomfort after surgery. We strongly suggest that you use them as directed. If you anticipate needing a refill, please contact our office before 3 PM Friday. Our call coverage will not renew narcotic prescriptions over the weekend.
11. If you have had a general anesthesia:
    a. Do not drive or operate complicated machinery for 24 hours.
    b. Avoid making important decisions or signing important papers for 24 hours.
    c. Do not drink alcoholic beverages for 24 hours.
    d. Adhere to a diet of liquids or light nourishment for your first meal. If you tolerate this, you may resume your normal diet.
12. If you develop any of the following symptoms, notify your doctor immediately:
    a. Temperature greater than 100° Fahrenheit
    b. Intolerable pain, swelling, or bleeding

If problems arise or if you are unable to urinate or tolerate liquids by mouth within 6 hours, please call your doctor. If you are unable to contact your doctor, please go to the emergency room at MEDICAL CENTER at 123 Elm Street or your nearest emergency room.

Discharge medication: _____

Special instructions: _____

_____, MD

Return to doctor's office: _____Phone: _____

A copy of these instructions have been given to the patient and/or patient's representative.

_____, RN/LVN   Date _____

Patient/Legal Guardian Signature: _____

If signed by other than patient, indicate relationship: _____

POSTOPERATIVE INSTRUCTIONS FOLLOWING TISSUE BIOPSY OR MINOR SURGERY—LOCAL ANESTHESIA

1. Unless your doctor has said otherwise, limit your physical activities for at least the first 24 hours.
2. Try to keep movement and straining in the area to a minimum for 2 to 3 days.
3. Try to keep your dressing clean and dry. You may remove the outer bandage after 24 hours.
4. You may bathe as usual after 48 hours.
5. If your operative site is an extremity, elevate that extremity for 24 hours. This will minimize pain and/or swelling.
6. With local anesthesia you may resume your normal diet.
7. If you develop any of the following symptoms, notify your doctor immediately:
   a. Temperature greater than 100° Fahrenheit
   b. Intolerable pain, swelling, or bleeding

IF PROBLEMS ARISE, PLEASE CALL YOUR DOCTOR. IF YOU ARE UNABLE TO LOCATE YOUR DOCTOR, CALL (123) 456-7890, AND ASK FOR THE PHYSICIAN ON CALL.

Discharge medication: _____

Special instructions: _____

_____, MD

Return to doctor's office: _____Phone: _____

A copy of these instructions have been given to the patient and/or patient's representative.

_____, RN/CMA   Date _____

PROCEDURE 6-5

ASSISTING WITH MINOR SURGERY

Objective

Understand and demonstrate the correct procedures for selecting and preparing the correct equipment for a minor surgical procedure using aseptic technique; preparing and assisting the patient, and assisting the physician during a minor surgical procedure.

PROCEDURE

1. Check that the room is spotlessly clean, well ventilated, and well lit.

2. Wash your hands. Use appropriate personal protective equipment (PPE) as dictated by facility.

3. If electrical or battery-run equipment is to be used, check it for working order.

4. Assemble and prepare supplies and equipment.
  a. Open and place a sterile drape towel on a clean and dry tray or Mayo stand. This will be used as a sterile field.
  b. Place the required supplies and instruments on this sterile field. Sterile supplies are to be handled with sterile transfer forceps or sterile gloved hands (refer to the section on handling sterile supplies).

   When the required instruments come wrapped in the same package or in a commercially prepared package, open the wrapper and use it for the sterile field. Then, with individually wrapped sterilized hemostats or gloved hands, organize the instruments for use (Figure 6-17, *A*). Refer to the previous section on opening sterile packages.

5. Cover this sterile setup with a sterile towel until ready to use (Figure 6-17, *B*).

6. Obtain any medications or solutions that will be required during the procedure.

RATIONALE

Avoid contamination to the sterile setup.

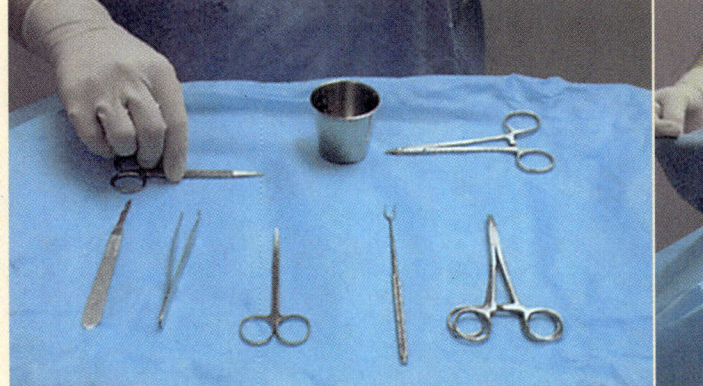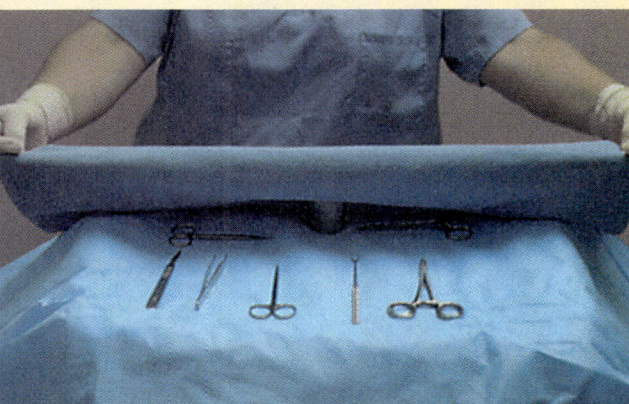

FIGURE 6-17 **A,** Use sterile gloves to organize instruments for minor surgery. **B,** Cover sterile setup with a sterile towel until ready to use.

Continued

PROCEDURE 6-5

ASSISTING WITH MINOR SURGERY—cont'd

7. Open outer wrap of the sterile glove pack for the physician.

8. Prepare the patient. Refer to the preceding discussion on preparing the patient for minor surgery.

   a. Explain the procedure. Have the necessary consent forms ready for the patient to sign.

   b. Provide a gown and instruct on clothing that must be removed.

   c. Have the patient void if necessary.

   d. Position the patient according to the type and location of surgery that is to be performed. The patient must be made comfortable, whether sitting or in a prone or supine position.

Avoid any undue tension or movement during the operation.

   e. If required, wash the operative site with soap and water and shave the area. (Materials for preparing the skin are listed on p. 317.)

The skin cannot be sterilized. Washing helps to reduce the risk of contamination. Microorganisms can also grow on hair; therefore the physician may request that you shave the operative area and surrounding skin.

SKIN PREPARATION

   a. Pull skin taut to shave (Figure 6-18).

   b. Rinse and dry the shaved area.

   c. Wash area with an antiseptic soap, using a firm, circular motion. Start at the center and move outward (Figure 6-19). Do not return to the washed area.

   d. Rinse and blot dry with sterile gauze.

9. Summon the physician. The physician dons gloves, injects the local anesthetic (when one is required), paints the skin with an antiseptic solution such as povidone-iodine, and drapes the operative area with sterile drapes.

These drapes provide a sterile area around the operative area, thus helping to reduce contamination to the surgical wound.

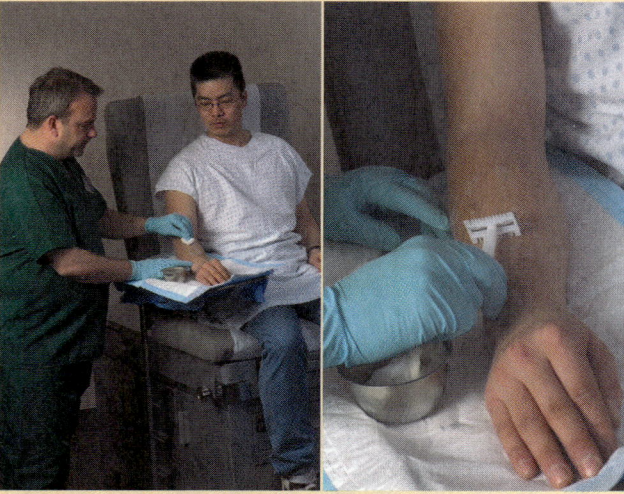

FIGURE 6-18   When shaving the skin in preparation for minor surgery, pull the skin taut and be careful not to cut it.

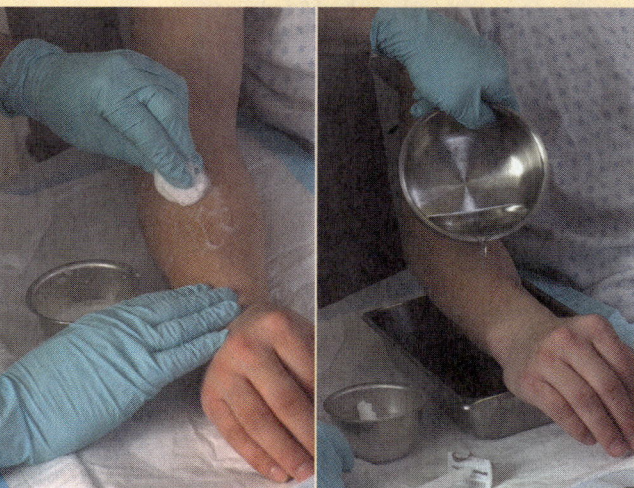

FIGURE 6-19   Using an antiseptic soap, wash operative area with a firm circular motion. Start at the center and move outward. Rinse area.

PROCEDURE 6-5

ASSISTING WITH MINOR SURGERY—cont'd

10. When the physician has donned the sterile gloves, remove the sterile towel that is covering the tray of instruments. Standing behind or to the side of the instrument tray, carefully grasp the two distal corners of the towel. Slowly lift the towel off by lifting it toward you. You must not touch anything but the two distal ends of the towel.

If you touch anything, you may contaminate the sterile setup.

11. Assist the physician as requested. If additional supplies are needed, you must use surgical aseptic technique when handing them to the physician or placing them on the sterile field. (Refer to the previous section on handling sterile supplies.)

12. Offer the patient physical and emotional support. It may be necessary for you to steady the patient's arm, hand, leg, head, or any body part to prevent moving or jerking while the physician is operating. Casually and calmly talk to the patient.

Casual and calm conversation may help to direct attention from any pain or discomfort being experienced and may help the patient relax.

13. Do not stand between the patient and the physician, between the physician and the light source, or too near the sterile setup.

The operative area must not be obstructed. Sterile supplies must not be contaminated.

14. **If you actually help the physician and handle the sterile supplies during the procedure, you must again scrub your hands thoroughly before the procedure begins, don sterile gloves, and sometimes also don a sterile gown.** During the procedure, you are expected to hand the instruments to the physician and to receive them after use. When directly assisting the physician with the instruments, you must anticipate the physician's needs (that is, you must know when the physician will need an instrument or other supplies). You must hand an instrument over so that when the physician grasps it, it is ready to use without need for adjustments.

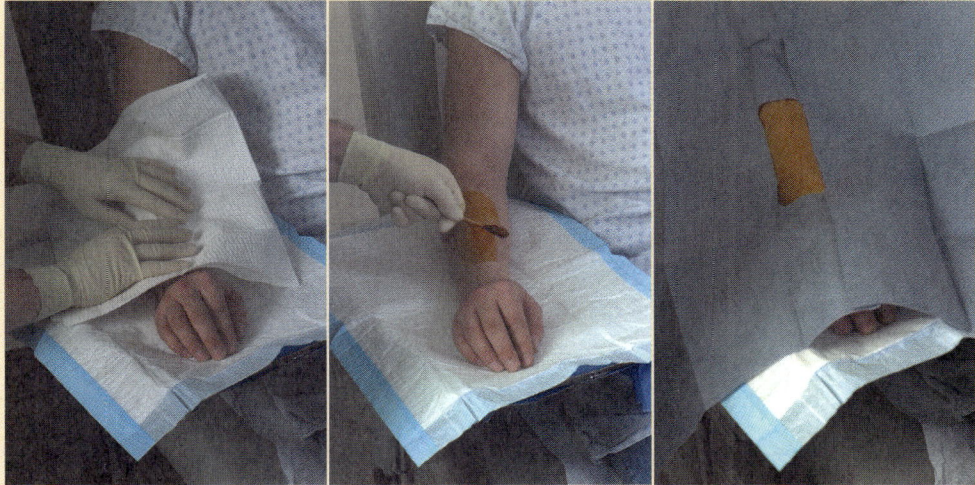

FIGURE 6-19—cont'd   Blot area dry with sterile gauze. Paint the skin with antiseptic solution and drape the operative site with a sterile drape.

Continued

PROCEDURE 6-5

ASSISTING WITH MINOR SURGERY—cont'd

15. Hold containers for collecting specimens, drainage, or discharge near the work area when needed (Figure 6-20). Wear disposable, single-use examination gloves when there is any chance that you will have direct contact with a specimen or drainage.

Wear gloves for your protection.

16. Place soiled instruments in a basin or container, out of the patient's view, when they are no longer needed. Avoid contaminating the remaining sterile supplies.

17. Place soiled sponges and dressings in a plastic bag. Do not allow wet items to sit on a sterile field.

Contamination will result.

18. When a biopsy is obtained, immediately place it into the designated jar containing a preservative solution (see Figure 6-20). Hold the lid of the container so that the underside of the lid is facing down.

Do not touch the inside of a specimen jar because it is sterile. Holding the lid in this position helps to prevent contamination of the underside of the sterile lid by microorganisms in air currents or by objects touching it.

19. Label the specimen jar with the patient's name, the date, and the source of the specimen. Ensure that the lid of the jar is closed securely.

20. After the surgery, it is often advisable to allow the patient to rest for a short while. When sedation has been administered, never leave the patient alone on the examining table unless it has guard rails.

21. Help the patient prepare to leave the office. Do not allow the patient to leave the office without the physician's knowledge. Check with the physician regarding future treatments, medications, and appointments. Often the physician gives the patient instructions regarding postoperative care to be performed at home (see Health Matters on p. 312).

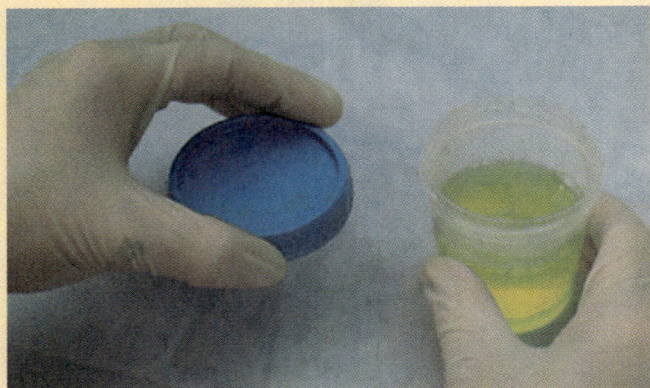

FIGURE 6-20   Hold container for receiving specimens or discarding near the work area.

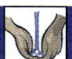

PROCEDURE 6-5

ASSISTING WITH MINOR SURGERY—cont'd

22. Provide clear and concise postoperative instructions to the patient, when necessary. When indicated, make sure that the patient knows and understands about the following:

   a. Compresses

   b. Elevation of the affected part(s)

   c. Presence of a drain

   d. Changing dressing—how often, how it should be done, what to look for (drainage, healing, and so on), and how long to continue

   e. The possibility of pain and the use of medications ordered for this

23. Send any specimen(s) collected to the laboratory along with a properly completed laboratory requisition. (See Chapter 11, Collecting and Handling Specimens.) Record in the patient's chart the date and time that the specimen was sent to the laboratory.

This provides documentation that the specimen was properly attended to.

24. When the patient has left, sanitize reusable instruments and supplies, discard disposables properly, and clean and prepare the room for the next patient. When time permits, clean all instruments for sterilization, sterilize, and return them to the proper storage area, following the procedures presented in Chapter 2.

25. Wash your hands.

Materials for Office Surgeries

The following are sample lists of equipment used for minor office surgeries that may vary with the individual physicians' preferences and the case. Supplies and instruments can be added or deleted to meet the requirements of the particular situation. Once you learn the physician's preferences, you can prepare lists for each procedure and use them as a reference when preparing for minor surgery. Figure 6-21 shows standard instruments used for medical-surgical purposes, Figure 6-22 shows supplies and instruments used for procedures involving incisions *without* suture closure, and Figure 6-23 shows supplies and instruments used for procedures involving an excision of tissue and closure *with* sutures. Figure 6-24 shows a setup for major surgery.

Materials basic to all procedures
- Individually wrapped sterile forceps
- Sterile gloves for the physician
- Sterile gloves for the assistant when directly assisting with the procedure

NOTE: When using instruments for the following setups that have been soaking in a chemical solution, rinse them in sterile water before using.

Materials for preparing the skin area
- Surgical detergent for washing the skin
- Sterile sponges (cotton balls and gauze—2 × 2 and 4 × 4 inch)
- Sterile forceps
- Antiseptic solution such as povidone-iodine (Betadine) for disinfecting the skin
- Razor and blade (if skin is to be shaved)
- Draping materials

Materials for administering local anesthesia
- Sterile antiseptic in sterile container such as povidone-iodine solution (Betadine)
- Applicators or cotton balls and a forceps to use when painting the skin to disinfect it; prepackaged sterile povidone-iodine applicators are available and may be used instead
- Sterile syringe (3 or 5 cc)
- Sterile needles: 25-gauge, $\frac{1}{2}$ inch, and 23- or 24- gauge, $1\frac{1}{2}$ inch (size and gauge vary with site to be infiltrated)
- Local anesthetic: ampules or vials of lidocaine 1% or 2% or procaine hydrochloride 1% or 2%. For a topical spray anesthetic, ethyl chloride may be used

FIGURE 6-21 Instruments used for medical-surgical purposes. **A,** Types of scissors. *Left to right,* Straight iris scissors, curved Iris scissors, suture scissors, curved Metzenbaum blunt blade scissors, disposable suture scissors, bandage scissors with the flat blunt tip to prevent puncturing skin when cutting away bandage; **B,** *Top (left to right),* punch biopsy forceps, No. 11 scalpel blade and handle. *Bottom (left to right),* Straight mosquito forceps, curved mosquito forceps, straight Kelly forceps, curved Kelly forceps, tissue forceps plain tipped, tissue forceps toothed tipped, Allis clamp, needle holder.

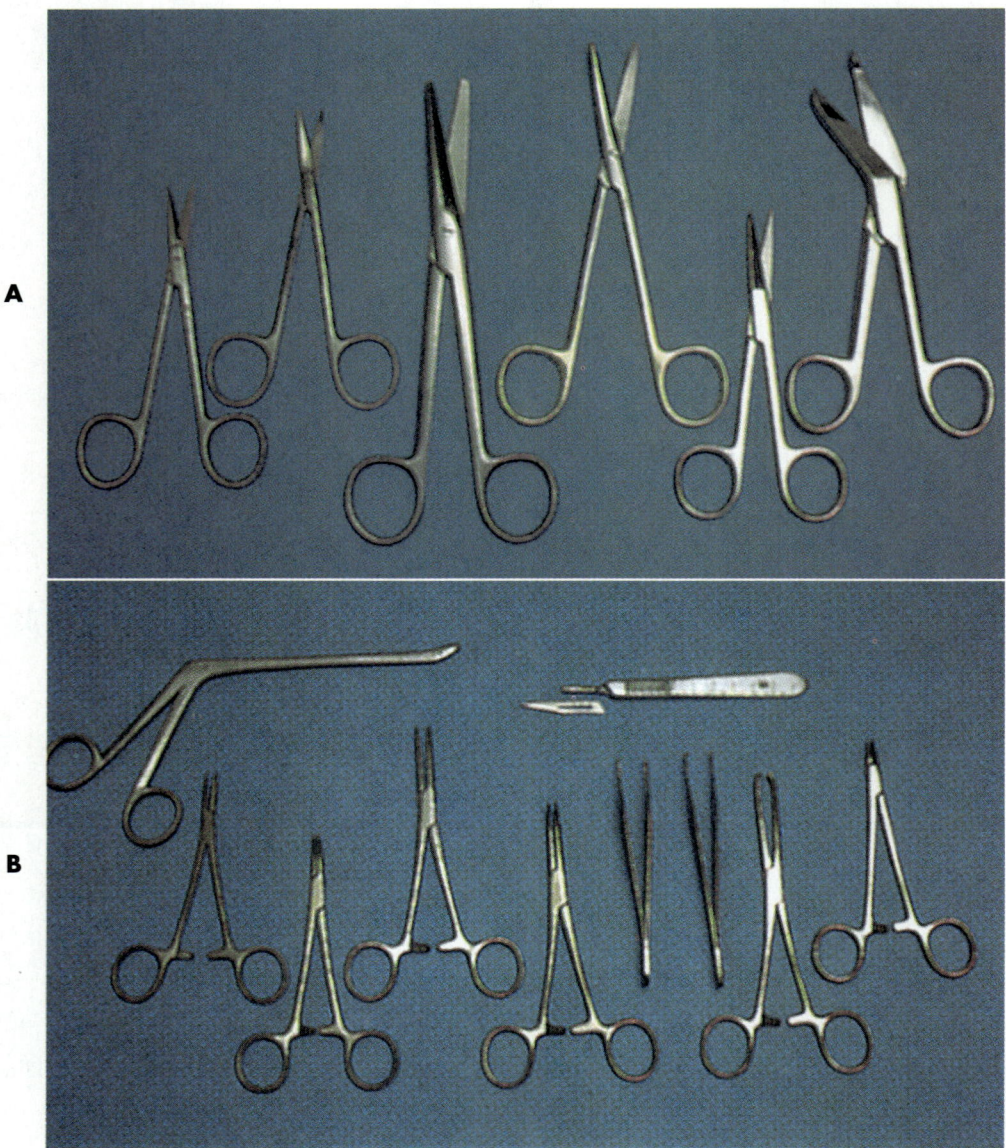

- Alcohol sponge to cleanse the vial top
- Sterile gloves (depending on physician's preference and procedure to be performed)

This setup may be prepared individually or added to the sterile setup used for the procedure.

Materials for suturing lacerations
- Materials for preparing the skin
- Local anesthetic setup
- Sterile gloves
- Toothed-tipped tissue forceps
- Hemostat
- Needle holder
- Suture scissors
- Suture material with suture needle
- Sterile gauze: 2 × 2 and 4 × 4 inch (for sponging and dressing wound; larger dressings are needed for lacerations larger than 3 inches)
- Adhesive or, preferably, hypoallergenic tape and bandage scissors to cut it
- Container for used instruments and sponges
- Biohazard bag or waste container for sponges and gloves

FIGURE 6-22   Supplies and instruments used for minor surgery involving incision **without** suture closure. Materials for preparing the skin: container with sponges in surgical detergent and razor with blade. Materials for local anesthesia: vial of local anesthetic medication, 3-cc syringe with needle, alcohol sponge (other antiseptic solutions could be used rather than alcohol sponge). Other supplies and instruments: sterile gloves for the surgeon; 4 × 4 and 2 × 2 inch sponges; and instruments *(left to right)*—No. 3 scalpel blade and handle, scalpel blades *(top to bottom,* No. 11, No. 10, No. 15), curved Iris scissors, straight mosquito forceps, tissue forceps (plain tipped).

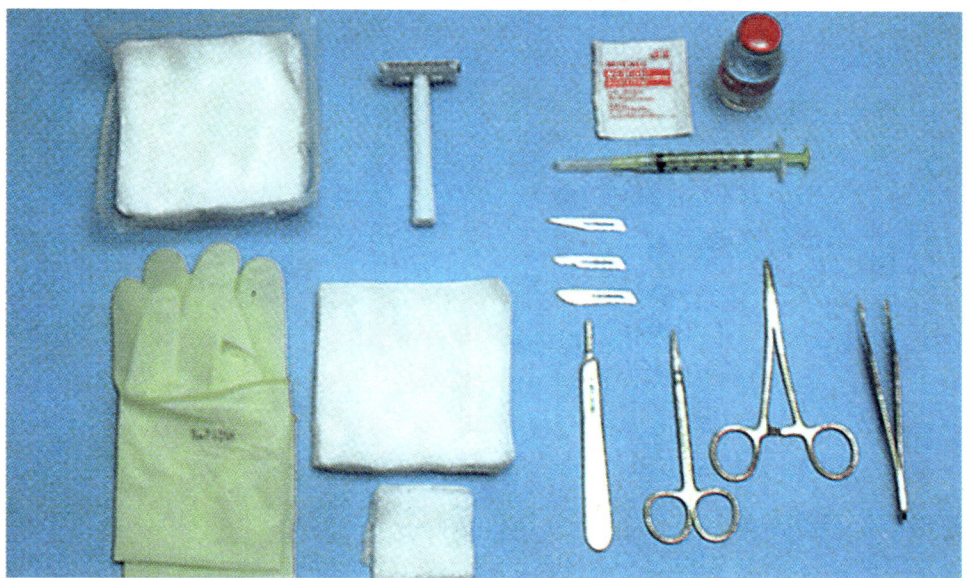

FIGURE 6-23   **A,** Supplies and instruments used for minor surgery when excising tissue and closing the skin **with** suture materials. *Left and along the top,* materials for preparing the skin and administering local anesthesia, sponges, and sterile gloves for the surgeon. Additional supplies and instruments *(left to right):* No. 3 scalpel blade handle, No. 10 *(top)* and No. 15 scalpel blades, toothed-tipped tissue forceps, curved Iris scissors, curved and straight mosquito forceps, straight and curved Kelly forceps, suture scissors, needle holder with mounted curved atraumatic needle with suture materials, and container for specimen with preservative solution.

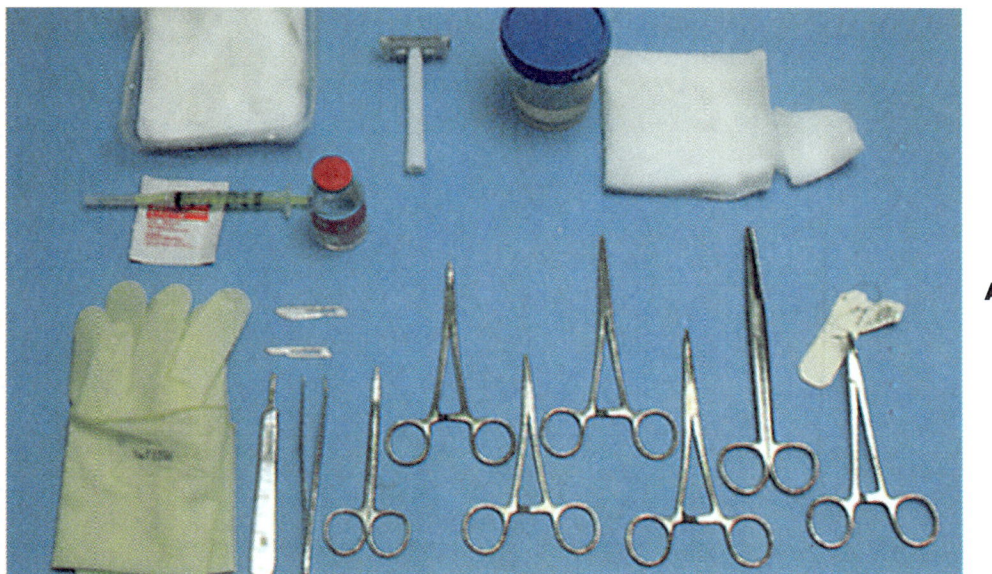

A

Continued

FIGURE 6-23—cont'd   **B,** Laboratory requisition to accompany tissue specimen for cytology and/or pathology testing.

B

OUTPATIENT CYTOLOGY/PATHOLOGY REQUISITION

M E D I C A L   C E N T E R

**SHADED AREA MUST BE COMPLETED FOR BILLING
PLEASE PRINT**

FOR LAB USE ONLY	BILL:
SPECIMEN NUMBER	☐ PHYSICIAN'S/INSTITUTION ACCOUNT

LAST NAME   FIRST NAME

BILL:
☐ PHYSICIAN'S/INSTITUTION ACCOUNT
☐ PATIENT
☐ PATIENT'S/INSURANCE (COMPLETE INFO BELOW OR ATTACH COPY OF CARD)

PREVIOUS NAME (IF DIFFERENT FROM ABOVE)   DATE OF BIRTH   SEX

PATIENT ADDRESS

MEDICARE #   MEDI-CAL #

CITY   STATE   ZIP

INSURANCE INFORMATION
PROVIDE AS MUCH AS POSSIBLE

TELEPHONE NO./PATIENT   SOCIAL SECURITY NO.

GUARANTOR (IF OTHER THAN PATIENTS)

CARRIER

CHIEF COMPLAINT

CARRIER ADDRESS

CLINICAL HISTORY   SERVICE DATE

INSURED'S NAME

IDENTIFICATION NO.

| LMP | HORMONES: (SPECIFY) | PREGNANCY ☐ NOW LAST ___/___/___ | POST MENOPAUSAL? ☐ | IRRADIATION DATES | GROUP NO. |
| | | | HYSTERECTOMY? ☐ | | INSURED'S EMPLOYER |

☐ SEND COPY OF REPORT TO: ☐ CALL RESULTS TO:

PHONE:

CYTOLOGY

PAP SMEAR	☐ Cervix	☐ Endocervix	☐ Vagina
PREVIOUS SMEARS:	☐ MC	☐ Elsewhere	☐ None

Diagnosis: _____

☐ OTHER CYTOLOGY [Site:]

PATHOLOGY

☐ CERVICAL BIOPSY

☐ ENDOCERVICAL	☐ BIOPSY	☐ CURETTAGE
☐ ENDOMETRIAL	☐ BIOPSY	☐ CURETTAGE
☐ PRODUCTS OF CONCEPTION	☐ TAB	☐ SAB

☐ FINE NEEDLE ASPIRATE [Site:]

☐ BIOPSY, SKIN	☐ Punch	☐ Shave	☐ Excision

☐ BIOPSY, PROSTATE [Diagram site]

☐ BIOPSY, OTHER [Site:]

GENERAL INSTRUCTIONS FOR CERVICAL/VAGINAL PAP SMEARS:
1. Please fill out history completely.
2. Label all specimen containers and slides with patient's FULL name.
3. Prepare one or two smears of material from scraping and brushing of cervical canal and/or cervical os.
4. Fix slide(s) immediately.

Department of Pathology
Paul Wilson, MD, Director

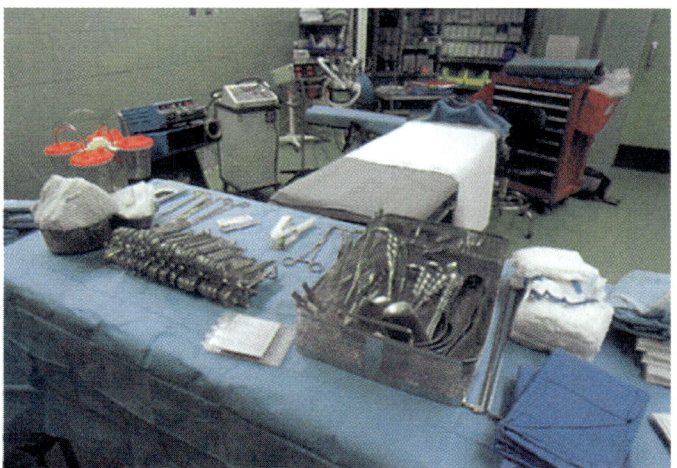

FIGURE 6-24 Setup for major surgery. Note the difference in the instrument setup required for major surgery versus that presented in Figures 6-21 and 6-22 for minor surgery.

NOTE: If the wound is infected or abscesses are to be incised, suture material is not needed because infected wounds are usually not sutured.

Materials for incision and drainage (I & D) of an abscess or cyst (see Figure 6-22)

- Materials for preparing the skin
- Local anesthetic setup
- Sterile gloves
- No. 3 scalpel handle and blade; usually a No. 11 blade or a No. 15 blade for finer and smaller incisions
- Iris (small) sharp scissors to dissect and cut with; sometimes larger blunt scissors are also needed
- Tissue forceps
- Hemostat
- Rubber drain to be inserted to provide drainage during healing, when indicated. (Size varies with the size of the incision and area drained. If the drain is sutured to the skin for support, suture material, suture needle, and needle holder are needed.)
- Sterile gauze for sponging and dressing the wound (2 × 2 and 4 × 4 inch)
- Adhesive or, preferably, hypoallergenic tape and bandage scissors to cut it
- Container for used instruments and gauze sponges
- Biohazard bag or waste container for contaminated disposable articles

Materials for removing foreign bodies in subcutaneous tissues, small growths, and tissue biopsy specimens (see Figure 6-23)

- Materials for preparing the skin
- Local anesthetic setup
- Sterile gloves
- Mosquito forceps, straight and curved
- Kelly forceps, straight and curved
- No. 3 scalpel handle and blade (No. 10 or No. 15 blade) and the electrocautery unit, including a lubricated lead plate, that is placed under the patient for grounding purposes; this plate is not needed when the table is grounded; some tables are supplied with an electrical system that is grounded to an electrical wall outlet
- Iris scissors (small sharp scissors)
- Toothed-tipped tissue forceps
- Suture scissors
- Suture material and needle
- Needle holder
- Sterile gauze for sponging and dressing the wound (2 × 2 and 4 × 4 inch)
- Adhesive or, preferably, hypoallergenic tape and bandage scissors to cut it
- Container for used instruments and sponges
- Biohazard bag or waste container for contaminated disposable articles
- Specimen bottle containing a preservative solution for a tissue biopsy specimen; Zenker's solution or formalin 10% are the preferred solutions used to preserve small tissues, warts, and moles
- Biopsy forceps are also needed for obtaining a biopsy from certain body sites, such as the uterine cervix; in this case, dressing materials or tampons are needed to pack the area after the biopsy has been obtained, in addition to instruments used in pelvic examination (see Chapter 5)
- Laboratory requisition

Materials for a cervical biopsy

- Materials for preparing the skin—skin antiseptic solution
- Sterile gloves
- Vaginal speculum
- Uterine dressing forceps
- Cervical biopsy punch forceps
- Coagulant gel or foam
- Sponges
- Uterine tenaculum
- Vaginal packing or tampon
- Specimen bottle with preservative solution such as 10% formalin
- Laboratory requisition
- Biohazard bag or waste container for disposable contaminated articles

Colposcopy. A colposcopy is an examination of the vagina and cervix done with a colposcope. A colposcope is a lighted instrument with lenses that magnify and focus an intense light on the tissues of the vagina and cervix. This allows the physician to observe the anatomy of these tissues in greater detail. Through the colposcope the physician can see areas of abnormal tissue that can be removed by biopsy or cryosurgery. A colposcopy is performed to assess patients with cervical lesions that were observed during a pelvic examination, to assess the cervical cells and tissues when the results of a Pap smear fall within abnormal ranges, to visualize abnormalities, to assess patients who were exposed to diethylstilbestrol in utero, to obtain a biopsy specimen, and at times to substitute for a cone biopsy when the physician is evaluating the cause of abnormal cervical cytologic findings.

If biopsy specimens were taken, the patient may have some vaginal bleeding. Provide a perineal pad for the patient. Inform her that she may have a coffee-colored granular discharge for about 3 days. Also instruct her to call the physician if she has excessive bleeding or discharge. (See also Pelvic Examination and a Pap Smear in Chapter 5.)

Endocervical curettage.

Depending on the findings from a colposcopy and to further examine for precancerous conditions, the physician may perform an endocervical curettage (ECC), cryosurgery, or both. In an ECC, cells are scraped from inside the cervical canal. This is necessary when the physician cannot see this area during a colposcopy. The ECC can help the physician determine a more precise diagnosis and plan treatment accordingly.

Cryosurgery.

When the endocervical curettage shows that the cervical canal has no dysplasia (an alteration in the shape, size, and organization of cells or an abnormal development of cells), cryosurgery may be performed. Cryosurgery (also known as cryotherapy) in this area of the body is commonly used to treat any type of cervical erosion or chronic cervicitis. Freezing temperatures ($-40°$ to $-80°$ C) are used in this treatment method. The physician uses the colposcope to magnify the surface of the cervix. Then a low-temperature probe is applied to the affected area, freezing and destroying the involved cells. The patient may experience some cramping resembling menstrual cramps and may be given a mild analgesic, such as naproxen (Anaprox) or ibuprofen (Advil), before the procedure and a prescription for the same after the procedure. It is important that she use sanitary pads and not tampons because she would not want to irritate the tissues that had been treated. Explain to the patient that she will most likely have a clear, watery discharge for about the next 4 weeks, to report any foul odor or unusual discharge to the physician, to abstain from sexual intercourse for 4 weeks, to douche with a dilute vinegar and water solution, and to schedule a return visit in 6 weeks so that the physician can determine if the cervix is healing properly. The new cells that grow during healing are usually normal.

Endometrial biopsy.

An endometrial biopsy (EMB) is done for the following reasons:

- To detect endometrial carcinoma and precancerous conditions
- To monitor the effects of hormonal therapy on the uterine endometrium, including the effects of estrogen in patients with suspected ovarian dysfunction, or to determine adequate levels of circulating progesterone
- To routinely screen selected patients for early detection of endometrial carcinoma; the American Cancer Society recommends that women at high risk have this done at menopause; a woman is considered to be at high risk if she has a history of infertility, obesity, failure to ovulate, or abnormal bleeding or if she has had or is undergoing estrogen therapy
- To determine if ovulation has occurred

- To detect inflammatory conditions or polyps
- To assess abnormal uterine bleeding

As for the previous gynecologic procedures, the patient is placed in a lithotomy position (see Chapter 5), and the physician performs a bimanual pelvic examination by placing one hand on the woman's abdomen and one or two gloved fingers of the other hand in the woman's vagina to determine the position of the uterus (see Figure 5-20). The physician then administers the local anesthetic. After the anesthetic has taken effect, the physician inserts the uterine sound and then the Knovak suction tube curette into the uterus to obtain the specimens, *or* the physician may use an endometrial suction curette that has centimeter markings on it so that uterine sounding can be done with the same instrument. Specimens are obtained and placed in the specimen bottles containing 10% formalin and sent to the laboratory for histologic examination. After the procedure, provide the patient with a sanitary pad. Inform her that some vaginal bleeding is to be expected but, if excessive bleeding occurs, she must inform the physician. Also tell her that she should not douche or have sexual intercourse for the next 72 hours. A mild analgesic may be prescribed for any discomfort.

Materials for a colposcopy

- Sterile gloves
- Vaginal speculum
- Sterile gauze: 4×4 inch
- Long (8-inch), sterile cotton-tipped applicators
- Acetic acid 3% (some physicians may use Lygol's solution instead of or in addition to acetic acid)
- Kevorkian biopsy forceps (for a cervical biopsy)
- Endocervical curette (for an endocervix tissue sample)
- Two specimen bottles with 10% formalin preservative; label bottle No. 1 *cervical* and bottle No. 2 *endocervical*
- Coagulating agents (Monsel's solution or silver nitrate applicators may be used after a biopsy has been taken)
- Perineal pad
- Laboratory requisition
- Biohazard bag or waste container for contaminated disposable articles

Materials for a vulvar biopsy

- Sterile gloves
- Materials for preparing the skin area
- Sterile needle: 30 gauge, 1 inch
- Sterile syringe: 3 or 5 cc
- Lidocaine 1%
- Cervical punch biopsy forceps
- Coagulating agents (Monsel's solution on a 6-inch applicator or silver nitrate applicators)
- Perineal pad
- Laboratory requisition
- Biohazard bag or waste container for contaminated disposable articles

Materials for an endocervical curettage (ECC)

- Sterile gloves

- Povidone-iodine
- Long cotton-tipped applicators
- Cotton balls
- Sterile gauze: 4 × 4 inch
- Two specimen bottles with 10% formalin (one is used and labeled for the ECC and the second bottle is used and labeled for the EMB)
- Sanitary pad
- Vaginal speculum
- Kevorkian curette *or* a disposable Z-sampler (endometrial suction curette)
- Uterine tenaculum
- Laboratory requisitions
- Biohazard bag or waste container for contaminated disposable articles

Materials for an endometrial biopsy (EMB)
In addition to the materials needed for the endocervical curettage (ECC), add the following:

- Lidocaine 1%
- Spinal needle: 22 gauge
- Syringe: 10 cc
- Uterine sound
- Knovak suction curette with a 10-cc 3-ring syringe *or* an endometrial suction curette, such as the Z endometrial sampler or Pipelle
- Kidney stone or straight packing forceps

Materials for cervical cryosurgery
- Sterile gloves
- Vaginal speculum
- Acetic acid 3% solution
- Long cotton-tipped applicators
- Cryosurgery unit
- Sanitary pad
- Biohazard bag or waste container for disposable contaminated articles

Materials for a 6-mm skin biopsy
- Materials for preparing the skin—skin antiseptic solution or an alcohol sponge
- Local anesthetic setup—sterile needle: 25 gauge, ⅝ inch or 30 gauge, ½ inch; 3-cc syringe; 1% lidocaine
- Sterile gloves
- No. 3 scalpel handle and a No. 15 blade
- Biopsy punch: 6 mm
- Suture set with straight sharp scissors (scissors used to remove the top two layers of skin)
- Suture material: 5-0 black silk and curved needle
- Needle holder
- Sterile gauze: 2 × 2 and 4 × 4 inch
- Specimen bottle with 10% formalin
- Adhesive bandage (used for the dressing over surgical site)
- Laboratory requisition
- Biohazard bag or waste container for contaminated disposable articles

Materials for an aspiration (needle) biopsy of the breast
- Materials for preparing the skin
- Sterile gloves
- Topical spray anesthetic (ethyl chloride is often used)
- Syringe: 12-cc, No. 18 needle, and a sterile culture tube to receive the specimen; most laboratories prefer to receive the specimen in the culture tube because each laboratory may use different procedures for fixing, staining, and examining the specimen
- An adhesive bandage is usually sufficient for the dressing
- Laboratory requisition when a specimen is sent for cytologic or histologic examination

For a **fine-needle aspiration (FNA),** many use a No. 20 gauge 2½-inch needle with a 20-cc syringe.

For a **core biopsy**, add the following:

- Biopsy syringe gun
- Needle: No. 14 or 16 gauge
- Two or three microscopic slides
- Container with preservative and label for the slides
- Biohazard bag or waste container for contaminated disposable articles

Materials for electrocauterization (Figure 6-25)
- Materials for skin preparation
- Local anesthetic setup, depending on extent and site of area to be cauterized; at times this may not be required
- Sterile gloves
- Electrocautery unit
- Extension electrode for the cautery and instruments used for a pelvic examination (see p. 183) for cauterization of the uterine cervix
- Container for used instruments and sponges
- Dressing materials: size and type determined by size and type of area cauterized; an adhesive bandage may be applied to a small area to protect it from irritants; commonly dressings are not applied to small, superficial areas
- Biohazard bag or waste container for contaminated disposable articles

FIGURE 6-25 Supplies and instruments for electrocauterization.

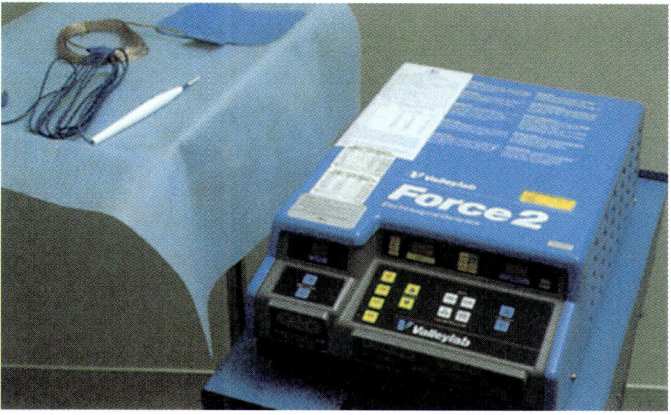

Insertion of an Intrauterine Device

An intrauterine device (IUD) is inserted into the uterus for the purpose of contraception. Only two types of IUDs are available in the United States: the Progestasert (a T-shaped IUD containing progesterone) and the Copper-T (ParaGard) (a T-shaped IUD wrapped with copper wire). The Progestasert IUD must be replaced every year, whereas the Copper-T can remain in place and be effective for 10 years. The physician inserts the IUD usually on the third day of the patient's menstrual period because at this time the cervix may be dilated some and the patient is assumed not to be pregnant. Before the insertion of an IUD, the patient should have had a Pap smear. On occasion, the physician may choose to insert an IUD 5 to 10 days after the patient's menstrual period. The patient is positioned and draped as for a pelvic examination. A consent form must be signed before an IUD is inserted (Figure 6-26).

SUTURE REMOVAL

After the physician has inspected a wound and suture line, the medical assistant may be directed to remove the sutures. (Agency policy and state law determine who can remove sutures.) The condition of the suture line and the progress of healing determine when suture materials can be removed. Depending on the location of the sutures and the progress of healing, sutures are generally removed from the third to the tenth or twelfth day postoperatively. Sutures that are left in place longer than necessary may be a source of infection.

FIGURE 6-26   Consent form for insertion of an IUD.

OB/GYN CLINIC
IUD CONSENT FORM

I have been informed by my physician of alternative methods of birth control and have chosen to use the IUD. I have received literature explaining the use of the IUD. I have read the literature and I understand it. I also understand the risks of insertion and use of an IUD. Some serious complications which may occur are an increased chance of infection, rarely leading to sterility, and possible uterine perforation. I understand that there is still a possibility of pregnancy with an increased risk of miscarriage or, rarely, a tubal pregnancy.

Signed_____
patient
Date_____

Date of insertion_____

Lot number of IUD_____

Name of IUD_____

Date to be changed_____

PROCEDURE 6-6

INSERTING AN IUD

Objective

Understand and demonstrate the correct procedure for preparing the equipment and assisting the patient and physician when the patient is having an IUD inserted.

Equipment (Figure 6-27)

Surgical soap and water
Alcohol or povidone-iodine
Sterile sponges

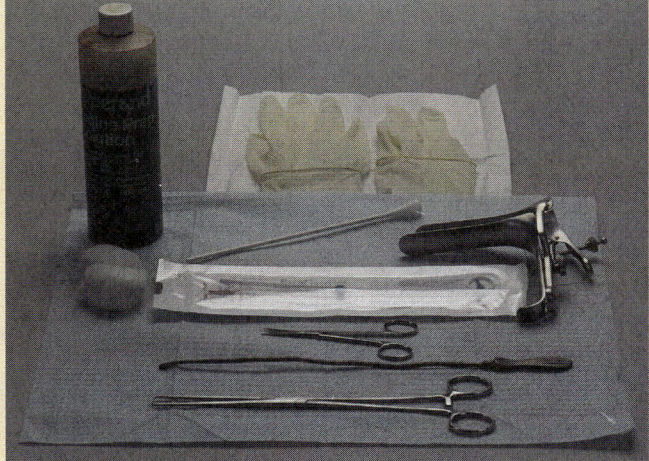 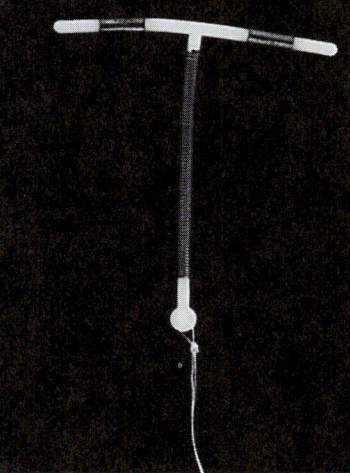

FIGURE 6-27   **A,** Equipment for insertion of an IUD. *Top to bottom,* Sterile gloves, vaginal speculum *(top),* sponge stick, IUD, suture scissors, uterine sound, and single-toothed tenaculum; **B,** Copper-T IUD.

PROCEDURE 6-6

INSERTING AN IUD—cont'd

Vaginal speculum
Sterile gloves
Sterile single-toothed tenaculum
Sterile uterine sound

Sterile sponge stick
Sterile suture scissors
IUD and inserter

PROCEDURE

The physician will:

1. Introduce the vaginal speculum into the vagina.

2. Perform a pelvic examination.

3. Prepare the cervix with surgical soap and water and then with alcohol or povidone-iodine.

4. Grasp the cervix with the single-toothed tenaculum.

5. Introduce the uterine sound into the uterus to check for depth.

6. Prepare and insert the IUD.

7. Withdraw the IUD inserter.

8. Cut the string attached to the IUD with suture scissors.

9. Perform a digital examination.

PROCEDURE

The medical assistant should now:

10. **Wash hands** and assemble the equipment. **Use appropriate personal protective equipment (PPE) as dictated by facility.** (Step 10 should be completed before patient's arrival.)

11. Help the patient assume a supine position for 5 to 10 minutes to prevent the state of shock.

12. Elevate the patient's head 45 to 50 degrees for 5 minutes.

13. Have the patient sit up with legs over the side of the table and maintain this position for a few minutes to ensure that the patient's condition is stable.

14. **Give the patient further instructions:**
    a. If bleeding, fever, or pain occurs, notify the physician.
    b. Check for the presence of the IUD string in the vagina once a month after her menstrual period. (If she cannot find the string, she should make an appointment to see the physician.)
    c. A yearly checkup with the physician is necessary.
    d. The Progestasert IUD must be changed every year because effectiveness decreases after that time span.
    e. Once dressed, she is free to leave.

15. Ask the patient if she has any questions; answer them adequately or refer the patient to the physician.

PROCEDURE 6-7

REMOVING SUTURES

Objective
Understand and demonstrate the correct method for removing sutures from a patient's skin; note the suture line; care of the suture line; give the patient any required instructions; and record the procedure.

Equipment (Figure 6-28)
Sterile gloves
Suture removal kit that includes suture scissors, plain-tipped

tissue forceps, sterile 4 × 4 inch gauze
Antiseptic solution in container (or disposable povidone-iodine applicators)
Sterile applicators or gauze or cotton balls
Container for removed sutures, used instruments, and sponges

Continued

PROCEDURE 6-7

REMOVING SUTURES—cont'd

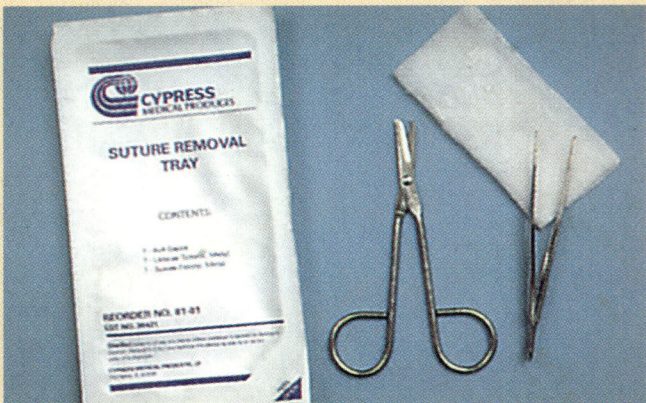

FIGURE 6-28   Sterile, disposable suture-removal kits.

PROCEDURE

1. **Wash your hands** and assemble the equipment. **Use appropriate personal protective equipment (PPE) as dictated by facility.**

2. Identify the patient and explain the procedure. Explain that the patient will feel a slight pulling sensation as the suture is removed.

3. Don sterile gloves.

4. Cleanse the suture line with an antiseptic (for example, povidone-iodine). Start from the incision line and work outward, with one stroke per cotton ball or applicator.

5. Using plain-tipped tissue forceps, grasp the knot of the suture and gently pull it away from the skin.

6. Using suture scissors, cut the suture below the knot (the part that is closest to the skin).

7. To remove the suture, pull it straight up from the skin and place it in the container. Pull gently to keep pain and tissue damage to a minimum.

8. Continue to remove all sutures in this manner.

9. Count the number of sutures that you removed.

10. Note the condition of the suture line.

11. Cleanse the suture line with an antiseptic.

12. Apply a sterile dressing or leave open to the air as applicable.

RATIONALE

Explanations provide reassurance and help the patient to relax.

Maintain surgical asepsis.

Remove bacteria from the incision line.

Cutting this way prevents pulling the knot through the skin.

Using a smooth continuous motion to remove the suture reduces tension on the suture line and patient discomfort. Cutting the suture as close as possible to the skin prevents pulling previously exposed contaminated suture through the skin.

Ensures that all sutures were removed.

A dressing would protect the wound site. Dressing may not be needed unless the patient's clothing would irritate the wound site.

PROCEDURE 6-7

REMOVING SUTURES—cont'd

12. Give the patient any instructions as needed.
Example: Notify the physician if the skin feels warmer than usual and is red, or if there is any drainage or opening of the incision.

14. Dispose of supplies properly.

15. Remove your gloves and **wash your hands**.

16. Record the procedure. Note the date, time, how many sutures were removed, the location of the wound, the condition of the wound site, and any directions given to the patient. Sign your name.

Charting Example

September 23, 20__, 4 PM
6 sutures removed from palm of right hand. Suture line is dry and appears to be healing well.
E. M. Day, CMA

FIGURE 6-29   Types of wounds.

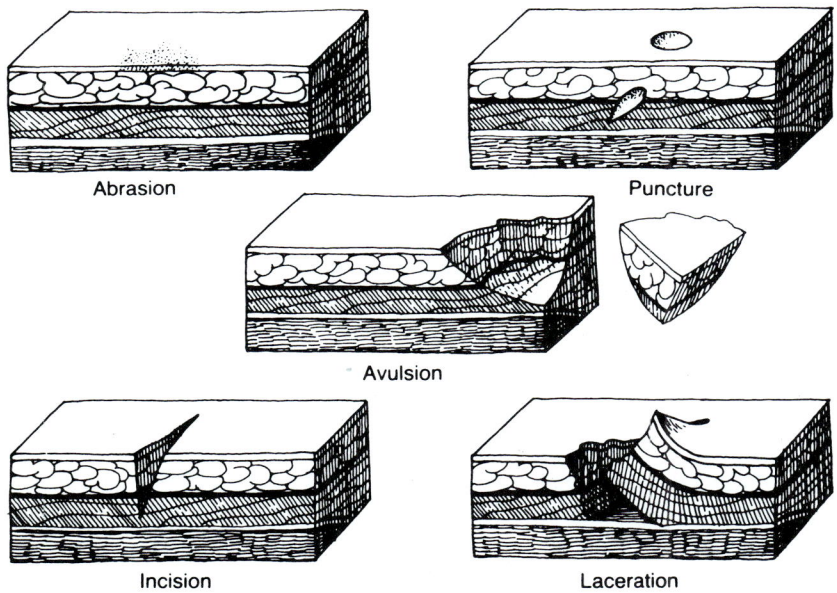

Abrasion

Puncture

Avulsion

Incision

Laceration

WOUNDS

A wound is a break in the continuity of external or internal soft body parts, caused by physical trauma to the tissues. An **open wound** is one in which the skin and mucous membranes are broken; in a **closed wound**, the skin is not broken, but there is a contusion (bruise) or a hematoma (hem-a-to′ma), a tumorlike mass of blood.

Types of open wounds include the following (Figure 6-29):

abrasion (ab-ra′zhun)—A scrape on the surface of the skin or on a mucous membrane (for example, a skinned knee)

avulsion (a-vul′shun)—A piece of soft tissue torn loose or left hanging as a flap

incision—A straight cut caused by a cutting instrument, such as a scalpel (surgical knife), for surgical purposes

laceration (las′e-ra′shun)—A tear or jagged-edged wound of body tissues

puncture—A small, external opening in the skin made by a sharp, pointed object, such as a needle or nail

Microorganisms can invade both open and closed wounds, and an infection can result. **Signs and symptoms that indicate**

the presence of an infection include redness, heat, pain, swelling, and, at times, the presence of pus and a throbbing sensation at the wound site. Fever often accompanies infection. As the temperature rises, pulse and respiration rates also rise. An indication that an infection is spreading from a wound caused by needle pricks, splinters, or small cuts is the presence of a red streak running up the extremity from the wound site.

Wounds that are most susceptible to infection are those in which blood cannot flow freely; those in which tissues are crushed; and those in which the break in the skin closes or falls back in place, thus preventing entrance of air, as seen in puncture wounds.

Common pathogenic organisms causing a wound infection include the following:

staphylococci (staf-il-o-kok′si)—Bacteria that occur in grape-like clusters; gram-positive cocci. Pathogenic species cause suppurative (pus-producing) conditions.

streptococci (strep″to-kok-si)—A type of bacteria occurring in chains; gram-positive cocci.

colon bacillus (*Escherichia coli*)—A type of bacteria; a normal inhabitant of the intestinal tract; gram-negative bacteria. Pathogenic *E. coli* are responsible for many infections of the urinary tract and for many epidemic diarrheal diseases, especially in infants.

gas bacillus (*Clostridium perfringens*)—A type of bacteria; gram-positive bacteria; anaerobic; the most common cause of gas gangrene. (Gas gangrene is a condition often resulting from dirty lacerated wounds in which the muscles and subcutaneous tissue become filled with gas and serosanguineous exudate. It is caused by the species of *Clostridium* that breaks down tissue by gas production and toxins. An exudate is material that has escaped from blood vessels and has been deposited in a body cavity, in tissues, or on the surface of tissues, usually as a result of inflammation.)

tetanus bacillus (*Clostridium tetani*)—A type of bacteria; gram-positive bacteria; anaerobic; spore-forming rods; the causative organism of tetanus or lockjaw. This organism enters the body through a break in the skin, especially through puncture wounds. In this case infection is often obvious. Tetanus and gas bacilli are common in puncture wounds because they are anaerobic (that is, they grow in the absence of oxygen).

One of the body's natural defense mechanisms against infection or trauma is the inflammatory process. It works to limit damage to the tissue, remove injured cells, and repair injured tissues (see also p. 42).

The Healing Process

Wounds heal by first intention or by second intention, depending on damage or loss of tissue. When the edges of wounds can be brought together, as in sutured surgical incisions, or when a minimal amount of tissue is lost or damaged, as in a relatively clean and small cut, they heal by first intention. There will be little inflammation and minimal scarring, if any.

When the wound edges cannot be approximated because of extensive tissue loss or damage, healing by second intention occurs. This is seen in open and infected trauma or surgical wounds, such as after the incision and drainage of abscesses or in major lacerations. Because large amounts of granulation tissue form to fill the gap between the wound edges and to allow epithelial cells to migrate across the wound surfaces from the edges, this healing process is also known as healing by granulation or indirect healing. This is a slower process than healing by first intention; thus it involves a greater risk of infection and usually produces greater scarring.

The healing process normally occurs in the following three stages:

1. Lag phase: Blood serum and cells form a fibrin network in the wound. A clot is formed that fills the wound and begins to knot the edges together with shreds of fibrin. Dried proteins then form a scab.
2. Fibroplasia: Granulation tissue (fragile, pinkish red tissue) forms as the fibrin network absorbs and epithelial cells start forming from the edges to form a scar.
3. Contraction phase: Small blood vessels are absorbed, fibroblasts (cells from which connective tissue develops) contract, and the scar begins to shrink and changes in color from red to white.

The body's ability to heal after any trauma is affected by the general health status of the individual. Good health helps the body deal successfully with injuries and infections.

Care of Wounds

The goals of wound care are to promote healing and prevent additional injury. There are two schools of thought regarding the care of a wound: some prefer to leave the wound undressed, and others prefer to dress a wound.

Most closed wounds are left undressed, as well as some wounds that have sealed and can be protected from additional injury, irritation, and contamination. Exposure to the air helps keep the wound dry and can promote healing. Open wounds covered with a dressing provide a warm, dark, moist area that is suitable for growth of microorganisms. Dressings applied incorrectly can interfere with adequate circulation to the area, which will interfere with the healing process; also, if a dressing does not stay in place, it can cause further irritation to the wound and possibly cross-contamination.

Regardless of the method used (dressed or undressed), a wound must be kept clean, have dead tissue removed, and then be allowed to drain freely.

When a dressing is changed, it and the wound must be inspected for the amount and character of **drainage**, if present. The **amount** is best described as scant, moderate, or large; the **character** refers to the color, odor, and consistency of the drainage. **Common terms that describe drainage are as follows:**

serous—Consisting of serum (clear, straw-colored liquid)
sanguineous—Consisting of blood or blood in abundance

serosanguineous—Consisting of blood and serum
purulent—Consisting of or containing pus (a pale, yellow, creamy, yellow-green sticky fluid exudate)

The condition of the wound, the degree of healing, and the integrity of sutures and drains must also be observed during a dressing change.

DRESSINGS AND BANDAGES

Techniques of applying dressings and bandages vary according to the extent and location of wounds, injuries, or burns; the materials to be used; and the purpose for which they are applied.

Dressings

Dressings are materials of various types placed directly over wounds, open lesions, and burns as the immediate protective covering. When used correctly, dressings serve the following eight purposes:

1. To protect wounds from additional trauma
2. To help prevent contamination of the wound
3. To absorb drainage
4. To provide pressure for controlling hemorrhage, promoting drainage, and reducing edema
5. To immobilize and support the wound site
6. To ease pain
7. To provide a means for applying and keeping medications on the wound
8. To provide psychologic benefits for the patient by concealing, protecting, and giving support to the wound.

To prevent contamination and the possibility of an infection developing, sterile technique and sterile dressing materials must be used when applying or changing a dressing. The only exception is in emergency situations when the patient has serious bleeding. On those rare occasions, it is more important to stop the bleeding than to worry about contaminating the wound with unsterile materials.

Dressing materials.
Various types and sizes of commercial sterile dressings are available (Figure 6-30). Many are made of gauze, such as folded gauze sponges* available in various sizes (for example, 2 × 2 inch, 4 × 4 inch, and 3 × 4 inch) and gauze fluffs, which are loosely folded, large gauze squares used to absorb large amounts of drainage or to pack an opening. Some dressings are made from viscose rayon and cellulose materials such as folded Topper* sponges supplied in 3 × 3 inch, 4 × 3 inch, and 4 × 4 inch sizes; still others are made from a unique, nonwoven, binderless soft fabric called Sofwik,* (for example, Sof-wik dressing sponges, available in 4 × 4 and 2 × 2 inch sizes). Larger absorbent gauze and dressings made from similar materials are available for dressing

large wounds, major burns, or major surgical wounds (for example, Surgi-Pad Combine Dressing* supplied in 5 × 9, 8 × 7½, and 8 × 10 inch sizes) and ABDs, abdominal pads, supplied in 5 × 9 and 8 × 10 inch sizes.

Other dressing materials have a special covering over the gauze to prevent them from sticking to an open or draining skin area. These are called nonadhering dressings. Examples of these include the Band-Aid Surgical Dressing,* which is a complete dressing in a single package, consisting of a nonadherent facing, enclosing an absorbent filler, and backed by Dermicel* tape, available with 4 × 6 inch tape and 4 × 3 inch pad or 8 × 6 inch tape and 8 × 3 inch pad. Telfa† is a gauze dressing with a plasticlike covering on the side that is to be placed over the wound; it is also available in various sizes. Steripak is another complete dressing, made of layers of absorbent cellulose and covered with a nonadhering, perforated plastic material that is secured to a vented adhesive tape. Steripak is available in 4 × 8 inch, 4 × 4 inch, and 2 × 4½ inch sizes. The Adaptic* nonadhering single-layer dressing, made of a highly porous weave, is used as the immediate covering over a wound under an absorbent secondary dressing; it is available in a foil envelope in 3 × 3 inch, 3 × 8 inch, 3 × 16 inch sizes and in a bottle in dimensions of ½ inch × 4 yards for a packing strip. Vaseline‡ petrolatum gauze, a fine-mesh, absorbent gauze impregnated with white petrolatum, is a nonadhering dressing that clings and conforms to the wound. It is used over open or draining wounds to prevent the top dressing from sticking to the wound or disrupting newly formed tissue.

---

*Johnson & Johnson, New Brunswick, NJ.
†Kendall Co, Greenwich, Conn.
‡Chesebrough Pond's Inc, Greenwich, Conn.

FIGURE 6-30 Dressing materials representing a system of wound-management products for use in the care of lacerations and abrasions, multiple trauma, and burns.

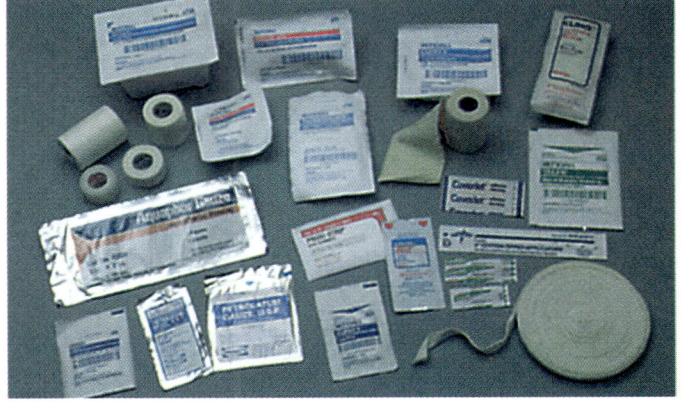

---

*Johnson & Johnson, New Brunswick, NJ.

A third type of dressing material is kept moist in a package; some are premedicated. These are used for debriding tissue, for treating open or ulcerated wounds, and sometimes for dermatologic conditions.

Spray-on dressing materials are also available that, when sprayed over the wound, form a transparent, protective film. These are nontoxic and somewhat bacteriostatic and allow for close observation of an incision or wound site. Fluff cotton or cotton balls are never to be used for dressings because the fibers may get embedded in the wound and are difficult to remove if they do.

To hold dressings in place securely, various types and sizes of tape are available. The types of tape include hypoallergenic cloth tape, hypoallergenic paper tape, transparent tape, elastic cloth tape, and adhesive tape; sizes range from $\frac{1}{2}$ inch to 3 inches.

When changing or applying an initial dressing, select the dressing materials according to the purposes to be accomplished; in other words, know why the wound is to be dressed. This enables you to select the proper types and amounts of dressing materials. Any dressing must be large enough to cover the wound completely and extend at least an inch or more beyond.

In addition to patients who have had minor surgery in the office, patients who have had surgery in the hospital may come to the physician's office for a dressing change or wound culture when necessary. You may assist the physician with these procedures or perform them alone.

Dressing change with a wound culture. When infection is suspected, a wound culture is taken to determine the presence and type of microscopic organism that is causing the infection. Cultures can be obtained from wounds on any part of the body. Soiled dressings are removed and replaced by a sterile dressing.

Current findings suggest that wounds should be **cleansed with sterile normal saline**. Betadine and other antiseptic solutions are cytotoxic (agents that destroy or damage tissue cells) and will not allow the wound to heal. Wound treatment specialists state, "Never clean or irrigate a wound with anything stronger than you would use to irrigate the eye." When the wound has normal serous or sanguineous or serosanguineous drainage, clean the wound with sterile normal saline and apply a dry dressing. If signs and symptoms of inflammation are noted, such as the wound area being red, tender, warm to touch, or swollen or causing any limitation of function, a culture is usually taken *before* the wound is cleansed and then covered with a sterile dry dressing. If the results of the culture indicate an infection, the physician may order an antibiotic for treatment. Antibiotic ointments may also be ordered. Ointments are applied to the dressing, and then the dressing is applied to the wound. Antiseptic solutions such as Betadine *may* be used to clean *closed dry* wounds. This treatment varies with the physician's preference for wound management.

Text continued on p. 336

PROCEDURE 6-8

DRESSING CHANGE WITH A WOUND CULTURE

Objective
Understand and demonstrate the correct procedure for changing a patient's dressing, obtain a wound culture and prepare it to be sent to the laboratory, and record the procedure. Provide education to the patient for changing a dressing at home and have the patient demonstrate to you how he or she will do it at home.

Equipment (Figure 6-31)
To obtain the culture
    Sterile applicator(s) in a sterile culture tube(s) or a Culturette.*
The type of culture tube varies, depending on the specific organism that is suspected. Check with your laboratory to ensure accuracy. Most laboratories request that an anaerobic Culturette be used for wound cultures. Always **check the expiration date** on the outside wrapper before using to ensure stability of the culture medium at the time of use. (See Chapter 11 for additional information on cultures and materials used.)
To change the dressing
    Sterile dressing or a prepackage sterile dressing set containing:
        Tissue forceps
        Hemostat
        Scissors
        Gauze sponges 2 × 2 inch, or cotton balls, or antiseptic swabs

Dry dressings (for example, 4 × 4 inch gauze, Topper sponges, Sof-wik sponges)
Small container for saline *or* antiseptic solution
Antiseptic solution of physician's choice *or* sterile normal saline

*Marion Scientific Corp.

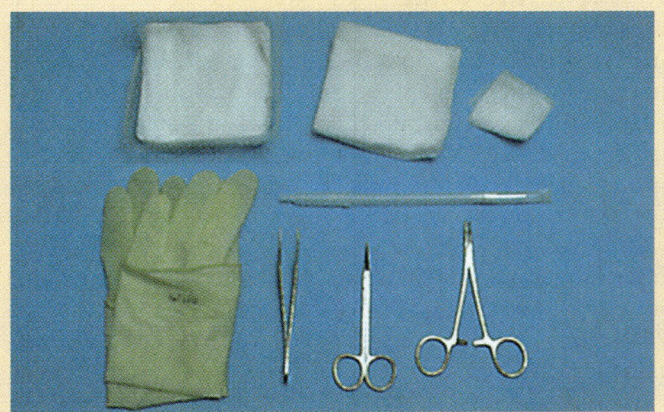
FIGURE 6-31 Supplies and instruments for dressing change with wound culture.

PROCEDURE 6-8

DRESSING CHANGE WITH A WOUND CULTURE—cont'd

Additional equipment

Antiseptic solution, if ordered and not supplied in the prepackaged dressing set, such as povidone-iodine, hydrogen peroxide, alcohol 70%

Tape, preferably hypoallergenic

Plastic bag for soiled dressing and disposable equipment

Disposable, single-use examination gloves

Disposable sterile gloves

Draping materials, as needed

Laboratory requisition

Biohazard bag or waste container for contaminated disposable articles

Sterile transfer forceps (may be used by some)

Optional equipment

Acetone or benzine or commercial tape remover to moisten tape on old dressing for easier removal

Sterile saline to moisten a dressing that has stuck to a wound to allow easier removal

Sterile towels

Additional dressing supplies appropriate to the condition of the wound site (for example, Telfa, adhesive bandages, Steripak, Surgi-Pads, Adaptic dressing, roller gauze bandage, Kling elastic gauze bandage)

PROCEDURE

RATIONALE

1. **Wash your hands. Use appropriate personal protective equipment (PPE) as dictated by facility.**

2. Assemble the equipment. Place the supplies on a flat, clean surface, convenient for use.

3. Identify the patient and explain the procedure. Explain that you will remove the soiled dressing, obtain a culture of the discharge from the wound, and apply a sterile dressing. The culture will then be sent to the laboratory for study. When the physician receives the laboratory report, the appropriate medication to eliminate the causative organism(s) of the infection may then be prescribed.

   Provide reassurance and gain the patient's cooperation.

4. Have the patient put on a patient gown, if necessary. Position the patient, providing for comfort and relaxation. Drape if and as needed, exposing the area where the wound is located. When the wound is on the arm or leg, place a towel under the area to be dressed. Remind the patient not to touch the open wound once the dressing has been removed and not to talk over it because microorganisms can spread into the wound. Gowning, positioning, and draping vary with the location of the wound.

   The important thing to remember is that the part of the body from which the culture is to be obtained and the dressing changed must be well supported and exposed. In addition, the patient's modesty must be protected.

5. **a.** Open the dressing set. Using sterile forceps, arrange supplies in their order of use.

   b. Open plastic bag. Place the bag in a convenient place to receive the soiled dressing and used disposable supplies. Use surgical aseptic technique at all times. The wrapper on the dressing set is used for the sterile field.

   c. Pour the sterile saline *or* antiseptic solution into the sterile container located on the sterile field.

      NOTE: When the antiseptic solution is supplied in the dressing tray set, do not pour the solution until after you have donned sterile gloves.

Continued

PROCEDURE 6-8

DRESSING CHANGE WITH A WOUND CULTURE—cont'd

    d. Cut pieces of tape that will be used to secure the clean sterile dressing when applied. These may be tagged onto the side of your dressing tray.

    e. Don disposable, single-use examination gloves.

6. Loosen tape on the present dressing (Figure 6-32). Loosen and pull tape gently, pulling toward the wound so you don't tear newly formed tissue. When the tape doesn't pull away easily, moisten it with a sponge soaked with acetone, benzine, baby oil, or a commercial tape remover.

7. Loosen and remove the soiled dressing with a sterile forceps (Figure 6-33) or a gloved hand. Do not pull on the dressing. A dressing can also be removed by placing your hand inside a plastic bag. Then grasp and lift the dressing off, inspect for drainage, and invert bag over the dressing. Handle all dressings as if they are contaminated. If you used forceps for this step, set it aside or if disposable, discard in the bag with the soiled dressing. If a dressing is difficult to remove, sterile saline may be applied to help loosen it.

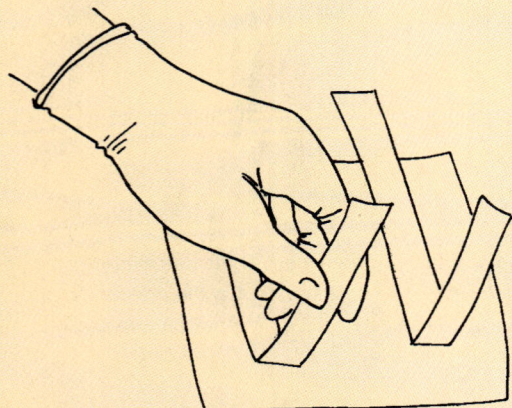

FIGURE 6-32 Technique for loosening tape on dressing.

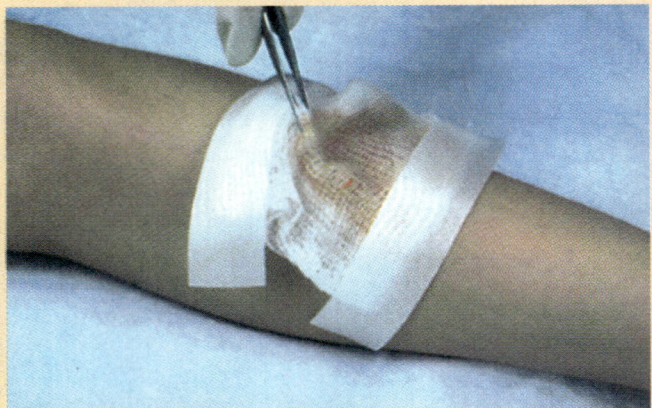

FIGURE 6-33 Remove soiled dressing with a forceps.

PROCEDURE 6-8

DRESSING CHANGE WITH A WOUND CULTURE—cont'd

8. Inspect the dressing and discard it in the plastic bag. Observe the amount and type of drainage on the dressing.

9. Observe the wound. Note the location, type, and amount of drainage coming from the wound and the presence of pus, necrosis, or a putrid odor. Note the degree of healing and when sutures are present, if they are intact.

Accurate observations must be made so that you will be able to chart adequate and accurate information.

10. Remove the sterile applicator from the sterile culture tube or Culturette.* Swab the drainage area of the wound once to obtain a specimen. If you need more of the drainage for culturing, you must use another applicator. Swab only the draining area of the wound. Do not spread the infection to a clean area on the wound. **Swab the wound only once in one direction. Never go back and forth over the area.**

11. Place the applicator(s) in the culture tube(s) and set aside. Secure the lid tightly to prevent air from getting into the tube.

Air causes the specimen to dry, thus destroying the microorganisms.

12. Remove disposable, single-use examination gloves. Dispose of them in the plastic bag.

13. Don sterile gloves as described previously to complete the dressing change.

Gloves are donned to prevent any microorganisms that may be on your hands from entering the wound and also to keep your hands clean.

14. Pick up gauze sponge with forceps or hemostat (whichever is most comfortable for you to use).

15. Dip the sponge into the sterile saline or antiseptic cleansing solution to wet through. Do not oversaturate the sponge. Keep sponge and forceps facing downward.

Many current standard guidelines for wound care state that topical antiseptics are not to be used on open wounds or ulcers.

16. Gently, but thoroughly, cleanse the wound using single strokes over and parallel to the incision, **one sponge per stroke.** Starting at the center of the wound, stroke toward the ends. Cleanse the side farthest from you, working outward from the incision, and then repeat on the side closest to you (Figure 6-34).

Bacterial count is usually lowest at the center of the incision and greatest at the edges. Always work from the least contaminated areas to most contaminated areas to avoid contaminating uncontaminated sites.

*Marion Scientific Corp.

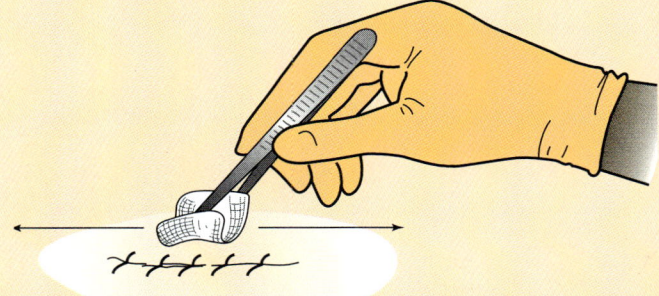

FIGURE 6-34   Cleanse wound, starting at center going toward the end. Use one sponge per stroke.

Continued

PROCEDURE 6-8

DRESSING CHANGE WITH A WOUND CULTURE—cont'd

17. Discard each sponge in the plastic bag for waste after use. Do not touch the bag with the forceps.

18. Repeat the process directly over the wound until it is cleansed to your satisfaction. Use a clean sponge for each single stroke.

19. When cleansing a drain site or a very small wound, move the sponge with sterile saline *or* antiseptic sponge in a circle around the site (Figure 6-35). Cleanse around and away from the wound in an ever-widening circle. Do not go back over a clean area.

20. Discard the sponge and repeat.

21. Apply the sterile dressing. Center it over the wound area. Forceps or gloved hands are used to apply the dressing. Additional layers of dressings are added as indicated by the type of wound and amount of drainage (when present).

22. Discard disposable forceps and gloves in plastic waste bag. Close the plastic bag by tying a knot in the top. Put reusable forceps to the side of the sterile field or in a container for used supplies. Remove gloves by pulling on the cuff and turning inside out.

23. Secure the dressing with tape applied so that it conforms to body contours and movement. Ensure that it is adequately spaced; do not cover the entire dressing with tape (Figure 6-36). Place each strip of tape over the middle of the dressing and press down gently on both sides, working toward the ends. Hypoallergenic tape is preferred. Have equal lengths of tape on both sides of the dressing—not too short or too long. Tape should not cover the entire dressing. Distribute tension away from the incision. Do not tape too snugly.

If tape covers the entire dressing, it interferes with air circulation; if tape is too snug, it may constrict blood flow to the wound and interfere with the healing process.

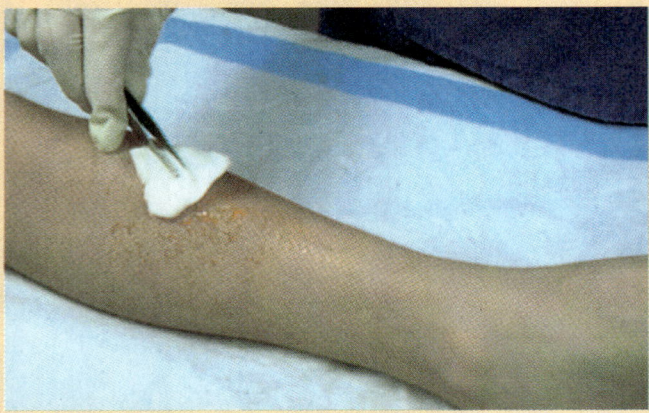
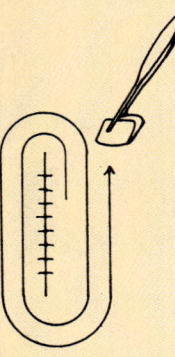

FIGURE 6-35 Cleanse small wound or drain site using circular strokes, working from center to outside portion of wound site.

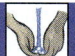

PROCEDURE 6-8

DRESSING CHANGE WITH A WOUND CULTURE—cont'd

24. Attend to the patient's comfort; you may reposition the patient if necessary. Observe the patient for any undue reaction. Provide further instructions as indicated or as ordered by physician. Check if the patient has any questions. Inform the patient if he or she is free to leave. Help the patient dress when necessary.

Patient education for changing a dressing at home:

- Discuss the importance of infection control.
- Demonstrate the correct technique for changing the dressing.
- Give adequate instructions:
  - **a.** Change the dressing in a bathroom near a sink.
  - **b.** Wash your hands.
  - **c.** Wear single-use, disposable gloves when changing the dressing.
  - **d.** Remove the dressing. Discard the dressing and gloves in a plastic bag.
  - **e.** Wash your hands.
  - **f.** Apply a new glove(s).
  - **g.** Cleanse the wound. Depending on the size of the wound, use sterile normal saline on a sterile Q-tip or on sterile gauze.
  - **h.** Apply a new dressing.
  - **i.** Secure the dressing with tape as needed.
  - **j.** Remove glove(s) and wash you hands.
- Remind the patient of any information the physician has discussed, such as signs and symptoms of wound infection, what to do if excessive bleeding occurs, how often to change the dressing, and if another appointment is necessary.

      NOTE: **It is advisable to have the patient demonstrate to you how he or she would change the dressing at home. This helps to ensure that correct techniques will be used.**

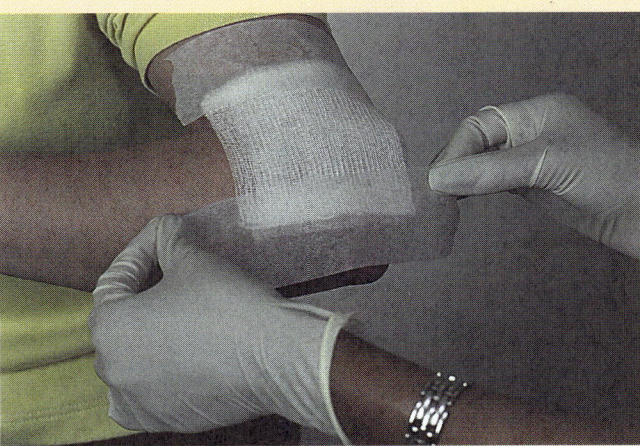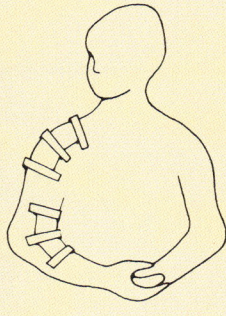

FIGURE 6-36 Correct method of securing a dressing to conform to body contour and movement.

Continued

PROCEDURE 6-8

DRESSING CHANGE WITH A WOUND CULTURE—cont'd

25. Label culture tube(s) or Culturette(s)* completely and accurately. Complete and attach the appropriate laboratory requisition. The label should include the following:
   Patient's name
   Physician's name
   Date
   Time
   Source of specimen
   Test requested

26. Take or send the culture to the laboratory. Avoid delay.

   Delay could cause drying of the specimen.

27. Remove used items from the treatment room; dispose of correctly, for example, in a red biohazard bag used for disposal of contaminated supplies. Discard soiled items and disposable equipment in a covered container according to agency policy. Wearing disposable, single-use examination gloves, rinse reusable instruments under running water and then soak in detergent and water until you are ready to prepare them for sterilization (see Chapter 2).

   Infection control guidelines must be followed.

28. **Wash your hands.**

29. Replace supplies as needed. Leave the treatment room clean and neat.

30. Record the procedure and observations on the patient's chart, using correct medical abbreviations.

   *Marion Scientific Corp.

Charting Example

March 4, 20__, 1 PM
Rt. forearm dressing changed.
Moderate amount of thick, yellow, purulent drainage on lower end of laceration.
Culture taken and sent to laboratory for C & S [culture and sensitivity].
Wound cleansed and dry sterile dressing applied.
Ann Michaelson, CMA

Bandages

Bandages are strips of soft, pliable materials used to wrap or cover a body part. When used correctly, bandages serve four basic purposes:

1. To hold dressings or splints in place
2. To immobilize or support body parts
3. To protect an injured body part
4. To apply pressure over an area

Bandaging materials should be clean, but not necessarily sterile, because they should never come into direct contact with an open wound, as do dressings.

Bandaging materials.   Several types of bandages are prepared commercially.

Adhesive and elastic tape.   Adhesive and elastic tape are supplied in rolls of various widths. When tape is used for a bandage, it is applied directly to the skin. When wrapping a body part with tape, be careful not to cut off circulation by wrapping too tightly. Elastoplast is an example of an elastic adhesive bandage.

Roller bandages.   Roller bandages are available in various widths and materials. *Gauze,* a porous, lightweight, nonstretch material, has little absorbency, does not self-adhere, and does

FIGURE 6-37   A, Triangular bandage; **B,** triangular bandage used for arm sling.

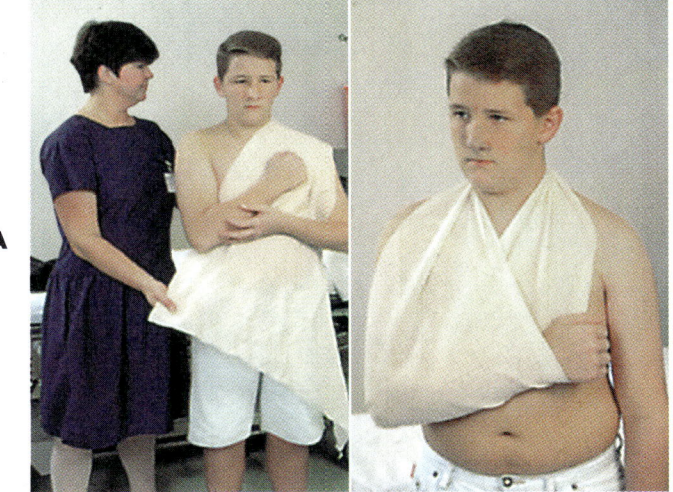

A   B

not conform readily to body contours. However, it is relatively inexpensive.

A preferred type of gauze bandage is the *elastic gauze bandage,* such as Kling. Kling conforms to all body contours, stretches, adheres to itself, and is absorbent; it does not slip with movement and therefore eliminates frequent rebandaging. It is nonocclusive, allowing wound aeration, and thus does not interfere with wound healing.

Elastic bandages.   Elastic bandages, made of woven cotton with elastic fibers, are particularly useful for bandaging areas that require firm support, immobilization, or the application of pressure. Commonly used are the Ace bandage or the Peg bandage, which is self-adhering. Once wrapped around a body part, nonadhering elastic bandages are secured with bandage clips or tape. (See Figure 6-39, which illustrates the application of a Peg bandage.)

Triangular bandages.   Triangular bandages are large pieces of cloth, usually cotton, in the shape of a triangle. These bandages are usually used for slings on an injured arm but can be adapted for use on almost any part of the body (Figure 6-37). A **cravat bandage** can be made by folding the point of a triangular bandage to the midpoint of the base and continuing to fold it lengthwise until the desired width is obtained (Figure 6-38). A cravat bandage can be used to hold a dressing in place, to help support an injured joint, to hold a splint in place, and if necessary, as a tourniquet.

Tubegauz.   Tubegauz, a seamless, tubular-knitted, cotton bandage, is adaptable and conformable to all body areas. Because Tubegauz is tubular, it stays in place with little or no adhesive tape. A finger or cage-type appliance is used to apply Tubegauz to provide a neat and strong bandage (see Figure 6-41 for instructions on applying this type of bandage). Tubegauz is supplied in various sizes from $\frac{5}{8}$ inch to 7 inches. The size of the

bandage to be used is determined by the size of the body part to which it will be applied (for example, a $\frac{5}{8}$-inch bandage can be used on small fingers and a toe of either infants or adults; 1 inch Tubegauz can be used on larger fingers and toes of adults and also on the hands and feet of infants; $1\frac{1}{2}$-inch Tubegauz may be used on the arms and legs of infants and on the arms and feet of children; $2\frac{5}{8}$ inches may be used on the arms and lower legs of adults or the legs and thighs of children; $3\frac{5}{8}$-inch Tubegauz may be used on the heads, arms, shoulders, legs, and thighs of adults and possibly on the trunks of infants; 5-inch Tubegauz is used on the heads and small trunks of adults, and the 7-inch Tubegauz can be used on the trunk of an adult).

Application of bandages.   Important criteria for acceptable bandaging techniques are that the bandage perform its function and that it not cause additional problems or pain. The following measures promote safety and comfort when applying bandages:

- Observe the principles and practices of medical asepsis when applying a bandage.
- Select a bandage of appropriate size for the area to be bandaged.
- Apply bandages to areas that are clean and dry. When an open wound is present, apply a bandage over a dressing.
- Do not have two skin surfaces touching each other under a bandage. Use absorbent material between touching skin surfaces (for example, when bandaging two fingers together, place a padding between them to prevent the skin from rubbing together). Other areas that necessitate similar techniques include the axillary areas (an individual's perspiration provides a moist environment that is conducive to the growth of microorganisms), the areas under the breasts, areas in the groin or folds of the abdomen, and areas between the toes.
- Pad bony prominences and joints over which a bandage must be placed to prevent skin irritation, provide comfort, and maintain equal pressure on body parts.
- Apply bandages on a body part while in its normal functioning position and when placed in a resting position (1) so that deformities will not result and (2) to avoid muscle strain. Joints should be slightly flexed rather than extended or hyperextended.
- Apply bandages with sufficient pressure to attain the intended function (that is, pressure, support, or immobilization) but do not apply the bandage too tightly because this interferes with circulation to the area. Ask the patient if the bandage feels comfortable.
- Wrap the bandage from the end of a limb toward the center of the body to avoid congestion and circulatory interferences in the distal part of the extremity.
- When possible, leave a small portion of an extremity, such as a finger or toe, exposed so that any change in circulation can be observed. Signs that indicate that the bandage is too tight include coldness and numbness to the part, pain, swelling, cyanosis, and pallor. If any of these signs occur, the bandage must be loosened immediately.

FIGURE 6-38 **A** to **D,** Cravat bandage.

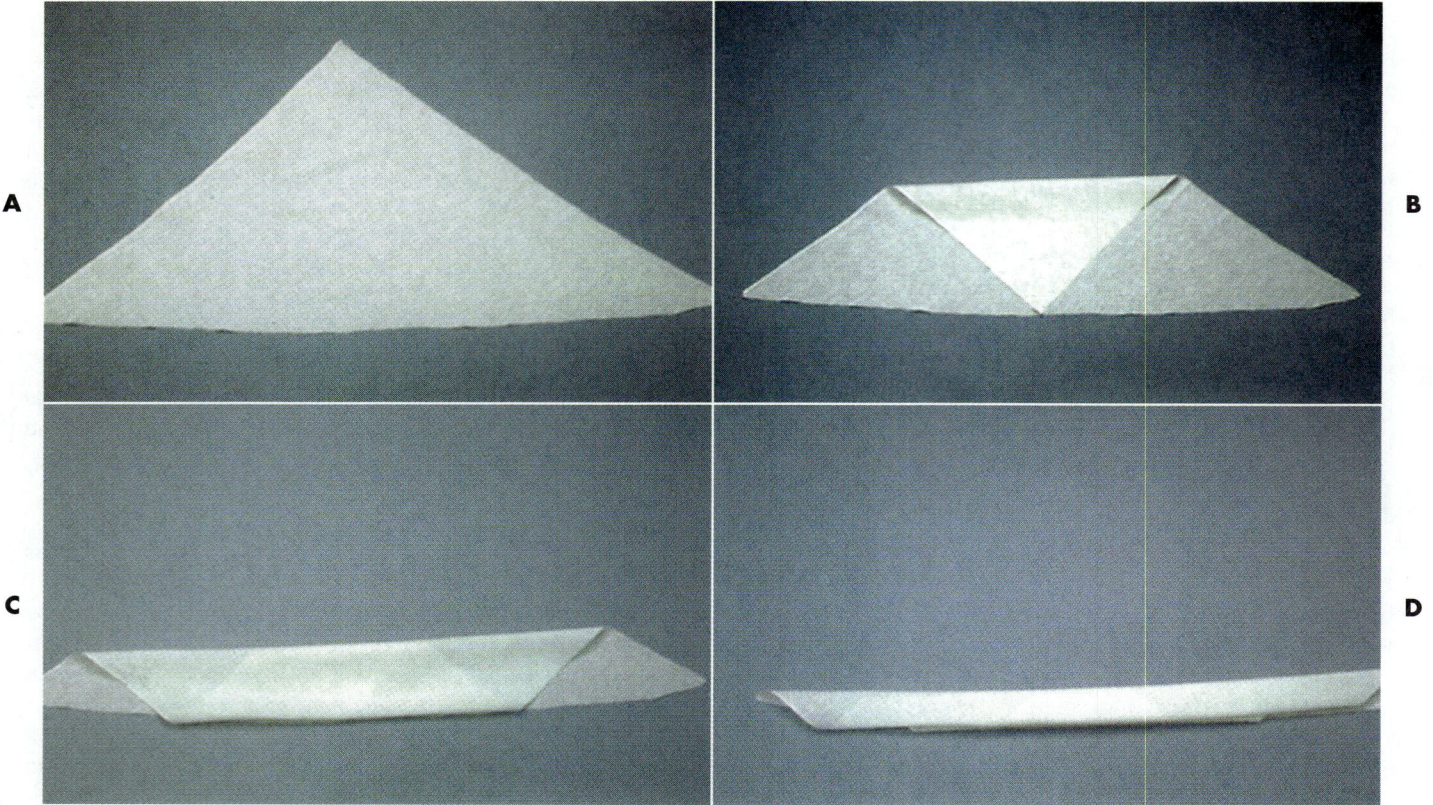

- Apply bandages so that they are secure and do not move about over the area, causing irritation or the need for re-bandaging frequently.
- Apply chest bandages so that they do not interfere with breathing.
- Avoid unnecessary layers of bandages; too many layers are uncomfortable. Use only the amount of bandage material needed to accomplish its purpose.
- Place securing materials, such as clips, pins, or knots, well away from the wound or inflamed area and off pressure points and bony prominences to avoid undue pressure and irritation to the area.
- Check (or inform the patient to check) the bandage at regular intervals to note the circulation to the part and to see if the bandage needs to be reapplied (for example, when it has slipped out of place or loosened to the point at which it is no longer accomplishing its purpose). Also, it is very important to check bandages frequently on injuries or burns involving swelling to ensure that they are not becoming too tight.
- Replace bandages as required. Many bandages can be washed or autoclaved and then reused. Gauze should be discarded and replaced with clean gauze.

Basic wrapping techniques.   There are five basic turns used alone or in combination when applying a roller bandage. The type of turn used depends on the purpose and the area being bandaged (Figure 6-39).

When beginning a wrap with a roller bandage, you may anchor it by placing the outer portion on a bias next to the patient's skin; the bandage is circled around the body part, allowing the corner edge to protrude; the protruding edge is then folded down over the first turn and covered with the second encircling turn of the bandage.

The **circular turn** encircles the part, with each layer of bandage overlapping the previous one. This turn is used most often for anchoring a bandage at the start and at the end and on body parts that are even in size, such as the hand, fingers, toes, and circumference of the head.

The **spiral turn** is applied by angling the turns of the bandage in a spiral fashion with each turn overlapping the previous one by one-third to one-half the width of the bandage. This turn is used on body parts that increase in size where circular turns are difficult to make and on cylindric parts, such as the forearm, fingers, legs, chest, and abdomen.

The **figure-eight turn** consists of diagonal turns that ascend and descend alternately around a part, making a figure eight. This turn is used over joint areas, such as the wrist, ankle, elbow, or knee to support the joint, support a dressing, or apply a pressure bandage.

Figure 6-39 illustrates the circular, spiral, and figure-eight turns, along with wrapping techniques for the Peg self-adhering, elastic bandage.

FIGURE 6-39   Bandage-wrapping techniques illustrating the circular, spiral, and figure-eight turns. The Peg self-adhering elastic bandage is used in these illustrations. (Courtesy Becton-Dickinson, Division Becton, Dickinson and Co, Rutherford, NJ.)

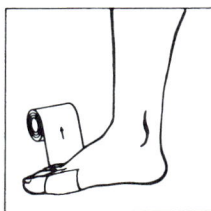

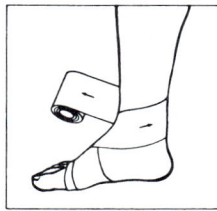

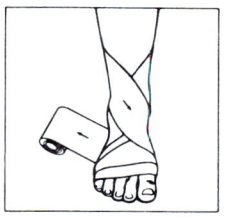

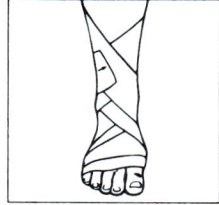

Foot and ankle   Use 3-inch width. Hold foot at right angle to leg. Start bandage on ridge of foot just back of the toes.

Pass bandage around foot from inside to outside. After two or three complete turns around foot, ascending toward the ankle on each turn, make a figure eight turn by bringing bandage up over

the arch—to the inside of the ankle—around the ankle—down over the arch—and under the foot

Repeat the figure eight wrapping two to three times. Fasten end by pressing the last 4 to 6 inches of <u>unstretched</u> bandage to the preceding layer.

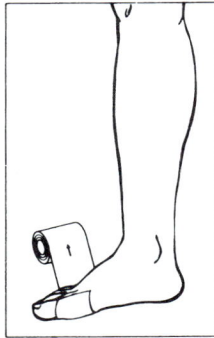

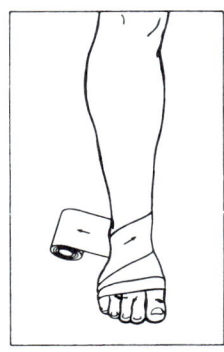

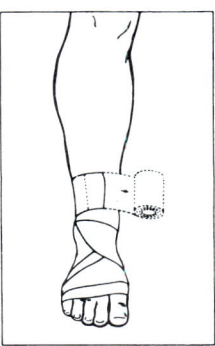

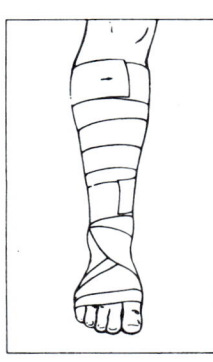

A

Lower leg: Use 3 to 4-inch width depending on the size of the leg. A leg wrap requires two rolls of bandage. Hold foot at right angle to leg. Start bandage on ridge of foot just back of the toes.

Pass bandage around foot from inside to outside. After two complete turns around foot, make a figure eight turn by bringing bandage up over the arch—to the inside of the ankle—around the ankle—

down over the arch—and under the foot. Start circular bandaging, making the first turn around the ankle. To begin the second roll of bandage, simply overlap the <u>unstretched</u> ends by 4 to 6 inches, press firmly, and continue wrapping.

Wrap bandage in spiral turns to just below the kneecap. Fasten end by pressing the last 4 to 6 inches of <u>unstretched</u> bandage to the preceding layer.

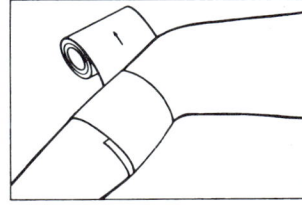

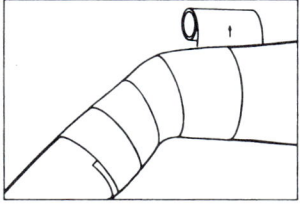

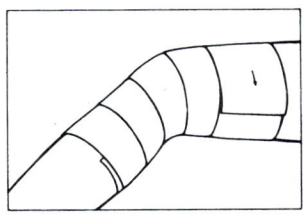

Knee   Use 4-inch width. Bend knee slightly. Start with one complete circular turn around the leg just below the knee.

Start circular bandaging, applying only comfortable tension. Cover kneecap completely.

Continue wrapping to thigh just above the knee. Fasten end by pressing the last 4 to 6 inches of <u>unstretched</u> bandage to the preceding layer.

Continued

FIGURE 6-39—cont'd   Bandage-wrapping techniques illustrating the circular, spiral, and figure-eight turns. The Peg self-adhering elastic bandage is used in these illustrations. (Courtesy Becton-Dickinson, Division Becton, Dickinson and Co, Rutherford, NJ.)

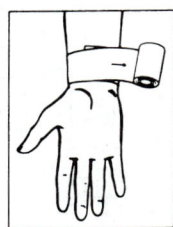 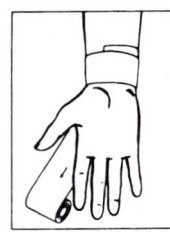 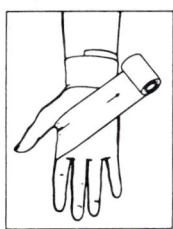 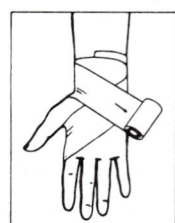 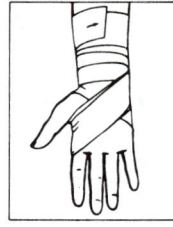

Wrist Use 2- or 3-inch width. Anchor bandage loosely at the wrist with one complete circular turn.

Carry the bandage across the back of the hand, through the web space between the thumb and index finger

and across palm to the wrist. Make a circular turn around the

wrist and once more carry the bandage through the web space and back to the wrist.

Start circular bandaging, ascending the wrist. Fasten end by pressing the last 4 to 6 inches of <u>unstretched</u> bandage to the preceding layer.

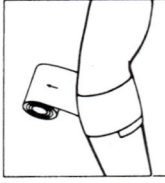 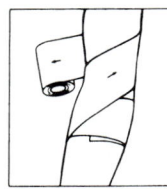 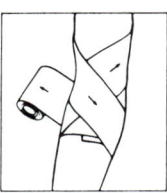 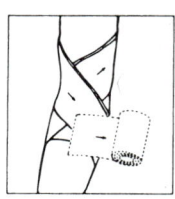 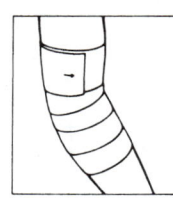

B

Elbow Use 3- or 4-inch width, depending on the size of the arm. Two rolls of bandage are required to complete the wrap. Start with a complete circular turn just below the elbow.

Wrap bandage in loose figure eights

to form a protective bridge across the front of the elbow joint.

Fasten end by pressing 4 to 6 inches of unstretched bandage to preceding layer. Start second bandage with a circular turn below the elbow

over the first wrap. Continue spiral bandaging over the elbow, ascending to the lower portion of the upper arm. Fasten end with a circular turn.

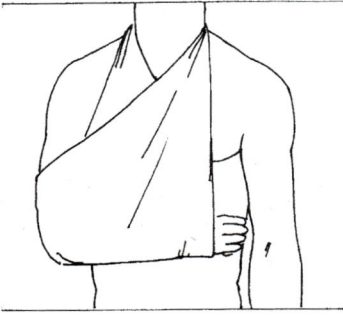 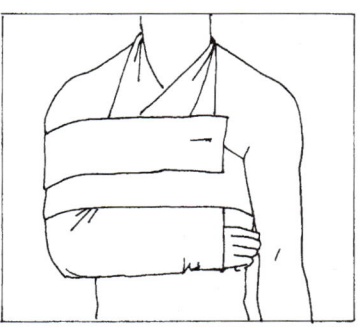 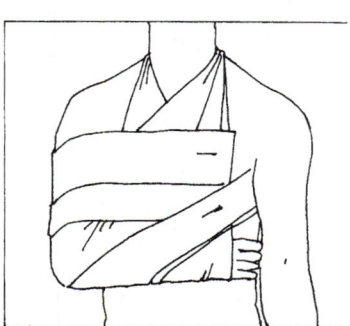

Shoulder A shoulder wrap is used to provide additional support for an arm in a sling. Use 4- or 6-inch width. One or two rolls of bandage may be used. Start under the free arm.

Carry the bandage across the back, over the arm in the sling, across the chest and back under the free arm in complete circular, overlapping turns. Fasten the end by pressing 4 to 6 inches of <u>unstretched</u> bandage to underlying bandage.

Additional support can be obtained with a second bandage. Start at the back just behind the flexed elbow in the sling. Carry the bandage under the elbow, up over the forearm, around the chest and back, and repeat. Fasten end.

The **spiral-reverse turn** is a spiral turn in which reverses are made halfway through each turn; the bandage is directed downward and folded on itself, wrapped around the part so that, when it circles around, it is parallel to the lower edge of the previous turn. Each turn overlaps the previous one by two-thirds the width of the bandage. Spiral-reverse turns create a neater fit because they take up the slack on the lower ends of the bandage applied to cone-shaped parts or parts that vary in width, such as the leg, thigh, or forearm.

The **recurrent turn** is a series of back-and-forth turns anchored by circular or spiral turns. After the bandage has been anchored, it is folded at right angles and passed across and back over the center of the part. Each subsequent fold is slightly angled and overlaps the previous fold by two-thirds the width of the bandage, first on one side and then on the other side of the center fold. To finish the bandage, a circular turn is made around the part and secured with tape, clips, pins, or a knot. The recurrent turn is used to bandage the head, fingers, toes, or the stump of an amputated limb (Figure 6-40).

Application of Tubegauz bandages.   When a Tubegauz bandage is applied, there is one basic method used for application to any body part being bandaged. Figure 6-41 illustrates areas where the Tubegauz may be applied, basic instructions for all its applications, and a simple arm or leg bandage.

FIGURE 6-40   Bandage-wrapping technique: recurrent turn used for head bandage.

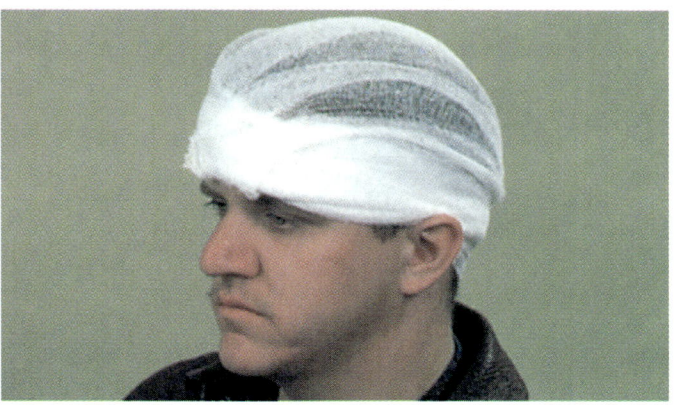

FIGURE 6-41   Tubegauz bandage applications.

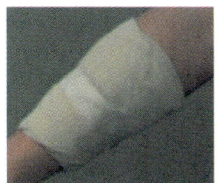

Arm or Leg

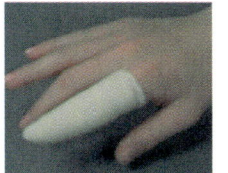

Finger

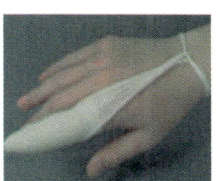

Finger Stall

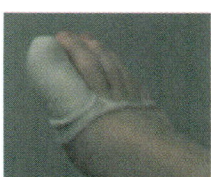

Toe

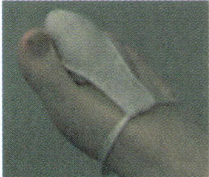

Toe Splint

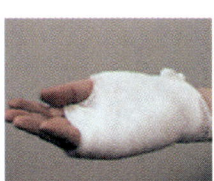

Palm of Hand

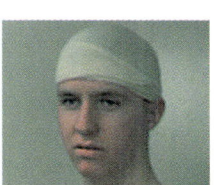

Head

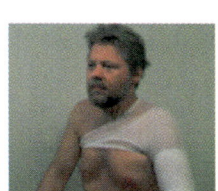

Shoulder

TUBEGAUZ

Tubegauz is a seamless, tubular-knitted cotton bandage designed as an improved method of bandaging.

Tubegauz is:
- Quick and easy to apply
- Efficient and neatly conformable
- Produced from quality cotton yarns
- Adaptable to all body areas
- Economical to use
- Strong yet soft in texture

Continued

FIGURE 6-41—cont'd Tubegauz bandage applications.

BASIC INSTRUCTIONS FOR ALL TUBEGAUZ APPLICATIONS

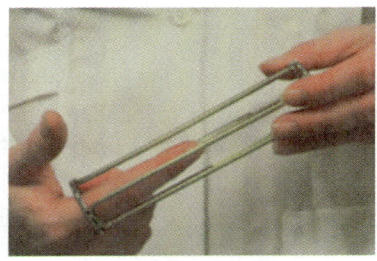

1 To apply any Tubegauz, first select a cage-type applicator that fits comfortably over the area to be bandaged.

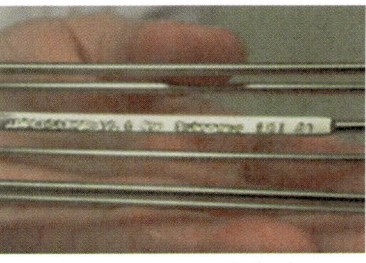

2 Next, select the size Tubegauz as printed on the cage-type applicator. For example, use Tubegauz size 01 for applicator No. 1.

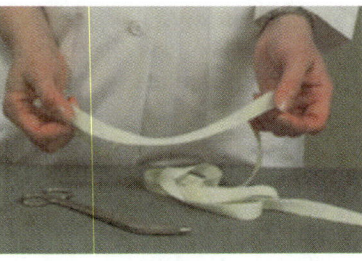

3 To load the Tubegauz onto the applicator, place the "channeled end" of the applicator on a flat surface and pull several feet of Tubegauz from the dispenser box.

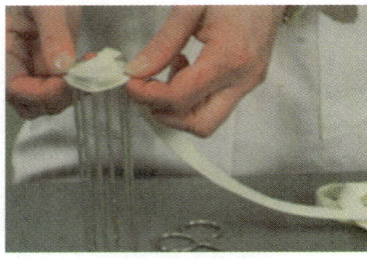

4 While spreading open the end of the tubular knit, slip the Tubegauz over the "smooth end" of the applicator.

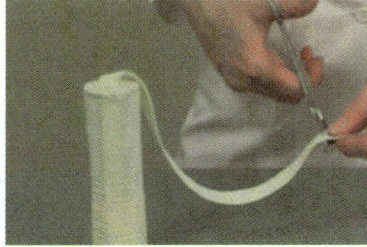

5 Complete loading by gathering sufficient Tubegauz to complete the bandage onto the applicator and cut off near the dispenser box opening.

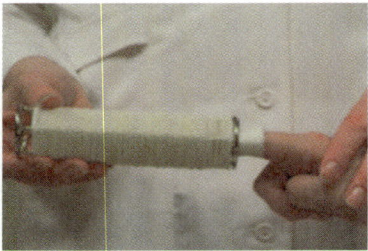

6 With the applicator loaded, pass the channeled end of the applicator over the limb to the middle of the dressing.

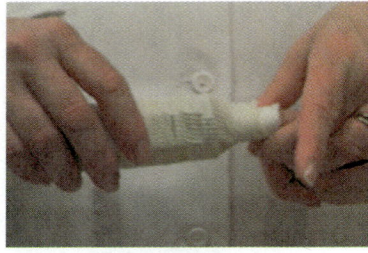

7 Pull the Tubegauz over the channeled end of the applicator, holding it lightly in place around the dressing.

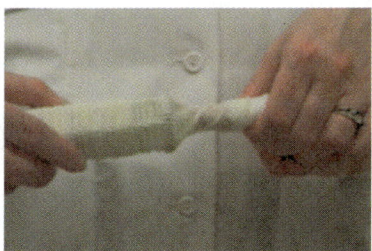

8 Continue to secure the dressing and Tubegauz end with one hand while slightly rotating clockwise to anchor as you withdraw the applicator over the limb.

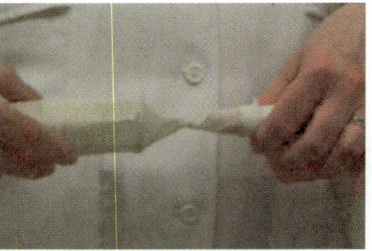

9 Withdraw the applicator several inches below the dressing or to the extremity, then rotate one full clockwise turn to anchor or close.

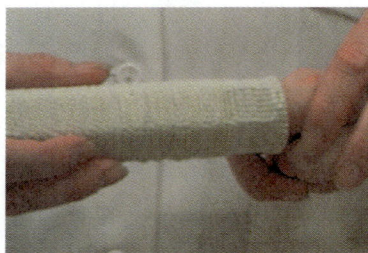

10 Move the applicator forward past the starting point and anchor with slight rotation several inches above the dressing.

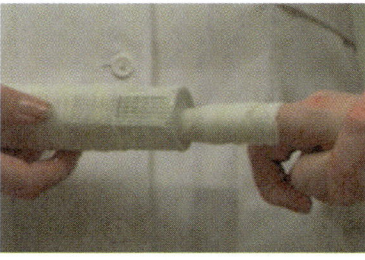

11 Continue this "back and forth" action until the desired layers of Tubegauz have been applied. Complete the last layer by stopping at the end of the bandage nearest the mesial plane.

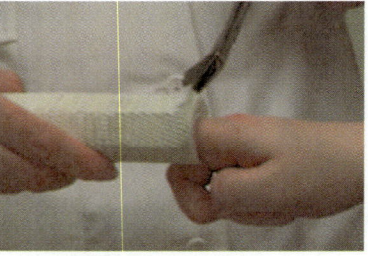

12 To finish, snip a small hole in the channeled rim, and continue cutting the Tubegauz from the applicator using the channeled rim as a cutting guide. If necessary, adhesive tape may be used to secure either end.

Remember . . .
  Tubegauz is often applied over a sterile dressing that covers broken skin. Tubegauz is not sterile, but can be autoclaved on or off a metal applicator if desired.
  Always load sufficient Tubegauz onto the applicator. It is difficult to complete a neat bandage when you have run out of Tubegauz in the middle of a procedure.

FIGURE 6-41—cont'd   Tubegauz bandage applications.

SIMPLE ARM OR LEG BANDAGE

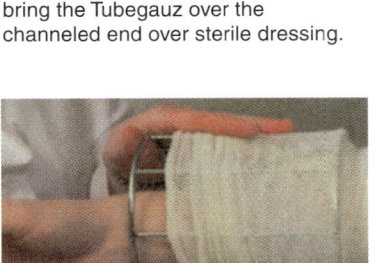

1 With applicator loaded as directed, bring the Tubegauz over the channeled end over sterile dressing.

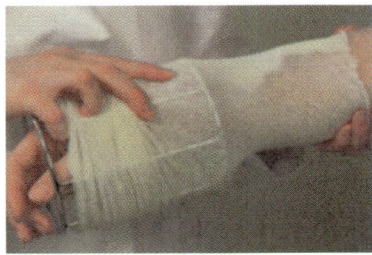

2 Hold the Tubegauz on the dressing with one hand and withdraw the applicator with the other hand letting the Tubegauz roll off the applicator to cover the desired area (usually just below the sterile dressing).

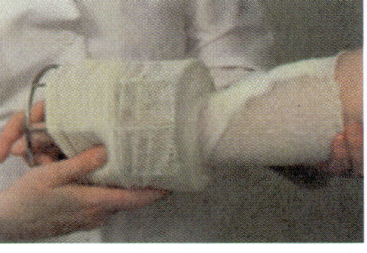

3 Rotate clockwise about 1/2 to 3/4 turn to anchor slightly and proceed in opposite direction to above dressing.

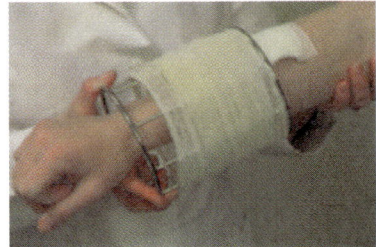

4 Rotate again in the same direction and return to base of bandage.

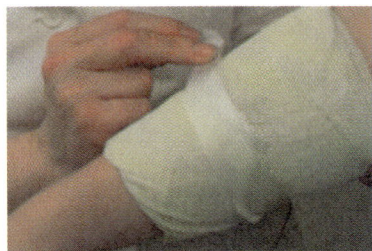

5 Cut Tubegauz off in channeled rim.

6 Secure with adhesive or slit and tie.

Adhesive tape may be applied at center of bandage by allowing a little more Tubegauz so that, after anchoring at base, the raw edge finishes in the center.

CASTS

Casts are a type of bandage made of either plaster of Paris or synthetic materials such as fiberglass, polyester, plastic, or other materials. The synthetic casts are stronger, lighter, and more resistant to water. However, they are more expensive and have a rough exterior. Casts are used to immobilize broken bones, injuries, joint disorders, or congenital disorders such as a dislocated hip or club foot. They are also used to protect the affected area and to reduce pain. Immobilization of a fractured bone holds bone fragments in place until healing takes place. Immobilization usually includes the joints immediately proximal and distal to the fractured bone. The healing time for a fracture depends on the type of fracture, the kind of bone affected, and the age of the person (see also Fractures in Chapter 17 and Figure 17-28). A child's bones generally heal much faster than those of an adult. Patients with simple fractures are often treated in the physician's office or clinic. The patient with a cast can generally carry on with most activities of daily living without causing any further damage to the injured site. However, a plaster-of-Paris cast may restrict some activities because of its weight and inflexibility. If a cast is not applied correctly or cared for properly, it can *cause* physical injury. Patients must be given instructions on the proper care of a cast and on signs to watch for that may indicate problems or complications. The medical assistant may be required to assist the physician when a cast is applied or removed and to give the patient important information and instructions.

Care of Casts

Plaster casts dry on their own. Thin casts may dry completely in several hours. Thick casts dry completely in 2 to 3 days, releasing heat and moisture. During this time, casts must be handled with care. Instruct the patient to lift or move the cast with the palms of the hands, not the fingers, and to support the entire length of the cast on a pillow to reduce the chance of denting. A dent on the outside of the cast causes a bump on the inside, which causes pressure on the skin. It is best to lie still until the cast dries to prevent misshaping the new cast. Instruct the patient to avoid resting the cast on hard or sharp surfaces (because dents can cause sores); to expose the cast to air to promote drying; to keep it uncovered, even at night (because it is still drying and needs air flow); and not to stand on a walking cast until it is completely dry. The cast is completely dry when it no longer feels damp or slightly soft to touch.

Ongoing care: instructions for the patient

- Keep the cast dry. Cover it with a waterproof cover whenever you are going to come in contact with water or while bathing (see Figure 6-45). Wrap plastic around the edges of the cast before you wash the surrounding skin. Plaster casts become soft and heavy when wet. Synthetic casts may cause skin softening if exposed to moisture frequently.
- Avoid excessive activity and hot rooms because heat causing perspiration can make the cast very uncomfortable.

- Whenever possible, elevate the limb in the cast to help prevent swelling.
- Avoid tight clothing that could restrict circulation.
- Do not put anything down a cast such as a ruler or a knitting needle. An itching sensation under the cast is normal. If it persists or becomes troublesome, consult the physician.
- Do not cut or trim the cast. See the physician if it causes discomfort. You can use masking tape to cover sharp edges.
- Never use powders or creams under a cast. You may use rubbing alcohol on the skin around the cast to protect and toughen the skin.
- If you have a cast on the leg, keep a sock or knit cap over the toes to keep them warm.

Contact the physician immediately if you notice any of the following:

- Broken, cracked, soft, or loose places on the cast
- Skin irritation caused by the cast rubbing the skin
- Raw or red skin under the edges of the cast
- A bad odor coming from the cast
- The feeling of the cast being too tight
- Prolonged swelling
- Fingers or toes below the cast becoming numb, difficult to move, discolored, or cold. (Casts are applied snugly but are fit to allow adequate circulation necessary for proper healing.)

- General discomfort because of constant or severe pain
- A burning sensation, especially over a bony prominence
- Bleeding or a red-pink discoloration on the cast

Cast Removal

Before the cast is removed, more x-ray films are usually taken to be sure that the bones have healed sufficiently for safe removal. A special tool, the manual or electric plaster cutter, or cast cutter, is used to cut the cast. The blade of the cast cutter vibrates instead of spinning. It can only cut hard surfaces such as casts and not soft things, like the skin. The patient needs to be reassured that the cast cutter will not cut his or her skin. Some pressure or vibration and heat will be felt, but it will not be painful. The cast is bivalved (opened or split) at a site away from an incision line or surgical area. The padding and stockinette are cut off with scissors. The skin under the cast is usually dry and scaly. You can instruct the patient to wash the skin with a mild soap and water and to use skin lotion or bath oil or both to help it return to normal. There is usually some stiffness in the joints; thus the limb should be moved gently. Exercises are usually prescribed for the joint and the extremity. When a leg cast has been removed, elastic bandages may also be prescribed to help prevent dependent edema. Always *remind patients* to check with the physician if, at a later time, they have any questions or problems about the body part from which the cast was removed. *Text continued on p. 349*

PROCEDURE 6-9

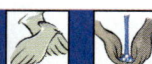

PLASTER-OF-PARIS CAST APPLICATION

Objective

Understand and demonstrate competency in preparing for and assisting the physician with the application of a cast, and attending to the patient as needed.

Equipment

Plaster-of-Paris bandages (appropriate width)—Various widths from 5 to 20 cm or 2, 3, 4, and 6 inches.

Webril (sheet wadding)—A thick, nonabsorbent cotton web covered with starch to hold it together. Used as padding for casts. Available in widths of 5 inches by 6 yards.

Felt or sponge rubber pads—Used over bony prominences to protect them from pressure if needed.

Tubular stockinette (appropriate width)—A seamless rib knit material of natural color. It is available in widths of 3, 6, 10, and 12 inches or 5 to 45 cm; used as a lining or thin padding for the cast.

Bandage scissors

Rubber gloves and rubber or plastic protective apron for the physician

Cast knife—Used for trimming the ends of the cast that may be rough after the cast has hardened.

Bucket of water lined with a cloth or plastic to catch waste plaster. The water should be warm—70° to 75° F (21° to 24° C).

After x-ray films have been taken to determine the extent of the injury, the physician reduces the fracture (returns the bone fragments to their normal position) and then applies the cast.

PROCEDURE

1. **Wash your hands** and assist with the procedure as required. **Use appropriate personal protective equipment (PPE) as dictated by facility.**

2. Place stockinette over the affected area (Figure 6-42).

3. Place felt or sponge rubber over bony prominences, such as the ankle.

RATIONALE

The stockinette helps to protect the skin.

This protects these areas from pressure.

PLASTER-OF-PARIS CAST APPLICATION—cont'd

4. Apply Webril padding. Apply it so that it extends over the edge to cover the round edges of the plaster.

    The sheet wadding padding serves as a lining for the cast.

5. When the physician is ready to apply the cast, you should:
    a. Place the bandage in the bucket of warm water for 5 seconds. Place only a few bandages in the water at a time.
    b. Carefully remove the bandage from the water. Hold it horizontally with an end in the palm of each hand and gently compress it to remove excess water (Figure 6-42, *F*).

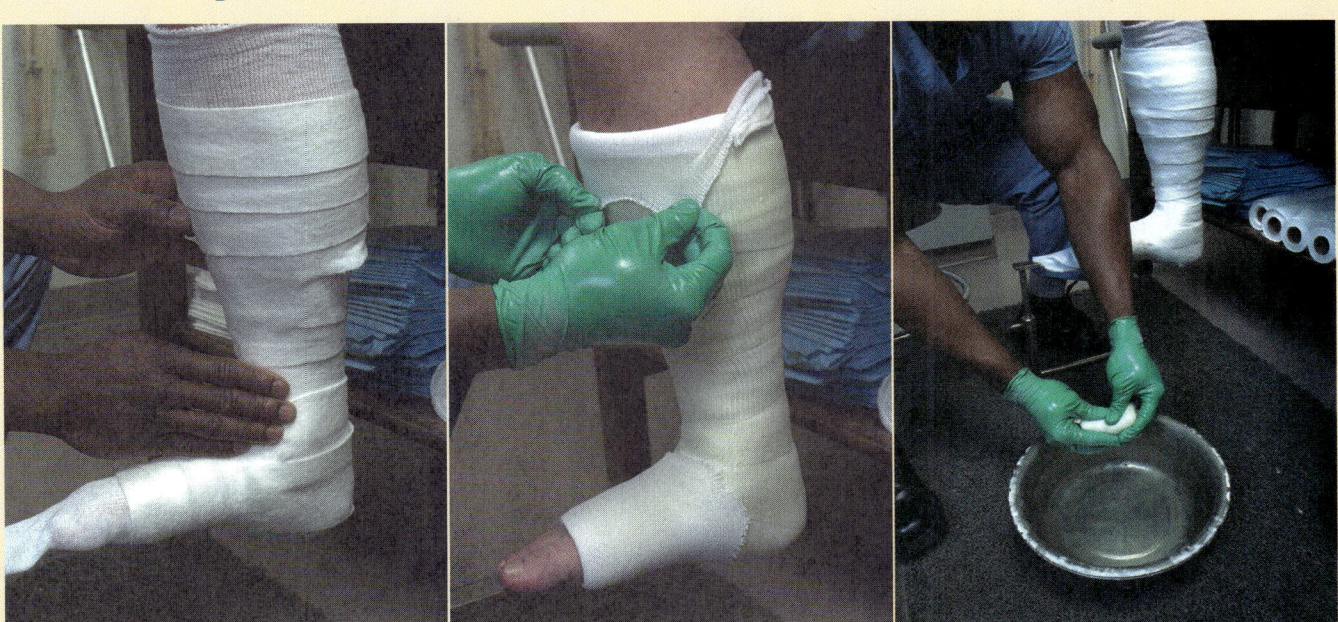

FIGURE 6-42 **A** through **E,** Preparation for cast application. **F,** Remove plaster bandage from the water; hold it horizontally, using both hands, and gently compress it to remove excess water. Quickly hand to the physician so it can be applied before it dries.

Continued

PROCEDURE 6-9

PLASTER-OF-PARIS CAST APPLICATION—cont'd

Remove it carefully so that none of the plaster is lost. *DO NOT* wring the cast material. Squeeze it at the ends, pushing toward the center.

c. Quickly hand the bandage to the physician so that it can be applied before it begins to set (Figure 6-43).

Plaster bandages start to harden within 3 to 7 minutes.

d. Continue to prepare as many bandages as needed. At the end, the physician will usually fold the excess stockinette and sheet wadding back over the cast and bind them down with a final roll of plaster (see No. 4 of this procedure). The physician will use the knife to trim any sharp or rough edges.

e. When the procedure is completed, remove and discard the cloth or plastic liner from the bucket. Any waste plaster will have collected in the liner of the bucket. Discard it in the regular garbage can.

f. Discard water down sink. Check that there is no plaster in the water.

Plaster in the water could clog the drain in the sink.

g. Attend to the patient's safety and comfort (Figure 6-44). Provide the patient with any further instructions if directed to do so by the physician. Explain that the cast will feel warm immediately after it is applied because the plaster was dipped in warm water to make it moldable to the limb. A chemical reaction between the plaster and water causes the cast to feel warm. See also earlier section, Ongoing Care: Instructions for the Patient (Figure 6-45).

h. Clean the work area.

i. **Wash your hands.**

j. Do any recording required of you. The physician usually records this procedure, along with other recordings regarding the fracture and the patient's condition.

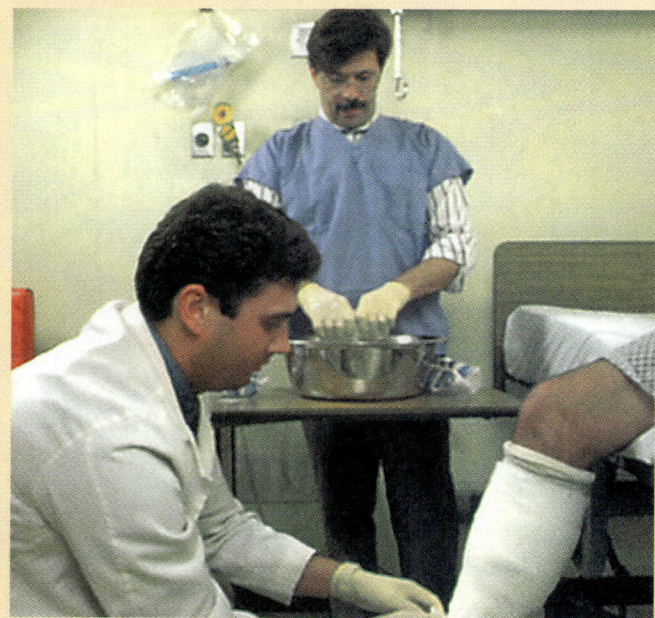

FIGURE 6-43 Physician applying cast to patient's leg.

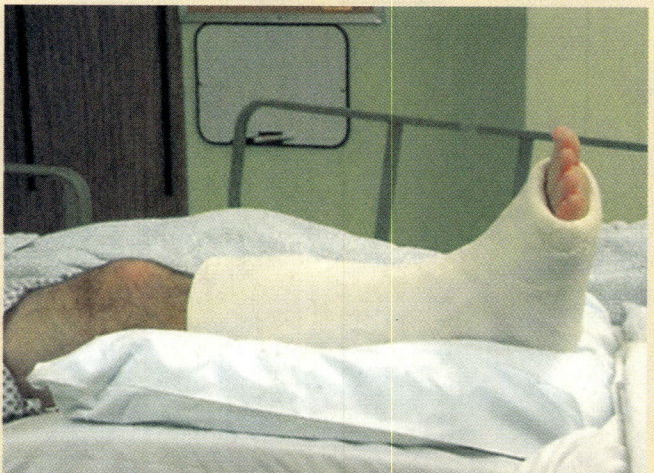

FIGURE 6-44 Plaster-of-Paris cast on leg.

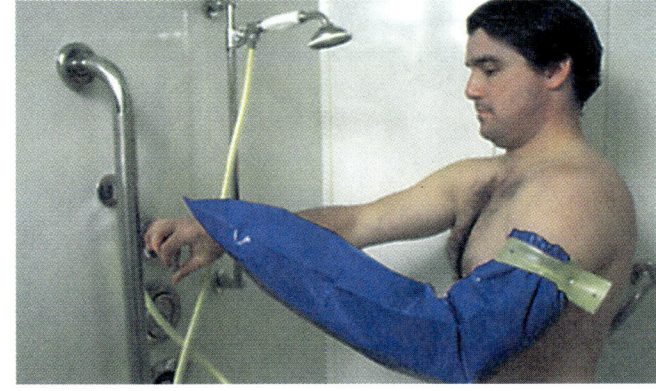

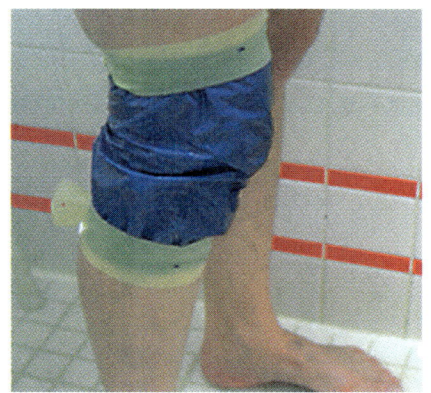

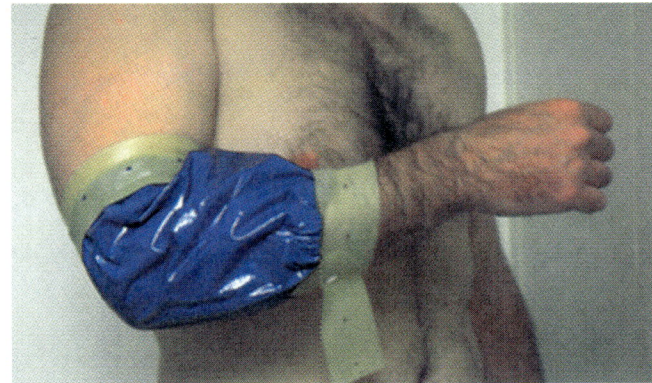

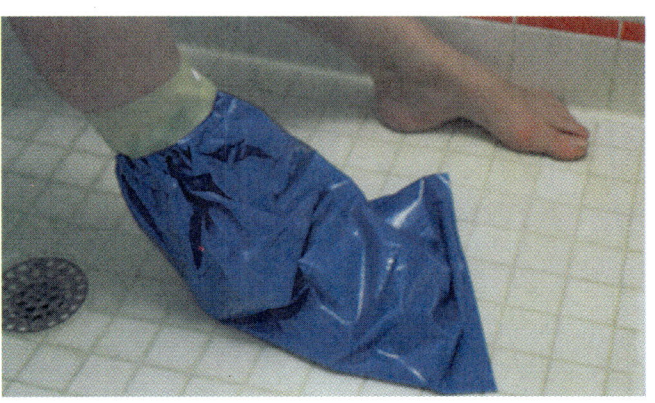

FIGURE 6-45   ShowerSafe waterproof cast and bandage cover. This is a durable, reusable, and pliable plastic covering used to keep casts, wounds, and bandages dry during showering or bathing. ShowerSafe reduces the risk of infection and preserves the integrity of a cast or bandage. **A,** Arm; **B,** elbow; **C,** knee; and **D,** foot and ankle. (Courtesy Trademark Corp, Fenton, Mo.)

PROCEDURE 6-10

FIBERGLASS CAST APPLICATION

Objective

Understand and demonstrate competency in preparing for and assisting the physician with the application of a fiberglass cast and attending to the patient as needed.

Equipment

Fiberglass bandages
Webril (sheet wadding)

Felt or sponge rubber pads
Tubular stockinette
Bandage scissors
Rubber gloves and rubber or plastic protective apron for the physician
Cast knife
Bucket and cold water

PROCEDURE

1. Follow steps 1 through 4 as outlined for application of a plaster cast.

RATIONALE

Continued

PROCEDURE 6-10

FIBERGLASS CAST APPLICATION—cont'd

2. When the physician is ready to apply the cast, you should:

    a. Place the bandage in a vertical position in the bucket of cold water. The water should be at least $\frac{1}{2}$ inch above the bandage. Only a few bandages should be placed in the water at a time.

    b. Carefully remove the bandage from the water when the water stops "bubbling." Shake water out of the bandage.

    c. Continue to prepare and hand the physician as many bandages as needed.

    d. When all the bandages are applied, the physician rubs the bandages a number of times to make sure that all the bandages adhere and that the bandage is smooth. It is vital that the cast be set correctly to maintain the correct support and body alignment required for proper healing of the bone(s) (Figure 6-46).

3. Attend to the patient as required. Provide the patient with instructions if directed to do so by the physician.

4. Clean the work area and discard any waste.

DO NOT squeeze water out of the bandage because fiberglass hardens very quickly and the physician needs enough time to apply the cast before it starts to harden.

NOTE: *A fiberglass cast commonly dries within 1 hour. A fan or air gun may be used to hasten the drying process. NEVER use a heat blower or heat lamp to dry a fiberglass cast because the fiberglass material becomes hot and could burn the patient's skin under the cast material.*

If a fiberglass cast becomes wet, it will swell. If swelling is excessive, it could compress tissue and cause problems. Therefore you must emphasize to the patient to keep the cast dry. You should also caution the patient against using a blow-dryer on the cast (should it become wet) to prevent burning the skin beneath the cast.

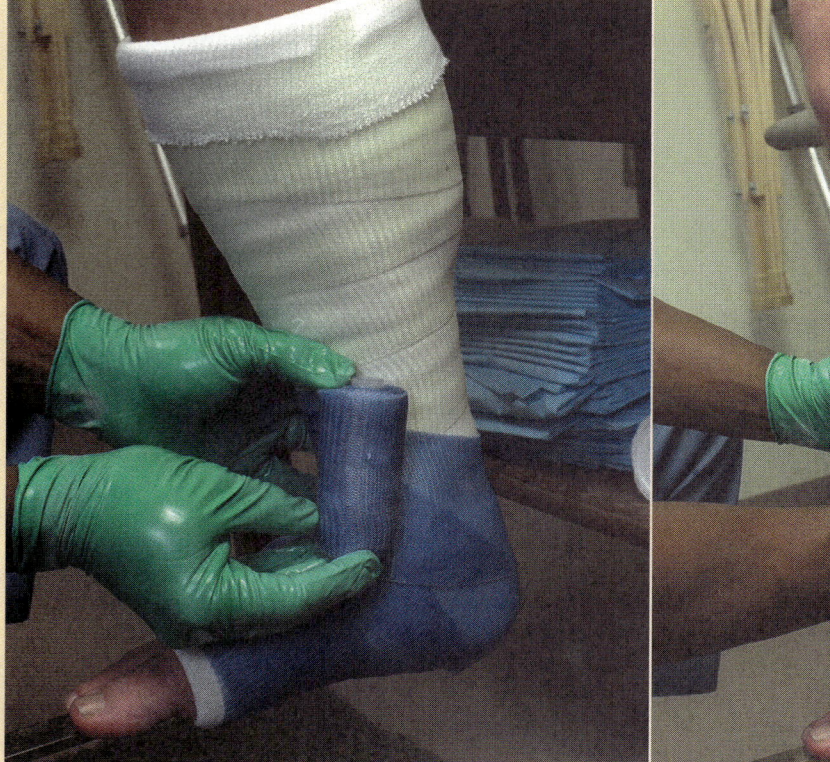
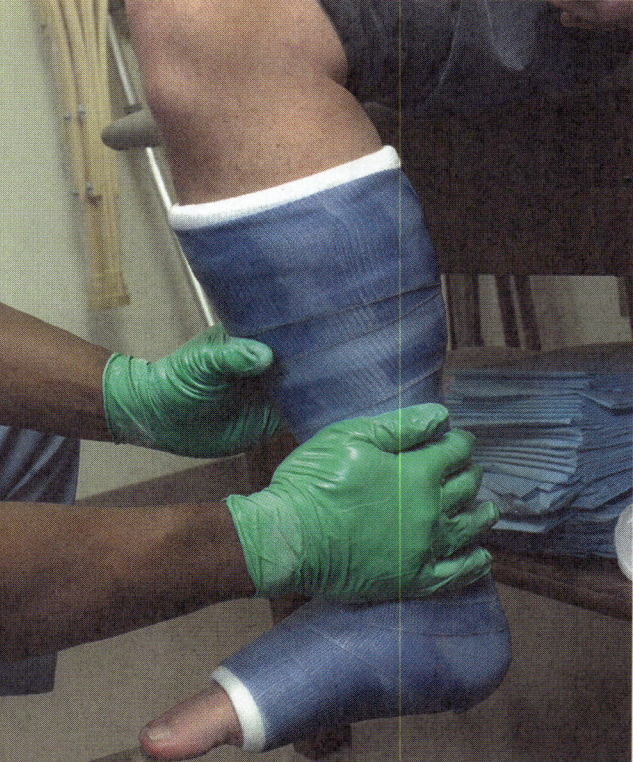

FIGURE 6-46 Fiberglass cast application.

CONCLUSION

Strict aseptic technique is necessary at all times when handling sterile supplies and assisting with sterile or surgical procedures. Never be reluctant to admit a possible break in technique.

Be honest and admit contamination of sterile equipment, even if you are the only one who realizes that the equipment is not sterile. It is no disgrace to contaminate sterile equipment. The only disgrace is to use it after you know it is contaminated because you would then subject the patient to the great danger of infection.

Learn the principles and practice the sterile techniques to be used when handling sterile supplies and equipment and when assisting with sterile procedures. Practice handing instruments so that the physician can grasp them in the way most convenient to use during a procedure. Be prepared to select and arrange the supplies and equipment required for the minor surgeries listed in this chapter.

When ready to accurately demonstrate your skills, arrange with your instructor to take the performance test.

REVIEW OF VOCABULARY

The following is a sample of a minor surgery report using terms that have been defined for you. Read it and be able to define or explain the terms that are italicized.

Operative report

DIAGNOSIS: Lipomas in right buttock and posterior thigh (Rt); large mole, right posterior thigh.
POSTOPERATIVE DIAGNOSIS: Same.
OPERATION: Excision of lipomas; *cauterization* of mole.
ANESTHESIA: *Local infiltration*—Lidocaine 1%
SURGEON: A. Joseph, MD
PROCEDURE: *Sterile field* and *setup* prepared. *Sterile gloves donned.* With the patient in a prone position, the usual *skin preparation* was performed, and then *sterile drapes* were applied. The *local anesthetic* was administered. The tumors were excised without any difficulty, and two *biopsy* specimens were sent to the laboratory for cytology studies. The tissues were approximated with *000 black silk.*
The *cautery* unit was then used to remove a questionable mole on the right posterior thigh.
Dry dressings were applied to the surgical sites.
POSTOPERATIVE STATUS: The patient left the office with minor complaints of discomfort in the surgical areas.
Patient to return in 1 week for removal of sutures and for follow-up care.

Andrew Joseph, MD

Pathology reports

The following minor surgery pathology reports were received in a physician's office. After reading these, you should be able to discuss the contents of these reports with your instructor. Reference sources may be used to obtain definitions of terms with which you are not familiar.

Patient No. 1
CLINICAL DATA: 63-year-old black male with sebaceous cyst of the left axilla and skin tag of the right arm.

CLINICAL DIAGNOSIS: Epidermoid inclusion cyst, left axilla, and right arm skin tag.
MATERIAL FROM: Excision of the above.
GROSS DESCRIPTION: The specimen is received in formalin in two parts:
Part 1, labeled "left axilla," consists of a soft, round lesion with an opaque, glistening serosal surface, measuring $1.5 \times 1.3 \times 0.7$ cm. Sectioning reveals a cystic character of the lesion with brown, friable contents. Representative sections are submitted.
Part 2, labeled "right upper arm," consists of a brown piece of tissue covered with skin and measuring $0.7 \times 0.3 \times 0.2$ cm. Sectioning reveals a pale, pinkish tan, fibrous core. Representative sections are submitted.
MICROSCOPIC: Sections show features listed in the diagnosis.
DIAGNOSIS
  1. Epidermal inclusion cyst (excision biopsy, left axilla).
  2. Fibroepithelial skin tag with hyperkeratosis (excision biopsy, right upper arm).

J. D. Wynn, MD

Patient No. 2
CLINICAL DATA: 29-year-old white female with a recent onset of a right breast mass with nipple retraction.
CLINICAL DIAGNOSIS: Right breast mass.
MATERIAL FROM: Breast biopsy.
GROSS DESCRIPTION: Received fresh, labeled "breast mass," are two pieces of fibrofatty tissue measuring $1.8 \times 1.3 \times 1.3$ cm and $1.7 \times 1.7 \times 0.6$ cm, weighing 2.1 and 1 g, respectively. Serial sections reveal homogeneous fibrofatty tissue. The specimen is submitted in its entirety.
MICROSCOPIC: Sections show features listed in the diagnosis.
DIAGNOSIS: Focally acute and chronically inflamed breast tissue with fat necrosis and fibrosis; see note (right breast biopsy).

NOTE: The peripheral nature of this inflammatory process suggests that it may represent the wall of an abscess.

J. D. Wynn, MD

Patient No. 3

CLINICAL DATA: 34-year-old white female with a lump in the upper outer left breast.

CLINICAL DIAGNOSIS: Same as above.

MATERIAL FROM: Left breast biopsy.

GROSS DESCRIPTION: Received in formalin are three pieces of pale tan, firm, fibrous tissue with attached yellow fat measuring $2.2 \times 1.4 \times 0.5$ cm, $1.1 \times 1.0 \times 0.3$ cm, and $0.4 \times 0.2 \times 0.1$ cm. Serial sectioning reveals similar homogenous, white, fibrous tissue. Representative sections are submitted.

MICROSCOPIC: Sections show features listed in the diagnosis.

DIAGNOSIS: Mammary dysplasia characterized by cyst, adenosis, and apocrine metaplasia (left breast biopsy).

J. D. Wynn, MD

Patient No. 4

The following three reports were received in a physician's office on a patient who initially came in for a breast examination complaining of feeling two painful lumps in her left breast.

The physician performed an FNA on one of the lumps and ordered a bilateral comprehensive mammogram and left breast ultrasound. Results indicated the need for an excisional biopsy, which was performed in the outpatient surgical clinic at the Medical Center.

After reading these, you should be able to discuss the contents of these reports with your instructor. Reference sources may be used to obtain definitions of terms with which you are not familiar.

Pathology/Cytology Report

Final Diagnosis

Fine-needle aspirate, left breast left lower outer quadrant—atypical mammary epithelial cells present, see microscopic.

Clinical History

Left breast lower outer quadrant, R/O fibroadenoma vs CA

Tissues

Breast—left lower outer quad

Gross Description

Received are two air-dried smears that are stained with Quik stain. WB 5/22/00

Microscopic Examination

Both smears show considerable artifact. There is seen on a bloody background groups of cells that vary somewhat in size and shape, are loosely coherent, have nuclei ranging 2 to 3 times red cell diameters. There is an occasional intact cell present. There are many disrupted cells present. This does not suggest to me a fibroadenoma, and it is atypical and biopsy is recommended.

Original report read and signed _____ **05/22/00**

John David, MD

Department of Radiology

Bilateral Comprehensive Mammogram and Left Ultrasound

Bilateral comprehensive mammogram (06/02/2000)

Left ultrasound (06/02/2000)

Compare: 7/30/99

The patient now reports two lumps in the left breast. BBs were placed on the overlying skin. Mammography shows no soft tissue mass or calcifications in those regions. There has been no change since 07/30/99. The two areas were evaluated sonographically. In the 6:00 location where there has recently been a fine-needle aspiration performed by Doctor James, no sonographic abnormality is identified. In the 4:00 position where the patient feels a second lump, there is a 3×5 mm in diameter simple cyst.

Elsewhere, the mammographic examination is normal and stable.

Impression

No significant change. No suspicious finding identified. 3×5 mm in diameter cyst in the 4:00-5:00 position of the left breast. Otherwise normal. Comprehensive bilateral mammographic follow-up is recommended in 1 year.

Findings and recommendations were reviewed directly with the patient.

Jack Bracken, MD

Pathology/Cytology Report

Final Diagnosis

Gross and microscopic diagnosis

Fibrocystic change with mild ductal epithelial hyperplasia and mild lobular hyperplasia, negative for atypia, with interlobular fibrosis, sclerosing adenosis, and microcyst formation with apocrine metaplasia (biopsy, left breast mass).

Comment

The left breast mass consists of breast tissue with interlobular fibrosis and other changes described above. Grossly and in section (B) there is hemorrhage consistent with prior fine-needle aspiration. Evidence of a fibroadenoma is absent. Although the biopsy findings of mild epithelial hyperplasia probably explain the atypical fine-needle aspirate findings of 5/22/00 (00-CS6499), close follow-up is suggested, as clinically warranted.

Clinical History

Left breast mass

Tissues

Breast—left tissue

Gross Description

Submitted fresh and labeled "left breast tissue" are two segments of tissue, the larger 5 × 3.5 × 1.8 and the smaller a disk 2.2 cm in diameter × 0.5 cm in thickness. Each is coated with India ink. On cut section, there is soft, grayish-white fibrosis, negative for suspicious areas. Focally, there is reddish hemorrhage, raising the question of a prior fine-needle aspiration. The tissue is near totally sampled in (A) through (F).

The smaller disk is bisected and sampled in (G).

FM 7/2/00

Original report read and signed _____ **07/06/00**

J. B. Brown, MD

CRITICAL THINKING SKILLS REVIEW

1. Having opened a sterile suture removal kit for use, the physician then decides not to remove the patient's sutures. What would you now do with these instruments?

2. When pouring a solution into a sterile container on a sterile field, you accidentally spill some of the solution on the sterile field. What would you do to remedy this contamination?

3. While directly assisting with a minor surgical procedure, you accidentally puncture your sterile glove with a needle. What should be your next actions?

4. Differentiate between a sterile field and a sterile setup.

5. When assisting with minor surgery, the physician asks for the thinnest black silk suture material. What size (number) would you provide?

6. Surgical asepsis is commonly referred to as sterile technique or surgical aseptic technique. Explain what is meant by these terms.

7. List 15 of the principles and practices of surgical aseptic (sterile) technique.

8. Why do you open envelope-wrapped sterile packages with the top flap going away from your body?

9. Before pouring a sterile solution for use, why do you first pour a small amount into a waste container?

10. List two reasons for wearing sterile gloves during a procedure.

11. Name and describe three methods used to administer a local anesthetic for a minor surgical procedure.

12. List the supplies and equipment that you would assemble and prepare when the physician is to:
    a. Incise and drain an abscess
    b. Remove sutures
    c. Repair a laceration by suturing
    d. Obtain an aspiration (needle) biopsy of breast tissue
    e. Remove a wart on the patient's left hand
    f. Insert an IUD

13. Describe how to prepare a patient for minor surgery.

14. State the purpose of an IUD.

15. List and explain four terms that describe the character of drainage from a wound.

16. Describe the five types of open wounds and explain the healing process.

17. List eight purposes of dressings and four purposes of bandages.

18. List and explain the five basic turns used to apply roller bandages, indicating when each may be most appropriately used.

19. List and briefly describe four types of dressing materials and four types of bandage materials.

20. State the purpose of casts.

PERFORMANCE TEST

In a skills laboratory, a simulation of a joblike environment, the medical assistant student will demonstrate skill and knowledge when performing the following activities without reference to source materials. Time limits for the performance of each procedure are to be assigned by the instructor (see also p. 104).

1. Given a sterile syringe in a peel-down package and a sterile envelope-wrapped pack of instruments, open these packs and with a sterile transfer forceps arrange the contents for use, avoiding contamination.
2. Given a sterile solution and a sterile container, pour the solution into the container, avoiding contamination.
3. Given a pair of sterile gloves, don them, avoiding contamination, and then remove.
4. Given the choice of a variety of sterile instruments and prepackaged instrument sets, select, identify by name, and prepare for use those that will be used for:
   a. Preparing the patient's skin for minor surgery
   b. Administering a local anesthetic
   c. Suturing a laceration
   d. Incision and drainage of an abscess or cyst
   e. Removal of a foreign body in subcutaneous tissue, a wart and a mole, and a tissue biopsy from the skin surface
   f. Cervical biopsy
   g. Aspiration (needle) biopsy of breast tissue
   h. Insertion of an IUD
   i. Vulvar biopsy
   j. Endocervical curettage
   k. Endometrial biopsy
   l. Cryosurgery
   m. Colposcopy
   n. A 6-mm skin biopsy
   o. Suture removal
   p. Dressing change with a wound culture
   q. Application of a plaster-of-Paris cast
   r. Application of a fiberglass cast
5. Given a sterile hemostat, while gloved, hand it to the physician in the most convenient way for immediate use.
6. Demonstrate the proper procedures for:
   a. Preparing the skin for a minor surgical procedure
   b. Removing sutures
   c. Assisting with the application of a plaster-of-Paris cast
7. Demonstrate the proper procedure for changing a dressing and obtaining a wound culture.
8. Demonstrate the application of a roller, triangular, and Tubegauz bandage.
9. At the completion of the preceding activities, be able to discuss with the instructor at least 10 of the principles of surgical aseptic technique, how to prepare a patient physically and mentally for minor surgery, and how to assist the physician during a minor surgical procedure.

The student must be able to perform these activities with 100% accuracy 90% of the time. If the student contaminates any item during the performance of these skills, the correct actions to remedy the contaminated site must be employed 100% of the time.

The successful completion of each procedure will demonstrate competency levels as required by the AAMA, AMT, and future employers.

INTERNET RESOURCES

MedScape
www.medscape.com

CBS HealthWatch
www.cbshealthwatch.medscape.com

Wound Care Strategies
www.woundcarestrategies.com

National Association for Healthcare Quality
www.nahq.org

The World Foundation for Medical Studies in Female Health
www.wffh.org

Life Link
www.lifelinkfound.org

TransWeb
www.transweb.org

National Cancer Institute
www.nci.nih.gov

National Institutes of Health
www.nih.gov

Columbia University's Health Education Site
www.goaskalice.columbia.edu/index.html

Principles of Pharmacology and Drug Administration

7

CHAPTER

◼ Cognitive Objectives

On completion of Chapter 7, the medical assistant student should be able to:

1. Define, spell, and pronounce the terms listed in the vocabulary.
2. List and briefly describe the uses, sources, names, classifications, and types of drugs.
3. Select and name official and other reference books on drugs.
4. Differentiate between a controlled substance, a prescription drug, and a nonprescription drug.
5. Define "prescription"; list and explain the seven parts of a prescription.
6. Differentiate between administering, dispensing, and prescribing medications.
7. Interpret abbreviations and symbols commonly used when administering medications.
8. State and discuss drug standards and the laws governing drug usage.
9. State and describe the various types of pharmaceutical preparations.
10. Explain how drugs should be stored, handled, and labeled.
11. List examples of drugs that may be kept on an emergency tray.
12. List additional supplies that should be kept near the emergency tray for emergency situations.
13. List eight signs and symptoms of hypoxemia.
14. Describe the difference between an oxygen mask and a nasal cannula. Discuss how each should be placed on a patient when oxygen is to be administered.
15. State the usual amount of oxygen administered through an oxygen mask and through a nasal cannula.
16. State and discuss the legal requirements for controlled substances inventory and the prescriber's record.
17. List 12 routes by which medication may be administered, briefly describing each.
18. List at least 15 rules for administering medications and 15 specific rules for administering injections.

19. Calculate the correct dose of a medication to be administered.
20. List the five rights for preparing and administering medications. State a sixth right that has been added by many medical authorities.
21. State the correct size needle and syringe for intramuscular and subcutaneous injections; list factors that influence these choices.
22. List at least eight factors that influence drug dosage and action.
23. Discuss aspects of patient education when drug therapy is initiated.
24. State six reasons why medication is administered by an injection.
25. List six to eight dangers involved when giving injections and the sites that are to be avoided.
26. List anatomic sites for administering an intramuscular injection, a subcutaneous injection, and an intradermal injection.
27. Describe how drugs are placed into a syringe from a vial, from an ampule, and from a prefilled sterile cartridge-needle unit.
28. Explain how the skin is prepared before an injection is administered.
29. Explain why the skin disinfectant should be allowed to dry before giving an injection.
30. Explain why it is recommended that the needle be inserted and removed quickly and the medication be injected slowly when giving an injection.
31. Discuss eight guidelines suggested for use to prevent needlesticks.
32. Discuss the protocol to follow after an accidental needlestick and occupational exposure to blood.
33. List four sites used for administering an insulin injection.
34. Discuss the concepts of rotating injection sites for insulin injections.
35. State four factors that influence the absorption of insulin.

36. State at least 10 points to consider for the administration of insulin.

37. Explain what to do with a syringe and needle after use.

38. List three reasons for the administration of solutions by an intradermal injection.

39. Discuss reasons why patients may not follow the directions given for taking medications. List some tips that may help patients to follow the directions given.

■ Terminal Performance Objectives

On completion of Chapter 7, the medical assistant student should be able to:

1. Given medication orders, interpret these, and calculate the dose of the drug to be administered.

2. Given a medication order, prepare and administer safely and efficiently a subcutaneous and an intramuscular injection using (a) a sterile disposable syringe and needle of the correct sizes and (b) a reusable injector (for example, Tubex injector) with a prefilled sterile cartridge-needle unit.

3. Given a medication order, prepare and administer safely and efficiently an intramuscular injection using the Z-track technique.

4. Demonstrate how to identify the correct sites for administering a subcutaneous and an intramuscular injection by palpating definite anatomic landmarks.

5. Demonstrate how to fill a syringe with a medication from a vial; from an ampule.

6. Demonstrate how to reconstitute a powdered drug for administration by injection.

7. Demonstrate how to administer insulin using the correct insulin syringe for the insulin preparation available.

8. Demonstrate how to place an oxygen mask and a nasal cannula on a patient for the administration of oxygen.

9. Given the *PDR* or other reference pharmacology book, obtain information on a variety of drugs.

10. Provide instructions and patient education that is within the professional scope of a medical assistant's training and responsibilities as assigned.

The student is to perform these objectives with 100% accuracy.

VOCABULARY

addiction (ah-dik'shun)—An acquired physiologic or psychologic dependence on a drug with tendencies to increase its use.

adulteration (ah-dul'ter-a'shun), **adulterated**—The addition or substitution of an impure or weaker and usually cheaper substance in a formulation or product.

AMA—American Medical Association.

anaphylactic (an"ah-fi-lak'tik) **shock**—An intense state of shock brought on by hypersensitivity to a drug, foreign toxin, or protein. Early symptoms resemble an allergic reaction, then increase in severity rapidly to dyspnea, cyanosis, and shock. This can be fatal if emergency measures are not taken immediately (see also the section on First Aid for allergic reaction to drugs in Chapter 17).

BNDD—Bureau of Narcotics and Dangerous Drugs (a federal government agency of the DEA).

broad-spectrum—Adjective describing the ability of an agent to be effective against a wide range of microorganisms (for example, a broad-spectrum antibiotic such as tetracycline).

chemotherapy (ke"mo-ther'ah-pe)—The use of drugs (chemicals) to treat disease; a type of therapy used for cancer patients in which powerful drugs are used to interfere with the reproduction of the fast-multiplying cancer cells.

contraindication (kon'tra-in"di-ka'shun)—Condition in which the use of certain drugs or treatments should be withheld or limited.

cross-tolerance—Cross-tolerance can develop when tolerance to one drug increases the body's tolerance to drugs in the same category (for example, a tolerance to one depressant drug leads to a tolerance of other depressant drugs).

crude drug—An unrefined drug.

cumulative action of a drug—A drug accumulates in the body; it is eliminated more slowly than it is absorbed.

DEA—Drug Enforcement Administration. This is the federal law enforcement agency charged with the responsibility of combating drug diversion.

dilute—To weaken the strength of a substance by adding something else.

drug idiosyncrasy (id"e-o-sing'krah-se)—An unusual or abnormal response or susceptibility to a drug that is peculiar to the individual.

drug tolerance—The decreased susceptibility to the effects of a drug after continued use. In this case an increased dosage would be required to produce the desired effects because the initial dose would be ineffective.

FDA—Food and Drug Administration (a federal government agency).

habituation—Emotional dependence on a drug caused by repeated use, but without tendencies to increase the amount of the drug.

HHS—Health and Human Services (a federal government agency).

parenteral (pah-ren'ter-al)—Not through or in the digestive tract, for example, intramuscular, subcutaneous, intravenous, or intradermal injection.

parenteral dosage—A drug given by injection; administering a drug by a route that bypasses the digestive tract.

PDR—*Physicians' Desk Reference,* a book on drugs.

placebo (plah-se'bo)—An inactive substance resembling and given in place of a medication for its psychologic effects to satisfy the patient's need for the drug; it hopefully will produce the same effect as the real medication through psychologic means. A placebo may be used experimentally.

prophylaxis (pro"fi-lak'sis)—Prevention of disease.

pure drug—A refined drug; one that has been processed to remove all impurities.

The consistent use of Universal/Standard Precautions is required by all health care professionals in all health care settings as a method of infection control. It is assumed that these precautions are used in all of the following procedures. Review Chapter 1 if you have any questions on methods to use because the methods or techniques are not repeated in detail in each procedure presented in this chapter.

Be sure to consult the latest guidelines issued by the Centers for Disease Control and Prevention (CDC) and consult with infection control practitioners when necessary to identify specific precautions that pertain to your particular work situation.

Of the many duties of a medical assistant, administering medications responsibly is extremely important. As a member of a professional team involved with the medical care of the public, the medical assistant must seek all possible knowledge of a drug—its use or abuse, correct dosage, methods and routes of administration, symptoms of overdose, and abnormal reactions that may occur when it is administered—before administering it to a patient. Although this book does not provide a detailed presentation of pharmacology, it does include general concepts, basic information on drugs, and procedures for the correct methods of administration. Reference sources for more detailed information on drugs are cited.

PHARMACOLOGY AND DRUGS

Pharmacon is Greek for drugs. Pharmacology is the science that deals with the study of drugs—their origin, properties, uses, and actions. Drugs are any medicinal substances or mixtures of substances that are used for therapeutic, prophylactic, or diagnostic purposes. Drugs are either medicinal, therefore therapeutic, or poisonous, depending on dosage and use. The therapeutic use of drugs includes the application of these substances to treat or cure a disease or condition, to relieve undesirable symptoms such as pain, and to provide substances that the body is not producing or not producing in sufficient amounts (for example, insulin, used for diabetes mellitus, and thyroid extract, used for hypothyroidism). Prophylactically, drugs are used to prevent diseases, such as vaccinations given to prevent communicable diseases. Drugs can also help a physician diagnose an illness, as seen when a contrast medium is given to a patient in a diagnostic x-ray film procedure or when antigens are used to detect skin allergies in a patient.

Pharmacology has undergone tremendous changes during the past few decades and continues to be dynamic. Through constant study and research, new drugs arrive on the market, and some old ones are withdrawn, either because newer ones are more effective or because complications arising from the use of the older drugs prove to be too hazardous to the patient's health.

Drugs are derived from the following four main sources:

1. Plant sources—Obtained from plant parts or products. Seeds, stem, roots, leaves, resin, and other parts yield these drugs; examples include digitalis and opium.
2. Animal sources—Glandular products from animals such as insulin and thyroid.
3. Mineral sources—Some drugs are prepared from minerals (for example, potassium chloride and lithium carbonate [an antipsychotic]).
4. Synthetic sources—Laboratories duplicate natural processes. Often side effects can be eliminated and potency of the drug increased (for example, barbiturates, sulfonamides, and aspirin).

Drug Name: Brand (Trade), Generic, and Chemical

A typical drug may be known by as many as three names, as follows:

1. A brand or trade (proprietary) name
2. The generic name
3. The chemical name

When a drug is developed and marketed, it is assigned a specific name that is patented by the pharmaceutical company that has manufactured it. This is called the **trade** or **brand name** of the drug and is the exclusive property of the manufacturer. The first letter of a brand name of a drug is capitalized. After a patent has expired (drug patents run 17 years), other companies may manufacture and sell the drug either under different brand names or under the drug's generic name. These exact copies of the original drug are often called generic drugs. Each drug has an official or nonproprietary name, which is also called the **generic name.** This name is often descriptive of the chemical composition or class of the drug and is assigned to the drug in the early stages of its development for general recognition purposes. Thus every drug has a generic name. Generic names are established by the U. S. Adopted Name Council (USAN). Except in the case of older drugs, the generic (USAN) name is identical to the USP *(United States Pharmacopeia)* or NF *(National Formulary)* name. A generic drug may be manufactured by any number of companies and placed on the market under a different brand or trade name (see Table 7-1 for examples). Brand names are prominently used in advertising a drug to the medical profession, although the generic name must appear in advertising and labeling in letters at least half as big as that of the brand name. The first letter of the name of a generic drug *is not* capitalized.

When prescribing a drug, the physician may use either the generic or the trade name. Currently the trend is to write more prescriptions using the generic name, if one is marketed (many trade names are still under patent protection and are not available from other manufacturers by the generic name), because it is generally less expensive for the patient to purchase. Sometimes the physician orders a specific trade name; however, most states now have laws that entitle the patient to ask the pharmacist for the medication under its generic name unless the physician has specifically directed otherwise, either orally or in handwriting. Also, the pharmacist filling the prescription order for a drug product prescribed by its trade or brand name may select another drug product of the same generic drug type (that is, the generic or chemical name of the drug that is considered to be therapeutically equivalent or "bioequivalent"), unless the physician has specifically directed otherwise either orally or in handwriting, and can do so only when the drug product selected costs the patient less than the prescribed drug product. Because both trade- and generic-named drugs represent the same chemical formula and must heed the same Food and Drug Administration (FDA) standards, they can be used interchangeably according to most state laws. "In approving a generic drug product, the FDA requires rigorous tests and procedures to assure that the generic drug is interchangeable with the brand-name drug under all approved indications and conditions of use," wrote Stuart Nightingale, MD, an FDA associate commissioner. When the substitution is made, the use of the cost-saving drug product dispensed must be communicated to the patient, and the name of the dispensed drug product must be indicated on the prescription label, except when the prescriber orders otherwise.

The third name a drug may be assigned is the **chemical name.** This represents the drug's exact formula (that is, the chemical makeup or molecular structure). Generally this name is used only by the manufacturer and on occasion by the pharmacy when compounding a drug because for most drugs, the chemical name is long and complex.

References and Official Books on Drugs

Established standards and up-to-date information on drugs are published in various books; some of the more common ones follow.

United States Pharmacopeia–National Formulary.
Once two individual books, the *USP* and *NF* are now published as a single volume. The *National Formulary* was acquired by the U. S. Pharmacopeial Convention, Inc., in 1975 and now publishes the USP-NF approximately every 5 years. This is an authoritative book establishing the standards for drugs. Only "official" drugs are listed in this book. All drugs sold under the name listed in the USP-NF must legally conform to the standards set forth. Detailed information is provided on the description of drugs; standards for purity, strength, and composition; storage; use; and dosage. Drugs that meet the standards set by the *Pharmacopeia* bear the initials *USP* on their labels. Some drugs listed in the USP section of the book are cross-referenced to the NF chapter. The NF chapter of the book deals primarily with the pharmaceutical ingredients of the drugs.

AMA Drug Evaluations.
AMA Drug Evaluations is a book published annually by the American Medical Association (AMA). New drugs that are not yet listed in the USP but that have been evaluated by the Council on Drugs of the AMA are presented.

Physicians' Desk Reference.
Although not official, the *Physicians' Desk Reference* (PDR) is a common reference book used by most medical personnel. It is published annually by Medical Economics, Inc., and is automatically distributed free of charge to medical offices, agencies, and hospitals. The PDR has seven sections that list the following:

1. Names, addresses, emergency telephone numbers, and a partial list of products available from the manufacturers who have provided information for the PDR
2. Products by brand name in alphabetic order
3. Products according to an appropriate drug category or classification
4. Products under generic or chemical name headings
5. Products shown in color and actual size under company headings
6. An alphabetic arrangement by manufacturer of over 2500 products; each is described regarding composition, use and action, administration and dosage, precautions, contraindications, side effects, form in which each is supplied, and

TABLE 7–1   Examples of Drug Names

Generic Name	Brand or Trade Name	Pharmaceutical Company
hydrocodone bitartrate	Vicodin	Knoll
diazepam	Valium	Roche
naproxen	Naprosyn	Roche

the common names and generic compositions or chemical names

7. An alphabetic arrangement by manufacturer of diagnostic products with descriptions for use
8. Name, address, and telephone numbers of Certified Poison Control Centers
9. Key to Controlled Substances Categories
10. Information on Vaccine Adverse Event Reporting System

Supplements that provide new or revised product information developed after the PDR was published for the current year are published and distributed as necessary.

American Hospital Formulary Service.   The American Hospital Formulary Service (AHFS) publishes a book that is subscribed to by all hospital pharmacists. It contains extensive, unbiased drug information kept current by periodic supplements. The AHFS arranges drugs into therapeutic or pharmacologic classes according to official (generic) names.

Medical assistants should be familiar with these publications and always keep one or more up-to-date copies in the physician's office as a reference source, for both the physician and themselves.

Drug Standards and Laws Governing Use

When physicians or other qualified medical practitioners prescribe, administer, or dispense drugs, including narcotics, they must comply with federal and state laws that regulate such transactions. Comprehensive laws have been passed by the U. S. Congress and individual state legislatures to regulate the manufacture, sale, possession, administration, dispensing, and prescribing of a range of drugs.

To assist physicians in complying with legal obligations, medical assistants should know and understand the laws regulating drugs and narcotics in the state in which they are employed because individual states may supplement federal legislation with their own laws.

All drugs available for legal use are controlled by the Federal Food, Drug and Cosmetic Act of 1938. This act contains detailed regulations to ensure the purity, strength, and composition of food, drugs, and cosmetics. The general purpose of this act, which is based on interstate commerce, is to control movement of impure and adulterated food and drugs. Amended periodically, the Federal Food, Drug and Cosmetic Act is enforced by the Food and Drug Administration (FDA), a department within the Department of Health and Human Services (HHS), formerly the Department of Health, Education and Welfare (HEW). There are also other federal and differing state laws that regulate the development, sale, and use of drugs.

Legal Classification of Drugs

Controlled substances.   Drugs having the potential for addiction and abuse, including narcotics, stimulants, and depressants, are termed **controlled substances**. Control of these drugs at all levels of manufacturing, distribution, and use

is mandatory. Federal legislation that outlines these controls is the Controlled Substances Act of 1970 (the Comprehensive Drug Abuse Prevention and Control Act), which became effective May 1, 1971, and supersedes the Harrison Narcotic Act of 1914. This act is enforced by the Drug Enforcement Administration (DEA) in the U. S. Department of Justice. It is designed to improve the administration and regulation of the manufacturing, distribution, and dispensing of controlled substances by providing a "closed" system for legitimate handlers of these drugs. Such a closed system should help reduce the widespread diversion of these substances out of legitimate channels into the illicit market. Under this act, drugs that are under federal control are classified into one of five schedules. Each schedule (Schedule I through Schedule V) reflects decreasing levels of addiction and abuse potential, with Schedule I being the classification with highest potential for drug addiction and abuse. Complete listings of the drugs in each schedule are available from district DEA offices. Only a few examples are included here. All controlled substances listed in the PDR are indicated by the symbol C, with the Roman numeral II, III, IV, or V printed inside the C to designate the schedule in which the substance is classified.

- **Schedule I**—These drugs, having the highest potential for addiction and abuse, have not been accepted for medical use in the United States. Their use is limited to research purposes only after the research facility has obtained government approval and agreement to research protocol to test drugs for medical indications. Examples are heroin, marijuana, lysergic acid diethylamide (LSD), and mescaline.
- **Schedule II**—These drugs have a high potential for abuse and addiction but are acceptable for medical use for treatment in the United States. Examples are amobarbital, amphetamine, cocaine, codeine, meperidine, methadone, methamphetamine, morphine, opium, and secobarbital.
- **Schedule III**—These drugs have less potential for abuse than the drugs in Schedules I or II and have a moderate or low addiction potential. They are acceptable for medical use for treatment in the United States. Examples are APC (*a*cetylsalicylic acid, *p*henacetin, and *c*affeine) with codeine, butabarbital, methyprylon, nalorphine, and paregoric. Anabolic steroids became a Schedule III controlled substance in 1991. These drugs are synthetic preparations of the male hormone, testosterone. They have been used by some for a muscle-building effect.
- **Schedule IV**—These drugs have a lower potential for abuse and a more limited addiction liability than those in Schedule III. They are acceptable for medical use for treatment in the United States. Examples are chloral hydrate, diazepam, meprobamate, paraldehyde, and phenobarbital.
- **Schedule V**—These drugs have a low potential for abuse and a limited addiction liability relative to drugs in Schedule IV. They are acceptable for medical use for treatment in the United States. Examples are drugs of primarily low-strength codeine (less than those compounds included in

Schedule III) combined with other medicinal ingredients, as well as preparations containing limited quantities of certain narcotic drugs generally used for antitussive (to suppress coughing) and antidiarrheal purposes.

For a complete listing of all the controlled substances, contact any office of the DEA.

Under federal law, every practitioner who administers, dispenses, or prescribes a controlled substance (with the exception of interns, residents, law enforcement officials, and civil defense personnel who meet special conditions outlined in the Federal Code of Regulations) must be registered with the DEA. Medical practitioners must also have a valid license to practice medicine in their chosen state. The practitioner's office location from which controlled substances are handled must be registered, and the certificate of registration must be kept at this location and available for official inspection. Applications for this registration can be obtained from any DEA regional office or from the DEA Section, PO Box 28083, Central Station, Washington, DC 20005. Registration must be renewed every 3 years.

Only DEA-registered practitioners can order and purchase controlled substances. Schedule II substances must be ordered with the Federal Triplicate Order Form DEA-222. For example, the physician must fill out a Triplicate Order Form to obtain Demerol from the normal source of supply. Orders for Schedules III, IV, and V substances require only the practitioner's DEA registration number. In some states, when ordering Schedule II substances from out-of-state companies, a copy of the purchase agreement (*not* the Federal Triplicate Order Form) must be sent within 24 hours of placing the order to the office of the state attorney general.

Physicians who discontinue practice must return their Registration Certificate and any unused order forms to the nearest DEA office. It is suggested that the word *VOID* be written across the face of the order form before it is sent to the DEA. Physicians having controlled substances in their possession when they discontinue their practice should obtain information from the nearest field office of the DEA and from the responsible state agency on how to dispose of these drugs.

Some important duties of the medical assistant are to ensure that the physician is *currently* registered with the DEA, to obtain the correct federal forms for ordering and purchasing controlled substances, and to keep appropriate records of all transactions. Failure of the physician to comply with the laws regulating the use of controlled substances and other drugs can lead to considerable civil and criminal liability, in addition to the loss of the right to dispense or prescribe medications.

Prescription drugs. Prescription drugs may be obtained only when prescribed, administered, or dispensed by practitioners licensed by state law to prescribe drugs. The Federal Food, Drug and Cosmetic Act requires that these drugs bear on the label the legend *"Caution: Federal Law prohibits dispensing without prescription."* Examples include digoxin and penicillin.

Nonprescription drugs. Drugs easily accessible to the general public fall into the nonprescription drug category. They are often referred to as "over-the-counter" (OTC) drugs because they can be obtained without a prescription (for example, vitamin tablets and aspirin).

Classification of Drugs

Drugs are classified in various ways, including the following:

- Drugs that have a principal action on the body (for example, analgesics and antidiarrheals)
- Drugs used to treat or prevent specific diseases or conditions (for example, hormones and vaccines)
- Drugs that act on specific organs or body systems (for example, cardiovascular drugs and gastrointestinal drugs)
- Forms of drug preparations (for example, solids or liquids)

You should be aware that often one drug may be used to treat different conditions either because it has multiple effects in addition to its primary effects or because it can affect different body systems by exerting its primary effect. For example, a broad-spectrum antibiotic can be used to treat various types of infectious processes, or a diuretic may be used to exert an effect on the cardiovascular system or on the urinary system.

Table 7-2 is a classification of drugs on the basis of their primary actions or effects on the body. Table 7-3 lists 50 of the most commonly used prescription drugs. The accompanying box discusses an emergency tray and emergency tray drugs.

Text continued on p. 364

TABLE 7–2 **Classification of Drugs Based on Actions or Effects on Body**

Drug	Action	Examples*
Amphetamine	Acts as stimulant on central nervous system; has temporary effect of increasing energy and mental alertness; sometimes used to depress the appetite	amphetamine (Benzedrine), dextroamphetamine (Dexedrine)
Analgesic	Relieves pain	aspirin, Empirin with codeine, codeine, acetaminophen (Tylenol); ibuprofen (Advil), naproxen (Aleve)

*Drug names that are capitalized or in parentheses are the trade/brand names.

TABLE 7–2 Classification of Drugs Based on Actions or Effects on Body—cont'd

Drug	Action	Examples*
Anesthetic	Produces generalized or local loss of feeling	thiopental sodium (Pentothal Sodium), tetracaine hydrochloride (Pontocaine Hydrochloride), lidocaine hydrochloride (Xylocaine Hydrochloride)
Angiotensin-converting enzyme inhibitors	Used for hypertension	Capoten, Vasotec, Prinivil
Antacid	Counteracts acidity in stomach	sodium bicarbonate, Maalox, Mylanta, Prilosec, Zantac
Anthelminthics	Destructive to worms	mebendazole (Vermox), Mintezol
Antianginal	Dilates coronary arteries or increases blood flow through collateral coronary vessels	nitroglycerin (Nitrostat), isosorbide (Isordil), amyl nitrite, and drugs listed under calcium channel blockers and beta-adrenergic receptor antagonists
Antianxiety	See sedative/hypnotic	see sedative/hypnotic on page 361
Antiarrhythmic	Prevents harmful atrial and ventricular rhythms	amiodarone hydrochloride (Cordarone), procainamide hydrochloride (Pronestyl), quinidine
Antibiotic	Inhibits growth and reproduction of or eliminates pathogenic bacterial microorganisms	penicillin, ampicillin, tetracycline, Rocephin
Antidiabetic agents	Used to treat type I diabetes, insulin-dependent diabetes	regular insulin (Humulin R, Novolin R), NPH insulin, Lente Insulin, Humulin N Insulin, Ultralente Insulin, Humulin 50/50 and 70/30 Insulins
Antidiarrheal	Counteracts diarrhea	Lomotil, Kaopectate, codeine, paregoric, Imodium, tincture of opium
Anticoagulant	Inhibits blood-clotting mechanism	heparin sodium, dicumarol, warfarin sodium (Coumadin)
Anticonvulsant	Inhibits convulsions, as in epilepsy; prevents or reduces the frequency or severity of seizures related to idiopathic epilepsy, as well as seizures secondary to drug reactions, hypoglycemia, eclampsia, alcohol withdrawal, or traumatic brain injury	phenytoin (Dilantin), phenobarbital, Tegretol, Neurontin, Depakote
Antidepressant	Relieves depression; often called mood elevator or modifier	*Tricyclic antidepressants:* imipramine (Tofranil), amitriptyline (Elavil), doxepin (Sinequan), desipramine (Norpramin) *Monoamine oxidase inhibitors (MAO):* phenelzine sulfate (Nardil), tranylcypromine sulfate (Parnate) *Antimanic agents:* lithium (Eskalith) *Serotonin uptake inhibitors:* fluoxetine hydrochloride (Prozac), Zoloft, Paxil *Miscellaneous:* Serzone, Effexor, Wellbutrin
Antidote	Neutralizes or acts as an antagonist to a poison or drug overdose	Lorfan, naloxone (Narcan) (narcotic antagonists)
Antiemetic	Counteracts nausea and vomiting	dimenhydrinate (Dramamine), prochlorperazine (Compazine), triethobenzamide (Tigan)
Antifungal	Destroys or checks the growth of fungi; controls *Candida (Monilia)* infections in vagina	Mycostatin, nystatin, Lamisil (not for vaginal use), miconazole (Mycelex), Lotrimin
Antihistamine	Counteracts effect of histamine in the body; given to relieve symptoms of allergic reactions such as hay fever and also to relieve symptoms of common cold	diphenhydramine (Benadryl), promethazine (Phenergan), chlorpheniramine (Chlor-Trimeton), loratadine (Claritin), fexofenadine (Allegra)
Antihypertensive (also referred to as hypotensive)	Reduces high blood pressure	reserpine (Serpasil), guanethidine (Ismelin), hydrochlorothiazide (Esidrix)

*Drug names that are capitalized or in parentheses are the trade/brand names.

Continued

TABLE 7-2 **Classification of Drugs Based on Actions or Effects on Body—cont'd**

Drug	Action	Examples*
Antiinflammatory agent and non-steroidal antiinflammatory drug (NSAID)	Reduces or relieves inflammation	*Nonsteroidal agents:* Arthrotec, indomethacin (Indocin), aspirin, naproxen (Naprosyn), piroxicam (Feldene), Lodine, Relafen *Steroids:* triamcinolone (Kenacort), triamcinolone acetonide (Kenalog), prednisone
Antiarthritic preparation	Acts against arthritic symptoms	indomethacin (Indocin), phenylbutazone (Butazolidin), prednisone, piroxicam, (Feldene), naproxen (Naprosyn)
Antiseptic Skin antiseptic Urinary antiseptic to be taken internally	Inhibits growth of microorganisms	70% alcohol nitrofurantoin (Macrodantin), nalidixic acid (NegGram)
Antineoplastic	Inhibits growth and spread of malignant cells	chlorambucil (Leukeran), busulfan (Myleran), melphalan (Alkeran), fluorouracil or 5-FU (Adrucil), megestrol acetate (Megace), tamoxifen citrate (Tamofen)
Antitussive	Inhibits cough reflex	codeine, Benylin cough syrup, Benadryl, Sucrets Cough Control Lozenge
Astringent	Constricts tissue and arrests discharges or bleeding	silver nitrate, alum, zinc oxide
Beta-adrenergic blockers	Used to treat angina, hypertension, cardiac arrhythmias, myocardial infarctions. Act as a shield against excessive stimulation to the sympathetic nerve endings in the heart tissue. Slow down the heartbeat besides making the heart less responsive to stimulations. Thus the heart performs more work with less oxygen demand and pain can be prevented	Inderal, Corgard, Lopressor, Tenormin, Visken
Bronchodilator	Causes dilation of bronchi, eases breathing	aminophylline, albuterol, isoproterenol (Isuprel), epinephrine (Adrenalin)
Calcium channel blockers	Used for hypertension, angina, and tachycardia	diltiazem (Cardizem), Nifedipine, Nicardipine, verapamil (Isoptin)
Cardiogenic (heart stimulator)	Strengthens heart muscle action	digoxin (Lanoxin)
Cathartic	Relieves constipation and promotes defecation; often classified according to the increased intensity of their action as laxatives, purgatives, and drastic purgatives	Cascara, mineral oil, castor oil, bisacodyl (Dulcolax), Fleet enema, Citrate of magnesia
Contraceptive	Prevents or diminishes likelihood of conception	Enovid, Ortho-Novum, Ovulen, Nordette, Desogen, Norplant (an implant)
Cytotoxins	Toxic to certain cells. Used for treatment of cancer	Cytoxan, 6-mercaptopurine
Decongestant	Relieves swelling and congestion in upper respiratory tract	(Actifed combination decongestant and antihistamine); pseudoephedrine (Sudafed), phenylephrine (Neo-Synephrine)
Diuretic	Increases urinary output	hydrochlorothiazide (HydroDiuril), furosemide (Lasix)
Emetic	Stimulates vomiting	Ipecac syrup
Estrogens	Used as oral contraceptives (see above); used in replacement therapy for conditions resulting from estrogen deficiency; also used to treat certain breast carcinomas and prostate cancer and some breast cancer in men	estradiol (Estrace), conjugated estrogens (Premarin), estrone (Theelin and Femogen), ethinyl estradiol (Estinyl and Feminone), Estraderm

*Drug names that are capitalized or in parentheses are the trade/brand names.

TABLE 7–2 **Classification of Drugs Based on Actions or Effects on Body—cont'd**

Drug	Action	Examples*
Expectorant	Liquefies mucus in bronchi and aids in the expectoration of sputum, mucus, or phlegm	terpin hydrate, potassium iodide, guaifenesin (Robitussin)
Hemostatic	Arrests flow of blood by helping coagulation	vitamin K, thrombin
Hormone	Endocrine system produces hormones and secretes them directly into bloodstream; commercial preparations are available for patients whose own glands are malfunctioning	cortisone, insulin, thyroxin
Hypnotic	Produces sleep	Restoril, Ambien, glutethimide (Doriden), chloral hydrate, Dalmane
Immunosuppressive	Prevents rejection of transplanted organ	cyclosporine (Sandimmune), azathioprine (Imuran)
Laxative	Promotes movement of bowels	mineral oil, senna (Senokot)
Miotic	Contracts pupils of eye	Pilacar ophthalmic solutions
Muscle relaxant	Relaxes muscles	diazepam (Valium), carisoprodol (Soma) compound
Mydriatic	Dilates pupils of eye	phenylephrine (Neo-Synephrine) solution, atropine sulfate ointment
Narcotic	Produces sound sleep, stupor, and relief of pain	Drugs derived from opium; morphine, codeine; meperidine (Demerol) (a synthetic narcotic); Percodan, and Dilaudid (semisynthetics)
Psychedelic	Produces feelings of relaxation, freedom from anxiety, highly creative thought patterns, and perceptual changes; causes hallucinations, alters mental functions; highly controversial, potentially very dangerous, and used only under controlled supervision for experimental purposes	LSD, mescaline
Sedative	Quiets and relaxes patient without producing sleep	phenobarbital
Sedative/hypnotic	Calms or quiets patients who are anxious or disturbed	**Antianxiety (anxiolytic)**
	Act pharmacologically as general depressants of the central nervous system	*Benzodiazepines:* Librium, diazepam (Valium), Ativan, Serax, Halcion, Xanax, Dalmane *Nonbenzodiazepines:* meprobamate (Equanil and Miltown)
	Used for treating schizophrenia and other major affective disorders	**Antipsychotic (neuroleptic)** *Phenothiazines:* chlorpromazine (Thorazine), Mellaril, Haldol, Navane, Stelazine, Trilafon
Stimulant	Increases activity of an organ or body system	caffeine, amphetamine (Benzedrine)
Styptic	Checks bleeding by means of astringent quality	Styptic pencil
Sulfa preparations	Antibacterial	sulfisoxazole (Gantrisin), Bactrim, Septra
Vaccine	Prevents infectious diseases	Salk polio vaccine, tetanus and typhoid vaccines, measles, mumps, and hepatitis A and B vaccines
Vasoconstrictor	Constricts blood vessels to increase force of heartbeat, relieve nasal congestion, raise blood pressure, or stop superficial hemorrhage	epinephrine (Adrenalin), norepinephrine (Levophed), ephedrine sulfate
Vasodilator	Dilates blood vessels and reduces blood pressure	nitroglycerin, reserpine (Serpasil), amyl nitrite, nimodipine (Nimotop), Persantine
Vitamins	Organic substances found in foods that are necessary for body to grow and maintain health; commercial preparations of all these vitamins are available	Fat-soluble vitamins: A, D, E, K Water-soluble vitamins: B, C

*Drug names that are capitalized or in parentheses are the trade/brand names.

TABLE 7–3 **Top 50 Prescription Drugs, 2000**

Rank	Trade Name	Generic	Pharmacologic Classification
1.	Premarin	estrogen, conjugated	Female hormone
2.	Synthroid	levothyroxine	Thyroid hormone
3.	Lipitor	artovastatin	Lipid lowering agent
4.	Prilosec	omeprazole	Antiulcer
5.	Vicodin	hydrocodone & acetaminophen	Analgesic
6.	Proventil	albuterol	Bronchodilator
7.	Norvasc	amlodipine	Antihypertensive
8.	Claritin	loratadine	Antihistamine
9.	Trimox	amoxicillin	Antibiotic
10.	Prozac	fluoxetine	Antidepressant
11.	Zoloft	sertraline	Antidepressant
12.	Glucophage	metformin	Hypoglycemic
13.	Lanoxin	digoxin	Cardiotonic
14.	Prempro	estrogen & medroxyprogesterone	Female hormone
15.	Paxil	paroxetine	Antidepressant
16.	Zithromax Z-Pak	azithromycin	Antibiotic
17.	Zestril	lisinopril	Antihypertensive
18.	Zocor	simvastatin	Lipid lowering agent
19.	Augmentin	amoxicillin & clavulanate	Antibiotic
20.	Celebrex	celecoxib	Analgesic, arthritis
21.	Coumadin	warfarin	Anticoagulant
22.	Vasotec	enalapril	Antihypertensive
23.	Amoxil	amoxicillin	Antibiotic
24.	Lasix	furosemide	Diuretic
25.	Levoxyl	levothyroxine	Thyroid hormone
26.	Cipro	ciprofloxacin	Antibiotic
27.	Keflex	cephalexin	Antibiotic
28.	K-Dur	potassium chloride	Electrolyte
29.	Deltrasone	prednisone	Glucocorticoids
30.	Pravachol	pravastatin	Lipid lowering agent
31.	Bactrim	trimethoprim-sulfamethoxazole	Antibiotic
32.	Biaxin	clarithromycin	Antibiotic
33.	Tylenol #3	codeine & acetaminophen	Analgesic
34.	Tenormin	atenolol	Antihypertensive
35.	Zyrtec	cetirizine	Antihistamine
36.	Ambien	zolpidem	Hypnotic
37.	Darvocet-N	propoxyphene & acetaminophen	Analgesic
38.	Xanax	alprazolam	Tranquilizer
39.	Ultram	tramadol	Analgesic
40.	Accupril	quinapril	Antihypertensive
41.	Prinivil	lisinopril	Antihypertensive
42.	Cardizem CD	diltiazem	Antianginal
43.	Glucotrol XL	glipizide	Antidiabetic
44.	Allegra	fexofenadine	Antihistamine
45.	Toprol-XL	metoprolol	Antihypertensive
46.	Dyazide	triamterene & hydrochlorothiazide	Diuretic
47.	Flonase	flutacasone	Glucocorticoids
48.	Cardura	doxazosin	Antihypertensive
49.	Fosamax	alendronate	Bone resorption inhibitor
50.	Lotensin	benazepril	Antihypertensive

From the Redbook 2000.

Emergency Tray and Emergency Drugs

Emergency Tray

Keep a special container or tray with drugs needed for emergencies in a readily accessible location. Also keep sterile syringes, needles, alcohol sponges, diluents, and a tourniquet in this container. In most offices and clinics, the physician makes a checklist of the drugs and supplies to be kept in the emergency tray, varying with the need of the office and the physician's preference. You should be familiar with these specific drugs, knowing the use, usual dosage, and method of administration for each. Check this container or tray frequently to replace items that have been used and to discard outdated drugs or sterile supplies.

Listed in the text that follows are examples of drugs that may be kept on the emergency tray. These vary according to the type of patient and possible emergency that you may encounter at your facility.

Additional supplies that may be kept near this tray for emergency situations include the following:

- Airway equipment (Ambu bag, laryngoscopes and airways of different sizes, and resuscitation masks of various sizes to fit adults, children, and infants; see Figure 17-5)
- Defibrillator and/or an automated external defibrillator (see Chapter 17)
- Electrocardiogram machine
- Intubation equipment and other related materials
- Oxygen tank, mask, and/or nasal cannula with tubing
- Intravenous (IV) sets
- IV solutions (bottles or bags)
- Suction equipment

You should check this equipment daily to make sure that it is in proper working order and to ascertain that there is sufficient oxygen in the tank.

NOTE: For emergencies in each treatment room, some offices and clinics have a plastic bag hanging on the wall containing a single-use resuscitator with mask, filter, and one-way valve.

Emergency Tray Drugs

albuterol (Proventil)—A bronchodilator; an inhalant used to ease breathing, as for asthmatic patients

Benadryl—An antihistamine; used to relieve symptoms of allergic reactions, itching, and anaphylactic shock

Compazine—An antiemetic; used to counteract nausea and vomiting

Dextrose 50%—Used for severe hypoglycemia

diazepam (Valium)—A muscular relaxant and an antianxiety, minor tranquilizer; used to relax muscles or calm and quiet extremely anxious patients

NOTE: Valium must be kept in a locked drawer or cabinet.

digoxin (Lanoxin)—A cardiac glycoside; used for congestive heart failure and certain cardiac arrhythmias

epinephrine (Adrenalin)—A vasoconstrictor and antispasmodic; used to counteract anaphylactic shock, to relieve symptoms of allergic reactions, and as an emergency heart stimulant

Ipecac—An emetic; used to stimulate vomiting in some poisoning cases

Lasix—A diuretic; used to promote the formation and excretion of urine

Narcan—A narcotic antagonist; used in emergency situations for narcotic overdose

nitroglycerin—A vasodilator; used commonly for angina patients

phenytoin (Dilantin)—An anticonvulsant; used to control seizures

Pitocin—A hypothalamic hormone; stimulates uterine contractions to control postpartum bleeding in obstetric patients

steroids—such as hydrocortisone (Solu-Cortef) or methylprednisolone (Solu-Medrol)—Used for their antiinflammatory action

The following drugs may be used during cardiac arrest:

sodium bicarbonate—Used during resuscitation to help correct metabolic acidosis

calcium gluconate or **chloride**—Used for cardiac resuscitation to increase myocardial contractility when epinephrine has failed

isoproterenol (Isuprel)—Used to increase heart rate and cardiac output

lidocaine (Xylocaine)—Used to control ventricular tachycardia

procainamide (Pronestyl)—Used for premature ventricular contractions, ventricular tachycardia, atrial arrhythmias, and paroxysmal atrial tachycardia

verapamil (Isoptin)—Used in arrhythmias to delay conduction through the atrioventricular (AV) node

PRESCRIPTIONS

A prescription is an order written by a licensed physician giving instructions to a pharmacist to supply a certain patient with a particular drug of specific quantity, prepared according to the physician's directions. It is a *legal document*. A prescription consists of the following seven parts (Figure 7-1):

1. Date and patient's name and address (for children, age should be given)
2. Superscription, consisting of the symbol ℞, from the Latin *recipe*, meaning "take thou"
3. Inscription, specifying the ingredients and the quantities; the name of the drug, the dosage form, and the amount per dose
4. Subscription, directing the pharmacist how to compound the drug(s). It generally designates the number of doses to be dispensed.
5. Signa (Sig), from Latin, meaning "mark," which gives instructions to the patient indicating when and how to take the drug and in what quantities
6. Physician's signature, address and phone number, registry number (this is the physician's license number), and, when prescribing controlled substances, the Bureau of Narcotics and Dangerous Drugs (BNDD) number (this is the same as the DEA number)
7. Number of times, if any, that the prescription may be refilled

Some state regulations require that the prescription form have a statement indicating that a generic equivalent may be dispensed. If this is not acceptable, the physician must write out "No substitutions" *or* "dispense as written" *or* initial a box that states "Do not substitute" or "Dispense as written." The pharmacist puts the name of the drug dispensed on the label of the container.

Current prescription writing has been greatly simplified, as pharmaceutical companies now prepare most drugs ready for administration. These preparations have largely eliminated the need for the pharmacist to compound or mix drugs and solutions.

When the physician writes a prescription, he or she gives it to the patient to take to a pharmacist, who dispenses the required medication. Once the prescription has been filled, the pharmacist must keep a record of that sale for 2 years (3 years in four states).

These records are subject to inspection and copying at any time by authorized employees of state and federal law enforcement and regulatory agencies. When a prescription is written for a Schedule II controlled substance (narcotic), a few states require the physician to use an official triplicate prescription blank. In this case, one copy is kept for the physician's office files, and the original and other copy are given to the patient to take to the pharmacist. After filling the prescription, the pharmacist retains the original and endorses the copy, which is forwarded to the Department of Justice at the end of the month in which the prescription was filled.

All prescriptions written for controlled substances in Schedule II must be wholly written in ink or indelible pencil or typewritten, and they must be signed by hand by the physician. A separate prescription blank must be used for each controlled substance ordered. These prescriptions must contain the following information:

- Name and address of the patient
- Date of prescription
- Name and quantity of controlled substance prescribed
- Directions for use
- Physician's DEA registration number (the BNDD number)
- Signature, address, and phone number of physician

Prescriptions for controlled substances in Schedule II cannot be refilled, and some states require that they be filled within 7 days from the date written.

In a bona fide emergency, the physician may telephone a prescription order to a pharmacist for a Schedule II controlled substance. In these cases, the prescribed drug must be limited to the amount required to treat the patient during the emergency period. Within 72 hours the physician must furnish a written, signed prescription order to the pharmacy for the controlled substance prescribed. Pharmacies are required by law to notify the DEA if they have not received the written prescription order within the 72 hours. ("Emergency" means that the drug must be administered immediately for treatment, that there is no alternative treatment available, and that it is not possible for the physician to provide a written prescription form for the drug at that time.)

Prescriptions for controlled substances in Schedules III, IV, and V are written on the physician's standard prescription blank and need only to be signed by the prescriber. These prescriptions are limited to five refills within a 6-month period with proper authorization. A prescription for any controlled substance must be issued for a legitimate medical purpose by physicians acting in good faith in the course of their professional practice. Keep in mind that regulations for prescribing and dispensing controlled substances differ for each of the five schedules and may also be subject to stricter controls passed by many states. Therefore it is vital for you to learn the laws that apply for your state.

FIGURE 7-1   Sample of a prescription.

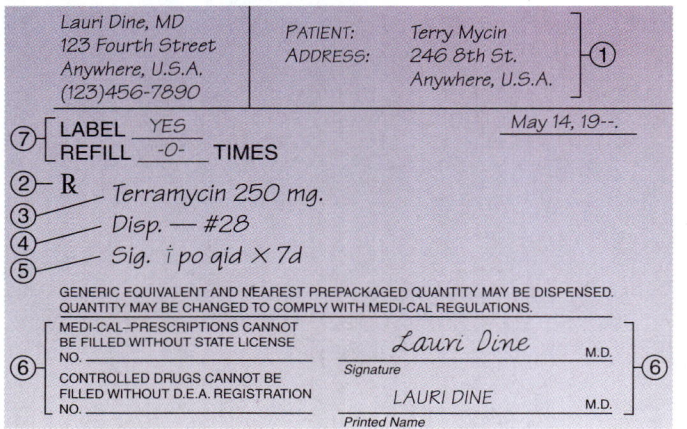

Prescription pads should be kept in a safe place where they cannot be picked up easily by patients. Minimize the number of pads in use at one time. Use them only for writing prescriptions; *do not* use them for notes or memos. A drug abuser could easily erase the note and use the blank to forge a prescription. The DEA and the local police department are to be contacted if your office experiences any theft or loss of controlled substances or official order forms. Contact a local police department if you are aware of forged prescriptions.

Although medical assistants do not write prescriptions, a knowledge of prescription abbreviations and terms used is valuable and may be required to carry out the physician's orders, transcribe medical notes, take telephone messages, answer questions for a patient regarding a prescription, verify information for a pharmacist, and understand instructions for the administration of medications. Table 7-4 is a list of the more common abbreviations and symbols used.

At times the medical assistant may be required to telephone a pharmacy to order a prescription drug that the doctor has prescribed for a patient. When this is done, the following information must be given to the pharmacy:

- The spelling of the patient's name and his or her address and telephone number.
- The name, dose, and quantity (for example, how many tablets) of the drug to be dispensed.
- The instructions to the patient for taking the drug.
- The prescribing doctor's name and telephone number.
- The doctor's license number.
- The doctor's DEA number. Many HMOs require this number to be on *this* record before they will pay for the prescription. This may vary with individual insurance plans and from state to state.

TABLE 7–4   Common Prescription Abbreviations and Symbols*

Abbreviation or Symbol	Meaning	Abbreviation or Symbol	Meaning	Abbreviation or Symbol	Meaning
ā	before	L	liter	qam	every morning
āā	of each	liq	liquid	qd	every day
ac	before meals	m or min	minim	qh	every hour
ad lib	as desired	mcg or μg	microgram	q2h or q2°	every 2 hours
amt	amount	mEq	millequivalent	(q3h or q3° and	every 3 hours
aq	aqueous	mEq/L	milliequivalents per	so on)	
bid	twice a day		liter	qhs	every night
c̄	with	mg	milligram	qid	four times a day
cap(s)	capsule(s)	ml	milliliter	qod	every other day
cc	cubic centimeter	mm	millimeter	qs	quantity sufficient
dil	dilute	npo (NPO)	nothing by mouth	℞	take thou
Dx or Diag	diagnosis	NS	normal saline	s̄	without
D/C or d/c	discontinue	noc(t)	night	sc or subq or SubQ	subcutaneous
D/W	dextrose in water	od	daily or once a day	Sig	directions
dr	dram	OD	right eye	sol	solution
ʒ	dram	oint	ointment	ss or s̄s̄	one half
ʒi	one dram	OS	left eye	subling	sublingual (under the
d	day	OU	both eyes		tongue)
Dr	doctor	oz	ounce	stat	immediately
fl or fld	fluid	ʒ or oz	ounce	S/W	saline in water
g or gm	gram	p̄	after, past	tid	three times a day
gal	gallon	per	by or with	tinc or tr or tinct	tincture
gr	grain	pc	after meals	tab	tablet
gt or gtt	drop(s)	po (per os)	by mouth	tsp	teaspoon
H or hr	hour	prn	whenever necessary	Tbsp	tablespoon
hs	hour of sleep or bedtime	pt	pint (or patient)	ung or ungt	ointment
IM	intramuscular	pulv	powder	U	units
IU	international units	q	every	wt	weight
IV	intravenous				
kg	kilogram				

*According to the style of the American Medical Association, medical and pharmaceutical abbreviations are to be written without the use of periods. For example, rather than writing *b.i.d.* as was done in the past, you will now write *bid,* and so on.

- The number of times the prescription can be refilled, if any. Orders to refill the prescription can be given for 6 to 15 months, depending on the drug.
- The name of the person making this call and his or her affiliation and title.

Patients may also telephone the pharmacy to request a refill of their medication(s). If no refill order is on file, the pharmacy calls the physician's office to request a refill order. The pharmacy gives the patient's name, the name of the drug, the last dose given, and when the last prescription was dispensed. The medial assistant provides this information to the physician and then calls the pharmacy with the physician's decision. Schedule II controlled substances *cannot* be refilled with a telephone order. Refill orders for drugs in Schedules III, IV, and V may be given over the telephone.

ADMINISTER, DISPENSE, PRESCRIBE

In the physician's office, medications may be handled in one of three ways: they may be administered, dispensed, or prescribed. A medication is administered when it is actually given to the patient to take by mouth or when it is injected, inserted, or given by any other method used for administering medications. It is dispensed when it is given to a patient by the physician or pharmacist at the pharmacy to be taken at a later time. It is prescribed when the physician gives the patient a written order, the prescription, to have filled by the pharmacist. Only the physician is licensed to prescribe medications, and in some states under *specific protocols,* certain classifications of nurses can write and sign *some* prescriptions. Depending on state law, various medical personnel may administer medications, and the physician and pharmacist dispense them. On occasion, under the physician's order and supervision, the medical assistant may also dispense stock medications to a patient in the physician's office or health agency.

PHARMACEUTICAL PREPARATIONS

Because of the various properties and uses of different drugs, they are prepared in different ways for patient use. Drugs are supplied in either a solid or liquid state.

Solid state (Figure 7-2)

pills—Small, hard, molded objects of medication, either oval or round.

tablets—Dried, powdered medications compressed into a round or disk-shaped object. Some are scored across the middle so that they can easily be broken in half.

caplets—Tablets shaped like capsules with a special coating to make them easy to swallow. Like tablets, they are said to be virtually tamperproof.

capsules—Liquid or powdered medication enclosed in a rod-shaped gelatin container.

gelcaps—Soft gelatin capsules that cannot be opened. Inside the capsule is an oil-based medication, for example, Tylenol Gelcap or Mylanta Gelcap.

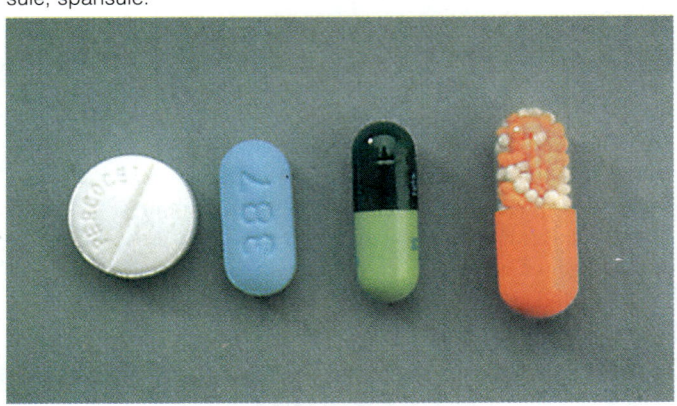

FIGURE 7-2 Solid forms of drugs; *Left to right,* tablet, caplet, capsule, spansule.

spansules—Granules of medication enclosed in a capsule that is prepared so that the medication will be released at various times after being ingested; a sustained-release capsule such as Dexedrine, Contac, or Ornade (for cough or cold).

powders—Medications or mixtures of medications ground into a powder.

lozenges (also called troche [tro′ke]) —Small, round, oval or oblong tablets that release a drug while dissolving in the mouth. The lozenge contains a drug incorporated in a flavored, sweetened base made of sugar and mucilage or a fruit base.

skin patch (transdermal patch)—An adhesive disk impregnated with a medication that is absorbed through the skin into the bloodstream over time.

thin, silicone-rubber capsules or rods (subdermal implants)—Thin capsules or rods of medication that are implanted under the skin. These are used for a slow release of a medication over an extended period.

suppositories—Molded cone-shaped mixtures of medication dispersed in a firm base such as cocoa butter that dissolves and is absorbed when inserted into a body cavity such as the rectum or vagina.

Liquid state

solutions—Liquid preparations consisting of one or more substances **(solutes)** that are dissolved or suspended in a substance (the **solvent**). The most commonly used solvents are distilled water, sterile water, normal saline, and alcohol. Solutes may be (1) a 100% full strength or pure drug in a solid, liquid, or powder form; (2) tablets of a known specific amount of drug; or (3) stock solutions that are strong solutions of known strength used to prepare a weaker solution. To obtain a **true solution,** the solute must be completely dissolved in the solvent. If the solute is evenly dispersed throughout the solution but not dissolved, it is called a **suspension** or a **colloidal solution.** The difference between a true solution and a colloidal solution is determined by the molecular size of the particles of the solute; the colloidal solution contains very small particles. Drugs that are supplied in a suspension *must* be shaken before being administered; the label bears the instruction, *"Shake well."*

diluent—A solution that is added to another to reduce the strength of the initial solution or mixture or to make it more liquid, or thinner, less viscous. Percentages or ratios are used to describe solutions. For example, a 15% solution means that 15 parts of the solute are mixed with 85 parts of the solvent. Some solutions come prepared for immediate use; others have to be mixed before they are suitable for use. When a solution must be prepared for use, it may be necessary to convert the apothecary system of weights and measures to the metric equivalents. Tables 7-6 and 7-8 contain equivalents for these two systems and the preparation of solutions. Some solutions may be administered by injection, mouth, inhalation, irrigation, or lavage; others may be used topically on the skin, on dressings, or for cleansing purposes.

emulsion—An oily substance suspended in a liquid with which it does not mix or in which it does not dissolve, such as fat globules in water with an emulsifying agent (for example, various ointments, Petrogalar [a laxative], and homogenized milk).

tincture—An alcohol solution prepared from drugs or chemicals such as tincture of iodine, tincture of thimerosal (Merthiolate), or tincture of benzalkonium (Zephiran).

lotions—Aqueous preparations containing suspended particles used for local applications intended for soothing (for example, calamine lotion or Caladryl lotion).

elixirs—Solutions containing water, alcohol, and sugar used often as flavoring agents or solvents (for example, terpin hydrate elixir or phenobarbital elixir).

liniment—A liquid or soft mixture of drugs with soap, alcohol, oil, or water used for external application by rubbing it into the skin (for example, camphor liniment, or chloroform liniment).

ointment—A mixture of drugs with a fatty substance used for external application (for example, A & D ointment, zinc oxide ointment, and various antibiotic ointments).

aerosol—A suspension of a drug that is administered in a fine mist or spray. It can be inhaled for treatment of respiratory conditions; others are sprayed on topically. Examples include Alevaire, Bronkosol, and Mucomyst.

spray—*See* Aerosol.

syrup—A thick, concentrated solution of a sugar in water or a watery liquid. A syrup can be used as a flavored vehicle for a medication.

PROFESSIONAL RESPONSIBILITIES

Storage and Handling of Drugs

If a physician keeps medications in the office, certain rules and precautions should be followed. Ideally, all medications should be stored in a separate room in a locked cabinet, and all *must* be kept in their original containers. Many medications must be stored in dark containers or dark areas or refrigerated. Some *must* also be in glass containers because the chemical composition of the drug may react with plastic. Drugs that must be refrigerated are labeled as such. Because drugs deteriorate, it is necessary to have a review schedule so that outdated drugs can be discarded and replaced with a new supply. When discarding outdated, opened drugs, pour liquids down the sink; crush drugs that are in the solid form and flush them down the sink. You should also use this method if you have taken a drug out of its original container and then are unable to use it because it is *never* to be replaced in the container once removed. This method of disposal of medications eliminates the possible chance of drug abuse (that is, persons taking medications out of garbage containers and administering the drug to themselves or dispensing it to others). For unopened drug containers, consult pharmaceutical distributors for possible exchange policy. If no policy exists, dispose of unopened drugs in the same fashion as opened drugs.

To avoid medication errors, keep drugs for external use well separated from those to be used internally. Store disinfectants, cleansing preparations, and all drugs that are poisonous if taken internally in a location well separated from the other drugs. To facilitate easy access to the drugs, organize the central storage area. You may organize the drugs alphabetically or according to drug substance or classification (for example, antibiotics, contraceptives, diuretics, hormones, vaccines). It is also recommended to label storage areas as **external use only** and **internal use**. You can further label areas such as drugs to be used for oral administration and those for parenteral administration.

In addition, **federal law requires that all controlled substances be kept in a substantially constructed, separate, securely locked cabinet or safe.** Some states require that these drugs be kept in a locked cupboard in a locked room. Extra security precautions must also be taken for the needles and syringes that are used for administering parenteral medications. Any loss or theft of controlled substances must be reported by the physician on discovery to the local police department and to the DEA field office in the area. The field office can provide information on what reports are required of the physician.

Labeling

All drugs and solutions must be clearly labeled. Poisons should be clearly labeled as such and kept separate from other medications. Leave all drugs and solutions in the original labeled containers until they are administered or dispensed. Never use, but rather discard, medications or substances that are not clearly labeled or those in unlabeled containers. **When pouring liquids from bottles,** hold the bottle so that the label is facing the palm of your hand. Using this technique prevents soiling or obliterating the label if any of the liquid runs down the side of the bottle (Figure 7-3, *A*; see also p. 370). If a label becomes loose, soiled, or torn, type a new label with the exact information that was provided on the original. It is advisable to have someone else in the office check the new label for accuracy before you affix it to the container.

FIGURE 7-3 **A,** Hold the medicine or graduate at eye level so that you can measure accurately as you pour the medication; **B,** shake or drop tablet into the cap of container.

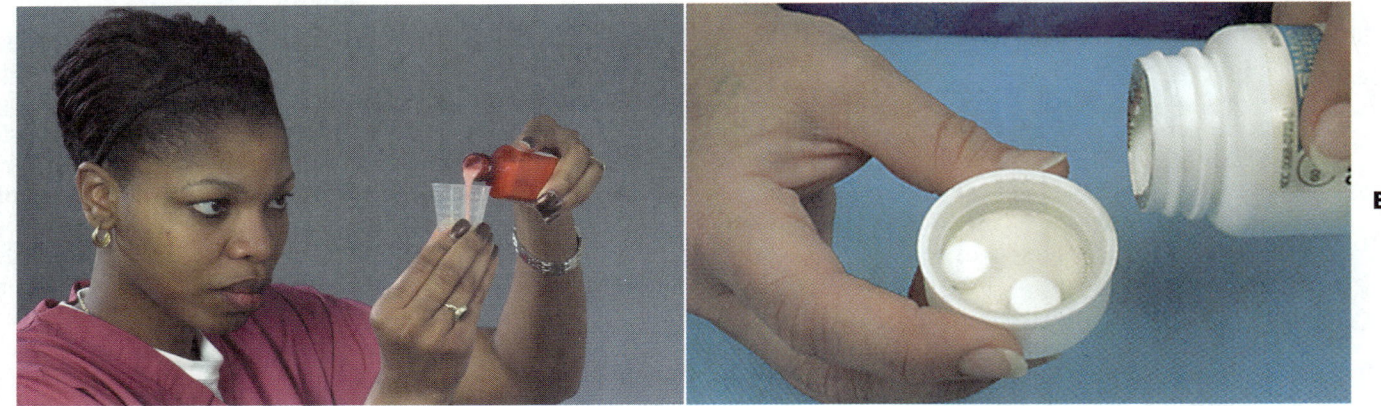

Controlled Substances Inventory and Prescriber's Record

In addition to keeping a running inventory of all narcotics and controlled substances, a physician who dispenses or regularly engages in administering controlled substances is required to maintain a special record, either a card for each type of drug or a daily log book. All these records are to be kept for 2 years (3 years in some states) and are subject to inspection and copying by authorized employees of state and federal law enforcement and regulatory agencies. The physician must also take an inventory every 2 years of *all* stock of the substances on hand.

Records kept on all Schedule II controlled substances dispensed, administered, or prescribed must show the date, name and address of the patient, character and quantity of the drug provided, and pathologic condition and purpose for which the drug was provided. *All records and inventories for controlled substances in Schedule II must be stored separately from other files.*

Records kept on all Schedule III, IV, and V controlled substances administered or dispensed from the office or medical bag must show the date, the name and address of the patient, and the quantity of the drug dispensed or administered. Schedule III, IV, and V records and inventories may be stored separately from other files or in such form that the information is readily retrievable from the practitioner's other business and professional records.

Medical assistants should play a major role in helping the physician keep all the appropriate records, guarding prescription pads, securing medication storage areas to prevent theft, ensuring the proper type of storage and correct labeling for all medications, and discarding and destroying outdated drugs.

ROUTES AND METHODS OF DRUG ADMINISTRATION

Drugs are supplied in various forms for different purposes (Table 7-5). Certain drugs can be administered in a variety of ways, and others must be administered in a specific way to be effective. Methods of administration are divided into two general categories: (1) drugs used for local effect, which are applied directly to the skin, tissue, or mucous membrane involved, and (2) drugs used for a systemic or general effect. A drug applied in this manner must be absorbed and circulate through the bloodstream to produce an effect on the body cells or tissues.

Rules for Administering Medication

Certain rules are to be followed when preparing and administering medications. Additional guidelines and rules that apply specifically to medications given parenterally (by injection) are described later in this chapter.

You must know and always adhere to the five rights of proper medication administration, which are as follows:

- *Right* drug
- *Right* dose
- *Right* route for administration
- *Right* time
- *Right* patient

It is the patient's *right* to expect the five *rights*.

A *sixth* right has been added by many medical authorities to the traditional five rights.

- *Right* documentation

It is the patient's *right* to expect all six of the *rights*.

General instructions

1. Wash your hands before preparing medications.
2. Give only medications and the correct dosage for which you have the physician's written order. A safe practice is to follow only *written* orders that are *complete.*
3. Prepare the medication in a well-lit area away from distractions and interruptions. Give full attention to what you are doing.

TABLE 7–5 Routes and Methods Used for Administering Medications

Route of Administration	Method of Administration	Form of Drug
Oral	The patient is given the drug by mouth to swallow. This is the simplest method and the method most desirable to patients.	Pills, tablets, capsules, spansules, or solutions supplied in bulk form or as a unit dose
Sublingual	The drug is placed under the patient's tongue and left to dissolve and be absorbed. It is not to be chewed or swallowed.	Tablets
Buccal	The drug is placed between the cheek and gum to dissolve and be absorbed.	Tablets
Inhalation	The drug is given via the respiratory tract. The patient inhales the drug using a nebulizer or a special mechanical apparatus.	Aerosols, sprays, mists, or steams medicated with drugs; also oxygen
Rectal	The drug is inserted into the rectum. This method is used when a patient cannot tolerate the drug orally; if unconscious; or if the drug would be destroyed by digestive enzymes. Also may be administered by proctoclysis, a drip method.	Suppositories, enemas, or other solutions
Inunction or topical	The drug is applied or rubbed into the skin. Disposable single-use, examination gloves or tongue depressors should be used when applying drugs such as nitroglycerin or those containing mercury to a patient. This prevents absorption of the drug into your system.	Ointments, lotions, sprays, solutions, powders, tinctures, liniments
Vaginal	The drug is inserted into or applied to the vagina.	Suppository; solution, as in a douche; or liquids or ointments to be applied for local effect on the cervix or vaginal canal; also contraceptive foams and creams
Instillation	The drug is applied in drops to a membrane (e.g., eye or ear).	Solutions
Irrigation	The drug is flushed through a membrane or body cavity.	Solutions
Parenteral	The drug is given by injection through a needle. Types of injections include: • *Subcutaneous:* under the skin • *Intramuscular:* into a muscle • *Intradermal* or *intracutaneous:* into the upper layers of the skin. Used chiefly for skin reactions, as in allergy or tuberculosis testing • *Intraarticular:* into a joint for local effects • *Intraarterial:* into an artery; used in certain diagnostic procedures • *Lumbar puncture* or *intraspinal:* into the spinal canal between two vertebrae; used to administer drugs for diagnostic techniques or for spinal anesthetics • *Intravenous:* into a vein; used for immediate effect of a drug, for blood transfusions, or for parenteral feeding	A drug solution supplied in ampules for single use; in vials for single or multiple use; and in syringes or cartridges prefilled by the manufacturer. Drugs that deteriorate in solutions may be supplied in vials in powdered form to which a specified amount of diluent is to be added when prepared for use. Sterile hypodermic tablets that are to be dissolved before the drug is administered are also available. Larger amounts of solutions for intravenous use are supplied in bottles of 250 ml, 500 ml, or 1000 ml, such as dextrose in water and normal saline, to which other drugs may be added. Plasma and blood are also used for intravenous transfusions.
Transdermal patch (Figure 7-4)	The patch, an adhesive disk impregnated with medication, is applied to a clean dry skin area on the upper arms and legs, chest, and back (e.g., nitroglycerin—a vasodilator used for heart patients); or behind the ear (e.g., Transderm Scop used for motion sickness); or on the trunk of the body, including the abdomen and buttocks but not the breasts (e.g., Estraderm patch—a type of estrogen); or to a nonhairy site on the trunk or upper arm (e.g., Habitrol—a nicotine system used to help people stop smoking). The patches release a controlled amount of drug over time. The drug is absorbed through the skin into the bloodstream.	Single-unit adhesive skin patch in a foil packet
Subdermal implant (Figure 7-5)	A thin capsule or rod of medication is implanted under the skin, commonly in the upper or lower arm. A local anesthetic is given before the implant is placed under the skin.	Thin silicone rubber capsules or rods (e.g., Norplant—a method of birth control)

4. **Read the label of the medication three times:**
   a. When removing from the storage area
   b. Before pouring the desired amount
   c. When replacing the container in the storage area
   Do not use unlabeled or illegibly labeled medications.

5. Know the drug that you are giving. Check the PDR or other reference books if you are unsure of the usual actions, uses, dosage, route of administration, and undesirable side effects.

6. Calculate a dose accurately, when this is necessary. Consult the physician or another competent person for verification when you doubt your answer.

7. **ADMINISTRATION OF LIQUID ORAL MEDICATIONS**—Shake well any medication that is in the form of an emulsion or suspension.
   a. Do not use medications that have changed color, turned cloudy, or have sediment at the bottom (except suspensions).
   b. Hold the bottle with the label in the palm of your hand to avoid damaging the label if the liquid runs or spills.
   c. Hold the medicine or graduate at eye level so that you can measure accurately as you pour the medication (see Figure 7-3, *A*).

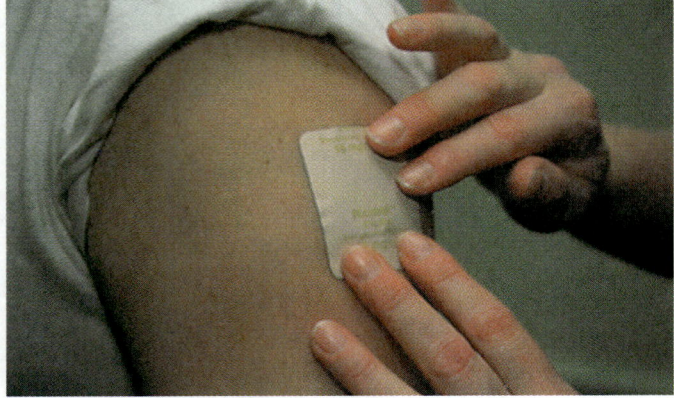

FIGURE 7-4 Transdermal patch on patient's arm.

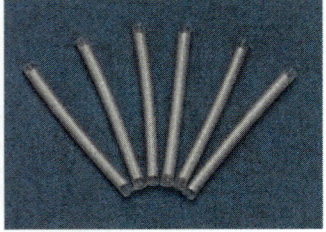

FIGURE 7-5 Six subdermal implants (Norplant) filled with synthetic progesterone used as a form of birth control.

d. Wipe the neck of the container before replacing the cap.
   e. Do not mix liquid medications unless specifically ordered to do so.

8. **ADMINISTRATION OF SOLID ORAL MEDICATIONS**—Tablets, caplets, capsules, or spansules: Shake or drop the tablet or other preparation into the cap of the container; then drop it into a medicine cup. You must *not* handle the medication with your fingers (see Figure 7-3, *B*).

9. *Do not* leave poured medications unattended.

10. Do not administer medications prepared by others. If an error is made, the person administering the medication is responsible.

11. Take both the drug and container to the physician for additional identification when you have prepared the medication to be administered by the physician.

12. Know your patient. You may ask the patient to state his or her name to ensure correct identification.

13. Make sure that the patient is not allergic to the medication before you administer it. Check the chart for any record of allergies and also ask the patient.

14. Stay with the patient until you are certain that an oral medication has been swallowed.

15. **ADMINISTRATION OF RECTAL SUPPOSITORY**—Have the patient assume the Sims' position on the left side. Don gloves. Lubricate the suppository with a water-soluble lubricant, for example, K-Y jelly. Spread the patient's buttocks and insert the suppository about 2 inches into the rectum. The anal canal of an adult is about 1 inch long. Inserting the suppository 2 inches into the rectum facilitates retention. The drug is absorbed through the mucous membrane when the suppository melts. It takes about 10 minutes for the suppository to melt.

16. Observe the patient for any unusual reactions to the drug administered.

17. Discard a medication that the patient refuses. Never replace a medication into the original container once it has been removed.

18. Report immediately to the physician if the patient refuses the medication or if an error was made so that appropriate action can be taken promptly or adjustments made for the patient's care. Follow any new orders that the physician may provide. Prompt corrective action is an important responsibility of the medical assistant if any error is made.

19. Record as soon as possible on the correct patient's chart the date, time, drug and amount given, route of administration, and your signature. *(Errors in administering drugs must also be recorded, describing the incident in full.)* Body locations must be recorded for drugs administered parenterally, by transdermal patch, or when implanted under the skin by the physician. In addition, if the medication administered was a narcotic or other controlled substance, you must record this information in the physician's controlled substances records.

Dosage: Weights, Measurements, Calculations

A complete understanding of basic arithmetic is essential when preparing solutions or administering medications. A review of mathematic calculations is recommended at this time before you prepare to calculate doses and administer medications.

The two primary systems of weights and measures used for describing dosages for medications are the apothecary system and the metric system. The **apothecary system** is our oldest system of measurement, the term being an ancient word meaning pharmacist or druggist. Today the trend is to eliminate the use of the apothecary system and to use the **metric system**, the standard system of weights and measurements set up by the International Bureau of Weights and Measures, although it has not been completely adopted for use by everyone at this time. Therefore you must have an understanding of both systems.

The apothecary system units of fluid measurement are the minim, fluid dram, fluid ounce, pint, quart, and gallon. The units of solid measurement are the grain, dram, ounce, and pound. Roman numerals and fractions are used with this system (for example, HCI gtt X [hydrochloric acid drops ten]; or nitroglycerin gr 1/150 [nitroglycerin grains one/one hundred fifty]).

In the metric system, the units of fluid or volume measurements are the milliliter, or cubic centimeter, and liter. Units of weight or solid measurements are the kilogram, milligram, and gram. Arabic numbers and the decimal system are used with this system. Example: $1/1000 = 0.001$, $1/100 = 0.01$, $1/10 = 0.1$ (for example, tetracycline 250 mg/ml or cc).

See Tables 7-6 through 7-9 for the equivalent values of apothecary and metric measurements for liquids and solids, and the equivalents of common household weights and measurements for these systems.

At times you may be required to calculate the dose of a medication that you are to administer. A simple formula to use is:

$$\frac{\text{Dose you want}}{\text{Dose you have}} \times \text{Quantity on hand} = \text{Quantity to administer}$$

Example: The physician has ordered 500 mg tetracycline, by mouth (po). The dose of tetracycline that you have on hand is labeled 250 mg/tablet.

Therefore:

$$\frac{\text{Dose you want (500 mg)}}{\text{Dose you have (250 mg)}}$$
$$\times \text{Quantity on hand (1 tablet)} = \text{Tablets to give (2)}$$

You would therefore give the patient two tablets of tetracycline 250 mg/tablet so that the patient would receive 500 mg of tetracycline as ordered.

The same formula can be used when preparing drugs supplied in a solution form.

Example: The physician has ordered 500 mg tetracycline to be given intramuscularly (IM). The bottle you have on hand is labeled tetracycline 250 mg/ml. Therefore:

$$\frac{\text{Dose you want (500 mg)}}{\text{Dose you have (250 mg/ml)}}$$
$$\times \text{Quantity on hand (1 ml)} = \text{Dose in ml that you give (2 ml)}$$

When this formula is used, both the dose you want to give and the dose you have on hand must be expressed in the same measurements; that is, to give so many milligrams, the dose on hand must be in milligrams per milliliter for a solution, or in milligrams per tablet or capsule for drugs supplied in the solid form. If this is not the case, you have to convert one measurement into the equivalent value of the other. You should be familiar with the methods used for converting one system of measurements into the other. See Table 7-10 for conversion techniques for calculation of drug doses and the formula for calculating pediatric doses using *Clark's rule*.

To gain competence in this procedure, you should refer to some of the many books available with practice problems in the mathematics of drugs, solutions, and dosages. Use the tables of weights and measurements for a reference. When you doubt your calculations, always seek help from another competent person or the physician.

TABLE 7–6 Metric System Equivalents

Dry weights	
100 micrograms (μg)	= 1 milligram (mg)
1000 mg	= 1 gram (g)
1000 g	= 1 kilogram (kg)

Liquid volume	
1000 milliliters (ml)	= 1 liter (L)
1000 cubic centimeters (cc)	= 1 L
1 ml	= 1 cc
1000 L	= 1 kiloliter

TABLE 7–7 Household System Equivalents

60 drops (gtt) = 1 teaspoon (tsp)
4 tsp = 1 tablespoon (Tbsp) = 1/2 ounce (oz)
2 Tbsp = 1 fluid (fl) oz = 30 cc
8 fl oz = 1 cup (C) = 16 Tbsp
1 pint (pt) = 2 C = 16 oz = 480 cc (approximately)
1 quart (pt) = 4 C = 32 oz
1 gallon (gal) = 4 qt = 128 oz
16 oz = 1 pound (lb)

TABLE 7–8 Metric Doses With Approximate Apothecary Equivalents*

Weights				Liquid Measures†	
Metric	**Approximate Apothecary Equivalents**	**Metric**	**Approximate Apothecary Equivalents**	**Metric**	**Approximate Apothecary Equivalents**
1 gram	= 15 grains	15 mg	= $\frac{1}{4}$ gr	1000 ml	= 1 quart (qt)
2 grams (g)	= 30 grains (gr)	12 mg	= $\frac{1}{5}$ gr	750 ml	= 1$\frac{1}{2}$ pints
1.5 g	= 22 gr	10 mg	= $\frac{1}{6}$ gr	500 ml	= 1 pint (pt)
1 g	= 15 gr	8 mg	= $\frac{1}{8}$ gr	250 ml	= 8 fl ounces
1000 mg	= 15 gr	6 mg	= $\frac{1}{10}$ gr	200 ml	= 7 fl ounces
0.75 g or 750 mg	= 12 gr	5 mg	= $\frac{1}{12}$ gr	100 ml	= 3$\frac{1}{2}$ fl ounces
0.6 g or 600 mg	= 10 gr	4 mg	= $\frac{1}{16}$ gr	50 ml	= 1$\frac{3}{4}$ fl ounces
0.5 g or 500 mg	= 7$\frac{1}{2}$ gr	3 mg	= $\frac{1}{20}$ gr	30 ml	= 1 fl ounces
450 mg	= 7 gr	1.5 mg	= $\frac{1}{40}$ gr	15 ml	= $\frac{1}{2}$ fl ounce (4 fl drams)
300 mg	= 5 gr	1.2 mg	= $\frac{1}{50}$ gr	10 ml	= 2$\frac{1}{2}$ fl drams
0.25 g or 250 mg	= 4 gr	1 mg	= $\frac{1}{60}$ gr	8 ml	= 2 fl drams
200 mg	= 3 gr	0.8 mg	= $\frac{1}{80}$ gr	5 ml	= 75 minims (1$\frac{1}{4}$ fl drams)
0.15 g or 150 mg	= 2$\frac{1}{2}$ gr	0.6 mg	= $\frac{1}{100}$ gr	4 ml	= 1 fl drams
120 mg	= 2 gr	0.5 mg	= $\frac{1}{120}$ gr	3 ml	= 45 minims
0.1 g or 100 mg	= 1$\frac{1}{2}$ gr	0.4 mg	= $\frac{1}{150}$ gr	2 ml	= 30 minims
75 mg	= 1$\frac{1}{4}$ gr	0.3 mg	= $\frac{1}{200}$ gr	1 ml	= 15 minims
60 mg	= 1 gr	0.25 mg	= $\frac{1}{250}$ gr	0.75 ml	= 12 minims
50 mg	= $\frac{3}{4}$ gr	0.2 mg	= $\frac{1}{300}$ gr	0.6 ml	= 10 minims
40 mg	= $\frac{2}{3}$ gr	0.15 mg	= $\frac{1}{400}$ gr	0.5 ml	= 8 minims
30 mg	= $\frac{1}{2}$ gr	0.1 mg	= $\frac{1}{600}$ gr	0.3 ml	= 5 minims
25 mg	= $\frac{3}{8}$ gr			0.25 ml	= 4 minims
20 mg	= $\frac{1}{3}$ gr			0.2 ml	= 3 minims
				0.1 ml	= 1$\frac{1}{2}$ minim
				0.06 ml	= 1 minim

*The approximate dose equivalents in this table represent the quantities that would be prescribed, under identical conditions, by physicians trained, respectively, in the metric or in the apothecary system of weights and measures.

†A milliliter (ml) is the approximate equivalent of a cubic centimeter (cc).

TABLE 7–9 Common Household Weights and Measurements With Metric and Apothecary Equivalents and Preparation of Solutions

Household	Metric and Apothecary Equivalents	
	Metric	**Apothecary**
Liquid		
1 drop (gtts)		= 1 minim (m)
15 drops	= 1 milliliter (ml or cc)	= 15 minims
1 teaspoon (tsp) or (t)	= 4 ml	= 1 fluid dram (fl dr)
1 dessert spoon	= 8 ml	= 2 fl dr
6 teaspoons or 2 tablespoons (tbsp) or (T)	= 30 ml	= 1 fluid ounce
1 measuring cup	= 240 ml	= 8 fl ounces
2 measuring cups	= 500 ml	= 1 pint (pt) (16 fl oz)
4 measuring cups	= 1000 ml	= 1 quart (qt) or 2 pts or 32 oz
1 tbsp	= 15 ml	= 4 drams ($\frac{1}{2}$ oz)
Dry		
$\frac{1}{8}$ teaspoon	= 0.5 gram (g)	= 7$\frac{1}{2}$ grains (gr)
$\frac{1}{4}$ teaspoon	= 1 g	= 15 gr
1 teaspoon	= 4 g	= 60 gr or 1 dram
1 tablespoon	= 15 g	= 4 drams
2 tablespoons	= 30 g	= 1 ounce

TABLE 7–9   Common Household Weights and Measurements With Metric and Apothecary Equivalents and Preparation of Solutions—cont'd

	Preparation of Solutions	
Prescribed Strength	**Amount of Full-Strength Drug**	**Amount of Fluid**
1:1000	1 teaspoonful	1 gallon (gal)
1:1000	15 drops	1 quart
$\frac{1}{10}$ of 1%	15 drops	1 quart (qt)
1:500	2 teaspoonsful	1 gallon
1:500	30 drops	1 quart
$\frac{1}{5}$ of 1%	30 drops	1 quart
1:200	5 teaspoonsful	1 gallon
1:200	1¼ teaspoonsful	1 quart
$\frac{1}{2}$ of 1%	1¼ teaspoonsful	1 quart
1:100 (1%)	2¼ teaspoonsful	1 quart
1:50 (2%)	5 teaspoonsful	1 quart
1:25 (4%)	2½ tablespoonsful	1 quart
1:20 (5%)	3 tablespoonsful	1 quart

TABLE 7–10   Conversion Techniques for Calculation of Drug Dosages

Metric measurements to apothecary measurements
1. *Grams to grains:* Multiply the number of grams by 15
2. *Milligrams to grains:* Divide the number of milligrams by 60
3. *Grams to ounces:* Divide the number of grams by 30
4. *Milliliters to fluid ounces:* Divide the number of milliliters by 30
5. *Milliliters to minims:* Multiply the number of milliliters by 15

Apothecary measurements to metric measurements
1. *Grains to grams:* Divide the number of grains by 15
2. *Grains to milligrams:* Multiply the number of grains by 60
3. *Ounces to grams:* Multiply the number of ounces by 30
4. *Fluid ounces to milliliters:* Multiply the number of fluid ounces by 30
5. *Minims to milliliters:* Divide the number of minims by 15

Metric measurements to metric measurements
1. *Grams to milligrams:* Multiply grams by 1000
2. *Milligrams to grams:* Divide milligrams by 1000
3. *Liters to milliliters:* Multiply liters by 1000
4. *Milliliters to liters:* Divide milliliters by 1000

Pediatric Dose Calculation

The formula for calculating a pediatric dose is different. The calculation of a pediatric dose is based on the body weight of the child. The formula, called *Clark's rule,* is as follows:

$$\frac{\text{Weight of child in points} \times \text{Usual adult dose}}{\text{divided by 150}} = \text{Safe dose for a child}$$

Example: The physician has ordered aspirin for a child that weighs 22.5 pounds. Knowing that the usual adult dose of aspirin is 10 grains, you would calculate as follows:

$$\frac{22.5 \text{ lb} \times 10 \text{ gr}}{150} = \frac{225}{150} = 1.5 \text{ grain}$$

You would therefore give the child 1.5 gr of aspirin, which is a safe dose for a child.

For some drugs the pediatric dose is stated by the manufacturer in the literature accompanying the drug.

More examples and conversion problems are included in the *Student Mastery Manual* that accompanies this textbook.

FACTORS INFLUENCING DOSAGE AND DRUG ACTION

Not all individuals respond to a given medication in the same manner. When prescribing a drug for a patient, the physician takes into account the following factors that influence the prescribed dosage and anticipated action.

Age

Infants, young children (see Table 7-10), and the elderly usually require a smaller dosage of a medication.

Sex

The average woman is given a smaller dosage than the average man because of the difference in body structure and overall weight. Also, when a woman is pregnant, drugs and the dosage are monitored very closely to prevent harmful effects to the fetus.

Weight

The usual rule is the smaller or lighter the patient, the smaller the dosage of drug. Certain medication dosages are determined according to the weight of the patient.

Past Medical History and Drug Tolerance

If a patient has been taking a medication regularly for an extended period, a tolerance to the drug may have developed, and a larger dosage may be required to obtain the desired results. This is often seen with the use of narcotics, barbiturates, sedatives, and analgesics.

Physical or Emotional Condition of the Patient

A patient who has excruciating pain requires a larger dose of an analgesic than a patient who experiences intermittent pain. A severely depressed patient requires a larger dosage of an antidepressant than a patient suffering from mild depression.

Drug Idiosyncrasies or Allergies

At times the patient may experience an abnormal susceptibility or reaction to a drug. Alternative drugs with similar actions can then be prescribed.

Type of Action Desired or Produced

Drugs can produce local, systemic, selective, or cumulative actions. A **local action** occurs when the drug is absorbed and produces an effect at the site to which it was administered (for example, a local anesthetic administered to deaden sensation in the body area to be treated). A **systemic action** occurs when the drug is absorbed and circulates in the bloodstream to produce a general effect (for example, central nervous system stimulants and depressants). A **selective action** is a more specific effect of a drug on one special body area than on other areas (for example, bronchodilators). A **cumulative action** occurs when a drug accumulates in the body and exerts a greater effect than the initial dose; the drug accumulates in the body faster than it can be

metabolized and excreted, such as alcohol does when a person drinks two or three drinks in 1 hour.

Route of Administration

Although there are exceptions, generally medications administered parenterally are given in smaller dosages than those given by mouth. Larger amounts of medications are used for topical application than for internal administration. Drugs administered parenterally produce their effects much more rapidly than drugs administered orally. When a systemic effect is desired from a drug that would have an irritating or undesirable effect on certain tissues, it should be given intramuscularly rather than by other parenteral routes.

Time of Administration

For optimal effects, some drugs must be taken before meals; two, three, or four times a day; or after meals to avoid irritating the lining of the stomach. Drugs will be absorbed more quickly and have a more rapid effect if taken on an empty stomach.

Interactions of Drugs

Some drugs, when taken together, may enhance or counteract the effect of the other.

Interactions are described as follows:

- **Synergistic:** One drug augments the activity of the other drug; the action of the drugs is such that their combined effect is greater than the sum of their individual effects. For example, barbiturates taken with alcohol have up to four times the depressant effect than either drug would have if taken alone.
- **Potentiating:** A synergistic action in which one drug increases the effect of another drug when taken simultaneously, producing a combined effect that is greater than the sum of the effects of each drug taken separately.
- **Antagonistic:** One drug neutralizes or counteracts the action of the other drug when they are taken together.
- **Additive:** When the combined effect produced by the action of two or more drugs is equal to the sum of their separate effects.

Thus it is vital to know if the patient is taking any other medication and, in some cases, any alcoholic beverage, before a new medication is prescribed. It is also important to ask if the patient takes nonprescription drugs or herbs. Often patients do not consider drugs that they purchase over the counter to be medications; nonetheless, these are medications that may possibly interact adversely with a prescription drug.

Summary

Drugs are potent substances that can provide individuals with extremely beneficial results when used properly and with care, but they are also capable of producing hazardous or fatal results when used indiscreetly. Toxic effects such as allergic reactions, adverse effects on the blood or blood-producing tissues, drug dependence, accidental poisoning, or drug overdose can be the result of careless or uninformed use of any drug on the market for legal use or from illegal drugs obtained in the streets. Always handle and administer drugs with extreme care because a life may depend on their proper use.

PATIENT EDUCATION

Patient education is a vital part of all medical care and treatment. When drug therapy is initiated, certain considerations and drug safety precautions must be brought to the patient's attention. The physician or medical assistant should instruct the patient to do the following:

- Inform the physician of **all** drugs, including prescription and over-the-counter drugs, herbal preparations, or street drugs, currently being taken or taken periodically. If the patient has more than one physician, tell each of them what drugs are being taken.

   This information is important because some drugs (as well as some foods and medical conditions) can alter another drug's effect. Today interest in herbs is expanding as claims made for their healing powers are growing. Herbs interact with each other and with many prescription drugs; therefore it may be necessary to adjust the dosage of a prescription medication for a patient who is taking herbal preparations. Herbs can be as strong as any other drug, so patients need to be just as careful about using them as they would any other drug on the market. The FDA classifies herbs as foods, not drugs, and as such, they are not subject to the rigorous testing and monitoring done to other drugs on the market. When buying any herbal product, one should always look for the word "standardized" on the label. This means that the manufacturer guarantees the presence of an effective percentage of the active ingredient in the product.

   The more doctors a patient sees and the more medications taken, the more important it is to be careful.
- Always obtain medications from the same pharmacy. Most pharmacies now have computer systems that keep continuous records of your prescriptions and have programs that warn of harmful interactions or unusual dosages.
- Organize all medications.
- Inform each physician of any reactions or allergies that he or she has to drugs.
- Know the *name, dosage,* and *purpose* of each medication that he or she is taking.
- Know how, how often, and for how long the drug is to be taken.

   The patient should follow the instructions for taking the drug as prescribed. At times a drug should be taken with food, before or after meals, or on an empty stomach. These directions must be followed precisely because there are sound medical reasons for these directions. Some drugs should be taken with food to avoid or minimize gastrointestinal irritation and reactions. Others should not be taken within 2 hours of certain foods, such as dairy products, or

should be taken on an empty stomach for proper metabolism and absorption. When drugs are to be taken 3 or 4 times a day, or every 6 hours, be sure that the patient understands the time schedule to be followed. Again, based on sound scientific reasoning, drugs should be taken according to a specific schedule to maximize treatment.
- Know the possible dangers of exceeding the recommended dosages.
- If necessary, devise a calendar or diary as a reminder of what drug to take and when.
- Call the physician if *any* unusual reaction(s) occur. (The patient should be informed of possible side effects.) Recommended doses can cause undesirable and even potentially dangerous side effects or adverse reactions in some people.
- Do not stop taking the medication unless directed to do so by the physician. Some drugs, such as antibiotics, must be taken for 7 to 10 days to be effective; other drugs, such as prednisone or levothyroxine (Synthroid), should be tapered off slowly under the direction of the physician.
- Do not skip taking medication(s).
- **NEVER** share medications.
- Be aware that some drugs may lead to a dependency if misused or abused, and understand the dangers of dependency.
- Do not save old prescriptions. Look for the expiration date on all drugs being used. Old or outdated drugs should be flushed down the sink or toilet.
- *Never* give medications to anyone else. They are only for *his or her* condition.
- Do not use alcohol when taking medications unless the physician or pharmacist says it is safe.
- Avoid certain activities such as driving a motor vehicle when taking drugs that cause drowsiness.
- Check with the pharmacist regarding where to store medications. Some drugs must be kept in a refrigerator. Others should be kept in a dry, cool atmosphere. Usually medications should not be kept in a hot, damp bathroom cabinet.
- Do not keep medications in a bedside stand. Take medications in a well-lit area to read the label and be sure that the medication and dosage are correct.
- **Always** read the label of the container from which he or she removes the medication before taking it. **Never** assume that he or she is taking the right medication without reading the label on the container.
- Be alert for special labels with added directions or warnings added to the medication container (see the accompanying Health Matters box).
- If the patient has poor vision, ask the physician or pharmacist to print the name of the drug and the treatment schedule out clearly on a separate piece of paper or card.
- Keep all drugs out of the reach of children.
- Always ask or call the physician if he or she has any additional questions regarding the medication therapy.
- **Be aware that all of the preceding directions are vital to a successful program of medical care. Directions must be followed to use drugs safely.** (See the box on Compliance Issues and Tips.)

HEALTH **MATTERS**

KEEPING YOUR PATIENTS INFORMED

Some medications will carry one or more of the following additional labels. It is vital that the patient understand the importance of adhering to these directions.

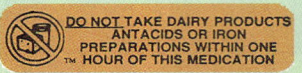

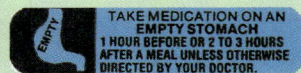

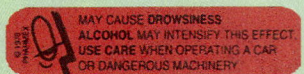

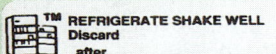

Swallow Whole. Do Not Chew Or Crush.

Do Not Take Aspirin Or Aspirin Containing Products Without Knowledge And Consent Of Your Physician.

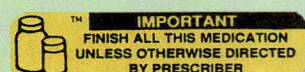

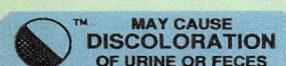

Do Not Drink Alcoholic Beverages While Taking This Medicine.

Take This Medicine With A Snack Or Small Meal If Stomach Upset Occurs

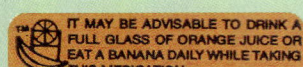

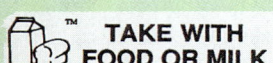

Do Not Use This Medicine If You Are Pregnant, Plan To Become Pregnant, Or Are Breastfeeding. Check With Your Doctor Or Pharmacist.

Read The Patient Information Leaflet That Came With This Medicine

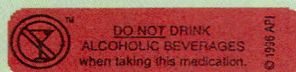

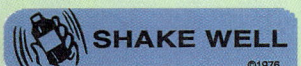

Take Or Use This Medicine Exactly As Directed. Do Not Skip Doses Or Discontinue Unless Directed By Your Doctor.

Obtain Medical Advice Before Taking Nonprescription Drugs. Some May Affect The Action Of This Medication.

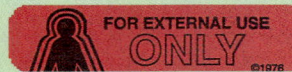

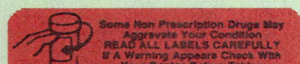

Take Or Use This Medicine Exactly As Directed. Do Not Skip Doses Or Discontinue Unless Directed By Your Doctor.

Some Nonprescription Drugs May Aggravate Your Condition. If You Have Questions, Check With Your Doctor Or Pharmacist.

HEALTH **MATTERS**

COMPLIANCE ISSUES AND TIPS

Never assume that all patients understand the instructions given and that there isn't any problem with the medication regimen. Many times prescription medications are not taken the way they should be, and millions just are not taken. There are dangers of *noncompliance,* that is, not taking the medications as prescribed. These dangers could include serious medical problems; recurrent infections; the development of drug-resistant conditions, such as some tuberculosis cases and some sexually transmitted diseases; and possibly emergency situations and early deaths. Researchers also attribute new, drug-resistant strains of HIV to patients who do not follow their complex medication regimen and attribute the misuse of antibiotics over extended periods to creating forms of previously treatable diseases that now cannot be treated even with the most advanced medications.

When assisting with obtaining medical histories, you can ask patients if they have been taking their medication(s) and specifically if they have missed any doses in the past week or more. Often patients don't understand instructions or don't understand how important the medication is, or they are embarrassed to discuss side effects, such as constipation, diarrhea, or erectile dysfunction (ED) (impotence). Some patients don't follow directions because they simply forget to take the medication, they find it inconvenient to take the medication as directed, or they find it too expensive to take the prescribed amount. Some even deny that they have a medical problem that necessitates taking medications, and others just don't want to take drugs but haven't expressed this to the physician. Some patients, especially older patients, may find it hard to swallow a tablet, so rather than possibly choking on it, they just don't take it; again, they don't mention this to the physician because they are embarrassed to express their fear of choking. Patients with asymptomatic diseases, such as high blood pressure, often think that they don't need the medication unless they have symptoms, so they stop taking the drug when they begin to feel better or when they don't have any apparent symptoms. Other drugs that often are not taken as directed are those with unpleasant side effects and those used for treating psychiatric conditions. All of these issues should be addressed.

Once you have developed a good rapport with patients, they often will discuss many of their concerns with you; in turn, you can relate this information to the physician. You may also ask patients to bring all of their medications to their next appointment or to bring at least a list of the medications that are currently prescribed for them and a list of those that they are taking as scheduled. When they come for their appointment, ask them to tell you what each drug is for and how much and when each should be taken. This allows you to find out if patients are following and understanding directions. The list can then be reviewed with the physician to make sure that all of the medications are still needed. If patients are not taking their medications as prescribed, ask them why they haven't been doing so. The reason(s) will enable the physician and you to work with patients to solve the problem(s).

HEALTH **MATTERS—cont'd**

TIPS

- Give patients written information to take home about their treatment program and instructions for taking their medications.
- Have patients repeat the instructions given to ensure that they understand them.
- For patients having trouble swallowing pills or complaining that the pill isn't going down when they swallow it, suggest the following:

Get a liquid form of the medication if one is available.

Split tablets that are scored down the middle in half. Smaller pieces may be easier to swallow.

Eat a piece of banana after swallowing the pill. The soft bulk of the banana will push the pill down often better than more liquid.

- Ask patients how they are going to remember to take their medication(s). You could suggest that they create a medicine record form, as the following example shows, which would include writing down the name of each medicine, the reason for taking it, the amount (dosage), and the time(s) of day each should be taken. They could also record each time they take a dose. Medicines should be added to the record as they get new prescriptions or when they take over-the-counter drugs, including herbal preparations. Also suggest that they link taking their medication(s) to some everyday activity, such as taking the pill when they brush their teeth, before getting dressed, after lunch, when they watch a regular TV news or other regular show, and so on.

Prescription Medicines

Name of medicine (Example)	Reason taken	Dosage	Time(s) of day
Penicillin VK 250 mg	To treat my strep throat	1 tablet, 4 times a day	9 am, 1 pm, 5 pm, 9 pm

Over-the-Counter Medicines

(Check here if you use any of these)

[ ] Laxatives
[ ] Diet pills
[ ] Vitamins
[ ] Minerals
[ ] Cold medicine
[ ] Aspirin/other pain, headache, or fever medicine
[ ] Cough medicine
[ ] Allergy relief medicine
[ ] Antacids
[ ] Sleeping pills
[ ] Herbal preparations
[ ] Others (names):

_____

_____

- Encourage patients to ask the pharmacist any questions they may have when they pick up their prescription or to call the pharmacist later from home if that would make them feel more comfortable.

- Ensure that patients understand the meanings of "generic" and "brand" names of drugs.
- Make sure patients understand that they are not "bothering" you or the physician with any of their concerns and questions and that you and the physician are happy to help them. Patients must understand and feel comfortable with the treatment program. Encourage patients to ask the following questions:

    What is the medicine's name?
    Is there a generic form available?
    Why am I taking this medicine?
    When should I take it?
    Should I take this on an empty stomach or with food?
    Is it safe to drink alcohol with it?
    If I forget to take it, what should I do?
    How much should I take?
    How long am I to take it?
    What problems should I watch for?

- **Remember, medicines can only help if taken the correct way.**

INJECTIONS

Injections are an important means of administering drugs for various forms of treatment. Because two foreign objects, the medication and the needle, are being introduced into the patient's body, these procedures must be performed with extreme care and excellent technique. The effectiveness of the medication is influenced by the correct choice of injection site and the use of precise technique. Any injection administered into an inappropriate body site or with incorrect technique may interfere with the body's use of the medication and, more importantly, may cause irreparable damage. The practices of aseptic (sterile) technique (see Chapter 6) must be observed when administering injections to minimize the danger of causing an infectious process.

Reasons Physicians Order Injections

1. To achieve a rapid response to the medication. When injected, a medication enters the bloodstream quickly and therefore is more effective.
2. To guarantee the accuracy of the amount of medication given.
3. To concentrate the medication in a specific area of the body, such as into a joint cavity, fracture, or lumbar puncture.
4. To produce local anesthesia to a specific part of the body.
5. To administer the medication when it cannot be given by mouth or by other methods, either because of the physical or mental condition of the patient or the nature of the drug.
6. When the effect of the medication would be destroyed by the digestive tract or lost through vomiting or when it would irritate the digestive system.

Dangers and Complications Associated With Injections

1. Injury to superficial nerves or to a vessel
2. Introduction of infection resulting from the improper disinfection of the injection site, from a contaminated needle or syringe, or from an operator with unclean hands
3. Breaking a needle in a tissue
4. Injecting a blood vessel rather than a muscle or subcutaneous tissue
5. Hitting a bone in a very thin patient
6. Allergic reactions that may be mild, severe, or even fatal
7. Toxic effects produced by the medication
8. Too much air entering the bloodstream in a venipuncture

Body Areas to Avoid When Administering Injections

1. Burned areas
2. Scar tissue
3. Edematous areas
4. Cyanotic areas
5. Traumatized areas
6. Areas near large blood vessels, nerves, and bones
7. Areas where there have been a change in skin texture or pigmentation
8. Areas where there are other tissue growths such as a mole or wart

Supplies and Equipment for Administering Injections

Syringes. Disposable plastic or glass and nondisposable glass syringes are available in several standard sizes and shapes. The most common sizes used in the physician's office are 2, 3, 5, or 10 cc or ml. The parts of the syringe are the **barrel,** the outside portion, with calibrated markings used to measure the amount of solution to be drawn into the barrel; the **plunger,** the portion that fits inside the barrel; the **flange,** a rim at the end of the barrel used by some when pushing on the plunger when injecting a drug; and the **tip,** the point at which the needle will be attached, which is either a plain or a Luer-Lok tip. A solution is drawn up into the barrel by suction when the plunger is pulled out and injected by pushing the plunger

back into the barrel (Figures 7-6 and 7-7). Other variations of syringes include the insulin syringe (Figure 7-8), tuberculin syringe (Figure 7-9), Tubex injector for use with a disposable needle-cartridge unit, and a disposable syringe unit-dose system.

FIGURE 7-6 **A,** Parts of a syringe; **B,** Safety-Lok syringe.

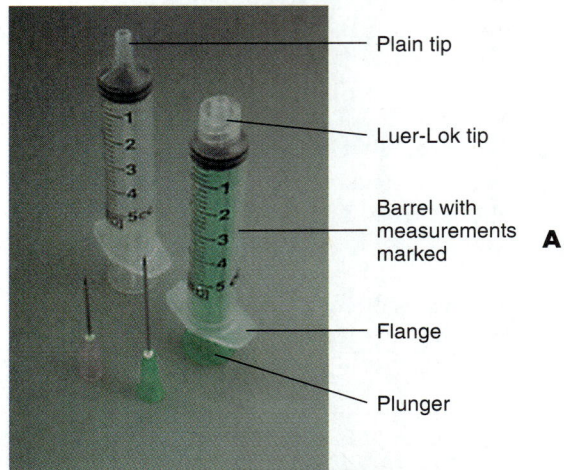

Plain tip
Luer-Lok tip
Barrel with measurements marked **A**
Flange
Plunger

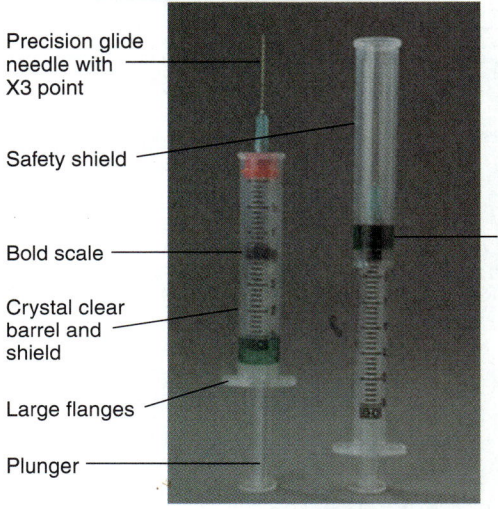

Precision glide needle with X3 point
Safety shield
Bold scale
Crystal clear barrel and shield
Large flanges
Plunger

Safety lock indicator (turns green to visibly confirm the shield is safely locked) **B**

FIGURE 7-7 Syringes, 5 cc and 10 cc, with needles attached. Calibrations are marked in cubic centimeters.

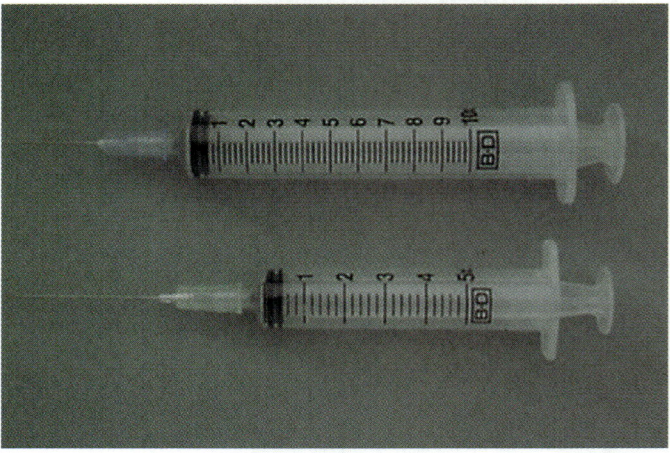

A variety of systems are available with a safety shield that is pulled up and over the needle after use. The purpose of the safety shield is to cover the needle without having to recap the needle after use. This provides protection for the user from a possible needlestick and/or contamination before the syringe is discarded (see Figure 7-6, *B*; Figures 7-10 to 7-12). Sterile disposable syringes come supplied in a paper wrapper or a rigid plastic container. Calibrations, usually in cubic centimeters (cc) or milliliters (ml) and minims, are marked on the barrel of the syringe.

See Figure 7-10 for the procedure for using the Safety-Lok syringe and Figure 7-12 for a procedure for using the Monoject safety syringe.

Needles.   Needles come in various lengths, ranging from $\frac{1}{4}$ to 6 inches, and with various gauges, ranging from 13 to 30. The gauge of the needle and the length are indicated on the outside of the sterile protective cover or wrapper. Some manufacturers also color code the wrappers for quick and easy identification of the gauge. The parts of a needle are the **point;** the **bevel,** which is the slanted part of the opening; the **cannula** or **shaft;** and the **hub,** which fits onto the tip of a syringe (Figure 7-13). The smaller the gauge of the needle, the larger the **lumen** or inside diameter. For example, an 18-gauge needle has a large lumen, whereas a 26-gauge needle has a small lumen. The size and length of a needle govern its use.

Today most practitioners use disposable needles and syringes to prevent all danger of cross-infection, although the reusable type is still available.

Skin antiseptic.   Before an injection is administered, the skin must be cleaned with an antiseptic. The most commonly used is isopropyl alcohol placed on a clean cotton ball or a prepackaged sterile alcohol sponge.

Medications and diluents.   Most medications for parenteral use are in an aqueous solution or in a suspension; although some are in an oil solution or in a suspension, and a few are in tablet or powdered form. When a sterile hypodermic tablet or powdered drug is to be dissolved before parenteral use, sterile water for injection or sterile normal saline is used as the diluent. The type and amount to be used are indicated on the container in which the drug is supplied.

Medication solutions are supplied in single- or multiple-dose form. Those for **single use** are supplied (1) in syringes or cartridges that are prefilled by the manufacturer; (2) in an ampule, a small glass container with a constricted neck that is to be broken off when the drug is to be used; or (3) in a single-dose vial.

Containers with **multiple doses** of a medication are called vials. These are small bottles containing from 10 to 50 ml of a drug solution. Vials are usually covered with a soft metal cover and have a rubber, self-sealing stopper. At the time of use, this rubber stopper is cleansed with an alcohol sponge and then punctured with the needle to inject air and withdraw an equal amount of drug (Figure 7-14). Procedures to withdraw solutions from an ampule and vial are discussed later under Administration of an Intramuscular Injection.

Reconstitution of a Powdered Drug

Some medications deteriorate or remain stable for only a short time when mixed in certain solutions. These medications are supplied as a powder in a sterile field. This powder has to be made into a solution before the medication can be administered. Sometimes a special diluent is provided with the medication; at other times sterile water or sterile normal saline is used to reconstitute the medication. **Reconstitution** is the process of adding a liquid to a powdered drug in preparation for administration. The manufacturer's directions for reconstituting the medication must be followed precisely to avoid overdosing or underdosing the patient. When the powder and diluent are mixed, the solution should appear clear (or cloudy if it is a suspension) without any clumps of powder left in it. *Read* the manufacturer's description of the medication to be certain if it should appear clear or cloudy. Examples of drugs supplied in a powdered form that need to be reconstituted before use include potassium penicillin G; the measles, mumps, and rubella vaccination; and ceftriaxone (Rocephin), a broad-spectrum antibiotic.

FIGURE 7-8   Insulin syringes. Calibrations are marked in units per cubic centimeters.

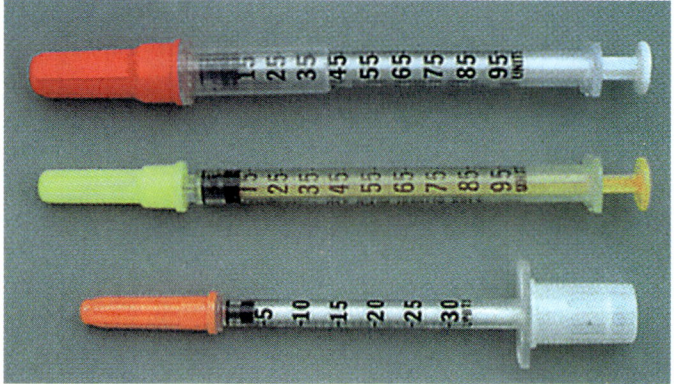

FIGURE 7-9   Tuberculin syringe with fine calibrations up to 1 cc.

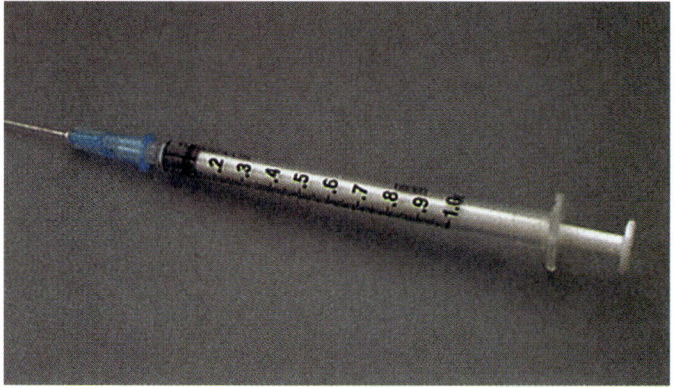

FIGURE 7-10 Procedure for using the Safety-Lok syringe. (Courtesy Becton-Dickinson, Division of Becton, Dickinson and Co., Rutherford, NJ.)

Drawing the Medication

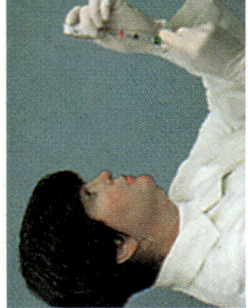

- Using your usual aseptic technique, prepare and draw up medication into the syringe.

- **Note:** The SAFETY-LOK Syringe requires no technique change for drawing medication.

Giving the Injection

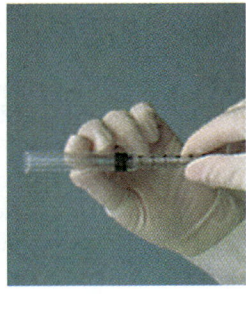

- Proceed to administer the injection following established technique.

- The SAFETY-LOK Syringe is primarily designed for IM and SUB-Q injections but can also be used for most IV port injections.

Locking the Shield

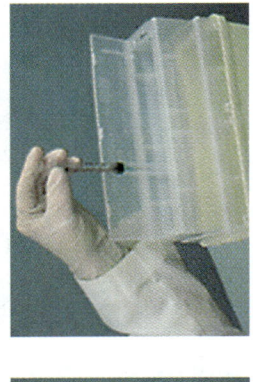

- After completing your injection, hold syringe with needle pointed away from you.

- Grasp the syringe flanges with one hand and position other hand over safety shield.

- Twist safety shield to loosen from syringe barrel by breaking seal.

- Push safety shield forward over needle until you hear an audible click. A slight twisting action may facilitate locking.

- The safety shield is now locked firmly in place.

Discarding the Used Syringe

- Proceed to nearest sharps collector and discard.

- All sharps should be safely discarded after use in an approved sharps collector.

FIGURE 7-11   Monoject safety syringes. (Courtesy Sherwood Medical, St. Louis, Mo.)

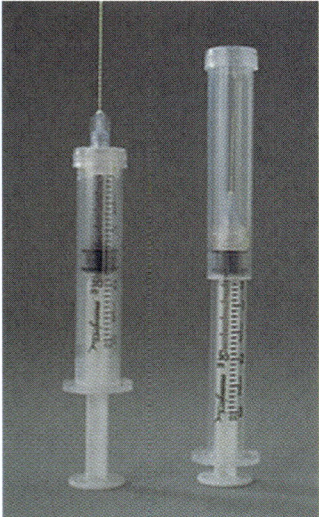

Procedure for reconstituting a powdered drug for administration

1. Using a syringe and needle, insert the needle through the cleansed rubber stopper of the vial containing the diluent.
2. Withdraw the amount of liquid diluent that is to be added to the powdered drug. (See step 6 under Administration of an Intramuscular Injection for the procedure for withdrawing a solution from a vial.)
3. Add this liquid to the vial containing the powdered drug.
4. With the needle above the fluid level in the vial, withdraw an amount of air equal to the amount of liquid diluent just added.
5. Remove the needle from the vial.
6. Discard the syringe and needle in the used sharps container.
7. Roll the vial between your hands. This mixes the liquid with the powdered drug.
8. Observe the solution obtained to make sure that all of the powdered drug has been mixed and dissolved. The solution should be clear (or cloudy if it is a suspension).
9. Label a multiple-dose vial with the date and time of preparation, the expiration date according to the drug, the dilution/strength of the medication prepared, and your initials. Labeling as stated is very important because reconstituted drugs are stable for only a short time.
10. Store any remaining drug according to the manufacturer's directions. Some drugs may have to be placed in a refrigerator.

Selection of Syringe and Needle Size

The smaller the amount of medication to be given, the smaller the size of syringe to use. In special circumstances such as the administration of insulin, it is essential that an insulin syringe be used. For measuring a very small amount of drug, use a tuberculin syringe, which is a 1-cc or 1-ml syringe marked in tenths (0.1) and hundredths (0.01) of a cubic centimeter or milliliter on one side of the scale and minims on the other side.

Needles with large lumens (for example, 18 to 20 gauge) are required when the medication to be injected is oily or very thick. Needles with small lumens (for example, 23 to 25 gauge) are used for aqueous, or thin, "watery" solutions.

The site and route of the injection help determine the length of the needle that you should use. The patient's muscle size and thickness of overlying fatty tissue must be taken into consideration when giving an intramuscular injection.

Shorter needles with a large-gauge number may be used on children and very thin patients; longer needles may be required for obese patients to ensure that the needle reaches muscular or subcutaneous tissue.

To restate, consider the following when selecting a needle for an injection:

- Patient's age and weight
- Condition and turgor (resiliency) of the tissue
- Route of administration
- Site to be used for the injection
- Thickness of the medication
- Thickness of both the muscle and fatty tissue

Common sizes of syringes and needles used for various injections are shown in Table 7-11.

Anatomic Selection of the Injection Sites

Intramuscular Injections.   The main objective when administering an intramuscular medication is to inject it deep into the muscle for gradual and optimal absorption into the bloodstream. The usual amount of solution to be given by this method is 2 to 5 ml, *except* to the mid-deltoid, where the usual amount is 0.5 to 2 ml. It is recommended to divide a 4- or 5-ml dose in half, using two different sites for injecting the medication. Identification of suitable sites for an injection is based on the use of definite anatomic landmarks, located by palpation. Four anatomic sites commonly used follow.

Gluteus medius or dorsogluteal.   The most common site for intramuscular injections, the gluteus medius, or dorsogluteal, site is located in the upper outer quadrant (UOQ) of the buttock. Have the patient assume a prone position, toes pointed inward, with the buttock clearly exposed. This position allows for best relaxation of the muscles and best exposure of the area. Injecting a needle into a tense muscle causes pain. Undergarments must be completely removed. Under no circumstances must you deviate from using the correct technique. Palpate for and then draw a diagonal line from the greater trochanter of the femur to the posterior superior iliac spine. The injection is to be given *well above and outside* of this diagonal line. The upper limit of the site is an area several inches below the iliac crest. These landmarks must be palpated to ensure the correct location for the injection. Extreme care must be taken to locate the correct site to avoid hitting the sciatic nerve or the superior gluteal artery (Figure 7-15).

A

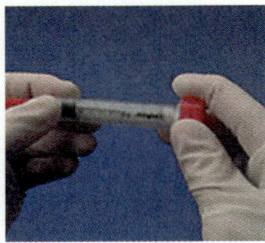

1. Select desired size from convenient Monoject dispenser. Color-coding makes it quick, easy. Check sterility (see that the heat stake has not been broken).

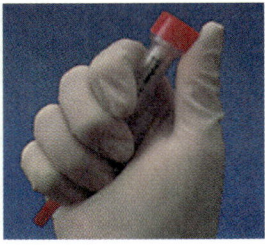

2. Open hard pack by breaking heat stake. Press area of cap directly above heat stake with thumb. Or lightly grasp and twist cap. Or tap cap against hard surface. Then remove cap.

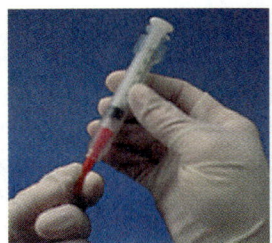

3. Hold sleeve firmly with one hand; then push needle sheath with other hand until syringe end protrudes from sleeve about 1 inch.

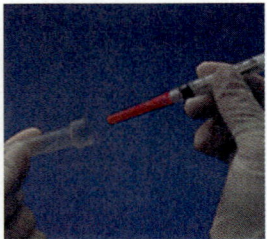

4. Remove syringe and needle from sleeve.

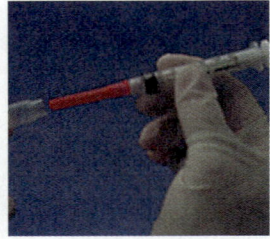

5. Reverse sleeve so small opening is facing the needle sheath end of syringe.

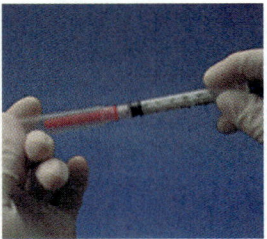

6. Firmly insert needle sheath into sleeve. Hold sleeve in stationary position. Then twist syringe clockwise to seat needle.

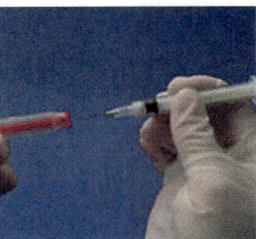

7. Pull syringe with attached needle straight out of needle sheath. Keep the sleeve containing sheath nearby. It's your Mini-safety platform or Mini-container.

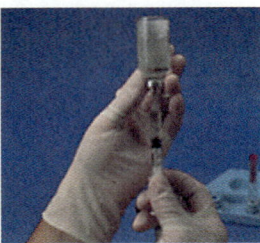

8. Insert needle into medication vial and draw prescribed amount of medication. You're ready to resheath with virtually no change of needlestick.

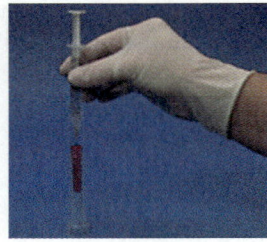

9. Resheath filled syringe in Mini-container. It's perfect for single-use situations.

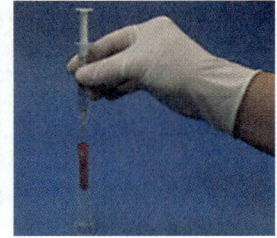

10. Or use handy Stat Tray. Holds two syringes and their Mini-containers. Fits conveniently on patient tray tables and unit dose carts.

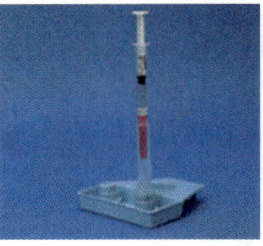

11. After administration, resheath contaminated needle into Mini-container, Stat, or Monotray Medication Tray using just one hand. Your hands don't get near the needle.

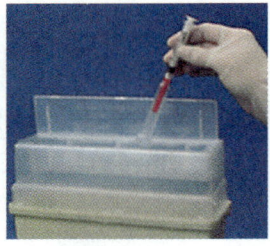

12. Discard entire unit into a puncture-resistant Monoject Sharps Container. That's the Monoject System of Safety.

B

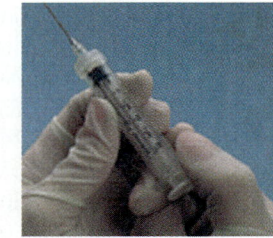

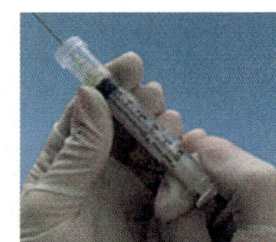

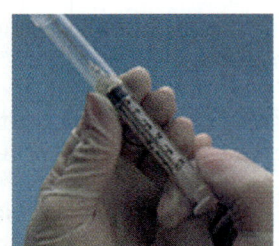

After giving the injection, hold syringe flanges and push safety shield forward over the needle. You will hear a click. The shield is now locked over the needle. Discard the whole unit into the sharps container.

FIGURE 7-13   **A,** Various-sized needles; **B,** needle point and bevel; **C,** types of needle walls and bevels.

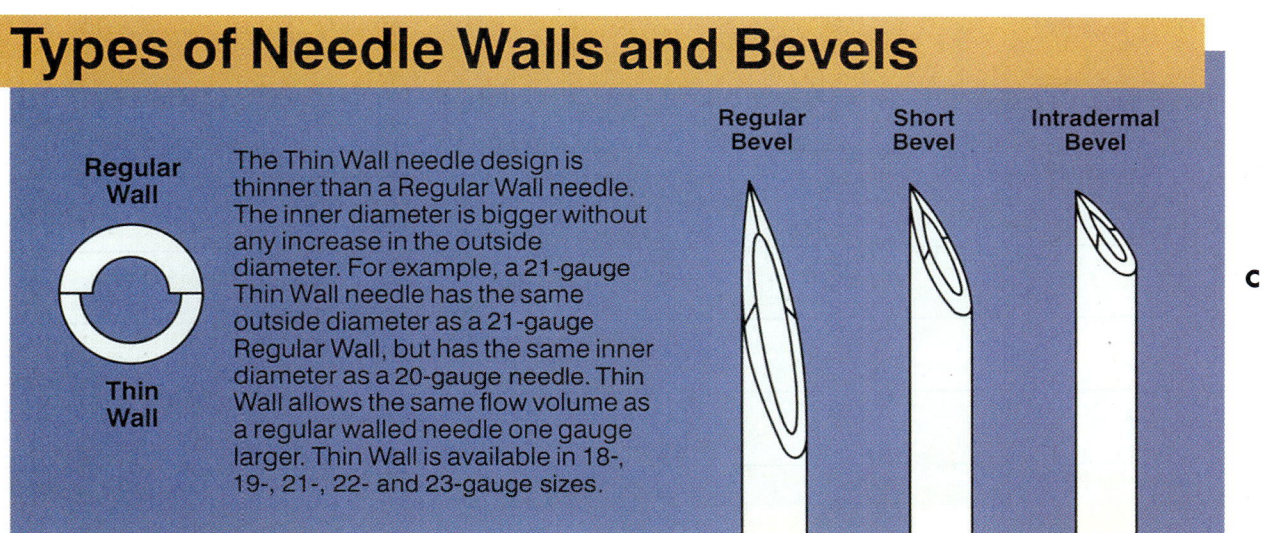

A

Bevel
Lumen
Point
Cannula or shaft
Hub

B

Point
Lumen (the opening in the shaft)
Bevel (the slant/angle between the top side and the bottom side of the needle)

Types of Needle Walls and Bevels

Regular Wall

Thin Wall

The Thin Wall needle design is thinner than a Regular Wall needle. The inner diameter is bigger without any increase in the outside diameter. For example, a 21-gauge Thin Wall needle has the same outside diameter as a 21-gauge Regular Wall, but has the same inner diameter as a 20-gauge needle. Thin Wall allows the same flow volume as a regular walled needle one gauge larger. Thin Wall is available in 18-, 19-, 21-, 22- and 23-gauge sizes.

Regular Bevel   Short Bevel   Intradermal Bevel

C

FIGURE 7-14   Drugs supplied in liquid form. *Left to right,* Cartridge, vial, ampule.

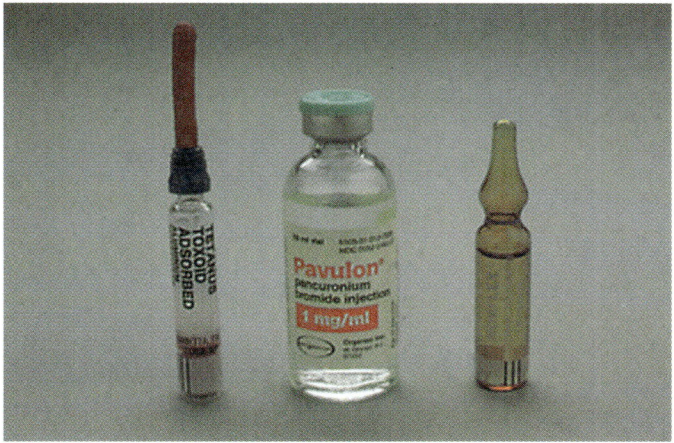

TABLE 7–11   Common Sizes of Syringes and Needles and Uses

Type of Injection	Size of Syringe	Size of Needle	Example for Use
Subcutaneous	2, 2½, or 3 cc	½ inch (in) or ⅝ in, 23- or 26-gauge	Immunizations, heparin
Intramuscular	2 to 5 cc	1½ in (1 in for thin or small patients, 2-3 in for obese patients), 21- or 22-gauge	Analgesics, vitamins, various antibiotics, and hormones
		1½ in, 20-gauge	Penicillin and thick solutions
Intradermal	1 cc	¼ in, 1/2 in, ⅜ in, 26- or 27-gauge	Schick, Dick, tuberculin, and allergy skin tests
Insulin	⅜ cc, ½ cc, 0.5 cc, or 1 cc calibrated in units	½ in or ⅝ in, 27- to 29-gauge	Insulin
Intravenous (IV)	10, 20, or 50 cc	1¼ in, 1½ in, 22-gauge	Penicillin IV drip, transfusions
		1 to 1½ in, 18-, 19-, 20-, or 21-gauge	Glucose, blood tests

FIGURE 7-15   **A,** Gluteus medius IM injection site; **B,** dorsogluteal—adult; posterior view of gluteal region and thigh; **C,** dorsogluteal-pediatric; posterior view of gluteal region and thigh.

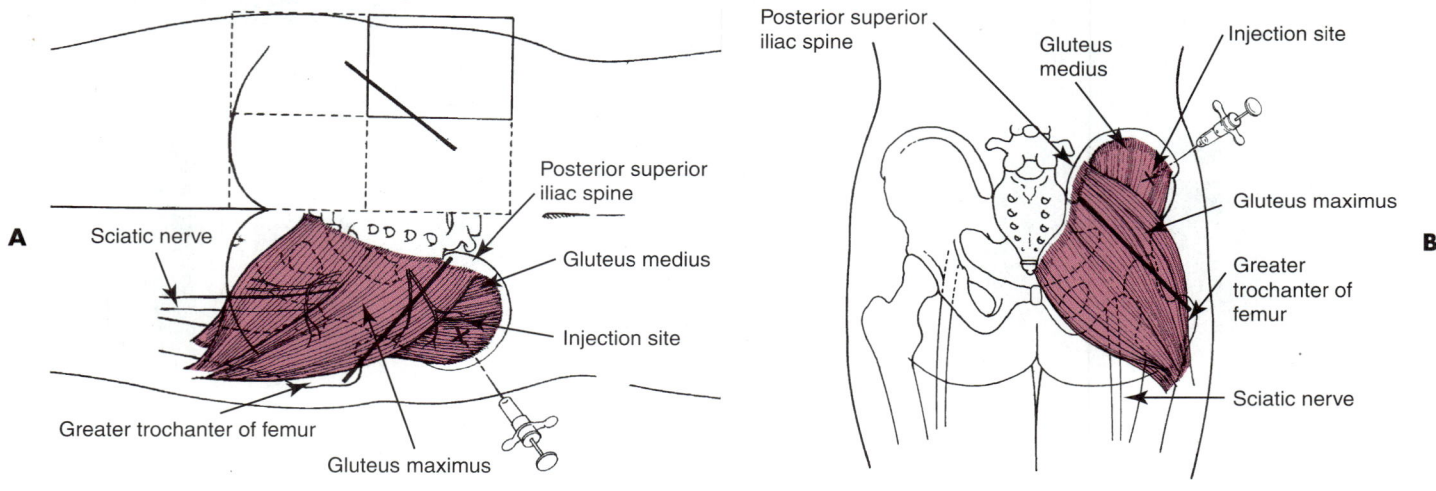

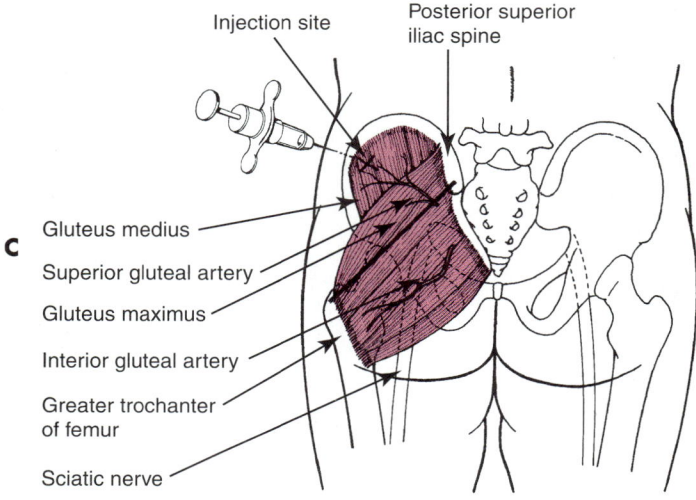

Mid-deltoid area.   The mid-deltoid site is located on the upper, outer aspect of the arm, below the lower edge of the acromion and above the axilla. Although this site is easy to access when the patient is standing, sitting, or in a prone or supine position, the actual area that can be used for the injection is limited because of major vessels, nerves, and bones in the upper arm that must be avoided. Therefore the use of this site for injections is limited because this small area can tolerate only small amounts of medication and infrequent injections. In addition, patients often experience more pain and tenderness in this area (Figure 7-16).

The mid-deltoid area is often a preferred site by some for giving vaccinations and some lipid-soluble analgesics, but it is generally not considered to be the first choice for other drugs.

Ventrogluteal area (von Hochstetter's site).   The ventrogluteal area has grown in recognition for use because this site is removed from major blood vessels and nerves. To locate this site, have the patient in a supine or side position. Palpate for the greater trochanter of the femur, the iliac crest, and the anterior-superior iliac spine. Then place the palm of your right hand on the patient's left greater trochanter and your index finger on the anterior superior iliac spine and move your middle finger posteriorly along the iliac crest as far as possible. (Do this with your left hand when injecting into the patient's right side.) A V space is now formed between your index and middle finger. The injection is to be given in the middle of this V space (Figures 7-17 and 7-18).

Vastus lateralis.* The vastus lateralis, the thick muscle on the upper side of the leg, is also being used more often because it is free of major blood vessels and nerves. With the patient in a supine position, locate this site by palpating the greater

---

*When intramuscular injections are administered to children, both the ventrogluteal and the vastus lateralis sites are recommended. See also Figure 5-56.

FIGURE 7-16   Mid-deltoid IM injection site. **A,** Deltoid—adult; lateral view of shoulder and arm; **B,** deltoid—pediatric; anterior view of shoulder and arm.

FIGURE 7-17   **A,** Ventrogluteal IM injection site; **B,** ventrogluteal—pediatric; lateral view of gluteal region and thigh.

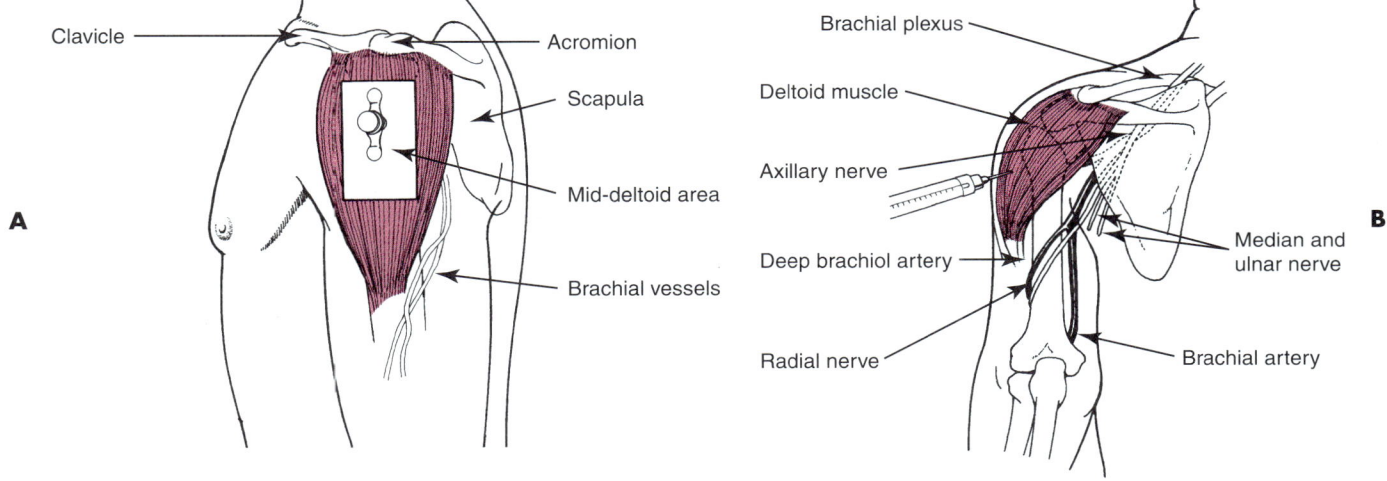

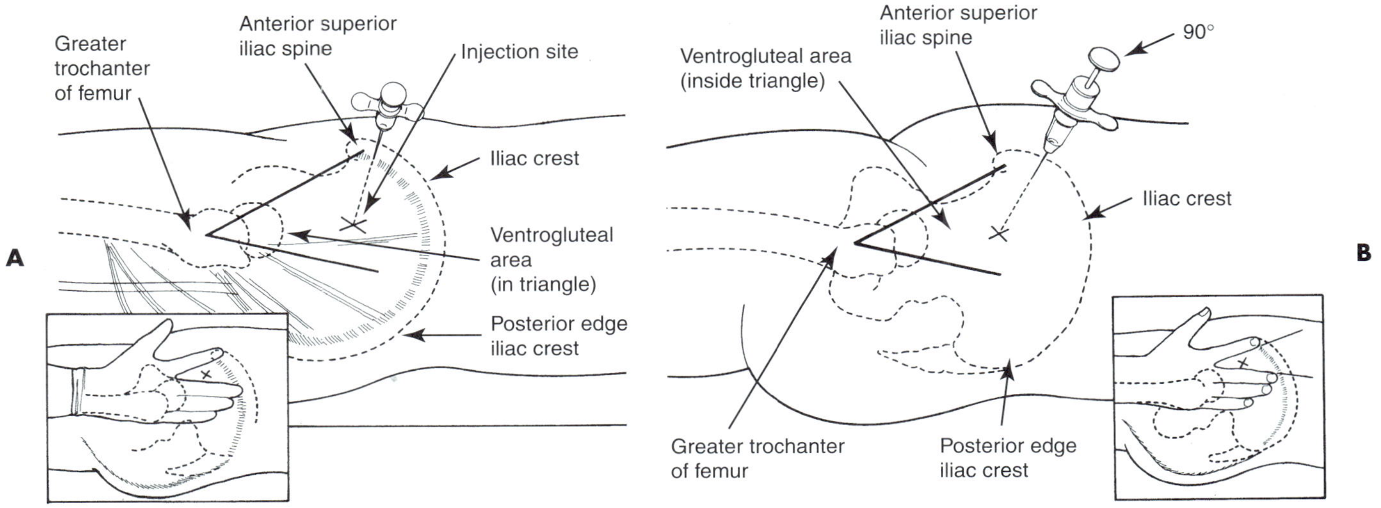

FIGURE 7-18   Ventrgluteal area on a 130-lb boy.

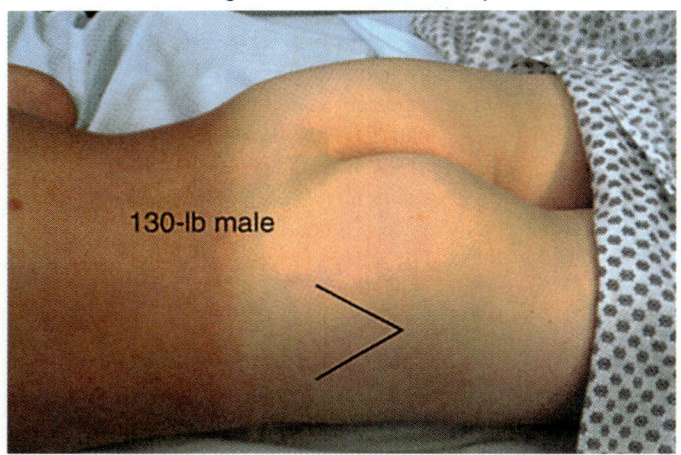

130-lb male

FIGURE 7-19   **A,** Vastus lateralis IM injection site; **B,** vastus later-alis—pediatric; anterior view of the thigh.

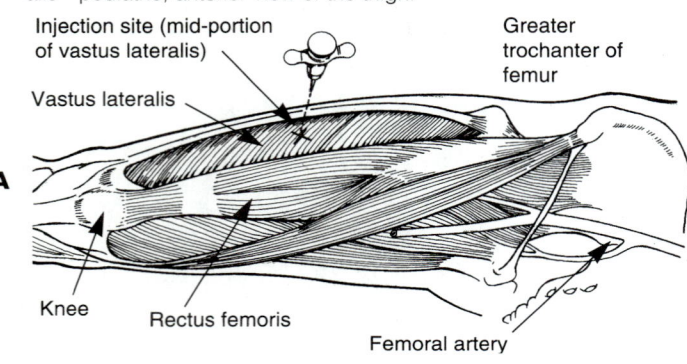

Injection site (mid-portion of vastus lateralis)

Greater trochanter of femur

Vastus lateralis

A

Knee   Rectus femoris

Femoral artery

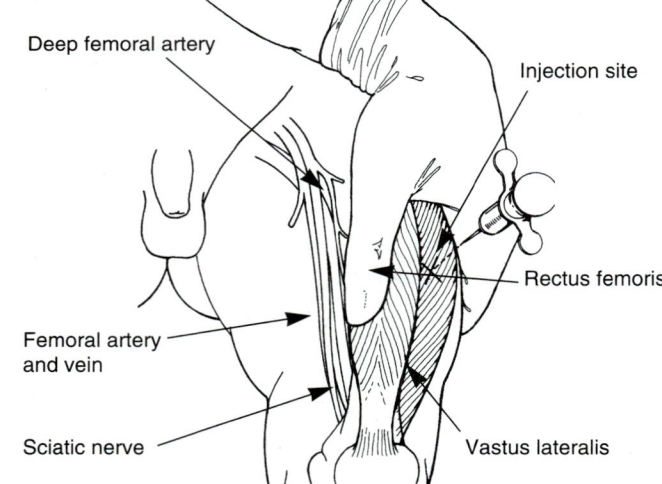

Deep femoral artery

Injection site

B

Rectus femoris

Femoral artery and vein

Sciatic nerve   Vastus lateralis

FIGURE 7-20   **A,** Right vastus lateralis area on 135-lb female; **B,** right vastus lateralis area on 180-lb male.

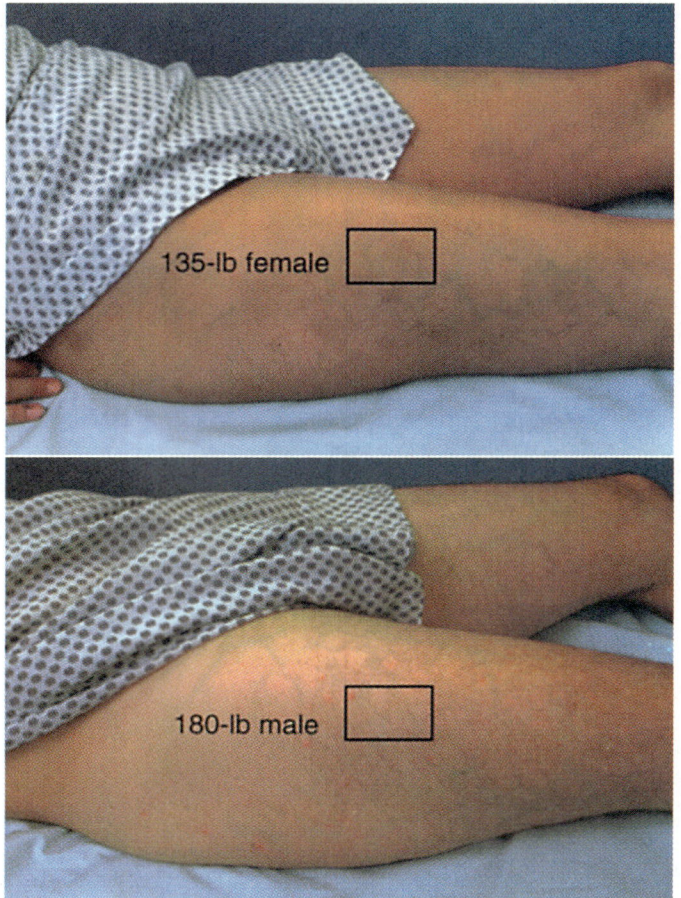

135-lb female   **A**

180-lb male   **B**

trochanter of the femur and the lateral aspect of the patella. Divide the distance between these two landmarks into thirds. The needle is to be inserted into the middle third of this area (Figures 7-19 and 7-20).

Subcutaneous injections.
The objective of a subcutaneous (sc) injection is to deposit a relatively small amount of an aqueous solution under the skin for fairly rapid absorption into the bloodstream. The amount of the solution given by this method should not exceed 2 ml. To avoid overdistention of the tissues, the medication should be administered slowly. The most common and preferred sites for a subcutaneous injection are the following:

- Outer surface of the upper arm, usually halfway between the shoulder and elbow
- Lateral aspect of the thigh
- Upper two thirds of the back

Additional sites that may be used, especially when the medication is self-administered, as a diabetic may do, include the following:

- Areas on the abdomen
- Front aspect of the thigh

When frequent subcutaneous injections are given, sites of administration should be rotated to prevent damage of a tissue, excessive pain, and possible disfigurement (Figure 7-21).

FIGURE 7-21   Subcutaneous injection sites

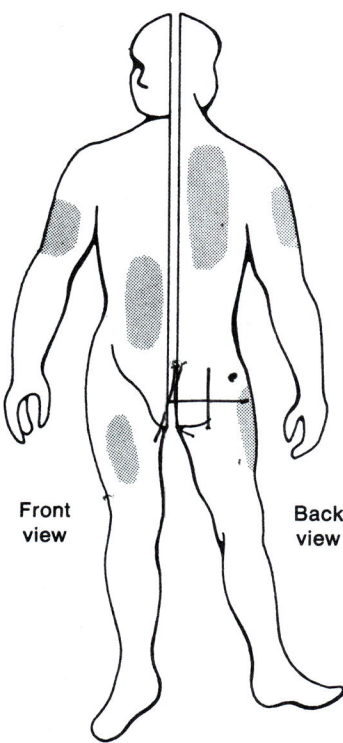

Front view   Back view

FIGURE 7-22   Packaged sterile syringes and needles labeled according to contents.

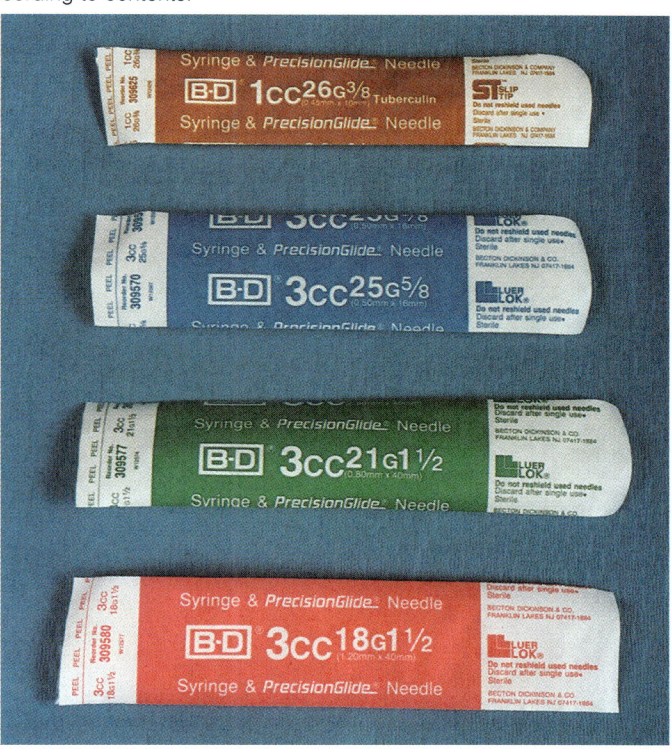

Intradermal injections.   The objective of the intradermal injection is to inject a minute amount of solution between the layers of the skin. The amount of drug given by this method is usually 0.1 to 0.3 ml. A tuberculin syringe (see Figure 7-9) is used because of the fine calibrations, which provide the best means for measuring minute amounts of a drug. Drugs must be administered slowly in this method; they produce a small, pale bump on the skin when given correctly.

The most common and preferred site for intradermal injections is the ventral surface of the forearm, approximately 4 inches below the elbow. The lateral and posterior sides of the arm can also be used if and when required because they can be easily observed for reactions to the drug injected and they also can be kept free of irritation from clothing. Intradermal injections are used for various skin tests to determine allergies (sensitivities) to drugs and various other foreign substances, such as food substances, dust, and grass; to determine the patient's susceptibility to an infectious disease, such as tuberculosis (the Mantoux test) and diphtheria (the Schick test); or to aid in the diagnosis of infectious diseases. In addition to their common use for these tests, intradermal tests are used in the diagnosis of parasitic infections, such as schistosomiasis and fungal diseases.

Because intradermal injections are used for skin tests, the procedure for administering the injection is discussed and outlined in Chapter 8, p. 415. Preparation of the syringe and needle and withdrawal of the drug into the syringe are the same as for the intramuscular and subcutaneous injections, *except* that a ³⁄₈- or ½-inch, 26- or 27-gauge needle, and a tuberculin syringe are used. The needle is inserted, bevel facing up, only about ⅛ inch (or until just the bevel is under the surface of the skin).

Instructions for Administering Injections

In addition to the rules listed on pp. 368-370, the following apply to injections:

1. Select the injection site carefully. You must avoid major blood vessels, nerves, and bones.
2. Use only sterile, preferably disposable, syringes and needles (Figure 7-22).
3. Select the correct size of syringe according to the amount of medication to be given and the appropriate size and length of needle, depending on the type of solution to be given and the size and condition of the patient.
4. Insert the needle, using the correct angle (Figure 7-23).
5. After inserting the needle, but before injecting the medication, always pull the plunger back to determine if you have entered a blood vessel (except when injecting heparin or insulin subcutaneously or when giving a drug intradermally).
6. If you have entered a blood vessel, you may withdraw the needle a bit, redirect, and again insert the needle. Pull the plunger back to determine if you have entered a second blood vessel, **or** some recommend removing the needle and beginning the procedure over again as stated in No. 7.
7. If a large amount of blood returns in the syringe when you pull back on the plunger, remove the needle and begin the procedure again, using new medication, syringe, and needle.

FIGURE 7-23 Angles of insertion for parenteral injections.

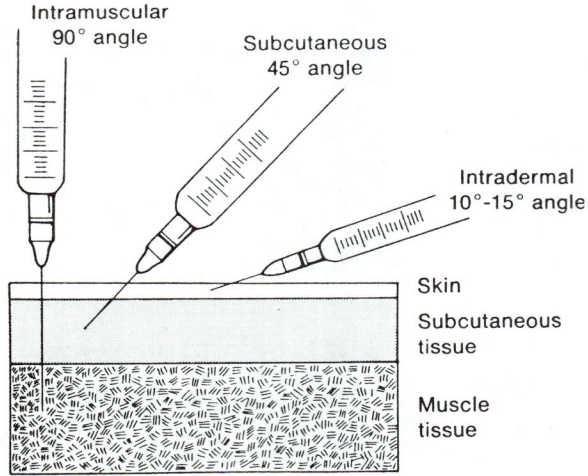

FIGURE 7-24 When you have to cap a needle, place needle cap on its side on a flat surface. Insert needle into cap without holding the cap. Secure the cap on the needle by pushing it against a vertical surface such as a closet door or the wall. Keep your other hand behind your back during this procedure. This technique has been approved by OSHA.

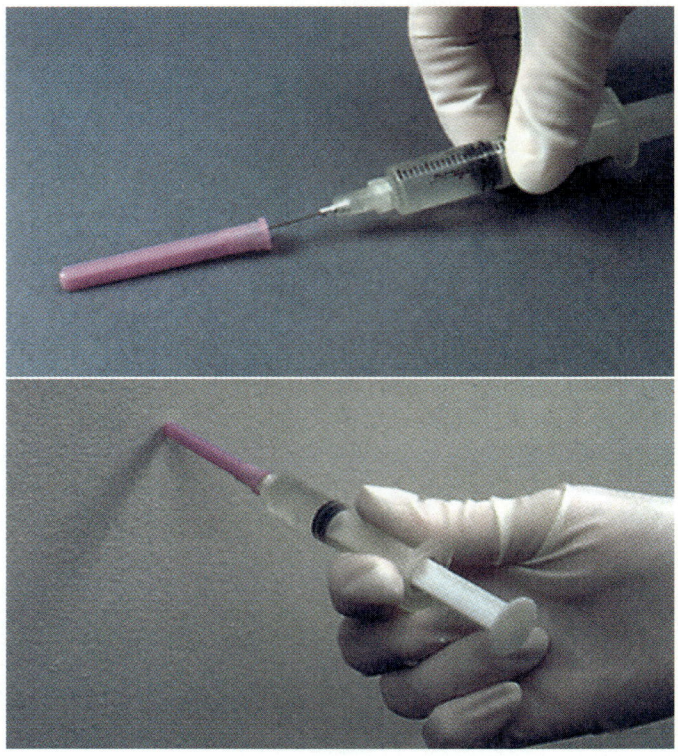

8. Rotate injection sites on patients receiving frequent injections.

9. Aseptic technique must be used when administering all injections.

10. The Occupational Safety and Health Administration (OSHA) has set Universal/Standard Precautions that state: "Gloves shall be worn when it can be reasonably anticipated that the employee may have hand contact with blood, other potentially infectious materials, mucous membranes, and nonintact skin; when performing vascular access procedures; and when handling or touching contaminated items or surfaces." Therefore wearing gloves for administering an injection is highly recommended by most professionals. You have to make this decision on the basis of each situation and patient and according to agency policy. The employer must have gloves readily accessible for your use if you decide to wear gloves for administering injections.

11. Dispose of used needles and sharps into the puncture-resistant containers immediately.

12. Allow refrigerated drugs to warm to room temperature before injecting (unless otherwise instructed by the manufacturer's literature).

13. Allow the skin disinfectant to dry before giving the injection. If the skin is not dry before the injection is given, some of the disinfectant can be forced into subcutaneous tissue and cause more discomfort to the patient.

14. To help in reducing pain to the patient, insert and remove the needle quickly.

15. Inject the medication slowly. Rapid injection can cause sudden distention of the tissue and more discomfort.

Guidelines for Preventing Needlesticks

1. Slow down and *think* when using or disposing of needles.

2. *DO NOT recap* needles unless absolutely necessary. If necessary, place cap on table top before inserting needle (insert needle into cap without holding cap) (Figure 7-24).

3. When using syringes that have a safety shield, learn how to use them proficiently before you use them. After giving an injection, slide the cover over the needle and lock it in place (see Figures 7-6, 7-10, and 7-11).

4. *Never* put a needle down—dispose of it promptly in approved container.

5. *Never* put needles or other sharp instruments in trash cans, your pocket, or linen containers.

6. *Never* leave needles or other sharp instruments on countertops, examination tables, or disposable procedure trays.

7. *Never* push a needle into the sharps container with your hand. If the needle does not go into the opening easily, use a large syringe to push it in.

8. *Never* try to remove a needle or syringe from the sharps container.

9. Pick up improperly discarded needles with extreme caution and dispose of them in the nearest sharps container. Do not attempt to cap the needle; use tongs or forceps to pick up sharps. Wash your hands after you dispose of the needle.

More than two dozen needlestick-prevention devices are available on the market. Hospitals and health care agencies are starting to test and adopt some of the new technologies. When you encounter any of these devices, make sure that you are proficient in the technique before you use it to ensure safety.

CAUTION: Some authorities believe that some of the devices may even increase needlesticks by giving the user a false sense of security and a feeling that he or she does not have to be vigilant about proper technique. **There is no substitution for proper technique. This must not be forgotten regardless of any device on the market.**

Accidental Needlestick and Occupational Exposure to Blood

When giving injections, you are at risk for an accidental needlestick and exposure to the human immunodeficiency virus (HIV) and the hepatitis viruses from an infected patient's blood. **Most** exposures **do not** result in infection. The risk of infection varies with the amount of blood in the exposure, the amount of the virus(es) in the patient's blood at the time of exposure, and whether postexposure treatment was obtained. Your employer should have a system for reporting exposures to quickly evaluate the risk of infection from the exposure, counsel you about recommendations for treatments available to prevent infection, and monitor you for side effects of treatments and determine if infection occurs. This may involve testing your blood and that of the source patient and offering appropriate postexposure care (Figure 7-25).

Immediately following an exposure to blood from a needlestick, wash the area with soap and water. No scientific evidence shows that the use of antiseptics for wound care or squeezing the wound would reduce the risk of transmission of HIV or hepatitis. The use of a caustic agent such as bleach is not recommended. Inform your supervisor or employer of the incident. Fill out an incident report completely, stating only the facts (Figure 7-26). Prompt reporting is essential because in some cases, HIV **postexposure treatment** may be recommended and should be started as soon as possible—preferably *within 1 to 2 hours.* The possible risks of acquiring hepatitis B and hepatitis C should be discussed with your health care provider. You should have already received the hepatitis B vaccine (see Chapter 1), which is extremely safe and effective in preventing hepatitis B. **The risk of HIV infection after an occupational exposure is very low but is not zero.** HIV infection has been reported after occupational exposures to HIV-infected blood through needlesticks or cuts. (The average risk is 0.3%, that is, about 1 in 300.) Studies have suggested that postexposure treatment with certain antiviral drugs *may* prevent infection with HIV. Both risk of infection and possible side effects of drugs must be carefully considered when deciding whether to take postexposure treatment. Exposures with a lower infection risk may not be worth the risk of the side effects associated with these drugs. If the source individual cannot be identified or tested, decisions regarding follow-up should be based on the exposure risk and whether the source is likely to be a person who is HIV positive. **Follow-up HIV testing and counseling** should be available to all workers who are concerned about possible HIV infection through occupational exposure. Counseling is also available from the National Clinicians' PEPline (Post Exposure Prophylaxis line) at 1-888-448-4911.

Follow-up after exposure. You should be tested for HIV antibody as soon as possible after exposure (baseline) and periodically for at least 6 months after the exposure (for example, at 6 weeks, 12 weeks, and 6 months). If you take antiviral drugs for postexposure treatment, you should be checked for drug toxicity, including a complete blood count and kidney and liver function tests just before starting treatment and 2 weeks after starting treatment. Any sudden or severe flulike illness that occurs during the follow-up period must be reported, especially if it involves fever, rash, muscle aches, tiredness, malaise, or swollen glands. These signs and symptoms may suggest HIV infection, drug reaction, or other medical conditions. *You should contact your health care provider if you have any questions or problems during the follow-up period.*

NOTE: **The preceding information also applies to exposures that occur through cuts from sharp instruments contaminated with an infected patient's blood or through contact of the eye, nose, or mouth (mucous membrane) or skin with a patient's blood. Cuts should be washed with soap and water; splashes to the nose, mouth, or skin should be flushed with water; and eyes should be irrigated with clean, saline, or sterile solutions.**

The **risk for HIV infection** after exposure of the eye, nose, or mouth to HIV-infected blood is estimated to be, on average, 0.1% (1 in 1000).

The risk after exposure of the skin to HIV-infected blood is estimated to be less than 0.1%. A small amount of blood on intact skin *probably* poses no risk at all. The risk may be higher if the skin is damaged (for example, by a recent cut) or if the contact involves a large area of skin or is prolonged.

Public health service guidelines for the management of health care worker exposures to HIV and recommendations for postexposure prophylaxis.*

Assessments of the risk for infection resulting from the exposure and the infectivity of the exposure source are key determinants of offering postexposure prophylaxis (PEP). Systems should be in place for the timely evaluation and management of exposed health care workers (HCWs) and for consultation with experts in the treatment of HIV when using PEP.

Recommendations for PEP were modified in 1998 to include a basic 4-week regimen of the two drugs zidovudine (AZT) and lamivudine (Epivir) for most HIV exposures and an expanded regimen that includes the addition of a protease inhibitor indinavir (Crixivan) or nelfinavir (Viracept) for HIV exposures that pose an increased risk for transmission or when resistance to one or more of the antiretroviral agents recommended for PEP is known or suspected. The CDC provides flowcharts to guide clinicians and exposed HCWs in deciding when to consider PEP.

Occupational exposures should be considered urgent medical concerns to ensure timely administration of PEP. Health care organizations should have protocols that promote prompt

---

*U.S. Department of Health and Human Services, CDC, Atlanta, Ga., updated May 1998.

FIGURE 7-25   Sample occupational health and injury clinics worksheet.

OCCUPATIONAL HEALTH AND INJURY CLINICS WORKSHEET

Date: _____   Date/Time of Exposure: _____ / _____ AM/PM

HEALTH CARE WORKER INFORMATION

Name (Print): _____   Date of Birth: _____

Employer: _____

Department: _____   Job Title: _____

Work phone/extension: _____   Home phone: (_____) _____

Vaccinated for Hepatitis B? ___ Yes ___ No   Year series was completed: _____

HBsAb result, if known: _____   Date of titer: _____

Last DT booster (for punctures only): _____ (year)

Current Meds: _____

_____   Drug Allergies: _____

EXPOSURE INFORMATION

Brief description of how exposure occurred _____

_____

Type: ___ Needlestick ___ Mucous Membrane Splash ___ Puncture with contaminated instrument or device ___ Blood to non-intact skin or wound

Type of body fluid: ___ Blood ___ Other body fluid (please check): ___ Vaginal secretions ___ Amniotic fluid ___ CSF ___ Peritoneal fluid ___ Pleural fluid ___ Saliva ___ Semen ___ Other _____

Was body fluid visibly contaminated with blood? ___ Yes ___ No

Part of worker's body involved: _____ Left/Right (circle)

Device that caused injury: ___ Needle (gauge): ___   Scalpel/blade ___ Tenderlet/Lancet ___ Glass ___ Other: _____

Depth of puncture: ___ <3 mm ___ >3 mm

Type of needle (If Applicable): ___ Injection ___ Vacutainer ___ Butterfly ___ Suture ___ LP needle/stylet ___ Tubex (cartridge) _____ Other _____

Personal Protective Equipment Worn: ___ gloves (single/double) ___ goggles/glasses ___ face shield ___ mask ___ gown

Wound decontaminated? ___ Yes ___ No ___ Soap/water ___ Other antiseptics used (please indicated): _____

Mucous Membrane(s) flushed? ___ Yes ___ No ___ Tap water ___ Saline (amt): _____

SOURCE PATIENT INFORMATION

Name: _____   Physician: _____

Diagnosis: _____

HIV Status: ___ Negative ___ Positive ___ Unknown   Date of test: _____

HBsAg: ___ Negative ___ Positive ___ Unknown   Date of test: _____

Hep. C Ab: ___ Negative ___ Positive ___ Unknown   Date of test: _____

TREATMENT AND FOLLOW-UP

National Clinicians' PEPline Consulted? (1-888-448-4911): ___ Yes ___ No

PEP medications given: ___ Yes ___ No   Time of first dose: _____ AM/PM

___ Consent obtained ___ Counseling Sheet given

___ Combivir only (ī tablet BID) # _____

___ Combivir (ī BID) # ___ & Viracept (250 mg īīī capsules TID with food) # ___

Labs Ordered on Source Patient: ___ HIV (consent) ___ HBsAg ___ Hep. C Ab

Results: _____ HIV _____ HBsAg _____ Hep. C Ab

Labs Ordered on Health Care Worker: ___ HIV (consent) ___ HBsAg ___ Hep. C Ab ___ Chemistry panel-12 ___ CBC ___ Amylase

Code no. for HIV _____

___ DT 0.5 ml IM (R or L deltoid) ___ H-BIG (0.06 ml/kg) Dose: _____ IM (RUOQ or LUOQ) ___ Hepatitis B vaccine 1.0 ml IM (R or L deltoid)

Dates for Follow-up Appts:

If PEP given: 2 wks _____ 4 wks _____ 6 wks _____

HIV testing: 6 wks _____ 3 mos _____ 6 mos _____ 12 mos _____

Hep. C testing: 3 mos _____ Hep B vaccine: 1 mo _____ 6 mos _____

Additional comments: _____

_____

Clinician (Please Print): _____

Signature: _____   Title: _____

Any person who makes or causes to be made any knowingly false or fraudulent material statement or material representation for the purpose of obtaining or denying workers' compensation benefits or payments is guilty of a felony.	**EMPLOYEE REPORT OF OCCUPATIONAL INCIDENT, INJURY OR ILLNESS** EMPLOYEE CASE NO

FORM TO BE COMPLETED IMMEDIATELY AFTER INCIDENT.   Please type or print clearly and firmly.

EMPLOYEE INFO

NAME: LAST FIRST M.I.	SOCIAL SECURITY NUMBER	SEX □ MALE □ FEMALE	BIRTH DATE (MM/DD/YY)

HOME ADDRESS	CITY	STATE	ZIP CODE	HOME PHONE NUMBER ( )

DEPARTMENT	JOB TITLE	HIRE DATE (MM/DD/YY)

EMPLOYEE STATUS □ VOLUNTEER □ FULL TIME □ PART TIME □ TEMPORARY □ PER DIEM	DEPT. EXTENSION NUMBER	OTHER EMPLOYMENT - GIVE EMPLOYER NAME, ADDRESS, PHONE NUMBER □ NO □ YES

SHIFT USUALLY WORKED □ DAYS □ EVENINGS □ NIGHTS □ ROTATING	HOURS USUALLY WORKED ___ HOURS PER DAY ___ DAYS PER WEEK ___ TOTAL WEEKLY HOURS	WERE YOU PERFORMING YOUR REGULAR WORK DUTIES

DATE OF INCIDENT (MM/DD/YY)	TIME OF INCIDENT _____ A.M. _____ P.M.	TIME BEGAN WORK _____ A.M. _____ P.M.	ABLE TO WORK AT LEAST ONE FULL DAY AFTER INCIDENT? ___ YES ___ NO	DATE LAST WORKED (MM/DD/YY)

ADDRESS WHERE INCIDENT OCCURRED (NUMBER, STREET, CITY, ZIP)	DEPARTMENT WHERE INCIDENT OCCURRED (GIVE BLDG, FLOOR, ROOM NO.)

DID INCIDENT INVOLVE A PATIENT? (E.G. GIVING INJECTION, LIFTING PATIENT) □ NO □ YES - GIVE PT. NAME AND ROOM NO.	TO YOUR KNOWLEDGE WERE OTHER EMPLOYEES INJURED IN THIS INCIDENT? □ NO □ YES

INCIDENT REPORTED TO IMMEDIATE SUPERVISOR NAME: DATE:	CLAIM FOR WORKERS' COMPENSATION BENEFITS FORM RECEIVED? □ NO □ YES - RECEIVED FROM _____ ON _____ NAME OF PERSON DATE

CAUSE OF INCIDENT

WHAT WERE YOU DOING WHEN THE INCIDENT OCCURRED?

HOW DID THE INCIDENT HAPPEN? WHAT WAS THE CAUSE?

WHAT MACHINE, TOOL, PIECE OF EQUIPMENT OR CHEMICAL WERE YOU USING THAT WAS MOST CLOSELY CONNECTED TO THE INCIDENT/EXPOSURE?

WHAT WOULD YOU RECOMMEND TO PREVENT THIS TYPE OF INCIDENT?

DID ANYONE WITNESS YOUR INCIDENT?
□ NO   □ YES - GIVE NAME(S):

NATURE OF INCIDENT

NATURE OF INCIDENT (CHECK ONE)
□ NO APPARENT INJURY/ILLNESS/EXPOSURE
□ NO INJURY/ILLNESS/EXPOSURE
□ NEAR MISS
□ SPECIFY EXACT TYPE OF INJURY BELOW
   (E.G. CUT, STRAIN, BURN)
	BODY PART
	NAME SPECIFIC PART(S) OF BODY INJURED (E.G. RIGHT MIDDLE FINGER, RIGHT KNEE)
	
	BODY PART _____
	    □ RIGHT □ LEFT
	□ I DECLINE TREATMENT REGARDING THIS INCIDENT AT THIS TIME.
	
	_____ DATE _____ TIME _____ INITIAL
		NOTE AREA(S) OF PAIN/INJURY USING "X" MARKS AS APPROPRIATE

HAVE YOU EVER HAD THIS TYPE OF INJURY OR ILLNESS BEFORE?
□ NO   □ YES - LIST PRIOR INJURY DATES

NAME OF PRIMARY CARE PHYSICIAN

I CERTIFY THAT ALL OF THE FOREGOING INFORMATION IS TRUE, CORRECT AND COMPLETE, AND THAT I HAVE NOT OMITTED ANY PERTINENT INFORMATION.

EMPLOYEE SIGNATURE: DATE:

TO BE COMPLETED BY EMERGENCY UNIT OR OCCUPATIONAL HEALTH SERVICES STAFF.

TREATMENT

DATE OF EXAM: _____
 	
TIME OF EXAM: _____ A.M. _____ P.M.
 	
DIAGNOSIS AND TREATMENT GIVEN:
	DISPOSITION
	□ SENT HOME
	□ HOSPITALIZED
	□ CLEARED TO RETURN TO
	  □ FULL WORK ON _____
	           DATE
	  □ MODIFIED WORK ON _____
	    (LIST RESTRICTIONS) DATE
	□ EMPLOYEE DECLINED TREATMENT
		REFERRED TO:
		□ OCCUPATIONAL HEALTH SERVICES
		□ OCCUPATIONAL INJURY CLINIC
		□ OTHER (SPECIFY):

EMERGENCY UNIT SIGNATURE: DATE:	OCCUPATIONAL HEALTH SERVICES SIGNATURE: DATE:

reporting and facilitate access to postexposure care. Enrollment of HCWs in registries designed to assess side effects in health care workers (HCWs) who take PEP is encouraged.

Exposure report. If an occupational exposure occurs, the circumstances and postexposure management should be recorded in the HCW's confidential medical record (usually on a form that the facility designates for this purpose; see Figures 7-25 and 7-26). Relevant information includes the following:

- Date and time of exposure
- Details of the procedure being performed, including where and how the exposure occurred, and if the exposure was related to a sharp device, the type of device, and how and when in the course of handling the device the exposure occurred

- Details of the exposure, including the type and amount of fluid or material and the severity of the exposure (for example, for a percutaneous exposure, depth of injury and whether fluid was injected; or for a skin or mucous membrane exposure, the estimated volume of material, duration of contact, and the condition of the skin [for example, chapped, abraded, or intact])
- Details about the exposure source (that is, whether the source material contained HIV or other bloodborne pathogen[s]) and if the source is an HIV-infected person, the stage of disease, history of antiretroviral therapy, and viral load, if known
- Details about counseling, postexposure management, and follow-up

Text continued on p. 398

PROCEDURE 7-1

ADMINISTRATION OF AN INTRAMUSCULAR INJECTION

Objective
Understand and demonstrate the correct procedure for filling a syringe with medication from an ampule and from a vial; then prepare the patient, administer the drug by giving an IM injection, and chart the procedure.

Equipment
Appropriate-sized sterile needle and syringe, depending on amount and type of drug to be given (usually a 2- or 3-cc syringe and a 21- or

22-gauge, 1½-inch needle), or when the medication is supplied in a prefilled sterile Tubex cartridge-needle unit, use the Tubex injector.
    A 23-gauge, 1-inch needle may be used when administering the drug into the deltoid muscle.
    Sterile alcohol sponges
    Medication ordered
    Small tray
    Disposable, single-use examination gloves

PROCEDURE	RATIONALE
1. Wash your hands. Use appropriate personal protective equipment (PPE) as dictated by facility.	
2. Assemble the equipment.	
3. Prepare the syringe and needle for use. When using a separate syringe and needle, remove them from the wrappers and leave the cover (sheath) on the needle intact. Grasping the hub of the needle and the barrel of the syringe, attach the hub of the needle to the tip of the syringe. Secure by turning the hub ¼ inch clockwise. Avoid touching the tip of the syringe and the open end of the hub of the needle with your fingers.	*The tip of the syringe and the open end of the needle are to remain sterile.*
4. Compare the physician's order with the label on the medication.	*These must be the same. At times you may have to calculate the dose to be given.*

5. Check the label of the medication three times during the preparation of the medication to ensure that you have the correct medication and strength:
  • When removing the medication from storage area
  • When filling the syringe
  • When replacing the medication in the storage area
	The same medication is often supplied in different strengths.

6. Take an alcohol sponge to cleanse the rubber stopper of the vial or the neck of the ampule; then discard this sponge. Withdraw medication into the syringe.	*Cleansing helps prevent the introduction of microorganisms into the vial and prevents contamination of the needle.*

PROCEDURE 7-1

ADMINISTRATION OF AN INTRAMUSCULAR INJECTION—cont'd

If an ampule is used:

a. Tap the tip of the ampule to dislodge any medication there.

b. Cleanse the neck at the marked line.

c. Hold the ampule; with your other hand, cover the top end with a sponge and break the top off going away from you (Figure 7-27). The medication is now ready for use.

The sponge is used to protect your fingers when the top is broken off.

d. Remove the needle cover (sheath). Do not touch the opening of the ampule with the needle.

The needle is contaminated if it touches the outside or entrance of the ampule. In this instance, you must obtain another sterile needle for use.

e. Insert the needle into the ampule (Figure 7-28).

f. Pull back on the plunger of the syringe to withdraw the required amount of medication.

g. Remove the needle from the ampule.

h. Replace the needle cover (sheath) over the needle, using the one-handed method (see Figure 7-24) or a recapping device.

i. Place this unit on a small tray.

j. Check the label and then discard the ampule, or keep the ampule with the syringe until after the medication has been administered and then discard both in the used sharps container.

Keeping the ampule with the syringe containing the drug is good for identification purposes.

k. Proceed to the patient, carrying this medication and a sterile alcohol sponge on the small tray.

If a vial is used:

a. Take the syringe and pull the plunger back to obtain a measured amount of air equal to the amount of medication to be withdrawn from the vial.

b. Remove the needle cover.

c. Insert the needle through the cleansed rubber stopper, keeping it above the solution (Figure 7-29, *A*).

d. Push the plunger of the syringe down to the bottom of the barrel (see Figure 7-29, *A*).

This gives air replacement, which prevents the creation of a vacuum in the vial when the medication is withdrawn. If a vacuum is created, it makes it difficult to withdraw the medication. Do not inject more air than is required because the pressure in the vial then forces the solution into the syringe, making it difficult to obtain an accurate dose.

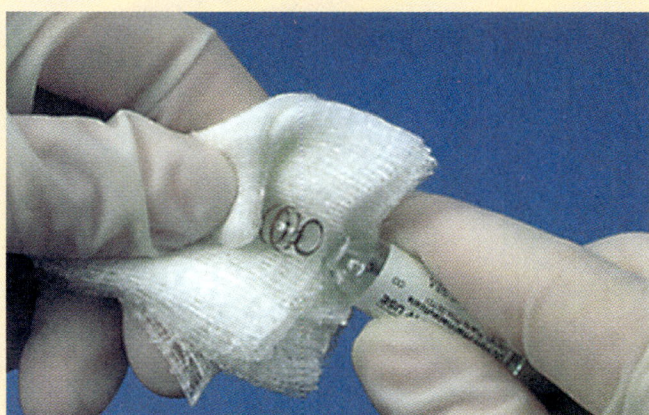

FIGURE 7-27   Techniques for breaking top off ampule.

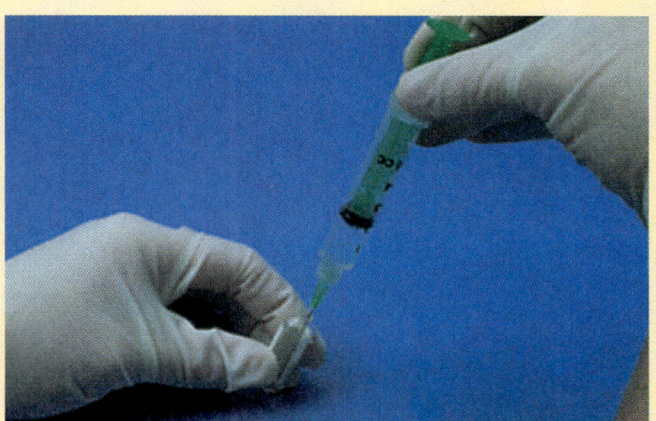

FIGURE 7-28   Insert needle into ampule and pull back on syringe plunger to withdraw the medication.

PROCEDURE 7-1

ADMINISTRATION OF AN INTRAMUSCULAR INJECTION—cont'd

e. Invert the vial; have the vial and syringe at eye level (see Figure 7-29, *B*).

f. With the needle opening in the solution, pull the plunger of the syringe back gently until the required amount of medication has been obtained (see Figure 7-29, *B*).

g. Remove any air bubbles in the syringe by tapping the barrel with your fingertips until all of the air bubbles have disappeared (see Figure 7-29, *C*). Check again to make sure that you have the required amount of drug in the syringe before removing the needle from the vial.

h. Remove the needle from the vial.

i. Replace the needle cover over the needle, using a recapping device or a one-hand method.

j. Place the filled syringe with the covered needle on a small tray.

k. Check the label on the vial, and replace it in the correct storage area or keep the vial with the syringe until the drug has been given.

l. Proceed to the patient, carrying the medication and a sterile alcohol sponge on the small tray.

7. Identify the patient and explain the procedure.

8. Select the injection site and position the patient accordingly, exposing the site clearly. Refer to earlier section, Anatomic Selection of the Injection Sites, p. 381. Your view of and accessibility to the injection site must not be obstructed by the patient's clothing or any drape sheet. Be sure that you have ample lighting when administering the injection.

Keep the vial and syringe at eye level to ensure correct measurement of the drug withdrawn.

Prevent contamination of the needle.

Ensure that the correct medication will be administered.

Correct patient identification is crucial. Explanations help gain the patient's cooperation and relaxation.

FIGURE 7-29 Withdrawing medication from vial. **A,** Insert needle through cleaned rubber stopper; keep needle above level of solution; push plunger down. **B,** Hold syringe at eye level to ensure correct measurement of medication. **C,** Keep syringe in a vertical position; tap barrel to remove any air bubbles.

PROCEDURE 7-1

ADMINISTRATION OF AN INTRAMUSCULAR INJECTION—cont'd

9. Don disposable, single-use examination gloves.

10. With the alcohol sponge, cleanse the injection site, starting at a central point and moving out to an area approximately 2 inches square; allow it to dry.

11. Remove the needle cover.

12. Hold the syringe with the needle facing upward; slowly push on the plunger until a tiny drop of medication comes to the needle tip.

This helps get rid of air bubbles, which must be expelled from the syringe before injecting the medication. Also, the tiny drop of medication obtained at the top of the syringe ensures that the needle is clear and not plugged.

13. Using the index finger and thumb of your nondominant hand, spread or tense the skin around the injection site. For the deltoid and vastus lateralis sites, grasp the skin. This technique works best on these muscles.

Spreading the skin will make the skin taut. This makes needle insertion easier.

14. Using your **dominant hand,** hold the syringe and needle as if you were holding a pencil, with the bevel of the needle facing up (Figure 7-30). Your index finger and second finger may surround the top part of the needle hub with your thumb placed on the end of the syringe; or all three fingers may surround the bottom end of the syringe near the needle, but not touching the needle.

15. With a quick thrust, insert the needle at a 90-degree angle to about three fourths of the needle length. *Do not* hit the skin with the hub of the needle (see Figure 7-30). Hold the needle perpendicular to the skin and insert quickly in a dartlike thrust.

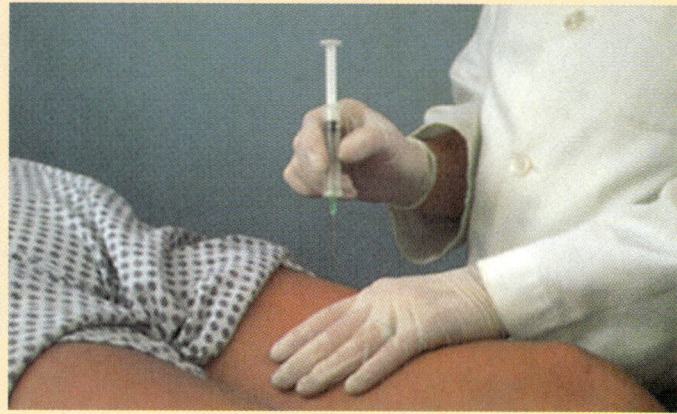

FIGURE 7-30   Giving intramuscular injection. With your dominant hand, hold syringe and needle in pencil or dartlike grip; insert at 90-degree angle. Do not hit skin with hub of needle.

Continued

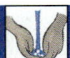

PROCEDURE 7-1

ADMINISTRATION OF AN INTRAMUSCULAR INJECTION—cont'd

16. Steady the syringe with your **dominant hand.** Using your other hand, pull back on the plunger to see if any blood can be aspirated into the syringe (Figure 7-31). If you have entered a blood vessel, withdraw the needle slightly, redirect, and reinsert; then pull back on the plunger again to check for blood. *Some recommend completely withdrawing the needle if a blood vessel is entered and beginning the procedure again with a new needle, syringe, and medication.*

Aspiration must be done to check if you have entered a blood vessel. Supporting the syringe and needle with your dominant hand prevents movement of the unit. Movement of the unit would cause extra discomfort/pain for the patient.

17. Continue to steady the syringe with your dominant hand. With your other hand, push on the plunger slowly to inject the medication.

Injection of the medication slowly allows the solution to disperse into the tissues. Discomfort caused by pressure will result if the medication is injected too quickly.

18. Using your **nondominant hand,** apply pressure at the injection site with the alcohol sponge and quickly remove the needle with your **dominant hand (the hand that has constantly been on the syringe and needle unit).**

*Applied pressure and the quick withdrawal of the needle reduces discomfort and the risk of medication leaking into the subcutaneous tissues and possibly forming abscesses. **NOTE:** By keeping your dominant hand in constant contact with the syringe and needle unit rather than switching hands after inserting the needle as some sug-*

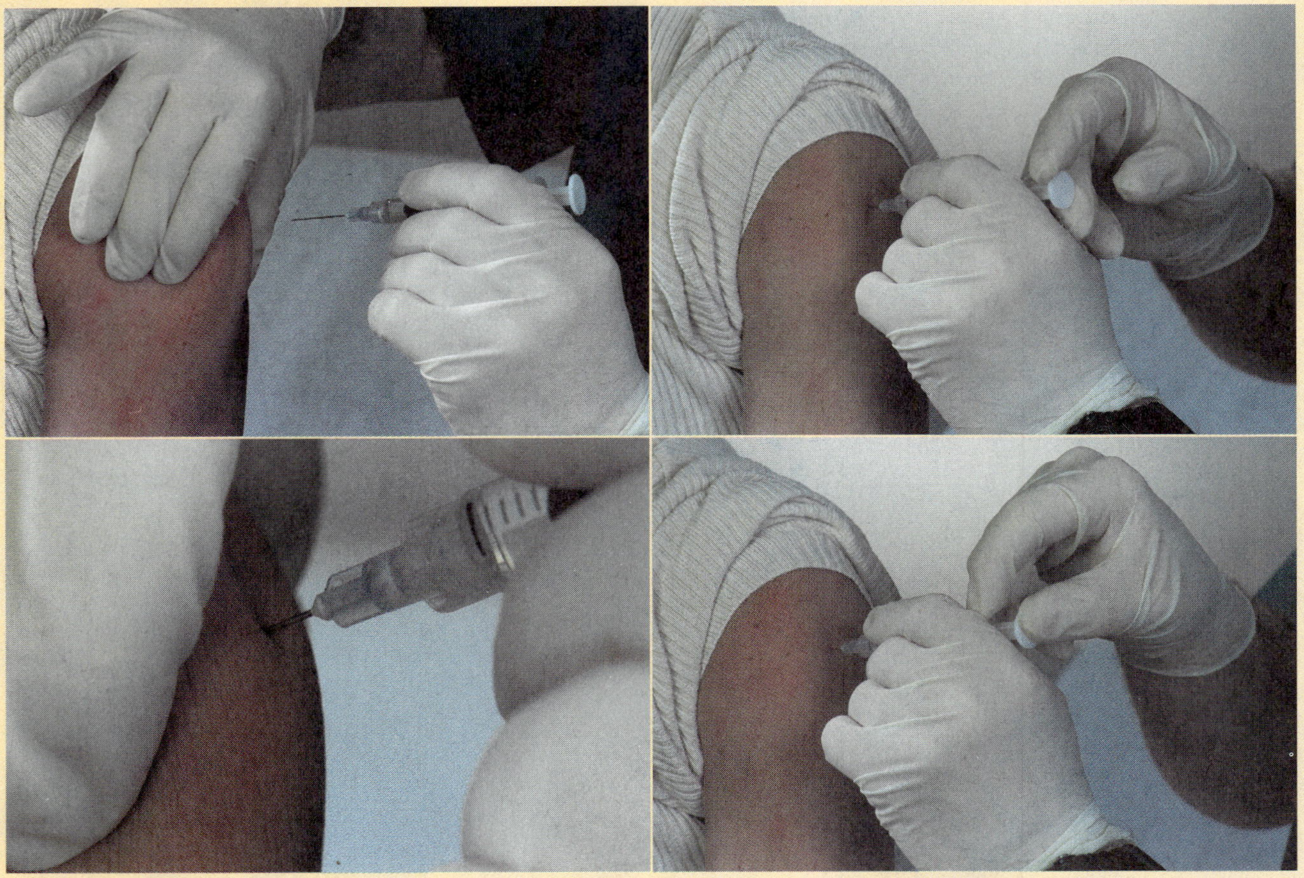

FIGURE 7-31   **A,** Insert needle with a quick trust. **Do not** hit skin with hub of needle. **B,** Pull back on plunger to determine if the needle entered a blood vessel. **C,** Inject the medication slowly by pushing the plunger down. **These photos show technique with the LEFT hand being the dominant hand.**

PROCEDURE 7·1

ADMINISTRATION OF AN INTRAMUSCULAR INJECTION—cont'd

gest (that is, inserting the needle with your dominant hand, then changing hands and steadying the syringe with your nondominant hand, then using your dominant hand to aspirate and push on the plunger), you help prevent further discomfort to the patient and tissue irritation that may occur if the syringe is jiggled or moved during a hand change.

19. Massage the injection site. Move the tissue as you massage, not merely the sponge (Figure 7-32). If rapid absorption is desired, continue to massage the area for about 2 minutes.

Massaging the area helps spread the medication in the tissue.

20. Help the patient assume a comfortable and safe position.

21. Observe the patient for any unusual reactions, such as a rash or shock.

22. Inform the patient if he or she is free to leave or if the physician requires additional consultation time.

23. Place a disposable needle and syringe in a puncture-resistant container without breaking or recapping the needle. The needle box should be in the room or as close as possible to the area of use (Figure 7-33). After using a reusable syringe and needle, flush tap water through both until clean. Separate the needle, barrel, and plunger and place each in a designated cleansing solution until ready to prepare all for sterilization.

To protect the physician, medical assistant, and janitorial staff. Needle recapping and disposal are frequent causes of needlesticks.

24. Remove gloves.

25. Wash your hands.

26. Record the procedure on the patient's chart.

Charting Example

June 3, 20__ 4 PM
Penbritin-S 500 mg IM in ROQ [right outer quadrant] of buttock.
Brook Thomas, CMA

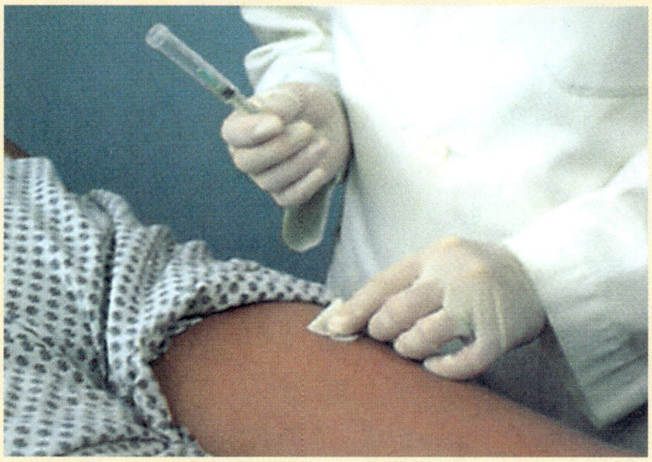

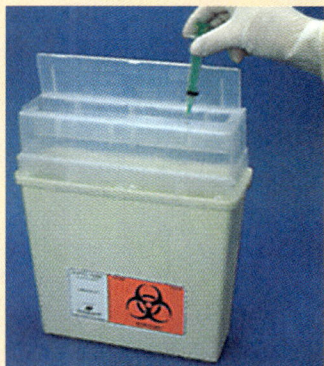

FIGURE 7-33 Puncture-resistant containers marked "Biohazard" must be used to dispose of used syringes.

FIGURE 7-32 After the injection has been administered, massage and cleanse injection site with sponge to remove any blood or medication that might be present.

Using the Tubex Injector

For the procedure for using this newer type of injector and sterile cartridge-needle unit, see Figure 7-34.

If a reusable injector and medication in a prefilled sterile cartridge-needle unit are used, the method for giving the medication is basically the same as when using a disposable or reusable syringe. After use, you should clean the reusable injector with an antiseptic solution. Sterilization is not required because the injector does not come in direct contact with the patient.

Text continued on p. 402

FIGURE 7-34   Technique for using the Tubex injector (closed injection system). Method of administration is the same as with conventional syringe. Remove needle cover by grasping it securely; twist and pull. Introduce needle into patient, aspirate by pulling back slightly on the plunger, and inject.

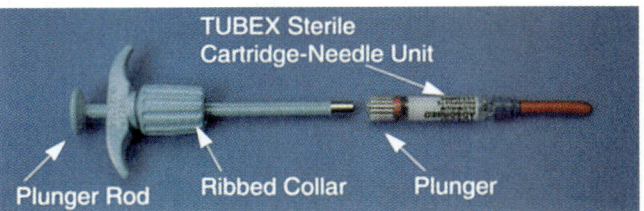

HOW TO LOAD

HOW TO UNLOAD AND
DISCARD USED UNIT

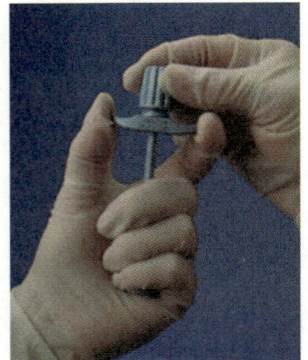

1. Turn the ribbed collar to the "OPEN" position until it stops.

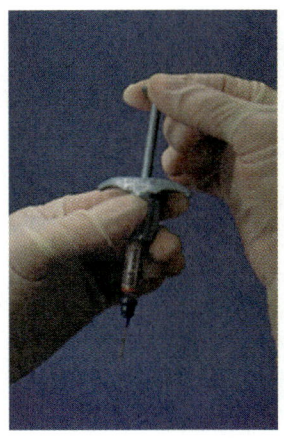

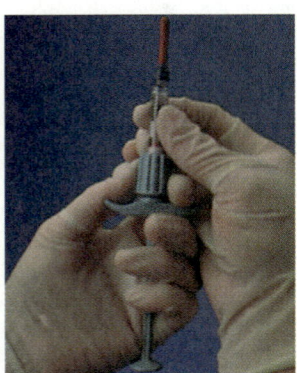

2. Hold injector with the open end up and fully insert the TUBEX sterile cartridge-needle until.

Firmly tighten the

1. Do not recap the needle. Disengage the plunger rod.

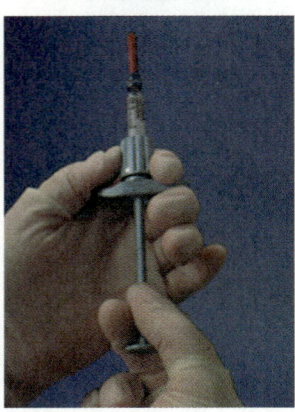

3. Thread the plunger rod into the plunger of the TUBEX sterile cartridge-needle until slight resistance is felt.

The injector is now ready for use in the usual manner.

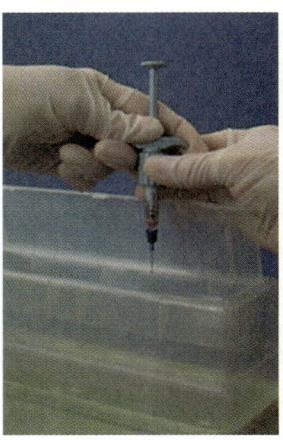

2. Hold the injector, needle down, over a needle disposal container and loosen the ribbed collar. Tubex cartridge-needle unit will drop into the container. The TUBEX Injector is reusable; do not discard.

PROCEDURE 7-2

INTRAMUSCULAR Z-TRACK TECHNIQUE

Objective
Understand and demonstrate the correct procedure for administering a medication using the IM **Z**-track technique.

The alternative intramuscular injection technique is called the **Z**-track technique. It can be used for an iron injection, which may cause irritation of subcutaneous tissue and discoloration from leaking medications, or when complete absorption of the medication by the muscle tissue is crucial. The preferred site for this technique is the upper outer quadrant of the buttock.

In this technique the tissue is pulled down and toward the median before, during, and after the injection. When the tissue is released, the needle track that is created is a **Z** pattern rather than the straight needle track that is created in other intramuscular injections. The **Z**-pattern track keeps the medication deep in the muscle and prevents seepage up through the tissues.

Use a 2-inch needle if the patient weighs approximately 200 pounds. If you don't use a needle 2 inches long on a patient of this weight, you will need to insert the needle its full length and then indent the tissue with the hub of the needle to ensure deep muscle penetration.

Use a 1¼- to 1½-inch needle if the patient weighs around 100 pounds. Use a ¾- to 1-inch needle on children weighing around 50 pounds.

Follow steps **1** through **12** as outlined on pp. 392-395, under Administration of an Intramuscular Injection, *except* that you should *change needles* after you have drawn the medication into the syringe. This eliminates the chance of medication left in the needle leaking into the tissue during the injection or of an extra "needle's worth" of medication being given. This minute extra amount of drug is of less concern with adult patients than it is with children, for whom even minute quantities of drug may be significant. Now use the following procedure (Figure 7-35).

An example of a drug administered using the Z-track technique is Interferon 5 ml.

PROCEDURE

13. Move the skin downward and toward the median.

14. Insert the needle at a 90-degree angle while maintaining traction on the tissue.

RATIONALE

The skin and subcutaneous tissue of an average adult moves about 1 to 1.6 inches. The underlying muscle within the selected injection site remains stationary.

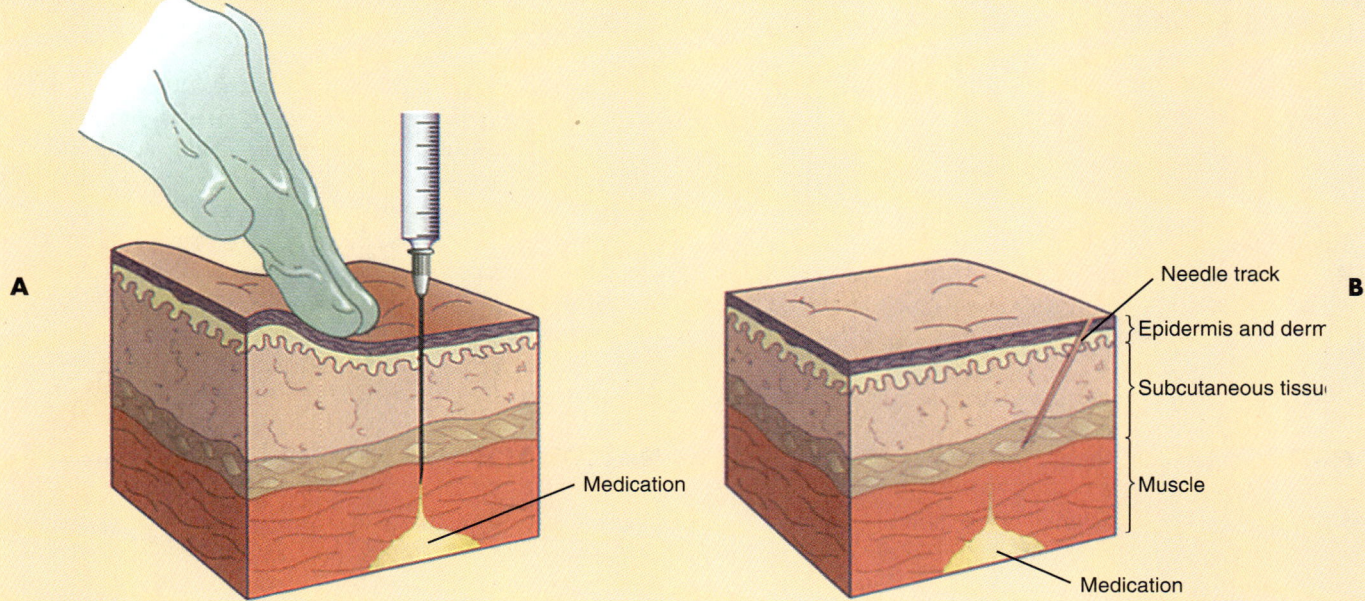

FIGURE 7-35   Intramuscular Z-track injection. **A,** Pull skin to one side, insert needle, aspirate, and inject the medication. Wait 10 seconds, then withdraw the needle. Release the pull on the skin. **B,** This seals off the injection site, preventing leakage or tracking of the drug from the muscle into other layers of tissue. (From Bonewit-West K: *Clinical procedures for medical assistants,* ed 5, Philadelphia, 2000, WB Saunders.)

Continued

PROCEDURE 7-2

INTRAMUSCULAR Z-TRACK TECHNIQUE—cont'd

15. Extend the thumb and index finger of the hand that is displacing the tissue to support the base of the syringe and aspirate by pulling back on the plunger with your other hand.

Maintain traction on the tissue. If blood appears, select a new site and use a new needle, syringe, and medication.

You may damage subcutaneous tissue and cause pain if traction is released while the needle is in place.

16. Inject slowly and smoothly while maintaining traction on the tissue.

17. Wait 10 seconds; then withdraw the needle and immediately release the skin, creating a **Z** pattern, which blocks any infiltration of the medication into the subcutaneous tissue.

Waiting provides time for the medication to disperse into the muscle and gives the muscle time to relax.

18. DO NOT MASSAGE THE INJECTION SITE. If bleeding occurs, gently wipe the area with a dry sterile cotton ball or gauze.

This minimizes the chance of the medication spreading into other layers of tissue. Massaging could cause the medication to seep back into the zigzag track and cause the patient pain.

19. Advise the patient not to exercise or wear tight clothing immediately after the injection.

20. Continue with steps 20 through 26 of Administration of an Intramuscular Injection on p. 397.

PROCEDURE 7-3

ADMINISTRATION OF A SUBCUTANEOUS INJECTION

Objective

Understand and demonstrate the correct procedure for preparing a medication, administering it by a subcutaneous injection, and charting the procedure.

Equipment

Sterile needle and syringe; usually a 2-cc syringe, ½- or ⅝-inch, 25-gauge needle (a 23- or 27-gauge needle could be also be used)

Sterile alcohol sponges

Medication ordered

Small tray to transport prepared medication to the patient

Disposable, single-use examination gloves

Preparation of the needle, syringe, and medication follows the same procedure that was outlined under Administration of an Intramuscular Injection. Remember to wash your hands before beginning the procedure, check the medication label three times, measure dosage accurately, identify the patient and explain the procedure, position the patient, and select the injection site correctly before administering the medication.

Follow steps **1** through **12** as outlined under Administration of an Intramuscular Injection on pp. 392-395 and then continue as follows.

PROCEDURE

13. Grasp the skin surrounding the injection area between your thumb and index finger or spread the skin and hold it taut.

14. Hold the barrel of the syringe between your thumb and the other fingers of **your dominant hand,** letting the hub of the needle rest on your index finger. The bevel of the needle should be facing upward.

RATIONALE

The decision of which method to use depends on the size of the patient and the size of the needle. You may grasp the skin on small, very thin, or dehydrated patients; you may spread the skin on large, well-nourished patients. Whichever method you use, be sure that you enter subcutaneous tissue when inserting the needle.

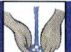

PROCEDURE 7-3

ADMINISTRATION OF A SUBCUTANEOUS INJECTION—cont'd

15. Insert the needle at a 45-degree angle into the skin, using a quick, forward thrust (Figure 7-36). The needle should be inserted almost to its full length. Do not touch the skin with the hub of the needle.

16. Release the skin.

17. Keep your dominant hand on the syringe for support. With your other hand, pull back on the plunger to see if you aspirate any blood. Refer to steps 16 through 23 under Administering an Intramuscular Injection for full explanations of the remaining steps.

18. Inject the medication slowly.

19. With an alcohol sponge, apply gentle pressure to the injection site, and quickly remove the needle.

Applying gentle pressure prevents the skin from being pulled along with the needle.

20. Massage the injection site with the alcohol sponge and observe the patient for any unusual reaction.

   NOTE: ***Do not*** massage the injection site after administering allergy injections or heparin. Only apply pressure for these injections.

Massaging the tissue after giving heparin can cause dispersal of the heparin, resulting in a hematoma.

21. Leave the patient safe and comfortable, providing any further instructions.

22. Remove and dispose of used equipment properly. Do *not* recap the needle. Place disposable syringe and needle in a puncture-resistant container for used sharps. See step 23 on p. 397.

23. Remove gloves.

24. Wash hands.

25. Record the procedure on the patient's chart.

Charting Example

June 2, 20__, 2 PM
Lovenox 40 mg, sc in left upper arm.
Kathy Kron, CMA

NOTE: *Lovenox is a new preparation of heparin, an anticoagulant.*

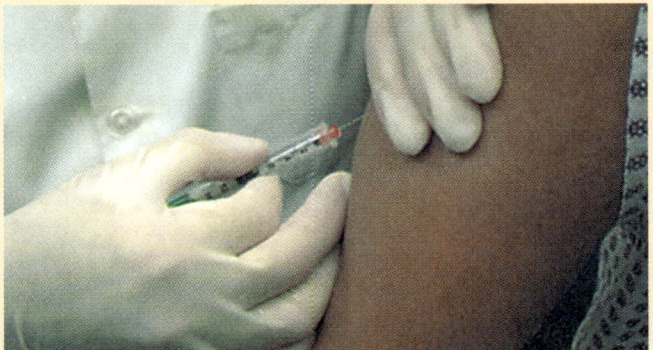

FIGURE 7-36 Technique for administering a subcutaneous injection. Insert needle at a 45-degree angle.

Insulin Injections

Insulin is a hormone produced in the body by the beta cells of the islands of Langerhans in the pancreas. It is secreted in response to increased levels of glucose in the bloodstream. Insulin takes part in the regulation of the processes necessary for the metabolism of proteins, fats, and carbohydrates and regulates the metabolism of glucose. Insulin lowers blood glucose levels and aids in the transport of glucose from the blood to the muscle cells and other tissues. Insulin deficiency results in hyperglycemia and can also result in diabetes mellitus.

Insulin preparations are used to treat all type I (insulin-dependent, formerly called juvenile-onset diabetes) diabetes patients and some type II (non–insulin-dependent, formerly called mature or adult-onset) diabetes patients. It may also be used temporarily for type II diabetics whose blood glucose levels are acutely elevated (as may be seen during an infection or trauma), who become pregnant, or who need insulin only until they lose enough weight *or* for type III—gestational diabetes.

Insulin use is a type of replacement therapy; it restores the ability of the cells to use glucose as an energy source and to correct the metabolic derangements seen in the different types of diabetes. The goal is to mimic the body's normal production and use of insulin. Special regimens are designed for each patient according to his or her needs. In addition to taking insulin, the patient must be educated about diabetes; the special care, diet, and treatment needed; and the complications that can occur if the program of therapy is not followed diligently. The patient's family should also receive diabetic education so that they can provide support to the patient and care if needed in time of emergency. (See also section on insulin reaction and diabetic coma in Chapter 17).

Insulin preparations and concentrations.

Different types of insulin preparations and concentrations are available (Figure 7-37). The most common types are listed in Table 7-12. In the United States, the most common concentration of insulin is U-100 (100 units of insulin per milliliter).

However, U-500 is also available (see Figure 7-8 for different types of insulin syringes).

Injection sites and factors that influence absorption of insulin.

Insulin is administered by a subcutaneous injection given into the abdomen, arms, thighs, or buttocks.

Insulin absorption rates and timing can vary for a patient. Insulin is absorbed at different rates, varying with the injection site. For example, the timing of insulin injected into the thigh can vary as much as 50% from the same amount of insulin given into the abdomen, resulting in variable insulin effects and blood glucose levels. Therefore *rotating injection sites is no longer recommended.* However, *it is recommended* that each injection site be about 1 inch from the last site used in the *same body area* (that is, if given in the abdomen, the next injection would be given in the abdomen 1 inch away from that site). This method not only prevents tissue damage that may result if the same site is used repeatedly but also increases the predictability of the effects of the insulin action because it is given in the same body area. Each site should not be used more than once every 30 days.

Other factors that affect the absorption rate of insulin include the following:

- Angle and depth of the injection
- Vascularity of the injection site
- Physical activity (for example, jogging after an injection into the thigh)
- Temperature (for example, increased after jogging or taking a hot bath)

The abdominal sites are preferred because absorption from these sites is rapid and unaffected by exercise. The arms are the second sites that provide the fastest absorption rate of insulin, followed by the thighs and buttocks. These last three areas are acceptable, especially for pregnant patients and for those who are taking more than two injections per day. For patients who wish to use more than the abdominal sites and who are taking more than two injections per day, the recommendation is to be consistent in the use of one area for each injection time. For example, insulin taken before breakfast would always be given in the abdomen, and insulin taken before lunch would always be given in the arm.

Procedure for insulin injections

1. Insulin should always be given 30 minutes *before* a meal.
2. Each injection site should be 1 inch away from the last site used.
3. Cleanse skin with alcohol and allow it to dry before inserting the needle.
4. Inject at a 90-degree angle *unless* the patient is very thin or is a child; then inject the needle at a 45-degree angle.
5. Insert the needle *quickly*. This minimizes discomfort.
6. If you grasped the tissue to insert the needle, let go of the skin *before* you inject the insulin. Pressure from the grasp can lead to insulin leakage.

FIGURE 7-37 Insulin label shows brand name, concentration, type species, and expiration date.

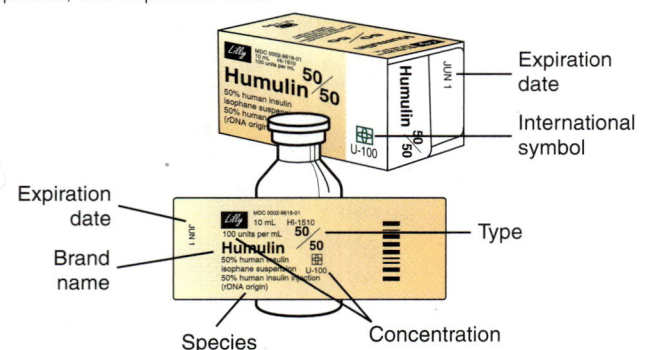

TABLE 7–12   Insulin Preparations

Type (Classification)	Onset of Action*	Peak Action*	Duration of Action*
1. Humalog (rapid acting)	Within 15 minutes	90 to 95 minutes	Less than 5 hours
2. Regular (short acting)	Within 1 hour (15 to 60 minutes)	2 to 4 hours	5 to 8 hours
3. Semilente (short acting)	30 to 60 minutes	4 to 6 hours	8 to 12 hours
4. Lente (intermediate acting)	1 to 4 hours	6 to 10 hours	12 to 24 hours
5. NPH (intermediate acting)	1 to 4 hours	6 to 10 hours	12 to 24 hours
6. Human Ultralente (intermediate acting)	1 to 4 hours	6 to 10 hours	12 to 24 hours
7. Animal Ultralente (long acting)	3 to 6 hours	14 to 20 hours	24 to 36 hours
8. 70/30: mixture of NPH (70%) and Regular (30%)	See timing for each above.		
9. 50/50: mixture of NPH (50%) and Regular (50%)	See timing for each above.		

*Approximate ranges only.

NOTE: Insulin should be stored in a refrigerator. Some bottles that are currently used can be stored at room temperature out of direct sunlight for 1 month. Read the manufacturer's directions carefully.

Regular insulin should be clear. All other types should be uniformly cloudy after rolled in your hands before use. DO NOT use the insulin if it looks clumpy or stays in precipitation after you roll it in your hands.

HEALTH MATTERS

KEEPING YOUR PATIENTS INFORMED

It is estimated that over 16 million people in the United States have *diabetes* and of these, *half* are unaware of their disease. Roughly, 700,000 people have Type I diabetes, and the other 15.3 million (90% to 95%) have Type II diabetes.

Many people are unaware of their disease until severe symptoms develop or until they are treated for one of its serious complications (see Chapter 17). Diabetes has been listed as the fourth-leading cause of death *by disease* in America as a result of the serious nature of some of the complications, such as heart disease, stroke, and kidney disease. Each year, at least 178,000 people die as a result of diabetes and its complications. See also Chapter 5, page 174, "Foot Care Guidelines for Patients with Diabetes."

As with many situations in life, information and knowledge can promote health. Numerous booklets, books, charts, and other materials are available for patient education programs and diabetic care. Information about daily health maintenance, diet and nutrition, exercise, long-term complications, emergency situations, and more can be obtained from the following agencies and others:

- The American Diabetic Association at 1-800-342-2383 or 1-800-232-3472
- Novo Nordisk Pharmaceuticals, Inc., at 1-800-727-6500
- Eli Lilly and Company at 1-800-545-5979

Having a variety of educational materials readily available for patients is a part of total patient care. Patients can also call these agencies and others for answers to many of their questions relating to diabetes.

REMEMBER, EDUCATION IS THE MOST BASIC TOOL OF DIABETES CARE.

---

7. Inject the insulin slowly. This allows tissue expansion and minimizes pressure that could cause leakage of some of the insulin.
8. Withdraw the needle quickly. Quick withdrawal minimizes a track for insulin leakage.
9. ***Do not* rub** the injection site after withdrawing the needle. Rubbing the injection site can vary the absorption rate.
10. *Do not* use the same site more than once every 30 days.
11. *Do not* rotate injection sites.
12. When mixing Regular Insulin with a longer-acting insulin, you must follow the manufacturer's recommendation, which states that you must **always** first draw up the clear Regular Insulin into the syringe and then draw up the second insulin (for example, NPH).

OXYGEN ADMINISTRATION

Oxygen is commonly used as a drug for patients with hypoxia (oxygen deficiency) or hypoxemia (deficiency of oxygen in the blood). We cannot live without oxygen. Room air that we normally breathe is approximately 21% oxygen.

Signs and Symptoms of Hypoxemia
- Anxiety or a feeling of impending doom
- Confusion
- Cyanosis
- Dyspnea
- Increased blood pressure
- Pale, cool extremities (caused by vasoconstriction)
- Restlessness
- Tachycardia

Conditions for Which Oxygen Administration May Be Required

- Apnea
- Carbon monoxide poisoning
- Congestive heart disease
- Chronic obstructive pulmonary disease (COPD)
- During surgical procedures
- Myocardial infarction
- Pulmonary edema
- Pneumonia
- Shock

Methods of Oxygen Administration

Before oxygen is administered, the patient's respiratory condition must be assessed. This includes observing the respiratory rate and rhythm and the amount or nature of the difficulty in breathing that the patient is experiencing. When feasible, obtain and record baseline vital signs. Two methods used to administer oxygen in the physician's office or clinic are by using the face mask or the nasal cannula (Figure 7-38). Check the physician's order for the method and rate of oxygen administration.

Face mask. The face mask is a device that is shaped to fit snugly over the patient's mouth and nose. It can be secured in place with a strap that goes around the head, or it can be held with the hand. The mask has valves that allow oxygen to be inhaled or pumped into the respiratory tract and carbon dioxide exhaled into the environment. Oxygen flows at a prescribed rate through a tubing to the mask. A flow rate of 8 to 15 liters per minute delivers 45% to 60% oxygen concentration.

Nasal cannula. The nasal cannula is a device that consists of two pronglike tubes that are placed into the nostrils to deliver oxygen. The nasal tubes should curve with the nasal passage to

FIGURE 7-38 **A,** Oxygen being administered through a nasal cannula; **B,** oxygen tank; **C,** mask, nasal cannula, and tubing; **D,** oxygen being administered through a face mask.

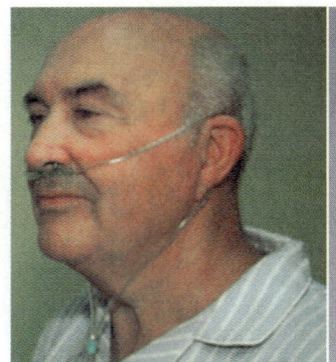
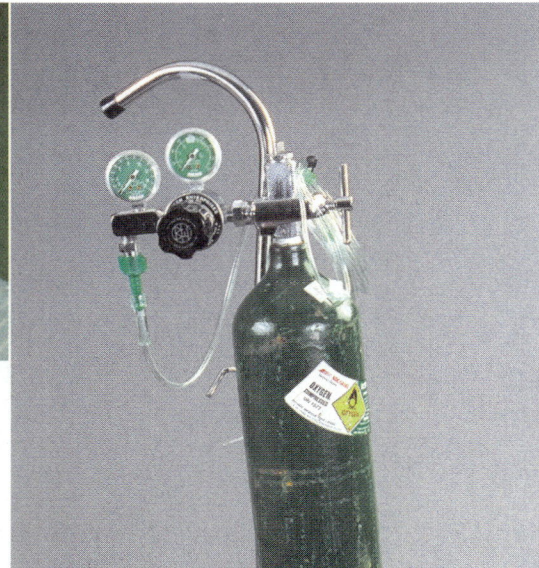
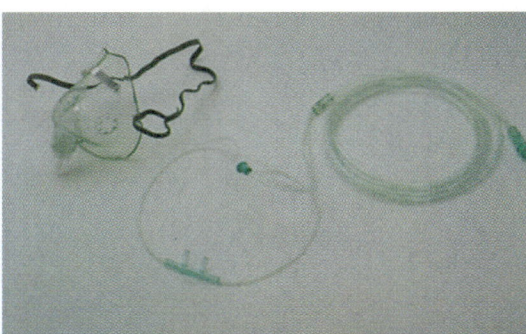
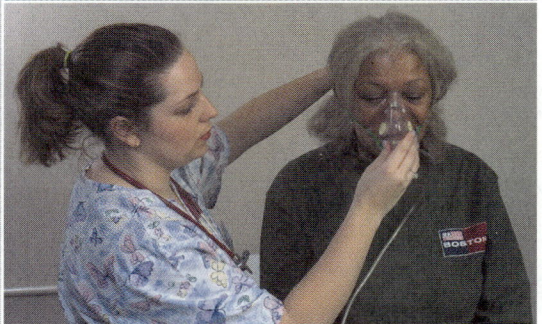

ensure delivery of the correct amount of oxygen. The patient must be instructed to breathe through the nose so that oxygen is not lost. Oxygen flows at a prescribed rate through a tubing to the nasal cannula. A flow rate of 2 liters per minute delivers 24% oxygen concentration. Flow rates higher than 5 liters per minute dry the nasal membranes if used for any length of time.

Keep the following points in mind when administering oxygen:

- Do not use electrical appliances when oxygen is being administered. Do not connect or disconnect plugs when oxygen is in use.
- Do not use acetone and alcohol in the presence of oxygen.

- Do not use oil or grease on oxygen equipment. Your hands must also be free of grease when you are turning oxygen equipment on or off.
- Do not use oxygen tanks as a clothes rack.
- Keep all flammable substances away from the area where oxygen is in use.
- Post "No Smoking, Oxygen in Use" signs in areas where oxygen is being used.
- Patients *should not be allowed* to have cigarettes, lighters, or matches with them while oxygen is being used because they may forget that these items should not be used while oxygen is being administered.
- When transporting an oxygen tank, fasten it to the platform of a carrier designed for that purpose.

CONCLUSION

Having completed this chapter, you should be able to discuss the laws regulating the distribution and administration of medication, in addition to the responsibilities and rules governing the administration of all types of medication. Certain legal stipulations are set forth that a physician must meet before using narcotics. You should be familiar with the special laws of your state and know how you can best help your physician comply with the state and federal laws applying to the dispensing, administering, and prescribing of medications, including narcotics and controlled substances. Knowledge of and familiarity with resource reference books on drugs are necessary to ensure adequate knowledge of any medication you are required to administer. Numerous references provide information on improved

medication techniques and current pharmacologic products. Check with your instructor for additional assignments and reference sources in areas of your own particular interest and need.

A variety of ways in which medications may be administered has been discussed in this chapter. You must be able to describe all 12 routes of administration and demonstrate your ability to administer an intramuscular and a subcutaneous injection. When you think you are competent, arrange with your instructor to take the performance tests. You are expected to accurately demonstrate your ability to prepare for and administer subcutaneous and intramuscular injections to a patient, in addition to identifying the equipment used and the care of such equipment after use.

REVIEW OF VOCABULARY

Read and define the italicized terms that have been presented in this unit.

Addiction and habituation of many drugs are major health problems in present-day society. To add to this problem, many use *crude drugs* rather than *pure drugs,* which may exert increasing *toxicity* in those who partake. Many individuals are unaware of the many *side effects* that drugs may produce, such as drug *tolerance* or the more severe reaction of *anaphylactic shock. Chemotherapy* used correctly in medical situations can produce marvelous results. At times there are *contraindications* to administering certain drugs to a patient. *Drug idiosyncrasies* or *side effects* may occur in patients receiving certain drugs. It is vital that you report this information to the physician so that this particular *prophylactic treatment may be altered.*

A *cumulative action of a drug* may be desired at times and at other times, contraindicated; thus any prolonged drug therapy must be monitored closely for various medical reasons.

The *HHS, FDA,* and *DEA* are all governmental agencies involved with the regulations controlling the commerce and administration of drugs.

Useful pharmacology book resources include the *PDR* and *USP-NF.* Familiarity with these sources is vital when knowledge of approved drugs, their dosages, actions, and contraindications is sought.

When you take an inventory of the *stock supply of drugs* in the office, you must discard *outdated drugs* and reorder a new supply. At times you may receive medications in a *unit dose.* An accurate inventory of all medications on hand is the responsibility of the medical assistant. Always know the drug before administering it to a patient. It is also important for a medical assistant to be familiar with drugs that have been *dispensed, administered, or prescribed* to the patient by the physician.

The following are sample patient reports. Read and define the italicized terms and abbreviations and state the classifications and uses for the drugs listed.

Patient No. 82647
Date: 1/28/01

CHIEF COMPLAINT

Ms. Day developed some pain in her left hand about November 19, 2000, while trying to E-mail on her computer. Since then, she has had continuing pain *focalized* near the wrist.

On examination, *adductor pollicis longus* and *extensor pollicis brevis tendons* are nontender. Her *tenderness* is over the *first carpometacarpal joint*. This area has been *injected* with *triamcinolone* and *1% Xylocaine*. The patient has been given a *prescription* for 25 tablets of *Vicodin*, tab 1 *q3h prn* pain. She has been sent for *x-rays* of her left hand and will be seen again in 2 weeks for reevaluation.

Impression:

Synovitis, first carpometacarpal joint, left hand.

B. Tren, MD
BT/tek

Patient No. 82647
Date: 2/25/01

PROGRESS REPORT
Date: 2/25/01

Ms. Day returns, and she is much better after the injection at the *first carpometacarpal joint*.

On examination today, there is no *tenderness* or *inflammation*. The patient has been instructed to not overdo it, and at the first signs of symptoms, she should resume taking *Naprosyn*. She has been given a *prescription* for *Naprosyn 375 mg,* total of 25 tablets, with instructions to take one twice a day with a meal, should she become *symptomatic*. She may return to the clinic on a *prn* basis.

B. Tren, MD
BT/tek

Patient No. 35728
Date: 8/2/01

PROBLEM: Medication reaction

S: Comes in complaining of a dry cough and irritated throat for 3 weeks and is now beginning to feel somewhat SOB, but hasn't really heard any wheezing. There is no sneezing or other URI symptoms. He is taking his Vasotec 10 mg qd.

O: Vital signs stable w/BP 130/80. Temp: 99.4°. TMs are clear w/some cerumen but TMs are not occluded. Nasal mucosa: normal. Pharynx: unable to visualize due to extreme gag reflex. Cervical nodes: nontender, nonpalpable. Chest: clear w/good aeration throughout.

A: Doubt infectious etiology even though temp is 99.4° today, most likely a reaction to Vasotec. BP is currently well controlled.

P: D/C Vasotec, begin Norvasc 5 mg po qd. He has a return visit scheduled for 8/11 at which time his BP will be reassessed as well as the cough and irritation in his throat. All of this was carefully reviewed w/pt.

Patient No. 97601
Date: 8/4/01

PROBLEM: Cracked tooth

S: Pt cracked a lower molar on the L side and had a root canal, 10/16. She took Pen VK 500 qid from 9/15 to 9/22. She is concerned now because she has a persistent lymph node in the L anterior cervical area.

O: Lymph node is about 1 × 1 cm, not particularly painful. It is soft. It seems like a reactive node. Dr. Burney examined it as well.

A: Reactive lymph node secondary to cracked tooth w/abscess.

P: Follow. No antibiotic treatment at this time. Told to return if it doesn't get any better. Pen VK 500 mg 1 qid × 10d will then be prescribed.

CRITICAL THINKING SKILLS REVIEW

1. Explain what a drug is; list three uses and four sources from which drugs are derived.
2. Describe the difference between the trade name and the generic name of a drug and give two examples of each.
3. Describe the difference between the following three classifications of drugs: (a) controlled substances, (b) prescription drugs, (c) nonprescription drugs.
4. List one use for each of the following: (a) analgesics, (b) anticoagulants, (c) antidotes, (d) antiseptics, (e) bronchodilators, (f) diuretics, (g) emetics, (h) hemostatics, (i) miotics, (j) narcotics, (k) antianxiety drugs, (l) vasodilators, (m) insulin.
5. List seven parts of a prescription.
6. Drugs are supplied in either a solid or liquid form. List five types of solid preparations and five types of liquid preparations.
7. Describe how and where medications should be stored.
8. When the label of a medication is torn and soiled so that the name of the drug cannot be clearly identified, what should you do with it?

9. List the information that must be kept on the office record for Schedule II controlled substances after they have been administered to a patient in the office.

10. List and briefly describe 12 routes by which medications can be administered.

11. List the five rights of proper medication administration. List one additional right added by many medical authorities.

12. When preparing medication to be administered, the label should be checked three times. List the three times when you should read the label of the medication.

13. Discuss at least 10 rules and responsibilities that you must be concerned with when administering medications.

14. Discuss five factors that influence dosage and drug action.

15. List six reasons for administering a medication by injection.

16. Discuss dangers involved and areas to avoid when giving medication by injection.

17. When asked to give a patient a subcutaneous injection, what size needle and syringe will you use? What sizes would be used for an intramuscular injection? Into which body sites would you administer each of these injections?

18. You have inserted the needle into the patient's right gluteus medius. As you withdraw the plunger of the syringe, a large amount of blood returns. What does this indicate, and what would be your next action?

19. The following orders have been written by the physician for patients. Using the abbreviation lists, transcribe these orders into English.
   a. Compazine 15 mg × 12 caps
      Sig i̅ cap po, tid, ac & hs, prn
   b. Digoxin 0.25 mg × 30 tabs
      Sig i̅ cap po, od

   c. Digoxin 0.25 mg × 30 tabs
      Sig i̅ tab po, bid for 10 days, then ½ tab bid
   d. Benadryl 50 mg × 8 caps
      Sig i̅ cap po, qid for 2d
   e. Naprosyn 500 mg × 60 tabs
      Sig i̅ tab po bid pc
   f. Vitamin B₁₂ 200 mcg, IM, qd
   g. Ampicillin 500 mg × 28 caps
      Sig 500 mg po, q6h for 7 days
   h. Amoxil 500 mg po, qd for 7 days
   i. Tetracycline 250 mg × 28 caps
      Sig i̅ po, 1 hr ac c̅ H₂O
   j. Keflin 0.5 gm IM stat and then q6h for 7 days
   k. Regular insulin 1 vial 100 IU/cc
      Sig 20 IU sc, ac and 40 IU, hs, sc
   l. Demerol 100 mg IM stat
   m. Seconal 50 mg po, hs, may repeat × 1, prn

20. Solve the following problems to determine the amount of drug that is to be administered.
   a. Give ASA gr 10 po; bottle reads 5 gr/tablet
   b. Give Compazine 10 mg IM; ampule reads 5 mg/ml
   c. Give ascorbic acid 0.5 g po; bottle reads 500 mg/tablet
   d. Give Kantrex 15 gr IM; bottle reads 1 g = 3 ml
   e. Give Maalox 1 ounce. How many ml do you give?
   f. Give tetracycline 500 mg, po; bottle reads 250 mg/capsule
   g. Give Valium 5 mg po; bottle reads 10 mg/tablet

21. After giving Mrs. Jones an IM injection, you accidentally stick your finger with the needle. Discuss what action you *must* take.

PERFORMANCE TEST

In a skills laboratory, a simulation of a joblike environment, the medical assistant student will demonstrate skill and knowledge in preparing for and administering medication safely and efficiently by accomplishing the following without reference to source materials. For these activities, the student needs a person to play the role of the patient to demonstrate the correct positioning of the patient and to locate the correct anatomic site to be used for the injection. An artificial limb may be used for performing the actual injection. Time limits for the performance of each procedure are to be assigned by the instructor (see also p. 104).

1. Intramuscular injection in one of the four sites discussed in this unit; IM injection using the **Z**-track technique.
2. Subcutaneous injection in the upper, outer part of the arm.
3. Loading and using a Tubex injector with a prefilled sterile cartridge-needle unit for an IM injection.
4. Reconstituting a powdered drug for administration.

The student is expected to perform these skills and record the procedures on the patient's chart with 100% accuracy.

The successful completion of each procedure will demonstrate competency levels as required by the AAMA, AMT, and future employers.

INTERNET RESOURCES

INFORMATION ON DRUGS

Drugs: How to use; side effects; objective information
www.safemedication.com (sanctioned by pharmacists)
www.healthtouch.com/level1/p_dri/htm

Drugs: Clinical trials
www.centerwatch.com

Site to identify medication (pill, tablet, etc.)
www.rxlist.com

Articles on medications (effects, trials, etc.)
www.rxmed.com

Occupational Safety and Health Administration (OSHA) directive
www.osha-slc.gov/OshDoc/Directive_data/CPL_2-2_44D.html

The Institute for Safe Medication Practices
www.ismp.org

The U.S. Pharmacopeia (USP)
www.usp.org/information/programs/pgrams/form.htm

Medic Alert
www.medicalert.org

National Association for Healthcare Quality
www.nahq.org

Poison Control Center
www.calpoison.org

American Cancer Society
www.cancer.org

American Diabetes Association
www.diabetes.org

National Institute on Drug Abuse
www.nida.hih.gov

The Food and Drug Administration
www.fda.gov

Drug Enforcement Administration (DEA)
www.usdoj.gov/dea/index.htm

Health Touch (prescription and OTC drug uses and side effects, plus other health topics)
www.healthtouch.com

Diagnostic Allergy Tests, Intradermal Skin Tests, and Tuberculosis

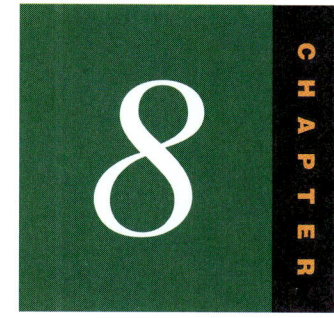

CHAPTER 8

■ Cognitive Objectives

On completion of Chapter 8, the medical assistant student should be able to:

1. Define, spell, and pronounce the terms listed in the vocabulary.
2. Discuss the nature, causes, signs, and symptoms of allergies. Differentiate between symptoms of a cold and symptoms of allergies.
3. List methods used for the diagnosis and treatment of allergies.
4. Describe and differentiate between the following tests:
   a. Patch test
   b. Scratch test
   c. Intradermal skin test
   d. Mantoux test for tuberculosis
   e. Tine tuberculin test
   f. Radioallergosorbent test (RAST)
   g. Immunoglobulin electrophoresis
5. Describe how to determine the results of the tests (a) through (e) given in No. 4.
6. Explain how tuberculosis (TB) is transmitted from person to person.
7. Differentiate between TB infection and TB disease.
8. List the signs and symptoms of TB disease.
9. Differentiate between pulmonary TB and extrapulmonary TB.
10. List the risk factors for the development of TB.
11. State the groups of people who are more likely to be exposed to or infected with *Mycobacterium tuberculosis*.
12. State the groups of people who are more likely to develop TB disease once they are infected with the bacteria.
13. Explain the purpose of the tuberculin skin test.
14. Describe how the Mantoux tuberculin skin test is given.
15. State when the results of the tuberculin skin test are determined and how the induration is measured.
16. Describe why the Mantoux skin test is preferred over the multiple-puncture test (tine test).
17. Discuss how the reaction to the Mantoux test is classified.
18. Describe the factors that determine the infectiousness of a TB patient.
19. Discuss when a TB patient would be considered *noninfectious*.
20. Discuss the main goal of a TB infection control program.
21. Discuss eight recommendations that should be observed in medical offices and clinics because of the potential for TB transmission.

■ Terminal Performance Objectives

On completion of Chapter 8, the medical assistant student should be able to:

1. Select the correct equipment and supplies needed to perform diagnostic allergy and intradermal skin tests.
2. Correctly perform and read and record the results of the following tests:
   a. Patch test
   b. Scratch test
   c. Intradermal skin test
   d. Mantoux test for tuberculosis
   e. Tine tuberculin test
3. Prepare the patient and the equipment and administer an intradermal injection in the correct body site.
4. Provide instructions and patient education that is within the professional scope of a medical assistant's training and responsibilities as assigned.

The student is to perform these activities with 100% accuracy before passing this chapter.

The consistent use of Universal/Standard Precautions is required by all health care professionals in all health care settings as a method of infection control. It is assumed that these precautions are used in all of the following procedures. Review Chapter 1 if you have any questions on methods to use because the methods or techniques are not repeated in detail in each procedure presented in this chapter.

Be sure to consult the latest guidelines issued by the Centers for Disease Control and Prevention (CDC) and consult with infection control practitioners when necessary to identify specific precautions that pertain to your particular work situation.

VOCABULARY

allergen (al'-er-jen)—Any substance that induces hypersensitivity.

allergy (al'er-je)—An unusual and increased sensitivity (hypersensitivity) to specific substances that are ordinarily harmless.

anaphylaxis (an"ah-fi-lak'sis)—An unusual or hypersensitive reaction of the body to foreign protein and other substances; often caused by drugs, foreign serum (for example, tetanus), and insect stings and bites.

atopy (at'o-pe)—A hypersensitive state that is subject to hereditary influences (for example, hay fever, asthma, and eczema).

contact dermatitis—Dermatitis caused by an allergic reaction resulting from contact of the skin with various substances (for ex-

ample, poison ivy or chemical, physical, and mechanical agents).

dermatitis (der"mah-ti'tis)—Inflammation of the skin.

induration (in"du-ra'shun)—An abnormally hard spot; a process of hardening.

vesicle (ves'i'kl)—A circular, blisterlike elevation on the skin containing fluid.

wheal (hwel)—A temporary, round elevation on the skin that is white in the center and often accompanied by itching.

ALLERGIES

The study and diagnosis of allergies are closely related to the field of immunity (review pp. 37-39). When a foreign agent (antigen) enters the body, antibodies are produced that attack and render the antigen harmless. This reaction is part of the body's natural defense mechanisms. However, in some instances, when the same antigen enters the body again, the antibodies, rather than protecting the body, set up an antigen-antibody reaction, producing harmful or uncomfortable results such as the signs and symptoms of an allergy.

An **allergy** is the abnormal individual hypersensitivity to substances (allergens) that are usually harmless. **Allergens**, substances capable of inducing hypersensitivity, can be almost any substance in the environment. Examples of allergens to which patients have become sensitive are dust, animal hairs, plant and tree pollens, mold spores, soaps, detergents, cosmetics, dyes, food, feathers, plastics, and even some valuable medicines. However, caution must be exercised when potential drug allergies are assessed because a drug reaction may not always be an allergic response. It could be an interaction with another drug that the patient is taking, a misdose, a side effect, and even an adverse effect of the drug.

Specialists agree that the symptoms of allergy and asthma increase along with the amount of pollutants both indoors and outdoors. One of the most common offenders is the house dust mite (a microscopic organism that lives in bedding, carpets, cushions, and stuffed toys). Cat hair follows as the second most common cause, and in the northeastern United States, the number-one allergen is the cockroach.

When the allergen comes in contact with or enters the body, it sets off a chain of events that brings about the allergic reaction. The allergen itself is not directly responsible for the allergic reaction. An allergy does not develop on the first contact with the allergen but can develop on the second contact or even years later after repeated contact with the allergen.

Signs and symptoms of allergies include sneezing, stuffed-up and runny nose, watery eyes, itching, coughing, shortness of breath, wheezing, rashes, skin eruptions, slight local edema, vomiting and diarrhea (from food allergies), and also mild-to-severe anaphylactic shock, which can be fatal unless treated.

Although allergy symptoms are often difficult to ignore, parents often mistake allergies for cold symptoms. The symptoms of allergies are usually more prolonged. Characteristic symptoms of colds are a stuffy nose, sneezing, a sore throat, a cough, mild chest discomfort, and slight weakness. Colds usually last from 2 days to 1 week, whereas, depending on the allergy, symptoms can last days, a week, or indefinitely. Allergies frequently "flare up" when the allergen is present and also at certain times of the year, depending on the allergen.

Diagnosis and Treatment of Allergies

For the physician to correctly treat the patient's condition, the allergen responsible for the reaction must be identified. After obtaining a detailed case history from the patient, the physician may order one of three skin tests: (1) patch test, (2) scratch test, or (3) intradermal test. The medical assistant may perform these tests or prepare the equipment and assist the physician with the procedure. The principle involved is that when a minute amount of various suspected allergens is applied to the skin in these tests, a mild allergic reaction occurs at the site of the offending allergen without causing any serious symptoms.

The size of the response correlates roughly with the severity of symptoms produced by natural exposure to the same allergen. As many as 20 to 30 tests may be necessary before the offending allergen or allergens are identified. Control tests using the diluent without the active allergen are essential in each type of testing. Positive reactions at the other test sites can be compared with the appearance at the control site to verify that they are a true allergic reaction and not merely an irritating reaction to the diluent or trauma to the skin area. Ready-made bottled preparations of allergen materials or diagnostic sets with vials containing up to 39 various allergens are available for testing.

Once the offending allergen has been identified, the first step in treatment is to avoid it. At times a special diet may have to be designed for the patient, or special antiallergic cosmetics may have to be used. When the allergen is animal hair, the patient has to avoid the animal and may have to give away a household pet. Patients with hay fever or asthma often have to move to a different locale or plan a trip to a place free from the offending pollen during certain seasons of the year. Often patients can be cured of allergies by receiving a series of **desensitization treatments** (immunotherapy). For these treatments, patients are given the allergen(s) in gradually increasing amounts to reduce their sensitivity to those substances or to build up their resistance to the point of immunity. Allergies that are resistant to cure may be controlled with certain medications such as antihistamines, epinephrine, aminophylline, and cortisone preparation.

Medications used to relieve the itching, sneezing, and sniffing often make people drowsy. New antihistamines now available have the advantage of being longer acting and nonsedating so that people can continue with daily activities much easier. For people that cannot take or are not helped with antihistamines, prescription corticosteroid nasal sprays are available. The nasal sprays do not appear to cause the potential serious side effects that are sometimes seen with other forms of steroid treatment. Both types of these newer drugs have been found to be effective and safe when used properly and as directed. However, long-term use of nasal corticosteroids in children is still debatable.

Skin testing and desensitization treatments for allergies are generally safe, but severe and even fatal reactions could occur, depending on the patient's sensitivity to the allergen being used. Therefore *a physician must be in the office or clinic when these tests are done because the patient could experience respiratory distress or anaphylaxis.*

Although not common, these conditions can be extremely serious. The medical assistant must be able to recognize any signs of distress in the patient being tested for allergies and alert the physician immediately. The onset of a reaction may be gradual. Initial mild signs may include pallor, flushing, shortness of breath, local pruritus (itching), dyspnea, cough, cyanosis, and even malaise and abdominal pain. These local reactions must not be ignored because they could rapidly escalate into a systemic response involving cells throughout the body.

As the process continues the patient may then have generalized pruritus, swelling, or hives. Respiration could become impaired because of laryngeal edema and bronchospasm (airway obstruction). If an open airway is not maintained and oxygen provided, the patient could die from respiratory failure. Other serious events could be hypotension, tachycardia, and decreasing levels of consciousness. Without treatment, these problems could progress to a serious state of shock and even death. *Emergency equipment and drugs (for example, epinephrine [Adrenalin] and oxygen) must always be readily available in the medical facility in areas where diagnostic agents and drugs are given that could lead to an anaphylactic reaction.* People with known allergies should wear a medical identification bracelet or necklace. Also, some may carry a kit with prescribed medication to be used in cases of systemic allergic reactions. Medical records of patients who have allergies should be clearly and explicitly labeled with information on all substances to which the patient is allergic (see also Allergic Reaction in Chapter 17).

Patch test.

Formerly used to detect tuberculosis, the patch test has been proven to be unreliable for that use. Today the patch test is most often used to diagnose skin allergies, especially contact dermatitis, and is the simplest type of skin test. To determine tissue hypersensitivity, gauze is impregnated with the substance to be tested and then applied and left in contact with an intact skin surface for 24 to 72 hours (usually 48 hours).

Scratch Test

In the scratch test, one or more scratches are made in the skin, and a drop of the substance to be tested is placed in the scratch and left for 20 minutes. The scratch test is often used for detecting types of allergies. Kits to be used for this test come in various sizes with various numbers of allergens. Some physicians may keep multiple-dose bottles of allergens for common allergies rather than using the test kits. The history obtained from the patient usually indicates the type and number of tests to be performed (Figure 8-1).

Intradermal skin tests.

In intradermal (intracutaneous) tests, a small amount of the substance under study is injected underneath the outer layer of skin (that is, the dermis—the layer of skin just below the epidermis). These tests are used to determine allergies; to determine the patient's susceptibility

FIGURE 8-1   Scratch test on patient's back; used for determining allergies.

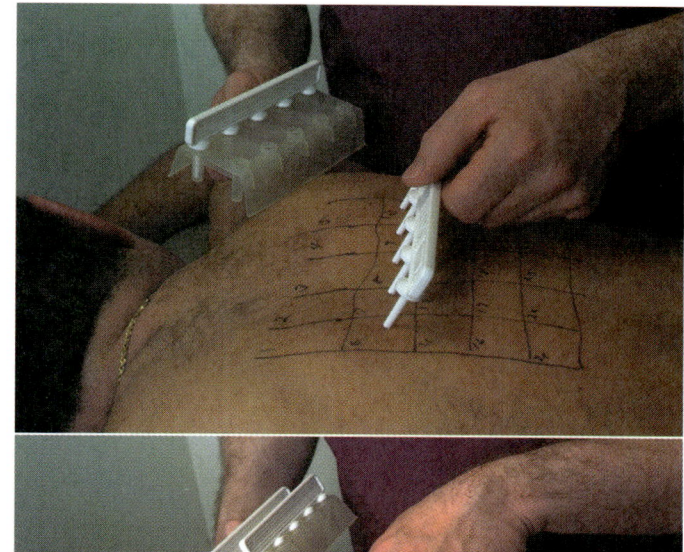

A

B

to an infectious disease; and to diagnose infectious diseases, such as tuberculosis (the Mantoux test) and diphtheria (the Schick test). For all these tests the general rules for administering injections apply (refer to pp. 387-388, Intradermal Injections and Instructions for Administering Injections). Commercial trays of prepackaged sterile syringes are available for intradermal allergy tests (Figure 8-2). Intradermal testing tends to be more accurate than the scratch test and is often performed if scratch test results are negative or unclear.

The American Academy of Allergy and Immunology recommends that patients having skin tests and/or desensitization treatments for allergies remain under observation for at least 20 minutes after injection (or for a longer time for high-risk patients) to minimize the risk of any severe reactions from the allergens.

Radioallergosorbent testing.   The radioallergosorbent test (RAST) is a radioimmunoassay test used to identify and quantify immunoglobulin E (IgE) antibodies in serum that has been mixed with any of 45 known allergens (IgE is one of five classes of humoral antibodies produced by the body). If an atopic allergy to a substance exists, an antigen-antibody reaction occurs. IgE often mediates an allergic response and is measured to detect allergic reactions and diseases. The general agreement is that this test should be used as a supplemental test rather than a screening test and as such is not used that often. However, it is useful for testing persons who have severe skin disease or eczema (commonly seen in children) for whom skin testing may be difficult to determine and may likely be

Text continued on p. 419

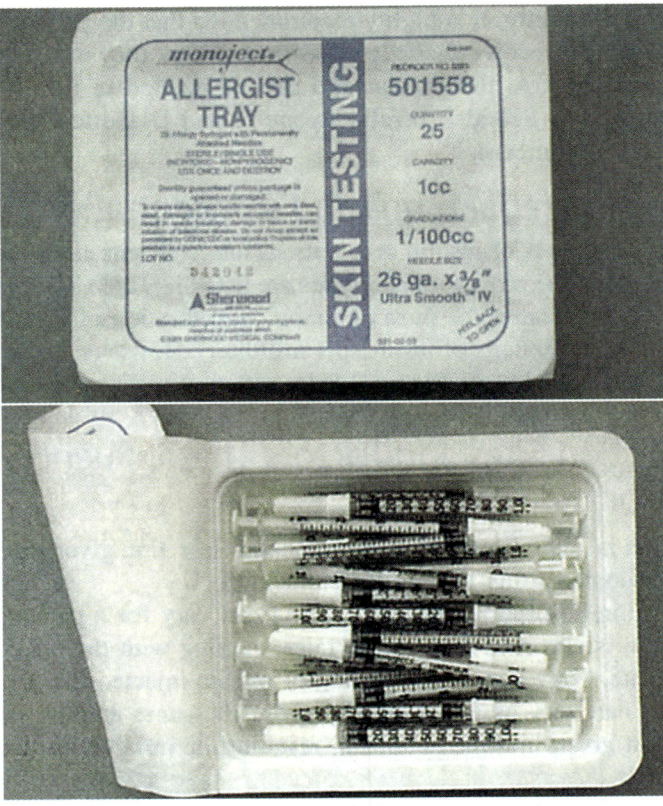

FIGURE 8-2   Prepackaged tray of sterile intradermal syringes for allergy testing.

PROCEDURE 8-1

PATCH TEST

Objective
Understand and demonstrate the correct procedure for performing a patch test and reading and recording the test and results.

Equipment
Antiseptic sponge to cleanse the skin or an alcohol sponge
Containers with the allergen(s) to be tested
Small gauze dressing(s) and square(s) of plastic wrap or commercially prepared protective covering patch(es)
Adhesive or paper tape

PROCEDURE

1. Check physician's order.

2. **Wash your hands. Use appropriate personal protective equipment (PPE) as dictated by facility.**

3. Assemble supplies.

4. Identify and prepare the patient.
   a. Explain the procedure.
   b. Provide a patient gown if needed.

RATIONALE

Explanations help gain the patient's cooperation, help alleviate fear of the unknown, and help the patient to relax.

PROCEDURE 8-1

PATCH TEST—cont'd

c. Position in a comfortable sitting position with the arm exposed and well supported or the back exposed if the patch is to be applied there.

5. Cleanse the skin site to be used and allow it to dry. The anterior forearm or the upper back are common test sites. The forearm is the preferred site for adults, and the back is the preferred site for children.

6. Place a drop or two of the specific allergen on the gauze dressing; cover this with a square of plastic wrap.

7. Place the gauze on the skin site and attach with tape. Commercially prepared covering patches come ready to be applied and do not need the plastic wrap covering.

8. Write the name of the test substance on the tape or write a number on the tape and in the patient's record with the name of the allergen used.

When a positive reaction occurs, it is vital that the correct allergen be identified. Correct record keeping is a must. As many as 20 to 30 patches may be applied at one time on the back.

9. Instruct the patient. Explain to the patient that if intense itching occurs, he or she should remove the patch and contact the physician immediately for further instructions. Also tell the patient to avoid wetting or scratching the test site until the patch is removed so that the allergen is not spread over a large area.

The patch is to be kept in place for varying lengths of time, depending on the allergen used and the physician's order (minimum 24 hours, up to 72 hours). Commonly it is left in place for 48 hours.

10. Record the test on the patient's record.

11. Remove the patch at the specified time and read the results (observe the reaction). Discard the patch in a designated covered container. The test result is negative when there is no reaction on the skin; the test result is positive when the skin is reddened (erythematous) or swollen or when vesicles are present.

12. Instruct the patient when and if to return for another appointment.

13. Leave the treatment room clean.

14. Wash your hands.

15. Record the reaction on the patient's record.

Charting Example

August 4, 20__, 1 PM
Patch tests done on forearm ×2.
Ari Sabir, CMA

Charting Example

August 6, 20__, 1 PM
Skin patches removed.
Results of the test—negative. Results confirmed with Dr. Allen.
Ari Sabir, CMA

PROCEDURE 8-2

SCRATCH TEST

Objective
Understand and demonstrate the correct procedure for performing a scratch test, and reading and recording the test and results.

Equipment
Commercially prepared kit with needles for each test and the allergen solutions, either in a capillary tube or bottle; when the prepared kit is not used, you will need the bottles containing the allergens to be tested and 26-gauge needles (a lancet or a dull sterile knife may also be used).
Two small towels
Washable ink pen
Toothpick or medicine dropper (to be used when the substance is provided in a bottle)
Patient gown
Disposable, single-use examination gloves

PROCEDURE

1. Check physician's orders.

2. **Wash your hands. Use appropriate personal protective equipment (PPE) as dictated by facility.**

3. Assemble the equipment.

4. Identify and prepare the patient:
   a. Explain the procedure.
   b. Ask the patient to disrobe to the waist and put the gown on with opening in back.
   c. Position the patient in a prone position (face down) on the examining table with the back exposed or sitting with the arm well supported and exposed.

5. Don gloves. Wash the back (or arm) with soap and water; dry thoroughly.

6. Write test numbers 2 inches apart on sections of the skin to correspond with the allergen container numbers. Use a pen with washable ink.

7. Make a ⅛-inch, superficial scratch with the needle supplied in the kit *or* with a 26-gauge needle *or* with a dull, sterile knife. *Do not penetrate the skin or cause bleeding.*

8. Place a drop of the allergen on the scratch. For solutions supplied in a capillary tube, break the tube in two and allow the solution to drop onto the scratch. For solutions supplied in separate bottles, use a toothpick end or a medicine dropper to pick up a drop of the solution and drop it onto the scratch. If the first scratch is used as a control test site, place a drop of normal saline on it (see Figure 8-1).

9. Make each additional scratch with a separate needle. Use a clean toothpick or medicine dropper for each solution to be tested.

10. Allow the allergen solution to set for 20 minutes with the back or arm exposed to the air. Provide for the patient's comfort.

RATIONALE

Explanations help gain the patient's cooperation and help the patient to relax.

The skin must be thoroughly cleansed and dried before the scratches are made. Gloves protect you against contamination.

Each allergen container is numbered to correspond with the numbered section on the skin to eliminate the possibility of incorrect readings.

Use only a minute quantity of the allergen solution to avoid severe allergic reactions. When placed on the scratch, some of the solution is absorbed into deeper layers of tissue.

Make sure that the patient is not chilled; provide extra covering over areas of the body not used for testing.

PROCEDURE 8-2

SCRATCH TEST—cont'd

11. Wipe the excess solution from each scratch separately.

12. Read the results (observe the skin reactions). NOTE: You may also read the test results 24 hours later to check for delayed reactions. You must have the physician check the results with you.

13. Give the patient further instructions:

   a. To dress and feel free to leave

   b. To return in 24 hours for a delayed reaction reading

   c. To schedule a future appointment for consultation

14. Remove used supplies from the treatment room and dispose of in designated covered containers for used supplies and laundry; put needles in a rigid, puncture-resistant container used for contaminated sharps. Leave the treatment room clean and neat.

15. Remove gloves and wash your hands.

16. Record the test and results on the patient's chart.

Avoid spreading the solution in one scratch to another scratch.

Test results are interpreted as follows:
   NEGATIVE: No reaction has occurred after 20 minutes.
   POSITIVE: The appearance of redness or swelling or a wheal at the test site. Positive results are designated as slight (1+), moderate (2+), or marked (3+).

Charting Example

August 4, 20__, 1 PM
20 scratch tests administered. Results—positive reactions to dust, cat hair, and plant pollen. Negative to other substances. Results confirmed with Dr. Allen.
Mary Donovan, CMA

PROCEDURE 8-3

ADMINISTRATION OF AN INTRADERMAL INJECTION

Objective
Understand and demonstrate the correct procedure for giving an intradermal injection, and reading and recording the test and results.

Equipment
Alcohol sponge or skin antiseptic and cotton ball

Tuberculin syringe because fine calibrations are needed (0.5 or 1 ml)
Needle: ⅜- or ½-inch, 26- or 27-gauge (see Figure 7-9 on p. 379)
Solution to be injected
Disposable, single-use examination gloves

PROCEDURE

1. Wash your hands. Use appropriate personal protective equipment (PPE) as dictated by facility. Steps 1 through 11 listed here correspond to steps 1 to 11 of Administration of an Intramuscular Injection, pp. 392-395.

RATIONALE

Continued

PROCEDURE 8-3

ADMINISTRATION OF AN INTRADERMAL INJECTION—cont'd

2. Assemble the equipment.

3. Prepare the syringe and needle for use.

4. Compare the physician's order with the medication label.

5. Check the medication label three times during preparation: when removing drug from the storage area, before measuring the desired amount, and when replacing container in the storage area.

6. Cleanse the vial rubber stopper, insert the needle, and withdraw the needed amount of solution into the syringe.

7. Identify the patient and explain the procedure.

Explanations help to reassure and relax the patient.

8. Select the injection site and position the patient comfortably. For intradermal injections, use the anterior surface of the forearm, about 4 inches below the elbow. In patients over 60 years of age, inject the solution into the area over the trapezius muscle (on the back), just below the acromial process (Figure 8-3).

For patients over 60 years of age, loss of skin turgor in the forearm can contribute to bruising or to extravasation of the testing solution.

9. Don gloves. Cleanse the injection site with the alcohol sponge and allow to dry thoroughly.

Gloves provide protection against possible contamination.

10. Remove the needle cover.

11. Expel any excess air that may have entered the syringe.

12. Stand in front of the patient. With your nondominant hand, grasp the middle of the patient's forearm on the posterior side and pull the anterior skin taut.

Pulling the skin taut allows for easier insertion of the needle.

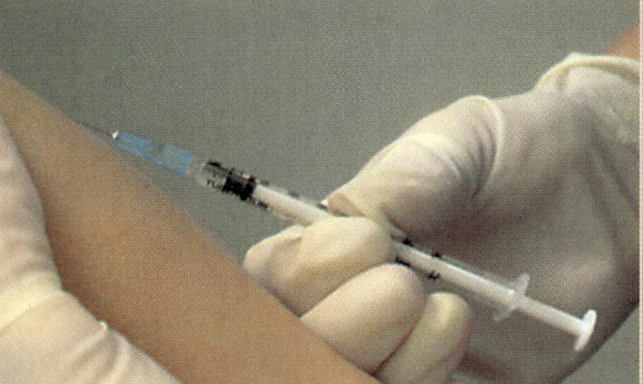
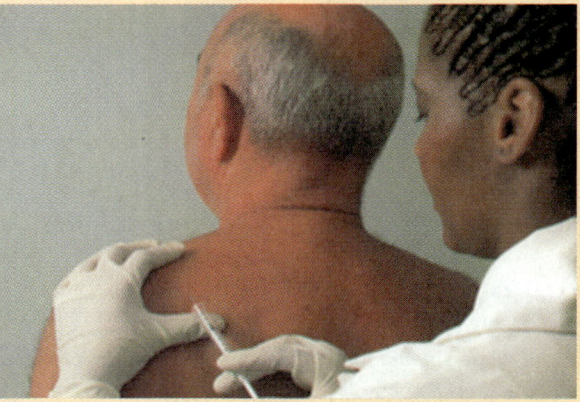

FIGURE 8-3 **A,** Administering an intradermal injection at a 10- to 15-degree angle on dorsal surface of forearm, about 4 inches below elbow. **B,** Administering intradermal skin test over the trapezius muscle just below the acromial process on elderly patients.

PROCEDURE 8-3

ADMINISTRATION OF AN INTRADERMAL INJECTION—cont'd

13. Hold the barrel of the syringe between your thumb and other fingers of your dominant hand; have the bevel of the needle facing upward.

14. Insert the needle into the skin at a 10- to 15-degree angle (see Figures 7-23 and 8-3). The angle used to insert the needle is almost parallel to the skin. Insert the point of the needle into the most superficial layers of the skin.

15. Inject the solution slowly. NOTE: This type of injection does not require aspiration before the solution is injected. As the drug is injected, a small pale bump (Figure 8-3, *C*) will rise over the point of the needle in the skin. If the injection is given subcutaneously (that is, no bump forms) or if a significant part of the solution leaks from the injection site, repeat the test immediately at another site at least 2 inches (5 cm) away.

16. Withdraw the needle and wipe the injection site gently with the alcohol sponge. Do not apply pressure or massage the skin.

17. Observe the patient for any unusual reaction, such as general febrile reaction, faint feeling, and shock.

18. Position the patient for safety and comfort and provide further instructions. If the patient feels faint, have him or her lie down or sit for a few minutes.

19. Tell the patient when the test results will be read. Schedule a future appointment when necessary. The patient may be dismissed if the results are not read until a day or two later. If the test result is to be determined within the next half hour or so, let the patient rest comfortable and safely. The skin reaction is read at various times, depending on the test done. Check with the physician or the literature that accompanies the drug used. Most allergy skin tests are read within 20 to 30 minutes, the Mantoux test for tuberculosis is read within 48 to 72 hours, and other tests are read at varying times within 48 hours.

20. Remove and dispose of the used syringe and needle correctly. Place a disposable syringe and needle in a puncture-resistant, disposable container without breaking or recapping the needle.

21. Remove gloves.

22. Wash your hands.

23. Record the procedure on the patient's chart. When several skin tests are given, record the site of each injection and the name of the substance injected.

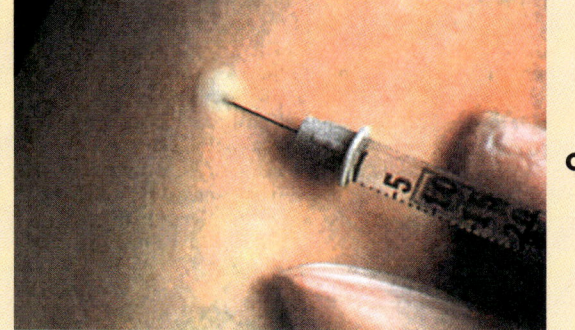

FIGURE 8-3—cont'd   C, Formation of bleb following intradermal injection.

The medication must not be dispersed into the underlying tissues.

Ensure that no unusual reaction occurs.

This avoids confusion when the results are read.

Continued

PROCEDURE 8-3

ADMINISTRATION OF AN INTRADERMAL INJECTION—cont'd

24. Read the skin reaction. Many tests are read as either positive or negative, depending on the amount of redness (erythema) or hardening (induration). For some tests the areas of redness or induration must be measured in millimeters. Follow the directions provided with the test solution (Figure 8-4).

25. Record the reaction on the patient's chart.

Charting Example

August 5, 20__, 4 PM
Reaction of Mantoux test given August 3, 20__, 4 PM, is negative—induration 0 mm. Results confirmed by Dr. Allen.
M.E. Burgdorf, CMA

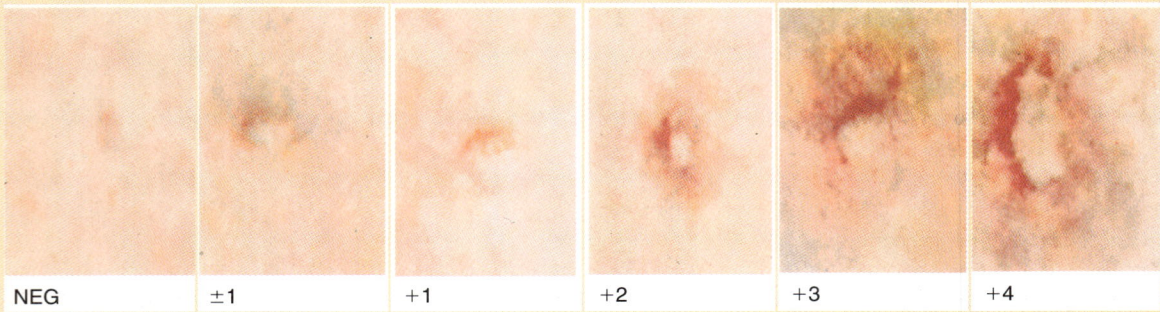

| NEG | ±1 | +1 | +2 | +3 | +4 |

FIGURE 8-4   Skin test results. The diameter of the *induration* is measured in millimeters and recorded.

TUBERCULOSIS VOCABULARY

The definitions given are those most applicable to usage relating to tuberculosis (TB) as stated by the CDC.

acid-fast bacilli (AFB)—Bacteria that retain certain dyes after being washed in an acid solution. Most acid-fast organisms are mycobacteria. When AFB are seen on a stained smear of sputum or other clinical specimen, a diagnosis of TB should be suspected; however, the diagnosis of TB is not confirmed until a culture is grown and identified as *M. tuberculosis*.

anergy—The inability of a person to react to skin-test antigens (even if the person is infected with the organisms tested) because of a weakened immune system, often caused by HIV infection or severe illness.

anergy testing—Giving skin tests using two substances other than tuberculin; done to determine whether a person is anergic. People who do not react to any of the substances, including tuberculin, after 48 to 72 hours (that is, people who have less than 3 mm of induration to all of the skin tests), are considered anergic.

cavity—A hole in the lung resulting from the destruction of pulmonary tissue by TB or other pulmonary infections or conditions. TB patients who have cavities in their lungs are referred to as having cavitary disease, and they are often more infectious than TB patients without cavitary disease.

culture—The process of growing bacteria in the laboratory so that organisms can be identified.

drug resistance, acquired—A resistance to one or more anti-TB drugs that develops while a patient is receiving therapy and that usually results from the patient's nonadherence to therapy or the prescription of an inadequate regimen by a health care provider.

drug resistance, primary—A resistance to one or more anti-TB drugs that exists before a patient is treated with the drug(s). Primary resistance occurs in persons exposed to and infected with a drug-resistant strain of *M. tuberculosis*.

engineering controls—Engineering systems used to prevent the transmission of TB in health care facilities, including ventilation, high-efficiency particulate air (HEPA) filtration, and ultraviolet germicidal irradiation.

false-negative reaction—A negative reaction to the tuberculin skin test in a person who has TB infection; may be caused by anergy, recent infection (within the past 10 weeks), or very young age (younger than 6 months old).

TUBERCULOSIS VOCABULARY—cont'd

false-positive reaction—A positive reaction to the tuberculin skin test in a person who does not have TB infection; may be caused by infection with nontuberculous mycobacteria or by vaccination with bacille Calmette-Guérin (BCG).

first-line drugs—The most often used anti-TB drugs (that is, isoniazid [INH], rifampin, pyrazinamide, ethambutol, and streptomycin).

induration—An area of swelling produced by an immune response to an antigen. In tuberculin skin testing or anergy testing, the diameter of the indurated area is measured 48 to 72 hours after the injection, and the result is recorded in millimeters.

isoniazid (INH) —A first-line, oral drug used either alone as preventive therapy or in combination with several other drugs to treat TB disease.

latent TB infection—Infection with *M. tuberculosis,* usually detected by a positive purified protein derivative (PPD) skin-test result, in a person who has no symptoms of active TB and who is not infectious.

multidrug-resistant tuberculosis (MDR-TB)—Active TB caused by *M. tuberculosis* organisms that are resistant to more than one anti-TB drug; in practice, often refers to organisms that are resistant to both INH and rifampin with or without resistance to other

drugs (*see* Drug Resistance, Acquired, and Drug Resistance, Primary).

positive PPD reaction—A reaction to the purified protein derivative (PPD)–tuberculin skin test that suggests the person tested is infected with *M. tuberculosis.* The person interpreting the skin-test reaction determines whether it is positive on the basis of the size of the induration and the medical history and risk factors of the person being tested.

preventive therapy—Treatment of latent TB infection used to prevent the progression of latent infection to clinically active disease.

second-line drugs—Anti-TB drugs used when the first-line drugs cannot be used (for example, for drug-resistant TB or because of adverse reactions to the first-line drugs). Examples are cycloserine, ethionamide, and capreomycin.

ultraviolet germicidal irradiation—The use of special lamps that give off ultraviolet light, which kills the tubercle bacilli contained in droplet nuclei.

ventilation systems—Air systems designed to maintain negative pressure and to exhaust the air properly; designed to minimize the spread of TB in a health care facility.

unreliable. Also, with RAST there is no danger of problematic allergic reactions occurring with test allergens because it is performed on a blood sample.

Immunoglobulin electrophoresis. Serum electrophoresis is another blood test that can be used to detect diseases of hypersensitivity and other conditions. In this test, increased levels of IgE are found in the serum of someone with allergies such as hay fever or asthma and also in anaphylaxis.

TUBERCULOSIS

Tuberculosis (TB) is an infectious disease caused by the tubercle bacillus *Mycobacterium tuberculosis.* TB is spread from person to person through the air. When a person with TB disease of the lungs or throat coughs, sneezes, laughs, sings, and even talks, tiny particles containing *M. tuberculosis* may be expelled into the air. These tiny particles are called *droplet nuclei* and can remain suspended in the air for several hours, depending on the environment. When another person inhales the air that contains the droplet nuclei, some of these bacteria may reach the alveoli in the lungs (Figure 8-5). It is here in the lungs that the infection begins. The bacteria start to multiply, and some will enter the bloodstream, spreading throughout the body to areas that TB disease may develop. These areas include the upper portions of the lungs, the larynx, the kidneys, the brain, bones, and joints. Normally, within 2 to 10 weeks the body's immune system will stop the further multiplication and spread of the bacteria. The bacteria become inactive, but they

remain alive in the body and can become active later. This is called **TB infection**. The immune system is keeping the bacteria under control. People with TB infection:

* Have no symptoms
* Do not feel sick
* Cannot spread TB to other people (they are not infectious)
* *Usually* have a *positive* skin-test reaction
* Usually have a normal chest x-ray examination
* Have negative sputum smears and cultures
* Are *not* a case of TB
* Can develop TB disease later in life if they are in a high-risk group and do not receive preventive therapy (see the Health Matters box)
* May never develop TB disease

Some people with TB infection develop **TB disease**. If their immune system cannot stop the bacteria from becoming active and keep them under control, the bacteria begin to multiply rapidly. TB disease can develop very soon after infection or many years after infection. Presently in the United States, 10% of all people who have TB infection will develop TB disease at some point. Because about half the risk of developing TB disease is concentrated in the first 2 years after infection, it is vital to detect new infection early. Treatment can be given to people with infection so that they will never develop TB disease. This is a very important aspect of **preventive medicine**. People with TB disease are most likely to transmit TB before the disease has been diagnosed and treatment has started.

FIGURE 8-5   Transmission of TB. TB is spread from person to person through the air. The dots in the air represent droplet nuclei containing tubercle bacilli. The bacilli are inhaled, enter the lungs, and travel to the alveoli, where they multiply.

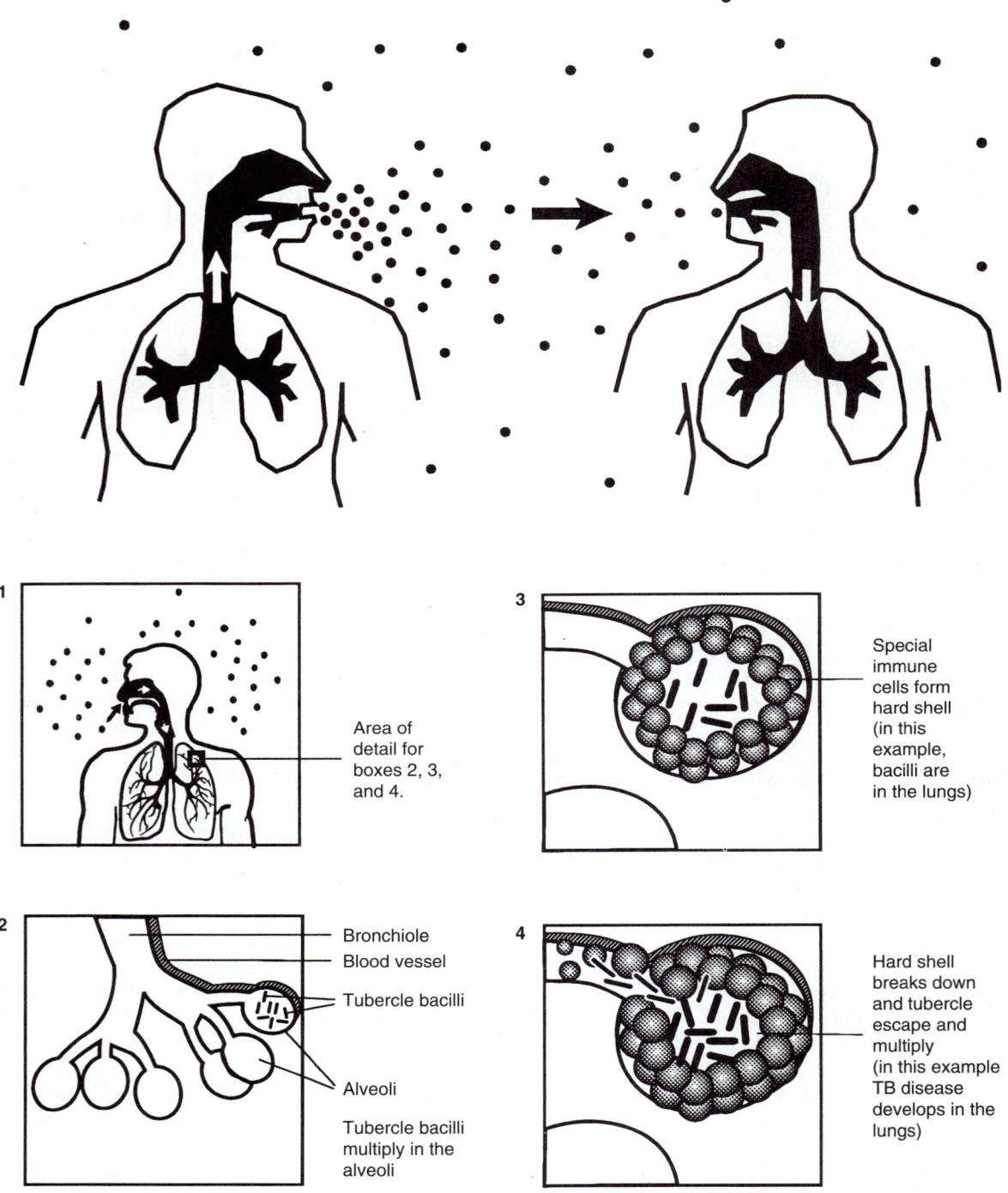

1 Area of detail for boxes 2, 3, and 4.

3 Special immune cells form hard shell (in this example, bacilli are in the lungs)

2 Bronchiole
Blood vessel
Tubercle bacilli
Alveoli
Tubercle bacilli multiply in the alveoli

4 Hard shell breaks down and tubercle escape and multiply (in this example TB disease develops in the lungs)

Usually only people with pulmonary or laryngeal TB are infectious because they may cough and expel the bacteria into the air. People with extrapulmonary TB usually are not infectious, and TB patients who are receiving treatment are less likely to be infectious. Infectiousness appears to decline rapidly after adequate treatment is started, but this result can vary from patient to patient. After 2 to 3 weeks of adequate treatment, if symptoms have improved *and* if three consecutive sputum smears collected on different days are negative, the person can be considered *noninfectious.*

HEALTH MATTERS

PEOPLE AT HIGHER RISK FOR EXPOSURE, INFECTION, OR TB DISEASE

Some groups of people are at higher risk for TB disease because they are more likely to be exposed to or infected with *M. tuberculosis.* This category includes those in close contact with people who have infectious TB disease, people born in areas of the world where TB is common (Asia, Africa, and Latin America), elderly people, the homeless, low-income groups with poor access to health care, and people who inject illicit drugs. This category also includes people who live or work in certain settings (for example, nursing homes, correctional facilities, homeless shelters, and drug treatment centers) and other people who may be exposed to TB on the job, such as health care workers.

Other groups of people are at higher risk for TB disease because they are more likely to develop the disease once infected—for example, people with certain medical conditions, especially HIV infection. For people infected with *M. tuberculosis* and HIV, the risk of developing TB disease is about 7% to 10% **each year.** In contrast, for people infected only with *M. tuberculosis,* the risk of developing TB disease is 10% **over a lifetime.**

Studies show a connection between the HIV epidemic and the increasing rates of TB. *First,* the areas that have been the most affected by the HIV epidemic have also reported the largest increases in TB cases. *Second,* the largest increase in TB cases has occurred among people of ages 25 to 44—the age group most affected by AIDS. *Third,* TB is common among AIDS patients. *Fourth,* HIV infection is common among TB patients.

Other conditions that place people at a higher risk for developing TB disease once infected include the following:

* Alcohol abuse and drug injection
* Recent TB infection (within the past 2 years)
* Diabetes mellitus
* Prolonged therapy with corticosteroids
* Immunosuppressive therapy
* Certain types of cancer (leukemia, Hodgkin's disease, or cancer of the head or neck)
* Severe kidney disease
* Low body weight (10% or more below the ideal weight)
* Poor nutrition
* High stress

Signs and Symptoms of TB Disease

Signs and symptoms of TB disease depend on where in the body the TB bacteria are growing. The *signs and symptoms of pulmonary TB* include coughing, pain in the chest when breathing or coughing, and coughing up sputum or blood. *General symptoms* of TB disease (pulmonary or extrapulmonary—outside of the lungs) include fatigue or weakness, malaise, loss of appetite, weight loss, chills, fever, and night sweats. The symptoms of extrapulmonary TB disease vary, depending on the area of the body that is infected with the disease. For example, TB of the spine may cause back pain; TB of the kidney may cause blood in the urine. *All these symptoms may be caused by other diseases, but they should lead the physician to suspect TB disease.*

Some people with TB disease may not have any signs and symptoms. However, most people with TB disease experience one or more symptoms that led them to seek medical care. Usually if symptoms are present, they have developed gradually and may have been present for weeks or months before the person seeks medical advice. Any person with signs and symptoms of TB should be evaluated for TB disease right away, at the same time the tuberculin skin test is given. Also, anyone who has a positive tuberculin skin test reaction should be evaluated for TB disease.

Diagnosis of TB *Infection*

A tuberculin skin test is the only way to determine if the person has TB infection *before* the infection has progressed to TB disease. The immune system of a person who has TB infection

will recognize the tuberculin because it is similar to the bacteria (tubercle bacilli) that caused the infection. Tuberculin testing is useful for the following:

* Examining a person who is not sick but who may have TB infection, such as a person who has been exposed to someone with TB
* Screening groups of people for TB infection
* Examining a person who has symptoms of TB

Different types of tuberculin tests are available, such as the Mantoux tuberculin skin test and the multiple-puncture tests, such as the tine test. The Mantoux test is the preferred method because it is more accurate and the amount of tuberculin given can always be measured. In multiple-puncture tests, the actual amount of tuberculin that enters the skin cannot be measured.

Tuberculin skin testing is contraindicated *only* for people who have had a necrotic reaction to a previous tuberculin skin test. It is *not* contraindicated for any other people, including infants, children, pregnant women, people who are HIV positive, or people who have been vaccinated with bacille Calmette-Guérin (BCG)—the vaccine for TB disease that is used in many countries but rarely in the United States.

Diagnosis of TB *Disease*

Anyone with symptoms of TB or who has a positive skin test should be evaluated for TB disease. The four steps for diagnosing TB include the following:

1. Medical history. This will include asking the patient if he or she has:
   - Been exposed to someone who has TB infection or disease
   - Experienced any of the symptoms of TB
   - Had TB infection or disease before
   - Any of the conditions that put a person at a higher risk for TB (see the Health Matters box)
2. Tuberculin skin test. After TB has been transmitted, it takes 2 to 10 weeks before TB infection can be detected by this test.
3. Chest x-ray study. If TB disease is in the lungs, the chest x-ray film usually shows signs of the disease.
4. Bacteriologic examination and drug sensitivity testing. Sputum is collected if TB of the lungs is suspected. If other parts of the body are thought to be infected, different specimens are obtained. For example, if TB of the kidneys is suspected, a urine sample would be examined; if TB meningitis is suspected, cerebral spinal fluid would be examined.

Smears and bacteriologic cultures are examined for the presence of acid-fast bacilli (AFB). TB is suspected if a smear is AFB positive; however, it is not excluded if AFB are not present because only 50% to 80% of patients with TB of the lung have AFB-positive smears. A diagnosis is confirmed when the culture demonstrates the growth of *M. tuberculosis*. A confirmed diagnosis may take 3 to 6 weeks because of the time it takes for these bacteria to grow in a culture. Other tests that provide quicker results are currently being evaluated but are not available for routine use.

Drug sensitivity tests are done to determine which drugs can kill the tubercle bacilli that are causing the patient's disease. This identification is very important because some strains of tubercle bacilli are resistant to the commonly used drugs.

The new drug Rifater, a combination pill (rifampin 120 mg, isoniazid 50 mg, and pyrazinamide 300 mg), was approved for use in the summer of 1998. Its use decreases the number of pills that patients have to take and also decreases the risk of bacteria becoming resistant to the drug.

Smear examinations and cultures should be done periodically to monitor the patient's response to therapy. Drug sensitivity tests should be repeated if the culture results are still positive after the patient has received 3 months of therapy or if the patient does not seem to be responding to therapy. (Also see Bacterial Culture and Sensitivity [C & S] Testing in Chapter 11 and the accompanying figures.)

With early diagnosis and appropriate treatment, TB can usually be cured. In 1989 the Department of Health and Human Services predicted that by the year 2010, tuberculosis would be eliminated. Unfortunately the opposite is occurring; the cases of TB are increasing. Even more alarming is an increase in tuberculosis cases that are resistant to the common anti-TB drugs used to cure this disease (see earlier Health Matters box).

Infection Control and TB Precautions for the Medical Office*

The main goal of an infection control program is to detect TB disease early and to promptly isolate and treat people who have TB disease.

In general, the symptoms of active TB are symptoms for which patients are likely to seek treatment in a medical office. Because of the potential for *M. tuberculosis* transmission, the following recommendations should be observed:

- A risk assessment should be conducted periodically, and TB infection-control policies based on results of the risk assessment should be developed for the medical office. The policies should include provisions for identifying and managing patients who may have undiagnosed active TB; managing patients who have active TB; and educating, training, counseling, and screening all personnel.
- While taking patient's initial medical histories and at periodic updates, medical assistants who work in medical offices should routinely ask all patients whether they have a history of TB disease or have had symptoms suggestive of TB.
- Patients with a medical history and symptoms suggestive of active TB should receive an appropriate diagnostic evaluation for TB and be evaluated *promptly* for possible infectiousness. Ideally, this evaluation should be done in a facility that has TB isolation capability.
- TB precautions in medical offices that provide evaluation or treatment services for TB patients should include (1) placing these patients in a separate area apart from other patients and not in open waiting areas (ideally, in a room or enclosure meeting TB isolation requirements); (2) giving these patients surgical masks† to wear and instructing them to keep their masks on; and (3) giving these patients tissues and instructing them to cover their mouths and noses with the tissues when coughing or sneezing.
- TB precautions should be followed for patients who are known to have active TB and who have not completed therapy until a determination has been made that they are noninfectious.
- Patients with active TB who need to attend a health care clinic or office should have appointments scheduled to avoid exposing HIV-infected or otherwise severely immunocompromised persons to *M. tuberculosis*. This recommendation could be accomplished by designating certain times of the day for appointments for these patients or by treating them in areas where immunocompromised persons are not treated.

---

*Guidelines for Preventing the Transmission of TB in Health Care Facilities, U.S. Department of Health and Human Services, PHS, CDC, Atlanta, Ga.
†Surgical masks are designed to prevent the respiratory secretions of the person wearing the mask from entering the air. When not in a TB isolation room, patients suspected of having TB should wear surgical masks to reduce the expulsion of droplet nuclei into the air.

- If cough-inducing procedures are to be administered in a medical office to patients who may have active TB, they should be performed using local exhaust ventilation devices (for example, booths or special enclosures [Figure 8-6]) or, if this is not feasible, in a room that meets the ventilation requirements for TB isolation.
- Office personnel should wear respiratory protection when present in rooms or enclosures in which cough-inducing procedures are being performed on patients who may have infectious TB.
- After completion of cough-inducing procedures, patients who may have infectious TB should remain in their isolation rooms or enclosures and not return to common waiting areas until coughing subsides. They should be given tissues and instructed to cover their mouths and noses with the tissues when coughing.
- Office personnel who have a persistent cough (that is, a cough lasting more than 3 weeks), especially in the presence of other signs or symptoms compatible with active TB (for example, weight loss, night sweats, bloody sputum, anorexia, or fever), should be evaluated promptly for TB. Personnel with such signs or symptoms should not return to the workplace until a diagnosis of TB has been excluded or until they are receiving therapy and a determination has been made that they are noninfectious.
- Personnel who work in medical offices in which there is a likelihood of exposure to patients who have infectious TB should be included in employer-sponsored education, training, counseling, and purified protein derivative (PPD) testing programs appropriate to the level of risk in the office.

- In medical offices that provide care to populations at relatively high risk for active TB, use of engineering controls for ventilation, filtration, and ultraviolet germicidal irradiation for general-use areas (for example, waiting rooms) should meet any applicable federal, state, and local requirements.

Criteria for Reporting TB Cases

All 50 states, the District of Columbia, New York City, U.S. dependencies and possessions, and independent nations in free association with the United States* report TB cases to the Centers for Disease Control and Prevention (CDC) based on certain criteria. Each reported TB case is checked to make sure that it meets the criteria. All cases that meet the criteria, called **verified TB cases,** are counted each year.

Cases that meet **one** of these three sets of criteria are counted as verified TB cases:

1. The patient has a *positive culture* for *M. tuberculosis.*
2. The patient has a *positive smear for AFB,* but a *culture* has not been done or cannot be done.
3. The patient has a *positive tuberculin skin test reaction,* has other signs and symptoms of *TB disease,* is being treated with two or more TB drugs, and has been given a complete diagnostic evaluation.

---

*The dependencies, possessions, and independent nations include Puerto Rico, the U.S. Virgin Islands, Guam, American Samoa, the Republic of the Marshall Islands, the Commonwealth of the Northern Mariana Islands, and the Federated States of Micronesia.

FIGURE 8-6   TB patient sitting in a special booth used when the patient needs to cough up sputum for testing. Patient expectorates sputum into a sterile container. Using this special booth helps prevent the spread of tubercle bacilli.

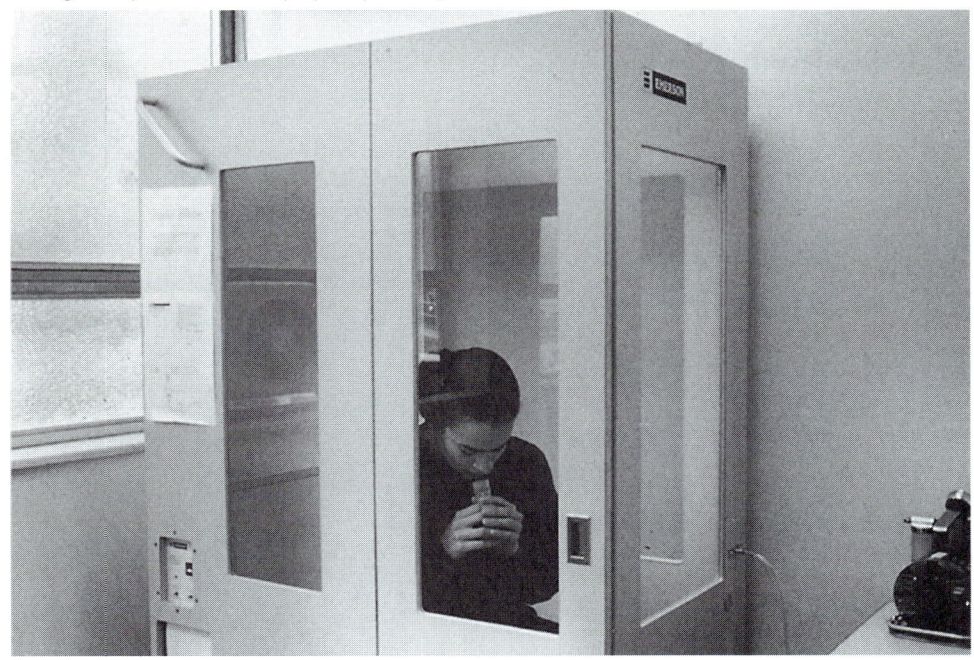

In addition, cases that do not meet any of these criteria (for example, a patient who is *anergic* and has a *negative culture* for *M. tuberculosis* but who has *signs and symptoms of TB disease*) may be counted as a verified TB case if a health care provider has reported the case and decided to treat the patient for TB disease.

Mantoux Test

The standard and preferred test recommended by the American Lung Association and the CDC to help detect people exposed to and infected with *M. tuberculosis* is the Mantoux test (also called the tuberculin or purified protein derivative (PPD) skin test or PPD intermediate [5 TU]). The Mantoux test is performed by injecting intradermally exactly 0.1 ml of tuberculin PPD. This dose contains 5 tuberculin units (TUs) of tuberculin PPD. The reaction is read 48 to 72 hours later. Only induration is considered when interpreting the test results. The Mantoux test should only be given to patients who have never had a positive PPD test in the past. Additional exposure to the tuberculin may cause skin necrosis at the site of the intradermal injection.

Equipment
- Alcohol sponge
- Tuberculin syringe (0.5 or 1 ml) with a $\frac{3}{8}$- or $\frac{1}{2}$-inch, 26- or 27-gauge needle
- Tuberculin PPD, 5 TU (intermediate) strength
- Disposable, single-use examination gloves

Procedure. Follow the intradermal injection technique described in previous paragraphs, measuring 0.1 ml of tuberculin PPD 5 TU into the syringe for administration. Record the date, time, manufacturer, lot number, amount of PPD administered, site and route of administration, and your signature.

Reading mantoux skin reactions
- Read 48 to 72 hours after the injection.
- Consider **only** induration (area of hardened tissue; swelling that can be felt) around the site of the injection when interpreting the results.
- Measure the diameter of induration transversely (lying in crosswise direction) to the long axis of the forearm and record in millimeters.
- Disregard erythema (redness).
- Disregard erythema greater than 10 mm if induration is absent because the injection may have been made too deeply. In this case, repeat testing.
- *All* reactions, even those classified as negative, should be recorded in millimeters.

Interpreting tuberculin reaction
Positive reaction. Induration measuring 10 mm or more indicates hypersensitivity to the tuberculin PPD and is interpreted as positive for present or past infection with *M. tuberculosis*. A positive reaction does not necessarily signify active disease. Further diagnostic procedures must be performed before a di-

agnosis of TB is made. NOTE: In parts of the United States where TB is *highly unlikely,* an induration of 15 mm or more is considered positive for people who do not have *any* risk factors for TB.

Doubtful reaction. Induration measuring 5 to 9 mm means that retesting may be indicated using a different test site.

Negative reaction. Induration of less than 5 mm indicates a lack of hypersensitivity to the tuberculin; thus tuberculosis infection is highly unlikely.

NOTE: The CDC has recommended that 5 mm or more induration should be the value used to interpret this skin test in HIV-positive individuals because when it is interpreted in HIV-infected individuals using the standard 10-mm induration measurement, it has been found to be less reliable. Induration of 5 mm or more is also considered positive for close contacts of people with infectious TB, people who have abnormal chest x-rays, and people who inject drugs and whose HIV status is unknown.

NOTE: To detect people who have been exposed to TB but test negative to the PPD skin test because they have very low antibody levels to the tuberculin, a second PPD test, called a booster dose, should be given 1 week after the first test.

Tine Tuberculin Test

NOTE: The intradermal tine tuberculin test is no longer recommended by most public health authorities. However, the test is still performed by health care providers in some areas of the United States.

The intradermal tine tuberculin test provides a convenient *screening* method for skin tuberculin reactivity in individuals and in large population groups. It does not diagnose TB. The reactivity of this test is comparable to, or more potent than, the intermediate-strength Mantoux test (5 TU) administered intradermally. The disposable tine unit used for this test consists of a stainless steel disk, with four tines or prongs 2 mm long attached to a plastic handle. The tines have been dipped in a solution of *Old tuberculin*–containing stabilizers and then dried. The entire unit is sterile as long as the plastic cap is not removed (Figure 8-7, *A*).

FIGURE 8-7 **A,** Tine unit for tuberculin testing; **B,** administering the tine tuberculin test.

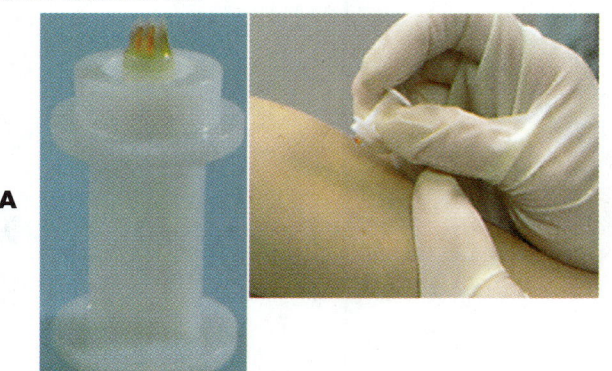

HEALTH MATTERS

KEEPING YOUR PATIENTS INFORMED

- A skin test is the only way to find out if you have TB infection.
- A positive tuberculin skin test reaction *usually* means you have TB infection.
- If you have a positive reaction to the skin test, the physician may do other tests to determine if you have TB disease.
- If you have recently spent time with someone with infectious TB, your skin test reaction may not be positive until 10 to 12 weeks after the last time you spent with the infectious person. This delay is because it can take that long for your immune system to react to the skin test.
- If you were vaccinated with BCG, you may have a positive reaction to the TB skin test. The physician will determine if you have TB infection by evaluating your medical history and why the skin test may be positive. If you do have a positive tuberculin reaction, you should be evaluated for preventive therapy.
- If you have TB infection and you are in one of the high-risk groups, you need to take a medication to prevent the development of TB disease. This is called **preventive therapy.**

- If you are younger than 35 years and you have TB infection, you may benefit from preventive therapy even if you are not in a high-risk group.
- If you do not take preventive therapy, you must be aware of the signs and symptoms of TB disease. Symptoms could develop at a later time, and in this case, you need to see the physician immediately.
- It is extremely important that you take all of the pills given to you so that your preventive therapy is effective.
- If you have TB disease, you will be given several drugs or the new combination pill. Taking a combination of drugs will work better in killing the bacteria that are causing your disease.
- If you have TB of the lungs or throat, you are probably infectious. After taking the medication for a few weeks, you should feel better. The physician will order a few tests to determine if you are still infectious.
- When you are no longer infectious or feeling sick, you can do the same things that you were doing before you got sick.

PROCEDURE 8-4

ADMINISTRATION OF THE TINE TUBERCULIN TEST

Objective
Understand and demonstrate the correct procedure for performing the tine tuberculin test and reading and recording the test and results.

Equipment
Disposable, single-use examination gloves
Alcohol sponge (acetone or soap and water can also be used)
Tine unit
Millimeter ruler (supplied with tine unit)

PROCEDURE

RATIONALE

1. **Wash your hands. Use appropriate personal protective equipment (PPE) as dictated by facility.**

2. Assemble the equipment.

3. Identify the patient and explain the procedure (also see the Health Matters box above).

   Explanations help to gain the patient's cooperation and alleviate any apprehension.

4. Don gloves; explain what is to occur and how it may feel.

5. Expose the patient's forearm, cleanse the skin with the alcohol sponge, and *allow the skin to dry thoroughly.* The preferred site for the administration of this test is the volar surface of the upper third of the forearm, over a muscle belly. Avoid hairy areas and areas without adequate subcutaneous tissue, such as over a tendon or a bone.

   The skin area must be thoroughly dry *before application of the tine test. The tuberculin must not be mixed with the skin cleanser.*

PROCEDURE 8-4

ADMINISTRATION OF THE TINE TUBERCULIN TEST—cont'd

6. Remove the protective cap on the tine unit while holding the plastic handle.

The protective cap is removed to expose the four impregnated tines.

7. With your nondominant hand, grasp the upper third of the patient's forearm on the posterior side firmly and stretch the anterior skin tightly (see Figure 8-7, *B*).

A firm grasp of the patient's forearm is necessary because the sharp momentary sting from the tine unit may cause the patient to jerk the arm and cause scratching.

8. With your dominant hand, apply the disk by puncturing the skin. Hold approximately 1 second before withdrawing.

Sufficient pressure must be exerted so that the four puncture sites and a circular depression of the skin from the plastic base are visible on the patient's skin.

9. Discard the tine test unit in the appropriate rigid, puncture-resistant sharps disposal container. The tine test unit must never be reused.

10. Instruct the patient when to return for the reading of the test results. Tests should be read in 48 to 72 hours.

> NOTE: **For both the Mantoux and tine tuberculin skin tests the following may apply in some clinics or offices:** Instruct the patient how to determine a negative result and mail the test card result back to you. Provide the patient with written instructions (Figure 8-8).

PATIENT INFORMATION: TUBERCULOSIS SKIN TEST

A

A Tuberculosis skin test has been placed on your right forearm. This test detects previous exposure to the tuberculosis organism. A positive test may or may **not** indicate disease.

A positive test is detected by a swelling and unusual redness at 48–72 hours after the test. If you have either of these findings 2–3 days after the test it is very important that you return to the Medical Clinic (M–F, 9–5), phone #223-4567, to have the test interpreted. If the 48–72 hour period falls on the weekend, please call the Urgent Care Department, #223-9786, so arrangements can be made to have your skin test interpreted there.

If the test is negative, please mail in the card attached to this paper so that we may record it in your chart.

If this test is being required for work purposes you **must** return for formal interpretation regardless of the results of the test.

Thank you.

B

TB TEST RESULT

☐ NEGATIVE

Check above box if negative and return card to Health Plan.

Name: _____

Health Plan Number:_____

Any redness or swelling at the site of the test in 48–72 hours, please call and make an appointment with the Medical Clinic #223-4567.

FIGURE 8-8 **A,** Written instructions for the patient for tuberculosis skin test. **B,** TB test result card to be returned by patient if skin test is negative.

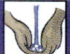

PROCEDURE 8-4

ADMINISTRATION OF THE TINE TUBERCULIN TEST—cont'd

11. Remove gloves.

12. Wash your hands.

13. Record the test on the patient's medical record.

Charting Example

August 27, 20__, 11 AM
Tine test administered in left anterior forearm. Patient to re-
turn August 29, 20__, 11 AM, for reading of the reaction.
Sissy Block, CMA

14. Read the reaction in a good light with the patient's forearm slightly flexed. Tests should be read in 48 to 72 hours. The extent of induration is the sole criterion; erythema without induration is insignificant. Determine the size of the induration in millimeters by inspecting the site and palpating with gentle finger stroking. Measure with a millimeter ruler the diameter of the largest single reaction around one of the puncture sites (Figure 8-9).

Interpretation of tuberculin test reactions as recommended by the American Lung Association follow.

- *POSITIVE REACTION: Induration measuring 5 mm or more. The significance of this test and the management of the patient are the same as for one who reacts with 10 mm or more of induration to the standard Mantoux test. Further diagnostic procedures must be considered, such as a chest x-ray film, laboratory*

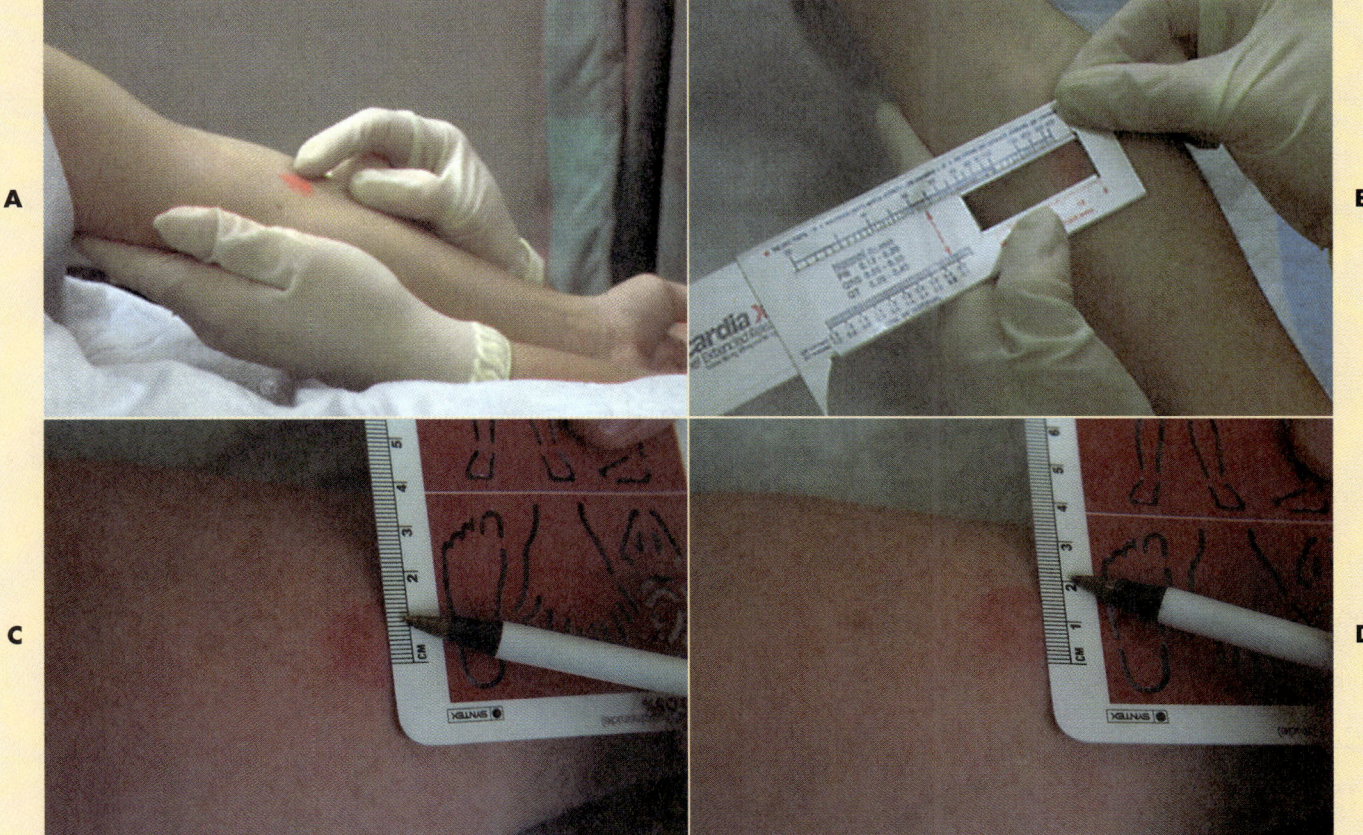

FIGURE 8-9 Reading the reaction of a tine tuberculin test. **A,** Palpate the area for presence of induration. **B,** Using a millimeter ruler, measure the largest single reaction around one of the puncture sites. **C,** Measure *only* induration. **D,** Measuring erythema and induration—this is INCORRECT.

Continued

PROCEDURE 8-4

ADMINISTRATION OF THE TINE TUBERCULIN TEST—cont'd

examinations of sputum and other specimens, and confirmation using the Mantoux method. Chemotherapy should not be started solely on the basis of a single positive tine test result.

- *DOUBTFUL REACTION: Induration of 2 to 4 mm. Patients in this group should have a Mantoux test done, and management should be based on the Mantoux reaction.*

- *NEGATIVE REACTION: Induration of less than 2 mm. Patients in this group do not need to be retested unless they are in contact with someone who has tuberculosis or if clinical evidence suggests the disease.*

15. Record the time and results on the patient's record.

Charting Example

August 29, 20__, 11 AM
Results of the tine test administered August 27, 20__, at 11 AM are negative. Induration 0 mm. Results confirmed with Dr. Allen.
Sissy Block, CMA

CONCLUSION

You have now completed the chapter on Diagnostic Allergy Tests and Intradermal Skin Tests. When you are familiar with the contents of this chapter, arrange with your instructor to take a performance test. You are expected to demonstrate accurately your skill in preparing for and performing all of the procedures outlined in this chapter.

REVIEW OF VOCABULARY

Read the following report and define the italicized terms.

Ms. Amy Fenster came to the office with an obvious case of *contact dermatitis.* Patient stated that she had been working in her garden when the signs and symptoms started and thinks that poison ivy may be the *allergen.*

Patient has no other known *allergies* and has never experienced *anaphylaxis* nor any previous *dermatitis.*

Family history includes the presence of various *atopies* in both her mother and father.

Further studies will include a *scratch test,* in addition to a *Mantoux test* that is required by her present employment.

A. Belman, MD

The following are two reports and samples of TB Registration Forms from charts in the physician's office. After reading these, you should be able to discuss the contents with your instructor. Be prepared to define and explain any medical terms that are used. A medical dictionary, other reference books, and information given in other chapters of this book may be used as references for obtaining definitions or explanations of the contents of this report.

Progress Notes

Name: John Dobson

DOB: 3/14/50

9/17/00

Problem: Pneumonia

S: 50-year-old smoker, diagnosed with left lower lobe (LLL) infiltrate pneumonia 9/16/00 and was treated with Ceftin 500 mg bid × 10 days. Patient complaining of itching, being dizzy, and sleeping longer after taking Ceftin. Denies rash. Itching relieved by Benadryl. Complaining of nausea with medication. No known allergy to Ceftin. Still slightly short of breath but overall improved. Still coughing with dark-colored sputum. Denies fever, throat swelling, or dysphagia. Believe itching is probably caused by mosquito bite. Is improving. Took second dose of Ceftin today. Has not smoked in 3 days. Wants to return to work on Monday.

O: BP 120/80; Heart rate 76; T 97°; wt 163. *General:* No appreciable disease. Patient is coughing. *HEENT:* WNL. *Chest:* scattered rales LLL, remaining fields clear to auscultation, no wheezes. Slightly coarse breath sounds over bronchi. No retractions, no dullness to percussion. *Heart:* regular rate and rhythm. *Skin:* scattered bumps on hands and feet, appearance consistent with mosquito bites. No macular or papular rash on trunk, lower extremities, or upper extremities; no rash on face.

A: LLL pneumonia per chest x-ray, 9/16/00, in smoker. Improving with Ceftin. Still with some shortness of breath and fatigue. Doubt Ceftin allergy. Still waiting for sputum culture results that are due 9/21/00.

P: Continue Ceftin, add albuterol inhaler 2 puffs q4h or prn for wheezing or chest tightness. Signs of drug allergy explained to patient. Additional self-care recommended to patient. Advised not to return to work until 9/23 if possible. To telephone if no improvement over the weekend or if fever increased, short of breath, or cough. Strongly encouraged permanent smoking cessation. Will discuss this at the next visit. Also follow-up visit requested for 7 to 10 days from today.

J.B. Fletcher, MD

Progress Notes

NAME: K.P. Lam

DOB: 4/6/81

K.P. is a 19-year-old man from the Philippines. He originally presented with a 15-lb weight loss, profound fatigue, and sneezing × 4 months. He denies fever, night sweats, and productive cough. He cannot recall a history of allergies and attributes the fatigue to his busy schedule of work and school. The physical examination was unremarkable, and he was initially treated for allergic rhinitis.

K.P. did not improve with antihistamines. Subsequently, a PPD was placed with a 20-mm induration. He was sent for a chest x-ray that ultimately showed a large, right upper lobe cavity. This finding immediately prompted the TB experts to get sputum smears. These smears came back positive for acid fast bacillus (AFB), indicative of active tuberculosis. Once the diagnosis of active TB was established, public health investigators began the process of screening all his contacts. This meant going to all his classes and workplace to perform PPD placements on his contacts.

K.P. was placed on ethambutol, pyrazinamide (PZA), isoniazid (INH), and rifampin with vitamin B_6. Because of the severity of his case, he was put on direct observed therapy for 2 weeks until his sputum smears became negative for AFB. His regimen will continue for another 11 months with periodic chest x-ray films to monitor his recovery.

NOTE: *The above case illustrates the need to be aware of TB and how it may present. Clearly, K.P. did not have pulmonary symptoms at the initial visit, yet he had a particularly active case of TB that may have been missed. Being aware of the possibility that TB may cause a number of constitutional symptoms, such as weight loss, fever, night sweats, and fatigue, may help to detect less classic cases of TB.*

TB REGISTRATION FORM

DATE OPENED: _____

DATE CLOSED: _____

PATIENT: _____   DOB: _____   CC#: _____

ADDRESS: _____   SEX: _____   B#: _____

BIRTHPLACE: _____   RACE/ETHNICITY: _____

TEL #1: _____   US SINCE: _____   LANGUAGE: _____

TEL #2: _____   SSN: _____   WEIGHT: _____

MEDI-CAL #: _____

- -

- -

REFERRAL SOURCE: _____   CONTACT TO: _____

PMD: _____   SMEAR: Date: _____   Pos: ____ Neg: ____

CULTURE: Date: _____   Pos: ____ Neg: ____

RESISTANCE: Yes: ____ No: ____

PAST DX TB: Yes ____ No ____ Unk ____   (date/place) _____

PAST TX TB: Yes ____ No ____ Unk ____   (date/place) _____

(details) _____

PPD: Date: _____   Result: _____ mm

Date: _____   Result: _____ mm

CXR: Date: _____ NL ____, ABNL ____, INF ____ (R/L), CAV ____ (R/L), EFF ____ (R/L), NOD ____ (R/L)

Date: _____ NL ____, ABNL ____, INF ____ (R/L), CAV ____ (R/L), EFF ____ (R/L), NOD ____ (R/L)

HIV STATUS: ____ HOMELESS WITHIN PAST YEAR (Including SRO): Yes ____ No ____ Unknown ____ Declined ____

SYMPTOMS: None ____, Cough (duration) ____, Hemoptysis ____, Fever ____, Nightsweats ____

Wt loss (amount lost), ____,   Other _____

OTHER MEDICAL PROBLEMS: None ____,   Present: _____

Hx of hepatitis: Yes, ____, No ____ .

MEDICATION CURRENTLY TAKING: (check) None ____, Birth-control pills ____, Phenytoin ____, Methadone ____, Antabuse ____,

Glucocorticoids ____, Other _____

ALCOHOL INTAKE: _____

IDU: _____   OTHER: _____

PERTINENT PHYSICAL FINDINGS: _____

_____

_____

INITIAL DIAGNOSIS: TB = 0   1   2   3   4   5

Dispo: CLOSE - PREVENTIVE TX - CHEMO TX - NO RX/STUDIES PENDING

COMMENTS/M.D. ORDERS/SPUTUM RESULTS:

Date: _____ MD Signature: _____

ABNL, Abnormal lung; *CAV,* cavity; *CXR,* chest x-ray; *DX,* diagnosis; *EFF,* effusion; *EMB,* ethambutol; *IDU,* intravenous drug use; *INF,* infusion; *INH,* Isoniazid; *NL,* normal lung; *NOD,* nodular; *PZA,* pyrazinamide; *RIF,* rifampin; *R/L,* right/left; *TX,* treatment.

TB REGISTRATION FORM FOR PATIENTS BEGINNING INH OR MULTIDRUG RX

PATIENT: _____   CC#: _____

DIAGNOSIS FOR WHICH ANTI-TB DRUGS ARE BEING PRESCRIBED:

TB-1   Contact

TB-2   Less than 21 years old _____,   Contact _____,   Converter _____,   Postpartum _____,
Newcomer _____,   Special clinical circumstances _____

TB-3   Pulmonary _____,   Extrapulmonary _____,   (give site) _____

TB-4   Inadequate prior Rx _____

TB-5   Suspect _____   Probability of TB: High _____,   Moderate _____,   Low _____

MEDS ORDERED: INH _____ mg qd, _____ 6 mo, RIF _____ mg qd, _____ 6 mo
_____ 12 mo,   _____ 12 mo

PZA _____ mg qd, _____ 6 mo, EMB _____ mg qd, _____ 6 mo
_____ 12 mo   _____ 12 mo

Others _____

DIRECTLY OBSERVED THERAPY: Yes _____,   No _____

SIDE EFFECTS/TOXICITY OF ANTI-TB DRUGS EXPLAINED TO PATIENT: Yes _____,   No _____

OTHER ORDERS: _____

_____

_____

_____

MD Signature: _____   Date: _____

FINAL DIAGNOSIS: TB = 0   1   2   3   4   5

Chemo TX Status: _____

Dispo: Close _____   Follow-up _____ & MD Orders: _____

Date: _____   MD Signature: _____

As patient, parent, or legal guardian, I authorize
necessary exams, tests, and/or treatment.   Signature: _____

CRITICAL THINKING SKILLS REVIEW

1. Define the term *allergy* and list six signs and symptoms of an allergy.
2. A patch test is left in place for a minimum of __ hours, up to a maximum of __ hours.
3. List two body sites that are often used to apply a patch test. Which is the preferred site for adults? For children?
4. Describe how you would read and record the results of the following:
   a. Patch test
   b. Scratch test
   c. Mantoux test
   d. Tine tuberculin test
5. What body site would you use to administer an intradermal injection?
6. Why don't you massage the skin after administering an intradermal injection?
7. Where would you administer the tine tuberculin test? What is the purpose of this test?

8. Why are control tests essential in each type of allergy skin test?

9. What is the tuberculin skin test used for?

10. Describe how the Mantoux tuberculin skin test is given.

11. With the Mantoux skin test, when is the patient's arm examined? How is the tuberculin reaction determined?

12. Why is the Mantoux skin test preferable to multiple-puncture tests?

13. Why does the site of disease affect the infectiousness of a TB patient?

14. List three criteria used to determine when a TB patient can be considered noninfectious.

15. What is the main goal of a TB infection control program?

16. What would make you suspect that a patient has TB disease?

17. In the physician's office an elderly man comes to the desk and says he wants to be checked for TB because one of his friends was just hospitalized with TB. You notice that he is coughing and spitting up sputum frequently and looks tired and thin. The waiting room is full of patients, and you know that it will be at least an hour before the physician can see him. What should you do?

PERFORMANCE TEST

In a skills laboratory, the medical assistant student will demonstrate skill in performing the following activities without reference to source materials. Time limits for the performance of each procedure are to be assigned by the instructor (see also p. 104).

1. Select and prepare the supplies and equipment and then perform the following procedures:
   a. Patch test
   b. Scratch test
   c. Intradermal skin test (intradermal injection)
   d. Mantoux test
   e. Tine tuberculin test
2. Read and record the results of these tests.

The student is expected to perform these skills with 100% accuracy before passing this chapter. **The successful completion of each procedure will demonstrate competency levels as required by the AAMA, AMT, and future employers.**

🖳 INTERNET RESOURCES

Centers for Disease Control and Prevention (CDC)
www.cdc.gov

Medic Alert
www.medicalert.org

National Institutes of Health, National Heart, Lung and Blood Institute
www.nhibi.nih.gov

Poison Control Center
www.calpoison.org

Center for Science in the Public Interest
www.cspinet.org

American Association for Respiratory Care
www.aarc.org

American Lung Association
www.lungusa.org

Allergy, Asthma, & Immunology Online
www.allergy.mcg.edu

American Academy of Allergy, Asthma, and Immunology
www.aaaai.org

National Institute of Allergy and Infectious Diseases
www.niaid.gov

Drug Enforcement Administration (DEA)
www.usdoj.gov/dea

Instillations and Irrigations of the Ear and Eye

9

CHAPTER

■ Cognitive Objectives

On completion of Chapter 9, the medical assistant student should be able to:

1. Define, spell, and pronounce the terms listed in the vocabulary.
2. Describe how to instill drops into the ear and eye and explain the reason for the actions taken.
3. Describe how to irrigate the ear and eye and explain the reasons for the steps taken.
4. Explain the difference between an instillation and an irrigation.
5. List:
   a. Two purposes for an ear instillation
   b. Four purposes for an eye instillation
   c. Four purposes for an ear irrigation
   d. Four purposes for an eye irrigation

■ Terminal Performance Objectives

On completion of Chapter 9, the medical assistant student should be able to:

1. Demonstrate the proper procedure for performing an ear instillation and irrigation.

2. Demonstrate the proper procedure for performing an eye instillation and irrigation.
3. Provide instructions and patient education that is within the professional scope of a medical assistant's training and responsibilities as assigned.

The student is to perform these objectives with 100% accuracy 95% of the time.

The consistent use of Universal/Standard Precautions is required by all health care professionals in all health care settings as a method of infection control. It is assumed that these precautions are used in all of the following procedures. Review Chapter 1 if you have any questions on methods to use because the methods or techniques are not repeated in detail in each procedure presented in this chapter.

Be sure to consult the latest guidelines issued by the Centers for Disease Control and Prevention and consult with infection control practitioners when necessary to identify specific precautions that pertain to your particular work situation.

VOCABULARY

auricle (aw′ri-kl)—The outer projection of the ear; also known as the pinna (pin′nah).

canthus (kan′thus)—The inner canthus is the angle of the eyelids near the nose; the outer canthus is the angle of the eyelids at the outside corner of the eyes (see Figure 9-2).

cerumen (se-roo′men)—Ear wax secreted by the glands of the external auditory meatus.

conjunctiva (kon-junk′ti-vah)—The delicate membrane lining the eyelids and reflected onto the front of the eyeball.

cornea (kor′ne-ah)—The transparent section of the eyeball that permits light to enter the eye. It is part of the focusing system of the eye.

external ear—Includes the auricle, or pinna, and the external auditory meatus.

external auditory meatus (me-a′tus)—The canal or passage leading from the outside opening of the ear to the eardrum; also called the external acoustic meatus.

miotic (mi-ot′ik)—A medication that causes the pupil of the eye to contract.

mydriatic (mid″re-at′ik)—A medication that causes the pupil of the eye to dilate.

ocular (ok′u-lar)—Pertaining to the eye.

ophthalmic (of-thal′mik)—Pertaining to the eye.

ophthalmology (of″thal-mol′o-je)—The study and science of the eye and its diseases.

otic (o′tik)—Pertaining to the ear.

otology (o-tol′o-je)—The study and science of the ear and its diseases.

otoscope (o′to-skop)—An instrument used for visual inspection of the ear.

sclera (skler′ah)—The white outer layer of the eyeball. It is touch sensitive and is transparent over the front of the eyeball.

tear (lacrimal) glands—The glands of the underside of the upper lids that secrete a fluid to keep the eyes moist.

tympanic (tim-pan′ik) **membrane (TM)**—The eardrum; it serves as the membrane that separates the external auditory meatus from the middle ear cavity.

As a medical assistant, you may be asked to perform ear and eye instillations and irrigations. These procedures differ slightly. An instillation is the dropping of a fluid into a body cavity; an irrigation is the flushing or washing of a body cavity with a stream of fluid. Observe practices of medical asepsis (as outlined in Chapter 2) when performing these procedures. If the area being treated has an open wound, be sure to use sterile technique.

To understand ear and eye instillations and irrigations and to be of most help to the patient and physician, you should be familiar with the anatomy and physiology of these two special sense organs. You should review these topics before studying and practicing the procedures in this chapter. The ear is diagrammed in Figure 9-1, and the eye is diagrammed in Figures 9-2 and 9-3.

EAR INSTILLATION

When instilling solutions into the ear, keep in mind that the direction of the external ear canal in adults differs from that in children. To straighten the ear canal so that the medication will be effective, slightly different techniques are used for each age group.

Use medical aseptic technique when instilling solutions into the ear because the outer ear is not sterile. However, if the tympanic membrane is not intact, you must use sterile technique. To lessen discomfort for the patient, warm the medications slightly before using. Solutions that are either too cold or too hot may cause a feeling of dizziness in addition to pain. You can warm a bottle of eardrops by placing the bottle in a plastic bag to protect the label and then placing the bag and bottle in a basin of warm water for a few minutes. You can check the temperature of the medication by placing a drop or two on your inner wrist; it should feel warm, not hot.

Ear instillations are performed to accomplish the following:

1. Soften cerumen (ear wax) so that it can be removed easily later
2. Instill an antibiotic solution to combat an infection in the ear canal or eardrum
3. Instill an antiinflammatory medication, for example, a steroid, to combat inflammation

EAR IRRIGATION

An ear irrigation, the washing out of the external auditory canal with a stream of fluid, is performed to accomplish the following:

1. Cleanse the external auditory canal (external acoustic meatus)
2. Relieve inflammation of the ear
3. Dislodge impacted cerumen or foreign bodies from the external auditory canal
4. Apply antiseptics to combat infection
5. Apply heat to the tissues of the ear canal

Before an irrigation is done, ask the patient if he or she has a history of drainage from the ear and if he or she has ever had a perforation or other complications from a previous irrigation. If the answer to either question is "yes," notify the physician before giving this treatment. Also, before the irrigation, visually examine the ear canal with an otoscope. When the purpose of the irrigation is to cleanse the ear canal or to remove

FIGURE 9-1   Diagram of the ear. (From Thibodeau GA: *Anatomy and physiology,* ed 2, St Louis, 1993, Mosby.)

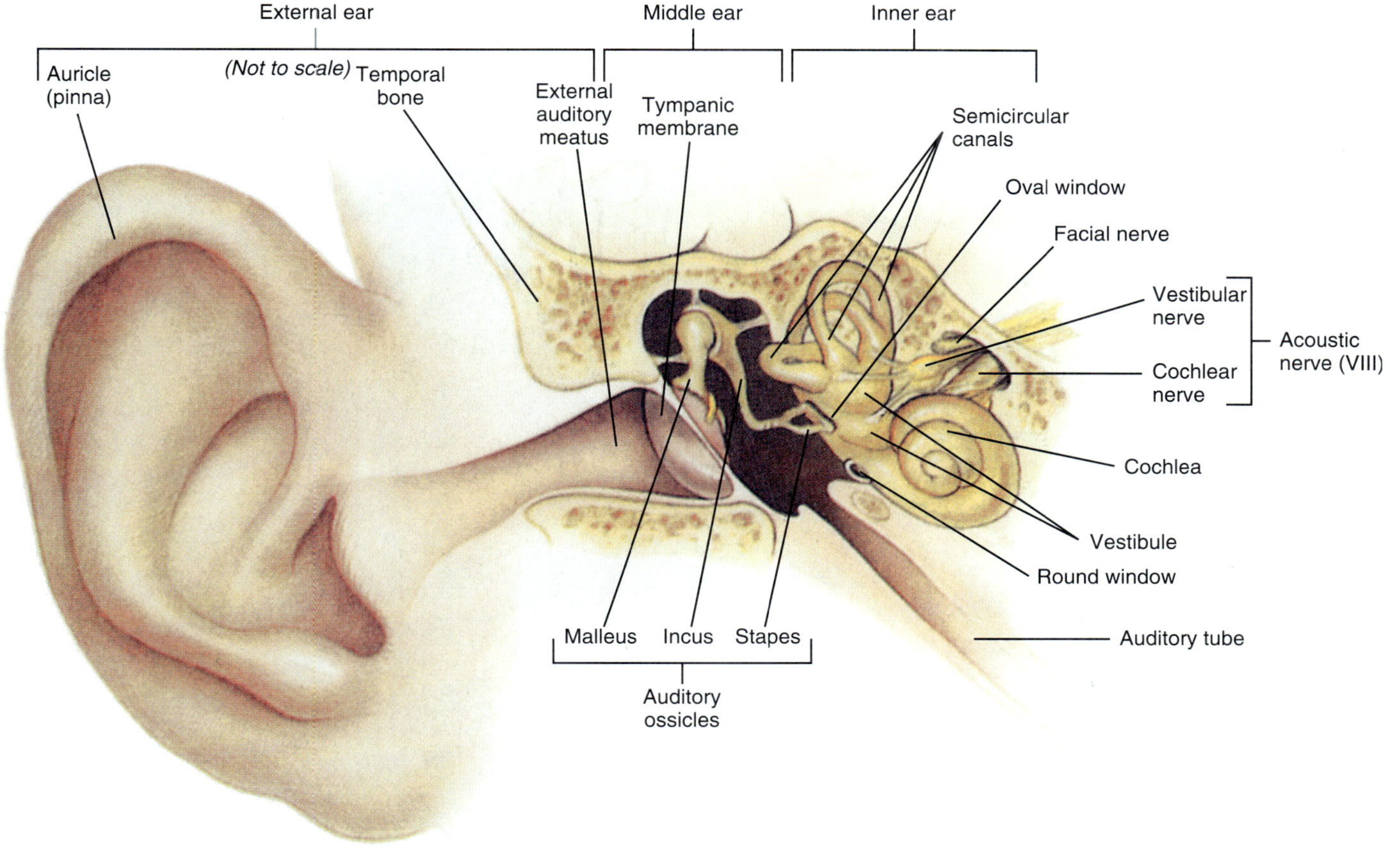

cerumen or foreign bodies, also perform a visual examination after the irrigation to determine if the results are satisfactory.

When this procedure is done, take extreme care to prevent injury to the tympanic membrane and the spread of any infection to the mastoid cavity.

EYE INSTILLATION

Eye instillations are performed to do the following:

1. Dilate the pupil of the eye
2. Constrict the pupil of the eye
3. Relieve pain in the eye
4. Treat eye infections; relieve inflammation
5. Anesthetize the eye
6. Stimulate circulation in the eye

Medications instilled into the eye are supplied either in a sterile liquid form as eyedrops or in a sterile ointment form.

EYE IRRIGATION

Eye irrigations are performed to do the following:

1. Relieve inflammation of the conjunctiva

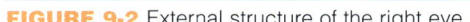

FIGURE 9-2 External structure of the right eye.

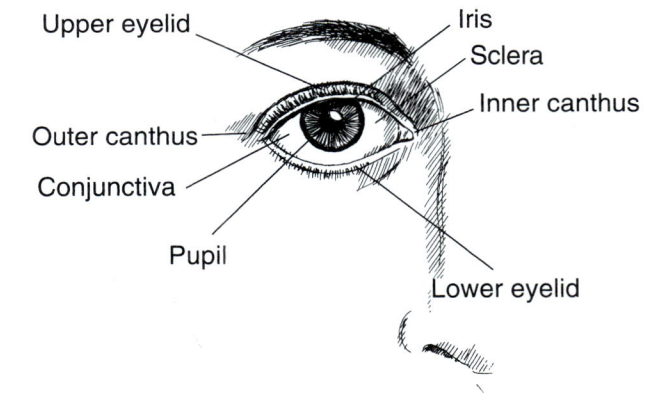

2. Remove inflammatory secretions
3. Prepare the eye for surgery
4. Wash away foreign material or injurious chemicals
5. Provide antibacterial and antifungal effects

FIGURE 9-3 Diagram of the eye.

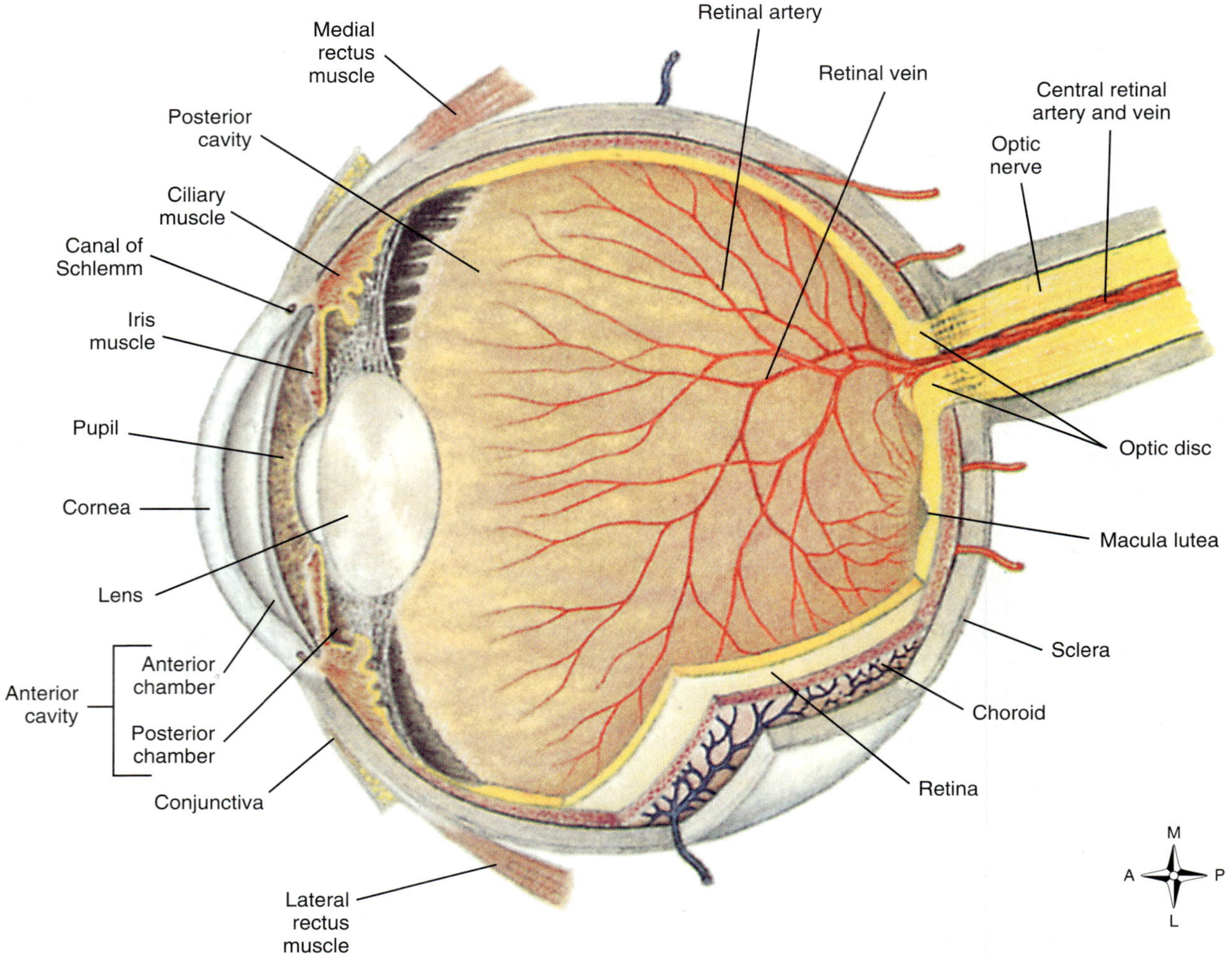

Medial rectus muscle

Posterior cavity

Ciliary muscle

Canal of Schlemm

Iris muscle

Pupil

Cornea

Lens

Anterior cavity
- Anterior chamber
- Posterior chamber

Conjunctiva

Lateral rectus muscle

Retinal artery

Retinal vein

Central retinal artery and vein

Optic nerve

Optic disc

Macula lutea

Sclera

Choroid

Retina

M
A — P
L

PROCEDURE 9-1

EAR INSTILLATION

Objective

Understand and demonstrate the correct procedure for performing an ear instillation and recording the procedure on the patient's chart.

Equipment

Prescribed medication and eardropper
Cotton balls
Disposable, single-use examination gloves

PROCEDURE

1. Check the medication order carefully (that is, the name and amount of medication and which ear requires treatment).

2. **Wash your hands. Use appropriate personal protective equipment (PPE) as dictated by facility.**

3. Assemble supplies.

RATIONALE

Avoid medication errors.

PROCEDURE 9-1

EAR INSTILLATION—cont'd

4. Read the medication label carefully three times and check with the order. Warm the solution.

The label must be checked to avoid the possibility of any mistake.

5. Identify the patient and explain the nature of the procedure and the purpose.

Prevent giving a drug to the wrong patient. Explanations help gain the patient's full cooperation.

6. Place the patient in a sitting or side-lying position.

7. Don disposable, single-use examination gloves.

8. Instruct the patient to tilt the head toward the unaffected side.

9. Stand at the patient's head.

10. Withdraw the medication into the dropper and examine the dropper for any defects.

A safe vehicle must be used to administer the medication.

11. Straighten the external ear canal. For adults, gently pull the top of the earlobe upward and backward. For children, gently pull the bottom of the earlobe downward and backward (Figure 9-4).

The direction of the external ear canal differs in adults and children.

12. Place the tip of the dropper just slightly inside the external meatus (external ear canal) and instill the correct amount of medication. Do not touch the ear canal. Position the dropper so that the drops are instilled along the side of the ear canal.

13. Instruct the patient to keep the head tilted or to remain on the unaffected side for a few minutes.

This position prevents leakage of the medication from the ear and helps the medication flow to the inside of the ear to the infected eardrum.

14. Place a cotton ball over the opening of the ear only if ordered.

A cotton ball is placed over the ear opening only when ordered because it may absorb some of the medication and prevent the desired action on the ear tissue. Also, cotton balls may prevent drainage from escaping when present.

15. Discard unused medication in the dropper and replace the dropper into the bottle, avoiding contamination. When the dropper is contaminated, it must be replaced with a clean dropper.

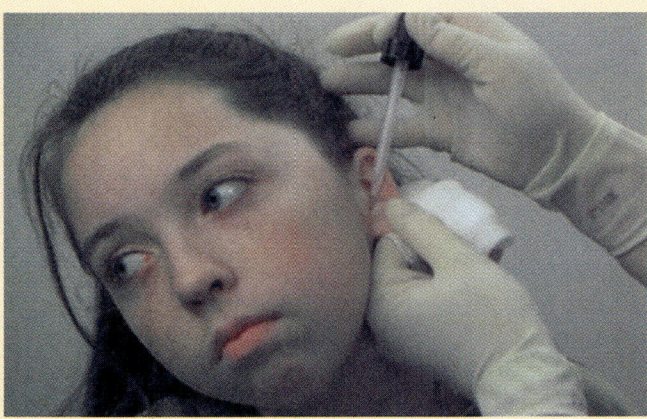

FIGURE 9-4 Instillation of eardrops.

Continued

PROCEDURE 9-1

EAR INSTILLATION—cont'd

16. Remove and discard gloves.

17. Provide for the patient's safety and comfort. Give further instructions as required. Tell the patient to notify the physician if the original complaints persist, if there is any drainage from the ear, how much and the color of any drainage, and/or if there is any change in hearing.

18. Return supplies to designated area.

19. Wash your hands.

20. Record the procedure on the patient's chart.

Charting Example

October 10, 20__, 11 AM
5 gtt Cerumenex instilled to left ear. Cotton ball placed in external ear canal and left for 15 minutes, then left ear irrigated with warm normal saline. Large amount of cerumen returned.
Sarah Dolan, CMA

PROCEDURE 9-2

EAR IRRIGATION

ObjectiveObjective
Understand and demonstrate the correct procedure for performing an ear irrigation and recording the procedure on the patient's chart.

Equipment
Drapes: towel, and a small rubber sheet, if available, or a waterproof pad
Kidney or ear basin for drainage
Syringe—either a metal ear syringe (such as a Pomeroy syringe), an Asepto bulb syringe (Figure 9-5), or a rubber bulb syringe

Warm sterile solution/medication, as ordered by the physician, in a container; solutions commonly used include:
  Normal saline
  Sterile water
  Antiseptic solutions
    Amount: 500 to 1000 ml, as ordered
    Temperature: 100° F (approximately 38° C) (near body temperature)
Sterile cotton balls
Sterile applicators
Disposable, single-use examination gloves

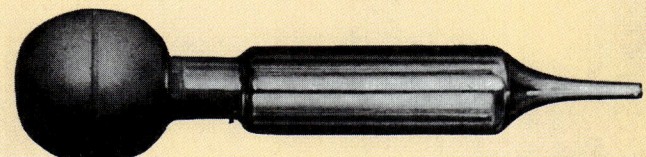

FIGURE 9-5 Asepto bulb syringe.

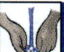

PROCEDURE 9-2

EAR IRRIGATION—cont'd

PROCEDURE

1. Follow the procedure as outlined for an ear instillation in Steps 1 through 5:
   a. Check the medication order.
   b. **Wash your hands. Use appropriate personal protective equipment (PPE) as dictated by facility.**
   c. Assemble the supplies.
   d. Check the solution/medication label three times; warm solution.
   e. Identify the patient and explain the procedure and purpose.

2. Position the patient sitting with the head slightly tilted toward the affected side.

3. Place a small rubber sheet (when available) or a waterproof pad and a towel over the patient's shoulder.

4. Don gloves.

5. Instruct the patient to hold the kidney or ear basin under the ear and firmly against the neck (Figure 9-6).

6. Cleanse the outer ear and external auditory meatus as necessary (to remove any discharge or debris present) with the irrigating solution or normal saline.

RATIONALE

This position allows gravity to help the irrigating solution to flow from the ear to the basin.

Protect the patient's clothing from any drainage.

The basin provides a receptacle to receive the irrigating solution and to prevent it from running down the patient's neck.

Cleansing the outer parts of the ear is necessary to prevent the introduction of foreign materials into the ear canal during the irrigation.

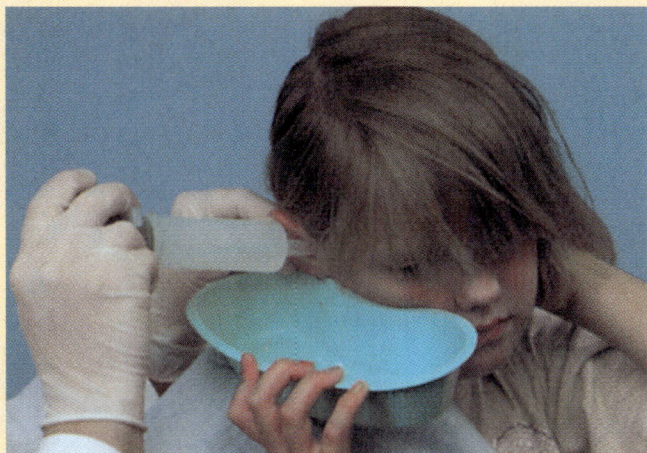

FIGURE 9-6 Ear irrigation. Have patient hold kidney or ear basin under ear and against the neck. Head should be tilted toward the affected side. Pull earlobe up and backward for an adult or down and back for children. Place tip of syringe in ear pointing up and back and gently direct a steady, slow stream of solution against the roof of the ear canal (see procedure on p. 437 of Ear Instillation, Step 11).

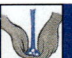

EAR IRRIGATION—cont'd

7. Test the temperature of the solution by putting a few drops on the inner aspect of your wrist and on the patient's wrist. The solution should feel warm.

Warm solutions are more comfortable for the patient. Cold or too hot solutions may cause more discomfort and a feeling of dizziness. Anxiety is reduced when the patient knows the temperature of the solution.

8. Fill the syringe with the irrigating solution; expel any air present.

Air forced into the ear canal produces excessive discomfort for the patient.

9. Straighten the ear canal by gently pulling the earlobe downward and backward for infants and children or upward and backward for adults.

Straightening the ear canal allows the irrigating solution to reach all areas of the canal.

10. Place the tip of the syringe at the opening of the ear. With the tip pointing upward and toward the posterior end of the canal, gently direct a steady slow stream of solution against the roof of the canal. Use only enough force to accomplish the purpose of irrigation (see Figure 9-6).

Direct the solution at the roof of the canal to prevent injury to the tympanic membrane, to prevent pushing material farther into the canal, and to facilitate directing the inflow and outflow of the solution.

11. Do not obstruct the opening of the ear canal with the syringe tip.

The solution must be able to flow freely in and out of the ear canal.

12. Observe the returning solution to see if anything is removed, such as cerumen, a foreign object, or discharge.

13. Observe the patient for any signs of discomfort or dizziness. If these occur, discontinue irrigation and report to the physician. Irritation to the semicircular canals may cause dizziness and nausea. Have a glass of water for the patient.

A drink of water may help to reduce any dizziness.

14. Continue the irrigation until the desired results appear or the prescribed amount of solution has been used.

15. On completion of the treatment, dry the external ear with a cotton ball; dry the neck when required.

Drying promotes patient comfort.

16. Have the patient keep the head tilted toward the affected side or lie on the affected side for a few minutes.

This allows any remaining solution in the ear canal to escape from the ear.

17. Remove the soiled towel and rubber sheet (if used). Give further instructions as indicated. Patient may resume normal level of activity.

Provide for the patient's safety and comfort.

18. Return supplies to designated area. Remove and dispose of gloves.

19. Wash your hands.

20. Record the procedure on the patient's chart.

Charting Example

October 11, 20__, 12 PM
Left ear irrigated with normal saline. Large amount of cerumen returned. Patient stated that she felt much relief on completion of the irrigation.
Jane Evans, CMA

PROCEDURE 9-3

EYEDROP INSTILLATION

Objective

Understand and demonstrate the correct procedure for performing an eyedrop instillation and recording the procedure on the patient's chart.

Equipment

Sterile eyedropper
Sterile medication *or* sterile medication in bottle with sterile eyedropper
Cotton balls or tissue
Disposable, single-use examination gloves

PROCEDURE

RATIONALE

1. Check the medication order carefully (that is, the name and amount of medication and which eye requires medication). Know the abbreviations:
   OD—right eye *(oculus dexter)*
   OS—left eye *(oculus sinister)*
   OU—both eyes or each eye *(oculus uterque)*

   Avoid medication errors.

2. **Wash your hands. Use appropriate personal protective equipment (PPE) as dictated by facility.**

3. Assemble supplies.

4. Read the medication label carefully three times and check with the order.

   The label must be checked to avoid the possibility of any mistake because an error could have serious results.

5. Identify the patient and explain the procedure and the purpose. Warn the patient that the medication may feel cold and to avoid flinching or squeezing the eye when it is instilled.

   The patient must be identified to avoid giving the drug to the wrong patient. Explanations help gain the patient's full cooperation.

6. Have the patient assume a supine or a sitting position with the head tilted slightly backward.

7. Don disposable, single-use examination gloves.

8. Stand at the patient's head.

9. Withdraw medication into the dropper. Examine the dropper carefully for any defects.

   A safe vehicle must be used for administering the medication.

10. Using the index and middle finger over a tissue, draw the lower lid down gently, *or* draw the lower lid down with index finger and the brow up with the middle finger; have the patient look up (Figure 9-7). Do not touch any part of the eye during the procedure except the lower lid, especially in patients who have had eye surgery.

    The tissue prevents your fingers from slipping when instilling the drops.

11. Hold the dropper parallel to the eye about ½ inch away from the inner canthus (the inner angle of the eyelids near the nose), and instill the drop(s) into the center of the conjunctival sac of the lower lid (see Figure 9-7).

    To avoid injuring the eye, never point the dropper toward it; never allow the dropper to touch the eyeball or the eyelids. Be extremely careful to support the head well if the patient is restless or jerking the head.

Continued

PROCEDURE 9-3

EYEDROP INSTILLATION—cont'd

12. Instruct the patient to close the eyelids and move the eye but not to squeeze the eyelids.

This movement helps distribute the medication over the eyeball; squeezing would cause some of the medication to be forced out.

13. Wipe off the excess medication that overflows onto the cheek or eyelids with cotton balls or tissue.

14. Discard the unused solution and replace the dropper into the bottle without touching the sides or outside of the bottle with the dropper.

Avoid contaminating the dropper. When the dropper is contaminated, a new bottle of eyedrops must be ordered.

15. Provide for the patient's safety and comfort. At times an eye pad may be applied as a dressing over the eye for protection (Figure 9-8). Give further instructions as required. Tell the patient how long to leave the eye pad in place (this will vary with the physician's decision) and to notify the physician if original complaints persist or return.

16. Return supplies to designated area.

17. Remove and dispose of gloves.

18. Wash your hands.

19. Record the procedure on the patient's chart.

Charting Example

October 9, 20__, 10:30 AM
Neosporin Ophthalmic Solution 2 gtt given in OD.
Nancy Brown, CMA

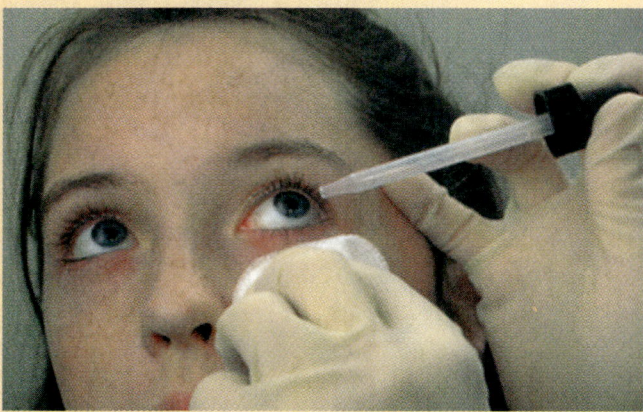

FIGURE 9-7 Instilling eyedrops. Hold eyedropper parallel to eye to avoid injury to patient's eye.

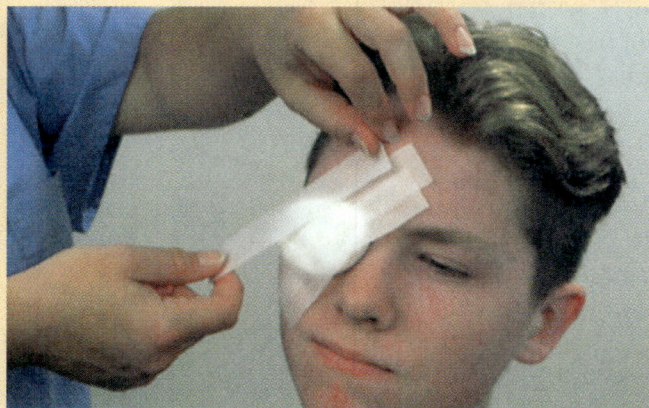

FIGURE 9-8 Application of eye pad.

PROCEDURE 9-4

EYE OINTMENT INSTILLATION

Objective
Understand and demonstrate the correct procedure for instilling eye ointment and recording the procedure on the patient's chart.

Equipment
Sterile eye ointment in tube
Cotton balls or tissue
Disposable, single-use examination gloves

PROCEDURE

RATIONALE

Same as for instilling eyedrops *except omit Step 9 and follow Step 11 as stated here:*

11. Gently squeeze a thin strip of ointment from the tube along the lower lid without touching the lid.

NOTE: When instilling eyedrops and ointment at the same time *instill the eyedrops first,* ointment last.

If the patient's eyedropper or tube touches the eyelid and is contaminated, do not use it again until it is resterilized.

Discard the contaminated tube unless it is being used by only one patient.

PROCEDURE 9-5

EYE IRRIGATION

Objective
Understand and demonstrate the correct procedure for performing an eye irrigation and recording the procedure on the patient's chart.

Equipment
Towel
Sterile eyedropper for small amounts of solution; rubber bulb or Asepto syringe for larger amounts of solution; sterile eye cup for home use

Small basin for solution
Sterile cotton balls
Kidney basin to catch the solution
Sterile solution as ordered by the physician, usually boric acid or normal saline, 30 to 240 ml (1 to 8 ounces) at 98.6° F (37° C) (that is, near body temperature)
Disposable, single-use examination gloves

PROCEDURE

RATIONALE

1. Check the medication order carefully (that is, the name and amount of solution to be used and which eye is to be treated). Know the abbreviations:
OD—right eye
OS—left eye
OU—both eyes

2. Wash your hands. Use appropriate personal protective equipment (PPE) as dictated by facility.

3. Assemble supplies.

4. Check the label of the solution three times.   *Prevent drug errors (see Chapter 7).*

PROCEDURE 9-5

EYE IRRIGATION—cont'd

5. Identify the patient and explain the procedure and the purpose of the irrigation. Instruct the patient not to squeeze the eyes during the treatment.

Gain the patient's cooperation by providing an explanation and adequate instructions.

6. Have the patient assume a lying or sitting position with the head tilted backward and toward the side being treated.

The head is tilted to the side so that the solution does not run toward the inner canthus of the eye or over to the unaffected eye, which could then result in cross-infection (when the eye treated is infected).

7. Place or have the patient hold the kidney basin in position to receive the solution from the eye. Place a towel under the basin (Figure 9-9).

Avoid getting the solution on the patient or on the examining table when the patient is lying down.

8. Don disposable, single-use examination gloves.

Gloves protect your hands from exposure to pathogens if the patient's eye is infected.

9. Stand in front of or at the side of the patient.

10. Cleanse the eyelid with a cotton ball moistened with the irrigating solution. Start at the inner canthus and wipe toward the outer canthus.

All materials (crusts, discharge, and so on) on the lids or lashes must be washed away before exposing the conjunctiva.

11. Fill the irrigating dropper or syringe with the solution. Warm solutions are most comfortable to the patient (that is, the solution temperature should be close to normal body temperature).

12. Pull the lower lid down gently and the brow up. Instruct the patient to look up, but not to squeeze the eyelids (see Figure 9-9). Do not apply pressure over the eye. If the patient has had intraocular surgery, do not ask the patient to look up because this may cause injury.

Supporting the eyelids minimizes blinking and exposes the upper and lower conjunctival membranes for irrigation. Pressure on the internal eye structures could cause injury.

13. Holding the dropper or syringe parallel to the eye, squeeze the solution into the eye, allowing it to flow away from the nose. Hold the dropper or syringe ½ inch from the eye and allow the solution to flow in a steady stream but at low pressure (see Figure 9-9).

The solution is directed away from the nose so that it does not enter the nasolacrimal duct or spill over into the unaffected eye, which could result in transmission of an infection, if it is present. Too much pressure may be injurious to the eye tissues.

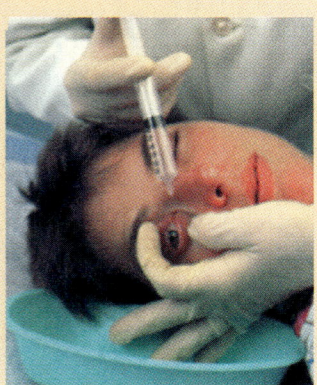

FIGURE 9-9 Eye irrigation. Hold dropper or syringe parallel to eye and squeeze solution into eye at inner canthus, allowing it to flow away from the nose.

PROCEDURE 9·5

EYE IRRIGATION—cont'd

14. Do not allow the dropper or syringe to touch the eye or eyelids.

Prevent injury to the eye. Dropper or syringe becomes contaminated if it touches the eye.

15. Continue the procedure until the eye is free of secretions, or the desired results occur, or the prescribed amount of solution has been used.

16. Gently dry the eye and cheek with sterile cotton balls; discard the cotton balls in designated container.

Remove excess solution. Provide for the patient's comfort.

17. Provide for the patient's safety and comfort; provide further instructions as indicated; allow the patient to rest for a few minutes.

18. Observe the drainage in the basin, then discard. Discard soiled disposable items; return reusable items to designated area for used supplies.

19. Remove and dispose of gloves.

20. Wash your hands.

21. Record the procedure, the type and amount of solution used, and the results on the patient's chart.

Charting Example

October 11, 20__, 1 PM
OD irrigated with 100 ml 5% boric acid.
Redness in OD has markedly decreased.
Patient stated that the treatment felt soothing.
Patient instructed to continue treatments at home for 1 week, as ordered by Dr. McArthur, and then to return for examination.
Shannon Lee, CMA

CONCLUSION

When you have practiced the procedures outlined in this chapter and feel competent with your knowledge and skills, arrange with your instructor to take the performance test. You will be expected to prepare for and perform ear and eye instillations and irrigations.

When treating the eye, keep in mind that it is a delicate sense organ that must be treated gently. Solutions and medications instilled into the eye should be applied to the lower conjunctiva and *not* on the corneal surface.

When irrigating the ear, you must gently direct a steady, slow stream of solution against the roof of the canal to prevent injury to the tympanic membrane, to prevent pushing material further into the canal, and to permit the solution to flow in and out of the ear freely.

REVIEW OF VOCABULARY

Using the information presented in this chapter and other reference sources of your own choice, define the following terms.

Terms pertaining to the ear

1. *Auricle*
2. *Cerumen*
3. *External acoustic meatus*
4. *Semicircular canals*
5. *Pinna*
6. *Tinnitus*
7. *Otopyorrhea*
8. *Otitis media*
9. *Audiometer*
10. *Ménière's syndrome*
11. *Tympanic membrane (TM)*
12. *Otoscope*
13. *Otology*
14. *Myringoplasty*

Terms pertaining to the eye

1. *Canthus*
2. *Cataract*
3. *Pupil*
4. *Conjunctivitis*
5. *Mydriatic*
6. *Miotic*
7. *Presbyopia*
8. *Glaucoma*
9. *Hyperopia*
10. *Errors of refraction*
11. *Ophthalmoscope*
12. *Lacrimal duct*
13. *Intraocular*
14. *Cornea*

The following are reports from charts in the physician's office. After reading these, you should be able to discuss the contents with your instructor. Be prepared to define and explain any medical terms that are used. A medical dictionary, other reference books, and information given in preceding chapters of this book may be used as references for obtaining definitions or explanations of the contents of these reports.

Children commonly insert small objects into their ears and up their noses. These foreign bodies may be removed in the physician's office, an ambulatory surgical center, or outpatient department of the hospital if general anesthesia is required. The following is an example of an operative note dictated at the conclusion of a procedure performed on a young child. Read it and be prepared to discuss the italicized terminology. (See the report on p. 447.)

Patient No. 1

DATE: 12/13/00

PROBLEM: Cerumen impaction

S: 45-year-old white woman is concerned that she has occluded eardrums again and has found that this problem has been increasing. She was previously advised not to use Q-tips. She has been using some type of vegetable oil for 2 nights in her ears to soften the wax because Cerumenex is irritating to her ear canals. She has not done any other preventive care.

O: BP 150/90, heart rate 72, Wt 162. HEENT: both tympanic membranes are totally occluded. Bilateral lavage done, and tympanic membranes then normal with good light reflex. Large amounts of cerumen removed.

A: Bilateral cerumen impaction.

P: Lavage and told to use oil or Debrox drops once per week to keep from developing an impaction. Recommended that she use a hair dryer for drying her ears and avoid using Q-tips.

Patient No. 2

DATE: 6/7/00

PROBLEM: Cerumen impaction

S: 58 y/o male has a continual problem with clogged R ear. He was seen on 4/00 for this problem and had a lavage at that time; was advised to use Debrox at home once per week thereafter and could lavage with bulb syringe if needed. Patient thinks that he has decreased hearing today.

O: HEENT: Left tympanic membrane negative; right tympanic membrane occluded with pale, yellow/whitish wax. After lavage, somewhat more clear, but now there is a small perforation in the inferior portion of the right tympanic membrane. No obvious signs of infection.

A: 1. Right cerumen impaction.
    2. Small perforation of right tympanic membrane.

P: Lavage as above and referred patient to Dr. John Grant. Started patient on Cortisporin eardrops, 2 drops 3×/d until he sees Dr. Grant.

PROBLEM: Hypertension

S: Patient has been on Vasotec 5 mg since 5/2/00. He had a BP of 190/108 about 1 month ago. It is better today. Denies chest pain, SOB, or dizziness.

O: BP 150/90. Chest clear. Heart rate: 76 and regular. Extremities: no edema.

A: Hypertension, inadequate control.

P: Increase Vasotec 5 mg to 2 qd., finish out this Rx and then he may change to 10 mg tabs, 1 qd. To return for BP check in 3 weeks.

Operative report

PATIENT: John Brown

PREOPERATIVE DIAGNOSIS: Foreign body *bilaterally* of the ear canal and right *serous otitis media*.

POSTOPERATIVE DIAGNOSIS: Same.

OPERATION: Removal of *foreign body* both ears, *cerumen*, and right *myringotomy*.

FINDINGS: The *external ear* was examined for signs of inflammation or trauma. Examination of the *external audi-*tory meatus revealed a piece of dry popcorn in the right ear; this was removed and myringotomy performed; glue-like fluid was aspirated. A piece of Styrofoam was removed from the left ear canal. The *left tympanic membrane* was normal.

Jack Klein, MD

CRITICAL THINKING SKILLS REVIEW

1. Explain the difference between an instillation and an irrigation.
2. State the reason for pulling an adult's earlobe upward and backward when giving an ear instillation or irrigation.
3. List three reasons why an ear irrigation is done with a steady, slow stream of solution and not a fast, high-pressure flow.
4. Explain how cerumen can be softened for later removal.
5. Explain to a mother how she should instill eardrops into her 5-year-old son's left ear.
6. Describe the position you would have a patient assume for an ear irrigation. Explain the reason for your answer.
7. The physician has asked you to prepare a patient for an eye irrigation. List the supplies you would need and explain how you would prepare and position the patient for this procedure.
8. List four purposes for which an eye irrigation may be performed.
9. Explain how you would put eye ointment into a patient's eye.
10. When eyedrops and eye ointment are both ordered for the patient at the same time, which agent would you instill into the eye first?
11. Name the region of the eye into which eyedrops should be instilled.

PERFORMANCE TEST

In a skills laboratory, the medical assistant student, with a partner, will assemble supplies and demonstrate the correct procedure for the following without reference to source materials. Time limits for the performance of each procedure are to be assigned by the instructor (see also p. 104).

1. Ear instillation
2. Ear irrigation
3. Eye instillation
4. Eye irrigation

The student is expected to perform these skills and record the procedures on the patient's chart with 100% accuracy.

The successful completion of each procedure will demonstrate competency levels as required by the AAMA, AMT, and future employers.

INTERNET RESOURCES

OnHealth
www.onhealth.com

drkoop.com
www.drkoop.com

Healthfinder
www.healthfinder.gov

MedScape
www.medscape.com

CBS HealthWatch
www.cbshealthwatch.medscape.com

United States National Library of Medicine (information on general health)
www.nlm.nih.gov/medlineplus

National Eye Institute
www.eyeinstitute.net

University of Ottawa (Eye Institute)
http://iyop-aipa.ic.gc.ca

Eye Institute of the Medical Center of Wisconsin
http://eyeinstitute.ncw.edu

National Ear Institute
www.hearinginstitute.org

Better Hearing Institute
Cynthia L. Compton MSC. CCCA
Director of Gallaudet University Assistive Devices Center
www.betterhearing.org

Columbia University's Health Education Site
www.goaskalice.columbia.edu/index.html

National Institutes of Heatlh
www.nih.gov

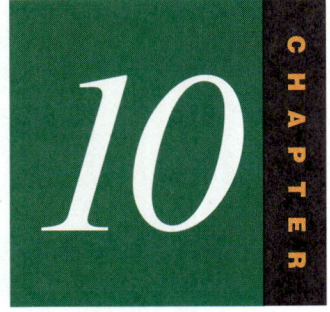
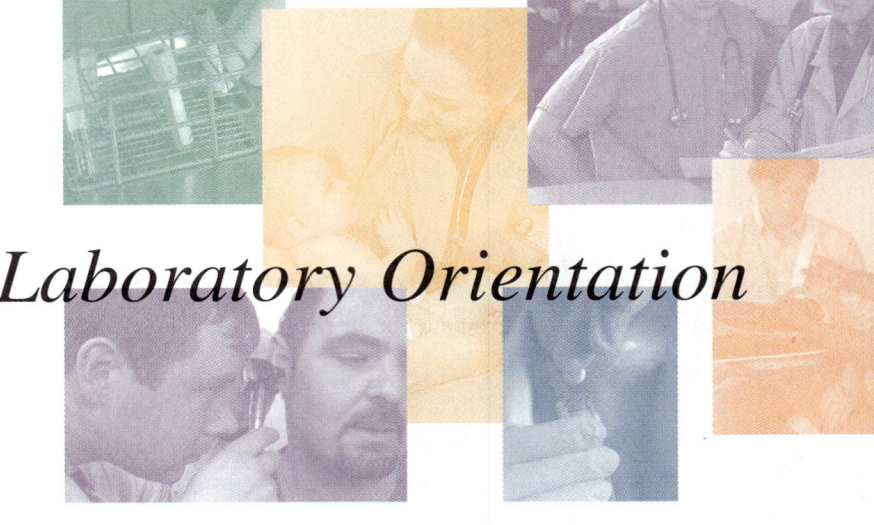

10 CHAPTER

Laboratory Orientation

■ Cognitive Objectives

On completion of Chapter 10, the medical assistant student should be able to:

1. Define, pronounce, and spell the vocabulary terms given.
2. State the importance of the information gathered from clinical laboratory tests.
3. List and discuss three formats that may be used to organize the recordings of various diagnostic procedures.
4. State the reason why most laboratory tests are performed in a commercial clinical laboratory rather than in a physician's office or in a health care agency.
5. List six types of workers in a clinical laboratory, indicating the basic responsibilities of each.
6. List six specialized departments common to all clinical laboratories and describe the function of each department.
7. List five additional special departments that may be part of some clinical laboratories and describe the function of each department.
8. Discuss the medical assistant's responsibilities when dealing with a clinical laboratory.
9. Discuss the Clinical Laboratory Improvement Amendments (CLIA) of 1988, stating the primary purpose of CLIA.
10. State how CLIA classifies all laboratory tests.
11. List the three levels of laboratory tests as identified by CLIA.
12. Explain what is meant by proficiency testing (PT) under CLIA regulations.
13. State the purpose of a laboratory test directory.
14. List the information that is customarily provided in a laboratory test directory.
15. List the information given on a laboratory report.
16. Discuss the purpose of a laboratory report form.
17. List seven items that are to be included on a laboratory requisition that accompanies a specimen to the laboratory.
18. List three reasons for the performance of diagnostic studies.
19. Discuss the organization of diagnostic reports that are to be placed in the patient's chart.
20. Discuss the concept and the purpose of quality control in the laboratory.
21. List 20 safety rules that should be followed when using laboratory equipment and chemicals and when around specimens.

■ Terminal Performance Objectives

On completion of Chapter 10, the medical assistant student should be able to:

1. Demonstrate safe practices when working with laboratory equipment and specimens.
2. Demonstrate proficiency in using a microscope.
3. Identify by name the parts of a microscope.
4. Demonstrate proficiency in using a clinical centrifuge.
5. Provide instructions and patient education that is within the professional scope of a medical assistant's training and responsibilities as assigned.

The student is to perform these objectives with 100% accuracy 95% of the time.

The consistent use of Universal/Standard Precautions is required by all health care professionals in all health care settings as a method of infection control. It is assumed that these precautions are used in all of the following procedures. Review Chapter 1 if you have any questions on methods to use because the methods or techniques are not repeated in detail in each procedure presented in this chapter.

Be sure to consult the latest guidelines issued by the Centers for Disease Control and Prevention and consult with infection control practitioners when necessary to identify specific precautions that pertain to your particular work situation.

Medical practice is based on information obtained from various sources. Chapter 4 discussed information obtained from a patient history and from a general or specific physical examination. Another important source of information to help diagnose and treat disease processes is gathered from clinical laboratory tests. It is important to remember that the physician evaluates all data gathered before making a diagnosis or initiating treatment. Often, information from a combination of sources is required because one source may not be sufficient (see Summary of Studies Used for Diagnosing Conditions Affecting Body Organs and Systems in the *Student Mastery Manual*). Repeat tests may be necessary to confirm initial findings and establish the progress of a disease process or its elimination.

Scientific and technologic discoveries have aided medicine tremendously by making accessible abundant data on numerous types of body specimens with a speed and accuracy that previously were not available. Laboratory medicine can determine changes in the chemical or physical characteristics of body fluids, excretions, and tissues and in turn reflect changes in the anatomy and physiology of various organs. Changes noted may indicate a disease process at the site from which the specimen was obtained (for example, a wound culture may identify the presence of bacteria and an infectious process). At other times, the changes in the characteristics of the specimen may indicate a disease process in another part of the body (for example, the presence of excessive sugar in the urine may indicate diabetes mellitus, a disorder in carbohydrate metabolism, and not a disorder of the urinary system; elevated levels of certain blood enzymes may indicate a heart attack or a liver disease).

Thus with laboratory techniques, specific data concerning the status of certain body functions and conditions may be determined. Normal values for the physical and chemical characteristics of body substances have been predetermined; each technique used has its own normal value ratio. Deviations from these set norms aid in the diagnosis and treatment of abnormal disturbances in body function and structure.

THE TYPICAL LABORATORY

Initially, many clinical laboratory procedures were performed in the physician's office. Over the years, as numerous tests have been developed that are more time consuming and require more specialized equipment, specially trained personnel have become necessary. Although many physicians still perform basic routine tests in their offices, they usually find it more economical, efficient, and accurate to have most tests performed by the trained personnel in a hospital or a private or public health department laboratory.

A clinical laboratory employs various types of workers. These may include a **physician** who is certified as a **pathologist** acting as the director of the laboratory; **clinical laboratory scientists** (CLSs) (formerly called medical technologists), who are trained at a college for 4 years (who may also have a 1-year internship) and are able to perform specialized tests; and **medical technicians,** trained for 2 years at a junior or community college, who assist and perform tests under the supervision of the CLSs. In addition, a **cytotechnologist,** trained for 2 years at a college (plus a 1- to 2-year program in cytotechnology), is a highly specialized worker who examines cells and tissues microscopically for the presence of cancer. A **histological technician,** trained for 1 or 2 years in a technical training program, is also a specialized worker who is involved with the preparation of various types of tissues for microscopic examination performed by the pathologist. The **clinical laboratory assistant,** usually trained at a technical level or below that of a 2-year college program, performs basic and routine tests under the direct supervision of the CLS or the director of the laboratory. Often, CLSs become specialized in one or two fields in the clinical laboratory and devote all their working time to the area of their expertise.

All clinical laboratories have certain specialized departments in common. They are divided into areas on the basis of function and types of tests performed. These areas usually include hematology, urinalysis, serology, blood banking, medical microbiology, and clinical chemistry. Parasitology and examination of feces may be special departments, or they may be included in one of the other departments. Some laboratories may also have special areas for histology, mycology, immunochemistry, and cytology.

Hematology deals with the study of blood. Examination for the total cell number, the types and number of different cells, cell morphology (shape and size), and the important aspects of the functions of blood, in addition to coagulation studies, are all part of hematology (see also Tables 13-2 and 13-3).

Urinalysis deals with the examination of the physical, chemical, and microscopic properties of urine (see also Tables 12-1, 12-2, and 12-4 to 12-10).

Serology involves laboratory tests that examine blood serum. Reactions involving antibodies and antigens are observed and used to determine various types of infections, such as tests for infectious mononucleosis (Monospot). The tests for pregnancy, hepatitis B surface antigen, and syphilis are also serology tests because they involve immunologic reactions (see also Table 13-5).

Blood banking deals with the processing of blood and blood products that will be used for transfusions. It is also known as immunohematology because antigen-antibody reactions are involved in the typing of blood (see also Tables 13-5 and 13-6).

Medical microbiology deals with isolation and culture, microscopic identification, and biochemical tests to detect microorganisms that cause disease. Depending on the classification of the microorganisms under investigation, the field of medical microbiology is generally divided into areas of specialization that include the following (see also Tables 12-1, 12-7, 12-9, and 13-3):

bacteriology (bak-te″-re-ol′o-je)—The study of bacteria
virology (vi-rol′ -o-je)—The study of viruses
mycology (mi-kol′ o-je)—The study of fungi
rickettsiology (ri-ket″si-ol′o-je)—The study of rickettsiae
protozoology (pro″to-zo-ol′o-je)—The study of protozoa, the simplest forms of animals
phycology (fi-kol′je)—The study of algae
parasitology (par′ah-si-tol′o-je)—The study of parasites. These may be protozoans or even larger organisms that have microscopic stages in their development.

Parasitology may be an area apart from microbiology. Stool and blood specimens are examined for the presence of eggs or parts of a variety of roundworms, tapeworms, and flukes.

Clinical chemistry examines body fluids, such as blood, urine, and cerebrospinal fluid, for any change in their chemical content. Glucose and electrolyte levels are determined, as well as the presence of uric acid or urea in the urine or blood (see also Tables 12-1, 12-2, 12-4, and 13-4).

Histology involves the study of specimens of tissue from any source in the body. Form and structural changes are observed microscopically.

Immunochemistry is the study of the chemistry involved with immunity.

Cytology involves the microscopic study of cells to detect any abnormal or malignant changes. Examples include the Pap test and chromosome studies.

Cost Containment

Cost containment is a factor that must be considered when ordering or performing laboratory tests. Generally speaking, it is least expensive for the patient if simple routine laboratory tests are performed in the physician's office or health care agency, for two rea-

sons. *First,* the physician or you can collect and perform simple laboratory tests with relative ease on samples collected when the patient is in the office. *Second,* the physician or health care agency can avoid the costs of extensive laboratory equipment and the high salary of laboratory technicians or technologists. The next least expensive situation for patients is when you obtain the sample in your facility and forward it to a commercial laboratory or to refer patients directly to a commercial laboratory to have the test performed. The larger the laboratory or organization, the less expensive the procedure is for the patient because large laboratories perform tests on a large volume of samples using more sophisticated equipment. The specialized instruments available in large laboratories can perform multiple tests at the same time, thereby reducing the cost to each patient. The most expensive situation for patients is for the physician to refer them to a hospital laboratory to have the required test performed because the general high cost of operating a hospital must be shared by all departments. For example, when a laboratory test is performed in the physician's office or in a health care agency, it may cost the patient $10. When the same test is performed at a commercial clinical laboratory, it may cost the patient $15; and when the test is performed at a hospital laboratory, it may cost $20. Thus when laboratory tests other than the very simple procedures that the physician can easily perform or have performed in his or her facility are ordered, it is suggested that patients be referred to a commercial laboratory that is qualified and with which the physician has established a business relationship. This is the most cost-efficient procedure to follow. It is also important that the patient be referred to a laboratory that accepts payment under his or her insurance plan.

CLINICAL LABORATORY IMPROVEMENT AMENDMENTS

Passed by Congress in 1988, the Clinical Laboratory Improvement Amendments (CLIA) focused specifically on standards set for laboratory test performance. CLIA set standards designed to improve the quality of all laboratory testing (except research) in every laboratory and testing site in the United States, including facilities that perform only basic tests and those that perform the most complex tests. CLIA regulations, developed by the Department of Health and Human Services, apply to *all* laboratory testing that is used when assessing the health of a patient, when making a diagnosis, or when aiding the prevention or treatment of disease. Regulations have been established for the following:

- Laboratory standards
- Application and user fees
- Enforcement procedures
- Approval of programs for accreditation

Classification and Requirements for Laboratory Tests

CLIA classifies all laboratory tests according to the nature and complexity of the test. The three levels of tests established include low-complexity or waived tests, moderate-complexity tests, and high-complexity tests. In total, CLIA covers approximately 165,000 laboratory entities.

Low-complexity or waived tests. Low-complexity or waived tests are simple laboratory tests, including those that can be performed by patients at home. These tests are waived from specific CLIA requirements. All laboratories and testing sites that perform only these tests must apply for a certificate of waiver. They are still expected to follow proper laboratory procedures and the manufacturer's instructions for each test performed. These sites will not be inspected routinely but could be inspected on a random basis to determine if they are performing only the waived tests as stated. See the accompanying box for a list of some of the waived tests. Originally, there were only six tests that were waived. These were (1) hematocrit; (2) hemoglobin; (3) whole blood glucose;

Samples of CLIA Waived Tests*

Dipstick or tablet urinalysis (nonautomated)

Bayer Clinitek 50 Urine (automated)

Chemstrip Mini UA qualitative dipstick (automated)

Fecal occult blood

Ovulation test—visual color comparison tests for human luteinizing hormone

Urine pregnancy test—visual color comparison tests

Erythrocyte sedimentation rate (nonautomated)

Hemoglobin–copper sulfate (nonautomated)

Blood glucose, by glucose-monitoring devices cleared by FDA specifically for home use

HemoCue B-Glucose or Cholestech LDX System for glucose

LXN Duet Glucose Control Monitoring System (OR) 82985QW

LXN Fructosamine Test System

Bayer DCA 2000-glycosylate hemoglobin (HgbA1C)

Spun microhematocrit

Hemoglobin by single analyte instruments with self-contained or component features to perform specimen/reagent interaction, providing direct measurement and readout

Wampole STAT-CRIT Hct

Mico Diagnostics Spuncrit Model DRC-40 Infrared Analyzer for hematocrit

Blood cholesterol test, by cholesterol-monitoring device approved by FDA for home use

AccuChek InstantPlus Cholesterol (Boehringer Mannheim)

Cholestech LDX System for: Total cholesterol

Cholesterol, Total by Advanced Care (Johnson & Johnson)

Cholestech LDX System for: HDL cholesterol

Cholestech LDX System for: Triglycerides

Cholestech LDX System for: Lipid panel

ENA C.T. Total Cholesterol Test

Quidel QuickVue In-Line One-Step Strep A test (25 test kit ONLY— controls to be tested with each change in testing personnel)

Binox NOW Strep A Test *or* SmithKline Icon Fx Strep A Test

Wyntek Diagnostics OSOM Strep A test *or* Abbott Signify Strep A Test

BioStar Acceva Strep A Test (direct specimen only)

Applied Biotech SureStep Strep A (II) (direct from throat swab)

Meridian Diagnostics ImmunoCard STAT Strep A (direct from throat swab)

Jant Pharmacal AccuStrip Strep A (II) (direct from throat swab)

Quidel QuickVue One-Step *H. Pylori* Test for Whole Blood (30 test kit ONLY—controls to be tested with each change in testing personnel)

SmithKline Diagnostic FlexSure HP test for IgG—*H. pylori*

FlexPak HP Test for whole blood (IgG Ab for *H. pylori*)

GI Supply HP-FAST (presumptive ID of *H. pylori* in gastric biopsy tissue) 86318QW

Serim PyloriTek kit

Delta West CLOtest

SmithKline Gastroccult test

ChemTrak AccuMeter *H. pylori* Test (for whole blood)

ITC Protime Microcoagulation System (contact your Medicare carrier for payment instructions)

CoaguChek PST (Prothrombin Time) Boehringer Mannheim Corp (BMC) (contact your Medicare carrier for payment instructions) NOTE: Does not apply to any other BMC device for prothrombin time.

Nitrazine (pH) paper for body fluids pH

Microalbumin—Boehringer Mannheim Chemstrip Micral

Litmus Concepts FemExam TestCard (from vaginal swab)

Wyntek Diagnostics OSOM Mono Test (whole blood)

Wampole Mono-Plus WB

Seradyn Color Q Mono (whole blood)

BioStar Acceava Mono Test (whole blood)

Genzyme Contrast Mono (whole blood)

STC Diagnostics Q.E.D.A150—Saliva Alcohol Test

STC Diagnostics Q.E.D.A350—Saliva Alcohol Test

Provider-Performed Microscopy Procedures

Wet mounts, including preparation of vaginal, cervical, or skin specimens

All potassium hydroxide (KOH) preparations

Pinworm examination

Fern test

Postcoital direct, qualitative examination of vaginal or cervical mucus

Urinalysis; microscopic only

Urinalysis with microscopy (NOTE: May be used when only reading dipstick/tablet reagents nonautomative)

Urinalysis with microscopy (NOTE: May only be used when the laboratory is using an automated dipstick urinalysis instrument approved as waived)

Nasal smear for eosinophils

Fecal leukocyte examination

Semen analysis: presence and/or motility of sperm—excluding Huhner test

Urinalysis; two or three glass test (fractional urinalysis)

*California law (Business and Professions Code, Section 1265 [a][2]) recognizes only PHYSICIAN-Performed Microscopic Procedures to be eligible for registration rather than state licensure. A laboratory that uses personnel other than a physician to perform these procedures MUST be state licensed.

(4) dipstick urinalysis; (5) fecal occult blood; and (6) pregnancy test using a color change indicator. Currently there are more than 200 tests waived. This list should be checked periodically because additional tests may be added. The list is updated on the first Friday of each month. The FDA is responsible for advising and making recommendations to Health Care Financing Authority (HCFA), which then categorizes the tests.

For the list of waived tests, visit the following Web sites:

1. www.cdc.gov:80/phppo/dls/waived.htm (Centers for Disease Control and Prevention)
2. www.HCFA.gov/medicaid/CLIA/ (HCFA's home page)

Moderate-complexity tests and high-complexity tests.   All tests not listed as waived are divided into either one of two classifications, moderate complexity or high complexity (see the accompanying boxes), based on the nature of the testing procedure. Both of these classifications have specific requirements as set by CLIA regulations for personnel, quality control, proficiency testing, quality assurance, patient test management, and inspections. Most testing done in physi-

Samples of CLIA Moderate-Complexity Tests
- Microscopic analysis of urinary sediment
- Direct-antigen strep A tests
- Cervical and urethral Gram stains
- Hematology tests conducted on fully automated equipment that do not require operator intervention during the analytical process
- Chemistry tests conducted on fully automated equipment that do not require operator intervention during the analytic process
- Throat cultures
- Urine culture

CLIA High-Complexity Tests
Procedures related to the following:

- Cytogenics (branch of genetics dealing with the cellular constituents concerned with heredity, especially the origin, structures, and function of chromosomes)
- Histopathology (study of disease involving the tissue cells)
- Histocompatibility (study of the compatibility of the antigens of donor and recipient of transplanted tissue)
- Cytology (study of cells; types of cytology are aspiration biopsy cytology and exfoliative cytology, both of which involve the microscopic examination of cells)

These tests are usually not performed in medical offices or clinics but rather in large laboratories already subject to federal regulations.

cian office laboratories (POLs) is classified as moderate complexity unless it is waived. The *major* differences in requirements for moderate- and high-complexity testing concern personnel standards and quality control.

Personnel standards.   Regulations are provided for the various levels of personnel needed for maintaining a testing site. These could include a laboratory director, clinical and technical consultants, and testing personnel. The testing personnel for moderate-complexity testing must have, at minimum, a high school diploma and documentation of satisfactory completion of training appropriate to the testing performed in the testing facility. This training may have been obtained either formally or informally on the job. Personnel standards for high-complexity testing are more rigorous, and in general, the personnel need more education and experience than those performing moderate-complexity testing. Different states may have additional requirements.

Quality control.   Testing sites conducting tests that are not waived must perform routine quality control procedures and document the results. These procedures monitor and evaluate the quality and the accuracy of the tests performed. **Quality control procedures** include following the manufacturer's instructions, performing and documenting calibration procedures at least once every 6 months, running two levels of controls daily, performing applicable specialty and subspecialty quality control procedures, performing and documenting remedial action taken when errors are identified, preparing a procedural manual, and documenting all quality control procedures. For tests cleared by the Food and Drug Administration (FDA) as meeting CLIA quality control requirements, quality control requirements can be met by following the manufacturer's test instructions.

Proficiency testing.   Proficiency testing (PT) is an evaluation of the quality of a laboratory's performance by an approved proficiency test program. The PT program sends control samples to the laboratories to be tested in the same manner that patient's specimens are tested. The test results are returned to the testing program, and the laboratory's results are compared with the testing program's results for accuracy. These testing events occur three times a year, with five samples for each test performed. PT results are sent to the Health Care Financing Administration (HCFA), where they are reviewed for compliance with CLIA.

Quality assurance.   All testing sites must establish and follow written policies, procedures, and quality control procedures for monitoring and evaluating the quality of the testing process of each method to ensure accuracy and reliability of patient test results and reports.

Patient test management.   A system must be in place in all testing sites to ensure proper handling and testing of all specimens and to ensure that proper records and reports are maintained and provided.

All physician office laboratories (POLs) must obtain either a certificate of waiver, or, if the laboratory performs nonwaived tests, a registration certificate. Information and applications can be obtained from a regional office of the HCFA. In addition, in states with federally approved licensure programs, a laboratory may obtain a state license in lieu of a certificate or certificate of accreditation. Laboratories with state licenses only have to comply with the state rules, not the federal CLIA regulations.

LIASION AND RESPONSIBILITIES OF THE MEDICAL ASSISTANT WITH LABORATORIES

Because the information obtained from laboratory tests is an important source of data for the physician when treating a patient, as a medical assistant, you must have an understanding of and establish good communication with this branch of clinical medicine.

You have certain responsibilities when dealing with a laboratory, which include having a basic knowledge of the various tests available, properly collecting and handling specimens to be forwarded to a laboratory, instructing patients when preparing for certain tests (see Chapters 6 and 11), and handling completed reports as they return to the office. To help prevent errors, good communication among all parties involved is vital. When you are not sure of the procedure for collecting or handling a specimen or not sure of instructions that should be given to a patient, never hesitate to contact the laboratory for this information. By doing so, you avoid errors and inconvenience to the patient, who would have to return to give another specimen if the initial procedure had been performed incorrectly.

In addition, many laboratories provide manuals called **laboratory test directories.** These directories include the names of the tests that they perform; the normal values or normal ranges for each test; patient preparation; supplies needed; the amount and type of specimen required; the collection method to use; and instructions for the proper handling, storage, and transporting of the specimen for each test. A sample laboratory requisition form and billing codes may also be included.

Correctly labeling the specimen and completing the laboratory requisition are other important responsibilities. Always label the container in which the specimen has been collected with the date, the patient's name, and the source of the specimen. **On the laboratory requisition that accompanies the specimen, include the following:**

- The patient's full name, age, sex, and address
- The physician's full name (also address when sending specimens to outside laboratories)
- Date the specimen was collected, date the specimen was sent to the laboratory if this differs from the date of collection, and time the specimen was collected
- Source of the specimen

- Test(s) required*
- Possible diagnosis when feasible (this alerts the laboratory for specifics for which to watch and also alerts them of the possibility of pathogens being present in the specimen. For laboratories to be in compliance with Medicare and other insurance payments, they must have a diagnosis or the medical necessity or reason for the test and also the ICD-9 code when billing for the work performed.)
- Medications or treatments the patient is receiving that may interfere with test results

At times the physician requires test results immediately. In these situations, "STAT" (immediately) should be checked off on the laboratory requisition or printed in large bold letters on the requisition. Some laboratories provide you with **"STAT" stickers;** these should be placed on the specimen container and on the laboratory requisition.

Most laboratories provide specific requisitions for the various types of tests that are to be performed in different areas of the laboratory (see sample requisitions in Chapters 11 and 13). Be certain that you use the correct requisition for the test(s) requested on the specimen. For example, a blood specimen is sent to the hematology department when the test ordered is a complete blood count; therefore you must complete the hematology requisition. A cytology requisition is sent with a cervical smear for a Pap test.

Many laboratories find it more convenient to have one form that lists all the tests that they perform. Others may have one form for all blood/serum tests and another form for urine/other fluids (Figure 10-1, *A* and *B*). Cytology studies generally are on a separate form.

Medical assistants should know the normal ranges of test results so that when abnormal results are reported, they can be brought to the physician's attention immediately. Depending on the policy of the office or health agency, you may circle or underline abnormal results in red to bring them to the physician's attention quickly. In many cases, computerized reports automatically identify abnormal results on the report. Commonly, physicians sign or put a check on a laboratory report after viewing it. This gives you an indication that it may be filed in the patient's chart. *Never* file a report before it has been reviewed by the physician. To hasten the physician's awareness of abnormal test results, many laboratories report these by telephone

---

*At times, more than one test is performed at the same time to study a specific organ, body system, or disease or to be used as a screening process. This grouping of specific tests is referred to as **profiles** or **panels.** They provide the physician with an overview of the patient's status that a single test could not provide (for example, a kidney function profile that may entail 12 different tests or a cardiac profile that may entail 10 different tests). Different laboratories may include different tests in their profiles or panels, as discussed in Chapter 13 under Automation in the Clinical Laboratory and as given in Figures 13-24 and 13-25 and Table 13-4. The tests included in each profile or panel would be listed in the laboratory's test directory. Some laboratories have this information listed on the back of their requisition forms. A space designated as *other tests* provides an area to write in tests needed that are not printed on the requisition form used.

FIGURE 10-1 **A,** Laboratory requisition for blood/serum tests.

BLOOD/SERUM
MAIN LABORATORY (2M) REQUISITION
General Hospital
Clinical Laboratories
(TUBE STATION E-9)

DRAWING STATION 1C33

LAB USE ONLY

DATE, TIME RECEIVED

ACC#

TECH CODE:

PHYSICIAN NAME (Print), I.D. #, BEEPER/EXT.

COLLECTED BY   DATE   TIME

LOCATION

PATIENT NAME:
MEDICAL RECORDS NUMBER:
BILLING:
BIRTHDATE:
SEX: M F

PHLEBOTOMY DRAW: Date _____
AM / PM   0600 1100 1600 2100

FINGERSTICK GLUCOSE
0600 1100 1600 2100

CHECK BLOOD TUBE TYPE (COLOR)
- GEL
- RED (PLAIN)
- GREY
- GREEN GEL
- GREEN
- BLUE
- ROYAL BLUE
- LAVENDER
- MICRO (GEL)
- MICRO (LAVENDER)
(FOR URINES AND FLUIDS, USE URINE/FLUID REQUISITION)

DIAGNOSIS/HISTORY - (REQUIRED FOR IMMUNOLOGY. REQUIRED FOR SEROLOGY SENDOUT TESTS. INCLUDE DATE OF ONSET, SYMPTOMS, LABS, THERAPY.)

ICD - 9 CODE:

MEDICATION: (Indicate time of last dose):

PHONE SPECIMEN PROBLEMS OR CRITICAL VALUES TO:
DR. _____
PHONE # _____

STAT TEST - INDICATE BY
1) Checking Red Box after test, or
2) Writing "STAT" after test.
(RESIDENT APPROVAL MAY BE NEEDED)

TUBE TYPE IS GEL UNLESS OTHERWISE NOTED

Code	Test
AAP	Acetaminophen
ALB	Albumin
AFP	Alpha Fetoprotein (Tumor)
ALT	ALT (SGPT)
AMEB	Amebiasis Antibody
NH3	Ammonia - Green Top on Ice
AMY	Amylase
DNA	Anti-Double Stranded DNA
ADB	Anti-DNase B
AHT	Anti-Hyaluronidase
AMA	Anti-Mitochondrial Antibody
ANA	Anti-Nuclear Antibody
ASO	Anti-Streptolysin-O
ASMA	Anti-Smooth Muscle Antibody
ASPP	Aspergillus Immunodiffusion
AST	AST (SGOT)
B12	B12, Vitamin
DBIL	Bilirubin, Direct
TBIL	Bilirubin, Total
BRUC	Brucella Agglutinins
CA	Calcium
CBZ	Carbamazepine (Tegretol)
CO2	Carbon Dioxide
CEAG	Carcinoembryonic Antigen (CEA)
CP	CBC with Platelets - Lav

Code	Test
CDP	CBC with Platelets & Differential - Lav
MSS	Slide Review - Lav
C34I	CD4 T Cells - Lav
C4BI	CD4 CD8 T Cells - Lav
CL	Chloride
HDL	Cholesterol, HDL + Total
CHOL	Cholesterol, Total
CK	CK (Creatine Phosphokinase)
CKMB	CKMB
CMVG	CMV, IgG
COID	Coccidioides Immunodiff.
CAGG	Cold Agglutinins
C3	Complement, C3
C4	Complement, C4
CU	Copper - Royal Blue
CORT	Cortisol - ___ PRE - ___ POST
CREA	Creatinine
CRAG	Cryptococcal Antigen (Blood only; for CSF use Microbiology requisition)
DIG	Digoxin
LYTE	Electrolyte Panel (NA, K, CL, CO2)
QUAL	Electrophoresis, HGB - Lav
SPIF	Electrophoresis, Immunofixation
SPEL	Electrophoresis, Protein
ETHL	Ethanol
FERR	Ferritin
FIBR	Fibrinogen - Blue
FDD	Fibrin D-Dimer - Blue

Code	Test
RFOU/HCT	Folate, RBC - Lav
FEP	Free Erythrocyte Protopor. - Lav
FSH	FSH
GPDQ	G6PD, Quantitative - Lav
GENA	Gentamicin - ___ Peak - ___ Trough
GGT	GGT
GLUF	Glucose, Fasting - Grey
GLUC	Glucose, Random - Grey
GLUP	Glucose, 1 Hr Post 50gm Load - Grey
GLU2	Glucose, 2 Hr Post Prand - Grey
GTOR	Glucose, Oral (HR ___) - Grey
GLUS	Glucose, Serum
HAPT	Haptoglobin
BHCG	HCG, Serum
HPYI	Helicobacter Pylori, IgG
HA1C	Hemoglobin A1C
HAIM	Hepatitis A Ab-IgM (Acute exposure)
HBCM	Hepatitis B Core Antibody IgM (Acute exposure)
HBSB	Hepatitis B Surface Antibody (Prior Exposure/ Immunity)
HBAG	Hepatitis B Surface Antigen
HBTC	Hepatitis B Core Antibody Total
HCV	Hepatitis C Antibody
HID	Histoplasma Immunodiff.
HVL	HIV Viral Load - Lav (x3)
IGA	IgA
IGG	IgG
IGM	IgM

Code	Test
MONO	Infectious Mononucleosis Absorbed
FE	Iron
LACT	Lactate - Grey
LD	Lactate Dehydrogenase
BPB/BPBC	Lead (CHDP - ___) - Lead Tube
LDCH	Lipid Panel-Fasting (CHOL, HDL, TRIG, and LDL CALC)
LH	LH (Lutein, Hormone)
LPSE	Lipase
LI	Lithium
LIVP	Liver Panel (Alb, Bili, Alk Phos, ALT, AST)
METB	Metabolic, Basic (Lyte + BUN, Crea, Gluc)
METC	Metabolic, Comp (METB-CO2 + Alb, Alkp, AST, Ca, Tbil, TP)
MG	Magnesium
MIXS	Mixing Study PT, PTT, or TT - Blue
OSMO	Osmolality
PBAR	Phenobarbital
DPH	Phenytoin (Dilantin)
ALKP	Phosphatase, Alkaline
PO4	Phosphorus, Inorganic
K	Potassium
PRL	Prolactin
PSG	Prostate Specific AG
TP	Protein, Total
PT	Prothrombin Time (PT + INR) - Blue
PTT	Partial Thromboplastin Time (Activated) - Blue
RETH/CP	Reticulocytes (Incl. CBC/PLT) - Lav
RF	Rheumatoid Factor

Code	Test
	RUBELLA SEROLOGY
RUBE	Immune Status Screen
RUBP	Immune Status Prenatal Screen
	Diagnostic - ___ Acute - ___ Conv Acute/Convalescent Serum Required
RVVT	Russell's Viper Venom - Blue
	SYPHILIS SEROLOGY (RPR TITER AND MHA-TP TESTS ADDED BY LAB IF RPR REACTIVE)
RPR	Routine
RPRP	Prenatal
RPRC	Cord Blood
	Hx of SYPHILIS (SYHX) SYMPTOMATIC (SYM) TREATED < 1 YR (SYL) TREATED > 1 YR (SYG)
SAL	Salicylate
ESR	Sedimentation Rate - Lav
NA	Sodium
TES	Testosterone
THEO	Theophylline
TT	Thrombin Time - Blue
	OTHER TESTS:

Code	Test
ATMA	Thyroid Microsomal Antibody
TT3	T3 (Triiodothyronine)
FT4	T4, Free (Thyroxine)
TSH	TSH
TOBA	Tobramycin ___ Peak ___ Trough
TOXE	Toxoplasma IgG
TRSF	Transferrin
TRIG	Triglycerides, Fasting
TRPI	Troponin I
BUN	Urea Nitrogen
URIC	Uric Acid
VPA	Valproic Acid
VANA	Vancomycin ___ Peak ___ Trough
VZS	Varicella Immune Status
VOLS	Volatile Screen (Ethanol, Methanol, Isopropanol, Acetone)
ZN	Zinc - Royal Blue
	TESTS SENT TO THE CALIF. DEPT. OF HEALTH LAB OR CDC LAB. PROVIDE HISTORY ABOVE. INDICATE TEST BELOW.
PHLE	Lab Phlebotomy Outpatient

FIGURE 10-1, cont'd **B,** Laboratory requisitions for urine/fluids tests.

DATE, TIME RECEIVED　　ACC#　　PHYSICIAN NAME (Print),　　I.D.#,　　BEEPER/EXT.

TECH CODE:

LAB USE ONLY

URINE/FLUIDS
MAIN LABORATORY (2M) REQUISITION
General Hospital
Clinical Laboratories
(TUBE STATION E-9)

PATIENT NAME:

MEDICAL RECORDS NUMBER:

BILLING:

BIRTHDATE:

SEX: M F

DIAGNOSIS/HISTORY (REQUIRED FOR TOXICOLOGY).

MEDICATION: (Indicate time of last dose):　ICD-9 CODE

PHONE SPECIMEN PROBLEMS, OR CRITICAL VALUES TO:
DR.
PHONE#
PHONE STATS

STAT TEST - INDICATE BY
1) Checking Red Box after test,
or
2) Writing "STAT" after test.
(RESIDENT APPROVAL MAY BE NEEDED)

COLLECTED BY　　DATE　　TIME　　AM / PM

LOCATION

BODY FLUID TYPE
- CSF
- GASTRIC
- PERITONEAL
- PLEURAL
- SYNOVIAL
- URINE
　OTHER ___

(FOR BLOOD AND SERUM USE BLOOD/SERUM REQUISITION)

CSF

Code	Test
CSFC	CSF Chem (Tube # ___)
CALB	Albumin, CSF
CSFG	Glucose (STAT), CSF
CIGG	IgG, CSF
INDX	IgG Index, CSF (Serum also Required)
CSFP	Protein, CSF
GLUT	Glutamine, CSF
SCSF	CSF Cell Count (Tube # ___)
CSVD	VDRL for Syphilis, CSF TEST PERFORMED ONLY IF SERUM POSITIVE

(CHECK SPECIMEN TYPE ABOVE) PLAIN TUBE UNLESS NOTED

Code	Test
FALK	Alkaline Phosphatase
FAMY	Amylase
SFCC	Cell Count, Fluid (Lavender)
FCRE	Creatinine
FGLU	Glucose
FLDH	LD (Lactate Dehydrogenase)
FPH	pH (On Ice)
FTP	Protein, Total
SSYN	Synovial Cell Count (Lavender)

FECES

Code	Test
FECW	Fecal WBC
FATS	Fecal Fat, Qualitative
OCX	Occult Blood

URINE

* 24 HOUR COLLECTION PREFERRED
** PROTECT FROM LIGHT

Date/Time: Start:
Stop:

Code	Test
u	Random
UAMY	Amylase
UCA	Calcium *
UCL	Chloride
UCUB	Copper *
UCRE	Creatinine
CCLR	Creatinine Clearance * (Serum Also Required) HT ___ (IN) WT ___ (LBS)
CYS	Cystine - Qualitative
UPEP	Electrophoresis, Protein (Serum Also Required)
UGLU	Glucose *
HSID	Hemosiderin
	Iron
UPEI	Light Chains - Qualitative
UOSM	Osmolality
UPO4	Phosphorus, Inorganic *
POR	Porphyrin **
PBG	Porphobilinogen **
UPRG	Pregnancy Test

Code	Test
UK	Potassium
UPRO	Protein *
UNA	Sodium
UUN	Urea Nitrogen
UURI	Uric Acid *
UDIP	Urinalysis Routine
UFAT	Urine Fat

OTHER TESTS

TOXICOLOGY

SUSPECTED DRUGS:

TIME/DATE OF INGESTION:

DAU　Drug of Abuse Screen
Includes following or check individual drug class

AMP	Amphetamine Like Drugs
BARB	Barbiturates
BENZ	Benzodiazepine/Metabolites
COCA	Cocaine/Metabolites
OPIA	Opiates
PCP	Phencyclidine
ETOH	Ethanol

CDS　**COMPREHENSIVE DRUG SCREEN**
Includes above Drugs plus over 50 Drugs of Abuse
and Pharmaceuticals: **SEE LAB MANUAL**

immediately and forward the written report later, signed by the laboratory worker who performed the test.

Often laboratories supply the physician's office with special **telephone reporting pads** to use to record results given over the telephone, thereby establishing some consistency for such reports. These should include a place to record the patient's name and identification number or medical record number, the laboratory accession number, and test results. After the permanent laboratory report has been received, it should be compared with the telephone report page. If everything is the same, the telephone report page can be destroyed. Physicians can also access computer-recorded laboratory results for tests performed on their patients from many hospital laboratories using their special computer identification code that they have established with the hospital laboratory. Many physicians' offices have a direct line to a commercial or hospital laboratory and can obtain computerized printouts of computerized reports.

Accuracy in reporting test results cannot be stressed enough because often the diagnosis and treatment for a patient are contingent on these reports.

Laboratory Reports

Laboratory reports are either a computer printout (Figure 10-2) or a preprinted form with handwritten or typed results signed by the clinical laboratory scientist who performed the test(s) and recorded the results.

The following information is generally included on the report:

1. Name, address, telephone number, and the name of the director of the laboratory.
2. Name and address of the physician who ordered the test(s) and the physician's computer code on a computer-generated report.
3. Patient's name, date of birth, sex, and medical record number or identification number. This identifying information is very important because a physician may have more than one patient with the same name, for example, common names such as Robert Smith or Joe Lee.
4. Date and time the specimen was collected.
5. Date and time the specimen was received by the laboratory.
6. Laboratory accession number. This is a number that the *laboratory* assigns a specimen when it is received by them. This provides identification for the specimen in the laboratory. In large laboratories, this number is often generated by a computer and reused every 2 months because of the great number of specimens that they deal with on a daily basis.
7. Date the test(s) results were obtained.
8. Normal ranges for the results of each test.
9. Name and result of each test.

DIAGNOSTIC AND THERAPEUTIC PROCEDURES

As mentioned earlier in Chapter 4, the physician arrives at a diagnosis by using and reviewing multiple factors and information obtained on the patient's condition (that is, the physician uses various studies to arrive at a diagnosis). Three reasons for diagnostic studies follow:

1. To determine (diagnose) the condition from which the patient is suffering so that treatment, if feasible, may be initiated.
2. To discover disease in its early stage before the patient experiences any signs or symptoms, a process called **screening**. Screening for disease often permits the cure of the disease because treatment can be started in the early stages of the disease process (for example, cancer) or early treatment can delay the progression of the disease (for example, hypertension).
3. To evaluate past or ongoing treatment and to regulate ongoing treatment received by the patient.

As the field of medical science continues to expand, newer and more accurate and sophisticated techniques are continually made available to help physicians diagnose disease processes. Diagnostic procedures and studies include but are not limited to physical examinations, surgical intervention, and laboratory technology. Other procedures used when diagnosing and treating disease processes require some elaboration. These involve the areas of radiology (roentgenology), the specialized field of nuclear medicine, special skin tests, physical medicine and physiotherapy, and electrocardiography.

To completely understand all of these diagnostic and therapeutic procedures, special courses of study are necessary. Nevertheless, the following chapters expose you to various additional tests that the physician may order for a patient. (Physical examinations, minor surgery, and special skin tests were discussed in preceding chapters of this book.) The descriptions of the following diagnostic and therapeutic studies and procedures are given to help you understand the nature and purpose(s) of the numerous clinical entities available to health care practitioners for the treatment and care of patients.

Various studies, related vocabulary, and procedures are presented, along with special patient preparation when required. *You are not expected to also be a laboratory, x-ray, nuclear medicine, or electrocardiography technician or a physical therapist, but you are expected to be familiar with the vocabulary and the nature and purpose(s) of diagnostic or therapeutic procedures and studies performed by these specialists.* At times you may be called on to assist with procedures performed by these medical specialists or to perform the more routine and simplified procedures, such as routine urinalysis, skin tests, the application of hot or cold, and electrocardiograms. In addition, you may be responsible for explaining the nature and purpose of the procedure to the patient, giving the patient special instructions when needed, recording the procedure on the patient's medical record, and filing or storing the reports and films received after the test or treatment has been completed.

This chapter and Chapters 14 and 15 present an opportunity for students to design their own step-by-step procedures and performance checklists. The *Student Mastery Manual* provides a summary of studies used for diagnosing conditions affecting body organs and systems.

FIGURE 10-2   **A** and **B,** Computer-generated laboratory reports. Note all the information given on the report.

EXAMPLE

–NO GREEN BAR–
GOES TO UNIT OR PHYSICIAN

REPORT PRINTING
DATE 06/15/98
TIME 11:38

NAME OF HOSPITAL OR LAB
CLINICAL LABORATORIES

CUMULATIVE SUMMARY

Pt unique number

PATIENT'S NAME

MEDICAL RECORD NUMBER

ACCT:	BILLING ACCT #	LOC:	7D	SERVICE:	DOB: 04/04/77
AGE:	21Y	SEX:	M	DR.: **NAME OF PHYSICIAN**	
ADM:	04/11/98				CODE:
DSC:	04/15/98				

Name of test   Physician
                                                          computer code

= AFB-RESPIRATORY CULTURES =

Specimen collect date   LAB accession #

04/11/98

R1634   ACC. NO.:   TRANSPORT TIME: UNKNOWN HRS   * * *   STATUS: FINAL 06/10/98   * * *

Time received in LAB

SPECIMEN DESCRIPTION: SPUTUM
COMMENT: NONE

Name of test

MICROSCOPIC EXAM: 1. NO ACID FAST BACILLI SEEN (CONCENTRATED SMEAR)

Test results

RESULT: 1. NO ACID FAST BACILLI RECOVERED AT 60 DAYS

As above

04/13/98
R1446   ACC. NO.:   TRANSPORT TIME: UNKNOWN HRS   * * *   STATUS: FINAL 06/10/98   * * *

SPECIMEN DESCRIPTION: SPUTUM
COMMENT: NONE

MICROSCOPIC EXAM: 1. NO ACID FAST BACILLI SEEN (CONCENTRATED SMEAR)

RESULT: 1. NO ACID FAST BACILLI RECOVERED AT 58 DAYS

As above

04/14/98
0630   ACC. NO.:   TRANSPORT TIME: 1.8 HRS   * * *   STATUS: FINAL 06/10/98   * * *

Time collected

SPECIMEN DESCRIPTION: SPUTUM
COMMENT: NONE

MICROSCOPIC EXAM: 1. NO ACID FAST BACILLI SEEN (CONCENTRATED SMEAR)

RESULT: 1. NO ACID FAST BACILLI RECOVERED AT 57 DAYS

A

PT NAME
06/15/98 11:38

CONTINUED   PAGE
CHART COPY CUMULATIVE SUMMARY

HOSPITAL LOGO
HOSPITAL NAME AND ADDRESS
PHONE NUMBER

CLINICAL LABORATORIES REPORT
Name of Director ——— JAMES LAWRENCE, MD, DIRECTOR

Continued

FIGURE 10-2—cont'd **A** and **B,** Computer-generated laboratory reports. Note all the information given on the report.

EXAMPLE

Printing date

06/14/98
15:50

Printing time

NAME OF HOSPITAL
CLINICAL LABORATORIES

CUMULATIVE SUMMARY

= PHYSICIAN COPY FOR: =

Unique number

PATIENT'S NAME

MEDICAL RECORD NUMBER

| ACCT: | BILLING ACCT # | | LOC: | PT LOCATION | SERVICE: | | DOB: 02/28/40 | |
| AGE: | 58Y | | SEX: | M | DR.: PHYSICIAN NAME | | | CODE: — Physician computer ID code |

= CHEMISTRY =

TEST:	IRON	TRANSF	%SAT	FERRITIN, SERUM
UNITS:	MCG/DL	MG/DL	%	NG/ML
LO-HI:	50-150	180-335	16-60	20-415

Value range

06/09 + 1030   23*   246   8*   44

Collect date   Collect time   Abnormal result

= MISCELLANEOUS HEMATOLOGY =

TEST: FEP
UNITS: UG/DL
LO-HI: <35

06/09 + 1030   PEND   (Test pending, no result, just test value range)

= HGB ELECTROPHORESIS =

06/09 + 1030   HGB A2   2.1   [<3]   %

        + 1030   HGB F, QUANT   0.8   [<1.1]   %

= OTHER TESTS =

06/09 + 1030   HGB ELECTROPHORESIS
               HGB ELECTROPHORESIS
                              PEND

"R" plus time = time received in LAB

REPORTS ON GREEN BAR ARE FOR MEDICAL PT RECORD

| PT NAME | END OF REPORT | PAGE |
| 06/14/98 15:50 | | NEW DATA 0 |

| HOSPITAL LOGO | CLINICAL LABORATORIES REPORT |
| NAME AND ADDRESS OF HOSPITAL | NAME OF DIRECTOR |

B

HEALTH **MATTERS**

KEEPING YOUR PATIENTS INFORMED

Be an organ donor. . . . It's the chance of a lifetime!*

You probably already know somebody who has benefited from having a transplant. In fact, you or someone close to you may need a transplant someday because it can happen to anyone at any age. Organ and tissue transplantation is one of this century's medical triumphs. It has become a routine practice that can dramatically improve—and even save—the lives of those suffering from vital organ failure or those suffering from bone defects, burns, and blindness. Thanks to people like you, who make the commitment to give others a second chance, transplant recipients return to living normal, productive lives.

The most precious gift that you can give someone is the gift of life itself. That's exactly what you do by becoming an organ and tissue donor. Yet, the simple truth is that there are not enough people who are making this life-giving choice.

Every year in the United States, more than 100,000 children and adults are forced to wait and hope for a chance to live normal, healthy lives. When you make an organ and tissue donation, you are providing these mothers, fathers, sons, and daughters with a second chance for life.

IMPORTANT FACTS ABOUT ORGAN AND TISSUE DONATION

Anyone can become an organ donor. Just by making your wishes known to your family, you can become an organ and tissue donor. Old age or a history of disease does not mean you can't donate. Organs and tissues that can't be used for transplants can often be used to help scientists find cures for serious illnesses.

Many organs and tissues can be donated. The heart, lungs, liver, kidneys and pancreas, as well as corneas, bone, skin, heart valves and blood vessels, are some of the organs and tissues that can be used to help improve the quality of life for people needing transplants and other surgical procedures.

Signing a donor card will not affect the care you receive at the hospital. If you are injured and brought to an emergency room, you will receive the best possible care, whether or not you have signed a donor card. Donation procedures begin only after all efforts to save your life have been exhausted, and death has been declared.

The organ transplant system is fair. The distribution of donated organs allows equal access for all patients awaiting a transplant in the United States. The National Transplant Act mandated the establishment of a national computer system for organ sharing that is based on need and availability.

Major religions support organ and tissue donation. Many faiths openly encourage it, seeing this as a final act of giving and as an expression of hope on the part of the donor.

*California Transplant Donor Network, San Francisco, Calif: 1-800-553-6667.

Organ and tissue donation does not eliminate the possibility of a regular funeral service. A traditional, open casket funeral service can still take place even though many organs and tissues have been donated. The surgical procedures used are performed by highly skilled professionals, and the appearance of the donor's body is unchanged.

The donor family incurs no expenses for the donation. After the determination of death has been made, all the costs associated with the donation are covered. The donor family does not bear any expense.

Follow these simple steps to become an organ and tissue donor. First discuss organ and tissue donation with your family. It is important that your loved ones are informed of your decision. Then sign a donor card in the presence of two witnesses and carry it with you at all times.

MAKE A VERY IMPORTANT DIFFERENCE IN SOMEONE'S LIFE.

Signing a donor card signifies your commitment to renewing the life and health of others in need. In the event of your death, your family will be asked what your wishes were. Now is the time to discuss this important issue with them. The gift of organ and tissue donation can truly be a gift of life for someone else.

1. Talk to your family about this important decision.
2. Fill out this donor card in the presence of two witnesses and sign your name in the space provided.
3. Have both witnesses sign their names in the spaces provided.
4. Carry this card in your purse or wallet where it can be easily found.

This is to inform you that I want to be an organ and tissue donor if the occasion ever arises. Please see that my wishes are carried out by informing the attending medical personnel that I am a donor. My desires are indicated below:

In the hopes that I may help others, I hereby make this gift for the purpose of transplant, medical study, or education to take effect upon my death. I give:

[ ] Any needed organs/tissues

[ ] Only the following organs/tissues

_____

Specify the organ(s)/tissue(s)

_____

_____

Limitations or special wishes if any

_____

_____

Donor's signature

Detach your donor card and give the above portion to your family.

Continued

HEALTH **MATTERS—cont'd**

Donor Card

This is a legal document under the Uniform Anatomical Gift Act or similar laws, signed by the donor and the following two witnesses in the presence of each other.

_____

Donor's signature

_____

Donor's date of birth   City & State

_____

Witness   Witness

_____

Next of kin   Telephone

(front)

Please type or print full name of donor.

In the hope that I may help others, I hereby make this gift for the purpose of transplant, medical study, or education to take effect upon my death.

I give: [ ] Any needed organs/tissues
       [ ] Only the following organs/tissues

_____

Specify the organ(s)/tissue(s)

_____

_____

Limitations or special wishes if any

(back)

Organizing the Recordings of Diagnostic Procedures

A patient's medical record should be maintained in an organized manner to facilitate easy accessibility to the information. Regular-sized paper or preprinted forms are customarily used when recording all information relevant to the patient's care. If you receive reports on small sheets, affix them to standard-sized sheets before filing them in the patient's medical record.

Various methods are used when filing laboratory reports in a patient's medical record. Some office or health care agencies have a certain order for compiling medical records, so that the laboratory report papers follow or precede other entries. One common method is to use a special standard-size sheet of paper designated specifically for staggering these reports. The first report is placed on the lower portion on this sheet, and each additional report is placed on top of the preceding one, allowing the bottom $\frac{1}{2}$ inch or so of each report to be visible, as this is where the date of the test is recorded. With this method, the most recent report is on top, which facilitates a quick review of current information (Figure 10-3).

One of three formats can be used for recording and organizing information and test results in the patient's record: the source-oriented format, the integrated format, or the problem-oriented format.

In the **source-oriented** medical record, all reports are filed chronologically according to their specialty (for example, all laboratory reports are filed together, x-ray film reports are filed together, and electrocardiogram records are kept together). The latest information is placed on top because it is the most important for the patient's current care and treatment.

In the **integrated** record, all information is recorded in strict chronologic order as the physician sees the patient, gives care, and orders various tests (that is, the physician dates and enters the patient's history, physical examination results, and the treatment given and ordered; the laboratory, electrocardiogram, and x-ray film reports are filed in the medical record immediately following the physician's notes for this particular situation; progress notes and future laboratory or x-ray reports continue to be entered in strict chronologic order).

In the **problem-oriented** medical record, all test results (laboratory, x-ray film, and physical) are entered and recorded in the "Objective" part of the progress notes, preceded by the number and title of the particular problem.

At times, a radiologist's office, an outside laboratory, or hospital **telephones test results** before mailing a written report. The information received in this manner should be labeled as a verbal report and recorded accurately and attached to the patient's medical record until the actual report is received.

You must ensure that all reports are received for diagnostic tests performed on the patient outside the physician's office. Only after the physician reviews them should you file them in the patient's medical record.

Develop a follow-through procedure for pending reports from outside sources. Usable methods include the following:

1. Use individual sheets for laboratory tests, x-ray film reports, electrocardiograms, and consultations from outside sources; they can be kept in separate files or in a binder. Each entry should be made on a separate line, giving the date, patient's name, and the test(s) ordered. As the reports are received, enter the date and check off the entry to indicate that it has been received.

2. Keep the patient's medical record in a special file until all outstanding reports have been received.

FIGURE 10-3 Laboratory report records. The first report is placed on the lower portion where indicated. Each additional report is placed on top of the preceding one, allowing the bottom ½ inch of each report to be visible. This area is where the date is recorded. The most recent report is on top, allowing for quick review of current information.

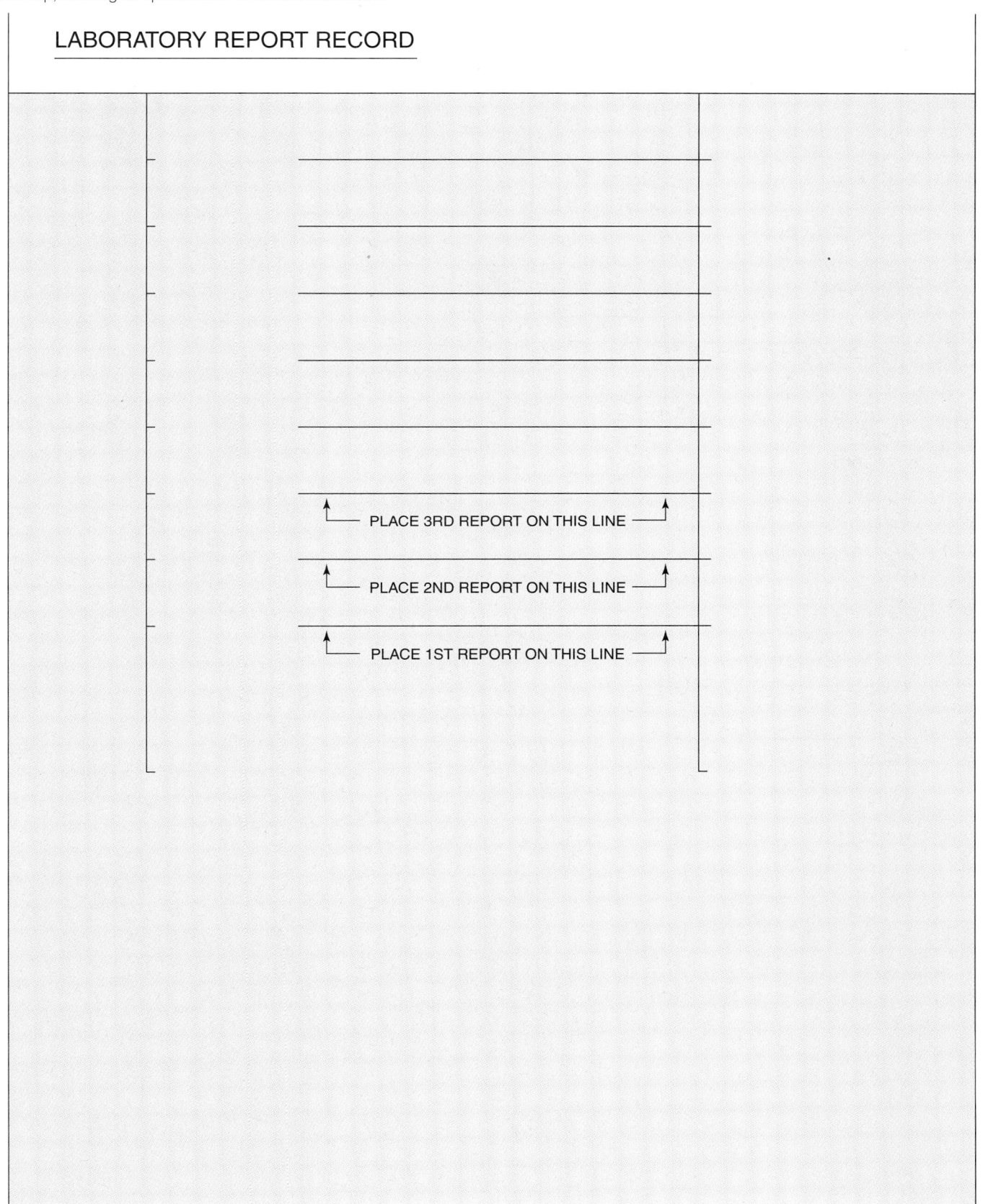

Continued

FIGURE 10-3—cont'd   Laboratory report records. The first report is placed on the lower portion where indicated. Each additional report is placed on top of the preceding one, allowing the bottom ½ inch of each report to be visible. This area is where the date is recorded. The most recent report is on top, allowing for quick review of current information.

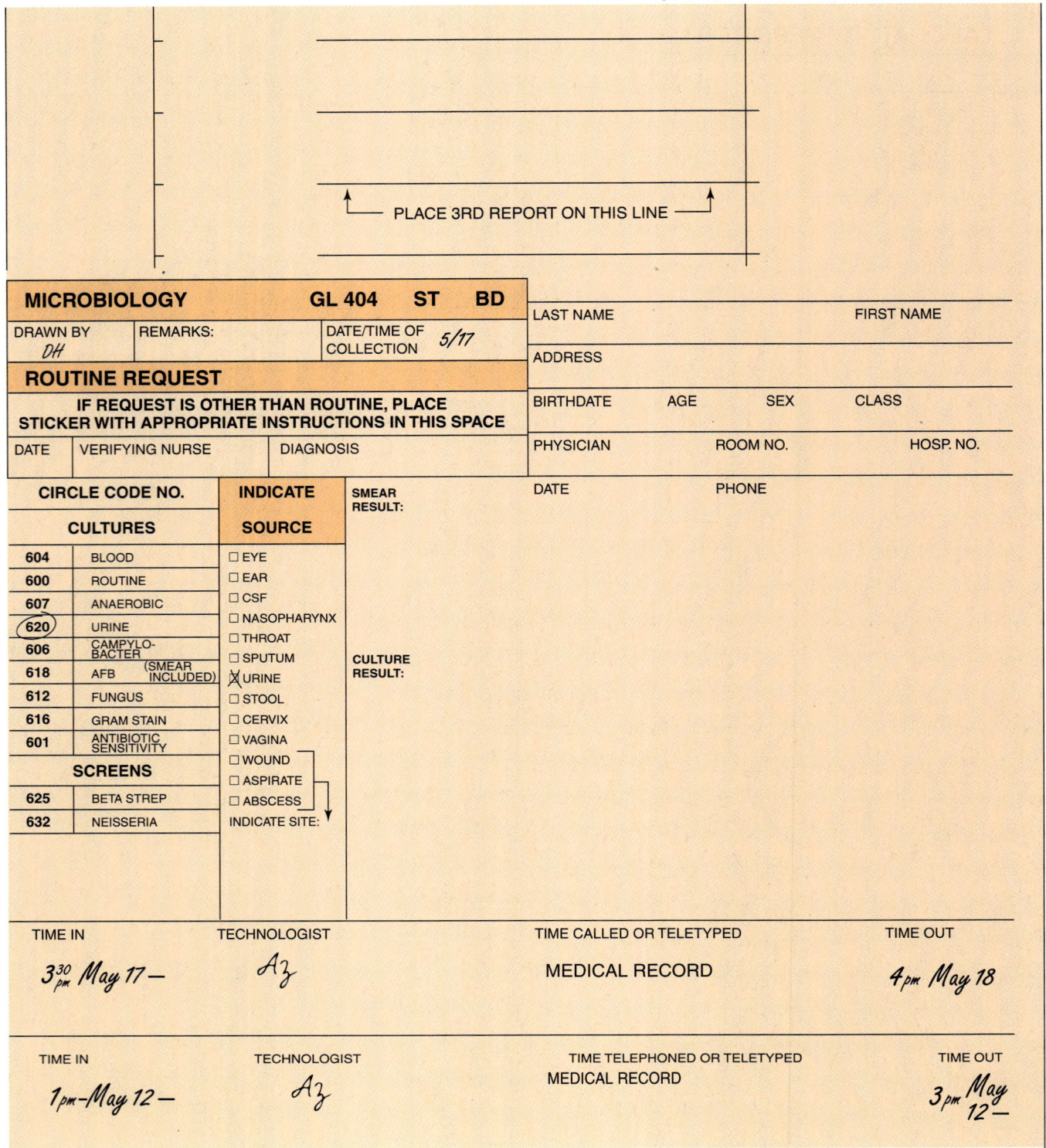

3. Place the patient's record back in the usual file with a colored flag attached to indicate that reports are yet to be received.

Regardless of the method, use a consistent follow-through procedure to ensure that all test results are received on a regular basis.

The next three chapters are devoted to information on the collection of various types of specimens and on urinalysis and hematology because urine and blood are the two most abundant body fluids and provide a wealth of information on an individual's health. Reference tables for various urine and blood tests with related information and the normal evaluation ranges for their results are also presented.

This book does not give detailed instructions for the procedures involved when performing all of these laboratory tests *because most* **must** *only be performed by certified laboratory personnel or physicians.* The purposes of the following information, as well as Chapters 11 through 13, are to prepare you for performing basic routine procedures that may be done in the physician's office or health care agency and to make you aware of some of the many laboratory tests, special equipment, and supplies that are available, along with the normal ranges for test results. You are expected to know how to collect and handle specimens. When applicable, you must also know the special instructions to give to the patient before the collection of a specimen and the normal test results expected. By attaining this knowledge and these skills, you can enhance patient care and increase your value to the physician, patient, and laboratory.

The remainder of this chapter discusses quality control and laboratory safety and two major pieces of laboratory equipment: the microscope and centrifuge. You should be familiar with this information and equipment if simple laboratory procedures are performed in the physician's office or health care agency and also when specimens and blood samples are to be prepared for transport to a commercial laboratory.

Collecting, Handling, Transporting, and Storing Specimens

See Chapter 11, p. 476, and also review Chapter 1.

QUALITY CONTROL AND LABORATORY SAFETY

Quality Control

Quality control and laboratory safety are vital aspects of laboratory technology. They are directly related to the collection, handling, processing, and testing of all specimens. Quality control involves methods used to ensure the **reliability** (the extent to which a test measurement, instrument, or reagent produces the same results with different personnel or performance of the test over time) and **accuracy** of the tests performed and tests results obtained. This begins with proper preparation of the patient, proper care and handling of specimens as discussed in Chapter 11, and evaluation of the techniques and equipment used to perform the tests.

Even the smallest laboratory *must* use methods to determine the accuracy of test results. Many **commercial control products** are available to check the reliability of test products and results. These products test for the same substance(s) for which you would be testing a patient's specimen. They are available in both normal and abnormal ranges and give the range of valid results. You should use both types to ensure test accuracy. Results differing from the normal ranges of the control indicate that your test is inaccurate. In this situation, repeat the control test. If the results are still out of the valid control range, do not use these supplies for testing specimens from patients until the problem has been identified and corrected. Machines must be calibrated frequently to ensure that they are working properly. Many are **calibrated** automatically with the aid of a computer. Keep a record of the results and dates of all the control tests you run. State laws usually require the records (see Controls for Routine Urinalysis on p. 545 in Chapter 12 and Tables 12-4 through 12-6.) *Ensuring that your equipment is functioning accurately is vital to quality control.*

Controls provide the laboratory worker with the capability to evaluate the changes or errors that are commonly associated with routine clinical chemistry. The controls should be used to establish confidence that the variables that cause errors are in check or within a range of acceptability as established by the laboratory. Guidelines have been established to aid the laboratory to initiate a quality control program using solutions of known values. By understanding the trends established by responsible interpretation of control values, better results are obtained with clinical procedures. Controls are tested often, usually in duplicate, to control laboratory error. By realizing that quality control assesses the sources of variables, from specimen transporting to recording of results, better values are obtained—with a high degree of confidence in the procedures used. An example of controls used for routine urinalysis is given in Chapter 12 on pp. 546-549.

Laboratory Safety

Laboratory testing involves certain safety hazards, such as exposure to strong chemicals and infectious materials. Thus laboratory workers must use safe, proper techniques when around and using laboratory equipment, chemicals, and specimens. The following *safety rules* should assist you in working in a safe manner. (Also review Universal/Standard Precautions and Laboratory Specimens in Chapter 1 regarding bloodborne pathogens.) Laboratory safety is also vital to quality control.

General instructions
- Do not eat, drink, or smoke in the laboratory.
- Use protective equipment such as rubber gloves, eye goggles, and apron when required.
- Keep pens, pencils, and fingers away from your mouth.
- **Wash your hands frequently and thoroughly. Use appropriate personal protective equipment (PPE) as dictated by facility.**
- If you are pregnant, you should not be exposed to potential or known pathogenic agents.

- If you are inexperienced, you should be well supervised.
- When you have an open wound or an eczematous skin condition, you should not handle pathogenic material unless the risks involved can be avoided by protective equipment.
- Process specimens from known infectious material separately from other specimens. Disinfect nondisposable equipment used for these specimens after use. Place all used disposable equipment in biohazardous waste containers.
- Clean your work area with a disinfectant at the end of the day and at least one other time during the day.

Chemicals and reagents

- Current inventory control is important. Discard chemical reagents in accordance with their expiration dates.
- Store labeled chemicals and reagents under nonreactive conditions with respect to light, moisture, and temperature. Follow the manufacturer's recommended storage procedures.
- You must not pipette by mouth. Mouth pipetting is prohibited under Universal/Standard Precautions set by the Occupational Safety and Health Administration (OSHA). Use a commercial pipetting device.
- You must use disposable gloves when handling specimens and disinfectants and when cleaning automatic blood-analyzing equipment.

Equipment

- Clean automatic blood- and serum-analyzing systems after each use according to the manufacturer's directions.
- Unplug electric appliances before cleaning or washing them.
- Unplug major appliances when lights stay dim or unusually bright.
- Use properly grounded three-pronged Underwriter's Laboratory (UL)-approved, double-insulated electrical equipment.
- Discard materials used to wipe machine parts during operation and cleaning with other biohazardous waste.
- Do not wear loose-fitting clothing when working around a Bunsen burner.
- Do not use Bunsen burners near areas where oxygen is in use or where flammables are stored.
- Know emergency fire procedures if use of a Bunsen burner is required.
- Do not leave Bunsen burners unattended when they are lit.
- Position centrifuges in areas where their vibrations do not cause items to fall off nearby shelves.
- Always balance the load in a centrifuge to avoid damage to the equipment and injury to yourself.
- Cover centrifuges when in use.
- Take care when loading and unloading a centrifuge to avoid spilling the specimens.
- Turn the centrifuge off before opening the lid (if it is not equipped with an interlocking device).

Glassware

- Take a regular inventory of all glassware. Discard all chipped or cracked pieces.
- Handle and store all glassware carefully to avoid breakage.

Identification of materials (chemicals and reagents)

- Label **all** materials clearly. Replace soiled labels immediately.
- Do not use but discard any unlabeled item according to Material Safety Data Sheets (MSDSs) in your area.
- When affixing a label, moisten it with a damp sponge. Do not lick the label.
- Make sure that poisons, corrosives, and flammable materials are labeled as such. Have a proper storage area for these items away from other solutions that you may have in the office or clinic. Consult the Environmental Protection Agency and the Hazard Communications Act in your area regarding regulations concerning MSDSs, labeling requirements, and posting of notices. These materials must be placed in special, approved containers when being transferred from the storage area to the work space.

THE MICROSCOPE

The microscope (Figure 10-4) is a precise scientific instrument used in the laboratory when an enlarged image of a small (microscopic) object is required. Using a microscope allows details of structure not otherwise distinguishable to be revealed. Microscopes vary greatly in quality. For maximum efficiency, the operation of a microscope must be studied carefully. Complete instructions for assembling and using the microscope are provided by each manufacturer. Read these instructions completely before you use the microscope for laboratory procedures.

Parts of the Microscope

Eyepieces. Eyepieces fit into the eyepiece tubes. The eyepieces in common use today are marked 5×, 6×, or 10×. The 10× eyepiece has the greatest magnifying power. Because the exterior surface of the eyepiece is exposed, it is likely to become dusty; therefore it should be carefully cleaned before use. You can clean it with a special lens paper or with a soft cloth.

Nosepiece and objectives. The microscope is provided with a revolving nosepiece into which the various objectives are screwed. Care must be used in properly attaching the objectives to the nosepiece. Follow the procedure provided by the manufacturer of the microscope. The objectives make up the lens system on the nosepiece. *Never* at any time force the objective or allow its lower end (the lens) to touch the metal stage. Lenses are very expensive and are easily damaged by contact with any other objects—slides, cover glasses, or specimens.

Objectives have different magnifying powers. The following are commonly used (Table 10-1):

- The lowest power objective, marked 16 mm or 10×
- The intermediate power (often called the high dry power) marked 4 mm, 43×, or 45×
- The highest power, the oil-immersion objective, marked 1.8 mm, 97×, or 100×

FIGURE 10-4   A, Nikon Labophot microscope; **B,** Nikon Optiphot microscope. (Courtesy Nikon Inc, Instrument Division, Garden City, NY.)

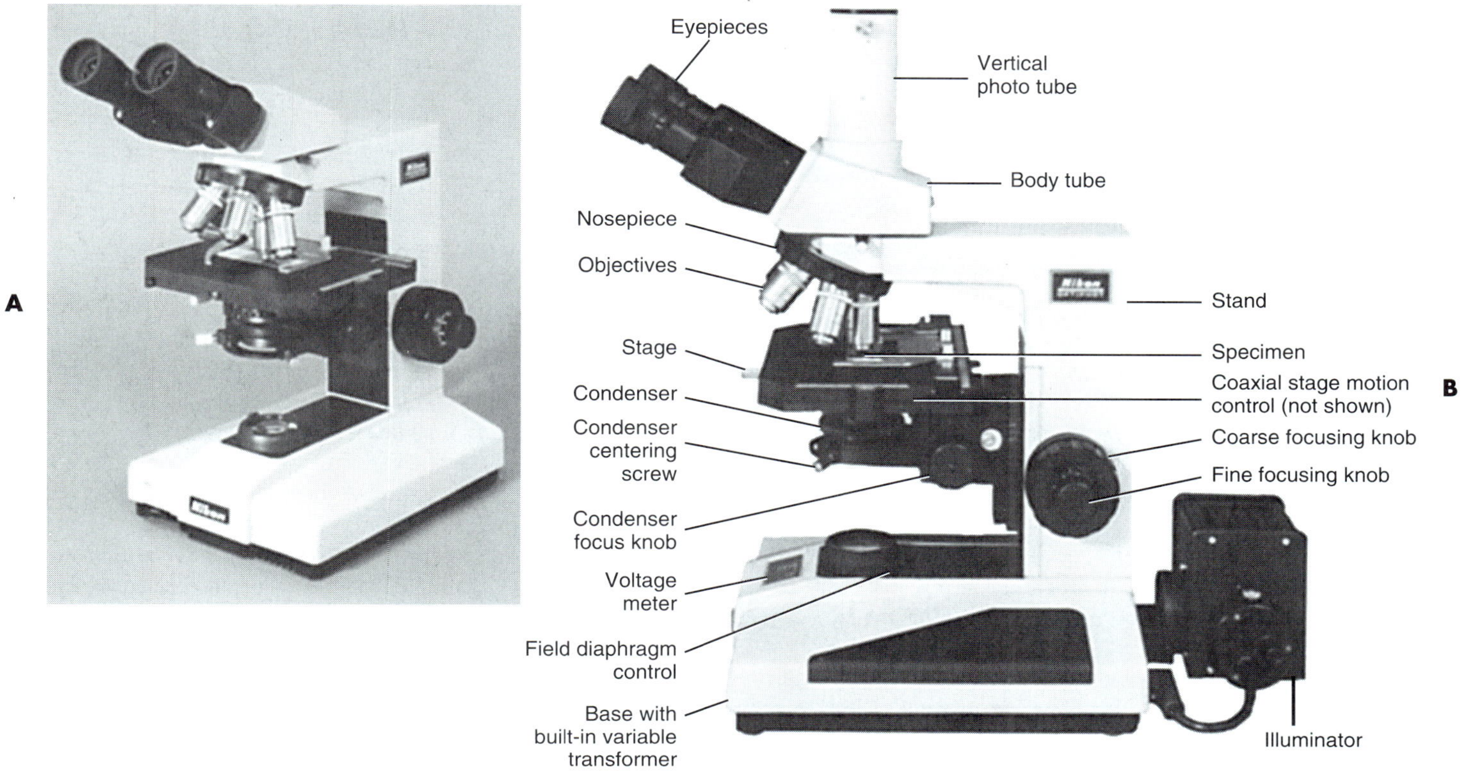

A

B

Labels (left side): Eyepieces, Nosepiece, Objectives, Stage, Condenser, Condenser centering screw, Condenser focus knob, Voltage meter, Field diaphragm control, Base with built-in variable transformer

Labels (right side): Vertical photo tube, Body tube, Stand, Specimen, Coaxial stage motion control (not shown), Coarse focusing knob, Fine focusing knob, Illuminator

TABLE 10–1   Microscope Objectives and Uses

Objective	Focal Length	Magnifying Power	Uses
Low power	16 mm	10×	Initial focusing
			Initial light adjustment
			Initial scanning of urine sediment and blood smears
			Manual counting of white blood cells
High power (or high dry power)	4 mm	43× or 45×	Study of cells and sediment in more detail
			Study of wet preparations such as urine sediment
			Manual counting of red blood cells
Oil immersion	1.8 mm	97× or 100×	Viewing of very small structures
			Viewing blood films such as the differential white blood cell count or the reticulocyte count
			Viewing microorganisms
			Viewing a Gram stain to identify different types of bacteria

In becoming familiar with the different objectives, remember that the low power is the shortest of the three objectives, whereas the oil immersion is the longest of the three. Another point of differentiation is the size of the opening in the smaller end of the objectives. The objective with the widest lens is the lowest power, and conversely, the one with the smallest lens is the highest power—the oil-immersion lens. Some examples of magnification power are given in Table 10-2.

Arm or stand.   The arm or stand (see Figure 10-4) is used for carrying the microscope. When carrying the microscope, place one hand on the arm and support the base of the microscope with your other hand.

Body tube.   The body tube directs the path of light from the light source to the eyepieces.

TABLE 10–2 Examples of Magnification

Eyepiece	Objective	Magnification
5×	10×	50
10×	10×	100
5×	45×	225
10×	45×	450
5×	100×	500
10×	100×	1000

Stage. The stage is the flat heavy part on which slides are placed for examination. On the stage are found two slide clips. In place of these clips, it is more convenient to apply an attachable mechanical stage, which is used to move the slides more precisely. This mechanical stage is almost indispensable in laboratory work, especially when the work requires high-power magnification.

Substage. Fitting into the opening on the stage and immediately below it is the substage. This part holds the **substage condenser,** a necessity in microscopic work. Its purpose is to direct, focus, and condense the light on the object under examination. For best results, focus the proper amount of light onto the object by lowering and raising the substage by means of the pinion adjustment (or condenser focus knob). On the lower part of the substage condenser is found the **shutter or diaphragm.** This shutter or diaphragm is used to close off light or to admit more light. Because the amount of light required varies, adjustment of the substage in connection with specific uses of the microscope is described in a later paragraph.

Other parts of the microscope. The larger of the two knobs, the **pinion head** or **coarse-focusing knob,** is used for coarse adjustment of the microscope. The smaller knob, the **fine-focusing knob,** is used in fine adjustment and focusing. These two knobs are important because they must be used every time the instrument is used. When you are looking for the field, you must always lower the head of the microscope by means of the coarse adjustment. You then use the fine adjustment. This is absolutely essential when using high-power magnification. Another part of the microscope is the **light source** or **illuminator,** which is part of the system providing a source of light for viewing a slide. You can direct the light precisely to obtain the clearest possible image. The light source is a built-in light bulb (illuminator) located at the base of the microscope directly under the center of the stage. The light is directed to the condenser above it, which directs/condenses the light on the object under examination. Two other parts of the illumination or light system are the condenser and the diaphragm, which were explained earlier under Substage.

Care, cautions, and maintenance

1. When carrying the microscope, hold it by the arm with one hand, supporting the bottom of the microscope base with the other.

2. Handle the microscope gently, taking care to avoid sharp knocks.

3. Do not try to adjust the microscope yourself if you do not fully understand its mechanism. You may throw the instrument out of balance and adjustment or damage the lens by hitting it on the stage.

4. Never force the adjustment knobs if they do not turn easily. They may need oiling or simple adjustment.

5. Never force a high-powered objective on a microscope slide. Doing so may break the slide, scratch the objective, or damage the lens.

6. Be sure that the lens of the objective is clean before attempting to do microscopic work. Do not leave dust, dirt, or finger marks on the lens surfaces. To clean the lens surfaces, remove dust with a soft-haired brush or gauze. Use a soft cotton cloth, lens tissue, or gauze lightly moistened with absolute alcohol (methanol or ethanol) only for removing finger marks or grease. For cleaning the objectives and immersion oil, use only xylene. For cleaning the surface of the entrance lens of the eyepiece tube, use absolute alcohol. Observe sufficient caution in handling alcohol and xylene.

7. Avoid the use of any organic solvent (for example, thinner, ether, alcohol, or xylene) for cleaning the painted surfaces and plastic parts of the instrument. Mild soap and water may be used on these parts.

8. Avoid using the microscope in a dusty place or where it is subject to vibrations or exposed to high temperatures, moisture, or direct sunlight.

9. To avoid the possibility of impairing its operational efficiency and accuracy, never attempt to dismantle the instrument.

10. Direct your attention to protecting the objective lenses. Never leave immersion oil on the objective when the instrument is not being used. Before you put the microscope away, rotate the nosepiece so that the low-power objective is in position.

11. Remove the eye lens at regular intervals to clean out the dust and dirt particles that may have collected.

12. When the microscope is not in use, cover it with the accessory vinyl cover and store it in a place free from moisture and fungus. Keeping the objectives and eyepieces in an airtight container containing desiccant (a substance that promotes dryness) is especially recommended.

13. Contact the salesperson for any serious problems you may have with the instrument.

Space for Using the Microscope

The microscope should be kept set up and ready for use. However limited the office laboratory area is, sufficient space must be allotted exclusively for the use of the microscope. It need be no more than a shelf wide enough to accommodate the equipment. Added to this should be a convenient seat of *proper height*. A kitchen stool will suffice. Trying to work with the microscope handicapped by improper relationship between the height of the worktable and stool is fatiguing and may lead to unreliable work.

FIGURE 10-5   Technologist using microscope.

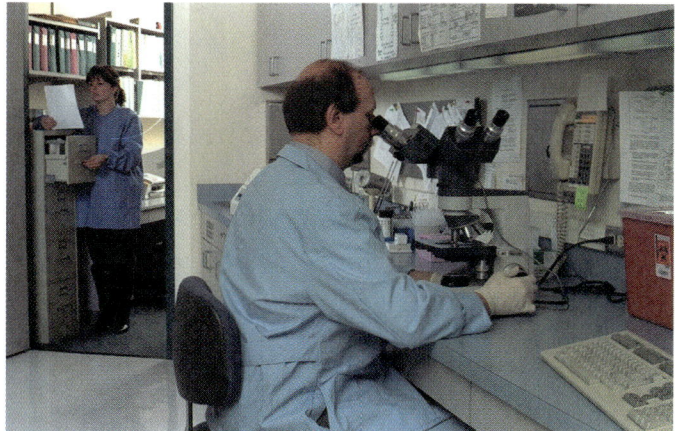

FIGURE 10-5   Technologist using microscope.

Use of the Microscope (Figure 10-5)

Place the material to be examined under the microscope on a glass slide. Place the slide on the microscope stage and fasten it with the clips or hold it in place by the mechanical stage. Using the lowest power objective and a 10× eyepiece, slowly lower the microscope head by using the coarse-focusing knob. When you find the field, adjust the light by raising or lowering the pinion attached to the substage. Next, open or close the diaphragm to admit just the proper amount of light to give a clear, distinct field. To make the field of vision clear, use the fine-adjustment knob. From this point on, you can obtain a higher power of magnification by changing the objective.

Proper Adjustment of Illumination

The problem of obtaining maximum efficiency of illumination remains. Two factors enter into this problem: the light itself and the manipulation of the diaphragm, which controls the amount of light admitted to the condenser.

To know when the illumination has been properly adjusted, place a slide on the microscope and focus the low-power lens on it. Remove the ocular and look down the tube of the microscope at the lenses of the objective. If shadows appear in this field, try to eliminate them by raising and lowering the condenser.

The most difficult part of illumination seems to be the proper manipulation of the iris diaphragm. Two cardinal principles should be remembered. First, the lower the power of the objective used, the more the light should be cut. In using the 16-mm lens to examine urine sediment or to count leukocytes, the diaphragm should be closed almost completely; when the 4-mm objective is brought into play, the opening should be slightly increased; and when using the oil-immersion objective, the diaphragm may be opened wide. Second, the more brilliantly stained the object being viewed, the more light you can admit. As an example, if a differential blood count is being made with the 4-mm lens (the high dry power), the diaphragm may be at least half open; whereas during the examination of urinary sediment, especially if seeking hyaline casts, the light should be cut almost completely off. If this is not done, these hyaline structures will not be seen. *The diaphragm should be*

constantly adjusted while an examination is being made to obtain the most revealing picture. It is controlled by a little lever below the condenser. You should learn to locate this lever and manipulate it subconsciously because the fine adjustment is kept in constant use while focusing. If you are having trouble with an examination and things are not seen as clearly as they should be, examine the amount of light being admitted. The trouble is not infrequently caused by improper adjustment of the diaphragm.

Focusing

In the microscopes illustrated in Figure 10-4, a coarse- and a fine-adjustment control are seen; the larger, coarse-adjustment knob is placed behind the smaller, which is for fine adjustment. The coarse adjustment is for finding the relative focus; the fine adjustment is for bringing out the details clearly. **Do not use these interchangeably.** Using the coarse adjustment for fine focusing results in broken cover glasses and slides; *trying to find a field with the fine adjustment places too much strain on it and quickly wears it out.*

Place a slide on the stage and bring the low or high dry power objective down until it almost touches. Then, while looking into the microscope, slowly raise it with the coarse adjustment until the image is seen. Using the fine adjustment, bring out the details as described. A good technique is to never turn the fine adjustment more than two thirds of one revolution. Keeping the slide moving on the stage while attempting to focus is often helpful. If this is not done, you may find that you are trying to focus on a spot where there is no material.

If a clear image cannot be obtained even though the illumination has been found satisfactory, rotate the eyepiece. If the blur is seen to rotate, the eyepiece is the source of the trouble. Remove it and wipe it thoroughly. Clean the upper portion frequently because it becomes soiled from contact with the eyelashes. If the difficulty is not in the ocular, then the back of the objective may have become fogged. This is not an infrequent occurrence if the instrument has been brought into a warm room from a cold one. Another possibility is that the objective has been dipped into some fluid—immersion oil or water—and this has dried and caused fogging. Water can be removed with moistened lens tissue, and the lens can then be polished dry. If oil has dried on the lens, remove it cautiously with the smallest possible amount of xylene and wipe away the excess of this reagent lens tissue.

Never focus down while looking through the microscope. This is inviting disaster to slides and cover glasses, as well as possible damage to the lens. Observe from one side when you do focus down.

Use of Objectives

Of the three objectives, which are designated 16 mm, 4 mm, and 1.8 mm, respectively, the 16-mm is the shortest in length and has the widest lens. The objective is used for low-power work, principally examining urine sediment, counting leukocytes, and inspecting the counting chamber of red cells for irregularity of distribution *(but only an expert should use it for counting these cells).* The 4-mm lens, the high dry, is mostly used for close inspection of the urinary sediment, counting red blood cells, and making routine differential blood cell counts.

Always use a cover glass when using the high dry power objective for examining urinary sediment. Do not dip the lens into the fluid without this protection. When using the 4-mm objective for differential blood counts, spread a thin film of immersion oil on the slide, over the stained blood, before making the examination.

The oil-immersion lens (1.8 mm) is used for obtaining the highest magnification in a conventional light microscope. Used with the eyepiece that gives a magnification of 10 diameters (marked 10×), the object as seen is about 1000 times its actual size. To use this lens, place a drop of immersion oil (such as Nujol) on the slide and focus down with coarse adjustment until the tip of the lens just touches the oil. Now, look through the microscope and focus upward very slowly with the coarse adjustment. When the object is seen, bring it into proper detail by use of the fine adjustment. This lens is used for all types of bacteriologic work, for seeking parasites, and for all other purposes demanding high magnification (see Table 10-1).

Practical Pointers for Microscope Use

If a single-tube microscope is used, learn to work with both eyes open. Squinting or closing one eye causes unnecessary strain. If much work is done, frequently shift from one eye to the other.

If you wear glasses, learn to do microscopy without them if possible. The instrument can focus to compensate for your visual defects if you are nearsighted or farsighted. On the other hand, if astigmatism is your difficulty, you have to wear glasses because this difficulty cannot be corrected by the microscopic lens.

CENTRIFUGES

Centrifuges are motorized devices that rotate at a high speed (Figure l0-6). The speed is stated as **revolutions per minute (rpm).** Centrifuges are used to separate components of varying densities contained in liquids by spinning them at high speeds. Through centrifugal (moving away from a center) force, heavier or solid components move to the lower part of the container, and lighter substances move to the upper part of the container. By this process the two substances, solid material and fluid supernatant, are separated. The supernatant is the clear upper portion of the mixture after it has been centrifuged.

Centrifuges are used in every department of a clinical laboratory. In a physician's office or health care agency, centrifuges are used if a microscopic analysis of urine is performed and also when serum or plasma is required for hematology or blood chemistry laboratory tests.

Numerous types of centrifuges are available. Each must be selected according to the intended use. Centrifuges commonly used in a physician's office or clinic are table models. One type is used for routine blood and urine separations (see Figure 10-6), and another type is used for microhematocrit applications. The **speed** at which these centrifuges operate varies from

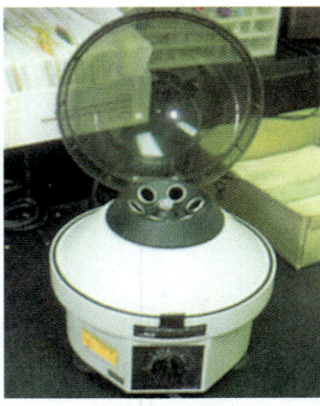

FIGURE 10-6 Centrifuge used for blood and urine separations.

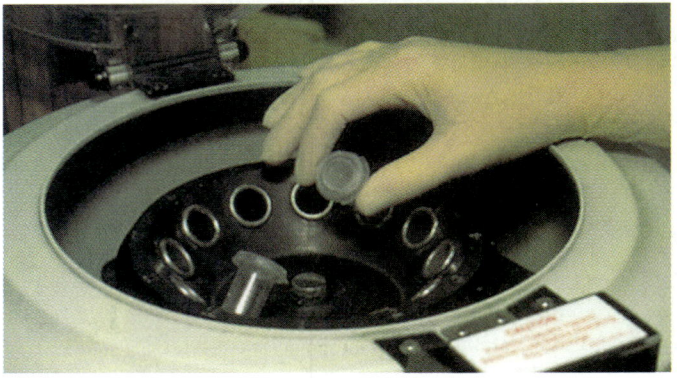

FIGURE 10-7 Placing specimen tubes in centrifuge.

3200 rpm for the routine blood and urine separations to 11,500 to 15,000 rpm for the microhematocrit centrifuges. You should use special **centrifuge tubes** in the centrifuges for serum or urine separations. These tubes are either conical or round-bottomed and made of a special quality glass. You can also put some Vacutainer tubes used for blood collection into the centrifuge. Use capillary tubes in the microhematocrit centrifuges. Remember to *always* use tubes that are the correct size and strength for the required application.

The centrifuge contains special centrifuge cups with rubber cushions that are used to hold the tubes containing the blood or urine samples. Be certain that the cushions are at the bottom of the holders before you place the tubes into them.

Placement of Tubes in the Centrifuge

When you place a tube containing a specimen into the centrifuge, you must counterbalance it with a tube of similar design and weight. The other tube must be placed directly opposite the tube containing the specimen and should contain a liquid of equal weight. Water can usually be used for this purpose (Figure 10-7). If you do not balance the load in a centrifuge, the centrifuge may vibrate severely, and you may lose the specimens. *Do not* use tubes that are cracked or badly scratched because they may break under the stress of the centrifugal force. If the tubes do break, immediately turn off the centrifuge. Don rubber gloves and clean the centrifuge cushion and cup. You must clean these areas before using the centrifuge again to avoid additional breakage.

Operating the Centrifuge

When you operate the centrifuge, you must close the cover. (Many newer models will not work if you do not close the cover.) If you are using an older-model centrifuge, do not open the cover until the rotor has completely stopped. Do not brake sharply when using centrifuges that operate with hand brakes. Always use tubes that are the correct size and strength for the required application. Electrical appliances such as the centrifuge should have three-pronged grounding plugs, and sufficiently grounded outlets should be available. Frequent lubrication, calibration, and cleaning are necessary for the proper operation of all centrifuges. Specific instructions for operating each centrifuge are provided by the manufacturer. Read these instructions completely and carefully before you operate any centrifuge.

CONCLUSION

With the advances in the knowledge of physiology and improved technology, scientific, diagnostic and therapeutic procedures have increasingly become valuable aids to the physician and the patient. From all the diagnostic and therapeutic procedures presented in the preceding chapters and in Chapters 11 through 16, you can see that modern medicine offers many methods to physicians for arriving at a diagnosis and treating disease processes. The functional and structural alterations of body tissues, organs, and systems in disease can be studied and treated. Great strides have been made and even greater achievements are expected as the mysteries of scientific research continue to unfold. At the opposite end of the spectrum from the concept of disease is health. For the body to remain healthy, the functions of the body systems must be normal. A primary requirement for survival of the human organism is the maintenance and safeguarding of the anatomic and physiologic equilibrium of the individual cells that make up the sum of the body and its parts.

Numerous sources are available for expanding your knowledge on the topics discussed in the following chapters. Check with your instructor for additional enrichment assignments and references in areas of your own particular need and interest.

REVIEW OF VOCABULARY

Using the information presented in this chapter and other reference sources of your own choice, read and define the italicized terms.

All clinical laboratories have certain specialized departments in common. They are divided into areas on the basis of function and types of tests performed. These areas usually include *hematology, urinalysis, serology, blood banking, medical microbiology, and clinical chemistry. Parasitology* and examination of feces may be special departments, or they may be included in one previously mentioned. Some laboratories may also have special areas for *histology, mycology, immunochemistry, and cytology.*

Correct labeling of a specimen and completing a *laboratory requisition* are important duties of the medical assistant when sending specimens to *outside laboratories.*

One of three formats can be used for recording and organizing information and test results in the patient's record: the *source-oriented format, the integrated format, or the problem-oriented format.*

Special care must be given to the *microscope* and *centrifuge* when using these pieces of equipment for laboratory work.

CLIA 1988 focuses specifically on *standards* set for *laboratory test performance.*

The following are two cumulative laboratory reports received in the physician's office. Identify the following information that should be included in all laboratory reports.

1. Name and address of the physician that ordered the laboratory work
2. Patient's name and medical record number
3. Date the specimen was collected
4. Time that the specimen was received by the laboratory
5. Laboratory accession number
6. Type of specimen
7. Name and result of the laboratory test performed

Clinical Laboratory Report

SAWYER-WESTMAN CLINICAL LABORATORIES

08/15/00   CUMULATIVE SUMMARY

11:39

                                                                PATIENT'S NAME

                                                                Jack Green

                                                                MEDICAL RECORD NUMBER

                                                                857621

ACCT: 9899   LOC: SERVICE: DOB: 09/21/47

AGE: 50Y   SEX: M   DR.: Clint Barry, MD   CODE: 7691

                        PARASITOLOGY (CONTINUED)

07/24/00

R1210   ACC. NO.:00129   TRANSPORT TIME: UNKNOWN HRS   *** STATUS: FINAL 07/29/00 ***

SPECIMEN DESCRIPTION: STOOL

COMMENT: NONE

EXAMINED BY: 1. CONCENTRATION AND PERMANENT STAIN

RESULT: 1. NO OVA OR PARASITES SEEN.

07/24/00

R1210   ACC. NO.:00130   TRANSPORT TIME: UNKNOWN HRS   *** STATUS: FINAL 07/29/00 ***

SPECIMEN DESCRIPTION: STOOL

COMMENT: NONE

EXAMINED BY: 1. CONCENTRATION AND PERMANENT STAIN

RESULT: 1. NO OVA OR PARASITES SEEN.

07/29/00

R1535   ACC. NO.:01020   TRANSPORT TIME: UNKNOWN HRS   *** STATUS: FINAL 08/05/00 ***

SPECIMEN DESCRIPTION: STOOL

COMMENT: NONE

EXAMINED BY: 1. CONCENTRATION AND PERMANENT STAIN

RESULT: 1. NO OVA OR PARASITES SEEN.

                              CONTINUED

08/15/00 11:39   CUMULATIVE SUMMARY

Sawyer-Westman

Clinical Laboratories   CLINICAL LABORATORIES REPORT

                                                   James Lawrence, MD, DIRECTOR

Clinical Laboratory Report

SAWYER-WESTMAN CLINICAL LABORATORIES

06/15/00   CUMULATIVE SUMMARY

11:38

                                                                    PATIENT'S NAME

                                                                    James White

                                                                    MEDICAL RECORD NUMBER

                                                                    89638

ACCT: 98956   LOC: 7D   SERVICE: DOB: 04/04/77

AGE: 21Y   SEX: M   DR.: Donald Wise, MD   CODE: 5629

ADM: 04/11/00

DSC: 04/15/00

AFB-RESPIRATORY CULTURES

04/11/00

R1634 ACC. NO.:123 TRANSPORT TIME: UNKNOWN HRS   *** STATUS: FINAL 06/10/00 ***

SPECIMEN DESCRIPTION: SPUTUM

COMMENT: NONE

MICROSCOPIC EXAM: 1. NO ACID FAST BACILLI SEEN (CONCENTRATED SMEAR)

RESULT: 1. NO ACID FAST BACILLI RECOVERED AT 60 DAYS

04/13/00

R1446 ACC. NO.: 899 TRANSPORT TIME: UNKNOWN HRS   *** STATUS: FINAL 06/10/00 ***

SPECIMEN DESCRIPTION: SPUTUM

COMMENT: NONE

MICROSCOPIC EXAM: 1. NO ACID FAST BACILLI SEEN (CONCENTRATED SMEAR)

RESULT: 1. NO ACID FAST BACILLI RECOVERED AT 58 DAYS

04/14/00

0630   ACC. NO.: 979   TRANSPORT TIME: 1.8 HRS   *** STATUS: FINAL 06/10/00 ***

SPECIMEN DESCRIPTION: SPUTUM

COMMENT: NONE

MICROSCOPIC EXAM: 1. NO ACID FAST BACILLI SEEN (CONCENTRATED SMEAR)

RESULT: 1. NO ACID FAST BACILLI RECOVERED AT 57 DAYS

                                    CONTINUED

James White

06/15/00 11:38   CHART COPY CUMULATIVE SUMMARY

Sawyer-Westman   CLINICAL LABORATORIES REPORT Clinical Laboratories

Clinical Laboratories   James Lawrence, MD, DIRECTOR

CRITICAL THINKING SKILLS REVIEW

1. State the importance of the information gathered from clinical laboratory tests.
2. List six specialized departments common to all clinical laboratories. Describe the function of each department.
3. Describe the medical assistant's responsibilities when dealing with a commercial clinical laboratory.
4. List seven items that are to be included on a laboratory requisition that accompanies a specimen to the laboratory.
5. Explain to a new staff member when you would use a laboratory test directory.
6. Discuss the Clinical Laboratory Improvement Amendments (CLIA) of 1988. State the primary purpose of CLIA.
7. State the three levels of tests that were established by CLIA for laboratory tests.
8. Explain the concept of quality control to a new member on staff at the clinic where you are working.
9. Discuss proficiency testing with another medical assistant.
10. If a physician's office laboratory *only* performs waived tests, what type of certificate must it apply for before laboratory tests are performed?
11. Describe how reports would be filed in the source-oriented record.
12. List seven safety rules that should be adhered to when working with laboratory equipment and specimens.
13. State how you should carry a microscope.
14. State what type of tubes should be used in a centrifuge.

PERFORMANCE TEST

In a skills laboratory, a simulation of a joblike environment, the medical assistant student is to demonstrate the correct procedure for the following without reference to source materials.

1. Demonstrate proper use and care of a microscope.
2. Demonstrate proper use and care of a centrifuge.
3. Given sample laboratory requisitions and physician's orders, correctly complete each requisition to be sent to the laboratory along with a specimen.
4. Demonstrate the use of safety rules when working with laboratory equipment and specimens.
5. Demonstrate the use of commercial control products to check the reliability of test products and test results.

The student is expected to perform these skills with 100% accuracy 90% of the time.

The successful completion of each procedure will demonstrate competency levels as required by the AAMA, AMT, and future employers.

INTERNET RESOURCES

National Association for Healthcare Quality
www.nahq.org

American Liver Foundation
www.info@liverfoundation.org

United Network for Organ Sharing
www.unos.org

Bugs in the News (information about microbiology in a user-friendly style)
http://falcon.cc.ukans.edu/~jbrown/bugs.html

United States National Library of Medicine (information on general health)
www.nlm.nih.gov/medlineplus

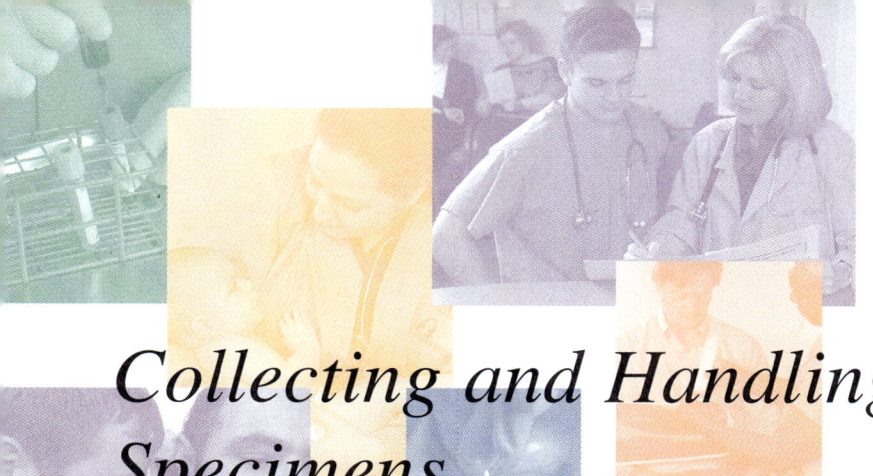

Collecting and Handling Specimens

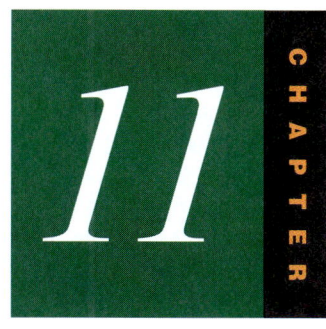

11 CHAPTER

■ Cognitive Objectives

On completion of Chapter 11, the medical assistant student should be able to:

1. Define, spell, and pronounce the vocabulary terms listed.
2. Discuss the proper care, handling, transporting, and storing of all specimens.
3. List the information that must be included on a laboratory requisition when sending a specimen for examination.
4. Explain how a specimen should be prepared for transportation through the mail to an outside laboratory.
5. List the purposes, basic equipment, and supplies required and the medical assistant's usual assisting responsibilities for each procedure described in this chapter.
6. Discuss the definition of "fasting" with reference to the collection of a specimen from a patient.
7. Discuss steps and precautionary measures that should be used to prevent infection from a specimen.
8. Discuss techniques and methods that must be used to prevent contamination of a patient specimen.
9. State and define seven types of urine specimens and discuss at least 10 general facts relating to the collection of urine for examination.
10. Discuss the hemoccult slide test for stool specimens, stating why and how it is done; the special diagnostic diet that the patient may be on before and during the test; and medications that would interfere with the test.
11. Differentiate between upper and lower respiratory tract specimens.
12. Differentiate between a smear, a culture, and a culture medium.
13. Briefly discuss the Gram stain and the culture and sensitivity tests performed for bacteriologic studies.
14. List seven types of smears that may be done to detect vaginal disorders and diseases.
15. Discuss patient care before and after a lumbar puncture.
16. State the cause and list at least four common signs and symptoms of a strep throat infection. Discuss complications that could result if not treated in the early stages of infection.
17. Discuss an example of a screening laboratory test that may be used to diagnose strep throat while the patient is in the physician's office or clinic.
18. Briefly discuss the causes, signs and symptoms, diagnostic methods used, treatment, and complications that can result for the sexually transmitted diseases discussed in this chapter.
19. Explain what the OraSure test is, what it is used for, and how it is performed.

■ Terminal Performance Objectives

On completion of Chapter 11, the medical assistant student should be able to:

1. Demonstrate correct technique and proper communication to the patient for collecting the following specimens, preparing them to be sent to the laboratory, and completing the appropriate requisition form for the tests that are ordered:
   a. Urine specimen
   b. Stool specimen
   c. Sputum specimen
   d. Throat culture
   e. Nasopharyngeal culture
   f. Wound culture
   g. Vaginal smears and cultures
2. Demonstrate the correct technique for making a smear for cytology studies and a smear for bacteriology studies.
3. Demonstrate the correct technique for performing a QuickVue In-Line One-Step Strep A diagnostic test that is used to diagnose strep throat.
4. Demonstrate the correct procedure for performing a Gram stain.
5. Demonstrate the correct procedure for performing a hemoccult slide test on a stool specimen.
6. Demonstrate the correct technique for inoculating a culture medium with a specimen obtained on a cotton-tipped applicator.

7. Demonstrate the proper procedure for assisting with a lumbar puncture.

8. Demonstrate the correct method for recording information on a patient's medical record after the specimen has been sent to the laboratory.

9. Demonstrate the correct method for completing various types of laboratory requisition forms that accompany a specimen that is sent to the laboratory.

10. Provide instructions and patient education that is within the professional scope of a medical assistant's training and responsibilities as assigned.

The student is to perform these objectives with 100% accuracy 95% of the time.

The consistent use of Universal/Standard Precautions is required by all health care professionals in all health care settings as a method of infection control. It is assumed that these precautions are used in all of the following procedures. Review Chapter 1 if you have any questions on methods to use because the methods or techniques are not repeated in detail in each procedure presented in this chapter.

Be sure to consult the latest guidelines issued by the Centers for Disease Control and Prevention and consult with infection control practitioners when necessary to identify specific precautions that pertain to your particular work situation.

VOCABULARY

aerobe (a'er-ob)—A microorganism that lives and grows in the presence of free oxygen.

aerobic (aero'bic)—Capable of living and functioning in the presence of free oxygen.

anaerobe (an-a'er-ob)—A microorganism that lives and grows in the absence of oxygen.

anaerobic (an'aero'bik)—Capable of living and functioning without oxygen or air.

bacteriology (bak-te"e-ol'o-je)—The study of bacteria.

bacteriolysis (bak-te"re-ol'i-sis)—The destruction of bacteria.

biochemistry (bi"o-kem'is-tre)—The study of chemical changes occurring in living organisms.

culture (kul'tur)—The reproduction or growth of microorganisms or of living tissue cells in special laboratory media (the material on which the organisms grow) conducive to (to promote) their growth. Various types of cultures include the following:

blood culture—Used in the diagnosis of specific infectious diseases. Blood is withdrawn from a vein and placed in or on suitable culture media; then it is determined whether pathogens grow in the media. If organisms do grow, they are identified by bacteriologic methods.

gelatin culture—A culture of bacteria on gelatin.

hanging drop culture—A culture in which the bacteria are inoculated into a drop of fluid on a coverglass and then mounted into the depression on a concave slide.

negative culture—A culture made from suspected material that fails to reveal the suspected microorganism.

positive culture—A culture that reveals the suspected microorganism.

pure culture—A culture of a single microorganism.

smear culture—A culture prepared by smearing the specimen across the surface of the culture medium.

stab culture—A bacterial culture made by thrusting a needle inoculated with the microorganisms under examination deep into the culture medium.

streak culture—A bacterial culture in which the infectious material is implanted in streaks across the culture medium.

tissue culture—The growing of tissue cells in artificial nutrient medium.

type culture—A culture that is generally agreed to represent microorganisms of a particular species.

culture medium—A commercial preparation used for the growth of microorganisms or other cells. (Types of culture media are described in this chapter.)

Culturette—A commercially prepared bacterial culture collection/transport system, consisting of a sterile plastic tube with applicator. Modified Stuart's transport medium is held in a glass ampule at the bottom end to ensure stability of medium at the time of use. Transport medium is released only after the sample is taken, by crushing the ampule. A moist environment (not immersion) is maintained up to 72 hours to preserve the specimen (see Figure 11-8).

Culturette II culture collection system—Identical to the Culturette, with the exception that the plastic tube contains two applicators and the ampule contains twice the medium (1 ml) (see Figure 11-8).

anaerobic Culturette culture collection system—This system offers the same basic properties of the Culturette, plus a standardized and dependable anaerobic environment for transport of anaerobic bacteria. Once released, the transport medium maintains an anaerobic environment for up to 48 hours. Many laboratories request that the anaerobic culture system be used when taking a wound culture.

cytology (si-tol'o-je)—The study of the structure and function of cells.

dysplasia (dis-pla'ze-ah)—An abnormal development of tissue.

fixation of a smear—Spraying with or immersing a slide into a special solution, or drying the slide over a flame, or air-drying to harden and preserve the bacteria for future microscopic examination.

histology (his-tol'o-je)—The study of the microscopic form and structure of tissue.

incubation (in-ku-ba'shun)—When pertaining to bacteriology, this term refers to the period of culture development.

VOCABULARY—cont'd

inoculate (i-nok'u-lat)—In microbiology, this refers to the introduction of infectious matter into a culture medium in an effort to produce growth of the causative organism.

macroscopic (mak-ro-skop'ik) **examination**—An examination in which the specimen is large enough to be seen by the naked eye.

medical microbiology—The study and identification of pathogens and the development of effective methods for their control or elimination (see also Chapter 2).

microorganism (mi-kro-or'gan-ism)—A minute, living body not visible to the naked eye, especially a bacterium or protozoan; these are viewed with a microscope.

microscopic (mi-kro-skop'ik) **examination**—An examination in which the specimen is visible only with the aid of a microscope.

pathogen (path'o-jen)—A disease-producing substance or microorganism.

pathogenic (path'o-jen'ic)—Pertaining to a disease-producing microorganism or substance.

serologic (se-ro-loj'ik) **test**—A laboratory test involving the examination and study of blood serum.

smear (smer)—Material spread thinly across a slide or culture medium with a swab, loop, or another slide in preparation for microscopic study.

specimen (spec'i-men)—A small part or sample taken to show kind and quality of the whole (for example, a specimen of urine, blood, or other body excretions) or a small piece of tissue for macroscopic and microscopic examinations.

sputum (spu'tum)—A mucous secretion from the trachea, bronchi, and lungs ejected through the mouth, in contrast with saliva, which is the secretion of the salivary glands.

stool (stool)—Body waste material discharged from the large intestine; also called feces or bowel movement.

swab (swob)—A small piece of cotton or gauze wrapped around the end of a slender stick used for applying medications, cleansing cavities, or obtaining a piece of tissue or body secretion for bacteriologic examination; also called cotton-tipped applicator.

urine (u'rine)—The fluid containing certain waste products and water that is secreted by the kidneys, stored in the bladder, and excreted through the urethra.

viable (vi'ah-bl)—Able to maintain an independent existence.

The science of laboratory technology is becoming increasingly sophisticated in methods used to process specimens obtained from a patient. Thus rarely will you be required to perform the actual tests on collected specimens in a physician's office or health agency, other than simple tests that may be performed several times a day, such as a routine urinalysis. The Clinical Laboratory Improvement Amendments (CLIA) of 1988 have established three categories of laboratory tests on the basis of the complexity of the test. To perform tests under each category, the laboratory must meet certain personnel standards, and each state may establish stricter standards. These regulations in each state determine which laboratory tests you can perform. (See also Chapter 10, pp. 450-453, and Boxes 10-1 through 10-3.) Most physicians use the services of professional laboratories, which can perform tests under controlled conditions with expensive equipment that is impractical for the physician's office. Often the patient is referred to a clinical laboratory, where the specimen is obtained and processed and the results prepared for report to the physician. At other times, the medical assistant must collect the specimen or assist the physician when obtaining the specimen. Once the specimen has been properly obtained, your responsibility is to ensure that it is preserved and labeled correctly for submission to the laboratory for examination. Therefore it is imperative that you know how to collect various types of specimens and prepare a smear or culture from the specimen so that specimens arrive at the laboratory in good condition for processing. When collecting specimens, you must also be aware of any special preparation that is required by the patient, ensure that the patient is thoroughly informed and understands the instructions (for example, collect the first morning specimen or fast 12 hours before collection of the specimen), ascertain that this preparation has been followed, and be certain that the correct equipment is used for the specimen obtained. Most professional laboratories furnish manuals, often called laboratory test directories, on request, which outline the specific requirements for each study to be performed. In this chapter, you learn techniques for obtaining and for helping the physician obtain different types of specimens, smears, and cultures, in addition to the care and handling of specimens.

Before beginning this chapter, review the infectious disease process, Universal/Standard Precautions, infection control, and medical and surgical aseptic techniques presented in Chapters 1, 2, and 6.

SPECIMENS

Samples of body fluids, secretions, excretions, or tissues can be removed from a patient's body for laboratory study. These materials, once removed, are called **specimens**. Serologic, biochemical, and microscopic tests can be performed on all body specimens. These tests provide a means for evaluating the patient's health status and identifying pathogenic microorganisms and other abnormalities present. Once the suspected cause of a disease process is determined, appropriate methods of treatment can be provided.

Instructions to the Patient and Special Preparation

A specimen should be collected at the onset of a disease or condition and, when possible, before the administration of any antibiotics when an infectious process is suspected. Often the active participation of a patient is required to obtain a specimen; therefore you must give appropriate instructions. Explain the procedure that is to be used in collecting the specimen (such as urine, sputum, or stool) completely and accurately.

Some tests require **special preparation** by the patient, and again you must give the appropriate instructions, along with an explanation of the necessity for following these instructions. An informed patient usually is more cooperative in following specific directions, which in turn facilitates accurate test results. Special preparation usually means a modification in diet, or a period of fasting before the specimen collection, or medication restrictions. The time of day the specimen is to be collected may be specific; that is, the first morning urine is to be collected. **Fasting** means abstaining from *all* food, gum, cigarettes, and fluids except water for usually 12 to 14 hours before the specimen is collected. Fasting specimens are generally collected in the morning for the patient's convenience.

Some medications interfere with test results. When feasible, a patient may be advised by the physician to discontinue the medication for 48 to 72 hours before certain urine tests and for 4 to 24 hours before some blood tests. When it is not medically advisable for the patient to go without the medication for any length of time, a notation must be made on the laboratory requisition regarding what drug and the amount of drug that the patient is taking. This information alerts the laboratory to the presence of the drug. At times the laboratory may be able to use a different method of testing that would not be altered by the presence of the medication. For women, the use of vaginal medications, douches, or the time of the menstrual flow should be avoided when vaginal specimens are to be obtained.

It is often advisable to write out the specific directions for patients so that they have an accurate reminder of the special requirements for each test to be performed in addition to the time and date of the test. For some tests you may have preprinted instruction forms to give to the patient.

Caring for, Handling, Transporting, and Storing Specimens

Essential considerations to remember with regard to each specimen follow. See earlier Vocabulary section for types of collection and transport systems used.

1. *Review and follow the Centers for Disease Control and Prevention Universal/Standard Precautions in Chapter 1. Universal/Standard Precautions* is an approach to infection control. According to this concept, all human blood and other body fluids (such as semen, vaginal secretions, cerebrospinal fluid, pleural fluid, pericardial fluid, peritoneal fluid, amniotic fluid, saliva in dental procedures, any body fluid that is visibly contaminated with blood, and *all* body fluids, secretions, and excretions except sweat) in situations in which it is difficult or impossible to differentiate between body fluids are treated as if known to be infectious for human immunodeficiency virus (HIV), hepatitis B virus (HBV), and other bloodborne and other pathogens. Wear gloves for handling specimens at all times.

2. *The specimen must be properly labeled and placed in the correct container.* Place each specimen in the proper container or solution that is designed for the type of material collected with the lid fastened securely. Label the container with the specimen with the patient's name, the date, the source of the specimen, and the attending physician's name.

   Place specimens of blood or other potentially infectious materials in containers that prevent leakage during collection, handling, processing, storage, transport, or shipping. Label or color-code these containers before they leave your facility unless you place them in red bags or red containers, which may substitute for labels. The label must bear the legend *BIOHAZARD* and must be fluorescent orange or orange-red or predominantly so, with lettering or symbols in a contrasting color. Affix the labels as close as possible to the container by adhesive, wire, string, or other method that prevents their loss or unintentional removal. You must also affix these warning labels to refrigerators and freezers that contain blood or other potentially infectious materials (Figure 11-1).

3. *The specimen must be protected when it is sent to outside laboratories or through the mail.* Most outside laboratories provide specific instructions for transporting specimens to them. You must place and secure specimens that are sent to outside laboratories through the mail in a proper transport container. This special container protects and preserves the specimen for examination. Close the container securely and wrap it in a protective covering, such as corrugated cardboard or cotton, which absorbs shock or possible leakage. Place the wrapped specimen container in a watertight metal container (Figure 11-2), which is then placed with a laboratory requisition into a stiff cardboard mailing container that has shock-resistant insulating material (Figure 11-3). The outside of this container must have a label that identifies it as a medical specimen.

4. *The specimen must be uncontaminated.* To prevent addition of microorganisms to the specimen obtained from the patient, use sterile containers, sterile applicators, or other

FIGURE 11-1 Biohazard label in fluorescent orange or orange-red with lettering or symbols in a contrasting color.

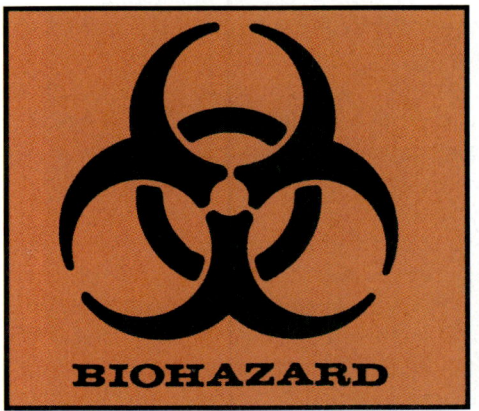

sterile devices, as well as clean or sterile techniques to collect the specimen.

a. Do *not* use cracked or broken containers and applicators.

b. Use only regulation tops or plugs on stopper bottles and test tubes. Do *not* use cotton balls or gauze as a substitute. Many laboratories now use plastic-capped tubes, screw caps, and metal closure tubes; special vials or tubes with rubber stoppers are used for transporting suspected anaerobic organisms.

c. Discard plugs or the inner surface of tops that come in contact with an unsterile surface.

d. Fill containers only halfway. Do not allow the top or plug to become wet, either from the specimen or other sources, to prevent contamination to the specimen and to personnel handling it.

e. Do not spill specimen material on the outside of the container or on any surface. If outside contamination of the primary container occurs, place the primary container into a second container that prevents leakage during handling, processing, storage, transport, or shipping, and label or color-code it as discussed in

FIGURE 11-2 Wrap specimen container for mailing in corrugated cardboard or cotton and place in watertight metal container.

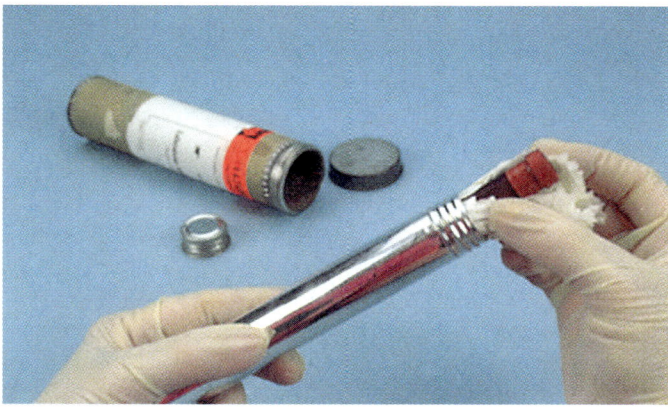

FIGURE 11-3 Place watertight metal container containing specimen and laboratory requisition into a stiff cardboard mailing container.

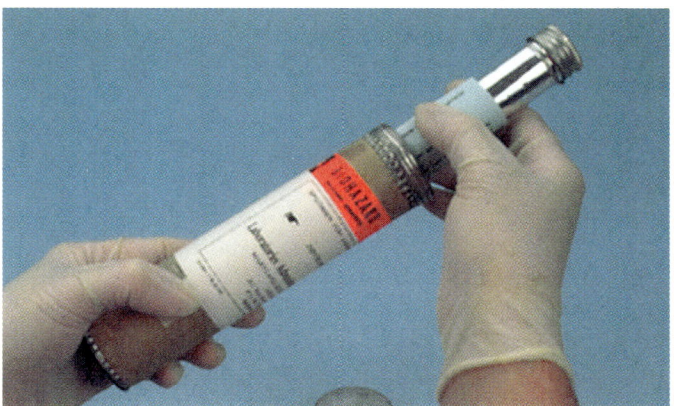

No. 2. This is for the protection of everyone handling the specimen or near the area. If a specimen is accidentally spilled, call the laboratory to inquire how to destroy the pathogens that may be in the specimen and what to use. You must clean the work area immediately. A disinfectant such as a 1:10 dilution of sodium hypochlorite (household bleach) or Bytech solution is often used to clean the area.

5. *Spills of blood and other body secretions:* Clean spills promptly. Wear gloves to clean up large spills; use paper towels, then place them in an infectious waste container. Then use 5.25% sodium hypochlorite (household bleach) diluted 1:10 to disinfect the area. Do not place sodium hypochlorite directly on large amounts of protein matter (for example, urine, stool, blood, or sputum) to protect yourself from noxious fumes. You may order a 1:10 dilution of bleach for the office or clinic from a hospital pharmacy.

6. *Laboratory procedures* should be adopted to prevent the formation of aerosols. Biologic safety cabinets (Class I or II) and other primary containment devices (for example, centrifuge safety cups) are advised whenever you conduct procedures that have a high potential for creating aerosols or infectious droplets. Follow other standard laboratory safety practices.

7. *The specimen must contain living organisms collected from the proper source and reach the laboratory in a condition suitable for culturing, incubating, or examining.* Specimens collected for a smear or culture may be taken from any body opening, whether natural, surgical, or accidental; for example, material may be collected from the ear, eye, nose, throat, urethra, vagina, rectum, or a wound. **Body fluids** such as urine, blood, and cerebrospinal fluid, as well as **samples of tissue** (biopsy), may also be obtained. To make sure that the pathogens remain viable (living), send all specimens to the laboratory for processing without delay. If there is a delay, keep most specimens in a refrigerator for a few hours. Generally you may store swabs from the throat, rectum, and wounds, as well as fecal (except do *not* refrigerate feces that are to be examined for the presence of ova and parasites) and sputum samples, in a refrigerator for several hours. Spinal fluid may contain organisms that are sensitive to cold; therefore place this specimen in a bacteriologic incubator and *not* in a refrigerator.

Swabs of infectious matter must be prevented from drying before they are processed in the laboratory. Sometimes the sterile swab is moistened with a broth or placed into tubes containing broth or a selected holding medium to prevent drying of the specimen. The broth is used to keep the air around the swab moist and is *not* a culture medium.

Use special procedures for preservation and growth when an anaerobic organism (one able to live in the absence of oxygen) is believed to be the causative agent. Processing these specimens *immediately* is vital to maintaining the organism in a viable state. When there is a delay, you may place inoculated culture plates, for example, cultures for gonorrhea, in a candle jar (see Figure 11-18) and then send them to the laboratory.

Urine specimens should be examined or sent to the laboratory immediately. If this is not possible, you must refrigerate them (see Nos. 8 and 9 under General Facts Relating to Urine Collection, which follows later in this chapter, and also Chapter 12).

Most **blood specimens** must be examined within 8 hours or less from the time they were collected—preferably, within 2 to 4 hours from the time they were collected. Blood for bacteriologic studies must be collected in special containers and must not be left unattended for any length of time. These specimens must be examined as soon as possible. Blood drawn for an electrolyte panel should be refrigerated if it is not tested immediately. Other blood samples may be left standing on the counter for 2 to 4 hours before testing, although some results may vary if the blood is left standing for 2 or more hours (see Chapter 13).

When a specimen is to be examined in the physician's office or clinic, it should be tested, cultured, or examined microscopically immediately.

8. *The specimen should be handled and transported in an upright position and should not be shaken.* Remember that failure to successfully identify pathogens may result from improper collection, care, and handling techniques.

9. *Avoid and prevent contamination to yourself and other personnel who will be handling the specimen.* All specimens obtained for microbiologic study are presumed to contain potentially dangerous pathogens. Always keep in mind the possibility of spreading the infectious pathogen, know the necessary protective measures that must be adhered to (as listed), and use excellent aseptic technique when obtaining the specimen. Disposable, single-use examination gloves must be worn for handling all specimens. In addition, adhere to the following rules:

   a. *Do not* eat, drink, or smoke while handling specimens because you could transmit pathogens to yourself by hand-to-mouth contact.

   b. *Do not* lick the label that will be placed on the specimen container.

   c. Wear gloves to cover any cut or scratch that you have.

   d. If you accidentally touch some of the specimen collected, immediately wash the contact area thoroughly with an antiseptic soap. If the contact area was on a cut or scratch, apply tincture of iodine or another antiseptic solution to the area. Report the incident to your supervisor or employer.

   e. At the end of each workday, clean the work area with a disinfectant solution.

10. *A laboratory requisition to accompany the specimen must always be filled out completely and accurately.* **The following information must be included:**

    a. Date (time of day if relevant; for example, an early morning specimen)

    b. Name of the patient, address, age, and sex

    c. Name of the attending physician and address

    d. Source of the specimen

    e. Name of laboratory test(s) to be performed

    f. A notation if the patient is already taking antibiotics. (False-negative results could be obtained if the antibiotic has suppressed the growth of the microorganism[s].)

    Additional information depends on the type of specimen obtained and may include the following:

    g. Clinical history

    h. Previous normal or abnormal results

    i. Previous surgery

    j. X-ray film treatment

    k. Clinical diagnosis

    For vaginal and cervical specimens, the following, if applicable, are also added:

    l. Hormone treatment

    m. Date of last menstrual period (LMP)

    n. Postpartum

    o. Postmenopausal

    p. Pregnant

    q. DES child (that is, if the mother took DES [diethylstilbestrol] when pregnant with the patient)

11. **All specimens from all patients, whether known to be infected or not, should be handled with caution** (see also Chapter 1).

URINE SPECIMEN COLLECTION

A specimen of urine is collected to perform a urinalysis (u″rinal′i-sis), which is an analysis of the physical, chemical, and microscopic properties of urine. The results of these examinations help determine renal (kidney) functions of the body, which in turn helps the physician diagnose and provide the appropriate treatment required for a disease process.

Many types of tests are used in analyzing urine to determine whether it contains abnormal substances indicative of disease (see Chapter 12 for urinalysis procedures). The most significant substances normally absent from urine and detected by a urinalysis are protein, glucose, acetone, blood, pus, casts, and bacteria.

Types of Urine Specimens

Random or spot specimen. To collect a random or spot specimen, the patient voids at any time of the day or night, collecting a portion of the urine in a clean container.

Fasting specimen. To collect a fasting specimen, the patient voids 4 or more hours after ingestion of food and discards this urine. The next voided specimen is collected and regarded as the fasting specimen.

First morning specimen. To collect a first morning specimen, the patient voids and discards the specimen before going to bed. On arising the next morning, the patient collects the first morning specimen.

Postprandial specimen. To collect a postprandial specimen, the patient voids after eating and collects this specimen.

urination (u-"ri-na'shun), **voiding, micturition** (mik"tu-rish'un)—The act of passing urine from the body.

diuresis (di"ur-re'sis)—An abnormal, increased secretion of urine as seen in diabetes mellitus, diabetes insipidus, or when large amounts of fluid have been drunk; this can be artificially produced by drugs with diuretic properties.

enuresis (en"u-re'sis)—The involuntary excretion of urine, especially at night during sleep; bedwetting; most often seen in children with either physical or emotional problems.

frequency—The need to urinate frequently. Urination at frequent short intervals without an increase in daily output. This is seen in cystitis and also with reduced bladder capacity.

incontinence (in-kon'ti-nens)—The inability to refrain from the urge to urinate. This may occur in times of stress, anxiety, anger, postoperatively; from obstructions that prevent the normal emptying of the urinary bladder, spasms of the bladder, irritation caused by injury or inflammation of the urinary tract, damage to the spinal cord or brain; or from the development of a fistula (an abnormal tubelike passage) between the bladder and the vagina or urethra.

urgency—A feeling of the need to urinate *immediately*.

Midstream specimen.

To collect a midstream specimen, the patient starts to void into the toilet or bedpan; then, without stopping the process of voiding, a portion of the urine is collected in a clean container. The last part of the urine flow is passed into the toilet or bedpan.

Clean-catch specimen.

To collect a clean-catch specimen, the patient washes the external genitalia with soap and water or some mild antiseptic solution. Then a midstream urine specimen is collected in a clean, dry container or in a sterile container if the specimen is being collected for bacterial examination. This yields a specimen with limited contamination by skin bacteria.

Multiple-glass specimens.

The multiple-glass test is performed on men to evaluate a lower urinary tract infection. The man must have a full bladder because three samples of urine are collected. To collect a multiple-glass specimen, the patient washes the area around the urinary meatus with an antiseptic solution. He then voids about 100 ml (approximately 3½ ounces) into a clean, dry container. This specimen contains microorganisms and sediment "washed" from the urethra. Without interrupting the voiding process, he then voids another 100 ml of urine into a second clean, dry container. This specimen contains microorganisms and sediment representative of that in the bladder and kidney. Then the man stops voiding, and the physician gently massages the prostate gland. After this, the third urine specimen is collected in a clean, dry container. This last specimen contains secretions from the prostate gland.

Timed specimen (24-hour specimen).

To collect a timed specimen, the patient discards the first morning specimen and then collects all urine for exactly 24 hours. (See No. 12, under General Facts Relating to Urine Collection.) Other timed specimens could be for 12 hours or as requested by the laboratory for specific examinations.

Drug screen specimen (urine toxicology screening).

A random urine specimen may be collected. Some laboratories require a midstream specimen. Only a small amount of urine is needed. For some tests the laboratory uses only 7 drops, but you should collect at least 1 ml. Always check with the laboratory for their requirements. Obtain as much information about the type and amount of drug taken and the time it was consumed (see Figure 10-1, *B,* on p. 455). **If the test is for medicolegal testing purposes, the patient must sign a consent form.**

Choice of collection type.

A specific type of urine collection can provide optimum information when performing certain tests; for example, postprandial urine can be used for testing sugar content, and first morning specimens can be used for testing protein content.

General Facts Relating to Urine Collection

1. To minimize bacterial and chemical contamination, use only clean, dry, or sterile collection containers. Disposable containers are ideal.

2. The early morning urine specimen is the most concentrated; therefore, if at all possible, this is the specimen that should be obtained for simple routine testing. The concentration of urine varies during a 24-hour period, partly as a result of the patient's food and water intake and level of activity.

3. A freshly voided specimen is adequate for *most* urinalyses when the first morning specimen cannot be obtained, although collection of a clean-catch midstream specimen is the method of choice.

4. To collect a freshly voided specimen in the office, give the patient a clean, wide-mouthed bottle and instruct him or her to void directly into it. Inform the patient how much urine you want in the bottle (that is, up to what point in the bottle you want collected). Usually 2 to 4 ounces is sufficient.

5. When urine is required for **bacterial cultures,** collect a clean-catch midstream specimen in a sterile container and submit it to the bacteriology laboratory department as soon as possible for testing.

6. Ask patients if they are taking any medications, and if so what type, and if they are on a special diet because certain medications and diets affect the findings of a urinalysis. NOTE: A note of medications or special diet should be recorded on the laboratory requisition and the patient's chart. When feasible, the physician may advise the patient to stop taking the medication for 48 to 72 hours before the test.

7. Inquire if a female patient is menstruating when a urine specimen is collected because if blood is found in the

urine, it may be from the vaginal canal rather than from the urinary tract. A note of this must also be recorded, and another specimen may be required when the patient has finished menstruating.

8. Voided specimens should not be left standing at room temperature because they become alkaline as a result of contamination by urea-splitting bacteria from the environment. Explain to the patient that refrigeration of the specimen is necessary if collected at home, until time to submit it for analysis. If examination is delayed in your office or the laboratory, the specimen should also be refrigerated.

9. **Microscopic and chemical examination** of urine should be performed *within 1 hour* after collection. Waiting for longer than 1 hour causes dissolution of cellular elements and casts and bacterial overgrowth, unless the specimen was obtained under sterile conditions.

    An increase in bacteria can cause changes that result in the pH measurement of urine changing from acidic to alkaline. The alkaline pH may lead to a false-positive protein test. If glucose was in the urine, it will decrease because when bacteria are present, they will use the glucose as food. If the specimen cannot be refrigerated or examined within 1 hour of urinating, preservatives can be used to prevent deterioration of the specimen.

10. When more than one specimen is required, number each specimen according to its sequence.

11. If the patient is **to collect the specimen at home,** you should have explained the following procedure previously.
    a. Use a thoroughly clean, 3- to 4-ounce container in which to collect the specimen.
    b. Boil the container that will be used for the collection for 20 minutes before using it.
    c. Do not use a container that has held drugs or other solutions that may make the specimen unsuitable for examination. Medical facilities that have specimen containers readily available may provide them to the patient.

12. When a **24-hour specimen** is required, it is vital that the patient understand the procedure. All urine must be collected within a 24-hour period.
    a. The first early morning specimen is discarded.
    b. All subsequent specimens are collected, including the first early morning specimen the next day.
    c. The last specimen is collected 24 hours after collection was started.
    d. Urine is collected in a clean bottle into which a preservative has been added. (Preservative is prescribed by the laboratory.) This bottle must be refrigerated or kept cold by placing it in a bucket of ice. Instruct the patient not to sniff the contents of the container, and if male, not to void directly into the container.

PROCEDURE 11-1

CLEAN-CATCH, MIDSTREAM, VOIDED SPECIMEN

Objective
Understand and demonstrate the correct procedure for instructing the patient how to obtain a clean-catch midstream urine specimen; prepare the specimen to be sent to the laboratory; and record the procedure on the patient's chart.

Equipment
Antiseptic solution or antiseptic wipes (such as povidone-iodine wipes) or soap and water
Washcloth

Sterile gauze sponges: 4 × 4 inch
Sterile specimen container (with cover) NOTE: Commercially prepared kits for collecting a midstream specimen are available. These kits contain a sterile specimen container and label, antiseptic wipes, and absorbent tissues.
Tissues
Laboratory requisition
Disposable, single-use examination gloves (if you will be handling specimen)

PROCEDURE

1. **Wash your hands. Use appropriate personal protective equipment (PPE) as dictated by facility.**

2. Assemble supplies and equipment.

3. Identify the patient and explain the procedure.

RATIONALE

Explanations help gain full cooperation from the patient, which is required to obtain a specimen successfully.

CLEAN-CATCH, MIDSTREAM, VOIDED SPECIMEN—cont'd

For a female patient:

a. Ask patient to wash her perineal area using soap, water, and washcloth; separate labia and cleanse the area around the urinary meatus.

Careful cleansing is necessary to obtain a satisfactory specimen. The urethral orifice is colonized by bacteria. Urine readily becomes contaminated during voiding.

b. Repeat step (a) using water and 4 × 4 inch sponges. NOTE: Rather than using soap and water, the patient may wash herself with 4 × 4 inch sponges soaked with a mild antiseptic solution such as povidone-iodine.

It is important to remove all the soap because a soap residue changes the results of the specimen analysis.

c. Instruct patient to start voiding into the toilet and, after she has voided for a few seconds, to move the specimen container into the urinary stream to catch the midstream specimen in the sterile container. Instruct the patient to fill the container no more than three-fourths full.

This helps wash away urethral contaminants.
You need approximately 2 to 4 ounces of urine for analysis.

d. Instruct the patient to finish voiding into the toilet bowl. Provide tissues for the patient to wipe herself and to wash the outside of the container if spillage should occur after collecting the specimen.

For a male patient:

a. Instruct the patient to take the penis, retract the foreskin (if uncircumcised) to expose the urinary meatus, and cleanse thoroughly with soap and water using the washcloth.

Careful cleansing is necessary to obtain a satisfactory specimen. The urethral orifice is colonized by bacteria. Urine readily becomes contaminated during voiding.

b. Repeat step (a) using 4 × 4 inch sponges and water. NOTE: Rather than using soap and water, the patient may wash himself with 4 × 4 inch sponges soaked with a mild antiseptic solution such as povidone-iodine.

It is important to remove all soap because a soap residue changes the results of the specimen analysis.

c. Instruct the patient to start voiding into the toilet and, after he has voided for a few seconds, to move the specimen container into the urinary stream to catch the midstream specimen. Instruct the patient to fill the container no more than three-fourths full.

This helps cleanse the urethral canal.
You need only 2 to 4 ounces for the analysis.

d. Instruct the patient to then finish voiding into the toilet. The patient is to avoid collecting the last few drops of urine.

Prostatic secretions may be introduced into the urine at the end of the urinary stream.

4. Have the patient signal you when the specimen has been obtained or instruct the patient where to place the specimen container.

5. Send properly labeled specimen, with the correct laboratory requisition, to appropriate laboratory or refrigerate it until it can either be tested or sent to the laboratory (Figure 11-4). Do not allow a urine specimen to stand at room temperature for any length of time. It is best to put a cover on the container.

An unrefrigerated urine specimen becomes worthless if left at room temperature for any length of time. Chemical and microscopic examination of urine should be performed within 1 hour of collection. If this is not possible, it should be preserved in the refrigerator.

6. Don single-use, disposable examination gloves.

7. Perform the urinalysis if this is required of you. See Chapter 12 for this procedure.

Continued

PROCEDURE 11-1

CLEAN-CATCH, MIDSTREAM, VOIDED SPECIMEN—cont'd

URINALYSIS		G/L 410	ST	SP	LAST NAME		FIRST NAME	
REMARKS:		TIIME OF COLLECTION:			ADDRESS			
ROUTINE REQUEST	ROUTINE – SPECIMENS NOT ACCEPTED AFTER 4:00 P.M. PRE-OP – SPECIMENS NOT ACCEPTED AFTER 8:00 P.M.				BIRTHDATE	AGE	SEX	CLASS
IF REQUEST IS OTHER THAN ROUTINE, PLACE STICKER WITH APPROPRIATE INSTRUCTIONS IN THIS SPACE					PHYSICIAN			
DATE	VERIFYING NURSE	DIAGNOSIS			DATE		PHONE	

URINALYSIS — *PLEASE PRINT – PRESS HARD*

CODE 800	ROUTINE URINALYSIS (INCLUDES ALL TESTS LISTED)				
	COLOR		**820**	WBC/HPF	
	CHARACTER		**M**	RBC/HPF	
836	SPECIFIC GRAVITY	1.0	**I**	BACTERIA/HPF	
	pH		**C**	MUCUS/LPF	
830	PROTEIN		**R** **O**	EPITHELIAL CELLS/LPF	
814	GLUCOSE		**S**	CRYSTALS/LPF	
818	KETONES		**C** **O**	CASTS/LPF	
822	OCCULT BLOOD		**P**	OTHER:	
814	REDUCING SUBSTANCES		**I**		
815	GALACTOSE		**C**		
TIME IN		TECHNOLOGIST		TIME CALLED OR TELETYPED	TIME OUT

FIGURE 11-4   Sample urinalysis laboratory requisition that is sent with urine specimen to the laboratory.

8. Remove gloves.

9. Wash your hands.   *Avoid contamination.*

10. Record on the chart the appropriate information. Always record on the chart if the urine appeared abnormal (for example, if blood appeared to be present or if the urine was cloudy). Record the results if you have performed the analysis (as described in Chapter 12).

Charting Example

February 25, 20__, 4 PM
Clean-catch urine specimen obtained and sent to the laboratory for routine UA [urinalysis].
Betty Bittinger, CMA

STOOL SPECIMEN COLLECTION

A stool specimen is collected for macroscopic, microscopic, and chemical examination to help diagnose the presence of parasites and ova, occult blood, fecal urobilinogen, pus or mucus, membranous shreds, worms, infectious diseases, and foreign bodies and to detect the amount of fat being eliminated and various disorders of metabolism.

The stool is examined **macroscopically** for its amount, consistency, color, and odor. Normal color varies from light to dark brown, depending on urobilin content, a product formed from bilirubin. Various foods, medications, and conditions affect the color of the stool. For example, when a person has ingested the following, the color of the stool may be affected:

- Meat protein—The stool may be dark brown.
- Spinach—The stool may be green.
- Beets—The stool may be red.
- Cocoa—The stool may be dark red or brown.
- Bismuth, iron, or charcoal—The stool may be black.
- Barium—The stool may be milky white.

In conditions in which a patient is having upper gastrointestinal bleeding, the stool is tarry black; in lower gastrointestinal bleeding, it is bright red or bloody; and in biliary obstruction, it is clay colored. Other clinical conditions in which the stool has certain characteristics include the following:

- Steatorrhea (excess fat in the feces resulting from a malabsorption state caused by disease of the intestinal mucosa or pancreatic enzyme deficiency)—The stool appears bulky, greasy, foamy, foul in odor, and gray or clay colored with a silvery sheen.
- Chronic ulcerative colitis—Mucus or pus may be visible in the stool.
- Constipation, obstipation, and fecal obstruction—The stool appears as small, dry, rocky-hard masses.

As with most specimens, a fresh specimen is absolutely necessary and should be obtained before the administration of antibiotic therapy. Stool containing barium, mineral oils, or magnesia is usually unsuitable for diagnosis.

To best demonstrate **parasitic infection,** three fresh specimens collected on three different days are usually necessary. These must be sent to the laboratory immediately so that the parasites can be observed under the microscope while they are fresh, viable, and warm. Stool for **occult blood testing** should not be more than 1 hour old.

Some laboratories now prefer the new collection system that no longer requires that specimens be warm. The specimens are placed into two separate vials, each containing a special preservative, and then are sent to the laboratory as soon as possible.

When forwarding the specimen to a hospital or large laboratory, send specimens to be tested for occult blood to the hematology laboratory, specimens for culture and acid-fast bacilli to the bacteriology laboratory, and specimens for parasites and ova to the parasitology laboratory. Accompany all specimens with the appropriate clinical laboratory slips with accurate and completed information.

Hemoccult Slide Test on a Stool Specimen

The Hemoccult slide test is a rapid, noninvasive, convenient, and virtually odorless method for detecting the presence of **fecal occult (hidden) blood** as an aid to diagnosis of various gastrointestinal conditions, including polyps, peptic ulcers, hemorrhoids, hiatal hernia, and cancer of the colon or rectum. This test is performed in the following situations:

- During routine physical examinations
- In newly admitted hospital patients
- In postoperative patients
- In newborn infants
- In screening programs for colorectal cancer

Because Hemoccult tests require only a small stool specimen, offensive odors are minimized, and storage or transport of large stool specimens is unnecessary. Figure 11-6 contains more information, special instructions for the patient, and the equipment and procedure for performing this test. The American Cancer Society recommends that a stool blood test be performed every year on patients of ages 50 years and older. This

Text continued on p. 489

VOCABULARY

bowel movement—The elimination/excretion of fecal material from the intestinal tract.

constipation (kon-sti-pa'shun)—A condition in which the waste material in the intestine is too hard to pass easily or in which bowel movements are so infrequent that discomfort results.

diarrhea (di-a-re'a)—Rapid movement of fecal material through the intestine, resulting in poor absorption and producing frequent, watery stools.

excrete (ek-skret')—To eliminate useless matter such as feces and urine.

excreta (ek-skre'tah)—Waste material excreted or eliminated from the body. Feces, urine, perspiration, and also mucus and carbon dioxide (CO_2) can be considered excreta.

excretion (ek-skre'shun)—The elimination of waste materials from the body. Ordinarily, what is meant by excretion is the elimination of feces, but it can refer to the material eliminated from any part of the body.

feces (fe'sez)—Body waste excreted from the intestine; also called stool, excreta, or excrement.

flatulence (flat'u-lens)—Excessive formation of gases in the stomach or intestine.

flatus (fla'tus)—Air or gas in the stomach or intestine.

guaiac (gwi'ak) **test**—The preferred chemical test to determine the presence of occult blood in feces.

melena (mel-e'nah)—Darkening of stool by blood pigments.

obstipation (ob'sti-pa'shun)—Extreme constipation caused by an obstruction.

occult blood—Obscure or hidden from view.

occult blood test—A microscopic or a chemical test performed on a specimen to determine the presence of blood not otherwise detectable. Stool is tested when intestinal bleeding is suspected but blood is not visible in the stool.

parasite (par'ah-sit)—An organism that lives on or in another organism, known as the host, from which it gains its nourishment (for example, fungi, bacteria, and single-celled and multicelled animals).

stool—The fecal discharge from the bowels (*see also* Feces).

lienteric stool—Feces containing much undigested food.

urobilinogen—A colorless compound formed in the intestines by the reduction of bilirubin.

STOOL SPECIMEN

Objective

Understand and demonstrate the correct procedure for obtaining a stool specimen from a patient; prepare the specimen to be sent to the laboratory; and record the necessary information on the patient's chart.

Equipment

Stool specimen container of waxed cardboard with a lid or of plastic with a lid

Wooden tongue depressor or spatula

Clean bedpan with cover

Label for container

Small plastic bag

Laboratory requisition

Disposable, single-use examination gloves

PROCEDURE

RATIONALE

1. **Wash your hands. Use appropriate personal protective equipment (PPE) as dictated by facility.** Obtain a clean bedpan with a clean cover to give to the patient for use.

2. Identify the patient. Explain to the patient that a stool specimen is needed and that a bedpan must be used. Have the patient empty the bladder first if necessary because urine should not be collected in the bedpan with the stool specimen.

   Explanations help gain the patient's full cooperation, which is essential for proper specimen collection.

3. Prepare the label for the specimen container. Fill out the laboratory requisition accurately and completely. You can do this while the patient is collecting the specimen.

4. Don gloves.

5. After the patient has used the bedpan, cover it and remove it to your work area. Provide means for the patient to wash the hands.

6. Transfer a portion (1 to 2 teaspoons) of the stool into the specimen container by using the clean tongue depressor or spatula as a spoon. Place the lid on the container securely. Be sure that there is no toilet tissue in the stool specimen. Do not smear the specimen on the edge or outside of the container. You may scrape the tongue depressor or spatula only on the inside of the container to rid it of feces.

7. Place the tongue depressor or spatula in the plastic bag and wrap it securely for proper disposal. Do not throw it in the wastebasket. You should have a special container for used equipment such as this.

   The tongue depressor may be contaminated with infectious disease organisms.

8. Empty and clean the bedpan. Avoid contaminating yourself or your work area. Before emptying the bedpan, observe the feces for anything that appears abnormal to you; if so, report it at once.

9. Remove gloves.

10. **Wash your hands thoroughly.**

11. Label the container and attach the correct completed laboratory requisition to the container (Figure 11-5). The purpose of the examination must be stated on the requisition.

STOOL SPECIMEN—cont'd

12. Send or take the labeled specimen to the laboratory immediately. If there is a delay, try to place the specimen for parasite examination in a warm place until it can be delivered to or picked up by the laboratory. Refrigerate specimens for other examinations until delivered to the laboratory. NOTE: If more than one specimen is to be sent, indicate No. 1, No. 2, and so on. A stool specimen should be warm when it arrives in the laboratory for examination. This is especially important when looking for parasites so that they may be examined under the microscope while viable, fresh, and warm. Specimens for tests other than parasite detection can generally be refrigerated for a few hours when not sent immediately to the laboratory.

13. Wash your hands again.

Because of the chance of having disease organisms on your hands, wash them again to be safe.

14. Record on the patient's chart. If relevant, describe the appearance of the stool when charting.

Charting Example

February 27, 20__, 10 AM
Stool specimen No. 1 sent to laboratory for ova and parasites and fat content examinations.
Connie Hanks, CMA

FECES - SEMEN

FECES – SEMEN LABORATORY

DATE   Feb. 27, 20__ .
Patient's name
Physician's name
and address

Routine Feces Consists Of • Gross Description • Ova & Parasites • Occult Blood
☐ CULTURE REQUIRED   (ALSO SUBMIT BACTERIOLOGY REQUEST)

☐ ROUTINE FECES   ☐ UROBILINOGEN (QUAL.)   ☐ SEMEN ANALYSIS
☑ OVA & PARASITES   ☑ FAT (QUAL.)   ☐
☐ OCCULT BLOOD   ☐ STARCH   ☐
☐ BILE PIGMENT (QUAL.)   ☐ TRYPSIN   ☐

COMMENTS: *Stool spec #1*

FECES – SEMEN

FINDINGS	STOOL EXAMINATION		FINDINGS			FINDINGS	SEMEN ANALYSIS
	COLOR		OVA & HELMINTHS	PARASITES			APPEARANCE
	CONSISTENCY		DIRECT				VOLUME (cc)
	MUCUS		CONC.				COUNT 100-150 M/cc
	PUS CELLS		TROPHOZOITES	AMEBAE			RBC
	RED BLOOD CELLS		CYSTS				WBC
	BENZIDINE	OCCULT BLOOD	NEUTRAL FAT	Fats			CRYSTALS
	GUAIAC		STARCH				% MOTILITY (INIT.)
	UROBILIN	BILE PIGMENT	TRYPSIN				MORPHOLOGY
	BILIRUBIN						
	UROBILINOGEN (QUAL.)						

ADDITIONAL RESULTS:

DATE	TECHNOLOGIST'S SIGNATURE

FIGURE 11-5   Sample laboratory requisition for fecal specimen.

FIGURE 11-6 **A,** Hemoccult slides procedure. (Courtesy SmithKline Diagnostics, Inc, Sunnyvale, Calif.)

Hemoccult Single Slides are convenient for use when single stool specimens are to be tested.

Hemoccult II Slides, in cards of three tests, are designed so your patient can collect serial specimens at home over the course of three bowel movements. After the patient collects the specimens, the Hemoccult II test may be returned to a laboratory, a hospital, or a medical office for developing and evaluation. Serial fecal specimen analysis is recommended when screening asymptomatic patients (**B** and **D**).

Hemoccult Tape is designed to complement Hemoccult slides and is best suited for "on-the-spot" testing for occult blood during rectal or sigmoidoscopic examinations. The Hemoccult test and other unmodified guaiac tests are *not recommended* for use with gastric specimens.

SUMMARY, EXPLANATION AND LIMITATIONS OF THE TEST

The Hemoccult test is a simplified, standardized variation of the guaiac test for occult blood. It contains specially prepared guaiac-impregnated paper and is ready for use without additional preparation.

When a small stool specimen containing occult blood is applied to Hemoccult test paper, the hemoglobin comes in contact with the guaiac. Application of Hemoccult Developer (a stablized hydrogen peroxide solution) creates a guaiac/peroxidase-like reaction which turns the test paper blue within 60 seconds if occult blood is present.

The test reacts with hemoglobin released from lysed cells. When blood is present, hemolysis is promoted by substances in the stool, primarily water and salts. Typical positive reactions for occult blood are shown under READING AND INTERPRETATION OF THE HEMOCCULT TEST. As with any occult blood test, results with the Hemoccult test cannot be considered conclusive evidence of the presence or absence of gastrointestinal bleeding or pathology. *Hemoccult tests are designed for preliminary screening as a diagnostic aid and are not intended to replace other diagnostic procedures such as proctosigmoidoscopic examination, barium enema, or other x-ray studies.*

BIOLOGICAL PRINCIPLE

The discovery that gum guaiac was a useful indicator for occult blood is generally credited to Van Deen. The test depends on the oxidation of a phenolic, compound, alpha guaiaconic acid, which yields a blue-covered, highly conjugated quinone structure. Hemoglobin exerts a peroxidase-like activity and facilitates the oxidation of this phenolic compound by hydrogen peroxide.

REAGENTS

Natural guaiac resin impregnated into standardized, high-quality filter paper.

A developing solution containing a stabilized dilute mixture of hydrogen peroxide (less than 6%) and 75% denatured ethyl alcohol in aqueous solution.

PERFORMANCE MONITORS

The function and stability of the slides and Developer can be tested using the on-slide Performance Monitor. Both a positive and negative Performance Monitor are located under the flap and below the specimen windows on the back of the Hemoccult II and Hemoccult single slides.

The positive Performance Monitor contains a hemoglobin-derived catalyst which, upon application of Developer, will turn blue within 10 seconds.

The negative Performance Monitor contains no such catalyst and should not turn blue upon application of Developer.

The Performance Monitors provide additional assurance that the guaiac-impregnated paper and Developer are functional. In the unlikely event that the Performance Monitors do not react as expected after application of Developer, the test results should be regarded as invalid. The manufacturer will provide further assistance should this occur.

Precautions

- For *In Vitro* Diagnostic Use.
- Because this test is visually read and requires color differentiation, it should not be interpreted by people who are color-blind or visually impaired.
- Patient specimens and all materials that come in contact with them, should be handled as potentially infectious and disposed of with proper precautions.

Hemoccult Slides (yellow and green card)

- Do not use after the expiration date which appears on each slide.

Hemoccult Developer (yellow label and bottle cap)

- Hemoccult Developer is an irritant and is flammable.

Avoid contact with eyes and skin. If developer comes in contact with eyes or skin, rinse promptly with water. Do not leave uncapped or expose to heat.

- Do not use after expiration date on the bottle.

IMPORTANT: Use Hemoccult Developer (yellow label and cap) only with Hemoccult slides and tape. *Do not interchange Hemoccult with Hemoccult SENSA test reagents, which are identified by blue and green packaging.*

Storage and Stability

Store Hemoccult test components at controlled room temperture, 15 - 30°C (59 - 86°F), in original packaging. Do not refrigerate or freeze.

Protect Hemoccult slides from heat and light. Do not store near volatile chemicals (e.g., iodine, chlorine, bromine, or ammonia).

Store Hemoccult Developer at 15° to 30°C (59° to 86°F); protect from heat. Keep bottle tightly capped when not in use to prevent evaporation.

Sample Collection

The Hemoccult test requires only a small fecal sample. The sample is applied as a **thin smear** to the guaiac paper of the Hemoccult slide or tape using the applicator stick provided. The sample may be collected from the toilet bowl with the aid of a container, toilet tissue, or collection tissue (provided with Hemoccult II Dispensapak™ Plus).

Hemoccult slides may be prepared and developed immediately, or prepared and stored for up to 14 days at controlled room temperature, 15-30° (59-86°F), before developing.

Patients using the Hemoccult II test should be instructed to return all slides to the physician or laboratory immediately after preparing the last test. IMPORTANT NOTE: *Current U.S. Postal Regulations prohibit mailing completed test slides in standard paper envelopes. Physicians who wish their patients to return slides by mail, must instruct their patients to use only U.S. Postal Service approved mailing pouches.**

Fecal samples **should not be collected** if hematuria or obvious rectal bleeding, such as from hemorrhoids, is present. Pre-menopausal women must be instructed to avoid collecting fecal samples during or in the first three days after a menstrual period.

Since bleeding from gastrointestinal lesions may be intermittent, *fecal samples for testing should be collected from three consecutive bowel movements or three bowel movements closely spaced in time.* To further increase the probability of detecting occult blood, separate samples should be taken from two different sections of each fecal specimen.

INTERFERING SUBSTANCES

In general, patients should not ingest foods, drugs, vitamins or other substances which can cause false-positive or false-negative test results for at least 48 hours before and continuing through the test period. Aspirin and other non-steroidal anti-inflammatory drugs should be avoided for at least seven days prior to and continuing through the test period.

Foods that can cause false-positive test results include red meat (beef, lamb) as well as processed meats and liver. In addition, some raw fruits and vegetables which are high in peroxidase, can cause false-positive results when fecal samples are tested immediately after collection. However, plant peroxidases are relatively unstable and when slides are developed several days after sample preparation, as is the case in a typical take-home or screening situation, even large quantities of raw fruits and vegetables have been observed to have no significant effect on test results.

Substances which can irritate the gastrointestinal tract and cause bleeding, such as aspirin, corticosteroids, indomethacin, zomepirac, naproxen, tolmetin, phenylbutazone, reserpine, anticoagulants, antimetabolites, cancer chemotherapeutic drugs, and alcohol in excess may produce positive test results. However, because acetaminophen has not been observed to cause substantial gastrointestinal tract bleeding, the use of acetaminophen is not expected to significantly affect test results.

The application of antiseptic preparations containing iodine, such as povidone iodine mixtures, to the anal area can also cause false-positive results.

False-negative test results can be caused by ascorbic acid (vitamin C) intake of more than 250 mg/day or by the consumption of excessive amounts of vitamin C enriched foods, such as citrus fruits and juices.

PROCEDURE

Materials Supplied: (see Panel E)
- Hemoccult Slides (or tape in plastic dispenser)
- Hemoccult Developer (yellow label and cap)
- Applicator sticks
- Patient envelopes with instructions for diet and sample collection
- Mailing Pouch for returning completed slides†
- Collection tissues†
- Hemoccult Product Instructions

*Mailing Pouches are included in HemoccultII Dispensapak Plus and may be ordered separately; refer to ORDERING INFORMATION.

†In Dispensapak# Plus configuration only.

FIGURE 11-6 **A,** Hemoccult slides procedure; **B,** reading and interpreting the Hemocult test; **C,** on-slide performance monitor feature; **D,** hemoccult tape preparation and development. (Courtesy SmithKline Diagnostics, Inc, Sunnyvale, Calif.)

A. PROCEDURE: HEMOCCULT SLIDES

Identification	Preparation	Development of Test	Development of Performance Monitors

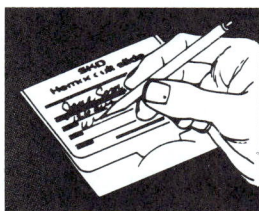 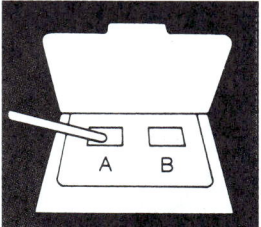 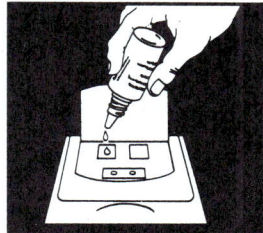 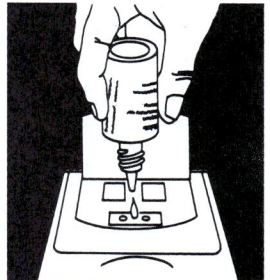

Write, or have patient write his or her name, age, address, phone number, and date specimen was collected in space provided on front of each slide.

1. Collect small stool sample on one end of applicator.
2. Apply thin smear inside box A.
3. Reuse applicator to obtain second sample from different part of stool. Apply thin smear inside box B.
4. Close cover. Return slide to physician.
CAUTION: Protect from heat.
5. If testing immediately, wait 3-5 minutes before developing. Otherwise, store slides as directed for up to 14 days until ready to develop.

1. Open flap in back of slide and apply two drops of Hemoccult Developer to guaiac paper directly over each smear.
2. Read results within 60 seconds.
ANY TRACE OF BLUE ON OR AT THE EDGE OF THE SMEAR IS POSITIVE FOR OCCULT BLOOD.

1. Apply ONE DROP ONLY of Hemoccult Developer between the positive and negative Performance Monitors.
2. Read results within 10 seconds.
A BLUE COLOR WILL APPEAR IN THE POSITIVE PERFORMANCE MONITOR, AND NO BLUE WILL APPEAR IN THE NEGATIVE PERFORMANCE MONITOR, IF THE SLIDES AND DEVELOPER ARE FUNCTIONAL.

IMPORTANT NOTE: Follow the procedure exactly as outlined above. Always develop the test, read the results, interpret them and make a decision as to whether the fecal specimen is positive or negative for occult blood BEFORE you develop the Performance Monitors. Do not apply Developer to Performance Monitors before interpreting test results. Any blue originating from the Performance Monitors should be ignored in the reading of the specimen test results.

B. READING AND INTERPRETATION OF THE HEMOCCULT TEST

Negative Smears*	Negative and Positive Smears*	Positive Smears*

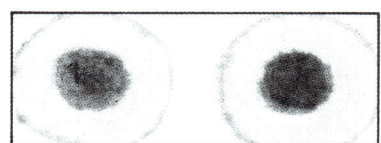 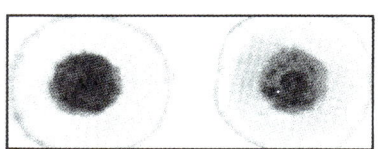 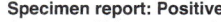

Specimen report: negative
No detectable blue on or at the edge of the smears indicates test is negative for occult blood.

Specimen report: Positive
Any trace of blue on or at the edge of one or more of the smears indicates test is positive for occult blood.

C. On-Slide Performance Monitors Feature*

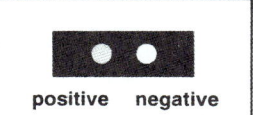

positive   negative

A blue color in the positive Performance Monitor will appear within 10 seconds if test system is functional.

No blue color will appear in the negative Performance Monitor if the test system is functional.

Neither the intensity nor the shade of the blue from the positive Performance Monitor should be regarded as an indication of what the blue from a positive fecal specimen should look like.

*The illustrations are an artist's rendition. Each specimen illustration is of two smears from a single stool specimen as displayed on a single Hemoccult test slide. A reaction on Hemoccult Tape may appear as any one of the illustrated smears.

D. Hemoccult Tape

Preparation	Development

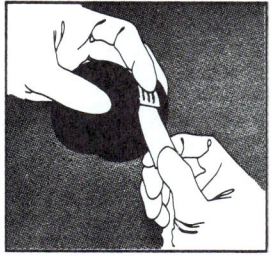 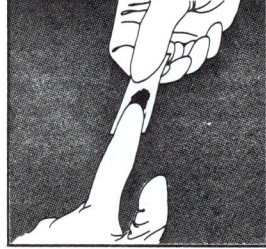 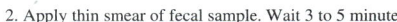 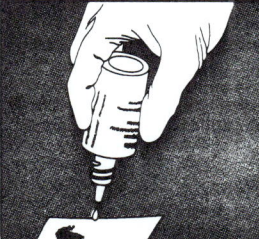

1. Apply two drops of Hemoccult Developer to side opposite smear.
2. Read results on side opposite smear within 60 seconds.
ANY TRACE OF BLUE ON OR AT THE EDGE OF THE SMEAR IS POSITIVE FOR OCCULT BLOOD.

1. Tear strip of tape from dispenser.   2. Apply thin smear of fecal sample. Wait 3 to 5 minutes.

FIGURE 11-6 **E,** Hemoccult II Slides. **F,** Hemoccult II Dispensapak with on-slide performance monitors. **G,** Instructions to the patient for collecting fecal specimens for Hemoccult II slide test and Hemoccult II procedure. (Courtesy SmithKline Diagnostics, Inc, Sunnyvale, Calif.)

E. SATISFACTORY LIMITS OF PERFORMANCE; EXPECTED RESULTS

Results with the Hemocult test are visually determined. The Hemoccult guaiac test paper should be observed for color change within 60 seconds after Developer has been applied.

This reading time is important because the color reaction may fade after two to four minutes.

If any trace of blue on or at the edge of the smear is seen, the test is positive for occult blood. For typical positive reaction, see READING AND INTERPRETATION OF THE HEMOCCULT TEST.

NOTE: Because this test is visually read and requires color differentiation, it should not be read by the visually impaired.

The function and stability of the Hemoccult slides and Developer can be tested using the on-slide Performance Monitors. The Hemoccult Tape may be tested by applying a drop of diluted whole blood (1:5,000 in distilled water) to an unused portion of the tape. Add Developer to opposite side. If any blue appears, the guaiac-impregnated paper and Developer are functional.

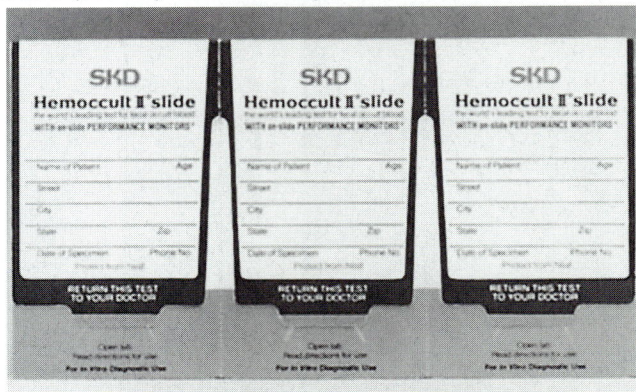

F. INSTRUCTIONS TO THE PATIENT FOR COLLECTING FECAL SPECIMENS FOR THE HEMOCCULT II SLIDE TEST

Hemoccult slides are used routinely to check the intestinal tract.

Please follow these instructions carefully.

Before beginning the Test Procedure, please read Sample Collection Instructions. For accurate test results, it is important to follow the diet below for at least 48 hours before collecting the first stool sample. Remain on this diet until you have completed all three slides.

1. Use a ball-point pen to write your name, age and address on the front of each slide.
2. After a bowel movement, open the front of Slide 1. Use one applicator to collect a small stool sample from the toilet bowl.
3. Apply sample inside Box A. Collect a second sample from a different part of the stool using the same applicator. Apply this sample inside Box B. Discard applicator in a waste container. Do not flush wooden applicator.
4. Close the cover flap. Fill in the date on the front of the slide; place slide in the paper envelope; allowing slide to air-dry overnight.
5. Repeat Steps 2-4 for your next 2 bowel movements. After last completed slide has air-dried overnight, immediately return all slides to your doctor or laboratory. NOTE: Current U.S. Postal Regulations prohibit mailing completed test slides in a standard paper envelope. If you wish to return your slides by mail, ask your doctor for a U.S. Postal Service approved mailing pouch.

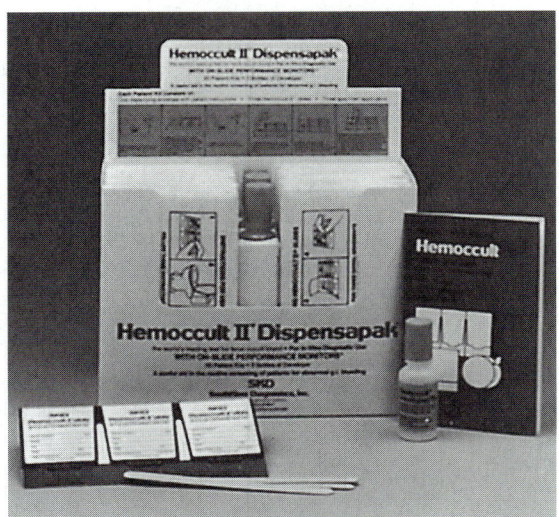

G. SAMPLE COLLECTION INSTRUCTIONS

Do not collect samples during, or until three days after your menstrual period, or while you have bleeding hemorrhoids or blood in your urine.

Do collect samples from three consecutive bowel movements or three bowel movements closely spaced in time.

Do protect slides from heat, light, and volatile chemicals (e.g., iodine or bleach).

Do keep slides closed when not in use

Do follow the Special Diagnostic Diet Instructions (below) for 48 hours before proceeding.

Special Diagnostic Diet Instructions
Foods To Eat

- Well-cooked, pork, poultry, and fish
- Any cooked fruits and vegetables
- High-fiber foods (e.g., whole wheat bread, bran cereal, popcorn)

If following any part of the Special Diagnostic Diet is a problem, talk to your doctor.

Foods, Vitamins, And Drugs To Avoid

- Red meat (beef, lamb), including processed meats and liver
- Any raw fruits and vegetables (especially melons, radishes, turnips and horse-radish)
- Vitamin C in excess of 250 mg per day
- Aspirin or other nonsteroidal anti-inflammatory drugs (avoid for 7 days prior to and during the testing period)

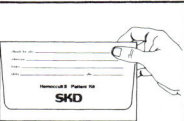
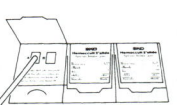
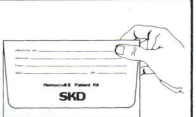

1. Fill in patient information on Hemoccult II* test. Give kit to patient.

2. **Patient,** at home, opens a cover flap and applies thin stool smear to Box A, a second smear from a different site to Box B. Patient performs procedure for three consecutive bowel movements.

3. **Patient** returns prepared slides to doctor's office or lab.

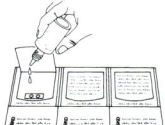
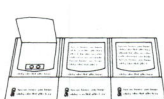
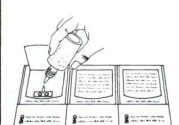

4. **Doctor or medical assistant** applies two drops of Developer on the back of the slide directly over each smear.

5. **Doctor or medical assistant** reads results within 60 seconds. Any trace of blue on or at the edge of the smear is positive for blood.

6. **Doctor or medical assistant** applies ONE DROP ONLY of Developer between the positive and negative Performance Monitors*. A blue color will appear within 10 seconds in the positive Performance Monitor, no blue in the negative Performance Monitor, if the slides and Developer are functional.

(Text material adapted with permission of SmithKline Diagnostics, Inc., Sunnyvale, Calif.)

test indicates hidden (occult) blood in feces, which may be an early indicator of colorectal cancer. The risk of developing colorectal cancer increases after age 50 for both men and women. Anyone with a personal or family history of colorectal cancer, ulcerative colitis, polyps in the colon or rectum, or a personal history of inflammatory bowel disease has a higher chance of developing this cancer.

The American Cancer Society estimated that 93,800 people (43,400 males and 50,400 females) would develop colorectal cancer in the year 2000. These figures are updated every year. When colorectal cancer is detected in its early stages, up to 92% of these people may be treated successfully. When cancer is detected after symptoms appear and has spread to other parts of the body, only 46% to 58% may be treated successfully. Thus earlier detection could save thousands of lives each year (see the Health Matters box and also Figure 5-22).

Millions of people have the Hemoccult screening test performed each year *because* early detection and treatment of colorectal cancer has proven effective in saving lives.

RESPIRATORY TRACT SPECIMENS

Sputum Specimen Collection

Sputum specimens are examined to help determine the presence of infectious organisms or to identify tumor cells in the respiratory tract. The laboratory findings provide relevant information to the physician when making a diagnosis and initiating treatment.

Other specimens that may be obtained if a patient is unable to produce sputum include tracheal aspirates collected by aspiration with a suction catheter and bronchial washings and transtracheal aspirates collected by the physician or a pulmonary technician. These specimens are of more value diagnostically than sputum because they are not likely to become as contaminated with oropharyngeal flora. Nevertheless, because sputum is easy to collect and causes little discomfort to the patient, it is usually the first type of lower respiratory tract specimen to be obtained for examination and culture.

Procedures ordered on sputum specimens when sent to the laboratory include direct smears, routine culture and sensitivities, cultures for acid-fast bacilli (tuberculosis), fungus cultures, and sputum cytology (exfoliative cytology), which is performed to identify tumor cells.

Periodic sputum examinations may also be done on patients receiving antibiotics, steroids, and immunosuppressive agents for prolonged periods because these agents give rise to opportunistic pulmonary infections.

When collecting sputum specimens, your understanding of the physician's order is essential. For example, if the order states "sputum cultures × 3," this means that you should collect three different specimens at different times or on 3 successive days. This order *does not* mean that you collect one specimen and divide it into three different containers. Even though these specimens would each be cultured, the findings would show that they were duplicates; thus the whole procedure would have to be repeated.

VOCABULARY

exfoliative cytology—Microscopic examination of cells desquamated (shedding) from a body surface as a means of detecting malignant change.
expectorate—The ejection of sputum and other materials from the air passages.
hemoptysis (he-mop′ti-sis)—Coughing up blood as a result of bleeding from any part of the respiratory tract. The appearance

of the secretion in true hemoptysis is bright red and frothy with air bubbles.
immunosuppressive agents—Drugs that inhibit the formation of antibodies to antigens that may be present.
saliva (sah-li′vah)—The enzyme-containing secretion of the salivary glands in the mouth.

PROCEDURE 11-3

SPUTUM SPECIMEN

Objective
Understand and demonstrate the correct procedure used to obtain a sputum specimen from the patient; prepare the specimen to be sent to the laboratory; and record the necessary information on the patient's chart.

Equipment
Disposable, single-use examination gloves, laboratory coat, and face shield or eye protection

Sterile specimen container
Glass jar for acid-fast bacilli culture
Cardboard sputum container may be used for other studies
Label
Laboratory requisition
Plastic bag and tape

PROCEDURE

1. **Wash your hands. Use appropriate personal protective equipment (PPE) as dictated by facility.** Don gloves and laboratory coat and assemble the supplies.

2. Identify the patient and explain the procedure. Give the sterile specimen container to the patient. Instruct the patient not to touch the inside of the container with the hands. Put face shield on. If feasible, the specimen should be collected in the morning before eating or drinking. Usually a minimum of 5 ml of sputum is required by the laboratory for testing.

3. Instruct the patient to cough deeply and expectorate directly into the container, avoiding contamination to the outside of the container with the sputum.

4. Label the container, and indicate test(s) required on the laboratory requisition (Figure 11-7). Accurate, complete information is always required: date, time, patient's name, type of specimen, test(s) to be performed, name of attending physician, and when available, the probable diagnosis.

5. Send the specimen to the laboratory.
   a. Secure the sputum container lid with tape.
   b. Place the container in a plastic bag and attach the laboratory requisition.
   c. Place all into a secure transport container for delivery to an outside laboratory. Specimens for culture and cytology should be sent to the laboratory within 30 minutes of collection. Refrigerate the specimen when it is not sent to the laboratory immediately.
      NOTE: Specimens must be as fresh as possible, except when accumulation over a specific length of time is ordered. Clearly mark on the label if the specimen is a 24-hour collection.

6. Remove gloves, laboratory coat, and face shield.

7. **Wash your hands.**

RATIONALE

This laboratory coat is to be worn only when collecting specimens. This protects your uniform.

Obtain freshly expectorated sputum.

Sputum (lung and bronchial specimen) is produced by a deep cough. You do not want a specimen of saliva from the mouth.

Any delay can cause organisms to multiply, which would result in misleading findings. Refrigerate to prevent bacteria overgrowth.

If a 24-hour specimen is to be obtained, instruct the patient to wrap a paper towel around the jar and secure it with a rubber band. Always keep the lid of the container closed except when in use.

Avoid contamination.

PROCEDURE 11-3

SPUTUM SPECIMEN—cont'd

8. Record on chart. Note any abnormal quality that you may have observed, such as sputum that appears to be blood tinged.

Charting Example

February 25, 20__, 8 AM

    Sputum specimen obtained; sent to laboratory for C & S [culture and sensitivity].

    Marjory Alvory, CMA

MICROBIOLOGY	GL 404	ST	BD

MICROBIOLOGY — PLEASE PRINT • PRESS HARD

DRAWN BY	REMARKS:	DATE/TIME OF COLLECTION

ROUTINE REQUEST

IF REQUEST IS OTHER THAN ROUTINE, PLACE STICKER WITH APPROPRIATE INSTRUCTIONS IN THIS SPACE

DATE	VERIFYING NURSE	DIAGNOSIS

LAST NAME / FIRST NAME / ADDRESS / BIRTHDATE / AGE / SEX / CLASS / PHYSICIAN / ROOM NO. / HOSP. NO. / DATE / PHONE

CIRCLE CODE NO. — **CULTURES**

604	BLOOD
(600)	ROUTINE
607	ANAEROBIC
620	URINE
606	CAMPYLO-BACTER
618	AFB (SMEAR INCLUDED)
612	FUNGUS
616	GRAM STAIN
(601)	ANTIBIOTIC SENSITIVITY

SCREENS

| 625 | BETA STREP |
| 632 | NEISSERIA |

INDICATE SOURCE

☐ EYE ☐ EAR ☐ CSF ☐ NASOPHARYNX ☐ THROAT ☑ SPUTUM ☐ URINE ☐ STOOL ☐ CERVIX ☐ VAGINA ☐ WOUND ☐ ASPIRATE ☐ ABSCESS INDICATE SITE:

SMEAR RESULT: CULTURE RESULT:

TIME IN / TECHNOLOGIST / TIME CALLED OR TELETYPED / TIME OUT

MEDICAL RECORD

FIGURE 11-7 A, Sample laboratory requisition for sputum specimen for culture and sensitivity tests.

Continued

PROCEDURE 11-3

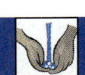

SPUTUM SPECIMEN—cont'd

MICROBIOLOGY REQUISITION

GENERAL HOSPITAL
CLINICAL LABORATORIES

DOUGLAS A. BLACK, M.D., DIRECTOR

DATE, TIME RECEIVED   ACC #

LAB USE ONLY

PHYSICIAN NAME (Print)
I.D. NUMBER
BEEPER/EXTENSION
COLLECTED BY   DATE   TIME   A.M.   P.M.
WARD OR LOCATION

PATIENT NAME:
MEDICAL RECORD NUMBER:
BILLING:
BIRTHDATE:
SEX: M   F
PATIENT HISTORY / DIAGNOSIS / SUSPECTED INFECTIOUS AGENT.
ICD - 9 CODE:
DATE OF ONSET
ANTIMICROBIAL THERAPY

THIS REQUISITION MAY BE USED FOR MORE THAN ONE
TYPE OF CULTURE OR TEST PER SPECIMEN.

USE ONE REQUISITION FOR EACH SPECIMEN.

SOURCE OF SPECIMEN

- BLOOD
- CSF
- FLUID (specify source) ___
- THROAT
- TRACHEAL ASPIRATE
- SPUTUM, expectorated
- SPUTUM, induced
- BRONCHOALVEOLAR LAVAGE (BAL)
- URINE, clean catch midstream
- URINE, first stream (for chlamydia LCR only)
- URINE, indwelling CATH
- URINE, straight (in & out) CATH
- URINE, entire first morning (for AFB only)
- URINE: other (specify) ___
- STOOL
  - Bloody diarrhea   Yes   No
- GU SITE   Cervix   Urethra
  - Other (specify) ___
- ABSCESS (specify site) ___
- TISSUE (specify site) ___
- ULCER (specify site) ___
- WOUND (specify site) ___
- STERILIZER TEST
- OTHER (specify site) ___

TEST(S) REQUESTED

BACTERIAL

- Routine culture. If source of specimen & type of collection received are appropriate, work-up will include Gram stain, anaerobic culture, and susceptibility testing. Throats done for Group A strep only unless other specific organism requested.
- Gram stain only
- Add Legionella culture
- Other Non-Routine Cultures - please check:
  - E. coli 0157   Vibrio   Yersinia
  - H. ducreyi (chancroid)   B. pertussis
  - Bartonella (Rochalimaea) blood culture
    Requires culture kit with instructions. Call Lab x 8576
  - Other (specify) ___

Screening cultures
- Gonococci (GC) only
- Group A strep only   Group B strep only
- Culture & smear (smear not done on blood, clear CSF, gastric, or urine)
- Add M. haemophilum culture
- Add other (specify) ___

AFB
- Culture (includes cryptococcal antigen test on CSF)
- Other (specify) ___

FUNGAL
- Cryptococcal antigen (CSF only; if specimen is blood, use Blood/Serum Main Lab requisition)
- Routine culture (Specify virus) ___

VIRAL
- Herpes simplex only culture
- Direct FA for Herpes simplex virus (HSV)
- Direct FA for Varicella-zoster virus (VZV)
- Rapid test for respiratory syncytial virus (RSV)
- Rapid test for Influenza A virus
- Other (specify) ___

CHLAMYDIA

PARASITOLOGY
- Exam for intestinal parasites (O & P)
- Giardia antigen test - requires approval of Lab Medicine Resident, x 8576, or LMR on call
- Cryptosporidia, Isospora, Cyclospora
- Microsporidia
- Pinworm prep
- Blood parasites
- Filaria concentration
- Trichomonas
- Other (specify) ___
- Clostridium difficile

TOXIN ASSAY

ALL TESTS LISTED BELOW REQUIRE APPROVAL OF LAB MEDICINE RESIDENT. CALL EX. 8576 OR BEEP LMR ON CALL

SPECIAL TESTS
- Bacterial antigens
  Specify organisms ___
- Direct FA for Bordetella pertussis/ parapertussis
- Direct FA for T. pallidum / Dark field exam
- Direct FA for Legionella pneumophila
- Antimicrobial tests - (e.g. combination antimicrobials, serum killing levels, or MLCs)
  Specify test ___

FIGURE 11-7—cont'd   B, Microbiology laboratory requisition for various specimens and tests.

Throat and Nasopharyngeal Cultures

Upper respiratory secretions most often obtained for examination are throat and nasopharyngeal cultures.

The throat is defined as the area of the body that includes the larynx and pharynx, passageways that link the nose and mouth with the respiratory and digestive systems. A sore throat is caused by inflammation, irritation, or infection of tissue in one or more of the areas in the pharynx or larynx. The common cause of throat infection is the invasion of the tissues by bacteria, such as streptococci, staphylococci, or pneumococci. Inflammation and discomfort in the throat are often caused by tonsillitis, as well as by just an overuse of the voice or excessive smoking.

Throat cultures are performed to determine the presence and the type of microscopic organism that is the cause of an in-fection. They are often ordered for patients suspected of having streptococcal pharyngitis and also for those with suspected cases of pertussis (whopping cough), diphtheria, and gonococcal pharyngitis. The nasopharynx (na′zo-far′ingks) is the part of the pharynx above the soft palate that is connected with the nasal cavities and provides a passage for air during breathing.

Usually nasopharyngeal cultures are ordered on infants and children (when a sputum specimen cannot be obtained) who are suspected of having whooping cough, pneumonia, or croup. They may also be ordered for patients thought to be carriers of pathogenic organisms that cause meningitis, diphtheria, scarlet fever, pneumonia, rheumatic fever, and other diseases.

Cultures should be obtained *before* antibiotic therapy is started because antibiotics may interfere with the growth of the microorganism in the laboratory.

PROCEDURE 11-4

THROAT CULTURE

Objective

Understand and demonstrate the correct procedures for obtaining a specimen for a throat culture; prepare the specimen to be sent to the laboratory; and record the procedure on the patient's chart.

Equipment

Sterile cotton-tipped applicator(s) in a sterile culture tube(s) or Culturette(s) (Figure 11-8)
Clean tongue depressor
Laboratory requisition(s)
Disposable, single-use examination gloves

PROCEDURE

1. **Wash your hands. Use appropriate personal protective equipment (PPE) as dictated by facility.**

2. **Assemble the required equipment.**

3. **Identify the patient and explain the procedure. Tell the patient that you are going to swab the back of the throat with the cotton-tipped applicator to obtain a specimen that will then be examined in the laboratory.**

RATIONALE

Avoid contamination.

This helps determine the cause of the patient's sore throat.

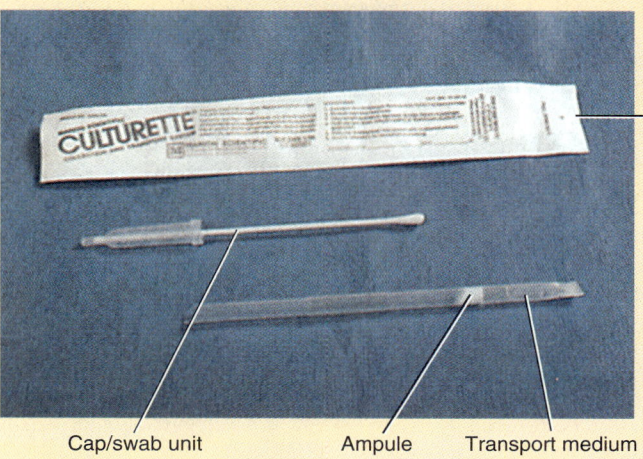

Peel-apart envelope

Cap/swab unit   Ampule   Transport medium

FIGURE 11-8 Culturette II and Culturette bacterial collection/transport systems. (See Vocabulary, p. 474, for an explanation of these systems.) (Courtesy Marion Scientific Corp, Kansas City, Mo.)

PROCEDURE 11-4

THROAT CULTURE—cont'd

4. Have the patient assume an upright sitting position facing you. The area where you are working should be well lit. You may use an examination light that is positioned to give maximal illumination of the patient's throat.

5. Don gloves.

6. Ask the patient to open the mouth as wide as possible, to extend the tongue, and to say "ah."   *Saying "ah" helps relax the patient's throat muscle and minimizes the gag reflex.*

7. Remove the sterile, cotton-tipped applicator(s) from the culture tube or from the Culturette tube. Commercially prepared culture tubes are available in which the applicator stick is secured in the lid of the tube.

8. Depress the patient's extended tongue with the tongue blade until the back of the throat is clearly visible (Figures 11-9 and 11-10). Place the tongue blade over two thirds of the tongue.   *This helps prevent the patient's tongue from touching the applicators as you are obtaining the throat specimen.*

9. Using the cotton-tipped applicator, swab the area at the very back of the throat on both sides. Pay particular attention to swabbing any red, raw, or raised bumps along the side and any areas coated with pus. Take care not to swab the tongue but only the part of the throat from which the specimen should be obtained. Saliva must be avoided. Heavy mucus draining down the back of the throat from the nose is also undesirable culture material.   *Saliva dilutes the specimen, leads to overgrowth of nonpathogens, or inhibits the growth of the pharyngeal flora.*

10. Remove the applicator quickly but gently and place it into the culture tube, securing the lid. If a Culturette has been used, release the transport medium by crushing the ampule with your fingers.

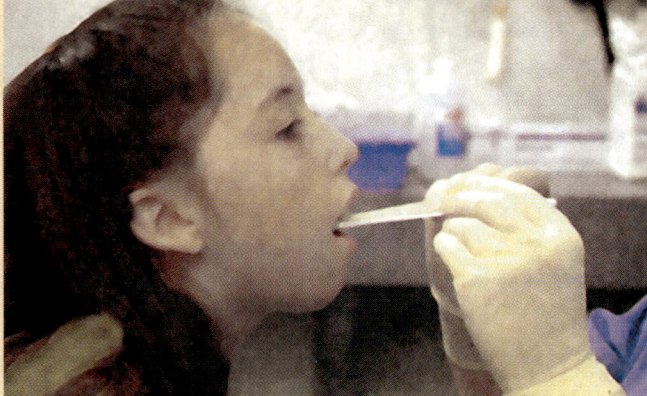

FIGURE 11-9 Obtaining a throat culture.

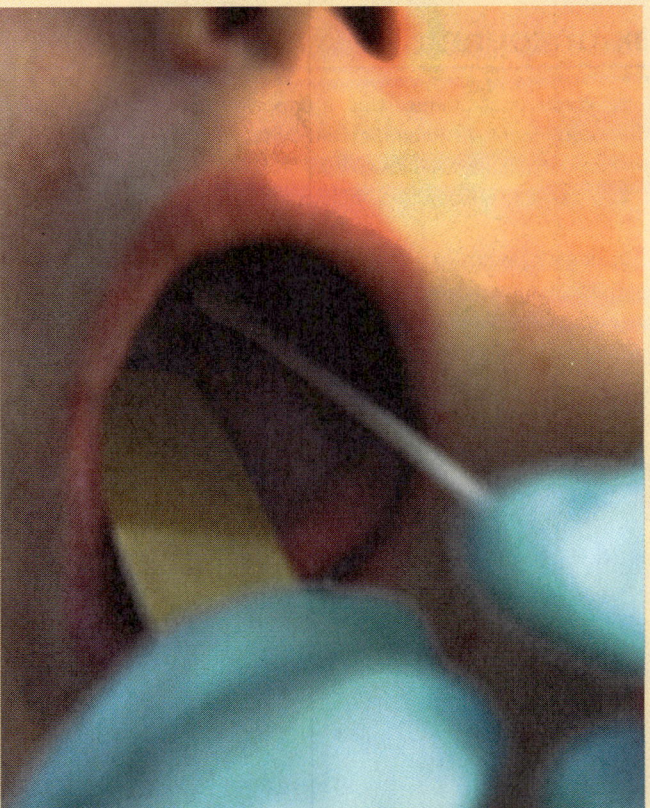

FIGURE 11-10 Area of the mouth in which to swab for the throat culture.

PROCEDURE 11-4

THROAT CULTURE

NOTE: On occasion, two cultures are required—one each from the right and left tonsillar areas. Use two culture tubes with applicators when doing this and label each specifically. Use a quick, downward stroke, first on one side and then, with *another* applicator, on the opposite side. Keep the tongue depressed while obtaining both specimens.

11. Remove the tongue blade and discard into covered waste container.

12. Attend to the patient's comfort; you may reposition the patient if necessary.

13. Remove gloves.

14. Wash your hands.

15. Label the culture tube(s) completely and accurately: patient's name, doctor's name, date, and source of culture.

16. Complete and attach the appropriate laboratory requisition. The information in No. 15 is to be included, as well as the type of examination required.

17. Send the culture tube to the laboratory. Avoid delay. In the laboratory the culture is transferred by the technician to a culture medium.

18. Record on chart.

Your specimen must not dry out before the laboratory can transfer it to a culture medium. A culture medium enables growth of the infectious organism for future examination.

Charting Example

February 27, 20__, 1 PM
Throat culture obtained and sent to laboratory for C & S [culture and sensitivity].
Marcia Edwards, CMA

PROCEDURE 11-5

NASOPHARYNGEAL CULTURE

Objective

Understand and demonstrate the correct procedure for obtaining a nasopharyngeal specimen for a culture; prepare the specimen to be sent to the laboratory; and record the procedure on the patient's chart.

To obtain a better specimen with more organisms, you may induce the patient to cough by taking a throat culture first. Coughing can force organisms from the lower respiratory tract up to the nasopharyngeal area.

PROCEDURE

RATIONALE

1. Obtain a throat culture first (if desired).

Continued

PROCEDURE 11-5

NASOPHARYNGEAL CULTURE—cont'd

2. Insert a sterile cotton-tipped applicator through the nose into the nasopharyngeal area. ·

3. Gently rotate the applicator to obtain the specimen.

4. Remove the applicator and place it into the sterile culture tube; secure the lid.

5. Label and send the specimen to the laboratory with the correct laboratory requisition.

To prevent the drying of the specimen on the applicator, avoid delay.

6. Record the procedure on the patient's chart.

Charting Example

February 27, 20___, 1 PM

    Throat and nasopharyngeal specimens obtained and sent to the laboratory for C & S [culture and sensitivity].

    Abby Nelson, CMA

STREPTOCOCCUS SCREENING

A very common infection, especially in children and young adults, is streptococcal pharyngitis, commonly referred to as strep throat. This infection is caused by group A beta-hemolytic strep-tococci. These pathogens are the most common bacterial agents associated with infections of the upper respiratory tract and of the skin. Common signs and symptoms of strep throat include a sore throat, fever, chills, swollen lymph nodes in the neck, and, on occasion, nausea and vomiting. The tonsils are often covered with a white or yellow exudate, and the throat is diffusely red. Treatment generally includes penicillin or erythromycin for patients allergic to penicillin. Prompt diagnosis and treatment of strep throat are important because complications such as rheumatic fever, otitis media, acute glomerulonephritis, or sinusitis may develop.

Several commercial kits can be used to screen for group A streptococci in 4 to 8 minutes in the physician's office or clinic. A throat specimen is needed to perform all of these tests. The manufacturer's directions for each test must be followed precisely to ensure accurate and reliable results. (See also discussion of Gram stain on p. 501).

QuickVue In-Line One-Step Strep A Test. The QuickVue In-Line One-Step Strep A test is used as an aid in the diagnosis of group A streptococcal infections. It provides quick

Text continued on p. 498

PROCEDURE 11-6

QUICKVUE IN-LINE ONE-STEP STREP A TEST*

Objective

Understand and demonstrate the correct procedure for performing a Strep A test and interpreting the test results.

Important:

- Wash your hands before and after performing the test.
- Gloves should be worn when handling human samples.

- Do not use the extraction solution if it is green before breaking the ampule.

Before Testing:

- Only use the swabs provided in the kit.

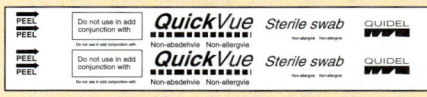

QUICKVUE IN-LINE ONE-STEP STREP A TEST*—cont'd

1. Remove the test cassette from foil pouch and place on a clean, dry, level surface. Using the notch at the back of the chamber as a guide, insert the swab **completely** into the swab chamber.

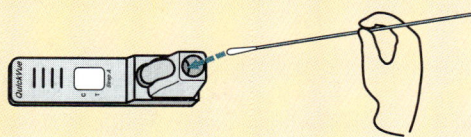

2. Squeeze to crush the glass ampule inside the extraction solution bottle.

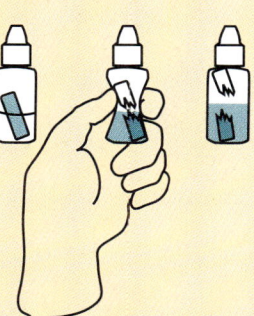

Perform the Assay:

3. Vigorously shake the bottle 5 times to mix the solutions. Solution should turn green after the ampule is broken. **Solution must be used immediately.**

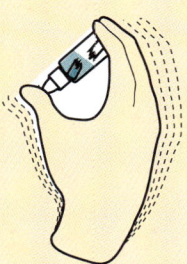

4. Remove the cap. Quickly fill the chamber to the rim (approximately 10 drops).

Quickly → fill to rim

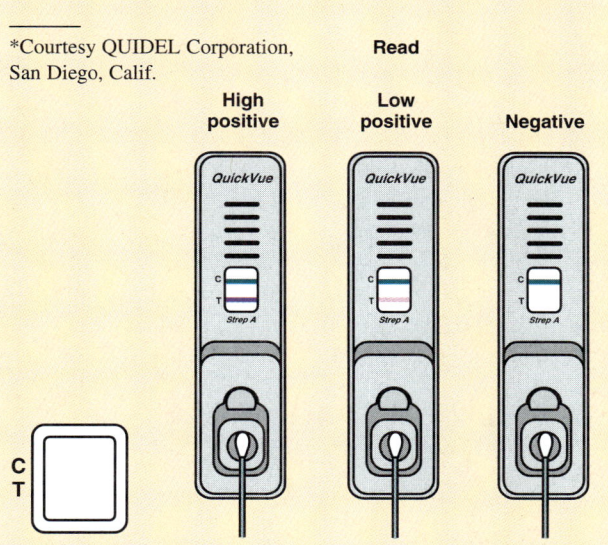

5. Begin timing.

   If liquid has not moved across the result window in 1 minute, completely remove the swab and reinsert. If liquid still does not move across, retest with a new specimen, test cassette, and extraction solution bottle.

   The test cassette should not be moved until the assay is complete.

6. **READ RESULTS AT 5 MINUTES.** SOME POSITIVE RESULTS MAY BE SEEN EARLIER.

7. **Interpretation of Results**

   Positive result:

   The appearance of any pink-to-purple line next to the letter "T" in the result window, along with a blue control line next to the letter "C," means that the test is positive for group A streptococcus.

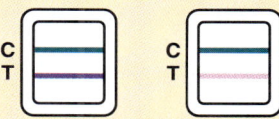

   Negative result:

   The appearance of only the blue control line next to the letter "C" in the Result Window means that the test is negative. A negative QuickVue result means that the swab is presumptive negative for group A streptococcus.

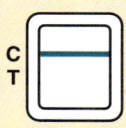

   Invalid result:

   If the blue control line does not appear next to the letter "C" at 5 minutes, the test is considered INVALID, and the test result cannot be used. If this occurs, retest using a fresh swab and a new Quick-Vue test cassette or contact Technical Assistance.

---

*Courtesy QUIDEL Corporation, San Diego, Calif.

detection of group A streptococcal antigens from a patient's throat swab specimen. Obtain a specimen by following standard throat swab collection methods, *using the swab provided with the kit.*

Handling swab specimens. Because group A streptococcus is an infectious agent, follow standard precautions for infectious agents such as wearing disposable rubber gloves while handling swab specimens. Swabs may be disposed of according to the usual procedure of your facility.

WOUND CULTURE

When a wound is thought to be infected, a wound culture is done to determine the presence and the type of microorganism that is causing the infection. Cultures can be obtained from wounds on any part of the body.

The procedure for obtaining a wound culture is described on pp. 331-336 in Chapter 6.

SMEARS FOR CYTOLOGY STUDIES

PROCEDURE 11-7

CYTOLOGY SMEARS

Objective
Understand and demonstrate the correct procedures for making a smear with a specimen obtained by the physician for cytology studies, and preparing the smear to be sent to the laboratory.

Equipment
　　Sterile cotton-tipped applicators or Ayer spatulas (number depending on the number of smears to be obtained)
　　Frosted-end glass slide(s)

　　Fixative spray such as Cyto-Fix (a water-soluble antiseptic), Spray-Cyte, or bottle of fixative solution (solution of 95% isopropyl alcohol preferred; however, formalin 10% may also be used)
Cardboard or plastic slide holder, rubber band, and envelope provided by the laboratory if the slide is to be mailed
Laboratory requisition
Disposable, single-use examination gloves

PROCEDURE

1. **Wash your hands. Use appropriate personal protective equipment (PPE) as dictated by facility.**

2. Write the patient's name and the date on the frosted end of the slide.

3. Don gloves.

4. When a physician has obtained the specimen on the applicator or spatula, be prepared to hold the slide while the physician makes the smear.
　　or
　　Take the applicator from the physician with your dominant hand, grasping the distal end of the stick.

5. Hold the glass slide between your thumb and the index finger of your nondominant hand.

6. Starting near the unfrosted end of the slide, spread the specimen longitudinally along the slide by rotating the applicator in the opposite direction of spreading motion (that is, when spreading the specimen from right to left over the slide, rotate the cotton applicator clockwise [Figure 11-11]).

7. Spread the specimen onto the slide evenly and moderately thin so that individual cells can be identified under a microscope.

RATIONALE

Provides protection for yourself from possible contamination.

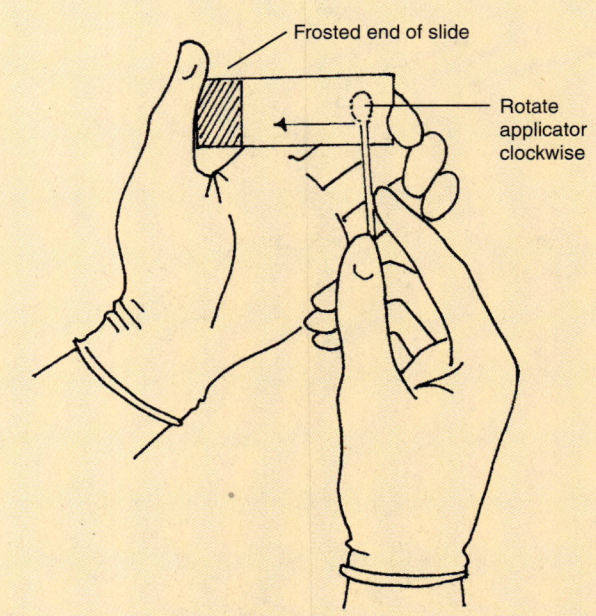

FIGURE 11-11 Making a smear for cytology studies.

PROCEDURE 11-7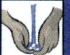

CYTOLOGY SMEARS

8. Discard the applicator in a biohazardous waste container.

9. Fix the smear by immediately spraying it with the fixative spray or by immersing it in the bottle of fixative solution obtained from the laboratory. This should be done within 4 seconds. Spray 5 to 6 inches away. With a continuous flow, make a stroke from left to right, then right to left. Allow to dry 4 to 6 minutes.

Use fixative spray to prevent drying and death of cells. The smear must be fixed within 4 seconds to prevent drying and death of cells.

10. Remove gloves. **Wash your hands.**

11. Send the smear in the designated container to the laboratory for cytologic tests with the correct and completed requisition (Figure 11-12).

NOTE: If you are to mail the slide to a particular laboratory, place the slide inside the cardboard slide holder provided, once the fixative is dry. Close it with a rubber band.

Fill out the requisition, giving the patient's name, age, LMP (last menstrual period), hormonal or other medication or treatment, pertinent clinical data, and history of any previous atypical Pap smears if this is a vaginal or cervical smear. Insert the slide and requisition into the envelope provided, seal, and mail (see Figure 5-19).

In the laboratory, the smear will be incubated for a prescribed time (24 to 72 hours) at 37° C (98.6° F) or room temperature because excessive heating of the smear destroys the microorganisms. To identify specific organisms, the laboratory personnel will use various staining procedures and then examine the smear microscopically.

CYTOLOGY— SURGICAL PATHOLOGY REQUISITION. SEE BACK PAGE FOR INSTRUCTIONS

FOR LAB USE ONLY

CYTOLOGY - SLIDE NUMBER _____

PREVIOUS SMEARS: ☐ NO ☐ YES GRADE_____

PERTINENT HISTORY: (MUST BE COMPLETED)

| LMP | HORMONES | LAST PREG. | PREGNANT NOW? ☐ YES ☐ NO | IRRAD-IATION | SURGERY? | POST-MENO-PAUSAL |
| / / | | | | | | |

MATERIAL SOURCE

☐ CERVIX
  ☐ GASTIC
☐ VAGINA
  ☐ BREAST
☐ SPUTUM
  ☐ CSF
☐ URINE
☐ FLUID
OTHER _____

DATE & TIME OF COLLECT

PLEASE PRINT

LAST NAME   FIRST NAME

ADDRESS

| BIRTHDATE | AGE | SEX | CLASS |

| PHYSICIAN | ROOM NO. | HOSP. NO. |

| DATE | PHONE |

NAME OF INSURANCE CO.

A

MISCELLANEOUS FINDINGS					ESTROGEN EFFECT		HORMONAL PROFILE		
TEST	MANY	MOD-ERATE	FEW	NONE	HIGH			PB	I	S
RBC										
WBC					MODERATE		MI			
TRICHOMONAS					LOW		☐ SPECIMEN UNSATISFACTORY			
CANDIDA					ATROPHY					
BACTERIA					INVALID DUE TO INFLAMMATION	SCANTY ☐ DRIED ☐	EXCESSIVE INFLAM. EXUDATE ☐			
ENDOCERVICAL CELLS										

NAME OF INSURED & I.D. NO.   (ATTACH MEDI-CAL STICKER TO GREEN COPY)

CHARGE TO: ☐ PATIENT   ☐ PHYSICIAN

☐ NEGATIVE   ☐ ABNORMAL   SEE REPORT BELOW

TECHNOLOGIST/ PATHOLOGIST _____

TIME IN   TIME OUT

FIGURE 11-12   Sample laboratory requisition for cytology studies. **A,** Front side of requisition.

PROCEDURE 11-7

GENERAL INSTRUCTIONS:	1. Fill out history 2. Label specimen containers and slides with patient's FULL name. 3. Deliver sputum, fluid and urine specimens within 1 hour of collection; REFRIGERATE until delivery
CERVICAL/VAGINAL PAP SMEAR	1. Prepare 1 or 2 smears of material from scraping of cervical canal and/or cervical os. 2. Place slides in fixative* immediately for a minimum of 10 minutes.
SPUTUM	1. Obtain first morning, deep-cough specimen. 2. Instruct patient to rinse mouth with water before stimulating cough. 3. Collect specimen in container with tightly fitted lid. 4. 50% Alcohol may be added as a preservative if specimen cannot be delivered to laboratory within 2 hours of collection.
BREAST (Nipple Secretion, Cyst Fluid)	1. Prepare 1 or 2 direct smears on a Dakin all-frosted slide. 2. Place slides in fixative* immediately.
BRONCHIAL WASH PERICARDIAL FLUID PERITONEAL FLUID PLEURAL FLUID	1. Collect fluid in vacuum bottle or Vacu-Bag.
GASTRIC WASH	Contact Cytology 24 hours in advance for detailed instructions.
SPINAL FLUID	1. Collect 5 to 7 ml of fluid.
URINE	1. Collect 1st morning, clean catch specimen. A catherized specimen is suggested from female patients.

B

FLUIDS — DELIVER TO LAB IMMEDIATELY

*Fixative in bottle can be obtained in Cytology Lab.

FIGURE 11-12—cont'd   Sample laboratory requisition for cytology studies. **B,** Back side of requisition.

SMEARS FOR BACTERIOLOGY STUDIES

PROCEDURE 11-8

BACTERIOLOGY SMEARS

Objective

Understand and demonstrate the correct procedure for making a smear for bacteriology studies and preparing the smear to send to the laboratory.

The procedure for making a smear for bacteriology studies is the same as that for cytology smears (Steps **1** to **8**, pp. 498-499), except to fix the smear.

PROCEDURE

9. Place the smear on a flat surface and allow to air-dry for approximately a half hour.

10. Grasp the slide with forceps and pass it quickly through the flame of a Bunsen burner 3 or 4 times to *heat fix* the slide. *Do not* overheat the slide because this will distort the cells present.

11. Forward the slide to the laboratory in the container provided with the completed laboratory requisition.

RATIONALE

Air-drying allows the specimens cells to dry slowly.

Microorganisms are killed with the heat and attached to the slide so that they will not wash off when the slide is stained in preparation for examination.

GRAM STAIN

Once a smear is sent to the laboratory, it will be treated in various ways so that visualization of microorganisms under a microscope is possible. A method commonly used to identify bacterial organisms is the Gram stain. This staining method permits the classification of bacteria into four groups: gram-positive or gram-negative rods and gram-positive or gram-negative cocci. The technique involves the treatment of the smear with Gram crystal violet, Gram iodine solution, 95% ethyl alcohol-acetone decolorizer, and safranin counterstain, after which the forms and structure of the microorganisms can be visualized. Bacteria are differentiated on the basis of their color reaction to the aforementioned stains. Gram-positive organisms stain purple (for example, staphylococci, streptococci, and pneumococci). Gram-negative organisms are decolorized with the alcohol-acetone solution and retain only the red color of the counterstain, safranin (for example, gonococci, meningococci, and *Escherichia coli).* Such a classification has important clinical implications because it immediately narrows down the differential diagnosis, thus guiding treatment until additional tests such as culture and sensitivity are completed. The type of groups in which bacteria are arranged, such as chains, pairs, and clusters, can also be seen on the Gram stain. This is another important guide for treatment.

The Gram stain is usually followed by a culture and sensitivity test to help determine definitive diagnosis and appropriate treatment of an infectious process.

Often the physician will want to start antibiotic therapy for an infectious process before the culture and sensitivity test results are available. In this case the results of the Gram stain are most useful. With the results of the Gram stain, the physician can start a reasonable antibiotic regimen on the basis of past experience as to what drug(s) work against the identified microorganism. For example, this protocol is used when it is suspected that the patient may have streptococcal pharyngitis (strep throat) caused by a group A beta-hemolytic streptococci. This type of streptococcal pharyngitis most often affects young children between the ages of 3 and 15 years and young adults. Early diagnosis and treatment of this condition are important because it can be followed by serious conditions such as rheumatic fever or glomerulonephritis.

PROCEDURE 11-9

  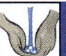

GRAM STAIN

Objective
Understand and demonstrate the correct procedures for performing a Gram stain on a smear on a glass slide and prepare the slide for microscopic examination.

Equipment
Smear on a glass slide that has been heat fixed
Slide forceps

Staining rack
Wash bottle containing distilled water
Gram crystal violet
Gram iodine solution
95% ethyl alcohol-acetone decolorizer
Safranin counterstain
Bibulous paper pad (absorbent paper pad)
Disposable, single-use examination gloves

PROCEDURE

1. After making the smear and heat fixing it as described earlier, place the slide on the staining rack, with smear side facing up.

2. Cover the slide with Gram crystal violet. Allow it to react for 1 minute (Figure 11-13, *A*).

PROCEDURE

3. Grasp the slide with slide forceps and tilt it about 45 degrees to allow the Gram crystal violet to drain off (Figure 11-13, *B*).

4. Rinse the slide thoroughly with distilled water for about 5 seconds (Figure 11-13, *C*).

A   **B**   **C**

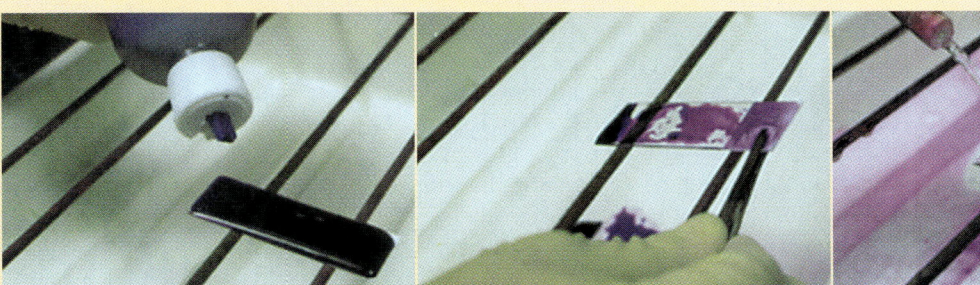

FIGURE 11-13   Gram stain procedure.

Continued

PROCEDURE 11-9

GRAM STAIN—cont'd

PROCEDURE

5. Replace the slide on the staining rack.

6. Cover the smear with Gram iodine solution, allowing it to react for 1 to 2 minutes.

7. Grasp the slide with the slide forceps and tilt it to a 45-degree angle to allow the Gram iodine solution to drain off.

8. Rinse the slide in this position with distilled water from the wash bottle for 5 seconds.

9. With the slide still tilted at a 45-degree angle, slowly pour the alcohol-acetone solution over it. This decolorizes the smear. Gram-positive bacteria are resistant to decolorization and retain the Gram crystal violet stain. These bacteria remain purple. Gram-negative bacteria are now clear or colorless because they are unable to retain the stain.

10. Rinse the slide with distilled water for 5 seconds.

11. Replace the slide on the staining rack, cover it with the safranin counterstain, and allow it to react for 30 to 60 seconds. The

PROCEDURE

gram-negative bacteria must be counterstained to be seen under the microscope. The safranin counterstain stains them pink or red.

12. Grasp the slide with the slide forceps and tilt it to a 45-degree angle to allow the safranin counterstain to drain off.

13. Rinse the slide thoroughly with distilled water for 5 seconds.

14. Blot the smear dry between the pages of the bibulous paper pad with the smear side facing down. Do not rub the slide because you could rub the smear off the slide (Figure 11-13, D).

15. The slide is now ready to be examined microscopically. Position the slide on the microscope using the oil-immersion objective. Adjust the microscope for the examination of the smear, ensuring that the slide was prepared properly (Figure 11-13, E). (Refer to Chapter 10 for instructions on using a microscope.)

16. Notify the physician that the smear is ready to be examined.

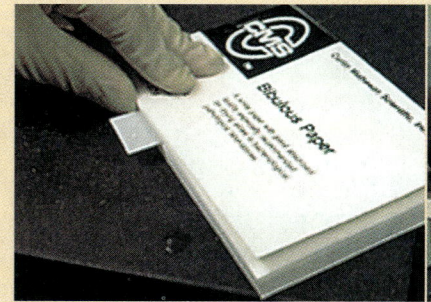
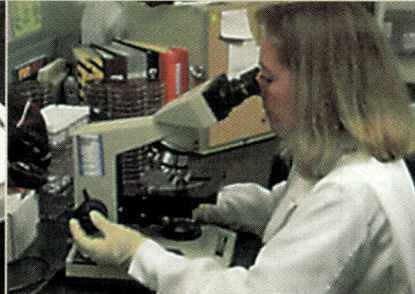

FIGURE 11-13 Gram stain procedure.

BACTERIAL CULTURE AND SENSITIVITY (C & S) TESTING

Bacteria may be identified by means of a culture. A specimen is put on a culture medium that is conducive to the growth of microorganisms (Figure 11-14). The culture is then incubated for 24 to 48 hours to allow the growth of the microorganisms. After this period, the appropriate tests are performed to identify the microorganisms present. Commonly, the identification of a specific microorganism is accompanied by a sensitivity study, which determines the sensitivity of bacteria to

antibiotics. The disk-plate method is most commonly used clinically (Figure 11-15). This method measures the inhibition of growth of a microorganism, on the surface of an inoculated culture medium plate, by an antibiotic diffusing into the surrounding medium from an impregnated disk. The organism is reported as being sensitive, intermediate, or resistant to the antibiotic. The results obtained from a C & S provide the physician with information used to determine which antibiotic can be used to destroy pathogens causing a patient's infectious condition.

FIGURE 11-14   Blood agar culture media contained in a Petri dish showing growth of bacterial colonies.

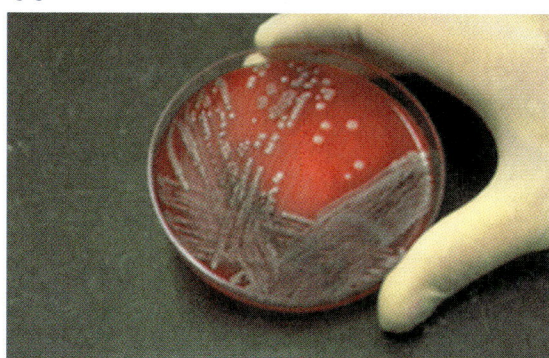

FIGURE 11-15   Disk-plate method for sensitivity test. Microorganism being tested is inoculated on the agar medium. Paper disks containing antibiotics are placed on the medium. Clear zones represent inhibition of growth of the microorganism by the specific antibiotic. Zone size is significant. If zone size is smaller than prescribed for clinical effectiveness, the microorganism is reported to be resistant to the drug. Growth around the impregnated disk indicates that the organism cannot be destroyed or inhibited by that antibiotic. When the microorganism is sensitive to the antibiotic, there is a clear zone around the impregnated disk, indicating that the antibiotic was effective in destroying the organism.

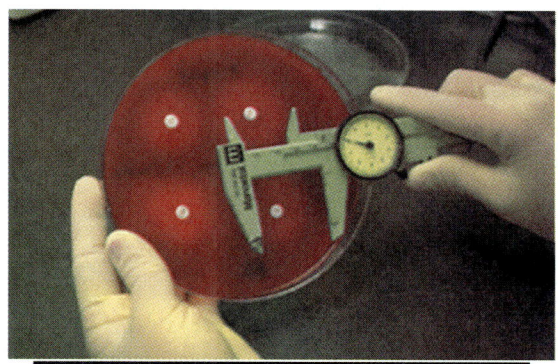

A

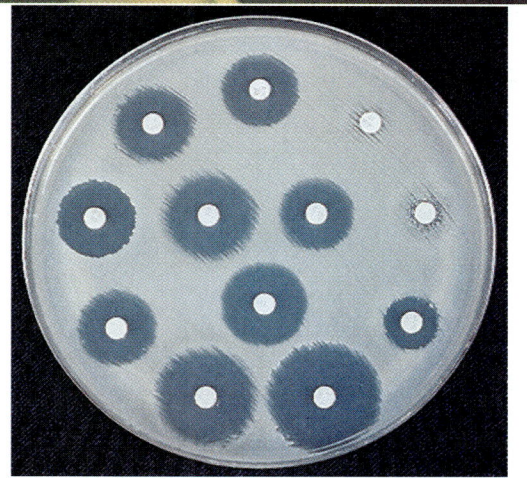

B

CULTURE MEDIA

A **culture medium** is a sterile, commercial preparation used for the growth of microorganisms or other cells. The most commonly used media are broths (liquids), gelatin (solid), and agar (solid). The **liquid media** are usually prepared in test tubes; **solid media** are prepared in test tubes or in Petri dishes or plates (round, flat, covered dishes) (see Figure 11-14).

Liquid media (broths) may be used for the growth of most organisms and for studying the production of gas, odor, and pH changes. Solid media (agar and gelatin base) are used for the growth of organisms, which then allows the observation of colony size, shape, and color.

The classification of media according to their function and content follows:

- **Enrichment media.** These contain substances that inhibit the growth of various bacteria. They are used especially to isolate organisms that grow in the intestines and to prepare cultures from stool specimens. Examples include chocolate agar and blood agar.
- **Selective media.** These contain substances that suppress the growth of some organisms while enhancing the growth of others. They are used to examine stool and sputum specimens (for example, mannitol salt agar and the modified Thayer-

Text continued on p. 506

PROCEDURE 11-10

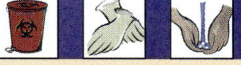

INOCULATING A CULTURE MEDIUM

Objective
Understand and demonstrate the correct procedures for inoculating a culture medium with a specimen obtained on an applicator; prepare the culture plate to send to the laboratory; and record the procedure on the patient's chart.

Equipment
Sterile cotton-tipped applicators in a sterile tube or Culturettes

Culture medium—this varies with the type of specimen collected and the laboratory's preference; for example, Thayer-Martin (TM) culture medium is used most often for vaginal, cervical, and rectal cultures
Bunsen burner and match
Sterile wire loop in container
Candle jar (see Figure 11-18)
Disposable, single-use examination gloves

PROCEDURE 11-10

INOCULATING A CULTURE MEDIUM—cont'd

PROCEDURE	RATIONALE
1. Wash your hands. Use appropriate personal protective equipment (PPE) as dictated by facility. Don disposable, single-use examination gloves.	*Prevent contamination.*
2. When you or the physician has obtained the specimen, remove the top cover lid of the culture plate and place it upside down on a flat surface.	*Placing the lid in this manner avoids contamination to the inner surface of the lid, which covers the culture.*
3. Inoculate the culture plate by rolling the applicator in a large Z pattern on the culture medium (Figure 11-16).	*This pattern provides adequate exposure of the organisms on the medium.*
4. Discard the applicator in a covered container for waste materials.	
5. Replace the cover lid on the culture plate.	
6. Obtain the wire loop and the Bunsen burner.	
7. Light the burner and place the wire loop over the flame until it is red hot.	*Heating the loop destroys unwanted organisms. If these organisms were not destroyed, a contaminated growth of organisms would be found in the culture medium.*
8. Allow the loop to cool.	*If the loop is too hot, it destroys the organisms that were inoculated on the medium.*
9. Remove the lid of the plate, placing it upside down on a flat surface.	
10. Cross-streak the inoculated medium with the wire loop. With moderate pressure, crisscross the Z with the wire loop (Figure 11-17). Cross-streaking may be done in the laboratory.	*Cross-streaking spreads the organisms and isolates the colonies from the few contaminants that occasionally grow on selective media.*
11. Replace the lid on the culture plate.	

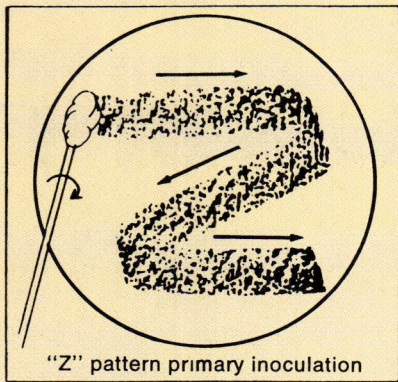

"Z" pattern primary inoculation

FIGURE 11-16   Method for inoculating culture medium. (From *Criteria and techniques for diagnosis of gonorrhea*, U.S. Department of HEW/Public Health Service, Centers for Disease Control and Prevention, Atlanta, Ga.)

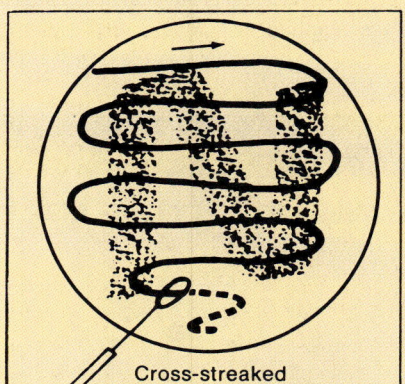

Cross-streaked

FIGURE 11-17   Cross-streaking inoculated medium with sterile wire loop. (From *Criteria and techniques for diagnosis of gonorrhea*, U.S. Department of HEW/Public Health Service, Centers for Disease Control and Prevention, Atlanta, Ga.)

PROCEDURE 11-10

INOCULATING A CULTURE MEDIUM—cont'd

12. Reflame the loop to destroy any organisms that were picked up during the streaking process.

13. Return the loop to the storage place. Store the loop with the wire extending out of the container.

Protect the delicate wire so that it is not destroyed.

14. Label the cover plate with the patient's name, date, and source of specimen.

15. Place the culture plate in a candle jar, with the medium on the top side of the plate (Figure 11-18).
   NOTE: A candle jar is a large, gallon jar with a candle burning in it. The lid is tightly closed after the culture plate has been placed in it. When the oxygen in the jar is depleted, the candle goes out. An appropriate carbon dioxide environment is thus established. The gonococcus bacteria grow best in an environment enriched with carbon dioxide. Each time you place a culture plate in this jar or remove a plate, the candle must be relit.

16. Remove gloves.

17. Wash your hands.

18. Send the culture plate in the candle jar to the laboratory for incubation, along with the appropriate laboratory requisition completed correctly. The jar is kept at room temperature or 35° to 36° C (95° to 96.8° F). Incubation period is usually 20 to 24 hours. After this period, the laboratory worker will examine the culture growth.

19. Record the procedure completely and accurately.

20. NOTE: Following the determination of the type of organism that has grown on a culture plate, sensitivity tests are usually performed to determine the appropriate antibiotic to use for treatment. The organism grown is subjected to a special plate containing various samples of antibiotics. After a period of incubation, this plate is examined. When no growth is observed around a particular antibiotic sample, this indicates that the particular drug is effective in destroying or controlling the infectious organism causing the disease process in the patient (see Figure 11-15).

Charting Example

February 20, 20__, 5 PM
Cervical and rectal specimens obtained by Dr. Edwards. Culture made and sent to the laboratory for C & S.
Judy Dansie, CMA

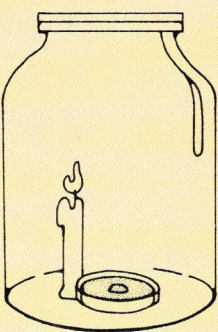

FIGURE 11-18 Inoculated culture medium plate placed in a candle jar for incubation. The jar provides an environment in which bacterial colonies can grow.

Martin media, which are used mainly for suspected gonorrhea specimens and sometimes for detection of meningitis).

- **Differential media.** These contain substances that are used to distinguish between one microorganism and another. They are used to differentiate between forms of colony growth; for example, MacConkey agar is used for routine culturing of stool specimens, and eosin-methylene blue (EMB) agar is used for routine culturing of urine specimens.

Culture media are stored in a refrigerator and warmed to room temperature before being used. If the culture media are cold when used, the microorganisms placed on them will be destroyed. Petri plates are placed in the refrigerator with the media side facing up. Commercial plates come packaged in plastic bags that prevent the media from drying out. These plates have an expiration date on them. If the expiration date has passed, these plates must not be used.

VAGINAL SMEARS AND CULTURE COLLECTION

To assist the physician in diagnosing various gynecologic conditions (for example, cancer of the uterus or cervix, dysplasia, infections, sexually transmitted diseases (STDs), and estrogen levels), smears and cultures for cytologic and bacteriologic tests are obtained from the vagina, cervix, and sometimes the rectum. Some of the more **common gynecologic laboratory tests** include the Papanicolaou (Pap) smear, vaginal smears for trichomoniasis and candidiasis (moniliasis) (common vaginal infections), vaginal smears to determine estrogen levels, and smears and cultures for sexually transmitted diseases (STDs) (for example, gonorrhea, herpes simplex virus type II, and *Chlamydia trachomatis*) (Table 11-1).

HEALTH MATTERS

KEEPING YOUR PATIENTS INFORMED

BEHAVIORAL MESSAGE FOR YOUTH AND SEX PARTNERS OF PATIENTS*

DISEASE PREVENTION

Syphilis, gonorrhea, and chlamydia
- Refer sex partners for prompt medical evaluation
- Avoid sexual activity until treatment is completed and partners are cured
- Use condoms to prevent future infections

Genital warts (human papilloma virus [HPV])
- Return for weekly treatment and follow-up until lesions have resolved
- Women should have annual Pap smears
- Abstain from sex or use condoms during sex while receiving therapy

Genital herpes
- Keep involved area clean and dry
- Abstain from sex while symptomatic
- Use condoms to offer some protection
- All patients should be aware of the risk of fetal infection

Trichomoniasis (TRICH)
- Continue taking vaginally administered medications even during period
- Return to doctor if not cured or problem recurs
- Avoid all alcohol until 3 days following completion of therapy (metronidazole)
- Sex partners of women with trichomoniasis should be treated
- Use condoms to avoid infections

Hepatitis B
- All pregnant women should be screened for Hepatitis B during pregnancy to ensure optimum management of the newborn
- Use condoms to prevent sexual transmission to others

AIDS/HIV
- Inform sex partners and needle-sharing partners of seropositivity
- Women of childbearing age should be counseled about risk of perinatal transmission and about contraception options
- STD-causing ulcers and inflammation have been associated with an increased risk of acquiring or transmitting HIV infection
- Use condoms to avoid infection

Nongonococcal urethritis (NGU)
- Return to doctor if symptoms persist or recur after treatment
- Avoid sexual activity until treatment is completed and partners are cured
- Use condoms to avoid future infections

Pelvic inflammatory disease (PID)
- Receive medical evaluation in 2 to 3 days after therapy has begun
- Refer sex partners for medical examination and treatment
- Avoid sexual activity until treatment is completed and partners are cured
- If an intrauterine device is used, some doctors may recommend removal
- Use condoms to avoid future infections

PROTECT YOURSELF—YOU HAVE CHOICES
Risk Reduction
- Wait to have sex
- Limit number of sex partners
- Learn how to negotiate safer sex with partners

*Taken from Centers for Disease Control and Prevention (CDC) recommendations.

TABLE 11–1 Sexually Transmitted Diseases

	HIV Infection/Disease Acquired Immune Deficiency Syndrome (AIDS)	Cervicitis	Chlamydia
What is it?	An infection by a virus that damages the body's ability to fight infections Most at risk: • Gay and bisexual males • Intravenous (IV) drug users • Recipients of certain blood products • Sexual partners of these groups • Infants born to mothers at risk	An infection of the cervix caused by gonorrhea, chlamydia, or herpes	An infection caused by a bacterium • In women, can cause cervicitis, urethritis, and PID • In men, may cause nongonococcal urethritis (NGU) or infection of the prostate and epididymis
How do you get it?	• Sexual contact with semen, blood, or vaginal secretions of someone with HIV infection • Sharing unsterile IV needles • Breast milk	• Sexual contact with someone who carries the organisms	• Sexual contact with someone who carries the organism
How long after contact will it infect your body? (even if you don't have symptoms)	2 weeks-6 months: symptoms may not develop for 15 or more years	Gonorrhea: 3-5 days Chlamydia: 1-3 weeks Herpes: 2-20 days	1-3 weeks
What are the symptoms?	• Constant fatigue • Unexplained fever, chills, or night sweats • Unexplained weight loss greater than 10 pounds • Unexplained swollen glands • Pink/purple flat or raised blotches on or under skin • Constant diarrhea • Persistent white spots in mouth • Dry cough, shortness of breath	• Green, yellow, or white vaginal discharge in some women • Light bleeding or spotting after intercourse • Occasionally mild pelvic pain or painful intercourse • MOST WOMEN HAVE NO SYMPTOMS	WOMEN: • Pelvic pain, painful or frequent urination • Vaginal discharge • Bleeding after intercourse • MANY WOMEN HAVE NO SYMPTOMS MEN: • Discharge from the penis • Painful urination • MAY HAVE NO SYMPTOMS
How to know for sure?	• Symptoms reviewed by a clinician • Examination performed • Blood tests performed • Oral HIV test	• Pelvic examination to look at cervix • Sample of cervical discharge examined under microscope and sent for laboratory tests	• Sample of discharge examined under a microscope and sent for laboratory tests • Urine tests
How is it treated?	• There is no known cure for AIDS • Treatments focus on the secondary diseases that take advantage of the body's inability to fight infection; AIDS patients should consult a counselor for long-range health planning • Drugs are available to help fight the spread of infection.	• Gonorrhea treated with ampicillin or similar antibiotic • Chlamydia treated with tetracycline or similar antibiotic • Usually both drugs are given to treat both organisms	• Tetracycline or other antibiotics
What can happen if you don't take care of it?	• Persons with AIDS can develop certain life-threatening diseases, which healthy persons with functioning immune systems can ward off • If a woman has HIV, she can pass the virus to her fetus who can then develop AIDS • Can spread infection to sexual partner(s)	• Gonorrhea and chlamydia can spread to cause pelvic inflammatory disease (PID) • Infertility (inability to have children) • All three organisms can be passed to newborn at birth • Can spread organisms to sexual partner(s)	• Severe infection of the reproductive organs • Infertility (inability to have children) • If a woman has cervical chlamydia when she gives birth, the infection can be passed to newborn • Can spread infection to sexual partner(s)
What should you do if you think you might have it?	1. Go to your doctor, local health department, STD or family planning clinic for tests and treatment. GO AS SOON AS POSSIBLE. 2. If you have an infection, be sure to contact all of your recent sexual partners so that they can be tested and treated. 3. Avoid sexual contact until you've taken all of your medication and all symptoms are gone. You might have to return to your doctor or clinic for a test to be sure that your infection is cured.		

Reproduced with permission of Planned Parenthood. Alameda/San Francisco, revised 1999.

Continued

TABLE 11-1 **Sexually Transmitted Diseases—cont'd**

	Genital Warts/ Condylomata	Gonorrhea	Genital Herpes
What is it?	Warts caused by a virus called the human papilloma virus (HPV)	An infection by a bacterium • In women, can infect the cervix, urethra, uterus, and tubes • In men, can infect the urethra, prostate, and epididymis	An infection by a virus called herpes simplex virus (HSV)
How do you get it?	• Skin-to-skin contact with genital warts	• Sexual contact with someone who has gonorrhea	• Sexual contact with someone who has herpes • Direct contact with a herpes sore or discharge from a sore • Herpes can be spread even when no sores are present
How long after contact will it infect your body? (even if you don't have symptoms)	1-6 months	1-10 days	Usually 2-20 days
What are the symptoms?	• Small, painless, cauliflower-like bumps that grow around the sex organs or rectum • There might be slight itching, burning, or irritation, especially with many sores • Warts may be found on the cervix (inside the vagina) where the woman may not notice them	WOMEN: • Pelvic pain, painful urination, vaginal discharge, or fever • 8 of 10 WOMEN WITH GONORRHEA HAVE NO SYMPTOMS MEN: • Painful urination • Drip or discharge from the penis • MAY HAVE NO SYMPTOMS	• Painful blisters that break into open sores • Sores usually appear on or near the mouth, sex organs, or rectum. They may be found on a woman's cervix (inside her vagina) where she may not notice them • Sores will dry up and disappear in 5-21 days
How to know for sure?	• Sores examined • Pap smear may detect presence • Colposcopy may be used to examine tissue	• Sample of discharge examined under a microscope and sent for laboratory tests • Urine tests	• Sores examined • Fluid may be taken from a sore and sent to a laboratory • Blood test may be taken
How is it treated?	Can be removed by: • Burning them off with chemicals, electric current, or laser • Freezing them off • Minor surgery (only if nothing else works)	• Penicillin or other antibiotics	• Once infected, the virus stays in the body; there is no known cure for herpes • Acyclovir is used to treat outbreaks or can be used continuously for up to 6 months to prevent new outbreaks
What can happen if you don't take care of it?	• They can grow larger in size or spread to new areas and become harder to remove • Cervical warts are associated with abnormal Pap smears and can lead to more serious problems • If a woman has cervical or vaginal warts when she gives birth, they can be passed to newborn • Can spread warts to sexual partner(s)	• Severe infection of the reproductive organs • Infertility (inability to have children) • Heart trouble • Skin disease • Arthritis (joint problems) • If a women has gonorrhea when she gives birth, the infection can be passed to newborn and cause eye damage • Can spread infection to sexual partner(s)	• The sores will go away on their own, but they can return, often when ill or under stress • If a woman has herpes sores when she gives birth, the infection can be passed to newborn, causing it serious illness or death • Can spread infection to sexual partner(s) even when no sores are present

TABLE 11–1   **Sexually Transmitted Diseases—cont'd**

Pelvic Inflammatory Disease (PID)	Syphilis	Urethritis	Vaginitis
An infection of the uterus, tubes, and pelvic organs caused by gonorrhea, chlamydia, or other bacteria	An infection from a bacterium	An infection of the urethra caused by gonorrhea, chlamydia, trichomonas, or other organisms • In men, urethritis without gonorrhea is called NGU (nongonococcal urethritis)	An infection of the vagina that has many causes Most common infections: • Yeast • Trichomonas • Gardnerella
• Sexual contact with someone who carries the organisms	• Sexual contact with someone who carries the organisms • Any contact with a syphilis sore	• Sexual contact with someone who carries the organisms	• Sexual contact with someone who carries the organisms • Yeast infections can also occur in women who have not had sexual contact
Varies: organisms can be carried in cervix for months before PID develops	10-90 days	Gonorrhea: 3-5 days NGU: 1-3 weeks	Varies
• Lower abdominal pain, painful intercourse, burning on urination, heavy periods or irregular bleeding, fever, chills • SOME WOMEN HAVE MILD OR NO SYMPTOMS	• EARLY STAGE: A painless sore on the mouth, sex organs, or elsewhere on the body. If left untreated, the sore will go away in a couple of weeks, but syphillis is still present in the body • Many people with syphilis do not notice the sores	WOMEN: • Painful or frequent urination MEN: • Painful or frequent urination • Drip or discharge from penis	• Change in vaginal discharge (more than usual, different color, bad odor) • Itching or burning in or near vagina • Painful urination
• Pelvic examination to feel uterus and tubes • Sample of cervical discharge examined under a microscope and sent for laboratory tests • Blood tests • Pregnancy test to exclude ectopic pregnancy	• A doctor may take a sample from a sore and look at it under a microscope • A blood test will be taken • If the first blood test is negative, another may be necessary in 6 weeks	• Sample of urethral discharge or urine is examined under a microscope and sent for laboratory tests	• Sample of discharge examined under a microscope
• Ampicillin or similar antibiotic followed by tetracycline or doxycycline • Bed rest and "pelvic rest"	• Penicillin or other antibiotic medicine	• Gonorrhea treated with ampicillin or similar antibiotic • Chlamydia treated with tetracycline or similar antibiotic • Usually both drugs are given to treat both organisms	Depending on type of infection: • Vaginal creams, tablets, douches, suppositories • Oral antibiotic medicine
• Pelvic abscess, which may require surgery • Infertility (inability to have children) • Repeat episodes of PID • Chronic pelvic pain • Increased risk of tubal pregnancy • Can spread organisms to sexual partner(s)	SECOND STAGE • (6 weeks-4 months after contact): new sores, rash, fever, hair loss, body aches, sore throat, enlarged lymph nodes THIRD STAGE • (Years later): damage to heart, blood vessels, brain, eyes • A pregnant woman with syphilis can pass it on to the unborn child, causing it severe damage or death • Can cause PID	• In men, urethritis organisms can infect the reproductive organs • Infertility (inability to have children) • Can spread organisms to sexual partner(s)	• Extreme discomfort that will get worse • Can spread to sexual partner(s)

General Instructions

1. Instruct the patient not to douche or use vaginal medication or have sexual intercourse for 24 hours before having a specimen taken (some physicians request abstinence for 48 hours or up to 3 days before the specimen is obtained).
2. Do not collect vaginal or cervical smears when a woman is menstruating because the blood cells that are produced during that period can invalidate the microscopic readings.
3. Avoid doing a Pap smear for at least 6 weeks if the cervix has been cauterized and for a longer period if the woman has undergone radiation therapy because these procedures cause distortion to the cervical cells.
4. Call the laboratory for specific instructions when in doubt on how to collect a particular specimen. Many laboratories provide all the necessary equipment and instructions.
5. Always wash your hands extremely well before and after assisting with any of these procedures. **Always wear gloves when obtaining and handling ALL specimens.**
6. General preparatory and assisting techniques required are the same as those outlined for assisting with a pelvic examination (see Chapter 5, pp. 183-190).
7. Always adhere to proper and accurate procedures to help the physician make a correct diagnosis and initiate the best treatment possible. It is your responsibility to see that specimens are handled and labeled correctly after the physician has collected them.

Papanicolaou Smear or Test

The Pap smear is probably the most common vaginal and cervical smear done because the specimen is easily obtained at the same time that a woman is having a pelvic examination. The Pap test is used to detect cervical cancer. **The American Cancer Society recommends the following:**

- All asymptomatic women age 18 to 40, and those under 18 who are sexually active, have a Pap test annually for three negative examinations. After three or more consecutive satisfactory normal annual examinations, the Pap test may be performed less frequently at the discretion of the physician.
- All asymptomatic women age 40 and over have a Pap test annually for three negative examinations. After three or more consecutive satisfactory normal annual examinations, the Pap test may be performed less frequently at the discretion of the physician.
- Women who are at high risk of developing cervical cancer because of early age of first intercourse, multiple sexual partners, or other risk factors may need to be tested more frequently.
- A pelvic examination should be done as part of a general physical examination every 3 years from age 18 to 40 and annually thereafter.*

Refer to Pelvic Examination and Pap Smear in Chapter 5, pp. 183-190, for more specific information about the procedure, method, and assisting techniques used when obtaining this smear for examination.

Vaginal secretions for hormone evaluation.
Used to determine a woman's estrogen level, the specimen is obtained from the midlateral vaginal wall on a cotton-tipped applicator or spatula. A smear is then made and sent to the laboratory.

Smear for trichomoniasis vaginitis. *Trichomonas* is a genus of parasitic protozoa that occurs in vaginal secretions, causing a vaginal discharge, pruritus (itching), and sometimes a burning sensation when voiding. When trichomoniasis is diagnosed, specific medication, such as metronidazole (Flagyl), is prescribed for treatment. This organism is generally passed from one person to another through sexual contact; therefore the patient's partner, who may be a carrier of the infection but is presenting no symptoms, should also be treated.

When obtaining a smear to diagnose this condition, follow the procedure for assembling equipment and preparing and assisting the patient as outlined for a Pelvic Examination and Pap Smear in Chapter 5, *except* that a vaginal aspirator may be used rather than an applicator to collect the vaginal discharge, depending on the physician's preference. Follow Steps 1 through 13(b), as outlined on pp. 183-185, and then perform the steps in the following procedure on obtaining a smear for trichomoniasis vaginitis.

Smear for candidiasis (monilial vaginitis).
Monilia, now commonly called *Candida*, is a yeastlike fungus. Referred to simply as **a yeast infection** by the general public, it is often in the female's vagina without causing any symptoms; at other times, it produces an uncomfortable white, cheesy or curdlike vaginal discharge, itching, and irritation of the vulva.

Yeast infections are not commonly transmitted by sexual contact; the organisms are found everywhere. However, male sexual partners are advised to wear condoms during outbreaks of candidiasis. Often, infections tend to recur. The **treatment** generally includes the use of vaginal suppositories or creams that the physician prescribes. Over-the-counter (OTC) vaginal medications, such as miconazole (Monistat) and clotrimazole (Gyne-Lotrimin), provide effective treatment for women with recurrent infections. The procedure for obtaining this smear is identical to the one described for trichomoniasis, *except* that the following three steps should be done first.

1. Place a small amount of saline on a slide.
2. Add (mix) 10% potassium hydroxide (KOH) to the saline.
3. Proceed as was described in Steps 2 through 9 on p. 511.

NOTE: If the *Candida (Monilia)* organism is present on the smear, the laboratory technician will observe the branching arms of the fungus when it is viewed under a microscope.

---

*The American Cancer Society: Cancer-related checkup, 1998.

PROCEDURE 11-11

SMEAR FOR TRICHOMONIASIS VAGINITIS (WET MOUNT METHOD)

Objective
Understand and demonstrate the correct procedures for making a smear for Trichomoniasis vaginitis using a specimen obtained by a physician on a cotton-tipped applicator; preparing the smear to send to the laboratory; and recording the required information on the patient's chart.

PROCEDURE	RATIONALE
1. Wearing disposable, single-use examination gloves, place a small amount of normal saline on a slide. The physician obtains a vaginal specimen by saturating the cotton-tipped applicator with the vaginal discharge (or collects the fluid with the vaginal aspirator).	
2. You or the physician then dip the saturated cotton-tipped applicator into the saline solution on the slide (or place the fluid in the aspirator into the saline).	
3. Discard the applicator in a covered container for waste disposal.	
4. Place a cover glass over the depressed section in the middle of the slide. A cover glass is a small, thin piece of glass that covers the saline and the specimen obtained on the glass slide so that any movement of the live cells can be viewed when the slide is examined under a microscope.	
5. Send the smear to the laboratory at once. If the *Trichomonas* organism is present, the laboratory technician will observe a moving, flagellated organism when the slide is viewed under the microscope.	*If the organism is present, it has to be identified immediately.*
6. Assist the patient as required.	
7. Assemble used equipment and dispose of it according to office or agency policy. Refer to Steps 14 to 25 as outlined in the Pelvic Examination procedure in Chapter 5, pp. 183-190.	
8. Remove gloves.	
9. **Wash your hands.** Resupply clean equipment as necessary.	
10. Record on the patient's chart accurate and complete information.	

Charting Example

February 9, 20__, 1:15 PM
Vaginal smear for *Trichomonas* obtained by Dr. Rouse.
Specimen sent to the laboratory immediately.
Patient sent home with a prescription to be filled, pending positive test results from the lab and notification from the doctor.
Susan King, CMA

Smears and cultures to detect gonorrhea.

Gonorrhea is a highly contagious STD caused by the bacterial organism *Neisseria gonorrhoeae,* or gonococcus. **Symptoms** in a man usually occur within 1 week after exposure; a woman experiences no early symptoms. A man has a burning sensation when voiding and a whitish fluid discharge or pus from the penis. Women may experience pain in the lower abdomen, with or without a whitish vaginal discharge or a burning sensation when voiding. Penicillin and other antibiotics or the sulfonamide drugs are all effective treatment. Cure for gonorrhea occurs relatively rapidly, although the patient is not considered cured until cultures taken of the discharge are negative for 3 to 4 weeks. Although gonorrhea is contracted through sexual contact, the gonococcus bacteria can infect the eyes (gonorrheal conjunctivitis), a break in the skin, or an open wound. Thus the importance of preventing contamination to yourself and others with specimens obtained from patients suspected of having gonorrhea cannot be overemphasized. Avoid touching your eyes, always wear gloves, and then wash your hands extremely well after assisting the physician when a specimen is obtained.

Procedure.   For direct smears to be examined, urethral, endocervical, and vaginal specimens are collected and smeared evenly and moderately thinly on two glass slides and then fixed and dried for 4 to 6 minutes (as described previously). Some physicians may obtain a specimen from the anal canal and also from the oropharynx, a common local source for disseminated gonococcal infection. The anal specimen is obtained by inserting a sterile, cotton-tipped applicator approximately 1 inch into the anal canal. The applicator is moved from side to side; 10 to 30 seconds are allowed for absorption of the organisms on the applicator. A smear is then made and fixed. The oropharynx culture is obtained by swabbing the posterior pharynx and tonsillar crypts with a cotton-tipped applicator.

When a culture is desired, two sterile, cotton-tipped applicators or Culturettes are used to collect the specimen. One is placed in a sterile culture tube or Culturette. The second applicator with the specimen is streaked across a special culture medium such as the Thayer-Martin medium. Both specimens are sent to the laboratory together.

CHLAMYDIA TRACHOMATIS: THE DIRECT SPECIMEN TEST*

Chlamydiae are a large group of obligate (able to survive only in a particular environment), intracellular parasites closely related to gram-negative bacteria. The two species are *Chlamydia trachomatis,* primarily a human pathogen, and *Chlamydia psittaci,* primarily an animal pathogen.

The chlamydial infections of trachoma, inclusion conjunctivitis, and lymphogranuloma venereum have been recognized and studied for many years. However, the chlamydiae bacteria have only recently been identified as important etiologic agents in sexually transmissible diseases. The prevalence of these chlamydia-related diseases and the population at risk are thought to exceed those of gonorrhea. *C. trachomatis,* the nation's **most common STD,** is now known to cause urethritis, epididymitis, proctitis, cervicitis, pelvic inflammatory disease, infant pneumonia, and conjunctivitis. It has also been implicated in Reiter's syndrome and premature birth. In both sexes, the infection *may be asymptomatic.*

Females risk the most serious complication of chlamydial infection—acute salpingitis—and they can pass the infection to their newborn infants and sexual partners. Because of these risks, specific diagnosis of *C. trachomatis* in the large population of asymptomatic women is critical.

In addition to being undetected in large proportions of the female population, the organism is masked in another large population: men and women who have gonorrhea. Often chlamydia cannot be differentiated from gonorrhea on the basis of symptoms alone. The result is that gonorrhea is treated, but the *C. trachomatis* goes undetected. Moreover, chlamydia and gonorrhea may require different antibiotic treatment.

The common thread running through all of these aspects, and the most significant element in terms of control, has been the difficulty of diagnosis. Clinically visible signs (for example, macroscopic appearance of cervix, amount of vaginal discharge) are not specific for chlamydial infection, nor are cellular changes seen on Pap smears. Tissue culture, although extremely sensitive and specific, requires a considerable technical and financial commitment and hence is unavailable to most physicians. Also, results from tissue cultures are not available until 4 to 6 days later.

Current efforts to control chlamydial infections have been limited by this lack of adequate diagnosis. Asymptomatic and recurrent infections have gone undetected, and coinfections have been treated inappropriately.

Practical Screening: The Direct Specimen Test*

Screening for chlamydial infections in asymptomatic women requires a diagnostic method that is less costly, less complex, and more available than tissue culture. *The MicroTrak Direct Specimen Test* meets these criteria, while retaining the sensitivity and specificity of tissue culture.

Using monoclonal antibodies labeled with fluorescein, the direct specimen test can detect and identify the smallest forms of the organisms, elementary and reticulate bodies, in direct urethral or cervical smears. Diagnosis can be made within 30 minutes after specimen receipt in the laboratory. No cell culture is required.

Procedure.   As simple a procedure for a physician to perform as a Pap smear, the cervix (or, in the male, the urethra) is swabbed to remove a smear specimen. The specimen is rolled onto a glass slide fixed with methanol and sent to the laboratory at room temperature. In the laboratory, the slide is stained with the MicroTrak antibody solution, causing *Chlamydia,* if present, to appear as individual, bright apple-green pinpoints on a

---

*Courtesy MicroTrak/Syva Co, Palo Alto, Calif.

*Courtesy MicroTrak/Syva Co, Palo Alto, Calif.

background of reddish cells when viewed through a fluorescence microscope, a typical item available in most large laboratories. MicroTrak Mounting Fluid contains photobleaching retardant to inhibit fading of fluorescence during examination of the specimen (Figure 11-19).

This simple test design allows specific diagnosis of *C. trachomatis* in exactly the screening situations that must be tapped: prenatal clinics, family planning clinics, gynecologic offices, and abortion clinics. Furthermore, any routine pelvic examination during which a Pap smear is taken can now be seen as an opportunity to screen for *C. trachomatis*. In populations of women under 25 years of age, in which *C. trachomatis* is about 40 times more prevalent than abnormal cytology, the rationale for such Pap/MicroTrak testing is apparent. With the rapid results afforded by the new test, physicians can prevent further spread to sexual partners or neonates by beginning specific treatment immediately, even while patients are still in the clinic. Follow-up testing to document cure also becomes more convenient.

These advances will undoubtedly contribute to a more targeted therapy and an eventual reduction in the number of chlamydial infections. Similar applications of monoclonal antibody technology are being developed for herpes simplex virus, gonorrhea, and other infectious diseases. The promise for improved diagnosis in these areas is equally great.

FIGURE 11-19   Procedure for *Chlamydia trachomatis* direct specimen test. (Courtesy MicroTrak/Syva Co, Palo Alto, Calif.)

Chlamydia trachomatis and Neisseria gonorrhoeae

Single-swab specimens.   The Gen-Probe PACE 2 direct specimen assay is one system available to test for **both** gonorrhea and chlamydia from a single-swab specimen (two tests, one swab). Specimen collection kits containing swabs and a transport tube are available to test for both gonorrhea and chlamydia from an endocervical or a urethral specimen and to test for chlamydia from a conjunctival specimen. When a urethral sample is needed, the patient should not have voided for at least 1 hour before the sample is obtained. After the specimen has been collected on the swab, the swab must be fully inserted into the transport tube. Once the swab is in the tube, the shaft is to be cut off or snapped off at the score line. Care must be taken not to splash the liquid transport media contents of the tube. A cap is to be applied tightly. The tube is now ready to be transported to the laboratory. The tube is to be kept at 2° to 25° C (10° to 51.4° F) and tested within 7 days (Figure 11-20). The laboratory test that will be performed on the specimen swab takes about 2 hours to be completed. This testing system eliminates the need to prepare slides or culture media, thus being much more convenient in most situations.

Urine specimens.   Urine specimens can also be used to detect gonorrhea and chlamydia infection(s). The patient should not have voided for at least 1 hour before collecting a urine specimen. Give the patient a sterile, preservative-free collection cup. Instruct the patient to collect the *first* 15 to 20 ml of voided urine in the cup (the first part of the stream) and then cap the cup securely. Label the specimen and complete the laboratory requisition. Refrigerate the specimen immediately at 2° to 8° C (10° to 20.8° F). Specimens stored and shipped at this temperature must arrive at the test site within 24 hours of shipment, and many of the available tests must be processed within 4 days of specimen collection. Specimens can also be frozen at minus 20° C or below and must be processed within 60 days of specimen collection. Once frozen, specimens should not be thawed until ready for testing.

Collection

The specimen is swabbed from the urethra, endocervical canal, rectum or neonatal conjunctiva and applied directly to the slide, where it is fixed and sent to the laboratory. (Recommended: MicroTrak™ Specimen Collection Kit containing 2 swabs, slide with 8 mm well, acetone fixative, and transport pack.)

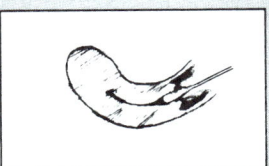

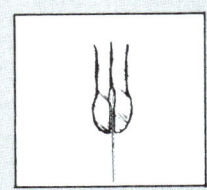

Staining

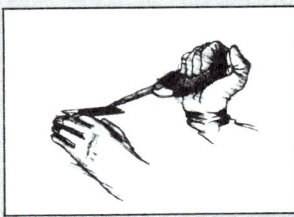

The fixed specimen is stained with MicroTrak™ Reagent and incubated at room temperature for 15 minutes.

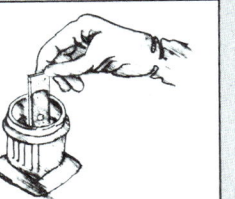

A rinse step removes unbound antibody. The slide is allowed to dry.

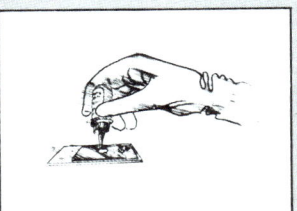

Mounting fluid (provided) is added and the coverslip is applied.

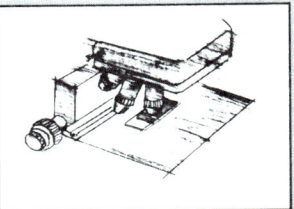

Viewed under the fluorescence microscope, positive specimens contain fluorescent apple-green chlamydial organisms.

See package insert for full instructions

FIGURE 11-20 **A,** Gen-Probe specimen collection kit for urethral or conjunctival specimens and for female endocervical specimens. These kits contain swabs and a transport tube containing liquid transport media. **B,** Collecting female endocervical specimen. **C,** Collecting male urethral specimen. **D,** Collecting conjunctival specimen. **E,** Place specimen swab in tube and cut or snap off shaft of swab at score line; then cap tube. The specimen is now ready to be sent to the laboratory for testing.

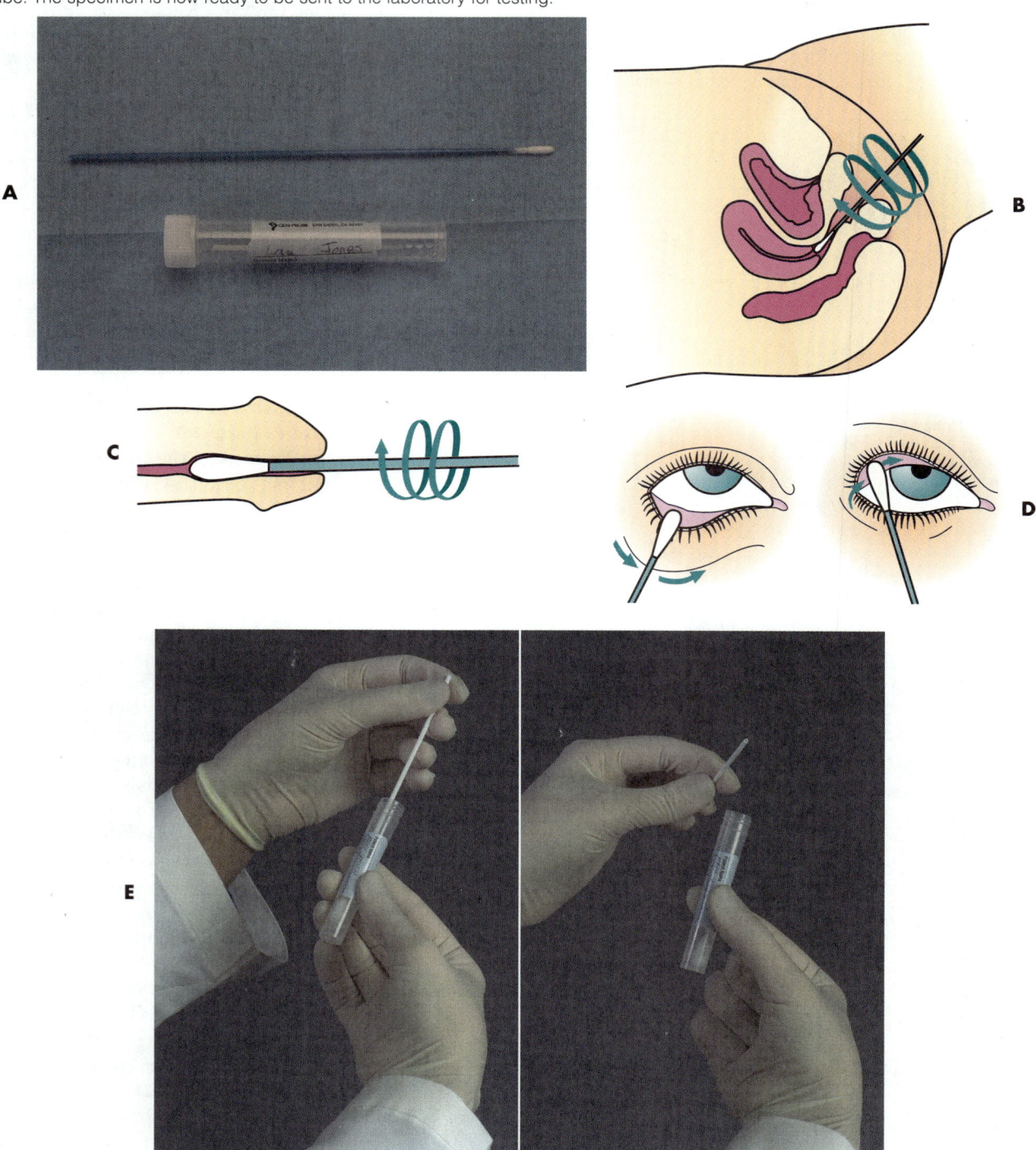

HEALTH MATTERS

KEEPING YOUR PATIENTS INFORMED

CHLAMYDIA FACTS*

- Chlamydia is the most common bacterial STD.
- Greatest number of cases is in people under the age of 25 years.
- Of sexually active females, 15% to 28% are infected.
- Of college students and military personnel, 10% are infected.
- Chlamydia causes 35% to 60% of nongonococcal urethritis (NGU) in heterosexual men.
- Of men with chlamydia, 40% to 50% are *asymptomatic*.
- Of women with chlamydia, 60% to 80% are *asymptomatic*.

GONORRHEA FACTS†

- Gonorrhea is the *most commonly reported* communicable disease in the United States.
- Greatest number of cases is in people under the age of 25 years.
- The chance of reinfection increases with each new infection.

- Gonorrhea can be transmitted *to and from* the pharynx (throat) or penis.

PELVIC INFLAMMATORY DISEASE (PID) FACTS‡

- There are 1 million new cases of PID per year.
- In the United States, 250,000 women are hospitalized per year.
- One fourth of women with PID will develop infertility or ectopic pregnancy.
- PID is the cause of 30% to 40% of all cases of female infertility.
- Costs run over *$4.2 billion per year* for treating PID and sequelae.
- Of women with PID, 20% to 25% will have another episode.

Data from:
*Jon Ellen, MD, Assistant Adjunct Professor, Adolescent Medicine, University of California, San Francisco, Calif.
†Deborah Dean, MD, Assistant Professor of Medicine, University of California, San Francisco, Calif.
‡Abner Korn, MD, Director of Gynecology, Department of OB/Gyn, San Francisco General Hospital, Calif.

HERPES SIMPLEX VIRUSES: DISEASES, DIAGNOSIS, AND TYPING*

Herpes simplex viruses (HSVs) are ubiquitous among humans. Once acquired, HSV can remain latent in the regional sensory ganglia and, when reactivated, move back along the sensory nerves to produce recurrent infections. HSV infections include genital lesions, cold sores, pharyngitis, ocular keratitis, and encephalitis.

The viruses are classified as type 1 or 2 according to their genetic and antigenic composition. Although each type has been associated with a characteristic pattern of infection (oral HSV-1 and genital HSV-2), the site of infection is not an accurate predictor of the virus type. For example, HSV-1 is now suspected to cause a significant proportion of primary genital herpes.

Specific diagnosis of HSV infection is required in many situations, including infections of neonates, immunocompromised patients, or individuals suspected of having herpes encephalitis. In addition, specific diagnosis is useful in counseling sexually active individuals. Typing may be useful in (1) prognosis, because it has been reported that the recurrence rate of genital HSV-1 infection is less than that of genital HSV-2; (2) treatment, because it has been reported that the antiviral activity of chemotherapeutic agents can differ between the two HSV types; and (3) epidemiologic research, in which an association of HSV infection with other disease processes, such as cervical carcinoma, is being studied.

Virus isolation in tissue culture is routinely used for diagnosing HSV infections. Although tissue culture amplifies small numbers of infectious organisms for detection, it requires special facilities and 1 to 7 days before a result can be reported. Culture has stood as a generally recognized reference method, but recovery is recognized to be less than 100%.

Direct examination of viral antigen in cells obtained from lesions provides results more rapidly. A poorly prepared slide can be rapidly identified so that another specimen can be obtained promptly. However, it must be recognized that viral antigen is identified by stained specimens and no direct association with infectivity can be made.

Several laboratory methods of typing HSV have been reported, including plaque size, pock size on chorionic membrane, neutralization, enzyme-linked immunosorbent assay (ELISA), restriction endonuclease analysis, BVDU [E-5-(2-bromovinyl)-2′-deoxyuridine] sensitivity, and immunofluorescence.

The Syva MicroTrak HSV-1/HSV-2 Direct Specimen Identification/Typing Test and Culture Confirmation/Typing Test*

The Syva MicroTrak HSV-1/HSV-2 Direct Specimen Identification/Typing Test can provide typing results within 30 minutes of specimen receipt. The test can easily be used for the identification and typing of HSV in clinical specimens taken directly from external lesions (Figure 11-21).

Cell culture must be initiated at the same time the direct specimen is taken. This allows recourse to the culture results if a direct specimen is negative or inadequate for analysis.

---

*Courtesy MicroTrak/Syva Co, Palo Alto, Calif.

*Courtesy MicroTrak/Syva Co, Palo Alto, Calif.

FIGURE 11-21   A, Syva MicroTrak specimen collection kit; **B,** HSV-1/HSV-2 Direct Specimen Identification/Typing Test. (Courtesy MicroTrak/Syva Co, Palo Alto, Calif.)

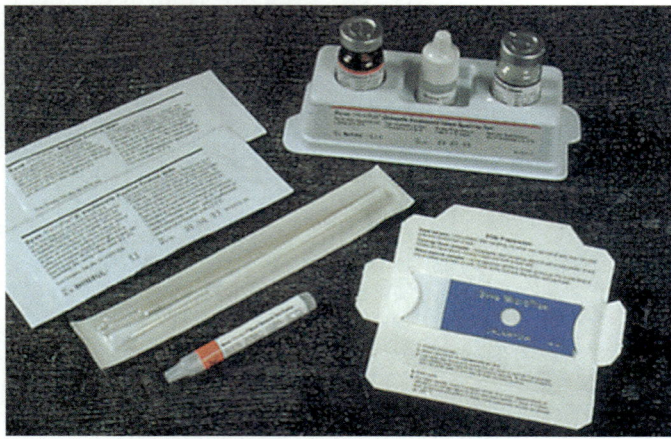

A

Procedure

Collection

The specimen is swabbed from the base of the lesion and applied directly to two slide wells, which are then fixed and sent to the laboratory. (Recommended: MicroTrak™ Specimen Collection Kit containing 2 swabs, slide with 8 mm wells, acetone fixative, and transport pack.)

Samples of poor quality may result in false negative determinations. A sample for isolation in cell culture must therefore be taken at the same time as the direct specimen. This allows recourse to the culture if a direct specimen is negative or inadequate for analysis.

Staining

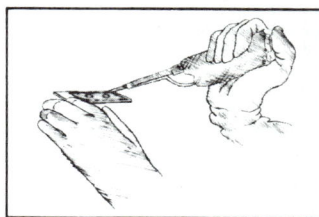

One fixed specimen is stained with HSV 1 Reagent and the other is stained with HSV 2 Reagent. The slide is incubated either at room temperature for 30 minutes or at 37 °C for 15 minutes.   **B**

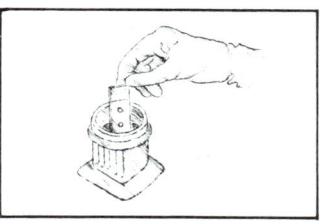

A rinse step removes unbound antibody. The slide is allowed to dry.

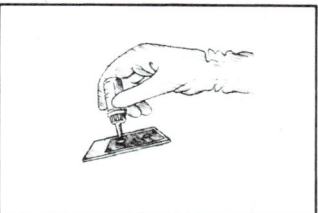

Mounting fluid (provided) is added and the coverslip is applied.

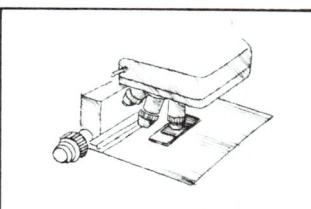

Viewed under the fluorescence microscope, positive cells display characteristic fluorescent apple-green staining. (Specimen quality is checked by evaluating the counterstained cells.)

Procedure.   Samples are taken by swabbing the base of the lesion with two Dacron-tipped swabs simultaneously. One swab is used to apply the specimen directly to a dual-well microscope slide, which is then air-dried and fixed with acetone. The other swab is placed in a transport medium, and both specimens are sent to the laboratory. Monoclonal antibodies that react specifically with HSV-1 or HSV-2 have been prepared and labeled with fluorescein isothiocyanate. At the laboratory, one well on the dual-well slide is stained with HSV-1 reagent and the other well with HSV-2 reagent.

The labeled antibodies bind specifically to their respective viral antigens, and rinse step removes unbound antibody. When slides are viewed under a fluorescence microscope, cells that are positive for the particular viral type show apple-green fluorescent staining that is characteristic of infection with HSV-1 and HSV-2, as demonstrated in the positive control wells; negative cells show only counterstaining, as demonstrated in the negative control wells. The absence of positive cells in the specimen wells should be interpreted cautiously.

In the culture procedure, the transport medium is inoculated into two tissue culture tubes. After the specimens have been cultured, cells are transferred to two slide wells, air-dried, fixed with acetone, and tested with the Syva MicroTrak HSV-1/HSV-2 culture confirmation/typing reagents.

ORASURE HIV-1 ANTIBODY TESTING SYSTEM

Human immunodeficiency virus (HIV) infection and acquired immunodeficiency syndrome (AIDS) are endemic in the United States. Once seen as conditions affecting primarily homosexual men and injecting drug users, HIV and AIDS are increasingly common in young people, women, and minority races. HIV has become the leading cause of death among Americans of ages 25 to 44. People with HIV infection can benefit from the early start of antiretroviral therapy (see also Chapter 1). **Oral HIV testing** in people 13 years of age or older is an alternative to the

HEALTH **MATTERS**

KEEPING YOUR PATIENTS INFORMED

SHOULD I BE TESTED?

HIV is the virus that causes AIDS. These questions will help you decide about taking the HIV test. You will also learn about HIV and AIDS prevention. The HIV test is confidential, and results of the test will be placed in the confidential section of your medical record. Your answers to these questions and the test results will not be shared with anyone outside of the Health Center without your written permission.

Age: ___ Ethnicity/Race: _____ Country of Origin: _____

Gender: ☐ Male ☐ Female ☐ Other, specify _____

Circle your answer:

YES	NO	DON'T KNOW	1. Have you ever been tested for HIV (the AIDS virus)?
YES	NO	DON'T KNOW	2. Did you or any of your sex partner(s) have a blood transfusion or get blood products (for hemophilia) between 1978-1985?
YES	NO	DON'T KNOW	3. Have you or any of your sex partner(s) ever used or shared needles for injecting drugs or other substances?
YES	NO	DON'T KNOW	4. Have you or any of your sex partner(s) had sex while high on drugs or alcohol?
YES	NO	DON'T KNOW	5. Have you had any partners in the past 12 months? If yes, how many? _____
YES	NO	DON'T KNOW	6. Since 1978, have you or any of your sex partner(s) ever traded sex for money or drugs?
YES	NO	DON'T KNOW	7 Has (have) your sex partner(s) had other sex partners in the past?
			8. Does (do) your current sex partner(s) have other sex partners now?
YES	NO	DON'T KNOW	9. Do you have sex with men? (if no, skip to #11)

10. If you have sex with men, have your male partners had sex with (check one):
    - ☐ men only?
    - ☐ women only?
    - ☐ both men and women?
    - ☐ don't know

YES	NO	DON'T KNOW	11. Do you have sex with women? (if no, skip to #13)
YES	NO	DON'T KNOW	12. If you have sex with women, have your female partners had sex with (check one):

   - ☐ men only?
   - ☐ women only?
   - ☐ both men and women?
   - ☐ don't know

YES	NO	DON'T KNOW	13. Have you ever had a sexually transmitted disease (VD)? For example, gonorrhea, chlamydia, herpes, warts, etc.
YES	NO	SOMETIMES	14. Have you ever used condoms/latex barriers to protect yourself and your partner(s) from sexually transmitted diseases, HIV, or pregnancy?
YES	NO	DON'T KNOW	15. Do you have any children who had a positive HIV test or have AIDS?
YES	NO	DON'T KNOW	16. Have any of your sex partner(s) had a positive HIV test or have AIDS?
YES	NO	DON'T KNOW	17. Do you think you may have been exposed to HIV?
YES	NO	DON'T KNOW	18. Would you like to be tested for HIV (the AIDS virus) in our clinic today?
YES	NO	DON'T KNOW	19. Did you know that we offer the HIV oral test?
YES	NO	DON'T KNOW	20. Is OraSure a deciding factor for taking the test?

FOR WOMEN ONLY:

YES	NO	DON'T KNOW	21. Are you now pregnant or trying to get pregnant?

FOR OFFICE USE ONLY:

Date of Assessment: ____/____/____   # _____

____FP____Perinatal____Primary Care___Other   Site # _____

Comments: _____

blood tests that are currently available for determining HIV infection. Oral testing also offers a highly accurate, noninvasive technique and an approach that may be more accessible and available to many people who possibly have been exposed to HIV. The oral sample being collected is known as the oral mucosal transudate (OMT). The OMT contains large amounts of immunoglobulin G (IgG), the type of antibody used to detect HIV. OMT fluid testing is preferable to blood samples because there is no risk of blood exposure occurring from needlestick accidents or during testing and disposal of equipment and specimens. Patients seem more willing to give a sample of oral fluid

rather than a sample of blood most likely because collection is painless and noninvasive. Numerous studies have concluded that HIV is not transmitted by oral fluids in the mouths of people with HIV infection.

An approved noninvasive HIV-1 antibody test shown to be more than 99% accurate is the OraSure HIV-1 oral specimen collection device. The OraSure device consists of an absorbent cotton fiber pad treated with specific nontoxic chemicals that is attached to a nylon stick, along with a specimen vial containing a preservative solution (Figure 11-22). The pad absorbs antibodies, if present, from the blood vessels in the mucous membranes of the cheek and gums in the mouth. IT IS NOT A SALIVA TEST. The OraSure test determines the presence of HIV-1 antibodies, *not* the presence of the virus itself (blood tests determine the same). Diseases, oral conditions, medications, and any non-HIV–related medical condition will not affect the accuracy of the OraSure test. **The OraSure device is to be used *only* for diagnostic purposes and *not* for screening blood donors.** Use of the OraSure device is restricted to people who have been trained in its use. Training manuals and patient information pamphlets are available from the manufacturer.

A patient **must** sign a consent form (Figure 11-23) before being tested. The patient **must** also receive appropriate precounseling and postcounseling because this test and the results present complex issues. The physician or other trained person designated by the physician **must** provide the patient with the pamphlet "Testing for HIV Antibodies With OraSure," which is provided by the manufacturer with the OraSure device. It contains information about the OraSure test, HIV, and AIDS. This

Text continued on p. 521

FIGURE 11-22   OraSure collection device consists of a pad treated with nontoxic chemicals attached to a nylon stick and a vial containing a preservative solution. Pad is placed in the mouth and held in place between the lower gum and cheek for 2 minutes, then placed in the vial.

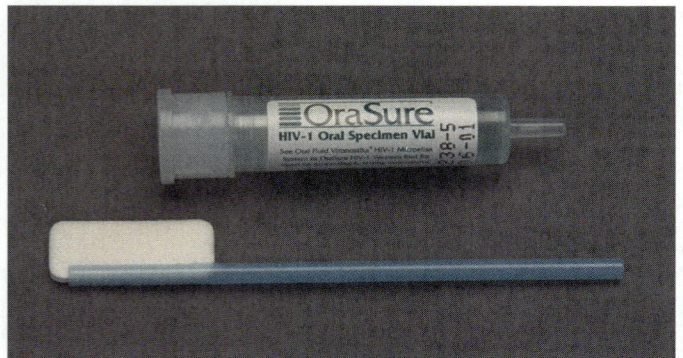

FIGURE 11-23   **A,** Consent form to be signed before HIV testing.

A

HEALTH SERVICES

Phone: 231-5746

HIV TESTING & COUNSELING PROGRAM

CONSENT FOR TESTING
TO DETECT ANTIBODIES TO THE
HUMAN IMMUNODEFICIENCY VIRUS (HIV)

I have been informed that the oral mucosal fluid will be tested for the antibodies to the Human Immunodeficiency Virus (HIV), the probable causative agent of AIDS. I have been informed about the implications and limitations of the test. I have had a chance to ask questions which were answered to my satisfaction. I understand that the test's accuracy and reliability are not 100% certain.

By my signature below, I acknowledge that I have been given information concerning the benefits and risks and I consent to be tested for the antibodies to HIV.

Date: _____

_____
Signature

_____
Printed Name

FIGURE 11-23—cont'd **B,** HIV counseling and testing data form.

HIV COUNSELING and TESTING DATA FORM

ADMINISTRATIVE INFORMATION

SESSION DATE __ __ / __ __ / __ __   SITE No. __ __ __ __
(mm / dd / yy)

UNIQUE TESTING CODE

Place Laboratory Sticker Here

CLIENT INFORMATION

Race/Ethnicity

1st	2nd	
☐	☐	White (not Hispanic)
☐	☐	African American / Black
☐	☐	Native American / Alaskan Native
☐	☐	Mexican
☐	☐	Central American
☐	☐	South American
☐	☐	Other Hispanic / Latino
☐	☐	Filipino
☐	☐	Chinese
☐	☐	Other Asian / Pacific Islander
☐	☐	Other, Specify_____

Age __ __

Gender: ☐ Male   ☐ Transgendered : Male to Female
☐ Female   ☐ Transgendered : Female to Male
☐ Other, Specify_____

Sexual Orientation: ☐ Heterosexual   ☐ Bisexual
☐ Gay Male   ☐ Lesbian/Gay Female
☐ Other, Specify_____

Residence County_____

Residence Zip Code __ __ __ __ __

Is the client pregnant? ☐ Yes   ☐ No   ☐ Not sure

Referred by:

☐ HIV+ Partner Referral
☐ Partner Notification by Health Worker
☐ Outreach Worker
☐ HIV Education Program
☐ AIDS Hotline
☐ Other AIDS Agency
☐ Alcohol/Drug Treatment Program
☐ M.D./ Health Clinic
☐ Friend/Relative
☐ Media
☐ No Specific Referral Source
☐ Other, Specify _____

Reason for testing :

☐ Reconfirming HIV+ result
☐ Reports HIV/AIDS-like symptoms
☐ Has current HIV+ partner
☐ Had past HIV+ partner
☐ TB diagnosis   ☐ PPD reactive
☐ Worried about infecting others
☐ Pregnancy
☐ Risk behavior
☐ New relationship
☐ Just wanted to know
☐ New exposure
☐ At request of partner
☐ Immigration
☐ Rape/Assault
☐ Other, Specify_____

TEST RESULTS   ☐ Positive   ☐ Negative   ☐ Inconclusive

COUNSELING

	Date Service Provided	Counselor Initials
Risk Assessment	__ __ / __ __ / __ __ (mm / dd / yy)	__ __ __
Disclosure Session	__ __ / __ __ / __ __ (mm / dd / yy)	__ __ __
Mail / Phone Client Contact	__ __ / __ __ / __ __ (mm / dd / yy)	

CLIENT SEXUAL RISK HISTORY

(1) **Number of client's sex partners in the last 12 months** ☐☐☐ (000-999 partners)

For ALL partner items below, please enter the most recent occurrence as follows:
0=NEVER **6**=within the last 6 months **D**=Client declined to provide information
1=within the last year **2**=within the last 2 years
3=within the last 3 or more years ago.

Leave blank only to indicate that the risk was not assessed.

Has client ever had sex with:

(2) **One or more partners who had other partners.** (within the last) ☐ months/year(s)

(3) **Male partner(s).** (within the last) ☐ months/year(s)

Sexual Activity	Condom or Latex Barrier Protection		
Oral	☐ Never	☐ Sometimes	☐ Always
Vaginal	☐ Never	☐ Sometimes	☐ Always
Anal Insertive	☐ Never	☐ Sometimes	☐ Always
Anal Receptive	☐ Never	☐ Sometimes	☐ Always

(4) **Female partner(s).** (within the last) ☐ months/year(s)

Sexual Activity	Condom or Latex Barrier Protection		
Oral	☐ Never	☐ Sometimes	☐ Always
Vaginal	☐ Never	☐ Sometimes	☐ Always
Anal Insertive	☐ Never	☐ Sometimes	☐ Always

(5) **Sex with prostitute / sex worker.** (within the last) ☐ months/year(s)

Sexual Activity	Condom or Latex Barrier Protection		
Oral	☐ Never	☐ Sometimes	☐ Always
Vaginal	☐ Never	☐ Sometimes	☐ Always
Anal Insertive	☐ Never	☐ Sometimes	☐ Always
Anal Receptive	☐ Never	☐ Sometimes	☐ Always

(6) **Partner who injected drugs or other substances.** (within the last) ☐ months/year(s)

Sexual Activity	Condom or Latex Barrier Protection		
Oral	☐ Never	☐ Sometimes	☐ Always
Vaginal	☐ Never	☐ Sometimes	☐ Always
Anal Insertive	☐ Never	☐ Sometimes	☐ Always
Anal Receptive	☐ Never	☐ Sometimes	☐ Always

(7) **HIV infected partner.** (within the last) ☐ months/year(s)

Sexual Activity	Condom or Latex Barrier Protection		
Oral	☐ Never	☐ Sometimes	☐ Always
Vaginal	☐ Never	☐ Sometimes	☐ Always
Anal Insertive	☐ Never	☐ Sometimes	☐ Always
Anal Receptive	☐ Never	☐ Sometimes	☐ Always

(check as needed): ☐ **Client knew of partner's HIV+ status prior to sexual activity.**

(8) *(female client only)* **Male partner who has had sex with a male.** (within the last) ☐ months/year(s)

Sexual Activity	Condom or Latex Barrier Protection		
Oral	☐ Never	☐ Sometimes	☐ Always
Vaginal	☐ Never	☐ Sometimes	☐ Always
Anal Receptive	☐ Never	☐ Sometimes	☐ Always

B

TURN OVER →
Continued

FIGURE 11-23—cont'd B, HIV counseling and testing data form.

OTHER CLIENT RISK HISTORY

0=NEVER   6=within the last 6 months   D=Client declined to provide information
1=within the last year   2=within the last 2 years
3=within the last 3 or more years ago.   Leave blank only to indicate that the risk was not assessed.

(9) Drug use. (within the last) ☐ months/year(s)   (if #9 is Zero, go to # 10, else, mark as many as apply below)

☐ alcohol   ☐ crack   ☐ PCP
☐ marijuana   ☐ ampethamines   ☐ LSD
☐ heroin, etc. ☐ cocaine   ☐ psilocybin
☐ barbiturates ☐ nitrates/ites ☐ other hallucins.
☐ tranquilizers ☐ ecstasy   ☐ other, specify:

Used drugs before sex. ☐ Never   ☐ Sometimes   ☐ Always

(10) Injected drugs or other substances. (within the last) ☐ months/year(s)

(if #10 is Zero, go to # 11, else , mark one each below.)

IDU Treatment   ☐ Never   ☐ Past   ☐ Current
Shared Needles   ☐ Never   ☐ Sometimes ☐ Always
Bleached works   ☐ Never   ☐ Sometimes ☐ Always
Needle Exchange ☐ Never   ☐ Sometimes ☐ Always

(11) Diagnosed with STD. (within the last) ☐ months/year(s) Specify STD_____

(12) Received money/other items or services for sex. (within the last) ☐ months/year(s)

(13) Received drugs for sex. (within the last) ☐ months/year(s)

(14) Behavior resulting in other blood to blood contact (s/m, tattoing, piercing, cuts, etc)

or that allows blood contact with mouth, vagina or anus. (within the last) ☐ months/year(s)

(15) Shared objects/fingers inserted in mouth, vagina or anus. (within the last) ☐ months/year(s)

(16) Blood to blood exposure on the job. (within the last) ☐ months/year(s)

(17) Job exposure blood known to be HIV+. (within the last) ☐ months/year(s)

(18) Blood/blood product transfusion before 1985. ☐   for items #18, #19 and #20

(19) Child of HIV infected woman. ☐   check box as appropriate

(20) Other behavior.   Specify_____ ☐

B

REFERRALS

RA Disc
☐   ☐   None, Client refused
☐   ☐   None, Client getting services
☐   ☐   None, Reason: _____
☐   ☐   Referral list only
☐   ☐   HIV Prevention/Education
☐   ☐   Medical Care
☐   ☐   Mental Health
☐   ☐   Drug Treatment / Needle Exchange
☐   ☐   Social Services
☐   ☐   Pregnancy Evaluation
☐   ☐   Other, specify _____
☐   ☐   Other, specify _____
☐   ☐   Other, specify _____

CLIENT HIV TESTING HISTORY

Number of prior H I V tests

☐0 ☐1 ☐2 ☐3 ☐4 ☐5 ☐6 ☐7 ☐8 ☐9+

☐ Check here if client has used home test kit.

Last test result (check one)

☐ Positive   Inconclusive ☐
☐ Negative   Did not return for result ☐

____/____/____ Date:(mm/yy)

GOALS

☐ No Negotiated Behavior Change ← mark this box only if there are no other boxes marked below.

Disclosure

Columns: Risk Assessment / Achieved / Attempted / No Effort made / No opportunity

☐ ☐☐☐☐ Reduce number of partners.
☐ ☐☐☐☐ Increase condom / barrier use.
☐ ☐☐☐☐ Reduce drug use.
☐ ☐☐☐☐ Reduce IDU. *
☐ ☐☐☐☐ Increase bleaching works.
☐ ☐☐☐☐ Utilize needle exchange.
☐ ☐☐☐☐ Increase needle exchange.
☐ ☐☐☐☐ Other (1)_____
_____
_____
_____
_____
☐ ☐☐☐☐ (2)_____
_____
_____
_____
☐ ☐☐☐☐ (3)_____
_____
_____
_____

OPTIONAL DATA

(1)_____   (2)_____
(3)_____   (4)_____

COUNSELOR POINTS TO COVER WITH CLIENT

● Focus on small, realistic changes the client can make.
● Focus on client's perception of their risk(s).
● Ask client to state what behavior(s) they believe they could change to reduce their HIV risk(s) while waiting for results.
● Reinforce and praise positive risk changes the client has already made.
● Problem solve with the client to help them implement their chosen plan.

COUNSELOR NOTES: _____
_____
_____
_____

*Intravenous drug use

information must be read to people who cannot read. Patients must also be informed about other methods used for HIV testing and be encouraged to ask questions. After all this has been completed, the OMT sample can be collected.

Procedure

1. Check the expiration date on the package. *Never* use a device from an expired package. Open the OraSure HIV-1 package containing the collection pad and the specimen vial.
2. Peel open the pad package far enough so that the stick handle on the device can be easily grasped for removing the pad from the package (Figure 11-24).
3. Instruct the patient to take hold of the stick and remove the test collection pad from the package.
4. Instruct the patient to hold the test collection stick with the pad facing *downward* (Figure 11-25), to place the collection pad in his or her mouth between the lower gum and cheek, and to gently rub the pad back and forth along the gum line until the pad is moist.

5. Begin timing for 2 minutes. Instruct the patient to leave the pad in place for 2 minutes (5 minutes maximum).
6. Remove the specimen vial from the package. Record patient identification and date of collection on the vial.
7. Carefully open the vial in an upright position to avoid spilling contents.
8. Give the opened vial to the patient **or** hold it in your gloved hand.
9. At the end of 2 minutes, instruct the patient to remove the pad from his or her mouth and to place the pad into the specimen vial. The pad is to be pushed *all the way to the bottom of the vial* (Figure 11-26).
10. Instruct the patient to break the collection pad stick by snapping it against the side of the specimen vial and to return the vial to you if he or she was holding it (Figure 11-27). (The stick is scored to enable easy breakage.)
11. Cap the vial securely. The cap *snaps* into place when it is placed securely on the vial.
12. Follow the physician's orders for handling the specimen. You may wrap the laboratory requisition around the specimen vial, secure it with a rubber band, and place it into a sealable plastic bag before it is sent to a laboratory that is qualified to test this special specimen.

Specimens may be stored at 4° to 37° C (39° to 98° F) for a maximum of 21 days. This includes the time needed for shipping and testing. Local, state, and federal regulations regarding transportation must be followed (see also Chapter 1 and p. 476 in this chapter). Test results can be obtained *only* by the physician who ordered the test or by someone under the supervision of the physician.

LUMBAR PUNCTURE

A lumbar puncture (LP) is the insertion of a thin, hollow needle into the subarachnoid space of the spinal canal, usually between the third and fourth (L3-4) or between the fourth and fifth (L4-5) lumbar vertebrae, to withdraw cerebrospinal fluid (CSF) or to inject air or a radiopaque contrast medium into this

FIGURE 11-24 Peel the device package open and have patient remove the pad by holding onto the stick handle.

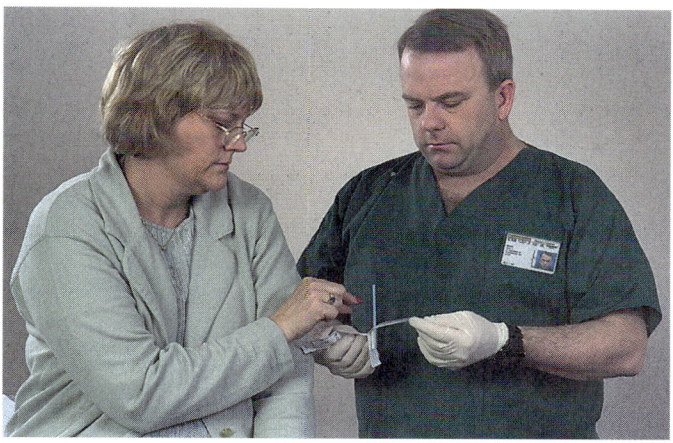

FIGURE 11-25 Hold test pad collection stick with pad facing down and insert between gum and cheek.

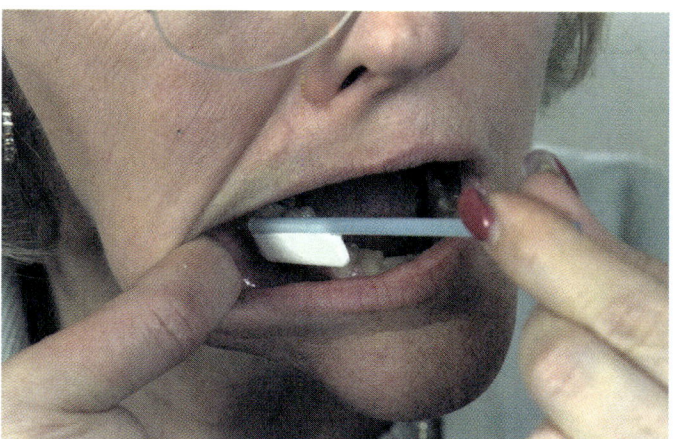

FIGURE 11-26 Collection pad with the specimen is placed in the vial and inserted to the bottom.

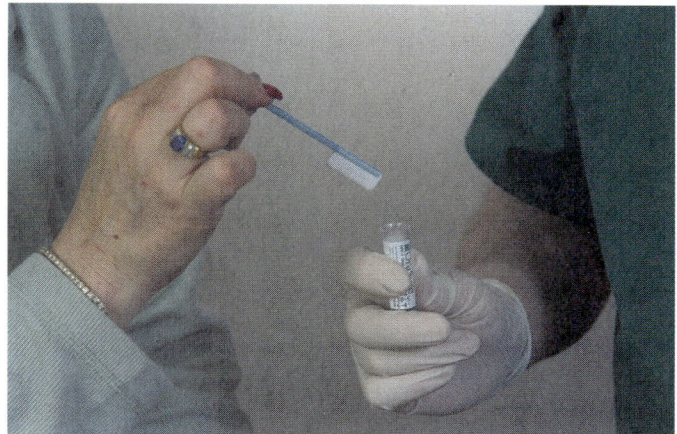

FIGURE 11-27   Patient is instructed to break the collection pad stick by snapping it against the side of the specimen vial.

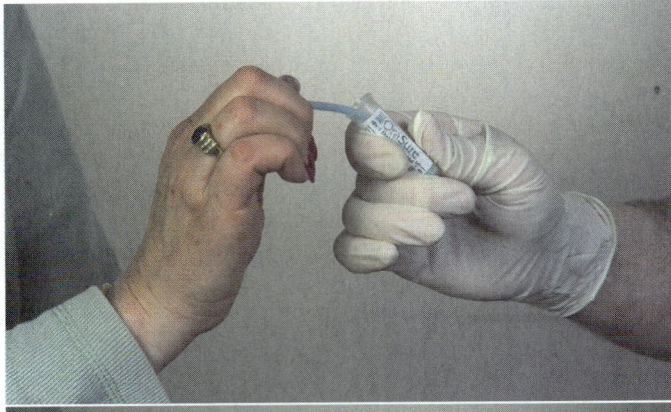

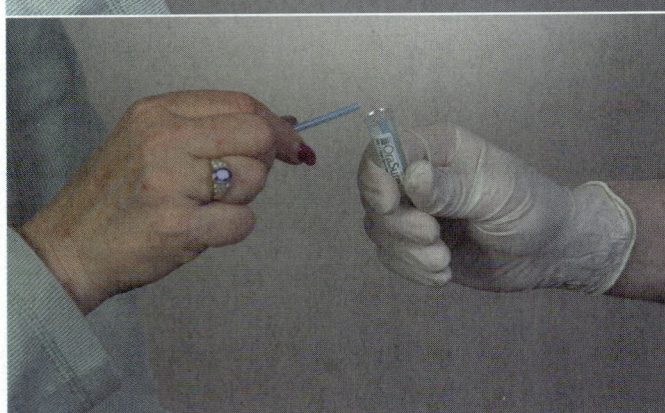

space. This procedure, also called a **spinal puncture** or **spinal tap,** is done under aseptic conditions for both diagnostic and therapeutic purposes.

For *diagnostic purposes,* an LP is done to:

- Obtain a specimen of CSF for laboratory examination (for example, microscopic examination to determine the presence of white blood cells, red blood cells, neoplastic cells, and microorganisms; chemical determinations for sugar and protein; and serology tests to detect syphilis and certain viral infections)
- Determine the presence of an obstruction to the flow of the CSF
- Measure the pressure within the cerebrospinal cavities
- Inject a radiopaque contrast medium into the subarachnoid space for an x-ray film examination of the spinal canal and cord (myelogram)

For *therapeutic purposes,* an LP may be performed to relieve cerebrospinal pressure or to remove pus or blood from the subarachnoid space. It is also necessary for the injection of a spinal anesthetic. **The patient must sign a consent form before an LP is performed.**

PROCEDURE 11-12

 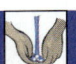

LUMBAR PUNCTURE

Objective
Understand and demonstrate the correct procedure for assisting the physician performing a lumbar puncture; attending to the patient; preparing the specimens to be sent to the laboratory; and record relevant information on the patient's chart.

Equipment
A sterile prepackaged or disposable set containing the following:
  Lumbar puncture needles, 20- to 22-gauge, 3 to 5 inches long (size may be specified by the physician)
  Three-way stopcock
  Needles, 22-gauge, 1½-inch and 25-gauge, ½-inch; and a 3-ml (or 3-cc) syringe for injecting a local anesthetic
  Spinal fluid manometer for measuring CSF pressure
  Local anesthetic—usually 1% lidocaine (Xylocaine) 10 mg/ml, or procaine
  Three sterile gauze sponges, 2 × 2 inch
  Sterile drape towel
  Sterile fenestrated drape (drape sheet with an open window or hole in it)

  Three swab sticks (stick with a small sponge on the end)
  Three sterile test tubes fitted with snap-top or screw-on caps, for the collection of the CSF
  Small sterile container for antiseptic solution, which is used on the patient's skin
  Adhesive bandage or gauze and tape for dressing at site of puncture when the needle is withdrawn
Additional supplies needed:
  Sterile gloves
  Local anesthetic, if not on sterile tray
  Skin antiseptic such as Betadine
  Soap and water
  Blood pressure cuff (may be used if a Queckenstedt test is to be performed)
  Laboratory requisition
  This is a sterile procedure; excellent aseptic technique must be carried out to avoid any possibility of introducing microorganisms into the spinal canal. It is more commonly done in a hospital or clinic where the patient may rest, lying flat for at least 6 hours after the procedure has been completed.

PROCEDURE 11-12

LUMBAR PUNCTURE—cont'd

PROCEDURE

1. **Wash your hands. Use appropriate personal protective equipment (PPE) as dictated by facility.**

2. Assemble the required supplies and equipment.

3. Identify the patient and explain the procedure. Ensure that the consent form has been signed. Explain what is to occur and how it may feel. You may explain to the patient that there is no danger of injury to the spinal cord because it does not extend past the second lumbar vertebra, and the physician will be inserting the needle at a location that is lower than that level.

4. Have the patient void; save a specimen if required. A full bladder only makes the patient more uncomfortable.

5. Provide a patient gown and have the patient disrobe completely. The gown should be put on with the opening in the back.

6. Summon the physician into the room.

7. Using aseptic technique, open the sterile glove pack and the outer wraps of the LP tray for the physician. The physician dons the sterile gloves and prepares the supplies on the tray for use. The tray and all contents are sterile on all surfaces.

8. Position the patient on the side with a pillow under the head. The knees must be drawn up toward the chest, and the head bent forward as close as possible to the knees (Figure 11-28).

9. Cleanse the skin with soap and water at and around the site to be entered; then prepare (swab) this area with the antiseptic solution by taking a sterile swab stick soaked in the desired antiseptic solution. It is best to start at the area that will be punctured and cleanse and prepare in a circular outward fashion. The physician may choose to do the skin preparation after donning sterile gloves. In this case, you pour the antiseptic solution into the small sterile container on the tray.

   After the skin is prepared, the physician drapes the area with the fenestrated drape and the towel.

10. Assist the physician as required. When using a stock supply of local anesthetic solution, hold the vial, check the label, and repeat the name and dosage of the drug aloud so that the physician hears what you are saying. Then hold the vial so that the physician can also read the label before withdrawing the solution into the needle and syringe. This step is omitted if the drug ampule is supplied on the tray because the physician alone checks the label and withdraws the drug.

RATIONALE

Explanations help alleviate some fear of the unknown, thus allowing the patient to relax somewhat and cooperate during the procedure.

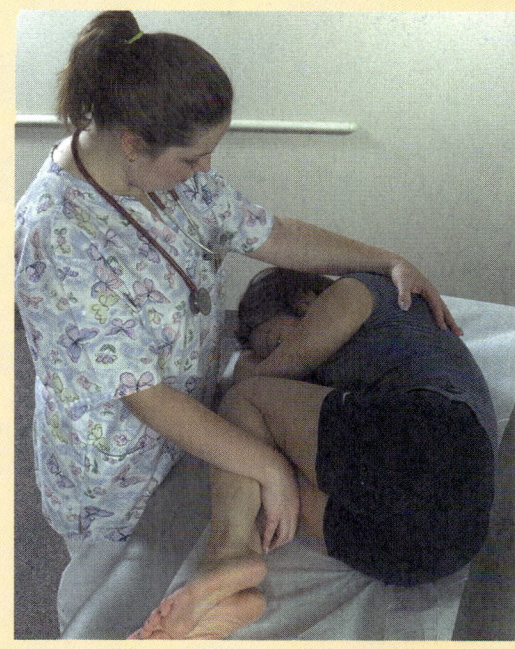

FIGURE 11-28   Patient positioned for a lumbar puncture.

Because the patient's skin is the most likely source of contamination, it must be disinfected before the puncture is done.

LUMBAR PUNCTURE—cont'd

11. Help the patient maintain the correct position. Explain to the patient the importance of remaining very still. You may stand on the side facing the patient's front and hold onto the back of the knees and shoulder. Tell the patient to breathe slowly and deeply through the mouth. Using the 3-ml syringe with the 25-gauge needle, the physician administers the local anesthetic. For deep infiltration, the 22-gauge, 1½-inch needle is used. The usual dose of lidocaine is 1 to 2 ml.

Supporting the patient helps prevent sudden moves that (1) make it more difficult for the physician to insert the spinal needle, (2) cause the needle to break, or (3) cause trauma to the surrounding tissues.

12. Once the spinal needle is in place, instruct and help the patient to slowly straighten the legs (this prevents a false increase in intraspinal pressure) and to breathe normally (that is, not to hold the breath or strain). The spinal puncture needle is introduced into the L3-4 or L4-5 interspace, which is below the level of the spinal cord. To take a pressure reading, the physician attaches the stopcock to the spinal needle and the manometer into the stopcock. At this time you may be asked to record the pressure reading.

13. Don gloves and be ready to receive the specimens of CSF once the physician has obtained them. Check that the caps are secured tightly; stand tubes upright, after securing the caps on tightly. Approximately 2 ml of fluid is collected in each of the three test tubes for observation, comparison, and analysis. Normal CSF is clear, colorless, and sterile. Some disposable trays have depressions in which the physician places the tubes upright, after securing the caps on tightly.

14. Date and label the tubes: CSF No. 1, No. 2, and No. 3, respectively.

 If asked to assist with a Queckenstedt test, which is done when a spinal tumor is suspected, follow this procedure.

Numbering the tubes is important to the laboratory because it considers the contents of tube No. 3 to be the cleanest specimen. This specimen is used by the laboratory for bacteriology and microbiology examinations. The first specimen obtained (tube No. 1) contains the first amount of fluid obtained. Because this is the first amount of fluid obtained after the needle punctured the skin, it is considered by the laboratory to be the most likely specimen to be contaminated.

15. Place a blood pressure cuff around the patient's neck and inflate it to a pressure of 22 mm Hg (the physician attaches the manometer).

 or

 You may be asked to compress the jugular veins for 10 seconds and then release either the cuff or your own pressure on the jugular veins.

 Normally, there is a rapid rise in pressure of the CSF when the veins are compressed and a rapid return to normal when compression is released. When the pressure rises and falls slowly, this indicates a blockage caused by a lesion or tumor that is compressing the spinal subarachnoid pathways.

 These pressure readings are done at 10-second intervals and measured each time the veins are compressed.

16. Note any unusual reaction in the patient (for example, a change in patient's color, respiratory rate, or pulse rate). If you do note any of these changes, inform the physician in a manner that does not alarm the patient.

PROCEDURE 11-12

LUMBAR PUNCTURE—cont'd

17. After the needle is withdrawn, you may place an adhesive bandage or gauze dressing over the puncture site.

18. Assist the patient as required. It is highly advisable to keep the patient lying flat for 6 to 12 hours (up to 24 hours is recommended) to help avoid headaches. If this procedure was done in the office or clinic, keep the patient lying flat for as long as possible before sending him or her home. Encourage the patient to take a liberal amount of fluids. Inform the patient of any special instructions. Often glucose or saline is administered intravenously to a patient with a severe headache. An ice cap and aspirin may also be given to alleviate a headache.

19. Label and send specimens obtained to the laboratory with the completed requisition. Spinal fluid is to be stored in an incubator, not a refrigerator.

Spinal fluid may contain organisms that are sensitive to cold.

20. Return to the examining room to assemble all used supplies and equipment, dispose of them properly, and replace with clean equipment as necessary.

21. Remove gloves.

22. Wash your hands.

23. Do any recording required of you accurately and completely.
NOTE: Physicians may wish to vary the procedural details according to their technique and judgment.

Charting Example

February 11, 20__, 2 PM
Lumbar puncture done by Dr. Cox. Three CSF specimens sent to lab for examination. Opening pressure reading was 250 mm H_2O. Spinal fluid appeared slightly blood tinged.
Patient had no complaints at this time and is resting quietly in the office bed.
Susan Oliver, CMA

CONCLUSION

When you have practiced the procedures in this chapter sufficiently, arrange with your instructor to take the performance test. You are expected to demonstrate accurately your ability to prepare for and to assist with all the procedures outlined in this chapter and to perform some of them. In addition, you are expected to identify accurately the supplies and equipment by the proper name when questioned by your instructor.

REVIEW OF VOCABULARY

The following are samples of information seen on various patient charts. In each of these samples, words that have been defined for you are used. Read them and define the italicized terms.

1. Chief complaint: *Diuresis* and *frequency* for the past 2 months. Laboratory data: urine specimen obtained for *C & S*, and a routine urinalysis. Results: *C & S* showed no growth and no cells; *routine urinalysis*—sugar 4 plus; acetone, moderate.

2. History: This 35-year-old white female accountant has approximately nine *bowel movements* a day times 4 months, increased by activity and eating either fatty or sugary foods. The *stools* are loose and have no form. There is some mucus in the stools and some *melena*. She had problems with *constipation* up until 4 months ago. Stools are extremely foul smelling. *Tarry stools* were followed with *guaiac tests; occult blood stools* were noted. Question of *GI bleeding*.

3. History: This 54-year-old gentleman stated that he first coughed up some bright red blood in his *sputum* about 3 weeks ago. The *hemoptysis* occurred again 1 week ago. He has a chronic cough and has smoked two packs of cigarettes daily for the past 15 years.

    Sputum exfoliative cytology: There was a single group of highly atypical cells present, with nuclear features strongly suggestive of malignancy, although the nuclei are partially obscured by the blood and show some degenerative changes.

4. This patient was first seen 1 week ago, at which time she complained of lower abdominal pain and *dysuria*. The patient also indicated that she had noted progressive *vaginal discharge* during the past week. The patient had previously been followed in the *GYN* clinic at City Hospital because of repeated *Pap smears* that showed *dysplasia* consistent with malignancy. A cervical biopsy was done, but the pathology specimen showed no malignancy. *Vaginal and endocervical smears* were obtained and sent to the lab for *Trichomonas* and *Monilia examinations*. Treatment pending positive laboratory results.

5. This patient complained of severe, persistent pain in the lower back radiating down the right leg. After a complete examination was done, this patient was referred to the x-ray department for a *myelogram*.

6. *Rectal, cervical,* and *throat cultures* showed no *gonorrhea*.

7. *Vaginitis,* secondary to the steroid treatment. The patient has had well-documented *Candida* growth in her vaginal mucosa and has been treated with Mycostatin suppositories.

PATHOLOGY REPORT

The following is a pathology report received in the physician's office after the patient had surgery because of an abnormal Pap smear and postmenopausal bleeding. After reading this, you should be able to discuss the contents with your instructor. A dictionary or other reference book may be used to define terms that are not familiar to you.

PATIENT: Pat Lewis
DATE OF BIRTH: 7-09-33
DATE RECEIVED: 12-12-00
PREOPERATIVE DIAGNOSIS: Abnormal Pap smear, postmenopausal bleeding.
POSTOPERATIVE DIAGNOSIS: Same.
SOURCE OF TISSUE: **A,** D & C curettings; **B,** cold cone biopsy.
OPERATION: Biopsy.
GROSS DESCRIPTION: **A,** Specimen consists of bits of glistening mucoid pink-to-reddish material, totaling about 1 cm in aggregate. Totally embedded in one cassette. **B,** Specimen consists of a somewhat cone-shaped piece of pink, rubbery tissue, 1.8 cm in maximum diameter and varying from 1 to 1.7 cm in height. A widely patulous, round external os, 1 cm in diameter, occupies the cervical aspect.
MICROSCOPIC DESCRIPTION: **A,** Sections show one intact fragment of endometrial tissue with a single nonsecretory gland and compact stroma, along with fragments of glandular tissues lined usually by low-columnar, inactive cells. A rare gland shows slightly taller lining and some perinuclear vacuoles within the cytoplasm. **B,** Sections show a moderately severe chronic and subacute cervicitis and endocervicitis with many of the endocervical glands located in the ectocervical tissues and opening almost up to the surface. Some of these glands are lined by atypical reactive cells. The overlying squamous epithelium shows thickening and areas of parakeratosis and rather marked hyperkeratosis. Occasional granular cell layer is present, and the epithelium is infiltrated with occasional inflammatory cells. The endocervical mucosa is denuded, covered with fibrin and fresh blood. Stroma shows infiltrated chronic inflammatory cells along with an occasional lymphoid follicle. No evidence of malignancy.
DIAGNOSIS: **A,** Fragments of nonsecretory endometrial glands. **B,** Severe chronic and subacute cervicitis and endocervicitis, conization.

M.L. McArthur, MD

CRITICAL THINKING SKILLS REVIEW

1. List four types of materials that can be obtained from a patient's body for laboratory examination.
2. What is meant by "special preparation" of the patient before collecting a specimen?
3. List three types of specimens for which active participation of the patient is required.
4. After obtaining a throat culture, you accidentally drop the lid of the culture tube on the floor. What action would you take before sending the specimen to the laboratory?
5. What specimens should be kept refrigerated if you cannot send them to the laboratory immediately, and why do you refrigerate them?
6. Itemize all the information that should be written on a laboratory requisition when submitting a specimen to the laboratory for examination.
7. You have obtained a wound culture and have sent it to the laboratory for a C & S. Explain what types of testing will be performed on the culture and the purpose of these tests.
8. Why is it important for you to wash your hands before and after obtaining any type of specimen from a patient?
9. List information that you should provide to patients when they are collecting a urine specimen at home.
10. Explain the procedure for fixing a smear; state the value and use of smears.
11. Explain the procedure for inoculating culture media.
12. In what position would you place a patient who is to have a vaginal smear taken? Why?
13. When a physician is doing a lumbar puncture on the patient, where would the spinal needle be inserted, and why at this location?
14. List and compare the three classifications of culture media as described in this chapter.
15. What is the purpose of performing an occult blood test on a stool specimen?
16. List three substances that may affect the color of a stool specimen.
17. What is the purpose(s) of obtaining a sputum specimen from a patient? Describe the explanation that you would give to a patient who is to collect a sputum specimen.
18. Name two common vaginal infections that are diagnosed by means of vaginal smears.

PERFORMANCE TEST

In a skills laboratory, a simulation of a joblike environment, the medical assistant student is to demonstrate skill and knowledge in performing the following procedures without reference to source materials. For these activities the student needs a person to play the role of the patient. Time limits for the performance of each procedure are to be assigned by the instructor (see also p. 104).

1. Given an ambulatory patient and the appropriate supplies, prepare for, give explanations to the patient for, and obtain the following: (a) urine specimen, (b) stool specimen, (c) sputum specimen, (d) throat culture, (e) nasopharyngeal culture, (f) wound culture.
2. Given an ambulatory patient and the required equipment, prepare for, give explanations to the patient for, and assist with the following procedure: (a) vaginal smears and cultures, (b) preparing a smear from the specimen obtained by the physician, (c) lumbar puncture.
3. Having obtained the aforementioned specimens, smears, and cultures, complete the appropriate laboratory requisition form, forward all to the laboratory for examination, and record the procedure on the patient's chart.
4. Given the required supplies, demonstrate the correct procedure for staining a smear using the Gram stain.
5. Given the required supplies, demonstrate the proper procedure for performing a hemoccult slide test on a stool specimen.
6. Given the required supplies, demonstrate how to inoculate a culture medium.

The student is expected to perform these skills with 100% accuracy 95% of the time.

The successful completion of each procedure will demonstrate competency levels as required by the AAMA, AMT, and future employers.

🖥 INTERNET RESOURCES

Men's Health
www.healthfinder.gov

The World Foundation for Medical Studies in Female Health
www.wffh.org

Centers for Disease Control and Prevention (CDC)
www.cdc.gov

Female Health
www.wwfh.org

Women's Health
www.healthfinder.gov/justforyou/women/default.htm

National Association for Women's Health
www.nawh.org

Planned Parenthood
www.ppfa.org/ppfa

American Cancer Society
www.cancer.org

CDC AIDS Clearinghouse
www.cdcnac.org

CDC Hepatitis Branch
www.cdc.gov/ncidod/diseases/hepatitis/hepatitis.htm

The Johns Hopkins University School of Medicine STD Research Group
www.med.jhu.edu/jhustd/stdpage2.htm

JAMA Sexually Transmitted Disease Information Center
www.ama-assn.org/special/std/std.htm

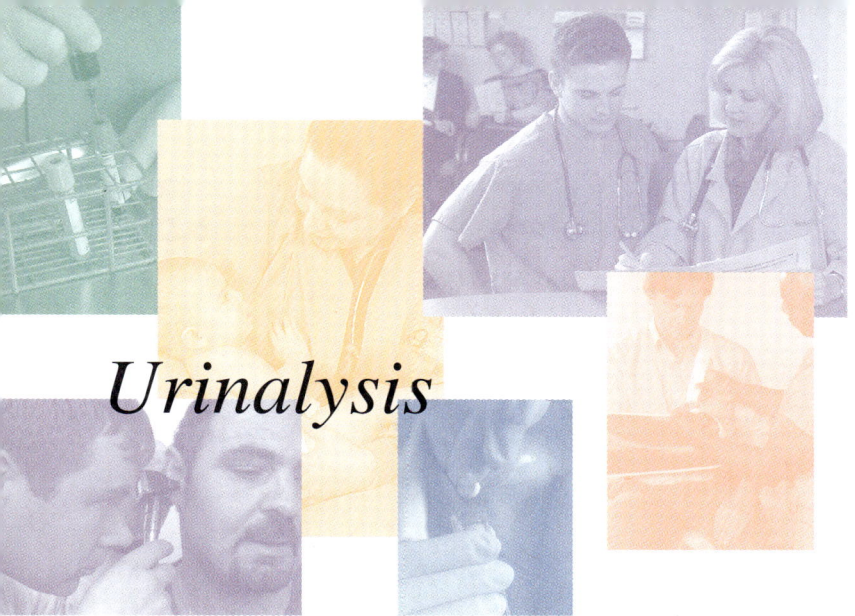

Urinalysis

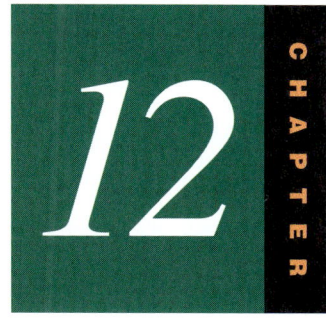

12 CHAPTER

■ Cognitive Objectives

On completion of Chapter 12, the medical assistant student should be able to:

1. Define, spell, and pronounce the vocabulary terms listed.
2. Briefly describe the formation of urine, list the main normal components of urine, and give a description of normal urine.
3. Define "routine urinalysis," listing the three basic categories into which it is divided, along with the major observations and examinations made in each category.
4. Describe the fourth category of tests that may now be included in a routine urinalysis.
5. Describe the standard procedure to follow when performing a routine urinalysis.
6. Identify normal and abnormal findings obtained on a complete urinalysis. Relate the abnormal findings to the most probable or possible causes.
7. Describe a reagent strip that is used for doing chemical tests on a urine specimen.
8. Explain how reagent tablets are to be stored.
9. Discuss the advantage and use of the Dipper and Dropper quality control systems for the chemical analysis of urine.
10. List the organized and unorganized sediment that may be present in a urine specimen, indicating if they are normal or abnormal findings.
11. Identify urine tests other than those performed on a routine urinalysis.

■ Terminal Performance Objectives

On completion of Chapter 12, the medical assistant student should be able to:

1. Demonstrate the correct procedure for performing a physical and chemical analysis of a urine specimen.

2. Demonstrate the correct procedure for preparing a urine specimen for a microscopic examination.
3. Demonstrate the correct procedure for testing a urine specimen for the presence of glucose, acetone, and bilirubin using the Clinitest, Acetest, and Ictotest reagent tablets.
4. Demonstrate the correct procedure for testing a clean-catch midstream urine specimen for bacteriuria using the Microstix-3 reagent strip.
5. Demonstrate the correct methods for using the Dipper and the Dropper quality control systems.
6. Demonstrate the correct procedure for testing a urine specimen to determine a pregnancy.
7. Demonstrate the correct procedure for testing urine for phenylketonuria (PKU).
8. Provide instructions and patient education that is within the professional scope of a medical assistant's training and responsibilities as assigned.

The student is expected to perform these objectives with 100% accuracy.

The consistent use of Universal/Standard Precautions is required by all health care professionals in all health care settings as a method of infection control. It is assumed that these precautions are used in all of the following procedures. Review Chapter 1 if you have any questions on methods to use because the methods or techniques are not repeated in detail in each procedure presented in this chapter.

Be sure to consult the latest guidelines issued by the Centers for Disease Control and Prevention and consult with infection control practitioners when necessary to identify specific precautions that pertain to your particular work situation.

URINARY SYSTEM: FORMATION AND COMPONENTS OF NORMAL URINE

The organs of the urinary system include the **two kidneys, two ureters, one bladder,** and **one urethra** (see also Chapter 18). Urine is formed in the kidneys and passes through the ureters into the bladder, where it remains until the individual voids; then it is excreted through the urethra. The kidneys, located in the retroperitoneal cavity (which means they lie behind the peritoneum), lie anterior and lateral to the twelfth thoracic and first three lumbar vertebrae; they are relatively small, approximately $4\frac{1}{2}$ inches long, 2 inches wide, and $1\frac{1}{4}$ inches thick. Being highly complex and discriminatory organs, they help maintain the state of homeostasis in the internal environment by selectively excreting or reabsorbing various substances according to the needs of the body. From your studies in anatomy and physiology, you should recall the nephron unit, which is the functional unit of the kidney. Each kidney has approximately 1,000,000 nephron units working together to selectively retain or excrete the substances passing through them. Blood, entering the kidneys by way of the renal arteries, eventually reaches the nephron unit for this process to occur. Approximately 1200 ml (30 ml = 1 fluid ounce) of blood flows through the kidneys each minute. This represents about one fourth of the total blood volume in an adult. As blood enters the glomerulus of the nephron, water and the low-molecular-weight components of the plasma filter through to Bowman's capsule, then to Bowman's space, and on through the various parts of the tubules. It is in the tubules that reabsorption of some substances, secretion of others, and the concentration of the urine occur as mechanisms for conserving body water. Many components of the plasma filtrate, such as water, glucose, and amino acids, are partially or completely reabsorbed; and potassium, hydrogen ions, and other substances are secreted. On the average, nearly all the water that passes through this network is reabsorbed; approximately 1 liter (1000 ml) or so is secreted as the largest component of urine (Figure 12-1). **The main normal components of urine follow:**

1. Water—About 95% of urine is water.
2. Nitrogenous waste substances or the organic compounds (that is, urea, uric acid, and creatinine).
3. Mineral salts or the inorganic compounds such as sodium chloride, sulfates, and phosphates of different kinds.
4. Pigment—Derived from certain bile compounds, it gives color to the urine.

Many physiologic changes in the body can lead to an upset in the normal functions carried out by the kidneys. Urine, which is continuously formed in and excreted from the body, provides important information with regard to many diseases and disorders. Accordingly, it is widely studied as an aid in diagnosis, in monitoring the course of treatment of disease, and also in providing a profile of the patient's health status. Urine has been referred to as a mirror that reflects activities within the body and, as such, provides much varied information as a result of many chemical, physical, and microscopic measurements. The analysis of urine can provide information about the whole body, as well as its many parts. Kidney disorders modify the composition of urine and may also affect many other body functions. The study of urine may also reflect the situation in which kidney function is normal but other parts of the body are functioning incorrectly.

ROUTINE URINALYSIS

A routine urinalysis, or basic urinalysis as it is often called, can be easily and quickly performed. It is a basic test, but it provides the physician with a tremendous amount of information when a disease process is present. This test can help confirm or rule out a suspected diagnosis. All patients having a physical examination or entering the hospital for treatment have a urinalysis performed. Often it is a routine test for many patients seen in the physician's office or clinic and is repeated annually or as frequently as necessary to evaluate the patient's health status.

A routine urinalysis is divided into three basic categories. (A fourth category—detection and semiquantitation of bacteriuria—can now also be done easily in the microbiology and urinalysis laboratories). These categories, the major observations, and the examinations for each follow.

1. General physical characteristics and measurements
   a. Appearance
   b. Color
   c. Odor
   d. Quantity
   e. Specific gravity
2. Chemical examinations
   a. Reaction (pH)
   b. Protein
   c. Glucose
   d. Ketone
   e. Bilirubin
   f. Blood
   g. Nitrate
   h. Urobilinogen
   i. Special tests when indicated, such as for pregnancy, phenylketonuria, and porphyrinuria

3. Microscopic examination of centrifuged sediment
   a. Cells (epithelial, red, and white blood cells)
   b. Casts
   c. Bacteria
   d. Parasites and yeasts
   e. Spermatozoa
   f. Crystals
   g. Artifacts and contaminants
4. Detection and semiquantitation of bacteriuria
   a. Culture plate methods—this requires the special facilities and personnel of a microbiology laboratory. Tests should be done immediately, or the specimen should be refrigerated.
   b. Nitrite test and culture strip methods—this can now be done in the urinalysis laboratory.

Standard Procedures

A freshly voided, random urine specimen is collected in a dry, clean container. (Review types of urine specimens outlined in Chapter 11; also review Chapter 10.) This specimen should be examined within 1 hour to avoid changes or deterioration to the contents. If the examination cannot be performed within this time, the specimen should be refrigerated at 5° C (41° F) to preserve the specimen.

When you are doing the examination, the **first** procedure is to note the physical characteristics of the urine; the **second** is to measure the specific gravity; the **third** is to perform a series of

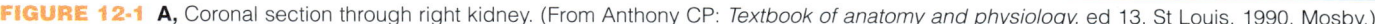

FIGURE 12-1 **A,** Coronal section through right kidney. (From Anthony CP: *Textbook of anatomy and physiology,* ed 13, St Louis, 1990, Mosby.)

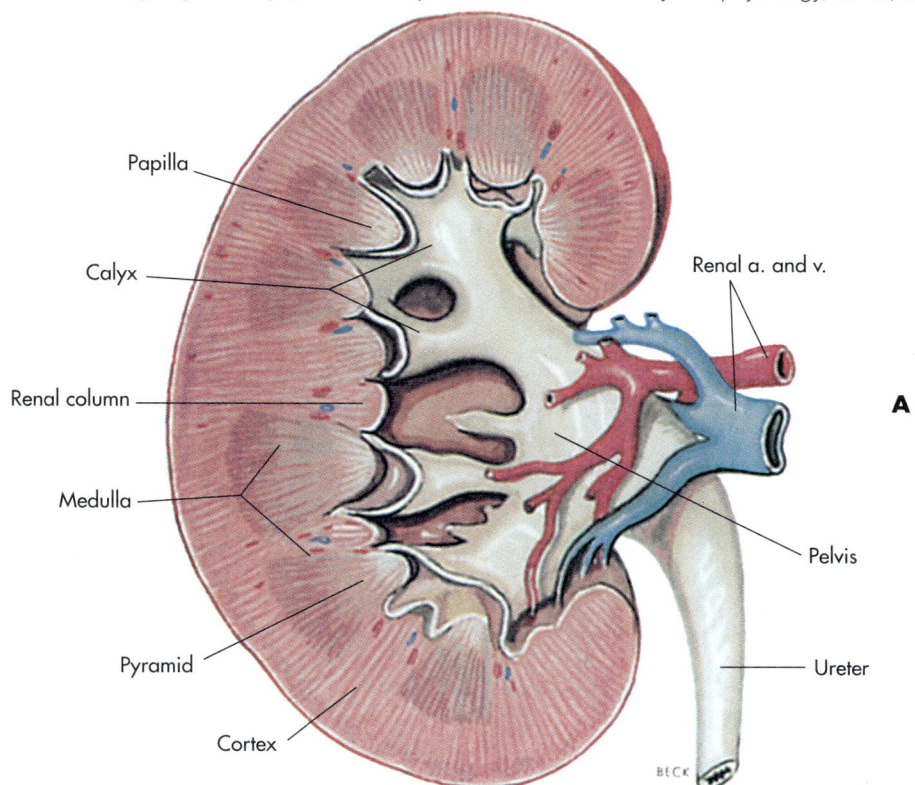

Papilla

Calyx

Renal column

Medulla

Pyramid

Cortex

Renal a. and v.

A

Pelvis

Ureter

BECK

Continued

FIGURE 12-1—cont'd B, Nephron unit with its blood vessels. Blood flows through nephron vessels as follows: intralobular artery → afferent arteriole → glomerulus → efferent arteriole → peritubular capillaries (around tubules) → venules → intralobular vein. (From Anthony CP: *Textbook of anatomy and physiology,* ed 13, St Louis, 1990, Mosby.)

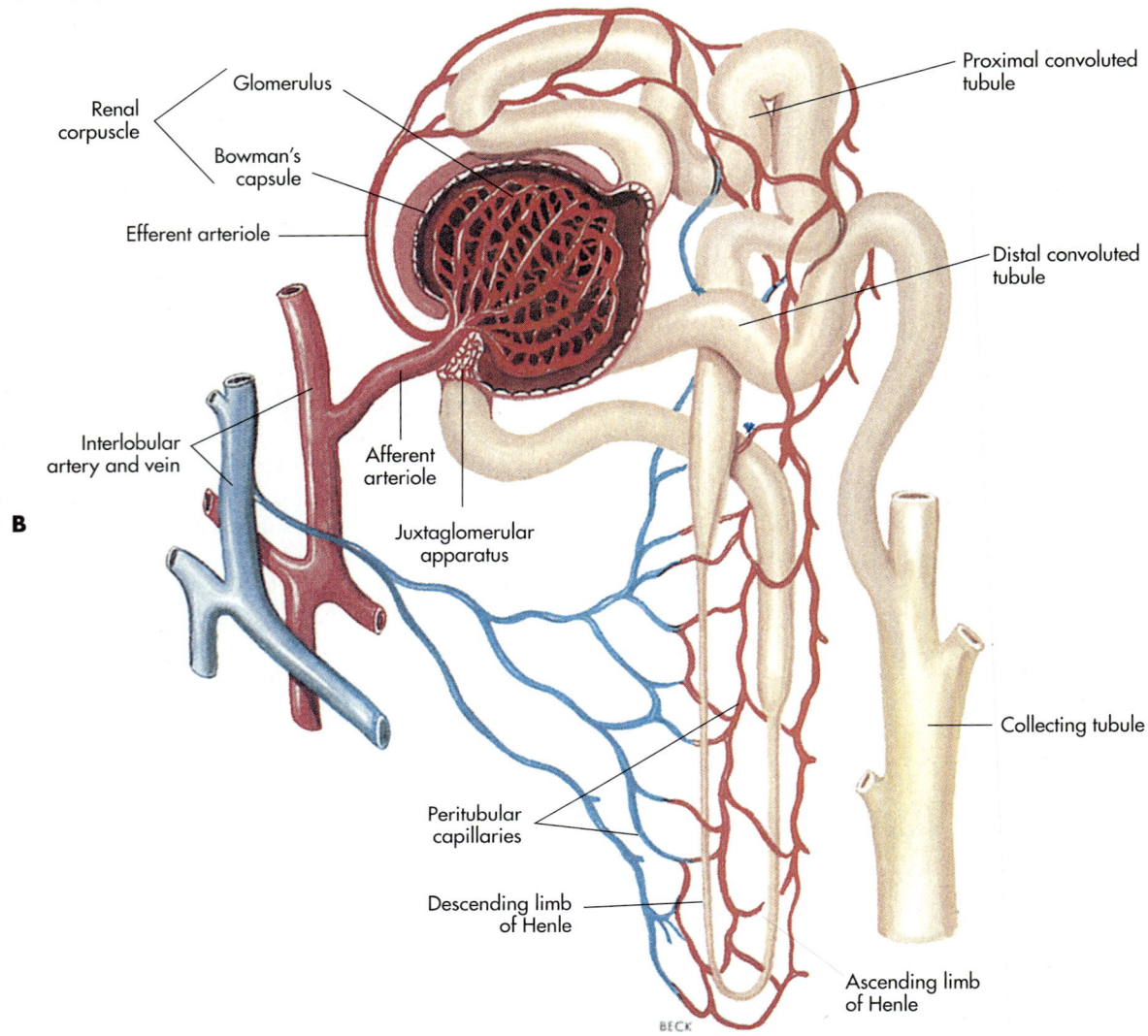

chemical tests; and the **fourth** is to prepare the specimen for the microscopic examination. This fourth step is accomplished by centrifuging 10 to 12 ml of a thoroughly mixed urine specimen; then the residual sediment is resuspended in 0.25 to 1 ml of urine on a slide for the microscopic examination. The remainder of the urine specimen should be kept until all the procedures are completed, in case any of the tests have to be repeated, or if other special tests have to be performed.

Tests performed on a random specimen of urine are **qualitative**. Only the concentration of a substance in this particular specimen can be measured. The total amount of a substance excreted can be measured only when urine is collected over an accurately measured period, such as when collecting a 24-hour specimen.

General Physical Characteristics and Measurements

Appearance. The appearance is generally the first observation made on a urine specimen by virtue of just handling the specimen.

Normal, fresh urine is usually transparent or clear. If the specimen is alkaline, it may appear white and cloudy because of the presence of carbonates and phosphates, but it will clear when a small amount of acid is added to the urine. Urate crystals may be present in an acid urine, giving the specimen a pinkish, cloudy appearance, which usually clears on heating to 60° C (140° F). Both of these appearances are normal.

Abnormal cloudiness in urine may be seen in patients who have a urinary tract infection. This may be caused by the presence of pus cells, leukocytes, and bacteria or by the alkalinity of the urine. Also important to note when observing the appearance of urine is the presence of any sediment (solid particles) in the urine. The presence of red blood cells, white blood cells, or casts in large amounts could indicate renal disease or bladder or urinary tract infection.

Color. Normal fresh urine color ranges are described as straw colored, yellow, or amber—the result of the presence of the yellow pigment, urochrome. The concentration of normal urine determines the degree of the color: highly concentrated urine is dark; dilute urine is pale. Various other factors affect the color of urine (for example, medications, dyes, blood, and food pigments). In many disease states, color changes are caused by the presence of pigments that normally do not appear.

Medications such as multivitamins may make the urine a very pronounced dark yellow; nitrofurantoin (Furadantin) (used in the treatment of urinary tract infections) may make the urine brown; and phenazopyridine (Pyridium) (an analgesic used for relief of pain, frequency, urgency, and other discomforts arising from irritation of the lower urinary tract mucosa) produces a red-orange discoloration of the urine. The presence of hemoglobin in the urine may make it red-brown; bile pigments may turn urine yellow to yellow-brown or greenish. Melanins (dark pigments that occur abnormally in certain tumors), when excreted in urine, cause it to turn brown-black if left standing. If the patient is eating large amounts of carrots, the urine may turn a bright yellow. In hepatitis the urine may be a pronounced orange (when the urine is shaken, even the bubbles are orange if the patient has hepatitis). Also, when an individual eats a fair amount of rhubarb, the urine may be red to red-brown.

Odor. Normal urine has a characteristic aroma that is thought to be caused by the presence of certain acids. An ammonia-like odor develops when urine is left standing for any length of time because of the decomposition of urea in the specimen.

Urine containing acetone, as seen in patients with diabetes mellitus, may have a fruity odor. Urinary tract infections may cause the urine to be foul smelling or putrid.

Although the odor of the urine is usually recorded for a routine analysis, it is generally thought to be of little significance in diagnosing a patient's condition.

Quantity. The normal quantity of urine voided by an adult in a 24-hour period varies somewhat, depending on the individual's fluid intake, the temperature and climate, the amount of fluid output through the intestines (as in diarrhea), and the amount of perspiration. The average quantity is about 1500 ml and ranges from 750 to 2000 ml. The quantity voided by children is somewhat smaller than the amount excreted by adults, but the total volume is greater in proportion to body size.

To measure the quantity of urine, pour the specimen into a large graduated cylinder and record the quantity in cubic centimeters or milliliters. The amount recorded is reported as urine quantity per unit of time (usually 24 hours). Measuring the quantity of urine output is an important aid in diagnosing conditions or diseases related to polyuria, oliguria, or anuria.

Anuria is the absence of urine. At times it may be described as the diminution of urine secretion to 100 ml or less in 24 hours. This may be seen in shock, severe dehydration, and urinary system disease.

Oliguria is the diminution of urinary secretions to between 100 and 400 ml in 24 hours, more commonly defined as scanty amounts of urine. This is seen in drug poisoning, deep coma, and cardiac insufficiency and after profuse bleeding, vomiting, diarrhea, and perspiration. Oliguria is also present with decreased fluid intake and with an increased ingestion of salt.

Polyuria is an excessive excretion of urine. This occurs in diabetes mellitus, diabetes insipidus, chronic nephritis, and following the use of diuretic medications or an excessive intake of fluids. It also may be present during periods of anxiety or nervousness.

Dysuria is painful or difficult urination, symptomatic of many conditions such as cystitis, prolapse of the uterus, enlargement of the prostate, and urethritis.

Specific gravity. The specific gravity of urine is its weight compared with the universal standard weight of an equal amount of distilled water (expressed as 1.000). This measurement indicates the relative degree of concentration of dilution of the specimen, which in turn helps determine the kidney's ability to concentrate and dilute urine.

Normal specific gravity of urine is generally between 1.010 and 1.025, although it may range from 1.003 to 1.030, depending on the concentration of the urine. The first morning specimen has the highest specific gravity, generally being greater than 1.020. It then varies throughout the day, depending largely on the individual's fluid intake.

Abnormally low specific gravity values may be seen in patients who have diabetes insipidus, pyelonephritis, glomerulonephritis, and various kidney anomalies. In these conditions, the kidneys have lost effective concentrating abilities. Values lower than 1.009 are seen in alkalosis, hypercalcemia, hypothermia, potassium deficiency, and increased fluid intake.

Abnormally high values are seen in patients with diabetes mellitus, congestive heart failure, hepatic disease, and adrenal insufficiency. The specific gravity is also elevated when the patient has lost an excessive amount of water through the gastrointestinal tract, as with diarrhea and vomiting, or through the skin during excessive perspiration. High amounts of glucose and protein in the urine, as seen in patients with diabetes mellitus, also increase this value.

Several methods are available for measuring the specific gravity of urine. The newest and easiest method is by using one of five of the Bayer Corporation's Multistix reagent strips. The strip is dipped into the urine specimen and then is compared with the color chart. The test strip reflects specific gravity as it changes color from blue (low specific gravity) through shades of green to yellow (high specific gravity). (See also Chemical Examinations of Urine Using Reagent Strips.)

Specific gravity can also be measured by using a refractometer—Total Solids (TS) Meter—a delicate, handheld instrument that requires calibration daily. Only 1 to 2 drops of urine are required when using this meter.

Procedure for determining the specific gravity of urine using the refractometer

1. Clean and dry the surface of the prism and cover and close the cover.
2. Using an eyedropper, place a drop of urine at the notched end of the cover (Figure 12-2, *A*). The urine should be drawn over the prism by capillary action.
3. Pointing the meter toward a light source, rotate the eyepiece to focus on the calibrated scale (Figure 12-2, *B*). You will observe a light and a dark area.
4. Read the results on the specific gravity scale at the line that divides the light and dark areas (Figure 12-2, *C*). The specific gravity of this specimen is 1.020.
5. Record the results.
6. Clean the prism with a damp cloth and dry it.

The specific gravity of urine can also be determined by using a **urinometer,** a weighted, bulb-shaped instrument that has a stem with a scale calibrated from 1.000 to 1.040. The procedure for using the urinometer follows on p. 535.

The urinometer should be placed in distilled water and checked daily to test its reliability. If it does not read 1.000 when in the distilled water, the urinometer must be replaced. Also, if an unusually high reading is found when testing a urine specimen, remove the urinometer and rinse it under cool water to remove all urine residual; test in distilled water and then retest the urine specimen. These extra steps are important in case someone had previously left an unclean urinometer, which would lead to abnormal test results when used again.

Chemical Examination of Urine Using Reagent Strips

Chemically impregnated reagent strips have virtually replaced older, more cumbersome methods for performing a urinalysis. They provide an easy and rapid method for obtaining the results of tests done in a routine or basic urinalysis; thus they are es-

FIGURE 12-2 A to **C,** Using a refractometer to determine the specific gravity of urine. The specific gravity of this specimen is 1.020.

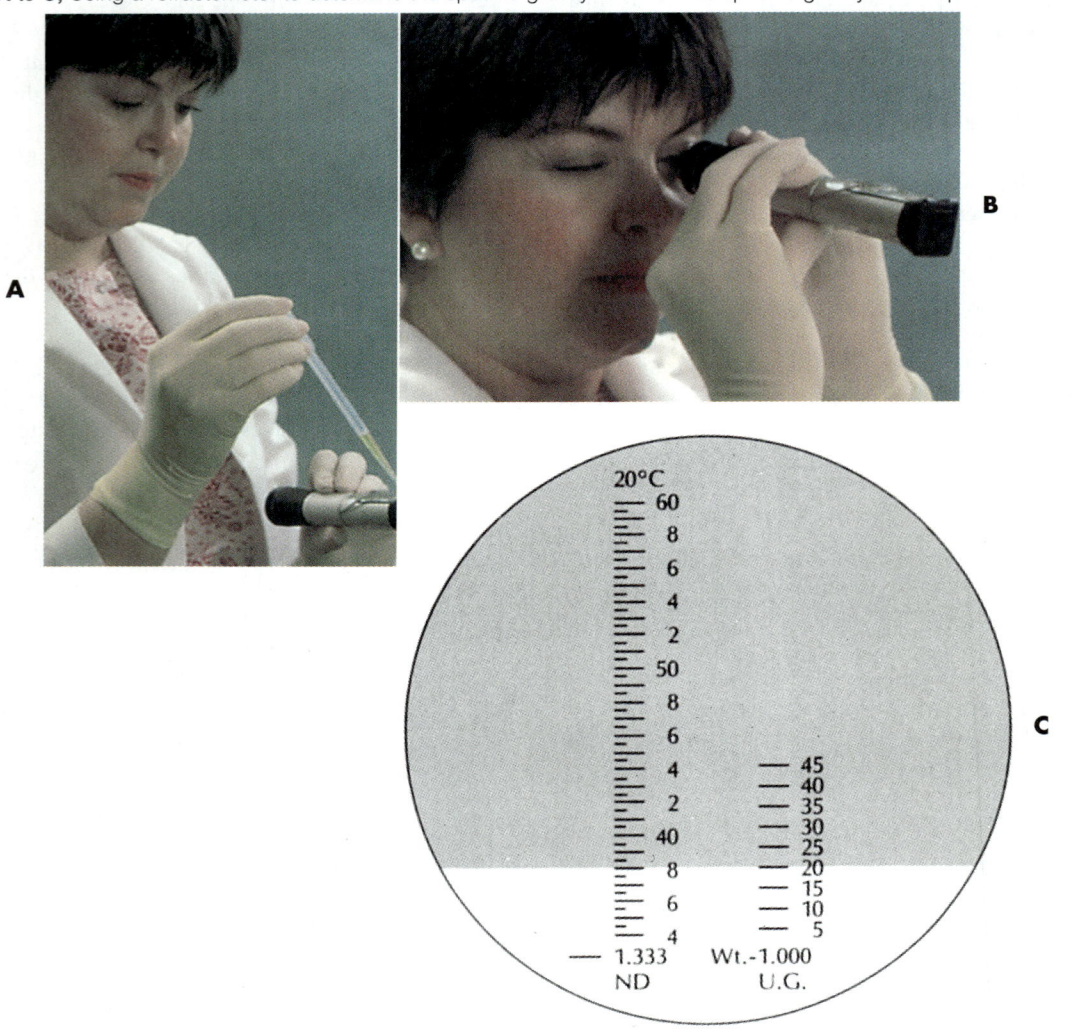

pecially practical and convenient for use in a physician's office or clinic. In addition to these strips, other special paper tapes, chemical tablets, selectively treated slides, and simplified culture tests are available for special examinations.

The pH of urine and several other components can be easily and rapidly determined with the use of a variety of specially prepared reagent strips and a color chart. The reagent strip is a clear plastic strip with up to 10 pieces of colored filter paper attached, each used to identify different components in the urine. Every piece of filter paper is impregnated with various chemicals and changes color when dipped in the urine. Color changes on the filter papers depend on the presence and amount of the substance that is being measured.

The most complete reagent strip is the Multistix 10 SG,* which is used for determining the pH and specific gravity, as well as the presence and amount of urobilinogen, nitrite, blood, bilirubin, ketone, glucose, protein, and the presence of intact and lysed leukocytes (white blood cells) in urine. Various other Multistix reagent strips are available. The Multistix product name includes a number suffix that indicates the number of urine tests on the strip. In addition, strips that test specific gravity have an *SG* suffix.

———————
*Bayer Corp, Elkhart, Ind.

PROCEDURE 12-1

DETERMINING THE SPECIFIC GRAVITY OF URINE (URINOMETER)

Objective
Understand and demonstrate the correct procedure to determine the specific gravity of a urine specimen using an urinometer; and record the results on the patient's chart.

Equipment (Figure 12-3)
One 5-inch-high glass cylinder
One urinometer
Disposable single-use exam gloves

PROCEDURE

1. **Wash your hands. Use appropriate personal protective equipment (PPE) as dictated by facility.** Assemble the equipment and don disposable, single-use examination gloves.

2. Pour well-mixed urine into the cylinder to the three-quarter mark (to within 1 inch from the top of the cylinder). Have the cylinder on a flat surface.

3. Place the urinometer in the urine and spin it gently (Figure 12-4, *A*). The urinometer floats in the urine.

4. Place the cylinder so that the lower line of the meniscus is at eye level (Figure 12-4, *B*). The meniscus is a crescent-shaped line appearing at the surface of a liquid column.

5. Read the specific gravity by noting the point where the lower middle part of the meniscus crossed the urinometer scale. Do not allow the urinometer to touch the sides of the cylinder.

6. Discard the urine. Rinse the urinometer and cylinder with water. Wipe the urinometer dry before using it again.

7. **Remove gloves and wash your hands.**

8. Record the reading.

RATIONALE

When there is insufficient urine to float the urinometer, the specific gravity cannot be read. You would then simply record "Quantity insufficient."

An inaccurate reading results if the urinometer touches the sides of the cylinder.

Charting Example

October 10, 20__ 9 AM
Urine specific gravity 1.017
D. Day, CMA

Continued

PROCEDURE 12-1

DETERMINING THE SPECIFIC GRAVITY OF URINE (URINOMETER)—cont'd

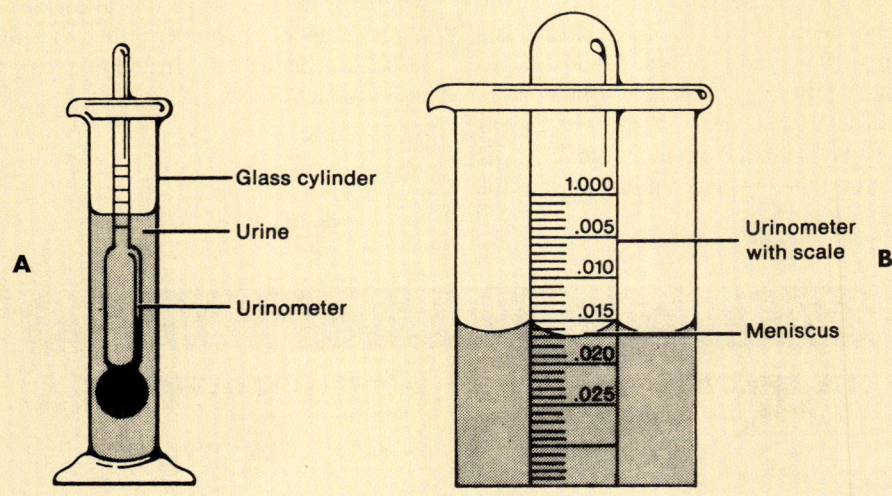

FIGURE 12-3 **A,** Items for determining specific gravity of urine; **B,** urinometer scale for determining specific gravity of urine. Specific gravity as shown would be 1.017.

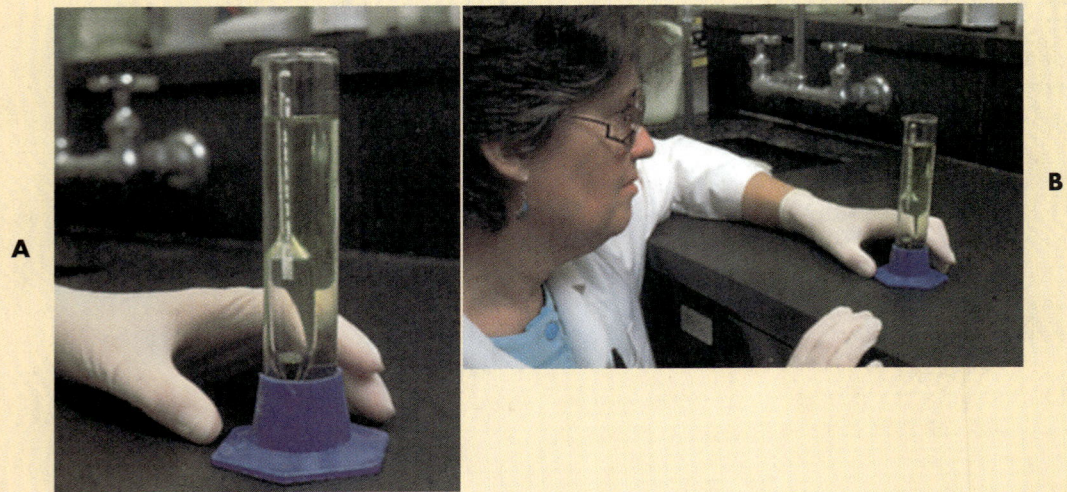

FIGURE 12-4 **A,** Place urinometer in the urine and spin it gently. **B,** To read specific gravity, place the cylinder so that the lower line of the meniscus is at eye level.

Reagent strips are supplied in dark plastic bottles containing 100 strips with directions for use (Figure 12-5, *A*). The color chart and specified times used to read the results of the tests are presented on the sides of the bottle. Both open and unopened product **expiration dates** are established for these strips to ensure maximum product quality. **Always** check the expiration date before using.

Because the pH of urine is usually determined as part of a complete urinalysis, it is desirable to use a multiple reagent strip such as one of the Multistix or one of the other reagent strips. Table 12-1 shows the wide range of Bayer reagent strips and tablets that are readily available for use.

Procedure for using a reagent strip

1. Don disposable, single-use examination gloves.
2. Dip the test areas of the strip into a freshly voided urine specimen (Figure 12-6, *A*); remove immediately and tap to remove excess urine (Figure 12-6, *B*).

FIGURE 12-5 **A,** Multistix 10 SG reagent strips; **B,** Multistix 10 SG chart used for determining amounts of 10 factors when performing urinalysis.

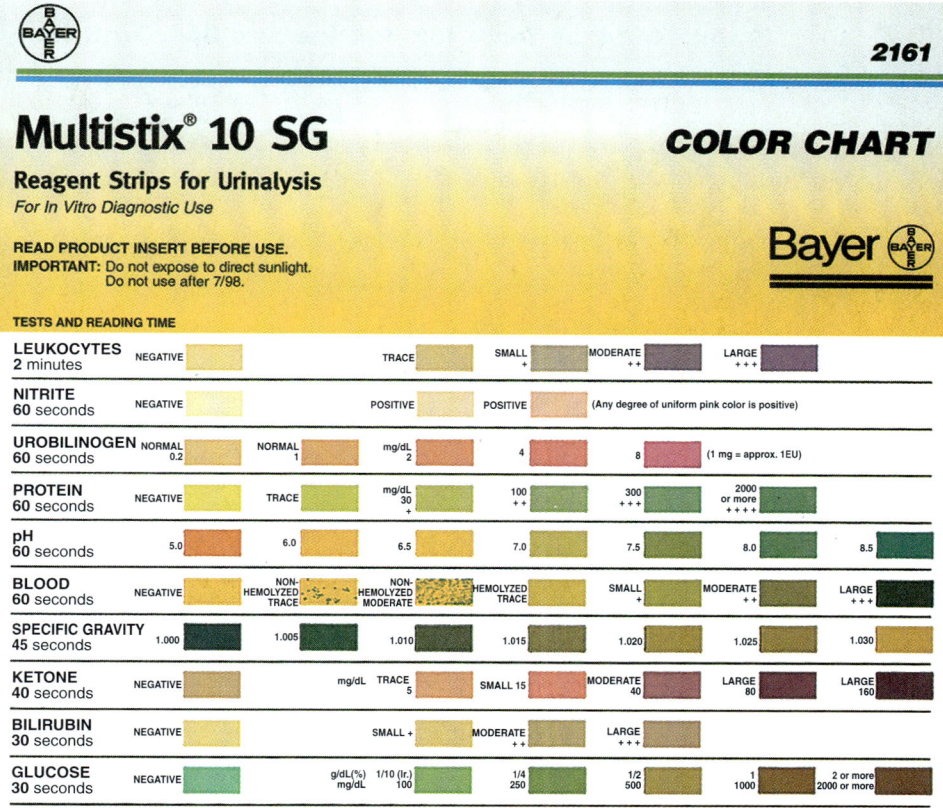

TABLE 12–1   Rapid Reagent Tests for Routine and Special Urinalyses

Reagent Test	Substances Determined	Technique*
N-Multistix	pH, protein, glucose, ketones, bilirubin, blood, nitrite, and urobilinogen	Use fresh, uncentrifuged urine. Preservatives may be added. Dip reagent strip in specimen, remove, and compare each reagent area with corresponding color chart on bottle label at the number of seconds specified.
Multistix	pH, protein, glucose, ketones, bilirubin, blood, and urobilinogen	As above
Multistix 10 SG	Glucose, bilirubin, ketone, specific gravity, blood, pH, protein, urobilinogen, nitrite, leukocytes	As above
Multistix 9	Glucose, bilirubin, ketone, blood, pH, protein, urobilinogen, nitrite, leukocytes	As above
Multistix 9 SG	Glucose, bilirubin, ketone, specific gravity, blood, pH, protein, nitrite, leukocytes	As above
Multistix 8	Glucose, bilirubin, ketone, blood, pH, protein, nitrite, leukocytes	As above
Multistix 8 SG	Glucose, ketone, specific gravity, blood, pH, protein, nitrite, leukocytes	As above
Multistix 7	Glucose, ketone, blood, pH, protein, nitrite, leukocytes	As above
Uristix 4	Glucose, protein, nitrite, leukocytes	As above
Multistix 2	Nitrite, leukocytes	As above
N-Multistix SG	Glucose, bilirubin, ketone, specific gravity, blood, pH, protein, urobilinogen, nitrite	As above
Bili-Labstix	pH, protein, glucose, ketones, bilirubin, and blood	As above

Courtesy Bayer Corp, Diagnostics Division, Elkhart, Ind.

*See package inserts for proper procedures.

Continued

TABLE 12–1   Rapid Reagent Tests for Routine and Special Urinalyses—cont'd

Reagent Test	Substances Determined	Technique*
Labstix	pH, protein, glucose, ketones, and blood	As above
Hema-Combistix	pH, protein, glucose, and blood	As above
Combistix	pH, protein, and glucose	As above
N-Uristix	Protein, glucose, and nitrite	As above
Uristix	Protein and glucose	As above
Clinistix	Glucose	As above
Albustix	Protein	As above
Hemastix	Blood	As above
Microstix-nitrite	Nitrite	As above
Urobilistix	Urobilinogen	As above, but preferably using a 2-hour urine specimen collected in early afternoon (between 2 PM and 4 PM).
Microstix-3	Bacteriuria	Dip culture-reagent strip in specimen for 5 seconds, remove, read nitrite test area after 30 seconds. Insert and seal strip in sterilized plastic pouch provided, incubate for 18 to 24 hours. Compare color densities on total and gram-negative culture pads with chart provided, without removing strip from pouch. Incinerate pouch with strip still sealed inside. (Some facilities may autoclave the pouch and then dispose of according to their policies.)
Ictotest	Bilirubin	Place 5 drops of urine on the special mat. Cover with the reagent tablet. Flow 2 drops of water onto tablet. Compare the color reaction with the color chart.
Diastix	Glucose	Use fresh, uncentrifuged urine. Do not use preservative containing formaldehyde. Dip reagent strip in specimen, remove, and compare with color chart on bottle label.
Ketostix	Ketones (principally acetoacetic acid)	As above, but urine must be at least at room temperature at the time of testing.
Keto-Diastix	Glucose and ketones (principally acetoacetic acid)	As above for Diastix and Ketostix.
Clinitest	Reducing substances, including sugars	Add Clinitest tablet to test tube containing mixture of 5 drops of urine and 10 drops of water. Spontaneous boiling occurs; after it stops, compare color in tube with color chart.

Courtesy Bayer Corp, Diagnostics Division, Elkhart, Ind.

*See package inserts for proper procedures.

3. Compare the test areas to the appropriate color chart on the bottle at the specified times (Figure 12-6, *C*).
4. Remove gloves and wash your hands.
5. Record the results.

For best results, reading urine tests at the proper time is critical. Multistix reagent areas are designed to be read from the bottom up. After removing the Multistix 10 SG reagent strip from the urine, read the results at the following specified times (see Figure 12-5, *B*):

Glucose—read at 30 seconds
Bilirubin—read at 30 seconds
Ketone—read at 40 seconds
Specific gravity—read at 45 seconds
Blood—read at 60 seconds
pH—read at 60 seconds
Protein—read at 60 seconds
Urobilinogen—read at 60 seconds
Nitrite—read at 60 seconds
Leukocytes—read at 2 minutes

For screening positive from negative specimens only, all reagent areas except leukocytes may be read between 1 and 2 minutes.

The addition of a leukocyte test to dry reagent strips may reduce the need for microscopic analysis. Chemical testing for leukocyte esterase detects lysed white blood cells that cannot be detected microscopically. Because leukocyte esterase will be present hours after sample collection, false-negative results are reduced.

Microscopic analysis of urine is not indicated when negative findings are obtained for leukocytes, nitrite, protein, and occult blood. Time-consuming microscopies can be reduced to those specimens for which positive chemical results suggest that more specific information is needed.

FIGURE 12-6   **A** to **C,** Using a reagent strip.

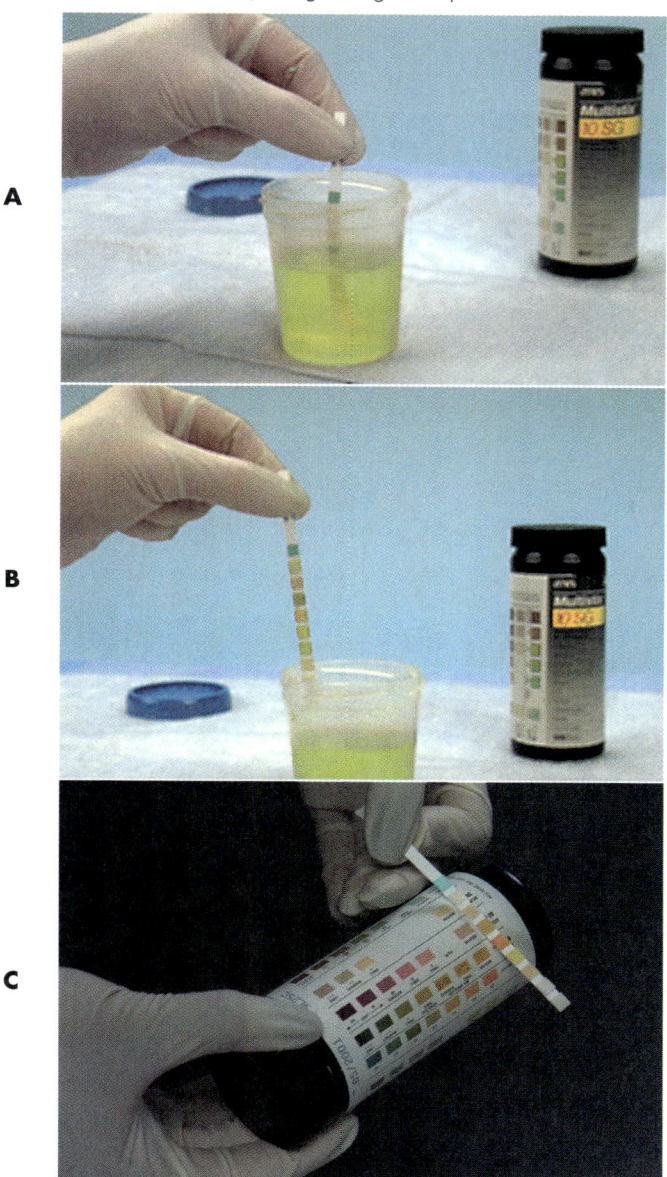

FIGURE 12-7   Clinitek 200 semiautomated urine chemistry analyzer for moderate- to large-volume urine testing. It is designed to read strips; results are printed on a paper printout. (Courtesy Bayer Corp, Elkhart, Ind.)

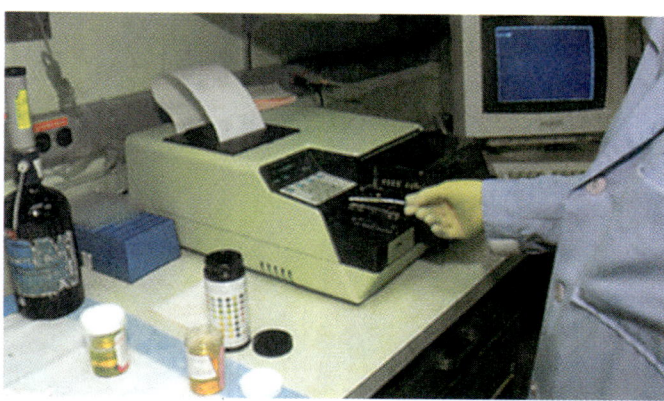

Urine Chemistry Analyzers for Use With Reagent Strips

The Bayer Multistix reagent strips are also designed for use with instrumentation, such as with the Clinitek 200 or Clinitek 200+ semiautomated urine chemistry analyzers for moderate-to large-volume urine testing (Figure 12-7) or the Clinitek 10 or Clinitek 50 urine chemistry analyzers for small- to medium-volume urine testing (Figure 12-8). These instruments are semiautomated and are designed to *read* the reagent strips. Readings are standardized for improved precision through the elimination of visual color discrepancies and operator and environmental variables. Both of these analyzers are easy to use. Directions for use are supplied with the instruments, and they must be followed explicitly. To ensure quality control, daily calibration is recommended for these analyzers. (See also Chapter 10 for additional information on quality control.)

Clinitek 10 and Clinitek 50.
When the Clinitek 10 or Clinitek 50 analyzer is turned on, the feed table automatically moves out to the *load* position; then the instrument goes through a self-test cycle. After this cycle is completed, the name of the Bayer strip programmed to be read is displayed (see Figure 12-8).

After properly immersing the reagent strip in urine and removing the excess urine by blotting, slide the strip onto the feed table, pad side up, within 10 seconds after pressing the *Start* button. Be sure that the tip of the strip lies flat on the table and is touching the end stop of the feed table insert.

Record the test results shown on the display panel; then remove and discard the used reagent strip. The Clinitek 50 analyzes, displays, and prints results at the rate of one test per minute.

Computerized results.
The newer urine chemistry analyzers, the Clinitek 200+ and Clinitek 50, may be interfaced with a computer so that results are automatically uploaded to the computer. Abnormal results can be highlighted on the printed report to simplify reviewing results. There are also computer programs designed to interface with the chemistry analyzers and a compatible computer. These allow the operator to store, access, and collate patient identification data, specimen physical characteristics, confirmatory tests, and microscopic evaluation data. All information can be entered or retrieved easily.

Significance of Test Results

Multistix 10 SG reagent strips (see Figure 12-5) may provide diagnostically useful information about the status of carbohydrate metabolism, kidney and liver function, acid-base balance, bacteriuria-pyuria, and many other conditions.

Reaction (pH).
pH is the symbol for the hydrogen-ion concentration that expresses the degree of acidity or alkalinity of a solution. The pH is measured on a scale ranging from 0 to 14, with 7 being neutral, 0 to 7 acidic, and 7 to 14 alkaline. Usually freshly voided normal urine from patients on normal

FIGURE 12-8 Clinitek 50 urine chemistry analyzer. A semiautomated instrument designed to read the reagent strip. Results show up on the display panel and are printed on a paper printout.

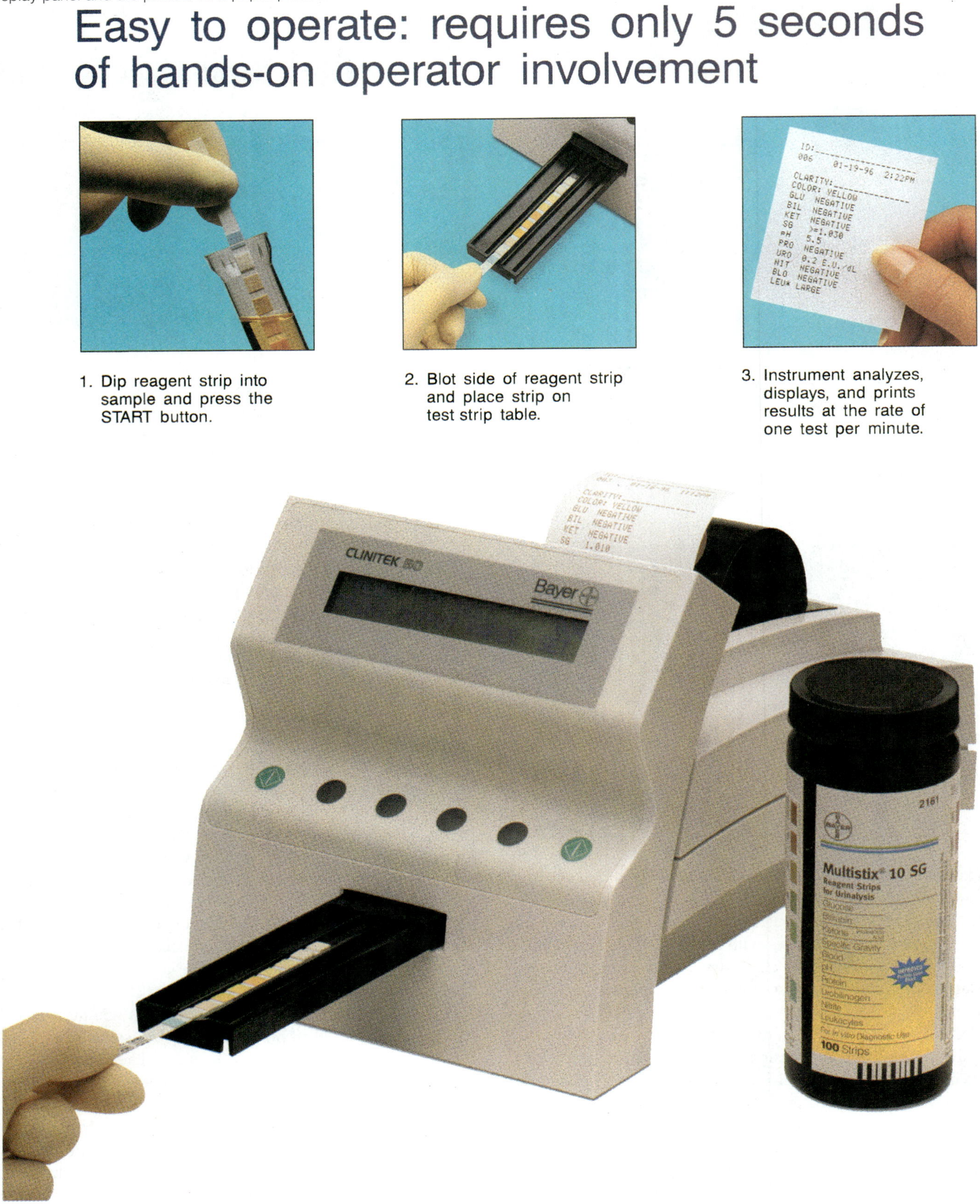

Easy to operate: requires only 5 seconds of hands-on operator involvement

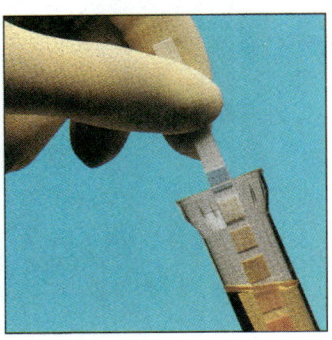

1. Dip reagent strip into sample and press the START button.

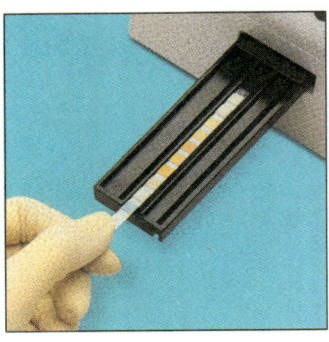

2. Blot side of reagent strip and place strip on test strip table.

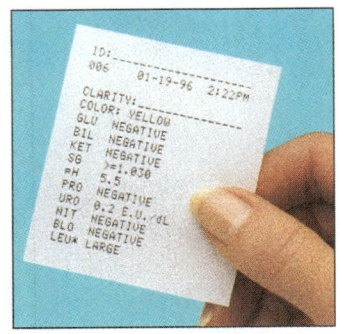

3. Instrument analyzes, displays, and prints results at the rate of one test per minute.

diets is acidic, having a pH of 6.0, although normal kidneys are capable of secreting urine that may vary in pH from 4.5 to slightly higher than 8.0.

Excessively acid urine may be obtained from patients on a high-protein diet or those who are taking certain medications such as vitamin C or ammonium chloride and from patients who are retaining a large amount of sodium. In the conditions of uncontrolled diabetes mellitus and acidosis, the patient's urine is also very acidic.

Alkaline urine is seen in patients who have ingested a large meal and in those who consume a diet high in milk and other dairy products, citrus fruits, and vegetables. Certain medications such as sodium bicarbonate help produce alkaline urine. Urinary tract infections, specimens contaminated by bacteria, and specimens left standing for any length of time also produce highly alkaline urine (Table 12-2).

Protein.   Normal urine may contain protein, mostly albumin, after exposure to cold, excessive muscular activity, or ingestion of large amounts of protein (see Table 12-2).

Albuminuria (al″bu-mi-nu′re-ah) is the presence of serum albumin or serum globulin in the urine. It is usually a sign of renal impairment; however, it can also occur in healthy individuals after vigorous exercise.

Proteinuria (pro″te-in-u′re-ah) is an abnormal increase of protein in the urine and is an important indicator of renal disease. Also, it is seen in congestive heart disease, constrictive pericarditis, multiple myeloma, and toxemia of pregnancy. Functional proteinuria is seen in fever, excessive exercise, emotional stress, exposure to heat or cold, and fad diets.

Renal damage and proteinuria may also result from acute and chronic glomerulonephritis, nephrotic syndrome, venous congestion in the kidney, renal tubular disease, tumors, pyelonephritis, toxic irritation of the kidney, polycystic kidney disease, hyperthyroidism, lupus erythematosus, central nervous system lesions, convulsions, stress, hematologic disorders, septicemia, infections, hepatic disease, high-protein diet, salt depletion, dehydration, and diabetes insipidus.

Glucose.   Normal urine does not contain any detectable glucose unless the concentration of blood glucose exceeds 160 to 180 mg/dl; at that point, glucose begins to spill into the urine (see Table 12-2).

Glucosuria (gloo″ko-su′re-ah) or **glycosuria** (gli″ko-su′re-ah) is abnormally high sugar content in the urine. The major cause of this condition is diabetes mellitus. Other common causes of glucosuria include an excessive carbohydrate intake, pain, excitement, liver damage, shock, and sometimes general anesthesia. Ingestion of large amounts of vitamin C may interfere with glucose testing and produce a false-positive result.

Other causes of above-normal ranges of glucose include central nervous system damage, endocrine imbalance, intracranial injury, infections, stress, pregnancy, pancreatitis, and renal tubular damage.

Ketone.   Normally ketone bodies do not appear in urine unless the patient is on a carbohydrate-deficient diet or a diet that is extremely rich in fat content (see Table 12-2).

Acetonuria (as″e-to-nu′re-ah) or **ketonuria** (ke″to-nur′re-ah) is the presence of acetone or ketone bodies in the urine. This condition is an important symptom in diabetes mellitus. Ketonuria is also seen in patients whose carbohydrate intake is decreased, such as with fasting, anorexia, or starvation; in gastrointestinal disturbances; following general anesthesia; in cyclic vomiting, dietary imbalance, eclampsia, exposure to cold, excessive insulin, fever, pyloric stenosis, or severe diarrhea; and with strenuous exercise.

Bilirubin.   Normally, no bilirubin appears in the urine (see Table 12-2). **Bilirubinuria** (bil″i-roo″bi-nu′re-ah) is the presence of bilirubin in the urine. It occurs in liver disease, bile duct obstruction, cancer of the head of the pancreas, hyperthyroidism, infectious mononucleosis, and septicemia. The presence of bilirubin in the urine aids in the diagnosis of jaundice, because bilirubin is not present in hemolytic jaundice but is present in obstructive or hepatic jaundice.

Blood.   A few red blood cells noted in urine when examined under the microscope are normal. The Multistix 10 SG does not determine the number of red blood cells present but provides an indication of the presence of occult blood conditions, trauma, hemorrhage, or infection (see Table 12-2). It also detects the presence of free hemoglobin and myoglobin. The presence of hemoglobin indicates rapid or extensive intravascular destruction of the red blood cells. *Hemoglobinuria* is seen in transfusion reactions, hemolytic anemia, infections, drug ingestion, and malaria and in the presence of toxins and venoms.

Myoglobinuria is seen in alcoholic polymyopathy, progressive muscle disease, trauma, burns, convulsions, hyperthermia, electrical shock, infection, and infarction of muscle tissue and in the presence of toxins and venoms.

Hematuria (hem″ah′tu-re-ah) is the presence of blood in the urine. The urine may be slightly blood tinged, grossly bloody, or a smoky brown color. Hematuria is symptomatic of injury, disease, or calculi in the urinary system. Certain drugs such as anticoagulants or sulfonamides may also cause hematuria.

Nitrite.   Normal urine should yield negative results; a positive result is a reliable indication of significant bacteriuria (see Table 12-2). **Bacteriuria** (bak-te″re-u′re-ah) is the presence of bacteria in the urine. A positive nitrite test is indicative of a urinary tract infection or a contaminated specimen. When an infection is suspected and the nitrite test yields negative results, it could be that the urine has not been in the bladder long enough for the nitrates (which are normal in urine) to be reduced to nitrites (pathogens would cause this change).

Urobilinogen.   Normal urine contains a small amount of urobilinogen. Biliary obstruction leads to the absence of urobilinogen in the urine; reduced amounts are seen during antibiotic therapy, in the absence of intestinal bacteria, in acid urine,

Text continued on p. 544

TABLE 12-2   Urine Profile of Differential Disease Findings*

N = Normal   I = Increased   D = Decreased

Multistix Urine Reagent Strip Tests	Renal	Hepatic	Pancreatic	Gastrointestinal	Cardiovascular	Other
pH	Renal tubular acidosis—D Bacterial infections—I Chronic renal failure—I		Diabetic acidosis—D	Diarrhea—D Pyloric obstruction—I Vomiting—I Malabsorption—N or D	Congestive heart failure—N	Dehydration—D Starvation—D Low-carbohydrate diets—I Acetazolamide therapy—I Metabolic acidosis—D Metabolic alkalosis—I Emphysema—D
Protein	Nephrotic syndrome—I Pyelonephritis—I Glomerulonephritis—I Kimmelstiel-Wilson syndrome—I Malignant hypertension—I				Benign hypertension—I Congestive heart failure—I Subacute bacterial endocarditis—I	Toxemia of pregnancy—I Gout—I Brown-spider bite—I Acute febrile state—I Carbon tetrachloride poisoning—I Electric-current injury—I Potassium depletion—I Orthostatic proteinuria—I
Glucose	Lowered renal threshold—I Renal tubular disease—I		Pancreatitis—I Diabetes mellitus—I	Alimentary glycosuria—I	Coronary thrombosis—I	Pheochromocytoma—I Hyperthyroidism—I Acromegaly—I Shock—I Pain—I Excitement—I
Ketones		von Gierke's disease (glycogen storage disease)—I	Diabetic acidosis	Vomiting—I Diarrhea—I		Starvation—I Low-carbohydrate diets—I Eclampsia—I Trauma—I Chloroform or ether anesthesia—I Hyperthyroidism—I
Specific gravity	Glomerulonephritis—D Pyelonephritis—D	Hepatic disease—I		Vomiting—I Diarrhea—I	Congestive heart failure—I	Diabetes insipidus—D Fever—I

Nitrite	Urinary tract infection				
Bilirubin	Complete and partial obstructive jaundice—I Viral and drug-induced hepatitis—I Cirrhosis—I	Carcinoma of the head of the pancreas—I	Choledocho-lithiasis—I	Congestive heart failure in the presence of jaundice—I	Recurrent idiopathic jaundice of pregnancy—I Noxious fumes—I Chlorpromazine hepatitis—I
Blood	*Hematuria in:* Acute nephritis Passive congestion of the kidneys Calculi Malignant papilloma Renal carcinoma Nephrotic syndrome Polycystic kidneys	*Hemoglobinuria in:* Kimmelstiel-Wilson syndrome	*Hematuria in:* Diverticulosis of the colon	*Hematuria in:* Bacterial endocarditis *Hemoglobinuria in:* Intravascular hemolysis Hypertension with renal involvement	*Hematuria in:* Chronic infections Chronic phenacetin ingestion Sulfonamide therapy Sickle cell disease *Hemoglobinuria in:* Severe burns Hemolytic anemias Transfusion reaction Sudden cold Eclampsia Allergic reactions Multiple myeloma Alkaloids—poisonous mushrooms
	Hematuria in: Cirrhosis (impaired prothrombin function)				
Urobilinogen	Obstruction of the bile duct—D Liver cell damage—I Cirrhosis—I	Carcinoma of the head of the pancreas—D	Suppression of the gut flora—D (antibiotic therapy)	Congestive heart failure—I Extravascular hemolysis—I	Noxious fumes—I Hepatitis associated with infectious mononucleosis—I Thalassemia—I Pernicious anemia—I Hemolytic anemias—I Chlorpromazine hepatitis—D

Courtesy Ames Co., Inc., Division Miles Laboratories, Inc., Elkhart, Ind.

*These findings are characteristic of the conditions listed, but are not necessarily found consistently in all cases. Definitive diagnosis must rely upon clinical acumen and the results of other indicated procedures.

and in biliary obstruction; and increased amounts of urobilinogen in the urine are present in liver tissue damage, congestive heart failure, reduced renal function, starvation, alkaline urine, and hemolytic anemia and when there is bacteria growth in the small intestine (see Table 12-2).

Leukocytes. Positive results are clinically significant. Positive and repeat trace results indicate that further testing of the patient and/or sample is needed, according to the medically accepted procedures for pyuria. The presence of leukocytes in the urine could indicate and could be seen in acute pyelonephritis, cystitis, salicylate toxicity, drug therapy (ampicillin, allopurinol, kanamycin, methicillin), tuberculosis infection, fevers, bladder tumor(s), and systemic lupus erythematosus and after strenuous exercise (see Table 12-7).

Specific gravity. See p. 533 and Table 12-2.

Tests for Glucose, Acetone, and Bilirubin Using Chemical Reagent Tablets
Clinitest*

When the presence of glucose is determined by use of a reagent strip, a more quantitative determination may be required. This can be accomplished by using the Clinitest reagent tablet 5-drop method (Figure 12-9).

1. Don disposable, single-use examination gloves.
2. Place 5 drops of urine into a test tube.
3. Rinse dropper; add 10 drops of water to the test tube.
4. Add one Clinitest tablet to the test tube.
5. Wait 15 seconds while the spontaneous boiling occurs; this is the normal action seen when the tablet is added to the urine and water mixture. Do not touch the bottom of the test tube because intense heat is generated during this reaction.
6. Once the boiling stops, shake the tube gently and compare the color of the contents with the color chart that accompanies the bottle of tablets. Do not wait longer than 15 seconds to compare the colors because results seen after this period are invalid. There are six color blocks ranging from dark blue (indicating a negative reading) through green and tan and up to orange, which is read as 2% or 4+, indicating the presence of large amounts of sugar. The results are interpreted and recorded as negative, trace, 1+, 2+, 3+, or 4+, or 0%, ¼%, ½%, ¾%, 1%, or 2%.

   Observe the solution in the test tube carefully during the reaction and the 15-second waiting period to detect rapid, pass-through color changes caused by large amounts of sugar (over 2%). Should the color *rapidly* pass through green, tan, and orange to a dark green-brown, record as over 2% (4+) sugar without comparing the final color development with the color chart.
7. Remove gloves and wash your hands.
8. Record the results.

---

*Bayer, Corp, Elkhart, Ind.

FIGURE 12-9 Clinitest procedure. **A,** Place 10 drops of water into test tube containing 5 drops of urine. **B,** Add one Clinitest tablet to test tube. **C,** Compare contents in test tube with color chart.

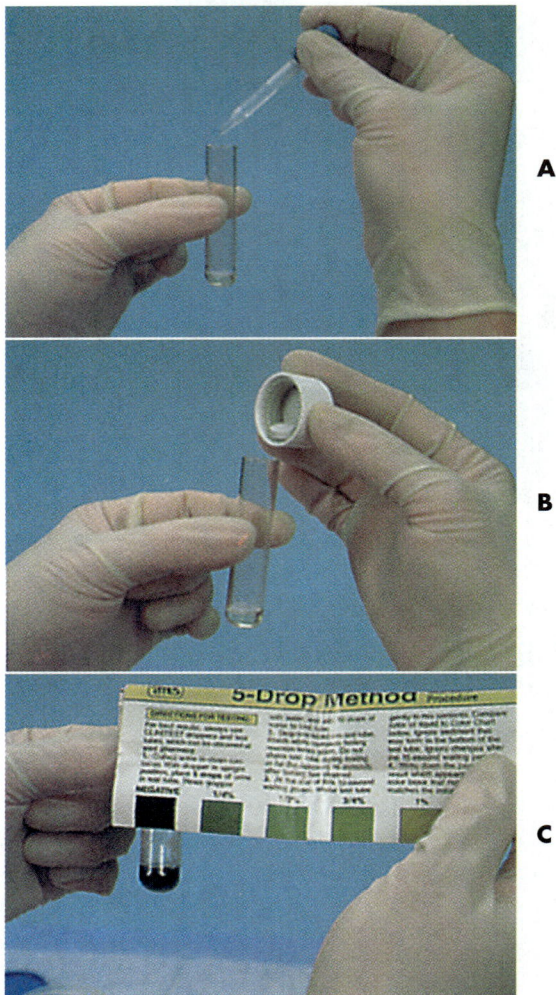

TABLE 12-3

Test Result	Color Change	Interpretation
Negative (0%)	Dark blue	No glucose present
Trace (¼%)	Green	250 mg/dl*
1+ (½%)	Olive green	500 mg/dl
2+ (¾%)	Green-brown	750 mg/dl
3+ (1%)	Tan	1000 mg/dl
4+ (2%)	Orange	2000 mg/dl

*1 deciliter (dl) = 100 milliliters (ml).

NOTE: The use of this method is not advisable for patients receiving the drugs nalidixic acid (NegGram), cephalothin (Keflin), cephalexin monohydrate (Keflex), cephaloridine (Loridine), probenecid (Benemid), or large amounts of ascorbic acid because they may cause a false-positive result. The preferred method in these situations is testing the urine using the Diastix or other reagent strips used for testing the presence of glucose in the urine.

A modification of the standard (5-drop) procedure is the *Clinitest reagent tablet 2-drop method,* also used for quantitative determination of reducing sugars, generally glucose, in urine. Directions for use are identical to the standard procedure, except 2 drops of urine and 10 drops of water are used. For this specific tablet, the results are identified by comparing the contents in the test tube with a color chart having seven color blocks ranging from dark blue through green and tan up to orange. The results are interpreted and recorded as 0, trace, 1/2%, 1%, 2%, 3%, or 5% or more.

Acetest*

To detect the presence of acetone and acetoacetic acid in urine, you may use the Acetest reagent tablet.

1. Don disposable, single-use examination gloves.
2. Place one tablet on a clean piece of paper, preferably white (Figure 12-10, *A*).
3. Place 1 drop of urine on the tablet (Figure 12-10, *B*).
4. At 30 seconds, compare the test results with the color chart. Colors will range from buff to lavender to purple. The four color blocks indicate negative, small, moderate, or large concentrations being present (Figure 12-10, *C*).
5. Remove gloves and wash your hands.
6. Record the results.

NOTE: This tablet may also be used to test serum, plasma, or whole blood. Serum or plasma ketone readings are made 2 minutes after application of the specimen to the tablet. When testing whole blood for ketones, apply the specimen to the tablet, wait 10 minutes, and then remove clotted blood and read the results immediately.

Ictotest*

To detect liver function, a simple test on urine to determine the presence of bilirubin may be done with the use of the Ictotest reagent tablet.

1. Don disposable, single-use examination gloves.
2. Place 5 drops of urine on the piece of special mat that is provided with the tablets.
3. Place a tablet in the center of the wet area.
4. Put 2 drops of water on the tablet.
5. Determine any color change on the mat around the table within 30 seconds and compare with the color chart. The presence of a blue or purple color indicates a positive reaction.
6. Remove gloves and wash your hands.
7. Record the results.

Summary

These three reagent tablets and the reagent strips must be kept in the bottles in which they are supplied, with the cap secured tightly. Exposure to the air or moisture for any length of time causes them to deteriorate, and they would then be unfit to use for testing urine. Do not remove the desiccants from the bottles. A **desiccant** is an

*Bayer Corp, Elkhart, Ind.

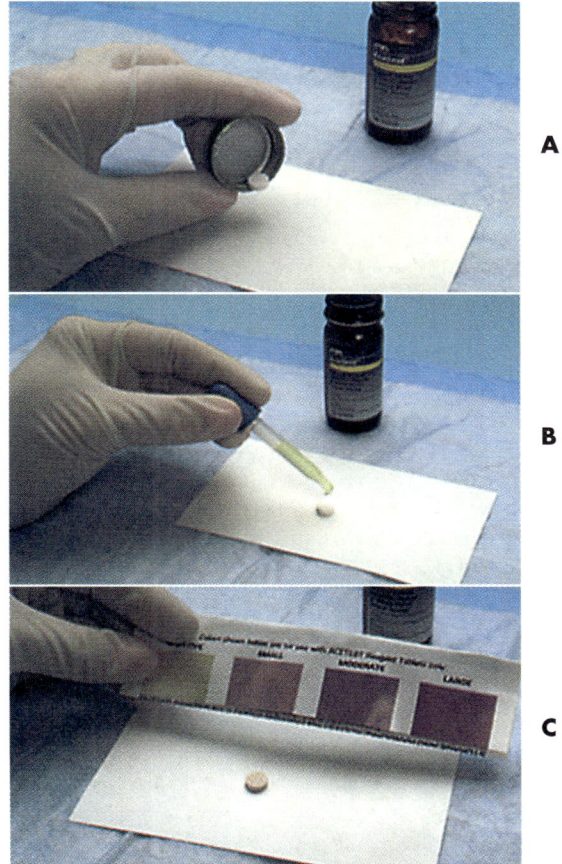

FIGURE 12-10 Using the Acetest reagent tablet to detect the presence of acetone and acetoacetic acid in urine. **A,** Place tablet on clean paper. **B,** Place 1 drop of urine of the tablet. **C,** Compare contents in test tube with color chart.

agent usually provided in a small pack in the bottle. Its function is to help keep the tablets or reagent strips dry. Store at temperatures under 30° C (86° F), and do not store in a refrigerator. Do not use after the expiration date indicated on the bottle.

CONTROLS FOR ROUTINE URINALYSIS

The various qualitative (or semiquantitative) tests for urinary pH, protein, blood, glucose, ketones, bilirubin, nitrite, urobilinogen, and specific gravity should be checked daily, using solutions containing known quantities of these substances. Two convenient quality control systems to help determine if tests are properly performed and interpreted are available: the Dipper and the Dropper—Quantimetrix urine dipstick controls. They are particularly valuable in instituting a quality control system or making an existing system more convenient by the use of ready-made controls.

Implementation of a quality control program is essential to ensure accuracy of urinalysis results. Performance of dipsticks and reagent tablets should be validated by testing with known positive and negative controls. Daily monitoring of control values establishes intralaboratory parameters for accuracy and precision of the test method. The Dipper and the Dropper Quantimetrix urine dipstick controls (Tables 12-4 and 12-5) are

Text continued on p. 550

TABLE 12–4   Urine Dipstick Control Kit—The Dipper

The Dipper

Product Description

The Quantimetrix Urine Dipstick Controls are supplied liquid, ready-to-use, requiring no reconstitution or dilution. They are prepared from human urine fortified to target levels with selected compounds that produce the desired reaction when tested by the methods indicated below in the **Intended Use** section. Preservatives including sodium azide have been added to inhibit microbial growth.

Intended Use

Control materials having known component concentrations are an integral part of diagnostic procedures. Daily monitoring of control values established intralaboratory parameters for accuracy and precision of the test method. The Quantimetrix urine Dipstick Control is intended to validate the performance of the **Multistix, Chemstrip,** and **Rapignost** dipsticks, and as a control for confirmatory tests such as **Acetest, Clinitest,** and **Ictotest** reagent tablets, and for hCG methods.

FOR IN VITRO DIAGNOSTIC USE ONLY

Procedure for Dipstick Testing

NOTE: Each tube of the Level 1 Control can be used as a normal control for dipsticks.

Each tube of the level 2 Control can be used as an abnormal control for dipsticks.

1. Remove the controls from the refrigerator and allow them to come to room temperature.
2. Immerse the dipstick in the control vial as if it were a patient specimen. **(Chemstrip users see limitations section).**
3. Read the urine dipsticks, visually or with an instrumental reader, in accordance with the manufacturer's instructions.
4. Immediately recap the controls and return them to 2°-8° C when not in use.

Procedure for hCG Testing

NOTE: The tubes of Level 1 Control marked hCG negative are to be used as a negative control for hCG methods. The tube of Level 1 Control marked hCG positive is to be used as a positive control for hCG methods.

1. Remove the controls from the refrigerator and allow them to come to room temperature.
2. Use the Level 1 hCG positive and negative controls as if they were patient specimens in accordance with the hCG test kit manufacturer's instructions.
3. Immediately recap the controls and return them to 2°-8° C when not in use.

Storage and Stability

1. The Urine Dipstick Control Kit should be stored at 2°-8° C when not in use. **Do not freeze.**

   Discard the control if turbid or any evidence of microbial contamination is present.
2. When stored at 2°-8° C the controls are stable until the expiration date stated on the label or 20 immersions, whichever occurs first.

3. The level 1 Controls are suitable for use as positive and negative controls for hCG methods until the expiration date, **even after 20 uses as a dipstick control.**

Expected Values

For **visual readings,** the expected ranges have been established from interlaboratory data by comparing the dipstick reaction that occurs with the controls to the color comparison chart with multiple lots of each manufacturer's dipsticks or reagent tablets.

For **instrument readings,** the expected ranges have been established from interlaboratory data from multiple lots of each manufacturer's dipsticks. Each laboratory should establish its own precision parameters.

For **specific gravity,** the expected ranges by refractometer have been established from the interlaboratory data.

For **total protein confirmation,** the Urine Dipstick Control may be used with the sulfosalicylic acid method at the user's discretion. This method has not been validated in our laboratory.

For **hCG,** the positive and negative results were obtained by testing each lot number of the Level 1 control with multiple lot numbers of at least 10 different hCG test kits of various sensitivities.

Limitations

Any future changes made by the manufacturer of a test method may give different values from the indicated range. Detailed information on the limitations of each test method is included in the limitations section of the manufacturer's package insert.

Rapignost users: Colors produced by the **urobilinogen** and **bilirubin** reactions on the Rapignost Dipstick with the Urine Dipstick Control are not characteristic of those shown on the manufacturer's label. The Urine Dipstick Control is *not* recommended for visual use for **urobilinogen** and **bilirubin.**

Chemstrip users: Loss of sensitivity of the bilirubin reactions, resulting in a **negative** response for **bilirubin,** may occur **before** 20 immersions of the Chemstrip Dipstick in each tube of Level 2 control. Therefore it is recommended that the Urine Dipstick Control be transferred directly onto the Chemstrip Dipstick rather than immersing the dipstick into the Level 2 control.

Clinitest tablet test: Use of the Level 2 Urine Dipstick Control with the Ames Clinitest tablets for reducing sugars may give an atypical color response. Because of purple and orange color formation in the foam, a murky green to a Clinitest assay for the Urine Dipstick Control is best interpreted as a positive or negative response. A clearer color representation is achieved if the tube is not swirled during or after the boiling reaction.

WARNING AND PRECAUTIONS

POTENTIAL BIOHAZARDOUS MATERIAL

Contains human urine. The FDA recommends that such samples be handled at the Centers for Disease Control and Prevention's Bio-Safety Level 2.

DISPOSE OF PROPERLY

Sodium azide may form metal azides in plumbing and pose a threat of explosion.

From Poon R, Hinberg I: Reflectometric evaluaton of Quantimetrix urine dipstick controls, *Clin Chem* 35:6, 1989.

hCG, Human chorionic gonadotropin.

TABLE 12–4 **Urine Dipstick Control Kit—cont'd**

| | Bayer Multistix | | | |
| | Visual | | Clinitek | |
Analyze	Level 1 Lot No. 44091 N or P	Level 2 Lot No. 44092	Level 1 Lot No. 44091 N or P	Level 2 Lot No. 44092
Glucose	Negative	100 (tr)-250 mg/dl	Negative	100 (tr)-250 mg/dl
Bilirubin	Negative	small (+)-lg (+++)	Negative	small (+)-lg (+++)
Ketones	Negative	5(tr)-80(lg) mg/dl	Negative	5(54)-40(mod) mg/dl†
Specific gravity	1.025->1.030	1.010-1.015	1.025->1.030	1.010-1.015
Blood	Negative	mod (++)-lg (+++)	Negative	small (+)-lg (+++)
pH	5.0-6.0	6.0-7.0	5.0-6.0	6.0-7.0
Protein	Negative	trace-100(++) mg/dl	Negative	trace-100(++) mg/dl
Urobilinogen	Normal	1-4 mg/dl*	Normal	1-4 mg/dl
Nitrite	Negative	positive	Negative	positive
Leukocytes	Negative	mod (++)-lg (+++)	Negative	mod (++)-lg (+++)

*For nonnumbered Multistix SG and N-Multistix SG dipsticks visual or Clinitek readings are 8 - # 12 Eu/dl for urobilinogen in Level 2.

†Clinitek 200 and 200# instruments may give an occasional reading of # 80. Clinitek 2000 instrument gives readings of 40 - # 160.

| | Behring Rapignost | | | |
| | Visual | | Rapimat | |
Analyze	Level 1 Lot No. 44091 N or P	Level 2 Lot No. 44092	Level 1 Lot No. 44091 N or P	Level 2 Lot No. 44092
Leukocytes	Normal	25-75 Leuk/ml	0.00-20 Leuk/ml	25-75 Leuk/ml
Nitrite	Negative	Positive	0.00 mg/dl	0.05 mg/dl (+)
pH	5-6	6-7	5-6	6-7
Blood	Negative	(+)-(++)	0.00 Ery/ul	10(+)-60(++)Ery/ul
Protein	Negative	30-100 mg/dl	0.00 mg/dl	30-100 mg/dl
Glucose	Normal	50-500 mg/dl	0.00 mg/dl	50-500 mg/dl
Ascorbic acid	Negative	Negative	Negative	Negative
Ketones	Negative	(+)-(+++)	0.00 mg/dl	100(++)-300(+++) mg/dl
Urobilinogen	Normal	*	0.00 mg/dl	4-12 mg/dl
Bilirubin	Negative	*	0.00 mg/dl	0.00 mg/dl
		*See Limitations		

| | Boehringer Mannheim Chemstrip Visual | |
Analyze	Level 1 Lot No. 44091 N or P	Level 2 Lot No. 44092
Leukocytes	Negative	Trace-(++)
Nitrite	Negative	Positive
pH	5-6	6-7
Protein	Negative	30(+)-100(++) mg/dl
Glucose	Normal	1/10-1/2
Ketones	Negative	mod (++)-lg (+++)
Urobilinogen	Normal	1-8 mg/dl
Bilirubin	Negative	(++)-(+++)*
Blood	Negative	10-250 Ery/ul
Specific gravity	1.015-1.020	1.005-1.015
		*See Limitations

| Additional Available Tests | | |
Test	Level 1 Lot No. 44091 N or P	Level 2 Lot No. 44092
Acetest	Negative	Small-mod
Clinitest	Negative	¼-½%*
Ictotest	Negative	Positive
Specific gravity (Refractometer)	1.019-1.025	1.007-1.012
Total protein (Sulfosalicylic acid)	Negative	Positive† *See limitations †See expected values

Multistix, Clinitek, Acetest, Clinitest, and Ictotest are trademarks of Bayer Corp, Diagnostics Division, Elkhart, IN 46515.

Rapignost and Rapimat are trademarks of Behring Diagnostics Inc, Somerville, NJ 08876.

Chemstrip is a trademark of Boehringer Mannheim Diagnostics, Indianapolis, IN 46250.

HCG (method sensitivity # 50 mIU/ml)	Lot No. 44091 N negative	Lot No. 44091 P* positive

TABLE 12–5   Urine Dipstick Control Kit—The Dropper

The Dropper

Product Description

The Quantimetrix Urine Dipstick Controls are supplied liquid, ready-to-use, requiring no reconstitution or dilution. They are prepared from human urine fortified to target levels with selected compounds that produce the desired reaction when tested by the methods indicated below in the Intended Use section. Preservations including sodium azide have been added to inhibit microbial growth.

Intended Use

Control materials having known component concentrations are an integral part of diagnostic procedures. Daily monitoring of control values establishes intralaboratory parameters for accuracy and precision of the test method. The Quantimetrix Urine Dipstick Control is intended to validate the performance of the Multistix, Chemstrip, and Rapignost dipsticks, and as a control for confirmatory tests such as Acetest, Clinitest, and Ictotest reagent tablets, and for hCG methods.

FOR IN VITRO DIAGNOSTIC USE ONLY

Procedure

1. Remove the control from the refrigerator and allow to come to room temperature.
2. Remove cap and invert bottle. While holding dipstick, gently squeeze the sides of the dropper bottle, and touch the tip of the bottle to the dipstick. Draw across all of the reagent pads. Turn dipstick on its side and drain excess control onto absorbent material.
3. Read the urine dipsticks, visually or with an instrumental reader, in accordance with the manufacturer's instructions.
4. Wipe off dropper tips and recap controls. Return them to 2°-8° C when not in use. Discard the controls if turbid or any evidence of microbial contamination is present.

Storage and Stability

1. The Urine Dipstick Control Kit should be stored at 2°-8° C when not in use. Do not freeze.
2. When stored at 2°-8° C the controls are stable until the expiration date stated on the label.

WARNING AND PRECAUTIONS
POTENTIAL BIOHAZARDOUS MATERIAL
Contains human urine. The FDA recommends that
such samples be handled at the Centers for
Disease Control and Prevention's Bio-Safety Level 2.
DISPOSE OF PROPERLY
Sodium azide may form metal azides in plumbing
and pose a threat of explosion.

---

*Quantimetrix Corporation, 4955 West 145th Street, Hawthorne, CA 90250.
hCG, Human chorionic gonadotropin.

Expected Values

For **readings,** the expected ranges have been established from interlaboratory data by comparing the dipstick reaction that occurs with the controls to the color comparison chart with multiple lots of each manufacturer's dipsticks or reagent tablets.

For **instrument readings,** the expected ranges have been established from interlaboratory data from multiple lots of each manufacturer's dipsticks. Each laboratory should establish its own precision parameters.

For **specific gravity,** the expected ranges by refractometer have been established from interlaboratory data.

For **total protein** confirmation, the urine Dipstick Control may be used with the sulfosalicylic acid method at the user's discretion. This method has not been validated in our laboratory.

For **hCG,** the positive and negative results were obtained by testing each lot number of the Level 1 control with multiple lot numbers of at least 10 different hCG test kits of various sensitivities.

Limitations

Any future changes made by the manufacturer of a test method may give different values from the indicated range. Detailed information on the limitations of each test method is included in the limitations section of the manufacturers' package insert.

Rapignost users: Colors produced by the urobilinogen and bilirubin reactions on the Rapignost Dipstick with the Urine Dipstick Control are not characteristic of those shown on the manufacturer's label. The Urine Dipstick Control is not recommended for visual use for urobilinogen and bilirubin.

Clinitest tablet test: Use of the Level 2 Urine Dipstick Control with the Ames Clinitest tablets for reducing sugars may give an atypical color response. Because of purple and orange color formation in the foam, a murky green to a purple color response may occur. Therefore results of the Clinitest assay for the Urine Dipstick Control are best interpreted as a positive or negative response. A clearer color representation is achieved if the tube is not swirled during or after the boiling reaction.

*See also p. 547.

TABLE 12–6   Urine Dipstick Chart

| | | URINE DIPSTICK CONTROL | | | | | | | QUALITY CONTROL LOG | | | | | | | | | | | | | | |

DATE _____ URINE DIPSTICK CONTROL LEVEL _____ LOT # _____ EXPIRATION DATE _____

DATE	Reagent Strip _____ Lot# _____	DIPSTICK TESTS											CONFIRMATORY TESTS						ADD. TESTS			
		Leukocytes	Nitrites	Urobilinogen	Protein	pH	Blood	Specific Gravity	Ketones	Bilirubin	Glucose	Protein	Method/Lot #	Ketones	Method/Lot #	Glucose	Method/Lot #	Bilirubin	Method/Lot #	hCG	Method/Lot #	Specific Gravity Refractometer	INITIAL
Assayed Value																							

Courtesy Quantimetrix Corp., Hawthorne, Calif.

intended to be used to validate the performance of the Multistix, Chemstrip, and Rapignost dipsticks for both visual and instrument readings and as a control for confirmatory tests, such as Acetest, Clinitest, and Ictotest reagent tablets, and for human chorionic gonadotropin (hCG) methods. Each laboratory should establish its own standards of performance. Quality control data logs (Table 12-6), such as the one provided with the Dipper, should be maintained for all urine dipstick and reagent tablet tests. Each kit contains a summary of the controls, instructions for use, and the expected values that should be obtained when using the controls with the different products.

Microscopic Examination of Centrifuged Urine Sediment

The third part of the routine urinalysis is the microscopic examination of the sediment present in the urine. The purpose of this examination is to identify the type and the approximate number of formed elements present, which in turn helps the physician determine the presence of a disease process. The sediment in urine is usually classified as organized or unorganized sediment. **Organized sediment** includes red blood cells, white blood cells, epithelial cells, casts, bacteria, parasites, yeast, fungi, and spermatozoa. **Unorganized sediment** is usually chemical and includes crystals of various components and other amorphous (having no definite shape) material. The urine specimen to be used in the microscopic examination must be freshly voided, preferably a clean-catch voided specimen, and examined without excessive delay so that cellular deterioration is prevented. Microscopic examination of urine is performed after the urine is centrifuged. Centrifugation produces a solid portion called sediment.

PROCEDURE 12-2

PREPARATION AND MICROSCOPIC EXAMINATION OF SPECIMEN

Objective

Understand and demonstrate the correct procedure for preparing a urine specimen for microscopic examination; performing the microscopic examination; and recording your findings.

Equipment

   Disposable, single-use examination gloves
   Laboratory coat (used only when working with specimens)
   Eye protection (optional)

   Fresh urine specimen
   Conical centrifuge tubes
   Clinical centrifuge
   Droppers
   Glass slides
   Cover glass
   Microscope
   See Chapter 10 for information on microscopes and
     centrifuges

PROCEDURE

1. Don disposable, single-use examination gloves.

2. To obtain the sediment, place 10 to 15 ml of thoroughly mixed urine in a centrifuge tube and centrifuge for 5 minutes at the standard speed of 1500 revolutions per minute (rpm).

3. Pour off the supernatant fluid (Figure 12-11, A). The supernatant is the clear upper liquid in the tube after it has been centrifuged.

4. Allow the several drops of urine that remain along the side of the tube to flow back down into the sediment; then tap the tube with your finger to mix the contents.

5. Place a drop of this sediment on a slide and cover with a cover glass. The slide is now ready to be examined (Figure 12-11, B).

6. Position the slide on the microscope stage (Figure 12-11, C).

7. Remove gloves and wash your hands.

8. Adjust the **low-power objective** of the microscope and examine the slide for casts in at least 10 different fields; then examine for other elements that are present in just a few fields. Reduce the light to a minimum by almost completely closing the diaphragm beneath the stage on the microscope and scan the entire slide to obtain an overall picture of the sediment. You must vary the intensity of the light source on the microscope so that correct identification of the various components may be obtained.

9. Next adjust the microscope to the **high-power objective** to identify the specific types of cells, such as red blood cells, white blood cells, crystals, and other elements present in the sediment. Further identification of the various types of casts should also be done at this time.

10. Estimate the approximate number of the various structures identified. Casts are counted per low-power field; epithelial

PROCEDURE 12-2

PREPARATION AND MICROSCOPIC EXAMINATION OF SPECIMEN—cont'd

cells, white blood cells (WBCs), and red blood cells are reported in terms of cells per high-power field (hpf) (for example, 10 to 15 WBCs/hpf). To determine the number of elements present, count the number of each type seen in **at least 10 fields.**

The average of this number is then used for the reported value. The other elements (crystals, bacteria, parasites, and spermatozoa) are reported as none, rare, occasional, frequent, many, or numerous.

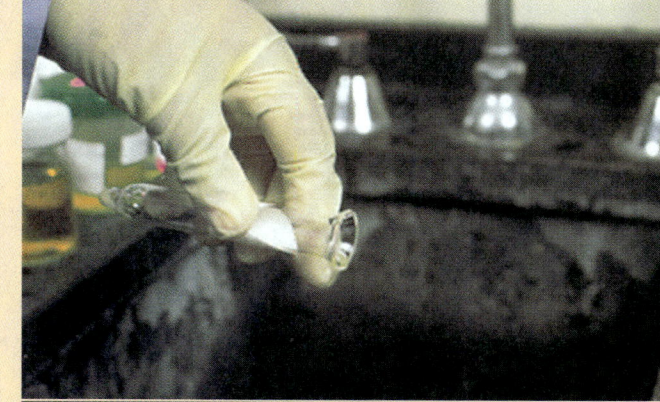

A

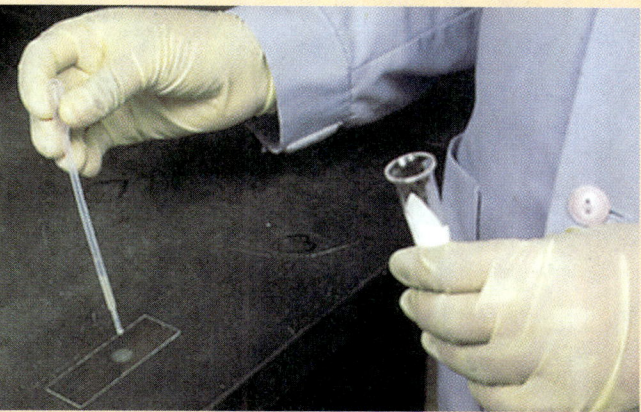

B

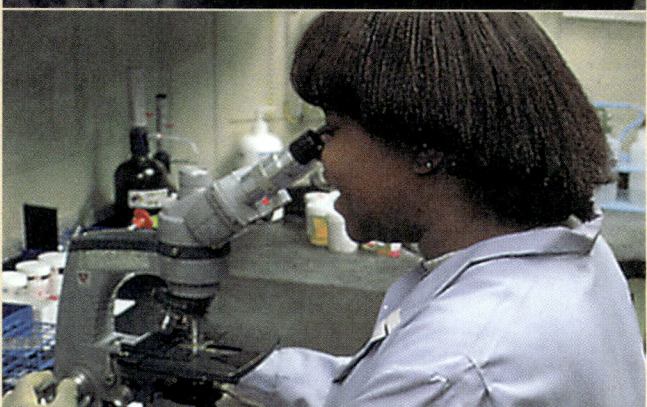

C

FIGURE 12-11 **A** to **C,** Microscopic examination of urine.

There is no easy way to learn how to identify these structures (Figure 12-12). A great deal of practice and training is required to master this skill. Reference charts and books should always be used without hesitation. *Usually this examination is performed by laboratory personnel; on occasion the physician may do it in the office or clinic laboratory. It is not commonly your responsibility to perform the actual examination, although in some instances, you may be required to prepare the slide for the examination* (see Figure 12-11).

Significance of microscopic test results.   Normal urine sediment contains a limited number of formed elements. The presence of one or two white and red blood cells and a few epithelial cells per high-power field is usually not considered abnormal. At times an occasional hyaline cast may also be considered a normal finding. Mucous threads in moderate amounts are normal.

Organized sediment (Tables 12-7 and 12-8)
1. Cells
   a.   Red blood cells (RBCs, or erythrocytes): The presence of more than one or two RBCs per high-power field is an abnormal finding. This may be caused by a variety of kidney and systemic diseases, as well as by trauma to the urinary system, violent exercise, or possible contamination from menstrual blood. Hemorrhagic diseases such as hemophilia may also produce hematuria. The presence of RBCs in the urine must always be reported because this is a significant finding.

FIGURE 12-12 Atlas of urine sediment. (Courtesy Bayer Corp, Elkhart, Ind.)

CELLS IN URINE

Epithelial Cells   Three types of epithelial cells may appear in urine sediment: renal tubular, transitional and/or squamous. Other types of cells may appear in urine but are difficult to identify due to morphologic changes caused by urine. Tubular cells are approximately 1/3 larger than white blood cells. Transitional epithelial cells may arise from the renal pelvis, ureters, bladder or urethra. They tend to be pear-shaped. Squamous cells are large and flat with a prominent nucleus. They originate in the urethra.

RENAL TUBULAR

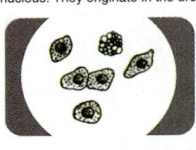 

TRANSITIONAL

SQUAMOUS

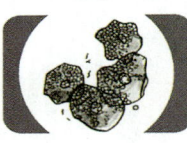 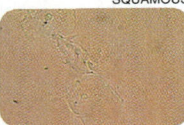

RBCs   Red blood cells may originate from any part of the renal system. The presence of large numbers of RBCs in the urine suggests infection, trauma, tumors, renal calculi, etc. However, the presence of 1 or 2 RBC/(HPF) in the urine sediment, or blood in the urine from menstrual contamination, should not be considered abnormal.

RBCs

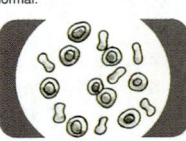 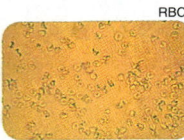

WBCs   White blood cells in the urine (pyuria) may originate from any part of the renal system. The presence of more than 5 WBCs per HPF may suggest infection, cystitis, or pyelonephritis.

RENAL TUBULAR & WBC (SEDI-STAIN*)

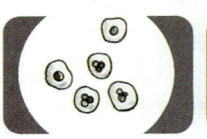 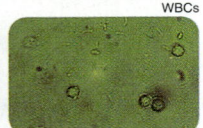

WBCs

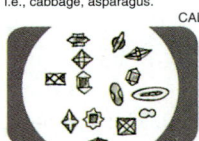 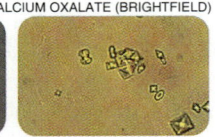

CRYSTALS FOUND IN ACID, NEUTRAL AND ALAKALINE URINE

Calcium Oxalate   Calcium oxalate crystals most frequently have an "envelope" shape and appear in acid, neutral or slightly alkaline urine. They appear in the urine after the ingestion of certain foods, i.e., cabbage, asparagus.

CALCIUM OXALATE (BRIGHTFIELD)

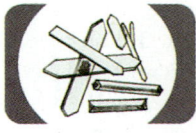 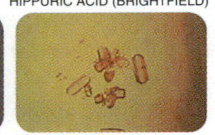

Hippuric Acid   Hippuric acid crystals are colorless or pale yellow. They occur as needles, six-sided prisms, or star-shaped clusters. They appear in urine after the ingestion of certain vegetables and fruits with benzoic acid content. They have little clinical significance.

HIPPURIC ACID (BRIGHTFIELD)

CASTS IN URINE

Hyaline Casts   Hyaline casts are formed from a protein gel in the renal tubule. Hyaline casts may contain cellular inclusions. Hyaline casts will dissolve very rapidly in alkaline urine. Normal urine sediment may contain 1 to 2 hyaline casts per low power field (LPF).

HYALINE

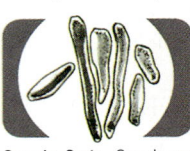 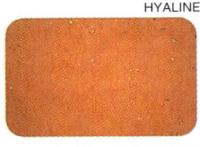

Granular Casts   Granular casts are casts with granules present throughout the cast matrix. They are quite refractile. If the granules are small, the cast is defined as a finely granular cast. If granules are large, it is termed a coarsely granular cast. Granular casts can appear in urine in normal or abnormal states.

GRANULAR

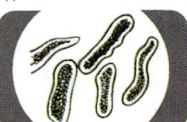 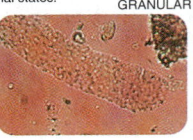

RBC Casts   RBC casts are pathologic and their presence is usually indicative of severe injury to the glomerulus. Rarely, transtubular bleeding may occur, forming RBC casts. RBC casts are found in acute glomerulonephritis, lupus, bacterial endocarditis and septicemias. "Blood" casts are granular and contain hemoglobin from degenerated RBCs.

RBC CASTS

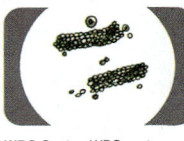 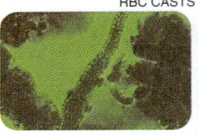

WBC Casts   WBC casts occur when leukocytes are incorporated within the cast matrix. WBC casts will usually indicate an infection, most commonly pyelonephritis. They may also be seen in glomerular diseases. WBC casts may be the only clue to pyelonephritis.

WBC CASTS

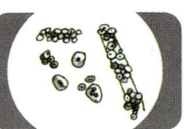 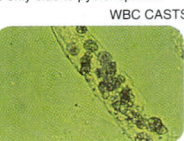

CRYSTALS FOUND IN ALKALINE URINE

Ammonium Blurate or Ammonium Urates   Ammonium urates are yellow-brown in appearance and occur in urine as spheres or spheres with spicules ("thorny apples"). Both forms are frequently seen together. They appear in urine when there is ammonia formation in the urine present in the bladder. They are considered to have little clinical significance.

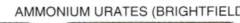

AMMONIUM URATES (BRIGHTFIELD)

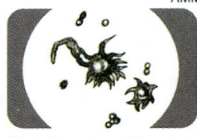 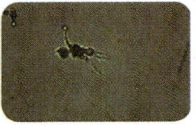

Triple Phosphate   Triple phosphate crystals are common in urine sediment. They have a "coffin-lid" shape, are colorless and appear in alkaline urine. The ingestion of fruit may cause triple phosphate to appear in urine.

TRIPLE PHOSPHATE (BRIGHTFIELD)

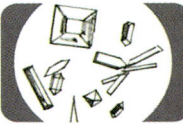 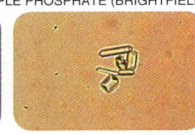

CRYSTALS FOUND IN ACID URINE

Uric Acid Crystals   Uric acid has birefringent characteristics; therefore, it polarizes light, giving multi-colors. Uric acid crystals are found in acid urine. Uric acid may assume various forms, e.g., rhombic, plates, rosettes, small crystals. The color may be red-brown, yellow or colorless. Although increased in 16% of patients with gout, and in patients with malignant lymphoma or leukemia, their presence does not usually indicate pathology or increased uric acid concentrations.

URIC ACID (BRIGHTFIELD)

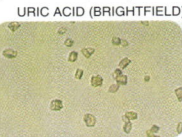

URIC ACID (POLARIZED)

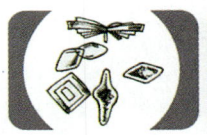 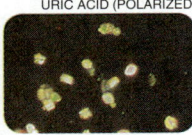

Leucine/Tyrosine Crystals   Leucine and tyrosine are amino acids which crystallize and often appear together in the urine of patients with severe liver disease. Tyrosine usually appears as fine needles arranged as sheaves or rosettes and appear yellow. Leucine is usually yellow, oily-appearing spheres with radial and concentric striations.

TYROSINE (BRIGHTFIELD)

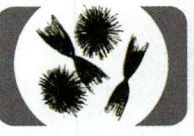 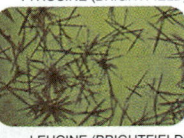

LEUCINE (BRIGHTFIELD)

Cystine Crystals   Cystine crystals are thin, hexagonal-shaped (6-sided) structures. They appear in the urine as a result of a genetic defect. Cystine crystals and stones will appear in the urine in cystinuria and homocystinuria. Cystine crystals are frequently confused with uric acid crystals. Cystine crystals do not polarize light.

CYSTINE (BRIGHTFIELD)

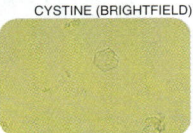
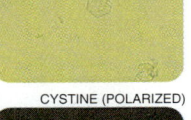

CYSTINE (POLARIZED)

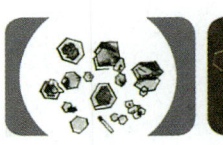 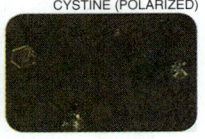

BACTERIA, FUNGI, PARASITES IN URINE

Bacteria   Bacteria in the urine (bacteriuria) can result from contaminants in collection vessels, from periurethral tissues, the urethra, or from fecal or vaginal contamination as well as from true urinary infection.

BACTERIA

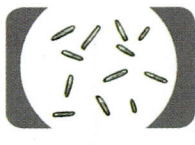 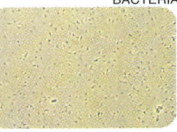

Yeast   Yeast cells vary in size, are colorless, ovoid, and are often budding. They are often confused with RBCs. *Candida albicans* is often seen in diabetes, pregnancy, obesity and other debilitating conditions.

YEAST

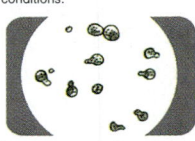 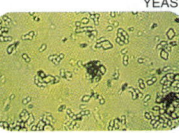

Trichomonas Vaginalis   Trichomonas vaginalis is a flagellate protozoan which affects both males (urethritis) and females (vaginitis).

TRICHOMONAS VAGINALIS

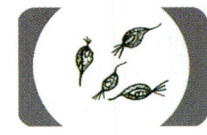 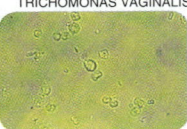

Selected Photomicrographs credited to Bowman Gray School of Medicine, Wake Forest University, N.C. and Rachel Lehman, MS, MT (ASCP).

FIGURE 12-13 Laboratory requisitions for urinalysis.

	ROUTINE URINALYSIS - 001			MICROSCOPIC - 022			QUANTITATIVE	
	APPEARANCE COLOR			WBC'S	/HPF	024	SULKOWITCH	
023	SPECIFIC GRAVITY			RBC'S	/HPF	026	BILE	
004	PH			CASTS (Hyaline)	/LPF		PHENYLPYRUVIC ACID	
	PROTEIN			CASTS (Granular)	/LPF	027	PHENESTIX	
	GLUCOSE			CASTS (Cellular)	/LPF	028	UROBILINOGEN	
007	KETONES (ACETONE)			CASTS (Waxy)	/LPF	029	PORPHOBILINOGEN	
3	OCCULT BLOOD			EPITHELIAL CELLS	/LPF	030	PORPHYRIN	
	BILE			BACTERIA		031	BENCE-JONES	
	UROBILINOGEN			MUCUS		025	TOTAL PROTEIN 24HR. SPECIMEN	
	LEUKOCYTE			CRYSTALS			TOTAL VOLUME REQUIRED:	
COMMENTS				AMORPHOUS				
				OTHER:			SIGNATURE:	
URINALYSIS			33	**F P N**			DATE:	

UR- **183900**
ICDA
REQUESTING PHYSICIAN
PHYSICIAN HAS SEEN-INITIAL

DMH-0067 (Rev. 3/83)

DMH-MedR-1065-A

b. White blood cells (WBCs, or leukocytes): The presence of large numbers of WBCs in the urine usually indicates the presence of a bacterial infection in the urinary tract and/or pyuria. Pyuria (pi-u´re-ah) is the excretion of urine containing pus. This indicates renal disease that may be either infection or lesions in the bladder, urethra, ureters, and kidneys.

c. Epithelial cells: The presence of large numbers of renal and bladder-type epithelial cells is abnormal and should always be reported. The presence of a large number of renal-epithelial cells may indicate degeneration of the renal tubules. Proteinuria and casts are often seen in this condition.

2. Casts

a. Correct identification of casts is essential because the presence of these structures is a most significant laboratory finding. Inflammatory disorders or damage to the glomerulus, tubules, or general renal tissue are usually associated with the presence of casts and are usually accompanied by albuminuria.

b. The various types of casts include RBC, WBC, epithelial cell, hyaline, granular, and waxy and fatty casts.

3. Bacteria (see Table 12-10): Normal urine does not contain bacteria unless the specimen was contaminated by improper collection techniques and handling or by vaginal secretions in the woman. The presence of numerous bacteria in the urine may indicate a urinary tract infection. A true infection can be differentiated from contamination if the specimen also contains WBCs.

4. Yeasts and parasites:

a. Yeast may be seen as a contaminant in the urine of women who have vaginal moniliasis, or it may indicate a urinary moniliasis, especially in patients who have diabetes mellitus.

b. Parasites seen in the urine are usually contaminants from vaginal or fecal excretions.

5. Spermatozoa: Spermatozoa may appear as contaminants in the urine. They often are present in urine after sexual intercourse or nocturnal emissions.

Unorganized sediment (Tables 12-9 and 12-10)

1. Crystals

a. The type and quantity of crystals in the urine vary with the pH of the specimen. Normally, most crystals are of little importance and form in urine as it cools.

b. Crystals seen in normal acid urine are uric acid, amorphous urates, hippuric acid, and calcium oxalate. Crystals seen in normal alkaline urine include triple phosphate, ammonium, magnesium, calcium phosphate, calcium carbonate, and ammonium urate. Abnormal crystals found in acid urine include cholesterin, cystine, leucine, and tyrosine.

2. Artifacts and contaminants: These include hair, cloth fibers, mucous threads, and other contaminants. It is important to differentiate these structures from other elements in the sediment that may indicate the presence of a disease process.

TABLE 12–7 Cells in Urine Sediment

Type	Presence in Normal Urine	Possible Causes of Abnormal Amounts of Cells in Urine
Red blood cells	0 to 2 cells/high-power field (depending on preparation of urinary sediment)	Inflammatory diseases Acute glomerulonephritis Pyelonephritis Hypertension Renal infarction Trauma Stones Tumor Bleeding diseases Use of anticoagulants
White blood cells	0 to 8 cells/high-power field (depending on preparation of urinary sediment) 0 to 4 cells/low-power field	Pyelonephritis Cystitis Urethritis Prostatitis Transplant rejection (manifested by lymphocytes in urine) Tissue injury accompanied by severe inflammation (manifested by monocytes in urine) Inflammation, immune mechanisms, and other host defense mechanisms (manifested by histiocytes in urine)
Squamous epithelial cells	Often present, depending on collection technique	Vaginal contamination
Transitional epithelial cells	Moderate number of cells present	Disease of bladder or renal pelvis Catheterization
Renal tubular epithelial cells	Present in small numbers; higher numbers in infants	Acute tubular necrosis Glomerulonephritis Acute infection Renal toxicity Viral infection
Cytomegalic inclusion bodies	Not normally present in urine	Cytomegalic inclusion disease
Tumor cells	Not normally present in urine	Tumors of • Renal pelvis • Renal parenchyma • Ureters • Bladder

Courtesy Boehringer Mannheim Diagnostics, Indianapolis, Ind.

DETECTION AND SEMIQUANTITATION OF BACTERIURIA

When obtaining a urine specimen for bacteriologic examination, you should collect a clean-catch midstream specimen in a sterile container (refer to Chapter 11 for this procedure). The first voided specimen of the day should be used whenever possible because bacteria will be more numerous. The examination should be done within 1 hour from the time of collection. When this is not possible, refrigerate the specimen to prevent the growth of microorganisms and test the specimen within 8 hours. *Never* add a preservative to a urine specimen that is to be used for bacteriologic culture tests because the preservative destroys the viability of most of the bacteria that may be present.

Culture Plate Methods

This technique requires the special facilities and trained personnel of a microbiology laboratory. There the identification

TABLE 12–8   Casts in Urine Sediment

Type	Description	Possible Causes
Hyaline casts	Colorless, transparent Low refractive index	Normal urine Strenuous exercise Acute glomerulonephritis Acute pyelonephritis Malignant hypertension Chronic renal disease
Red blood cell casts	Red cells in hyaline matrix Yellow-orange color High refractive index	Acute glomerulonephritis Lupus nephritis Severe nephritis Collagen diseases Renal infarction Malignant hypertension
White blood cell casts	Neutrophils in hyaline matrix High refractive index	Acute pyelonephritis Acute glomerulonephritis Chronic renal disease
Epithelial cell casts	Renal tubular epithelial cells in hyaline matrix High refractive index	Glomerulonephritis Vascular disease Toxin Virus
Granular casts	Opaque granules in matrix	Heavy proteinuria (nephrotic syndrome) Orthostatic proteinuria Congestive heart failure with proteinuria Acute or chronic renal disease
Waxy casts	Sharp, refractile outlines Irregular "broken off" ends Absence of differentiated structures	Severe chronic renal disease Malignant hypertension Kidney disease resulting from diabetes mellitus Acute renal disease
Fatty casts	Fat globules in transparent matrix	Nephrotic syndrome Diabetes mellitus Mercury poisoning Ethylene glycol poisoning
Broad casts	Larger diameter than other casts	Acute tubular necrosis Severe chronic renal disease Urinary tract obstruction
Mixed casts	Combination of any of the above	Any of the above, depending on cellular constituents

Courtesy of Boehringer Mannheim Diagnostics, Indianapolis, Ind.

and precise quantitation of bacterial species can be ascertained. If the specimen is not cultured immediately, refrigeration is mandatory.

Nitrite Test and Culture Strip Methods

A chemical test using a reagent strip, as discussed earlier in the section on chemical examination of urine, is used for the nitrite test. The culture strip method, a simplified semiquantitative culture test, provides greater precision than is possible with the nitrite test. Often used are the Microstix-3 reagent strips. This method is a three-way bacteriuria test. The strip contains three pads: (1) a nitrite reagent pad, (2) a dehydrated culture media pad that favors the growth of all types of bacteria commonly seen in urinary tract infections, and (3) a dehydrated culture media pad that supports growth of only gram-negative bacteria. A thermostatically controlled incubator specifically designed for use with the Microstix-3 is available. It is small, about the size of an average textbook, and relatively inexpensive; therefore it is very practical for use in a urinalysis laboratory in a physician's office or clinic.

TABLE 12–9 Urinary Crystals

Type of Urine	Type of Crystals	Description of Crystals	Significance When Found in Urine
Normal acid urine	Amorphous urate	Colorless or yellow-brown granules (pink macroscopically)	Nonpathologic
	Uric acid	Occur in many shapes; may be colorless, yellow-brown, or red-brown; and square, diamond shaped, wedge shaped, or grouped in rosettes	Usually nonpathologic; in large numbers, may indicate gout
	Calcium oxalate	Octahedral or dumbbell shaped; possess double refractive index	Usually nonpathologic, may be associated with stone formation
Normal alkaline urine	Amorphous phosphates	Small, colorless granules	Nonpathologic
	Triple phosphates	Colorless prisms with three to six sides ("coffin lids") or feathery, shaped like fern leaves	Usually nonpathologic; may be associated with stone formation
	Ammonium biurate	Yellow-brown "thorny apple" appearance or yellow-brown spheres	Nonpathologic
	Calcium phosphate	Colorless prisms or rosettes	Usually nonpathologic; may be associated with urine stasis or chronic urinary tract infection
	Calcium carbonate	Usually appear colorless and amorphous; may be shaped like dumbbells, rhombi, or needles	Usually nonpathologic; may be associated with inorganic calculi formation
Abnormal urine	Tyrosine	Thin, dark needles, arranged in sheaves or clumps; usually colorless, but may be pale yellow-brown	Liver disease or inherited metabolic disorder
	Leucine	Yellow-brown spheres with radial striations	Liver disease or inherited metabolic disorder
	Cystine	Clear, hexagonal plates	Cystinuria
	Hippuric acid	Star-shaped clusters of needles, rhombic plates, or elongated prisms; may be colorless or yellow-brown	Usually nonpathologic
	Bilirubin	Delicate needles or rhombic plates; red-brown in color; birefringent	Bilirubinuria
	Cholesterol	Colorless, transparent plates with regular or irregular corner notches	Chyluria, urinary tract infections, nephrotic syndrome
	Creatine	Pseudohexagonal plate with positive birefringence	Destruction of muscle tissue caused by muscular dystrophies, atrophies, and myositis
	Aspirin	Distinctive prismatic or starlike forms; usually colorless; show positive birefringence	Ingestion of aspirin or other salicylates
	Sulfonamide	Yellow-brown dumbbells, asymmetric sheaves, rosettes or hexagonal plates	Ingestion of sulfonamide drugs
	Ampicillin	Long, thin, clear crystals	Parenteral administration of ampicillin
	X-ray media	Long, thin rectangles or flat, four-sided, notched plates	X-ray procedure with contrast media

Courtesy Boehringer Mannheim Diagnostics, Indianapolis, Ind.

Procedure for Using the Microstix-3 Reagent Strip

1. Don disposable, single-use examination gloves.
2. Remove the strip from the wrapper; avoid contact of the test areas with anything.
3. Dip the strip in the urine specimen for 5 seconds and remove.
4. Read the nitrite test area 30 seconds later. Any degree of a pink color indicates the presence of 10^5 or more organisms per milliliter of urine.

TABLE 12–10   Microorganisms and Artifacts in Urine

Microorganisms/Artifacts	Significance When Found in Urine
Bacteria	More than 100,000 bacteria/ml indicates urinary tract infection
	10,000 to 100,000 bacteria/ml indicates that tests should be repeated
	Less than 10,000 bacteria/ml may signify urine in which any bacteria are due to urethral organisms or contamination
	Bacteria accompanied by white blood cells and/or white cell or mixed casts may indicate acute pyelonephritis
Fungi	May indicate contamination by yeasts from skin and hair
	May indicate diabetes mellitus or urinary tract infection
	Candida albicans may occur in patients with diabetes mellitus or in the contaminated urine of female patients with candidal vaginitis
Parasites and parasitic ova	Usually indicate fecal or vaginal contamination and should be reported
	Trichomonas may be found in patients with urethritis and in the contaminated urine of women with trichomonas vaginitis
	Pinworm is a common contaminant and should be reported
Spermatozoa	Nonpathologic
Urinary artifacts	Nonpathologic
Hair	May result from improper urine collection, improper slide preparation, or outside contamination
Starch from surgical gloves	
Pollen grains	
Bubbles	
Oil droplets	
Fibers	
Talc	
Dust	
Threads	
Glass particles	

Courtesy Boehringer Mannheim Diagnostics, Indianapolis, Ind.

5. Insert the strip in the sterile plastic pouch provided and seal.
6. Incubate the pouch for 12 to 18 hours.
7. Read the results without removing the strip from the transparent pouch. Compare the color densities on both culture pads with the chart provided. Magenta spots on the pads indicate bacterial locations.
8. Remove gloves and wash your hands.
9. Record the results and dispose of the still-sealed pouches by incineration (*or* autoclave pouches and then dispose of according to agency policy).

OTHER URINE TESTS

Protein Determinations

Bence Jones protein is the name of an abnormal protein in the urine that is commonly seen in patients who have multiple myeloma and a few other abnormalities. This protein is characterized by the fact that during special testing methods (the Bence Jones protein test), it precipitates (separates from the liquid) when urine is heated but disappears once the urine is cooled. Many believe that this is not a very sensitive test because it can miss detecting small amounts of the Bence Jones protein or other similar types of abnormal protein. Thus many laboratories have discontinued using this test and are now doing the urine-protein electrophoresis. This test determines the relative concentration and also the type of abnormal protein present in the urine. It can be performed on a random urine specimen, although it is preferable to collect a 24-hour specimen in most cases.

Hormone Determinations

Hormone determination urine tests help detect metabolic and endocrine conditions or disorders. One common test performed is the pregnancy test, in which urine is tested for the presence of the human chorionic gonadotropin (hCG) hormone. A wide range of tests is used for this purpose. Many are slide tests that provide results within a few minutes. Complete instructions for use are provided with the test equipment when purchased. Although these tests are highly reliable, incorrect results may be obtained at times because of the presence of protein or blood in the urine or when the urine is too dilute. For most reliable results, the urine should have a specific gravity of at least 1.015. The first morning specimen is preferred for testing.

Pregnancy Test

To determine if a woman is pregnant, blood or urine can be tested for the presence of the hCG hormone (Figure 12-14). Blood tests called radioisotope or radioimmunoassay (RIA) tests are more sensitive than urine tests. They use a radioactive substance to determine the presence of hCG in the blood. These tests can identify a pregnancy 7 days after conception. RIA tests take 1 to 2 hours to process in the laboratory. In the physician's office or clinic, urine tests are more commonly used to detect pregnancy. The urine pregnancy tests use an antigen-antibody response to determine the presence of hCG. Antibodies to the hCG bind with the hCG to produce either a clumping of cells or a color change that indicates pregnancy. Urine tests for pregnancy are usually recommended at least 2 weeks after the first missed menstrual period. A first voided morning specimen is preferred for testing because it usually contains the greatest concentration of hCG. The patient must be given a clean urine container and an explanation of how to collect the specimen. If the specimen is collected at home, direct the patient to keep the specimen in the refrigerator until she can bring it to the office or laboratory for testing.

Before the test is done, the specific gravity of the specimen must be measured. If the specific gravity is less than 1.010, the results of the hCG test may be false-negative because the urine is too dilute for testing. For the most reliable results, the urine should have a specific gravity of at least 1.015. The protein content should also be checked and noted if positive because protein can affect test results. **NOTE:** These tests are used to diagnose a pregnancy, but they do not necessarily indicate a normal pregnancy.

Quality controls.   Positive and negative controls should be performed routinely to check the reliability of the reagents and your technique. Commercial controls can be obtained, or you may use the urine from women who are known to be pregnant and those who are not pregnant. Check the expiration dates on the supplies so that outdated materials may be discarded and replaced with new supplies.

Phenylketonuria

Phenylketonuria (PKU) is an inherited disease that must be diagnosed early to avoid serious brain damage and mental retardation. A blood test may be performed 2 to 3 days after birth to aid in a diagnosis of PKU. A urine test can also be performed to diagnose or recheck the results of the first test. A urine test for PKU is generally performed at the infant's first checkup 6 weeks after birth. This test cannot be used before the sixth week of life because if performed earlier, it will produce invalid results. The urine test is the Diaper test, which uses 10% ferric chloride to determine color changes from the urine. PKU and the blood and urine tests performed are discussed further under Pediatric Examination in Chapter 5.

Diaper test

1. Drop 10% ferric chloride on a diaper that contains fresh urine.
2. Read the results. A green spot on the diaper is considered a positive result, which indicates the possibility of PKU.

Multiple-Glass Test

The multiple-glass test is performed on men to evaluate a lower urinary tract infection. See Chapter 11 for the procedure used to collect three specimens for this test.

Chlamydia and Gonorrhea

Urine specimens can also be used to detect gonorrhea and chlamydia infection(s). The patient should not have voided for at least 1 hour before collecting a urine specimen. Give the patient a sterile, preservative-free urine specimen collection cup. Instruct the patient to collect the *first* 15 to 20 ml of urine in the cup (the first part of the stream) and then cap the cup securely. Label the specimen and complete the laboratory requisition. Refrigerate the specimen immediately at 2° to 8° C (35.6° to 46.4° F). Specimens stored and shipped at this temperature must arrive at the test site within 24 hours of shipment, and many of the available tests must be processed within 4 days of specimen collection. Specimens can also be frozen at minus 20° C (−4° F) or below and must be processed within 60 days of specimen collection. Once frozen, specimens should not be thawed until ready for testing.

Other Tests

Numerous other tests can be performed on urine to aid the physician when diagnosing and treating a patient's condition. However, this book does not discuss all of them in detail. *Most must be performed in a laboratory by qualified personnel.* See Table 12-11 for additional urine tests, the average normal values, and the type of specimen that is required for testing.

FIGURE 12-14 A and **B,** Procedures for using a one-step hCG serum/urine pregnancy test. (**A,** Courtesy Pacific-Biotech, Inc, San Diego, Calif; **B,** courtesy Quidel Corp, San Diego, Calif.)

hCG TESTS — SERUM/URINE AND URINE ONLY

CARDS® Q.S.® hCG Serum/Urine Test Procedure Card

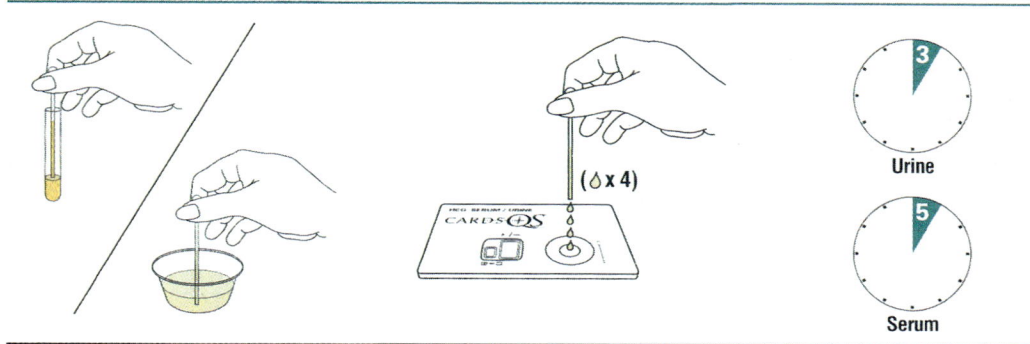

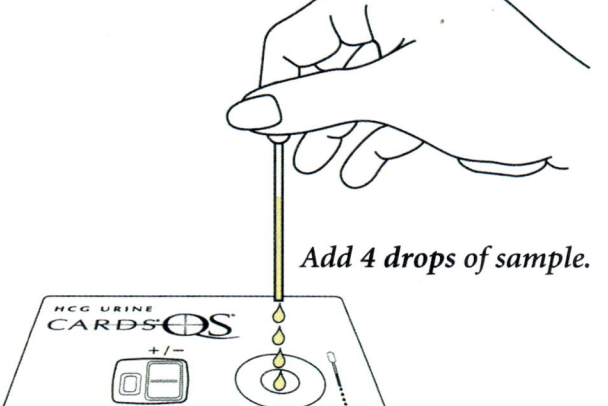

Add 4 drops of sample.

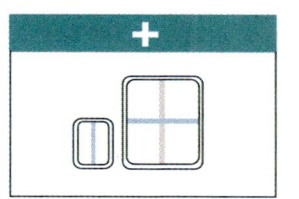 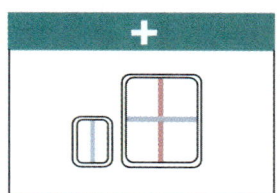

Pink and blue plus sign indicates a positive test result.

A

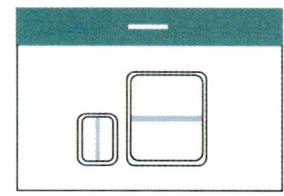

*A blue minus sign indicates
a negative test result.*

EASY TO USE

- Just add 4 drops of sample, serum or urine
- Two-color plus sign or minus sign for clearly distinguishable results
- Results in 3 minutes for urine / 5 minutes for serum; some positive results may appear **as soon as 1 minute** after sample addition

ACCURATE PERFORMANCE

- 10 mIU/mL sensitivity in serum; 20 mIU/mL sensitivity in urine
- Greater than 99% sensitivity and specificity
- Built-in procedural controls verify proper test and reagent performance

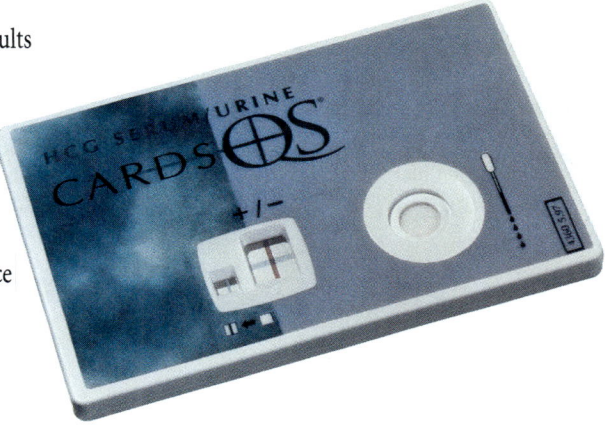

Continued

FIGURE 12-14—cont'd A and **B,** Procedures for using a one-step hCG serum/urine pregnancy test. (**A,** Courtesy Pacific-Biotech, Inc, San Diego, Calif; **B,** courtesy Quidel Corp, San Diego, Calif.)

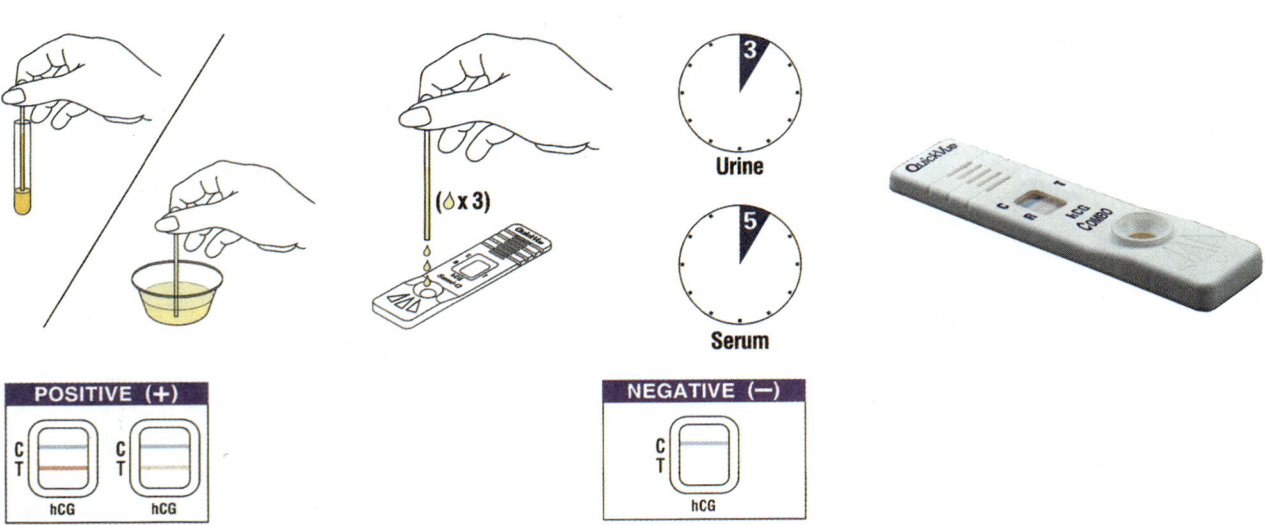

B

Intended Use
The QuickVue One-Step hCG-Combo Test is a sensitive immunoassay for the qualitative detection of human chorionic gonadotropin (hCG) in serum or urine for the early detection of pregnancy.

Summary and Explanation
Human chorionic gonadotropin is a hormone produced by the placenta shortly after implantation. Since hCG is present in the serum and urine of pregnant women, it is an excellent marker for confirming pregnancy. The QuickVue test uses a monoclonal antibody specific to the beta subunit of hCG in a single-step technology to accurately detect hCG.

Principle of the Test
Serum or urine is added to the Sample Well on the Test Cassette. If hCG is present in the specimen at a level of 10 mIU/mL with serum samples or 20 mIU/mL with urine samples, a pink-to-purple Test (T) Line will appear along with a blue Procedural Control (C) Line in the Result Window. If hCG is present at very low levels, or not present in the specimen, only a blue Procedural Control Line will appear in the Result Window.

Reagents and Materials Supplied
- Individually wrapped Test Cassette
  - Each cassette contains murine monoclonal antibody and caprine polyclonal antibody to hCG
- Disposable pipet
- 1 Package Insert

Materials Required but not Provided
- Watch or clock that measures minutes
- Specimen collection containers

Materials Recommended but not Provided
- External hCG controls traceable to WHO Standard (3rd IS 75/537).

Warnings and Precautions
- Kit contents are for *in vitro* diagnostic use.
- Do not use kit contents after the expiration date printed on the outside of the kit.

- Use appropriate precautions in the collection, handling, storage and disposal of the specimens and used kit contents.[1] Discard used pipets and test cassettes in a proper biohazard container.
- To obtain accurate results, you must follow the Package Insert instructions.

Kit Storage and Stability
Store kit at room temperature 59–86°F (15–30°C), out of direct sunlight. Kit contents are stable until the expiration date printed on the outer box carton. Do not freeze.

Specimen Collection and Storage
Serum
No special patient preparation is necessary. A whole blood specimen should be obtained by standard medical procedures. After clotting has occurred, the separated serum should be used for testing. Serum specimens may be stored refrigerated 36–46°F (2–8°C) for up to 48 hours prior to assay. If testing will be delayed for more than 48 hours, the sample may be frozen once at –20°C or below. If frozen, mix after thawing. Do not re-freeze. Do not chemically modify the serum in any way.

Urine
Collect specimens in clean container. First morning specimens generally contain the highest concentrations of hCG and are recommended for early detection of pregnancy. However, any urine sample is suitable for testing. Urine specimens may be kept at room temperature for 8 hours or stored at 36–46°F (2–8°C) for up to 3 days. Do not freeze specimens.

QUALITY CONTROL

Built-in Quality Control Features
The QuickVue test contains built-in control features. The development of the blue procedural Control Line next to the letter "C" is a positive procedural control. The procedural Control Line assures that the reagents were functioning properly and the assay procedure was followed properly. If this line does not develop, the test result is invalid. The absence of interfering background is a negative procedural control. If background color appears in the Result Window which interferes with your ability to read the test result, your result may be invalid. In this case, contact QUIDEL Technical Assistance.

FIGURE 12-14—cont'd A and **B,** Procedures for using a one-step hCG serum/urine pregnancy test. (**A,** Courtesy Pacific-Biotech, Inc, San Diego, Calif; **B,** courtesy Quidel Corp, San Diego, Calif.)

Optional Quality Control Feature
Good laboratory practice recommends the use of external controls to assure that the reagents and assay are preforming properly. For this purpose, we recommend the QuickVue hCG Controls (QUIDEL Catalog Number 0272), or the hCG Serum Control Set (QUIDEL Catalog Number 0281). External Controls should be tested with each new lot or shipment of test materials once for each 25-test kit, and as otherwise required by your laboratory's standard quality control procedures.

1. External Positive Control: Process the control as you would a patient sample. A positive signal is indicated by the appearance of a pink-to-purple Test Line, along with a blue procedural Control Line.
2. External Negative Control: Process the control as you would a patient specimen. A negative signal is indicated by the appearance of the blue procedural Control Line only.

Test Procedure
Use a new disposable pipet for each specimen.
• Remove the QuickVue Test Cassette from the foil pouch and place it on a clean, dry, level surface.
• Using one of the disposable pipets supplied, add **3 DROPS (125 μL)** of serum or urine to the **Round Sample Well** on the Test Cassette. The Test Cassette should not be moved again until the assay is complete and ready for interpretation.

• **FOR URINE:** Read result at **3 minutes**.
• **FOR SERUM:** Read result at **5 minutes**.
Note: Some positive results may be seen earlier.

Interpretation of Results
See Procedure Card for color result interpretation.

Positive:
The appearance of **any pink-to-purple line** next to the letter "T" in the Result Window, along with a blue Procedural Control Line next to the letter "C".

Negative:
The appearance of the blue Procedural Control Line next to the letter "C" **only** and no pink-to-purple Test Line next to the letter "T" at three minutes for urine or at 5 minutes for serum.

No Result:
If no blue Procedural Control Line appears, the test result is invalid and the specimen must be retested.

A specimen with a low level of hCG may show color development over time. If a negative result is obtained but pregnancy is suspected, another specimen should be collected after 48–72 hours and tested.

Limitations
• The contents of this kit are for use in the **qualitative** detection of hCG in serum or urine.
• Test results must always be evaluated with other data available to the physician.
• While pregnancy is the most likely reason for the presence of hCG in serum and urine, elevated hCG concentrations unrelated to pregnancy have been reported in some patients.[2,3] Patients with trophoblastic and nontrophoblastic disease may have elevated hCG levels, therefore, the possibility of hCG secreting neoplasms should be eliminated prior to the diagnosis of pregnancy.[8]
• hCG may remain detectable for a few days to several weeks after delivery, spontaneous abortion, or hCG injections.
• Very low levels of hCG are present in serum and in urine shortly after implantation. Positive test results from very early pregnancy may later prove negative due to natural termination of pregnancy. This is estimated to occur in 31% of pregnancies overall and 22% of clinically unrecognized pregnancies.[5] If a very low, faint positive serum result is obtained, another sample should be obtained in 48 hours and retested. If waiting 48 hours is not medically advisable, the test result should be confirmed with a quantitative hCG test.
• A normal pregnancy cannot be distinguished from ectopic pregnancy based on hCG levels alone. Abnormal pregnancies cannot be diagnosed by qualitative hCG results. The above conditions should be ruled out when diagnosing pregnancy.
• If a urine sample is too dilute, it may not contain a representative urinary hCG concentration. If a negative result is obtained and pregnancy is still suspected, a first morning urine sample should be obtained and tested.

Expected Values
Specimens containing as low as 10 mIU/mL (serum) or 20 mIU/mL (urine) (calibrated against the WHO 3rd IS 75/537) hCG will yield positive results when tested with the QuickVue test. In normal pregnancy, hCG can be detected as early as 6 days following conception with concentrations doubling every 32 to 48 hours, peaking in excess of 100,000 mIU/mL in approximately ten to twelve weeks. Levels of 25 mIU/mL are reportedly present in serum and urine as early as two to three days before expected menses. Serum hCG is rapidly cleared into the urine and the concentration of hCG in serum is approximately equal to the concentration in urine.

B

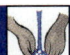

PROCEDURE 12-3

URINE PREGNANCY TEST: WAMPOLE 2-MINUTE SLIDE TEST

Objective
Understand and demonstrate the correct procedure for testing a urine specimen for the presence of a pregnancy.

Equipment
Timer
Pregnancy kit, which includes:
  Antiserum reagent
  Antigen reagent
  Clean glass slide with one or more raised circles on it
  Disposable stirrer
  Disposable pipet with rubber bulb
A good light source that the slide can be observed under
The urine specimen
Disposable, single-use examination gloves
Laboratory requisition

PROCEDURE

1. **Wash your hands. Use appropriate personal protective equipment (PPE) as dictated by facility.** Assemble equipment.

2. Remove reagents from the refrigerator and allow them to warm to room temperature.

3. Don disposable, single-use examination gloves.

4. Make sure that the urine specimen has been allowed to warm to room temperature if it had been stored in the refrigerator. If the urine is cloudy, centrifuge it and use the supernatant for the test. (The supernatant is the clear upper portion of a mixture after it has been centrifuged.)

5. Using the disposable pipet, place 1 drop of clear urine within one of the circles on the clean glass slide. The slide must be clean. Do not let the pipet touch the slide.

6. Add 1 drop of the antiserum reagent to the drop of urine. Hold the dropper at a 90-degree angle to the slide. Do not touch the urine with the dropper. Adding the reagents to the urine in the correct order is vital.

7. To mix the antigen reagent well, shake the bottle. Add 1 drop to the slide in the same circle with the urine and antiserum. Hold the reagent dropper at a 90-degree angle when adding the drop to the slide. Do not touch the specimen with the dropper.

8. Mix the reagents and urine with the stirrer. Spread the mixture over the entire circle.

9. Gently rock the slide for exactly 2 minutes. Set your timer. This rocking motion must be slow. Have the slide under a good light so that you can observe any agglutination (clumping together of cells).

10. Read the slide at 2 minutes. **If agglutination occurs,** the test is considered **negative** for pregnancy. Agglutination is recognized as a granular appearance to the solution. The test must be read at exactly 2 minutes.

RATIONALE

To ensure accurate results, all the fluids must be at room temperature.

Dirty slides can cause errors.

If the order is changed, the results can be inaccurate. Holding the dropper at a 90-degree angle allows you to squeeze out a standard-size drop.

Avoid contamination.

After 2 minutes, evaporation may occur and give the appearance of agglutination. Before 2 minutes, agglutination may occur and can be read as a negative result.

PROCEDURE 12-3

URINE PREGNANCY TEST: WAMPOLE 2-MINUTE SLIDE TEST—cont'd

11. **If agglutination does not occur,** the test is considered **positive** for pregnancy. Absence of agglutination is observed as a smooth, opaque suspension.

12. Thoroughly wash the glass slide, wipe dry, and replace in storage area. Return reagents to the refrigerator.

13. Remove your gloves and wash your hands before returning supplies to the storage area.

14. Record the results on the patient's chart. Include the date of the patient's last menstrual period (LMP).

Charting Example

October 10, 20__, 8 PM
Pregnancy slide test—positive
LMP—August 26, 20__
M.L. Johnson, CMA

TABLE 12–11   Average Normal Values for Urine Determinations

Test	Average Normal Value	Type of Specimen
Addis Count	WBC 1,800,000	12-hour
	RBC 500,000	
	Casts 0-5000	
Albumin		
Qualitative	Negative	Random
Quantitative	10-100 mg/24 hr	24-hour
Aldosterone	2-23 μg/24 hr	24-hour, refrigerated
Amino acid nitrogen	100-290 mg/24 hr	24-hour; refrigerated, collected in thymol
Ammonia	20-70 mEq/24 hr	24-hour
Ammonia nitrogen	0.14-1.47 g/24 hr	24-hour
Bence Jones protein	Negative	First morning specimen
Bilirubin	Negative	Random
Blood, occult	Negative	Random
Calcium		
Sulkowitch	Positive 1+	Random
Quantitative	100-250 mg/24 hr on an average diet	24-hour
Catecholamines	100-230 μg/24 hr	24-hour, preserve with 1 ml concentrated H_2SO_4
Chloride	110-250 mEq/24 hr	24-hour
Concentration test	Specific gravity of 1.025 or higher	Withholding fluids for the day before the test
Coproporphyrin	20 μg/100 ml	Random
Random	Adults: 50-200 μg/24 hr	24-hour; preserve with 5 g Na_2CO_3
24-hour	Children: 0-80 μg/24 hr	
Creatine	Men: 0-40 mg/24 hr	24-hour
	Women: 0-100 mg/24 hr	
	Higher in children	

Courtesy Ames Co., Division of Miles Laboratories, Inc, Elkhart, Ind, 1986. After Davidson I, Henry JB: *Todd-Sanford clinical diagnosis by laboratory methods,* Philadelphia, 1969, WB Saunders, and Goodale RH, Widmann FK: *Clinical interpretation of laboratory tests,* Philadelphia, 1969, Davis.

Continued

TABLE 12–11   **Average Normal Values for Urine Determinations—cont'd**

Test	Average Normal Value	Type of Specimen
Creatinine	Men: 1-1.9 mg/24 hr	24-hour
	Women 0.8-1.7 g/24 hr	
Dilution test	Specific gravity of 1.001 to 1.003	After 1200 ml water load
Estrogens	Men: 4-25 μg/24 hr	24-hours, refrigerate
	Women: 4-60 μg/24 hr	
Glucose		
Qualitative	Negative	Random
Quantitative	130 mg/24 hr	24-hour
Hemoglobin	Negative	Random
17-hydroxycorticosteroids	Men: 5.5-14.5 mg/24 hr	24-hour, tranquilizers interfere
	Women: 5-13 mg/24 hr	
17-ketosteroids	Men: 8-15 mg/24 hr	24-hour, tranquilizers interfere
	Women: 6-11.5 mg/24 hr	
	Children: 5 mg/24 hr	
Ketones	Negative	Random
Lead	100 μg/24 hr	24-hour, collect in lead-free bottle
Osmolality		
Normal fluid intake	500-800 mOsm/kg water	Random
Full range	38-1400 mOsm/kg water	Random
pH	4.6-8	Random
Phenylpyruvic acid	Negative	Random
Phosphorus	0.9-1.3 g/24 hr	24-hour
Porphobilinogen	Negative	Random
Potassium	25-100 mEq/24 hr	24-hour
Pregnanediol	Men: 0-1 mg/24 hr	24-hour, refrigerate
	Women: 1-8 mg/24 hr	
	Children: Negative	
Pregnanetriol	Men: 1-2 mg/24 hr	24-hour, refrigerate
	Women: 0.5-2 mg/24 hr	
	Children: <0.5 mg/24 hr	
Protein		
Qualitative	Negative	Random
Quantitative	10-150 mg/24 hr	24-hour
Bence Jones	Negative	**First morning specimen**
Sodium	110-260 mEq/24 hr	24-hour
Specific gravity		
Random	1.002-1.030	Random
24-Hour	1.015-1.025	24-hour
Sugars	Negative	Random
Tritratable acidity	200-500 ml of 0.1	24-hour, preserve with toluene
	NaOH/24 hr	
Urea nitrogen	6-17 g/24	24-hour
Uric acid	250-750 mg/24 hr	24-hour
Urobilinogen		
Semiquantitative	0.3-1 Ehrlich units/2 hr	2-hour afternoon specimen
Quantitative	1-4 mg/24 hr	24-hour, collect in dark bottle with 5 g Na_2CO_3, refrigerate
Uroporphyrin	10-30 μg/24 hr	24-hour, collect in dark bottle with 5 g Na_2CO_3
VMA (Vanilmandelic acid)	1-8 mg/24 hr	24-hour, preserve in 3 ml 25% H_2SO_4; no coffee or fruit for 2 days before test
Volume adults	600-1500 ml/24 hr	24-hour

*Courtesy Ames Co., Division of Miles Laboratories, Inc., Elkhart, Ind., 1986. After Davidson I, Henry JB: Todd-Sanford clinical diagnosis by laboratory methods, Philadelphia, 1969, Saunders, and Goodale RH, Widmann FK: *Clinical interpretation of laboratory tests,* Philadelphia, 1969, Davis.

KEEPING YOUR PATIENTS INFORMED

Millions of men and women suffer from **urinary incontinence** but often are too embarrassed to discuss the subject with their physician. Many resign themselves to thinking that this is a normal part of aging and start wearing adult diapers or pads. This condition affects women (20% to 40%) more often than men (10% to 20%) over 60 years of age. It is also commonly seen in women in their 40s and 50s. However, incontinence *should not* be seen as an eventual problem that comes with aging.

Those affected should be encouraged to speak to their physician regarding this condition, and literature should be readily available for them in the physician's office or clinic. Incontinence can be treated and even cured in most cases by learning how to strengthen the pelvic muscles, taking medication, or both. (Review the urinary system on p. 530.

Causes of urinary incontinence may be due to any of the following or a combination of more than one:

- Infections
- Weakened pelvic muscles that support the base of the bladder or weakened sphincter muscles in the wall of the urethra, at the base of the bladder. Both of these problems could result from childbirth.
- An overactive bladder
- Nerve damage
- Prostate enlargement
- In very rare cases, urinary incontinence could be associated with a spinal tumor, prostate cancer, or a herniated vertebral disk. In these circumstances, it is extremely important for the person to seek medical attention.

TYPES OF INCONTINENCE

1. **Stress incontinence:** Stress incontinence can develop when involuntary pressure is put on the bladder during lifting, straining, coughing, sneezing, or laughing. There is a weakening of the tissues supporting the bladder. This type is seen most often in women in their 40s and 50s.
2. **Urge incontinence:** Urge incontinence is most common in people over 60. It is usually due to involuntary contractions of the bladder muscle. People experience an urgent need to urinate and have a sudden loss of urine. Women often experience a combination of both stress and urge incontinence.
3. **Overflow incontinence:** Overflow incontinence is much less common. In this case the bladder is so full that it continually leaks urine. There is often weakened bladder muscles, a blocked urethra caused by prostate enlargement, or nerve damage.

TREATMENT

Patients will often be asked to keep a diary of urinary habits for at least 1 week before seeing the physician. This should include how much and how often they urinated or had leakage of urine.

A pelvic and/or rectal examination, a urinalysis to test for infection, and a noninvasive diagnostic imaging scan to check for residual urine in the bladder will usually be performed before treatment begins. Various approaches may be used for treatment. These include the following:

1. **Kegel's exercises** to strengthen the pelvic floor muscles have proven to be very effective in reducing urine leakage in 50% to 75% of women experiencing stress incontinence, and 20% of the cases have been cured with these exercises. Kegel's exercises are done simply by contracting and relaxing the pelvic floor muscles. The easiest way to identify these muscles is to have the person start to urinate and then stop the flow midstream. **Directions as follows should be given to the patient.**
    - Tighten the pelvic floor muscles and hold for a count of 10.
    - Relax the muscles completely for a count of 10.
    - Do these exercises 3 to 5 times a day in sets of 5 to 15 contractions.
    - Do not expect to experience results immediately. It may take 4 to 6 weeks for the first signs of improvement to be noticed.
    - These exercises must be continued indefinitely to keep these muscles strong and avoid urine leakage.

    At times these exercises may be more effective when weighted cones are inserted into the vagina.
2. A **pessary** (a stiff rubber ring) is inserted into the vagina. This ring puts pressure on the urethra, which results in less leakage. Some women use a tampon instead of the pessary.
3. **Collagen injections** can be administered near the sphincter. These increase the size of tissue and can help to strengthen the muscles.
4. **Bladder retraining** (timed urination) is used for people with urge incontinence because it helps to increase the bladder's storage capacity. Directions depend on how often the person is usually incontinent, for example, if he or she is usually incontinent every 4 hours, then he or she would be asked to urinate every 3 hours and then suppress any urgency. With improvement the time between urinating is extended.
5. **Biofeedback** is often used in combination with Kegel's exercises and bladder retraining. Special equipment, instructions, and patient training are required to perform biofeedback effectively. Studies have shown that using these techniques can be more effective than the use of drugs, but it is often difficult to find a physician with expertise in biofeedback.
6. Different **drugs** can be used successfully for urge and overflow incontinence.
7. **Cutting down on the use of caffeine and alcohol** is highly recommended because these products can irritate the bladder and trigger urinary frequency. This is also suggested for patients doing the pelvic exercises or using medication.
8. **Surgery** may be an option but is usually considered only as the last resort. Surgical procedures that would lift the bladder or strengthen the pelvic muscles can be used to treat stress incontinence.

Fortunately, most cases of incontinence can be helped and even cured by using one or more of these treatments.

Having completed the chapter on urinalysis, practice the procedures. When you think that you know the equipment and steps of the procedures, arrange with your instructor to take the performance tests. You are expected to demonstrate accurately your ability to prepare for and perform all of the procedures that have been presented.

The following is a sample of recorded patient information using words that have been presented in this chapter. Read it and define the italicized terms.

This patient, a 45-year-old man, was first seen in my office today with the chief complaint of *dysuria* for the past month. The patient stated that this was associated with *polyuria, gross hematuria*, weakness, back pain, and a high fever. He has never experienced *oliguria* and stated that he drinks copious amounts of water daily. One week ago he had an attack of dyspnea and coughing. The urinalysis today revealed marked *proteinuria, glycosuria*, and *ketonuria; specific gravity* of 1.030. *Microscopic* examination revealed *white cells* of 15 to 20/high-power field (hpf) and *red cells* of 10 to 15/hpf.

Pyuria was also detected in large amounts. Further study and examination were recommended for this patient. He will be admitted to the hospital at the end of this week.

M. Crossett, MD

The following are samples of progress notes from a patient's medical record. After reading these, you should be able to discuss the contents with your instructor. Be prepared to define and explain any medical terms that are used. A medical dictionary, other reference books, and information given in preceding chapters of this book may be used as references for obtaining definitions or explanations of the contents of these reports.

See also Problem-Oriented Medical Record in Chapter 4.

Progress Notes

10/23/00
PATIENT: Sally Jones
PROBLEM: Hematuria

S: 36 y/o F, w/asymptomatic hematuria. Smoker w/at least 12 pack year history. Very active aerobically. We had begun to refer her to Dr. Pauls in July and did a second urine culture, which showed some enterococcus, so we delayed the referral and treated her w/Macrobid 100 mg bid × 10 days. She comes today for a follow-up to see whether her urine has cleared. IVP was neg. Denies back pain, obvious blood in urine, or dysuria.

O: BP 100/70. Wt 159½. No CVA tenderness. Abdomen benign. UA shows repeated large amounts of blood w/no leukocytes or nitrites. WBCs 5-10, RBCs 20+, 3-4 epithelial cells.

A: 1. Persistent asymptomatic hematuria.

P: Copied most recent culture and UA. Sent another culture today. Referred to Dr. Pauls today for an evaluation.

PROBLEM: L breast tenderness.

S: LMP 10/10-10/15. Now having some tenderness in L inferior breast area.

O: Breast Exam: No obvious masses, but there is a tender area in the inferior portion of L breast w/what feels like very small cystic, soft lesions. No fixed, hardened lesions. Axilla w/o lymphadenopathy. No supraclavicular nodes.

A: 1. L breast tenderness w/possible small fibrocystic changes.

P: Referred to Dr. Jennings.

Progress Notes

PATIENT: Lee Ryan
9/20/00 BP 140/80 HR 76
PROBLEM: Hematuria

S: Pt was found, at her annual GYN exam on 9/11/00, to have moderate blood in her urine. Returns today to have urine checked again. She had come in the meantime, 9/16, and had another urinalysis, which showed a large amount of blood. She has no symptoms of flank pain, no dysuria. Pt is a runner and does a lot of aerobic exercise, which is important to her overall sense of well-being, and she doesn't want to d/c this activity. She has also had a possible hx of kidney stone in 1999. She was treated at the Medical Center in the ER w/fluids and pain meds. Pt is a smoker with at least a 20 pack-year Hx. She is unaware of the connection between smoking and bladder CA.

O: UA today shows large amounts of blood. Sediment spun but then inadvertently discarded by the nurses.

A: Hematuria-? etiology. Differential diagnosis: Benign postural (runner's) hematuria versus occult lesion in bladder v. possible residual stone.

P: Explained to the pt how to collect a 1st AM urine specimen immediately after arising from bed. She'll take the specimen directly to the lab. If there is persistent blood in her urine, I would recommend that she have a cystoscopy. Explained, at great length, the need to stop smoking.

9/27/00
left msg.—UA—(1st AM) still has blood
Plan: IVP—if negative, then to urologist
S. Dyer

10/14/00
Per phone call—IVP—positive
Cepro 250 mg ī bid × 3 weeks
S. Dyer

CRITICAL THINKING SKILLS REVIEW

1. List the four major components of normal urine.
2. Why and when is a routine urinalysis performed?
3. List five physical characteristics of urine and eight chemical examinations that are part of a routine urinalysis.
4. List and classify urine microscopic sediment as either organized or unorganized sediment.
5. Indicate if the following urinalysis results are normal or abnormal findings:
   a. Specific gravity of 1.035
   b. Red
   c. Glucose 4+
   d. Acetone, negative
   e. Numerous bacteria
   f. Foul odor
   g. Cloudy
   h. Quantity, 3500 ml in 24 hours
   i. pH 6.5
   j. Protein, trace amounts
   k. Ketones, large amount
   l. Blood, negative
   m. Urobilinogen 0.1 to 1, small amount
   n. Nitrite, positive
6. List two conditions or diseases in which each of the following may be detected:
   a. Albuminuria
   b. Glucosuria
   c. Acetonuria
   d. Bilirubinuria
   e. Hematuria
   f. Bacteriuria
   g. Polyuria
   h. Oliguria
   i. Anuria
   j. Dysuria
   k. Excessively acid urine
   l. Excessively alkaline urine
   m. Very low specific gravity
7. Name three items used for measuring the specific gravity of urine.
8. Differentiate between normal and abnormal sediment and contaminants that may be observed during a microscopic examination of urine.
9. You are asked to perform the chemical analysis on a urine specimen and find the bottle of reagent strips in the refrigerator with the cap removed. Is this the proper storage method for these reagent strips? Would you use one of these strips to perform the tests? Explain the reason for your answer.
10. A urine specimen that was collected at 10 AM for a microscopic examination was placed in your laboratory on the shelf. It is now 3 PM. What would you do with this specimen? Explain the reason for your answer.
11. Describe two tests for determining bacteriuria and three tests for determining glucosuria.
12. To determine if a woman is pregnant, urine may be tested to detect the presence of which hormone?

PERFORMANCE TEST

In a skills laboratory, a simulation of a joblike environment, the medical assistant student is to demonstrate skill in performing the following procedures without reference to source materials. For these activities the student requires a fresh urine specimen or a synthetic preparation of the same. Time limits for the performance of each procedure are to be assigned by the instructor (see also p. 104.)

1. Given a fresh urine specimen and the required supplies, perform a routine physical and chemical analysis on the specimen and record the results; then prepare the specimen for a microscopic examination.
2. Given a fresh urine specimen and the required supplies, perform a Clinitest, Acetest, Ictotest, and pregnancy test and record the results.
3. Given a fresh clean-catch midstream urine specimen and a Multistix-3 reagent strip, perform a semiquantitative culture test and record the results.
4. Given a Dipper or Dropper urinalysis control kit, determine if the test reagent strips are reacting properly.

The student is expected to perform these activities with 100% accuracy.

The successful completion of each procedure will demonstrate competency levels as required by the AAMA, AMT, and future employers.

 INTERNET RESOURCES

OnHealth
www.onhealth.com

drkoop.com
www.drkoop.com

Healthfinder
www.healthfinder.gov

The World Foundation for Medical Studies in Female Health
www.wffh.org

The National Institute of Diabetes and Digestive and Kidney Diseases of the National Institute of Health
www.niddk.nih.gov/health/diabetes/dylb/home/htm

Medline*plus*
www.nlm.nih.gov/medlineplus

Mayo Clinic Health Oasis
www.mayohealth.org

National Institutes of Health
www.nih.gov

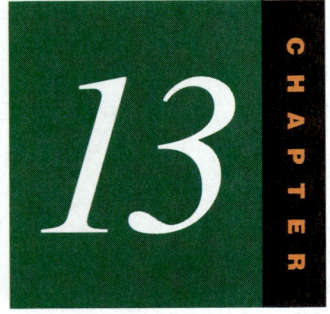

13 CHAPTER

Hematology and Blood Chemistry

Cognitive Objectives

On completion of Chapter 13, the medical assistant student should be able to*:

1. Define, spell, and pronounce the listed vocabulary terms and define the listed laboratory abbreviations.
2. List the components of blood; state where each is formed in the body and the functions of each.
3. Differentiate between granulocytes and agranulocytes.
4. List body sites used for obtaining capillary and venous blood for testing. List body sites to avoid when obtaining blood samples.
5. State three types of specimens that can be obtained from a venous blood sample.
6. Identify the use of different vacuum blood collection tubes by tube top color.
7. Explain the difference between a collection tube with an additive and one without an additive, indicating the preferred use for each.
8. List 12 factors that should be considered before performing a venipuncture.
9. List the general order of draw when more than one tube of blood is to be obtained during a venipuncture for various different tests.
10. Discuss how a blood specimen should be handled after collection.
11. Discuss patient preparation for blood tests.
12. List at least five blood tests that require the patient to be in a fasting state before having a blood sample drawn.
13. Give the laboratory results on blood tests that are presented in this chapter, determine if they represent normal values, and relate the abnormal findings to the most probable or possible causes.
14. Describe the steps for performing a blood glucose test using a blood glucose meter.

15. State three elements of quality assurance for blood glucose testing.
16. State seven possible causes of inaccurate blood glucose readings when using blood glucose meters.
17. Discuss the advantages of the Accu-Chek III and One Touch blood glucose meters used in monitoring blood glucose levels.
18. State six uses for the HemoCue blood glucose analyzer and explain how it is used.
19. Describe the steps for performing a blood cholesterol test using the AccuMeter.
20. State the three levels of cholesterol results and explain how each is classified.
21. State the two most routinely used systems for blood grouping and typing. List the blood types in each group and explain what the typing indicates.
22. List four components that can be obtained from a unit of whole blood for transfusion purposes.
23. State why it is important for a person receiving a blood transfusion to receive the same blood group that he or she has.
24. Discuss why it is important in pregnancy to identify cases in which the mother has Rh⁻ blood and the father has Rh⁺ blood type.
25. List eight blood tests that are performed for a complete blood count (CBC) and the normal values for each.
26. List blood tests that would be listed under the following classifications: hematology, chemistry, serology, thyroid function tests.
27. Explain the terms *multiphasic tests, test panels,* and *profiles.* Give examples of test panels and the reasons why they are done.
28. Discuss automation in the clinical laboratory and the advantages it provides.
29. Explain the purpose of a glycosylated hemoglobin test.
30. Discuss infectious mononucleosis, giving the signs and symptoms, incubation period, how it is diagnosed, and the treatment.

**It is suggested that you review Chapter 10 before proceeding with this chapter.

31. Discuss the blood donation process, and the blood donation eligibility guidelines.

Terminal Performance Objectives

On completion of Chapter 13, the medical assistant student should be able to:

1. Demonstrate the correct procedure for obtaining a blood sample from a patient by performing a skin puncture using (a) a lancet and (b) a Penlet II.

2. Demonstrate the correct procedure for obtaining a blood sample from a patient by performing a venipuncture using (a) a syringe and needle and (b) a Vacutainer needle and holder and vacuum tube.

3. Demonstrate the correct procedure for obtaining multiple blood samples using the Vacutainer holder and needle and evacuated blood collection tubes.

4. Demonstrate the correct procedure for using (a) the Unopette system and (b) the Microtainer capillary whole blood collector.

5. Demonstrate the correct procedure for performing (a) a copper sulfate relative density test used for screening anemia, (b) hematocrit test on capillary blood, and (c) blood hemoglobin test.

6. Demonstrate the correct procedure for determining the presence of glucose in blood by using (a) Dextrostix, (b) the Accu-Chek III and bG Chemstrip, (c) One Touch II blood glucose meter and test strip, and (c) HemoCue blood glucose analyzer.

7. Demonstrate the correct procedure for performing a blood cholesterol test using the AccuMeter.

8. Demonstrate the correct method for recording information relevant to the aforementioned procedures and findings.

9. Provide instructions and patient education that is within the professional scope of a medical assistant's training and responsibilities as assigned.

The student is expected to perform these objectives with 100% accuracy.

The consistent use of Universal/Standard Precautions is required by all health care professionals in all health care settings as a method of infection control. It is assumed that these precautions are used in all of the following procedures. Review Chapter 1 if you have any questions on methods to use because the methods or techniques are not repeated in detail in each procedure presented in the chapter.

Be sure to consult the latest guidelines issued by the Centers for Disease Control and Prevention and consult with infection control practitioners when necessary to identify specific precautions that pertain to your particular work situation.

VOCABULARY

agglutination (ah-gloo″tin-na′shun)—A clumping together of cells, as of blood cells or bacteria. An example is when red blood cells (RBCs) clump together as a result of an incompatible blood transfusion.

agranulocyte (a-gran′u-lo-sit″)—A white blood cell (WBC) with a clear or nongranular cytoplasm. There are two types, monocytes and lymphocytes.

anemia (ah-ne′me-ah)—There are various forms of anemia, but broadly speaking, it is a lack of RBCs in the circulating blood or a reduction of hemoglobin or both. Anemia is thought of as a symptom of a disease or disorder; it is not a disease.

anisocytosis (an-i″-so-si-to′sis)—A state of abnormal variations in the size of RBCs in the blood.

blood dyscrasia (dis-kra′ze-ah)—An abnormal or diseased condition of the blood.

electrolyte (e-lek′tro-lit)—Substances that separate into electrically charged particles, positive or negative, when dissolved in water; thus they are capable of conducting an electric current. They play an important part in maintaining fluid balance, in normal metabolism function, and in the functions of cells in the body. EXAMPLES: sodium, potassium, calcium, magnesium, chloride, and bicarbonate.

electrophoresis (e-lek″tro-fo-re′sis)—A laboratory method used to diagnose certain diseases by analyzing the plasma protein content.

erythrocytosis (e-rith″ro-si-to′sis)—Increased numbers of RBCs (erythrocytes).

granulocyte (gran′u-lo-sit″)—A WBC having granules in its cytoplasm. These types of WBCs are neutrophils, basophils, and eosinophils.

band-form granulocyte—A granular WBC in a stage of development.

hemoglobin (he″mo-glo′bin)—A protein in an RBC that carries oxygen and carbon dioxide. The pigment in hemoglobin is what gives the blood its red color. The protein in hemoglobin is globin; the red pigment is heme. For the body to make hemoglobin, it must have iron, which is derived from the food we eat.

hemolysis (he-mol′i-sis)—The destruction of RBCs with the release of hemoglobin into the plasma. This takes place normally at the end of the life span of a red blood cell (120 days). It can also occur when there is an antigen-antibody reaction, as seen in a blood transfusion reaction resulting from incompatible blood types being mixed, in hemolytic disease of the newborn (HDN; see pp. 629-630 in this chapter), or in metabolic abnormalities of the red blood cell that significantly shorten red cell life span.

hyperbilirubinemia (hy″per-bil″i-roo″bi-ne′me-ah)—Increased or excessive levels of bilirubin in the blood.

hypercalcemia (hi″per-kal-se′me-ah)—Increased or excessive levels of calcium in the blood.

hypercholesterolemia (hi′per-ko-les″ter-ol-e′me-ah)—Excessive levels of cholesterol in the blood.

hyperchromia (hi′per-kro′me-ah)—An abnormal increase of the hemoglobin levels in RBCs.

VOCABULARY—cont'd

hypercythemia (hy"per-si-the'me-ah)—An excessive number of RBCs in the circulating blood.

hyperemia (hi"per-e'me-ah)—An excessive amount of blood in a part.

hyperglycemia (hi"per-gli-se'me-ah)—Excessive amounts of glucose in the blood.

hyperkalemia (hi"per-kah-le'me-ah)—An excessive level of potassium in the blood.

hypernatremia (hi'per-na-tre'me-ah)—An excessive amount of sodium in the blood.

hyperoxemia (hi"per-ok-se'me-ah)—A condition in which the blood is excessively acidic. An increased oxygen content in the blood.

hyperproteinemia (hi"per-pro"te-i-ne'me-ah)—An excessive amount of protein in the blood.

hypo (hi'po)—A word part meaning an abnormal decrease or deficient amounts. If you replace this word element and definition for the word element "hyper" in all of the preceding terms (except in hyperemia and hyperoxemia), the correct meaning will be defined.

hypoxemia (h'pok-se'me-ah)—A deficient amount of oxygen (O_2) in the blood.

ischemia (is-ke'me-ah)—A deficient amount of blood in a body part as a result of an obstruction or a functional constriction of a blood vessel.

isocytosis (i"so-si-to'sis)—A state in which cells are equal in size; refers especially to equality of size of RBCs.

leukemia (lu-ke'me-ah)—A malignant disease of various types that is classified clinically as acute or chronic, depending on the character and duration of the disease; and myeloid, lymphoid, or monocytic, depending on the cells involved. This disease affects the tissues of the lymph nodes, spleen, or bone marrow. Symptoms include an uncontrolled increase of WBCs, accompanied by a decrease in RBCs and platelets. This results in anemia and an increased tendency to develop infection and hemorrhage. Other classic symptoms include pain in bones and joints; fever; and swelling of the liver, spleen, and lymph nodes. The precise cause is unknown.

leukocytosis (lu"ko-si-to'sis)—An increased number of circulating WBCs.

leukopenia (lu"ko-pe'ne-ah)—A deficient number of circulating WBCs.

macrocyte (mak'ro-sit)—The largest type of red blood cell; seen in cases of pernicious anemia (vitamin B_{12} deficiency) and folic acid deficiency.

microcyte (mi'kro-sit)—An abnormally small RBC, found in cases of iron deficiency anemia and thalassemia.

mononucleosis (mon"-o-nu"kle-o'sis)—An abnormal increase of the mononuclear WBCs in the blood.

infectious mononucleosis—Also called glandular fever, this is an acute infectious disease, caused by the Epstein-Barr virus (EBV).

phagocytosis (fag"o-si-to'sis)—The process by which WBCs destroy and engulf or ingest harmful microorganisms.

poikilocytosis (poi"ki-lo-si-to'sis)—The presence of RBCs in the blood that show abnormal variations in shape.

polycythemia (pol"e-si-the'me-ah)—An abnormally increased amount of RBCs or hemoglobin.

reticulocyte (re-tik'u-lo-sit)—A nonnucleated immature RBC. Generally, of all the RBCs in the circulating blood, less than 2% are reticulocytes.

septicemia (sep"ti-se'me-ah)—A condition in which there are toxins or bacteria in the blood.

serum (se'rum)—The clear, straw-colored liquid portion obtained after blood clots; it consists of plasma minus fibrinogen, which is removed in the process of clotting.

thrombocyte (throm'bo-sit)—A blood platelet.

thrombocytosis (throm'bosito'sis) or **thrombocythemia** (throm"bo-si-the'me-ah)—An abnormal increased number of platelets in the circulating blood.

thrombocytopenia (throm"bo-si"to-pe'ne-ah)—A decreased number of platelets in the circulating blood.

uremia (u-re'me-ah)—A toxic condition in which there are substances in the blood that should normally be eliminated in the urine.

venipuncture (ven"i-pungk'tur)—Puncturing a vein to collect a blood specimen or to administer medication.

vitamin K—A vitamin that is essential for the formation of prothrombin and the normal clotting of blood. A deficiency may result in hemorrhage because of a prolonged prothrombin time.

Hematology, the study of blood, covers vast areas and numerous tests. Today, in the physician's office or health care facility, most of the tests are performed by a trained laboratory worker, or blood samples are obtained and then sent to a larger clinical laboratory for testing. At other times, the patient is sent directly to the laboratory to have the blood sample drawn. Most laboratories use automated equipment when performing many of the tests. These modern advances in laboratory technology have made it possible to obtain quick and accurate results on a relatively small sample of blood.

For the most part, it is not your duty to perform blood tests, other than a few simple ones. Depending on the laws of the state in which you practice, you may be called on to perform a skin puncture or a venipuncture to obtain blood samples for testing at a clinical laboratory. Even though you may not perform these procedures, you should be familiar with the equipment and supplies that are needed, so that you are capable of assisting the physician as required or explaining the procedure to a patient. These procedures, supplies, and some of the routine and basic blood tests are discussed in this chapter.

BLOOD COMPONENTS, FUNCTIONS, AND FORMATION

Blood, a type of connective tissue, is composed of a clear, yellow, liquid portion (the plasma) in which the cellular or formed elements are suspended. **Plasma** makes up about 55% of the blood by volume. The remaining 45% consists of the **formed elements,** which are **red blood cells** (RBCs), **white blood cells**

(WBCs), and **platelets**. The average adult has approximately 5 to 6 quarts of blood.

Blood has at times been referred to as the *"river of life"* because it is by way of this special tissue that numerous substances are transported to all the cells in our body for nourishment and function and waste products are in turn carried to certain body systems for disposal. It is a transportation system in our body, helping also in the maintenance of acid-base, electrolyte, and fluid balance of the internal environment.

Plasma, which is 90% water, acts as the carrier for the formed elements and other substances, which include blood proteins, carbohydrates, fats, amino acids (proteins), mineral salts (the electrolytes), hormones, enzymes, gases, antibodies, and waste products such as urea and uric acid.

The formed elements all have special functions. The prime function of **RBCs, or erythrocytes,** is to transport oxygen from the lungs to the body cells and carbon dioxide from the cells back to the lungs to be exhaled. Each RBC contains a protein substance, **hemoglobin** (Hgb, or Hb), which gives red color to blood and also transports the oxygen and carbon dioxide to and from the body cells.

In each RBC there are about 300 million hemoglobin molecules. Each of these molecules can bind four molecules of oxygen. Normal hemoglobin molecules are saturated with oxygen. In hypoxemia, hemoglobin molecules are oxygen deficient. Anemia is the result of too few RBCs in the circulating blood, RBCs with reduced amounts of hemoglobin, or both.

The five types of **WBCs, or leukocytes,** are classified into general groups, the granular and agranular. **Granular** WBCs, sometimes called polymorphonuclear leukocytes, include the **eosinophils, basophils,** and **neutrophils.** They are characterized by their heavily granulated cytoplasm and segmented nuclei. The **agranular** leukocytes are the **monocytes** and **lymphocytes**, both having a solid nucleus and a clear cytoplasm. The prime function of WBCs is to protect the body against infection and disease; some fight invading bacteria by their phagocytic activity (destroying and ingesting harmful microorganisms), and others play an important role in producing immunity to disease. Infection in the body is indicated when there is a marked rise in the WBC count. In leukemia, the WBC count is also greatly increased.

Platelets (thrombocytes), the smallest of the formed elements in the blood, play a vital role in initiating the clotting process of blood. Thrombocytopenia may be accompanied by bleeding.

All blood cells are produced in hemopoietic (blood-forming) tissue. The agranular WBCs are produced mainly in lymph nodes and other lymphoid tissues. Granular WBCs, RBCs, and platelets are produced in the red bone marrow or myeloid tissue of bones, such as the femur, humerus, sternum vertebrae, and cranial bones (see Complete Blood Count: Hematology Test on p. 602).

OBTAINING BLOOD SAMPLES

Types and Sources

For most routine hematologic studies, there are two sources of blood for testing. **Capillary** or **peripheral blood** is obtained by performing a **skin puncture** on the palmar surface of the fin-

gertip or on the ear lobe. For infants, the skin puncture is done on the plantar surface of the great toe or heel. You *must* avoid areas that are cyanotic, scarred, traumatized, edematous, and heavily calloused. A minimal amount of blood, just a few drops, is obtained by this method, but it is sufficient to perform some of the routine tests, such as the complete blood count (CBC), some coagulation studies, and some of the chemistry tests.

The second source for obtaining blood is a vein. This is called **venous blood,** and the procedure by which it is obtained is called a **venipuncture.** The most common sites for obtaining blood by this method are the **basilic and cephalic veins** located in the **antecubital area of the arm,** which is at the inner aspect of the arm opposite the elbow. This is the more common method for obtaining a blood sample, and it is used when larger amounts of blood are needed to perform several different tests. When blood cannot be obtained from a vein in the antecubital space because of stenosed or collapsed veins or if the patient has plaster casts on both arms, **alternative sites** to use are the veins on the top of the hand, in the wrist, or even in the foot. In extreme situations, blood may be obtained from the femoral vein. However, this site must be used *only* by physicians.

Three types of specimens can be obtained from a venous blood sample.

1. **Serum.** Serum is obtained from a sample collected in a tube *without* an additive. Serum is most often used for most blood chemistry tests, pregnancy tests, viral studies, and the human immunodeficiency virus (HIV) antibody test.
2. **Whole blood.** Whole blood is obtained by collecting the blood sample with a tube *with* an anticoagulant additive. This specimen is most commonly used for hematology tests, such as the CBC, and sometimes coagulation studies, blood glucose, and some other blood chemistry tests that vary with the laboratory's preferences.
3. **Plasma.** Plasma is obtained from whole blood collected in a tube *with* an anticoagulant additive and then centrifuged. Centrifugation causes the specimen to separate into three layers. The top layer is plasma; the middle layer, called the buffy coat, contains WBCs and platelets; and the bottom layer contains RBCs. Hematology tests, coagulation studies, and some chemistry tests are performed on this type of specimen.

At times, special blood studies such as blood gases are ordered. In these circumstances, **arterial blood** (blood from an artery, usually the brachial or femoral) rather than venous blood is required. A physician or qualified laboratory personnel *must* obtain this blood sample. A situation in which this may be necessary in the physician's office is when an emphysemic patient has an acute episode of shortness of breath. The physician may draw arterial blood for blood gases while the patient is still breathing room air; then if oxygen is administered to the patient, the physician draws another arterial blood sample for examination. In the latter case, it is important to indicate on the laboratory requisition how many liters of oxygen were administered to the patient so that this can be considered when the test results are interpreted.

Commercial kits with required supplies are available. The blood sample must be collected in a heparinized vacuum tube or heparinized syringe. Heparin is used because unclotted blood is needed for analysis. Most laboratories require the needle to be removed from the syringe and the syringe to be capped with a rubber stopper. The specimen must be free from air contact because exposure to air affects the blood gases. Recapping or needle removal **must** be accomplished through the use of a mechanical device or a one-handed technique (see Chapter 7). The specimen must be placed in ice for delivery to the laboratory to maintain the viability of the blood as close to body conditions as possible. The specimen must be delivered to the laboratory as soon as possible, preferably within 5 to 10 minutes, for accurate testing to occur.

Collection Tubes and Proper Handling of a Venous Blood Sample

Because of the multitude of tests that can be performed on a blood sample, certain requirements must be met when collecting and handling the sample. Using excellent technique, the medical assistant will collect the samples in either a plain tube without additives or in a tube that contains anticoagulant additives. *The type of test to be performed, as well as the laboratory's preference, will govern this choice.*

Tubes without additives.
Generally speaking, a tube without an additive is used when a clot must form to obtain **serum** for testing. Once collected, the blood is left standing in an upright position at room temperature, usually for 30 to 60 minutes, to allow a clot to form. To separate the serum from the clot, the sample is then centrifuged for 10 minutes. After this, serum is removed from the tube and is ready for testing.

When serum is required for testing, it is more convenient to use a **serum separator tube** to collect the blood sample (Figure 13-1, *A* and *D*). Once collected, the sample is left standing at room temperature for 30 to 60 minutes and then centrifuged for 10 minutes. After centrifugation, a jellylike substance forms between the clot and the serum in the tube. The sample can then be sent to the laboratory in this tube. This sample is used most often for most blood chemistries (varying with

FIGURE 13-1 **A,** Vacutainer evacuated blood collection system. **B,** Vacutainer brand Safety-Lok needle holder. After venipuncture the yellow transplant shield is moved over the needle and locked into protective position. Then the whole unit is discarded in a biohazard sharps container. **C,** Vacutainer brand precision glide needles. These attach to a Vacutainer holder for use. The needle point exposed here is the point that punctures the rubber stopper of the vacuum tube when blood is collected. The part of the needle that has the cover on it is the point placed into the vein when obtaining a blood sample. (**B** and **C,** Courtesy Becton-Dickinson, Division of Becton, Dickinson & Co, Rutherford, NJ.)

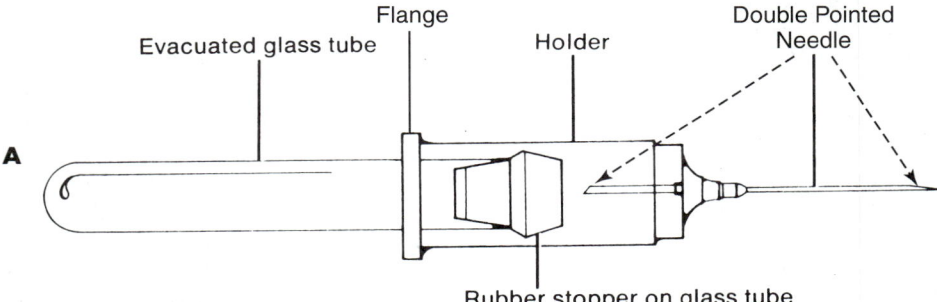

A

Evacuated glass tube — Flange — Holder — Double Pointed Needle

Rubber stopper on glass tube

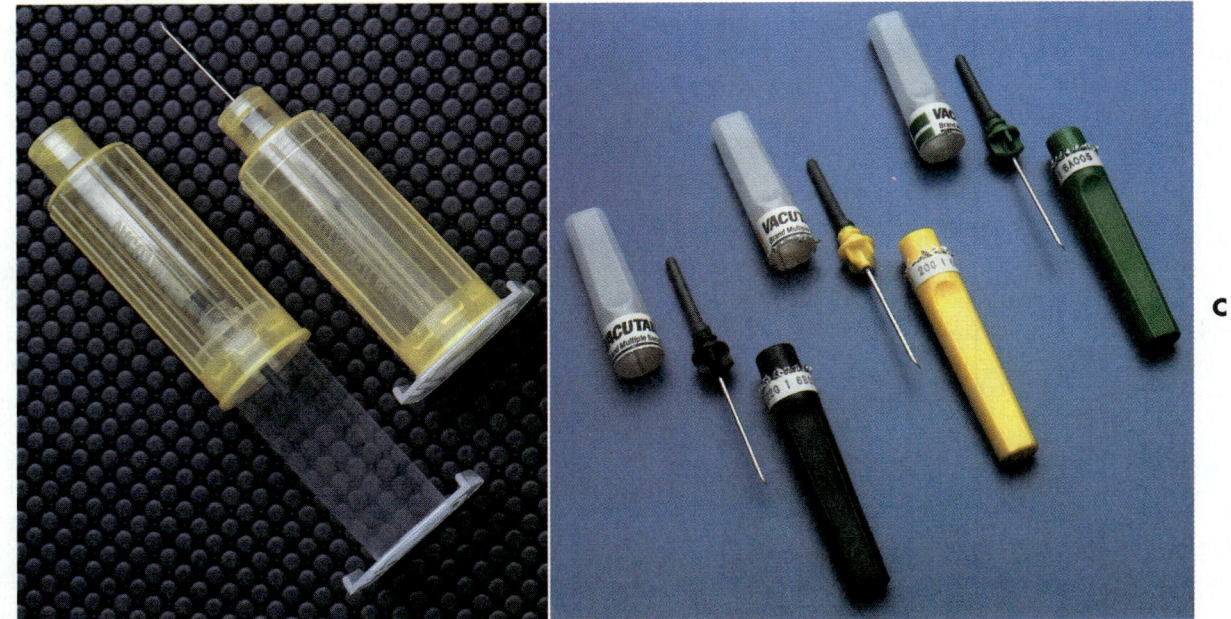

B

C

the laboratory's preference), serology tests, and Rh factor testing (see Chapter 10 for instructions for using a centrifuge).

Tubes with additives.

Tubes containing ethylenediaminetetraacetic acid (EDTA) anticoagulant additive are recommended for use when doing **hematology studies.** The WBCs and platelets are best preserved in this type of tube, and better red cell morphology results are then obtained. The additive has no adverse effects on the blood sample when a sufficient quantity of blood is obtained. Problems arise if too little blood is drawn into tubes containing anticoagulant additives. Misleading results, and therefore incorrect diagnoses occur (for example, the hematocrit is lowered and poor RBC morphology results because the RBC shrinks and produces a false appearance). All tubes with anticoagulant additives must be completely filled with blood to provide the proper ratio of blood to anticoagulant.

A tube containing an **anticoagulant additive,** such as heparin, prevents the blood from clotting. Depending on methods used by the laboratory when performing certain tests, this is generally the preferred tube to use when collecting a sample for blood chemistries, especially for potassium levels. This tube should not be used for hematology studies because the heparin additive distorts the cells and leads to false results.

Several other additives are used in tubes for collecting venous blood; however, the correct tube, plain or with an additive, must be used. Most laboratories supply these tubes with directions indicating which to use for various tests. *They are not interchangeable and must not be confused.* The laboratory's lab test directory also provides this information (also see Table 13-1 and Figure 13-2).

Vacutainer system.

Rather than using the conventional syringe, needle, and test tube when obtaining blood samples, newer, more convenient systems consisting of a disposable needle, a holder, and vacuum tubes are available. One such unit is the Vacutainer system, which consists of a holder-needle combination or separate needle and holder and evacuated glass tubes containing a premeasured vacuum to provide a controlled amount of blood draw. The tubes have **color-coded rubber stoppers** that indicate the type of test for which they are best suited and are supplied plain or with additives and sterile or nonsterile (Figure 13-2). (The trend today is to use sterile tubes for *all* collections.) All are available in a variety of sizes, the most common being 3-, 5-, 7-, 10-, and 15-ml capacities. Vacutainers are supplied in packages with labels that indicate the additives present in the tubes, the expiration date, and the approximate draw amount (see Figure 13-1, *E*).

Another type of tube is the Vacutainer brand tube with **Hemogard closure** (Figure 13-3). The rubber stopper that seals the tube is covered by a plastic shield—a shield that helps to protect laboratory personnel from contact with blood on the stopper or around the outer rim of the tube, as well as from blood splattering on opening the tube. The rubber stopper is recessed inside the plastic shield, so any drops left by a blood collection needle remain isolated from potential contact. To remove and to reinsert the Hemogard closure, see Figure 13-3.

The most commonly used vacuum tubes, classified according to the tube top color, additive content, average amount of blood drawn, and recommended use, are found in Table 13-1.

When you are to draw more than one tube of blood, the general order of draw is as follows:

- **First draw**—blood culture tubes (for example, sterile tubes with no additive; blood should be transferred to a culture medium within 5 minutes); tubes for sterile samples (for example, specimens for antibodies and sometimes special antibodies, such as for HIV, and for viral studies)
- **Second draw**—tubes with no additives (for example, red tops)
- **Third draw**—tubes for coagulation studies (for example, blue tops)
- **Last draw**—tubes with additives (for example, lavender, green, and gray tops)

FIGURE 13-1—cont'd   D, Serum separation tube (SST) used for various tests performed on serum. **E,** Sterile Vacutainer serum tubes of various sizes with and without additives used for hematology tests, chemistry tests, serology tests, blood typing, and other tests.

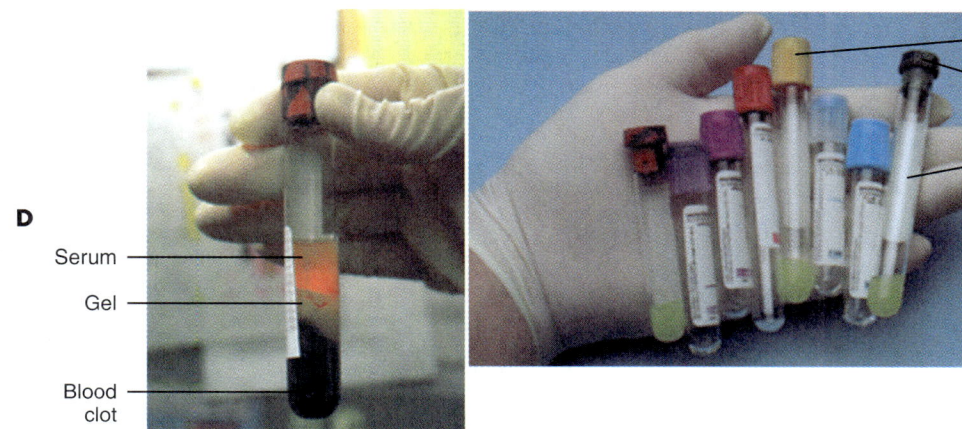

D

Serum

Gel

Blood
clot

Hemogard
closure

Rubber
stopper

Vacuum
tube

E

FIGURE 13-2 Vacutainer tube guide. (Courtesy Becton-Dickinson, Division of Becton, Dickinson & Co, Rutherford, NJ.)

VACUTAINER® Tubes with HEMOGARD Closure	VACUTAINER Tubes	Additive	Number of Inversions at Blood Collection (Invert gently, do not shake)	Laboratory Use	Volume Draw (ml.)	Remarks
Gold		• Clot activator and gel for serum separation	5	SST Brand Tube for serum determinations in chemistry. Tube inversions ensure mixing of clot activator with blood and clotting within 30 minutes.		
Light Green		• Lithium heparin and gel for plasma separation	8	PST Brand Tube for plasma determinations in chemistry. Tube inversions prevent clotting.		
Red		• None	0	For serum determinations in chemistry, serology and blood banking.		
Orange		• Thrombin	8	For stat serum determinations in chemistry. Tube inversions ensure complete clotting, usually in less than 5 minutes.		
Royal Blue		• Sodium heparin • Na$_2$EDTA • None	8 8 0	For trace element, toxicology and nutrient determinations. Special stopper formulation offers low levels of trace elements (see package insert).		
Green		• Sodium heparin • Lithium heparin • Ammonium heparin	8 8 8	For plasma determinations in chemistry. Tube inversions prevent clotting.		
Gray		• Potassium oxalate/ sodium fluoride • Sodium fluoride • Lithium iodoacetate • Lithium iodoacetate/ lithium heparin	8 8 8 8	For glucose determinations. Tube inversions ensure proper mixing of additive and blood. Oxalate and heparin, anticoagulants, will give plasma samples. Without them, samples are serum.		
Brown		• Sodium heparin	8	For lead determinations. This tube is certified to contain less than .01 µg/mL (ppm) lead. Tube inversions prevent clotting.		
Yellow		• Sodium polyanetholesulfonate (SPS) OR • ACD - Acid Citrate Dextrose Additions: Solution A - 22.0g/L trisodium citrate, 8.0g/L citric acid, 24.5g/L dextrose Solution B - 13.2g/L trisodium citrate, 4.8g/L citric acid, 14.7g/L dextrose	8 8 8	For blood culture specimen collections in microbiology. Tube inversions prevent clotting. For use in blood bank studies, HLA phenotyping, DNA and Paternity testing.		
Lavender		• Liquid K$_3$EDTA • Spray-dried K$_2$EDTA	8 8	For whole blood hematology determinations. Tube inversions prevent clotting.		
Light Blue		• 105M sodium citrate (3.2%) • 129M sodium citrate (3.8%)	8 8	For coagulation determinations on plasma specimens. Tube inversions prevent clotting. NOTE: Certain tests require chilled specimens. Follow recommended procedures for collection and transport of specimen.		
Small-volume Tubes (2ml and 3ml: 13 x 75 mm)	**Small-volume Tubes (2ml: 10.25 x 47 mm, 3ml: 10.25 x 64 mm)**					
Red		• None	0	For serum determinations in chemistry, serology and blood banking.		
Green		• Sodium heparin • Lithium heparin	8 8	For plasma determinations in chemistry. Tube inversions prevent clotting.		
Lavender		• Liquid K$_3$EDTA • Spray-dried K$_2$EDTA	8 8	For whole blood hematology determinations. Tube inversions prevent clotting.		
Light Blue		• .105M sodium citrate (3.2%) • .129M sodium citrate (3.8%)	8 8	For coagulation determinations on plasma specimens. Tube inversions prevent clotting. NOTE: Certain tests require chilled specimens. Follow recommended procedures for collection and transport of specimen.		

FIGURE 13-3 Vacutainer tubes with Hemogard closure. **A,** Closure cut away to demonstrate inside design. **B,** Procedure to remove and reinsert Hemogard closure. **Wear gloves for these procedures.** (Courtesy Becton-Dickinson, Division of Becton, Dickinson & Co, Rutherford, NJ.)

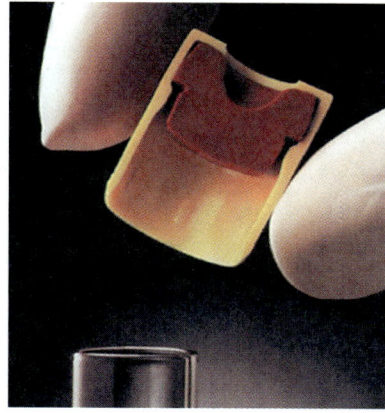

A

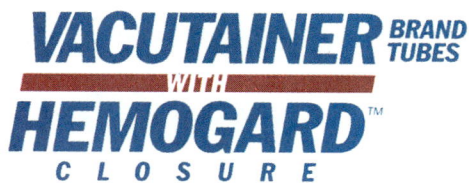

To remove HEMOGARD Closure

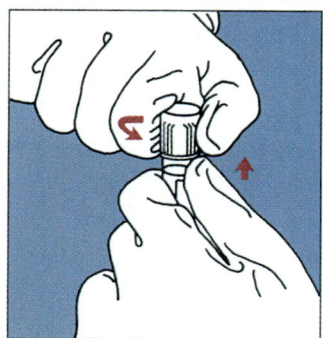

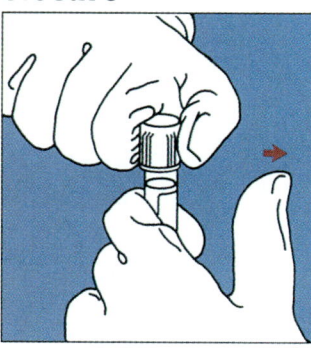

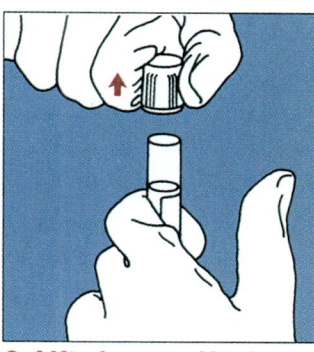

1. Twist and push upward

Grasp the VACUTAINER Tube with one hand, placing the thumb under the HEMOGARD Closure. (For added stability, place arm on solid surface.) With the other hand, twist the HEMOGARD Closure while simultaneously pushing up with the thumb of the other hand ONLY UNTIL THE RUBBER STOPPER IS LOOSENED.

2. Move thumb away before lifting closure

DO NOT use thumb to push closure off tube.
Caution: Any glass container has the potential to crack or break. To help prevent injury during closure removal, it is important that the thumb used to push upward on the closure be removed from contact with the tube as soon as the HEMOGARD closure is loosened.

3. Lift closure off tube

Note: In the unlikely event of the plastic shield separating from the rubber stopper, DO NOT REASSEMBLE THE CLOSURE. Carefully remove rubber stopper from the tube.

B

To reinsert HEMOGARD Closure

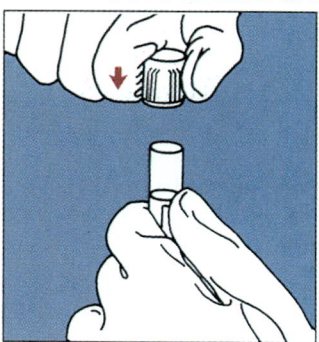

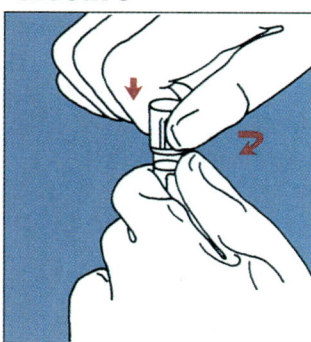

1. Replace closure over tube

2. Twist and push down firmly

Continue to twist and push down until stopper is fully reseated. Complete reinsertion of the stopper is necessary for the closure to remain securely on the tube during routine handling procedures.

CAUTION:
All biologic samples should be handled carefully. Exposure to such samples may transmit hepatitis, AIDS or other infectious diseases. All samples and collection materials should be handled and disposed of in accordnace with the Universal/standard Precautions recommended by the CDC,[1,2] OSHA,[3] the NCCLS[4] and the policies and procedures of your facility. In the event of exposure appropriate medical attention should be obtained.

TABLE 13–1   Commonly Used Vacuum Tubes

Tube Top Color	Additive	Average Amount of Blood Drawn	Common Blood Determination
Red (most common)	No additive	10 ml	Used for tests done on serum—Blood bank tests, e.g., blood typing (ABO and Rh factor) and cross-matching; serology tests; serum pregnancy test; most blood chemistries; immunology tests; viral studies; AIDS antibody (HIV antibody)
Lavender	Ethylenediamine tetraacetic acid, an anticoagulant (EDTA)	5 ml	Used for tests done on whole blood or plasma—Hematologic tests including a CBC, WBC, RBC, hematocrit, hemoglobin, platelet count, reticulocyte count, and sedimentation rate
Blue	Sodium citrate (an anti-coagulant)	5 ml	Used for tests done on whole blood—Coagulation studies including prothrombin time (PT), partial thromboplastin time (PTT), and thrombin time (TT)
Green	Sodium heparin	5 ml	Used for tests done on whole blood or plasma—Blood chemistry tests, especially potassium levels, electrolytes, blood gases
Gray	Potassium oxalate and sodium fluoride	5 ml	Used for tests done on whole blood or plasma—Blood glucose; blood alcohol; the coagulation study activated clotting time (ACT)
Gray and red (mottled top; serum separation tube)	Silicone serum separation material	5 ml	Used for tests done on serum—can be used for every test where you want the blood to clot **DO NOT USE FOR BLOOD BANK TESTS.**
Yellow	Sterile sodium polyanethole-sulfonate	5 ml	Used to collect whole blood for microbiology tests (blood culture tests)

After blood has been drawn, the tubes without an additive are *not* to be inverted or shaken but are to be centrifuged as discussed previously. Tubes that contain an additive should be gently inverted 8 to 10 times to mix the blood with the additive. *Do not shake these tubes* because vigorous mixing may cause **hemolysis**. The amount of blood drawn varies according to the size of the tube used.

Amount and handling of the specimen.

The amount of venous blood to be drawn is 3 to 30 ml, varying with the test(s) to be performed. The blood must be collected in the correct tube, and the tube must be at room temperature. Consult your laboratory for the exact amounts that are needed for each specific test that is to be performed. Often 1 to 2 ml more blood than required is drawn to avoid having a patient return for a second collection if the first battery of tests does not turn out.

A blood specimen must be tested on the same day of collection. When **serum** is needed for the test, it *must* be separated from the blood within 30 to 45 minutes after the sample has been collected. Blood collected in a tube containing an anticoagulant *must* be mixed gently with the anticoagulant immediately after collection.

Depending on the test(s) to be performed, blood should be examined within 8 hours or less from the time it was collected and preferably within 2 to 4 hours from the time that it was drawn. Blood for bacteriologic studies must be collected in spe-

cial containers and must not be left standing for any length of time. These specimens must be examined as soon as possible. Blood drawn for an electrolyte panel should be refrigerated if it is not tested immediately. Other blood samples may be left standing on the counter for 2 to 4 hours before testing, although some results may vary if the blood is left standing for 2 or more hours. *On request, your laboratory can provide schedules that list specific sample requirements for each test they perform.* The quality of a test is diminished if a blood sample stands for a long time before being tested; for example, glucose levels decrease within a couple of hours, and potassium levels rise if serum is allowed to stand on the cells; the sedimentation rate is lowered if left standing for over 2 hours, and the bacteria count increases.

When the specimen is to be sent to an outside laboratory, wrap it in protective materials and place it into the appropriate transport or mailing container. Always include the correctly completed laboratory requisition with the specimen. (Also see Chapter 1, Laboratory Specimens, on page 14.)

Labeling.

As with all specimens, you must accurately identify blood samples; label them with the patient's name, the date, your initials, and any other information required by the laboratory; and forward adequate amounts to the laboratory as soon as possible. You should also indicate on the laboratory requisition the time the sample was drawn. To prevent errors, patient identification on the collection tube must be identical to that on the requisition.

Patient preparation for blood tests.   Very few blood tests require any **special patient preparation.** Generally, special preparation means that the patient should fast (that is, abstain from all solid foods and liquids) for at least 8 hours and *up to* 12 to 14 hours before the blood sample is drawn. This preparation is required because food substances may alter the reliability of the test results. *Water may be taken before some tests (for example, for a fasting blood sugar). The laboratory can provide you with specific directions.* Usually you are to instruct the patient to take nothing by mouth (NPO) after midnight or NPO after dinner the night before the test is to be done. The tests for which the patient has to fast should be scheduled for the early morning to minimize the inconvenience that abstaining from food or fluids may cause the patient.

The principal tests that require the patient **to fast** beforehand include fasting blood sugar; glucose tolerance test; any type of lipid analysis, such as cholesterol and triglycerides, because fats from a meal flood the bloodstream and dramatically raise the triglycerides, and thus the results would be meaningless; and batteries or panels of blood chemistries, such as panels for liver, cardiac, or kidney function(s). Some laboratories also request that the patient be fasting before all enzyme and electrolyte tests. At other times fasting is done according to the individual orders of the physician. *Care must be taken to provide the patient with correct and adequate instructions in these situations.*

Some medications such as steroids, salicylates, or diuretics *may* interfere with test results. When feasible (that is, when health permits), the physician *may* advise a patient to discontinue *these* medications for 4 to 24 hours or up to 3 days before some blood tests. When discontinuing the medication is not medically advisable for the patient, the type and amount of drug that the patient is taking should be noted on the laboratory requisition. This alerts the laboratory to the presence of the drug, and at times, they may be able to use a different method of testing that would not be altered by the presence of the medication. Other tests require timed samples; that is, samples may be collected every hour for 3 consecutive hours, as in a glucose tolerance test. Patients must be made aware of these requirements.

Specific directions should be written out for patients so that they have an accurate reminder of the special requirements for each test to be performed, in addition to the time and date of the test. For some tests, you may have preprinted instruction forms to give the patient. Make sure that the patient understands the reasons for any special instructions. An informed patient usually is more cooperative in following specific directions, which in turn facilitates accurate test results.

Recording.   Proper recording on the patient's chart is essential. This includes the date, time, sample(s) obtained, test(s) to be performed, and when and how the sample was sent to the laboratory (see also Care, Handling, Transporting, and Storing Specimens in Chapter 11).

VENIPUNCTURE TECHNIQUE

Venipuncture is the preferred method for obtaining blood samples and must be used when a larger amount of blood is required for testing. From 3 to more than 30 ml may be drawn by this method. *Your goal* is to obtain an adequate blood specimen with minimal discomfort to the patient. To spare the patient the pain of unsuccessful punctures, consider the following before doing a venipuncture.

Venipuncture (troubleshooting) tips

1. Familiarize yourself with the laboratory's lab test directory containing information for collecting specimens and the equipment needed.
2. *Never* draw blood from a person who is standing.
3. Ask the patient if he or she has any preference regarding which vein you should puncture. Patients often know where their better veins are and which sites should be avoided.
4. Palpate the vein *before* inserting the needle to determine if the vein is patent (open, unobstructed).
5. Use a sturdy-walled vein for the puncture. The walls of sturdy veins feel firm when you touch them and exhibit elasticity and resilience when pressure is carefully applied.
6. If unable to enter a vein in the antecubital space, check for different sites, such as veins in the wrist or hand; however, *do not* use hand veins unless absolutely necessary because these veins move easily and can be more painful when punctured. Hand veins are also more fragile, and puncturing them can cause hematomas.
7. Stop the venipuncture if a hematoma develops.
8. Fragile veins are usually narrow veins. If you must puncture these veins, use a 23-gauge rather than a 21-gauge needle.
9. For small or fragile veins, you may use the **butterfly technique with a butterfly needle and tubing.** Insert the needle into the vein. When blood starts to flow into the tubing, insert the needle at the other end of the tubing into the vacuum tube. Leave the needle in position until the desired amount of blood is obtained.
10. Do not use a weak-walled vein. These veins are soft to the touch and lack the elasticity of a sturdy vein.
11. Do not use sclerosed veins. These veins are resistant to pressure, even if they do look like good veins.
12. Do not use a vacuum apparatus to draw blood from a small or constricted vein because this causes the vein to collapse.
13. **For obese patients,** put the tourniquet on fairly tight and feel for a vein deep in the antecubital space. A deep vein may be found in the center of this area. Be careful not to puncture an artery if going into deep tissue. If you find and feel an artery, you will feel it pulsate. A vein will feel like a tube, and you will not feel it pulsate. You may also check the veins in the wrist to use for the venipuncture site on an obese patient.
14. **For children,** have the parent leave the room before you do the venipuncture. Have someone assist you with the child. Another person can hold the child, hold his or her arm secure, and also talk to him or her. Perform the

procedure quickly. When someone is supporting the child and distracting his or her mind from the needle, you are better able to perform the venipuncture quickly.

15. **For the elderly,** having someone else hold the arm for support is sometimes advised because the patient could move his or her arm, which could interfere with the tests. This support is especially important if the patient is comatose. Be gentle if you tap the vein to encourage it to enlarge because tapping

too hard can traumatize the vein and nearby tissue. Also, to prevent trauma to the skin, apply the tourniquet carefully, making sure that it is snug but not too tight. You could put the tourniquet over the patient's sleeve to protect the skin.

16. ALWAYS explain who you are and what you will be doing, even if the patient has passed out or is comatose, because he or she may still be able to hear you or feel the needle prick.

PROCEDURE 13-1

VENIPUNCTURE USING A SYRINGE AND NEEDLE

Objective

Understand and demonstrate the correct procedures for obtaining a blood specimen using a syringe and needle; injecting the blood into a test tube and into a vacuum tube; preparing the tubes to be sent to the laboratory; and charting the procedure on the patient's chart.

Equipment

70% Alcohol and sterile cotton sponges *or* disposable alcohol sponges
- Do not use alcohol-based cleansing materials when samples are to be used for blood alcohol testing.
- When sterile collections are needed, such as for blood cultures, use tincture of iodine or other suitable alternative as designated by the laboratory for cleansing the skin.

Sterile cotton sponges

Tourniquet

Sterile disposable needle, usually 1-inch, 1¼-inch, or 1½-inch, 21-gauge

Sterile disposable syringe, either 5, 10, 20, or 30 ml (or cc), depending on the amount of blood to be obtained

Test tube(s) with proper patient identification, with or without additive, depending on the test that is to be performed, **or** a vacuum tube *(rather than the syringe and test tube, or vacuum tube, you may use the Vacutainer system with appropriate tube[s], needle, and holder; see Figure 13-1.)*

Adhesive bandage

Disposable, single-use examination gloves

Biohazard sharps container

PROCEDURE

1. **Wash your hands. Use appropriate personal protective equipment (PPE) as dictated by facility.**

2. Assemble required equipment.

3. Identify the patient and explain the procedure.

4. Have the patient sit with the arm well supported in a downward and extended position (Figure 13-4).

5. Prepare equipment for use: attach the needle to the syringe (or to the Vacutainer holder [see Figure 13-1, *A*]), leaving the needle shield in place. Label the collection tube with the patient's name, the date, and the time (Figure 13-5).

6. Select the site for venipuncture by palpating the antecubital space. This site is located on the inner aspect of the arm, opposite the elbow. You must avoid the artery. At the antecubital site, the basilic and cephalic veins are used for drawing blood samples.

7. Don gloves.

RATIONALE

Explanations help gain the patient's cooperation.

This avoids movement by the patient.

If you are drawing blood from more than one patient, it is best to label the tubes after you have drawn the blood. *Often when tubes are prelabeled, people have a tendency to use the wrong tube if they are in a rush or under pressure.*

VENIPUNCTURE USING A SYRINGE AND NEEDLE—cont'd

8. Apply the tourniquet around the patient's arm 3 to 4 inches above the elbow (Figure 13-6). The tourniquet must have enough tension to stop venous flow. Palpate the vein again (Figure 13-7). You may ask the patient to open and close the hand several times to help produce engorgement of the vein in the arm. The radial pulse should still be palpable.

9. Swab the venipuncture site with an alcohol sponge. Start at the intended puncture site and move out in a circular motion. *Do not palpate the venipuncture area after cleansing with alcohol.* Allow the site to air-dry.

10. Remove the needle shield.

Do not tie the tourniquet too tight because doing so obstructs arterial blood flow. If you cannot obtain a blood specimen within 2 minutes, loosen the tourniquet, wait a few minutes, and then reapply it. Do not keep the tourniquet tightened for more than 2 minutes.

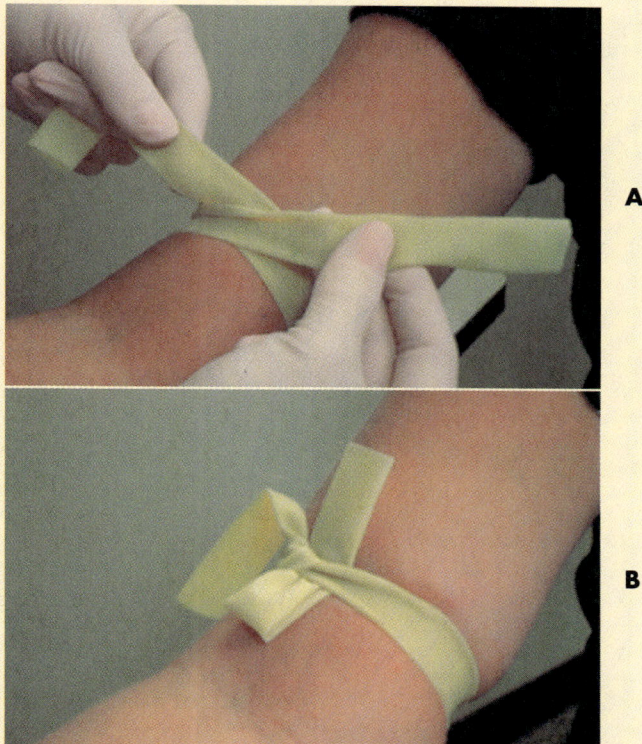

A

B

FIGURE 13-6   **A,** Apply the tourniquet around the patient's arm 3 to 4 inches above the elbow. Cross the ends of the tourniquet and pull the ends away from each other to create tension. **B,** Secure the tourniquet by tucking the upper end into the band to form a half-bow. The tourniquet must be tight enough to obstruct venous blood flow.

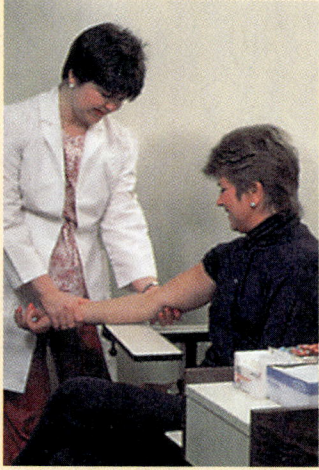

FIGURE 13-4   For a venipuncture, have the patient sit with the arm well supported in a downward and extended position.

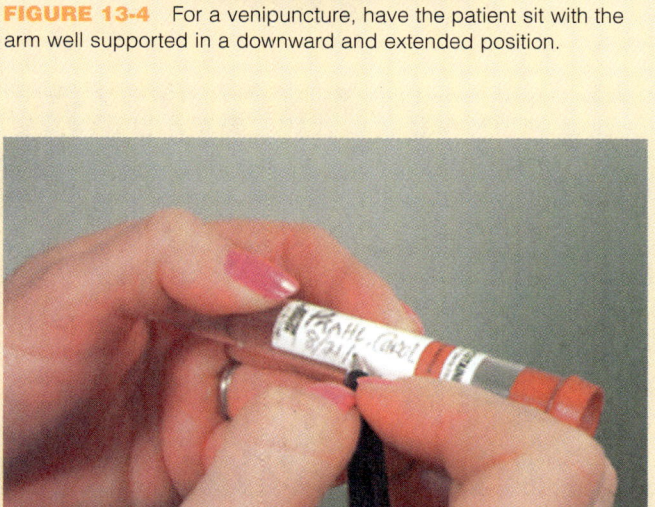

FIGURE 13-5   Label the collection tube with the patient's name, the date, and the time.

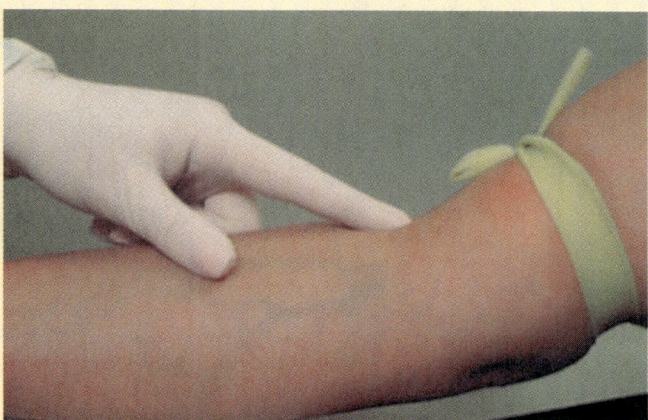

FIGURE 13-7   Palpate the vein once again after the tourniquet has been positioned.

Continued

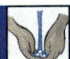

VENIPUNCTURE USING A SYRINGE AND NEEDLE—cont'd

11. Using your nondominant hand, draw the skin over the puncture site until tense. Gently and slowly insert the needle at a 15-degree angle through the skin into the vein (Figure 13-8).

Countertension immobilizes the vein and exerts tension in the opposite direction to that of the needle. Thus the needle goes in more easily and less painfully. You retain better control over the needle when the vein is immobilized by the countertension.

12. Having entered the vein using your dominant hand, now use your nondominant hand to slowly pull on the plunger of the syringe to withdraw blood. As soon as blood starts to flow into the syringe, release the tourniquet by pulling down on one of the ends. *Do not* pull up because that could separate the needle and vein prematurely (Figure 13-9; see Figure 13-11). Make sure that you do not move the needle and syringe after entering the vein.

The bevel of the needle should be facing upward so that the sharpest point of the needle is inserted first.

If you withdraw the blood too rapidly, you may cause the vein to collapse and thus will be unable to obtain the required sample. Keep in mind that a nontraumatic venipuncture produces the most reliable data because any tissue injury can falsely elevate some results, such an enzyme levels.

> **OR**
>
> Release the tourniquet *after* you have obtained the desired amount of blood and always *before* removing the needle. At times, when you release the tourniquet as soon as blood starts to flow into the syringe (or vacuum tube), the blood flows out very slowly. When this occurs, the procedure takes longer to complete.

13. When you have obtained the required amount of blood, place a dry sterile sponge over the puncture site and withdraw the needle, using a straight, downward motion. **The tourniquet must be off before the needle is withdrawn.**

14. Apply pressure with a sterile sponge over the puncture site for a few minutes; you may have the patient elevate the arm at this time. *Do not* apply pressure to the puncture site until the needle is completely removed. You may ask the patient to hold the sponge over the puncture site and apply the pressure.

Elevation prevents oozing of blood at the puncture site. Elevating rather than bending the arm helps to prevent possible bruising of the area. Do not apply pressure on the site before removing the needle because this would be painful and traumatize the vein unnecessarily.

15. Inject blood into the test tube(s) (Figure 13-10). **NOTE:** When injecting blood into a vacuum tube from a syringe and needle system, leave the needle on the syringe and gently insert the

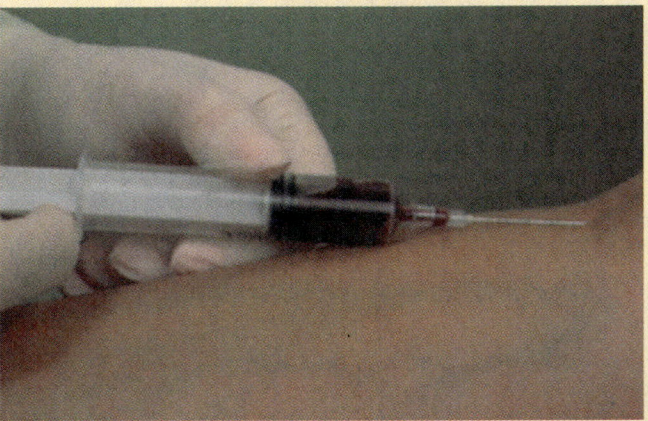

FIGURE 13-8   Gently and slowly, insert the needle at a 15-degree angle through the skin into the vein.

FIGURE 13-9   After entering the vein, use your nondominant hand to slowly pull on the plunger of the syringe to withdraw blood. Release the tourniquet as soon as blood starts to flow into the syringe.

PROCEDURE 13-1

VENIPUNCTURE USING A SYRINGE AND NEEDLE

needle through the rubber stopper on the tube that is positioned in a tube rack. *NEVER* hold the tube when puncturing the rubber stopper to fill the tube. The vacuum inside draws the required amount of blood into the tube. When using different tubes for multiple samples, first inject blood into the tubes that do not contain any additives, then into the coagulation tubes, and then into the tubes containing an additive.

16. Cap the tubes. Those that contain an additive should be *gently* inverted 8 to 10 times to mix the blood with the additive. Do not shake these tubes. Do not mix blood in the plain tubes (that is, tubes without an additive). Vigorous mixing may cause hemolysis.

17. Apply an adhesive bandage to the puncture site if desired.

18. Discard disposable syringe and needle in puncture-resistant containers designated for disposal (see Figures 7-32 and 13-13).

Proper disposal aids in preventing needlesticks and infection and is required by the OSHA bloodborne pathogen standard.

19. Remove gloves.

20. Wash your hands.

21. Complete the laboratory requisition, and send it to the laboratory with the blood sample(s) obtained.

22. Record on patient's chart.

Charting Example

May 18, 20__, 1 PM
Venipuncture done on left arm.
Two samples sent to lab for a CBC and blood chemistries.
Charles Rubin, CMA

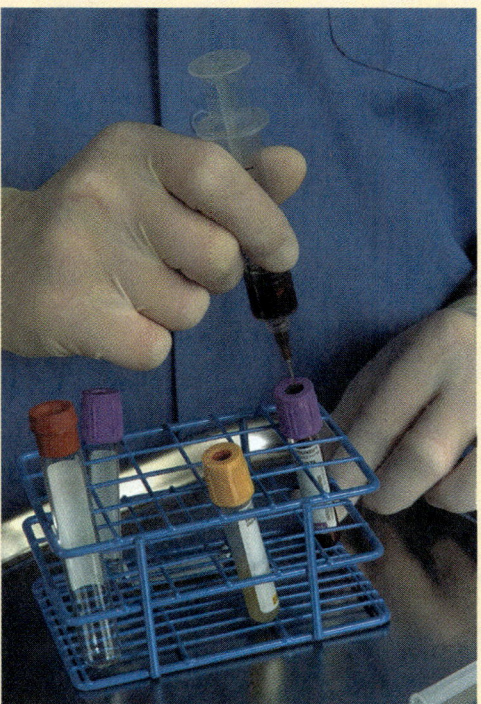

FIGURE 13-10   After obtaining the required amount of blood and removing the needle from the vein, inject blood into the test tube. When using a vacuum tube, leave the needle on the syringe and gently insert the needle through the rubber stopper on the tube that is standing in a tube rack.

Venipuncture Using the Vacutainer Evacuated Blood Collection Tube(s) for Drawing Single and Multiple Blood Samples (see Figure 13-1, *A*).

Objective: Understand and demonstrate the correct procedures to obtain single and multiple blood samples using the Vacutainer holder and needle, and vacuum tubes; and charting the procedure on the patient's chart.

1. **Wash your hands. Use appropriate personal protective equipment (PPE) as dictated by facility.**
2. Assemble required equipment.
3. Identify the patient and explain the procedure.
4. Have the patient sit with the arm well supported in a downward and extended position (see Figure 13-4).
5. Prepare equipment for use: attach the needle to the Vacutainer holder (see Figure 13-1, *A*), leaving the needle shield in place. Label the collection tube with the patient's name, the date, and the time (see Figure 13-5).
6. Select the correct tube for the type of sample required and label it. Gently tap tubes that contain additives to dislodge any additive that may be trapped around the stopper.
7. Insert the tube into the holder up to the guideline; push the tube stopper just to touch the needle inside the holder.
8. Perform the venipuncture in the usual manner (follow steps 6 through 11 in Venipuncture Using a Syringe and Needle).
9. Place two fingers at the end of the holder; with your thumb, push the tube onto the needle to the end of the holder. At the same time, stabilize the holder and needle with your other hand. Once the rubber stopper slides onto the needle, the vacuum pressure is accessed, and this draws blood from the vein into the collection tube (Figure 13-11).

10. **Release the tourniquet as soon as blood begins to fill the tube** (see Figure 13-11). Do not allow contents of tube to contact the stopper or the end of the needle during the procedure. NOTE: If blood doesn't flow into the tube or if the blood flow ceases before an adequate amount is collected, take the following steps:
    a. Check to see that the needle cannula is in the correct position in the vein.
    b. If a multiple sample needle is being used, remove the tube and place a new tube into the holder.
    c. Remove the needle and tube and discard. Start the procedure over again.

Continue with steps 11 through 20 for single-sample collections and steps 11 through 22 for multiple-sample collections.

Single-sample collection

11. Remove the needle from the vein when the vacuum is exhausted and blood stops flowing into the tube (Figure 13-12).
    OR
    Some specialists recommend disengaging the tube from the needle *before* removing the needle from the vein.
12. Apply pressure with a sterile sponge to the puncture site and have the patient elevate his or her arm for a few minutes to prevent oozing of blood (see Figure 13-12).
13. Remove the tube of blood from the holder.
14. For tubes that contain additives, *gently* invert 8 to 10 times to mix blood thoroughly with the additive. *Do not shake.*
15. Apply an adhesive bandage to the puncture site if required.
16. Discard the needle in a designated biohazard sharps container (Figure 13-13).
17. Remove gloves.
18. **Wash your hands.**
19. Complete the laboratory requisition and forward with the blood sample to the laboratory.

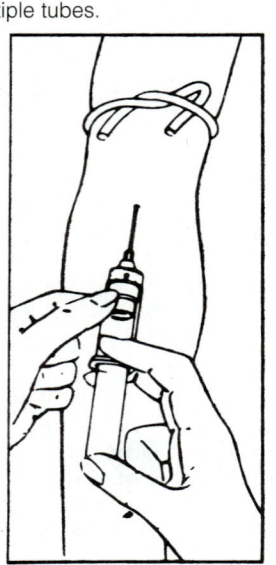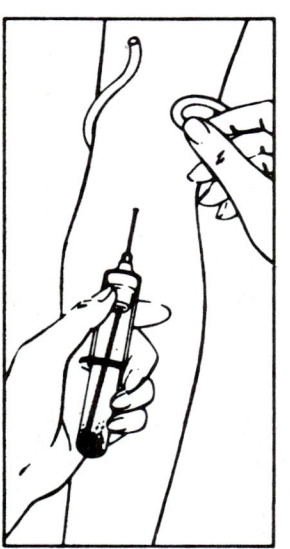

FIGURE 13-11 Correct position of patient's arm and tube assembly to prevent possibility of backflow. Tourniquet is released as soon as blood begins to flow or before the needle is removed if taking multiple tubes.

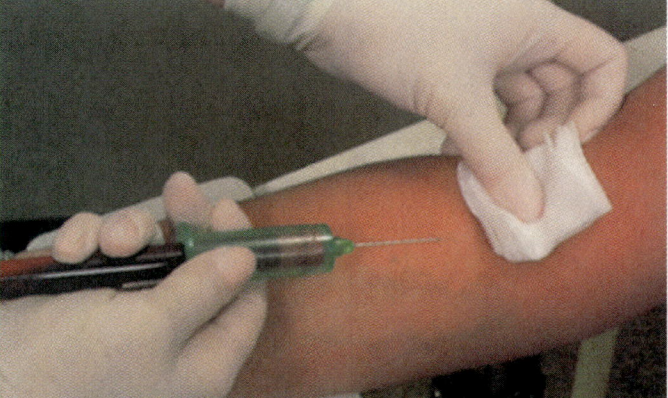

FIGURE 13-12 Remove needle from vein when vacuum is exhausted and blood stops flowing into tube. Apply pressure with a sterile sponge to the puncture site *after* the needle is completely removed.

20. Record on the patient's chart the date, time, procedure, and your signature.

Multiple-sample collection.   Complete Steps **1** through **10** on p. 582.

11. Remove the tube from the holder when the vacuum is exhausted and the blood stops flowing. Keep the needle holder steady.
12. Place the second and succeeding tubes into the holder, puncturing the diaphragm of the stopper to initiate blood

FIGURE 13-13   Vacutainer-type needle disposal container.

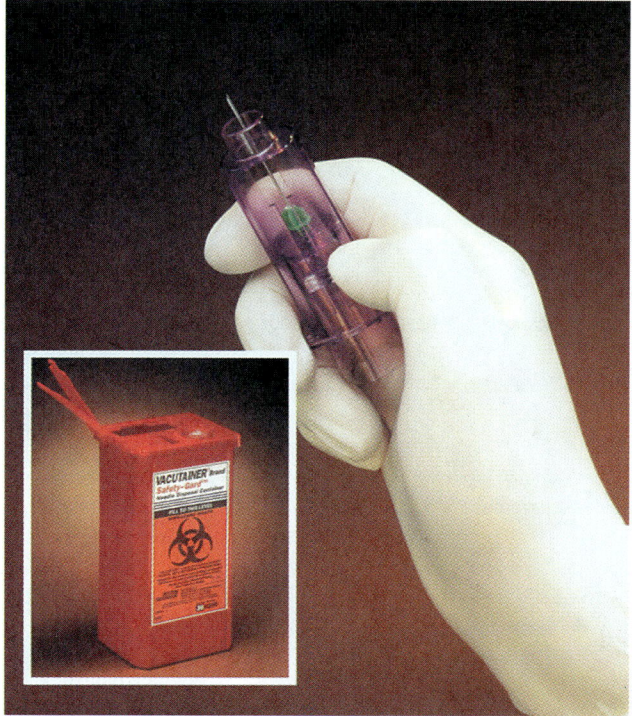

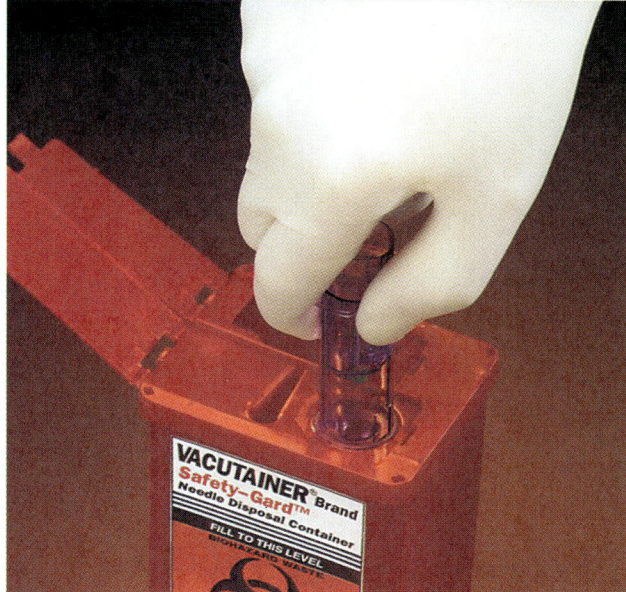

flow. Keep the needle holder steady. Tubes without additives are drawn first, then coagulation tubes, and then tubes with additives.

13. While blood is flowing into succeeding tubes, gently invert previously filled tubes that contain additives 8 to 10 times to mix the additive with the blood. *Do not shake.* Vigorous mixing may cause hemolysis.
14. Remove the needle from the vein when blood stops flowing into the last tube (see Figure 13-12).
15. Apply pressure with a sterile sponge to the puncture site (see Figure 13-12) and have the patient elevate the arm for a few minutes to prevent oozing of blood.
16. Remove the tube of blood from the holder. *Gently* invert the tube 8 to 10 times if it contains an additive. *Do not shake.*
17. Apply an adhesive bandage to the puncture site if required.
18. Discard the needle in a designated puncture-resistant biohazard sharps container (see Figure 13-13). If using the Vacutainer needle container, insert the needle into the slot on the top of the container and twist the holder counterclockwise until the needle is detached and falls into the container. *This type of Vacutainer holder is reusable.*

Any needle holder that becomes contaminated with blood is considered hazardous and *must* be decontaminated with bleach or disposed of in the **biohazard container.** The guidelines of the facility (where blood specimens are obtained) for reusing the holder must be known and followed precisely.

Other types of needles and holders are available for which the needle is self-capped after use. With these needles a protective shield is moved over the needle and locked into place after use. This type of needle holder *and* needle is to be discarded in the **biohazard sharps container** after use (see Figure 13-1, *B*).

The proper disposal of equipment after use is of the utmost importance and is required by OSHA's Universal/Standard Precautions to ensure that accidental needlestick and other injuries are prevented.

19. Remove gloves.
20. **Wash your hands.**
21. Complete the laboratory requisition and forward it with the blood sample to the laboratory.
22. Record on the patient's chart the date, the time, procedure, and your signature.

FINGERTIP SKIN PUNCTURE

Fingertip skin puncture using the Penlet II* (Figure 13-15)

Objective: Understand and demonstrate the correct procedure for obtaining a blood specimen by doing a fingertip skin puncture using the Penlet II; dispose of used equipment in appropriate containers.

Text continued on p. 585

_____
*Lifescan, Inc, Mountain View, Calif.

FINGERTIP SKIN PUNCTURE USING A LANCET

Objective

Understand and demonstrate the correct procedure for obtaining a blood specimen by the fingertip skin puncture method using a lancet; prepare the specimen to be sent to the laboratory; and record the procedure on the patient's chart.

Equipment

A sterile disposable lancet

70% Alcohol and cotton sponges *or* disposable alcohol sponges

Disposable, single-use examination gloves

Clean blood pipette *or* capillary tube *or* Unopette *or* Microtainer (this piece of equipment varies with your agency's preference, with the test(s) to be performed on the blood sample, and with the methods used by the laboratory)

or

A reagent strip if you are doing a simple test for blood glucose (see p. 617)

PROCEDURE

RATIONALE

1. **Wash your hands. Use appropriate personal protective equipment (PPE) as dictated by facility.**

2. Assemble equipment and supplies.

3. Identify the patient and explain the procedure.

   Explanations help gain the patient's cooperation.

4. Have the patient seated with the arm well supported.

   This avoids movement by the patient.

5. Select the lateral part of the tip of a *finger* or the *earlobe* for the puncture site; use the *heel* or *great toe for an infant.* Avoid the thumb and index finger.

   The thumb and index finger are usually more calloused than the other fingers. Using the lateral part of a fingertip rather than the palm side lessens discomfort to the patient.

6. "Milk" or gently rub the finger along the sides. If the patient's fingers are cold, you may rub them or apply a warm pack. You may also instruct the patient to dangle his or her hand toward the floor.

   Rubbing the finger promotes circulation. Dangling the hand helps force blood into the finger.

7. Clean the puncture site with an alcohol sponge; allow the area to dry. Do not blot or blow on the puncture site. Allow it to air-dry.

8. **Don gloves.**

9. Grasp the patient's finger on the sides near the puncture site with your nondominant thumb and forefinger.

10. Hold the lancet with your dominant fingers and make a quick in-and-out puncture on the side of the patient's fingertip. Hold the lancet at a right angle to the lines on the patient's finger (Figure 13-14). Lancets are usually designed so that you can make a puncture to a depth of 3 to 4 mm, which is sufficient to obtain drops of blood.

11. Wipe away the first drop of blood with a clean cotton sponge.

    The first drop of blood is not a desirable sample because it contains tissue fluid.

12. Apply gentle pressure above the puncture site to cause the blood to flow freely. Do not squeeze the finger.

    Squeezing the finger liberates tissue fluid, which in turn dilutes the blood and causes inaccurate results.

PROCEDURE 13-2

FINGERTIP SKIN PUNCTURE USING A LANCET—cont'd

13. Obtain the blood sample as required by the test to be performed. You may:

    a. Use the pipette to take up the blood sample. Take up the blood sample to the desired level in the pipette.

    OR

    b. Lightly touch the blood drop to the test pad on the reagent strip and continue the test according to the individual test directions.

14. When more than one sample is needed, wipe the finger with a clean cotton sponge and obtain fresh drops of blood in each pipette. You may have to apply gentle pressure to the finger to obtain more blood.

15. When using bulb pipettes and Unopettes, make dilutions according to instructions for the specific test to be performed. Do not dilute blood collected in Microtainers and capillary tubes; send it directly to the laboratory for testing.

16. Apply pressure to the puncture site with a dry cotton sponge. You may have the patient apply pressure with a cotton sponge over the puncture site.

17. Discard lancet in sharps container. Any sponge with blood on it must be disposed of in a container for biohazardous waste.

18. Label the blood samples and laboratory requisition correctly and forward to the laboratory for testing.

19. Remove gloves.

20. Wash your hands.

21. Record on the patient's chart the date, time, procedure, and your signature.

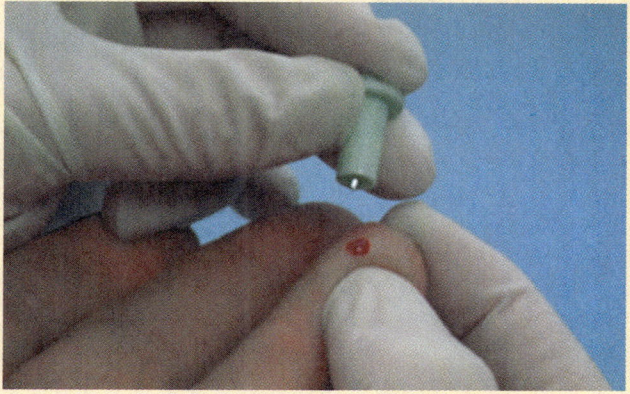

FIGURE 13-14   Fingertip skin puncture technique using a lancet.

Charting Example

April 21, 20___, 11 AM
    Finger puncture done on second finger, left hand. Blood sample sent to laboratory for a CBC (complete blood count).
    Ann Patterson, CMA

Fingertip Skin Puncture Using the Penlet II—cont'd

Equipment

Penlet II disposable caps (see Figure 13-15)

Sterile lancet

70% Alcohol and cotton sponges *or* disposable alcohol sponges

Disposable, single-use examination gloves

Procedure

1. Wash your hands. Use appropriate personal protective equipment (PPE) as dictated by facility.

2. Assemble equipment and supplies.

3. Identify the patient and explain the procedure.

4. Have the patient seated with the arm well supported.

5. Load the Penlet II with a sterile lancet. Remove the Penlet II cap by pulling it straight off. Insert a new, sterile lancet into the lancet holder. The lancet will slide into the lancet holder easier if you *do not* line up the ridges on the lancet with the slots in the lancet holder. Inserting the lancet may automatically cock the Penlet II (Figure 13-15, *B* and *C*).

FIGURE 13-15   **A,** Penlet II automatic blood sampling pen for obtaining a skin puncture blood sample. **B** through **J,** Technique for using the Penlet II puncture device.

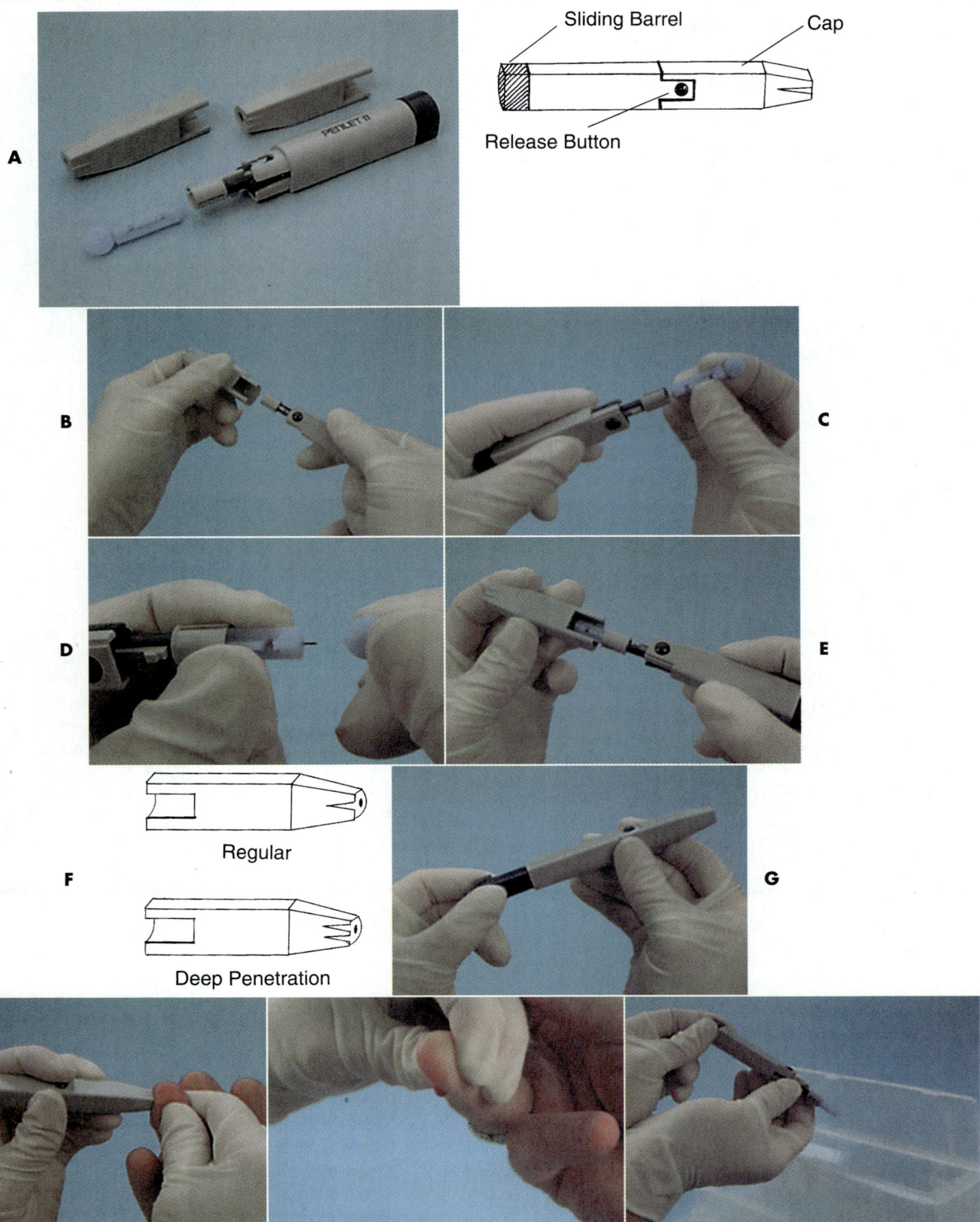

6. Select the lateral part of the tip of a finger for the puncture site.
7. "Milk" or gently rub the finger along the sides.
8. Clean the puncture site with alcohol sponge; allow the area to dry.
9. Don gloves.
10. Hold the end of the Penlet firmly with one hand, and with the other hand, twist off the lancet protective disk (Figure 13-15, *D*).
11. Replace the Penlet II cap (Figure 13-15, *E*). The Penlet II Sampler includes two caps. The cap that comes attached to the Penlet II Sampler has a *single line* on the flat side and works well for children and most adults. The other cap has *two lines* on the flat side and works well for very thick or calloused skin or when a deeper puncture is needed (Figure 13-15, *F*).
12. Cock the Penlet II. Holding the lower portion of the Penlet II, pull out the dark gray sliding barrel until it clicks. If it does not click, the Penlet II may have been cocked when the lancet was inserted (Figure 13-15, *G*).
13. Grasp the patient's finger on the sides near the puncture site with your nondominant thumb and forefinger.
14. Place the Penlet II firmly against the side of the finger, with the cap resting on the finger (Figure 13-15, *H*).
15. Press the dark gray release button. The depth of penetration of the lancet depends on the amount of pressure with which the Penlet II is held against the skin. The greater the pressure, the deeper the puncture (Figure 13-15, *I*).
16. Complete this procedure by following steps 11 through 20 in the Fingertip Skin Puncture Using a Lancet.
17. To remove the lancet from the Penlet II, take the cap off, insert the inside rim of the cap into the notched side of the lancet, and pull the lancet out. Grasp the dark gray T-shaped prongs. Point the lancet down and away from you. Pull back on the dark gray sliding barrel until the lancet drops out (Figure 13-15, *J*). Dispose of in a puncture-resistant container for used sharps.
18. Remove gloves.
19. **Wash your hands.**
20. Put a clean cap on the Penlet and replace in the proper storage area. Clean with soap and water as needed.

Unopette System

The Unopette system consists of a disposable, self-filling diluting pipette and a plastic reservoir prefilled with a precise amount of diluent. These systems serve as a collection and dilution unit for microblood samples. Various types of Unopette systems are available that contain the appropriate diluting substances required for hematology and chemistry tests (Figure 13-16).

Figure 13-17 shows the **Microtainer capillary whole blood collector.**

BLOOD TESTS

The results obtained from laboratory examinations performed on blood samples, combined with other clinical information,

help the physician in various aspects of patient care, such as screening for or diagnosing a condition, evaluating body functions, making therapeutic decisions, monitoring therapy provided, and monitoring the effects of medications.

Numerous blood tests can be performed to aid the physician when diagnosing, treating, or evaluating a patient's condition. Some of these tests are performed on whole blood, whereas others are performed on blood serum. A few simple procedures that may be performed in the physician's office or health agency and tables of many common tests done commonly in laboratories by certified personnel with the aid of automated equipment follow. The actual performance of these tests is usually not the medical assistant's responsibility because in general, *most state laws require that individuals performing laboratory procedures must be certified laboratory technicians, clinical laboratory scientists (formerly called medical technologists), or physicians certified or licensed in the state of their practice.* Nonetheless, it is important for you to be familiar with the type of tests available and the normal values for each and to have an understanding of the significance of normal and abnormal results. When aware of this information, you can better understand and appreciate the diagnosis, treatment, and evaluation of patients under the physician's care, and you are of greater value to the patient, physician, and laboratory.

At times, basic screening tests are performed in the physician's office; more detailed tests and precise results are obtained from larger laboratories using automated equipment.

All tests have **predetermined normal values or ranges** that establish the limits within which the results indicate the absence of any pathologic condition. Normal ranges are established on the basis of the procedures and equipment used by the laboratory. It is important to keep this in mind when reviewing laboratory reports received on specimens obtained from the patients under your physician's care. Often you may obtain a list of normal blood values from the laboratory that performs the procedures.

Generally, **hematology tests** are done on whole blood, and **serologic tests** and **blood chemistries** are done on serum or sometimes on plasma. **Blood banking** and **transfusion services** use cells and serum for testing.

A conscientious medical assistant should be alert for new techniques that may be valuable to the physician in the office. Manufacturers provide brochures and catalogues with information on the latest developments. Medically oriented magazines are another good source for obtaining this information.

AUTOMATION IN THE CLINICAL LABORATORY

Within the past 25 to 30 years, clinical laboratories have been confronted with an ever-increasing workload. An answer to this problem has been sought in automated instrumentation. These specialized modular systems *automate* or *semiautomate* the time-consuming, step-by-step procedures formerly performed by manual analysis. With refinement of instrumentation, fast and accurate methods have been developed for reporting a wide variety of laboratory information on body fluids, which include

Text continued on p. 590

FIGURE 13-16 Techniques for using the Unopette system for laboratory procedures. (Courtesy Becton-Dickinson, Division of Becton, Dickinson & Co, Rutherford, NJ.)

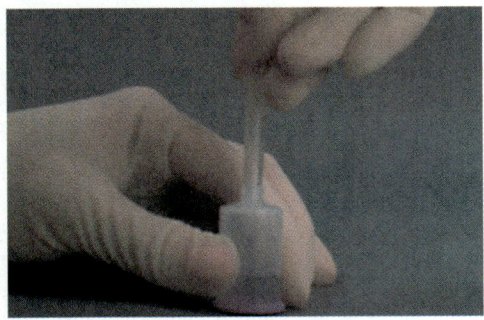

1. Puncture diaphragm

Using the protective shield on the capillary pipette, puncture the diaphragm of the reservoir as follows:

a. Place reservoir on a flat surface. Grasping reservoir in one hand, take pipette assembly in other hand. Push tip of pipette shield firmly through diaphragm in neck of reservoir, then remove.

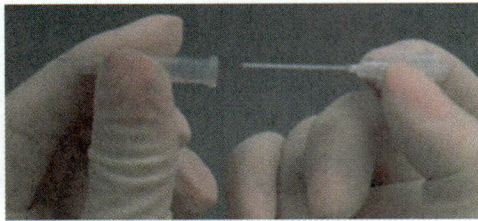

b. Remove shield from pipette assembly with a twist.

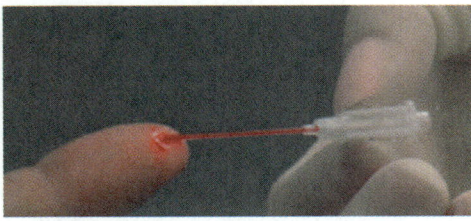

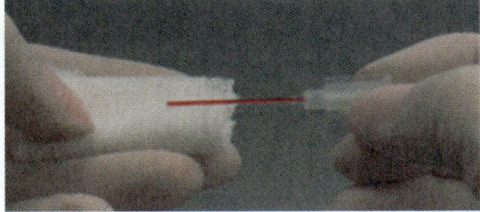

2. Add sample

Fill capillary with sample and transfer to reservoir as follows:

a. Holding pipette almost horizontally, touch tip of pipette to sample. (See alternate methods in illustrations above.) Pipette will fill by capillary action. Filling is complete and will stop automatically when sample reaches end of capillary bore in neck of pipette.

b. Wipe excess sample from outside of capillary pipette, making certain that no sample is removed from capillary bore.

c. Squeeze reservoir slightly to force out some air. Do not expel any liquid. Maintain pressure on reservoir.

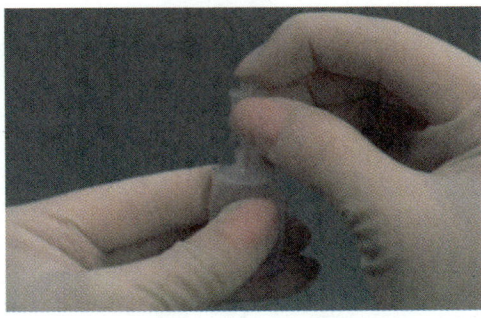

d. Cover opening of overflow chamber with index finger and seat pipette securely in reservoir neck.

e. Release pressure on reservoir. Then remove finger from pipette opening. Negative pressure will draw blood into diluent.

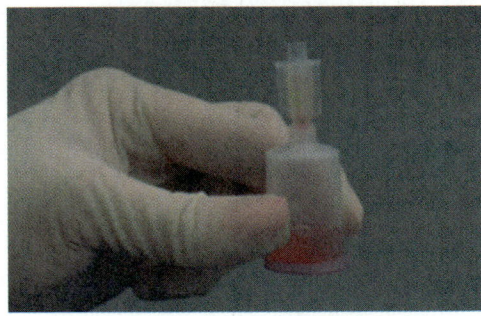

f. Squeeze reservoir gently two or three times to rinse capillary bore, forcing diluent into, but not out of, overflow chamber, releasing pressure each time to return mixture to reservoir.

CAUTION: If reservoir is squeezed too hard, some of the specimen may be expelled through the top of the overflow chamber.

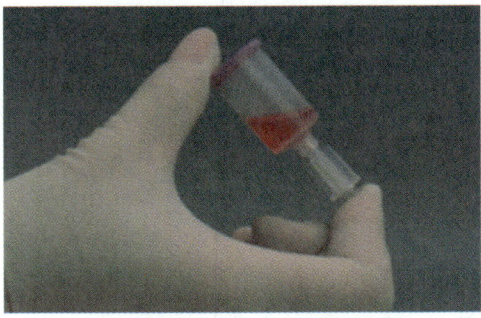

g. Place index finger over upper opening and gently invert several times to thoroughly mix sample with diluent.

FIGURE 13-16—cont'd   Techniques for using the Unopette system for laboratory procedures. (Courtesy Becton-Dickinson, Division of Becton, Dickinson & Co, Rutherford, NJ.)

3. Count cells (option 1)
Mix diluted blood thoroughly by inverting reservoir (see 2g) to resuspend cells immediately prior to actual count.

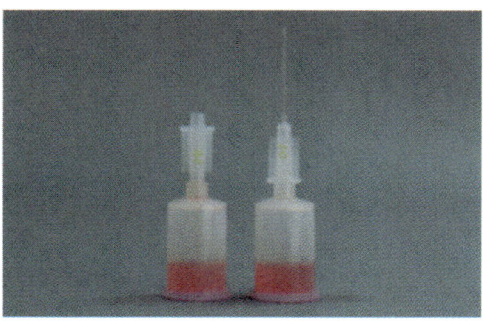

a. Convert to dropper assembly by withdrawing pipette from reservoir and reseating securely in reverse position.
b. Invert reservoir, gently squeeze sides and discard first three or four drops.

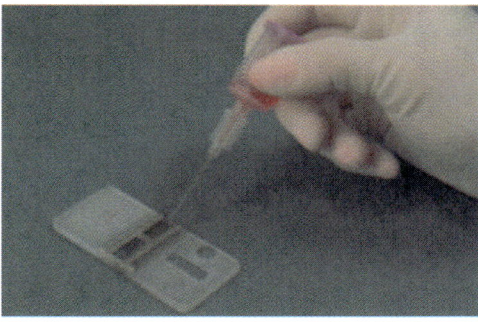

c. Carefully charge hemacytometer with diluted blood by gently squeezing sides of reservoir to expel contents until chamber is properly filled.

OR
3. Transfer contents (option 2)
Transfer thoroughly mixed contents of each reservoir to appropriately labeled test tubes or corresponding curvettes as follows:
a. Convert reservoir to dropper assembly by withdrawing pipette and reseating securely in reverse position as shown above.

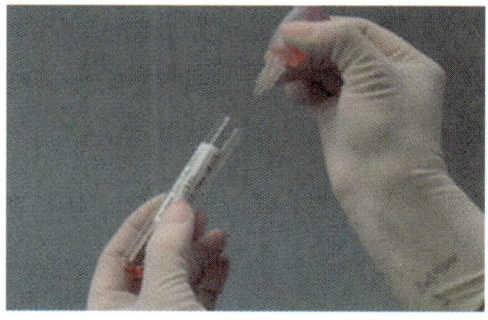

b. Place capillary tip into appropriately labeled test tube or curvette which will accommodate 5.0 ml of reagent and squeeze reservoir to expel entire contents.

OR
3. Store diluted specimen (option 3)

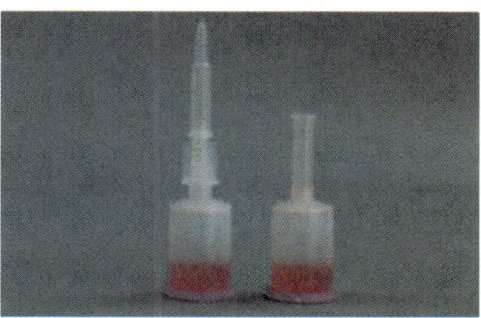

Cover overflow chamber with capillary shield or remove capillary and insert tip of shield firmly into reservoir opening. (Note time for which diluted specimen remains stable for each test.)

FIGURE 13-17   Microtainer capillary whole blood collector. (Courtesy Becton-Dickinson, Division of Becton, Dickinson & Co, Rutherford, NJ.)

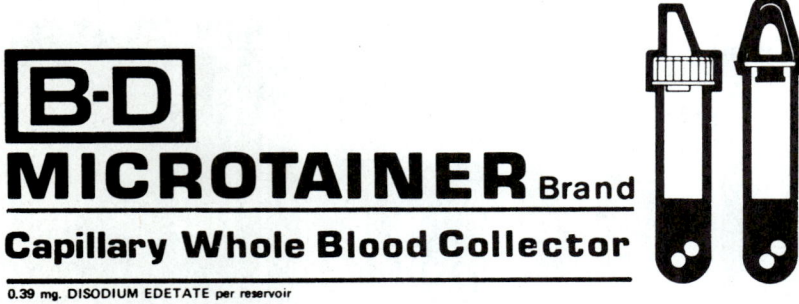

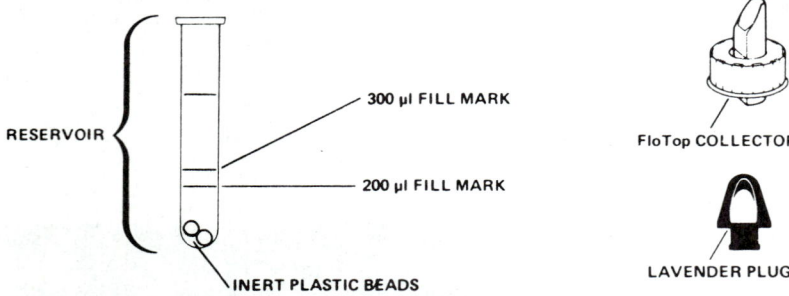

B-D MICROTAINER Brand
Capillary Whole Blood Collector

0.39 mg. DISODIUM EDETATE per reservoir

FOR LABORATORY USE ONLY · NON−STERILE · STORE BELOW 25ºC

THE FOLLOWING COMPONENTS ARE USED WITH THIS PROCEDURE:

RESERVOIR
300 µl FILL MARK
200 µl FILL MARK
INERT PLASTIC BEADS

FloTop COLLECTOR

LAVENDER PLUG

The MICROTAINER System for capillary whole blood samples provides a method for collecting, anticoagulating, storing and identifying the capillary blood sample. . . all in one unbreakable plastic tube.

ANTICOAGULANT

Each MICROTAINER Tube contains sufficient EDTA Na_2 (disodium edetate) to anticoagulate 300 microliters of capillary blood.

MIXING BEADS

Each MICROTAINER Tube contains two (2) inert plastic beads which aid in the dispersion of blood and anticoagulant for proper mixing of sample.

NON-INTERFERENCE WITH HEMATOLOGICAL DETERMINATIONS

Parallel comparisons of samples collected with the MICROTAINER Brand Capillary Whole Blood Collector and routine microcollection techniques have shown no significant differences for the following determination.[1]

WBC	MCH
RBC	MCHC
HGB	MCV
HCT	Platelets
Reticulocytes	
White Cell Differentials	

MICROTAINER Tubes for whole blood collections are to be used to collect and store capillary blood samples for outline hematological use. This system is composed of a one piece FloTop collector; a plastic tube containing an anticoagulant, EDTA Na_2 (disodium edetate), two (2) inert plastic mixing beads, and a lavender plug.

USERS SHOULD BE THOROUGHLY FAMILIAR WITH THE CONTENTS OF THIS PACKAGE INSERT PRIOR TO USE.

The FloTop collector directs the free flowing blood directly into the unbreakable plastic MICROTAINER

tube. The tubes are marked at the 200 and 300 microliter (µl) levels which indicate the desired filling range.

When the appropriate sample has been collected, the FloTop collector is removed from the tube and is replaced with the lavender plug and gently inverted, 8 to 10 times, to insure adequate anticoagulation of the specimen. The stoppered tube is now provided with protection against contamination, evaporation and spillage.

The anticoagulated whole blood samples can be directly pipetted from the MICROTAINER Tube and assayed for routine hematological parameters.

---

whole blood, plasma, serum, urine, and cerebrospinal fluid. The human element of error is virtually eliminated, ensuring the absolute objectivity of measurement that is so important to accurate diagnosis and monitoring. **Multiphasic tests or test panels or profiles** consist of a battery of automated tests performed on the same specimen at the same time. It has been found to be more useful and economical to subject every specimen to a battery or panel of automated tests than to limit the examination to one or two tests. Through this system of routine total blood counts and biochemical profiling, additional disease-screening tests may be routinely performed. Most hematology panels in laboratories that have any volume at all are done on automated systems. Numerous different machines are available; most of them automate or at least semiautomate the whole process, using only 1 ml of blood. Tests results are obtained visually on a digital display or video screen or on a hematology printout card (Figures 13-18 to 13-23). On some systems the computer can bring up each cell that has been

counted on a WBC differential count and display these cells on the screen of the machine.

The latest state-of-the-art systems use laser technology. Laser counters in hematology, such as the ELT-8, perform an automated CBC. The laser looks at the cells to determine the results. Traditionally the chemistry sections of laboratories are the most heavily automated. Most laboratories have at least some form of automation in chemistry if not in other departments. Often **biochemical panels** are used to determine liver, kidney, cardiac, and thyroid functions; also common are immunology panels, arthritis panels, obstetric panels, and so on.

Another panel is simply called a **Chemistry Screening Panel 12, 20,** or **24.** The numbers indicate how many tests are to be performed. These are general terms that are used; the type of tests run in these panels vary with the laboratory and how they have programmed the automated equipment for use. The tests that are performed in each panel are given on the laboratory's requisition so that the physician can determine which

FIGURE 13-18 COULTER STKS, a fully automated hematology system for CBCs and white cell differentials. In addition to WBC data, the STKS reports comprehensive RBC and platelet profiles with histograms. In all, 20 parameters are provided. (Courtesy Coulter Corp, Miami, Fla.)

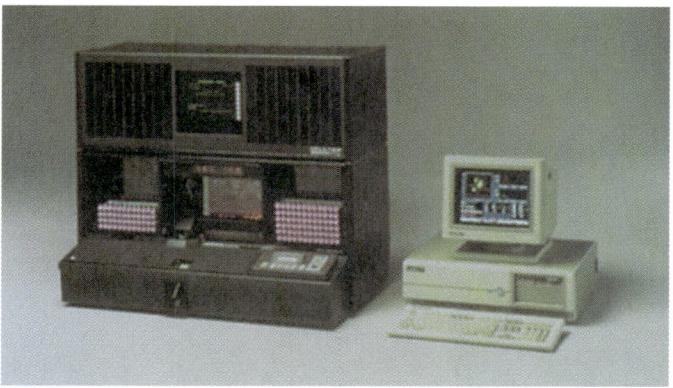

FIGURE 13-19 JT3 System provides a fully automated CBC, including the Coulter Histogram Differential with interpretive report, plus complete platelet and RBC profiles. Manual differentials are reduced by as much as 80%. Ideal for low-to-medium volume laboratory. (Courtesy Coulter Corp, Miami, Fla.)

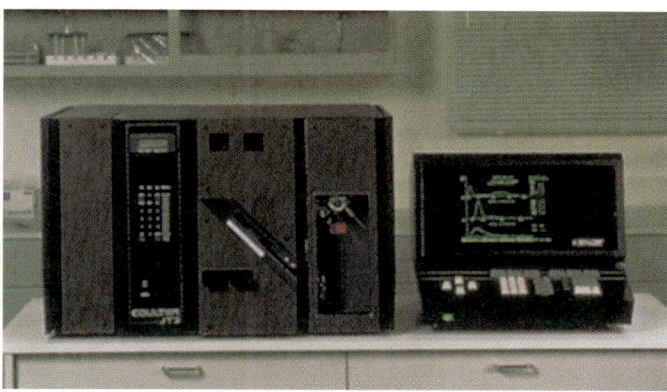

FIGURE 13-20 **A,** Automated flow cytometry system capable of processing samples at rates greater than 100 samples per hour. The system has an automated sample preparation, a multisample autoloader, and a high-speed flow cytometer. **B,** Histogram and report from the automated flow cytometer. (Courtesy Coulter Corp, Miami, Fla.)

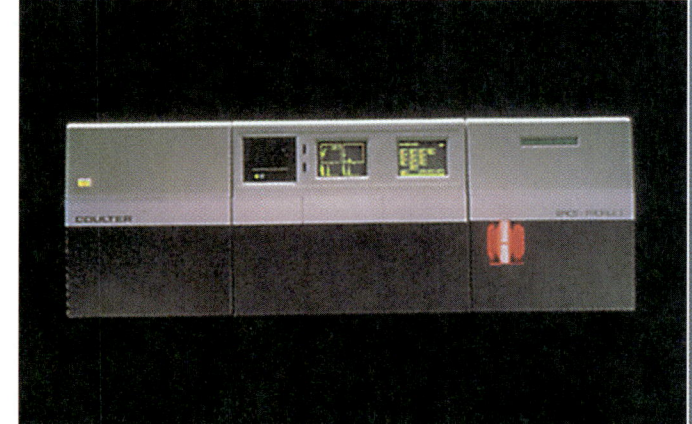

FIGURE 13-21 Compact Technicon H-2 hematology system provides accurate, comprehensive information on all cell types of clinical interest. It offers the choice of CBC with platelets, CBC and full differential plus RBC morphology, and lymphocyte subset analyses from a single aspiration of blood. Multiple report formats let the operator review a variety of results on the video screen, and any computer real-time (CRT) data can be printed out on a graphics printer. The Technicon H-2 provides a standard computer interface. Results may be automatically transmitted "live" to a remote laboratory computer, reducing data handling, transcription effort, and potential errors. (Courtesy Miles Inc, Diagnostics Division, Tarrytown, NY.)

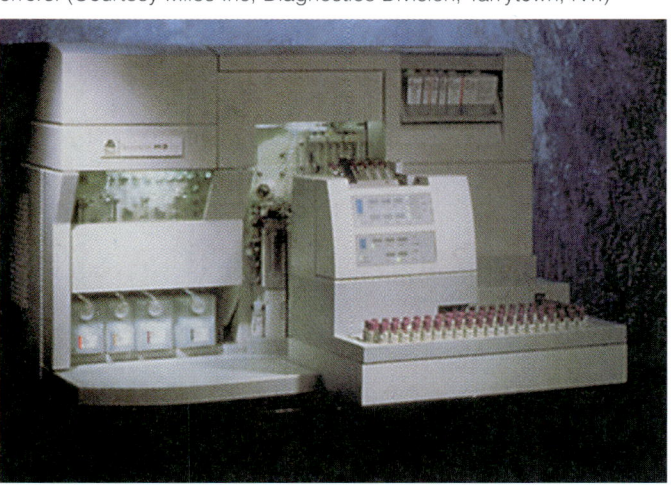

FIGURE 13-22 Technicon RA-2X system is a chemistry analyzer that can be programmed with 100 different tests. For chemistry profiles, one can select up to 27 tests at a time from this extensive menu, including immunoassays and electrolytes. Results are displayed on the computer screen and printed. (Courtesy Miles, Inc, Diagnostic Division, Tarrytown, NY.)

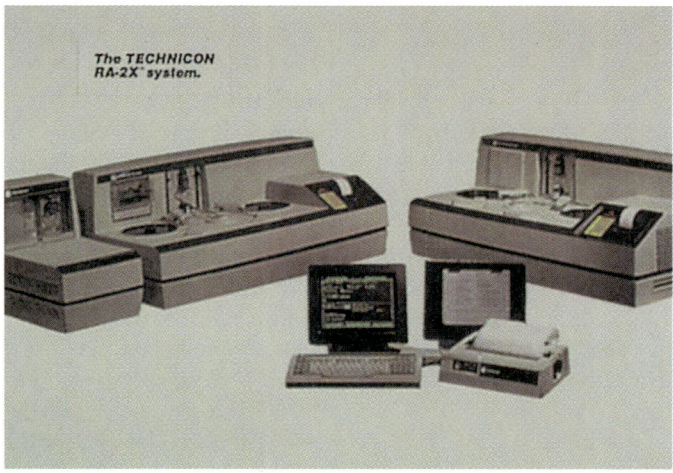

FIGURE 13-23 Serum Chemistry Graph displaying results from the SMA 12/60 on 12 biochemical tests. Results are presented in concentration terms on a precalibrated strip chart record. Normal test ranges for each parameter are printed as shaded areas; horizontal line crossing graph represents test results. Time from aspiration of given sample to finished chart is only 8 minutes—less time than it takes to complete any one of these test by any other methods. (Courtesy Miles, Inc, Diagnostic Division, Tarrytown, NY.)

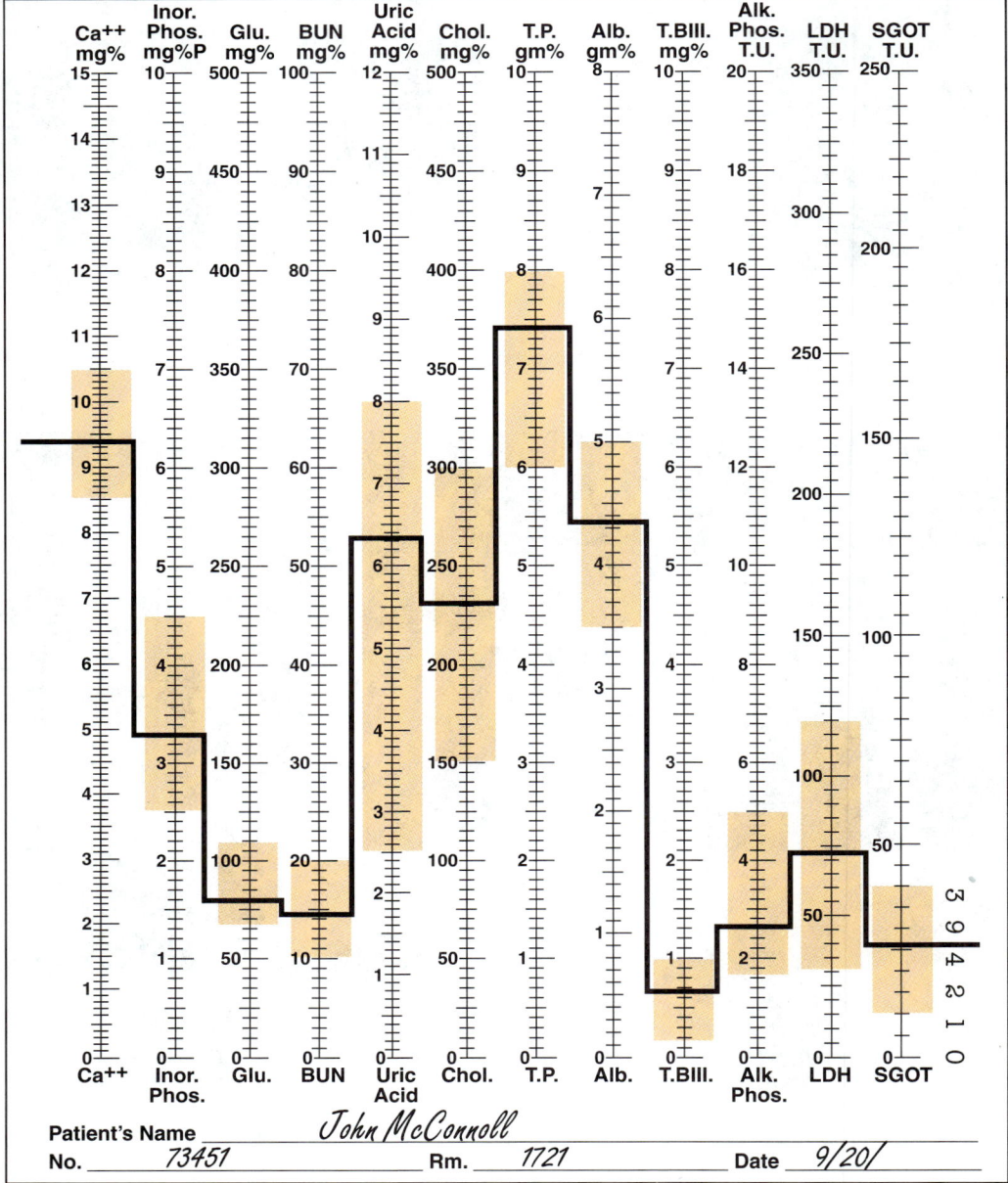

panel is most appropriate for the case (Figures 13-24 and 13-25). All of these panels are screening devices that allow the physician to focus on abnormal results for further study and investigation. Test results from the different systems can be reported on an 8½ × 11–inch sheet of precalibrated vertical graph paper called a serum chemistry graph (SCG), or on a similar horizontal graph for the other systems (see Figure 13-23). Rather than sending the physician the graph paper, most laboratories now have special computer printout forms that also record the results of the tests performed. The laboratory keeps the graph as its permanent record and sends the

computer printout to the physician. One example of the computer forms used is a sheet divided into columns. In different columns the names of the tests, the normal values or reference range, and the results of the tests performed are recorded (see Figure 13-26 and 13-27).

Physicians may view test results on their own computer by connecting to the laboratory's computer using a special individual computer code assigned to them by the laboratory. A printout of the results can also be obtained this way.

Many *multiphasic tests, panels, or profiles* are devised to provide information on particular body system disorders or

Text continued on p. 602

FIGURE 13-24   A, Clinical laboratories requisition form. Note the tests done in the different panels. (Courtesy SmithKline Beecham Clinical Laboratories, Dublin, Calif.)

SB SmithKline Beecham Clinical Laboratories

SelecTest™

LabBenefit™ ☐

BILL TO:
☐ ACCOUNT
☐ PATIENT
☐ OTHER

PRINT PATIENT NAME (LAST, FIRST, MIDDLE)

SBCL REGISTRATION # (IF APPLICABLE)   DOB (MM/DD/YYYY)   SEX

PATIENT SOCIAL SECURITY #   OFFICE / PATIENT ID #

ROOM #   LAB REFERENCE #   PATIENT PHONE # ( )

PRINT NAME OF INSURED/RESPONSIBLE PARTY (LAST, FIRST, MIDDLE) - IF OTHER THAN PATIENT

PATIENT STREET ADDRESS (OR INSURED/RESPONSIBLE PARTY)   APT. #   KEY #

CITY   STATE   ZIP

R E F E R R E D   B Y

DID YOU REMEMBER...

TO INCLUDE DIAGNOSIS CODE(S)?

TO REQUEST OR MARK TEST(S)?

TO PROVIDE ORDER CODE(S) FOR HANDWRITTEN TESTS?

TO CHECK "BILL TO" BOX ABOVE?

MEDICARE NUMBER   SUFFIX

MEDICAID NUMBER   STATE

RELATIONSHIP TO INSURED: ☐ SELF   ☐ SPOUSE   ☐ DEPENDENT

INSURANCE CO. NAME

MEMBER / INSURED ID #   GROUP #

INSURANCE ADDRESS

CITY   STATE   ZIP

EMPLOYER NAME/EMPLOYER #   INSURED SOCIAL SECURITY # (if not patient)

DATE COLLECTED   TIME   AM PM   TOTAL VOL/HRS. _____ ML _____ HR   ☐ Fasting

U.P.I.N. REFERRING PHYSICIAN AND/OR PAYORS

☐ ADDITIONAL PHYS.: Dr. _____   U.P.I.N. |__|__|__|__|__|

☐ Call Results to: ( )   ☐ Fax Results to: ( )   ☐ **STAT**

Send Duplicate Report to:

SBCL CLIENT # OR NAME: _____

ADDRESS: _____

CITY: _____   STATE _____   ZIP _____

ICD9 DIAGNOSIS CODE(S) FOR TESTS ORDERED (MUST BE PROVIDED)

PATIENT/RESPONSIBLE PARTY SIGNATURE (SEE ADVANCED BENEFICIARY NOTICE ON REVERSE) I have read the statement on the back of this requisition that Medicare is likely to deny payment for identified service(s) for the reason stated. If Medicare denies payment, I agree to be personally and fully responsible for payment.

X

A

AMA PANELS		
34392- 0	☐ ELECTROLYTE PANEL (4) (Na, K, Cl, CO2)	S
34388- 1	☐ BASIC METABOLIC PANEL (7) (Na, K, Cl, CO2, Glu, BUN, Cr)	S
@ 34391- 2	☐ HEPATIC FUNCTION PANEL (6) (Alb, TBili, DBili, AP, AST, ALT)	S
34389- 3	☐ COMP METABOLIC PANEL (12) (Na, K, Cl, Glu, BUN, Cr, Ca TP, Alb, TBili, AP, AST)	S
@ 7600- 4	☐ LIPID PANEL (Fasting Specimen) (TChol, Trig, HDL, calc LDL)	S
@ 20210- 5	☐ OBSTETRIC PANEL (ABO/Rh, Ind Coombs, CBC, RPR, HBsAg, Rubella IgG Ab)	1
@ 6462- 6	☐ HEPATITIS PANEL (HBsAg, HBs Ab, HBcAb (Total), HA Ab (Total), HC Ab)	S
@ 7020	☐ THYROID PANEL (T-4, T-3 UPTAKE & FTI)	S

TESTS		
7788- 7	☐ ABO GROUP & RH TYPE	1
223- 8	☐ ALBUMIN	S
234- 9	☐ ALKALINE PHOSPHATASE (AP)	S
823-10	☐ ALT (SGPT)	S
243-11	☐ AMYLASE	S
249-12	☐ ANTINUCLEAR AB (ANA)	S
822-13	☐ AST (SGOT)	S
285-14	☐ BILIRUBIN, DIRECT	S
287-15	☐ BILIRUBIN, TOTAL	1
4420-16	☐ C-REACTIVE PROTEIN	S
@ 29256-17	☐ CA 125	S

303-18	☐ CALCIUM (Ca)	S
310-19	☐ CARBON DIOXIDE (CO2)	S
6399-20	☐ CBC (includes DIFF/PLT)	L
978-21	☐ CEA	S
330-22	☐ CHLORIDE (Cl)	S
334-23	☐ CHOLESTEROL, TOTAL	S
374-24	☐ CK, TOTAL	S
795-25	☐ COOMBS, INDIRECT	1
375-26	☐ CREATININE (Cr)	S
418-27	☐ DIGOXIN	S
@ 457-28	☐ FERRITIN	S
466-29	☐ FOLIC ACID	1
470-30	☐ FSH	S
482-31	☐ GGT	S
8477-32	☐ GLUCOSE, GEST. SCR.	1
484-33	☐ GLUCOSE, PLASMA	G
483-34	☐ GLUCOSE, SERUM (Glu)	S
29407-35	☐ H. PYLORI IGG AB QL	S
8435-36	☐ HCG, SERUM, QUAL	S
8396-37	☐ HCG, SERUM, QUANT	S
@ 608-38	☐ HDL	S
496-39	☐ HEMOGLOBIN A1C	L
509-40	☐ HEMATOCRIT	L
510-41	☐ HEMOGLOBIN	L
7008-42	☐ HEMOGRAM (H/H, RBC, Indices, WBC)	L
1759-43	☐ HEMOGRAM/PLT	L
508-44	☐ HEP A AB - TOTAL	S
501-45	☐ HEP B CORE AB - TOTAL	S

499-46	☐ HEP B SURFACE AB QL	S
498-47	☐ HEP B SURFACE AG	S
8472-48	☐ HEP C VIRUS AB	S
6449-49	☐ HIV SCR-WB CONF	S
@ 7573-50	☐ IRON (TOT), IBC %SAT	S
@ 571-51	☐ IRON, TOTAL	S
593-52	☐ LDH	S
599-53	☐ LEAD (B)	1
615-54	☐ LH	S
613-55	☐ LITHIUM	1
@ 622-56	☐ MAGNESIUM	S
713-57	☐ PHENYTOIN	1
718-58	☐ PHOSPHORUS	S
723-59	☐ PLATELET COUNT	L
733-60	☐ POTASSIUM (K)	S
745-61	☐ PROGESTERONE	S
746-62	☐ PROLACTIN	S
754-63	☐ PROTEIN, TOTAL	S
@ 5363-64	☐ PSA (DX OR MONITOR)	S
8847-65	☐ PT WITH INR	1
763-66	☐ PTT, ACTIVATED	1
4418-67	☐ RHEUMATOID FACTOR	S
799-68	☐ RPR	S
802-69	☐ RUBELLA IGG AB	S
809-70	☐ SED RATE BY MOD WEST	1
836-71	☐ SODIUM (Na)	S
873-72	☐ TESTOSTERONE, TOTAL	S
@ 891-73	☐ TRANSFERRIN	S

@ 896-74	☐ TRIGLYCERIDES	1
@ 899-75	☐ TSH	S
859-76	☐ T-3, TOTAL	S
@ 867-77	☐ T-4 (THYROXINE)	S
866-78	☐ T-4, FREE	S
3020-80	☐ UA, CULTURE IF IND	1
6448-81	☐ UA, MACROSCOPIC	Y
7909-82	☐ UA, REFLEX	Y
294-83	☐ UREA NITROGEN (BUN)	S
905-84	☐ URIC ACID	S
916-85	☐ VALPROIC ACID	1
7065-86	☐ VIT B12/FOLIC ACID	1
927-87	☐ VITAMIN B12	S
937-88	☐ WBC	L
7064-89	☐ WBC & DIFF	L

MICROBIOLOGY		
SOURCE _____		
4558-90	☐ CULTURE, GENITAL	1
4485-91	☐ CULTURE, GP. A STREP	1
6649-92	☐ CULTURE, STOOL	1
394-93	☐ CULTURE, THROAT	1
395-94	☐ CULTURE, URINE, RTN	1
6919-95	☐ DNA PROBE, CHL & GC	1
8502-96	☐ DNA PROBE, CHLAMYDIA	1
8501-97	☐ DNA PROBE, GC	1
8625-98	☐ GIARDIA AG DETECTION	1
681-99	☐ OVA & PARASITES	1

ADDITIONAL TESTS: (MUST INCLUDE COMPLETE TEST NAME AND ORDER CODE. REFER TO SBCL DIRECTORY OF SERVICES.)

TOTAL TESTS ORDERED

@ = Medicare Limited Coverage Test

COMMENTS, CLINICAL INFORMATION:

Physician Signature

For any patient of any payor (including Medicare and Medicaid) that has a medical necessity requirement, you should only order those tests which are medically necessary for the diagnosis and treatment of the patient.

Continued

FIGURE 13-24—cont'd **B,** On the back side of the requisition is a list of the common ICD-9 diagnosis codes. Codes *must* be provided for *all* tests ordered. (Courtesy SmithKline Beecham Clinical Laboratories, Dublin, Calif.)

ADVANCE BENEFICIARY NOTICE

Medicare will only pay for services that it determines to be reasonable and necessary under section 1862 (a) (1) of the Medicare Law. If Medicare determines that a particular service, although it would otherwise be covered, is not reasonable and necessary under the Medicare Program standards, Medicare will deny payment for that service. Tests ordered by your physician and identified on the front of this requisition with an "@" or an "&" symbol are likely to be denied for payment. Those tests designated with the "@" symbol are likely to be denied for payment because Medicare usually does not pay for these tests for the reported diagnosis. Those tests designated with the "&" symbol are likely to be denied because the test is non-FDA approved/experimental. By signing the Patient/Responsible Party Signature on the front of this requisition, you are confirming your agreement to assume financial responsibility for the payment of these tests.   AMW

COMMON ICD-9 DIAGNOSIS CODES

To avoid unwarranted denials and subsequent rework for office staff, any requisitions sent to SBCL must include all medically appropriate ICD-9 diagnosis codes. ICD-9 codes are required by certain third party payors to confirm the medical necessity of the test(s) and/or profile(s) ordered. Below are ICD-9 codes most commonly received by SBCL. These codes were taken from the 1998 ICD-9 manual issued by the American Medical Association. While this list may be a useful reference tool depending upon the nature of your practice, *it is not complete. Please refer to the ICD-9 manual for a complete listing. The ultimate responsibility for correct coding lies with the ordering physician. Please place all medically appropriate ICD-9 code(s) on the front of the requisition in the designated diagnosis code field. If ordering testing solely for screening purposes, please provide the appropriate screening ICD-9 code(s).*

CODE	DIAGNOSIS (symptom, illness, injury, or complaint)
789.00	Abdominal pain, unspecified site
790.6	Abnormal blood chemistry, other
796.4	Abnormal clinical findings, other
706.1	Acne, other
496	Airway obstruction, chronic, not elsewhere classified
477.9	Allergic rhinitis, cause unspecified
280.9	Anemia, iron deficiency, unspecified
281.0	Anemia, pernicious
285.9	Anemia, unspecified
413.9	Angina pectoris, other & unspecified
424.1	Aortic valve disorders
716.90	Arthropathy, unspecified, site unspecified
493.90	Asthma, unspecified, without mention of status asthmaticus
427.31	Atrial fibrillation
724.5	Backache, unspecified
466.0	Bronchitis, acute
427.9	Cardiac dysrhythmia, unspecified
425.4	Cardiomyopathies, primary, other
429.2	Cardiovascular disease, unspecified
436	Cerebrovascular disease, acute but ill-defined (CVA NOS, stroke)
616.0	Cervicitis & endocervicitis
786.50	Chest pain, unspecified
286.9	Coagulation defects, other & unspecified
428.0	Congestive heart failure
780.31	Convulsions, febrile
780.39	Convulsions, other
414.01	Coronary atherosclerosis of native coronary artery
414.00	Coronary atherosclerosis of unspecified type of vessel, native or graft
786.2	Cough
311	Depressive disorder, not elsewhere classified
110.1	Dermatophytosis of nail
250.01	Diabetes mellitus, type I (IDDM), not stated as uncontrolled
250.00	Diabetes mellitus, type II (NIDDM) or unspecified type, not stated as uncontrolled
250.02	Diabetes mellitus, type II (NIDDM) or unspecified type, uncontrolled
787.91	Diarrhea
780.4	Dizziness & giddiness
995.2	Drug, medicinal & biological substance adverse effect, unspecified
622.1	Dysplasia of cervix (uteri)
786.09	Dyspnea & respiratory abnormalities, other
788.1	Dysuria
782.3	Edema
259.9	Endocrine disorder, unspecified
530.81	Esophageal reflux
625.9	Female genital organ symptom, unspecified
780.6	Fever
558.9	Gastroenteritis & colitis, noninfectious, other & unspecified
780.9	General symptoms, other
274.9	Gout, unspecified
784.0	Headache
599.7	Hematuria
569.3	Hemorrhage of rectum & anus
286.5	Hemorrhagic disorder due to circulating anticoagulants
573.3	Hepatitis, unspecified
042	Human immunodeficiency virus [HIV] disease
272.0	Hypercholesterolemia, pure
272.1	Hyperglyceridemia, pure
272.2	Hyperlipidemia, mixed
272.4	Hyperlipidemia, other & unspecified
401.1	Hypertension, essential, benign
401.0	Hypertension, essential, malignant
401.9	Hypertension, essential, unspecified
402.10	Hypertensive heart disease, benign, without congestive heart failure
402.90	Hypertensive heart disease, unspecified, without congestive heart failure
276.8	Hypopotassemia
244.9	Hypothyroidism, unspecified
607.84	Impotence of organic origin
564.1	Irritable colon
414.9	Ischemic heart disease, chronic, unspecified
719.40	Joint pain, site unspecified
593.9	Kidney & ureter disorder, unspecified
623.5	Leukorrhea, not specified as infective

CODE	DIAGNOSIS
272.9	Lipoid metabolism disorder, unspecified
794.8	Liver scan, abnormal
724.2	Lumbago
780.7	Malaise & fatigue
162.9	Malignant neoplasm of bronchus & lung, unspecified
153.9	Malignant neoplasm of colon, unspecified
174.9	Malignant neoplasm of female breast, unspecified
183.0	Malignant neoplasm of ovary
185	Malignant neoplasm of prostate
627.2	Menopausal or female climacteric states
626.4	Menstrual cycle, irregular
626.8	Menstruation, suppression of; dysfunc, uterine hemorrhage NOS
626.0	Menstruation, absence of
626.2	Menstruation, excessive or frequent
625.3	Menstruation, painful
424.0	Mitral valve disorders
799.9	Morbidity & mortality, other unknown and unspecified cause
729.1	Myalgia & myositis, unspecified
238.2	Neoplasm of uncertain behavior of skin
278.01	Obesity, morbid
278.00	Obesity, unspecified
715.09	Osteoarthrosis, generalized, multiple sites
715.90	Osteoarthrosis, unspecified whether generalized or localized, site unspecified
733.00	Osteoporosis, unspecified
785.1	Palpitations
795.0	Papanicolaou smear of cervix abnormality, nonspecific
443.9	Peripheral vascular disease, unspecified
462	Pharyngitis, acute
486	Pneumonia, organism unspecified
627.3	Postmenopausal atrophic vaginitis
790.93	Prostate specific antigen (PSA) elevation
600	Prostatic hyperplasia
601.9	Prostatitis, unspecified
585	Renal failure, chronic
714.0	Rheumatoid arthritis
461.9	Sinusitis, acute, unspecified
473.9	Sinusitis, chronic, unspecified
034.0	Streptococcal sore throat
780.2	Syncope & collapse
710.0	Systemic lupus erythematosus
246.9	Thyroid disorder, unspecified
463	Tonsillitis, acute
435.9	Transient cerebral ischemia, unspecified
465.9	Upper respiratory infection, acute, unspecified site
788.41	Urinary frequency
599.0	UTI (urinary tract infection), site not specified
616.10	Vaginitis & vulvovaginitis, unspecified
783.1	Weight gain, abnormal
783.2	Weight loss, abnormal
V28.8	Antenatal screening, other specified
V67.51	F/U exam for completed treatment w/high-risk meds, not elsewhere classified
V70.0	General medical examination (routine) at a health care facility
V70.9	General medical examination, unspecified
V72.3	Gynecological examination
V20.2	Infant or child health check, routine
V20.1	Infant or child (healthy) receiving care, other
V42.0	Kidney transplant
V72.6	Laboratory examination
V58.61	Long term (current) use of anticoagulants
V58.69	Long term (current) use of other medications
V70.3	Medical examination for administrative purposes, other
V22.0	Normal first pregnancy supervision
V22.1	Normal pregnancy (other) supervision
V71.9	Observation for unspecified suspected condition
V24.2	Postpartum follow-up, routine
V72.84	Pre-operative examination, unspecified
V22.2	Pregnant state, incidental
V74.5	Special screening examination for bacterial/spirochetal veneral disease
V72.9	Special investigation & examination, unspecified
V82.5	Special screening for chemical poisoning and other contamination
V76.2	Special screening for malignant neoplasms, cervix
V78.1	Special screening for other and unspecified deficiency anemia

B

FIGURE 13-25   **A,** Examples of laboratory test panels and individual laboratory tests.

PANELS / REQUEST FOR PATHOLOGIST CONSULTATION

			REQUEST FOR PATHOLOGIST CONSULTATION	
R ☐ Chemistry 6	R ☐ Chemistry 23	R ☐ Cardiovascular Evaluation	R ☐ Hepatitis Acute Panel	R ☐ Renal Panel
R ☐ Chemistry 8	R, L ☐ Anemia Panel	B, L ☐ Coagulation Panel I	R ☐ Liver Panel I	2L ☐ T and B Cell Evaluation
R ☐ Chemistry 10	R, L ☐ Arthritis I	B, L ☐ Coagulation Panel II	B, R ☐ Liver Panel II	R ☐ Thyroid Panel I
R ☐ Chemistry 15	R, L ☐ Arthritis II	U ☐ Drug Screen, Urine	R, RT* ☐ Prenatal Panel I	R ☐ Thyroid Panel II
R ☐ Chemistry 17	R, L ☐ Arthritis III	R ☐ Electrolytes	L, 2R, RT* ☐ Prenatal Panel II	
R ☐ Chemistry 17 with Thyroid I	R, L, U ☐ Basic Health Screen I	R ☐ Hepatitis A Panel	L, 2R, RT* ☐ Prenatal Panel III	
R ☐ Chemistry 20	R, L, U ☐ Basic Health Screen II	R ☐ Hepatitis B Panel	L, G, RT* ☐ Prenatal Panel IV	

For panel components please refer to our test directory.

INDIVIDUAL TESTS / REQUEST FOR PATHOLOGIST CONSULTATION

			REQUEST FOR PATHOLOGIST CONSULTATION	
R ☐ Acid Phosphatase, Prostatic	R ☐ Ferritin	R* ☐ HIV Antibody	R ☐ PSA	R ☐ Vitamin B-12
R ☐ Albumin	L ☐ FK 506: EIA	2L ☐ HIV1, RNA Quant.	B ☐ PTT	**BLOOD BANK**
R ☐ Alkaline Phosphatase	L ☐ FK 506: IMX	R ☐ P24 Antigen	RT ☐ Quinidine	RT* ☐ Blood Type & Rh
R ☐ Amylase	R ☐ Folic Acid	☐ HIV consent has been obtained	R ☐ RA Factor	RT* ☐ Antibody Screen
R ☐ ANA	R ☐ Free T-4	R ☐ Iron & Iron Binding	L ☐ Retic Count	**MICROBIOLOGY**
R ☐ Bilirubin, D & T	R ☐ FSH	R ☐ LDH	R ☐ RPR	Soource:
R ☐ BUN	R ☐ FTA (Hatts Test)	R ☐ Lithium	R ☐ Rubella	☐ Culture, AFB (TB)
R ☐ Calcium	R ☐ GGT	R ☐ Lutein, Hormone (LH)	L ☐ Sed Rate	☐ Culture, Bacterial
L ☐ CBC (includes Diff.)	R or G ☐ Glucose	R ☐ Magnesium	R ☐ Serum Protein Electro	☐ Culture, Fungus
R ☐ CEA	L ☐ GlycoHGB (AIC)	U ☐ Marijuana Screen	R ☐ SGOT (AST)	☐ Culture, G. C.
SMEAR ☐ Chlamydia Screen	R ☐ HCG, Quantitative	R ☐ Mono Test	R ☐ SGPT (ALT)	☐ Culture, Viral
R ☐ Cholesterol Total	R ☐ HDL, Cholesterol	R ☐ Phosphorus	R or G ☐ Sodium	☐ Strep Culture, Beta Strep
R ☐ Cholesterol, HDL	L ☐ Hemogram	L ☐ Platelet Count	R ☐ T-3 Uptake	☐ Strep Screen, Rapid
R ☐ CPK	R ☐ Hep. A Virus AB	R or G ☐ Potassium	R ☐ T-4	☐ Antibiotic Sensitivities
R ☐ C-Reactive Prot.	R ☐ Hep. B Core AB	R ☐ Preg. Test, Serum	R ☐ T-4, Free	☐ Gram Stain
R ☐ Creatinine, Serum	R ☐ Hep. B Surf, AB	U ☐ Preg. Test, Urine	R ☐ Testosterone	☐ Ova & Parasites
U ☐ Creatinine, Urine	R ☐ Hep. B Surf. Antig.	RT ☐ Procainamide/NAPA	RT ☐ Theophylline	☐ Occult Blood
L ☐ Cyclosporin	R ☐ Hep. C AB	R ☐ Progesterone	R ☐ Toxoplasma AB	☐ Cryptosporidium
R ☐ CMV Antibodies	SMEAR ☐ Herpes Simplex (FA)	R ☐ Prolactin	R ☐ Triglycerides	☐ Pinworm
RT ☐ Digoxin	R ☐ Herpes I-II AB	R ☐ Protein, Total	R ☐ TSH	☐ Rotavirus
R ☐ Estrogen		U ☐ Protein, Urine	R ☐ Uric Acid	☐ C. Difficile Toxin
R ☐ Epstein-Barr		B ☐ Prothrombin Time	U ☐ Urinalysis	☐ Fecal Fat Qualitative

OTHER TESTS/SPECIAL INSTRUCTIONS

A

TUBE SPECIMEN KEY
R = RED BARRIER   B = BLUE
RT = RED TOP, NO BARRIER   L = LAVENDER
G = GREEN BARRIER   U = URINE
* = MUST BE SIGNED, AND DATED, FULL NAME, D.O.B.—OTHERWISE REJECTED

Continued

FIGURE 13-25—cont'd **B,** Tests included in the different panels in Figure 13-25, *A,* on page 595.

PANELS

CHEMISTRY 6:

ANION GAP (CALCULATED)
BUN
CHLORIDE
CO2
GLUCOSE
POTASSIUM
SODIUM

CHEMISTRY 8:

ANION GAP (CALCULATED)
BUN
CALCIUM
CHLORIDE
CO2
CREATININE
GLUCOSE
POTASSIUM
SODIUM

CHEMISTRY 10 (NUTRITION PANEL):

ANION GAP (CALCULATED)
BUN
CALCIUM
CHLORIDE
CO2
CREATININE
GLUCOSE
MAGNESIUM
PHOSPHORUS
POTASSIUM
SODIUM

CHEMISTRY 15:

ALBUMIN
ALKALINE PHOSPHATASE
ANION GAP (CALCULATED)
BILIRUBIN, TOTAL
BUN
CALCIUM
CHLORIDE
CHOLESTEROL
CO2
CREATININE
GLUCOSE
PHOSPHORUS
POTASSIUM
PROTEIN, TOTAL
SGOT
SODIUM

CHEMISTRY 17:

A/G RATIO
ALBUMIN
ALKALINE PHOSPHATASE
BILIRUBIN, TOTAL
BUN
CALCIUM
CHOLESTEROL
CREATININE
GLUCOSE
LDH
POTASSIUM
PHOSPHORUS
PROTEIN, TOTAL
SGOT
TRIGLYCERIDES
URIC ACID

CHEMISTRY 17 WITH THYROID PANEL 1:

CHEMISTRY 17 (AS ABOVE)
THYROID PANEL 1 (T4, T3, FTI)

B

CHEMISTRY 20 OR CHEM 22AT:

A/G RATIO
ALBUMIN
ALKALINE PHOSPHATASE
ANION GAP (CALCULATED)
BILIRUBIN, TOTAL
BUN
CALCIUM
CHLORIDE
CHOLESTEROL
CO2
CREATININE
GLUCOSE
GGTP
IRON, TOTAL
LDH
PHOSPHORUS
POTASSIUM
PROTEIN, TOTAL
SGOT
SGPT
SODIUM
TRIGLYCERIDES
URIC ACID

CHEMISTRY 23:

A/G RATIO
ALBUMIN
ALKALINE PHOSPHATASE
ANION GAP (CALCULATED)
BILIRUBIN, TOTAL, DIRECT AND INDIRECT
BUN
CALCIUM
CHLORIDE
CHOLESTEROL
CO2
CREATININE
GLUCOSE
GGTP
LDH
PHOSPHORUS
POTASSIUM
PROTEIN, TOTAL
SGOT
SGPT
SODIUM
TRIGLYCERIDES
URIC ACID

ANEMIA PANEL:

CBC
IRON AND TIBC
RETICULOCYTE COUNT

ARTHRITIS PANEL I:

CBC
SEDIMENTATION RATE
RHEUMATOID FACTOR
URIC ACID

ARTHRITIS PANEL II:

ARTHRITIS PANEL 1
ANA

ARTHRITIS PANEL III:

ANA
SEDIMENTATION RATE
RHEUMATOID FACTOR

BASIC HEALTH SCREEN I:

CHEMISTRY 23
CBC
URINALYSIS

BASIC HEALTH SCREEN II:

CHEMISTRY 23
CBC
SEDIMENTATION RATE
THYROID PANEL I (T4, T3, FTI)
URINALYSIS

CARDIOVASCULAR EVALUATION:

CHOLESTEROL, TOTAL
HDL
CHOLESTEROL/HDL RATIO
LDL
TRIGLYCERIDES
VLDL
LDL/HDL RATIO

COAGULATION PANEL I:

PARTIAL PROTHROMBIN TIME
PLATELET COUNT
PROTHROMBIN TIME

COAGULATION PANEL II:

FIBRINOGEN
PARTIAL PROTHROMBIN TIME
PLATELET COUNT
PROTHROMBIN TIME

DRUG SCREEN, URINE:

PLEASE CALL LAB

ELECTROLYTE PANEL:

ANION GAP (CALCULATED)
CHLORIDE
CO2
POTASSIUM
SODIUM

HEPATITIS A PANEL:

HEPATITIS A ANTIBODY
HEPATITIS A, IGM

HEPATITIS B PANEL:

HEPATITIS B SURFACE ANTIGEN
HEPATITIS B SURFACE ANTIBODY
HEPATITIS B CORE ANTIBODY

HEPATITIS ACUTE:

HEPATITIS A ANTIBODY, IGM
HEPATITIS B SURFACE ANTIGEN
HEPATITIS B SURFACE ANTIBODY
HEPATITIS B CORE ANTIBODY

LIVER PANEL I:

ALKALINE PHOSPHATASE
BILIRUBIN, TOTAL, DIRECT
CHOLESTEROL
GGTP
LDH
SGOT
SGPT

LIVER PANEL II:

A/G RATIO
ALBUMIN
ALKALINE PHOSPHATASE
BILIRUBIN, TOTAL, DIRECT AND INDIRECT
GGTP
PROTHROMBIN TIME
PROTEIN, TOTAL
SGOT
SGPT

PRENATAL PANEL I:

ABO
ANTIBODY SCREEN
CBC
HEPATITIS B SURFACE ANTIGEN
RH TYPE
RPR
RUBELLA

PRENATAL PANEL II:

ABO
ANTIBODY SCREEN
CBC
HEPATITIS B SURFACE ANTIGEN
HIV
RPR
RUBELLA

PRENATAL PANEL III:

ABO
ANTIBODY SCREEN
CBC
HEPATITIS B SURFACE ANTIGEN
HEPATITIS C ANTIBODY
HIV
RPR
RUBELLA

PRENATAL PANEL IV:

ANTIBODY SCREEN
CBC
GLUCOSE LOAD

RENAL PANEL:

A/G RATIO
ALBUMIN
ALKALINE PHOSPHATASE
ANION GAP (CALCULATED)
BILIRUBIN, TOTAL
BUN
CALCIUM
CHLORIDE
CHOLESTEROL
CO2
CREATININE
GLUCOSE
LDH
PHOSPHORUS
POTASSIUM
SODIUM
PROTEIN, TOTAL
SGOT
URIC ACID

T AND B CELL EVALUATION:

WBC
LYMPH, % LYMPH
B CELLS
% B CELLS
TOTAL T CELLS (ACT3)
% T CELLS
T HELPER CELLS
% T HELPER CELLS
T SUPPRESSOR CELLS
T HELPER/SUPPRESSOR RATIO

THYROID PANEL I:

T-4
T-3
FTI

THYROID PANEL II:

T-4
T-3
FTI
TSH

FIGURE 13-26   Clinical laboratory computer-generated laboratory report.

DATE & TIME RECEIVED	ACCESSION NUMBER
10/ 20/ 2000 20: 45	
LOCATION	DATE REPORTED
	10/ 21/ 2000

PHYSICIAN	PATIENT INFORMATION

TEST		RESULTS	REFERENCE RANGE	UNITS
TYPE AND XMATCH - PACKED CELLS				
Specimen Id is "1"				
BLOOD BANK UNIT NUMBER		Y34612		
UNIT STATUS		RELEASED		
COMPONENT		PACKED RBC		
PATIENT ABO AND Rh		O NEG		
ANTIBODY SCREEN		NEGATIVE		
DONOR ABO AND Rh		O NEG		
CROSSMATCH EXPIRES IN 72 HOURS, UNLESS BLOOD BANK IS NOTIFIED.				
CHEMISTRY 23 - PANEL A				
SODIUM		141	133-145	ME@/L
POTASSIUM		4. 0	3. 5-5. 5	ME@/L
CHLORIDE	HI	111	98-105	ME@/L
CO2 CONTENT		29	24-32	ME@/L
ANION GAP	LO	1	7-14	
BLOOD UREA NITROGEN	HI	31	10-20	MG/DL
CREATININE, SERUM/PLASMA	LO	0.7	0. 9-1. 5	MG/DL
BUN/CREATININE RATIO	HI	44	12-20	MG/DL
GLUCOSE		110	80-125	MG/DL
FINAL Report		(Summary)	Page 1 of 2	

Continued

FIGURE 13-26—cont'd Clinical laboratory computer-generated laboratory report.

DATE & TIME RECEIVED	ACCESSION NUMBER
10/ 20/ 2000 20: 45	
LOCATION	DATE REPORTED
	10/ 21/ 2000

PHYSICIAN	PATIENTS INFORMATION

TEST		RESULTS	REFERENCE RANGE	UNITS
CHEMISTRY 23 - PANEL B				
CALCIUM, TOTAL, SERUM	LO	7. 4	8. 5-10. 5	MG/DL
PHOSPHORUS	LO	2. 8	3. 0-4. 6	MG/DL
URIC ACID	LO	3. 2	3. 5-7. 2	MG/DL
CHOLESTEROL	LO	123	151-240	MG/DL
TRIGLYCERIDE		121	58-258	MG/DL
LDH		217	118-242	IU/L
SGOT (AST)	HI	41	10-37	IU/L
SGPT (ALT)	HI	45	10-40	IU/L
GGTP	LO	8	11-51	IU/L
ALKALINE PHOSPHATASE		63	39-117	IU/L
BILIRUBIN, TOTAL		0. 3	0. 1-1. 5	MG/DL
ALBUMIN	LO	2. 4	3. 7-5. 2	G/DL
TOTAL PROTEIN	LO	3. 6	6. 0-8. 5	G/DL
ALBUMIN/GLOBULIN RATIO		2. 0	1. 0-2. 2	RATIO

FINAL Report   (Summary)   Page 2 of 2

FIGURE 13-26—cont'd   Clinical laboratory computer-generated laboratory report.

DATE & TIME RECEIVED	ACCESSION NUMBER
10/ 20/ 2000 20: 45	
LOCATION	DATE REPORTED
	10/ 21/ 2000

PHYSICIAN	PATIENT INFORMATION

TEST		RESULTS	REFERENCE RANGE	UNITS
HEMOGRAM	LO	2. 9	4. 5-10. 5	CU. MM.
WHITE BLOOD COUNT	LO	2. 39	4. 40-5. 90	CU. MM.
RED BLOOD COUNT	LO	7. 4	14. 0-18. 0	GM/ 100 ML
HEMOGLOBIN	LO	22. 3	40. 0-52. 0	%
MEAN CORPUSCULAR VOLUME		93	80-100	fL
MEAN CORPUSCULAR HGB		31. 0	27. 0-32. 0	PG
MEAN CORPUSCULAR HGB CONC		33. 2	31. 0-36. 0	%
DIFFERENTIAL, WBC				
SEGMENTED NEUTROPHILS		57	38-80	%
LYMPHOCYTE		29	15-45	%
MONOCYTES		7	1-10	%
EOSINOPHILS		1	0-4	%
BAND NEUTROPHILS	HI	6	0-5	%
ANISOCYTOSIS	ABN	SLIGHT		
HYPOCHROMIA	ABN	SLIGHT		
PLATELET ESTIMATE	ABN	DECREASED		
PARTIAL THROMBOPLASTIN TIME				
PARTIAL THROMBOPLASTIN TIME		31.7	20. 0-40. 0	SECONDS
CONTROL PTT		30. 4	20. 0-40. 0	SECONDS
PROTHROMBIN TIME				
PROTHROMBIN TIME		12. 2	10. 0-13. 5	SECONDS
CONTROL PT		12. 0	11. 0-13. 0	SECONDS
FINAL Report		(Summary)		

FIGURE 13-27   Computer-generated laboratory results for the requisition in Figure 13-24. (Courtesy SmithKline Beecham Clinical Laboratories, Dublin, Calif.)

LABORATORY REPORT

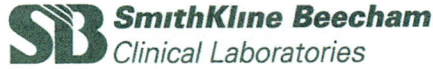
SmithKline Beecham Clinical Laboratories

```
          AREA/ROUTE/STOP: SFB0008
TEST ACCOUNT
6511 GOLDEN GATE DR
DUBLIN CA 94568
```

PATIENT NAME	PATIENT ID	ROOM NO.	AGE	SEX	PHYSICIAN
TEST,TEST					

PAGE	REQUISITION NO.	ACCESSION NO.	LAB REF. #	COLLECTION DATE & TIME	LOG-IN-DATE	REPORT DATE	& TIME
1	0123456	SF571697N			12092000	12092000	6:03PM

REMARKS

REPORT STATUS FINAL	TEST	RESULT IN RANGE	RESULT OUT OF RANGE	UNITS	REFERENCE RANGE	SITE CODE
Date of Birth: NG						
COMPREHENSIVE METABOLIC						SF
PANEL						
	GLUCOSE	98		MG/DL	70-115	
	UREA NITROGEN (BUN)	10		MG/DL	7-25	
	CREATININE	1.0		MG/DL	0.5-1.4	
	BUN/CREATININE RATIO	10		(CALC)	6-25	
	SODIUM	135		MEQ/L	135-146	
	POTASSIUM	4.3		MEQ/L	3.5-5.3	
	CHLORIDE	100		MEQ/L	95-108	
	CALCIUM	9.8		MG/DL	8.5-10.3	
	PROTEIN, TOTAL	8.0		G/DL	6.0-8.5	
	ALBUMIN	4.0		G/DL	3.2-5.0	
	GLOBULIN	4.0		G/DL (CALC)	2.2-4.2	
	ALBUMIN/GLOBULIN RATIO	1.0		(CALC)	0.8-2.0	
	BILIRUBIN, TOTAL	1.0		MG/DL	0.0-1.3	
	ALKALINE PHOSPHATASE	55		U/L	20-125	
	AST (SGOT)	23		U/L	0-42	
CBC (INCLUDES DIFF/PLT)						SF
	WHITE BLOOD CELL COUNT	6.2		THOUS/MCL	3.8-10.8	
	RED BLOOD CELL COUNT	4.80		MILL/MCL	4.40-5.20	
	HEMOGLOBIN	14.7		G/DL	13.8-15.6	
	HEMATOCRIT	43.5		%	41.0-46.0	
	MCV	90.6		FL	80.0-100.0	
	MCH	30.6		PG	27.0-33.0	
	MCHC	34.8		%	32.0-36.0	
	RDW	13.0		%	9.0-15.0	
	PLATELET COUNT	235		THOUS/MCL	130-400	
	ABSOLUTE NEUTROPHILS	4650		CELLS/MCL	1500-7800	
	NEUTROPHILS	75.0		%		
	ABSOLUTE LYMPHOCYTES	930		CELLS/MCL	850-4100	
	LYMPHOCYTES	15		%		
	ABSOLUTE MONOCYTES	434		CELLS/MCL	200-1100	
	MONOCYTES	7.0		%		
	ABSOLUTE EOSINOPHILS	124		CELLS/MCL	50-550	
	EOSINOPHILS	2.0		%		
	ABSOLUTE BASOPHILS	62		CELLS/MCL	0-200	
	BASOPHILS	1.0		%		
URINALYSIS, REFLEX						SF
	COLOR	YELLOW			YELLOW	
	APPEARANCE	CLEAR			CLEAR	
>> REPORT CONTINUED ON NEXT PAGE <<						

INDICATES TESTING SITE SEE REVERSE SIDE ▲

FIGURE 13-27—cont'd   Computer-generated laboratory results for the requisition in Figure 13-24. (Courtesy SmithKline Beecham Clinical Laboratories, Dublin, Calif.)

CONTINUED REPORT

LABORATORY REPORT

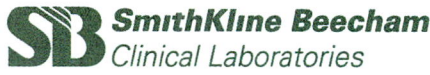

SmithKline Beecham
Clinical Laboratories

AREA/ROUTE/STOP: SFB0008
TEST ACCOUNT
6511 GOLDEN GATE DR
DUBLIN CA 94568

PATIENT NAME TEST, TEST	PATIENT ID	ROOM NO.	AGE	SEX	PHYSICIAN

PAGE 2	REQUISITION NO. 0123456	ACCESSION NO. SF571697N	LAB REF. #	COLLECTION DATE & TIME	LOG-IN-DATE 12092000	REPORT DATE 12092000	& TIME 6:03PM

REMARKS

REPORT STATUS FINAL	TEST	RESULT IN RANGE	OUT OF RANGE	UNITS	REFERENCE RANGE	SITE CODE
	Date of Birth: NG					
	URINALYSIS, REFLEX (CONTINUED)					
	SPECIFIC GRAVITY	1.020			1.001-1.035	
	PH	6.0			4.6-8.0	
	GLUCOSE	NEGATIVE			NEGATIVE	
	BILIRUBIN	NEGATIVE			NEGATIVE	
	KETONES	NEGATIVE			NEGATIVE	
	OCCULT BLOOD	NEGATIVE			NEGATIVE	
	PROTEIN	NEGATIVE			NEGATIVE	
	NITRITE	NEGATIVE			NEGATIVE	
	LEUKOCYTE ESTERASE	NEGATIVE			NEGATIVE	
	>> END OF REPORT <<					

INDICATES TESTING SITE SEE REVERSE SIDE

suspected conditions and also for screening purposes, some of which include a hepatobiliary profile, diabetes profile, cardiac screening, renal function, thyroid function, and arthritis. The grouping of specific tests provides the physician with an overall view of the patient's status that a single test could not provide. An example of a **cardiac profile (panel)** may include a serum aspartate aminotransferase (AST, formerly serum glutamic oxaloacetic transaminase [SGOT]), serum alanine aminotransferase (ALT, formerly serum glutamic pyruvic transaminase [SGPT]), lactic dehydrogenase (LDH), creatine phosphokinase (CPK), complete blood count (CBC), sedimentation rate, prothrombin time (PT), cholesterol, triglycerides, and potassium.

A **kidney function profile** may include total protein, albumin, globulin, albumin/globulin (A/G) ratio, creatinine, blood urea nitrogen (BUN), BUN/creatinine ratio, sodium, potassium, chloride, uric acid, and cholesterol. A **liver function profile** may include alkaline phosphatase, LDH, SGOT, SGPT, total bilirubin, total protein, albumin, globulin, and A/G ratio. (See Tables 13-2 to 13-4 for additional information on some of these tests and others. See also Figures 13-24 to 13-27 and 13-35, *C*.)

QUALITY CONTROL AND LABORATORY SAFETY

See Chapter 10, pp. 463-464.

HEMATOLOGY LABORATORY EXAMINATIONS

COMPLETE BLOOD COUNT: HEMATOLOGY TEST

Because the complete blood count (CBC) is the most common laboratory procedure ordered on blood, it is discussed more fully than other tests. A CBC gives a fairly complete look at the components in blood, providing a wealth of information on a patient's condition. The tests performed in a CBC include **red blood cell (RBC) count, hemoglobin (Hgb), hematocrit (Hct), white blood cell (WBC) count, differential (Diff) white cell count,** and a **stained red cell examination (red cell morphology).** The first four tests are quantitative measurements, and the last two are qualitative. All of these tests are performed on whole blood (Tables 13-2 and 13-3).

TABLE 13–2 Normal Values for a Complete Blood Count Performed on Whole Blood

Test	Values
Red cell count	
Females	4,000,000-5,500,000/mm³ blood
Males	4,500,000-6,000,000/mm³ blood
Hemoglobin	
Females	12-16 g/dl blood
Males	14-18 g/dl blood
Hematocrit	
Females	37%-47%
Males	40%-54%
White cell count	
(females and males)	5000-10,000/mm³ blood
Differential	
Polymorphonuclear neutrophils	60%-70%
Monocytes	2%-6%
Lymphocytes	20%-40%
Eosinophils	1%-4%
Basophils	0.5%-1%
Morphology (stained red cell examination)	Normal
Red blood cell indices	
Mean corpuscular volume (MCV)	80-95 μm³
Mean corpuscular hemoglobin (MCH)	27-31 pg/cell*
Mean corpuscular hemoglobin concentration (MCHC)	32-36 g/dl (or 32%-36%)
Red blood cell distribution width (RDW)	11%-14.5%
Platelets	150,000-400,000/mm³
	or
	200,000-400,000/mm³

*Picomole or micromicrogram.

mm³, Cubic millimeters; *dl*, deciliters (100 milliliters).

TABLE 13-3 Hematology Examinations Made on Blood

Test	Performed on	Normal Values*	Significance
Hematology blood tests			
1. Erythrocyte sedimentation rate (sedrate or ESR)	Whole blood	Wintrobe tubes: Female: 0-20 mm/hr Male: 0-9 mm/hr Westergren Female and male: 0-20 mm/hr	**Increased** in almost all infections, myocardial infarction, active rheumatoid arthritis, pulmonary infarction, shock, surgical operations, and pregnancy. **Decreased** in sickle cell anemia, polycythemia, cardiac decompensation, and newborn infants.
2. Microhematocrit (HCTM) or Hct	Whole blood	Female: 37%-47% Male: 40%-54%	Same as for regular hematocrit (see p. 604).
3. Reticulocytes (immature RBCs)	Whole blood	0.5%-1.55% of all RBCs in peripheral whole blood	**Increased** when bone marrow is manufacturing RBCs at an increased rate. May be seen in patients with acute or chronic hemorrhage or in sickle cell anemia. Normally elevated in infants and pregnant women. **Decreased** in aplastic and pernicious anemia.
4. Coagulation tests and platelets			
a. Bleeding time	Capillary whole blood	1-9 minutes (Ivy method)	**Increased** time indicates platelet deficiency, which may be due to pernicious anemia, aplastic anemia, acute leukemias, hemorrhagic disease of the newborn, multiple myeloma, chronic lymphocytic leukemia, and Hodgkin's disease.
b. Clot retraction time	Venous blood	30-60 min	**Prolonged** time seen in primary or secondary thrombocytopenia caused by aplastic or pernicious anemia, Hodgkin's disease, multiple myeloma, acute leukemia, and hemorrhagic disease of the newborn.
c. Coagulation or clotting time	Blood	Lee-White: 6-10 min Capillary tube: 3-7 min	Used as a measurement of ability of blood to clot properly. May indicate that vitamin K or calcium levels are inadequate for clotting of blood.
d. Fibrinogen (quantitative)	Blood plasma	200-600 mg/dl	**Increase** seen in inflammatory processes, infections, pregnancy, menstruation, and after x-ray treatment. **Decreases** noted in liver diseases, anemia, and severe malnutrition.
e. Platelet count	Whole blood	150,000 or 200,000-400,000/mm³ blood	**Decreased** numbers may indicate disease of the spleen; also will cause bleeding.
f. Partial thromboplastin test (PTT)	Blood plasma	Abnormal thromboplastin formation 60-70 seconds	This test is used to differentiate blood coagulation abnormalities. **Increased** in cirrhosis, Vitamin K deficiency, leukemia. **Decreased** in extensive cancer.
5. Prothrombin time (PT or Pro-Time)	Blood plasma	70%-110% of control value Average 11-12.5 seconds	Prolonged time may indicate vitamin K deficiency, liver disease, or an excessive use of dicumarol in treatment. When anticoagulation therapy used, PT kept at from 2 to 2½ times normal.
6. Bone marrow	Marrow aspirated from iliac crest or sternum, then placed on a slide and stained for examination	Various primitive cells are found	Abnormal cell findings may indicate a blood disorder such as leukemia.

dl, Deciliters (100 milliliters).

Additional tests that some laboratories include on a CBC are the **RBC indices** and a **platelet count.** The RBC indices include a mean corpuscular volume (MCV), a mean corpuscular hemoglobin (MCH), and a mean corpuscular hemoglobin concentration (MCHC) and a red blood cell distribution width (RDW) (see Table 13-2). The results of the RBC count, hemoglobin, and hematocrit are necessary to calculate the RBC indices.

Red Cell Count

The red cell count is the number of RBCs found in each cubic millimeter of blood. *Manual counting* may be used in some medical settings, but real care must be taken to minimize errors. *Determination with the automated counting equipment is considered more accurate.* **Elevated** red cell counts indicate **polycythemia** or that the patient has moved to a location with a higher altitude, where the air contains less oxygen. In the latter case, the body requires more red cells to carry sufficient oxygen to meet its needs. **Decreased** numbers of red cells are seen in patients with some form of **anemia,** after a hemorrhage, and also after the initial hemoconcentration of shock.

Hemoglobin

A hemoglobin test determines the oxygen-carrying ability of the blood. It is a simple and most efficient method to detect any **anemia** (pernicious, iron deficiency, sickle cell) and the severity of the condition. It also helps the physician determine the effectiveness of treatments administered to the patient. A patient is considered anemic if the hemoglobin value is below 12 mg/dl. **Low hemoglobin** values are also caused by hemorrhage. **Elevated concentrations** of hemoglobin may be seen in severely burned or dehydrated patients because the body has lost considerable amounts of fluid; thus the red cells are suspended in less fluid, and more hemoglobin is present in each deciliter (100 milliliters) of blood.

Hematocrit

The hematocrit, or packed-cell volume, represents the percentage of RBCs in the total blood volume. **Elevated hematocrits** are seen in patients with **polycythemia; a low hematocrit** is seen in **anemia** and **leukemia.** *Generally the hematocrit and hemoglobin concentrations are related.* Each 1% hematocrit contains 0.34 g of hemoglobin; the hematocrit should equal 3 times the hemoglobin within 3%. Thus if a patient's hemoglobin is 14 g/dl, the hematocrit should fall between 39% and 45% ($14 \times 3 = 42$, and plus or minus 3 = 39% to 45%). Deviation from this relationship usually indicates the presence of red cells of abnormal size or hemoglobin content.

White Blood Cell Count

The WBC count is the number of WBCs found in each cubic millimeter of blood. As with the red cell count, automated equipment now provides a more reliable count. A person's white count varies somewhat during a day because of exercise, emotional states, or digestion. Increases as great as 2000 WBC/mm³ may be seen in these situations. Pathologically, the WBC count **increases** in infections and leukemia. **Decreased** WBC count may be caused by radiation therapy, immunosuppressive therapy (chemotherapy) for cancer and transplant patients, toxic reactions, measles, typhoid fever, and infection hepatitis. This is the result of a depression of the bone marrow's blood-forming centers.

Differential White Cell Count

The differential is a test that determines the percentage of each of the five different types of WBCs in the blood. Each type of white cell has a specific function. Together with the degree of increase or decrease in the total number of white cells and with the percentage of each type of white cell, the physician is able to make a more definite diagnosis. Characteristic abnormal numbers and types of white cells are seen in various diseases (Figure 13-28).

Neutrophils. The body's **primary lines of defense** against infection are the neutrophils. They seek and destroy any invading bacteria by the process of phagocytosis. **Increased** numbers of neutrophils are seen in conditions such as appendicitis, tonsillitis, pneumonia, abscesses, granulocytic leukemia, and meningitis. A **decreased** neutrophil count (neutropenia) is seen in mumps, hepatitis, measles, aplastic anemia, agranulocytosis, and also in patients who are taking certain drugs such as certain antibiotics, antihistamines, anticonvulsants, and sulfonamides. In these cases the decease in the neutrophils causes an increase in one of the other WBCs, especially in the lymphocytes. Thus the actual value for each of the five types of WBCs must be known to determine if this is the case.

Monocytes. The body's **second line of defense** against invasion by foreign substances is the monocytes. These are also phagocytes because they ingest any foreign particles or bacteria that the neutrophils are unable to. The monocytes also clean up any cellular debris that remains after an infection or abscess subsides. **Increased** numbers of monocytes are seen in patients who have tuberculosis, amebic dysentery, typhoid fever, Rocky Mountain spotted fever, subacute bacterial endocarditis, or monocytic leukemia or in those patients who are recovering from a bacterial infection. Conditions with **decreased** numbers of monocytes are difficult to indicate because the normal count of the cells is so low.

Lymphocytes. The lymphocytes circulate through the body to destroy the toxic products of protein metabolism and to identify and produce antibodies against foreign cells. Recent studies are identifying new roles for these cells, especially in the field of immunology. **Increased** numbers of lymphocytes (lymphocytosis) are seen in viral diseases such as influenza, German measles, mumps, whooping cough, and infectious mononucleosis, as well as in lymphocytic leukemia. **Decreased** numbers are seen in patients who are taking cortisone, adrenocorticotropic hormone (ACTH), and epinephrine. Other types of leukemia and radiation also cause lymphopenia.

Eosinophils and Basophils. Little is known about the eosinophils and basophils. It is thought that the eosinophils

FIGURE 13-28 Main types of leukocytes. **A,** Granulocytes-neutrophils: segmented neutrophils are round or oval cells. The cytoplasm is a lavender or pink color, with pinkish or lavender granules. The nucleus is segmented, having from 2 to 12 segments, but usually 3 or 4, and it stains a purplish or lavender color. **B,** Stab neutrophils are round or oval, with a cytoplasm similar in color to that of the segmented neutrophils. It contains fine granules that are pinkish or reddish violet. The nucleus is one continuous piece that looks like a flexible rod. It commonly forms letter shapes such as C, N, S, and U. The nucleus is colored a dark purple or lavender and occupies about one fourth of the cell. **C,** Juvenile neutrophils are round or oval, and cytoplasm is usually a bluish pink, containing granules that may be definite or fine and purplish or reddish. The nucleus is bean shaped, usually purplish, and usually occupies about half the cell (juvenile neutrophil also appears at bottom of panel B). Not shown, myelocyte neutrophil cytoplasm often takes an almost neutral stain, tinged with blue; and it, as well as the nucleus, is dotted with definite pinkish or purple granules. The nucleus is round or oval, ordinarily stains bluish purple, and takes up about two thirds of the cell. **D,** Granulocytes-eosinophils. Eosinophil cytoplasm has light blue tinges and is covered with coarse, round, or oval bright pink or red granules. The nucleus is usually segmented and stains a deep lavender to light blue. **E,** Lymphocyte cytoplasm is usually a bright blue and at times may be almost negligible, as the purple or lavender nucleus may take up almost the entire cell. Immature lymphocytes are larger than mature cells, having much more cytoplasm, which generally stains a very pale, glasslike blue. Occasionally a few pink granules may appear in the cytoplasm. The nucleus is usually round or oval but may be indented as well. It stains a purple or lavender color. **F,** Monocytes are the largest of all the white cells. Often they are quite irregular in shape and usually take a pale stain. The cytoplasm is usually a smoky blue-gray, sometimes sprinkled with a fine pink dust. The nucleus generally is kidney shaped or round, often lobulated, staining a lavender color.

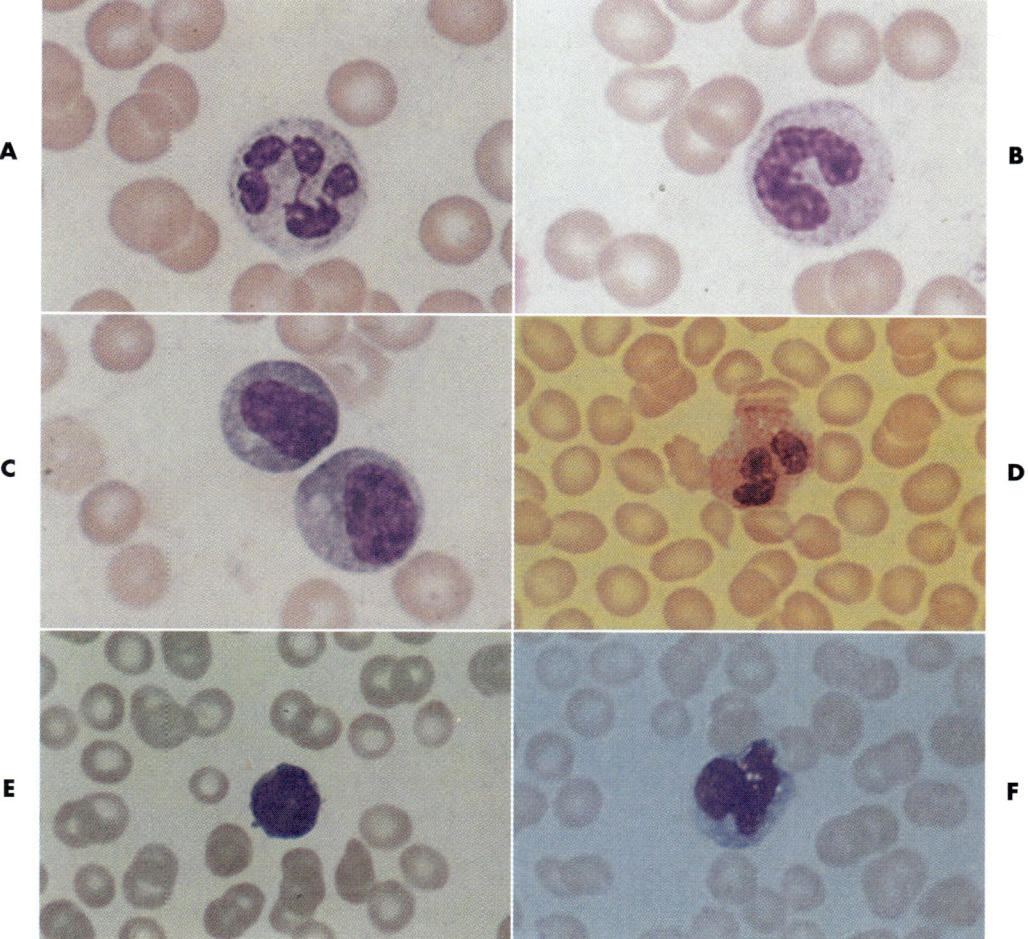

aid in detoxification by breaking down protein material and that they are associated with allergic reactions and production of antihistamine. **Increased** eosinophil counts are seen in patients who have hay fever, allergies, skin diseases, parasite infections, and asthma. **Decreased** counts are seen in patients who have increased levels of insulin, epinephrine, and ACTH. Stress following surgery may also cause eosinopenia.

Basophils are thought to produce heparin and histamine; thus some believe that they help prevent blood from clotting in inflamed tissues and play a role in clot breakdown. **Increased**

basophil counts are seen in patients who have hemolytic anemias or chronic granulocytic leukemia and who have had their spleen removed (splenectomy) and exposure to radiation. **Decreased** conditions have been identified in hyperthyroidism, acute allergic reactions, and in patients who are on steroid therapy.

Abnormal White Cells

The five types of white cells just discussed are all normal cells found in peripheral blood. In some disorders and diseases, immature neutrophils or atypical lymphocytes are seen. The *immature* neutrophils are myeloblasts, promyelocytes, myelocytes, metamyelocytes, and band cells. You will see these terms on some laboratory reports included with a differential report.

The first four types of these **immature neutrophils** are seen in certain forms of leukemia. The **band or stab cells** are immature forms of neutrophils that enter the circulation early when neutrophil production is stimulated significantly. The presence of these cells is referred to as a "shift to the left" in WBC production and indicates an ongoing acute bacterial infection.

Stained Red Cell Examination

Using the same stained slide that was used for determining the differential, the laboratory technologist then examines the RBCs for any variation in size, shape, structure, color, or content. **Anisocytosis** (variable and abnormal size[s]), **macrocytosis, microcytosis,** and **poikilocytosis** (abnormal degree of variation in shape) are reported as slight, moderate, or marked.

Classifying RBCs according to these variations is very helpful when determining the causes of anemia and other diseases. Small RBCs (**microcytes**) are seen in iron deficiencies and thalassemia; larger RBCs (**macrocytes**) are seen in vitamin B_{12} or folic acid deficiency and sometimes with liver disorders; **abnormal shapes** are present in sickle cell anemia, acquired immunohemolytic anemia, uremia, bleeding ulcer, and liver disease; color (pale) abnormalities are seen in cardiac disease, iron deficiency, and thalassemia, and more color will be seen with an increase of hemoglobin, as seen in dehydration.

Red Blood Cell Indices

The red blood cell indices include the **mean corpuscular volume (MCV),** the **mean corpuscular hemoglobin (MCH),** the **mean corpuscular hemoglobin concentration (MCHC),** and the **red blood cell distribution width (RDW).** These tests are valuable when classifying the different types of anemia. The red blood cell indices provide information about the average volume or size (MCV and RDW) of a single RBC, the average amount or weight of hemoglobin (MCH) within an RBC, and the average concentration or percentage of hemoglobin (MCHC) in a single RBC.

- An **increase** in the MCV is seen in liver disease, alcoholism, pernicious anemia, and folic acid deficiency. A **decrease** in MCV is seen in thalassemia (a hemolytic anemia) and iron deficiency anemia.
- An **increase** in MCH is seen in macrocytic anemia, and a **decrease** is seen in microcytic and hypochromic anemia.
- An **increase** in MCHC is seen in intravascular hemolysis, and a **decrease** occurs in iron deficiency anemia and thalassemia.
- An **increase** in RDW is seen in iron deficiency anemia, vitamin B_{12} or folate deficiency anemia, sickle cell anemia, hemolytic anemia, and posthemorrhagic anemia.

Platelets

The platelet count is the number of platelets (**thrombocytes**) per cubic millimeter of blood. Platelets are essential for the blood to clot. **Elevated** numbers of platelets are seen in malignant disorders, rheumatoid arthritis, iron deficiency anemia, and postsplenectomy syndrome. **Decreased** numbers of platelets are seen in hemorrhage, hemolytic anemia, infection, leukemia, cancer chemotherapy, and pernicious anemia.

Summary

As you can see, the significant findings obtained from a CBC are numerous. Evaluation of these findings, along with the total clinical picture of a patient's condition, provides the physician with valuable information for screening, diagnosing, treating, or evaluating and monitoring the progress of treatment for patient care.

Copper Sulfate Relative Density Test for Screening Anemia and a Hematocrit Test

Gross screening tests to determine if a patient has a sufficient volume of RBCs can be done by performing a relative density test with a few drops of blood in a copper sulfate solution. This test can indicate if a patient may have a reduced capacity to produce RBCs, a problem with any blood loss, or an insufficient diet for the adequate production and functioning of RBCs. This test is based on the fact that RBCs are the heaviest portion of blood. The copper sulfate solution is prepared so that the density of this solution is equal to that of blood, with 37% RBCs for women and 47% RBCs for men. These two figures are the normal lower limits for the percentage of RBCs in women and men, thus allowing you to divide all patients screened by this method into two groups—those above and those below the lower limit. When the results of this test indicate a volume of RBCs in the blood below the normal range, it should be followed by a more precise test (that is, a hematocrit). The hematocrit (Hct) represents the volume percentage of RBCs present in whole blood. The normal ranges for a hematocrit are 37% to 47% for women and 40% to 54% for men. Both of these tests are important aids to the physician when diagnosing and treating patients with anemia. They are relatively simple and can easily be performed in the physician's office or health agency.

Hemoglobin Determination With the HemoCue System

The HemoCue System is a portable instrument that uses a photometer to measure hemoglobin from a small volume of undiluted blood (0.01 ml). Venous, arterial, or capillary blood samples can be used. The measurement of whole blood hemoglobin is the most precise and useful laboratory test for distinguishing between **anemia,** normal hemoglobin, and **polycythemia.** Hemoglobin has been shown to be a more accurate and sensitive diagnostic tool than hematocrit in anemia detection. It is also the preferred procedure for following the status of a patient in various clinical situations, such as when monitoring the effects of epoetin alfa (a drug used for anemia secondary to chemotherapy, anemia secondary to zidovudine (AZT) treatment in HIV-positive patients, and anemia that is also seen in patients with chronic renal failure), in patients following transfusions, to determine hemoglobin levels in a person before he

Text continued on p. 610

HEALTH MATTERS

KEEPING YOUR PATIENTS INFORMED

IRON-DEFICIENT ANEMIA

Are you tired much of the time? Do you feel weak and have decreased activity tolerance? Do you constantly look pale? Do you have swollen and bleeding gums?

These are common complaints often heard from people who have iron deficiency anemia. Anemia is a decrease of hemoglobin in the blood to below the normal ranges (women: 12 to 16 g/dl; men: 14 to 18 g/dl). Any process that alters or decreases hemoglobin decreases the oxygen-carrying ability of the blood. Only about 3% of the required oxygen in the body is dissolved in the blood plasma. Hemoglobin carries the other 97% of the oxygen to the tissues.

Iron deficiency anemia is most often caused by inadequate supplies of iron in the blood, which is needed to synthesize hemoglobin. The shortage of iron could be caused by decreased intake of iron-rich foods, by an increased need for iron, by poor absorption of iron in the digestive tract, or by chronic blood loss. Iron deficiency anemia is the most common type of anemia worldwide and occurs most often in children, women, and the elderly, especially in underdeveloped countries.

As the condition develops, iron loss exceeds intake, and the iron stored in the bone marrow is used and depleted. This in turn leads to insufficient iron for red blood cell formation. With fewer red blood cells, there is decreased production of hemoglobin, smaller than normal red blood cells, and a decrease of oxygenation in the body tissues.

Diagnosis of iron deficiency anemia is confirmed with blood studies. Treatment is aimed at correcting the cause, which involves iron replacement with ferrous sulfate, the oral form being preferred (it can also be given by injection). It also includes increased dietary intake of iron-rich foods, such as meats, poultry, fish, green leafy vegetables, legumes such as lima beans and green peas, iron-enriched breads and cereals (also see Chapter 18), and nutritional education.

Ferrous sulfate should be taken with food because it can be irritating to the stomach and may cause some nausea. It also causes the stool to turn black and can be constipating. Increased intake of water and dietary fiber helps to prevent constipation. A list of foods rich in iron and written information about anemia should be provided to the patient.

Within 2 months the anemia is usually corrected, but often therapy is continued for another 4 months to replace tissue stores.

PROCEDURE 13-3

RELATIVE DENSITY TEST AND A HEMATOCRIT TEST

Objective

Understand and demonstrate the correct procedure for obtaining a blood specimen by doing a skin puncture; performing a copper sulfate relative density test and a hematocrit test; and recording the procedure and results on the patient's chart.

Equipment

- Sterile alcohol swabs
- Clean gauze pads
- Sterile disposable lancets
- Capillary tubes (heparinized and nonheparinized)

Copper sulfate ($CuSO_4$) solution for anemia testing for women and men
Clean containers to hold the $CuSO_4$ solution
Tray of a sealing compound (for example, Seal-ease or Critoseal)
Microhematocrit centrifuge
Microhematocrit reading card
Capillary bulbs (small rubber bulbs that fit over the capillary tube)
Disposable, single-use examination gloves

PROCEDURE

1. **Wash your hands. Use appropriate personal protective equipment (PPE) as dictated by facility.**

2. Assemble and prepare equipment and supplies for use. Fill a container approximately two-thirds full with the $CuSO_4$ solution. Cover the $CuSO_4$ solution when not in use; do not expose it to direct sunlight or freezing temperatures or allow it to evaporate. When doing multiple tests, change the solution after testing 15 patients.

3. Identify the patient and explain the procedure.

RATIONALE

Continued

PROCEDURE 13-3

RELATIVE DENSITY TEST AND A HEMATOCRIT TEST—cont'd

4. **Don gloves.**

5. Perform a skin puncture on the fingertip (see steps 1 to 12 in Fingertip Skin Puncture Using a Lancet, pp. 584-585).

6. Once blood flows freely, use a nonheparinized capillary tube to receive blood. Fill the tube to approximately three quarters. You may hold the tube in a horizontal position or slightly lower when filling the tube (Figure 13-29).

7. Apply pressure over the puncture site with a clean, dry gauze pad. Dispose of pad with blood on it in a container labeled for biohazardous waste. You may have the patient do this while you attend to the test.

8. Hold the capillary tube vertically over the container of $CuSO_4$ to allow the blood to drop into the solution. If the blood does not drop into the solution, apply the capillary bulb to the tube, then squeeze the bulb to force blood into the solution (Figure 13-30, *A* and *B*).

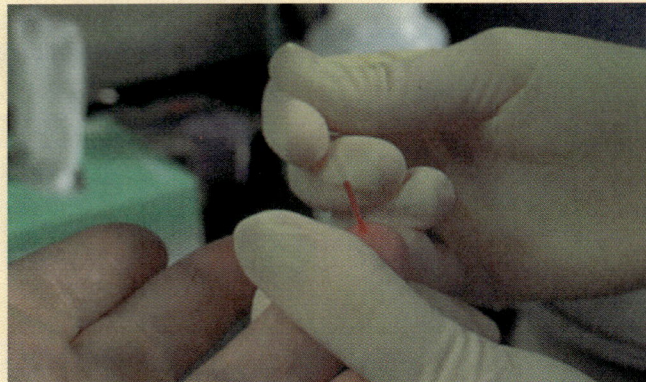

FIGURE 13-29 Use a nonheparinized capillary tube to receive blood. Hold the tube horizontally to or slightly lower than the blood on the finger.

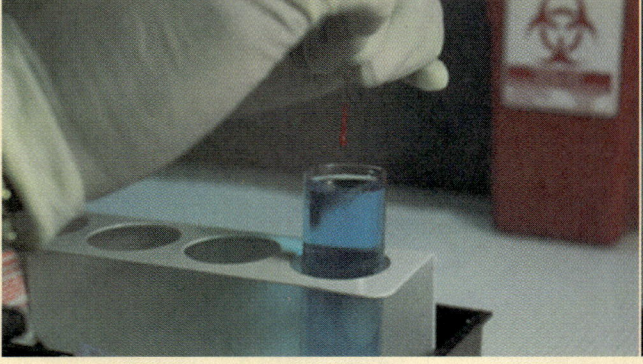
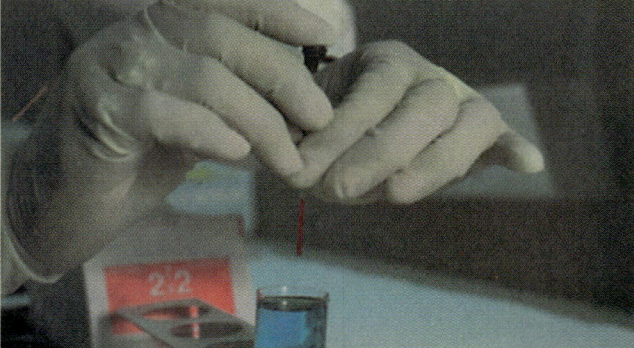

FIGURE 13-30 **A,** Hold the capillary tube vertically over the container of copper sulfate to allow the blood to drop into the solution. **B,** Apply a capillary bulb to the tube if the blood does not drop into the solution, then squeeze the bulb to force blood into the solution.

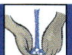

RELATIVE DENSITY TEST AND A HEMATOCRIT TEST—cont'd

9. Determine the test result. One of three reactions will occur:

  a. Blood drops through the solution without hesitating or rising.

  b. Blood hesitates and then drops through the solution.

  c. Blood hesitates, rises to the top of the solution, and eventually drops through the solution.

Result indication:

There are enough RBCs present in the blood. Record the results as "normal."

There may not be enough RBCs; a hematocrit test should be performed.

There are probably not enough RBCs present; a hematocrit test should be performed.

10. **When a hematocrit test is indicated:**

  a. Swab the finger with a sponge, then "milk" the finger, and, using the same puncture site, obtain another blood sample in a heparinized tube. Fill calibrated tubes to the calibration line. Fill uncalibrated tubes to approximately three quarters (within 10 to 20 mm of the end of the tube).

  b. Seal the dry end of the tube with a sealing compound by sticking it into the sealing compound tray (Figure 13-31).

The tube must be sealed to prevent blood leaking from the tube in the centrifuge. Sealing is not necessary when using a self-sealing microhematocrit tube.

  c. Place the tube into a slot in the microhematocrit centrifuge, with the sealed end down facing the outside of the centrifuge (sealed end toward the outer rim) (Figure 13-32). For balance, place another tube in a slot on the opposite side.

This tube position prevents leakage of blood when the centrifuge is turned on.

  d. Close and secure the lid of the centrifuge.

  e. Adjust the timer and spin down for 5 minutes at the speed of 10,000 rpm.

Centrifuging the blood samples causes the RBCs to settle at the bottom of the capillary tube.

  f. Using the scale provided on the centrifuge or the microhematocrit card, read the results as a percentage (Figure 13-33). Allow the centrifuge to come to a complete stop before you open the lid.

  g. Dispose of contaminated materials properly. Dispose of capillary tubes in puncture-resistant disposable sharps container labeled Biohazard. Any sponges with blood on them must be disposed of in a container for biohazardous waste.

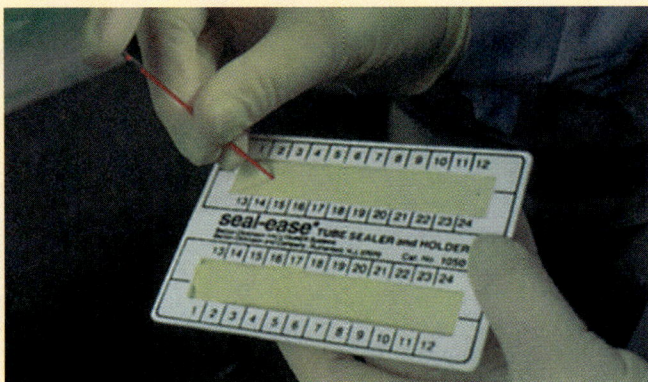

FIGURE 13-31   For a hematocrit test, take the capillary tube filled with blood and seal the dry end with a commercial sealing compound (for example, Seal-ease or Critoseal) or putty by sticking it into the clay tray.

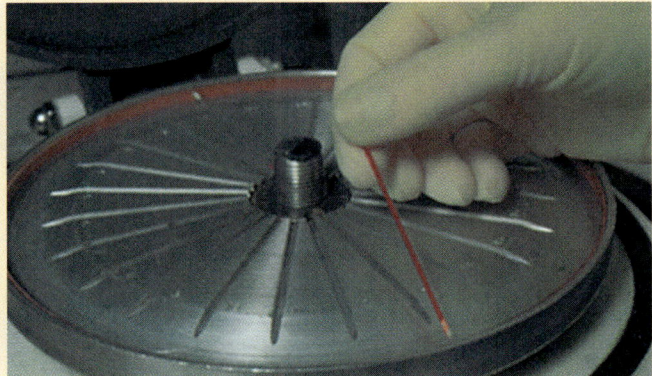

FIGURE 13-32   Place tube into a slot in the microhematocrit centrifuge. The sealed end of the tube should face the outside of the centrifuge.

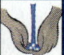

PROCEDURE 13-3

RELATIVE DENSITY TEST AND A HEMATOCRIT TEST—cont'd

11. Remove gloves.

12. Wash your hands.

13. Record the results.

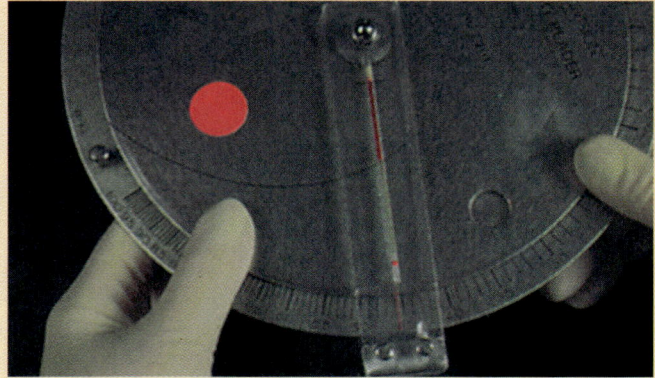

FIGURE 13-33   Read the results, using the scale on the centrifuge or on a microhematocrit card or reader.

Charting Example

April 26, 20__, 12 PM

Skin puncture done on second finger, left hand. CuSO^4 test done, and hematocrit was indicated. Hct: 34%

Anne Kaelberer, CMA

or

CuSO$_4$ test indicated need for Hct.

Hct: 34%

---

or she donates blood, in hemolysis, in hemorrhage, and also in dehydration or other shifts of plasma volume.

To measure the hemoglobin with this system, you fill a microcuvette with blood by capillary action and place this microcuvette on a slide, and the machine gives a digital readout in approximately 45 seconds. The HemoCue microcuvette is made of unbreakable plastic. Once used, you discard it in a biohazard waste container. The instrument is calibrated at the factory and is supplied with a control cuvette, which provides a simple check to ensure that the instrument is operating properly. See Figure 13-34 for the procedure for using the HemoCue instrument. The supplies and technique for performing the skin puncture are the same as was discussed previously in this chapter.

BLOOD CHEMISTRY LABORATORY EXAMINATIONS

BLOOD CHEMISTRIES

Some basic blood chemistries can be performed easily in the physician's office with the use of chemically impregnated reagent strips to determine the presence of blood glucose and blood urea nitrogen (BUN) (also see Table 13-4 and Table 13-5). (Blood glucose testing is more accurate than urine tests for glucose and is especially valuable in the management of diabetes.) In addition, compact and economical instruments are

available on the market, such as the *Ames Seralyzer Blood Chemistry Analyzer*. This instrument is a reflectance photometer that gives accurate quantitative results from blood serum or plasma for 15 routine diagnostic tests. Reflectance photometers measure light intensity to determine the exact amount of a substance present in a specimen. Blood chemistries, certain therapeutic drug assays (TDAs), and electrolytes are determined using special reagent test strips. The blood chemistry analyzer is particularly useful in the physician's office when on-site testing is desirable so that test results can be viewed as an aid to prompt decision making, often while the patient is still in the office. Most tests require less that 15 minutes of elapsed time, averaging 2 minutes of operator time. Once the test strip is placed on the specimen table, you can read the test results on the digital display in less than 2 minutes. Complete instructions for specimen collection, preparation, and use are supplied with the instrument. *Always* **check the expiration date** on the container of reagent strips because outdated reagent strips may produce false or inaccurate test results.

Another easy-to-operate, in-office chemistry analyzer performing 16 tests using reagent strips is the *Reflotron Plus System* (Figure 13-35). The Reflotron Plus System has a keyboard for entering patient data and test information and editing information to show patients how risks for certain conditions can be lowered by compliance with treatment recommendations. You place a drop of blood on the test pad on the reagent strip and insert the strip into the analyzer, and printed results are ready in

Text continued on p. 615

FIGURE 13-34   HemoCue test to determine blood hemoglobin and blood glucose. (Courtesy HemoCue, Mission Viejo, Calif.)

Capillary sampling technique using finger stick. Take the cuvette out of the container. **Reseal the container immediately.**

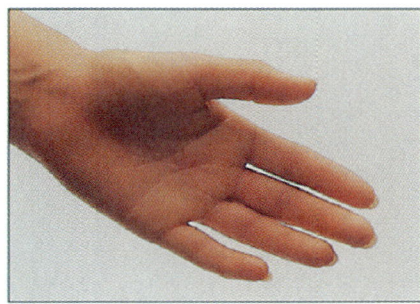

1. Make sure that the patient sits comfortably. The hand should be warm and relaxed. It is a good idea to heat cold hands in warm water before sampling. This increases the blood circulation. The patient´s fingers should be straight but not tense, to avoid stasis.

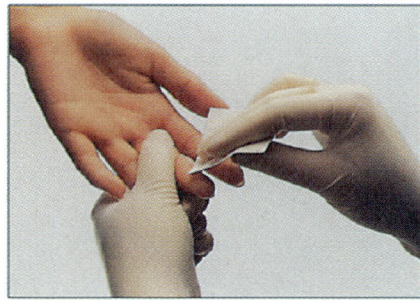

2. For best result use the middle finger or the ring finger for sampling. Avoid fingers with rings for sampling. Clean the puncture site with disinfectant and allow it to dry.

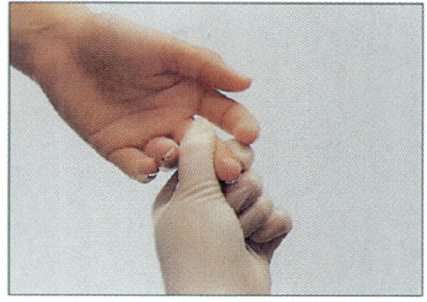

3. Using your thumb, lightly press the finger from the top of the knuckle to the tip. This stimulates the blood flow towards the sampling point.

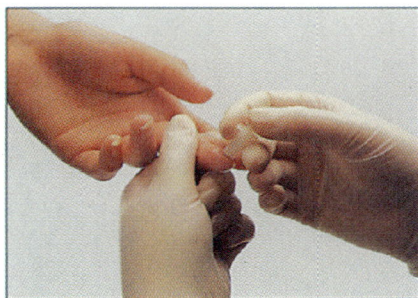

4. With the thumb's gentle pressure at the tip of the finger, prick at the side of the fingertip.
Not only is the blood flow at its best at this point, it also causes the least pain.

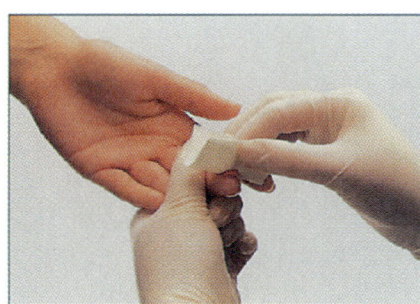

5. Wipe away the first two or three drops of blood. This stimulates the blood flow. If necessary, apply light pressure again, until another drop of blood appears. Avoid "milking."

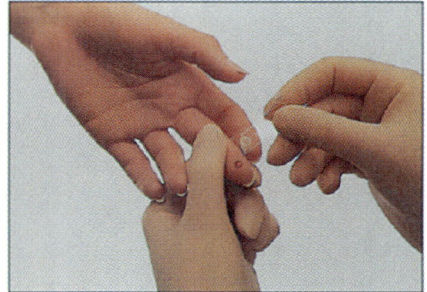

6. Make sure that the drop of blood is big enough to fill the cuvette completely. Introduce the cuvette tip into the middle of the drop.

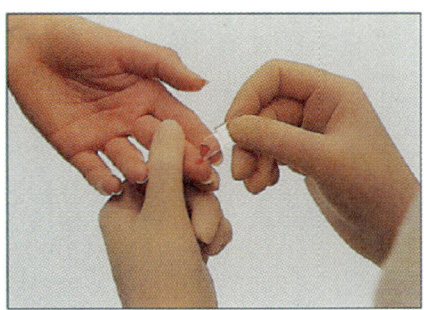

7. Fill the cuvette in one continuous process. It should never be topped up after the first filling.

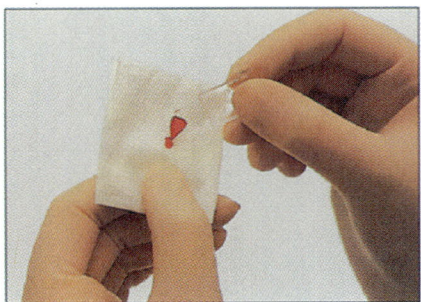

8. Wipe off the excess blood on the outside of the cuvette tip. Make sure that no blood is drawn out of the cuvette in this procedure.

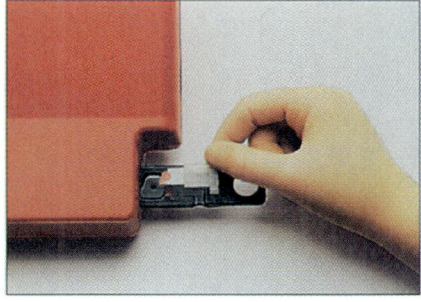

9. Place the filled cuvette into the cuvette holder immediately and push it into measuring position.

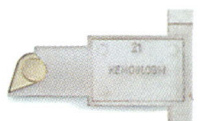

HemoCue Blood Hemoglobin Microcuvette.

The filled cuvette should be analyzed immediately and at the latest 10 minutes - after it has been filled.

Note: If a second sample is to be taken from the same fingerstick, it is important that this should be done immediately after the first sample has been taken. Wipe away the remains of the first drop of blood and take a second sample from a new drop of blood.

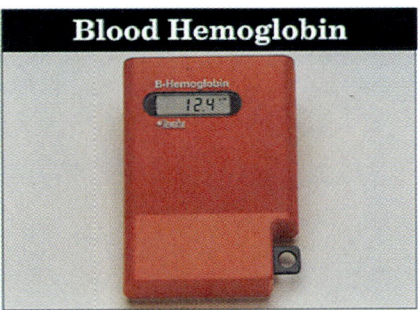

Blood Hemoglobin

10a. After approximately 15–45 seconds the result is displayed.

Blood Glucose

10b. Blood glucose results are displayed after 40-240 seconds.

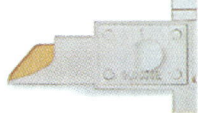

HemoCue Blood Glucose Microcuvette.

The cuvette should be analyzed within 40 seconds after being filled. It is not possible to remeasure a cuvette. Cuvette containers must be stored in a refrigerator when not in use.

TABLE 13-4   **Blood Chemistry Examinations**

Test	Performed on	Normal Values*	Significance
Blood chemistries			
1. Calcium (Ca++)	Blood serum	9-11.5 mg/dl	**Increased** in chronic nephritis with uremia, bone tumors including metastatic cancer of bone, hyperparathyroidism, Addison's disease, adenoma of parathyroids, emphysema, cardiac decompensation.
2. Inorganic phosphorus (Inor phos)	Blood serum	3-4.5 mg/dl	**Increased** in uremia, Bright's disease, excessive vitamin D intake, and hypoparathyroidism.
3. Glucose	Blood serum	80-120 mg/dl	**Increased** in diabetes mellitus. **Decreased** in hypoglycemia and after excessive insulin.
4. Blood urea nitrogen (BUN)	Blood serum	10-20 mg/dl	**Increased** in some kidney diseases, for example, glomerulonephritis, pyelonephritis, acute tubular necrosis, and urinary obstruction from a tumor or stones. Also increased in dehydration, gastrointestinal bleeding, shock, and gout. **Decreased levels** seen in liver damage, malnutrition, protein deficiency, and overhydration.
5. Uric acid	Blood serum	2.5-8 mg/dl	**Increased** in leukemia, gout, acidosis, toxemia, alcoholism, stress, lead poisoning, renal failure, diabetes mellitus.

6. Cholesterol	Blood serum	Up to 20 yr: 120-230 mg/dl
		30 yr: 120-240 mg/dl
		40 yr: 140-240 mg/dl
		50 yr: 150-240 mg/dl
		60 yr: 160-240 mg/dl
		100 yr: 160-240 mg/dl
		NATIONAL GUIDELINES
		Desirable: less than 200 mg/dl
		Borderline high: 200-239 mg/dl
		High: 240 mg/dl or higher
		Most physicians recommend that patients with levels higher than 200 take steps to reduce cholesterol to reduce the risk of coronary artery disease.
		BLOOD LIPIDS, LIPID PROFILE
		NOTE: These categories apply to people 20 years and older.
		• Total lipids: 400-1000 mg/dl
		• Cholesterol: 150-240 mg/dl
		• Triglycerides: 40-150 mg/dl
		• Phospholipids: 150-380 mg/dl
		• Cholesterol lipoproteins:
		  HDL: 45 mg/dl (men)
		     55 mg/dl (women)
		  VLDL: 25%-50%
		  LDL: 60-180 mg/dl
		• Cholesterol to HDL ratio
		  Male: ≤ 5.0 is desirable
		  Female: ≤ 4.4 is desirable
			Increased in cardiovascular disease, atherosclerosis, liver disease with obstructive jaundice, nephrosis, diabetes mellitus, hypothyroidism, and in diets too high in saturated fat or cholesterol. **Decreased** in anemia, malabsorption, hyperthyroidism, and hepatic failure.
			
			Increased HDL levels suggest a decreased risk of coronary artery disease. These tests are also used to help determine dietary treatment for heart patients.
			
			Increased LDL levels have been associated with coronary artery disease. Indicator of average risk for coronary heart disease.

	Test	Specimen	Normal Value	Clinical Significance
7.	Total protein (TP)	Blood serum	6-8 g/dl	**Increased** in dehydration, malignancy, hepatic disease, infection. **Decreased** levels in overhydration, hepatic insufficiency, burns, malnutrition, nephrosis.
8.	Albumin (Alb)	Blood serum	3.5-5.5 g/dl	**Increase** seen in dehydration. **Decreased** in overhydration, hepatic insufficiency, malnutrition, burns, nephrosis.
9.	Total bilirubin (indirect) (TB)	Blood serum	0.2-1.2 mg/dl	**Increase** seen in hemolysis, hepatic disease, obstructive jaundice, pulmonary infarct.
10.	Alkaline phosphatase (phos)	Blood serum	2-4.5 Bodansky units 4-13 King Armstrong units 20-90 IU/L	**Increased** in children and in women in the third trimester of pregnancy; in hepatic disease, obstructive jaundice, bone growth, osteoblastic bone tumors, peptic ulcer, and colitis. **Decreased** in hypothyroidism, anemia, malnutrition, pernicious anemia.
11.	Lactic dehydrogenase (LDH)	Blood serum	90-200 IU/L	**Increased** in myocardial infarction, muscle necrosis, hemolysis, kidney infarct, liver disease, and cerebral damage.
12.	Serum aspartate amino-transferase (AST), formerly SGOT (serum glutamic oxaloacetic transaminase)	Blood serum	10-49 IU/L or 12-36 U/ml	**Very high levels** seen 24 hr after a myocardial infarction, in liver disease, complete biliary obstruction and jaundice with hepatic cirrhosis. **Increased** in skeletal trauma, hemolysis, cerebral damage. **Lower levels** seen in pregnancy, chronic dialysis, beri beri.
13.	Serum alanine aminotrans-ferase (ALT), formerly serum glutamic pyruvic transaminase (SGPT)	Blood serum	5-35 IU/L	**Increased** in liver dysfunction. AST and ALT levels are frequently compared. The AST/ALT ratio is usually greater than one in alcoholic cirrhosis, metabolic tumor to the liver, and liver congestion. Ratios below one may occur in patients with viral hepatitis, acute hepatitis, and infectious mononucleosis.
14.	Serum phosphate (phosphorus)	Blood serum	Adults: 2.5-4.5 mg/dl Children: 3.5-5.8 mg/dl	**Increased** in renal failure, hypoparathyroidism, or increased dietary intake. **Decreased** in inadequate dietary intake, chronic antacid ingestion, hyperparathyroidism, and hypercalcemia.
15.	Potassium (K)	Blood serum	3.5-5.5 mEq/L	**Increased** in internal bleeding, renal failure, cell damage, acidosis, and Addison's disease. **Decreased** in chronic stress, diuretic administration, severe burns, diarrhea, starvation, pyloric obstruction, severe vomiting, liver disease, and malabsorption.
16.	Chloride (Cl)	Blood serum	96-110 mEq/L	**Increased** in anemia, eclampsia, dehydration, hyperventilation, and Cushing's syndrome. **Decreased** with severe vomiting, severe diarrhea, severe burns, ulcerative colitis, and pyloric obstruction.
17.	Triglycerides	Blood serum	40-150 mg/dl	**Increased** in diets too high in saturated fat or cholesterol. High level is a risk factor for heart attack. **Decreased** in anemia.
18.	Creatine phosphokinase (CPK)	Blood serum	1-10 U 0.2-1.42 U (two methods)	**Increased** in myocardial infarction, pulmonary edema, pulmonary infarction, DTs, and muscular dystrophy.
19.	Creatinine	Blood serum	0.7-1.7 mg/dl	**Increased** in nephritis and impaired kidney function.
20.	Icterus index	Blood serum	3-8 U	**Used** to discover early jaundice and for a liver function test.
21.	Sodium (Na)	Blood serum or plasma	136-145 mEq/L	**Increased** levels in excessive dietary intake, excessive sweating, extensive thermal burns, and diabetes insipidus. **Decreased** in deficient dietary intake, diarrhea, vomiting, diuretic therapy, chronic renal insufficiency, excessive water intake, congestive heart failure, peripheral edema, and ascites.

*For many years, laboratories have reported a number of their test results in milligrams (mg) percent, or milligrams (mg) per 100 milliliters (ml), or 100 cubic centimeters (cm³). A newer method, used by many, is the use of a deciliter (dl); 1 dl = 0.1 L or 100 ml or 100 cm³ (cubic centimeters). Thus in a report, mg/dl is the same as mg% or mg/100 ml. Keep in mind that test values *may differ*, depending on the methods and procedures used by the laboratory.

Continued

TABLE 13-4 Blood Chemistry Examinations—cont'd

Test	Performed on	Normal Values*	Significance
22. Thyroid function			
1. T₃ uptake (resin uptake/radioassay)	Blood serum	25%-35%	**Increased** in hyperthyroidism; **decreased** in hypothyroidism.
2. T₄ total thyroxin radio-immunoassay (T₄/RIA)	Blood serum	5.2-12.2 µg/dl	**Decreased** level of T₃ and **increased** level of T₄ if a woman is taking birth control pills.
3. T₃: T₄ ratio	Blood serum		The free thyroxin index is done in this case to confirm normal thyroid function.
4. Free thyroxin index (includes total T₄)	Blood serum	0.5-1.7	
Other tests			
23. Glucose tolerance test (standard test)	Blood serum	(Results per 100 ml blood) Fasting blood glucose: 80-120 mg After ingesting test doses of glucose: 30 min—150 mg 60 min—135 mg 2 hr—100 mg 2½ hr—80 mg	Used to detect abnormalities in carbohydrate metabolism such as occur in diabetes mellitus, hypoglycemia, and adrenocortical and liver dysfunction. In diabetes, fasting blood sugar (FBS) is around 120 mg/100 ml or higher. After 1 hr, level rises over 180 mg/100 ml, and does not return to normal in 2- and-3 hr specimens. Normally blood sugar will return to normal after 2 hr.
24. Glucose tolerance sum (GTS)			In older patients, diabetes is sometimes hard to diagnose. Some physicians will use the GTS. They will add the FBS, ½ hr, 1 hr, and 2 hr values obtained from the glucose tolerance test. If the sum of these values is less than 500 mg, the patient is not considered diabetic. When the sum is over 800 mg, the patient is considered diabetic. Various other tests will be done to confirm this diagnosis and rule out liver disease, chronic diseases, or potassium depletion.
25. Radioimmunoassay for serum pregnancy or human chorionic gonadotropin (HCG) Beta subunit for pregnancy	Serum	Quantitative results: First week: 20-60 mIU/ml Second wk: 60-200 mIU/ml Third wk: 200-2000 mIU/ml Second or third mo: 20,000-200,000 mIU/ml Second trimester: 12,000-60,000 mIU/ml Third trimester: 10,000-30,000 mIU/ml	Results reported as either positive or negative for pregnancy. A result of 5-15 mIU/ml may indicate an ectopic pregnancy. A result of less than 5 mIU/ml would be considered negative for an ectopic pregnancy.

less than 3 minutes. The hard copy printer eliminates the change of transcription errors and simplifies record keeping. In addition, **test profiles** can be obtained (Figure 13-35, *C*). Profiles provide information on particular body system disorders or suspected conditions and also can be used for screening purposes or to monitor chronic conditions. Complete instructions come with the instrument, and you can call the manufacturer with questions regarding the testing procedures. (NOTE: In addition to performing blood chemistry tests, the Reflotron and other similar reflectance photometers give results for a hemoglobin test. This eliminates the tedious and less accurate manual procedures that have been used in the past (see also p. 604, Hemoglobin).

Blood Glucose

Test for blood glucose using Dextrostix.*

The Dextrostix is a reagent strip that measures blood glucose levels over a range of 45 to 250 mg/dl of blood. It is supplied in glass bottles that have a color chart on the side that is used for determining test results. Only fresh blood is to be used on these strips because plasma and serum give false results.

Procedure

1. Wash hands. Don single-use, examination gloves.
2. Do a skin puncture on a fingertip. Allow a *large* drop of blood to form.
3. Place a large drop of blood on the test area of the strip. (This may be done by putting the strip on the blood over the puncture site.)
4. Wait 60 seconds exactly, holding the strip horizontally to avoid blood runoff from the test area.
5. Holding the strip vertically, wash the blood off, using a sharp stream of water from a wash bottle. No more than 1 to 2 seconds is required.
6. Compare the color on the test area with the color chart on the bottle. There are five color blocks representing 45, 90, 130, 175, and 250 mg/dl of blood.
7. Dispose lancet in puncture-resistant container used for sharps. Dispose test strip in container labeled "Biohazardous Waste."
8. Remove gloves.
9. Wash your hands.
10. Record the results.

NOTE: If you don't use enough blood, you will obtain lower values. If you overwash the strip, you can wash color off and obtain lower values.

To obtain more precise blood glucose results, the same manufacturer has marketed an instrument, the Eyetone Reflectance Colorimeter, to be used with the Dextrostix. From a precisely calibrated meter that covers the range of 10 to 400 mg/dl of blood glucose, rapid and accurate determination can be read. Complete instructions for use are provided with the instrument.

Blood Glucose Meters

There are many small, portable, easy-to-operate blood glucose meters on the market. Most use a specific reagent strip with a test pad area. When blood is applied to the test pad area, glucose in the blood reacts with the reagent in the test pad, and a color change occurs. This color change is read by the blood glucose meter as the concentration of glucose in the blood.

Timing of the test must be exact because both the amount of time the blood is on the test pad and the amount of glucose in the blood determine the test results. Newer meters begin timing automatically when blood is applied to the test pad, and/or the test pad does not require wiping or blotting.

To obtain a blood sample, you need a lancet. Many lancing devices are available on the market. The spring-loaded devices offer an advantage (that is, they provide a measured depth of lancet penetration for the finger puncture). Some manufacturers provide interchangeable endpieces that allow for different puncture depths (see Figure 13-15). You must not use endpieces or puncturing surfaces of the devices on more than one patient, or, if they are reusable, you must clean them with a bleach solution before reuse. This practice is followed to avoid the spread of infection.

Use each lancet only once and then discard it in the container for disposable sharps. *As with all procedures involving blood or body fluids, it is essential to follow the Universal/Standard Precautions presented in Chapter 1.*

Each blood glucose meter has specific operating instructions that must be followed precisely. Errors in technique or in use of the meter can cause inaccurate test results. Inaccurate readings are most often the result of operator error. **Common errors** include inaccurate timing, too much or too little blood, inaccurate calibration of the meter, and incorrect timing or method of wiping the blood from the reagent strip. These meters are designed for use with capillary (whole) blood; using venous blood or serum causes inaccurate readings. Other possible **causes of inaccurate readings** include a dirty meter, a outdated reagent strip, high altitudes, a high or low ascorbic acid blood level, and a high or low hematocrit. Remember that every instrument has limitations. If the blood glucose levels do not confirm other patient data, or when the results will have a critical impact on the physician's decision for treatment, a laboratory glucose level should be obtained.

Quality assurance is very important when using blood glucose meters. This includes regular cleaning and maintaining the instrument and using control solutions periodically to test the accuracy of the meter.

Test for blood glucose using the Accu-Chek III and Chemstrip bG.*

The Accu-Chek III is a battery-operated meter used to measure blood glucose (sugar). Chemstrip bG test strips are "read" by the Accu-Chek III to determine blood glucose levels. The Accu-Chek III provides blood glucose readings between 20 and 500 mg/dl. The Chemstrip bG

---

*Bayer Corp, Inc, Elkhart, Ind.

*Courtesy Boehringer Mannheim Corporation, 1992. Accu-Chek and Chemstrip are registered trademarks of Boehringer Mannheim GmbH, Indianapolis, Ind.

FIGURE 13-35 **A,** Reflotron Plus system; **B,** test results record; **C,** test profiles used to monitor chronic conditions. (Courtesy Boehringer Mannheim Corp, Indianapolis, Ind.)

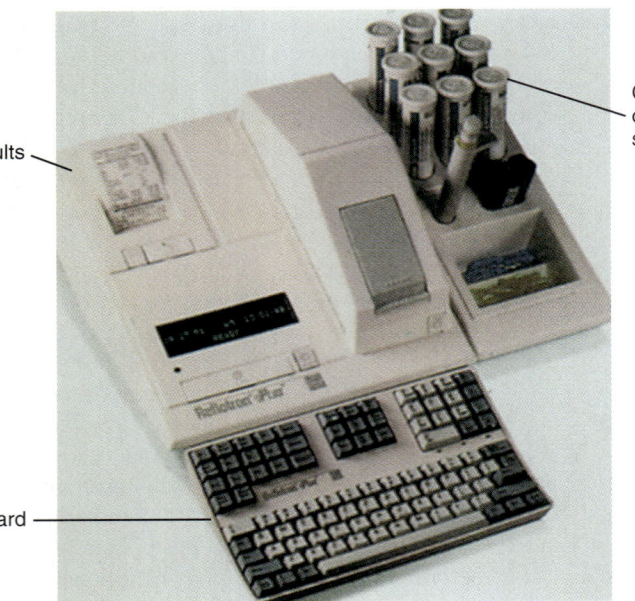

A

Printed results

Keyboard

Containers of test strips

Test pad   Test strip

16-test menu
- Hemoglobin
- Glucose
- Cholesterol
- Triglycerides
- HDL
- LDL (calculated)
- Uric Acid
- Bilirubin
- SGPT (ALT)
- SGOT (AST)
- GGT
- Amylase
- BUN
- Creatinine
- Potassium
- CK

B

```
******************************
09.17.00    AM   11:41:43
HEART HEALTH ASSESSMENT
        LOUIS KELLEY
******************************
CHOL        mg/dl  190.00
TG          mg/dl  150.00
HDL         mg/dl   38.00
SEX           M
AGE           45 years
SMOKING       No
DIABETES      No
CVD           Yes
ECG-LVH       No
SYSTOLIC    mmHg   145.00
DIASTOLIC   mmHg    98.00
LDL         mg/dl  122.00
CHOL/HDL RATIO      5.0
******************************
      FRAMINGHAM RISK
6 YR. CHD RISK         4.3%
RANGE         1.9% - 11.0%
CHD RISK MULT.         2.3
******************************
Hard  copy  test  results
```

An example of test results providing Heart Health Assessment which can be used to improve the effectiveness of your counseling efforts.

Run Total Cholesterol, Triglycerides and HDL Cholesterol tests.

Use the keyboard to input patient data at system prompt.

LDL and Total Cholesterol/HDL ratio calculated.

System calculates 6-year coronary heart disease (CHD) risk based on Framingham Study tables. CHD Risk Multiplier expresses patient risk in relation to the minimum risk (1.0) of the sex-related age group.

16-test menu makes it easier to monitor chronic conditions

C

Lipid/Coronary Risk
- Total cholesterol
- HDL cholesterol
- Triglycerides
- LDL (calculated)

Diabetes
- Glucose
- Triglycerides
- BUN
- Creatinine

Monitoring Hypertension Therapy
- Potassium
- Triglycerides

- Total cholesterol
- HDL cholesterol
- LDL (calculated)
- Uric acid
- Glucose
- BUN
- Creatinine

Anemia
- Hemoglobin

Arthritis/Musculoskeletal Disease
- CK
- Hemoglobin
- Uric acid

Gastrointestinal Disorders
- Amylase
- Total cholesterol
- GGT
- SGPT (ALT)
- SGOT (AST)
- Bilirubin
- Potassium

Renal Disease
- BUN
- Potassium
- Creatinine

may also be read visually without using the Accu-Chek III. The results are very close to those obtained when using the Accu-Chek III. This equipment can be used in the physician's office or by the patient at home (Figure 13-36, *A* to *C*). The purpose of testing with Chemstrip bG at home is to measure the amount of blood glucose in the blood. The results of this test help the patient determine how much insulin, food, and exercise are needed to control diabetes.

FIGURE 13-36 **A** and **B,** Accu-Chek and Chemstrip bG companion system for blood glucose testing; **C,** Accu-Chek III test guide. (Courtesy Boehringer Mannheim Corp, Indianapolis, Ind. Accu-Chek and Chemstrip are registered trademarks of Boehringer Mannheim GmbH).

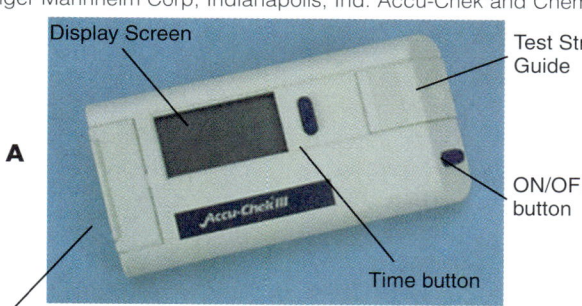

Display Screen

Test Strip Guide

A

ON/OFF button

Time button

Door covering RCL, Beep and SET buttons

Battery Compartment on back

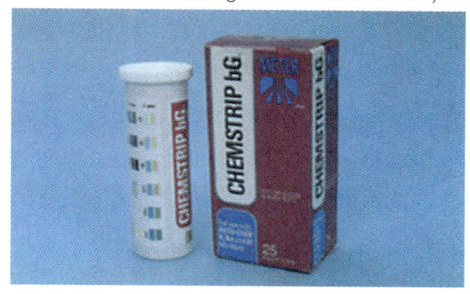

B

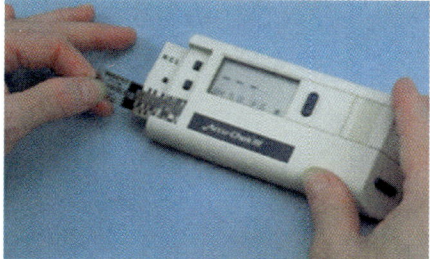

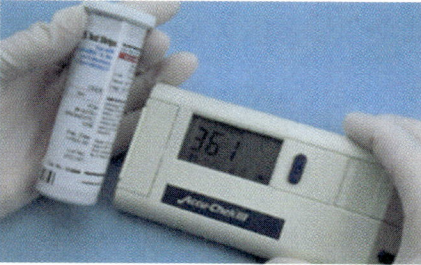

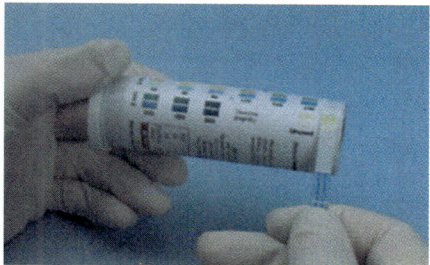

C

Insert code strip, pointed end first, as far as it will go.

Turn monitor ON.
Check that code number in display matches code on test strip vial label.

Remove unused test strip from vial and compare to "Unused" block on label. If strip pads are darker than label, follow directions in monitor *User's Manual.*

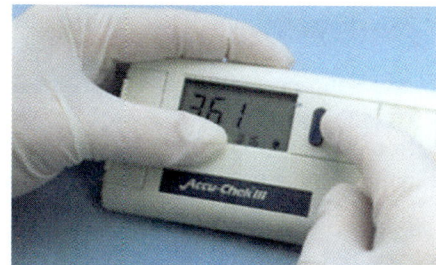

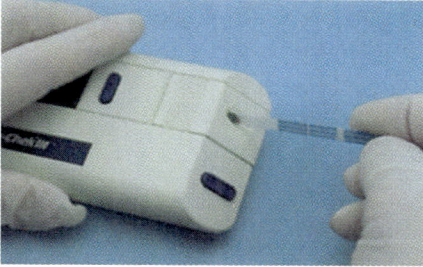

Press TIME button as soon as blood is on test strip.

Insert test strip in monitor as soon as you wipe it. Result appears at 120 seconds.

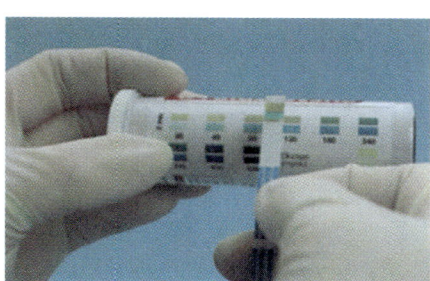

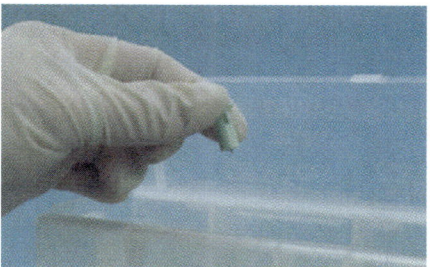

Compare colors on test pads to those on test strip vial label. If they do not agree, see "Problem Solving," page 18, in *Accu-Chek III User's Manual.*

Discard lancet in a puncture-proof container.

Equipment

Accu-Chek III Blood Glucose Monitor with a battery
Vial of Chemstrip bG 50 test strips (Cat. No. 00502)
Alcohol swab
Lancet or automatic finger skin puncture device
Dry cotton or rayon ball
Disposable, single-use examination gloves

Procedure for programming the Accu-Chek III

1. Open the box containing the vial of Chemstrip bGs. The box contains the package insert, a vial of 50 reagent strips, and a calibration strip that is wrapped in paper. Carefully remove the paper cover from the strip. This is the calibration strip that is used to program your Accu-Chek III meter for the new vial of strips. (Be sure that you are using Chemstrip bG 50, Cat. No. 00502.)
2. Compare the lot number on the calibration strip to the lot number on the side of the Chemstrip bG vial. These numbers must match exactly before proceeding to the next step.
3. Now you must program the meter. This step *must* be performed whenever you open a new vial of Chemstrip bG 50 test strips. *Programming of the meter is required only once per vial of test strips.* The capacity for memory enables the meter to retain the calibration curve until it is reprogrammed for use with a different vial of strips.
4. To start, place the meter with a battery in place on a flat surface with the calibration slot toward you.
5. Press the ON/OFF button once to turn the Accu-Chek III on.
6. Open door. Door is to the left of the display; press on outside left edge.
7. Insert code strip smoothly. Do not hesitate or pull back. Monitor beeps when code strip is in place. The code in the monitor display must match code on the vial of strips you are using. If not, repeat steps 6 to 8 with code strip that came with the test strips you are using.
8. Close the door.

   LEAVE THE CODE STRIP IN THE MONITOR. You can now turn the monitor off, or go on to do a test (see Figure 13-36).

Procedure for testing blood glucose with the Accu-Chek III

1. Turn the meter on by depressing the ON/OFF button once. The numeral "888" will appear on the display, followed by a three-digit code.
2. Lay an unused Chemstrip bG test strip on a flat work surface with the rest of the pads facing up.
3. Don gloves.
4. Do a skin puncture on the patient's fingertip using a lancet or an automatic finger-puncture device.
5. Lightly squeeze the fingertip, let go; repeat several times until a large droplet of blood has formed.
6. Lightly touch the blood onto the test pads of the Chemstrip bG strip. Make sure to cover both yellow and white squares completely. *Do not smear the blood.* Apply pressure over the puncture site with a clean, dry gauze pad or cotton ball.

7. Immediately press the TIME button. The meter will count to 60.
8. During the displays of 57, 58, and 59 the Accu-Chek III will emit three high beeps, and at 60, one low beep.
9. When the display reads 60 seconds, wipe the blood from the test pads with a clean, dry cotton ball using gentle pressure. Do not leave any blood on the test pads.
10. The Accu-Chek III will continue to count to 120 seconds. While the meter is counting, turn the test strip on its side with the test pads *facing* the ON/OFF button and insert the reacted test strip into the test strip adaptor. *The strip must be inserted before the display reads 120* (see Figure 13-36).
11. When the display reads 120, a high beep will be emitted, followed by the blood sugar value display in milligrams per deciliter. Read the blood sugar value on the display screen.

    NOTE: If "HHH" appears on the display screen, the blood sugar level is over 500 mg/dl, or the strip was not prepared correctly. Wait an additional minute, then take the reacted test strip out of the meter and compare it with the color chart on the side of the Chemstrip bG vial to estimate results up to 800 mg/dl.

    If "LLL" appears on the display screen, the blood glucose value is lower than the reading range of the instrument (less than 10 mg/dl). Values below 20 mg/dl have not been confirmed clinically. Consult the troubleshooting guide of the Accu-Chek III manual.
12. Record the test results.
13. Press the ON/OFF button to turn off the Accu-Chek III. Remove the test strip from the meter. Dispose of the lancet in biohazard container for used disposable sharps. Dispose of any sponge with blood on it and the test strip in the container for biohazardous waste.
14. Remove gloves and wash your hands.

How to change the battery in the Accu-Chek III monitor

1. Hold the Accu-Chek III face down in your hand.
2. Remove the battery compartment cover by placing your thumb on the grooved cover and sliding it toward you until it detaches from the instrument case.
3. Lightly press in and up on the edge of the battery to release it from the compartment. Tilt the instrument down until the battery slides out of the compartment.
4. Insert a new battery, making sure the plus signs on the battery and monitor case match.
5. Place the battery compartment cover on the meter and snap it into place.

   NOTE: The compartment cover will not fit on the meter correctly if the battery is not inserted properly.
6. The meter will have to be reprogrammed before it is used.

How to clean the Accu-Chek III monitor

1. The outer casing may be wiped with a slightly dampened cloth and a *mild* household cleaning agent. Dry thoroughly. You should also clean the test strip guide each time you calibrate the meter.

2. Remove the guide from the meter by placing your thumb on the grooved surface above the test strip chamber and sliding the cover toward you. Slide the cover away from the meter.
3. Pinch together the two small black tabs located behind the beige chamber cover.
4. Slide the test strip guide out of the cover.
5. Clean the inner surfaces of the channel of the test strip guide with soap and water. You may scrub it with a toothbrush. Rinse and dry.
6. To disinfect it, soak for 2 minutes in 70% alcohol or a 1:10 solution of sodium hypochlorite (household bleach). Rinse guide in water and dry.
7. Also clean the window surfaces on the side of the guide. Air-dry.
8. After the strip guide has dried completely, fold gray into black piece and replace it in the monitor. Slide the test strip guide back into monitor until it snaps into place. (Be sure serial numbers on the strip guide and monitor match if you are cleaning more than one monitor.)

Using the glucose control solution. Glucose Control Solution should be used for the following reasons:

- To practice correct technique
- To check for test strip deterioration (vial left uncapped, exposed to excessive heat or cold)
- To verify the performance of the Accu-Chek III (results are lower or higher than expected and don't agree with how the patient feels)

Instructions (see Figure 13-36)
1. Place a drop of the Glucose Control Solution on the Chemstrip bG instead of blood. *Use only Glucose Control Solution designed for use with Accu-Chek III.*
2. Follow steps 7 through 13 of the blood-testing procedure.
3. Record your value and make sure it is within the control range listed in the package insert.

Reading the Chemstrip bG visually
1. Follow steps 2 through 6 of the Procedure for Testing Blood Glucose With the Accu-Chek III.
2. Immediately start timing for 60 seconds.
3. At the end of the first 60 seconds, using gentle pressure, wipe blood from the test pads with a clean, dry cotton ball. Put cotton ball in container for "Biohazardous Waste."
4. Now wait another 60 seconds.
5. Compare the two reacted colors on the test pads with the color chart on the Chemstrip bG vial.
6. If the test pad matches 240, wait an additional 60 seconds before making a final reading.
7. Sometimes the colors on the treated area of the test strip will match a color block on the chart exactly. Colors range from beige through various shades of blue and green. At other times, you will find that the reacted colors fall between color blocks.

For example:
> The bottom (blue) square matches 180.
> The top (green) square matches 240.
> The results would be approximately 210.

$$\begin{array}{r} 180 \\ +\underline{240} \\ 420 \end{array} \div 2 = 210 \text{ mg/dl}$$

8. NOTE: If the patient has eyesight problems, this test cannot be used by the patient without the use of the Accu-Chek III meter.
9. Continue with steps 12 through 14 under Procedure for Testing Blood Glucose With the Accu-Chek III.

How to avoid inaccurate readings
1. Always carefully place a large drop of blood onto the test pads of the Chemstrip bG. Do not smear or rub the blood into the test pads.
2. Always use a drop of blood that is large enough to adequately cover both test pads simultaneously.
3. Always use a cotton ball to remove blood from the test pads. Wipe the pads with two or three even strokes, using a clean area of the cotton ball.
4. Always use a watch with a second hand to monitor the reaction times.
5. Always discard Chemstrip bG test strips on the expiration date shown on the vial. Use of expired strips may result in inaccurate readings.
6. Always use the color chart from the vial that corresponds to the strips. Use of a different vial color chart may result in inaccurate readings.
7. Do not cut or alter the strips in any way.

Storage of the Chemstrip bG. Chemstrip bG may be damaged if the strips are exposed to heat, light, or moisture. You should follow these suggestions:

- Keep the Chemstrip bG strips in the original vial. Do not transfer the strips into any other container.
- Store at room temperature under 86° F (30° C). Do not freeze.
- Always keep the vial capped tightly.

How to tell if the Chemstrip bG has spoiled
1. Check the expiration date, which is stamped on the side of every vial.
2. Throw away any strips you still have after the expiration date.
3. If in doubt, replace the strips with a new vial of Chemstrip bG.

Test for blood glucose using the One Touch blood glucose meters monitoring systems.
One Touch blood glucose meters are portable, battery-operated meters that are used with One Touch test strips to measure glucose concentrations in whole blood in a simple 45-second procedure (Figures 13-37 and 13-38). The *One Touch* meter

FIGURE 13-37 Abbreviated procedure; check strip procedure and steps for cleaning the One Touch Basic blood glucose monitoring systems. (Courtesy Lifescan Inc, Mountain View, Calif.)

ONE TOUCH®
BASIC™
BLOOD GLUCOSE MONITORING SYSTEM

Check Strip Procedure*

To check that the Meter is operating properly, the Check Strip must be used:
- **At least once per day.**
- **After cleaning the Meter.**
- **If the Meter has been dropped.**
- **When results do not reflect how the user feels.**
- **When ✓ NOT OK REDO ✓ appears on the display.**

STEP 1
Press On/Off Button.
- Last blood or Control Solution test result is displayed for 3 seconds.

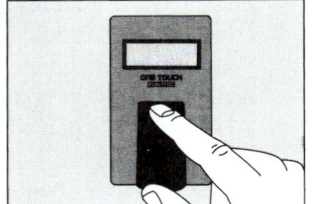

STEP 2
Insert Check Strip.
- While INSERT STRIP is displayed, insert Check Strip with Side 1 (purple) facing up.

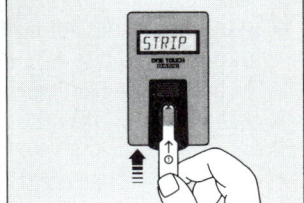

STEP 3
When APPLY SAMPLE appears, pull out the Check Strip.

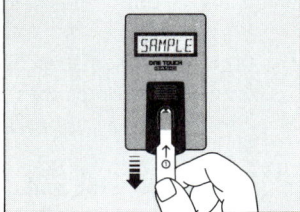

STEP 4
When INSERT SIDE 2 appears, turn the Check Strip over, with Side 2 (white) facing up, and insert Check Strip again.
- If ✓ 80 (example)
  ✓ OK

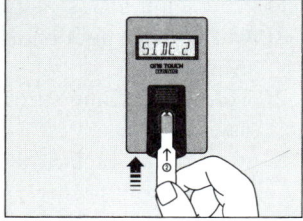

Cleaning the Meter*

STEP 1
Remove Test Strip Holder.

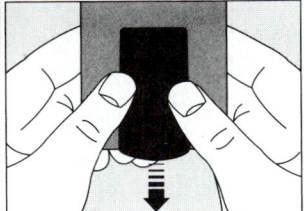

STEP 2
Wash and dry Test Strip Holder.

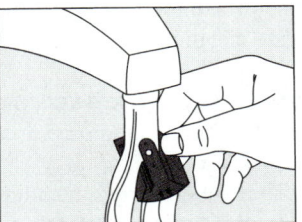

STEP 3
Clean Test Area. Use a cotton swab or soft cloth dampened with water to remove all blood, dirt, and lint from Test Area. **DO NOT USE:** Alcohol, cleansers with ammonia, glass cleaners, or abrasive cleansers.

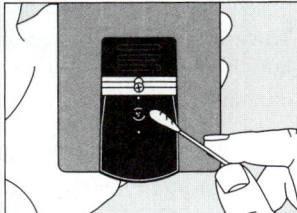

STEP 4
Dry Test Area with soft tissue or cloth. Remove any lint.

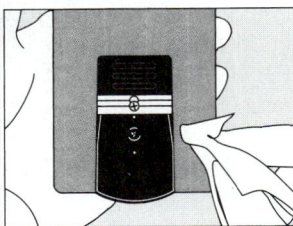

STEP 5
Replace Test Strip Holder.

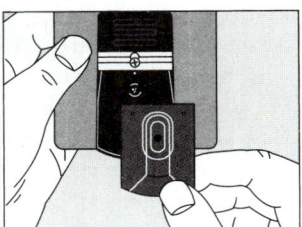

provides blood glucose readings between 0 and 600 mg/dl (0 and 33.3 mmol/L). Higher values are displayed as HIGH. This equipment can be used in the physician's office or by the patient at home. The purpose of testing with the One Touch at home is to measure the amount of blood glucose in the blood.

The results of this test help the patient determine how much insulin, food, and exercise are needed to control diabetes.

The new One Touch system makes reliable blood glucose monitoring easier than ever. With One Touch, results can be achieved by touching the reagent pad just once—to apply

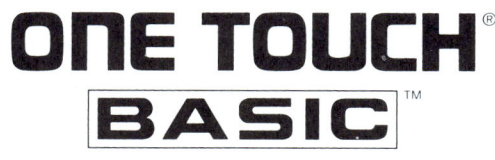

ONE TOUCH®
BASIC™
BLOOD GLUCOSE MONITORING SYSTEM

ABBREVIATED PROCEDURAL CHART*

STEP 1

Press On/Off Button.

- Last result, from either a blood glucose or Control Solution test, is displayed for 3 seconds.

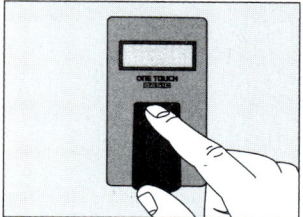

STEP 2

Match code numbers.

- Press C Button until code number on Meter <u>matches</u> code number on your current Test Strip package.

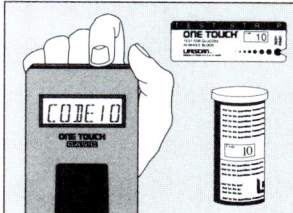

STEP 3

Insert Test Strip.

- While INSERT STRIP is displayed.

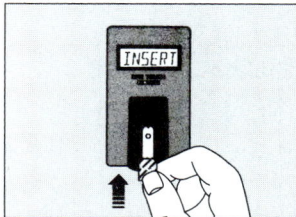

STEP 4

Obtain blood sample.

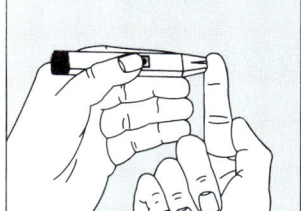

STEP 5

Apply blood sample to Test Spot.

- Check to make sure Meter is still on.
- Test Strip must be in Meter when you apply the blood.
- Blood should form a round, shiny drop and completely cover the Test Spot.

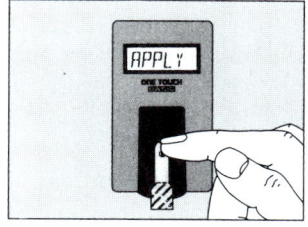

blood—because no wiping or blotting is required. One Touch eliminates three major stumbling blocks to reliable monitoring: starting the test, timing the test, and removing the blood. The opportunity for procedural error is virtually eliminated. To perform the test, insert the test strip into the meter, press the Power button, then apply a blood sample to the test spot on the reagent pad at any time. At this point the meter takes over, starting the test automatically when it detects blood on the reagent pad. No blood removal, timing, wiping, blotting, or washing is required. Test results appear in just 45 seconds. The One Touch meter provides a stable platform for the test strip while you are applying the blood sample. The test spot is smaller, so less blood is required, and the wider test strip is easier to handle.

FIGURE 13-38   One Touch II blood glucose meter. (Courtesy Lifescan Inc, Mountain View, Calif.)

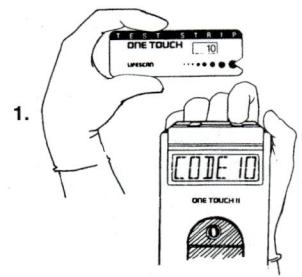

1. Press On/Off Button. CODE and a number will appear on display. Press C Button until code number on Meter *matches* code number on your current Test Strip package.

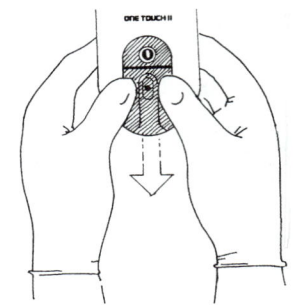

To Clean the Meter

1. Remove Test Strip Holder. Place thumbs on raised dots. Slide Holder toward you to remove. Wash and dry Test Strip Holder.

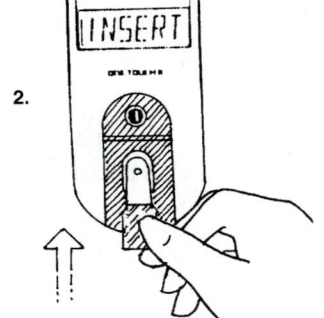

2. While INSERT STRIP is on the display, insert Test Strip with Test Spot facing up.

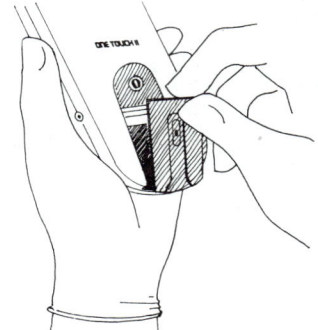

2. After cleaning and drying the Test Strip Holder and the Test Area—Hook bottom of Test Strip Holder to square notch at base of Meter. Push down on top of Holder until it snaps into place.

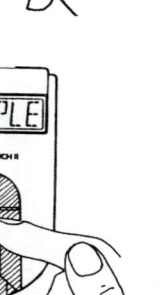

3. WAIT will appear; then APPLY SAMPLE. While APPLY SAMPLE is on the display and the Test Strip is in the Meter, obtain and apply blood sample to Test Spot. (NOTE: *Blood should form a round, shiny drop and completely cover the Test Spot.*) The Meter display counts down from 45—then the result appears.

An added feature for convenience is that the One Touch system is the first to provide "conversational" messages in plain English to guide you through the test. Messages and results are shown on a large, easy-to-read display. With each test, numerous system self-checks are automatically performed to ensure that the meter is working properly. In addition, 250 previous results can be easily recalled from its memory.

See Figure 13-37 for the procedure for using the *One Touch Basic* blood glucose meter. Easy-to-follow prompts guide you through three simple steps. You see accurate results in just 45 seconds. See Figure 13-38 for the new *One Touch II Meter*. Accurate results are obtained in 45 seconds. Easy-to-read prompts in English, Spanish, or seven other languages guide you through the simple three-step procedure. The new One Touch II Meter detects most errors in blood sample size and application, and it even notifies you when the meter must be cleaned.

All of these meters are very easy to use in the physician's office or by the patient at home or work. When using these me-

ters, you must read the Owner's Booklet for complete operating instructions and other important information. All One Touch meters are supplied with an Owner's Booklet that provides detailed information and instructions for use.

Inaccurate test results may be obtained from the meters for any of the following reasons:

1. An inadequate amount of blood was placed on the test strip; the entire reagent pad must be completely covered.
2. The wrong test strips were used; *only* One Touch test strips can be used with the One Touch meters. Test strips must not be cut or altered in any way.
3. The One Touch test strips used were:
   a. Beyond their expiration date printed on each foil wrapper on the outer package label.
   b. Discolored before use (normal reaction pad is ivory colored or light beige).
   c. Showing an abnormal color development during the test time (normal color development is blue/purple).

Blood Glucose Control for Diabetics

Test	Level for People Without Diabetes	Goal	Take Action if*:
Blood sugar before meals	Less than 110 mg/dl	80-120 mg/dl	Less than 80 or more than 140 mg/dl
Blood sugar at bedtime	Less than 120 mg/dl	100-140 mg/dl	Less than 100 or more than 160/dl
HbA$_{1c}$	Less than 6%	Less than 7%	More than 8%

*The action that should be taken may vary for different people. These test levels **are not for use** in pregnancy.

NOTE: The American Diabetes Association's standard for a diabetes diagnosis is a fasting blood glucose of 126 mg/dl. "Borderline" diabetes is an old term that is not currently used. People either have diabetes or they don't.

4. The One Touch test strip holder and window area are dirty.
5. The One Touch meter is out of calibration (for example, the calibration checkstrip result does not fall within the specified checkstrip range).
6. Inappropriate diagnostic use; One Touch test strips are for in vitro diagnostic use only.
7. Using the meter in intense direct sunlight may give low readings; shade the meter.

The Accu-Chek III and the One Touch series of blood glucose meters are particularly valuable to diabetic patients who have to monitor their blood glucose levels closely. These meters can be used virtually anywhere. In many situations, it is much easier for a person to obtain a small blood sample by a fingerprick than it is to obtain a urine sample. In addition, a blood glucose level provides more accurate information than does a urine glucose level. Even the most accurate urine-testing method does not reflect the exact status of blood glucose at a given time. Factors that can affect urine tests include the ability of the kidneys to reabsorb glucose back into the bloodstream. Also, the urine may have passed from the kidney to the bladder hours before the urine is tested. Both of these situations would not reflect the correct blood glucose level. Urine tests also require you or the patient to compare colors on the test strip with colors on a color chart to determine the percentage of glucose. People with visual disturbances or color blindness cannot accurately use these methods and must rely on others to verify the results. The portable blood glucose meters eliminate these problems, and accurate results can be obtained.

Quality assurance.   Quality control is a key element of all laboratory tests. Quality assurance areas for blood glucose monitoring with *all* of the blood glucose meters include the following.

- Training and periodic retraining of both health care workers and patients who perform their own tests in techniques for obtaining a blood specimen and using the monitors
- Periodic verification with the laboratory of the accuracy of the meter
- Regular cleaning and maintenance of the monitor

Test for blood glucose using the HemoCue Glucose Analyzer.   The HemoCue blood glucose analyzer is very useful when screening *and* diagnosing diabetes mellitus, screening for gestational diabetes, measuring blood glucose during oral glucose tolerance tests (OGTTs), and also for monitoring patients' glucose levels. Another recognized use is for *verifying* the function of patients' home glucose meters, which is recommended by leading authorities in diabetic care. The HemoCue blood glucose analyzer is a *diagnostic instrument* rather than a monitoring meter. The process for use is simple, has fewer steps, and is less prone to human errors. The three simple steps include the following:

1. Apply the microcuvette to a drop of blood obtained by a skin puncture. The microcuvette automatically draws up 5 µl of blood by capillary action. Capillary, venous, or arterial blood can be used.
2. Insert the microcuvette into the analyzer.
3. The result is displayed within 40 to 240 seconds. The results are given in mg/dl or mmol/L, as desired (see Figure 13-34 on p. 611).

GLYCOSYLATED HEMOGLOBIN TESTING (ALSO CALLED HB A$_{1c}$, GHb, GHB, GLYCOHEMOGLOBIN, DIABETIC CONTROL INDEX)

The glycosylated hemoglobin test is used to monitor diabetes mellitus treatment and control. This test measures the amount of hemoglobin A$_{1c}$ (Hb A$_{1c}$) in the blood. The result of this test gives an accurate picture of overall diabetes control by estimating the average blood glucose level for the preceding 2 to 3 months.

Hemoglobin in RBCs is mostly hemoglobin A. Some of this hemoglobin A consists of a type of hemoglobin (Hb A$_1$) that can combine with glucose in a process called *glycosylation*. Glucose that is not used for energy and is left in the bloodstream will attach itself to the hemoglobin in RBCs. This process results in glycosylated hemoglobin (GHb). RBCs live in the bloodstream for about 120 days. The amount of GHb depends on the amount of glucose available in the blood over the RBCs' life span. The more glucose available, the higher the GHb percentage will be. Therefore by determining the GHb or Hb A$_{1c}$, you can obtain the average blood glucose level over the past 100 to 120 days (the life span of RBCs).

One distinct advantage of this test is that a blood sample can be obtained at *any time* because it is not affected by short-term changes (that is, food intake, exercise, stress, or hypoglycemic agents) that do affect other blood glucose/sugar tests.

In other words, no special patient preparation is required. A major benefit of the Hb A_{1c} test is that it really can evaluate the success of and patient compliance with the diabetic treatment program. It also helps the diabetic feel confident that he or she is doing a good job overall in controlling his or her diabetes.

The Hb A_{1c} can be performed in a physician's office laboratory using capillary blood and a special blood analyzer. To have the test performed at an outside laboratory, collect approximately 5 ml of venous blood in a gray- or lavender-top tube.

This test is often ordered every 2 to 3 months. As the test is repeated over time, it provides the patient and the physician with comparison values so that they can see if the diabetes control is getting better, staying about the same, or getting worse. Hb A_{1c} test values may vary with the laboratory method used. The values in the table on page 623 are as stated in the American Diabetes Association standards of medical care for patients with diabetes mellitus. The values given refer to a range of 4% to 6% for people without diabetes (mean 5%, standard deviation 0.5%).

BLOOD CHOLESTEROL

AccuMeter Cholesterol Test*

The AccuMeter Cholesterol Test is a rapid, instrument-free enzyme assay for the *in vitro* quantitative determination of total cholesterol in whole blood. Cholesterol measurements are used in the diagnosis and monitoring of disorders involving excess cholesterol in the blood and of lipid and lipoprotein metabolism disorders. These conditions are often associated with coronary heart disease.

It is believed that lowering the mean value of cholesterol levels within the U. S. population will reduce the morbidity and mortality associated with coronary heart disease. This easy-to-use test system can assist medical professionals in the early identification and active monitoring of high-risk individuals.

Summary and explanation of the test. The AccuMeter Cholesterol Test is a fast, easy-to-use test system that combines the simplicity of visual result interpretation and proven enzymatic methods with the convenience of a cassette. The AccuMeter cassette is a self-contained chemical assay providing quantitative test results that are equivalent in accuracy, sensitivity, specificity, and reliability to complex, state-of-the-art, instrumented methods. The cassette combines a unique blood filtration device that separates plasma from RBCs and a mechanism that precisely meters sample volume. The assay is a solid-phase enzymatic method using a chromogenic complex for visual readout.

A drop of fingerstick blood is put directly into the Blood Well near the bottom of the cassette (see figure). After a few minutes, plasma is separated from whole blood by filtration. The tab is then pulled to initiate the reaction. Shortly thereafter

Before Blood Addition

the reagents start working, and a purple color appears in the Test Working Indicator. Over the next 15 minutes, a purple front advances up the Measurement Scale. The reaction is complete when a green color appears in the Complete Indicator. The test result is obtained by reading the height of the purple peak, as one would a thermometer, and determining the cholesterol concentration from a conversion chart.

Quality control for the AccuMeter. Each cassette has two built-in controls to make sure it is working properly. The Test Working Indicator turns light purple as the reagents begin functioning. The Complete Indicator turns green when the test is complete. Both controls must work properly to ensure the validity of the test results.

Good laboratory practice recommends the testing of a control reagent each day that patients are tested. Each site should establish standards of performance.

AccuMeter Cholesterol Controls can be ordered from ChemTrak.

Troubleshooting. If you have any problems performing the ChemTrak AccuMeter Cholesterol Test, the suggestions below may be helpful.

IF	THEN
The cassette is cracked or otherwise damaged.	Do not use the cassette.
The Measurement Scale of the cassette is blue or yellow.	The cassette has been exposed to excessive moisture or heat and should not be used.
You are not sure if you have put enough blood into the Blood Well.	Add one or two more drops of blood. The blood must fill the well to the black circle. If it takes longer than 5 minutes to prick the finger and add blood, the results of the test may be erroneous.
You pulled the tab on the cassette without waiting 2 minutes after the addition of blood to the Blood Well.	Discard the cassette and start over. Put blood into the Blood Well, wait 2 minutes, and initiate the test by pulling the tab to the right until it clicks into place and the red line is visible.

*Courtesy ChemTrak, Sunnyvale, California.

IF	THEN	IF	THEN
The tab does not click into place after being pulled to the right.	The test will not start working until the tab shows the red line. Pull the tab again to the right.	The matching *Cholesterol Result Chart* for the kit on hand is not available.	Use of an unmatched chart produces erroneous results. To obtain the matching *Cholesterol Result Chart,* call ChemTrak and specify the lot number of the AccuMeter Cholesterol Test on hand.
After 20 minutes, the Test Working and/or the Complete Indicator(s) do not turn color.	The test result is not valid unless both internal controls function properly. Disregard the result. Discard the cassette and start over.		

PROCEDURE 13-4

ACCUMETER CHOLESTEROL TEST

Objective
Understand and demonstrate the correct procedure for performing a blood cholesterol test using the Accumeter; and reading and recording the results on the patient's chart.

Equipment
Foil pouch containing an AccuMeter cassette and a desiccant packet

Two lancets
Alcohol pad
Gauze pad or clean tissues
Bandage
Procedure summary/Cholesterol result chart
Disposable, single-use examination gloves

PROCEDURE

1. Wash your hands. Use appropriate personal protective equipment (PPE) as dictated by facility.

2. Assemble and prepare equipment and supplies for use.

3. Identify the patient and explain the procedure.
NOTE: IT IS *NOT* REQUIRED THAT THE PATIENT FAST FOR THIS TEST.

4. Have the patient seated for at least 5 minutes before taking the blood sample.

5. Don gloves. Perform a skin puncture on the fingertip. (See steps 1 through 11 in Fingertip Skin Puncture Using a Lancet, pp. 584-585.) Use fresh whole blood obtained from a finger-prick. You need two or three large hanging drops for the test. You should complete fingerprick and blood addition within 5 minutes. Increase the blood flow to the fingers. Keep the hands below the heart and warm them by gently rubbing or by using a warm compress.

Choose the finger to be pricked. The ring or middle finger is recommended. *Avoid* pricking the center of the fingertip.

Clean the chosen finger with alcohol and dry thoroughly with a sterile pad.

RATIONALE

Sitting stabilizes the blood cholesterol.

Residual alcohol may interfere with the test.

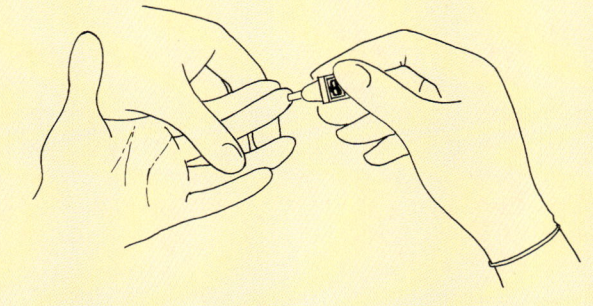

Continued

PROCEDURE 13-4

ACCUMETER CHOLESTEROL TEST—cont'd

6. Wipe away the first blood with a sterile pad. Hold the puncture point downward. Gently massage the finger from the base to the puncture point. Apply pressure just below puncture point to form hanging drops of blood. Do not excessively squeeze the finger. If you have trouble making large drops, prick another finger.

The first drop contains additional fluids from inside the finger. The blood that follows gives a more accurate result. Excessive squeezing and milking produce erroneous results. Hemolyzed samples should not be used. Residual alcohol may interfere with the test.

7. Touch two to three hanging drops of blood to the bottom of the Blood Well. The Blood Well must be filled to the black circle. Do not worry about overfilling the Blood Well. For best results, add blood as quickly as possible. Do not take longer than 5 minutes to add the necessary amount of blood.

   It is essential that at least 2 to 3 large hanging drops of fingerstick blood (~40 μl) be added to the Blood Well. If sufficient blood cannot be obtained from the first fingerprick, a second finger should be pricked to complete the test.

A low cholesterol value may be obtained if not enough blood is added to the cassette or if it has taken more than 5 minutes to add blood to the cassette.

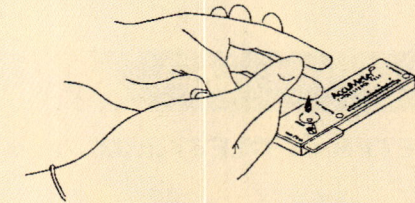

8. WAIT 2 BUT NOT MORE THAN 4 MINUTES AFTER ADDING BLOOD BEFORE PULLING TAB.

At least 2 minutes is needed for the blood to filter into the cassette.

9. Pick up the cassette in your left hand. Pull the tab firmly to the right with your other hand. Pull hard until the tab clicks into place. When the tab has been pulled out properly, a red line will be visible. The tab *can* be pulled very hard without breaking the tab or spilling blood.

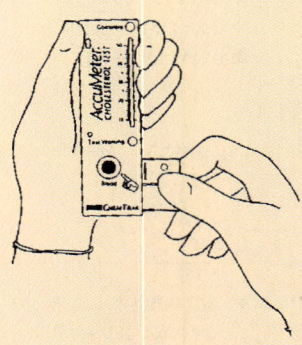

10. Leave the cassette on a flat surface undisturbed for about 15 minutes. During the first few minutes, the Test Working Indicator will turn light purple. The test is complete and ready to read when the Complete Indicator turns green.

11. Read results

   Results are not valid unless the Complete Indicator is green and the Test Working Indicator is purple.

   Read the result under good lighting. Find the peak of the purple color in the Measurement Scale. Read the peak at the farthest end of the color. The peak may resemble the tip of a feather. Read the mark to the left of the peak just as you would a thermometer. This is the test result number of the sample.

   If an unusually low or high reading is obtained, repeat the test with a new cassette and a fresh fingerprick sample.

Samples must be obtained from free-flowing fingerstick blood.

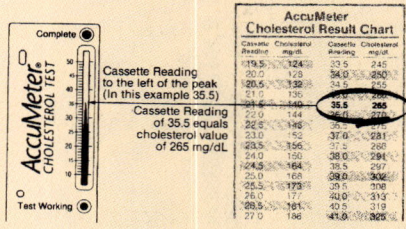

12. Evaluation of results

   The *Cholesterol Result Chart* is used to convert the color peak height to total cholesterol in milligrams per deciliter. Each *Cholesterol Result Chart* is specifically calibrated for the kit it accompanies. The lot number on the *Cholesterol Result Chart* must match the lot number of the cassette being used.

   Find the test result number in the "Cassette Reading" column. Just to the right of the test result number on the chart is the cholesterol value of the sample.

The test has been calibrated to measure cholesterol levels between 125 and 400 mg/dl. Patients with values below or above this level should be tested by another method. Elevated cholesterol levels should be confirmed by a clinical laboratory method. Use of an unmatched chart produces erroneous cholesterol values.

PROCEDURE 13-4

  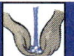

ACCUMETER CHOLESTEROL TEST—cont'd

EXPECTED VALUES

The Expert Panel of the National Cholesterol Education Program (NCEP) has established guidelines for the detection and treatment of high blood cholesterol in adults over 20 years of age to identify risk groups associated with various cholesterol levels. These levels are as follows:

NCEP Guidelines

Total Cholesterol	Classification
Less than 200 mg/dl	Desirable
200 to 239 mg/dl	Borderline high
240 mg/dl or greater	High

The Panel has made recommendations regarding the treatment of hypercholesterolemia. Recommendations include physician monitoring and changes in lifestyle to lower cholesterol values for individuals with values of 200 mg/dl or greater.

13. Dispose of contaminated materials properly. The used lancet should be placed in the disposable puncture-resistant sharps container. Place materials with blood on them in a container for "Biohazardous Waste."

14. Remove gloves.

15. Wash your hands.

16. Record the results.

Charting Example

December 22, 20__, 2 PM
    Skin puncture done on second finger, left hand. AccuMeter Cholesterol Test done. Results 186 mg/dl.
        J.A. Lee, CMA

OTHER BLOOD EXAMINATIONS

BLOOD GROUPS AND TYPES

Blood grouping and blood typing are classifications of blood based on the presence or absence of antigens on the surface of the RBCs. The presence or absence of these antigens is determined by the individual's inherited genetic code. Several different blood groups have been identified. The importance of the blood groups depend on their clinical significance in maternal-fetal compatibility, blood transfusion therapy, organ transplantation, disputed paternity cases, and genetic studies. The two most routinely used systems for blood grouping and typing are the **ABO system** and the **Rh factor or type**. The ABO blood group is identified by the presence or absence of the A antigen and/or the B antigen or the lack of both A and B antigens on the surface of the RBC. The **four blood types** in this blood grouping are determined by and named for these antigens. They are type A, B, AB, and O. Type O does *not* have either the A antigen or the B antigen. Corresponding antibodies, anti-A and anti-B agglutinins, are found in the plasma of some blood types (Tables 13-5 and 13-6).

The Rh factor is an antigenic substance that is present in the RBCs of most people. Someone who has the Rh factor is referred to as **Rh positive** (Rh$^+$); those that lack the factor in their RBCs are referred to as **Rh negative** (Rh$^-$). Eighty-five percent of the population is Rh$^+$. Rh stands for *Rhesus*. Because the Rh factor was discovered during studies on Rhesus monkeys in 1940, the factor was named using the first two letters of the word *Rhesus*.

Blood transfusions depend on the blood being classified as either Rh$^+$ or Rh$^-$ and on the ABO blood type classification. When receiving blood, it is vital that the recipient receive compatible blood (that is, blood that is the same type as the recipient's). If this does not happen, an antigen-antibody reaction occurs that could be harmful to the recipient. The reaction results in mild to serious illness, which can vary from mild fever to anaphylaxis with severe intravascular hemolysis, or even death. To safeguard against a transfusion reaction, donor blood is cross-matched (except in life-threatening emergencies) with the recipient's blood to ensure that the two are compatible.

All pregnant women should have ABO and Rh typing performed during pregnancy. If the mother's blood is Rh$^-$, further tests should be performed, and the father's blood type should be determined. If the father's blood is Rh$^+$, the mother's blood should be examined for the presence of Rh antibodies by the indirect Coombs' test (see Table 13-5). If the first test is negative, it should be repeated at weeks 30 and 36 of pregnancy. If these results are negative, no risk is involved to the fetus. If the test results are positive, the Rh antibodies may find their way over

TABLE 13–5 Serology, Special Chemistry, and Other Blood Examinations*

Test	Performed on:	Normal Values*	Significance
Serology (Certain special blood tests are covered in this item)			
1. STS (serologic test for syphilis) includes:			
a. Fluorescent treponemal antibody (FTA)	Blood serum	Negative	Used to confirm diagnosis of syphilis if VDRL or RPR is positive.
b. Rapid plasma reagin (RPR)	Blood serum or plasma	Negative	Both are screening tests for syphilis. Sometimes false positive results are obtained.
c. VDRL (Venereal Disease Research Laboratory)	Blood serum	Negative	Positive results confirmed with the FTA.
2. Special human antibodies			
a. Coombs' direct	Blood serum	Negative	Used to test newborn's blood for erythroblastosis fetalis (hemolytic disease of the newborn [HDN]). Also used in blood cross matching.
b. Coombs' indirect	Blood serum	Negative	Used to detect blood incompatibilities when cross matching; also to detect Rh incompatibility in maternal blood before delivery by demonstrating anti-Rh antibodies.
c. Heterophil antibody (MonoSpot test)	Blood serum	Concentrated to 1/28	Elevated in infectious mononucleosis and serum sickness.
d. LE test (lupus erythematosus)	Whole blood	Negative	A slide test for antinucleoproteins found in systemic lupus erythematosus (LE).
3. Bacterial and viral antibodies			
a. ASO (antistreptolysin) titer	Blood serum	To 400 U/ml	Increased values seen in rheumatic fever, and acute glomerulonephritis caused by hemolytic streptococcus.

b. Bacterial agglutinations
    Dysentery
    Brucellosis
    Paratyphoid A & B
    Typhoid O & H
    Typhus fever
    Leptospirosis
	Blood serum	No agglutination	Certain infections caused by viruses, bacilli, rickettsiae, and spirochetes, produce antibodies in the serum, which in turn cause agglutination (clumping) of these organisms.

c. Widal test	Blood serum	Negative	A test to diagnose typhoid and paratyphoid fevers.
4. Rheumatoid factors			
a. Latex slide agglutination	Blood serum	1:40 is uppermost serum dilution	Positive in rheumatoid arthritis and in some connective tissue diseases.
b. RA (rheumatoid arthritis) test	Blood serum	Negative	Results positive in 85%-90% of patients with rheumatoid arthritis.
Special Blood Chemistry			
5. HIV antibody for AIDS	Serum or plasma	Negative	A negative result indicates that the antibody is not in the blood. A positive result indicates that the antibody is in the blood.
NOTE: In many states it is a state regulation that the patient must sign a consent form before this test is performed (Figure 13-39)			

*NOTE: In some laboratories, serology will be under an area called special chemistry, and in other large laboratories, serology may be part of the blood bank department.

TABLE 13-5   Serology, Special Chemistry, and Other Blood Examinations—cont'd

Test	Performed on	Normal Values*	Significance
6. Hepatitis B surface antigen and hepatitis B core antibodies	Serum	Negative	The surface antigen test (HBsAg) is used to determine if a person is a carrier of the hepatitis B virus. The test for antibodies shows when there is active virus replication and may sometimes be detectable when the surface antigen is not.
7. Hepatitis A immunoglobulin M antibody (HA-IgM)	Serum	Negative	A positive result confirms a recent hepatitis A infection (usually within the past 3-6 months).
8. Hepatitis C virus (HCV) IgG antibodies	Serum	Negative	Used to detect exposure to hepatitis C virus. This assay reduced the incidence of posttransfusion hepatitis caused by the hepatitis C virus when used to screen donors.
9. Hepatitis D virus (HDV) antigen	Serum	Negative	Used to detect the HDV antigen a few days after infection. Antibodies are also detected early in the disease. A continuous elevation of these antibodies indicates a chronic or carrier state.
Microbiology			
1. Blood culture	Sample of blood grown on culture media	No growth after incubation period	Growth on culture media indicative of blood stream infection or septicemia.
Blood Bank			
1. Blood typing	Whole blood or blood serum	One of the following: Type O—45% of the population (Universal donor) Type A—40% of the population Type B—10% of the population Type AB—5% of the population (Universal recipient) And either: Rh positive—85% of population Rh negative—15% of population	Must be done before a patient receives a blood transfusion, to ensure a compatible transfusion; also important in pregnancy to help prevent erythroblastosis fetalis.

FIGURE 13-39   Signed consent form for HIV antibody blood test is required by some laboratories.

Department of Public Health

**CONSENT FOR TESTING BLOOD
TO DETECT ANTIBODIES TO THE
HUMAN IMMUNODEFICIENCY VIRUS (HIV)**

I have been informed that my blood will be tested for antibodies to the Human Immunodeficiency Virus (HIV), the probably causative agent of AIDS. I have been informed about the limitations and implications of the test. I have had a chance to ask questions that were answered to my satisfaction. I understand that the test's accuracy and reliability are not 100% certain.

I have been informed that the test is performed by withdrawing blood from my arm and testing that blood specimen.

By my signature below, I acknowledge that I have been given information concerning the benefits and risks and I consent that my blood be tested for antibodies to HIV.

Date: _____, 20 _____

_____
Signature

_____
Printed Name

TABLE 13–6   ABO Blood Groups

Blood Type	Type of Antigen Present on the Red Blood Cell	Type of Antibody Present in the Plasma
Group A	A	B
Group B	B	A
Group AB	A and B	None
Universal recipient		
Group O	None	A and B
Universal donor		

to the fetus's circulation and cause hemolysis (see Vocabulary on p. 569) of the fetal RBCs. This causes what is commonly referred to as hemolytic disease of the newborn (HDN). To determine the severity of the hemolytic anemia in the fetus, an amniocentesis can be performed. The amniotic fluid is evaluated for the quantity of bilirubin present.

It is also important in pregnancy to identify cases in which the mother is Rh$^-$ and the father is Rh$^+$. In these situations the mother should receive an injection of RhoGAM (Rh immunoglobulin) within 72 hours of each delivery to prevent any fetal hemolytic problems in subsequent pregnancies. RhoGAM prevents the mother's system from making Rh antibodies after the delivery.

In the medical laboratory, trained laboratory technologists can determine a person's blood type by doing either a slide test or a test tube test using commercially prepared antiserum. At times you may be required to obtain the blood specimen to be tested. In this case, you should collect approximately 7 to 14 ml of venous blood in a red-top tube. Some laboratories may also want 5 ml collected in a lavender-top tube. (This may vary among laboratories.) Eating and drinking do not affect this test.

Blood products.   When a person donates blood at a blood center, the blood is collected in a bag that contains an anticoagulant-preservative solution. This bag is called a **unit** and is labeled as **whole blood.** A unit of blood contains 500 ml (1 pint). Whole blood is needed for patients who are hemorrhaging, resulting in *severe* volume and RBC loss. However, few patients these days require whole blood, so blood centers divide the units of whole blood into **component parts,** which *are RBCs, platelets, fresh frozen plasma (FFP), and cryoprecipitate.*

To make a unit of **RBCs,** the blood bank technologists will centrifuge a unit of whole blood and remove the plasma. RBCs are given to patients to increase the oxygen-carrying capacity in their blood. Patients who are anemic from severe bleeding, from a decrease in RBC production, or from a decrease in RBC survival may receive RBCs depending on their hematocrit, underlying condition, and other signs and symptoms, such as weakness, extreme fatigue, or angina.

Platelets are given to patients who have a serious deficit in platelet function and number, such as that seen in patients who have thrombocytopenia following chemotherapy. However, the need to transfuse platelets also depends on the patient's overall condition. To obtain a unit of platelets from whole blood, platelets are extracted from 4 to 6 units of whole blood and combined in a single unit before they are transfused.

Fresh frozen plasma is given to provide clotting factors to patients who are bleeding because of coagulation deficiencies and also to patients who are about to have a major invasive procedure, such as major surgery.

Cryoprecipitate is used in patients with fibrinogen deficiencies to control bleeding. Cryoprecipitate is extracted from FFP after it has thawed. It is then refrozen until just before it is given to the patient (Table 13-7).

TABLE 13–7   **Blood Products for Transfusions and Recipient's Blood Types**

Recipient's Blood Type	Whole Blood From Donor	Red Blood Cells From Donor	Plasma From Donor
O	Type O	Type O	Any type
A	Type A	Type A Type O	Type A Type AB
B	Type B	Type B Type O	Type B Type AB
AB	Type AB	Any type	Type AB
Rh Factor			
Rh$^+$	Positive or negative	Positive or negative	Positive or negative
Rh$^-$	Negative	Negative	Positive or negative

HEALTH MATTERS

KEEPING YOUR PATIENTS INFORMED

ONE BLOOD DONATION CAN SAVE SEVERAL LIVES

Most patients in need of a transfusion do not need whole blood (except in the case of massive blood loss) but do need one or two of the components that can be separated from whole blood through a special spinning process done at blood banks. To answer the needs of these patients, blood donation centers can separate most whole blood donations into four components: plasma, red blood cells (RBCs), platelets, and cryoprecipitate.

- **Plasma** makes up approximately half of each pint of whole blood. It is used to restore blood volume, especially in patients who have a lot of bleeding during surgery.
- **Red blood cells** make up the other half of the pint of whole blood obtained for transfusions. Red cells are given to patients with severe anemia but whose blood volume is sufficient. Red cells carry nutrients and oxygen to the tissues and must be used within 42 days of donation.
- **Platelets** are needed for the blood to clot and are given to patients having heart surgery, those with leukemia, and also patients with bleeding problems. Platelets must be used within 5 days after being separated from whole blood.
- **Cryoprecipitate** is a small portion of the plasma that contains factors that help blood to clot. It is used primarily for patients with hemophilia.

By giving a patient only the blood component(s) needed, every single blood donation is used as efficiently as possible.

BLOOD DONATION PROCESS

Giving blood is safe and simple, and it saves lives. The donation process takes less than 1 hour. The following four steps are involved:

1. *Registration:* You must present valid identification, such as a driver's license, and give your name, address, phone number, and social security number.
2. *Medical history and miniphysical:* You will be asked a serious of medical questions to determine your eligibility. This information remains confidential. If you are eligible, your temperature, pulse rate, blood pressure, and hemoglobin level will be checked.
3. *The blood donation:* A nurse will cleanse an area on your arm, insert a sterile needle, and after 5 to 7 minutes, you will have donated 1 special pint of blood for a patient in need. It is impossible for you to contract *any* disease by donating blood. The needle that is used on you is sterile and is used only once, then discarded.
4. *Rest and refreshments:* After donating blood, you will be given a chance to relax and enjoy fruit juices and assorted snacks. Indulge yourself and feel very proud about giving a part of yourself so that someone in need may live.

Your blood donation will be tested, typed, and separated into various components that will be used for needy patients.

Support your community's blood drive programs. You can be a part of the team that saves lives.

BLOOD DONATION ELIGIBILITY GUIDELINES
General Requirements

Age: 17 (a 16-year-old can donate with written permission of parent or guardian and physician approval)

Weight: At least 110 pounds

Diet: A well-balanced meal is recommended within 4 hours of donation

Health: General good health

Identification: Valid identification such as a driver's license, DMV identification card, passport, social security number, and so on

HEALTH MATTERS—cont'd

DO NOT DONATE IF ANY OF THE FOLLOWING **APPLIES TO YOU:**

You are a man who has had sex with another man one or more times since 1977.

You are a past or present intravenous drug abuser.

You are a man or woman who has received money or drugs for engaging in sex since 1977.

You are a person with hemophilia who has received clotting factor concentrates.

You have been a sexual partner of any of the above within the past 12 months.

You were born/lived/had sexual contact with anyone from Cameroon, Central African Republic, Chad, Congo, Equatorial Guinea, Gabon, Niger, or Nigeria.

DO NOT DONATE IF THE FOLLOWING CONDITIONS APPLY TO YOU:

AIDS: You are a person with symptoms or laboratory evidence of HIV infection.

Cancer: Any type except for cured cancer of the skin or cervix. Five years cancer free and 5 years after completing radiation. People who have had chemotherapy for Hodgkin's disease, leukemia, and/or lymphomas should not donate.

Heart disease: Heart failure or coronary artery disease, such as angina pectoris or a heart attack (myocardial infarction).

Hepatitis: A history of the disease after the age of 10 or a positive laboratory test for the virus.

Organ failure: Kidney, lung, or liver failure.

Recreational drug use (by injection): Having injected yourself with drugs not prescribed by a physician.

YOU MUST WAIT BEFORE DONATION IF YOU HAVE ANY OF THESE CONDITIONS:

Condition

Allergy—No wait unless suffering from an allergy "attack"

Abortion/miscarriage—6-Week wait if pregnancy terminated in third trimester, otherwise no wait

Acupuncture: Depends on type of sterilization technique used

Alcohol consumption—No wait unless intoxicated

Anemia (past diagnosis)—No wait if corrected

Blood donation, apheresis—48 hours

Blood donation, whole—Every 8 weeks

Blood or plasma transfusion—12 months

Cough, cold, sore throat—Until well; no symptoms

Diabetes—No wait if medically controlled

Ear and body piercing—*See* Acupuncture

Electrolysis—*See* Acupuncture

Gonorrhea—12 months

Hepatitis contact—Depends on type

Herpes—No wait if not in active stage

High blood pressure—No wait if medically controlled

Malaria—3 years

    Immigration from malarial area—3 years

    Travel to malarial area:

        With use of antimalarial medicine—1 year

        Without use of antimalarial medicine—1 year

Nonspecific urethritis (NSU)—Until cured

Oral surgery and tooth extraction—72 hours

Pregnancy—6-Week wait after delivery

Recent surgery—When released from doctor's care

Syphilis—12 months

Tattoo—12 months

Immunizations/Vaccines (Shots)

Rubeola (measles), yellow fever, mumps, and oral polio—2 weeks

Rubella (German measles)—4 weeks

Hepatitis B vaccine—No wait

TB skin test—48 hours

Tetanus, diphtheria, typhoid, and cholera—No wait

Medications:

Retinoic acid (Accutane)—1 month

Allergy medications—No wait

Antabuse—72 hours

Antibiotics—3 days depending on indication

Metronidazole (Flagyl)—3 days

High blood pressure medicine—No wait

Oral contraceptives—No wait

Recreational drugs (without injection)—No wait

Etretinate (Tegison) (for psoriasis)—Permanently deferred

Tetracycline for acne—No wait

Vitamins—No wait

INFECTIOUS MONONUCLEOSIS

Infectious mononucleosis (IM) is an acute inflammatory disease caused by the Epstein-Barr virus (EBV). **Transmission** usually occurs by droplet infection and by direct oral contact. It is often referred to as the "kissing disease" because of the way it could be transmitted and because it most often affects young adults and also children. The disease is usually mild and may even go unnoticed in children. The older the person is, *usually* the more severe the symptoms will be.

The **incubation period** is of uncertain duration, but it is thought to be from 1 week to several weeks. **Signs and symp-**toms include physical and mental fatigue, severe weakness, headache, sore throat, swollen lymph glands, fever, enlargement of the spleen, and enlargement of the liver. In rare cases, complications may develop, including hemolytic anemia, severe thrombocytopenia, pericarditis, myocarditis, pneumonitis, Reye's syndrome, encephalitis, and other neurologic syndromes. Rupture of the spleen could occur, which would require immediate surgery and blood transfusions. **Treatment** for IM is primarily symptomatic. Bed rest is *extremely* important to prevent serious complications of the liver or spleen. Saline gargles are good for the sore throat, and aspirin or other analgesics are given for pain. Infection should provide permanent immunity.

FIGURE 13-40   CARDS O.S. MONO test used to detect infectious mononucleosis. (Courtesy Quidel Corporation, San Diego, Calif.)

MONO

IgM Heterophile Antibody Test
Using Serum, Plasma or Whole Blood

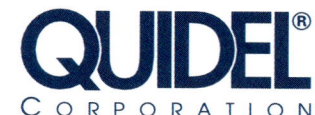

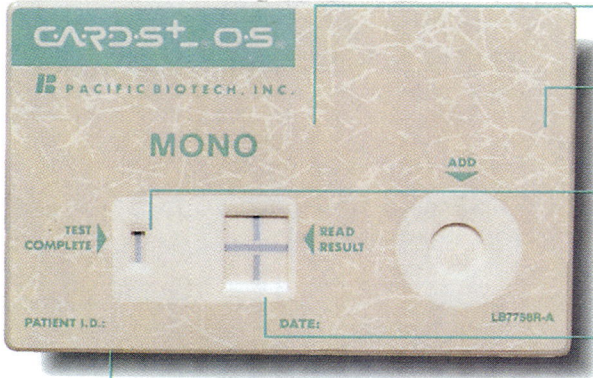

Label clearly identifies type of test – no potential mix-ups if other CARDS®O.S.® assays are also being performed.

Unique Reaction Unit functions as a stable workstation that is easy to handle and will not tip over.

"TEST COMPLETE" signal appears in approximately 5 minutes. Procedural control, meeting interim CLIA requirements, confirms the test is finished and the system has worked properly.

Easy-to-read result.

Markable space for writing patient information.

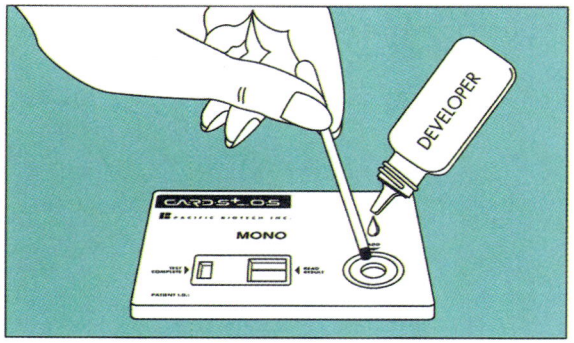

Dispense patient specimen and five drops of Developer into the "ADD" well.
Walk away.

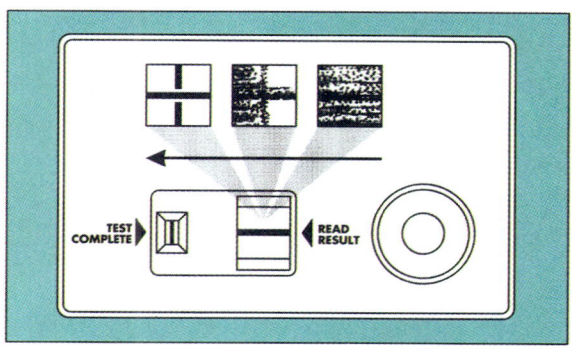

During the next few minutes, a blue color will be seen moving from right to left through the "READ RESULT" window. Test can be left for up to 20 minutes.

Read the result after the signal appears in the "TEST COMPLETE" window.

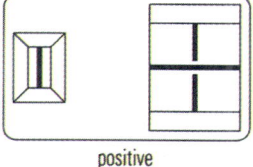

positive

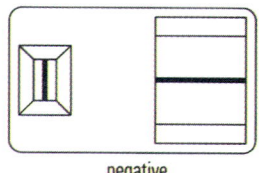

negative

Continued

Diagnosis of IM is made by laboratory blood tests. Hematology tests would show an increased number of lymphocytes and also an increased number of atypical lymphocytes. Other blood tests can determine the presence of the IM heterophile antibodies primarily of the immunoglobulin M (IgM) class. One such test is the CARDS O.S. MONO test. This test is used to aid in the diagnosis of IM by determining if IgM heterophile antibodies are present. If they are present, the test result would be reported as positive. If they are not present, the test result would be reported as negative. See Figure 13-40 for this test

FIGURE 13-40—cont'd   CARDS O.S. MONO test used to detect infectious mononucleosis. (Courtesy Quidel Corporation, San Diego, Calif.)

STORAGE

CARDS® O.S.® MONO can be stored at room or refrigerated temperature (2-30°C, 36-86°F). NOTE: Controls and Developer must be stored tightly capped.

PRECAUTIONS

1. For *in vitro* diagnostic use.
2. DO NOT use materials after expiration date. DO NOT mix components from different lots or different kits.
3. DO NOT interchange caps among reagents.
4. All patient samples and controls should be handled as if they were capable of transmitting disease. Observe established precautions against microbiological hazard throughout all procedures and follow the standard procedures for proper disposal of specimens.

SPECIMEN COLLECTION

1. Serum, plasma or whole blood (including fingertip blood) can be used. Specimens must be collected in a manner appropriate for laboratory testing.
2. Whole blood containing either EDTA or heparin as an anti-coagulant can be used immediately without centrifugation in this test.
3. Plasma specimens containing either EDTA or heparin as an anti-coagulant can be used.
4. Serum or plasma specimens can be stored at 2-8°C (36-46°F) for up to 72 hours, or below -20°C (-4°F) for three months. Specimens should not be repeatedly frozen and thawed. Thawed specimens should be inverted several times just prior to testing.
5. Whole blood specimens containing anti-coagulant can be stored at 2-8°C (36-46°F) for up to 72 hours. During storage, the red blood cells usually settle on the bottom of the tubes and the plasma fractions can be taken out and tested.
6. Fingertip blood should be tested immediately after the sample is taken.
7. Whole blood samples in which cell lysis has occurred will cause a red background to appear in the "Read Result" window. However, the result remains valid.

REAGENTS AND MATERIALS PROVIDED

1. Reaction Unit
2. Developer
3. Mono Negative Control
4. Mono Positive Control
5. Specimen Pipet
6. Heparinized capillary tubes 50 µL for fingertip blood procedure.
7. Capillary tube bulb
8. Directions for Use

MATERIALS REQUIRED BUT NOT PROVIDED

1. Vacutainer tubes:
   a. Plain for serum procedure
   b. EDTA or heparin for plasma and whole blood procedure
2. Finger Lancet for fingertip blood procedure
3. Centrifuge
4. Single-use disposable exam gloves

PROCEDURE

Read all of the procedural instructions before running patient samples.

External Quality Control

External Positive and Negative controls are provided in the kit for quality control.

1. **External Positive Control:** Put one drop of Positive Control in the "Add" well. Process the control as you would a patient specimen. A positive signal is indicated by a vertical blue line in the "Read Result" window, resulting in a positive sign (+).
2. **External Negative Control:** Put one drop of Negative Control in the "Add" well. Process the control as you would a patient specimen. A negative signal is indicated by a horizontal blue line (-), in the "Read Result" window.

Internal Procedural Control

1. **Internal Positive Procedural Control:** A blue line in the "Test Complete" window is considered an internal positive procedural control. If the test has been performed correctly and the Reaction Unit is working properly, this indicator will appear.
2. **Internal Negative Procedural Control:** A clear background in the "Read Result" window is considered an internal negative procedural control. If the test has been performed correctly and the Reaction Unit is working properly, the background will clear to give a discernible result.

Procedural Note

1. If specimens, Controls, Developer or Reaction Units have been stored in the refrigerator, allow them to warm to room temperature (18-30°C; 64-86°F) before testing.
2. DO NOT open the foil pouch until you are ready to perform the test.
3. Several tests may be run at one time.
4. To avoid cross-contamination, use a new disposable Specimen Pipet for each specimen.
5. To avoid contamination do not touch the tip of the bottle to the Reaction Unit.
6. Commercial controls other than Pacific Biotech's should not be used with CARDS® O.S.® MONO because they may contain additives which will interfere with the test performance. Contact Technical Service regarding the appropriate commercial controls. Outside the USA contact your local representative.

FIGURE 13-40—cont'd   CARDS O.S. MONO test used to detect infectious mononucleosis. (Courtesy Quidel Corporation, San Diego, Calif.)

QUALITATIVE TEST PROCEDURE

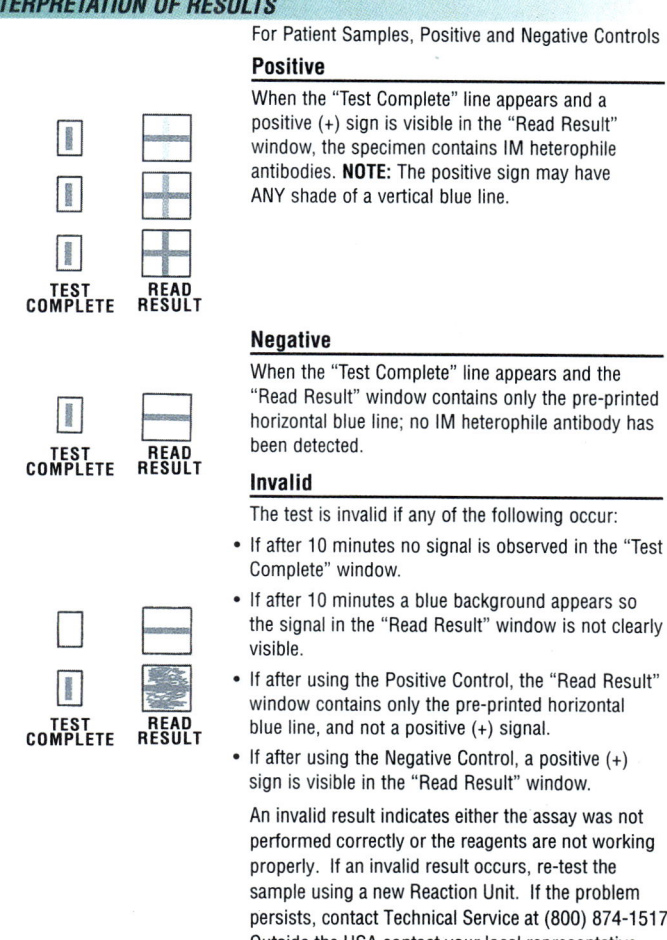

Figure I

Figure II

Figure III

1. Remove the Reaction Unit from the pouch and place it on a well lit level surface. The **"Read Result" window contains a horizontal blue line pre-printed on the membrane.**

2. Addition of Specimen: (Figure I)

   a. For serum, plasma or whole blood specimens in tubes: using the Specimen Pipet provided, place one drop of the specimen in the "Add" well.

   b. For fingertip blood: after filling capillary tube end to end (50 µL), dispense all blood into the "Add" well using the capillary tube bulb provided.

3. Hold the Developer bottle **vertically** and immediately add **5 drops** of Developer to the "Add" well. (Figure II)

4. Shortly after the specimen and Developer are added, a blue color will be seen moving through the "Read Result" window.

5. The test result can be read as soon as a distinct blue line appears in the "Test Complete" window. This will take approximately 5 minutes. (Figure III)

NOTE:

1. A signal will appear in the "Read Result" window before the test is completed. For maximum sensitivity or to confirm a negative result, interpret result only after the blue line appears in the "Test Complete" window.

2. The test result must be read within twenty (20) minutes from the addition of the Developer.

This product may also be marketed under the QuickVuet brand name.

INTERPRETATION OF RESULTS

For Patient Samples, Positive and Negative Controls

Positive

When the "Test Complete" line appears and a positive (+) sign is visible in the "Read Result" window, the specimen contains IM heterophile antibodies. **NOTE:** The positive sign may have ANY shade of a vertical blue line.

TEST COMPLETE   READ RESULT

Negative

When the "Test Complete" line appears and the "Read Result" window contains only the pre-printed horizontal blue line; no IM heterophile antibody has been detected.

TEST COMPLETE   READ RESULT

Invalid

The test is invalid if any of the following occur:

- If after 10 minutes no signal is observed in the "Test Complete" window.

- If after 10 minutes a blue background appears so the signal in the "Read Result" window is not clearly visible.

- If after using the Positive Control, the "Read Result" window contains only the pre-printed horizontal blue line, and not a positive (+) signal.

- If after using the Negative Control, a positive (+) sign is visible in the "Read Result" window.

TEST COMPLETE   READ RESULT

An invalid result indicates either the assay was not performed correctly or the reagents are not working properly. If an invalid result occurs, re-test the sample using a new Reaction Unit. If the problem persists, contact Technical Service at (800) 874-1517. Outside the USA contact your local representative.

---

procedure. Whole blood (including fingertip blood), plasma, or serum can be used for testing.

The IM heterophile antibodies are usually present 1 week after the onset of illness, peak at 2 to 4 weeks, and decline to low levels by 12 weeks. Heterophile antibodies have been detected in patients' serum over 1 year after the onset of the illness.

CONCLUSION

You have now completed the chapter on hematology. Practice the procedures, and when you think that you know the equipment and steps of the procedures, arrange with your instructor to take the performance tests. You will be expected to demonstrate accurately your ability to prepare for and perform all of the procedures that have been presented.

REVIEW OF VOCABULARY

The following are samples of patient information from medical charts. In each, terms that have been presented in this chapter are used. Read these and define the italicized terms. When laboratory values are given, determine if these are normal or abnormal results.

PATIENT NO. 1:

This patient has a history of various *blood dyscrasias*:

1990—*Anemia* and *anisocytosis*
1992—Both *hypernatremia* and *hypoglycemia* in different months
1993—*Septicemia* from undetermined causes

Present symptoms indicate *uremia* and *infectious mononucleosis*. Blood samples were obtained by *venipuncture* and sent to the laboratory for *multiphasic* tests.

PATIENT NO. 2:

Liver function studies showed minimal elevations of *SGOT* (AST) at 49.6 and 62 and then 41 units. *LDH* was not elevated, ranging at 100, 130, and 115. *Hypercholesterolemia* was revealed. *Serum electrolytes* showed slight *hypokalemia* of 3.4. With the use of potassium supplementation, the potassium rose to 4.1. The patient manifested some peripheral edema, which ultimately required the use of small doses of diuretics (Lasix 20 mg/day). This was thought to be the probable result of *hypoproteinemia*. *Serum albumin* was 3.0; total protein 6.4. *Bilirubin* remained minimally elevated at 1.4 and 1.2. *Alkaline phosphatase* was elevated at 278 and 288 IU/L (normal to 90). *CBC* showed a *hemoglobin* of 12.9 g, *hematocrit* of 37.6%, with *leukocytosis* of 14,000 and 13,500, and slight *poikilocytosis*. A *reticulocyte count* was 2.5%. *Prothrombin* time was 72%. *VDRL* was negative.

CRITICAL THINKING SKILLS REVIEW

1. Define blood.
2. List the WBCs that are classified as granulocytes and those that are classified as agranulocytes.
3. When asked to obtain a blood sample for a battery of 12 blood chemistry tests, what method and body site would you use to obtain this sample?
4. You have obtained a skin puncture blood sample. What tests might you perform in the office on this sample?
5. The following blood report has been sent to your office. Indicate which test results are normal and which are abnormal.
   WBCs—15,000/mm³
   Red blood cells—5.6 million/mm³
   Diff
        Lymphocytes—55%
        Eosinophils—8%
        Neutrophils—65%
   SGOT (AST)—65 U/ml
   Alkaline phosphatase—85 IU/L
   Prothrombin time—90% of control
   Hematocrit—45%
   Uric acid—13 mg/dl
   BUN—18 mg/dl
   Cholesterol—160 mg/dl
   VDRL—negative
   Coombs' indirect—negative
   Latex slide agglutination—positive
6. The physician has ordered a VDRL, a CBC, a Chemistry 15 panel, and a triglyceride test for a patient. Would you give this patient any special instructions before having a blood sample drawn? Could you collect one sample of blood in one tube? Would you use plain tube(s) or tube(s) with an anticoagulant additive? Explain the reasons for your answers.
7. The physician suspects that a patient may have hypothyroidism. What blood tests might be ordered to help diagnose this patient's condition?
8. What simplified tests might you do in the office to determine the presence of sugar in the blood?
9. Sexually transmitted diseases are on a constant rise at the present time. Often a physician orders a blood test to detect the presence of syphilis or uses one of these tests as a screening purpose for unsuspected cases. List three blood tests that may be performed to detect the presence of syphilis in a patient.
10. List the blood test(s) that a physician may order to help diagnose the following conditions and diseases:
    Liver disease
    Infection mononucleosis
    Myocardial infarction
    A diet too high in fat content
    Kidney disease
    Leukemia
    Chronic or acute infections
    Anemia
    Diabetes
    Rheumatoid arthritis
    Septicemia
11. List the tests performed when a CBC is ordered.
12. Define: multiphasic tests, test panel, and profile.
13. List three blood tests that require a patient to fast before the blood sample is drawn.

14. List the two most common veins used to obtain a blood specimen by venipuncture.

State/describe the anatomic location of these veins. State how much blood may be drawn from the patient by this method.

15. List three blood tests that would usually require you to use a collection tube without an additive.

State the color of the rubber stopper of the vacuum tube that you would use for this. Explain what you would do with this specimen after collection is completed (two steps).

16. State when you would use a collection tube with the additive EDTA. What color is the rubber stopper on this vacuum tube?

17. State when you would use a collection tube with the additive heparin. State the reason why you would not use this tube for hematology studies.

18. State four reasons why it is vital that the ordered blood test be performed within 8 hours or less once the blood sample has been drawn.

19. State when you would release the tourniquet on the patient when performing a venipuncture.

20. Describe what may happen if you withdraw blood too quickly when using a standard syringe and needle when performing a venipuncture.

21. State why you do not shake tubes containing an additive and blood specimen, and why you should just gently invert them 8 to 10 times.

PERFORMANCE TEST

In a skills laboratory, a simulation of a joblike environment, the medical assistant student is to demonstrate the correct procedure for the following without reference to source materials. For these activities, the student needs a person to play the role of a patient *or* an artificial appliance representing a human arm and hand, and a blood sample. Time limits for the performance of each procedure are to be assigned by the instructor (also see p. 104).

1. Given the required supplies and equipment, obtain blood samples from the patient by performing a fingertip skin puncture and a venipuncture. Then record these procedures on the patient's chart.

2. Having obtained a capillary blood sample in a nonheparinized capillary tube, perform a copper sulfate relative density test and record the results on the patient's chart.

3. Having obtained a capillary blood sample in a heparinized capillary tube, perform a hematocrit test using the microhematocrit centrifuge and record the results on the patient's chart.

4. Given a blood sample and a Dextrostix, test the sample for the presence of glucose and record the results on the patient's chart.

5. Having obtained a blood sample by performing a fingertip skin puncture, test the blood for the presence and amount of glucose using an Accu-Chek III and a Chemstrip bG; using a One Touch II blood glucose meter and a test strip; and using the HemoCue blood glucose analyzer and record the results on the patient's chart.

6. Having obtained a blood sample by performing a fingertip skin puncture, test the blood for the presence and amount of hemoglobin using a HemoCue hemoglobin analyzer and record the results on the patient's chart.

The student is expected to perform these skills with 100% accuracy.

The successful completion of each procedure will demonstrate competency levels as required by the AAMA, AMT, and future employers.

🖥 INTERNET RESOURCES

The World Foundation for Medical Studies in Female Health
www.wffh.org

Centers for Disease Control and Prevention (CDC)
www.cdc.gov

Orthoclinical Diagnostics (Clinical blood chemistry analyzers and blood banking; an interactive web site)
www.orthoclinical.com

National Institutes of Health, National Heart, Lung and Blood Institute
www.nhibi.nih.gov

American Heart Association
http://amhrt.org

Mayo Clinic Health Oasis
www.mayohealth.org

National Institutes of Health
www.nih.gov

American Diabetes Association
www.diabetes.org

Medline*plus*
www.nlm.nih.gov/medlineplus

American Liver Foundation
www.info@liverfoundation.org

14

CHAPTER

Diagnostic Medical Imaging, Radiation Therapy, and Nuclear Medicine

■ Cognitive Objectives

On completion of Chapter 14, the medical assistant student should be able to:

1. Define, spell, and pronounce the terms listed in the vocabulary and text of this chapter.
2. Explain the medical specialties of diagnostic radiology, radiation therapy, and nuclear medicine, listing examples of procedures performed by each.
3. Explain the nature and purpose of the diagnostic and therapeutic procedures outlined in this chapter.
4. Define the term *contrast medium* as used in radiology; state the function of contrast media and list at least three examples of these.
5. List and explain the nature of at least 10 radiologic procedures that use contrast media.
6. Discuss and distinguish between the special techniques of mammography, thermography, positron emission tomography (PET), tomography, computed tomography (CT), ultrasound, magnetic resonance imaging (MRI), digital radiography, and radiation therapy.
7. List and explain four basic positions used for proper exposure of the body part during radiography.
8. State and discuss the dangers, hazards, and safety precautions relevant to x-ray equipment and procedures.
9. List seven side effects that may be experienced by patients receiving high levels of radiation therapy.
10. List three body changes that may occur with overexposure to radiation.
11. Discuss the medical assistant's responsibilities relevant to radiologic procedures.
12. List at least eight x-ray examinations that do and eight that do not require special patient preparation.
13. Describe and discuss the possession, care, and storage of reports and x-ray films received in the physician's office.
14. Describe and discuss the steps involved in the processing of x-ray films.

■ Terminal Performance Objectives

On completion of Chapter 14, the medical assistant student should be able to:

1. Demonstrate proficiency in communicating proper preparation for x-rays to the patient.
2. Identify and demonstrate safety hazards and precautionary measures relevant to x-ray equipment.
3. Demonstrate the care and storage of the finished product when received in the physician's office.
4. Prepare and assist the patient for radiologic procedures.
5. Position the patient correctly for different x-ray film exposures (if licensed to do so).
6. Provide instructions and patient education that is within the professional scope of a medical assistant's training and responsibilities as assigned.

The student is to perform these objectives with 100% accuracy 95% of the time.

The consistent use of Universal/Standard Precautions is required by all health care professionals in all health care settings as a method of infection control. It is assumed that these precautions are used in all of the following procedures. Review Chapter 1 if you have any questions on methods to use because the methods or techniques are not repeated in detail in each procedure presented in this chapter.

Be sure to consult the latest guidelines issued by the Centers for Disease Control and Prevention and consult with infection control practitioners when needed to identify specific precautions that pertain to your particular work situation.

VOCABULARY

cassette (kah-set′)—A lightproof aluminum or Bakelite container with front and back intensifying screens, between which x-ray film is placed when used for x-ray examinations.

density—The quality of being dense or impenetrable. In radiology, density refers to how light or dark a film appears.

detail—The sharpness of the radiograph image.

enema (en′e-mah)—The introduction of a solution into the rectum; for an x-ray examination of the colon, a radiopaque solution is administered by enema.

fluoroscope (floo′or-o-skop″)—Equipment used during x-ray examinations for visual observation of the internal body structures by means of x-ray films. The body part to be viewed is placed between the x-ray tube and a fluorescent screen. As x-rays pass through the body, shadowy images of the internal organs are projected on the screen. Most fluoroscopic examinations require the use of a contrast medium to provide contrast (see p. 640).

fluoroscopy (floo″or-os′ko-pe)—Visual examination by means of an image intensifier.

ionizing (i″on-i-zing) **radiation**—Radiant energy given off by radioactive atoms and x-rays.

irradiate (i-ra″de-at)—To treat with radiant energy.

irradiation (i-ra″dē-ā′shun)—Exposure to radiation; the passage of penetrating rays through a substance or object.

oscilloscope (o-sil′o-skop)—An instrument for visualizing the shape or wave form of sound waves, as in ultrasonography, or of electric currents, as when monitoring heart action and other body functions.

radiation (ra″de-a′shun)—Electromagnetic waves of streams of atomic particles capable of penetrating and being absorbed into matter. Examples of electromagnetic waves are x-rays, gamma rays, ultraviolet rays, infrared rays, and rays of visible light. Atomic particles are alpha and beta particles.

radiograph (ra′de-o-graf″) or **roentgenograph** (rent′gen-o-graf) or **roentgenogram** (rent′gen-o-gram″)—The film or photographic record produced by radiography.

radiography (ra″de-og′rah-fe)—The taking of radiograms.

radioisotope (ra″de-o-i-so-top)—A radioactive form of an element consisting of unstable atoms that emit rays of energy or streams of atomic particles. Radioisotopes occur naturally, as in the case of radium, or can be created artificially, as in the case of cobalt.

radiologist (ra″de-ol′o-jist)—A physician specialist in the study of radiology.

radiolucent (ra″de-o-lu′sent)—That which permits the partial or complete passage of radiant energy such as x-rays. Dense objects appear white on the x-ray film because they absorb the radiation. An example of this is bone.

radionuclide (ra″de-o-nu′klid)—A radioactive substance.

radiopaque (ra″de-o-pak′)—That which is impenetrable by x-rays and other forms of radiant energy; matter that obstructs the passage of radiant energy, such as lead, which is often used as a protective device.

voltage (vol-tij)—The electromotive force measured in volts (the units of force for electricity to flow).

RADIOLOGIC PROCEDURES

Radiology (ra″de-ol′o-je) is the specialty of medical science that deals with the study, diagnosis, and treatment of disease by using x-rays, radioactive substances, and other forms of radiant energy, such as gamma rays, ultraviolet rays, alpha and beta particles, and sound and magnetic waves.

The procedures involved in radiology can be divided into three specialties: **diagnostic medical imaging, radiation therapy (radiation oncology),** and **nuclear medicine.**

The equipment used for radiologic procedures is very expensive and sophisticated; thus most physicians requisition these examinations or therapy from outside sources, such as a major treatment center, local hospital, or radiology office. However, some diagnostic radiology procedures, such as radiographs of the chest or skeletal fractures, may be performed in some larger offices or clinics or in physicians' offices in rural areas. It takes special training and great skill to do radiologic procedures and for physicians to accurately interpret the fluoroscopic, scanning, and x-ray images formed. Skilled radiologic technologists, called radiographers, prepare and position the patient and take the x-ray images. These individuals must be registered nationally to practice. In addition, those who practice in California, New York, and 28 other states must also

be licensed or certified by the state. The radiologist, a licensed physician specially trained in radiology, reads and interprets the films, scanning images, and fluoroscopic images.

For medical assistants to be well qualified and able to contribute to total patient care, it is imperative that they know the varied techniques, the purposes, and the nature of the specialized and highly technical radiology procedures. **Medical assistants are not legally allowed to perform radiologic procedures (unless licensed and registered to do so).** Descriptions of various x-ray, fluoroscopic, and nuclear medicine studies follow.

X-RAYS

X-rays are also called **roentgen rays,** after their discoverer, Wilhelm Konrad Roentgen (1845-1923), a physicist at the University of Würzberg, Germany, in 1895. They are a form of radiation that consists of energy waves of very short wavelength. This extremely short wavelength gives x-rays the special power of penetration. Although not visible to the human eye, x-rays can be captured on film as a visible image and can also be seen fluoroscopically by an image intensifier. The density of the matter at which x-rays are aimed and the voltage used determine the degree of x-ray penetration.

X-rays, capable of penetrating the body completely or in varying degrees and also of changing the basic structure of cells of the body, are used beneficially in the diagnosis of conditions and in the treatment of tumors and other medical conditions such as blood malignancies.

Various types of equipment are used for radiologic procedures. The equipment used for diagnostic procedures is of lower voltage than that used for radiation therapy.

Diagnostic Medical Imaging

By exposing body parts to x-rays, diagnostic medical imaging procedures create images on films or views on the **fluoroscope,** videotape, or videodisk that enable the physician to view the internal structures and functions of the body to pinpoint disease or anomalies. The observations made are then interpreted by the physician-radiologist, who then dictates the findings and radiologic diagnosis. The findings interpreted from these procedures help the physician make a diagnosis or evaluate ongoing treatment; they are also used to determine the effectiveness of a treatment program after therapy has been completed. In addition to the routine chest or skeletal films, many special diagnostic procedures and techniques can reveal more specific information about the function and structure of an organ.

Fluoroscopy: image intensification. **Fluoroscopy,** an image intensifier-television system, is an x-ray examination using an instrument that permits visual observation of deep structures of the body. X-rays from the x-ray tube pass through the patient's body and project shadowy images of organs and bones through an image intensifier. This information is fed to television monitors so that images can be readily observed during the procedure. Videotape and/or videodisk systems can record these images, which allows playback during the procedure or after it has been completed. A permanent recording of the fluoroscopic image can be made on 35-mm film. This is called **cinefluorography** and occurs simultaneously with television monitoring or image recording on a videotape and/or videodisk unit.

The major advantage of the fluoroscope over the usual type of x-ray film is that the action of organs, joints, or entire body systems can be observed in motion. The use of a contrast medium during fluoroscopy may be necessary in most procedures using this system.

Contrast medium techniques. A contrast medium is a **radiopaque substance** that is used in diagnostic radiology to permit a more accurate visualization of internal body parts and tissues in contrast to their adjacent structures.

Contrast media include liquids, powders, gas, air, or pills; these are administered orally, parenterally (by injection), or through an enema, each being specific for the examination of a particular organ or structure. The contrast medium opacifies the body part(s) under examination. Thus the structure and functions of the organ(s) can be observed and studied through x-ray films or fluoroscopy. **Positive contrast media** include barium sulfate and iodine compounds. Because these media have more density, they absorb more of the radiation, and they appear white on x-ray images. **Negative contrast media** include air, gas, and carbon dioxide and appear black on x-ray images.

Barium sulfate. This is a chalky compound, now available commercially in a premixed, flavored (such as cherry) liquid or paste. X-ray departments may also buy the powder form and mix it with water to the desired consistency.

Barium sulfate is an opaque medium used for two main types of x-ray and fluoroscopic examinations of the gastrointestinal (GI) tract. A barium meal or upper GI series is the oral ingestion of the barium mixture to outline the esophagus, stomach, and, if ordered, the small intestine, depending on the physician's request. A barium enema (BE), or lower GI series, outlines the colon for study after the instillation of the barium mixture through an enema. On occasion, a third examination, a barium swallow, is done to outline the esophagus (after the oral ingestion of the barium mixture) (Figures 14-1 and 14-2).

Iodine compounds. Containing up to 50% and more iodine, these radiopaque contrast media are used for the following tests on various body systems (see p. 641). If the patient is allergic to iodine, these examinations should not be performed. Other diagnostic techniques may then be used. The iodinated contrast media used for these procedures interfere with thyroid studies performed by the nuclear medicine department; therefore these

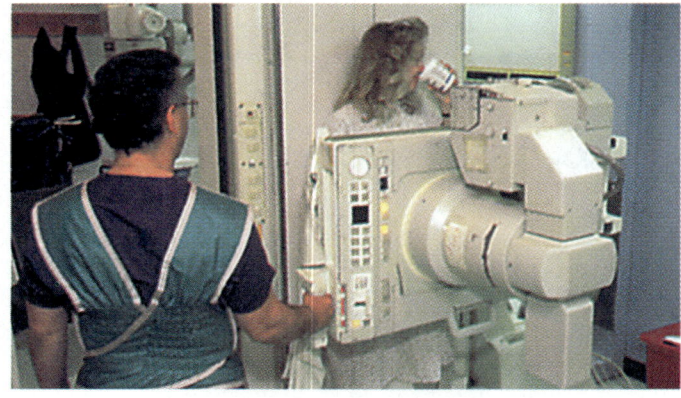

FIGURE 14-1 Upper GI barium study done under fluoroscopic control by technologist.

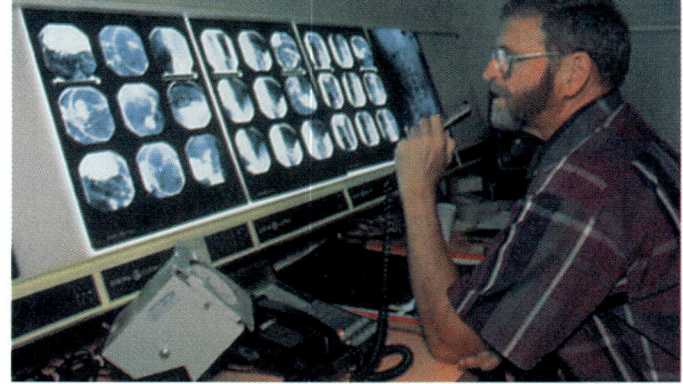

FIGURE 14-2 Physicians viewing gastrointestinal x-ray films.

procedures should not be performed when the patient is having thyroid function tests.

Air, oxygen (O₂), and carbon dioxide (CO₂).   Since the introduction of computed tomography and magnetic resonance imaging (see pp. 644 and 645), the frequency with which these negative contrast media have been used for cerebral pneumography (pneumoencephalography and pneumoventriculography) in radiology departments has essentially disappeared. Still, at times these negative media can be used for examination of the spinal cord, joints, and in combination with barium sulfate during a barium enema. Oxygen is rarely used. Carbon dioxide is used most often because it is absorbed by the body faster than

air or oxygen, thus limiting the duration of headaches that may follow a myelogram.

Mammography.   Mammography, an x-ray examination of the breast to identify breast lesions or tumors, involves detection of radiodense tissue or calcifications. Mammography is the most effective method for detecting early and curable breast cancer.

   Breast cancer is the leading cause of death in women under age 50 and is second only to lung cancer as the leading cause of death for older women. According to the American Cancer Society, one out of every nine women in the United States will develop breast cancer at some point during her lifetime. According to specialists, "It has been shown very clearly

---

VOCABULARY

Examinations using radiopaque contrast media

angiogram—X-ray record of blood vessels after injecting a contrast medium through a catheter inserted in the appropriate vessel (arteriogram, lymphangiogram, phlebogram) (Figure 14-3).

angiocardiogram—X-ray record of the heart and great vessels after injecting a contrast medium into a large peripheral vein or a chamber of the heart by direct heart catheterization.

arteriogram—X-ray record of an artery or arterial system after injecting a contrast medium through a catheter inserted in an artery.

arthrogram*—X-ray record of a joint after injecting a contrast medium into the joint or after injecting air or other gas into the articular capsule. Air can be combined with an iodine compound for double contrast studies.

bronchogram—X-ray record of the bronchial tree and lungs after instillation of a contrast medium into the bronchi via the trachea with a special instrument. This procedure is almost extinct since the introduction of new, more sophisticated modalities.

cerebral angiogram—X-ray record of the cerebral vessels after injecting a contrast medium into the common carotid artery; for x-ray records of the vessels in the posterior fossa or the occipital lobes, the medium is injected into the vertebral artery in the neck.

cholecystogram†—X-ray record of the gallbladder after oral ingestion of radiopaque granules or tablets taken the evening before the examination.

diskogram—X-ray record of the vertebral column after injecting a contrast medium into an intervertebral disk. This procedure is done infrequently.

hysterosalpingogram—X-ray record of the uterus and fallopian tubes after injecting a contrast medium through the vagina into the uterus.

intravenous cholangiogram†—X-ray record of the bile ducts after injecting a contrast medium intravenously. The contrast medium is excreted by the liver into the bile ducts; x-ray films are taken at intervals as the contrast medium is excreted through the hepatic, cystic, and common bile duct into the duodenum.

intravenous pyelogram (IVP)—X-ray records taken at intervals after intravenous injection of a contrast medium at intervals to ob-

serve the excretion rate and concentration of the dye in the renal pelves and the outline of the ureters and urinary bladder.

lymphangiogram—X-ray record of the lymphatic vessels after the injection of a contrast medium into the lymphatic system.

myelogram*—X-ray record of the spinal cord after injection of a water-soluble or an oily contrast medium, air, or gas (carbon dioxide) into the subarachnoid space through a lumbar puncture needle.

retrograde pyelogram—X-ray record of the urinary tract after introduction of a contrast medium through a urinary catheter into the ureters and pelves of the kidneys.

urogram—X-ray record of any part of the urinary tract after intravenous injection of a contrast medium. See also intravenous pyelogram.

---

*These examinations are rapidly being replaced by magnetic resonance imaging (see p. 645).

†In most facilities these procedures have been replaced by ultrasound examinations (sonography) of the gallbladder and bile ducts.

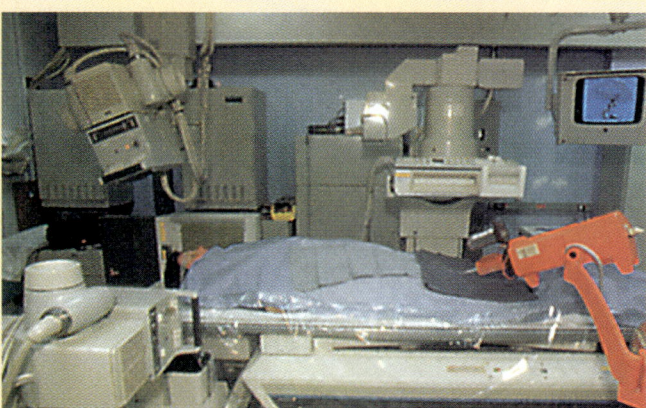

FIGURE 14-3 Vascular procedures suite. Patient is shown positioned for cerebral angiogram via femoral approach. Automatic injector and bilateral automatic film changers are used.

FIGURE 14-4   Mammographic unit.

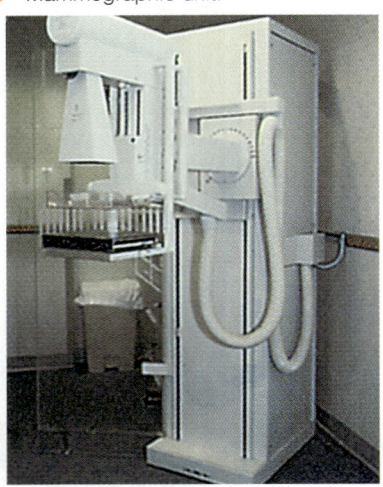

that a tumor can be seen with a mammogram as long as 2 years before either the patient or the physician is able to feel that tumor. The woman therefore has a 2-year head start on the treatment of her disease."

The new dedicated mammographic units (Figure 14-4) perform diagnostic x-ray examinations of the breast at radiation doses 5 to 10 times lower than the older units. Machines of this type provide enormous potential benefit for early cancer detection, and the minimal levels of radiation exposure have essentially removed any meaningful risk. Radiation physicists have estimated that the radiation risk of a low-dose mammogram may be equivalent to the lung cancer risk of smoking one cigarette. In addition, this "state-of-the-art" machine obtains magnified and grid images than can more optimally evaluate the young, dense, and small breast. Two films are taken from different angles: (1) the sitting or standing axillary and (2) the sitting or standing craniocaudal views (Figure 14-5).

FIGURE 14-5   A, Patient positioned for left craniocaudal view of breast for mammography. **B,** X-ray film of female breast (mammography showing entire breast back to rib cage). (Courtesy Picker Corporation, Cleveland, Ohio.)

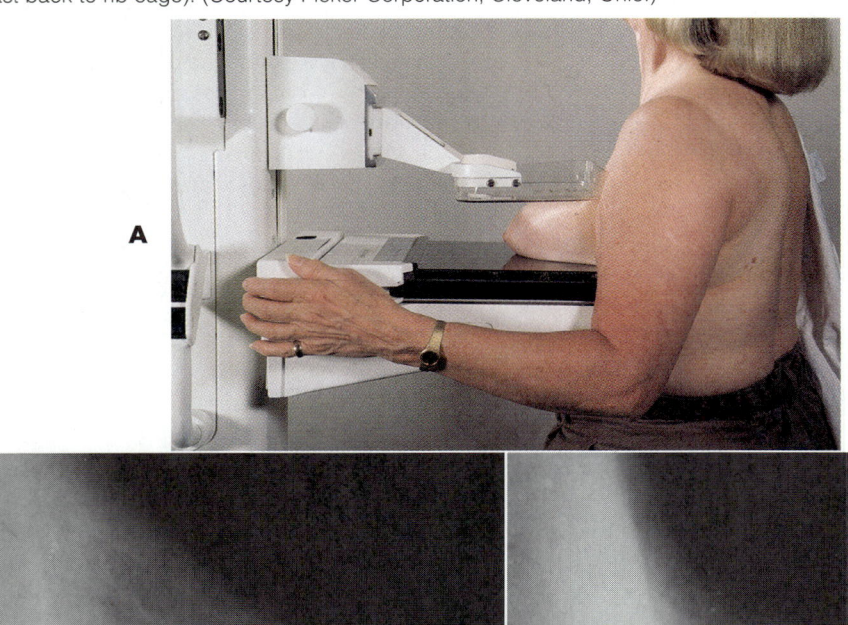

To achieve diagnostic x-ray images of the breasts at extremely low radiation doses, the breast must be compressed firmly by a clear plastic plate. Many women find this uncomfortable but tolerable. Some women find breast compression intolerable. For women with painful, tender breasts, it is suggested that they (1) schedule the examination during the time in the menstrual cycle when the breasts are least tender (this corresponds to the first 10 days of the cycle for many women); (2) avoid caffeine-containing products, such as coffee, tea, chocolate, cocoa, and soft drinks, for 1 week before the examination; (3) verbally cooperate with the radiographer to mutually arrive at a degree of compression that is tolerable to them and consistent with the technical requirements of the examination. The patient should be asked **not to wear** any powder, perfume, or deodorant on the day of the examination because these products sometimes show up as artifacts on the x-ray images.

The American Cancer Society's new recommendations state that "women without symptoms of breast cancer age 40 and over should have annual mammograms. All women are advised that monthly breast self-examination is an important health habit." (See Chapter 5.) Women ages 20 to 39 should have a breast physical examination done by a physician every 3 years, and women age 40 and over should have it done yearly, close to the time of the mammogram.

In cases in which a breast lump has been determined by a mammogram but is not clearly identifiable through palpation, a radiologist uses a *stereotactic Mammotest machine* to take "stereo" x-rays of the breast. With this machine, the radiologist can determine the exact location of a lesion within 1 mm of accuracy. A **fine-needle aspiration (FNA)** is then performed and evaluated by a cytopathologist. In an FNA, a thin needle is inserted into the lump, and a cell specimen is withdrawn. The patient's physician is informed of the results within a matter of hours.

New studies show that annual mammograms for women age 40 and over are safe and highly effective in reducing breast cancer risks. Specialists state that the benefits of an annual mammogram far outweigh the risks of radiation exposure. No woman has ever been shown to have developed breast cancer from mammography. Many specialists estimate that annual screenings would reduce breast cancer deaths by 35% in women of ages 40 to 49.

Breast ultrasound may also be done at the same time as a mammogram if the physician or radiologist determines that an ultrasound examination would provide valuable information. Ultrasonography is less sensitive than mammography as a screening tool for breast cancer but has a valuable diagnostic role in distinguishing cysts from solid masses in previously detected masses. Ultrasound is also useful in evaluating clinically palpable masses not visible on mammograms, especially in younger women.

Thermography. Thermography is a heat-sensing technique used in the detection of breast tumors. Essentially, an apparatus makes a photographic image of the varying skin temperatures. Body areas that are warm appear light; cool areas appear dark; and medium-temperature areas appear gray on the thermogram. Localized skin temperature elevations, such as those occurring over inflammatory or malignant lesions, are then sharply delineated against the temperatures of the surrounding tissues.

Although research continues, the majority opinion is that thermography is not a sufficiently reliable procedure to use for screening or detecting breast cancer. **Thus it is not recommended and is seldom used now,** except in institutions continuing investigative work. X-ray mammography is the superior diagnostic tool for detecting breast cancer.

Tomography. Tomography, or section roentgenography, has a special ability to penetrate dense shadows. X-ray pictures are taken in sections at different depths in the patient's body, focusing on the plane of the structure to be studied. Structures in front of and behind the plane under examination are blurred out.

Because of this, tomography can be a valuable diagnostic procedure when a definitive diagnosis cannot be made from conventional radiographs. Used to demonstrate and evaluate a number of different disease processes, traumatic injuries, and congenital abnormalities, tomography can be used in any part of the body, but it is most effective in areas of high contrast, such as the lungs and bones. Two of the most common uses are to demonstrate and evaluate benign and malignant processes in the lungs and for intravenous pyelograms.

Although computed tomography (CT) and magnetic resonance imaging (MRI) (see the following paragraphs through p. 646) have replaced the use of tomography to a great extent, at times, tomography is still the examination of choice. Many hospitals do not have the CT and MRI units because of the high cost. In addition, the cost to the patient is much higher for a CT or MRI examination. Tomography can often provide a satisfying diagnosis or at least screen the patient for further evaluation by more sophisticated modalities.

Positron emission tomography. Positron emission tomography (PET) is a computerized radiographic technique that uses radiopharmaceuticals (radioactive substances) to examine the metabolic activity of various body structures. The patient either inhales or is injected with a radiopharmaceutical. The computers and electronic circuitry of the PET device detect and convert gamma rays into color-coded images that indicate the intensity of the metabolic activity of the organ involved. Patients are exposed to very small amounts of radiation because the radioactive substances used are very short lived. Presently PET is used predominately as a research tool to study blood flow and the metabolism of the heart and the blood vessels and to detect early warning signs of heart problems and the stages of heart disease. With this knowledge a treatment program of diet, exercise, and certain medications, such as those used to lower blood cholesterol levels, can be started with life-saving results. PET is also used to determine local cerebral blood flow and the local cerebral metabolic rate of glucose. PET measures regional brain function that cannot be determined by any other diagnostic method, including CT and MRI. Current PET studies are used for patients with epilepsy, brain tumors, Alzheimer's disease, a stroke, spasmodic torticollis, and other movement disorders.

Computed tomography (CT scan).   The CT scanner, the developers of which were awarded the Nobel Prize for medicine in October 1979, has been a most significant breakthrough in medical technology.

CT is an advanced radiologic modality that provides valuable clinical information in the early detection, differentiation, and demarcation of diseases of the head and body. It often provides diagnostic information that cannot be obtained by any other method, especially in neurologic work.

Quick and noninvasive, the CT scan is particularly helpful in solving problems in which there is conflicting information from other radiologic or laboratory studies, and it may be necessary for planning radiation therapy for certain tumor masses. Its use has often replaced some examinations such as echoencephalography (see Diagnostic Ultrasound) and others, many of which (for example, the pneumoencephalogram and arteriogram) carry greater risk and discomfort to the patient. In addition, CT does, in certain cases, replace procedures that would require the patient to be hospitalized. This technique is used for neurologic procedures; to detect cerebral abnormalities (for example, tumors, lesions, hematomas, and bleeding in the brains of newborn infants); to search for childhood cancer; to detect masses in the chest, abdominal, and pelvic cavities; to examine the liver, spleen, pancreas, kidneys, adrenal glands, pituitary gland, and optic nerve; and for a generalized survey for lymphoma or metastases (Figure 14-6).

FIGURE 14-6   **A,** Technologist positioning patient for head scan with CT total body scanner. **B,** Control room for the CT Scanner. X-ray generation controls, scanning control console, and viewing monitors are found here. Main computer hardware is usually located in adjacent room.

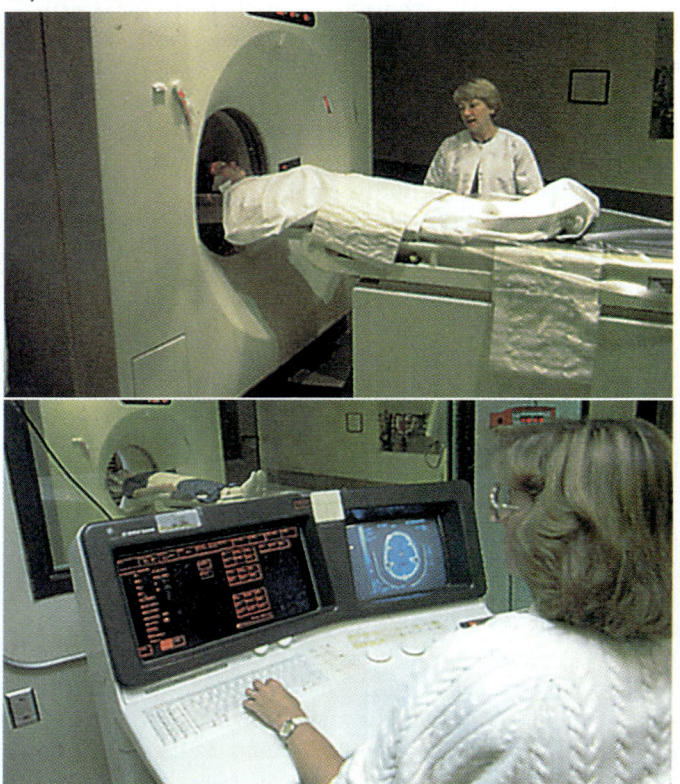

Machines called scanners (such as ACTA, CT/T, Synerview, Delta, Syntex) beam x-rays to scan the body site in a series of x-rays. The scanner combines the capabilities of traditional x-ray with that of a computer, providing an image of soft tissue in three dimensions. The x-ray tube and detector source rotate 360 degrees around the patient's head or body part being studied, taking multiple "slices"—cross-sectional readings. Thus every tissue and organ is x-rayed from all sides. As they pass through the body, the absorption rates of the x-rays are detected, and the density of the tissue is relayed to the computer. From the calculations performed by the computer, densities are translated into a picture of the body as if it were neatly cut into slices, each a fraction of an inch thick. This picture is projected on a screen for the radiologist to study (Figure 14-7).

The conventional x-ray film reveals only certain organs and tissues and requires multiple exposures to estimate the size and location of diseased areas. The CT scanner can distinguish nearly every type of tissue and has the ability to distinguish more minute differences in the various tissues. CT can determine the size and location of any pathologic condition with great accuracy. When first developed around the mid-1970s, CT scans were slow; however, now many machines in use can complete a scan in 4 to 5 seconds, and a more sophisticated machine can complete a scan in 1 second. Older, conventional scanners take 15 to 30 minutes or longer to complete all the slices required for a complete examination. These CT scanners can only be used for 15 to 20 examinations during an 8-hour workday.

The newest, most up-to-date scanner, the helical scanner, does volumetric scanning, taking a volume of areas rather than one image at a time. The scanned data are then reconstructed into three-dimensional images. Overall, the quality of the images produced is improved. The helical scanner can scan the

FIGURE 14-7   Images from a CT head scan. (Courtesy General Electric, Medical Systems, Milwaukee, Wisc.)

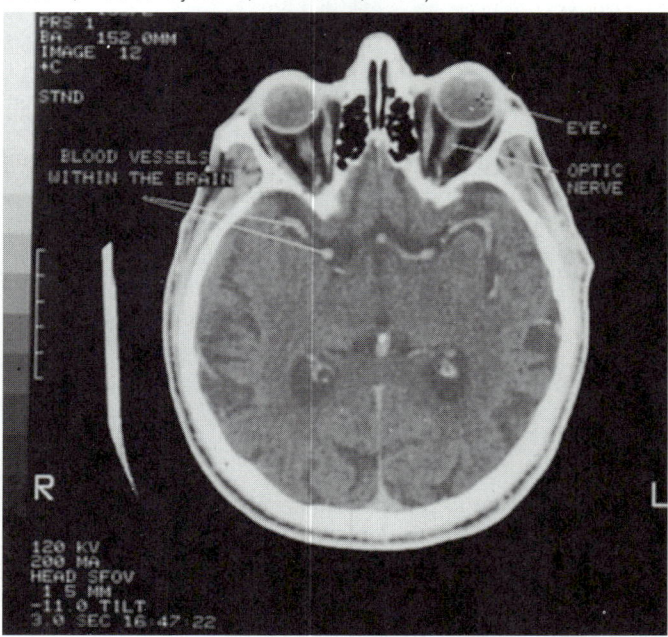

entire pelvis and abdomen in less than 40 seconds. These newer scanners can be used for 30 to 40 or more examinations during an 8-hour workday.

Minimal **patient preparation** is required for CT scans. Some facilities require the patient to have nothing by mouth for 4 hours before the examination if a contrast medium is used. For abdominal and pelvic scans, patient preparation is usually nothing by mouth. When a contrast medium is not used, patient preparation is not required. A contrast medium, which is almost always used for a CT scan, can be administered orally or intravenously.

An iodine-based contrast medium is used unless the patient is allergic to iodine-based products, is in renal failure, has multiple myeloma, or has abnormal blood urea nitrogen (BUN) and creatinine levels. In these situations the scan is done without the use of a contrast medium.

Insulin-dependent diabetics who are taking the new medication metformin (Glucophage) must cease taking this medication for at least 24 hours before having a scan using a contrast medium. Special arrangements must be made by the physician regarding this patient's medication regimen.

Research is continuing for a scanner that can make clear x-ray images of the fast-beating human heart. Some researchers are presently testing it as a noninvasive method to determine whether vein grafts installed in a coronary bypass surgery are allowing blood to flow freely or have become closed and useless. The National Aeronautics and Space Administration (NASA) is also interested in this device because it may be valuable in detecting the loss of calcium in bones, which is a serious consequence of weightlessness in space travel.

Although the use of the CT scan is superior in numerous situations, at times the findings obtained indicate the need for additional and invasive procedures for a conclusive diagnosis to be established.

Magnetic resonance imaging.

A newer and equally exciting technique for examining the body is magnetic resonance imaging (MRI). MRI is a computer-based, cross-sectional imaging modality that examines the interactions of magnetism and radio waves with tissue to obtain its images. Magnets, as the name suggests, are at the heart of this system. Many machines use superconducting magnets; the more powerful the magnets, the clearer the images produced.

An MRI has **major advantages,** such as the ability to examine properties of body tissue that have never before been visualized. Both anatomic and physiologic information can be obtained. No x-rays (that is, no ionizing radiation of any kind) are used to obtain an MRI, and it is a painless and usually noninvasive technique. On a few occasions a contrast medium may be used. There are no known harmful effects to the patient when exposed to the current levels of magnetic field strength and radio wave energy transmission.

Magnetic resonance is **used to** detect tumors in soft tissues because even in early stages, malignant tissue responds to the magnetic pull differently from normal tissue. No other imaging technique can detect such subtle differences in soft tissues. It is also used to examine the brain (it can distinguish brain tumors

from tiny blood clots and determine the chemical changes that cause dementia in the elderly); spinal cord tumors, cystic changes of the spine, and disk disease; the gastrointestinal tract; the heart muscle, septal defects, and cardiac valve leaflets; the lungs; the extremities (but bone lesions and calcium within tumors are seen better with CT); tumors of the liver and spleen; and pelvic structures (for example, bladder tumors, neoplasms in the female genital tract). It may detect prostate tumors, and it can outline the kidneys, adrenal glands, and retroperitoneal structures, such as lymph nodes (although there is limited evidence that MRI is superior to CT in this area).

New research suggests that by using MRI, two alterations in the brain's hippocampus, the center of memory and cognitive thinking, can be examined. The results could be used to increase the likelihood of an early diagnosis of Alzheimer's disease. Alzheimer's disease is incurable and irreversible, and it is a major cause of death among Americans, behind cancer and heart disease.

MRI of the heart after a heart attack may help determine which patients will do well and which ones will later suffer complications, such as another heart attack, congestive heart failure, stroke, or death. This new research found that patients who had heart attacks were more likely to suffer frequent heart complications within 2 years if the MRI scans showed that the heart's capillaries were partially blocked with dying blood cells and debris.

Two other major breakthroughs for MRIs are the use of an urgent MRI to determine if a patient is suffering from a stroke or another problem such as a migraine or a seizure. Also determined at this time is the area of the brain at risk. Time is of greatest essence—the faster a stroke is diagnosed, the faster treatment can be started, and thus the more brain tissue can be saved. This new MRI technique, known as diffusion-weighted imaging, is the first major clinical application of **functional magnetic imaging.** This new technology will enhance our understanding of how the human brain works. Another type of scan and a newer technique can identify levels of choline and other brain chemicals that are often altered by disease. Also, uses of functional MRI can help to explain the mechanics of addiction. These findings can be combined with other non-MRI methods to create even greater insights of the human brain.

However, MRI has its limitations. It cannot provide images of the hard part of the bones; thus we still need x-rays, CT, or other techniques to diagnose fractures and malformations in bones. Also, the strong magnetic field is potentially dangerous to patients with cardiac pacemakers and to those who have any type of metallic implants, such as aneurysm clips on blood vessels within the skull or clips tying off other blood vessels. The pull of the magnets could slip the clips out of place, and vessels could be torn. **It is therefore important to check that the patient does not have a pacemaker or metallic implants before an MRI is scheduled.**

The image produced by the computer can be viewed on a television monitor. If desired, the images can be photographed for further study. These images can also be stored on a computer disk temporarily and then transferred to an optical disk for permanent storage and retrieval (Figures 14-8 and 14-9).

FIGURE 14-8   MRI. **A,** Young child being assisted onto the table for an MRI procedure. People of all ages can have MRI examinations. **B,** Patient being positioned for an MRI of the head and neck. **C,** Control room for the MRI scanner. Technologist operating the MRI equipment. Note the image of the brain produced by the computer displayed on the television monitor.

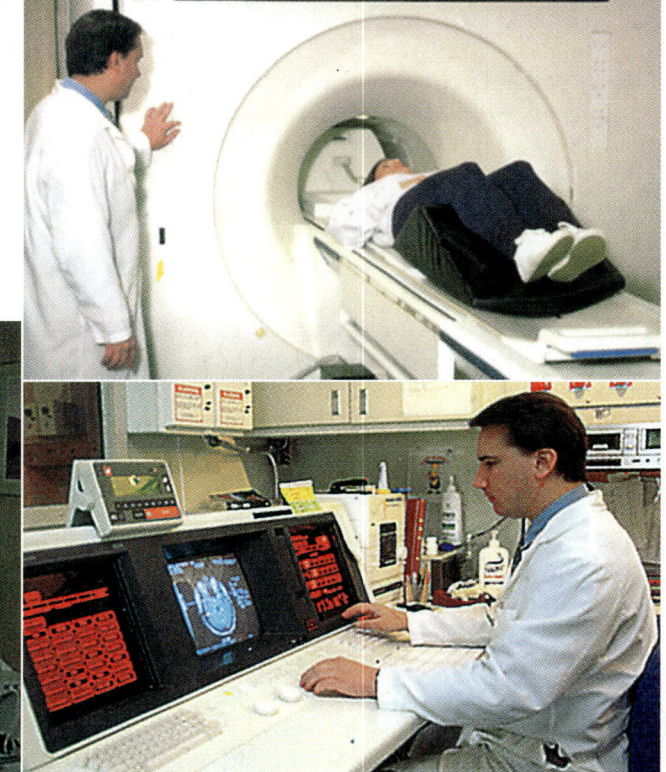

FIGURE 14-9   **A,** Image from MRI head and neck scan. (Courtesy General Electric, Medical Systems, Milwaukee, Wisc.)

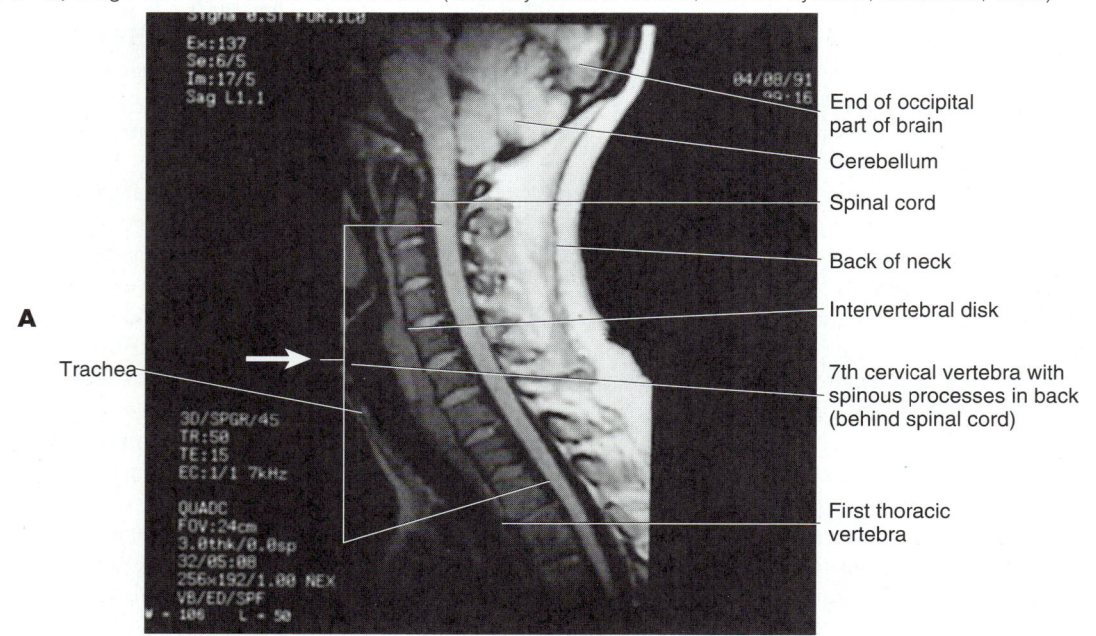

FIGURE 14-9—cont'd   **B,** Image from MRI knee scan. (Courtesy General Electric, Medical Systems, Milwaukee, Wisc.)

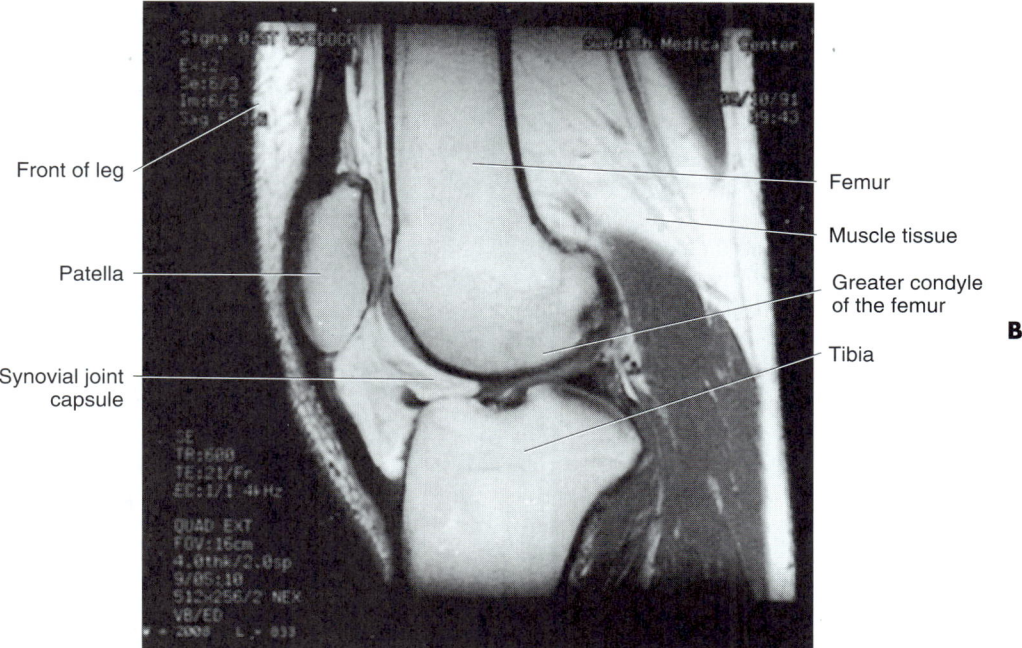

Front of leg

Patella

Synovial joint capsule

Femur

Muscle tissue

Greater condyle of the femur

Tibia

B

Digital radiography.   Digital radiography is the use of the conventional image intensifier-television system (fluoroscopy) in which the television signal is first digitized (information is stored in computer units called bits) and processed by the computer before the x-ray image is displayed on a standard television monitor.

The use of digital radiography has been successful in angiography. This procedure can replace the more complex and time-consuming procedure of arterial catheterization. Four advantages of this procedure are that it is safer for the patient, it is less painful, it uses a lower x-ray dose, and it requires a much smaller amount of contrast medium.

A **contrast medium** is injected through a catheter that is placed into a vein, preferably the basilic vein or alternately in the cephalic vein or the superior vena cava. As the x-ray images are taken, they are formed electronically and displayed on the television monitor. At the same time, the image is stored on a videotape, videodisk, or digital disk.

Digital angiography is used for head and neck angiograms and images of the pulmonary arteries and cardiac structures. Hospitalization of the patient is not required.

As digital radiographic devices and procedures expand, traditional studies in which film processing has been used may gradually be replaced by digital image processing.

Quantitative digital radiography (QDR), using the most advanced technology available, is used to screen patients for osteoporosis by measuring bone density. QDR provides the safest, quickest, most precise, and most reliable measurement of bone mineral content. It can be used to determine if osteoporosis is present and also is useful in following the effects of treatment for the disease. Cross-lateral and whole-body imaging can be obtained with the use of this examination.

Diagnostic ultrasound.   Diagnostic ultrasound, sometimes called **diagnostic medical sonography** or **ultrasonography,** *does not use ionizing radiation* to diagnose or treat disease but uses very high-frequency inaudible sound waves that bounce off the body to record information on the structure of internal organs.

In this examination, the patient's skin is covered with water, oil, or a special jelly that helps conduct the sound waves into the body. A special instrument, called a transducer, emitting sound waves is placed and moved on or near the patient's skin. Sound waves pass through the skin, strike the body tissues, and pass an echo reflection back to the instrument. These ultrasonic echoes are then recorded on the oscilloscope as a picture of a series of dots. This record produced is called an echogram or sonogram. The method of image recording in which the data are stored on film, paper, video, or other recording material is sometimes called hard copy.

Ultrasound can be **used to** detect abnormalities in the heart (echocardiography), major blood vessels, kidneys, abdominopelvic cavity, breast (it is the best method for distinguishing between solid and fluid-filled lumps in the breast and is often done when a mammogram or physical examination show positive results), scrotum, prostate, muscles, spine, and brain (echoencephalogram [EECG], although this has now been replaced by the CT scan, when available, because of the superiority of CT images of the entire cranial vault versus very limited knowledge available from the EECG).

Obstetric ultrasound screening during pregnancy has become very common usually between 16 to 22 weeks of gestation. Many women have come to expect an ultrasound as part of their prenatal care, but the American College of Obstetricians and Gynecologists states that ultrasounds are not always medically necessary. It is not a general screening tool and should not be used to merely determine the sex of the baby. The U. S. Department of Health and Human Services has listed 27 situations in which obstetric ultrasound is indicated. One of the most common indications is to determine the date of conception when it is unknown because this information is critical in deciding when to induce labor or to perform a cesarean section if necessary. Ultrasound is also indicated when vaginal bleeding occurs because this may indicate an impending miscarriage or fetal distress. Ultrasound can often reveal the nature and extent of a defect when the mother's blood level of alpha-fetoprotein is abnormal (this could indicate a neurologic problem, such as spina bifida) or if an amniocentesis has revealed a genetic defect, such as Down syndrome. It is also used to determine the presence of a pregnancy if other tests are unsuccessful; to differentiate between single and multiple pregnancies; to view placental position, various stages, and fetal positions during pregnancy; and for neonatal examinations (Figure 14-10). In some procedures, body structures such as the diaphragm, cardiac or fetal heart motion, or other organ structures that move with respiration are visible as they change position in time. This examination is often done with the mother positioned so that she is able to observe the fetal image on the display screen. The only patient preparation for this examination is that the woman have a full urinary bladder (see Table 14-4).

Ultrasound has the **advantages** of being a painless, noninvasive procedure that does not expose the patient to ionizing radiation. After 35 years of use, physicians have found no evidence that diagnostic ultrasound causes any untoward biologic effect. Therefore it has generally been accepted as a safe technique.

Ultrasound is also used for treatment in physical medicine (by physical therapists) for deep muscle or tension pain. In this case a different machine with a different sound wave intensity is used. (This is discussed in the chapter on physical therapy.)

Other diagnostic radiologic examinations

Abdomen. A survey film (flat plate) of the abdomen or kidney, ureter, and bladder (KUB) is ordered without the use of a contrast medium when abnormal conditions of the abdomen are suspected, such as tumors, abscesses, enlarged organs, bowel obstructions, or hematomas.

In the plain survey, three films are often taken. The patient may be placed in the erect, supine, prone, or lateral decubitus position, depending on the suspected pathologic condition to be studied (Figure 14-11). For perforated organs a flat plate and an upright or left lateral decubitus view is ordered.

Routine chest x-ray film. An x-ray record of the chest is obtained with the patient in the posteroanterior erect position. Generally, a left lateral view is also taken (Figure 14-12).

Kidney, ureter, bladder (KUB). A film of the abdomen is used to study the kidneys, flank area, gas patterns, abdominal wall, bones of the pelvis, and any unusual masses.

FIGURE 14-11 Radiologic technologist performing routine radiographic work (for example, pelvis or abdomen) with overhead tube mount.

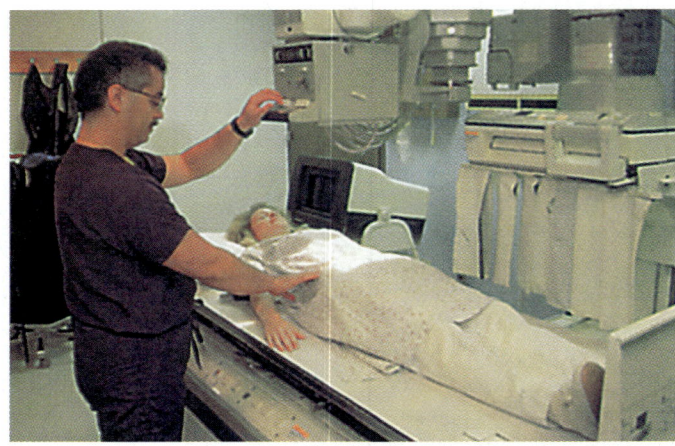

FIGURE 14-12 Physician interpreting and dictating the results of a chest x-ray film.

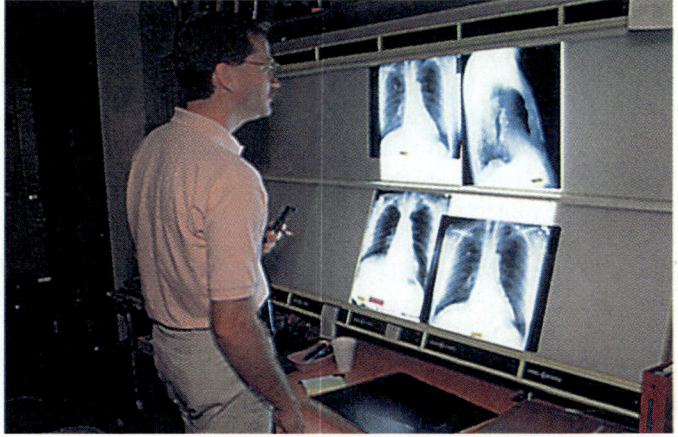

FIGURE 14-10 Obstetric ultrasound.

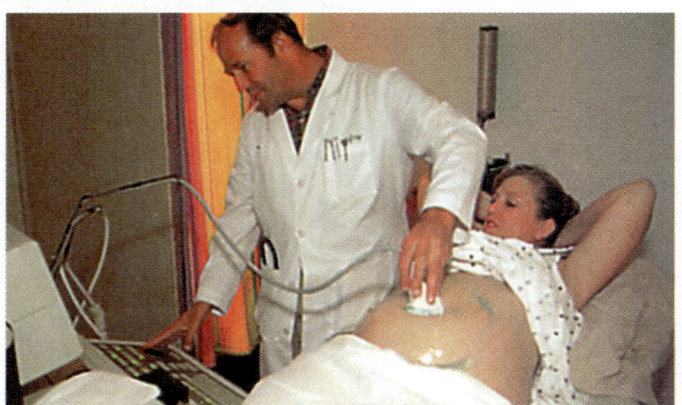

Skull series.   A series of radiographs of the skull is used to determine cranial injuries or the effects of trauma to the head and neck. CT has replaced the use of these films, except in cases of severe trauma.

Paranasal sinus films.   X-ray records are made of the paired sinuses within the frontal, ethmoid, sphenoid, and maxillary bones of the face. CT has often replaced the use of these films.

Bone x-ray films.   X-ray records are made of bones thought to have disease or trauma, such as tumors and fractures or displacement. X-ray studies of the vertebral column are common. Radiographs of the neck are called cervical x-ray films; those of the middle back are called thoracic x-ray films; and those of the lower back are called lumbosacral x-ray films.

RADIATION THERAPY

As a medical assistant, you should have some knowledge of radiation therapy because patients who are to receive or have experienced it may ask you questions. When radiation is applied for treatment of cancer and various other conditions by x-rays, beta rays, and gamma rays and other radioactive substances, it is called **radiation therapy, radiotherapy,** or **radiation oncology,** the purpose being to administer a definite amount of radiation to a specific location to irradiate diseased cells. Radiation therapy alters the diseased cell so that it cannot reproduce and will eventually age and die, leaving no new cells behind. Only the most extreme dose of radiation kills the cells directly.

The amount of energy that is deposited within the tissue and the condition of the biologic system determine the effectiveness of ionizing radiation in living tissue. The radiosensitivity of most tissues depends on the following:

- The number of undifferentiated (lack or absence of normal cell differentiation) cells in the tissue.
- The degree of mitotic activity (cell division that produces new cells) of the tissue. During mitosis, the human cells are most sensitive to radiation.
- The length of time that cells of the tissue continue to reproduce.
- The primary target of ionizing radiation is the DNA molecule and water molecule in the human cell. Water makes up about 80% to 85% of our bodies. When a water molecule is irradiated, the molecule disassociates into free radicals and will reconstitute at a later time into hydrogen peroxide, which is toxic to the cells. The end result is death of the malignant target cells.

Certain tumors are more radiosensitive than others. Some that are highly radiosensitive include tumors of the ovaries and testes, especially seminomas, lymphomas, Wilms' tumor of the kidney, retinoblastomas, and Hodgkin's disease. Those that are moderately radiosensitive include basal and squamous cell carcinomas of the skin, adenocarcinoma of the prostate, breast carcinoma, and Ewing's sarcoma of the bone. Tumors that are *relatively* radioresistant include sarcomas of the bone, connective tissue, and muscle and nerve tumors.

Certain sources of radioactivity are used for specific types or locations of cancer. Radium, for example, gives off rays (alpha, beta, and gamma) that affect the growth of tissue. In the form of seeds or needles (radium implants), radium can be implanted directly into a malignant tumor in the uterus or mouth for a prescribed period (possibly 3 to 4 days) to act on and destroy abnormal cells. This is called interstitial treatment. Permanent implant therapy may also be done using radon-222 seeds and iodine-125 seeds. These implants are left in the patient forever. Radioisotopes of cobalt can also be used for implantation, in addition to teletherapy or possible surgery. Teletherapy is radiation treatment administered by a radioactive isotope such as cobalt-60 or cesium-137, emitting high-energy gamma rays. These are housed in shielded units, similar to large x-ray units, which are placed at a distance from the patient. A beam of gamma radiation is aimed at the specific part of the body requiring treatment. Radiotherapy of this type is especially useful in the treatment of deep-seated malignancies not readily accessible for implantation. Radioisotopes are also available in a liquid form that can be used for local irradiation in the pleural or peritoneal cavities and also for the thyroid gland. **The use of radiation therapy in cancer is based on the fact that cancer cells are more sensitive to x-rays and other radioactive substances than other cells in surrounding normal tissue.**

Ionizing radiation affects both normal and diseased cells. The dose of radiation administered should be sufficient to treat the diseased area but not so great that it would permanently damage the surrounding normal tissues. Treatment techniques are designed to deliver a precise dose to the tumor, while limiting the amount of radiation delivered to the uninvolved portions of the tissue. Greater damage occurs to the abnormal cells because more of these cells are undergoing mitosis and are more poorly differentiated. Normal cells have a greater capability of repairing the resulting damage than do malignant cells. Low-voltage x-rays are used to treat conditions that require only surface penetration, such as skin lesions, whereas high-voltage radiation is used to treat deep-seated malignancies.

Effective treatment of cancer with radiation therapy depends on the following:

- The extent to which the disease has progressed

  What is the size of the initial tumor and are lymph nodes involved? Is there involvement or lack of involvement of the adjacent tissues, structures, or organs? For example, the tumor could attach itself to a blood vessel or nerve. Is there presence of metastases? The malignant cells could have traveled to a distant organ or site, such as seen in someone who has a breast tumor as the primary site of cancer and now has developed brain, lung, and bone cancer. At this stage it is very difficult to control the disease.
- The type of cells in the tumor
- The general health of the patient
- The location of the tumor
- The radiocurability of the tumor

- The services available at a given facility. Large hospitals have more equipment, have seen more cases, and know more of what is best for the prognosis.

For definitive treatment, the cancer must be in a tissue that is more radioresistant than the tumor.

Approximately 70% of all newly diagnosed cancer patients are treated with radiation therapy. Radiation therapy may be the only treatment used for some cancer, such as cancer of the larynx, skin, oral cavity, nasopharynx, cervix (although surgery may be the preferred treatment for cancer of the cervix), Hodgkin's disease, and malignant lymphoma (chemotherapy may also be used here).

Some of the **advantages** of this therapy are that it provides better cosmetic results over surgery; the body part is maintained; surgery can be saved for a later date, if needed; and this treatment is done on an outpatient basis, which allows the patient to maintain many of his or her everyday activities. However, the patient must make a time commitment for this therapy because the treatment often is scheduled for 5 days a week for 6 to 7 weeks.

Some **short-term adverse acute responses** do occur, but these go away once the treatment program has been completed. These responses commonly include the following:

- Erythema—a redness or inflammation of the skin or mucous membranes involved
- A decrease in complete blood count (CBC) values
- A generalized feeling of fatigue and tiredness
- Nausea when the treatment involves the abdominal area
- Hair loss in full brain irradiation

Long-term side effects may show up 1 to 2 years later. These could include cataracts of the eye, atrophy of the body part that was treated, and in the worse scenario, necrosis of tissues and organs involved and radiation myelitis when too much radiation was given to the spinal cord, which could lead to paralysis.

Great measures are taken to prevent all of these adverse side effects. Most can be avoided with a good treatment plan determined by a qualified licensed specialist working with the patient.

Often surgical interventions, chemotherapy, or a combination of the two are used in conjunction with radiation therapy for the treatment of cancer of the breast, uterus, lungs, and others. Other modalities such as CT and ultrasonography are used to locate the tumor(s) and to localize the boundaries of organs not involved. After therapy, these modalities can be used to record tumor regression and the effectiveness of the treatment program.

The advantageous role of radiation therapy for the treatment of cancer is well documented. It will likely continue to play an important and expanded role in the treatment of cancer.

NUCLEAR MEDICINE

Nuclear medicine is the medical specialty that deals with the diagnosis and treatment of disease processes with the use of radioactive substances, although it is used predominantly for diagnostic purposes. Radioactive pharmaceuticals are thought to be **radionuclides,** in which the nuclei of the atoms of that particular isotope are undergoing spontaneous disintegrations. These radionuclides are administered intravenously or orally to the patient, or a radioactive gas may be inhaled. Sophisticated measuring equipment and imaging devices that are interfaced with computers are used. A radiosensitive instrument known as a gamma camera or scintillation probe maps the area to be studied. To obtain the information desired, the gamma camera remains stationary over the organ of interest. This instrument records an image relating to the patterns of radioactivity concentrated within the organ being studied. This image is called a **scintigram** or **scintiscan** and is used by the physician to diagnose tumors or other disease processes. The scintillation probe is used primarily in the evaluation of hyperthyroidism. The probe is placed in close proximity to the skin over the organ being studied and records the concentration of radioactivity within the organ by giving a numeric printout.

When a radionuclide is used to make a medical diagnosis, the physician refers to the concentration of radionuclides as being **"hot spots"** or **"cold spots."** If the radionuclide concentrates in an abnormality, it is known as a hot spot within the scan; or, if the tumor does not concentrate the radionuclide, it is known as a cold spot within the surrounding tissue that has concentrated the radioactive pharmaceutical. Hot spots or cold spots can both denote abnormality, depending on the organ being studied. All radionuclides used for diagnostic procedures are short lived, which means that they remain radioactive only for a short time. Consequently, the radiation dose to the patient is small and usually does not cause any ill effects.

When radioisotopes are used in therapy doses, the effects are much like those seen when high-level radiation therapy is given to the patient. **The following are symptoms that may be seen when either radiation or radioisotope therapy is given:** loss of hair, shedding of skin, hemopoietic dysfunction, diarrhea, nausea, irritation of mucous membranes (such as in the mouth, throat, bladder, or vagina), and chromosomal changes.

All scans can usually be done on an outpatient basis. You should be aware of any special preparation required of the patient before having the scan and the approximate length of time of each scan so that the patient can be briefed on what to expect. Tables 14-1 and 14-2 outline the most common scans and the time required for each. Similar reference sheets should be available in the physician's office for your reference when necessary. Your responsibilities relating to the diagnostic studies presented in this chapter, as well as similar tables for x-ray examinations, are given on pp. 654, 655, 657, and 658.

POSITION OF PATIENT FOR X-RAY STUDIES

Radiograms are made by directing beams of x-rays through the x-ray tube toward a specific body part. The body part to be radiographed must be positioned correctly between the film-containing cassette and the x-ray source. The body part to be filmed is positioned closest to the cassette.

NUCLEAR MEDICINE VOCABULARY

Scanning studies used for diagnosis

bone scan—Used to detect osteogenic sarcoma and its metastases, bone neoplasms, localized lesions for biopsy, osteomyelitis, and stress fractures and to evaluate arthritis and Paget's disease.

bone marrow scan—Used to detect hemolytic and iron deficiency, to detect decreased marrow function secondary to radiation therapy, and to measure the functional marrow reserve in patients on chemotherapy.

brain scan—Used to detect, localize, or follow the course of suspected or proved vascular malformations, inflammatory diseases, abscesses, cerebrovascular accidents, metastatic brain tumor, and subdural hematomas.

cardiac scan—Used to detect myocardial infarctions and blood flow related to cardiac stress testing and cardiac artery stenosis. Sometimes used to evaluate pericardial effusion and localized ischemic scar damage.

cisternogram—Used to localize cerebrospinal fluid leaks, "normal pressure" hydrocephalus, and evaluation of the functional status of ventricular shunts. This procedure is done rarely.

hepatobiliary scan—Used to detect gallbladder patency and functioning.

kidney scan—Used to detect kidney disease, trauma, and tumors and to evaluate hypertension. Used to study patients with demonstrated or suspected sensitivity to iodinated radiographic contrast media.

liver scan—Used to detect primary and metastatic malignancy, biliary obstruction, abscesses, and cysts; sometimes used for the evaluation of hepatitis or cirrhosis, hepatomegaly, jaundice, and rupture.

lung perfusion—Used to detect a pulmonary embolus.

lung ventilation—Used to detect a pulmonary embolus. This procedure is usually done with a lung perfusion. Ventilation is done first and may be followed with the lung perfusion.

spleen scan—Used to detect splenomegaly and splenic rupture.

thyroid scan—Used to detect hyperthyroidism and the localization of nodules. Preoperative and postoperative scans are done for patients with thyroid carcinoma.

white blood cell scan—Used to determine the source of an infection in questionable cases. The image shows the destination of many of the labeled white blood cells (that is, they show the site of the infection).

TABLE 14–1 **Common Nuclear Medicine Scans That DO NOT Require Special Patient Preparation and Approximate Time Required for Each**

Scan	Procedure	Approximate Time Required
Brain scan	Intravenous (IV) injection and scan immediately. Wait 2 hr and take delayed scan.	Initial injection and flow study—15 min. Delayed scan—45 min
Bone scan	IV injection done and wait 3 hr, then scan.	1 hr plus 3-hr interval
Bone marrow scan	IV injection and begin scan in 15 min.	1 hr
Cisternogram	Injection into lumbar subarachnoid space via lumbar puncture.	Following injection, scans are done at 6-, 24-, 48-, and 72-hr intervals
Kidney and/or spleen scan	IV injection and scan immediately. For some kidney scans, hydration of patient will be necessary.	45-60 min
Liver scan	IV injection and wait 15 min for scan.	45 min
Lung perfusion scan	Inject and scan immediately.	45 min
Lung ventilation scan	Patient inhales radioactive xenon gas. Serial films are taken for 30 min while patient breathes inert xenon gas.	40 min
Thyroid scan*	IV injection of technetium 99m and scan; or patient is given iodine-123 orally and scanned either immediately or 4 to 24 hr later, respectively.	45 min
White blood cell (WBC) scan	Draw 50 ml blood; label WBC with indium III, then inject cells back into patient. Scan 24 hr later.	60 min

*X-ray intravenous iodionated dyes will interfere with the thyroid studies and must not have been done within 3 months of study. Vitamins with iodine interfere with thyroid studies and must be discontinued for at least 2 weeks before study. Synthroid or other thyroid medications must be stopped for at least 2 weeks before thyroid studies.

TABLE 14–2 **Nuclear Medicine Scans That DO Require Special Patient Preparation and Approximate Time Required for Each**

Scan	Procedure	Approximate Time Required
Cardiac scans	If patient is going to have thallium-201 heart scan, there should be nothing by mouth (NPO) for at least 3 hr before examination. Other cardiac scans need no special preparation.	
Thallium-201 heart scan	Intravenous (IV) injection and scan immediately. Scan is done with patient on a treadmill and at 85% stress. Delayed 6 and 24 hr films.	
Pyrophosphate heart scan	IV injection and scan immediately; then 1½ and 3 hr delayed films.	30-45 min
Cardiac wall motion scan	IV injection and scan immediately.	30-45 min
Gallium scan	For tumor localization and abscess. Patient is NPO for 6 hr before 24-hr examination. Does not have to be NPO for initial injection. Injection is given IV, and scans are taken at following times: 6 hr, 24 hr, 48 hr, 72 hr.	
Gallium scan, chest only	No preparation necessary, scan in 6 hr and 24 hr only.	
Gallium scan, abdomen (all orders should be obtained from physician)	NPO from midnight on evening of injection. Barium enema preparation evening of examination. Tap water enemas until clear on morning of 24-hr examination. Each day after 24-hr film, patient to have 30 ml milk of magnesia (light laxative) at hour of sleep to continue until examination is completed.	
Hepatobiliary scan	NPO 2 hr before. IV injection, then scan immediately.	60 min

FIGURE 14-13 Samples of various lead numbers and letters in different heights and thicknesses for radiographing directly on x-ray film.

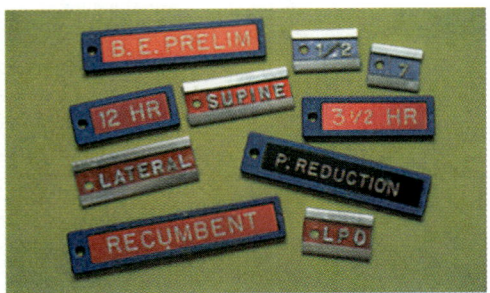

FIGURE 14-14 Technologist placing cassette with patient in position to obtain an anteroposterior (AP) view.

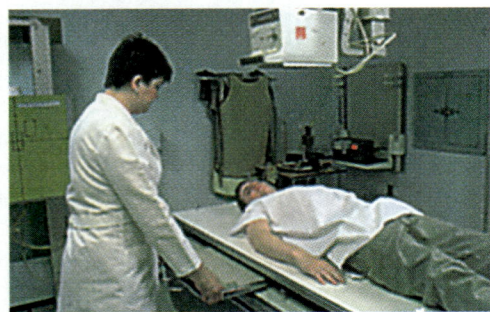

When the physician orders x-ray film to be taken, and when radiologists interpret the film, they use special terms to designate the position or direction of the x-ray beam and the patient's position. Before the x-ray film is taken, markers are placed on the film-containing cassette to indicate the position used, the patient's identification, and the date (Figures 14-13 and 14-14).

FIGURE 14-15 Anteroposterior (AP) position: The x-ray beam is directed from front to back.

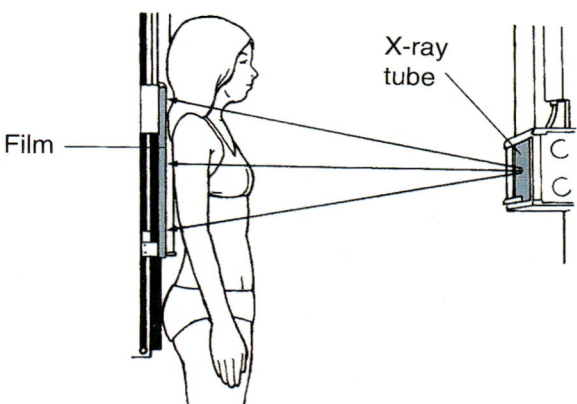

Basic Positions for Proper Exposure of Body Part

Anteroposterior (AP)—The x-ray beam is directed from front to back. The patient may be in a supine or standing position, having the back near the film and the front facing the x-ray tube (Figure 14-15).

Posteroanterior (PA)—The x-ray beam is directed from back to front. The patient is usually in an upright position, having the back facing the x-ray tube and the front near the film (Figure 14-16).

Lateral—The x-ray beam is directed from one side. In the right lateral (RL) view, the right side of the body is near the film, and the x-ray tube is pointed toward the left side (Figure 14-17). For the left lateral (LL) view, the left side of the body is nearest the film.

FIGURE 14-16 Posteroanterior (PA) position: The x-ray beam is directed from front to back

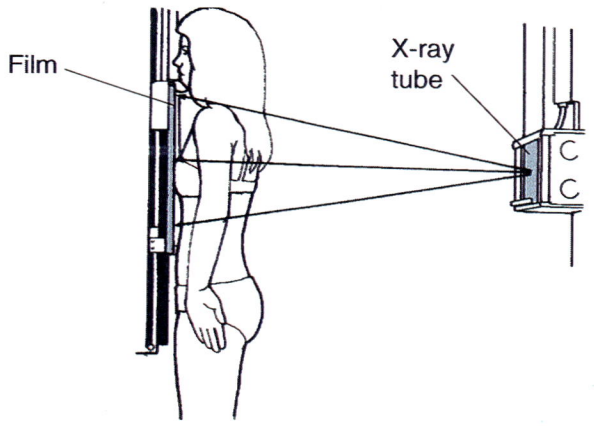

FIGURE 14-17 Lateral position: The x-ray beam is directed from one side.

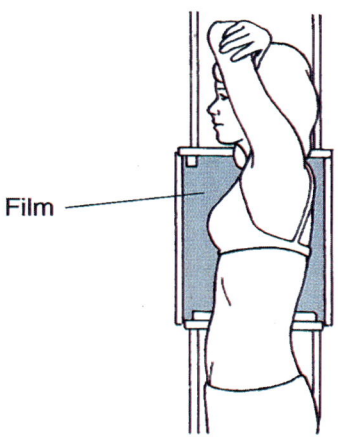

FIGURE 14-18 Oblique position: The x-ray beam is directed at an angle.

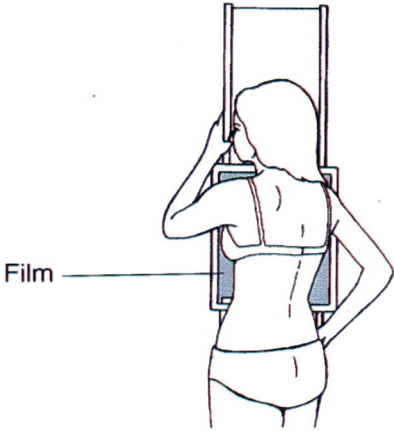

Oblique—These views are often used to outline areas that would be hidden and superimposed in the AP/PA and lateral positions. The patient is turned at an oblique angle (Figure 14-18).

Terms to Describe the Patient's Position

Supine—The patient is lying on the back, with face up.
Prone—The patient is lying on the abdomen, face downward.
Recumbent—The patient is lying down.
Erect—The patient is standing either facing the tube or facing away from the tube.

Other Terms to Describe Direction of X-ray Beam

Axial—The beam is angled.
Mediolateral—The x-ray beam is directed from the midline toward the side of the part being filmed. (This position is often used in mammography.)

Factors That Affect Images

Kilovoltage

There are two reasons kilovoltage has a profound effect on density:

1. The amount of x-rays produced is affected by tube kilovoltage.
2. The energy of the x-rays is affected by the kilovoltage. Kilovoltage determines the wavelength of radiation and thus its penetrating power. The greater the penetrating ability of the x-rays, the greater the amount of remnant radiation.

As mentioned earlier, the higher the kilovoltage, the greater the energy of the radiation, and more of the rays traverse the patient and exit on the other side to darken the film.

Milliamperage

The x-ray exposure rate is directly proportional to milliamperage. This is because milliamperage determines the amount of x-ray produced per unit of time. With all factors remaining the same, the greater the milliamperage, the greater the amount of radiation produced. If the milliamperage is halved, the amount of x-rays is reduced by half. Thus the amount of remnant radiation is directly proportional to the milliamperage.

Distance

Distance as discussed here relates to the distance from the radiation source (that is, from the x-ray tube to the radiographic file). X-rays emerge from the tube and diverge, proceeding in straight paths. Because of the divergence, they cover an increasingly larger area as they travel farther away from the tube. The radiation emitted from the tube remains the same, but because a larger area is covered as the distance increases, the amount of radiation per square inch is reduced.

The intensity of x-rays reaching the film varies inversely with the square of the distance. Therefore at twice the distance, the density is one fourth its original value; at half the distance, the density is four times greater.

The decrease in density at greater distances is solely a geometric factor relating to the divergent x-ray beam. The absorption of x-rays by intervening air is insignificant and can be totally disregarded.

From Gurley LT, Callaway WJ: *Introduction to radiologic technology*, ed 3, St Louis, 1992, Mosby.

Craniocaudal*—The x-ray beam is directed from the superior to inferior levels (from head to toe).

Decubitus—The x-ray beam is directed horizontally with the patient lying down.

RADIOLOGIC DANGERS, HAZARDS, AND SAFETY PRECAUTIONS

Dangers

X-rays do constitute a potential danger both to patients and health personnel; therefore proper precautions must be taken at all times.

Massive or excessive exposure to radiation can cause tissue damage and various side effects (see pp. 649 and 650). The purpose of radiotherapy is to destroy tissue in diseased areas, but in diagnostic radiology, exposure to radiation should be kept within safe limits because radiation has a cumulative effect over time. That is, the radiation a person receives today adds to the last dose received, and these in turn add to any future doses to accumulate a total radiation dosage. (Doses of radiation were measured in rads or rems or roentgens. According to the newer international standards set in the late 1980s, radiation units are now measured in grays (Gy), sieverts (Sv), or coulombs/kg. Rads = grays, rems = sieverts, and roentgens = coulombs/kg.)

Thus everyone should avoid all unnecessary radiation exposure. On the other hand, patients must be helped to realize the importance of any radiologic examination as an aid for the diagnosis and treatment of a disease process compared with the effects, if any, of the radiation dose that will be received. Newer machines and techniques have significantly reduced the amounts of radiation exposure compared with the same examination of 15 or more years ago.

When radiation goes beyond a safe limit, body tissues may begin to break down. Blood cells, skin, eyes, and reproductive cells are some of the tissues most sensitive to radiation. Overexposure to radiation can result in a lowered red blood cell and white blood cell counts because of disturbances of bone marrow and other blood-forming organs; burns on the skin and cancer; damage to the germinal cells in the ovaries and testes; and also damage to a fetus, especially in the first 3 months of pregnancy. Radiation also apparently predisposes individuals to the development of cataracts.

Studies have shown that massive and prolonged exposure to radiation can result in a higher incidence of cancer, especially of the lymph glands, and the various types of leukemia.

Hazards

Hazards of x-rays include the direct x-ray beam itself from the x-ray machine, which travels through an opening in the x-ray tube. Lead (which is able to stop x-rays from traveling) is in the x-ray tube housing to prevent the rays from escaping except through the opening.

A second hazard is scattered radiation of two types. **Leakage radiation** is radiation that may escape (leak) from the head of x-ray machines; this is dangerous to the operator. Therefore frequent inspection of all x-ray equipment is to be performed by a licensed radiation physicist. Once the primary beam of radiation strikes and reacts on the patient or anything else in its path, it is then called **secondary radiation,** which can be emitted in all directions. Secondary radiation is radiation that has deviated from its original path, being strongest close to the patient. Therefore distance is an important factor in radiation protection; that is, the farther one is away from the x-ray source, the better the protection one has from any form of radiation.

Lead screens or **shields** are used to separate x-ray personnel operating the controls of the machines from the patient receiving the radiation. These protect the personnel from secondary radiation. The walls of the x-ray room are also lined with lead, which absorbs secondary radiation when struck by it and thus prevents radiation from passing through the walls into adjacent areas, exposing others to the radiation. In most facilities, when x-ray machines are in use, a red light flashes on outside the room, indicating to others that radiation is being given and therefore not to enter the room. In some facilities there are interlocking devices by which the door won't open when radiation is being used. Sometimes these devices interact with the x-ray equipment so that the machines won't work unless the door is locked.

Safety Precautions

X-ray personnel and medical assistants exposed to possible radiation can control the potential dangers by adhering to the following prescribed safety precautionary measures:

1. Have the equipment inspected frequently by a qualified person to ensure that there is no leakage of radiation.
2. Stay behind the lead shield in a lead-lined room when the x-ray machine is being used.
3. Wear a lead apron and protective rubber-lead gloves if it is absolutely necessary to hold the patient or to remain in the room during any radiologic procedure. On these occasions, always face the patient so that the lead apron is closest to the patient or stay away from the patient. Never assume that you must hold or support the patient and do not do this routinely. Certain techniques can be used to maintain the patient in the correct position.
4. Wear a film badge (Figure 14-19) on outer clothing at the neck at all times when your job involves exposure to any type of radiation, including exposure to radionuclides. When pregnant also wear a film badge at the waist to record radiation exposure to the fetus in utero. A **film badge** is a small device that contains x-ray film that is sensitive to radiation and thus records the level and intensity of radiation exposure, which is measured in gray, sievert, or coulomb/kg. These badges are to be submitted periodically (weekly in some facilities) to a film badge service for evaluation, thus providing a means for warning personnel when dangerous levels of radiation exposure are near.
5. Have a periodic blood count performed to determine if a blood dyscrasia is present. Blood counts do not measure

---

*This position is often used in mammography.

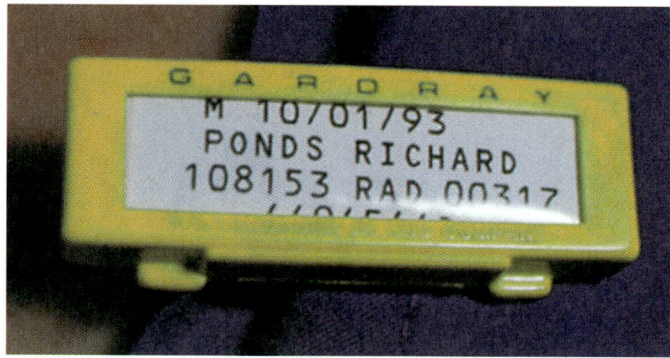

FIGURE 14-19 Film badge worn on outer clothing of radiographers to record the level and intensity of radiation exposure.

the amount of radiation but can indicate if radiation has damaged blood cells.

To protect the patient from unnecessary radiation exposure, adhere to the following:

1. Before making arrangements for a patient to have an x-ray examination, routinely ask:
   a. If and when the patient has had other x-ray studies or therapy and the nature of these.
   b. If the patient has been exposed to any radiation for other reasons, such as in employment or an experimental situation.
   c. If it is possible that a female patient is pregnant. These inquiries are important because the patient may have received excessive doses of radiation, and further exposure at that time may be detrimental to the patient's health status. When it appears that the patient has been exposed to a large amount of radiation recently and when a woman suspects that she is pregnant, inform the physician, without alarming the patient, and **before** making arrangements for the x-ray studies. The physician may want to change the order for x-ray studies at that time. The physician weighs the facts: that is, how urgent is the need for the x-ray examination versus the risk to the patient or fetus who will receive the additional radiation exposure.
2. Position the patient correctly for the x-ray film if licensed to do so (unlicensed personnel should not position patients for x-ray procedures) and when this is one of your assisting duties. Accuracy of the film requires that the patient assume and maintain the correct position without moving during the exposure time. If this is not attained, film distortion results, thus requiring the patient to be exposed to additional radiation while a repeat film is taken.
3. Shield the patient's abdomen and reproductive organs with a lead apron when appropriate, especially patients who are pregnant, patients of childbearing age, and children.

MEDICAL ASSISTANT'S RESPONSIBILITIES

Your responsibilities relating to radiologic procedures used in the physician's office are to prepare the patient, provide reassurance when needed, and use the safety measures relevant to x-ray equipment. When the physician employs a radiographer, you may not do any of these functions.

When outside sources are used, you are responsible for calling the radiologist's office or hospital x-ray department to schedule the examination and for furnishing the patient's name, type of insurance, the referring physician's name, and the type of examination.

One of the most important communications between the medical assistant and radiology department involves the scheduling of multiple x-ray procedures that are ordered at one time for the patient. Consultation is needed to sequence the procedures so that they do not interfere with each other and to decide how many procedures can be done on the same day. You should give all the information to the radiology department so that they can schedule the examinations in proper sequence. The general rule is that examinations **not** using a contrast medium are done **before** examinations that do use a contrast medium; for example, a chest x-ray would be done before a barium enema. **The patient is to take the physician's written requisition(s) to the x-ray department on the day of the examinations.**

In either situation, **before the scheduled date, patients should be informed** of the appropriate amount of time that the examination will take so they can schedule other activities accordingly and not get unduly upset or surprised if the examination takes an hour or so. Also, certain x-ray examinations require special patient preparation the day before, the morning of the study, or both. To **prepare the patient,** you must know and explain the instructions to the patient and ensure that they are understood and provide written instructions to be taken home. Remind the patient to *not wear* any jewelry or any metal, such as metal on a belt or in hairpins. Many physicians' offices have preprinted individual instructions to be followed before x-ray studies, or they may use product literature provided by pharmaceutical companies for patient use. **Written instructions** are essential because oral instructions can easily be forgotten. Repeat examinations required because of poorly given or misunderstood instructions cause unnecessary radiation exposure and expense for the patient.

For the x-ray studies discussed in this chapter, Tables 14-3 and 14-4 group those that do not require special patient preparation and those studies that do require individual patient preparation (listed as individual, because the specific preparation may vary among different radiology departments). The approximate amount of time required for each examination is also listed. Samples of individual patient preparations are given for common examinations. Similar reference sheets should be made available for you in the physician's office or clinic.

After the x-ray examination has been completed, you must check to ensure that a written report is received and then filed in the patient's chart after being reviewed by the physician and that the x-ray films, when sent to or when taken in the physician's office, are stored and handled correctly.

TABLE 14–3 **X-ray Examinations That DO NOT Require Special Patient Preparation**

Examination	Time Required
Barium swallow	½ to ¾ hr
Arthrogram	1½ hr
Diskogram, lumbar or cervical	1 hr
Hysterosalpingogram	1 hr
Lymphangiogram	6 hr
Mammogram	½ to ¾ hr
Thermography	Depends on area being studied (seldom used now)
Tomography	1 hr
Computed tomography	1 to 2 hr (no preparation if contrast medium not used)
Abdomen (flat plate)	20 min
Chest	20 min
Kidney, ureter, bladder (KUB)	10 min; 45 min when it includes intravenous urography
Skull series	20 to 30 min
Paranasal sinuses	20 to 30 min
Bone	15 min to 1 hr, depending on type and area being studied
Magnetic resonance imaging	1 hr (will vary with body part being examined)
Digital radiography	1 hr
Ultrasound of the gallbladder	1 hr

TABLE 14–4 **X-ray Examinations That DO Require Special Patient Preparation**

Examination	Time Required	Sample Preparation
Barium enema (BE)	30 to 60 min	Take 2 oz (4 tbs) castor oil at 4:00 PM the day preceding x-ray examination (may be taken in grape juice or root beer). No solid foods on day preceding examination; just liquids such as fruit juice, clear soup, jello, water, plain tea, or black coffee, but no milk products. NPO after midnight. No breakfast on day of examination. **or** Enemas till bowels are clear the evening before. NPO after midnight. Rectal suppository in the morning.
Barium meal (upper GI series)	30 to 60 min for stomach, but up to 90 min or 2 to 4 hr or more with small bowel examination; more films may be taken 6 hr or 24 hr later	Nothing to eat or drink after 10:00 PM the evening before examination. No breakfast, no fluids, no hard candy, and no cigarettes in the morning. Stomach must be empty. **or** Nothing to eat or drink after 8:00 PM. Do not eat breakfast. No water. Report to x-ray office.
Angiogram	1 to 3 hr	No breakfast when any of these examinations are done in the early morning; or no lunch if they are done in the afternoon.
Arteriogram	1 to 3 hr	
Angiocardiogram	2 hr	
Cerebral angiogram	2 to 3 hr	
Bronchogram	1 hr	NPO
Myelogram	1 hr	NPO
Computed tomography	1 to 2 hr	NPO for 4 hr before if a contrast medium is used.
Cholecystogram (gallbladder series)	1 to 2 hr	Evening before x-ray examination, eat a light supper, consisting of nonfatty foods such as lean meat (small portion) and fresh vegetables cooked without butter and no eggs, mayonnaise, French dressing, fried or fatty foods. After supper swallow gallbladder tablets with water, taking one at a time. Eat nothing after evening meal. Water, however, may be taken in moderate amounts until bedtime. Do not take a laxative. Do not eat breakfast. Report to x-ray department.

TABLE 14-4   **X-ray Examinations That DO Require Special Patient Preparation—cont'd**

Examination	Time Required	Sample Preparation
Cholecystogram—cont'd		**or**
		Low-fat evening meal. Telepaque tablets the evening before. NPO after midnight.
Intravenous cholangiogram	3 hr	NPO
Intravenous pyelogram (IVP)	1½ hr	Take 2 oz (4 tbs) of castor oil or 3 tablets bisacodyl (Dulcolax) at 4 PM the day before x-ray examination. Eat a clear liquid supper. Do not drink anything, even water, after midnight. Eat no breakfast, no fluids.
		or
		Same prep as for BE
		or
		Laxatives or enemas night before examination. NPO for 8 hr before examination
Retrograde pyelogram	1 to 1½ hr; usually done in operating room	NPO
Pneumoencephalo-myelogram	2 to 4 hr	NPO
Ultrasonography Pelvic ultrasound	25 to 45 min up to 2 hr	Afternoon before the examination, take 3 Dulcolax tablets and three glasses of water to clear the bowel. On the day of examination, use a Dulcolax rectal suppository 3 hr before examination. Then take three to four glasses of water 45 min before the examination and do not urinate. *A full urinary bladder is essential for this examination.*
		or
		A full urinary bladder is essential. Please do not empty your bladder for 1 to 2 hr before examination. Drink 4 to 6 glasses of any liquid 45 min before examination. Use 1 Dulcolax suppository 3 hr before examination.
Abdominal ultrasound		Take 1 dimethicone (Mylicon) tablet 4 times daily for 2 days before examination. Do not eat solid food after 8:00 AM on day of examination. You may take fluids as desired.
		or
		Take 10 oz. of citrate of magnesia and 3 glasses of water at noon the day before examination. Take 3 Dulcolax tablets at 6:00 PM with an additional 3 glasses of water. The evening meal should consist of clear fluids but no milk products. Have nothing other than liquids after midnight. Do not eat breakfast the day of examination.
		or
		NPO after midnight
Renal ultrasound		Drink 2 glasses of water 1 hr before examination.
Thyroid ultrasound		No preparation needed.
		Nothing by mouth 3 hr before examination.
Obstetrical ultrasound (see Figure 14-10)		*A full urinary bladder is essential.* Do not empty your bladder for at least 1 hr before examination. Drink 4 to 6 glasses of any liquid 45 min before examination.

PROCEDURE 14-1

PREPARATION OF PATIENT AND ASSISTING WITH RADIOGRAPHS

Objective

Understand and demonstrate how you would prepare and assist the patient who is having diagnostic medical imaging studies. Record the procedure on the patient's chart.

Continued

PREPARATION OF PATIENT AND ASSISTING WITH RADIOGRAPHS—cont'd

PROCEDURE	RATIONALE

PROCEDURE

1. Identify the patient, check if the special preparation was followed (when applicable), and explain the following:
   a. The value of the examination
   b. How the machine operates
   c. Whether it will hurt
   d. What clothing and other articles must be removed
   e. How to put on the patient gown (that is, with the opening in the front or back)
   f. What position will be required
   g. The importance of remaining still during the examination

2. Drape the patient as necessary. Shield the abdominal regions with a lead apron, especially for patients who are pregnant, patients of childbearing age, or children.

3. Reassure the patient as required. Radiographs are taken on either very sick patients or those who come in for diagnostic purposes, but they all must be given support and attention. Offer assistance to the patient when getting on and off the x-ray table. Remain calm and quietly cheerful.

4. Be empathetic and courteous; remain calm. The patient will be lying on or standing against a cold, hard plate. In an empathetic and courteous manner, emphasize the importance of remaining still in the proper position.

5. When the examination has been completed by the physician or x-ray technologist or radiographer, ask the patient to wait in the dressing room while the films are developed.

6. If it is necessary to obtain another film, explain to the patient that the physician requires another film for study.

7. Dismiss the patient after it has been determined that the films are satisfactory. If the x-ray film showed the presence of a fracture, make arrangements for immediate treatment. The physician will read the films later and notify the patient or schedule a future appointment for a time when the physician can review the results with the patient.

8. Record the procedure on the patient's chart.

RATIONALE

X-ray procedures performed in the office are used for diagnostic or screening purposes. If a required special preparation was not followed, the examination must be canceled and rescheduled. The patient can be told that x-ray examinations are painless, with the exception of those requiring the instillation of a contrast medium. On these occasions, when contrast media are used, an uncomfortable feeling can be expected, rather than pain. The patient is to remove clothes, watches, all metal, dentures, jewelry, and hairpins that may interfere with the accuracy of the x-ray film. These objects produce shadows on the film and may obscure details that should be observed.

The patient gown is usually put on with the opening in the back. For films of the breast, all clothing from the waist up is removed. The physician determines the position to be maintained by the patient; you tell the patient which position it will be (refer to pp. 652-653). Movement of the body during the examination causes distortion on the film. It is then necessary to repeat the examination, which provides additional radiation exposure for the patient.

Drapes may be used to provide warmth and to protect the patient's modesty, but they are not to interfere with the body part being filmed.

Careful and complete explanations to the patient help provide reassurance and reduce fear and confusion. Any reassurance of a nervous patient is helpful.

Distortion on the film occurs unless the required position is maintained.

The patient remains while films are developed to ensure that clear films have been obtained for study. This is much more convenient for everyone than to have the patient return later for retakes if the preliminary films are not clear.

Careful communication is important because you must avoid creating fears in the patient that unnecessary exposure to radiation will result or that the individual taking the x-ray was incompetent, thus necessitating another film.

Charting Example

August 1, 20__.
PA and lateral chest x-rays taken and read by Dr. Mouer.
Results—negative. Detailed report to follow.
Film No. 8179
Cassandra Quinn, CMA

FIGURE 14-20 **A,** Roller transport system of an automated x-ray film processor. Diagram showing how the roller transports films through the various sections of automated processor. The arrangement and number of components in the various assemblies may differ from model to model, but the basic plan is the same. **B,** Developing a radiograph using an automatic processor in the darkroom. (**A,** Courtesy Eastman Kodak Co, Rochester, NY.)

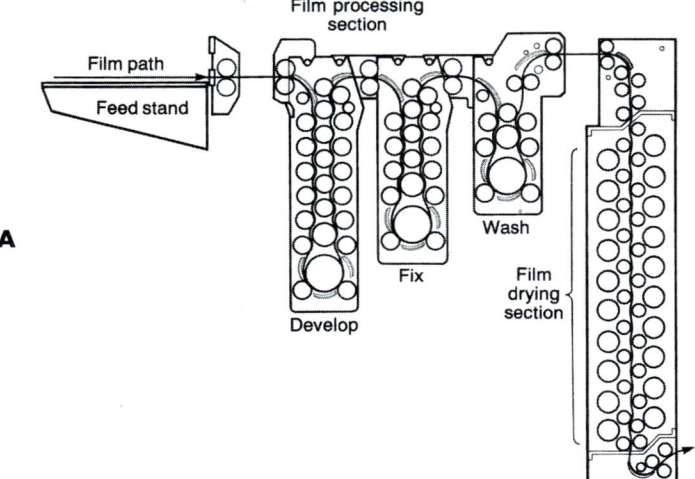

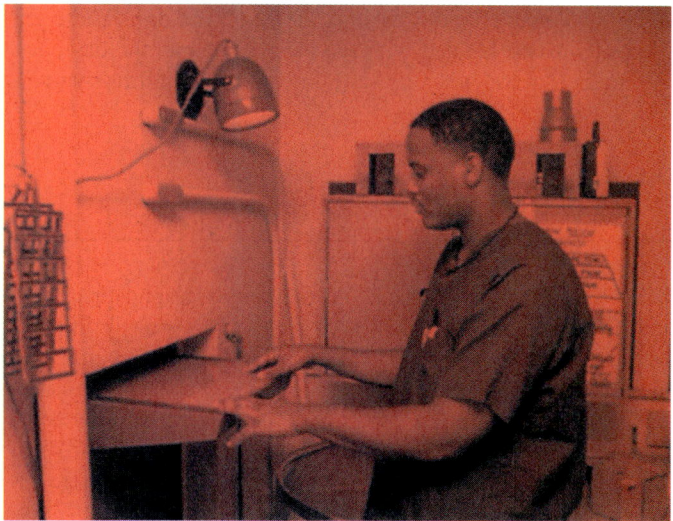

PROCESSING X-RAY FILM

Previously, processing x-ray film in a darkroom could be done by either manual methods or by mechanical methods using an automated film processor. Currently, because of the need for quality control procedures with emphasis on the developing equipment, state and federal guidelines require testing and consistency in developing, and only automated processing and developing meet these standards. The automated processing cycle produces a ready-to-read radiograph in as little as 90 seconds up to 10 minutes, depending on the processor used.

Three elements are required for proper automated processing. These include a processor, the correct film(s), and special chemicals. These components are designed to work together to produce a quality radiograph. Follow the manufacturer's recommendation for feeding the film into an automated processor. Usually you feed the film squarely into the processor and feed multiple films one after the other. The processor transports, processes, and dries the film and replenishes and recirculates the processing solutions (Figure 14-20).

After the automated processing procedure has been completed, the radiograph is ready for viewing on an illuminated viewbox (see Figure 14-12) or is to be placed in a special file envelope labeled with the patient's name, the date, and the x-ray number when used.

STORAGE AND MANAGEMENT IN THE OFFICE

Storage of X-ray Materials

When x-ray materials are used in the office, they require special storage attention. These supplies must be protected from damage caused by exposure to moisture, heat, and light. Unex-

posed film must be kept in a dry, cool place, preferably in a lead-lined box. The lead-lined box protects the film from any x-rays that may escape during filming.

When unexposed film is to be placed into a cassette for use, the film packets are to be opened only in the darkroom with only the darkroom light, called a safe light, on. Before development, the exposed film obtained after the radiologic procedure is completed must also be stored in a lead-lined box to protect it from secondary radiation, which would spoil the radiograph recorded on the film.

X-ray developer solutions must also be stored in a moisture-free, cool location because they are of extreme importance in processing quality radiographs.

Ownership of X-ray Films, Reports, and Records

There is often much controversy over the ownership of medical records, reports, and x-ray films. Note that this type of property legally belongs to the medical facility where it is made or recorded and does not belong to the patient. All x-ray films obtained on a patient are the sole property of the physician's office or hospital that performed the radiologic examination. Written x-ray reports from the radiologist are to be sent to the referring physician, but the actual films usually remain in the files of the office or hospital that did the filming. At times these films can be loaned out to the referring physician for further study, reference, or review as needed to confirm a diagnosis or to compare old films with current ones. At other times the radiologist's office routinely sends the films to the referring physician so that they may be kept as part of the patient's permanent medical record in the office, but they still remain as the legal property of the radiologist. Presently, in a few states patients can request, pay for, and obtain copies of the original x-ray film.

Radiologic films are permanent records for current or future reference (as opposed to fluoroscopy, which can be viewed only at the time of the examination unless the procedure was recorded on a videotape or 35-mm film). Special file envelopes are available in which to keep exposed film. These envelopes must be labeled with the patient's name, the date, and the number, if and when used. (Some places file films by number rather than by the patient's name. In this case, the number *must* be recorded on the patient's medical record for a cross-reference.)

X-ray films placed in filing envelopes should be filed in a dry, cool storage area, preferably in a metal cabinet; ones no longer needed for current reference should be filed in a permanent storage file so that they are available for future reference.

CONCLUSION

This chapter has introduced you to various diagnostic procedures used in the field of radiology. Your responsibilities in these fields, although limited, have been discussed. Numerous additional studies may be performed in these specialty areas of medicine for the diagnosis and treatment of disease processes; however, this book does not discuss all of them in detail. You may refer to various sources to expand your knowledge on these procedures. Check with your instructor for additional enrichment assignments and references in areas of your own particular need and interest. A tour through the radiology and nuclear medicine departments of a modern hospital, especially a large teaching hospital, would expose you to the dramatic progress that has been made in these fields of medicine.

When you think that you know the information presented in this chapter, arrange with your instructor to take a performance test.

REVIEW OF VOCABULARY

The following reports received in a physician's office pertain to some of the diagnostic examinations discussed in the preceding pages. Read these and be prepared to discuss the contents with your instructor. A dictionary or other reference books may be used to define the terms with which you are unfamiliar. In addition, you should read more on these examinations elsewhere to gain a more complete understanding of the procedures.

PATIENT NO. 1: Upper GI Series
Preliminary film reveals no significant soft tissue or osseous abnormality.

There is a small, lesser-curvature antral ulcer measuring 7 mm at its neck and 4 mm deep. No mass is identified, and peristalsis passes through the area with ease. No abnormalities are seen of the distal esophagus, remaining stomach, duodenal bulb, duodenal loop, or proximal small bowel.

CONCLUSION: Small lesser curvature antral ulcer.

Follow up x-ray studies done by another physician.

Comparison with previous study of 7-02-00 reveals near-complete clearing of the lesser-curvature antral ulcer. A tiny barium collection measuring about 2 to 3 mm remains in the same location with some adjacent thickened folds.

Duodenal bulb, duodenal loop, and proximal small bowel show no abnormalities.

Distal esophagus appeared normal without evidence of hiatus hernia or reflux.

Incomplete fusion of the L5 spinous process demonstrated.

CONCLUSION: Near-complete clearing of the lesser curvature antral ulcer. L5 spina bifida occulta.

PATIENT NO. 2: Barium Enema
Following a water-cleansing preliminary enema, the colon was filled quite readily from rectum to cecum, including terminal ileum.

The descending colon is displaced quite strikingly forward and toward the midline in the region of the previously described soft tissue mass closely related to the lower pole of the left kidney. There is no mucosal distortion, and the deformity is mainly that of extrinsic pressure rather than an intrinsic or invasive lesion.

The only other abnormality is a small area of kinking with slight narrowing of the lumen in the proximal transverse colon just distally to the hepatic flexure. That portion of the colon is quite redundant, and this is most likely a kink at the site of redundancy and not a true lesion; however, if surgery is contemplated, direct palpation of this area is suggested. The colon is otherwise normally outlined and so is the terminal ileum. It empties quite well.

CONCLUSION: Extrinsic pressure and displacement of the left colon by the previously described mass without evidence of any direct invasion. Small area of kinking and narrowing of the lumen at the proximal portion of the transverse colon, most likely normal and simply the result of local redundancy.

Otherwise normal study of the colon.

PATIENT NO. 3: Barium Enema
This is compared with similar study of 8/26/00. On the preliminary film there is some barium in the pelvis from previous

study. Gas pattern is unremarkable. The large bowel is filled in retrograde manner with barium. Free reflux into the terminal ileum was seen, and the appendix fills. There are a few diverticula deep in the sigmoid, which account for the retention of the barium seen on the scout film. The left colon now distends completely with no evidence of ischemic colitis and no residual stricture noted. The remainder of the colon is unchanged.

IMPRESSION: Normal barium enema without residual from the previously described ischemic colitis.

Diverticulosis of the sigmoid colon.

PATIENT NO. 4: Excretory Urography With Tomography

Preliminary examination demonstrates normal psoas and renal shadows.

There is an ovoid, homogeneous, increased density approximately 13 cm in maximum dimension in the left midabdomen.

Three calcified lymph nodes are in the right lower quadrant.

Opaque medium appears promptly and in good concentration demonstrating normal calyces, pelves, and ureters. The vesicle outline is normal, with minimal retention after voiding.

The left midabdominal mass moves independently from the lower pole of the left kidney, particularly noted in the erect position, and is separate from it. The mass has well-delineated margins and appears to be of homogeneous density. Ultrasound would readily distinguish a cystic from a solid lesion, separating such as a mesenteric cyst from a solid mesenchymal or epithelial tumor, or lymphoma. An ovarian tumor would be unusual in this location but possible.

CONCLUSION: Normal excretory urinary tract. Left midabdominal mass lesion, discussed previously.

PATIENT NO. 5: Ultrasound Consultation

CHIEF COMPLAINT: Right upper quadrant pain.

ULTRASOUND OF THE GALLBLADDER: The gallbladder is well seen. There is some slightly echogenic material in the dependent part of the gallbladder, but this is not definitely particulate, and there is no acoustic shadowing. Ducts are unremarkable.

IMPRESSION: The material in the gallbladder described previously most likely represents sludge. This is not considered definitely abnormal.

PATIENT NO. 6: Chest X-ray Report

In PA projection, there is a mild dextroconvex curvature of the lower thoracic spine. The bony thorax is otherwise unremarkable.

The heart, vessels, and mediastinal structures are normal.

Clear lungs are well expanded with sharp costophrenic angles. There is no evidence of active disease.

PATIENT NO. 7: Facial Bones X-ray Report

The facial bones, including the orbits, are intact.

A smooth, 1×1.5 cm soft tissue opacity lies about the posterior aspect of the roof of the left maxillary sinus.

CONCLUSION: Facial bones negative for fracture.

Soft-tissue mass about the roof of the left maxillary sinus. The possibility of a blow-out fracture of the orbit might be considered and should be clinically correlated.

Radiologic Consultation Report

PATIENT No. 8

THREE VIEWS OF THE LEFT HAND, 01/28/00

CLINICAL INFORMATION: Pain over the first carpometacarpal joint

COMPARISON STUDIES: There is no prior examination for comparison.

FINDINGS: There is mild spurring of the greater multangular at the first carpometacarpal joint. In addition, on the PA projection, there is suggestion of a 2-mm long osseous density adjacent to the radial aspect of the left greater multangular first metacarpal joint. Does this represent degenerative changes, or is there a history of prior trauma with a small avulsion fracture? There is, however, no evidence of subluxation. No acute fracture, bony destruction, or abnormal periosteal reaction is noted.

IMPRESSION:

1. Mild degenerative spurring at the greater multangular.
2. Small sliver of osseous density adjacent to the radial aspect of the first metacarpocarpal joint. Question etiology, question degenerative changes versus old healed avulsion fracture.

Dictated By:

Dan Brown, MD

CRITICAL THINKING SKILLS REVIEW

1. Mrs. G.B. Emerson, a 46-year-old, 164-lb woman, has been scheduled for a barium enema and a cholecystogram. Mrs. Emerson does not understand why she must have these tests.

   Explain the nature and purpose of these tests to her and the special directions that she must follow before having these tests performed.

2. The physician has ordered a PA and lateral chest x-ray film. Explain how the patient will be positioned when these films are taken.

3. Mrs. C.A. Lunatto has had extensive radiotherapy and now is experiencing diarrhea and some loss of scalp hair. List four other side effects that she may experience with continued radiation therapy.

4. Mr. K. Cole might have kidney disease. List five diagnostic studies that the physician may order to help diagnose the problem.

5. Ms. B. Milius has discovered several lumps in her breast while doing a breast self-examination and has now come to the physician for a checkup. List two studies that the physician may order for this patient to help diagnose the condition.

6. Mrs. Gwen Boyd is scheduled for an ultrasound to determine if is she is pregnant because other tests have proven unsuccessful. She feels apprehensive about having this test done and is fearful of the pain she expects to have during this test. Explain the nature and purpose of this test, indicating if pain is to be expected.

7. Explain the nature and purpose of computed tomography (CT). State the advantages of this technique and equipment over other types of radiologic examinations.

8. Explain the nature and purpose of magnetic resonance imaging. State the advantages of this technique over other types of radiologic equipment.

9. List four advantages of digital radiography.

10. What is a film badge, and why is it used?

11. List three ways to protect the patient from unnecessary radiation exposure when having x-ray examinations.

12. Discuss the medical assistant's responsibilities relevant to x-ray procedures performed in the physician's office; at an outside facility.

13. Describe how an x-ray film should be stored in the office.

14. Mr. B. Wingate had a myelogram performed last month and now is in your office, stating that he wants the x-ray films to take home. Define myelogram. Explain to Mr. Wingate why he cannot take the films home.

PERFORMANCE TEST

In a skills laboratory, a simulation of a joblike environment, the medical assistant student will demonstrate skill in performing the following activities without reference to source materials. Time limits for each of the following activities are to be assigned by the instructor (see also p. 104).

1. Communicate proper preparation for x-ray procedures to the patient.

2. Prepare the patient for and assist the patient during an x-ray examination.

3. Position the patient for the AP, PA, LL, and RL x-ray exposure, *only* if licensed to do so.

4. Care for and store an x-ray film in the office.

5. Demonstrate safety hazards and precautionary measures relevant to x-ray equipment.

The student is expected to perform these skills with 100% accuracy.

The successful completion of each procedure will demonstrate competency levels as required by the AAMA, AMT, and future employers.

🖥 INTERNET RESOURCES

American Cancer Society
www.cancer.org

National Cancer Institute
www.nci.nih.gov

The World Foundation for Medical Studies in Female Health
www.wffh.org

California Society of Radiological Technologists
www.csrt.org

National Action Plan on Breast Cancer
www.napbc.org

Susan G. Komen Breast Cancer Foundation
http://komen.org

Susan Love, M.D. (breast cancer)
www.susanlovemd.com

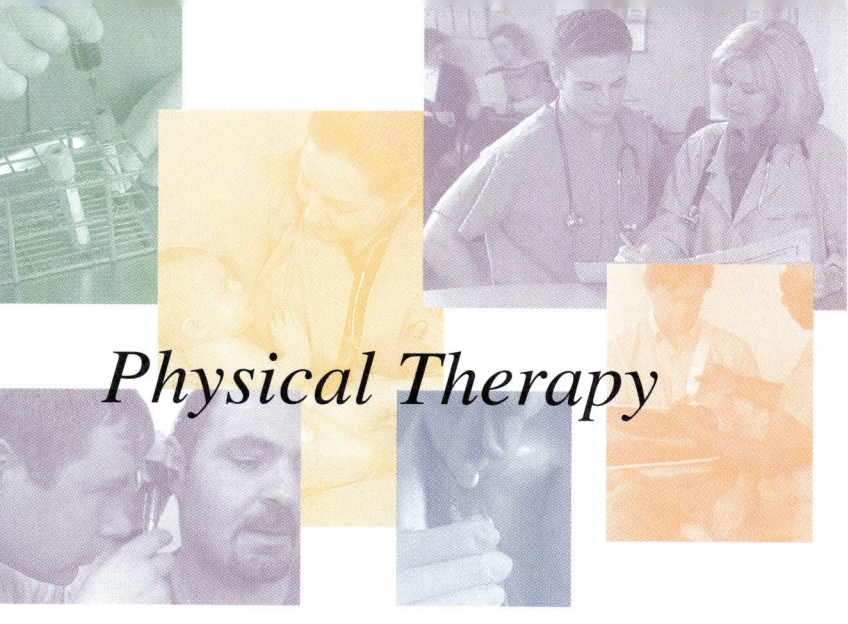

Physical Therapy

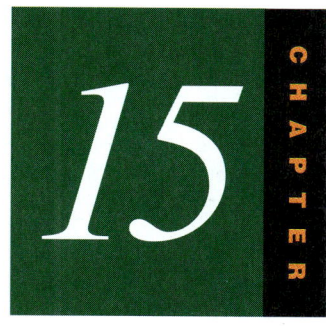

CHAPTER 15

■ Cognitive Objectives

On completion of Chapter 15, the medical assistant student should be able to:

1. Define, spell, and pronounce the terms listed in the vocabulary.
2. Differentiate between physical medicine and physical therapy; a physiatrist and a physical therapist.
3. List 11 modalities or techniques used for treatments in physical therapy, indicating the nature, purpose, or use of each.
4. Describe the differences between ultraviolet radiation, diathermy, ultrasound, and local applications of heat and cold.
5. State the physiologic reactions that occur with applications of heat and cold.
6. Discuss the principles of preparation and patient care for applications of heat and cold.
7. List examples of dry and moist applications of heat and cold and describe how to apply these to a patient.
8. Outline the types and uses of traction, massage, and exercises.
9. Differentiate between electrotherapy and electrodiagnostic techniques, explaining the nature and purpose of each.
10. Identify the medical assistant's responsibilities relevant to physical therapy procedures.
11. Outline the steps for performance checklists for the application of heat and cold treatments and other physical therapy modalities listed in this chapter.
12. Define and discuss the principles of body mechanics.
13. Discuss the safety precautions and techniques to use when helping patients get in and out of wheelchairs.
14. Define and state the goals of ergonomics.
15. Discuss and give examples of work-related musculoskeletal disorders (WMSDs).
16. Identify reasons for considering WMSDs a problem.
17. Discuss and identify 10 bad habits people often use when working on a computer or at a desk.
18. List and discuss 10 ways to change the habits identified in No. 17.

■ Terminal Performance Objectives

On completion of Chapter 15, the medical assistant student should be able to:

1. Assemble supplies and equipment necessary to correctly apply applications of heat and cold.
2. Apply the various hot and cold applications, using safety precautions to avoid injury to the patient or self.
3. Demonstrate proficiency in communicating proper preparation of the patient for physical therapy treatments.
4. Discuss with the instructor the desired and undesired effects of applications of heat and cold.
5. Design a teaching-instruction program for the patient who will be using the following modalities at home:
   a. Heating pad
   b. Moist cold compress
   c. Hot water bottle
   d. Ice pack
   e. Hot moist compress
   f. Alcohol sponge bath
   g. Chemical hot pack
   h. Chemical cold pack
   i. Ice bag
6. Design a performance checklist to be used for the application of the following:
   a. Dry heat applications
   b. Dry cold applications
   c. Moist heat applications
   d. Moist cold applications
7. Demonstrate correct standing, lifting, and bending techniques.
8. Demonstrate safe techniques when helping a patient get in and out of a wheelchair.
9. Assist patients in learning how to walk with crutches, a cane, and a walker.
10. Determine the correct size of crutches, a cane, and a walker for a patient.

11. Demonstrate and discuss body positions and other methods to use to help prevent physical problems when working at a computer and desk.

12. Demonstrate computer and desk stretches as given in this chapter.

13. Provide instructions and patient education that is within the professional scope of a medical assistant's training and responsibilities as assigned.

The student is to perform these activities with 100% accuracy.*

The consistent use of Universal/Standard Precautions is required by all health care professionals in all health care set- *tings as a method of infection control. It is assumed that these precautions are used in all of the following procedures. Review Chapter 1 if you have any questions on methods to use because the methods or techniques are not repeated in detail in each procedure presented in this chapter.*

Be sure to consult the latest guidelines issued by the Centers for Disease Control and Prevention and consult with infection control practitioners when needed to identify specific precautions that pertain to your particular work situation.

*Review Diagnostic and Therapeutic Procedures, as well as Organizing the Recordings of Diagnostic Procedures, in Chapter 10, pp. 456-463, before proceeding with this chapter.

VOCABULARY

arthritis (ar-thri′-tis)—Inflammation of a joint.

bursitis (bur-si′-tis)—Inflammation of a bursa. The most commonly affected is the bursa of the shoulder.

conduction (kon-duk′shun)—The passage or conveyance of energy, as of electricity, heat, or sound.

debridement (da-bred-ment′)—The process of removing foreign material and dead tissue.

hypothermia (hi-po-ther′me-ah)—Low body temperature.

light therapy or phototherapy (fo′to-ther′ah-pe)—The use of light rays in the treatment of disease processes. By custom, this includes the use of ultraviolet and infrared or heat rays (radiation).

modality (mo-dal′i-te)—Therapeutic agents used in physical medicine and physical therapy.

psoriasis (so-ri′ah-sis)—A chronic inflammatory recurrent skin disease characterized by scaly red patches on the body surfaces.

The lesions are seen most often on knees, elbows, scalp, and fingernails. Other areas often affected are the chest, abdomen, palms of the hands, soles of the feet, and backs of the arms and legs. The cause is unknown, although a hereditary factor is suggested.

sprain (spran)—A joint injury in which some fibers of a supporting ligament are torn or wrenched and partially ruptured, but continuity of the ligament remains intact. There may also be damage to the associated muscles, tendons, nerves, and blood vessels. A sprain is more serious than a strain.

strain (stran)—An overexertion or overstretching of some part of a muscle.

tendinitis (ten″di-ni′tis)—Inflammation of a tendon; one of the most common causes of acute pain in the shoulder.

Physical medicine or physiatrics (fiz′e-ah′triks) is the medical discipline that uses physical and mechanical agents in the diagnosis, treatment, and prevention of disease processes and bodily ailments. Physicians who specialize in this field are **physiatrists** (fiz″e-ah′trist). The therapeutic use of these agents in conjunction with patient education and rehabilitation programs (rather than by medicinal or surgical means) is called physical therapy (PT). **Physical therapists** are specially educated, licensed individuals skilled in the techniques of physical therapy and qualified to evaluate a patient's condition and complaints; to administer individualized treatments and tests, some of which could be prescribed by a physician; and to evaluate the patient's progress and test results. Licensed physical therapists can treat patients without a physician's referral, and some practice settings allow this type of direct access for care.

The **purpose and aim** of physical therapy are to relieve pain, increase circulation, restore and improve muscular function, normalize or improve movement patterns, build strength, and increase the range of motion or mobility of a joint. The **primary objective** of physical therapy is to promote optimum health and function for people of all ages. Aside from treating patients with neuromusculoskeletal conditions, physical therapy is involved with a significant number of physical conditioning programs, particularly for patients with cardiac and pulmonary conditions. Chest therapy is also given to patients with pulmonary conditions to help clear secretions and keep the air passageways open and clear. **Patient education** is a major area in physical therapy (that is, physical therapists teach and train patients how to perform essential activities that they can do themselves for their condition and how to avoid recurrences of certain problems).

A great variety of **modalities** and **techniques** using the properties of heat, cold, electricity, water, light, mechanical maneuvers, and exercise are used in physical therapy. Generally speaking, physical therapy treatments are given by physical therapists or the physician; therefore the medical assistant's duties may be limited. However, if you work in a physician's office, you are often required to administer some types of physical therapy treatments under the immediate direction and supervision of the physician. In addition, at the physician's request, you should be able to explain the nature and purpose of the treatment or test to the patient or provide adequate instructions to be followed by the patient at home. It is too often assumed that patients who are to use heat or cold applications at home know how to do so without assistance. You should ensure that these patients understand the dangers of using heat or cold to excess and the importance of using the correct solution at the proper temperature.

Some knowledge of the various modalities used in physical therapy is therefore a requirement for the well-trained medical assistant. The following pages discuss the various physical therapy modalities and techniques used, as well as their uses and purposes. Additional materials that may be studied or demonstrations for using the equipment are provided by the manufacturers of the modalities.

For any of the subsequent treatments that may fall within the scope of your job duties, you must implement the basic steps outlined in previous chapters for all procedures. You should now be able to organize the information that is presented on various treatments into the following briefly stated procedural steps. These steps can also be used as a guideline for a performance test checklist.

1. Check the physician's order.
2. **Wash your hands. Use appropriate personal protective equipment (PPE) as dictated by facility.**
3. Assemble the equipment and supplies needed.
4. Identify the patient and explain the nature and purpose of the treatment.
5. Prepare the patient: position correctly and comfortably and drape as necessary.
6. Prepare supplies for use.
7. Proceed with the treatment and time it accurately.
8. Observe the area to which the treatment has been applied frequently for desired or adverse reactions.
9. Remove the application used for the treatment.
10. Attend to the patient's safety and comfort; provide further instructions as indicated.
11. Properly care for the used equipment and supplies.
12. **Wash your hands.**
13. Record the treatment and the results obtained.
    Charting example
    September 9, 20__, 9 AM
    Hot moist compress applied to a wound on the inner aspect of the right forearm at 105° F (40.8° C) for 20 minutes. On completion of the treatment, the skin appeared pink, and the wound appeared clean; no evidence of suppuration present. Dry dressing was applied. Patient stated that most of the pain was relieved and that the compress provided much comfort.
    Kim Worth, CMA

ULTRAVIOLET LIGHT

Ultraviolet rays are rays beyond the violet end of the visible spectrum. They are produced by the sun and by sun lamps. Although ultraviolet rays produce very little heat, they can cause tanning on the skin or a sunburn (redness, erythema) and are capable of killing bacteria and other microorganisms and activating the formation of vitamin D.

Ultraviolet rays (light) are used therapeutically in the treatment of acne, psoriasis, pressure sores, and wound infections. The **purposes** of this treatment are to stimulate growing epithelial cells and cause capillary hyperemia and to increase cellular metabolism and vascular engorgement (an excess amount of blood in the vessels), which increases the skin's defenses against bacterial infections.

Various forms of apparatus provide ultraviolet rays. Before receiving ultraviolet treatment, the patient's sensitivity must first be determined. This is done by exposing different areas of the patient's skin to different doses of the rays for different time periods. The following day the patient returns so that the response can be determined. A little redness on the skin area is desired, but not a real burn. For example, if 20 seconds of exposure give the maximum coloration to the skin that is wanted without giving any more, the treatment is started with a 20-second exposure period to the ultraviolet light; then, depending on the light used, the exposure time is usually increased by 10-second intervals. The number of treatments to be given depends on how well the patient is responding.

When this treatment is given, the light must be placed at least 30 inches away from the patient and directed *only* on the area(s) to be treated.

Timing of the exposure period *must be exact* because excessive exposure can cause severe sunburn of up to second and third degree burns. Dark goggles should be worn by both the patient and the operator of the light to protect their eyes.

The patient *must never* be left unattended while being exposed to this light. If you are timing the exposure period and for some reason have to leave the room, you must disconnect the light and resume the treatment when you return. Some will turn off automatically, but it is still important for the operator to be present in the room when the patient is receiving this treatment to ensure that undesired burns do not result.

DIATHERMY

Diathermy is a heat-inducing wavelength that is part of the electromagnetic spectrum. It is the therapeutic use of a high-frequency current, the purpose being to generate heat within a part of the body. Diathermy works by inducing an electrical field, a conduction field in the tissues, and thereby heats the tissues and increases the circulation.

Diathermy is **used** in the treatment of muscular problems and sometimes for the treatment of arthritis, bursitis, and tendinitis. The term *diathermy* is also applied to the many different machines available for this purpose.

Depending on the machine used, the applicator is generally placed at least 1 inch away from the patient's skin. The heating element of some machines has a spacer built into it (that is, there is a space between the outside cover on the unit and the actual heating element). With these machines, the element is placed directly against the skin, because it is the outside cover of the unit and not the actual heating element that is in contact with the skin. The built-in spacer of these machines provides the required distance between the skin and the heating element.

Other machines have pads on the applicators. When these machines are used, towels (1-inch thickness) are placed between the pad and the patient's skin.

When giving diathermy treatments, you must watch for desensitized skin areas because patients have to be able to feel the heat; otherwise, they can get burned without realizing that they are getting burned. Areas of skin breakdown and other reactive areas, such as inflamed areas, must be avoided.

The electrical field of diathermy is attracted by metal. Therefore patients who have metal implants, such as joint implants, cannot receive diathermy treatments. In addition, patients cannot be wearing any jewelry or other metal objects, such as buckles and hairpins, and cannot be positioned on a metal table or chair but must be on wooden furniture. If these practices are not followed, the patient may receive severe burns because metal will become hot once the diathermy unit is turned on. Duration of the treatment is usually 15 to 20 minutes and should be timed carefully. You must explain to the patient that a warm, comfortable feeling should be experienced and if he or she becomes uncomfortable to inform the operator of the unit. If the patient complains that the treatment is becoming too hot, it must be stopped to avoid burning the patient. To operate any of the diathermy units available, you must carefully follow the instructions for use supplied by the manufacturers of each unit. Currently diathermy is seldom used in many facilities. It has been replaced by ultrasound.

ULTRASOUND

Ultrasound is also part of the electromagnetic spectrum. **Therapeutic ultrasound** is a very specific part of the sound spectrum that provides acoustic vibration with frequencies beyond human ear perception. This form of treatment uses high-frequency sound waves to penetrate deep tissue layers. Sound waves transform into heat whey they reach deep tissues. (Ultrasound is also used for diagnostic purposes. Review pp. 647-648 in Chapter 14).

Ultrasound vibrates on a molecular level. The two effects obtained from ultrasound are a mechanical effect and a heating effect. The mechanical effect, the vibration that causes the heating, is most noticeable on connective tissues, such as tendons and ligaments. A heating effect is produced on almost all tissues with the exception of bone because bone reflects ultrasound (that is, ultrasound is reflected from bone).

Ultrasound is of value for the treatment of pain syndromes to relax muscle spasms; to increase elasticity of tissues with collagen, such as tendons and ligaments so that they will respond better to stretching; and to provide deep penetration of heat and stimulate circulation in small areas, such as to increase blood supply to tissues in patients with vascular disorders. It is also used in breaking up calcium deposits and in loosening scars.

Ultrasound is applied by means of an applicator with a sound head, approximately 2 inches in diameter, that extends off from the special machine. Because ultrasound is not conducted through the air, a conducting medium must be spread on the patient's skin over the area to be treated. Special gels are

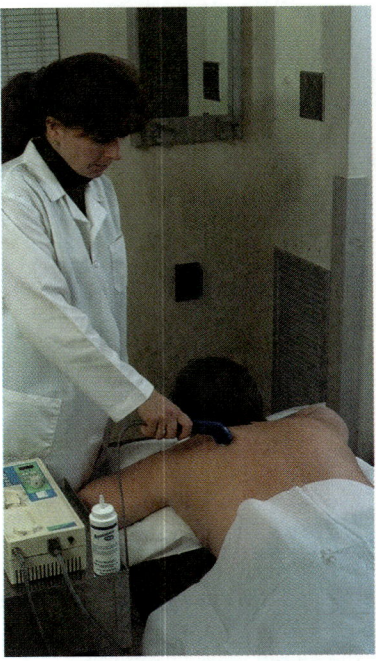

FIGURE 15-1 Ultrasound therapy applied to patient's shoulder in physical therapy.

available for this; mineral oil can also be used, but it is not as effective. After the gel is applied to the skin, the operator of the machine holds the sound head and moves it in a steady, up-and-down and rotary motion over the skin. The applicator must be in motion when used to prevent internal burns or tissue damage. Special care must also be taken when this treatment is used on patients with implants, such as joint implants, because ultrasound tends to vibrate and loosen the implant. In addition, heat builds up in the metal (Figure 15-1). Ultrasound can also be applied under water for treatment of the hands and feet. The water then acts as the conducting medium for the ultrasound. The length of any treatment depends on the size of the area being treated, but it is usually under 10 minutes. For example, ultrasound treatment to the lower back is applied for 6 to 7 minutes on one side. The minimal number of ultrasound treatments to be given to be effective varies from 5 to 12.

After use, the sound head should be cleansed with alcohol. Instructions for use of the ultrasound machines are supplied by the manufacturers and must be followed carefully.

LOCAL APPLICATIONS OF HEAT (THERMOTHERAPY) AND COLD (CRYOTHERAPY)

Dry and moist applications of heat and cold have been used universally as effective means of treatment by individuals in the home and by physicians, nurses, medical assistants, and physical therapists, either in an office or hospital setting. Tolerance for the temperature changes that occur when heat or cold is applied to the body varies with the individual and also varies in different parts of the body. Generally, the areas of the skin more

TABLE 15–1   **Physiologic Reactions Produced by Heat and Cold Applications**

Body Function	Heat	Cold
Blood vessels in area	Dilated (increasing circulation)	Constricted (decreasing circulation)
Heat production	Decreased	Increased (by shivering)
Blood pressure	Lowered	Elevated
Respiratory rate	Increased	Increased
Tissue metabolism	Increased	Decreased
Muscle spasm	Relaxed	Reduced
Temperature	Increased	Reduced

sensitive to these changes are those that are not usually exposed; the less sensitive areas are those that are exposed, usually having thicker and tougher layers of skin, such as areas on the soles of the feet or the palms of the hands.

Once heat or cold is applied to the skin, certain physiologic reactions occur in the body; heat has the opposite effect to that of cold, except for respiratory rate changes (Table 15-1).

Heat or cold modalities are to be placed on a bare body surface for only *short durations,* usually 15 to 20 minutes. An important fact to remember is that the prolonged use of heat (more than 1 hour) produces reverse secondary effects (that is, blood vessels then constrict, thus decreasing blood supply to the area). The prolonged use of cold (more than 1 hour) also has a reverse secondary effect (that is, blood vessels dilate, thus increasing circulation and tissue metabolism). In other words, the immediate effect of heat applications is vasodilation, whereas the prolonged effect is vasoconstriction; and the immediate effect of cold applications is vasoconstriction, whereas the prolonged effect is vasodilation. Therefore heat applications should not be left in place for long periods. Cold applications can be used for longer periods than heat, depending on the desired effects. The physician usually indicates the temperature (that is, warm or hot, tepid, cool, cold, or very cold) and the time to be used for the following applications of dry and moist hot and cold applications.

Principles for Preparation and Patient Care

Because applications of heat and cold are common treatments, you should keep in mind the following principles regarding preparation and patient care:

1. Learn exactly where and for how long the application is to be placed on the patient's body.
2. Position the patient comfortably so that the treatment can be maintained for the designated time.
3. Avoid accidents—be sure that the patient is positioned safely and will not fall. Place solutions in a convenient location and so that they will not spill.
4. Test the solution (with a bath thermometer) or the device you are using to be sure that it is at the exact temperature that the physician ordered or the recommended temperature for the method used.

5. Remove any dressings covering the area to be treated. (Review the procedure for a dressing change, pp. 330-336.) Apply a clean dressing, if ordered, when the treatment is completed.
6. Keep the application at the ordered temperature. Generally, compresses and packs cool off within 15 to 20 minutes and then have to be reheated and reapplied. If the temperature of the device or the solution changes, it will not accomplish its purpose and may even harm the patient.
7. Keep the patient warm during the application of heat; drape sheets or blankets can be used to cover the patient. When blood vessels dilate (as with the application of heat), more blood comes to the surface of the body, and the body is cooled by the surrounding air. Thus the patient can easily become chilled unless protected with covering.
8. Check the patient's skin frequently during the application to observe for any skin changes, as well as for any signs of burns or frostbite. Report any signs of burns or frostbite *immediately.*
9. Provide further instruction to the patient, as indicated, on completion of the treatment.

Thermotherapy

Superficial heat treatments can be administered with dry or moist heat applications. These local heat applications are used to relieve pain, to promote muscle relaxation and reduce spasm, to increase circulation to an area to relieve congestion and swelling by dilating the blood vessels, and to speed up the inflammatory process to promote suppuration (pus formation) and drainage from an infected area. In addition, dry heat applications are used to dry and heal surgical incisions and sutures, perineal lacerations, and skin ulcers.

Dry heat.   Dry heat applications often used include the following:

- Infrared radiation (heat lamps)
- Electric light bulbs
- Electric heating pads
- Hot water bottles
- Chemical hot pack
- Aquamatic (K- or K-matic) pad with cover and heating unit

Infrared radiation is dry heat application by means of a heat lamp. The term *infrared* usually refers to the heat lamp. Infrared rays from these lamps provide surface heat and penetrate the skin to a depth of about 5 to 10 mm. At times, a plain gooseneck lamp is used because the **incandescent light bulb** is a source of infrared rays. Heat lamps must be kept at least 2 to 4 feet away from the skin, varying with the type and intensity of the lamp used. The skin must be clean and free of any ointment or medicinal substances. The duration of the treatment is **usually 15 to 20 minutes** because prolonged or intense application can lead to burning and blistering of the skin.

Place **electric heating pads** in a protective covering, such as a towel or pillowcase, and then apply them to a dry area. Never use them over moist or wet areas or dressings by means of which moisture could come in contact with the electricity. Instruct patients not to lie on the pad because burns could result. The heat selector switch is usually set on the low or medium setting and left for an accurately timed period. (The amount of heat and time to be applied are designated by the physician.)

When using a **hot water bottle,** testing the temperature of the water accurately with a thermometer is essential before pouring it into the water bottle. Place hot tap water into a pitcher so that the temperature can be tested with a bath thermometer. Water not exceeding 125° F (52° C) is to be used. The accepted temperature ranges are from 115° to 125° F (46° to 52° C) for patients 2 years and older and from 105° to 115° F (41° to 46° C) for children under 2 years and for elderly patients. (The very young and the very old tend to be more sensitive to applications of heat and cold.)

Fill the hot water bottle only about half full and expel the air before you seal it. This allows the bottle to be lighter and more pliable so that it can be molded to the area on which it is to be applied. The outside of the hot water bottle must be dry and then placed into a protective covering, such as a pillowcase or towel, before it is applied to the patient. This protective covering should remain dry unless the hot water bottle is placed over moist dressings to keep them warm (Figure 15-2).

The patient should experience a feeling of warmth but not be uncomfortable; burns must be avoided. When the hot water bottle is left on for any length of time, it should be refilled with hot water to maintain the desired temperature. After use, wash the hot water bottle thoroughly with warm water and detergent, rinse it, and allow it to dry before being stored. Store the bottle with the stopper in place and air inside to prevent the sides from sticking.

Disposable chemical hot packs are prepared commercially in various sizes and shapes. When they are activated, they provide a specific amount of heat for a specific amount of time. They are pliable and can fit the contour of any body part. Follow the manufacturer's directions to activate the chemical reaction that produces the heat. The directions are usually to deliver a sharp blow to the pack or to knead it. Cover the pack with a cloth before applying it to the patient's skin.

The **Aquamatic (K- or K-matic) pad** is a rubber pad of tubular construction that is filled to about two-thirds full with distilled water. The water is heated and kept at an even temper-

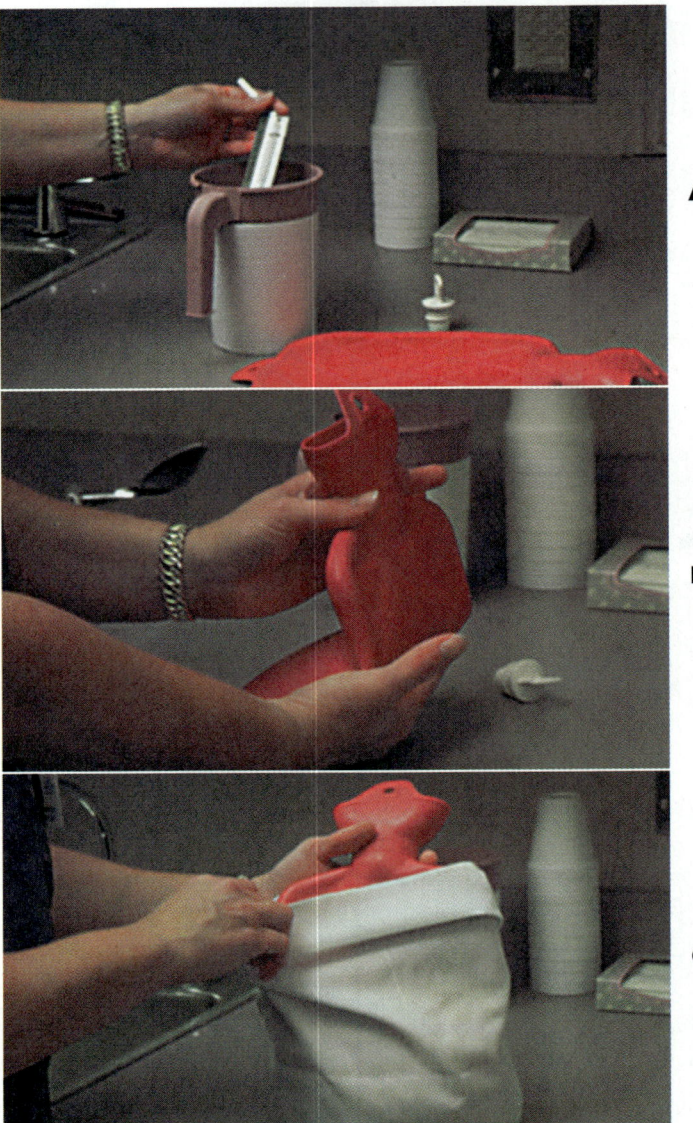

FIGURE 15-2 **A,** Test temperature of hot water before placing it into hot water bottle. **B,** Expel air from half-filled hot water bottle before using. **C,** Cover the hot water bottle before applying to patient.

ature by an electrical control unit. Cover the pad and place it around or over the body part or surface to be treated. It is usually left on the patient for 15 to 30 minutes. This pad is both more effective and safer than an electric heating pad or a hot water bottle because you can maintain a constant temperature by regulating the control unit (Figure 15-3).

Moist heat applications. Moist heat applications often used include the following:

- Hot soaks
- Hot compresses
- Hot packs

FIGURE 15-3   Aquamatic (K- or K-matic) pad and heating unit used for dry heat application.

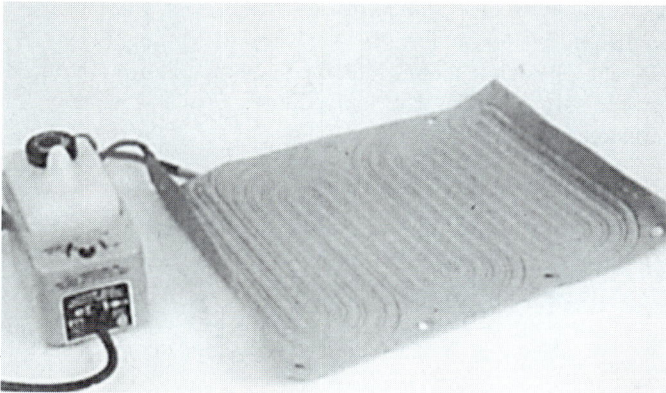

FIGURE 15-4   During a hot soak, add more hot solution to container at point farthest away from patient's skin and stir quickly into cooler solution.

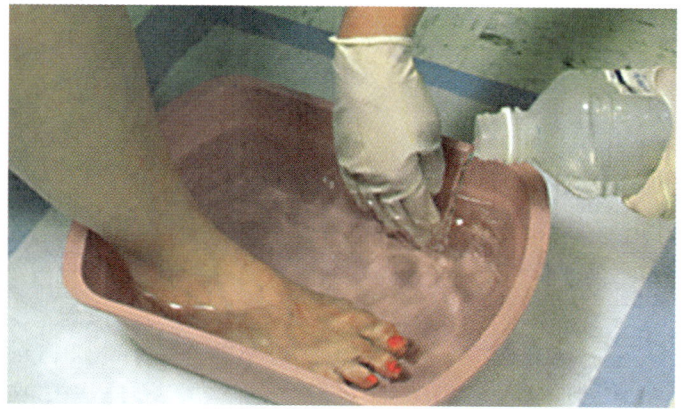

Hot soaks.   For a **hot soak,** the body part to be treated is immersed gradually (to allow the patient to become accustomed to the heat change) in tap water or a medicated solution of 105° to 110° F (41° to 44° C). *Unless otherwise ordered, the body part is kept immersed for 15 to 20 minutes.* This form of treatment can be used for heat application to the hands, arms, feet, or legs. The process of having the body from the neck down immersed in water in a special tank, called the Hubbard tank, or the body or a limb immersed in a whirlpool tank is more commonly referred to as **hydrotherapy** (see p. 672). Soaks applied to open wounds require the use of sterile technique, a sterile container, and a sterile solution. The water or solution temperature should be maintained as much as possible throughout the treatment. You can do this by removing some of the solution every 5 minutes or so and adding more hot solution. Take care to avoid burning the patient when the hot solution is added. Add the hot solution to the container at the point farthest away from the patient's skin and stir it quickly into the cooler solution (Figure 15-4).

Position the patient comfortably to prevent strain or pressure on the area treated and also to prevent fatigue. Observe the patient's skin during the treatment for excessive redness, at which time, remove the limb from the solution until it has cooled. Remember to record the observations made during the treatment on the patient's record. On completion of the treatment, dry the limb with a towel by patting, *not* rubbing. For an open wound, pat dry only the surrounding area. Do not allow the towel to touch the open wound. Observing the area after the treatment is necessary because you must record this information on the patient's record. **Soaks differ from compresses and packs in that soaks are used for shorter periods and usually at lower temperatures.**

Hot moist compresses and packs.   Two basic differences between compresses and packs are that (1) different materials are used for each and (2) a pack is usually applied to a more extensive body area than a compress.

A **compress** used for the application of moist heat is prepared by taking a soft square of gauze or similar absorbent material (a clean washcloth can also be used), soaking it in

FIGURE 15-5   **A,** Wring out hot compress to avoid excessive wetness before you apply it. **B,** Apply hot compress to body area.

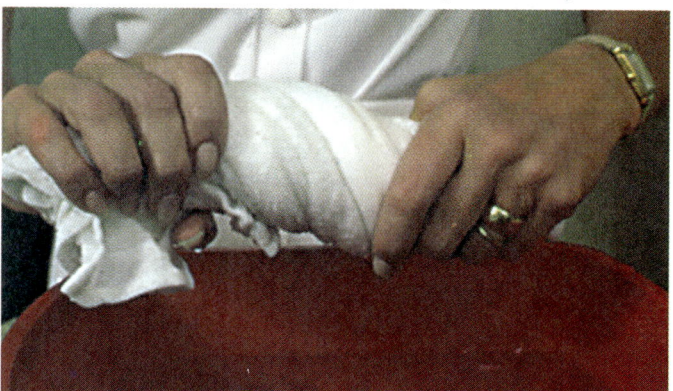

A

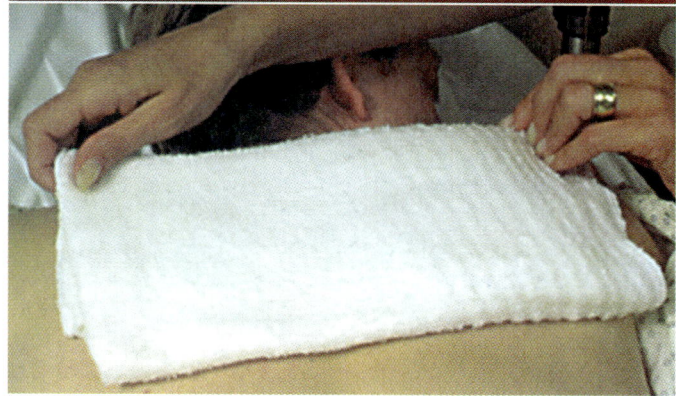

B

hot water, then wringing it out manually or with the use of forceps to avoid excessive wetness. This material is then applied to a limited body area, such as the finger or a small area on the arm, for a designated period (Figure 15-5). **Dry compresses** are used to apply pressure or medications to specific restricted areas.

A **pack** used for the application of moist heat is prepared in the same manner as a compress, except that flannel or similar materials are used. Commercially prepared hot packs filled with a silica gel (for example, Hydrocollator packs) are also used. Packs are usually applied to a more extensive body area.

Both *compresses and packs* are to be applied to the skin area slowly so that the patient can gradually adjust to the heat. The recommended water temperature for soaking gauze, flannel, or similar materials is 105° to 110° F (41° to 44° C). Commercially prepared packs are kept in a hot water bath at 140° to 160° F (60° to 71° C) until used and then wrapped in towels before being applied to the patient's skin. Both compresses and packs should be as hot as the patient can comfortably tolerate. A plastic covering can be placed over or wrapped around the compress or pack to concentrate and hold the heat over the area treated for as long a time as possible.

During these treatments, the patient's skin should be checked frequently to ensure that the skin is not burning and to observe for signs of increased redness or swelling. All observations must be recorded on completion of the treatment. If the patient experiences pain or is uncomfortable, the plastic covering should be removed or unwrapped to release some of the confined heat. If the area remains painful, the pack or compress is to be removed and cooled somewhat before being reapplied. This is done to prevent burning the skin.

Additional compresses or packs should be made ready for use when the applied one cools. The length of these treatments varies according to the physician's order. *Generally they are prescribed for 15 to 20 minutes,* but at times, they may be applied for 1 hour. On completion of the treatment, the compress or pack is removed, and the skin is patted dry. When these treatments have been applied to an open wound, *only* the surrounding area is to be patted dry. The open wound is *not* to be touched. A clean sterile dressing is applied to an open wound when ordered by the physician. Used equipment and supplies should be cared for properly, and the treatment and all observations should be recorded on the patient's record.

Cryotherapy

Cryotherapy, the therapeutic use of cold, is applied with dry or moist cold applications. Cold applications are used to:

1. Prevent edema or swelling
2. Relieve pain or tenderness (cold produces a topical anesthetic effect)
3. Reduce the inflammation and pus formation (cold inhibits microbial activity in the early stages of the infectious process)
4. Control bleeding (the peripheral vessels constrict with the application of cold, resulting in a decreased blood flow)
5. Reduce body temperature

Cold is commonly used following strain, sprains, and bruises and also for muscle spasm and tenderness. Any type of acute injury responds fairly well to cold. During the acute phase of an injury when there may be bleeding in the area, you should not use heat. The old rule of thumb for treating such injuries was to apply cold for the first 24 hours, then apply heat.

Currently, many health care practitioners often wait longer than 24 hours before using heat applications on patients and often use cold continually when positive results are being obtained.

The physician should indicate the temperature to be used for cold applications. The temperatures of the water are described as follows:

- Tepid: 80° to 93° F (26.7° to 33.9° C)
- Cool: 65° to 80° F (18.3° to 26.7° C)
- Cold: 55° to 65° F (12.3° to 18.3° C)
- Very cold: Below 55° F (below 12.5° C)

The selection of the temperature to use depends on the following:

- Condition of the patient
- Sensitivity of the patient's skin
- Area to be covered
- Method to be used

The duration of the application depends on the temperature (for example, an ice massage is given for a shorter period [5 minutes] than a cold compress or pack [20 or 32 minutes]). Colder temperatures can be tolerated best on small areas for a short time. Keeping skin temperatures below 40° F (4.4° C) for long periods is usually considered dangerous, except when ice is used for anesthesia.

Dry cold. Dry cold applications often used include the following:

- Ice bags
- Ice collars
- Chemical cold packs

Fill an **ice bag** one-half to two-thirds full with small pieces of ice; expel air from the bag by twisting the top and then capping (Figure 15-6). At this time, check the bag for leaks. Small

FIGURE 15-6 Expel air from ice bag by twisting the top and then the cap.

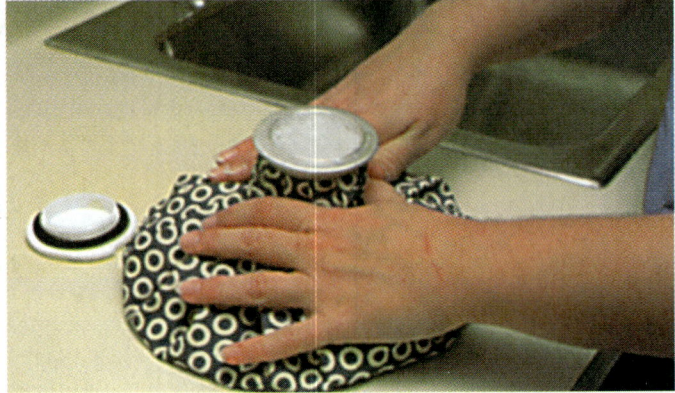

ice pieces reduce the amount of air spaces in the bag, which results in better conduction of cold and also allows the bag to mold better to the contour of the body part. Once the ice bag is sealed, dry it and place it in a protective covering, which provides comfort for the patient and absorbs moisture that condenses on the outside. For the ice bag to be effective, place it on the skin for 30 to 60 minutes, as designated by the physician. If the treatment is to be continuous, apply the ice bag for 30 to 60 minutes and then remove it for 1 hour. By doing the procedure in this manner, you allow the tissues to react to the immediate effects of the cold.

Check the patient's skin periodically for signs of decreased swelling or redness. When they are present, note signs of excessive coldness, which include mottled and pale skin and excessive numbness in the body part. When or if these signs occur, remove the ice bag and notify the physician.

Ice collars are rubber or plastic modalities that are smaller than ice bags and look like a medium-sized rectangle. They are used on the neck or on small areas or wrapped around a body part.

Chemical cold packs are rubberized, plasticized flat bags containing a chemical substance and a liquid. They are commercially prepared in various sizes and shapes and come with specific instructions that must be followed. Some are for one-time use, whereas others can be stored in a freezer for reuse. To activate the chemical reaction that produces the coldness, you must usually squeeze or knead the pack and then shake it to mix the contained granules and liquid. The pack remains cold for between 30 and 60 minutes, varying with the brand. Some packs are covered with a soft outer covering or wrap and therefore do not need an additional cover. Others have to be covered with a cloth before they are applied to the person's skin. They are pliable and can be molded to fit the contour of any body part (Figure 15-7, *A* and *B*).

Moist cold.
Moist cold applications often used include the following:

- Cold compresses
- Cold packs
- Ice massage
- Alcohol sponge baths

Moist cold compresses are generally applied to small areas, and cold packs are used on larger body areas, as are hot applications. Compresses may be used for treating a headache, a tooth extraction, or an eye injury. The area to which the compress is to be applied determines the type of material used. For example, a clean washcloth can be used on the head or face; surgical gauze dressings with a small amount of cotton filling can be used for eye compresses. Immerse the material used for the compress in a clean basin containing ice chips or small pieces of ice and a small amount of cold water. To avoid dripping, wring the material out manually or with the use of forceps and then place it on the skin for the amount of time designated by the physician (usually 20 to 30 minutes and then repeated every 2 hours). Change compresses frequently to maintain a cold application. Most patients will tell you when the compress no longer feels cold. Placing an ice bag over the compress helps keep the compress cold and reduces the number of times that it must be changed. Check the patient periodically during this treatment for any changes, such as a decrease or increase in swelling or redness on the area or a decrease or increase of pain. On completion of the treatment, pat the skin dry if necessary. Record the treatment and observations on the patient's record.

Cold packs (ice packs) may be applied to a small area but are generally used on larger areas, such as an arm or leg. At times they can be applied to the whole body to lower the temperature. In this case, hypothermia pads or blankets may be used rather than ice packs. These are used in hospitals with the patient under close observation for temperature and skin changes. Manufacturers of hypothermia units provide complete instructions for use, which must be followed precisely.

To apply a cold or ice pack, first wrap the extremity in wet toweling and then pack ice chips around it; place an additional towel over the ice to reduce the melting rate. Generally, these are applied for 20 to 30 minutes. Commercial cold packs are also available, which are kept in a freezer until used. They do not freeze stiff; thus they are pliable and can be molded to fit the contour of the body part.

FIGURE 15-7 **A,** Reusable chemical hot pack and cover; **B,** disposable chemical cold packs.

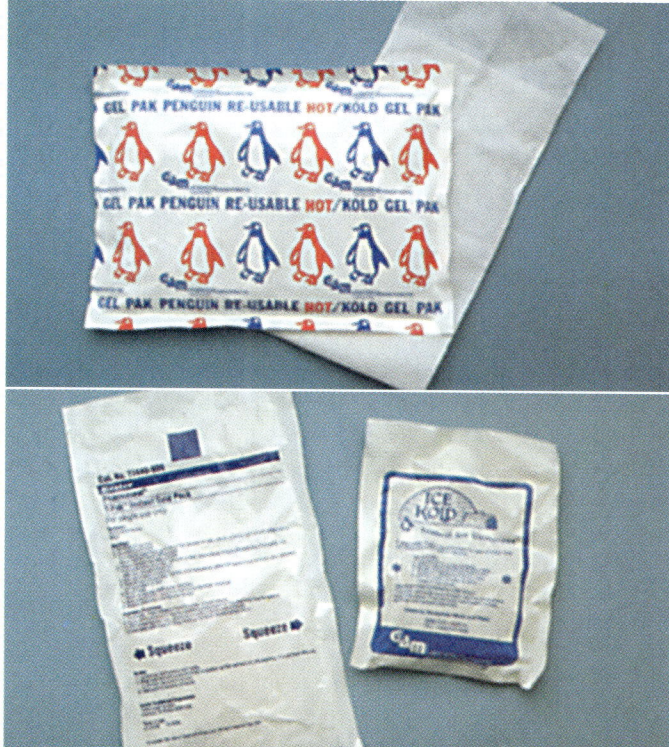

FIGURE 15-8   Ice massage is one form of cryotherapy that can be used to decrease pain. Use a chemical ice pack or freeze water in paper cup, cover cup, and rub it over affected area.

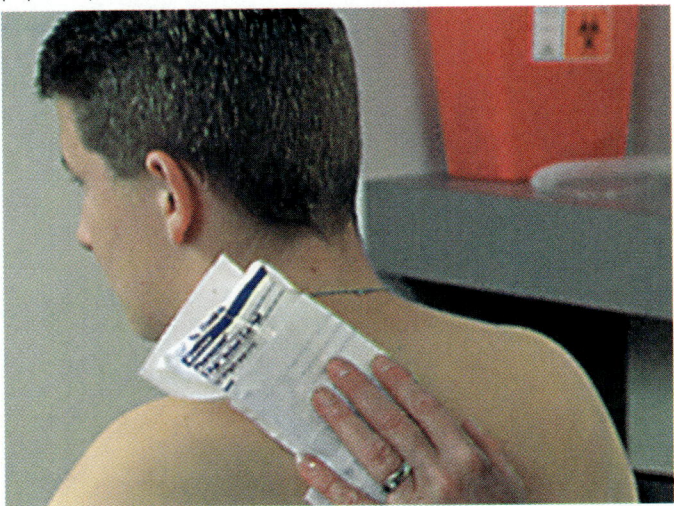

Ice massage is simply massaging the area with ice. This can be as simple as freezing water in a paper cup and then rubbing it over the affected area for approximately 3 to 5 minutes (Figure 15-8). Continue monitoring the skin for any changes.

In the past, **alcohol sponge baths** were recommended and used often, both in hospital and at home, for reducing a patient's elevated temperature. Presently they are more commonly done in a home situation because they have been replaced in many hospitals or health care facilities by hypothermia pads or blankets. A mixture of half alcohol and half tepid water is used for an alcohol sponge bath. Because alcohol vaporizes more quickly than water, heat is removed from the skin surface rapidly when this mixture is applied to the body in contrast to using just a cold bath.

An alcohol sponge bath should not exceed 30 minutes. Drape the patient with covers and apply a hot water bottle to the feet to avoid excessive chilling and shivering. Apply an ice bag to the head to promote comfort and relieve a headache, if present. Expose only the area being sponged. You need two clean washcloths—while one is being used, the other is to be cooling in the alcohol-water solution. Sponge each extremity for approximately 5 minutes, the back and buttocks for 5 to 10 minutes, and the trunk and abdomen for 5 minutes. Moist, cool cloths can be placed over large superficial blood vessels in the neck, axilla, and groin during the procedure as additional aids to lower the body temperature. Record the temperature 30 minutes after the sponge bath to determine if the treatment has been effective.

You should caution patients *not* to use alcohol sponge baths indiscriminately because alcohol has a tendency to dry out the skin. In addition, if a fever does not break after the application of two or three alcohol sponge baths given in the home, the physician should be notified.

HYDROTHERAPY

Hydrotherapy is the use of water in the treatment of disease processes. Because these treatments are usually not performed in the physician's office, the patient is referred to a physical therapy department in a hospital or to a physical therapist's office. On other occasions the patient may be instructed to apply hot or cold soaks, compresses, or packs at home.

Modalities used for hydrotherapy include the Hubbard tank, the whirlpool, and a larger pool, all with varying temperatures of hot or cold water, as designated by the physician for each patient's care.

These three modalities are used primarily to promote relaxation, circulation, and early motion (by exercising) of the injured body part. Other uses include those discussed previously under Local Applications of Heat and Cold on p. 666. Hydrotherapy is also used to cleanse and debride the skin (for example, in patients who have extensive burns). The **Hubbard tank** is a large tank in which the whole body can be immersed either in a sitting or lying position. It is basically a large whirlpool in which body exercises may also be done. The **whirlpool** is a tank of agitating water in which an arm, leg, or body can be immersed. The mechanical action of the water movement provides hydromassage, is very relaxing, and stimulates circulation. Body exercises cannot be done in the whirlpool tank because it is too small, but extremity exercises could be done. The pool used in physical therapy is like a medium-sized swimming pool. Many types of exercises can be performed in the pool because once in the pool, the effects of gravity can be reduced. For example, patients who are not strong enough to stand up alone can stand up in the pool because they are supported by the water. The water also produces a heating or cooling effect, depending on the temperature used.

PARAFFIN WAX HAND BATH

Another form of heat application used for patients with rheumatoid arthritis is the hot paraffin wax hand bath. The **purposes** of this treatment are to relieve pain; increase circulation; and decrease the duration of morning stiffness of the fingers, hands, and wrists. An advantage of this treatment over moist heat applications is the longer-lasting (2 to 3 hours) circulatory changes that it can produce. This procedure can be performed at home, in the physician's office, or in a physical therapy department. Special containers are available for storing and heating the wax; or in a home, a double boiler may be used. Commercial premixed preparations *with instructions* are available for home use. To use, rapidly dip the *dry* hand and wrist in the warm paraffin and remove. Do this repeatedly until a fairly thick coat of wax is allowed to harden, covering the area. Cover the wax-covered area with a plastic bag and a towel, which act as an insulator to help retain the heat. Do *not* move the fingers or hand after the initial coat of wax to avoid breaking the wax seal. Leave the wax (paraffin) in place for 15 to 20 minutes, then peel it off and replace it in the container for the next application. Put the fingers and wrist

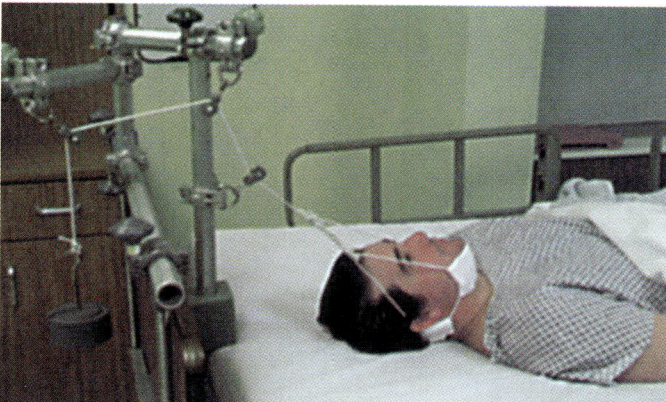

FIGURE 15-9   Weight or static traction as applied to head for cervical traction. The manufacturer's directions for use must be followed. The physician orders the number of pounds of traction to use.

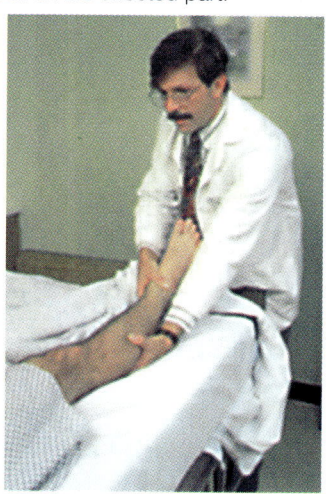

FIGURE 15-10   Manual traction applied by the therapist using the hands to exert a pull on the affected part.

through range-of-motion exercises because the heat relieves pain and thus enables the patient to exercise the fingers and wrist with greater mobility. NOTE: Be very careful that the hand and wrist are dry when placed in the warm paraffin wax. Moisture or water on the hand conducts heat much more quickly and can burn the area. Burns are prevented when the area immersed is dry and dipped and removed rapidly. Do *not* use this treatment if any wounds or cuts are on the area to be waxed.

TRACTION

Traction is the process of pulling or drawing, as applied to the musculoskeletal system for dislocated joints, fractured bones, or diseased peripheral joints (for example, arthritic joints). This therapy may be used in the orthopedic physician's office but more commonly is applied in sports medicine facilities and hospitals. Traction devices can also be set up for home use. **Traction is used in orthopedics to do the following:**

- Obtain and maintain proper position
- Correct or prevent a deformity
- Decrease or overcome muscle spasms
- Lessen or prevent contractures (an abnormal shortening of muscle tissue)
- Promote better movement of the area
- Lessen and prevent severe stiffening of peripheral joints
- Achieve relief of compression at vertebral joints
- Facilitate healing

Methods and Devices
Weight or static traction.   This method of traction is applied with weights of varied poundages that are connected to the end of a pulley mechanism. For example, the patient's head is placed in a head harness, which is attached to a rope with weights on the end. The rope is attached to a pole or door top

so that it stretches up over the head and then is displaced downward where the weights are attached. Units can be obtained for use at home (Figure 15-9).

Elastic traction.   Elastic traction is applied with elastic appliances that exert a pull on the affected limb.

Mechanical traction.   Mechanical traction is applied by means of units that give an intermittent type of traction primarily for spinal arthritis. They are set to pull and hold a set amount of tension for a set period and then to relax for a set period. They continue to pull and relax as long as they are set.

Manual traction.   Manual traction is applied by therapists using their hands to exert a pull on the affected part. In addition to other musculoskeletal problems, manual traction is used for treating peripheral joint disease, such as arthritic joints, to distract (slightly separate) the joint surface to obtain more movement and prevent severe stiffening or to treat stiffness in the neck or low back resulting from arthritis (Figure 15-10).

Skin traction.   Skin traction is applied by placing foam rubber pads or some other material with a weight attached to the end along the sides of the affected limb. For support, this application is wrapped with elastic bandages.

Skeletal traction.   Skeletal traction is applied **only** in the hospital. Surgically installed pins and wires or tongs (for example, head tongs) are used to apply a pulling force directly on a bone.

MASSAGE

Massage was probably the first form of physical therapy. Individuals instinctively rub or massage an area after incurring an injury or bruise. After administering an injection, the injection site is rubbed, which is also a type of massage. Massage can be that simple, but it is also a highly skilled technique. Massage is a systematic and methodic pressure applied to bare skin by stroking, rubbing, kneading or rolling, tapping or pounding with the fingers or cupped hand or by quick tappings with alternating fingertips. The type of massage used most often in physicians' offices and clinics is stroking. Also, tapotement, the pounding or cupping with a cupped hand on the back, is used on patients with chest congestion because this helps loosen the secretions to clear the congestion (Figure 15-11). Massages are also given to do the following:

- Aid circulation by removing blood and waste products from injured tissues and by bringing fresh blood to the injured part, which helps the healing process
- Relax muscles and relieve spasms
- Reduce pain
- Help restore motion and function to the affected part
- Decrease swelling
- Reduce edema

To apply massage effectively, the therapist or assistant must be in a comfortable position to avoid straining, and the hands should be warm to avoid discomfort to the patient. The patient must also be in a comfortable position so that beneficial results are more easily obtained.

EXERCISES

Therapeutic exercise is the performance of prescribed physical exertion to bring about the following:

- Improve one's general health status
- Improve one's general health status after being afflicted with disabilities affecting the neuromuscular, skeletal, cardiovascular, integumentary, respiratory, and urinary systems, in addition to treatment for congenital defects, prenatal and postnatal care, and psychiatric problems
- Correct a physical deformity
- Improve muscle tone and strengthen muscles
- Restore the strength of muscles that have atrophied or weakened because of disease processes

---

HEALTH **MATTERS**

STRONG MUSCLES PROVIDE PROTECTION FOR JOINTS

Exercise physiologists state that the best way to protect a joint is to strengthen the surrounding muscles. Everyone needs good strong muscles to help keep joints stable and to maintain flexibility. To achieve this, *regular exercise* and the *right kind* of exercise done the *right way* are needed. Regular exercise of any type will improve health in some way. Still, it is best to know what type of exercises to do for specific reasons, conditions, or problems that fit one's body type and capabilities. In addition to lowering the risk for heart disease, regular exercise improves the flexibility and mobility of joints and improves

muscle strength. With strong muscles, people are not as likely to fall and break a bone or injure a joint, and if someone does fall, he or she is better able to break the fall and avoid serious injury. One of the easiest and best exercises is walking. If someone walks regularly, there are definite benefits, *but* walking does not strengthen the muscles stabilizing the shoulder or the elbow joint. To accomplish this, *correct* weight-resistance exercise and stretching exercises are necessary. To learn specific exercises, proper techniques, and how to breathe properly and to be aware of posture throughout the exercise, we *must be taught*. Check community sources that provide classes on "Joint and Muscle Strengthening Exercises." As always, check with your physician before staring any extensive exercise program.

FIGURE 15-11 Tapotement form of massage used on people with chest congestion. Cup hands and pound or cup firmly and rapidly on the person's back over the lung area.

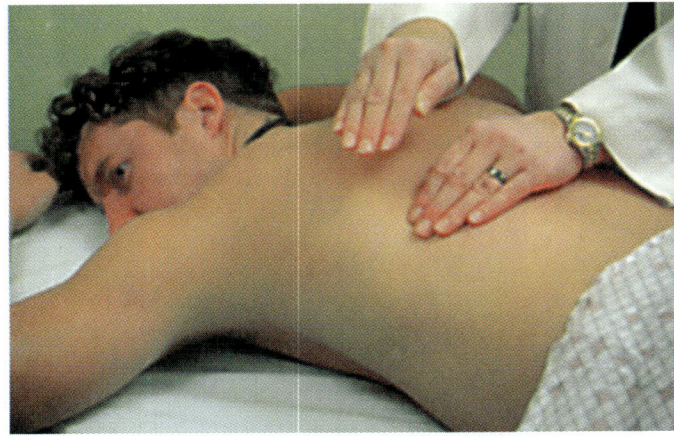

- Restore motion after a fracture, injury, or any form of immobilization
- Aid circulation
- Improve coordination

Exercises may be performed in the physician's office or in physical therapy departments, or the patient may be given instructions and taught the exercises to be performed at home. **Patients who are to do exercises at home must be *taught* how to do them and not just *told* what to do.** Reasons for the exercise program must also be explained to the patient. The medical assistant responsible for these duties should have the patient perform the exercises while in the office until the motions involved are fully understood to ensure that the patient is capable of performing the *prescribed* exercise program. (See the Health Matters box.)

Classification

Active exercises. All the motions involved in active exercise are performed totally by the patient and may involve the use of weights, pulleys, rubber balls, or similar appliances that the patient is to squeeze or manipulate.

Passive exercises. In passive exercises, movement to the part is done by another person or outside force without any voluntary participation from the patient (see Figures 15-13 through 15-15).

Aided exercises. In aided exercises, the patient is helped to move muscles that are too weak to move on their own strength. Exercises that are performed in a pool are also considered aided exercises.

Active resistance exercises. In active resistance exercises the patient voluntarily applies pressure or movement of the part, and another individual applies resistance to the motion.

Range-of-motion exercises. Range-of-motion exercises are designed to assist joint mobility and normal functioning (for example, bending the fingers, twisting the wrist around in a normal motion, or rotating the leg in a circumscribed fashion). They can be either active or passive exercises (Figures 15-12 through 15-15).

Text continued on p. 679

FIGURE 15-12   A, Range-of-motion exercises for the upper extremities.

NECK

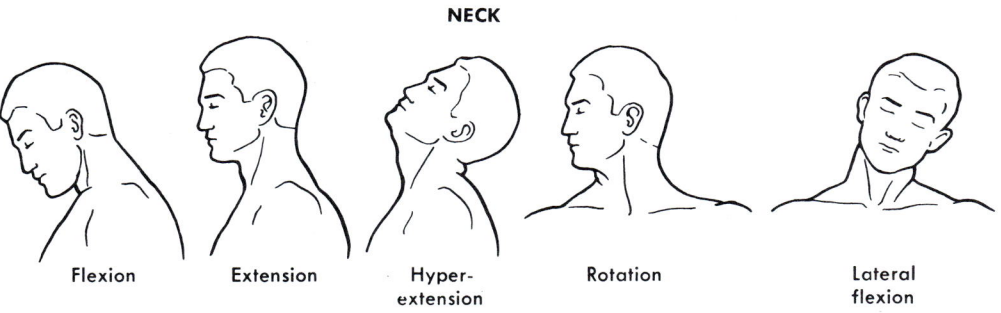

Flexion   Extension   Hyper-extension   Rotation   Lateral flexion

TRUNK

A

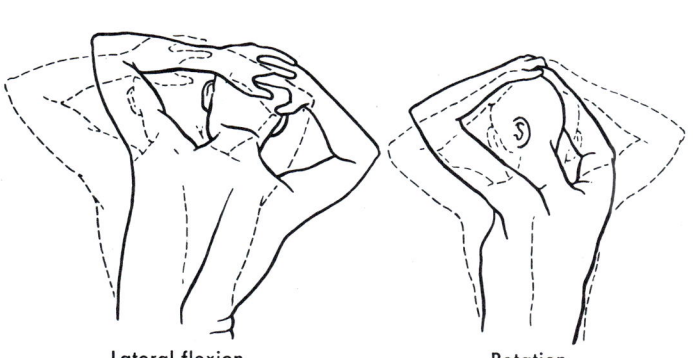

Lateral flexion   Rotation

Continued

FIGURE 15-12—cont'd **A,** Range-of-motion exercises for the upper extremities.

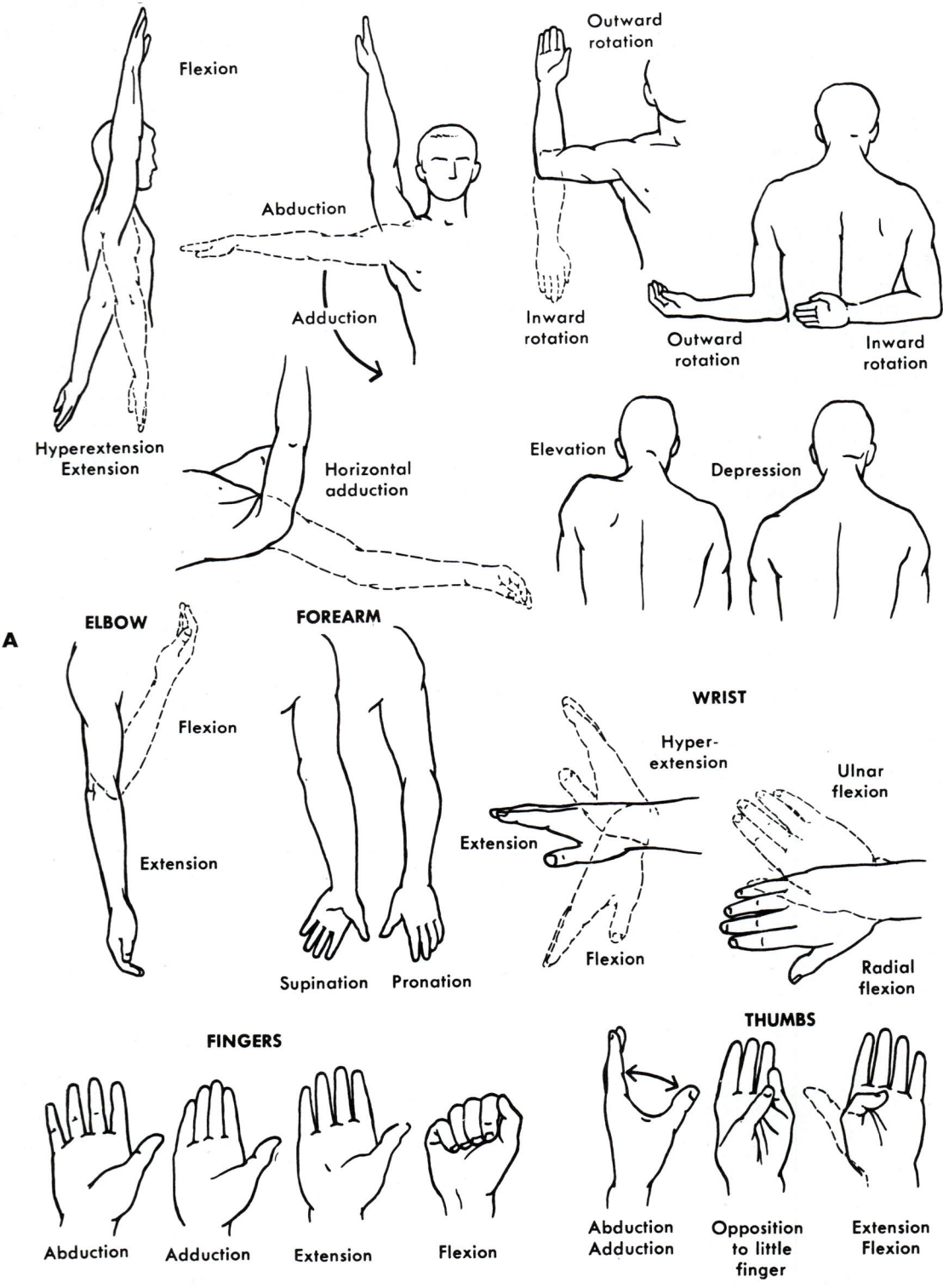

FIGURE 15-12—cont'd   **B,** Range-of-motion exercises for the lower extremities.

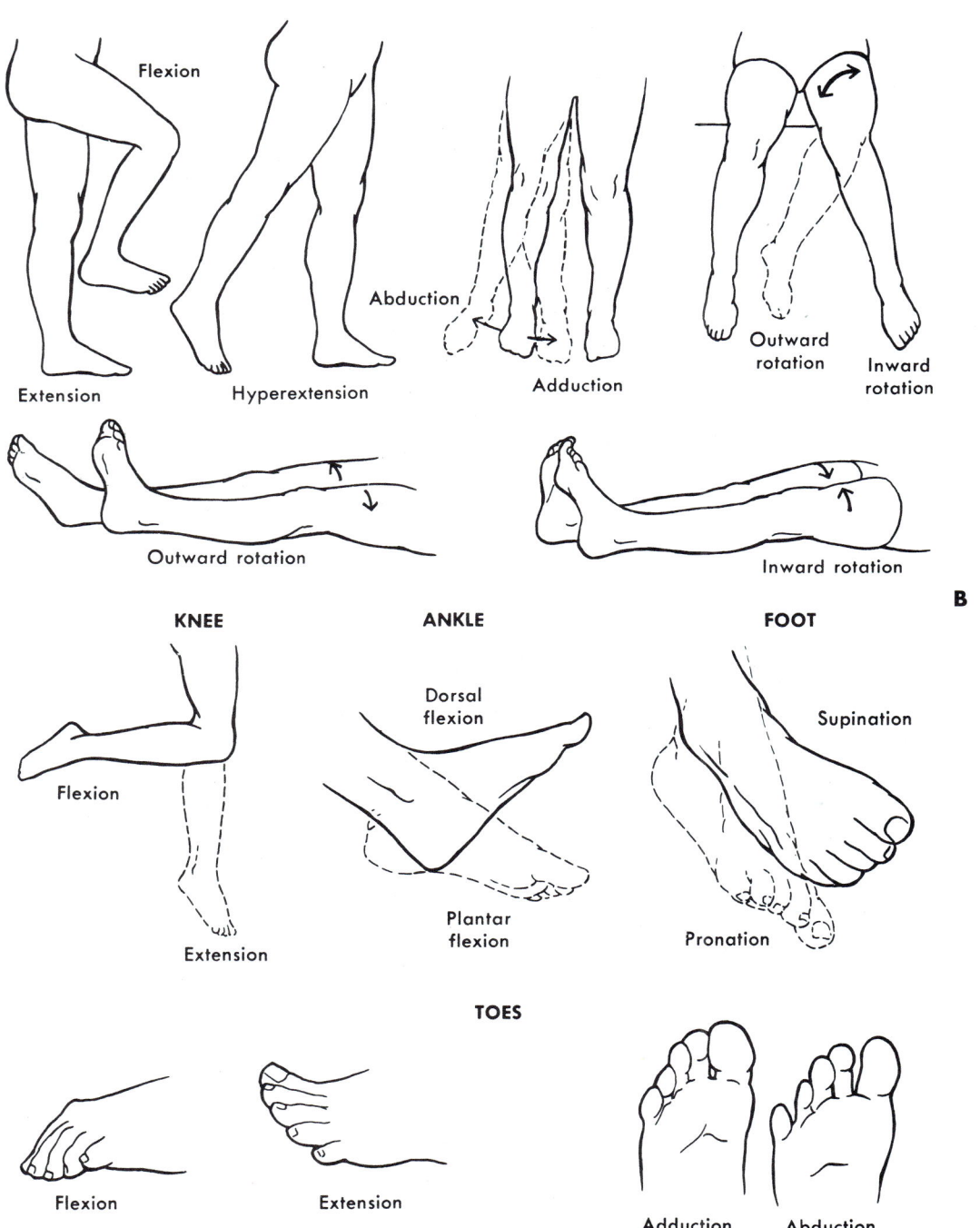

HIP

Flexion

Extension

Hyperextension

Abduction

Adduction

Outward rotation

Inward rotation

Outward rotation

Inward rotation

B

KNEE

Flexion

Extension

ANKLE

Dorsal flexion

Plantar flexion

FOOT

Supination

Pronation

TOES

Flexion

Extension

Adduction

Abduction

FIGURE 15-13 Abduction of thumb and finger extension. **A,** Hold the patient's fingers straight with one hand. Bend the patient's thumb toward the palm with your other hand. **B,** Move the patient's thumb back, pointing away from the hand. Repeat this movement. **C,** Rotate the thumb (in a circle). Perform these exercises on both the good and weak hands.

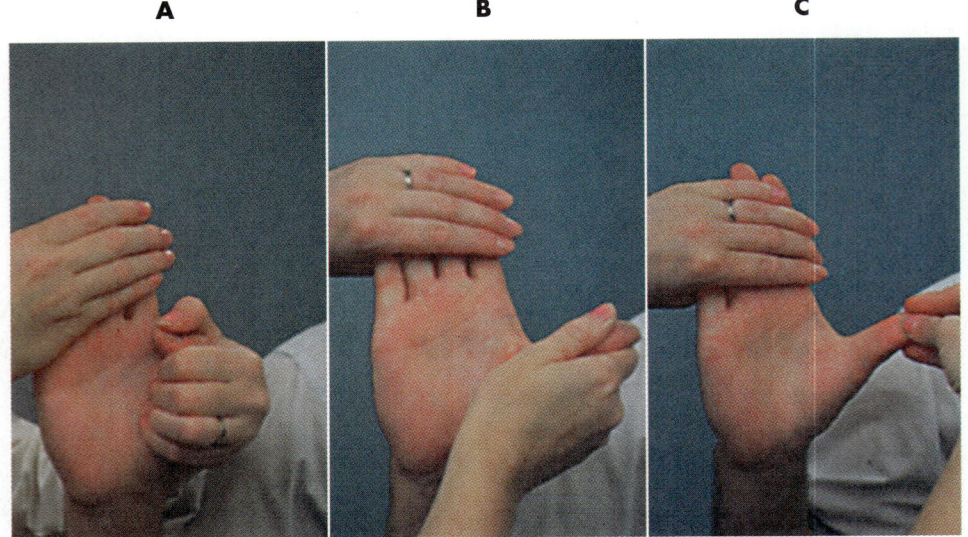

FIGURE 15-14 Toe extension and flexion. **A,** Support patient's foot and pull up on the toes. **B,** Support patient's foot and push toes down.

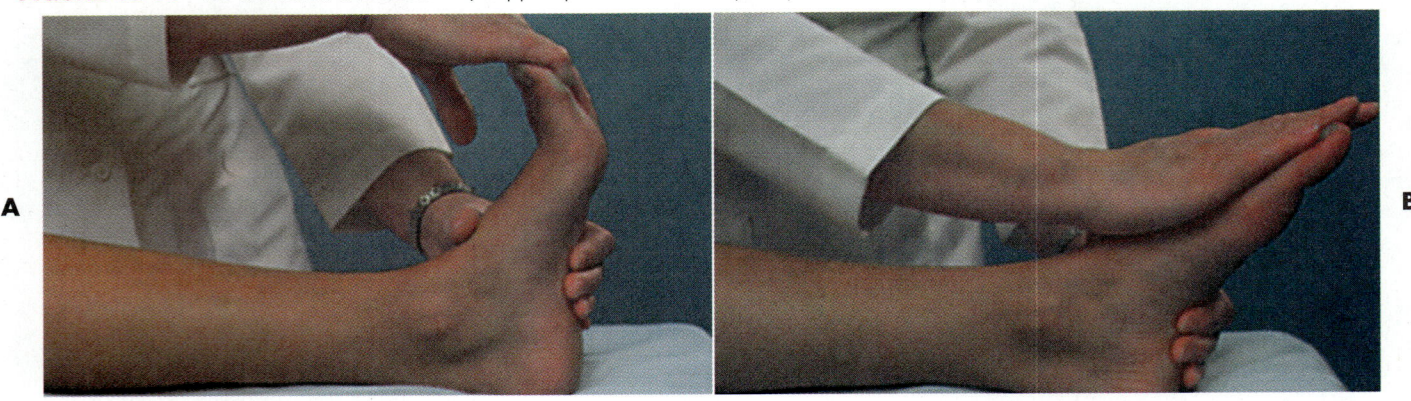

FIGURE 15-15 Eversion and inversion of foot. **A,** Support patient's foot and turn whole foot outward. **B,** Support patient's foot and turn whole foot inward.

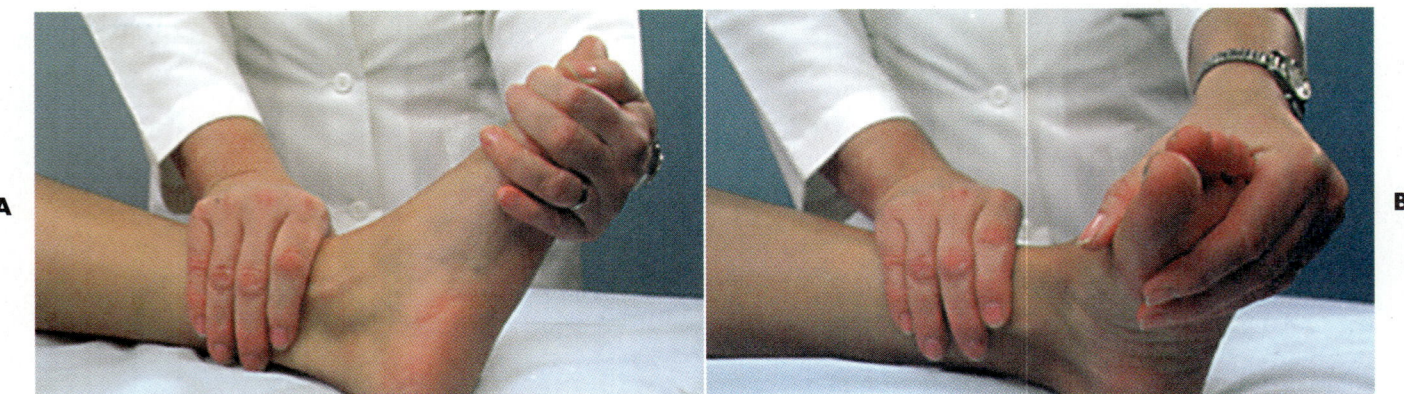

JOINT MOBILITY VOCABULARY

abduction—Movement of a body part away from the midline of the body, as when moving the arm out to the side (see Figure 15-13).

adduction—Movement of a body part toward the midline of the body, as when bringing a raised arm down to the side of the body. The opposite of abduction.

circumduction—Circular movement of a limb.

extension—Movement of a joint that opens it or that increases the angle between the bones (see Figures 15-12 to 15-14).

hyperextension—Extension of a limb or part beyond normal limits.

flexion—Bending of a joint so that the angle between bones is reduced, as in bending the arm at the elbow or the leg at the knee or the toes. Opposite of extension (see Figures 15-12 and 15-14).

dorsiflexion—Movement that bends a body part backward, as of the hand or foot.

eversion—Movement that turns a body part outward; movement of the ankle that turns the foot outward.

inversion—Movement that turns a body part inward; movement of the ankle that turns the foot inward (see Figure 15-15).

pronation—Movement of the arm to have the palm facing downward.

supination—Movement of the arm to have the palm facing upward. Opposite of pronation.

rotation—Process of turning around an axis, such as seen in rotation of the head, allowing the head to turn, extend, and flex. The rotation of a bone on its central axis.

    external rotation—Outward rotation.

    internal rotation—Inward rotation.

BODY MECHANICS

Body mechanics is the way you handle yourself safely and effectively. Essentially, it is how you hold yourself together to maintain good posture during function: when you are moving around, lifting, pulling, pushing, stooping, or carrying or when performing any type of manual labor. It is also how you use your body when sitting, standing, or lying down. Safe body mechanics include the principles of proper body alignment, balance, and movement. When you apply these principles, you minimize the amount of energy you expend, and you also improve your strength and flexibility when sitting, standing, and walking. An important aspect of using correct body mechanics is that you can prevent muscle and back fatigue, pain, strain, and injury.

Many individuals involved in the health care field often have to move or lift patients and equipment. Every time you lift, stand, sit, or even lie down, you are using your back. Therefore knowing how to use safe and effective methods for moving and lifting is crucial for your own protection and also for teaching patients how to use these methods for their own safety and protection. These methods apply to all activities involving body movement and posture in everyday life. **Safe and effective body mechanics** keep the spine balanced in a healthy position when you stand, sit, or lie down. This means using the spine as a total unit whenever possible and not as a series of loosely connected vertebrae. Try to keep your ears, shoulders, and hips in a straight line, the neck erect, the pelvis tipped forward, and the buttocks and stomach tucked in during most activities. These proper movements are extremely important both on the job and at home. **Good posture** is necessary because without it, the overall spinal structure can be weakened, and the back becomes more susceptible to injury.

You must develop, practice, and maintain correct standing, lifting, and bending habits. The following text provides a general guide for proper use of the body.

Standing

Good posture and muscles help to keep your spine balanced when standing. Stand with your feet apart and one foot slightly in front of the other to provide a stable and wide base of support. When you have to stand for a long time with little movement, place one foot on a low stool to help keep your spine in balance and alternate now and again. Strain on the lower back is relieved by lifting the foot to return the spine to its natural curve. Do not twist or lean forward when standing and lifting; move your feet instead, and keep your upper body in line with your hips.

Sitting

For the least strain and injury to your back, keep the three normal curves of your spine (cervical, thoracic, and lumbar) in balanced alignment. The lumbar curve must accommodate the most weight and movement and is commonly the area of most complaints. Sit straight in a chair that supports your lower back or add a support to your lumbar curve by placing a pillow or a towel rolled up to 4 to 6 inches behind that area. When sitting on a stool, lean forward and rest your upper body lightly on your elbows and arms on an elevated surface. *Do not* cross your legs. Crossed legs tilt the pelvis too far forward and aggravate bad backs. *Always attempt to sit with your knees level with or slightly higher than your hips.* Placing something under the feet such as a telephone book or a block of wood reduces back tension. When driving, position your seat so that your knees are level with your hips.

Lifting Techniques

1. Assess the load before beginning to lift. Get help when in doubt about lifting alone.
2. Clear the area where the lift will take place (for example, move chairs out of the way).

3. Explain the procedure to the patient (when the load you will be lifting is a patient) and continue to communicate during the procedure so that the patient can work with and not against you.

4. Keep the weight as close to your body as possible when lifting rather than reaching forward. This reduces the strain on your spine and places the weight in a position where the leg muscles can help lift.

5. Attain and maintain a firm grip on the object or patient throughout the lift.

6. Keep your back straight and body weight over your feet (if possible). Do not bend the lower back at the lumbosacral area. Engage your abdominal muscles to help you maintain a stable back position (Figure 15-16).

7. Use your leg muscles during the lift. Bend your knees and hips sufficiently (not your waist) so that your large leg muscles are used.

8. Establish a firm, stable foot position. Place your feet 10 to 12 inches apart and point them in the direction of the lift. One foot may be placed in front of the other for balance (see Figure 15-16).

9. Move feet with the direction of the lift. You must avoid twisting your back. Think of your spine as a fused unit and make turning movements with your feet and entire body in the direction you are moving. Twisting or pivoting on fixed feet can injure your back.

10. Avoid jerking and jolting. Use even, smooth movements.

11. When two people are required to perform the lift, one person is to act as the leader. The leader should set and call the signals for beginning the lift and subsequent moves.

12. Bend your knees and hips as much as possible when lowering the object or patient at the completion of the lift.

13. Use the appropriate type of lifting technique for the situation.

14. Use the "hip-bend" lift for loads that you must lift at a distance, such as when helping or lifting a patient from the examining table or when getting something from a place that is hard to reach. Once again, get as close to the load as possible. Then put your buttocks out behind you, keeping your head and back in a straight line (this helps to balance and protect your spine). Then bend your knees and hips (not your waist) and lift, using your leg, buttock, and abdominal muscles (Figure 15-17).

Remember that proper techniques are just as important when bending without lifting. Squat, don't bend (Figure 15-18).

Use both sides of your body when lifting, pushing, pulling, or carrying so that the weight does not pull your body into a strained position.

Pushing is easier on your back than pulling. When you push something, remember to bend your elbows, use your legs with one foot in front of the other, and keep the load close to your stomach when possible. Use a stool or ladder, if necessary, when you must reach for an item.

Wear comfortable, low-heeled shoes. Wearing high heels or clogs can throw your dynamic (functional or changing) posture off and make you compensate when trying to maintain balance.

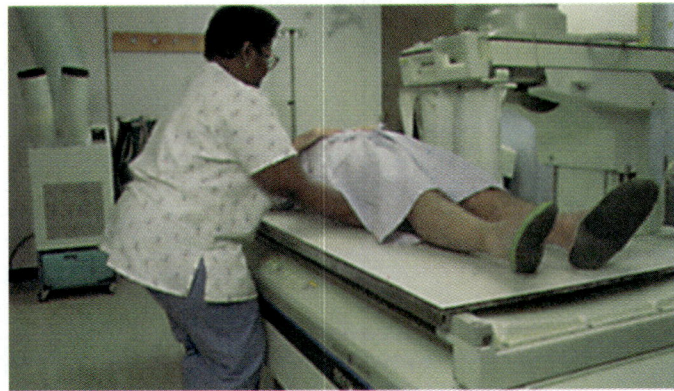

FIGURE 15-17 The hip-bend lift for loads that are hard to reach.

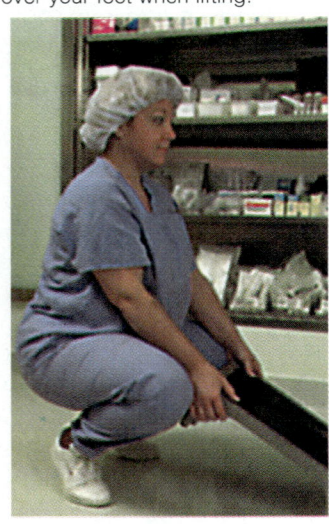

FIGURE 15-16 Proper body mechanics. Keep your back straight and body weight over your feet when lifting.

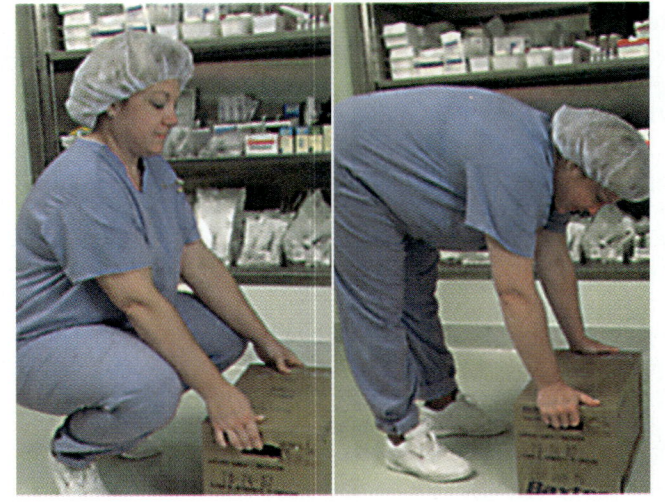

FIGURE 15-18 **A** and **B,** Squat, don't bend.

By using proper body mechanics and maintaining a healthy posture, you can encourage a stabilized and pain-free back. A variety of exercises, such as the partial sit-up and pelvic tilt, can strengthen the lower back and abdominal muscles. Strengthening these muscles greatly facilitates correct posture and proper body mechanics. Physical therapists can provide you with instructions for various abdominal and back-strengthening exercises, but remember that **an exercise program for back pain should not be initiated without a physician's recommendation.**

WHEELCHAIRS

Wheelchairs are mobile chairs of various shapes and sizes that are equipped with large wheels and brakes. Some are moved around manually, and others are motorized. When a patient will be using a wheelchair for a long time or permanently, the physical therapist works with a medical product store to obtain a wheelchair that meets the patient's needs. The therapist provides the store with all of the patient's information, such as size, disability, activities planned for the days ahead (for example, does the patient plan to go hiking in the wheelchair or use it just around the house), description of the patient's house and area where the chair will be used, what type of brakes are needed, and if the chair should have right- or left-handed propulsion.

Many patients who will be using the wheelchair forever are taught how to maintain it. For example, young patients who have spinal cord injuries are taught how to maintain the wheelchair just as they would be taught to maintain a bicycle (for example, how to fix a broken wheel or broken brakes). All patients are taught safety techniques for using a wheelchair, such as how to lock and unlock the brakes, how to kick the footrest out of the way, how to operate the different pieces of the wheelchair, and how to maneuver it in and out of different spaces. The patient practices using the wheelchair in the hospital before going home to ensure safe functioning at home.

Wheelchair Transfers

Transferring a patient from a wheelchair

- Obtain help from another person if you think that you will be unable to accomplish the transfer safely for yourself and the patient.
- Use your abdominal muscles and the strong muscles in your legs, not the weaker muscles in your back, when transferring a patient.
- Always move the patient toward the strong side if one side is stronger than the other.
- Support the patient's strong side when assisting with the move.
- Position the wheelchair parallel to the examining table to where the patient will be moving.
- Explain the procedure to the patient.
- Lock the wheels (Figure 15-19, *A*).
- Move the footrests out of the way (Figure 15-19, *B*).
- Position a step stool near the examining table.

- Stand facing the patient.
- Have the patient move forward in the chair. Stay directly in front of the patient. This is important so that you don't twist because twisting hurts your back.
- Bend down with your hips and knees. Do *not* bend your back. Then put your arms under the patient's arms and your hands firmly over the patient's scapulae. Have the patient's hands rest on your shoulders (Figure 15-20, *A*).
- Give a signal and lift upward so that the patient will rise to a standing position.
- Have the patient step up onto the stool and pivot with the back to the table (Figure 15-20, *B*).
- Ease the patient to a sitting position.
- Place one arm on the patient's shoulder and the other arm under the patient's knees (Figure 15-20, *C*).
- Using a *single* smooth move, raise the patient's legs onto the table and lower the head and trunk into the supine position.
- Attend to the patient's comfort and safety.

Transferring a patient from the examining table to a wheelchair

- Explain the procedure to the patient.
- Position the wheelchair parallel to the examining table.
- Lock the wheels and move the footrests out of the way (see Figure 15-19).

FIGURE 15-19   A, Lock the wheels of the wheelchair before helping a patient getting in or out of it. **B,** Move footrests of wheelchair out of the way before a patient gets in or out of it.

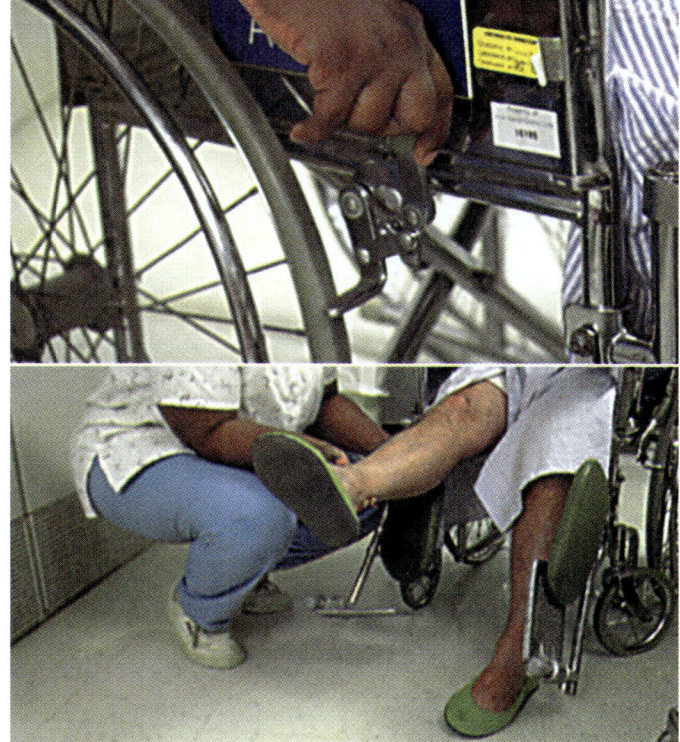

FIGURE 15-20 **A,** Assist patient out of wheelchair. **B,** Assist patient onto examining table. Have patient step up on stool and pivot with back to table. **C,** Assist patient to lie down on examining table. Place one arm on patient's shoulder and other arm under patient's knees.

A   B   C

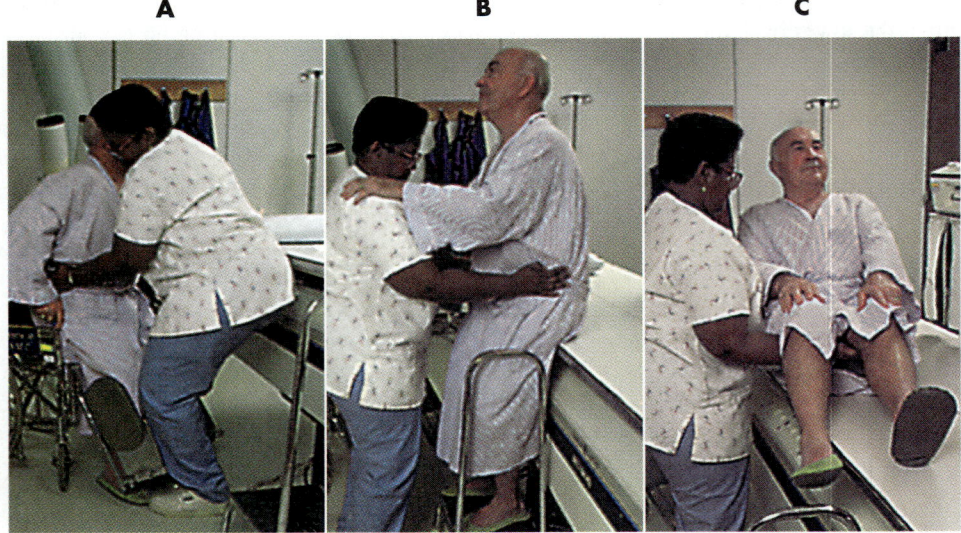

- If possible, assist the patient to turn onto the side, then help him or her at the shoulders and legs to sit up with the legs over the side of the table.
- Place one arm under the patient's shoulders and your other arm under the knees.
- Using a *single* smooth move, assist the patient to rise to a sitting position. At the same time, pivot a quarter of a turn so that the patient is sitting on the edge of the examining table with the feet dangling over the side.
- Stand facing the patient.
- Put your arms under the patient's arms and your hands firmly over the patient's scapulae. Have the patient's hands rest on your shoulders.
- Give a signal, lift upward, and raise the patient to a standing position.
- Pivot a quarter of a turn so that the back of the patient's knees touch the edge of the wheelchair.
- Ease the patient into the wheelchair.
- Position the footrests and the patient's feet on them.
- Attend to the patient's safety and comfort.

CRUTCHES

Crutches are wooden or metal supports used to aid a person in walking. The most common types are the tall crutch, which reaches from the ground up to the axillae (**axillary crutches**), and the Lofstrand or Canadian crutch (**forearm crutch**), which is a shorter crutch. The Lofstrand or Canadian crutch is an aluminum tube with a hand bar on which the patient supports his or her weight and a metal cuff that fits around the forearm. The metal forearm cuff supports the patient when he or she has to let go of the hand bar (for example, when grasping onto a handrail to climb stairs or when standing still). At the base of all crutches is a rubber tip that prevents slipping (Figure 15-21). The type of crutch used depends on the patient's disability. For

FIGURE 15-21 Two types of crutches: Lofstrand or Canadian *(left)* and axillary *(right)*. Note the rubber tip at the base of the crutch. This tip helps prevent slipping.

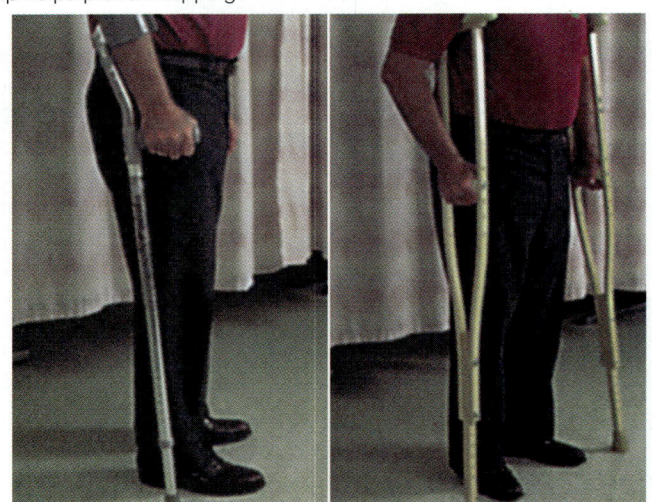

example, if the patient has broken or sprained one ankle, axillary crutches are used. When the patient will be on crutches for a long time, has only limited mobility in the legs, or is wearing leg braces or when he or she is a paraplegic, forearm crutches may be used. Patients with severe arthritis who have poor use of their hands may use platform crutches. When using these crutches, patients use their forearms to lean on the crutches (Figure 15-22).

Measuring for Axillary Crutches

Axillary crutches should be measured for each patient so that they do not cause pressure on the axillae. To determine the correct crutch height, have the patient wear walking shoes and stand erect. Position the crutch tips 2 inches (5 cm) in front of and 6 inches (15 cm) to the side of each foot. Adjust the crutch

FIGURE 15-22 Patient with platform crutches. Patient uses forearms to lean on crutches.

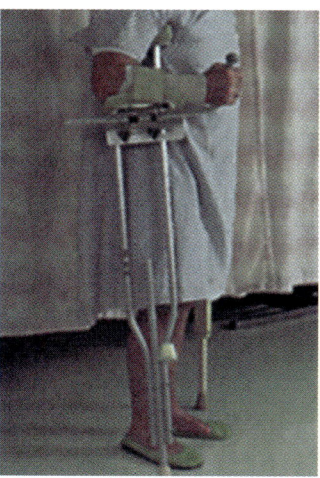

FIGURE 15-24 Verifying elbow flexion of a 30-degree angle using a goniometer.

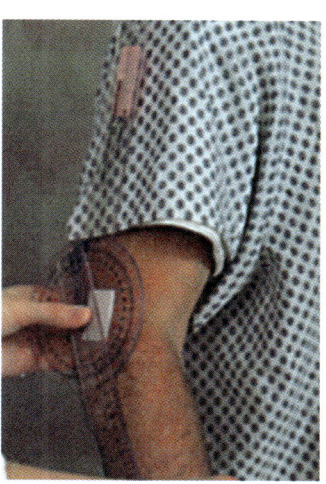

FIGURE 15-23 Measuring crutches. Axillary bars should be 3 fingerwidths below the axilla. Elbows should be flexed at a 30-degree angle when the patient's hands are on the handgrips.

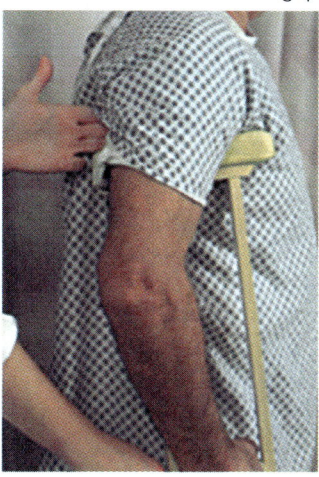

FIGURE 15-25 Basic crutch stance is the tripod position.

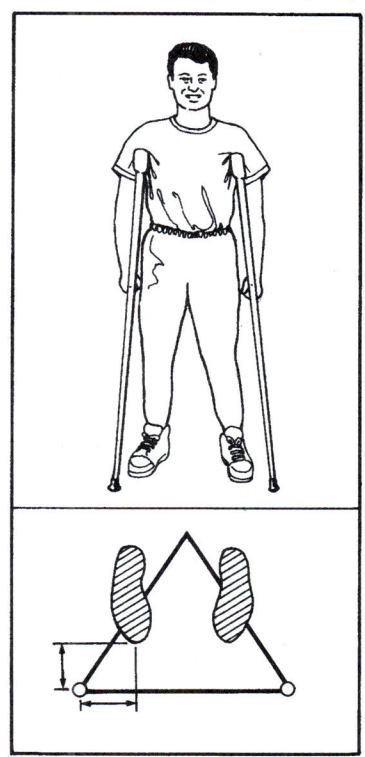

length so that the position of the axillary bars are at least 3 fingerwidths below the axilla. Adjust the handgrips on the crutches so that the patient's elbows are flexed at about a 30-degree angle and the hands on the handgrips are level with the greater trochanter of the femur when the crutches are in place (Figure 15-23). The angle of elbow flexion can be verified by using a measuring device called a goniometer (Figure 15-24).

Patient Teaching for Use of Crutches

Teaching the patient crutch-walking gaits may be the medical assistant's responsibility if a physical therapist is not available. **First,** you must instruct the patient in practicing correct standing posture, which is head and chest up, abdomen in, pelvis tilted inward, feet straight, and a 5-degree angle bend in the knee joint. Tell the patient not to look down at the feet.

The **basic crutch stance** is the tripod position (Figure 15-25). Have the patient stand erect with the feet slightly apart.

Place the tips of the crutches 6 inches in front of and 6 inches to the side of the toes to provide a broad base of support and balance. This position forms a triangle in which a line drawn between the two crutch tips forms the base of the triangle and the patient's feet are the apex. Standing correctly is essential for maintaining balance. Have the patient practice standing with the support of the crutches to become familiar with them and to bear weight on the palms of the hand and not on the axillae. Check the distance between the axilla and the axillary bar on the crutch. It should be at least 3 fingerwidths, or about 2 inches.

You must teach the patient *not* to rest the body's weight on the axillary bars of the crutch for more than a few minutes at a time because pressure on the axillae will cause pressure on the brachial plexus. Excessive pressure on the brachial plexus can cause numbness and tingling and can lead to severe and sometimes permanent paralysis in the arms. Teach the patient to bear weight on the palms of hands (see Figure 15-27). Check the angle of the patient's arms. When the hands are on the handgrips they are level with the greater trochanter of the femur and the crutches are in the walking position, the arms should be flexed at a 30-degree angle. Remind the patient that the arms are to support the body weight, not the axillae. Teach the patient to take small steps at first (that is, to move the crutches only about 12 inches forward with each step). If larger steps are taken, the crutches could slide forward, and the patient could fall. Demonstrate the proper hand and arm positions and gait before the patient tries to use the crutches. By doing this, you help the patient understand how the crutches are to be used. Concentration on a normal rhythmic gait must be accomplished.

Teach the patient to check the crutches for cracks and the rubber tips for wear and loose fit. The tips should be kept dry, and they should be replaced when they wear out. Wet or worn tips lessen surface tension and increase the likelihood of the patient falling.

Special concerns
- For some patients, especially the elderly, additional arm-strengthening exercises may be necessary before they can use crutches adequately.
- Pediatric crutches must be used for children.
- Provide the patient with a list of medical supply stores where repairs or parts for the crutches can be purchased.
- Discuss ways that the patient's home could be modified for easier mobility (for example, the elimination of throw rugs or waxed floors).

Gaits
In crutch-walking gaits, each foot and crutch is called a **point**. For example, in a two-point gait, two points of the total of four (two crutches and two legs) are in contact with the ground when taking one step. The type of gait to be used depends on the patient's condition.

Standing.   Before crutch walking begins the patient should assume the tripod position as discussed previously (see also Figure 15-25). From a sitting position, have the patient place the crutches in the hand on the strong side, move forward in the chair, grasp the arm of the chair with the other hand, and push himself or herself up to a standing position (Figure 15-26).

Two-point gait
1. The first type of two-point gait is when you put both crutches ahead of you and hop forward with one foot (Figure 15-27, *A*). This is a non–weight-bearing gait.
2. The second type of two-point gait is contralateral walking and a reciprocal walk. Put your left crutch and right foot forward; then put your right crutch and left foot forward, and repeat (Figure 15-27, *B*).

FIGURE 15-26   Using crutches to go from a sitting to a standing position.

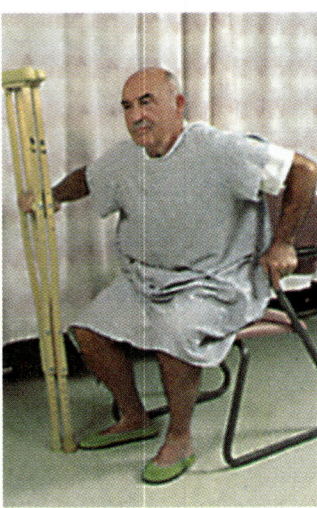

This is partial weight bearing on each foot and used for patients who can bear weight on each leg.

Three-point gait.   The three-point gait may be used when one leg is stronger than the other. Put your crutches forward and then bring the weaker leg through the crutches. Next bring the stronger leg forward, and then repeat, crutches out, then one leg, then the other leg. This is a partial weight-bearing gait (Figure 15-28, *A* and *B*).

Four-point gait.   For the four-point gait, put your right crutch forward, then the left foot, then the left crutch, and then the right foot, and repeat (Figure 15-29, *A* and *B*).

This type of gait is used for patients who can bear weight on the legs and also move each leg separately.

Swing-to gait.   For the swing-to gait, put the crutches forward and then swing the legs up to the same point (Figure 15-30, *A* and *B*).

Swing-through gait.   For the swing-through gait, put the crutches forward and then swing the legs past them (Figure 15-31, *A* and *B*).

The last two gaits are commonly used by paraplegics who are using forearm crutches and by paraplegics who wear weight-supporting braces on their legs. They can also be used for people with generalized weakness in the legs.

Sitting.   To go from a standing position to a sitting position, teach the patient to do the following:
1. Turn around and back into a well-supported chair until the legs touch the center of the chair seat.
2. Remove crutches from under the arms and place the crutches in the hand on the opposite side of the affected leg or on the stronger side of the body.
3. Grasp the chair arm with the other hand and lower the body into the chair.

FIGURE 15-27   **A** and **B,** Two-point gait.

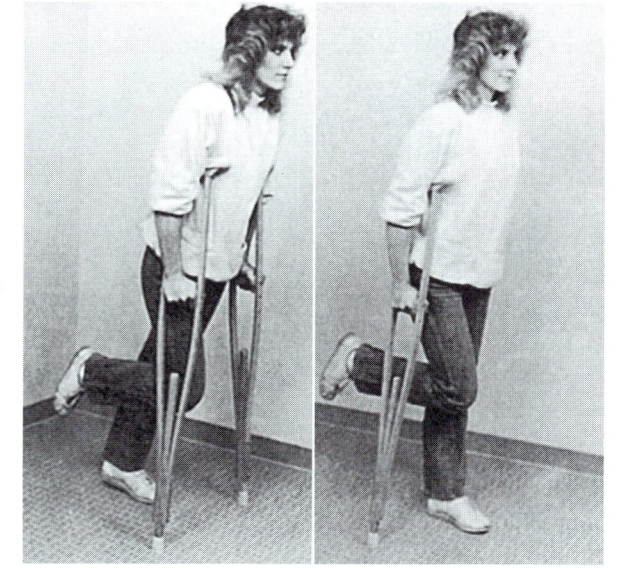

A

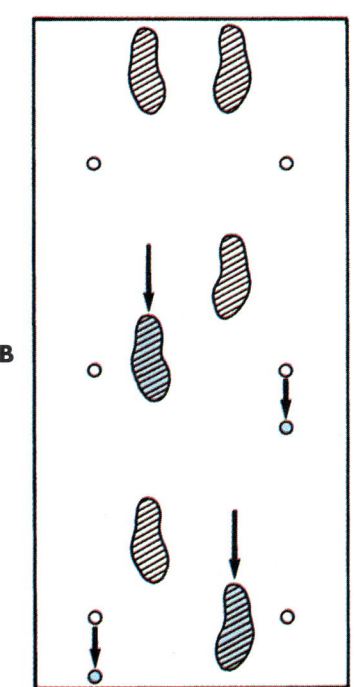

B

FIGURE 15-28   **A** and **B,** Three-point gait.

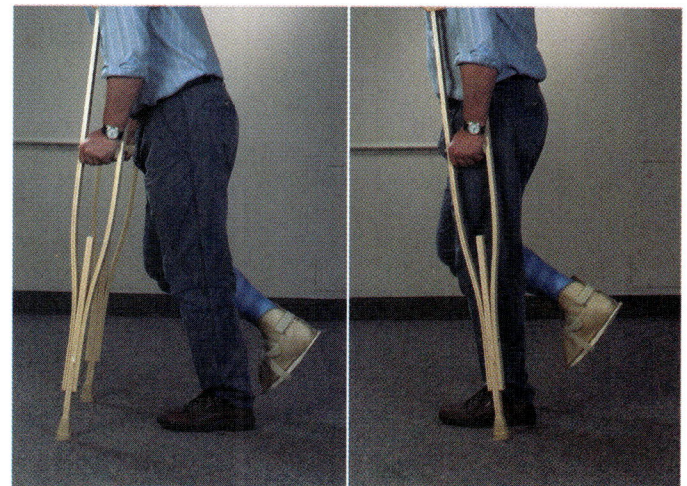

A

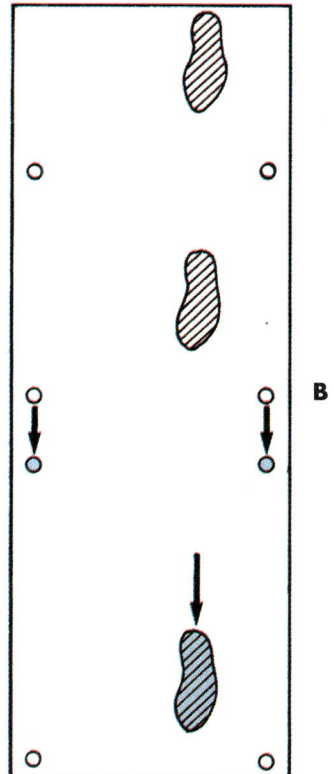

B

FIGURE 15-29 **A, B, C,** and **D,** Four-point gait.

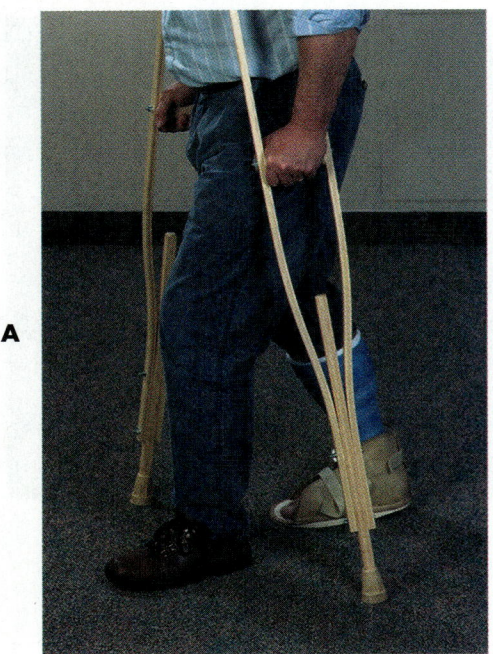

A

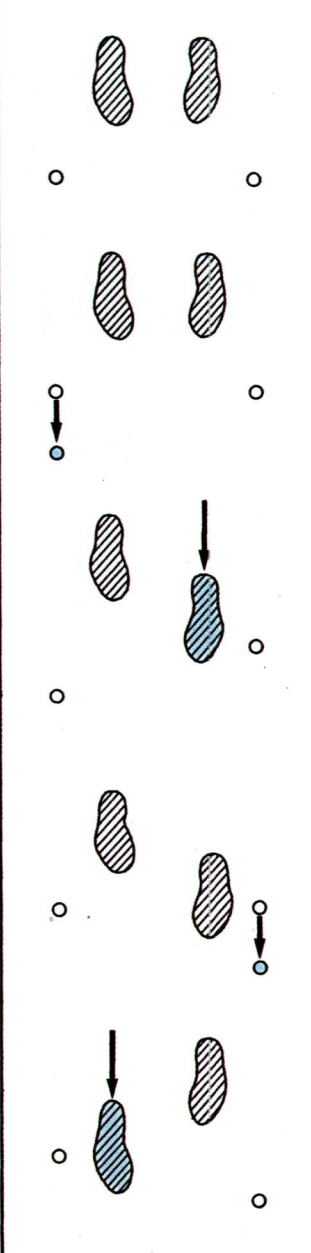

B

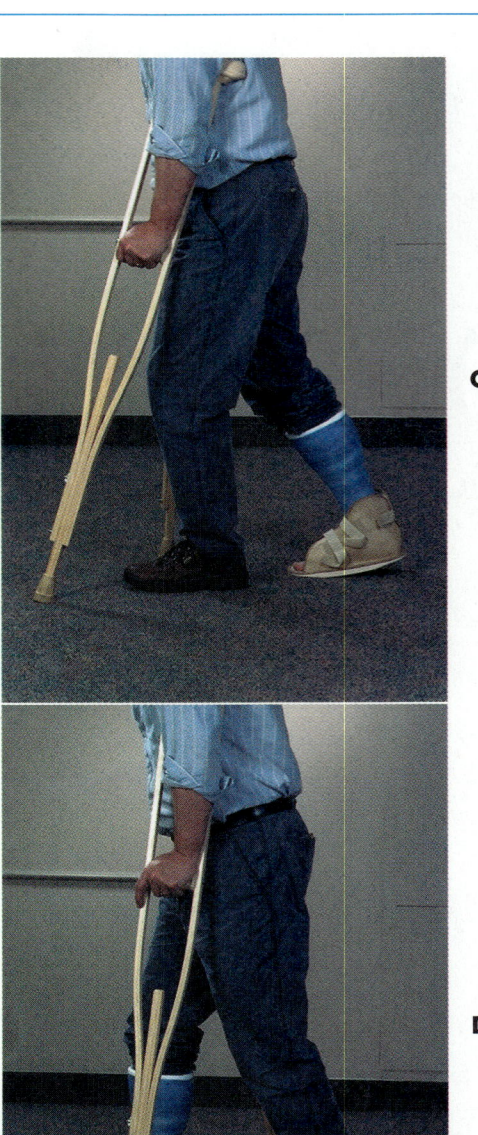

C

D

FIGURE 15-30   **A, B,** and **C,** Swing-to gait.

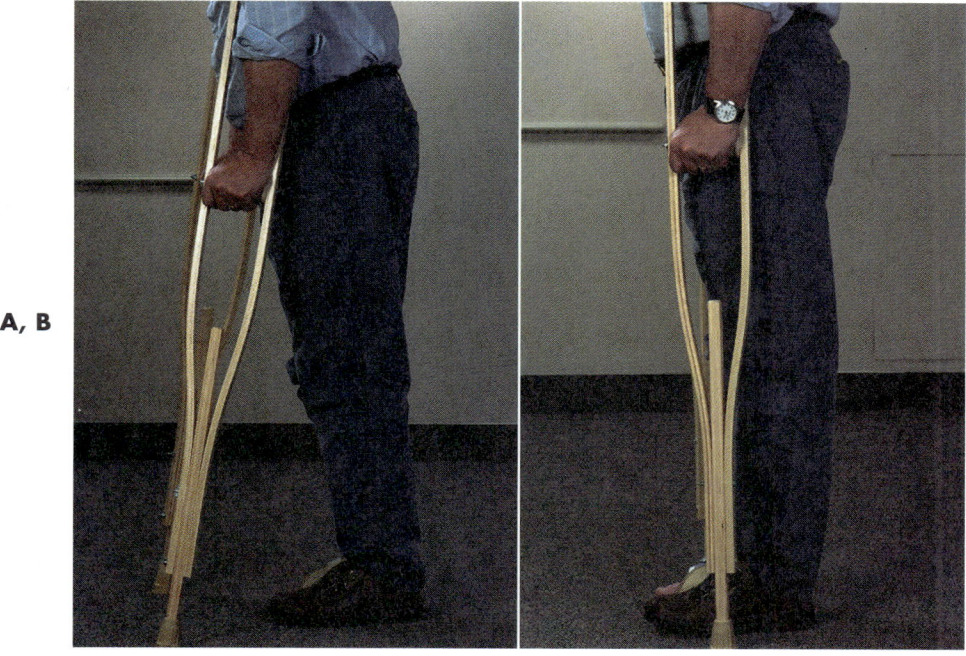
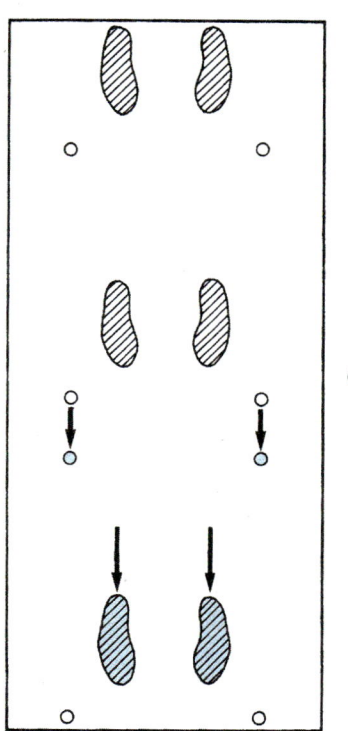

FIGURE 15-31   **A, B,** and **C,** Swing-through gait.

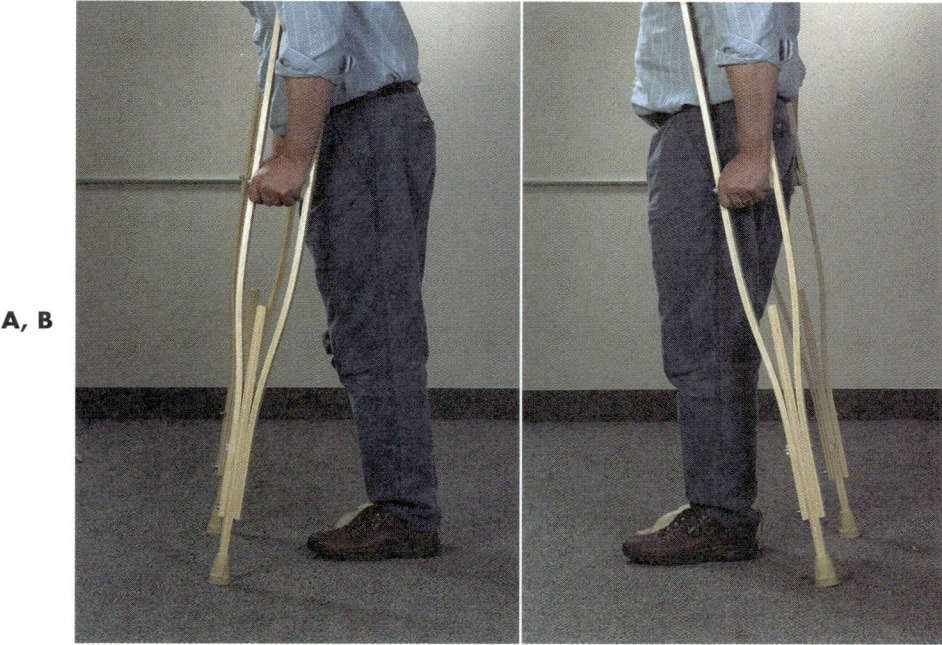
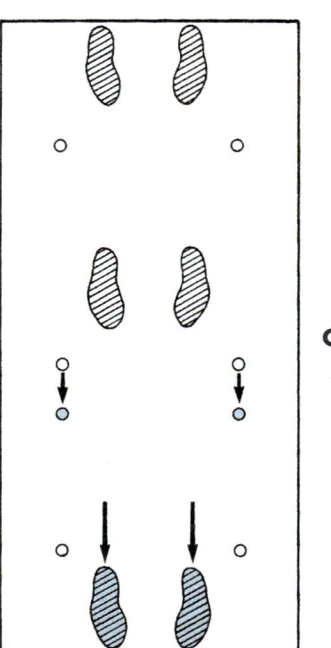

CANES

Canes of various sizes are made of aluminum or wood with a rubber-tipped end that helps to prevent sliding and provides support. Patients who need help with balance or who have one-sided weakness may use a cane to provide additional support. The patient's needs determine whether a single-tipped or a four-point (quad) cane is used (Figure 15-32). To ensure

maximum support, the cane length must be adjusted for each patient.

Instructions for Using a Single Crutch or Cane

1. Always hold a single crutch or cane on the *opposite* side of the injury. People normally walk contralaterally (that

FIGURE 15-32   **A,** Single-tipped and four-point (quad) canes; **B,** patient walking with a cane; **C,** patient walking with a single crutch.

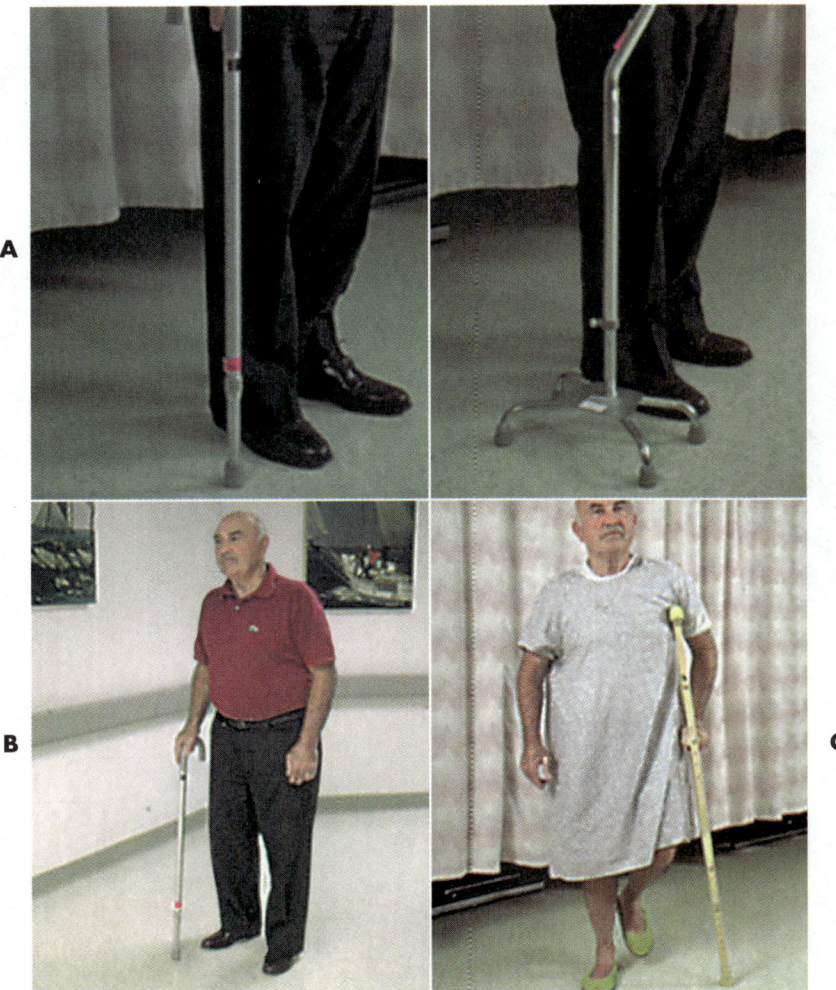

is, when the left arm swings out, the right leg goes out). Think of a crutch or cane as an extension of your arm. As your arm swings out, your opposite leg will go out. With the crutch or cane on the opposite side, it supports and takes the weight off of the injured leg (see Figure 15-32, *B* and *C*).

2. Place the cane 6 inches in front of and slightly to the side of the foot on the ***unaffected* side.**
3. The hand grip should be at the level of the hip joint (at the level of the greater trochanter of the femur).
4. Flex the elbow slightly during weight bearing.
5. Simultaneously move the cane and *affected* leg forward 6 to 10 inches (this varies with the patient's condition) and bear weight on the *unaffected* foot.
6. Transfer weight to the *affected foot and cane* while moving the *unaffected* foot forward. The cane provides support for weight bearing on the affected leg.
7. Repeat the procedure, taking small steps.

WALKERS

Walkers are four-legged assistive devices made of aluminum. The two types of walkers are the stationary walker, which has rubber tips on the legs, and the rolling walker, which has wheels on the two front legs. Walkers are used by patients who need help when standing or walking or who need help in maintaining balance. Patients who use walkers must have arms strong enough to bear partial weight.

Walkers are measured so that the height of the walker is just below the patient's waistline when the arms are flexed at a 30-degree angle while holding onto the handgrips.

To use the rolling walker, a patient just rolls it ahead as she or he walks with the walker. This type of walker can be dangerous for patients with balance or coordination problems. To use the stationary walker, the patient must lift it up and move it ahead a few inches or slide it forward and then step into the open side of the walker. This sequence is then repeated for the desired distance (Figure 15-33).

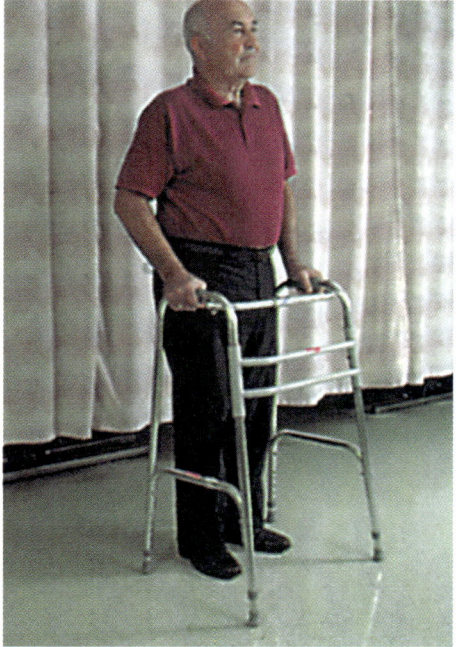

FIGURE 15-33   Patient using a stationary walker. Note the height of the walker and the position of the patient's arms.

ELECTROTHERAPY USING GALVANIC AND FARADIC CURRENTS

Galvanic current is a steady direct current; faradic current is alternating current produced by induction. Both are currents of low voltage that are used for many therapeutic purposes. The **basic use** for galvanic and faradic currents is for muscle stimulation, used to retrain patients when they have had nerve injuries. For example, as the injured nerve regenerates, the body may have forgotten how to contract a muscle; thus often these treatments are given to remind them and help them function once again.

Galvanic stimulation (or faradic if it works) can be used just to maintain the contractility of the muscle while waiting for the nerve to regenerate. Once the nerve is cut or degenerates, or if the nerve itself does not conduct stimuli, galvanic current (direct current) is the only thing that can be used. Direct current works directly on muscle tissue even when there is no intact nerve. Faradic current (alternating current) cannot be used because it will not work on muscle tissue in this case. Galvanic current is also used for *iontophoresis* (i-on′to-fo-re′sis). Iontophoresis or ionotherapy is the introduction of ions into the body through the skin by means of an electric current for therapeutic purposes. It is also used for the localized application of antiinflammatory drugs (for example, hydrocortisone applied to specific swollen or inflamed areas, rather than giving the drug by injection). (*Phonophoresis* is a similar modality using ultrasound instead of direct current.)

Faradic current is used mainly to stimulate weak muscles that have a normal nerve supply. This current causes contrac-tions, which in turn increase blood supply to the muscle and thus help the muscle gain strength. Increased circulation also helps to decrease edema. Faradic current is also used to decrease pain as it helps to block pain sensations.

These treatments can be applied in various ways. To stimulate muscles, the current must be interrupted. This is accomplished by a hand interrupter or an interrupter that is built into the equipment. Basically, to apply these currents, two electrodes padded with cotton that has been soaked in salt water are placed over the area to be treated. The soaked pads prevent the occurrence of severe wounds. When small muscles are treated, a very small applicator can be used. This has a push button on it so that specific jolts of current can be given. This apparatus can also be used when using what is called a surged current or a ramped current. These are currents that start out with nothing, then begin and increase up to a designated point, and then decrease. With these a smooth contraction and then a smooth relaxation is obtained. In addition to muscle stimulation, these currents can also be used on muscle spasms and on areas such as those around hematomas and bruises. Electrostimulation therapy is also used with biofeedback for muscle reeducation. The biofeedback machine allows the patient to hear the muscle contract and relax. This is especially helpful after surgery and for controlling chronic pain.

ELECTRODIAGNOSTIC EXAMINATIONS

Electrodiagnostic examinations used by physical therapy are performed by means of **electrical stimulation applied to muscles and nerves.** Various types of examinations are available, all having clinical value in the diagnosis and prognosis of some neuromuscular disorders. Two additional major electrodiagnostic examinations used for different clinical purposes are the electroencephalogram (EEG), which records the electrical impulses of the brain, and the electrocardiogram (ECG, or EKG), which records the electrical action of the heart. The ECG is discussed in Chapter 16.

Electromyographic examinations specifically measure the electrical activity in a muscle as a result of nerve conduction. A needle electrode is introduced into a muscle belly to study muscle action potentials. It also measures just the general electrical excitability of the muscle cells. The recording obtained (the electromyogram) can be most specific diagnostically because it not only tells you that something is wrong but will point out exactly what is wrong. It helps distinguish any weakness from neuropathy from that of other causes.

Other examinations available test the reaction time of a muscle to a shot of electricity; the threshold is tested (that is, how much electricity it takes to get a reaction from the muscle). The results obtained are compared with normal levels. Any deviation or fluctuation from the established norm helps diagnose certain problems such as damaged nerve and muscle tissues.

Nerve conduction studies are performed to test the speed with which the nerve is conducting; again, this helps the physician diagnose.

Special electrodiagnostic equipment is used for each of these tests, which are generally performed by a physical therapist or a physician. Medical assistants do not operate this equipment but may be expected to keep it clean and ready for use. You may also be expected to explain the nature and purpose of the examination to the patient.

DISABILITIES AND THERAPY

To provide a broader insight into the various types of patient conditions that benefit from physical therapy, Table 15-2 lists common disabilities with the common physical therapy modalities used for each.

TABLE 15–2 **Patient Conditions That Benefit From Physical Therapy and Occupational Therapy***

Disability	Therapy	Disability	Therapy
Amputations	Patient education for care of the residual limb Bed positioning Exercise Crutch training Prosthetic care and training	Cerebrovascular accident (CVA)—cont'd	**Occupational therapy:** Splinting, self-care instructions, such as dressing, training in one-handed activities
Arthritis and other rheumatic diseases	Heat Hot paraffin wax bath Exercise Pool Transfer techniques **Occupational therapy:** Splinting (Figure 15-34), functional exercise, self-care instructions, such as dressing	Congenital defects	Exercise Functional training
		Debility	Exercise Gait training
		Diabetes	Exercise
		Fractures of upper and lower extremity	Biofeedback and electrical stimulation therapy Exercise Gait training Modalities to control pain and edema (e.g., heat and/or cold applications)
Burns	Hubbard tank Heat Exercise Whirlpool Massage Splinting	General surgery	Graduated exercise program
		Heart surgery and pulmonary congestion	Bronchial hygiene that includes postural drainage and chest tapotement Breathing exercises Endurance exercises
		Infectious diseases	Graduated exercise program
Cardiovascular disease (cardiac and pulmonary rehabilitation)	Bronchial hygiene (e.g., postural drainage, chest tapotement) Graduated exercise program **Occupational therapy:** Packing activities: work simplification energy conservation	Low back pain	Pelvic traction (in bed and in clinic) Intermittent pelvic traction Ultrasound Heat Massage Pool Exercise Body mechanics instruction Mobilization of soft tissues and joints— manual therapy **Physical and occupational therapy:** Ergonomics—assessment and modification Industrial program for employee evaluation, work capacity, and modification training
Cerebral palsy	Exercise; neurologic facilitation exercises Functional training **Occupational therapy:** Self-care instruction, such as feeding and dressing		
Cerebrovascular accident (CVA)	Bed positioning Balance activities Bed mobility Exercise Balance exercises Neurologic facilitation exercises Transfer techniques Gait training	Lymphedema (after CVA, mastectomy, or sprain)	Jobst Intermittent Pressure Pump Exercise

Occupational therapy uses activities to maximize a person's independence, prevent disabilities, and maintain health.

TABLE 15–2   Patient Conditions That Benefit From Physical Therapy and Occupational Therapy—cont'd

Disability	Therapy	Disability	Therapy
Muscle spasm	Heat	Psychiatric	Pool
	Cold	problems—cont'd	Relaxation techniques
	Massage		**Occupational therapy:**
	Exercise		Therapeutic crafts and remedial games
Muscle disease	Pool	Pulmonary problems	Bronchial hygiene
	Exercise	(emphysema,	Breathing exercises
	Adaptive equipment	bronchitis, asthma)	Endurance exercises
Multiple sclerosis	Ice baths for relief of spasticity		Outpatient pulmonary rehabilitation clinic
	Exercise		Graduated rehabilitation with low flow
	Gait training		oxygen
	Transfer activities		**Occupational therapy:**
	Occupational therapy:		Pacing activities:
	Dressing training		work simplification
Neck pain	Intermittent cervical traction or collars		energy conservation
	Heat	Renal failure and	Graduated exercises
	Massage	transplants	Maintenance exercises
	Exercise	Scoliosis and other	Bracing
	Ice	postural defects	Exercise
	Ultrasound		Body mechanics instruction
	Joint mobilization or soft tissue		Posture instruction
	mobilization	Spinal cord injuries	Bracing
	Posture instruction		Exercise
	Also see Low back pain		Gait training
Osteoporosis	Bracing as indicated		Transfer activities
	Exercise		Wheelchair mobility
	Graduated weight bearing		**Occupational therapy:**
	Modalities for pain control		Self-care instruction, such as dressing
Parkinson's	Exercise		and splinting (Figure 15-34)
disease	Balance exercise	Sprains	Heat
	Gait training		Cold and compression
Peripheral nerve	Electrical stimulation		Exercise
injuries	Exercise		Gait training
	Splinting		Friction massage
	Occupational therapy		
Peripheral vascular	Buerger's exercises		
diseases	Gait training		
	General exercises		
Poliomyelitis	Bronchial hygiene		
	Exercise		
	Gait training with braces		
	Heat		
	Pool		
Pressure sores	Ultraviolet light (bacteriocidal)		
and wound	Bed positioning		
infections			
Prenatal and	Exercise		
postnatal	Breathing instruction		
situations			
Psoriasis	Ultraviolet light (bacteriocidal)		
Psychiatric	Exercise		
problems	Heat		

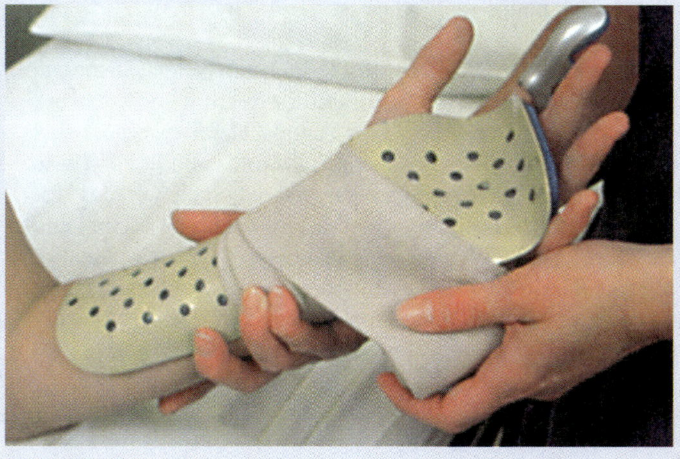

FIGURE 15-34   Examples of splints as applied to patient's finger, wrist, and forearm.

ERGONOMICS

Ergonomics (ur'gonom'iks) comes from the Greek words *ergon* meaning "work" and *nomos* meaning "law." It is a science devoted to the analysis and study of human work, especially as it is affected by individual psychology, anatomy, and other human factors. Dating back to the 1940s, ergonomics has gained momentum in the past decade or more as a result of the various work-related problems seen in the advanced industrialized and technological societies. Now ergonomics is viewed more precisely as the science of fitting workplace conditions and job demands to the capabilities of the working populations. The **goal of ergonomics** is to achieve effective and successful "fits" or interactions between the work and worker that will optimize and ensure high productivity, avoidance of illness and injury risks, and increased satisfaction among the workers. Many organizations have published manuals describing programs and techniques to control ergonomic hazards. The principles included in these programs aid employers in reducing the risk of work-related musculoskeletal disorders.

Work-Related Musculoskeletal Disorders (WMSDs)*

Although definitions vary, the general term *musculoskeletal disorders* describes the following:

- Disorders of the muscles, nerves, tendons, ligaments, joints, cartilage, or spinal disks
- Disorders that are not typically the result of any instantaneous or acute event (such as a slip, trip, or fall) but reflect a more gradual or chronic development (nevertheless, acute events such as slips and trips are very common causes of musculoskeletal problems, such as low back pain)
- Disorders diagnosed by a medical history, physical examination, or other medical tests that can range in severity from mild and intermittent to debilitating and chronic
- Disorders with several distinct features (such as carpal tunnel syndrome [see Health Matters box]) as well as disorders defined primarily by the location of the pain (that is, low back pain)

The term *WMSDs* refers to (1) musculoskeletal disorders to which the work environment and the performance of work contribute significantly or (2) musculoskeletal disorders that are made worse or longer lasting by work conditions. These workplace risk factors, along with personal characteristics (for example, physical limitations or existing health problems) and societal factors, are thought to contribute to the development of WMSDs. They also reduce worker productivity or cause worker dissatisfaction. Common examples are jobs requiring repetitive, forceful, or prolonged exertions of the hands; fre-

quent or heavy lifting, pushing, pulling, or carrying of heavy objects; and prolonged awkward postures. Vibration and cold may add risk to these work conditions. Jobs or work conditions presenting multiple risk factors have a higher probability of causing a musculoskeletal problem. The level of risk depends on the intensity, frequency, and duration of the exposure to these conditions and the individual's capacity to meet the force or other job demands that might be involved. These conditions are more correctly called "ergonomic risk factors for musculoskeletal disorders" rather than "ergonomic hazards" or "ergonomic problems." However, like the term *safety hazard,* these terms have popular acceptance.

Why are WMSDs a problem?   Many reasons exist for considering WMSDs a problem, including the following:

- WMSDs are among the most prevalent lost-time injuries and illnesses in almost every industry.
- WMSDs, specifically those involving the back, are among the most costly occupational problems.
- Job activities that may cause WMSDs span diverse workplaces and job operations.
- WMSDs may cause a great deal of pain and suffering among afflicted workers.
- WMSDs may decrease productivity and the quality of products and services. Workers experiencing aches and pains on the job may not be able to do quality work.
- Because musculoskeletal disorders have been associated with nonwork activities (for example, sports) and medical conditions (for example, renal disease, rheumatoid arthritis), it is difficult to determine the proportion related solely to occupation. For example, in the general population, nonoccupational causes of low back pain are probably more common than workplace causes. However, even in these cases, the musculoskeletal disorders may be aggravated by workplace factors.

Ergonomics for the Office

Today numerous jobs and many hobbies entail using a computer. Along with the advanced power of this technology has come numerous minor to major health problems. Millions of people who use a computer end the workday with stiff shoulders, pain in the neck, and even back pain. As many as three of four endure headaches and problems with their eyes, including temporary eye strain or blurred vision. Many suffer from problems that can become more serious, such as cumulative trauma disorders (injuries to the hands, arms, and shoulders) and repetitive strain injuries or disorders, such as carpal tunnel syndrome (see Health Matters box). **Carpal tunnel syndrome** is commonly diagnosed by the patient's complaints of pain, weakness, burning sensations, numbness, tingling, or a "pins and needles" feeling in the wrist and hand and by two tests done to elicit these same feelings when the patient is examined. In **Phalen's test** the patient is asked to flex the wrists and put the hands back-to-back for 1 minute (Figure 15-35). A positive finding called Phalen's sign is when the patient feels the numbness, tingling, burning, and other sensations over the pal-

---

*U.S. Department of Health and Human Services, Public Health Service, CDC, National Institute for Occupational Safety and Health, Cincinnati, OH. (1-800-356-4674; http://www.cdc.gov/niosh/homepage.html)

mar surface of the hand and the first three fingers and part of the fourth. The symptoms go away quickly after the hand returns to a resting position. The second test, **Tinel's test,** consists of tapping the palmar side of the wrist over the median nerve (Figure 15-36). A positive finding, the sensation of tingling or a prickly feeling, is called Tinel's sign.

HEALTH MATTERS

CARPAL TUNNEL SYNDROME

Elaine W. was a 14-year-old violin student when she first noticed troubling symptoms. After long practice sessions, she felt a strange tingling sensation in the fingers of her left hand. Soon, she was experiencing pain so severe that it woke her up at night. Then, she states, "I woke up one November morning, and I couldn't move my left hand at all." Frightened, she consulted her doctor, who diagnosed her with carpal tunnel syndrome. When rest and splinting did not alleviate her symptoms, Elaine had surgery to correct the problem. Although the surgery eliminated the pain and tingling, she still—some years later—has trouble holding things. "Wet dishes are the worst," she says. And at work, she uses a pencil to tap out words on her word processor.

Elaine is just one of 5 million Americans who suffer from carpal tunnel syndrome, a painful and debilitating irritation of the nerves and tendons in the wrist. The area for which the syndrome is named—the carpal tunnel—is the passageway formed by tendons and bones through which the nerves that supply the hand travel. When a person performs repetitive hand motion for long periods without rest, such as long typing sessions, assembly-line tasks, or in Elaine's case, practicing the violin, the nerves can become irritated, resulting in pain and numbness. Carpal tunnel syndrome is now the most commonly reported on-the-job injury. If untreated, it can cause permanent disability.

The first symptoms of carpal tunnel syndrome include hand and wrist pain and numbness. People with the syndrome describe the pain as an "electric" sensation that may radiate to the arm, shoulder, and back. Over 90% of carpal tunnel syndrome sufferers report that the pain is worse at night and so severe that it wakes them up from a sound sleep. In time, the sufferer may lose grip strength in the hand, making even everyday tasks awkward or impossible.

Although carpal tunnel syndrome is not a new condition (it was first described in 1854), it has only recently become a serious occupational hazard. One U. S. legislator describes carpal tunnel syndrome as "the industrial disease of the Information Age." If employers do not do something about it, some experts foresee that half of every dollar earned by companies may go toward treating carpal tunnel syndrome and its related disorders.

Many of today's occupations involve constant repetitive motions of the hand and wrist and at faster and faster speeds. Technical innovations—from grocery store scanners to computer keyboards—also contribute to the increase in carpal tunnel syndrome. For instance, typing on a typewriter requires the typist to take frequent breaks to insert paper and manually return the typewriter carriage at the end of each line. With today's computers, all these tasks are built in, with the result that computer typists spend long hours with their hands extended over a keyboard. Without frequent breaks, these typists are at risk for carpal tunnel syndrome.

What can be done to treat carpal tunnel syndrome? Individuals with the syndrome are treated with physical therapy and elaborate wrist splints that immobilize the affected area.

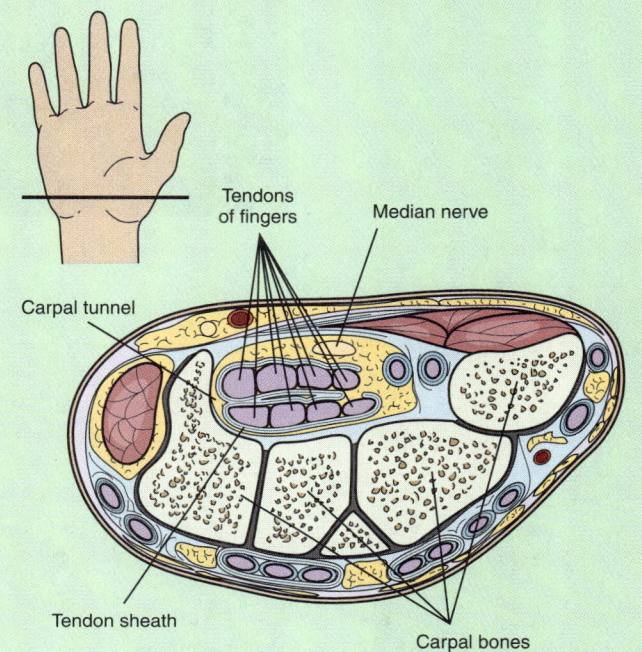

Sometimes surgery is necessary to correct the nerve damage. These treatments are often not effective in alleviating all the symptoms, and sufferers must learn to live with their disability.

Because of the surge in carpal tunnel syndrome cases, the Occupational Safety and Health Administration (OSHA) has drawn up guidelines for certain occupations, such as meatpacking, directed toward preventing the onset of the syndrome. Specially designed desks, chairs, and other office equipment for typists and data entry clerks take some of the stress off wrists and hands, and in some companies, typists are required to take rest breaks.

These guidelines make sense for those who find themselves stuck at a keyboard for long hours and who perform the same task over and over. Workers are advised to identify early signs and symptoms and to take steps to prevent wrist strain. They should also take frequent breaks and, for marathon typists, be sure their chair is comfortable and that they can reach the keyboard without straining.

From CTS: Relief at hand, *The University of California Berkeley Wellness Letter* 11(4):7, 1995; Gabor A: On-the-job straining: repetitive motion is the Information Age's hottest hazard, *US News and World Report* 108(20):51-53, 1990; Katz RT: Carpal tunnel syndrome: a practical review, *American Family Physician* 49(6):1371-1382, 1994; Treating for carpal tunnel syndrome, *Lancet* 338(8765):479-481, 1991.
Courtesy of the American Red Cross.

FIGURE 15-35   Phalen's test for carpal tunnel syndrome.

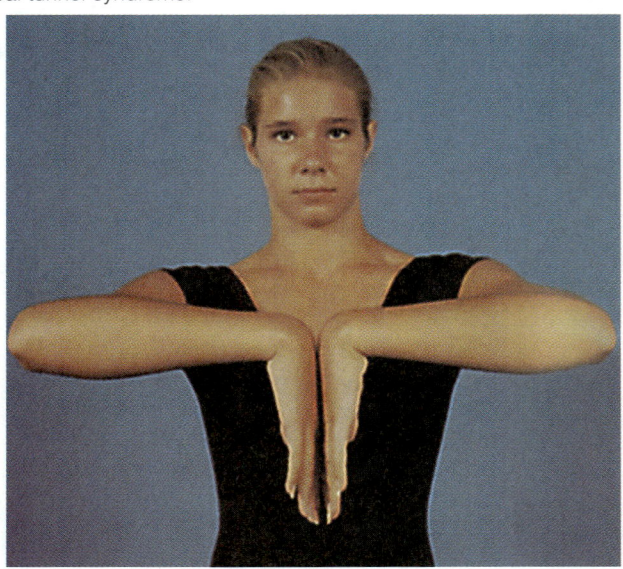

FIGURE 15-36   Elicitation of Tinel's sign used for diagnosing carpal tunnel syndrome.

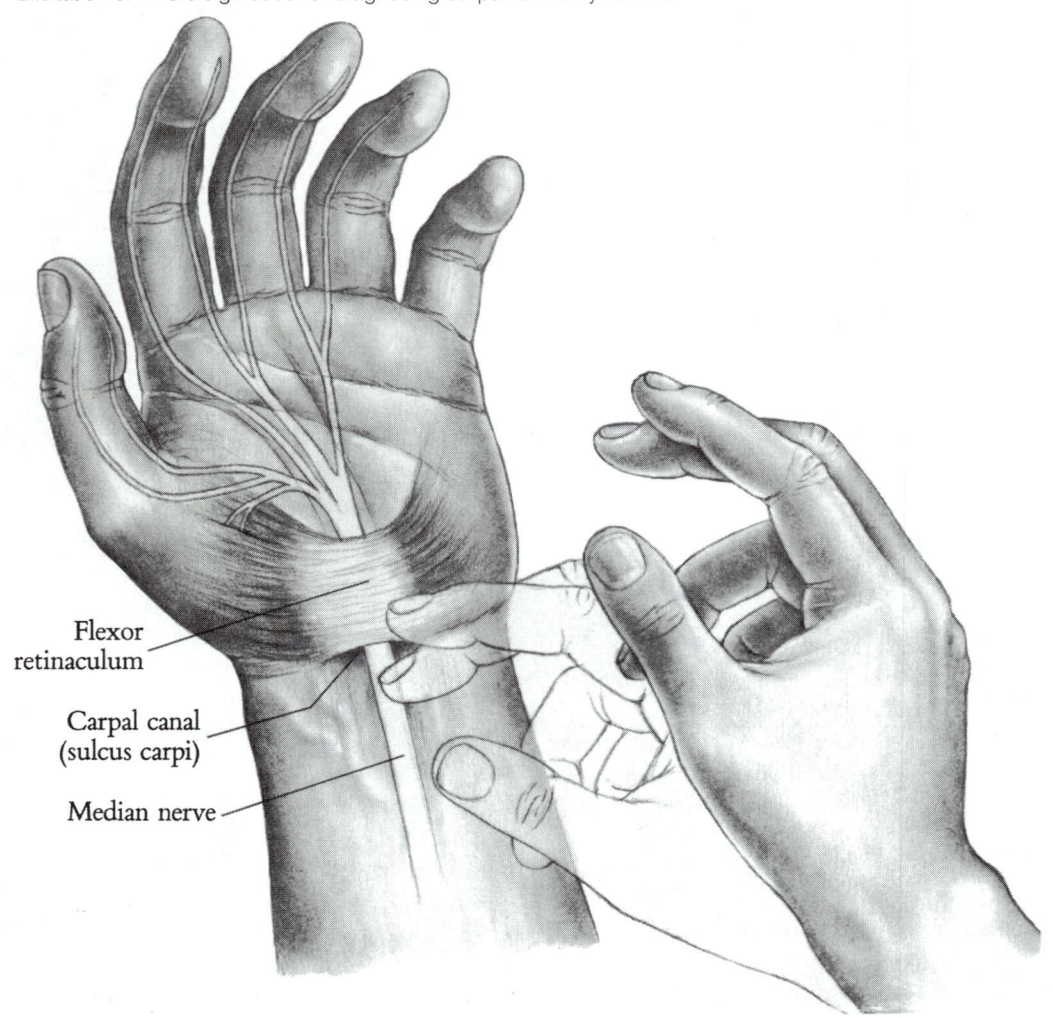

Flexor
retinaculum

Carpal canal
(sulcus carpi)

Median nerve

Unfortunately, various other joint problems and different types of nerve damage can affect all parts of the arms, elbows, wrists, hands, shoulders, and back. These injuries can be caused by simple things, such as improper use of a keyboard, improper position of computer equipment, improper body posture, improper handling of a telephone hand receiver, and failing to take stretch breaks and to look away from the computer screen periodically. The resulting medical problems can be very serious and can cause severe pain and even permanent disability. The answer to all of these problems is **prevention and education.** As the Surgeon General has recommended, *"Put Prevention Into Practice."* The following text discusses common (bad) habits that people use when working at a computer terminal and some solutions. Also see Figures 15-37 through 15-39; see Figure 15-40 for **computer and desk stretches**. By using these techniques and exercises yourself and sharing this advice with your patients, many painful and serious disabilities can be prevented.

Break these 10 bad computer habits*   Each year more and more people are developing computer-related work injuries. Computer-related injuries are one of the fastest growing

*Courtesy J. Martin Walsh, OTR, CHT, Davies Medical Center, San Francisco, Calif.

FIGURE 15-37   **A, Wrong**—Hands at an angle to the forearms. **B, Correct**—Hands aligned with the forearms.

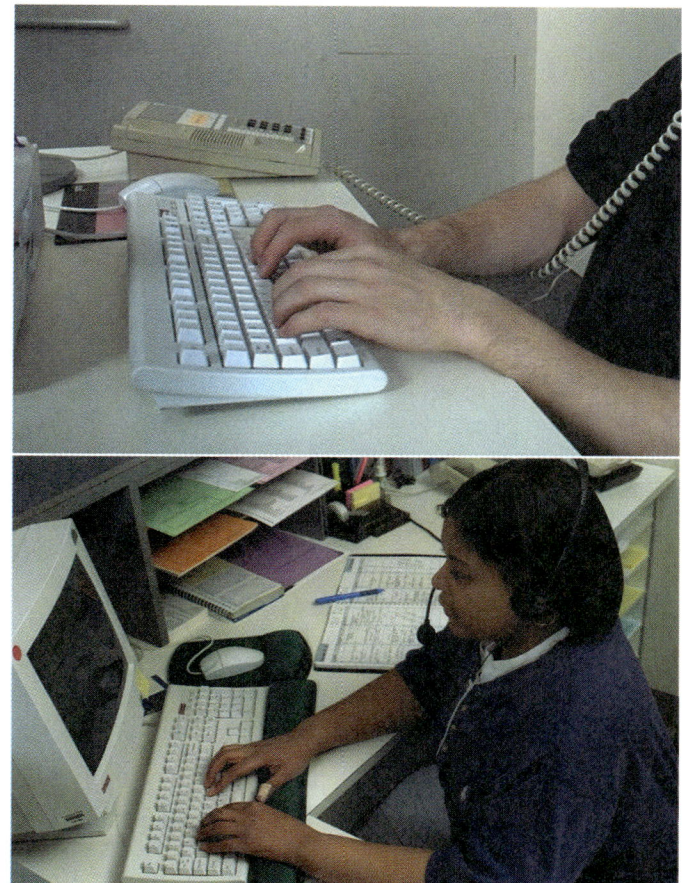

problems that businesses face today. It is not unusual for a worker to spend 6 or more hours a day on the keyboard, and if that worker were to type 60 words per minute, he or she would be making approximately 18,000 keystrokes per hour. If it takes about 1½ ounces of force to type one letter, in 6 hours of typing, that person would have delivered about 5 tons of force to the keyboard through the muscle of the forearms and hands. It is no wonder why computer injuries are becoming so widespread.

Computer-related injuries, or repetitive strain injuries or cumulative trauma disorders (as they are also known), are the result of prolonged static positions, repetitive movements, awkward hand positions, poor posture, faulty workstation designs, and fast-paced uninterrupted computer use. These injuries develop slowly and, as the name implies, are repetitive or cumulative in nature. The best treatment for computer-related injuries is prevention. By arranging your workstation properly, pacing and balancing your workday, stretching and exercising,

FIGURE 15-38   **A, Wrong**—Wrist resting on desktop. **B, Correct**—Wrists level with the keyboard

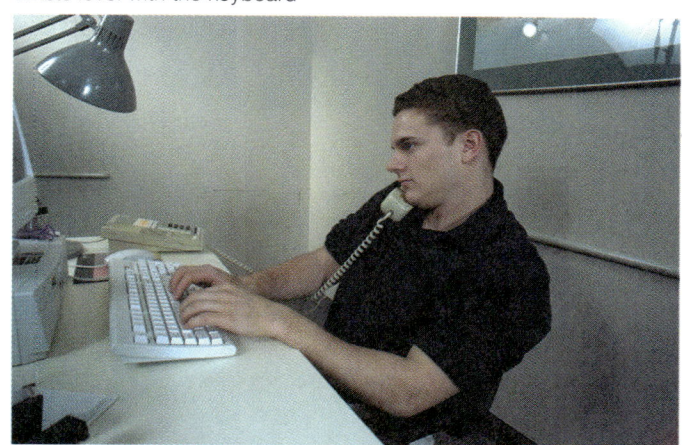

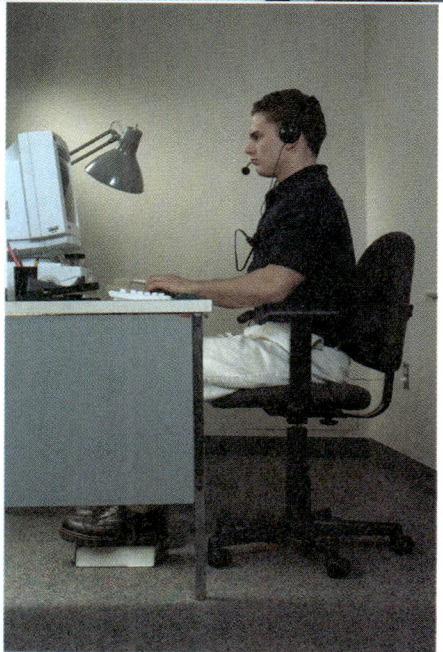

FIGURE 15-39 Ergonomics for the office. Showing correct position for back, arms, eye level to screen, and feet.

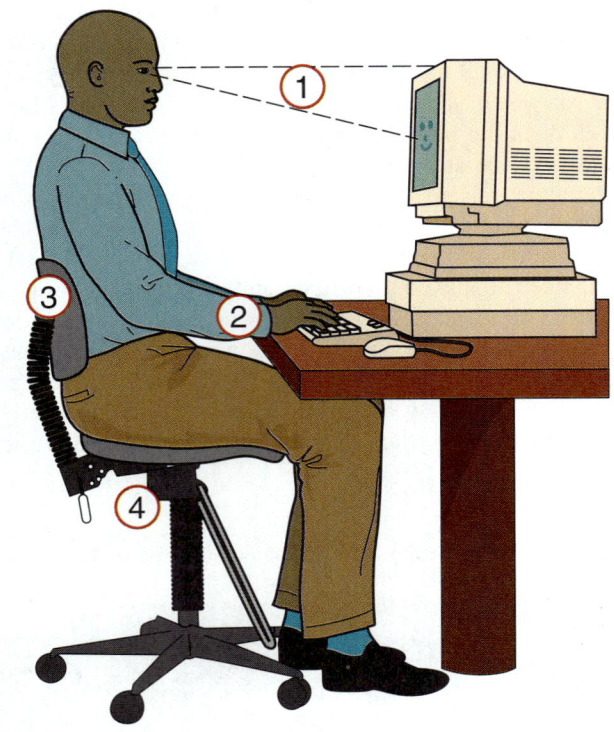

1. The top of your computer screen should be approximately at eye level, with the midpoint of the screen 4 to 9 inches below eye level.

2. Wrists should be held straight while you type, not flexed up or down.

3. The chair's backrest should provide comfortable but sturdy support, pressing firmly against your lower back.

4. Adjust chair height so that, with your feet resting squarely on the ground, your thighs are roughly parallel to the floor.

and learning some of the potential hazards of computer work, you can help prevent potential problems from developing.

The following text lists 10 common bad habits that can cause computer-related injuries and some simple solutions.

Bad habit no. 1: **Leaning your wrists on the desk.** Almost all computer users rest their hands or wrists on the edge of the desk. Resting your wrists on the desk causes the hands to be bent upward at the wrist to type and can cause overuse of the muscles on the top of the forearms. This position also can cause excessive pressure on nerves that run through the wrist. In addition, by locking the wrists down on the desk, the small tendons of the fingers are required to do the work that the larger shoulders muscles should do. Also, people tend to reach for keys by deviating the wrist instead of moving the whole hand over the keyboard. Using "wrist rests" can cause the same problems and are not recommended. Try keeping your wrists in a neutral or "straight" position and let your hands float over the keyboard so that your entire arm is working for you. This may require lowering your keyboard.

Bad habit no. 2: **Slouching and slumping.** Slouching causes you to compress your spine, which can cause lower back pain, throw your head forward, which can cause neck and arm pain, and round your shoulders, which causes shoulder pain. Instead of slouching, sit with your buttocks against the back of the chair. Support the normal curve of your lower back by using a lumbar support or adjusting the lumbar support on the chair if you have an adjustable chair. Work at an appropriate work height, which may involve raising or lowering your chair. Remember that computer keyboards are usually too high on standard desks and need to be lowered.

Bad habit no. 3: **Keeping your neck in a bent position.** Keeping your neck in a bent position to look down at the document you are typing or to view the monitor can cause neck pain and, eventually, problems radiating down your arms. To prevent excessive neck bending, purchase a copy holder and raise it so that it is even with the monitor. If your monitor is too low, causing you to keep your head bent forward, then raise the monitor either with a commercial monitor holder or by placing one or two phone books under the monitor. The top of the monitor screen should be parallel or even with your eyes.

Bad habit no. 4: **Twisting.** Twisting your neck or back frequently or maintaining them in a sustained twisted position can lead to neck and back pain. Remember to keep the computer keyboard and monitor directly in front of you. Many computer users have their monitors to one side of the desk and type on the keyboard while viewing the monitor with their heads turned to the side. Imagine watching a movie sideways with your head turned to the side to watch the movie. After a couple of hours, your neck would be very stiff and painful. So you can see how this can lead to neck pain if you type in this position for 6 to 8 hours a day. If you alternate between typing and writing throughout the day, consider getting an under-the-desk tray for your keyboard, which slides in and out. With this feature, you can slide the keyboard under the desk and free your desk space for writing.

Bad habit no. 5: **Overreaching.** Try to keep items that you use frequently close at hand to avoid repetitive or sustained reaching. Many people keep books and heavy files in book cases or cabinets over their desks. Consider moving these heavy items lower in a book case or file next to the desk. If it is not possible to lower these items, then stand up to retrieve these heavy items and use both hands to lift them from the shelves.

Bad habit no. 6: **Banging on the keyboard.** The harder you hit the keys on the keyboard, the more pressure that is being absorbed by your fingers and hands. The average person exerts at least $1\frac{1}{2}$ tons of force per day to the keyboard. Hitting the keyboard harder increases this force, so the gentler the touch the better.

Bad habit no. 7: **Work surface being placed too high.** As we mentioned before, most standard desks are too high for computer keyboards, so the keyboards must be lowered. The

FIGURE 15-40   Computer and desk stretches. (Excerpted from *COMPUTER & DESK STRETCHES.* Copyright 1996 by Bob Anderson, illustrated by Jean Anderson, Palmer Lake, Co. For a free catalog of Stretching Inc products/publications contact: PO Box 767, Palmer Lake, CO 80133-0767, 1-800-333-1307, http://www.stretching.com.)

Sitting at a desk or computer terminal can cause muscular tension and pain. Take a few minutes to do a series of stretches and your whole body will feel better. It is helpful to stretch spontaneously throughout the day, stretching any area of the body that feels tense. This will help greatly in reducing and controlling unwanted tension and pain. *(Most of these stretches may be done standing or sitting. When standing remember to keep your knees slightly bent to protect your back and to give you better balance.)*

How to Stretch:
•Stretch to a point where you feel a mild tension and relax as you hold the stretch.
•The feeling of stretch tells you whether you are stretching correctly or not.
•If you are stretching correctly, the feeling of stretch should slightly subside as you hold the stretch.
•Do not bounce.
•The long-sustained, mild stretch reduces unwanted muscle tension and tightness.
•Stretches should be held generally for 5-30 seconds, depending on which stretch you are doing.

•Breathe slowly, rhythmically, and under control.
•Relax your mind and body as much as possible.
•Always stretch within your comfort limits, never to the point of pain.
•Do not compare yourself to others. We are all different. Comparisons only lead to overstretching.
•Any stretch feeling that grows in intensity or becomes painful as you hold the stretch is an overstretch.

Note: If you have had any recent surgery, muscle, or joint problem, please consult your personal health care professional before starting a stretching or exercise program.

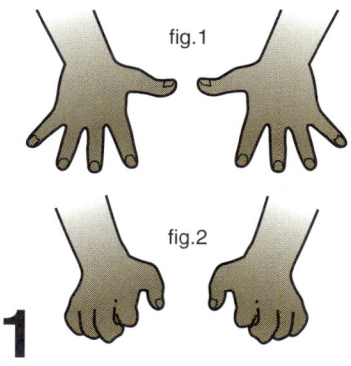

1

Separate and straighten your fingers until tension of a stretch is felt (fig.1). Hold for 10 seconds. Relax, then bend your fingers at the knuckles and hold for 10 seconds (fig.2). Repeat stretch in fig.1 once more.

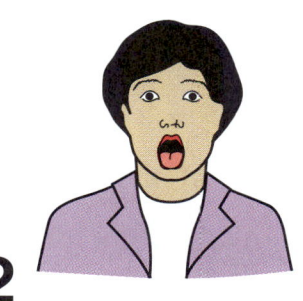

2

Raise your eyebrows and open your eyes as wide as possible. At the same time, open your mouth to stretch the muscles around your nose and chin and stick your tongue out. Hold this stretch for 5-10 seconds. **Caution: If your hear clicking or popping noises when opening mouth, check with your dentist before doing this stretch.**

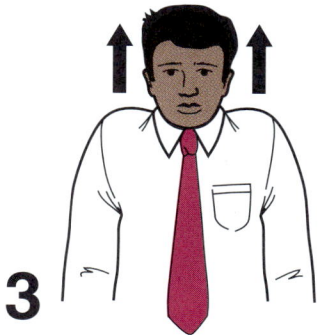

3

Shoulder shrug: Raise the top of your shoulders toward your ears until you feel slight tension in your neck and shoulders. Hold this feeling of tension for 3-5 seconds, then relax your shoulders downward. Do this 2-3 times. Good to use at the first signs of tightness or tension in the shoulder and neck area.

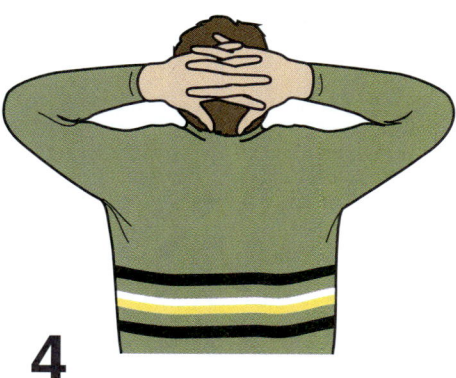

4

With fingers interlaced behind head, keep elbows straight out to side with upper body in a good aligned position. Pull your shoulder blades toward each other to create a feeling of tension through upper back and shoulder blades. Hold this feeling of mild tension for 8-10 seconds, then relax. Do several times.

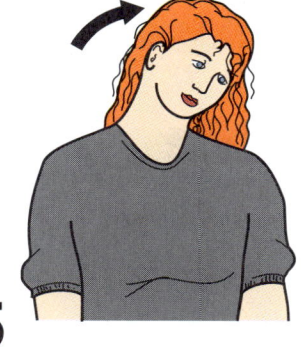

5

Start with head in a comfortable, aligned position. Slowly tilt head to left side to stretch muscles on the right side of neck. Hold stretch 5-10 seconds. Feel a good, even stretch. Do not overstretch. Then tilt head to right side and stretch. Do 2-3 times to each side.

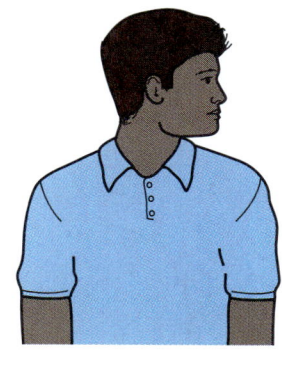

6

From a stable, aligned position turn your chin toward your left shoulder to create a stretch on the right side of your neck. Hold for 5-10 seconds. Repeat, each side twice.

FIGURE 15-40—cont'd Computer and desk stretches. (Excerpted from *COMPUTER & DESK STRETCHES*. Copyright 1996 by Bob Anderson, illustrated by Jean Anderson, Palmer Lake, Co. For a free catalog of Stretching Inc products/publications contact: PO Box 767, Palmer Lake, CO 80133-0767, 1-800-333-1307, http://www.stretching.com.)

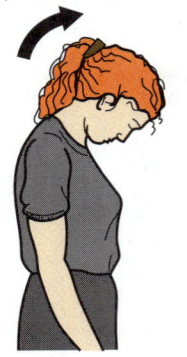

8

Repeat stretch #3

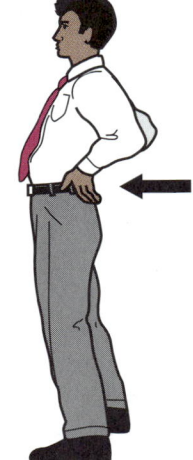

9

Standing with knees slightly bent, place your palms on lower back just above your hips, fingers pointing downward. Gently push your palms forward to create an extension in the lower back. Hold a comfortable stretch for 10-12 seconds. Repeat twice. Use this stretch after sitting for an extended peroid of time.

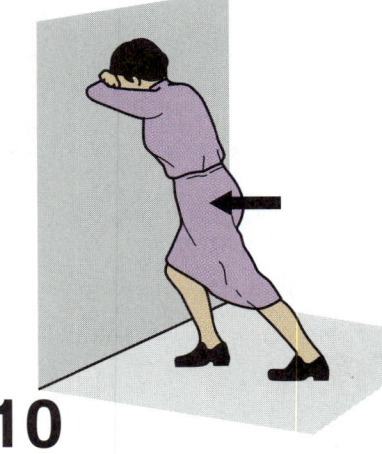

10

To stretch your calf, stand a little ways from a solid support and lean on it with your forearms, your head resting on your hands. Bend one leg and place your foot on the floor in front of you leaving the other leg straight, behind you. Slowly move your hips forward until you feel a stretch in the calf of your straight leg. Be sure to keep the heel of the foot of the straight leg on the floor and your toes pointed straight ahead. Hold an easy stretch for 10-30 seconds. Do not bounce. Stretch both legs.

7

Gently tilt your head forward to stretch the back of the neck. Hold for 5-10 seconds. Repeat 2-3 times. Hold only tensions that feel good. Do not stretch to the point of pain.

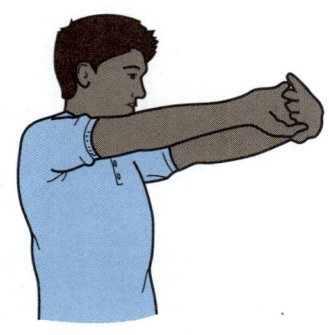

11

Interlace fingers, then straighten arms out in front of you, palms facing away from you. Hold stretch for 10-20 seconds. Do at least two times.

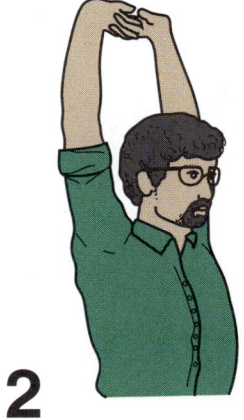

12

Interlace fingers then turn palms upwards above your head as you straighten your arms. Think of elongating your arms as you feel a stretch through arms and upper sides of rib cage. Hold for 10-20 seconds. Do three times.

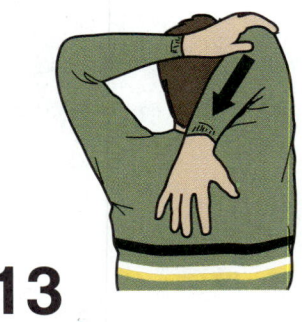

13

Hold right elbow with left hand, then gently pull elbow behind head until an easy tension-stretch is felt. Hold 10-15 seconds. Do not overstretch. Repeat for other side.

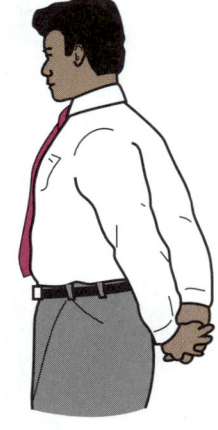

14

With fingers interlaced behind your back, slowly turn your elbows inward while straightening your arms. This is good to do when you find yourself slumping forward from your shoulders. Hold for 5-15 seconds. Do twice.

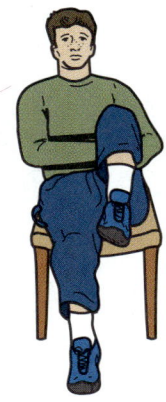

15

Hold onto the back of your upper leg just above the knee. Gently pull bent leg toward your chest until you feel an easy stretch. Hold for 10-30 seconds at easy stretch tension. Do both sides.

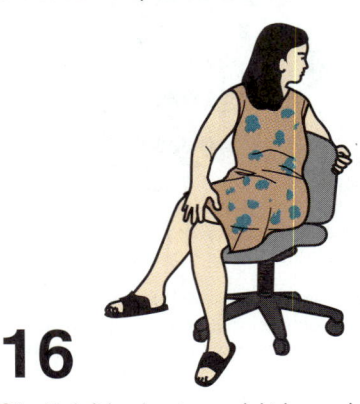

16

Sit with left leg bent over right leg and rest right hand on the outside of the upper thigh of the left leg. Now apply some controlled, steady pressure toward the right with your hand. As you do this look over your left shoulder to get the stretch feeling. Do both sides. Hold for 10-15 seconds.

keyboard should be lowered so that the elbows are at a 100- to 110-degree angle with the hands and wrists slightly lower than the elbows. This angle can be accomplished by installing a tray under your desk or sometimes by raising the height of your chair. If you raise the chair height, make sure your feet are still flat on the floor. If they are not flat to the floor, you will need a footrest to provide stability. A phone book often does the trick.

Bad habit no. 8: **Cradling the telephone.**   People who cradle the telephone by holding it up with their shoulders while they type or write risk serious neck problems. If you are on the phone all day and have to write or type while on the phone, switch to a telephone headset. Many headsets on the market are affordable, are easy to use, and are easy to disconnect if you often have to be up and down from your desk. Even if you are not on the phone all day, stop the habit of cradling the telephone. Instead, hold the telephone with one hand and type or write with the other. Leaning the elbows on the desk while holding the phone is also a bad habit because this position can lead to irritation of nerves that run through the elbow.

Bad habit no. 9: **Gripping the mouse too hard.**   Many people tend to grip the mouse too tightly or use too much force to click the mouse. Hold the mouse loosely; heavy gripping causes tension in the entire hand. Use a light touch when clicking and try not to raise your finger higher than necessary when clicking. Use your whole arm and shoulder to move the mouse, not just your wrist, and keep your wrist in a straight or neutral position. The mouse should also be at the same level as the keyboard, so if you lowered your keyboard, you should lower the mouse as well. Remember not to rest or lean your wrist and forearm on the table when using the mouse. If you are ambidextrous, try changing the mouse from one side to the other from time to time. Also, try to use the function keys as much as possible on the keyboard to avoid excessive mouse use.

Bad habit no. 10: **Skipping your breaks.**   Try not to work through your breaks and lunch. If you are typing and writing all day, your hands need the rest. Use your breaks as an opportunity to stretch your hands and arms. Better yet, taking a walk on your breaks or at lunch not only will be good for your body but also will help decrease your stress level.

CONCLUSION

You have now completed the chapter on physical therapy. After you have practiced the procedures and are ready to demonstrate your skills and knowledge attained, arrange with your instructor to take a performance test.

Various types of patient conditions and disabilities can benefit from physical therapy. Numerous other procedures, tests, and modalities are used in a physical therapy department; however, this book does not cover all of these in detail. Clinical experience or a field trip to a physical therapy facility would be most valuable for learning firsthand about the use of the various modalities and techniques.

REVIEW OF VOCABULARY

The following are statements taken from patient charts. Read these and be able to explain the nature of the types of treatment each patient has received.

PATIENT NO. 1

On January 14, the patient was working for the Webster Construction Co. in custodial activity. He was using a mop, and after pulling the mop through the wringer, he experienced right paralumbar pain. The next morning the patient couldn't move because of severe pain. He had an appointment at the Crossroads Clinic, and medications were prescribed. Later the patient saw Dr. Treadmill, who recognized the problem as one involving compensation. Furthermore, Dr. Treadmill obtained x-ray films and prescribed physical therapy. Physical therapy involved massages; ultrasound therapy; pelvic traction; and patient education in posture, body mechanics, and ROM exercises. Temporary relief came from these measures. About 8 or 9 days ago, however, because the trouble persisted, the patient was referred to me.

The patient stated that the pain in the right lower extremity prevents work. It is "static," by which the patient means it is not worsening or improving.

The patient in formative years had an occasional "kink" in the back but was never off work and never had professional attention.

PATIENT NO. 2

Patient brought in a prescription to continue treatment for 3 more weeks. The physician thinks that physiotherapy is helping and will see the patient at the end of 3 weeks. Patient states pain is gradually decreasing. Treatment: hot packs, ultrasound at 1.5 w/cm^2 for 7 minutes to left low back, and exercise progression to abdominal strengthening. Patient does exercises well and reports that she continues them at home.

Will Kerrigan, RPT

Documentation of Initial Evaluation in Physical Therapy

Patient No. 3

Date: 12/12/01

Medical Dx: DJD C-spine

History: 55-year-old male with 3-month history of right-sided neck pain of gradual onset, denies specific precipitating event or trauma. X-rays of C-spine unremarkable except for degenerative arthritic changes. This is his first referral to PT.

Patient reports prior whiplash injury to neck in motor vehicle accident 15 years ago; denies any residual problems from that injury prior to this recent onset of neck pain.

Subjective complaints: Patient complaining of constant pain radiating from his neck down his Rt arm to the elbow; also complaining of dropping things and occasional numbness/tingling in his hand that comes on usually with prolonged sitting. Pain is less on awakening in the AM; worsens as day progresses. Complaining of occasional discomforting sleep. Has had no relief from symptoms with NSAIDs or decreased work schedule; he does get a little relief of pain symptoms for a couple of hours with application of heat to the neck.

Objective findings:

- **ROM:** C-spine:

A/PROM*	Right	Left
Rotation	30° (end-feel leathery)	50° with pain Rt (end-feel muscular)
Lat flexion	20° (" ")	45° with pain Rt (end-feel muscular)

Flexion—25° (stiff): Extension—20° (end-range pain; no increase with repetitions)

Rt shoulder: A/PROM* WNL**

*Anterior/posterior range of motion

**Within normal limits

- **Strength:** C-spine: 3+/5 with no increase of pain with resistance. *Right upper extremity:* 4/5 except biceps, brachialis, and brachioradialis, which are 3/5. *Left upper extremity:* WNL except 4−/5 elbow flexors.
- **Sensation:** Hypesthesia over C5 distribution.
- **Special tests:** Negative TOS.
- **Posture:** Stands/sits with forward head, increase cervical lordosis, rounded/elevated shoulders, slight increase thoracic kyphosis.
- **Functional activity level:** Independent activities of daily living (ADL) although takes care with picking up fragile objects due to fear that he'll drop them. Drives only as necessary because of discomfort. Works only 4 hr/day in AM. Unable to do heavy household chores, gardening. When having the worst pain, his sleep is disrupted to 3 to 4 hours a night.

Goals:

Short-term goals—in 1 week:

- Patient able to correct cervical/thoracic posture in sitting and standing without verbal cues to improve cervical alignment.
- Patient able to position self for sleep to diminish irritation to neck to allow increased sleep time.
- Home program of postural exercises, heat, activity modification established.
- Pain no longer constant.

Long-term goals—in 4 weeks:

- Patient able to maintain correct cervical/thoracic posture 75% of the time in sitting and standing activities.

- Patient able to sleep through night without severe discomfort; awaken without severe pain 90% of the time.
- Patient able to tolerate 8-hr workday with pain level at 2-3/10 end of day 90% of the time.
- C-spine anterior/posterior range of motion Rt = Lt without pain in any direction end-range; pain-free driving.
- Pain occurs only occasionally and only at neck; no radiating pain to RUE.
- Residual occasional numbness Rt hand, no tingling.
- C-spine strength 4/5; RUE/LUE strength 4/5 bilaterally throughout.
- Resumption gardening, holding fragile objects without problems.

Plan: 2× / wk × 2 wks then 1× / wk × 2 wks.

- Patient education correct cervical/thoracic posture and alignment in sitting, standing, sleeping.
- Patient education home program including activity modification, ROM and isometric exercises C-spine, use of heat. Progress to strengthening exercises scapular stabilizers.
- Trial manual traction in clinic—possible progression to home traction unit if needed.

Follow-up treatment—third treatment session (1 week since initial evaluation):

S: Patient arrives in good spirits with significant decrease in pain especially at the end of the day (6/10 end of day; pain no longer constant; sleeping 6 hr/night × last 2 nights and awakens with pain at 2/10). Also notes pain radiating only to midhumerus. States he has been consistent with home program including postural correction qh, heat tid × 15 min, assisted ADL/function.

O: Pretreatment C-spine. Anterior ROM unchanged but with decrease in pain at end-ranges. After treatment, C-spine anterior ROM equal Rt and Lt (45° rot, 45° lat flex) without pain with pain-free C-spine and RUE. Able to demonstrate cervical ROM/isometric exercises added to home program.

Rx: Soft tissue mobilization paracervical mm; gentle manual traction to C-spine (constant × 5 min in C-spine flexion): patient education in cervical isometric and anterior ROM exercises; postural correction during functional activities (copy of home program in chart); ice massage to upper trapezius muscles × 5 min.

A: Patient making good progress; seems motivated to make needed postural changes. Short term goals (STG): In 1 week—

- Pain cont. no longer constant; radiating sx to shoulder.
- Patient able to maintain correct cervical/thoracic posture 50% of the time in sitting and standing activities.
- Patient able to sleep through night without discomfort; awakens w/ 0/10 pain 75% of the time.
- Patient able to tolerate 4-hr workday w/ pain level at 2-3/10 end of day 90% of the time.
- C-spine anterior/posterior ROM Rt = Lt w/o pain in any direction end-range; pain-free driving.
- Decrease numbness Rt hand, no tingling.
- C-spine strength 4−/5.

P: Continue treatment per initial plan—begin scapular stabilization exercises next session, reassess re: home traction next treatment session.

R. A. Wilmington, PT

CRITICAL THINKING SKILLS REVIEW

1. Define and state the purposes and time duration of application for each of the following:
   a. Ultraviolet light treatments
   b. Diathermy treatments
   c. Ultrasound treatments
   d. Application of moist and dry heat
   e. Application of moist and dry cold
2. How full should a hot water bottle be filled when applied to a patient? Why?
3. State the temperature of the water you would use when applying a hot water bottle to a 70-year-old man; to a 2-year-old child.
4. Define and discuss the principles of body mechanics.
5. Why should the patient's skin be checked frequently during any form of hot or cold application?
6. List five physiologic reactions produced by heat applications and five produced by cold applications.
7. List five situations in which cold applications may be used for treatment.

8. List five situations in which hot applications may be used for treatment.
9. List two modalities used in hydrotherapy. Explain each briefly. List two uses for each.
10. List five uses or purposes of exercises.
11. Differentiate between active and passive exercises.
12. State three purposes of traction and three purposes of massage.
13. State two types of electrodiagnostic examinations and explain each briefly.
14. Discuss the principles of electrotherapy using galvanic and faradic currents.
15. Define the term *ergonomics*. State the goal of ergonomics.
16. Describe and discuss the term *musculoskeletal disorders*.
17. State why work-related musculoskeletal disorders are a problem.
18. Differentiate between good and bad habits relating to body posture and habits when working at a desk or at a computer.

PERFORMANCE TEST

In a skills laboratory, the medical assistant student will demonstrate skill and knowledge in performing the following activities without reference to source materials. The student needs a partner to play the role of the patient. Time limits for the each of the following activities are to be assigned by the instructor (see also p. 104).

1. To the outer aspect of the patient's right forearm and to the inner aspect of the patient's left lower leg, prepare, apply, and remove the following:
   a. Hot water bottle
   b. Hot compress
   c. Ice bag
   d. Cold compress
2. Discuss the purpose and physiologic effects of hot and cold treatments with your instructor.
3. Demonstrate with a partner:
   a. Active exercises of the right arm
   b. Passive exercises to the right arm
   c. Active-resistant exercises to the patient's right hand
4. Using the information provided in this chapter, correctly write out the procedural steps and a performance checklist for the following applications of heat or cold:
   a. Heating pad
   b. Hot water bottle

   c. Hot moist compress
   d. Hot soak
   e. Ice bag
   f. Ice pack
   g. Moist cold compress
   h. Alcohol sponge bath
   i. Chemical cold pack
5. Using the information you outlined in No. 4, design a teaching-instruction sheet for the patient to use at home for each of the hot and cold applications listed.
6. Demonstrate safe and effective body mechanics when lifting a patient or heavy object.
7. Assist patients to learn how to walk with crutches and with a cane.
8. Assist patients to get in and out of a wheelchair.
9. Measure and determine the correct size of crutches, a cane, and a walker for a patient.
10. Demonstrate good body posture to maintain when working at a desk or computer terminal.
11. Demonstrate various computer and desk stretching exercises as given in this chapter.

The successful completion of each procedure will demonstrate competency levels as required by the AAMA, AMT, and future employers.

💻 INTERNET RESOURCES

The Arthritis Foundation
www.arthritis.org

Friends of Disabled Adults and Children (FODAC)
www.fodac.org

OSHA
www.osha.gov

MedScape
www.medscape.com

Assistive Technology Resources
curry.edschool.virginia.edu/go/cise/ose/resourses/asst_tech.html

Medline*plus*
www.nlm.nih.gov/medlineplus

Physical Activity and Health: A Report of the Surgeon General
www.cdc.gov/nccdphp/sgr/sgr.htm

American Academy of Orthopedic Surgeons Public Information
www.aaos.org/wordhtml/pat_educ.htm

Arthritis Advice
www.nih.gov/nia/health/pubpub/arthtis.htm

Doctors Guide to Osteoporosis
www.pslgroup.com/OSTEOPOROSIS.HTM

American College of Sports Medicine (ACSM)
www.a1.com/sportsmed

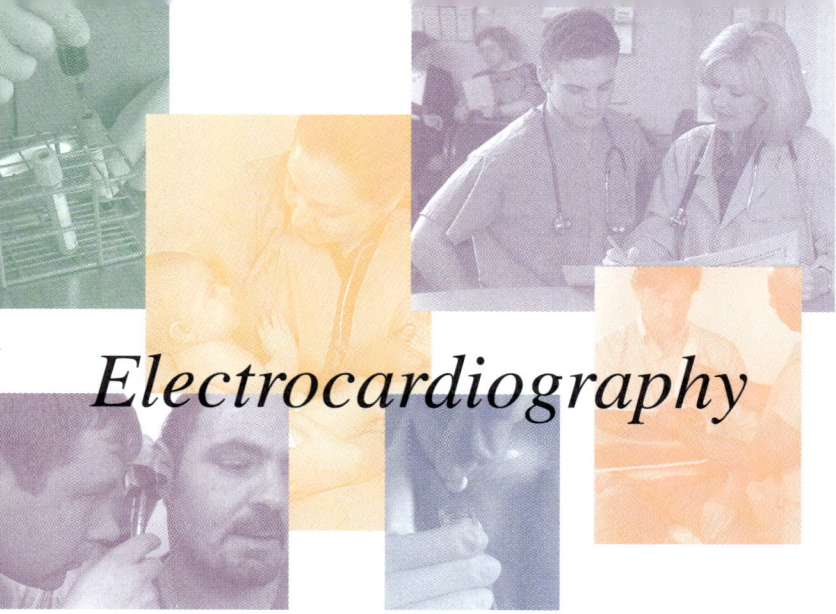

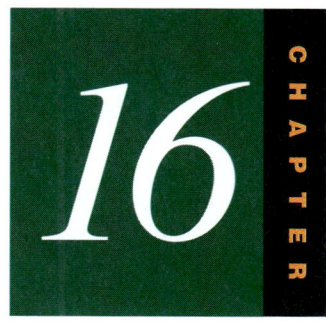

Electrocardiography

■ Cognitive Objectives

On completion of Chapter 16, the medical assistant student should be able to:

1. Define, spell, and pronounce the terms in the vocabulary and text of this chapter.
2. Explain the cardiac cycle and conduction system of the heart.
3. Explain how the heartbeat is controlled.
4. List eight components recorded on the electrocardiogram (ECG) cycle and relate these to the electrical activity of the heart.
5. State the normal time required for the cardiac cycle.
6. Describe electrocardiograph paper and indicate the significance of each small block and each large block.
7. List four factors that are interpreted from an ECG.
8. Describe how to monitor an ECG for abnormal and erratic tracings.
9. Briefly define and discuss three types of each of the following: sinus rhythms, atrial arrhythmias, and ventricular arrhythmias. State possible causes of each.
10. List three types of common artifacts that may be seen on an ECG and the causes for each.
11. Describe electrodes and electrolyte gel or paste and state the purpose of each.
12. List the 12 leads recorded on a standard ECG; state the electrical activity that each is recording; and recognize each recorded lead by interpreting the identification code used.
13. Discuss the phrase *standardizing the electrocardiograph,* indicating the importance of this. Illustrate and explain the universal standard of ECG measurement.
14. Discuss the concepts of the Phone-A-Gram, the computerized electrocardiograph.
15. Discuss the automatic electrocardiograph and state its advantages.
16. Explain what ambulatory cardiac monitoring (Holter monitoring) is and state why it is performed.
17. List eight instructions that should be given to a patient who will be wearing a Holter monitor.
18. Explain what is involved in a treadmill stress test.
19. State four reasons for a stress ECG test.

■ Terminal Performance Objectives

On completion of Chapter 16, the medical assistant student should be able to:

1. Demonstrate proficiency in communicating proper preparation of the patient for electrocardiography and in preparing the room and equipment.
2. Demonstrate the proper procedure for the application of the electrodes and lead wires to the patient for a standard 12-lead ECG and for a Holter monitor.
3. Locate and mark the six positions used to record the chest leads.
4. Demonstrate the proper procedure for recording the ECG with a standard electrocardiograph, mounting the finished product, and caring for the equipment after use.
5. Demonstrate the proper procedure for using a Holter monitor.
6. Provide instructions and patient education that is within the professional scope of a medical assistant's training and responsibilities as assigned.

The student is to perform these objectives with 100% accuracy 90% of the time (9 out of 10 times).

The consistent use of Universal/Standard Precautions is required by all health care professionals in all health care settings as a method of infection control. It is assumed that these precautions are used in all of the following procedures. Review Chapter 1 if you have any questions on methods to use because the methods or techniques are not repeated in detail in each procedure presented in this chapter.

Be sure to consult the latest guidelines issued by the Centers for Disease Control and Prevention and consult with infection control practitioners when necessary to identify specific precautions that pertain to your particular work situation.

VOCABULARY

amplify (am′pli-fi)—To enlarge, to extend.

arrhythmia (ah-rith′me-ah)—A variation from the normal or an irregular rhythm of the heartbeat. Used interchangeably with the term *dysrhythmia*.

atrium (a′tre-um)—One of the upper chambers of the heart. The right atrium receives deoxygenated blood from the body, whereas the left atrium receives oxygenated blood from the lungs. (The plural is *atria*.)

automaticity—The ability of the specialized heart cells (sinoatrial node, atrioventricular node, bundle of His, and Purkinje fibers) to spontaneously initiate an electrical impulse without stimulation from any other source, such as a nerve.

cardiac (kar′de-ak) **arrest**—The sudden and often unexpected cessation of the heartbeat. Permanent damage of vital organs and death are probable if treatment is not given immediately.

defibrillation (de-fi″bri-la′shun)—The application of electrical impulses to the heart to stop heart fibrillation or irregular contractions.

electrocardiograph (e-lek″tro-kar-de-o-graf″)—The instrument used in electrocardiography.

fibrillation (fi″bri-la-shun)—A cardiac arrhythmia characterized by rapid, irregular, and ineffective electrical activity in the heart. Ventricular fibrillation is a common cause of cardiac arrest.

myocardial infarction (mi″o-kar′de-al in-fark′shun) **(MI)**—The death of cells in an area of the heart muscle caused by oxygen deprivation, which in turn is caused by an interference of blood supply to the area. Commonly called a "heart attack."

myocardium (mi″o-kar-de-um)—The heart muscle.

oscilloscope (o-sil′o-skop)—An instrument used to display the shape or waveform of the electrical activity of the heart and other body organs (comparable to a television screen).

pacemaker (pas′mak-er)—The natural pacemaker of the heart is the sinoatrial (SA) node located in the right atrium. The normal

heartbeat results from an electrical impulse that originates in the SA node. The normal SA node normally paces the heartbeat, discharging impulses at a rhythmic rate of 60 to 100 beats per minute. See later section, Control of the Heartbeat: Conduction System of the Heart.

pericarditis (per″i-kar-di′tis)—Inflammation of the pericardium, the fibroserous sac enveloping the heart.

rhythm strip—An ECG recording of a single lead that is used to determine the *rhythm* of the heartbeat, such as a fast, slow, regular, or irregular rhythm, and ventricular fibrillation. It is also used to determine if the patient is experiencing any type of heart block (for example, third-degree heart block). The rhythm strip gives a one-dimensional picture of the beating of the heart to demonstrate the rhythm of the heartbeat *only,* in contrast to the 12-lead ECG, which can show damage to the heart and other conditions. Data from the rhythm strip can be a useful screening tool because frequent runs of arrhythmias can be more easily observed. The rhythm strip can also be used to confirm the basic assessment made on the 12-lead ECG. Current use of the rhythm strip is to record lead V_1, and possibly leads V_2 and V_5, although one could record any lead that is desired. Lead II is commonly used for cardiac monitoring. Rhythm strips are frequently recorded from a continuous cardiac monitor in intensive care units in the hospital and by paramedics in the field in emergency situations.

ventricle (ven′tri-kl)—One of the lower chambers of the heart. The right ventricle receives deoxygenated blood from the right atrium and pumps this blood through the pulmonary arteries to the lungs; the left ventricle receives oxygenated blood from the left atrium and pumps this blood out through the aorta to all body tissues.

Additional terms are defined within the text.

The science and art of electrocardiography combine advanced electromedical technology with the science and art of medical practice. Today, electrocardiographs present physicians with precise information by amplifying the minute electrical currents produced by the heart on a graphic record or tracing. This record or tracing is called an electrocardiogram (ECG, or EKG), defined simply as a graphic representation of the electrical activity (currents) produced by the heart during the processes of contraction and relaxation. More precisely, the ECG records the amount of electrical activity, the time required for this activity to travel through the heart during each complete heartbeat, and the rate and rhythm of the heartbeat. Many physicians now include an electrocardiogram as part of a complete physical examination, especially for patients 40 years of age or older. Many advise patients to have an ECG or a treadmill stress ECG before any serious jogging or other

exercise program is started (see Treadmill Stress Test at the end of this chapter).

Often physicians have medical assistants take the ECG. To be valuable members of the health team, those who take ECGs must acquire related knowledge and develop skills (that is, they must know what they are doing, why and how to do it, and then do it well).

The following pages are designed to help you acquire this knowledge and skill by discussing the nature and purpose of the ECG, the equipment and materials needed, preparation of the patient and equipment, ways to monitor the record for abnormal and erratic tracings, procedure for taking the ECG, and mounting the record obtained.

Before going further, you should review the anatomy of the heart to maximize your understanding of electrocardiography (Figure 16-1).

FIGURE 16-1   **A,** Your heart and how it works. (**A** courtesy the American Heart Association, Inc.)

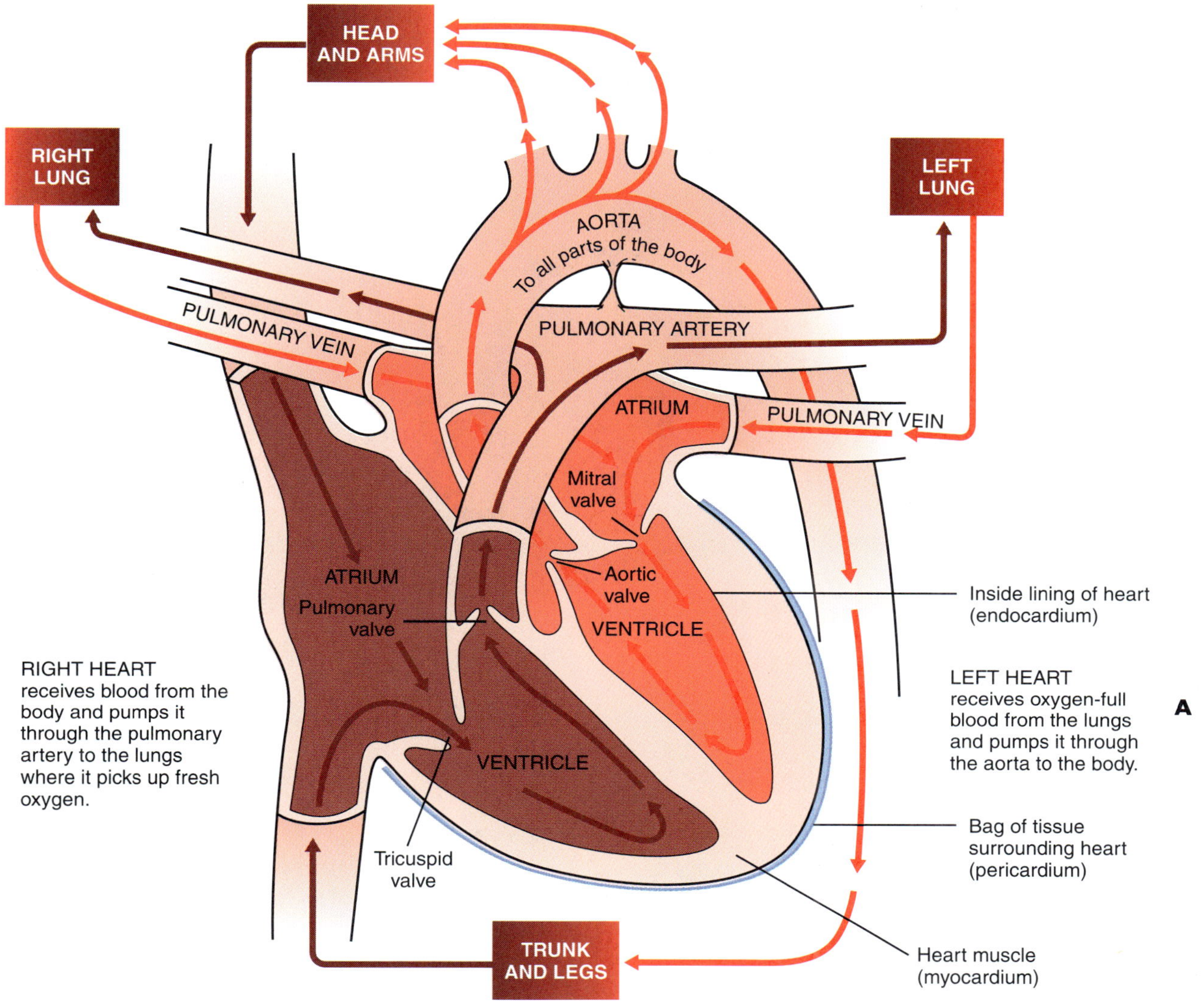

HEAD AND ARMS

RIGHT LUNG

LEFT LUNG

AORTA
To all parts of the body

PULMONARY VEIN

PULMONARY ARTERY

ATRIUM

PULMONARY VEIN

Mitral valve

ATRIUM
Pulmonary valve

Aortic valve

VENTRICLE

Inside lining of heart (endocardium)

RIGHT HEART
receives blood from the body and pumps it through the pulmonary artery to the lungs where it picks up fresh oxygen.

LEFT HEART
receives oxygen-full blood from the lungs and pumps it through the aorta to the body.

A

VENTRICLE

Tricuspid valve

Bag of tissue surrounding heart (pericardium)

TRUNK AND LEGS

Heart muscle (myocardium)

Your heart weighs well under a pound and is only a little larger than your fist, but it is a powerful, long working, hard working organ. Its job is to pump blood to the lungs and to all the body tissues.

The heart is a hollow organ. Its tough, muscular wall (myocardium) is surrounded by a fiberlike bag (pericardium) and is lined by a thin, strong membrane (endocardium). A wall (septum) divides the heart cavity down the middle into a "right heart" and a "left heart". Each side of the heart is divided again into an upper chamber (called an atrium or auricle) and a lower chamber (ventricle). Valves regulate the flow of blood through the heart and to the pulmonary artery and the aorta.

The heart is really a double pump. One pump (the right heart) receives blood that has just come from the body after delivering nutrients and oxygen to the body tissues. It pumps this dark red blood to the lungs where the blood gets rid of a waste gas (carbon dioxide) and picks up a fresh supply of oxygen that turns it a bright red again. The second pump (the left heart) receives this "reconditioned" blood from the lungs and pumps it out through the great trunk-artery (aorta) to be distributed by smaller arteries to all parts of the body.   *Continued*

FIGURE 16-1—cont'd **B,** Conduction system of the heart.

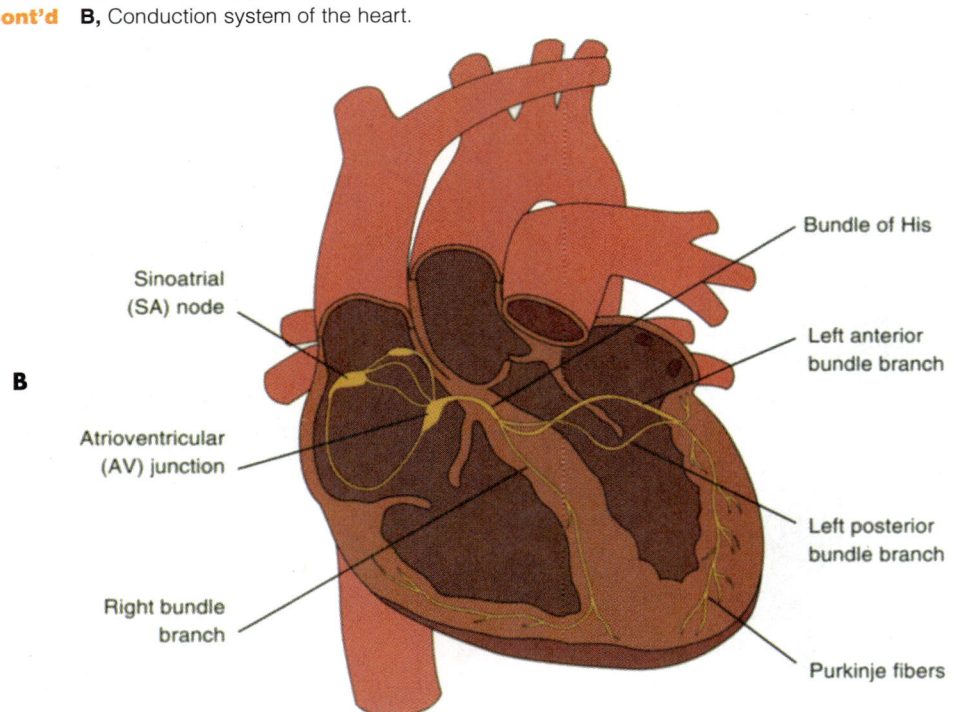

B

Sinoatrial
(SA) node

Atrioventricular
(AV) junction

Right bundle
branch

Bundle of His

Left anterior
bundle branch

Left posterior
bundle branch

Purkinje fibers

THE CARDIAC CYCLE AND ECG CYCLE

The term **cardiac cycle** refers to one complete heartbeat, which consists of contraction (systole) and relaxation (diastole) of both atria and both ventricles. The many cells of the heart are arranged so that they act together as one network or system. Throughout this network, two types of electrical processes, called **depolarization** and **repolarization**, are transmitted. When depolarization occurs, the cells are stimulated, and the **myocardium** (the heart muscle) contracts; as repolarization occurs, the myocardium relaxes. To understand the electrical activity of the heart, think of the heart as consisting of two separate cell networks, one being the **atria** and the other the **ventricles.** The two atria contract simultaneously; then as they relax, the two ventricles contract and relax, rather than the entire heart contracting as a unit. Any disturbance in the processes of the cardiac cycle cause a change in the electrical forces needed to maintain normal, rhythmic heartbeats and may produce an arrhythmia. Depending on the degree of disturbance, it could be a minor disruption of rhythm or a major life-threatening arrhythmia.

Each of these cell networks (the atria and the ventricles) is considered separately on the electrocardiogram, the graphic recording of these electrical forces produced by the heart; that is, the waves or deflections recorded on the electrocardiograph paper represent the sequence of events that occur during the cardiac cycle.

Waves

The normal ECG cycle consists of waves that have been arbitrarily labeled *P, QRS,* and *T waves.* Each wave corresponds to a particular part of the cardiac cycle (Figure 16-2). The **P wave** reflects contraction (depolarization) of the atria. The **QRS wave (QRS complex)** reflects the contraction (depolarization) of the ventricles. This wave follows the **P wave**. The **T wave** reflects ventricular recovery (repolarization of the ventricles). A T wave reflecting the repolarization of the atria is not visible because it is obscured by the QRS wave. A T wave follows every QRS wave. Occasionally, another wave, the **U wave,** appears after the T wave. It is a small wave and usually shows up on ECGs of patients who have a low serum potassium level. In some studies, U waves have been produced during the repolarization stages of the Purkinje fibers in the ventricle musculature.

Because the ventricles are much larger than the atria, the QRS and T waves are normally much larger than the P wave.

Intervals, Segments, and Baseline

P-R interval. The *P-R interval* reflects the time it takes from the beginning of the atrial contraction to the beginning of the ventricular contraction. The P-R interval is measured from the beginning of the P wave to the beginning of the QRS complex (Figure 16-3).

PR segment. The *PR segment* is part of the P-R interval. It reflects the time interval from the end of the P wave to the be-

FIGURE 16-2 Normal ECG deflections. (From Conover MB: *Understanding electrocardiography,* ed 4, St Louis, 1992, Mosby.)

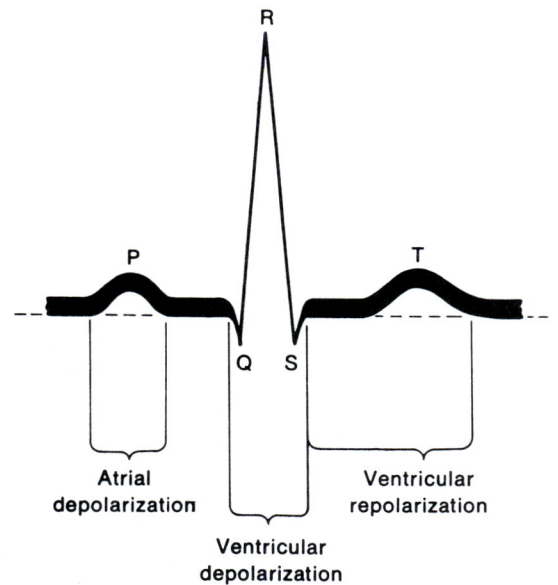

FIGURE 16-3 ECG intervals. (From Conover MB: *Understanding electrocardiography,* ed 4, St Louis, 1992, Mosby.)

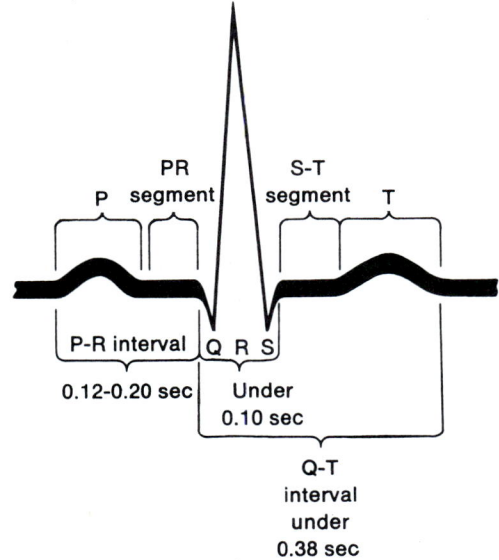

ginning of the QRS complex. It is the time it takes for the impulses to go from the atrioventricular (AV) node to the bundle of His, the bundle branches, and the Purkinje fibers in the ventricles. The PR segment is normally an isoelectric (flat) line.

ST segment.

The *ST segment* reflects the time interval from the end of the ventricular contraction (depolarization) to the beginning of ventricular recovery (repolarization). It is normally a flat (isoelectric) line that is measured from the end of the S wave (of the QRS complex) to the beginning of the T wave.

Q-T Interval.

The *Q-T interval* reflects the time it takes from the beginning of the ventricular depolarization to the end of the ventricular repolarization. This interval gives a better picture of the total ventricular activity. It is measured from the beginning of the QRS complex to the end of the T wave.

Baseline.

The *baseline,* a flat horizontal line that separates the waves, may be seen to run the length of the ECG tracing. This is known as the isoelectric line. The waves of the **ECG cycle** will deflect either upward (positive deflection) or downward (negative deflection) from the baseline (isoelectric line). This line is present when there is no current flowing in the heart, that is, after depolarization or after repolarization of the heart. The baseline present after the T wave reflects the period when the entire heart is resting or in its polarized state.

Observing and measuring the configuration and location of each wave in relation to the other waves and baseline, the intervals and the segments in each cycle, and then between each ECG cycle allows the physician to interpret and analyze the rate, rhythm, and conduction of the heart. Abnormalities detected in the ECG cycles help diagnose cardiac problems, for example, myocardial infarction (MI), pericarditis, myocarditis, left ventricular hypertrophy, atrial and ventricular arrhythmias, nodal block, and atrial and ventricular fibrillation, in addition to a variety of other conditions, such as acid-base imbalance, effects of various drugs, metabolic diseases, autonomic hyperactivity, and hyperventilation.

Control of the Heartbeat: Conduction System of the Heart

To understand the interpretation of an ECG, one must know the mechanism by which the heartbeat originates. Stimulation of the heartbeat originates in the sympathetic (acting to increase the heart rate) and parasympathetic (the vagus nerve, acting to slow the heart rate) branches of the autonomic nervous system. Although the heart is under the control of the nervous system, the myocardium (heart muscle) itself is capable of contracting rhythmically independently of this outside control. Despite this property of **automaticity,** impulses from the autonomic nervous system are required to produce a rapid enough beat to maintain circulation and life effectively. Without the nerve connection, the heart rate may be less than 40 beats per minute instead of the usual 70 to 90 beats per minute (average is 80 beats per minute).

Specialized masses of tissue in the heart form the conduction system, regulating the sequence of events of the cardiac cycle. These include the **sinoatrial (SA) node,** the **"pacemaker"** of the heart, located in the upper right-hand corner of the right atrium adjacent to the opening of the superior vena cava; the **atrioventricular (AV) node,** located near the intraventricular septum in the inferior wall of the right atrium and near the tricuspid valve; the **bundle of His** (or AV bundle), located in the interventricular septum, which then divides into the left and right bundles; and the **Purkinje fibers,** which terminate in the ventricles (see Figure 16-1, *B*).

The electrical impulse of the cardiac cycle is initiated by the SA node, from which wavelike impulses are sent through the atria, stimulating first the right and then the left atrium, and eventually sweep over the heart. In a comparable manner, if one drops a pebble in water, it will generate waves that travel outward from the point of origin.

When the atria have been stimulated, the impulse slows as it passes through the AV node. Slowing of the impulse at the AV node allows the resting ventricles (in diastole) to fill with blood from the atria. This wave of excitation (stimulation) then spreads down to the bundle of His, then to the right and left bundle branches, which then relay the impulse to the Purkinje fibers, an interlacing network terminating in the musculature of the ventricle. The Purkinje fibers distribute the impulse in the right and left ventricles, causing them to contract. Stimulation of the muscle of the ventricle begins in the intraventricular septum and moves downward, causing ventricular depolarization and contraction. Mechanically, the ventricles empty blood into the pulmonary (or lesser) circulation by way of the pulmonary artery and the right and left pulmonary branches, and into the systemic (or greater) circulation by way of the aorta. This stimulation or impulse must spread through the muscle of both atria and both ventricles before mechanical contraction can occur. To complete the cardiac cycle, the entire heart now relaxes momentarily, and then a new impulse is initiated by the SA node to repeat the whole cycle.

The electrical waveform that originates in the SA node and spreads throughout the heart then spreads through the body. From the body surface, it is possible to pick up these electrical impulses and record them on specialized paper (the electrocardiograph) or display them on an oscilloscope (comparable to a television screen).

Time Required for Cardiac Cycle

Each cardiac cycle takes approximately 0.8 second. With this time limit, there are 75 heartbeats per minute. When the heart beats more than 75 times per minute, the cycle requires less time. Conversely, when the heart beats less than 75 beats per minute, the cardiac cycle requires more than 0.8 second.

Heart Sounds During Cardiac Cycle

Typical sounds are elicited from the heart during each cardiac cycle. These sounds are described as *lubb dupp,* as heard through a stethoscope. The first sound, *lubb* (the systolic sound), is a longer and lower-pitched sound and is believed to be from the contraction of the ventricles and vibrations from the closing of the cuspid valves. The second sound, *dupp* (the diastolic sound), is shorter and sharper and occurs during the beginning of ventricular relaxation. It is thought to be due to the vibrations of the closure of the semilunar valves (pulmonic and aortic valves). Because these sounds provide information about the valves of the heart, they have clinical significance. Variations from normal in these sounds indicate imperfect functioning of the valves. Heart murmurs are one type of abnormal sound heard and may indicate stenosis or incomplete closing of the valves (valvular insufficiency). It is important to remember that the ECG does not record these sounds. They can be heard with a stethoscope that is put on the chest wall over the apex region of the heart.

HEALTH MATTERS

HEART HEALTH FACTS

The knowledge gained from the famous Framingham heart study has influenced and continues to influence the lives of millions of people.

- In 1959 studies showed that some heart attacks are "silent"— that is, they occur without warning. For some, the first and only symptoms could be death.
- In 1960 research showed that smoking increases the risk for heart disease.
- In 1961 studies showed that high blood pressure increases the risk for heart disease.
- In 1967 studies showed that overweight and obesity increase the risk for heart disease and that physical activity could reduce the risk.
- In 1976 the loss of estrogen associated with menopause was linked to an increased risk of heart disease in women.
- In 1978 atrial fibrillation (rapid irregular contractions in the upper chambers of the heart) was found to increase the risk of stroke fivefold.

- In 1988 more was learned about high-density lipoproteins (HDLs). High levels of HDLs were found to help protect people against heart disease.
- In 1991 weight fluctuations in people who diet, lose weight and then gain it back, then diet again, and so on, are at a greater risk for heart disease.
- In 1999 the Framingham researchers published a formula used to calculate your chance of getting a heart attack in the next 10 years. It uses your age, blood pressure, total cholesterol level, and HDL levels.

These numbers can be obtained from your physician after a routine checkup. Research and knowledge obtained from the Framingham studies have led to advances in the development of drugs needed to treat hypertension, stroke, and high blood cholesterol levels. Guidelines for preventing and treating heart disease have also been developed.

HEALTH MATTERS

KEEPING YOUR PATIENTS INFORMED

HEART DISEASE: WHO IS AT RISK?

Cardiac arrest: The heart stops beating.

Heart attack: Lack of blood supply to an area of the heart muscle, which leads to death of that tissue. This is also called a myocardial infarction.

Heart failure: A condition in which the heart fails to pump the required amount of blood needed by the body to maintain life.

Nearly three quarters of a million people die of heart disease each year. No one can tell if you have heart disease just by looking at you. However, certain factors can be checked to determine if you are at risk for developing heart disease.

RISK FACTORS YOU HAVE NO CONTROL OVER

1. *Gender.* More men than women develop heart disease.
2. *Age.* The older you get the more likely you are to develop heart disease.
3. *Heredity.* Genetic studies along with medical information collected over the past five decades will show which people are at a higher risk for cardiovascular disease.
4. *Family history.* A family history of heart attack, high blood pressure, or stroke puts you at a greater risk for the same problems. Although you can't change this risk, you can make a difference in your risk by having a healthy diet, not smoking, and doing regular exercise.
5. *Race.* African Americans are twice as likely to develop high blood pressure than white Americans and are also at a greater risk of developing heart disease. Factors such as medical care availability, diet, lifestyle, and stress may also have an effect on their risks for heart disease.

RISK FACTORS THAT CAN BE CONTROLLED MEDICALLY

1. *Hypertension (high blood pressure)* (see Chapter 3).
2. *Diabetes* (If diabetes is not treated, it can lead to blood vessel damage and thus a greater risk for heart disease (see also Chapter 17).
3. *Blood fats:* cholesterol, triglycerides, lipoproteins. Generally, the higher the blood cholesterol, triglyceride and LDL levels, the greater the risk for blood vessel and heart disease. (See also Chapters 13 and 18).
4. *Hormone replacement therapy (HRT) for postmenopausal women.* HRT is taking a combination of estrogen and progesterone, and estrogen replacement therapy (ERT) is taking only estrogen. Research studies have shown that HRT and ERT help protect postmenopausal women against cardiovascular diseases by increasing the levels of HDLs in the blood. HRT also lowers LDL levels and fibrinogen, a blood-clotting factor, in the blood. These therapies also relieve many menopausal symptoms and help protect women against osteoporosis. It is impor-

tant for women to discuss these therapies with their physician and to understand the benefits and risks of each before making a decision whether to use HRT or ERT.

RISK FACTORS THAT YOU CAN CHANGE

1. *Diet.* A high-fat and high-cholesterol diet puts you at a greater risk for developing atherosclerosis (fatty deposits along the walls of arteries). Slowly make dietary changes to include more vegetables, fruits, grains, poultry, fish, and other low-fat foods a part of your daily diet. (Also, see Chapter 18 for more information on nutrition.)
2. *Weight.* If you weigh more than you should, you are at greater risk for heart disease. Extra weight means extra work for the heart and in many cases contributes to high blood pressure, increased blood cholesterol, and increased risk of developing diabetes. Changing dietary habits and exercising will help you to maintain a healthy weight and your heart muscle in good shape.
3. *Exercise.* Physical activity has an effect on blood cholesterol. *Aerobic* exercise increases the HDL levels (high-density lipoproteins—the "good" lipoproteins), improves the heart's blood and oxygen supply, and strengthens the heart muscle. *Strength training* exercise builds muscle and may help to reduce the LDL levels (low-density lipoproteins—the "bad" lipoproteins). The combination of these exercises probably provides maximum protection to the heart. It is thought that the more you exercise and the greater the intensity used, the more you can reduce your risk for heart attack.
4. *Tobacco.* If you smoke or chew tobacco, you can greatly reduce your risk for heart disease by quitting—*now.* Heart disease is the number-one killer of smokers. Many programs are available to help people quit smoking. Also, medications can be prescribed by the physician to help you overcome the addiction to nicotine.
5. *Response to stress.* How you handle stress and anger also plays a role in your risk for heart disease. When you are overstressed and not handling it well, your heart has to work harder and faster, your blood pressure goes up, arteries narrow, levels of blood cholesterol and clotting factors increase, and abnormal heart rhythms can occur. These are all factors that increase your risk for heart disease over time. Exercise and various relaxation and stress management techniques can help reduce these risks.

More information on heart and blood vessel health can be obtained from the following resources:

American Heart Association

For information, contact your local American Heart Association or call: 1-800-242-8721

http://www.americanheart.org (Web site)

Continued

ELECTROCARDIOGRAM

Electrocardiogram Paper

To understand the significance of each wave and interval of various heights and widths recorded by an electrocardiograph, the medical assistant needs to know the significance of the small and large blocks on the ECG paper (Figure 16-4, *A*). On the horizontal line, which measures **time,** one small block represents 0.04 second (Figure 16-4, *B*). On the vertical axis, which measure **voltage** or **amplitude,** one small block represents 1 millimeter (mm). Because a large block is five small blocks wide and five deep, each large block represents 0.2 second (horizontal) and 5 mm (vertical).

Notice all the lines. Every fifth line (horizontal and vertical) is usually printed darker than other lines, producing blocks (squares) that are 5 × 5 mm. Thus two of the larger blocks equal 10 mm, or 1 cm.

These measurements, accepted internationally, allow physicians to interpret cardiac time (rate) on the horizontal line and cardiac voltage on the vertical axis and thus determine if the electrical activity of the heart is within normal limits.

ECG paper is heat sensitive and pressure sensitive. When the machine is on and running, a heated stylus moves over the paper to record the cardiac cycles. Because it is pressure sensitive, ECG paper must be handled carefully to avoid markings that would blemish the actual tracing.

Interpretation

When the physician interprets an ECG, the following factors are usually determined:

- **Rate**—How many beats per minute; determined are the atrial rate and the ventricular rate.
- **Rhythm**—Whether the heart rhythm is regular or irregular; determined are the atrial rhythm and the ventricular rhythm.
- **Conduction time**—How long it takes for the impulse originating at the SA node to stimulate ventricular contraction (review the conduction system, p. 707); determined are the P-R interval and the QRS duration.
- **Configuration and location**—Of each wave, the ST segment, the P-R interval, and sometimes the Q-T interval.

These findings are then recorded and reviewed by the physician to help establish a diagnosis or evaluate current treatment.

Because many physicians expect the medical assistant who takes a patient's ECG to monitor the graph for abnormal or erratic tracings, or artifacts (see p. 717), you should be aware of *heart rates and rhythms.*

Heart rate and rhythm. In a normal ECG, all heartbeats consist of three major units—the P wave, the QRS complex, and the T wave—and they appear as a similar pattern, equally spaced.

Briefly, the rate of a particular rhythm may be determined from the ECG simply by noting the distance between two R waves. As seen in Figure 16-4, *A,* two large squares between R waves indicate that the rate is 150 beats per minute; three large squares between R waves indicate that the rate is 100 beats per minute. Similarly, four large squares between R waves indicate a heart rate of 75 beats per minute. To obtain this rate per minute, divide the number of large squares between the R waves into 300. **NOTE:** If the rhythm is irregular, counting the squares in a single R-R interval gives an approximate rather than the precise rate that would be obtained with a perfectly regular rhythm. To calculate heart rate when the rhythm is *irregular,* count the number of cycles in a 6-second strip and multiply by 10. The ECG paper is marked along the top in intervals. Fifteen large squares equals 3 seconds. Thirty large squares equals 6 seconds (see Figure 16-13).

To determine if heart rhythm is regular or irregular, the distance between each P wave and then that between each R wave are measured. If the distance between all P waves is the same, atrial rhythm is regular; if the distance varies, rhythm is irregular. Similarly, if the distance between all R waves is the same, ventricular rhythm is regular; if not, it is irregular.

FIGURE 16-4 ECG paper with section enlarged. **A,** Number of large squares between recorded R waves indicate rate of heartbeat per minute; **B,** one large square enlarged; **C,** determining the heart rate.

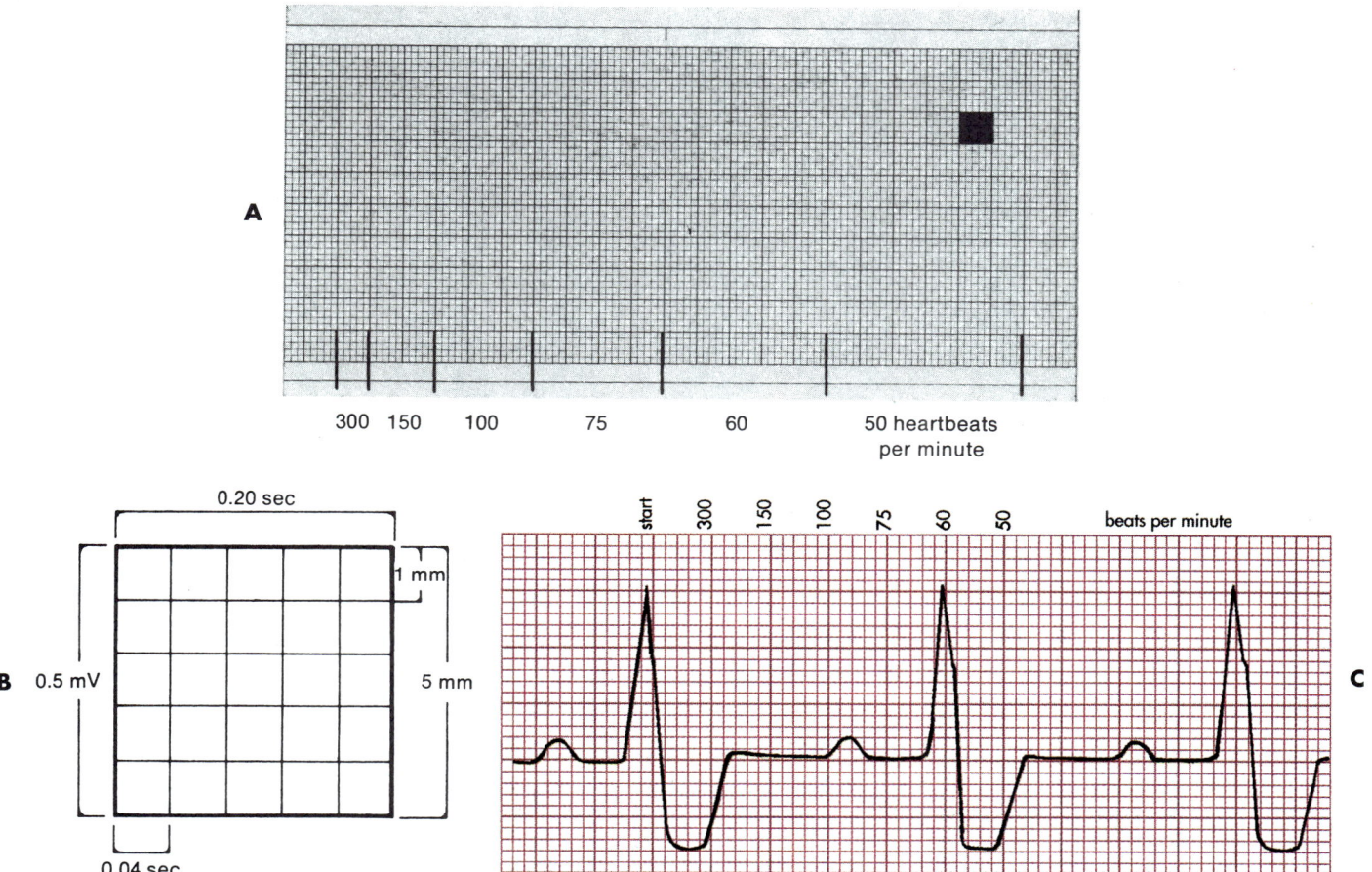

Normal sinus rhythm (Figure 16-5, *A*).

The term **normal sinus rhythm** refers to an ECG that is within normal limits. In normal sinus rhythm, the heart rate is 60 to 100 beats per minute, the rhythm is regular, P waves are present, QRS waves are of normal duration, and the P/QRS relationship and PR intervals are all within normal limits.

Normal sinus rhythm reflects normal electrical activity, that is, the rhythm originated in the SA node (the normal pacemaker of the heart) and followed normal pathways to the AV node, the bundle of His, the right and left bundle branches, and the Purkinje fibers, resulting in atrial and ventricular contraction (depolarization).

The **P waves** appear normal in shape (usually small and rounded) and uniform in appearance, followed by the QRS complex. The **P-R interval** is normally 0.12 to 0.20 second long. The **QRS complex** may be upright (positive) or downward (negative), depending on the monitoring lead and the conduction through the heart muscle. The width, measuring from the beginning to the end of the complex, should be between 0.06 and 0.12 second. If it goes over 0.12 second, it indicates prolonged contraction through the ventricles. The **T wave** is small and rounded and indicates ventricular recovery (repolarization). During this phase, the ventricles relax and refill with blood pumped from the atria. The **ST segment** is normally flat and varies according to heart rate—the faster the rate, the shorter the segment.

Common Rhythms (see Figure 16-5)

Sinus rhythms. Three arrhythmias that originate in the sinus or sinoatrial node are the following:

- **Sinus tachycardia**—A regular sinus rhythm of 100 to 180 beats per minute. It may be one of the first signs of congestive heart failure. It may also be seen when the patient has a fever; is anxious; has hypotension, hyperthyroidism, or chronic obstructive pulmonary disease; or is taking the drugs atropine, epinephrine, ephedrine, or Sudafed, or substances such as caffeine, nicotine, and cocaine.

- **Sinus bradycardia**—A regular sinus rhythm of less than 60 beats per minute. This may be seen in a patient with hypothyroidism, meningitis, disease of the SA node, or acute myocardial infarction (MI); in an athlete; or in a patient who is taking digitalis, propranolol, or verapamil.

- **Sinus arrhythmia** (dysrhythmia)—An irregular sinus rhythm in which the cycle lengths vary. It is a normal response of the heart to respiration in which the rate increases

Text continued on p. 717

FIGURE 16-5   Common cardiac rhythms and arrhythmias. **A,** Sinus rhythm; **B,** sinus bradycardia.

Sinus Rhythm.

Rate	60-100 beats per minute
Rhythm	Atrial regular Ventricular regular
P waves	Uniform in appearance, upright, normal shape, one preceding each QRS complex
PR interval	0.12-0.20 second
QRS	0.10 second or less. If greater than 0.10 second in duration, the QRS is termed "wide" since the existence of a bundle branch block or other intraventricular conduction defect cannot be accurately detected in a single-lead.

A

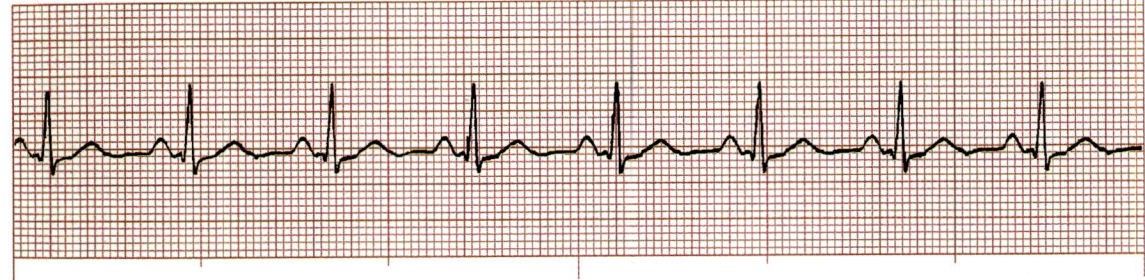

Sinus Bradycardia.

Rate	Less than 60 beats per minute
Rhythm	Atrial regular Ventricular regular
P waves	Uniform in appearance, upright, normal shape, one preceding each QRS complex
PR interval	0.12-0.20 second
QRS	Usually 0.10 second or less

B

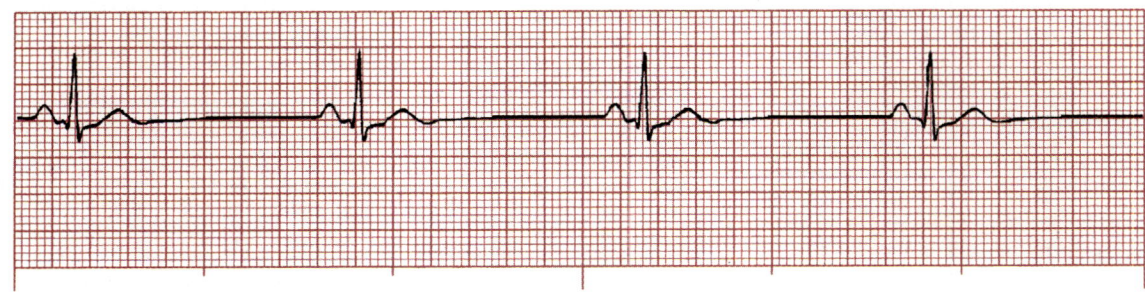

FIGURE 16-5—cont'd   Common cardiac rhythms and arrhythmias. **C,** Sinus tachycardia; **D,** sinus dysrhythmia.

Sinus Tachycardia.

Rate	Less than 100-160 beats per minute
Rhythm	Atrial regular Ventricular regular
P waves	Uniform in appearance, upright, normal shape, one preceding each QRS complex
PR interval	0.12-0.20 second
QRS	Usually 0.10 second or less

C

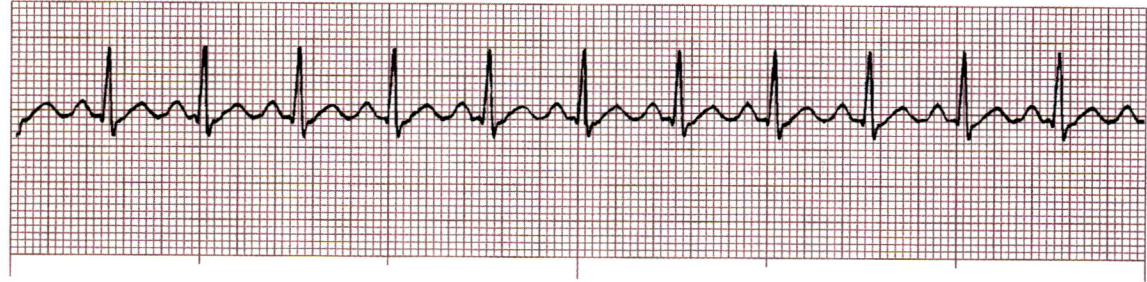

Sinus Dysrhythmia (Arrhythmia).

Rate	Usually 60-100 beats per minute but may be faster or slower
Rhythm	Irregular (R-R intervals shorten during inspiration and lengthen during expiration)
P waves	Uniform in appearance, upright, normal shape, one preceding each QRS complex
PR interval	0.12-0.20 second
QRS	Usually 0.10 second or less

D

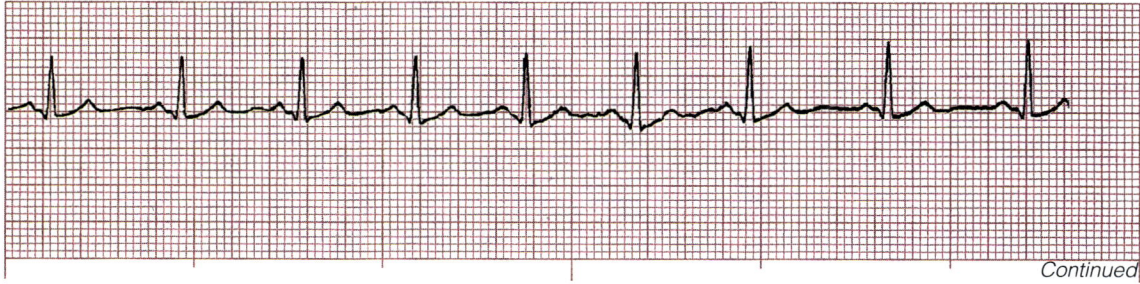

Continued

FIGURE 16-5—cont'd   Common cardiac rhythms and arrhythmias. **E,** Premature atrial complexes (PACs); **F,** paroxysmal atrial or supraventricular tachycardia.

Premature Atrial Complexes (PACs).

Rate	Usually normal, but depends on underlying rhythm.
Rhythm	Essentially regular with premature beats
P waves	Premature Differ from sinus P waves—may be flattened, notched, pointed, biphasic, or lost in the preceding T wave
PR interval	Varies from 0.12-0.20 second when the pacemaker site is near the SA node; 0.12 second when the pacemaker site is nearer the AV junction.
QRS	Usually less than 0.10 second but may be prolonged. The QRS of the PAC is similar to those of the underlying rhythm unless the PAC is abnormally conducted.

E

The fifth complex from the left is the PAC.

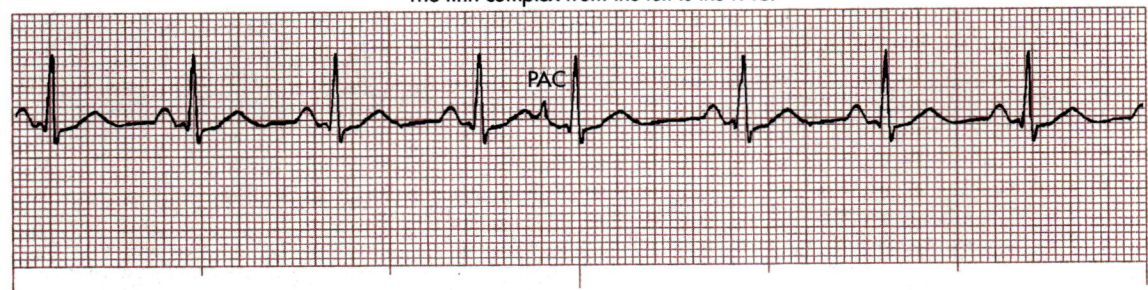

F

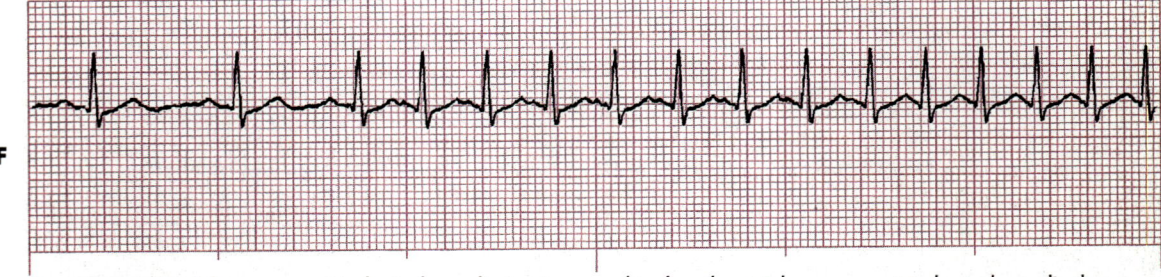

Paroxysmal atrial or supraventricular tachycardia is a term used to describe atrial or supraventricular tachycardia that starts and ends suddenly.

FIGURE 16-5—cont'd   Common cardiac rhythms and arrhythmias. **G,** Atrial fibrillation; **H,** premature ventricular complexes or ventricular premature beats.

Atrial Fibrillation.

Rate	Atrial rate usually greater than 350-400 beats per minute; ventricular rate variable
Rhythm	Ventricular rhythm usually very irregular; a regular ventricular rhythm may occur because of digitalis toxicity.
P waves	No identifiable P waves; fibrillatory waves present. Erratic, wavy baseline.
PR interval	Not measurable
QRS	Usually less than 0.10 second but may be widened if an intraventricular conduction defect exists

G

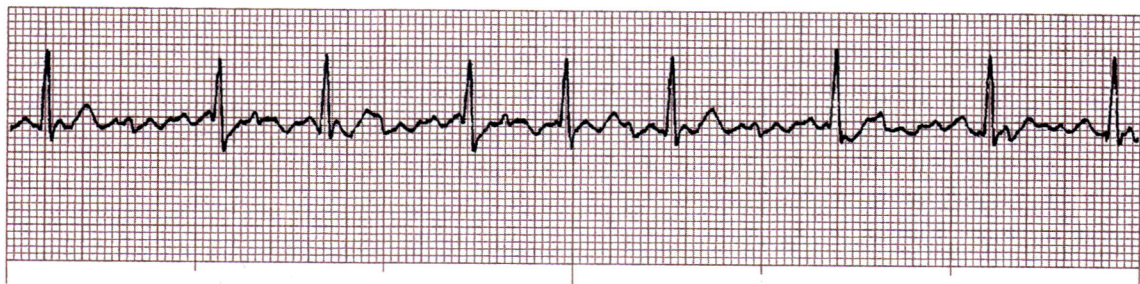

Premature Ventricular Complexes or Ventricular Premature Beats.

Rate	Usually normal, but depends on the underlying rhythm
Rhythm	Essentially regular with premature beats. If the PVC is an interpolated PVC, the rhythm will be regular.
P waves	There is no P wave associated with the PVC
PR interval	None with the PVC because the ectopic originates in the ventricles
QRS	Greater than 0.12 second. Wide and bizarre. T wave frequently in opposite direction of the QRS complex.

H

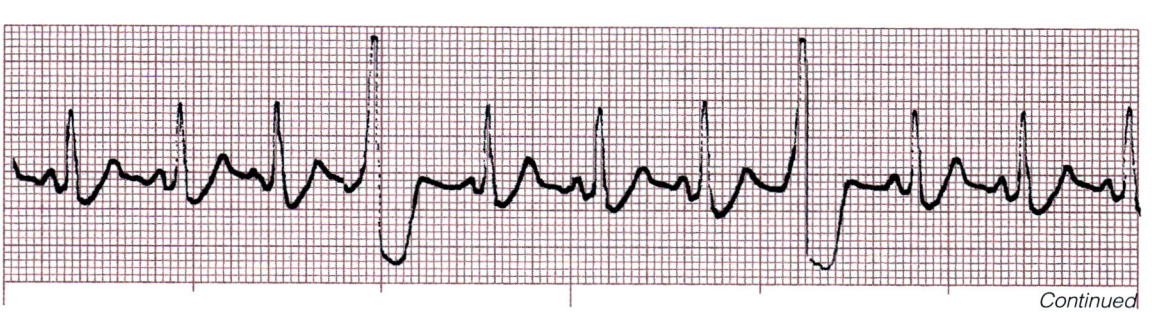

Continued

FIGURE 16-5—cont'd Common cardiac rhythms and arrhythmias. **I,** Ventricular tachycardia; **J,** ventricular fibrillation.

Ventricular Tachycardia (VT).

Rate	Atrial rate not discernable, ventricular rate 100-250 beats per minute
Rhythm	Atrial rhythm not discernible. Ventricular rhythm is essentially regular.
P waves	May be present or absent; if present they have no set relationship to the QRS complexes—appearing between the QRS's at a rate different from that of the VT.
PR interval	None
QRS	Greater than 0.12 second. Often difficult to differentiate between the QRS and the T wave.

I

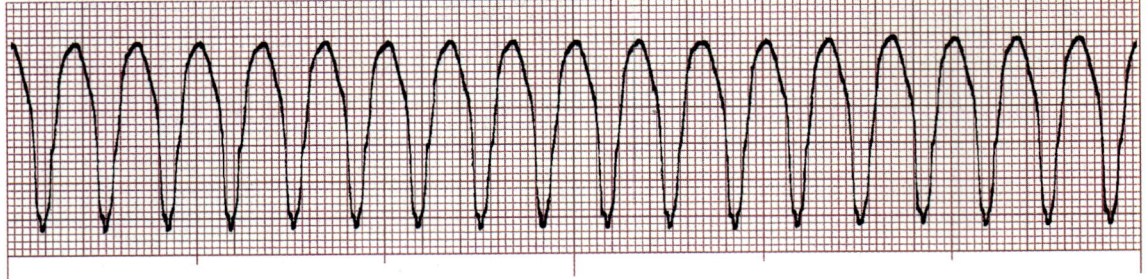

Ventricular Fibrillation.

Rate	Cannot be determined since there are no discernible waves or complexes to measure
Rhythm	Rapid and chaotic with no pattern or regularity
P waves	Not discernible
PR interval	Not discernible
QRS	Not discernible

J

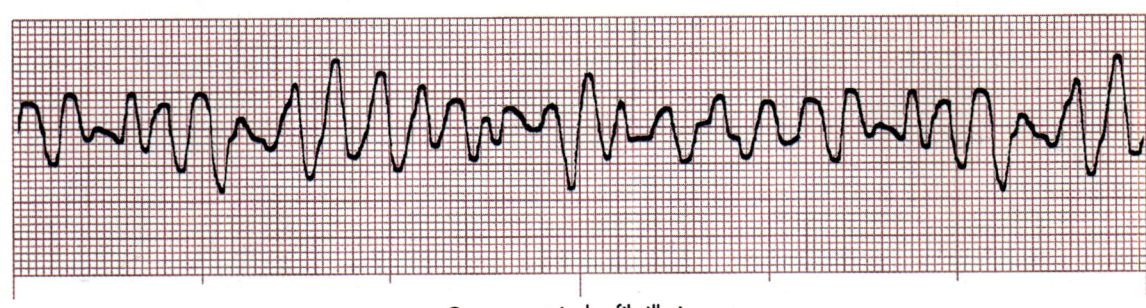

Coarse ventricular fibrillation

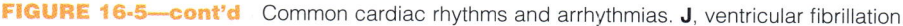

FIGURE 16-5—cont'd   Common cardiac rhythms and arrhythmias. **J**, ventricular fibrillation.

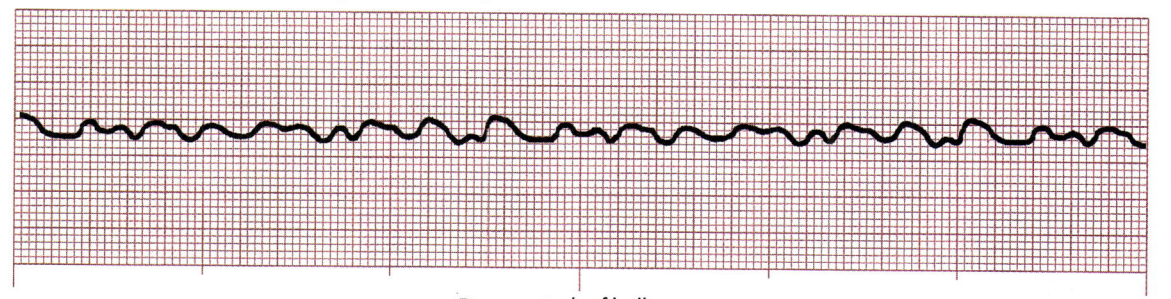

J

Fine ventricular fibrillation

with inspiration and decreases with expiration. It is commonly seen in the young and elderly and in a healthy heart during exercise or mental stress. Other causes include aging, postprandial hypotension, diabetes, and alcoholic cardiomyopathy.

Atrial arrhythmias.   Three arrhythmias that originate outside of the sinus node and above the branching portion of the bundle of His are the following (Figure 16-5):

- **Premature atrial contractions (complexes) (PACs)**—An irregular rhythm resulting from a premature atrial contraction originating within the atria but outside of the sinus node. PACs may be caused by a variety of stimuli, such as stress, caffeine, tobacco, hypoxia, electrolyte imbalance, or congestive heart failure (in MI), or with digitalis toxicity.
- **Paroxysmal atrial tachycardia (PAT)**—A regular rhythm of 140 to 250 beats per minute. This often has a sudden onset and terminates suddenly. It can occur in a healthy person or in a person who has heart disease. PAT also can be a sign of digitalis toxicity and can deteriorate into *atrial flutter* or *fibrillation*.
- **Atrial fibrillation**—An irregular rhythm of 150 to 200 beats per minute. This diagnosis is made because of an irregular ventricular rhythm and the absence of the P waves on the ECG. It is seen in patients with heart disease, pericarditis, mitral valve disease, hypertension, and pulmonary embolism.

Ventricular arrhythmias (Figure 16-5)
- **Premature ventricular contractions (complexes) (PVCs) or ventricular premature beat (VPB)**—An irregular rhythm with a distorted QRS complex and no P wave. PVCs are common after a myocardial infarction (MI) or in heart disease and are often associated with an increased incidence of ventricular fibrillation or tachycardia or sudden death. In people with healthy hearts, PVCs are

not associated with sudden death and are not treated. Anxiety, caffeine, and even anemia can cause PVCs.
- **Ventricular tachycardia**—A regular rhythm 75% of the time consisting of three or more PVCs at the rate of 120 to 250 beats per minute. Life-threatening ventricular tachycardia may lead to ventricular fibrillation. This is seen in patients with coronary artery disease or acute MI, digitalis toxicity, hypoxia, and anemia and with caffeine intake and also anxiety.
- **Ventricular fibrillation**—A disorganized activity in the ventricles. Ventricular fibrillation is very serious because the heart quivers and twitches but does not pump blood into the body. There is electrical chaos in the ventricles. It is caused by MI or ischemia and can be preceded by a PVC or ventricular tachycardia. It can result in cardiac arrest and death. (See Portable Automated External Defibrillator in Chapter 17.)

Artifacts.   Artifacts are defects (unwanted activity) on the electrocardiograph *not* caused by the electrical activity produced during the cardiac cycle. Because the ECG picks up and records every kind of electrical activity it can find, artifacts may appear, making the recording difficult to interpret. To remedy this situation, you should understand what causes artifacts and how they can be eliminated or greatly minimized and use the correct recording technique.

Of several **types of artifacts,** the most common are somatic tremor (muscle movement), wandering baseline (baseline shift), and alternating current (AC) interference.

Somatic tremor.   These artifacts can be identified by the unnatural baseline deflections, ranging from irregular vibrations in amplitude and frequency (jagged peaks of irregular height and spacing) to large shifting of the baseline (Figure 16-6, *A*). Muscle movement, which is either voluntary or involuntary, produces artifacts caused mainly when the patient:

- Is tense or apprehensive
- Moves or talks
- Is in an uncomfortable position
- Suffers from a nervous disorder that causes constant tremors, such as Parkinson's disease

The best way to avoid these patient-produced artifacts is to prepare the patient well, both emotionally and physically, preferably in a pleasant and relaxing atmosphere. The following will aid in patient preparation:

- Gain the full cooperation of the patient.
- Explain the procedure and what you will be doing.
- Position the patient comfortably, with limbs well supported.
- Offer assistance and reassurance as needed.
- Have patients suffering from a nervous disorder put their hands, palms down, under the buttocks or take a deep breath. This will help reduce artifacts (see also Preparation of Patient on p. 722).

Wandering baseline (baseline shift) (see Figure 16-6, B). Causes of this artifact include the following:

1. Electrodes that are applied too tightly or too loosely
2. Tension on an electrode as a result of an unsupported lead wire that is pulling the electrode away from the patient's skin

3. Too little or poor quality electrolyte gel or paste on an electrode
4. Corroded or dirty electrodes
5. Skin creams or lotions present on the area where the electrode is applied

To prevent artifacts, correct and attentive technique when applying the electrodes with the electrolyte gel or paste is a must. Wash the electrodes after each use and occasionally with kitchen cleanser but *never* use steel wool. Electrolyte gels or pastes that are left on the electrode can cause corrosion, which makes the electrode a poor conductor of cardiac electrical currents. The tips of the lead wires must also be kept clean.

Ensure that the patient's skin where the electrodes will be applied is clean; if necessary, wash the area briskly with alcohol or the presaturated electrolyte pads before applying the electrode.

Alternating current interference. Alternating current (AC) artifacts appear as a series of small regular peaks (or spiked lines) on the electrocardiogram (see Figure 16-6, C).

AC is our standard source for electrical power, and AC in electrical equipment or wires can radiate or leak a small amount of energy into the immediate area. When a patient is present in this area, some of the AC may be picked up by the body, which in turn is detected by the electrocardiograph. Thus an ECG with AC artifacts results. Common causes of AC interference artifacts include the following:

FIGURE 16-6 ECG artifacts. **A,** Somatic tremor artifact; **B,** wandering baseline; **C,** alternating current artifact. (From Conover MB: *Understanding electrocardiography,* ed 4, St Louis, 1992, Mosby.)

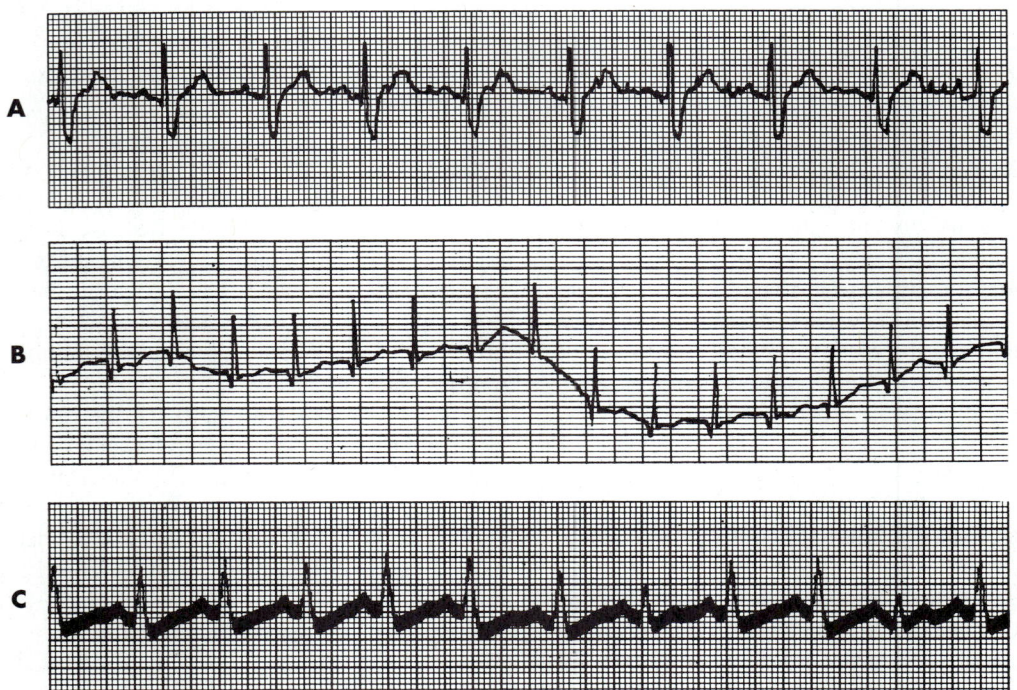

1. Improper grounding of the electrocardiograph
2. Presence of other electrical equipment in the room
3. Electrical wiring in walls or ceilings
4. X-ray or other large electrical equipment being used in adjacent rooms
5. Lead wires crossed and not following the contour of the patient's body
6. Corroded or dirty electrodes
7. Faulty technique of the operator

To minimize or eliminate AC interference, correct technique is required. The ECG unit must be properly grounded. Check the instructions in the operator's manual supplied with each unit by the manufacturer. Newer units have three-pronged plugs that are inserted into a properly grounded, three-receptacle outlet. Older units may have a two-pronged plug. In this case a ground wire from the unit is connected to a suitable ground, such as a cold water pipe.

Unplug other electrical equipment in the room. When x-ray equipment is being used in adjacent rooms, it may be necessary for you to wait until that procedure is completed or move to another room to record the ECG. Moving the patient table away from the wall may help minimize interference caused from electrical wiring. Lead wires must be straight and positioned to follow body contour; the line cord is to be away from the patient, and the unit should be near the patient's feet, not head. Electrodes must be cleaned after each use and occasionally should be scrubbed with a kitchen cleanser.

Additional problems.   When recording an ECG, you may encounter a few additional erratic tracings, which may appear as follows:

- An indistinct tracing usually caused by (1) the stylus heat being too low, (2) a bent stylus, (3) incorrect stylus pressure, or (4) a broken stylus heating element, which results in no tracing
- A straight line but no tracing, caused by the patient cable not being plugged in correctly
- A break between complexes, caused by a loose or broken lead wire

When you cannot correct the cause of an artifact, inform the physician and call the manufacturer or other repair service, according to office policy.

Electrocardiogram Electrodes and Electrolytes

Electrodes (also called **sensors**) are small metal plates or disposable self-adhesive conductive material pads placed on the patient to pick up the electrical activity of the heart and conduct it to the electrocardiograph. The standard 12-lead electrocardiograph has five electrodes: two to be attached to the fleshy part of the arms, two to be attached to the fleshy part of the legs, and one floating electrode that is placed in six different positions on the chest when recording the chest leads.

In the machine, this electrical current is changed into mechanical action, which is recorded on the ECG paper by a heated stylus. The small amount of electrical activity given off by the body is enlarged on the ECG paper by means of an **amplifier** inside the electrocardiograph. A **galvanometer,** also inside the ECG machine, changes the amplified voltages into mechanical action and records them on the paper. To help conduct this electric current, an **electrolyte** is applied to each electrode. These are used because skin is a poor conductor of electricity. Electrolytes are available in the form of gels, pastes, or flannel materials presaturated with an electrolyte solution. Electrolytes are not necessary when using disposable electrodes.

Once the electrodes are correctly secured to the patient with rubber straps, lead wires are fastened to them. These lead wires extend off the patient cable, which is attached to the electrocardiograph machine.

Electrocardiogram Leads

The standard 12-lead electrocardiograph system records electrical activity from the frontal and horizontal planes of the body by using 12 leads, as described in the text that follows.

Standard limb or bipolar leads.   The first three leads to be recorded on a standard ECG are known as leads I, II, and III. These are called bipolar leads because each of them uses two limb electrodes that record simultaneously the electrical forces of the heart from the frontal plane; that is, lead I records electrical activity between the right arm (RA) and left arm (LA); lead II records activity between the right arm and left leg; lead III records activity between the left arm (LA) and left leg (LL) (Figure 16-7, *A* and *B*).

FIGURE 16-7   **A,** Lead triangle showing position of standard limb leads; **B,** lead triangle showing position of augmented leads.

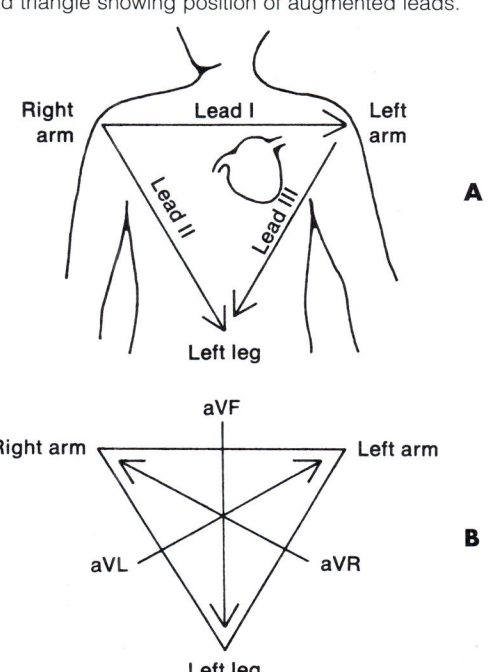

The right arm is considered a negative pole, and the left leg a positive pole. The left arm will either be negative or positive, depending on the lead; in lead I it is positive, and in lead III it is negative.

Upright (positive) deflections on the ECG indicate current flowing toward a positive pole; inverted (negative) wave deflections indicate current flowing toward a negative pole. For example, in lead I, the flow of current will be from a negative to a positive pole; thus the wave deflections on the recording will be upright.

Augmented leads. The next three leads are the augmented leads, designated as aV_R, aV_L, and aV_F. The *aV* stands for augmented voltage; the *R, L,* and *F* stand for right, left, and foot (leg), respectively. Augmented leads are unipolar and also record frontal plane activity.

Lead aV_R records electrical activity from the midpoint between the left arm and left leg to the right arm.

Lead aV_L records electrical activity from the midpoint between the right arm and left leg to the left arm.

Lead aV_F records electrical activity from the midpoint between the right arm and left arm to the left leg (Figure 16-7, *B*).

Chest or precordial leads. The last six leads of the standard 12-lead ECG are the chest or precordial leads. These leads are also unipolar and are designated as V_1, V_2, V_3, V_4, V_5, and V_6.

This third set of leads records electrical activity between six points on the chest wall and a point within the heart. To obtain these recordings, the chest electrode is moved to six predesignated positions on the chest. Figure 16-8 shows the location of these positions. The correct position *must* be used for each lead recording.

All 12 leads discussed can be interpreted separately or in combination. Each lead presents a picture of a different anatomic part of the heart, thus allowing the physician to determine areas of damage or problem areas.

When doing an ECG, the machine automatically connects the proper electrode potentials for leads I, II, III, aV_R, aV_L, and aV_F. To record the chest leads, the chest electrode must be moved manually to each of the assigned chest positions.

Suggested codes for marking leads. Certain codes are used to identify each lead recorded. Without these codes, determining which lead was being interpreted would be difficult and mounting the recording with proper lead identification would be impossible. An example of codes used is seen in Figure 16-8. On older machines the leads are coded (marked) by depressing the lead marker button. New machines automatically code for each lead as it is being recorded.

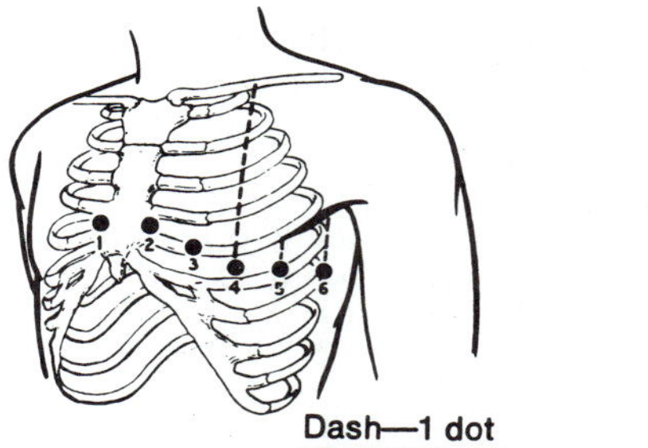

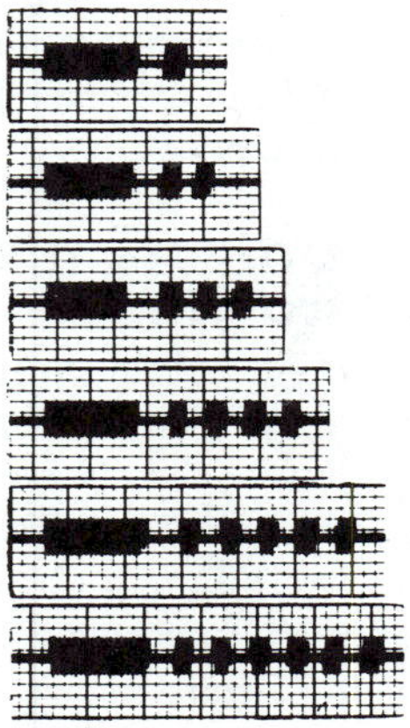

FIGURE 16-8 Leads of routine ECG. (Courtesy The Burdick Corporation, Milton, Wisc.)

Standardizing the Electrocardiograph

The diagnostic value of an ECG depends on an accurate recording. Standard techniques have been adopted to provide a recording that can be interpreted anywhere in the world, assuming the ECG machine used has been calibrated according to universal measurements.

The **universal standard** of ECG measurement is the following: 1 millivolt of cardiac electrical activity will deflect the stylus precisely 10 mm (1 cm) high (Figure 16-9, *A*). This is equal to 10 small blocks on the ECG paper.

Before any ECG is recorded, the machine must be standardized (that is, it must be checked to determine if it is set to record according to the universal measurement).

To standardize the machine, turn the main power switch on. The stylus should be positioned to run along on one of the dark horizontal lines. Set the lead selector switch to STD and the record switch to RUN. Quickly depress and release the standardization button. The standardization mark should reach 10 mm high and 2 mm wide. It appears as an open-ended rectangle (the open end being along the baseline). A slight slant may be seen in the top right corner, which is normal, but any other deviation is not normal and must be corrected. To correct any deviation, turn the standardization adjustment knob and repeat the procedure until the correct standardization mark is obtained.

You should consult the instruction manual provided by the manufacturer of each ECG machine because the aforementioned procedure may vary slightly among the various machines on the market.

When recording an ECG the R wave may have such a large amplitude that it goes off the ECG paper. One way to obtain a recording of the complete wave on the graph paper is to move the stylus to a different level on the paper. A **second method** is to set the standard at **one-half the usual size,** that is, set it at 5 mm rather than at the standard 10 mm high. By changing the standardization size the R wave is recorded at half the usual size or half the normal amplitude. This 5-mm standardization mark *must* be included with the lead when mounting the ECG so that the physician is be alerted to the change in amplitude (see Figure 16-9, *B*). At other times the waves being recorded may be extremely small, making the interpretation of the ECG very difficult. On these occasions the standardization mark can be **doubled in size,** that is, it can be made 20 mm high rather than the usual 10 mm high, which will double the size of the waves. *This changed standardization mark must be included with the wave(s) being recorded at this amplitude to allow for proper interpretation* (see Figure 16-9, *C*).

When the recording has been completed, the machine must be returned to the normal standard so that future recordings are not accidentally run at anything other than the normal standard of 10 mm high.

The **universal standard** for recording an ECG is at a **speed** of 25 mm per second. This can be increased on the machine to run the paper at 50 mm per second when segments of the ECG are close together or when heart rate is rapid. A notation of this change *must* be made so that the physician can accurately interpret the record.

Preparation and Procedure for Obtaining Electrocardiograms
Equipment
Bed or examining table (preferably without any metal
    attachments)
Linen sheet or blanket

FIGURE 16-9 **A,** Universal standard of ECG measurement 10 mm (1 cm) high. This is equal to 10 small blocks on the ECG paper; **B,** 5-mm high standardization mark one-half the universal standard; **C,** 20-mm high standardization mark, double the size of the universal standard of 10 mm.

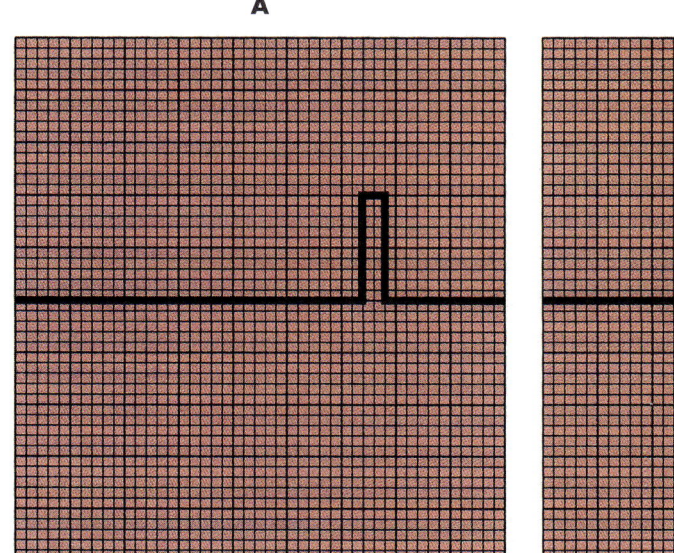
A

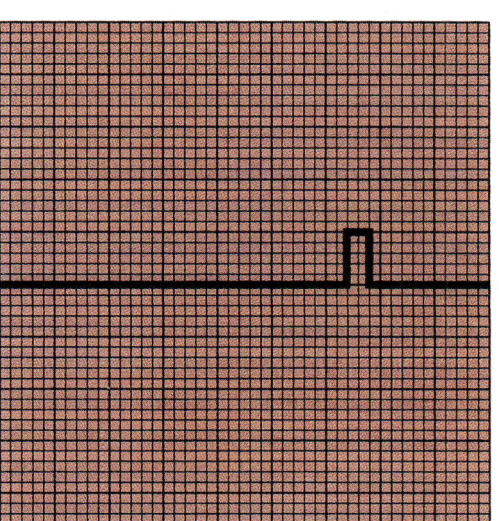
B

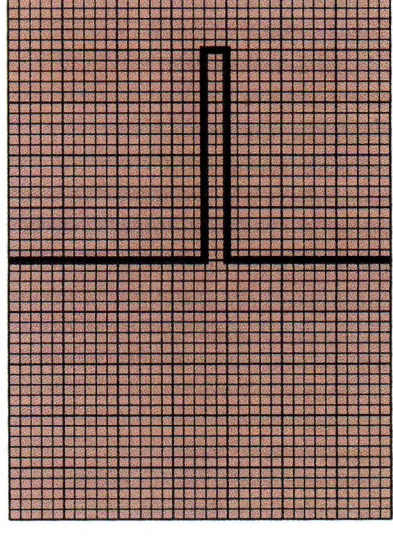
C

Electrocardiograph with patient cable lead wires
Electrolyte gel *or* paste *or* presaturated electrolyte pads
Electrodes and rubber straps
Gauze squares
Patient gown

Preparation of electrocardiograph room

1. The room should be as far away as possible from all x-ray and other electrical equipment that may cause artifacts on the ECG.
2. The room should be comfortably warm, quiet, pleasant, and not crowded with medical instruments, which may make the patient apprehensive.
3. The electrocardiograph (and patient) should be positioned away from wires, cords, and any other source of AC interference.
4. The bed or examining table must be wide enough so that the patient may rest comfortably with the extremities well supported; otherwise, muscle tension or tremors may cause artifacts.

Preparation of patient.

The quality of the record obtained is influenced by scrupulous attention to fundamental rules regarding the preparation of the patient. The medical assistant who is confident, but emphatic, will make it easier for the patient to relax, both mentally and physically.

1. Explain the nature and purpose of the electrocardiograph to the patient. Tactfully help the patient realize that full cooperation (that is, relaxing and not talking, moving, or chewing gum) helps to produce a reading that enables the physician to diagnose the patient's condition (when applicable).
2. Ensure the patient that no shock or other sensation will be felt.
3. Have the patient remove any jewelry that would interfere with the electrode placement or come in contact with the electrolyte.
4. Have the patient remove shoes and clothing from the forearms, lower legs, and chest; women may roll knee-hi stockings down. A patient gown should be put on with the opening in the front.

    NOTE: If a woman is wearing *sheer* nylons, saline- or alcohol-soaked pads can be placed over the stockings. This *cannot* be done over *thick* stockings because artifacts would result.
5. Help the patient assume a recumbent position on the table with arms at the sides and legs not touching. The extremities must be well supported on the table.
6. Place a cover over the patient with arms and lower legs exposed. Protecting the patient from cold or any other discomfort is very important. A small pillow can be placed under the head.
7. Locate and mark the six chest locations on the patient. (You can use a felt-tip pen and wash the markings off after the procedure with an alcohol sponge.) The patient gown over a woman's chest can be adjusted to avoid exposing the breasts and causing possible embarrassment and ap-

prehension, while still allowing you to adequately locate and record the chest lead positions.
8. Inquire if the patient has any questions before you begin the recording.

Application of electrodes and connection of lead wires

1. Expose the patient's arms and legs.
2. Attach one end of each rubber strap to each electrode (Figure 16-10, *A*). Disposable electrodes, when used properly, may be used for acceptable ECGs. Prepare the skin and carefully follow the manufacturer's instructions according to the type of electrode selected.
3. Place a small amount of electrolyte gel or paste, about the size of a pea, on the electrode (see Figure 16-10, *B*).
4. Using the side of the electrode, gently rub the electrolyte into the skin on the fleshy part of the right arm. Many cardiologists recommend that arm electrodes be placed on the upper arm because fewer muscle tremors are picked up from there. The area rubbed should not be much larger than the size of the electrode and should be slightly reddened by the rubbing. (If there is lotion or cream on the skin, remove it with an alcohol sponge before the electrolyte and electrode are applied.)
5. Place the electrode on this area; pull the rubber strap around and fasten it to the electrode. The electrode must not be pressing against the table or other body parts. The electrode must not be fastened too loosely or too tightly. Try to move the electrode about once secured in place. If it slips or slides on the limb, it is too loose and must be tightened; if the skin is pinched on either side of the electrode, the strap is too tight and must be loosened.
6. Using a gauze square, wipe away any excess gel or paste from around the electrode.
7. Follow this same procedure to apply the electrodes to the left arm and to the right and left legs over the fleshy part of the lower leg, *not* over the bone. By applying the electrodes to the fleshy areas on the limbs, the chance of undesirable muscle artifacts is minimized. Also use equal amounts of gel or paste on each electrode. Always follow the same pattern when applying electrodes to ensure consistency.
8. When using presaturated electrolyte pads rather than a gel or paste, rub the skin with the pad or a piece of gauze, then place the pad on the skin. The electrode is to be placed directly on top of the pad (see Figure 16-10, *C* and *D*).
9. *If taking an ECG on a patient who has a cast, amputation, or prosthesis, place the electrode above the affected area. The electrode for the other extremity must then be placed in the same location opposite the first. For example, if the patient has a cast extending from the knee to the ankle on the right leg, place the electrode on the inside of the upper right leg. The electrode for the left leg must then be placed on the inside of the upper left leg. If the electrodes are not placed in this manner (that is, if one electrode is placed on the upper part of the right limb above the cast and the other electrode is placed on the fleshy part of the lower left leg), the electric vector would be changed, and abnormal results would occur on the ECG.*

FIGURE 16-10 **A,** Attach rubber strap to electrode. **B,** Place small amount of electrolyte gel on electrode. **C,** Apply presaturated electrolyte pad and electrode to arm. **D,** Apply electrolyte pad, electrode, and rubber strap to arm. (Courtesy The Burdick Corporation, Milton, Wisc.)

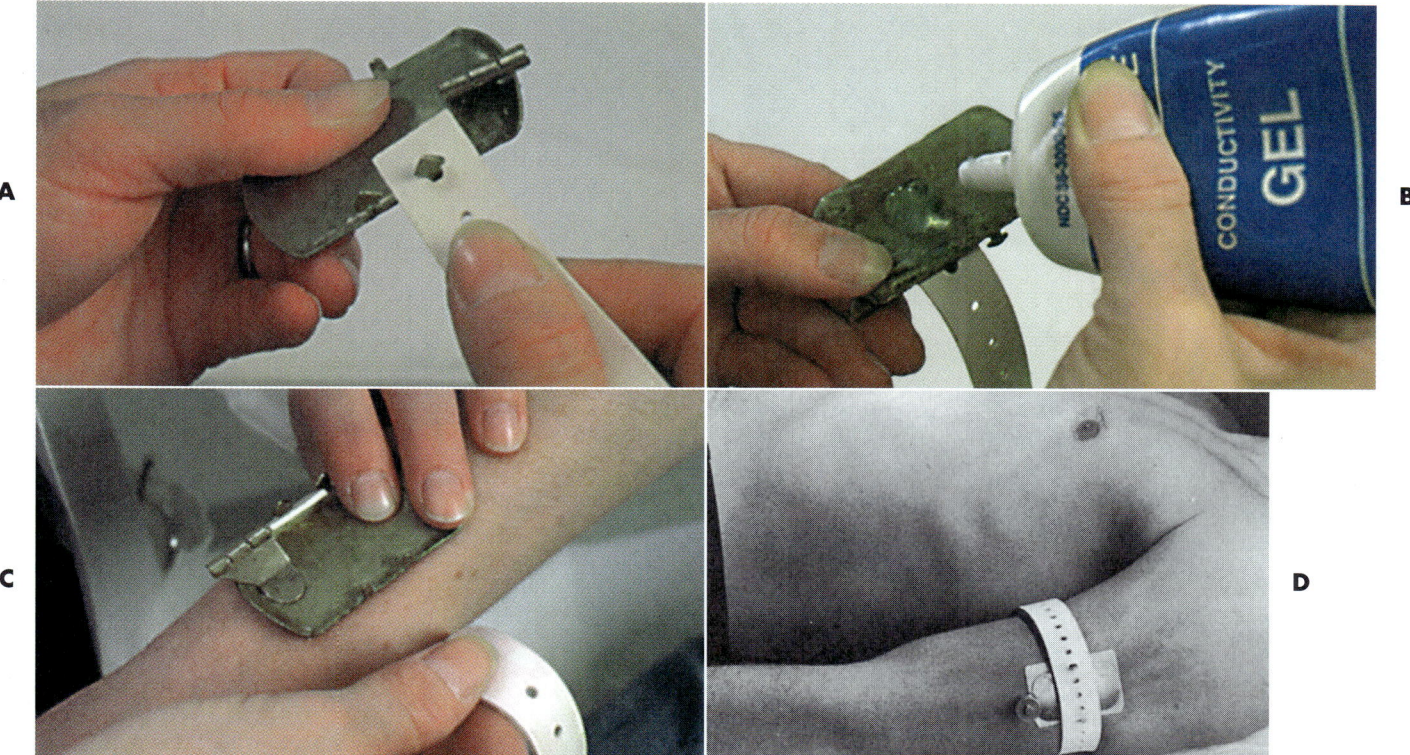

10. Leave the chest electrode unattached but not touching a direct surface *or* position it on the first chest position using the electrolyte of choice.
11. Firmly connect the patient cable lead wires to the proper electrodes so that the lead wire connector faces the patient's feet. Each wire is alphabetically coded: RA, right arm; LA, left arm; RL, right leg; LL, left leg; and C, chest. In addition, each lead wire is color coded to provide additional identification for the operator. The lead wires *must* be connected and arranged to follow the contour of the body without placing any strain on the electrodes so that the possibility of AC artifacts is minimized (Figure 16-11).
12. Plug the patient cable into the patient cable jack on the machine. Make sure that it is pushed in all the way.
13. Before beginning the recording, routinely check that all connections are secure, verify that the patient cable is supported on the table or over the patient's abdomen to prevent pulling of the cable, and see if the patient has any questions.

Recording the electrocardiogram (Figure 16-12)
Limb leads
1. Set the lead switch to STD (standard).
2. Turn recorder switch to ON. (Some machines require a warm-up period before recording. Check the instruction manual to determine if this is the case for the equipment you are using.)
3. Turn recorder switch to RUN.

FIGURE 16-11 Application of electrodes and connection to unit in correct positions. (Courtesy The Burdick Corporation, Milton, Wisc.)

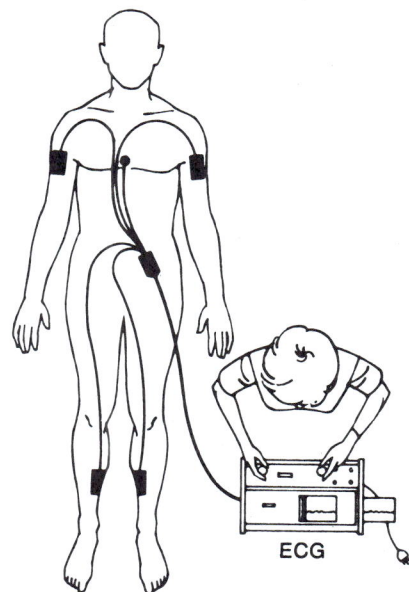

4. Center the baseline by turning the centering dial or position control knob.
5. Check the standardization; quickly depress and release the standardization button several times while the lead selector is on STD and the recorder switch is on RUN. The height of the standardization measurement should be 10 mm or two large squares from the baseline.

FIGURE 16-12 Single-channel electrocardiograph. Can be used in the manual mode or in the automatic mode. When used in automatic mode, the EK-10 records a complete 12-lead ECG in just 38 seconds. (Courtesy The Burdick Corporation, Milton, Wisc.)

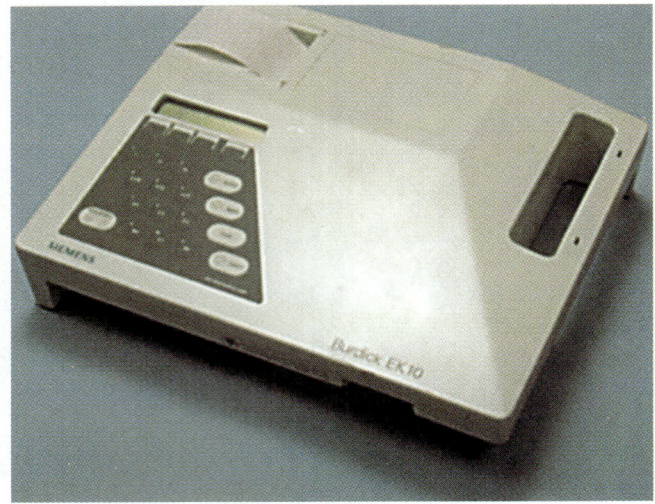

6. Turn the lead selector switch to lead I.
7. Mark the identification code for the lead immediately after it is selected, unless the machine does this automatically.
8. Run for a few heartbeats; depress the standardization button quickly if the physician requires proof of standardization for each lead. This standardization mark should be inserted between the T wave (or U wave when present) of one complex and the P wave of the next complex.
9. Record at least 8 to 10 inches to provide ample tracing of the lead.
10. Turn lead selector to lead II.
11. Repeat steps 7, 8, and 9.
12. Turn the lead selector to lead III and repeat steps, 7, 8, and 9.

Augmented leads: aV$_R$, aV$_L$, aV$_F$

13. Turn the lead selector to lead aV$_R$, mark the identification code, inset a standardization mark if required, and record 5 to 6 inches (see steps 7 and 8).
14. Turn the lead selector to lead aV$_L$ and repeat step 13.
15. Turn the lead selector to lead aV$_F$ and repeat step 13.
16. Turn off the machine.

Chest leads

17. Leave the limb electrodes and patient cable wires in place.
18. Position the chest electrode over the first chest position, V$_1$, applying the electrode with gel *or* paste *or* presaturated electrolyte pad in the same manner used for the limbs.
19. Turn the lead selector to STD, the recorder switch to RUN, and depress the standardization button.
20. Turn the recorder switch to OFF to prevent excessive movement of the stylus.
21. Turn the lead selector switch to V.
22. Turn the recorder switch to ON.
23. Mark the identification code for the lead and insert standardization marks as described in step 8, when required.

24. Record 5 to 6 inches.
25. Turn the recorder switch to OFF.
26. Move the chest electrode to the next position. Start again with step 21; repeat until all the chest leads have been recorded (that is, leads V$_1$ through V$_6$).
27. When all the leads have been recorded satisfactorily, turn the lead selector to STD and the recorder switch to OFF and unplug the power cord.
28. Disconnect the lead wires, unfasten the rubber straps, and remove the electrodes from the patient.
29. Wipe any electrolyte from the patient's skin.
30. Assist the patient as needed and provide further instructions as indicated. The patient may be free to leave *after* making a future appointment to review the results of the ECG with the physician, *or* the physician may wish to review the ECG with the patient at this time.
31. Label the recording with patient's name, date, and your initials.
32. Clean all equipment and return it to the proper storage area.
33. Wash your hands.
34. Record the procedure. Indicate if the patient was experiencing *any* chest pain during the recording. Chest pain could be correlated to an arrhythmia on the ECG.

    Charting Example

    October 3, 20__, 11 AM

    12-lead ECG done. Patient rested quietly during the procedure. Patient stated that he is taking verapamil and has brought his medication with him to review this therapy with Dr. Thomas.

    J.A. Lee, CMA

35. Mount the recording, using the preferred mount as indicated by the physician; record the required information on the mount. Sign your name to the mounted ECG.
36. Give the mounted ECG to the physician for review and interpretation.

Throughout the recording of the ECG, make sure that the stylus stays on the same baseline (Figure 16-13). Use the position control knob if any adjustment is necessary. Constantly watch for the appearance of any artifact. If an artifact does occur, determine the cause and correct the problem (refer to pp. 717-719).

Mounting an electrocardiogram. Mounting the ECG is important so that the recording can be protected, easily seen by the physician, and inserted into the patient's medical record after the physician has reviewed and interpreted it. A variety of commercially prepared mounts are available for use, or the recording can be mounted on a plain piece of paper. Regardless of the method chosen to mount the ECG, each lead must be correctly identified. In addition, the patient's name, address, age, sex, and the date of the recording must be documented. Other information may be included, varying with the physician's request, such as drugs the patient is taking (especially cardiac drugs such as digitalis and quinidine), height, weight, blood pressure, and occupation. See Figure 16-14 for sample mounts and specific directions for mounting the ECG.

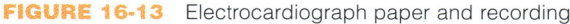

FIGURE 16-13   Electrocardiograph paper and recording.

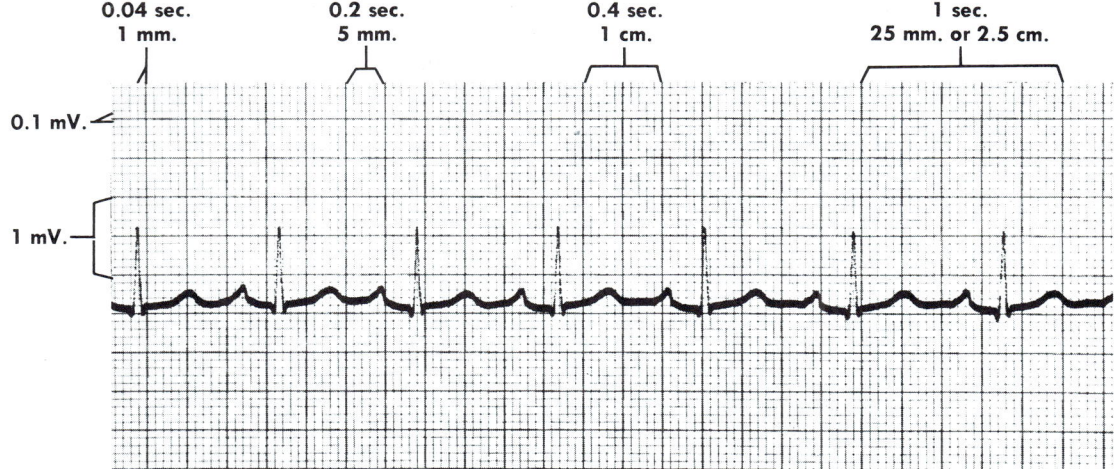

FIGURE 16-14   **A,** Sample ECG mount for mounting a three-channel electrocardiogram strip. Directions are given on the mount. (Courtesy Hewlett-Packard, Palo Alto, Calif.)

AGE _____ SEX _____ HT _____ WT _____ BP _____ OCCUPATION _____ WARD _____ PATIENT _____

DOCTOR _____   PATIENT NUMBER _____   DIGITALIS YES ☐ NO ☐   QUINIDINE _____ YES ☐ NO ☐   YES ☐ NO ☐   DATE _____ ECG NO. _____

ATRIAL RATE _____   P-R INTERVAL _____   VENTRICULAR RATE _____   Q-R-S INTERVAL _____   Q-T INTERVAL _____   S-T SEGMENT _____   ELEC. AXIS _____

RHYTHM _____   P WAVES _____   T WAVES _____

REMARKS _____

_____

_____

PATIENT/NUMBER

ADDITIONAL INFORMATION   OVER ☐

| LEADS 1-2-3 | AVR–AVL–AVF | V₁–V₂–V₃ | V₄–V₅–V₆ | CAL. 1 MV |

MOUNTING INSTRUCTIONS

1. CUT RECORD TO 11 INCHES.
2. REMOVE THIS PART OF THE PROTECTIVE PAPER BY BENDING THE CARD AT THE ARROW. LIFT THE CORNER OF THE PAPER AND PEEL IT OFF TO EXPOSE THE GUMMED SURFACE.

3. STARTING IN THE UPPER LEFT HAND CORNER, LINE UP THE TOP OF THE RECORD WITH THE TOP OF THE GUMMED SURFACE AND LIGHTLY PRESS DOWN.
4. WHEN ALIGNMENT IS SATISFACTORY, PEEL OFF THE REMAINING PROTECTIVE PAPER AND SMOOTH THE RECORD.

A

| LEADS 1-2-3 | AVR–AVL–AVF | V₁–V₂–V₃ | V₄–V₅–V₆ | CAL. 1 MV |

Continued

FIGURE 16-14—cont'd **B,** Sample ECG mount with instructions for use with single-strip ECG. (Courtesy Hewlett-Packard, Palo Alto, Calif.)

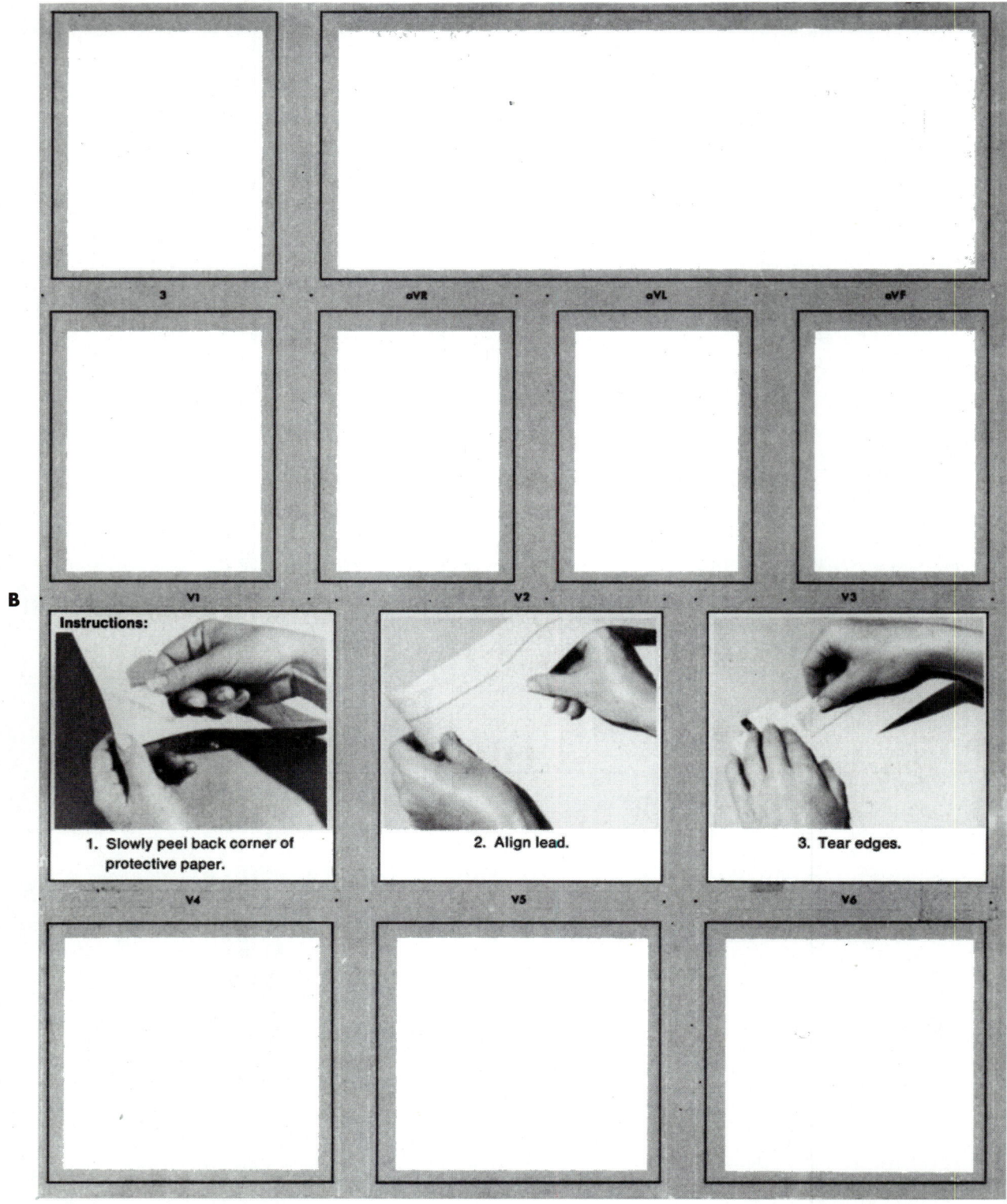

FIGURE 16-14—cont'd   **C,** Information to be recorded on back of single-strip ECG mount. (Courtesy Hewlett-Packard, Palo Alto, Calif.)

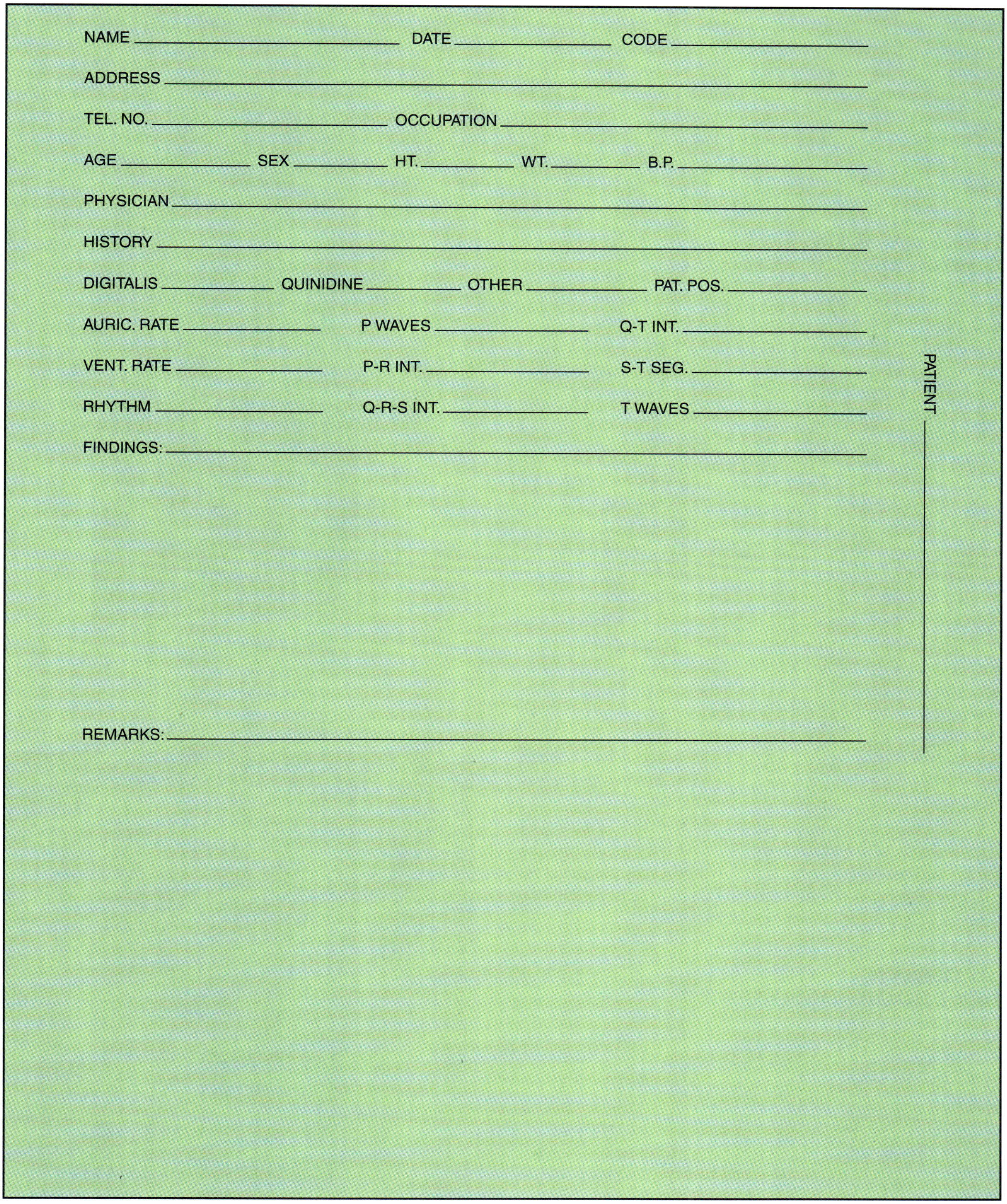

NAME _____ DATE _____ CODE _____

ADDRESS _____

TEL. NO. _____ OCCUPATION _____

AGE _____ SEX _____ HT. _____ WT. _____ B.P. _____

PHYSICIAN _____

HISTORY _____

DIGITALIS _____ QUINIDINE _____ OTHER _____ PAT. POS. _____

AURIC. RATE _____   P WAVES _____   Q-T INT. _____

VENT. RATE _____   P-R INT. _____   S-T SEG. _____

RHYTHM _____   Q-R-S INT. _____   T WAVES _____

FINDINGS: _____

REMARKS: _____

PATIENT

C

Cleaning Electrodes

All of the suction cup–type electrodes must be wiped clean immediately after each ECG is completed to prevent residual buildup and subsequent contact problems. Use only alcohol or soap and water to clean electrode surfaces, because polishes, commercial cleaners, and other such items if used can cause artifacts in the ECG tracing. Also, never use a scrub brush to clean the electrode surfaces because the metal plating is very thin and can be scraped away, thus rendering the electrodes useless.

PHONE-A-GRAM: THE COMPUTERIZED ECG

For over 2000 years, physicians from Hippocrates to Laënnec and Einthoven and many others have sought to improve diagnostic accuracy. By 1971 a computer-assisted ECG analysis program was developed. Phone-A-Gram is an example of a computerized ECG service providing all the necessary equipment and a second opinion for the diagnosis of a patient's condition.

This service includes a portable automatic ECG transmitter (a standard model, a scout model, or the strip-chart recorder model), all the auxiliary equipment, and a personal hookup into the national network (Data Center), which receives, converts, processes, analyzes, and prints out all ECG information for ready reference.

All ECG transmitting units are compact, portable, single-channel units with features of automatic lead switching and standardization across all 12 leads. The *standard model* is a battery-powered portable unit, but it does not provide a strip-chart. Like the standard model, the *scout model* is used in conjunction with a conventional electrocardiograph to produce an on-site tracing as the ECG is being transmitted.

The patient is prepared for the ECG in the usual manner, except all six chest lead electrodes must be applied to the patient's chest before you begin to record the ECG.

A standard telephone is used to dial the Data Center. The telephone handset is placed on the Phone-A-Gram unit, and the ECG is transmitted at the push of a button. The unit picks up signals from the patient and transmits them over the telephone to the Data Center for interpretation.

AUTOMATIC ELECTROCARDIOGRAPHS

The newer electrocardiographs have fewer operating controls and are much easier to use. With these new machines, you *don't* have to adjust controls such as position, sensitivity, heat, paper speed, run, and lead markers. You just set one switch to select the format that you want to record (Figure 16-15). Different *positions* on the electrocardiograph set it at different speeds and sensitivities. On most models, many different formats can be selected. Some electrocardiographs have a complete alphanumeric keyboard through which you can enter a wide range of patient data, including the patient's name, the requesting physi-

cian, name of the facility, and the operator's initials, on the ECG record. Other three-channel electrocardiographs can be operated manually or automatically by the push of a touch pad.

The **three-channel electrocardiograph** records three different leads at the same time. Leads I, II, and III are recorded simultaneously; then leads aV_R, aV_L, and aV_F; then leads V_1, V_2, and V_3; and then leads V_4, V_5, and V_6. The standardization mark is also recorded automatically. Length of each lead tracing and lead switching are controlled automatically. The tracing is produced on a three-channel paper, which can be a standard $8\frac{1}{2} \times 11$ inch page or an $8\frac{1}{2} \times 4$ inch page (Figure 16-16, *A* and *B*). Many of the electrocardiographs now come with a built-in computer program that analyzes the ECG tracing as it is being recorded. This provides the physician with additional information when he or she is interpreting the ECG.

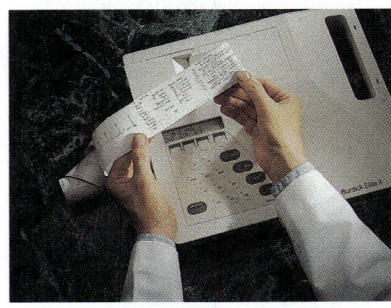

FIGURE 16-15   Simple one-step operation 12-lead ECG in a single-lead format. Simultaneous analysis of all 12 leads is provided. (Courtesy Burdick Inc, Milton, Wisc.)

FIGURE 16-16   **A,** Burdick's Portable Eclipse 850 three-channel electrocardiograph with a built-in computer program that interprets the tracing as it is being recorded. This information is printed above the lead recordings. This machine has storage for 40 ECGs and a fax option. (Courtesy Burdick Inc, Milton, Wisc.)

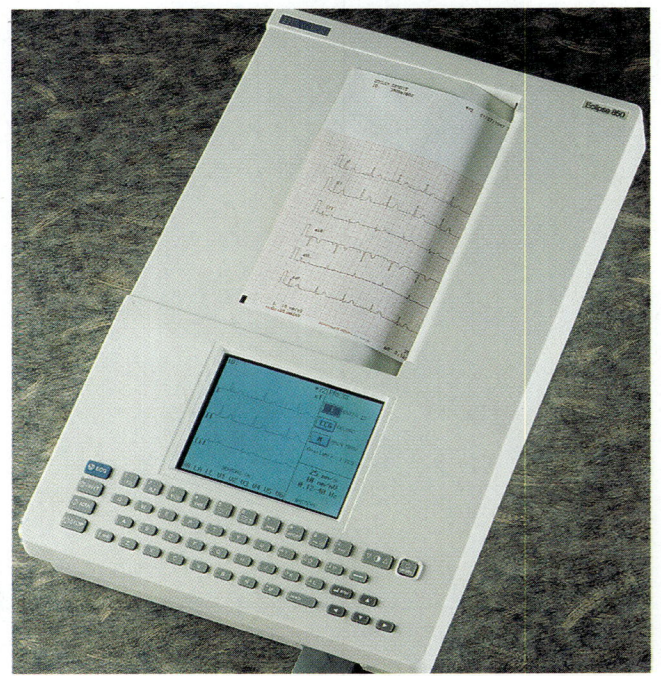

A

Continued

FIGURE 16-16—cont'd   **B,** Three-channel ECG recording. (Courtesy Burdick Inc, Milton, Wisc.)

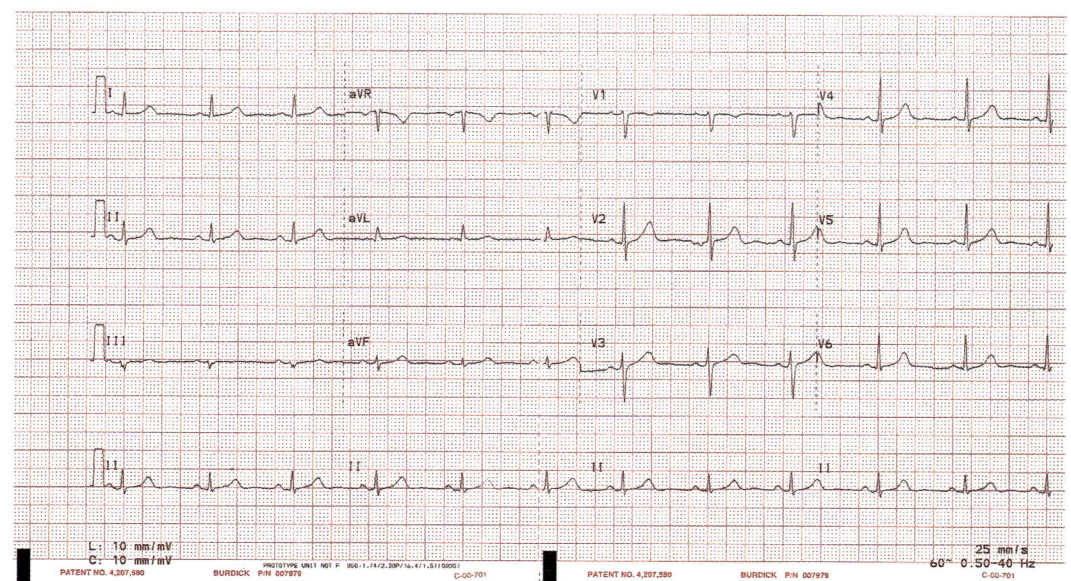

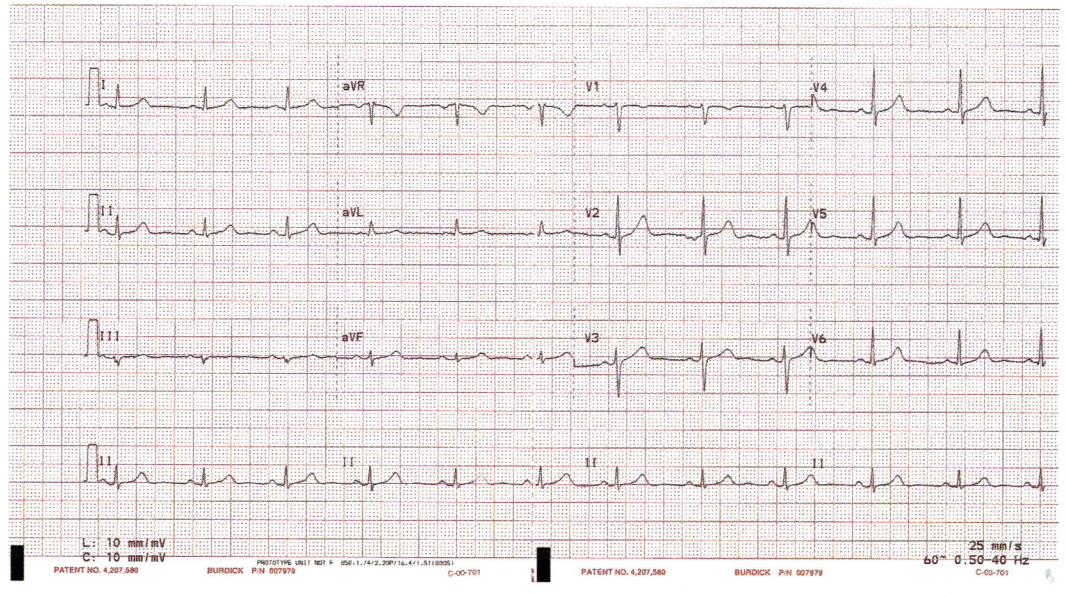

B

DIGITAL ELECTROCARDIOGRAPH FACSIMILE

Facsimile (fax) transmission of medical data is becoming an accepted practice for accessing off-site diagnostic expertise in a timely manner (see Figure 16-16). For instance, emergency rooms or private physicians may require quick, expert ECG diagnoses. Direct digital ECG fax transmits directly from the cardiograph to a fax machine and produces a faxed ECG copy of near-original quality. It eliminates the traditional intermediate step of copying the ECG report and sending via the traditional fax machine. A two-way, direct-digital ECG fax enhancement provides comments added by the physician, as well as a signature to be faxed back to the originating cardiograph. Physicians can receive the ECG anywhere with a fax machine; an internal modem and a software upgrade of the system are required.

AMBULATORY CARDIAC MONITORING (HOLTER MONITORING)

Ambulatory cardiac monitoring, often called Holter monitoring (named after the inventor), is a continuous recording of the electrical activity of the patient's heart (an ECG) for 24 to 48 hours (Figure 16-17). By means of a special monitor, the activity of the patient's heart can be recorded during unrestricted activity, rest, and sleep for future observation and study. Newer monitor models have a compact built-in computer that performs a wide range of sophisticated ECG recording functions. A typical Holter recording contains approximately 100,000 heartbeats. Ambulatory cardiac monitoring is done to correlate the activity of the patient with his or her heart activity and specifically for the following reasons:

1. To detect any cardiac rhythm disturbances and correlate them with patient symptoms of chest pain, palpitations, pulse irregularity, lightheadedness, dizziness, syncope, fatigue, shortness of breath, or sleep apnea

FIGURE 16-17 Ambulatory Holter cardiac monitor. (Courtesy Burdick Inc, Milton, Wisc.)

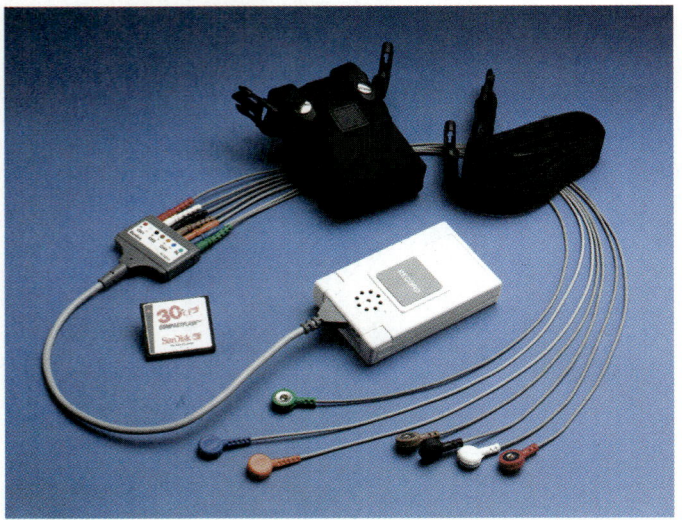

2. To assess the effectiveness of antiarrhythmic medication therapy
3. To assess the function of a new or old pacemaker

To record the activity of the heart, special electrodes are applied to the patient's chest. Lead wires are then attached to the electrodes. The lead wires are connected to a cable that is then connected to the portable monitor. The portable monitor, about the size of a small cassette recorder, is placed in a leather holder bag that is worn by the patient on a belt around the waist or over the shoulder. A diary is kept by the patient while the monitor is worn (see Figures 16-19 and 16-20). The patient's activities, along with the time of day, are to be recorded in the diary. Special notation is to be made of any stressful or significant event or any chest pain, palpitations, dizziness, or syncope, along with the time of day and the activity in which the patient is involved. Most of the monitors available have an **"event marker,"** which is a button that is to be pressed briefly at the time the patient experiences any unusual occurrence as just described. In addition, the patient is to record the event and the time of day in the diary. The monitors also have a clock that provides accurate time monitoring on the ECG recording. For this test, the best clothing for the patient to wear is a shirt or blouse that buttons in front and pants or a skirt so that the cable from the monitor can be comfortably placed at the waist. The procedure should be explained to the patient and instructions provided for the care of the monitor.

At the end of the prescribed period, the patient returns to the physician's office to have the electrodes removed and to turn in the monitor and diary. The monitor or tape (depending on the brand of equipment used) is then processed by a computer, and the ECG tracing, along with the interpretation, is generated. This report can then be matched and compared with the patient's diary. Times of recorded chest pain, palpitations, dizziness, syncope, or any other unusual occurrence are matched with the ECG to see if any abnormal heart rhythm was present at the same time (see also Common Rhythms discussed previously). Some equipment can store all of the data on a hard disk of a computer and also on diskettes. Other systems include an interface unit that provides immediate review of data via a liquid crystal display (LCD) screen while it transfers the complete 24-hour record to a computer diskette for remote analysis.

TREADMILL STRESS TEST

The *treadmill stress test* is used for noninvasive cardiac evaluation to aid physicians in patient diagnosis and prognosis with ECGs taken under controlled exercise stress conditions. During this test of increased stress and work, abnormal electrocardiographic tracings (that do not appear during an ECG taken when the patient is resting) may appear.

The stress test helps the physician to determine an appropriate exercise program for the patient. It is also used to assess cardiac function after heart surgery, to diagnose heart disorders, and to diagnose the possible cause of chest pain. It is an evaluation to aid physicians in patient diagnosis and prognosis with

Text continued on p. 735

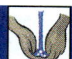

PROCEDURE 16-1

PROCEDURE AND PATIENT CARE FOR HOLTER MONITORING

Objective

Understand and demonstrate the correct procedure for using a Holter monitor, giving instructions to the patient, and recording the procedure in the patient's chart.

A variety of monitors are available on the market. The manufacturer's directions must be followed explicitly because the units are not interchangeable and they operate differently. **Three to seven electrodes** will be attached to the patient's chest; the number depends on how many ECG channels are to be recorded. Each channel uses two electrodes. The electrodes are connected to the lead wire set that plugs into the recorder. The following procedure presents the general guidelines that you use to prepare the patient for ambulatory cardiac monitoring. Make sure that you read the manufacturer's operating instructions thoroughly before starting any form of operation. In doing so, you will be able to use the equipment efficiently for the patient's welfare.

Equipment

Disposable electrodes (sensors)
Lead wires and cable
Monitor (recorder) with a new battery, leather holder bag, and belt for the patient's waist or a shoulder harness
Alcohol sponges
Gauze
Razor and blade (if the patient's skin has to be shaved)
Skin rasp (a rough material somewhat like sandpaper)
Nonallergenic adhesive tape
Patient diary for the unit that you are using
Interface unit and printer

PROCEDURE

1. **Wash your hands. Use appropriate personal protective equipment (PPE) as dictated by facility.**

2. Assemble and prepare equipment. Review the operating instructions if necessary. Insert a fully charged, new battery into the monitor. Make sure the poles on the battery are positioned correctly.

3. Identify the patient and explain the procedure. Give the patient the following instructions about caring for the monitor and assure him or her that he or she will not experience any electrical shock from the monitor.
   a. Maintain good contact of the electrodes with the skin.
   b. *Do not* bathe or shower with the monitor on under any circumstances.
   c. Unplug the ECG connector when changing clothes. An acoustic signal indicates that the device is disconnected.
   d. *Do not* take the monitor out of the carrying case and do not handle the monitor.
   e. *Do not* touch or move the electrodes during the monitoring time. This will help to avoid any artifacts from being recorded.
   f. Maintain the diary properly. You must stress the need to record significant symptoms and events and to record the day's events in the diary (for example, when the patient is awake, takes meals, takes medication, is under stress, smokes, exercises, has a bowel movement).
   g. If any pain or discomfort is experienced, press the event marker button briefly and record the time and the type of pain or discomfort in the diary.
   h. Minimize the use of electrical devices, such as shavers and electronic toothbrushes, and do not use an electric blanket.

RATIONALE

Only a new, fully charged alkaline battery guarantees a 24-hour monitoring period.

The electrical energy is coming from the patient and is being recorded by the monitor.

The electrodes and monitor must be kept dry.

These may cause an interference with an ECG recording.

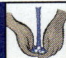

PROCEDURE 16-1

PROCEDURE AND PATIENT CARE FOR HOLTER MONITORING—cont'd

    i.   Call the physician's office if the electrodes become loose or detached or if the recorder stops or malfunctions.

4. Have the patient remove clothes from the waist up. A patient gown may be put on with the opening in the front.

Provide for the patient's comfort.

5. Have the patient lie down on the examining table.

6. Prepare the patient's skin for electrode placement.

    a.   Shave the patient's chest if necessary in the areas where the electrodes will be placed.

Skin preparation is recommended to avoid ECG signals with artifacts.

    b.   Thoroughly cleanse skin where the electrodes will be placed with an alcohol sponge.

Clean skin to remove any oil.

    c.   Allow skin to dry thoroughly.

    d.   Using the skin rasp (this is a fine abrasive), with medium pressure, rub the skin 3 or 4 times to remove the dead skin layer from the areas where the electrodes will be placed.

7. Remove the protective backing from the electrode and apply it to the chest position (Figure 16-18, *A* and *B*). **Select the elec-**

Pressing the center "gel cap" might cause the gel to move out onto the adhesive ring, and then it may not stay in place.

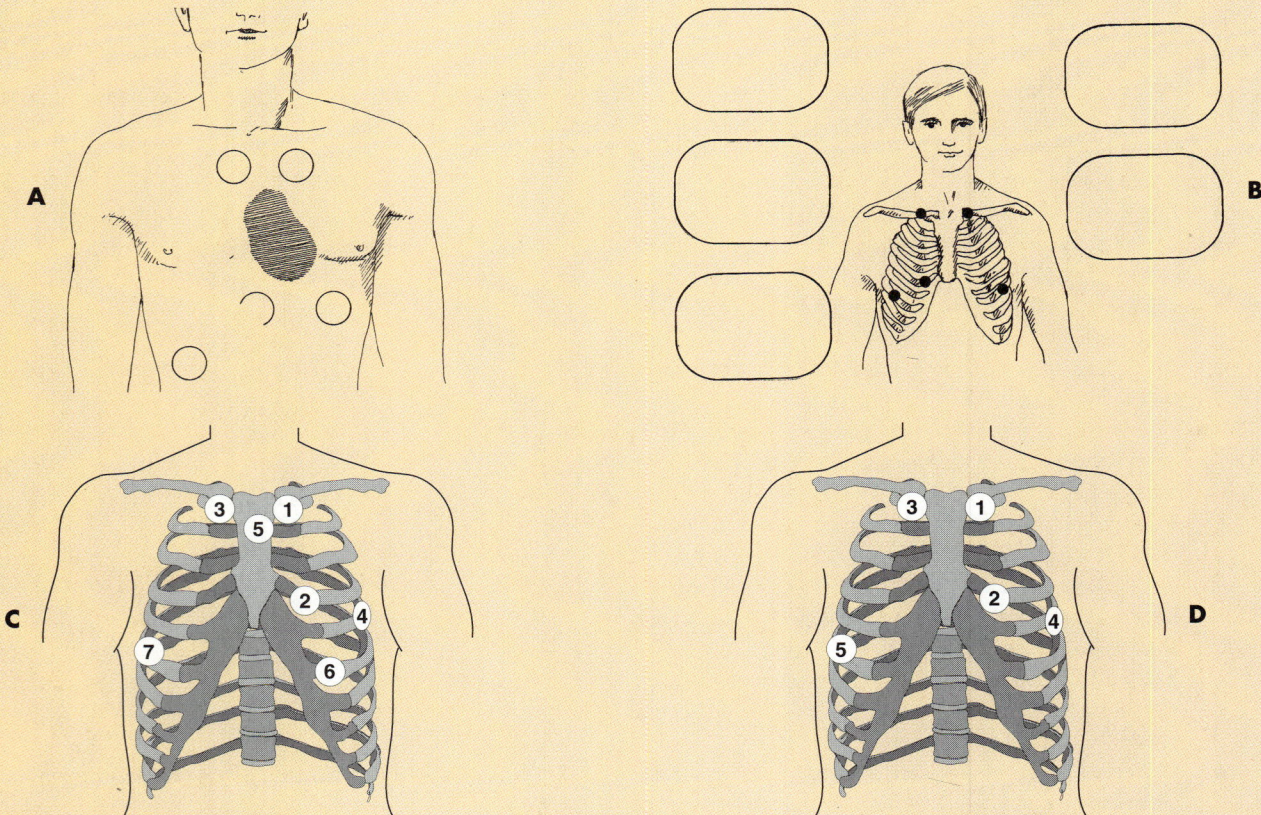

FIGURE 16-18 **A** through **D**, Suggested electrode (sensor) placement for Holter monitoring. (Courtesy Burdick Inc, Milton, Wisc.)

PROCEDURE 16-1

PROCEDURE AND PATIENT CARE FOR HOLTER MONITORING—cont'd

trode sites according to the diagram in the Holter manufacturer's manual. The electrodes have an adhesive backing that secures the electrodes to the skin. There is gel in the center of the back of the electrode to provide good conduction of the electrical impulses from the heart monitor. Press on the electrode's adhesive ring first. Avoid pressing the center "gel cap." Repeat until all electrodes are applied.

8. Attach the lead wires to the electrodes.

9. Place a strip of adhesive tape over the wire just below each electrode (Figure 16-19).

The tape helps to avoid tension and pressure on the electrodes.

10. Attach the ECG cable connector to the monitor.

11. Follow the start-up procedure for the system that you are using by following the directions given in the operator's guide. Examine the ECG printout and assess it with the criteria given with the system that you are using. Visually judge the quality of the ECG. If you do not obtain satisfactory results, check the placement of each electrode.

The start-up procedure for each system determines if the monitor is functioning correctly and recording an adequate ECG.

12. Most systems will then automatically switch over to monitoring.

13. Record the start time in the Patient Diary (Figure 16-20).

14. Have the patient redress.

15. Put the recorder in the holder bag and attach it to the patient's belt or to a shoulder harness (Figure 16-21). Make sure that the belt or harness is adjusted properly so that it does not pull or strain on the lead wires or cable connector.

The holder bag supports and protects the monitor. Pulling or putting tension on the lead wires and electrodes must be avoided to ensure a reliable recording. The electrodes must not be detached from the skin.

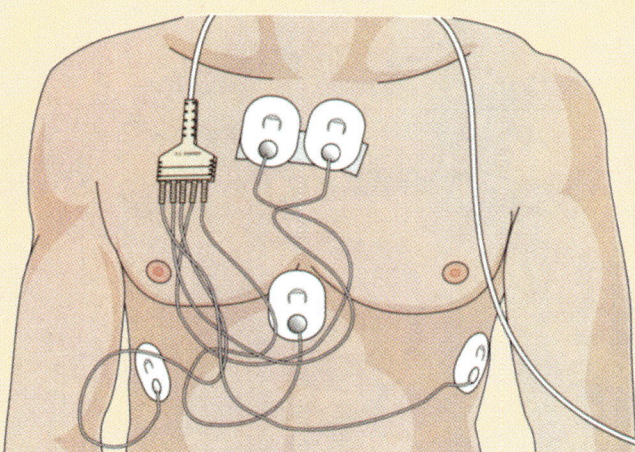

FIGURE 16-19   Electrodes are applied to the patient's chest. Lead wires connect the electrodes to a cable connector attached to the monitor. Adhesive tape is placed over the lead wire just below the electrode.

PROCEDURE AND PATIENT CARE FOR HOLTER MONITORING—cont'd

Burdick Custo-Kit

PATIENT DIARY

For Holter Electrocardiogram

Burdick

A Siemens Company
Milton, Wisconsin
800-777-1777

Reorder #097019

To The Patient:

Your physician needs to know more about your heart than he can learn from an ECG taken in his office. For this reason he has requested that you wear a **"Holter"** (named after Dr. Norman J. Holter) **Recorder** for a 24 hour period. This compact device records your heartbeat for 24 hours. When the test is complete the recorder will be returned for final printout and analysis by your physician.

This test is very valuable as it allows your physician to determine how your heart performs during the everyday situations you experience. This test is very common and the fact that your physician has ordered it **DOES NOT** mean that there is a problem with your heart. It is merely another useful tool in acquiring an accurate diagnosis. Try not to alter your daily routine because of this test. Your physician is trying to learn how **Your** heart responds to **Your** lifestyle.

What to Do During The Test

1. Keep an accurate diary. Indicate activities such as walking, running, sleeping, sexual activity, urinating, etc. Indicate symptoms such as pain (specify location), shortness of breath, dizziness, etc.

2. Do not tamper with the recorder.

3. Keep the recorder dry and avoid bumping or dropping it.

4. If the recorder stops or malfunctions or if an electrode comes loose, call your physician's office.

Impedance Value _____

Time Started _____

Time Completed _____

Recorder # _____
Medications:

TIME	ACTIVITY	SYMPTOMS

FIGURE 16-20 CUSTO-MEGA ambulatory ECG patient diary. (Courtesy The Burdick Corporation, Schaumburg, Ill.)

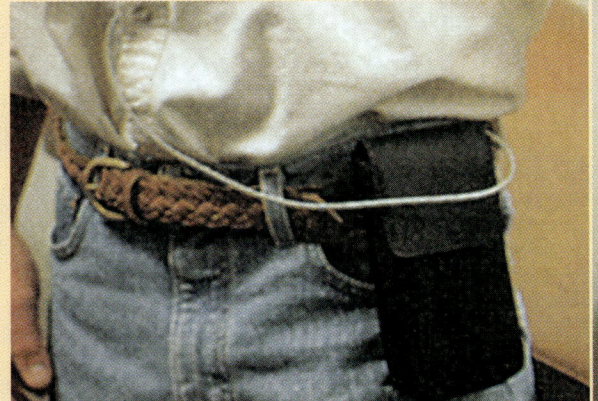

FIGURE 16-21 **A** and **B,** Monitor is placed in a holder bag that is worn on a belt around the patient's waist or on a shoulder harness.

PROCEDURE 16-1

PROCEDURE AND PATIENT CARE FOR HOLTER MONITORING—cont'd

16. Remind the patient of the special instructions that must be followed (review step 3).

17. Answer any questions that the patient may have.

18. Give the diary to the patient and review the instructions for maintaining this record.

19. Inform the patient when to return to have the monitor removed. The patient is not to remove the monitor. It is to remain in place until the scheduled time for removal.

20. Wash your hands.

21. Record the procedure in the patient's chart.

Charting Example

November 7, 20___, 1 PM
Holter monitor applied.
Monitoring commenced at 12:45 PM. Patient to return November 8 at 1 PM to have the monitor removed. Special instructions for care of the monitor and diary record provided.
J.A. Lee, CMA

---

electrocardiographic tracings (that do not appear during an ECG taken when the patient is resting).

The test is done in the presence of a physician, and the patient is constantly monitored. Systems used record and monitor the patient's ECG while it is being monitored by the physician (Figure 16-22).

Patient Preparation

The following information must be provided to the patient before the test is performed. An explanation of the test is given to help reduce any anxiety the patient may experience and to gain the patient's cooperation.

- Get adequate sleep the night before the test.
- Do not eat, smoke, or drink caffeinated beverages for 4 hours before the test. A light meal (without coffee, tea, or alcohol) may be eaten before that time.
- Wear comfortable clothing and flat walking shoes, preferably with rubber soles, for the test. To facilitate application of the ECG electrodes, wear a shirt that opens in the front.
- Discuss with the physician any medications that you are taking because they may or may not be allowed before the test is performed. For example, if taking a beta-blocker, such as propranolol (Inderal), the physician may direct you to discontinue taking the medication before the test.
- You must sign an informed consent form before the test can be performed.

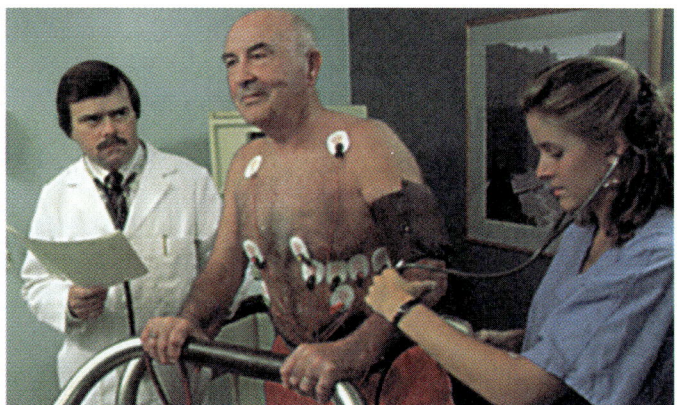

FIGURE 16-22   Treadmill stress test.

- Plan for the test to take about 45 minutes to 1 hour. It is performed by a cardiologist in a cardiology laboratory or clinic.
- You should not experience any pain during or as a result of the stress test. If excessive fatigue, chest pain, or breathing difficulties occur during the test, the physician will stop the test.

Report any complaints experienced after the test to the physician.

Procedure
- Electrodes are applied, and a baseline ECG is recorded.
- Vital signs are taken.
- The patient is asked to walk on a treadmill or pedal a bicycle at prescribed rates.
- During the exercises, heart activity is monitored, and the blood pressure is taken at the end of each testing interval.
- At the end of the test, the patient is asked to rest while monitoring continues until the vital signs and the ECG return to normal.
- The electrodes are removed, and the skin is cleansed of any electrolyte solution or gel.

Posttest Instructions to the Patient
- Rest for several hours.
- Avoid extreme temperature changes.
- Avoid stimulants.
- Do not take a hot shower or bath for at least 2 hours.
- Discuss the results and your feelings with the physician. Report if any physical symptoms were experienced after the test.

On rare occasions, complications, including a myocardial infarction (MI) or a fatal cardiac arrhythmia, may occur. Appropriate emergency equipment must always be available in the test room. This equipment should include antiarrhythmia drugs, a defibrillator, an Ambu bag, an airway, and intubation equipment (endotracheal tube and laryngoscope).

An assistant must stand near the patient during the test in case the patient becomes dizzy, faints, or falls. In these situations, support must be provided immediately.

CONCLUSION

Having completed the chapter on electrocardiography, you should have acquired a basic understanding of the technique for taking ECGs and the importance of this vital diagnostic procedure. After you have practiced the procedures and are ready to demonstrate your skills and knowledge attained, arrange with your instructor to take a performance test.

REVIEW OF VOCABULARY

The following are ECG reports received in the physician's office from a consulting cardiologist's office. These are presented to expose the medical assistant to ways in which the interpretation reports of the patient's ECG may be written. Normal and abnormal ECG findings are given.

Patient No. 1:
ECG OF 12-12-01 showed frequent PVCs (premature ventricular contractions). Rhythmic strip showed numerous PVCs.

Patient No. 2:
The patient's ECG showed normal sinus tachycardia of 145, with right axis; P pulmonale was noted inferior laterally; there were ST-T wave changes consistent with ischemia; no significant change since the reading on 9-30-01.

Gary Greaves, MD

Patient No. 3:
INTERPRETATION:
Rate: 75
Rhythm: sinus
P waves: normal
P-R interval: normal
Position: Intermediate heart
QRS waves: deep SV_{1-5}

T waves: normal
CONCLUSION: Intermediate heart within normal limits.

J. Dobbins, MD

Patient No. 4:
INTERPRETATION:
Rate: 60
Rhythm: sinus
P waves: normal
P-R interval: 0.16
Position: horizontal heart
QRS waves: deep SV_{1-4}
T waves: normal
CONCLUSION: Horizontal heart within normal limits.

Sally Eaton, MD

Patient No. 5:
INTERPRETATION:
Rate: 108
Rhythm: sinus tachycardia
P waves: normal
P-R interval: 0.18
Position: normal axis
QRS waves: deep SV_{1-4}

T waves: normal
CONCLUSION: Within normal limits except for mild sinus tachycardia.

Carol Overkamp, MD

Patient No. 6:

INTERPRETATION:
Rate: 52
Rhythm: sinus bradycardia
P waves: notched
P-R interval: 0.16
Position: left axis deviation
QRS waves: Deep Q_1, aV_L, V_{5-6}
T waves: low T waves
CONCLUSION: Sinus bradycardia, left atrial enlargement, and left ventricular hypertrophy.

Erik Evans, MD

Patient No. 7:

INTERPRETATION:
Rate: 60

Rhythm: sinus
P waves: notched
P-R interval: 0.18
Position: horizontal heart
QRS waves: slurred ST_1, aV_L, V_{5-6}
T waves: low T waves
CONCLUSION: Horizontal heart with left atrial enlargement, left anterior hemiblock, and old anterolateral myocardial damage.

John Dunn, MD

The following is a hospital discharge summary received in the office on one of the physician's patients. After reading this, you should be able to discuss the contents with your instructor. Be prepared to define and explain any medical terms that are used. A medical dictionary, other reference books, and information given in preceding chapters of this book may be used as references for obtaining definitions or explanations of the contents of this report.

Discharge Summary

Patient: Henry Jones   Med Rec #: 54321
                              Admitted: 09-13-01

Doctor: Ray Brown, MD   Discharged: 09-14-01
DISCHARGE DIAGNOSIS:
Coronary angioplasty

The patient underwent left and right heart catheterization and selective coronary arteriography and left ventricular cine angiography evaluation of very atypical chest pain syndrome. Left ventricular end-diastolic pressure was satisfactory, but left ventricular cine angiography demonstrated inferior wall hypokinesis that was actually a new finding compared with 1997. The distal circumflex artery demonstrated subtotal occlusion with fairly faint opacification of a distal obtuse marginal. This was mildly narrowed in 1997 and so had definitely demonstrated considerable progression. A relatively small diagonal branch had high-grade narrowing that was more pronounced than 1997. Otherwise, left anterior descending, a second diagonal, a first obtuse marginal and right coronary artery were satisfactorily patent and unchanged.

Because of these new findings and the patient's atypical chest pain, we attempted to open the distal obtuse marginal vessel and were unsuccessful, mainly because we could not manipulate the guidewire into the distal vessel. However, we did inflate the balloon for up to 5 minutes in this artery, and the patient had no chest pain syndrome, implying that the myocardium distal to this runoff is not dependent on a patent vessel. We then turned our attention to the diagonal and dilated this vessel satisfactorily. In this case, the patient did develop angina during the balloon inflations.

The patient was returned to the CCU and treated with heparin for several hours, and this was then discontinued and the sheaths withdrawn.

CPK level on the day of discharge was 94 U/L, hemoglobin was 14.6 g/dl, and creatinine was 1.1 mg/dl. The electrocardiogram after the procedure showed no changes from predilation.

The patient will be discharged home on the following medications:

1. Aspirin 5 grains a day.
2. Cardizem 240 CD each morning.
3. He will not take isosorbide or Lotensin for now.
4. He will resume Ticlid three times a day.

FOLLOW-UP: He will be seen in the office in 1 week.
ACTIVITY: He will resume normal activity.

FINAL DIAGNOSIS: Coronary artery disease

OPERATIONS/PROCEDURES:

1. Left and right heart catheterization, left ventricular cine angiography, selective coronary arteriography
2. Coronary artery angioplasty diagonal coronary artery

Ray Brown, MD

D: 09-14-01
T: 09-15-01
mdts, Job #4049

The following is a sample of a patient's medical history and physical examination. After reading this, you should be able to discuss the contents with your instructor. Be prepared to define and explain any medical terms that are used. A medical dictionary, other reference books, and information given in preceding chapters of this book may be used as references for obtaining definitions or explanations of the contents of this report.

History and Physical Examination

Patient: Henry Jones   Med. Rec. #: 12345
Doctor: Victor Sand, MD
Admitted: 09/12/01

CHIEF COMPLAINT: Two-vessel coronary artery disease and moderate left ventricular dysfunction per cardiac catheterization.

HISTORY OF PRESENT ILLNESS: Henry Jones is a 53-year-old gentleman with a history of hypercholesterolemia, left kidney stones, and hypothyroidism; otherwise in fairly good health. The patient denies hypertension, diabetes, and pulmonary or hepatic dysfunction.

Mr. Jones has been experiencing an unusual atypical generalized feeling of not quite being himself in the last 9 months. He has been experiencing fatigue and tiredness. The patient, however, denies having chest pain, jaw pain, arm pain, or dyspnea. The patient does admit to a 2-year history of GI discomfort, which he has associated with indigestion. The patient has been placed on Zantac for this discomfort. In July 2000 the patient went on vacation and experienced several episodes of atypical discomfort after eating and walking. He was placed on Propulsid and H2 blockers, which gave him no discomfort. In view of this, the patient was seen by a family physician following his return from surgery, and during the examination the patient was noted to have irregular heartbeat. The patient underwent a 12-lead EKG, which revealed left bundle branch block as well as some ST changes. Subsequently the patient was referred to Dr. Jones for cardiac evaluation. The patient subsequently underwent echocardiogram, which revealed dilated left ventricle with moderate left ventricular dysfunction. Follow-up thallium scan revealed an inferior septal ischemia. A small anterior septal scar was noted, and dilated left ventricle was also confirmed. In view of this, the patient was recommended for cardiac catheterization, and he underwent cardiac catheterization. This revealed two-vessel coronary artery disease with severe left ventricular dysfunction. The patient had total right coronary artery stenosis and moderately severe stenosis of the left anterior descending. In view of this finding, it was believed that the patient would be best served by having coronary artery bypass graft surgery and was referred to Dr. Joan Bennett.

The patient currently denies orthopnea, paroxysmal nocturnal dyspnea, palpitations, edema, or syncope.

Coronary risk factors include family history; uncle and aunt died in their 50s with myocardial infarction. The patient has hypercholesterolemia. He has a 70 pack-year history of smoking. Denies hypertension or diabetes.

PAST MEDICAL HISTORY: History of kidney stones, left, hypothyroidism, and peptic ulcer disease.
Surgery: Fractured right ankle. Left kidney stones. Tonsillectomy at age 26. Left knee scope.
Allergies: None known to medications.

Medications: Synthroid, 0.05 mg, and Zantac, 150 mg, once in a while for GI discomfort.

FAMILY HISTORY: Uncle, 52, with MI, and aunt in her 60s with MI.

REVIEW OF SYSTEMS: Unremarkable.

PHYSICAL EXAMINATION:
GENERAL: A 53-year-old male, well developed, well nourished, alert and oriented × 3, pleasant and cooperative, and tolerates the procedure well.
HEENT: Normocephalic, atraumatic. No evidence of mass lesions or pain. Sinus cavities nontender to palpation. Nasal passages patent bilaterally. Pupils are equal, round, reactive to light and accommodation. Extraocular movements are intact. No scleral icterus. Conjunctiva clear. No drainage or discharge noted. Buccal mucosa pink and moist, no erythema, exudates or excoriations. Teeth in good repair. Tongue protrudes in midline.
NECK: Supple. No evidence of jugular vein distention (JVD), no carotid bruits, no lymphadenopathy or thyromegaly noted. Trachea is midline and mobile.
CHEST: Symmetrical. No evidence of lesions. Resonant to percussion.
LUNGS: Clear to auscultation with no evidence of rales, rhonchi, or wheezes.
COR: Regular without gallop or rub noted.
ABDOMEN: Positive bowel sounds. Soft, nontender to palpation. No evidence of organomegaly.
EXTREMITIES: Full range of motion, muscle strength intact. No evidence of muscular atrophy, cyanosis, or digital clubbing. No pretibial edema noted. Peripheral pulses intact. There is granulation over the right femoral artery where the patient has undergone cardiac catheterization.
NEUROLOGIC: Both the motor and sensory examinations are grossly intact.

IMPRESSION:
1.   Two-vessel coronary artery disease involving total right coronary artery and severe left anterior descending stenosis with severe left ventricular dysfunction.
2.   History of hypercholesterolemia.
3.   Peptic ulcer disease.
4.   Hypothyroidism

PLAN: AM admit. The patient will undergo two-vessel coronary artery bypass graft surgery by Dr. Joan Bennett probably using bilateral internal mammary artery.

Victor Sand, MD

CRITICAL THINKING SKILLS REVIEW

1. Draw and label the waves, intervals, and segments of an ECG. Explain what each component signifies.
2. Explain what is happening in the heart during the process of depolarization and repolarization.
3. List eight abnormalities that may be detected on the ECG.
4. Mr. Perry Bloom is having an ECG done and wants to know if the record will pick up his heart sounds and what each of the little squares on the ECG paper mean. State and explain the answer that you give to this patient.
5. The physician expects you to monitor the recording of Mr. Bloom's ECG. List three items that you will look for.
6. During the recording of Max Sugar's ECG, he continually coughs and moves his hand to cover his mouth. What type of artifact would you expect to see on the record?
7. When recording Ms. Lillian Bell's ECG, the stylus continually wanders off the baseline. Describe the actions you would take to try to remedy this situation.
8. Explain to Ms. Maureen McArthur how and why the physician in your office can read her ECG taken on another machine by a different physician in another city.
9. Mrs. D. Bernstrom wants to know why you have to put that "gooey paste" on her body when you are applying the electrodes. State your reply to this patient.
10. Mrs. Sara Pace wants to know how you can tell if your ECG machine is working properly and what all those "funny little" waves on the ECG paper mean. What would you tell her?
11. State the purposes for the following items on the electrocardiograph:
    a. STD button
    b. Position control knob
    c. Lead selector knob
    d. Recorder switch
12. In the process of recording Mr. Dan Orlando's ECG, you suddenly notice that there is no tracing on the paper. What could cause this, and how would you remedy the situation?
13. Mrs. Colette Kelly's ECG tracing is very light and hard to distinguish. What could cause this, and how would you remedy the situation?
14. Illustrate identification codes for each of the 12 leads on a standard ECG.
15. List eight instructions that you should give to a patient who will be wearing a monitor.

PERFORMANCE TEST

In a skills laboratory, the medical assistant student will demonstrate skills in performing the following activities without reference to resource materials. For these activities the student will need five different individuals to play the role of the patient. Time limits for the performance of these skills are to be assigned by the instructor (also see p. 104).

1. Prepare the patient for an ECG.
2. Locate the six chest lead positions on at least five different individuals; then apply the electrodes and lead wires and record the ECGs of these individuals.
3. Mount the recordings obtained in No. 2.
4. Correctly care for the equipment after use.
5. Apply a monitor to a patient.
6. Give the patient instructions to follow when wearing a monitor.

The student is expected to perform these activities with 100% accuracy.

The successful completion of each procedure will demonstrate competency levels as required by the AAMA, AMT, and future employers.

INTERNET RESOURCES

American Heart Association
http://amhrt.org

American Red Cross
www.redcross.org

National Institutes of Health, National Heart, Lung and Blood Institute
www.nhibi.nih.gov

North American Association for the Study of Obesity
www.naaso.org

Heartstream: Forerunner Automatic external defibrillator (AED)
www.heartstream.com

American Dietetic Association
www.eatright.org

Determining Your Risk of Heart Disease
http://207.69.209.38/detrskm.htm

The Heart: An Outline Exploration
www.fi.edu/biosci/heart.html

Medline*plus*
www.nlm.nih.gov/medlineplus

Heart Information Network
www.heartinfo.org

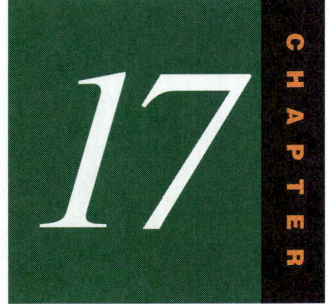

17 CHAPTER

Common Emergencies and First Aid

■ Cognitive Objectives

On completion of Chapter 17, the medical assistant student should be able to:

1. Define first aid and the related terminology presented in this chapter.
2. State the factors that constitute a medical emergency.
3. List four fundamental rules and general procedures to follow in a medical emergency.
4. Explain how to administer cardiopulmonary resuscitation (CPR).
5. Explain how to give first aid treatment for a victim who is choking.
6. List six common warning signals of a heart attack.
7. Discuss the 911 emergency telephone system.
8. Describe an automated external defibrillator and when it is used.
9. List three key points that must be considered if using a portable automated external defibrillator.
10. Discuss the term *cardiac defibrillation*.
11. State the average age that people most often experience a cardiac arrest.
12. Define ventricular fibrillation.
13. State the time frame during which defibrillation is most successful for victims of sudden cardiac arrest.
14. State the purpose of a poison control center.
15. Define and list eight signs and symptoms of a cerebral vascular accident (CVA). Discuss risk factors, prevention, and treatment for a stroke (CVA).
16. List six types of shock and the usual causes of each.
17. List at least 10 signs and symptoms of shock.
18. Differentiate between arterial, venous, and capillary bleeding.
19. List four methods used to control severe bleeding.
20. Explain what is meant by the pressure point method and list the seven pressure points used to control severe bleeding.
21. Differentiate between a superficial (first degree) burn, a partial-thickness (second-degree) burn, and a full-thickness (third-degree) burn.

22. Explain what is meant by the rule of nines in reference to burns.
23. Differentiate between hypoglycemia (insulin reaction) and hyperglycemia (diabetic coma) by stating the signs, symptoms, and causes of each.
24. List common symptoms of undiagnosed diabetes.
25. Explain when you should and should not induce vomiting when the victim has ingested a poisonous substance.
26. State and describe the first aid treatment for all the emergency situations discussed in this chapter.
27. List at least 15 items that should be included in a first aid kit.
28. Explain the Medic Alert system, how it works, and who should become members.

■ Terminal Performance Objectives

On completion of Chapter 17, the medical assistant student should be able to:

1. Demonstrate the proper first aid care to be used for all the medical emergencies presented in this chapter.
2. Demonstrate the proper application of a tourniquet.
3. Locate the seven pressure points and demonstrate how to use them to control severe bleeding.
4. Make appropriate decisions regarding care when given an example of an emergency.
5. Provide instructions and patient education that is within the professional scope of a medical assistant's training and responsibilities as assigned.

The student is expected to perform these objectives with 100% accuracy.

The consistent use of Universal/Standard Precautions is required by all health care professionals in all health care settings as a method of infection control. It is assumed that these precautions are used in all of the following procedures. Review Chapter 1 if you have any questions on methods to use because the methods or techniques are not repeated in detail in each procedure presented in this chapter.

Be sure to consult the latest guidelines issued by the Centers for Disease Control and Prevention and consult with infection control practitioners when necessary to identify *specific precautions that pertain to your particular work situation.*

VOCABULARY

antidote (an'ti-dot)—An agent used to counteract a poison.

biologic death—The condition that results when the brain has been deprived of oxygenated blood for a period of 6 minutes or more and irreversible damage has probably occurred.

clinical death—The state that results when breathing and circulation have stopped.

concussion (kon-kush'un)—The injury that results from a violent blow or shock.

concussion of the brain—A short or prolonged altered state of consciousness caused by a blow or fall. May be followed by dizziness, nausea, weak pulse, and transient amnesia.

contusion (kon-too'zhun)—A bruise, indicating injury to tissues without breakage in the skin. Discoloration appears because of blood seepage under the surface of the skin.

epinephrine (ep"i-nef"rin)—A hormone produced by the adrenal glands. Epinephrine can be administered parenterally, topically, or by inhalation. It is used as an emergency heart stimulant, to relieve symptoms in allergic conditions, and to counteract the lethal effects of anaphylactic shock.

tourniquet (toor'ni-ket)—A constricting device used to compress an artery or vein to stop excessive bleeding.

Additional terms are defined under their respective topics in this chapter.

When someone is injured or suddenly becomes ill, there is a critical period—before medical help is obtained—that is of the utmost importance to the victim. What you do or don't do during that time can mean the difference between life and death. For serious conditions, the victim *must* receive medical attention because first aid is not meant to resolve serious problems.

First aid is the immediate and temporary care given to the victim of an accident or sudden illness until the services of a physician can be obtained. It is the help that *you* can provide in emergencies until trained medical emergency personnel or a physician takes over. You owe it to yourself, the patients under the care of your physician-employer, your family, and the general public to know and understand the simple procedures that can be rendered quickly and intelligently in an emergency.

First aid is more than a dressing or a cold compress. The victim suddenly has new problems and needs, both emotional and physical, that must be cared for. Your contributions include offering well-chosen words of encouragement, a willingness to help, the uplifting effect of your evident capabilities and calmness, and the performance of temporary physical care to alleviate pain or a life-threatening situation.

It may be your responsibility to deal with an emergency before the physician or other emergency teams arrive. If you are familiar with the procedures for emergency care, can exercise good judgment, remain calm, and avoid panicking others, you can administer care in an orderly manner and thereby render great service to the patient and the physician. Whether you are in the physician's office, at home, or on the street, *you must take prompt action.*

Each year more than 1 million Americans die from sudden death. In many cases of sudden death, especially death from heart attacks, the victim could have been saved if the early warning signs of a heart attack were known, if someone close to the victim could have performed cardiopulmonary resuscitation (CPR), or if the victim had been transported quickly to a hospital or received first aid or medical attention at the scene of sudden illness or injury. *Time* is of the essence in any medical emergency in which breathing and heartbeat have ceased. Within 4 to 6 minutes after the heart stops, brain damage begins. Thus the importance of your knowledge and quick actions in a medical emergency cannot be overemphasized. **Know what constitutes an emergency, whom to call for help, and what to do.** An emergency exists when life is threatened, when situations develop that endanger a person's physical and/or psychologic well-being, or when pain and suffering occur.

When an emergency occurs in the physician's office, notify the physician. If the physician is not in the office and is not expected momentarily, call for a nearby physician; if none can be reached for immediate help, call the local emergency medical services (EMS) system, an ambulance, the fire and rescue squad, or the police department. You are *not* to assume the responsibility for making a diagnosis and providing medical treatment, but you *are* expected to make a reasonable judgment (that may require medical knowledge) of the situation and to provide immediate first aid care.

You should perform *only* those procedures that you have been trained to do and, when in the office or health care agency, only with the prior consent of the physician. An office policy should be established between you and the physician regarding what should be done in the case of office emergencies and in the case of emergency telephone calls from patients.

The following fundamental rules and general procedures to follow in an emergency are few, but very important:

1. Remain calm, reassure the patient, be empathetic, and do not panic. Act in an orderly, organized manner. Have a reason for what you do; avoid injury to yourself; know the limits of your capabilities; and avoid further injury to the patient.
2. Survey the situation to determine the nature of the emergency. A primary survey includes the ABCs for all emergencies (that is, check the patient for an open airway, for breathing, and for circulation). A secondary survey is done to examine the total body to determine what is wrong.
3. Take immediate steps to remedy the situation. Your responsibilities for the type of care to provide will vary in each situation and depend on the proximity of medical help, the seriousness of the injury or illness, and the immediate environment.
4. Seek medical help if needed and be able to describe the nature of the patient's condition. Think of yourself as a reporter who must obtain concise and relevant information and report it. Seek answers to questions that begin with who, what, when, where, why, and how.

This chapter provides important information in concise and convenient form on common emergencies and the first aid treatment to be administered. CPR, care for choking victims, and care for patients in shock are presented first. Other common emergencies are then discussed in alphabetic order. Read and study the contents of this chapter carefully and keep this or other first aid references in a convenient place where they will be on hand for quick reference when needed.

The purpose of this chapter is to provide a review and reference source for first aid treatment to use for common emergencies. It is not intended to be used as a substitute for a certified first aid program of study. Taking a certified First Aid and CPR course is highly recommended for medical assistants. Courses are offered by the American Red Cross and at many community colleges. Cardiopulmonary resuscitation courses for basic life support are also provided by the American Heart Association in numerous communities. All medical assistants should then take a refresher course in first aid every few years and in CPR every year.

CARDIOPULMONARY RESUSCITATION IN BASIC LIFE SUPPORT FOR CARDIAC ARREST

Cardiopulmonary resuscitation (CPR) is a combination of artificial respiration and artificial circulation. CPR should be started immediately by individuals **properly trained** to do so in emergency situations in which cardiac arrest occurs. The performance of CPR is *not recommended unless one has had proper training and practice in the procedure* because serious adverse consequences may result from faulty technique. Therefore the following information can serve as a review and reference source **after** you have completed a training course and before you take your next refresher course.

The *goal* of CPR is life support. When trained in CPR techniques, you must start life support techniques as quickly as possible and continue them until one of the following has occurred:

1. An effective respiration and pulse are restored to the victim.
2. You are completely exhausted and cannot continue CPR.
3. Care of the victim is turned over to medical or other properly trained personnel.
4. The victim is pronounced dead.

Basic and advanced life support. Life support is divided into two systems: basic and advanced life support. Basic life support (BLS) can be carried out by trained lay and medical persons and includes the following:

Basic ABC steps
A—Airway opened
B—Breathing restored
C—Circulation restored

Supplementary techniques
- Positioning—Position the victim properly (that is, in the supine position).
- Jaw thrust maneuver—May be required when the head-tilt alone is unsuccessful for opening the airway. This technique *without* the head-tilt is called the modified jaw thrust maneuver and is the safest to use on a victim who possibly has a neck injury.
- Opening the mouth—At times it may be necessary to force the mouth open for ventilation, to remove foreign bodies, or to allow drainage of vomitus or blood.
- Mouth-to-stoma resuscitation—When the victim has had a laryngectomy, he or she breathes through a stoma in the neck; in this case, mouth-to-stoma resuscitation must be performed.
- Adjunctive equipment—To be used only by those trained in its use.

Advanced life support is to be performed *only* by trained medical personnel and includes the following (Figure 17-1):

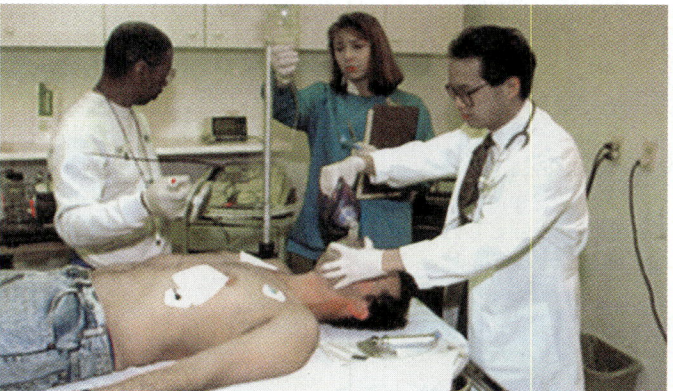

FIGURE 17-1 Advanced life support being administered to a patient by medical personnel in hospital emergency room.

- Definitive therapy
    - Diagnosis
    - Drugs
    - Defibrillation
- Cardiac monitoring and stabilization
- Transportation
- Communication

HEART ATTACK: SIGNALS AND ACTIONS FOR SURVIVAL*

Sudden death may be caused by poisoning, drowning, suffocation, choking, electrocution, and smoke inhalation; however, the most common cause is a heart attack. Everyone should know the usual early signals of heart attack and have an emergency plan of action. Early treatment often means the difference between life and death.

Signals.   The *most common signal* of a heart attack is an uncomfortable pressure, squeezing, fullness or pain in the center of the chest behind the breastbone, which may spread to the shoulder, neck, jaw, or arms (the pain may not be severe).

Other signals may include the following:

- Sweating
- Nausea, and maybe vomiting
- Shortness of breath *or* a feeling of weakness
- Apprehension

Sometimes these signals subside and return.

Actions
1. Recognize the "signals."
2. Stop activity and sit or lie down.
3. Act at once if pain lasts for 2 minutes or more—call the local emergency rescue service, usually 911, or go to the nearest hospital emergency room with 24-hour service.

CARDIOPULMONARY RESUSCITATION

Basic CPR is a simple procedure, as simple as A-B-C: Airway, breathing, and circulation. *The following brief review is based on the 1999 standards for CPR. It is to be used **only** for review purposes. It is not to be used for learning the procedure for performing CPR.*

Airway
If a person has collapsed, determine if he or she is conscious by shaking the shoulder and shouting, "Are you all right?" If the person does not respond, shout for help and have someone **contact the Emergency Medical Services (EMS), by calling 911 or a local emergency number.**

If you are alone, call the EMS before beginning CPR. If someone is with you, have that person call the EMS system while you begin CPR. Then open the airway (Figure 17-2). If

the victim is not lying flat on the back, roll him or her over, moving the entire body at one time as a total unit.

To open the victim's airway, use the head-tilt/chin-lift maneuver. Lift up the chin gently with one hand while pushing down on the forehead with the other to tilt the head back. Once the airway is open, place your ear close to the victim's mouth (Figure 17-3):

- **Look**—at the chest and abdomen for movement.
- **Listen**—for sounds of breathing.
- **Feel**—for breath on your cheek.

FIGURE 17-2   To open the airway, tilt the head back and lift the chin.

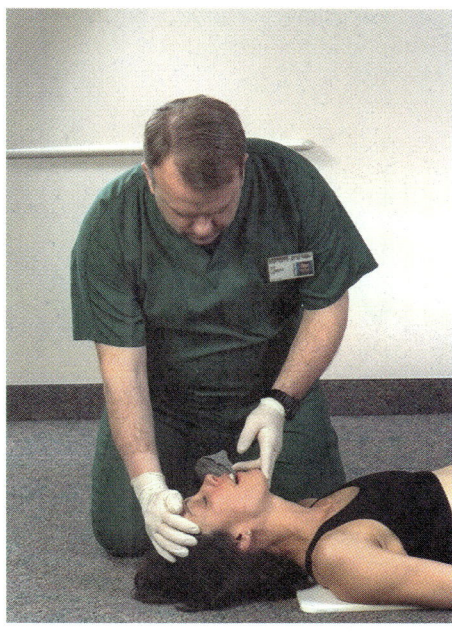

FIGURE 17-3   To check for breathing, look, listen, and feel.

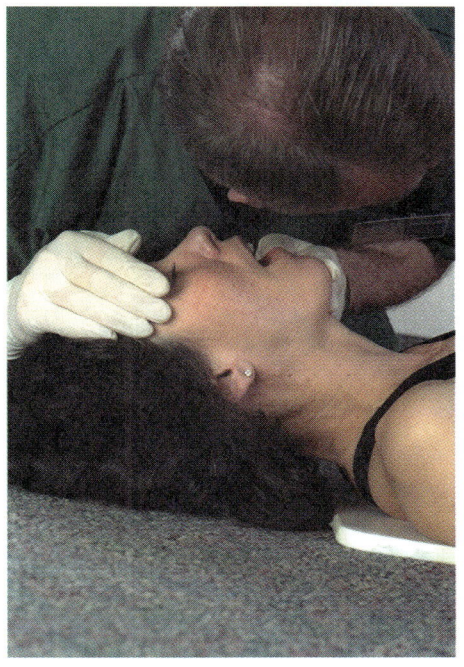

---

*Courtesy the American Heart Association.

If none of these signs is present, the victim is not breathing.

If opening the airway does not cause the victim to begin to breathe spontaneously, you must provide rescue breathing.

Breathing

The best way to provide rescue breathing is by using the mouth-to-mouth technique. Take your hand that is on the victim's forehead and turn it so that you can pinch the victim's nose shut while keeping the heel of the hand in place to maintain head tilt. Your index and middle fingers of your other hand should remain under the victim's chin, lifting up (Figure 17-4).

Immediately give two slow, full breaths (1.5 to 2 seconds per breath) using the mouth-to-mouth method while maintaining an airtight seal with your mouth on the victim's mouth. Watch the victim's chest to see that your breath goes in.

Breathing devices, such as face shields and resuscitation masks (Figure 17-5), are available to use when providing rescue breathing. These devices create a barrier between your mouth and nose and the victim's. In this way, you can have some protection from body fluids from the victim's nose, mouth, and face. Some resuscitation masks have one-way valves so that you are protected from contact with the air that the victim exhales. These devices are small and should be part of the emergency tray or first aid kit in the physician's office or clinic. They can also be part of a first aid kit that you keep in your car. When using a resuscitation mask or a face shield during rescue breathing, you may have to modify how you maintain the correct airway position, but the procedure remains the same.

FIGURE 17-4   Giving rescue breathing. Tilt the head back and pinch the nose shut with your thumb and index finger. Use the mouth-to-mouth method by breathing into the victim's mouth.

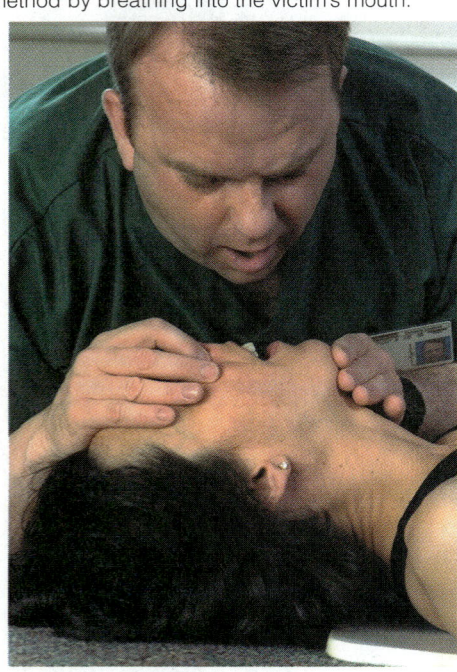

FIGURE 17-5   Face shields and resuscitation masks that can be used during rescue breathing to protect the rescuer from contact with any facial or oral secretions from the victim.

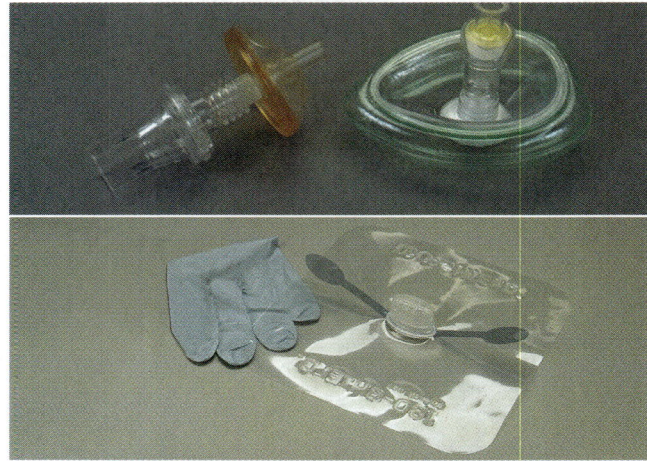

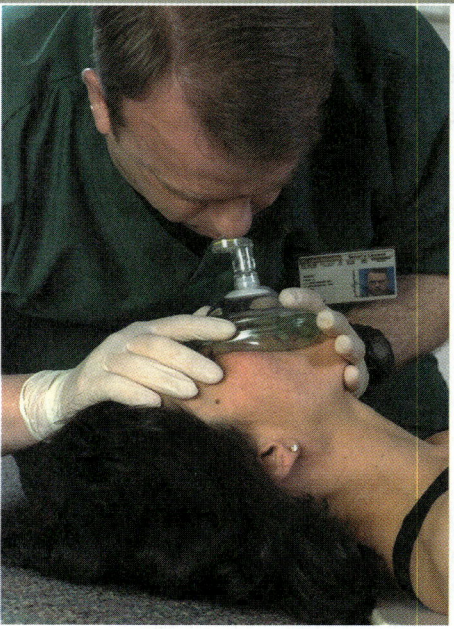

Check Pulse

After giving the two breaths, locate the victim's **carotid pulse** to see if the heart is beating. To find the carotid artery, take the hand that you are using on the victim's chin and locate the voice box. Slide the tips of your index and middle fingers into the groove beside the voice box. Feel for the carotid pulse (Figure 17-6). **Cardiac arrest** can be recognized by absent breathing and an absent pulse in the carotid artery in the neck.

If you cannot find the pulse, you must provide artificial circulation in addition to rescue breathing.

Cardiac Compression

Artificial circulation is provided by external cardiac compression. In effect, when you apply rhythmic pressure on the lower half of the victim's breastbone, you are forcing the heart to pump blood. To perform external cardiac compression prop-

erly, kneel at the victim's side near the chest at the level of the victim's shoulders. Locate the notch at the lowest portion of the sternum with the hand that was on the victim's chin. Put your middle finger on this notch and your index finger next to it. Place the heel of the hand that was on the victim's forehead on the lower half of the sternum, close to the index finger of your other hand (Figure 17-7). Place your other hand on top and parallel to the one that is in position. Be sure to keep your fingers off the chest wall. You may find it easier to do this if you interlock your fingers.

FIGURE 17-7   Locate correct hand position kneeling next to the victim.

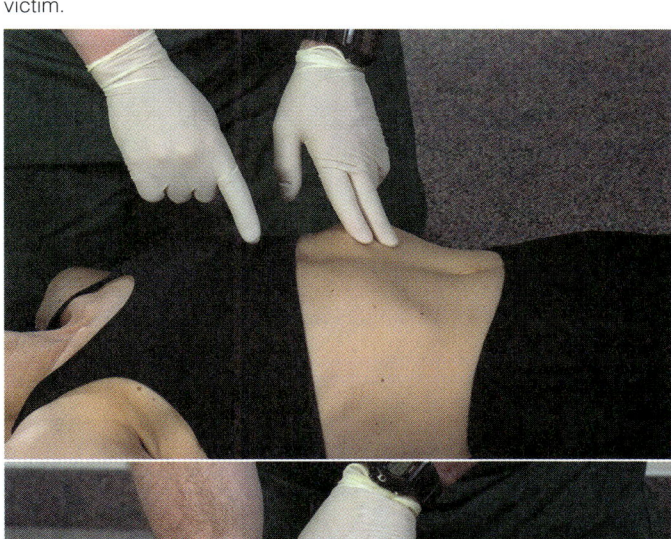

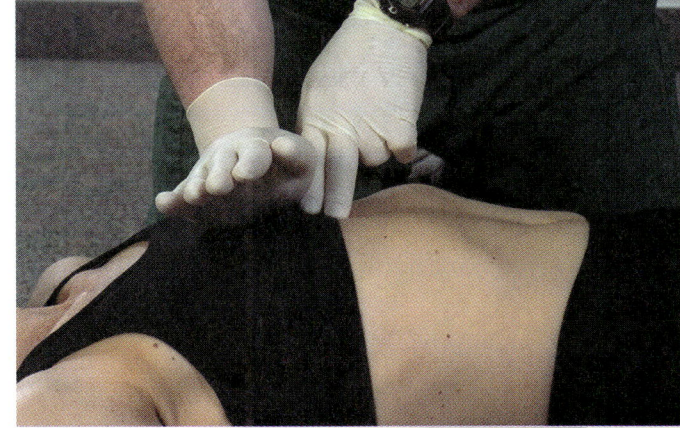

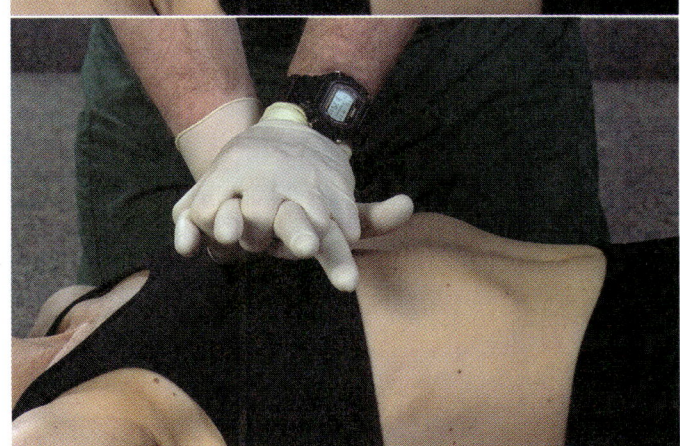

FIGURE 17-6   To determine if the heart is beating, check for carotid pulse on the side of the neck for both an adult and a child.

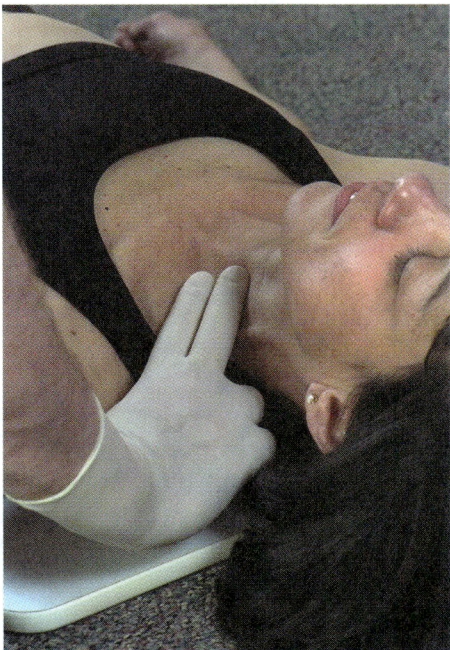

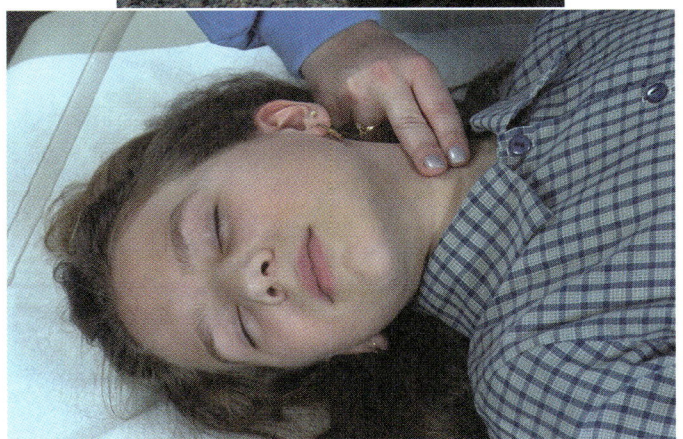

FIGURE 17-8   Give 15 chest compressions. Bring your shoulders directly over the victim's sternum, keep your arms straight, and compress down on the sternum 1½ to 2 inches for an adult victim.

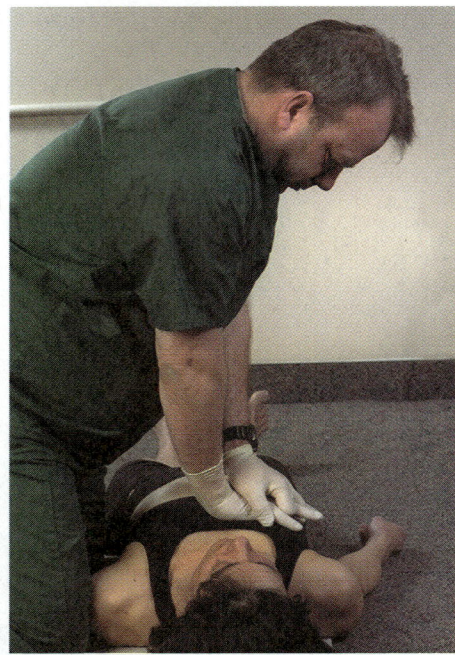

FIGURE 17-9   **A,** Once the need for rescue breathing has been established, seal your mouth completely around the victim's mouth while pinching the nose and maintaining an airway. Give 2 full slow breaths. **B,** The ratio is 15 chest compressions to 2 breaths. (From Henry M, Stapleton E: *EMT Prehospital Care,* ed 2, 1997, WB Saunders.)

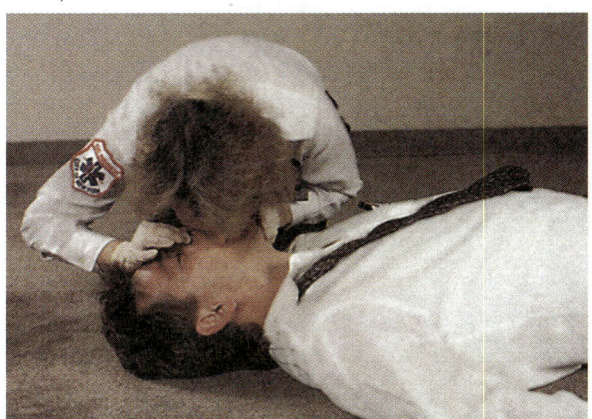

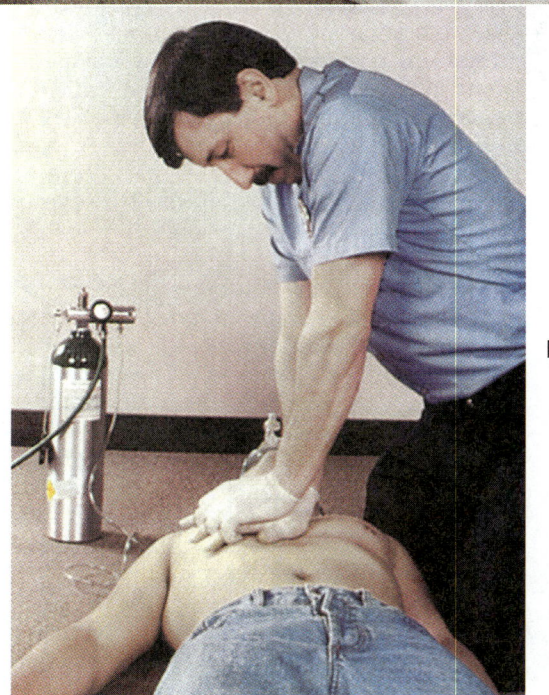

Bring your shoulders **directly over** the victim's sternum as you compress downward, keeping your arms straight (Figure 17-8). Depress the sternum about 1½ to 2 inches for an adult victim. Then relax pressure on the sternum completely. However, *do not* remove your hands from the victim's sternum but *do* allow the chest to return to its normal position between compressions. Relaxation and compression should be of equal duration.

If you are the only rescuer, you must provide both rescue breathing and cardiac compression (Figure 17-9). The proper ratio is 15 chest compressions to 2 full, slow breaths. You must compress at the rate of 80 to 100 times per minute when you are working alone because you will stop compressions when you take time to breathe.

When two rescuers are present, position yourselves on opposite sides of the victim, if possible. One of you should be responsible for interposing a breath (1.5 to 2 seconds) after each fifth compression, maintaining an open airway, and monitoring the carotid pulse for adequate chest compressions. The other rescuer, who compresses the chest, should use a rate of 80 to 100 compressions per minute.

Continue CPR until advanced life support is available (Figure 17-10).

CPR for Infants and Small Children

Basic life support for infants and small children is similar to that for adults. A few important differences to remember are as follows (Figure 17-11).

Activating the EMS system.   If you are alone with an infant or child, you *must* give about 1 minute of CPR *before* activating the EMS system, that is, do 20 cycles of compressions and rescue breaths; *then* activate the EMS system.

Airway.   When handling an infant, be careful that you do not exaggerate the backward position of the head tilt. An infant's neck is so pliable that forceful backward tilting might *block* breathing passage instead of opening them.

FIGURE 17-10   After 1 minute of CPR, check pulse and breathing. Continue with CPR if needed. While checking for the pulse, you **must** also be checking for breathing as shown in Figure 17-3. **Do both at the same time.**

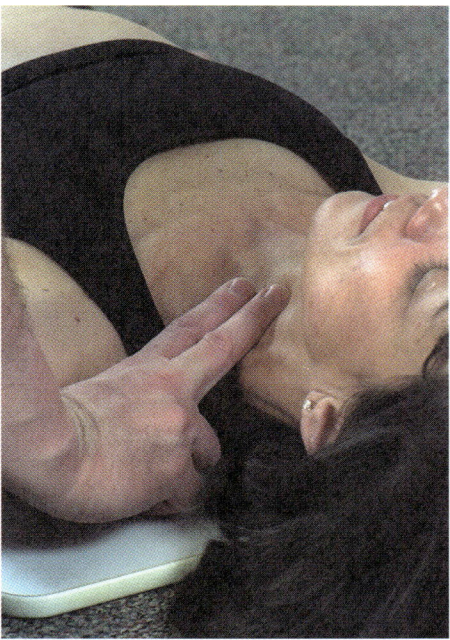

FIGURE 17-11   Different hand positions for giving chest compressions to an **A,** adult, **B,** child, and **C,** infant. (From Henry M, Stapleton E: *EMT prehospital care,* ed 2, 1997, WB Saunders.)

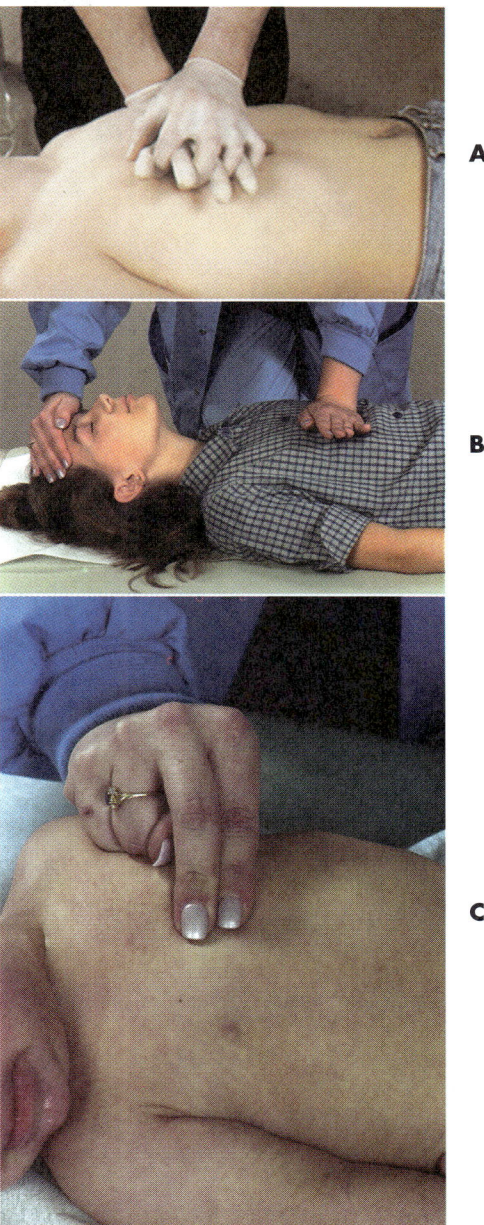

Rescuers	Ratio of Compressions to Breaths	Rate of Compressions	Depress Sternum
1	15:2	80 to 100 times/min	1½ to 2 inches
2	5:1	80 to 100 times/min	1½ to 2 inches

Breathing.   Don't try to pinch off the nose. Cover both the mouth and nose of an infant or *small* child who is not breathing with your mouth. Use small breaths with less volume to inflate the lungs. Give one small breath every 3 seconds for an infant (0 to 1 year) and one small breath every 4 seconds for a child (1 to 8 years). (For a child, a mouth-to-mouth seal should be made with the nose pinched tightly, as done for adults.)

Check pulse.   The absence of a pulse may be more easily determined by feeling for the **brachial pulse for infants** (0 to 1 years). Find this pulse by feeling on the inside of the upper arm midway between the elbow and the shoulder (Figure 17-12). (Locate the **carotid pulse for children** 1 to 8 years old as you would for an adult.)

Circulation.   The technique for cardiac compression is different for infants and small children. Only two fingers are used on an infant, and one hand is used for compression on a

child. The other hand may be slipped under the infant to provide a firm support for the back; or for both infant and child, the other hand is used to maintain the head position to maintain an open airway.

For **infants,** use only the *tips of two fingers* to compress the chest. Place the index finger of the hand nearest the infant's legs just under an imaginary line between the nipples where it intersects with the sternum. Compress the chest 1 fingerbreadth below this intersection, at the location of the middle and ring fingers. Depress the sternum between ½ to 1 inch at a fast rate of 100 times a minute. Make sure not to depress the tip of the sternum.

FIGURE 17-12   Location for checking for pulse on an infant. Feel on the inside of the upper arm midway between the elbow and shoulder.

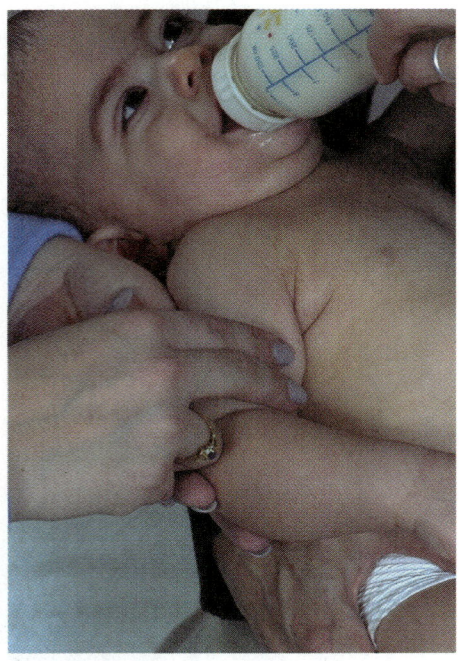

FIGURE 17-13   For suspected neck injuries, use the modified jaw thrust when checking for breathing. (From Henry M, Stapleton E: *EMT prehospital care,* ed 2, 1997, WB Saunders.)

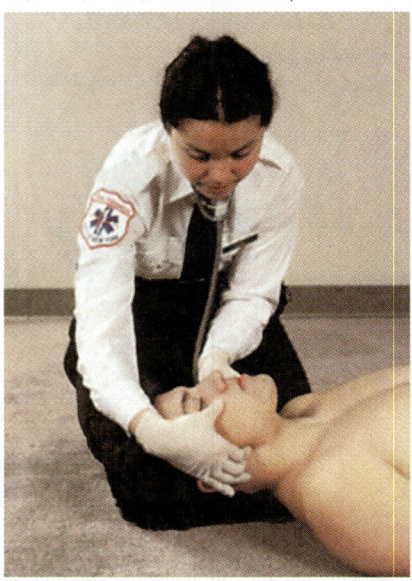

	Part of Hand	Depress Sternum	Rate of Compression	Ratio of Compressions to Breaths
Infants	Tips of two fingers	½ to 1 inch	At least 100 per minute	5:1
Children	Heel of hand	1 to 1½ inches	80 to 100 per minute	5:1

For **children 1 to 8 years old,** use only the *heel of one hand* to compress the chest. Depress the sternum between 1 and 1½ inches, depending on the size of the child. Use the same hand position as for adults. The rate should be 80 to 100 times per minute.

In the case of both infants and small children, breaths should be administered during the relaxation after every fifth chest compression.

CPR for children over 8 years old is the same as for adults.

Neck Injury

If you suspect that the victim has suffered a neck injury, you must not open the airway in the usual manner. If the victim is injured in a diving or automobile accident, you should consider the possibility of such a neck injury. In these cases, the airway should be opened by using a modified jaw thrust, keeping the victim's head in a fixed, neutral position (Figure 17-13). If the airway remains obstructed, tilt the head slowly and gently until the airway is open.

CHOKING

The urgency of choking cannot be overemphasized. Immediate recognition and proper action are essential. If the victim has good air exchange or only partial obstruction and is still able to speak or cough effectively, *do not interfere with his or her attempts to expel a foreign body*. The **distress signal for choking** is the gesture of clutching the neck between the thumb and index finger. *Prompt action is urgent in every case of choking*.

When you recognize complete airway obstruction by observing the conscious victim's inability to speak, breathe, or cough, the following sequence should be performed quickly on the victim in the sitting, standing, or lying position:

1. Manual thrusts (abdominal or chest) until effective or the person becomes unconscious.
2. Finger sweep if the victim is unconscious.
3. If the victim becomes unconscious, shout for help. Place the victim on the back, face up. Open the airway and attempt to ventilate. If unsuccessful, deliver up to five manual thrusts, probe the mouth with the finger, and attempt to ventilate. It may be necessary to repeat these steps. *Be persistent* (Figure 17-14).

FIGURE 17-14   Adult lifesaving steps. (Courtesy The American National Red Cross.)

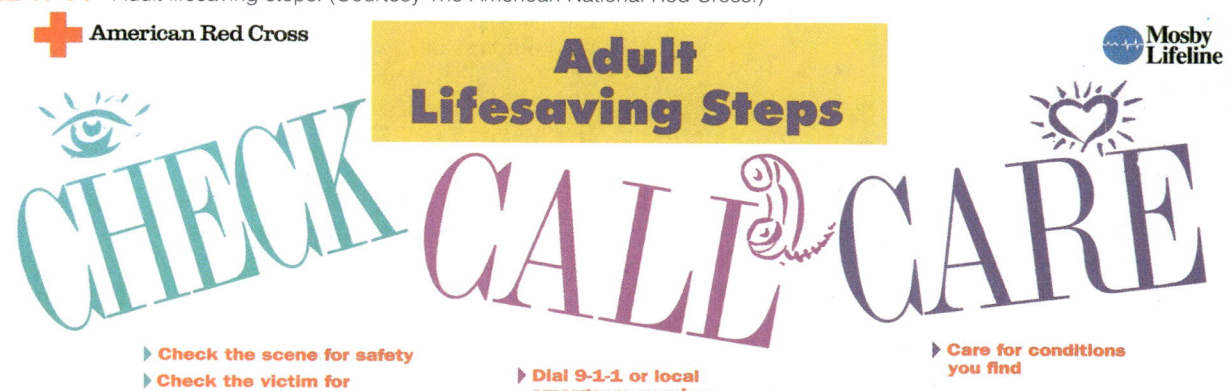

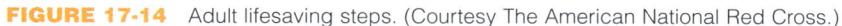

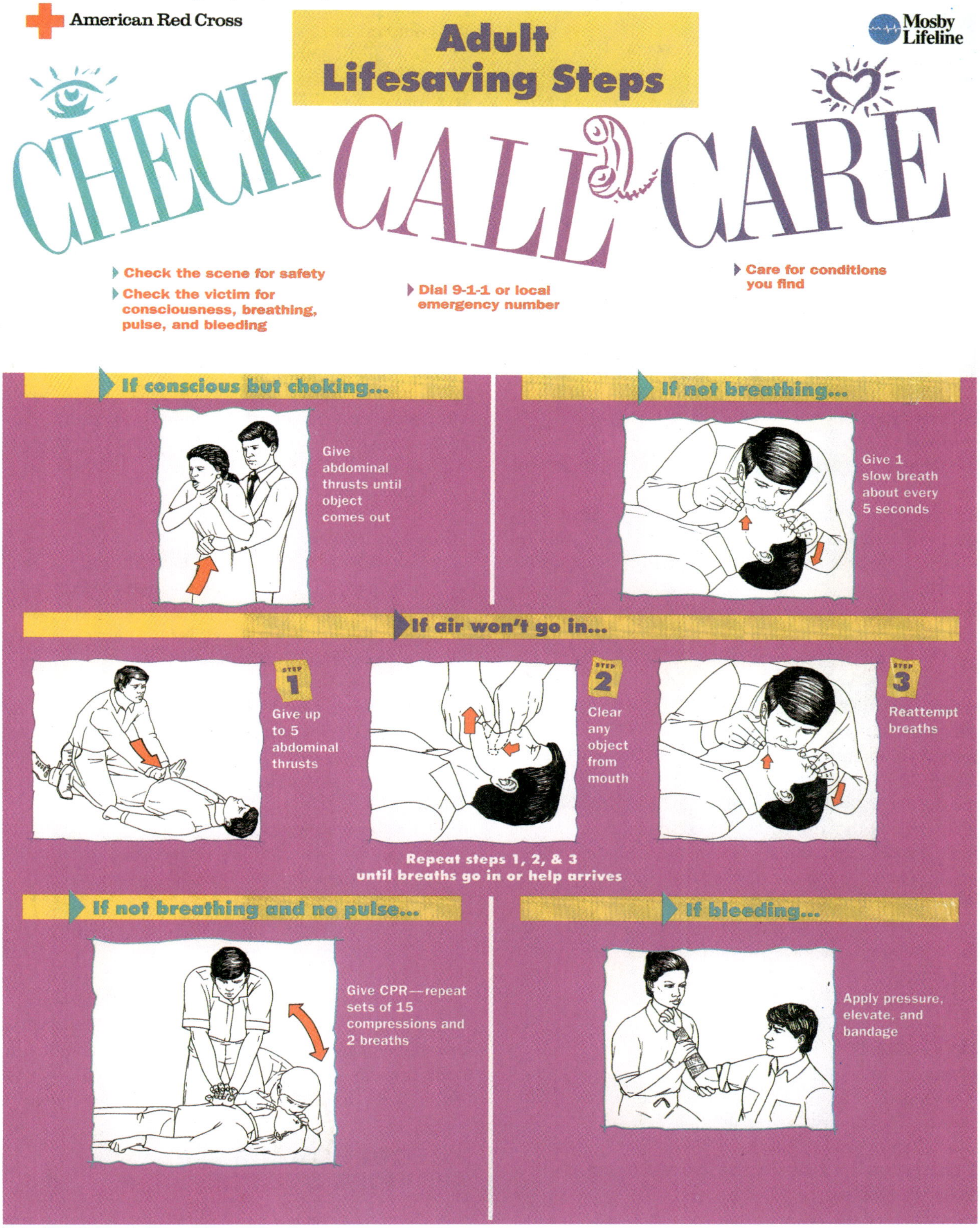

MANAGEMENT OF THE OBSTRUCTED AIRWAY

Abdominal Thrusts (Heimlich Maneuver)
Abdominal thrusts for the conscious victim.
Abdominal thrusts (subdiaphragmatic abdominal thrusts or abdominal thrusts), also called the Heimlich maneuver, is the technique recommended for relieving foreign-body airway obstruction. It may be necessary to repeat the thrust up to five times or continually until the victim's airway is cleared or the victim becomes unconscious. Never have your hands on the victim's xiphoid process of the sternum or on the lower margins of the victim's rib cage when performing this maneuver (Figure 17-15).

Manual thrusts are a rapid series of thrusts to the upper abdomen or chest that force air from the lungs.

Abdominal thrusts with victim sitting or standing
1. Stand behind the victim; wrap your arms around the waist.
2. Place the thumb side of your fist against the victim's abdomen in the midline slightly below the rib cage well below the tip of the xiphoid process and slightly above the umbilicus.
3. Grasp your fist with your other hand and press it into the victim's abdomen with a **quick upward thrust.**
4. Repeat if necessary.

Abdominal thrusts with victim in a lying position
1. Place the victim in a supine position; kneel astride the victim's hips/thighs.
2. Place the heel of your hand in the middle of the abdomen slightly below the rib cage well below the tip of the xiphoid process and slightly above the umbilicus. Place your other hand on top of your bottom hand.
3. Rock forward, having your shoulders directly over the victim's abdomen and press into the abdomen and toward the diaphragm with a **quick upward thrust.** *Do not* press to either side.
4. Repeat if necessary.

Chest Thrusts
Chest thrusts are to be used *only* when the victim is markedly obese or in the later stages of pregnancy. The downward thrusts will generate effective airway pressures.

Chest thrust with the conscious victim standing or sitting
1. Standing behind the victim, place your arms under the victim's armpits, and encircle the victim's chest.
2. Place the thumb side of your fist on the victim's sternum (breastbone), but not on the xiphoid process.
3. Grasp this fist with your other hand, and press on the victim's sternum with a quick backward thrust.

Chest thrust with the victim in a lying position
1. Place your hands in the same position used for closed chest compression.
2. Exert quick downward thrusts.

Infants and Children
For infants up to 1 year of age, the combination of five back blows and five chest thrusts continues to be recommended (Figure 17-16). Back blows are a rapid series of sharp whacks that are delivered with the heel of the hand over the spine and between the shoulder blades. The blows should be applied quickly, forcefully, and in rapid succession. For a child 1 to 8 years of age, abdominal thrusts are recommended.

Other Causes of Airway Obstruction
An adequate open airway must be maintained at all times in all unconscious patients.

Other conditions that may cause unconsciousness and airway obstruction include stroke, epilepsy, head injury, alcoholic intoxication, drug overdose, diabetes, swelling from infection or trauma, and coma.

Remember the following steps:

1. Is the victim unconscious?
2. If so, shout for help. Activate the EMS system: Send someone to call 911 or your local emergency number. If you are alone, call the EMS before starting CPR.
3. Open the airway, and check for breathing.
4. If not breathing, give two breaths.
5. Check carotid pulse.
6. If no pulse, begin external cardiac compression by depressing the lower half of the sternum 1½ to 2 inches (for adults).
7. Continue uninterrupted CPR until advanced life support is available.
   CPR for one rescuer:
   15:2 compressions to breaths at a rate of 80 to 100 compressions a minute (four cycles per minute)
   CPR for two rescuers:
   5:1 compressions to breaths at a rate of 80 to 100 compressions a minute

Periodic practice in CPR is essential to ensure a satisfactory level of proficiency. A life may depend on how well you have remembered the proper steps of CPR and how to apply them. You should be sure to have both your skill and knowledge of CPR tested at least once a year. *It could mean someone's life.*

EMERGENCY MEDICAL SERVICES SYSTEM
Any victim on whom you begin resuscitation must be considered as needing advanced life support. He or she will have the best chance of surviving if your community has a total Emergency Medical Services (EMS) system. This includes an efficient communications alert system, such as 911, with public awareness of how or where to call; well-trained rescue person-

FIGURE 17-15   Heimlich maneuver (abdominal thrusts).

A person choking on food will die in 4 minutes – you can save a life using the HEIMLICH MANEUVER*

Food-choking is caused by a piece of food lodging in the throat creating a blockage of the airway, making it impossible for the victim to breathe or speak. The victim will die of strangulation in four minutes if you do not act to save him.

Using the Heimlich Maneuver* (described in the accompanying diagrams), you exert pressure that forces the diaphragm upward, compresses the air in the lungs, and expels the object blocking the breathing passage.

The victim should see a physician immediately after the rescue. Performing the Maneuver* could result in injury to the victim. However, he will survive only if his airway is quickly cleared.

If no help is at hand, victims should attempt to perform the Heimlich Maneuver* on themselves by pressing their own fist upward into the abdomen as described.

WHAT TO LOOK FOR

The victim of food-choking:

1. Can Not Speak or Breathe.

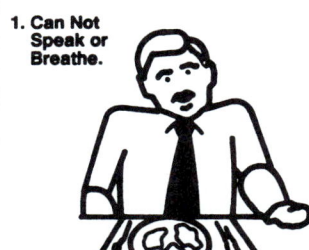

2. Turns Blue.

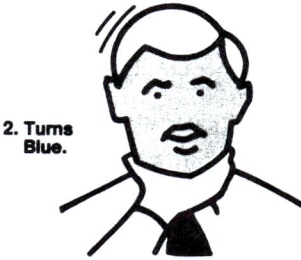

Heimlich Sign: Hand to neck signals: "I am choking!"

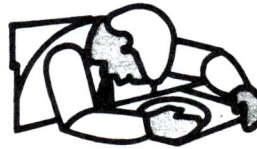

3. Collapses.

HEIMLICH MANEUVER*

RESCUER STANDING
Victim standing or sitting

□ Stand behind the victim and wrap your arms around his waist.

□ Place your thumb side against the victim's abdomen, slightly above the navel and below the rib cage.

□ Grasp your fist with your other hand and press into the victim's abdomen with a **quick upward thrust.**

□ Repeat several times if necessary.

When the victim is sitting, the rescuer stands behind the victim's chair and performs the maneuver in the same manner.

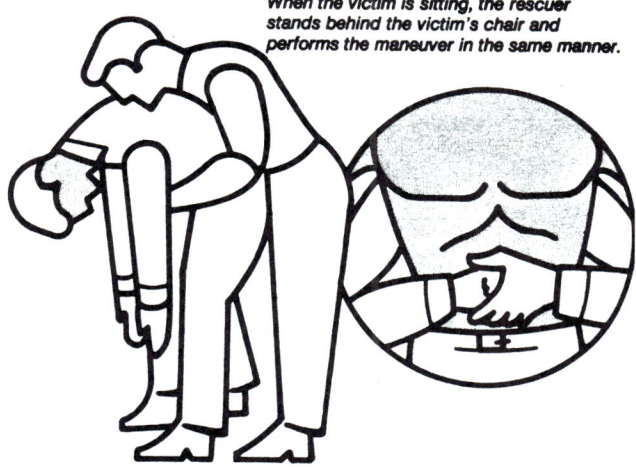

OR

RESCUER KNEELING
Victim lying face up

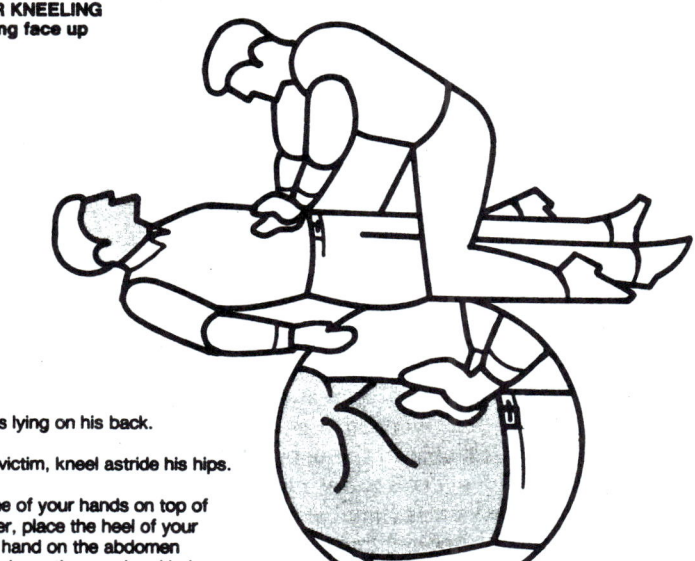

□ Victim is lying on his back.

□ Facing victim, kneel astride his hips.

□ With one of your hands on top of the other, place the heel of your bottom hand on the abdomen slightly above the navel and below the rib cage.

□ Press into the victim's abdomen with a **quick upward thrust.**

□ Repeat several times if necessary

FIGURE 17-16   Infant and child lifesaving steps. (Courtesy The American National Red Cross.)

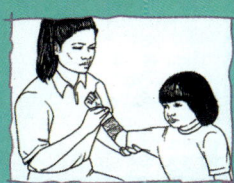

American Red Cross   **Mosby Lifeline**

Infant & Child Lifesaving Steps

CHECK CALL CARE

▶ Check the scene for safety

▶ Check the victim for consciousness, breathing, pulse, and bleeding

▶ Dial 9-1-1 or local emergency number

▶ Care for conditions you find

INFANTS
(birth to 1)

If conscious but choking...

Give 5 back blows ...

And 5 chest thrusts

Repeat blows and thrusts until object comes out

If not breathing...

Give 1 slow breath about every 3 seconds

If air won't go in...

STEP 1 Give 5 back blows ...

And 5 chest thrusts

STEP 2 Look for and clear any object from mouth

STEP 3 Reattempt breaths

If not breathing and no pulse...

Give CPR—repeat sets of 5 compressions and 1 breath

CHILDREN
(1-8)

If conscious but choking...

Give abdominal thrusts until object comes out

If not breathing...

Give 1 slow breath about every 3 seconds

If air won't go in...

STEP 1 Give up to 5 abdominal thrusts

STEP 2 Look for and clear any object from mouth

STEP 3 Reattempt breaths

Repeat steps 1, 2, & 3 until breaths go in or help arrives

If not breathing and no pulse...

Give CPR—repeat sets of 5 compressions and 1 breath

If bleeding...

Apply pressure, elevate, and bandage

Local Emergency Telephone Number: _____

Everyone should know what to do in an emergency. Call your local American Red Cross _____ for information on CPR and first aid courses.

Copyright © 1993 by
The American National Red Cross
Stock No. 652038
July, 1993
ISBN: 0-8016-7751-3
For ordering information,
please call 1-800-633-6699

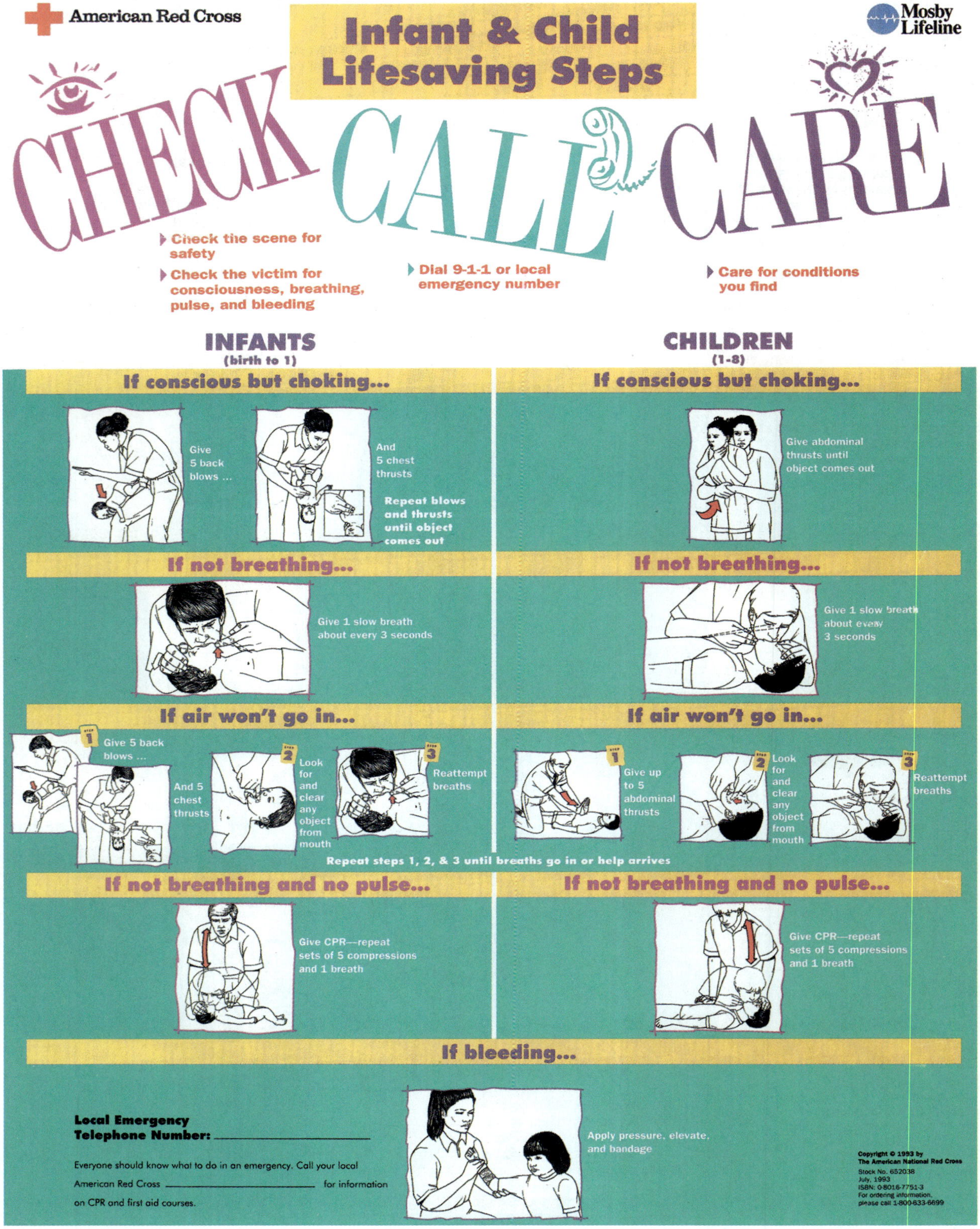

nel who can respond rapidly; vehicles that are properly equipped; an emergency facility that is open 24 hours a day to provide advanced life support; and an intensive care section in the hospital for the victims. You should work with all interested agencies to achieve such a system.

911: Emergency Telephone System

Many communities participate in the nationwide 911 emergency telephone system. To find out if it is in effect in your community, call information in your area.

The 911 telephone **system must be used only in emergency situations when you need help quickly.** Dial 911 only when you or someone nearby needs emergency medical help or an ambulance, when you see a fire or a crime in progress, or when you suspect that a stranger may be in your home or you see him or her trying to enter or leave. Because 911 is a local service in each area, it is not necessary to dial any special access codes before the number. You only need to use three telephone digits—911. You can dial 911 from any type of telephone, including coin-operated public telephones, without any charge (you don't have to put coins into a coin-operated telephone to dial 911). If you are calling for help for someone who does not live in your area, you should dial "0" for the operator instead of 911. This is because 911 is a *local* service and cannot be used to obtain help outside of your immediate area.

When you dial 911, you reach a specially trained emergency operator. This operator will ask you a few important questions so that the type of help you need will be obtained without delay. **Information that you will be asked includes the following:**

• What is the emergency?
• Where is the emergency? (Include cross-reference streets when applicable.)
• What is your name and address?

Even if you can't talk, **stay on the line.** In many communities, the special nature of the 911 system allows the emergency operator to know exactly where you are so that help can come quickly. The emergency operator immediately assesses the problem and by pressing a button, notifies the appropriate public emergency agency. The operator stays on the line to be sure that your problem is handled properly to get the fastest emergency service and to see if other emergency services are necessary. The emergency operator also serves to keep the caller calm while waiting for help to arrive. Callers who are disconnected after dialing 911 can be called right back and, in even greater emergencies, the operator can trace the location of the phone.

Remember to stay calm and do not hang up. The emergency operator should hang up before you do. Often people panic in an emergency situation. They may give the operator information in a hurried fashion and hang up to go back to the emergency scene before the operator has obtained adequate and correct information. When this happens, the proper help may not be able to reach you in an adequate time to meet the needs of the situation. In some communities, your line can be left open until the proper type of emergency help arrives. This would allow special instructions to be given for the emergency while you wait for help to arrive and, if necessary, to determine your address if you are unable to give it.

Remember, 911 must be used only to report "real" emergencies. It must not be used for every call that you may have to make to the police department, the fire department, or an ambulance service.

PORTABLE AUTOMATED EXTERNAL DEFIBRILLATORS (Figure 17-17)

Sudden cardiac arrest is a time-critical emergency. An estimated 350,000 Americans die each year from sudden cardiac arrest (SCA)—nearly 1000 each day. The average age of male and female victims is 65 years, but many are just in their 30s and 40s. The majority of arrests are due to **cardiac arrhythmias,** the most common being **ventricular fibrillation** (see Chapter 16). The heart's electrical signals become very chaotic, that is, "quivering" rather than beating with coordinated contractions; contractions cease, consciousness is lost, often without warning, and death follows within minutes if the condition is not reversed. To reverse this life-threatening condition, **external defibrillation,** the application of an electric shock to the heart muscle through the chest wall, is required. Defibrillation can end the irregular contractions and allow the heart to resume a coordinated rhythm.

Defibrillation given in less than 3 minutes after a cardiac arrest is most likely to be successful. For every minute that defibrillation is delayed, the likelihood of survival decreases by approximately 10%. Very few resuscitation attempts are successful after as little as 10 minutes (Figure 17-18).

FIGURE 17-17   Heartstream's ForeRunner portable external automated defibrillator. (Courtesy Hewlett-Packard, Heartstream, Seattle, Wash.)

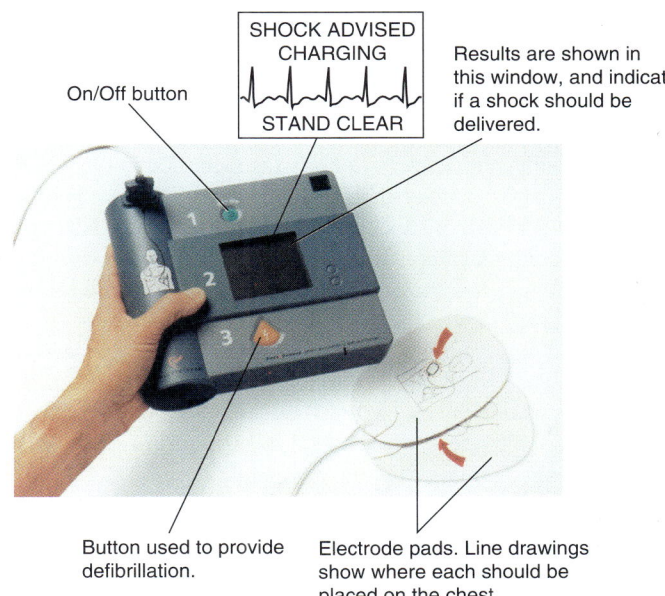

On/Off button

SHOCK ADVISED
CHARGING

STAND CLEAR

Results are shown in this window, and indicate if a shock should be delivered.

Button used to provide defibrillation.

Electrode pads. Line drawings show where each should be placed on the chest.

FIGURE 17-18 Relationship between sudden cardiac arrest *survival rate* and *time* to defibrillation. (Courtesy Hewlett Packard, Heartstream, Seattle, Washington).

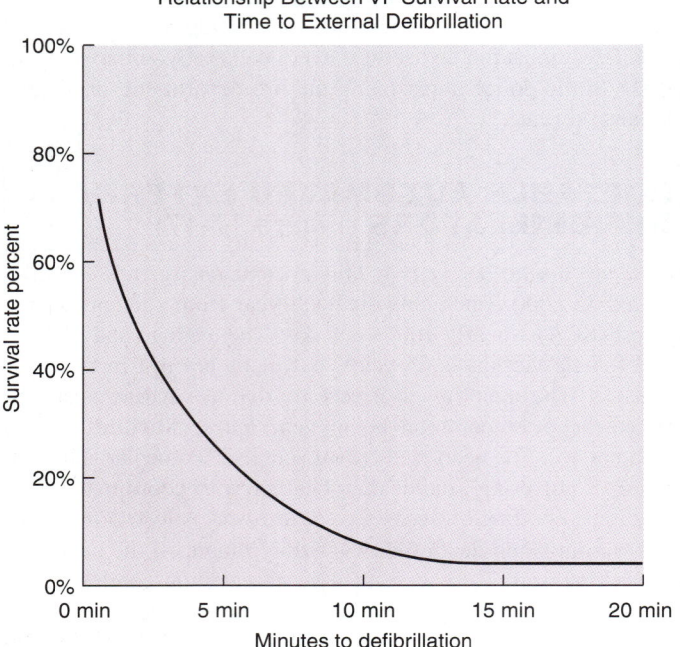

FIGURE 17-19 Heartstream's ForeRunner portable external automated defibrillator in use. Note the position of the electrodes on the chest. (Courtesy Hewlett Packard, Heartstream, Seattle, Washington).

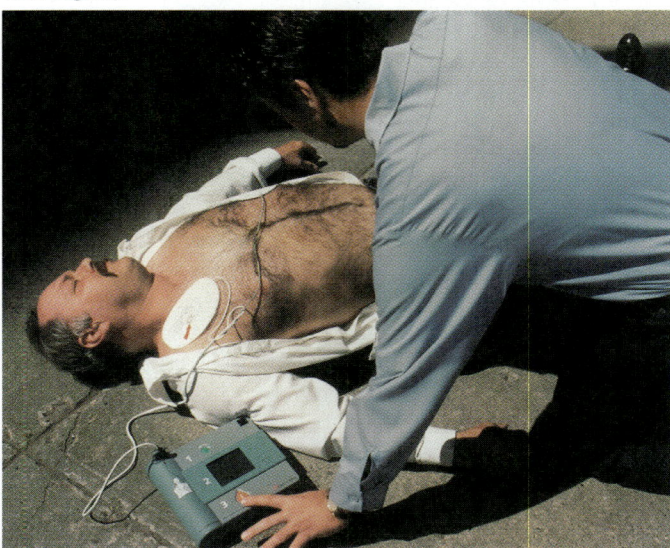

The American Heart Association has now included the use of portable automated external defibrillators (AEDs) as **standard care by all basic life support (BLS)** trained personnel who respond to a cardiac arrest. The built-in microcomputer in AEDs has the ability to accurately assess life-threatening, shockable ventricular arrhythmias (ventricular fibrillation and pulseless ventricular tachycardia) from normal rhythms or arrhythmias that should not be shocked in a cardiac arrest victim. The operator of the AED does not have to know how to recognize an arrhythmia or anything else on an ECG strip. **All that has to be done** is to apply the two electrodes to the chest of a patient who is unresponsive, pulseless, and not breathing. The chest positions where the electrodes should be placed are illustrated by line drawings on the electrode pads. **Safety controls** are built into the AED to guarantee that it will only activate the shock button when a life-threatening shockable arrhythmia is identified in the AED. The device *will not* activate the shock button and will not permit the operator to deliver a shock at any other time. **The AED will signal that defibrillation is indicated.** After the operator makes sure that no one is touching the patient, a preprogrammed shock can be delivered (Figure 17-19).

Training is required to learn how to operate the AED. These portable devices are becoming increasingly more common in various health care settings, as well as in industry, and will soon be considered the **initial treatment for patients older than age 8 in cardiac arrest.** Applying an AED to patients before giving CPR has little effect on the poor condition of patients who have nonshockable rhythms, such as asystole (a life-threatening condition involving an absence of electrical and mechanical activity in the heart).

Key Points for Using an Automated External Defibrillator

1. Use an AED only on patients who *are not* breathing and who have no pulse.
2. Give defibrillation before CPR. If you are the only first responder at the scene of a cardiac arrest, you must get, attach, and activate the AED. CPR is provided *only* if there is a delay in obtaining an AED or when the AED indicates that a shock to the heart is not advised.
3. Attention must be given to **safety factors.** All people must be clear of the patient before an AED is used for defibrillation because the defibrillator gives an electrical shock. Also, it is vital that the electrodes **not touch each other** when they are placed on a person with a small body frame (e.g., on a child).

Ultimately, improved outcomes and saving a person's life who has ventricular fibrillation depend specifically on more rapid access to defibrillation. Defibrillation must become part of lifesaving measures *at the scene* of a cardiac arrest. The American Heart Association estimates that 20,000 to 100,000 lives could be saved if AEDs were more readily available for first responders to use at the scene. By having a few hours of additional training along with CPR, many people responding to cardiac emergencies could qualify to provide lifesaving defibrillation for victims of sudden cardiac arrest. This technical advance in medical science has the potential to prevent tens of thousands of unnecessary deaths each year.

SHOCK

Shock, a state of collapse or a depressed condition of the circulatory system, occurs when the vital organs of the body are deprived of circulating blood flow necessary to sustain their normal cellular activity. It is a physiologic reaction of the body to severe injury or insult. Circulatory collapse may occur following hemorrhage, severe trauma, dehydration, massive infection, severe burns, surgery, increased peripheral resistance, decreased cardiac output, drug toxicity, pain, fear, or emotional distress.

Shock may be immediate or delayed, slight or severe, or even fatal. Every injury is accompanied by some degree of shock and should be treated promptly.

Types of Shock

Shock may be divided into six basic types. The exact cause of shock is not always the same for every patient.

Traumatic shock.   Traumatic shock is the direct result of extracellular fluid loss (for example, with extensive contusions or the loss of plasma from large burned areas).

Hemorrhagic or hypovolemic shock.   Hemorrhagic or hypovolemic shock is produced by a decrease in the circulating blood volume. The blood loss may be external or internal (into a body cavity where it is no longer accessible to the circulatory system).

Cardiogenic shock.   Cardiogenic shock is the result of conditions that interfere with the heart's function as a pump. This may be a result of cardiac failure, secondary to myocardial infarction, coronary thrombosis, or certain disorders of the rate and rhythm of the heart.

Septic shock.   Septic shock results from bacterial infection. It may occur from a massive infection of traumatized tissue or when toxic tissue products are absorbed. Gram-negative shock is a form of septic shock caused by infection with gram-negative bacteria (see Chapter 11).

Neurogenic shock.   Neurogenic shock is the result of loss of peripheral vascular tone with subsequent dilation of the blood vessels, decreased heart rate, and a drop in blood pressure to the point at which the supply of oxygen carried to the brain by the blood is insufficient. The patient then faints; thus this type of shock is often called fainting (syncope).

Anaphylactic shock.   Another type of shock is called *allergic* or *anaphylactic shock*. See "Allergic Reaction" on p. 756.

Signs and Symptoms of Shock

Five *P*'s denote the outstanding signs and symptoms of shock.

1. Prostration (extreme exhaustion; lack of energy)
2. Pallor (paleness)
3. Perspiration
4. Pulse (weak, rapid, and irregular)
5. Pulmonary deficiency

These vary in intensity, depending on the patient's condition and the injury or cause.

The most outstanding signs and symptoms of severe shock or the later stages of shock include the following:

1. The pulse is weak, rapid, and irregular.
2. Respirations increase in rate and are shallow.
3. Blood pressure is lowered—less than 90 mm Hg systolic.
4. The skin is markedly pale and may feel cold to the touch and moist with perspiration.
5. The lips, nailbeds, tips of the fingers, and lobes of the ears may be bluish (cyanosis).
6. The face may appear pinched and without expression.
7. The eyes may stare and often lose their characteristic luster.
8. The pupils may be dilated, especially in the late stages.
9. Occasionally the patient may be unusually anxious, restless, or excited.
10. When conscious, the patient appears disinterested in the surroundings and complains little of pain, although he or she may be groaning.
11. Later the patient may become apathetic and unresponsive. Eyes are sunken with a vacant expression.
12. If untreated, the patient eventually loses consciousness, vital signs drop, and death may occur.

First Aid Care

In any emergency situation, routinely evaluate the situation for the possibility of shock and take measures to prevent it. The following objectives for preventing or treating shock should be met:

1. Improve circulation of blood; control bleeding when necessary.
2. Ensure an open airway and an adequate supply of oxygen.
3. Maintain normal body temperature and keep the patient at rest.
4. Obtain medical assistance as and when required.

When treating a patient in shock, *the following steps apply:*

1. Do a quick primary survey of the situation. Ensure the ABCs of all emergencies; that is, maintain an open airway and check for breathing and circulation. Be prepared to give CPR if necessary.
2. Control severe bleeding if present.
3. Position the patient in a supine (lying) position with the lower extremities elevated 8 to 12 inches, *except* when there is a head injury, if breathing difficulty is thereby increased, if the patient complains of pain when this is attempted, or if the patient is vomiting. Keep a patient with a head injury lying flat or prop the head and shoulders up slightly.
4. Keep the patient warm but do not overheat.
5. Loosen tight clothing.
6. Do not move the patient unnecessarily.
7. Avoid disturbing the patient with noise and questions.
8. Do not give anything by mouth. When the patient has very dry lips or mouth, soak 4 × 4 gauze squares in cool water.

Have the patient suck on them. This helps to relieve some of the dryness.

9. When necessary, administer oxygen but only with the consent and directions of the physician (see Chapter 7, p. 403).

10. Provide constant, kindly, tactful encouragement and extreme gentleness when caring for the patient.

11. Call the physician or hospital promptly when the patient is going into or is in the state of shock.

12. Arrange for ambulance transport as indicated. Do not attempt to move the patient alone without explicit instructions from the physician unless the immediate surroundings would cause further harm to the patient.

ABDOMINAL PAIN

All abdominal pain should be investigated, especially unusual pain that occurs rather suddenly and is accompanied by fever. Treatment varies with the cause of pain. For pain caused by trauma, keep the patient lying flat if possible, in case of internal bleeding. For pain caused from metabolic or pathologic causes, keep the patient in a comfortable position until medical help arrives or the patient is transported to the hospital. The patient may flex the knees if moving the legs does not cause pain. Flexing the knees allows the abdominal muscles to relax. For any abdominal pain, remember the following:

- Keep the patient quiet and warm. Keep activity to a minimum.
- Do not apply heat.
- Do not give food, liquids, or laxatives.
- Place an emesis basin nearby in case the patient vomits.
- Check the patient frequently.
- Be empathetic.

Pathologic processes causing acute abdominal emergencies are inflammation, hemorrhage, perforation, obstruction, and ischemia (lack of adequate blood supply). These medical emergencies require immediate care by a physician because most often they require surgical intervention, although some may be treated medically.

ALLERGIC REACTION (ANAPHYLACTIC REACTION) TO DRUGS

Usually in an anaphylactic reaction or in any type of drug overdose reaction, the airway, breathing, and circulation will become impaired because of the effects of drugs on the central nervous system. Thus a **primary survey (the ABCs)** must be done.

A = *Airway*
Ensure that the airway is open.

B = *Breathing*
After you ensure that the airway is open, make sure that the breathing is spontaneous; in other words, make sure that the patient is breathing on his or her own.

C = *Circulation*
Check for a pulse beat. The best place to check the pulse rate is at the carotid artery.

When any of these areas requires stabilization, do nothing else except stabilize the ABCs and call or send for medical help. A **secondary survey** should also be made to ensure that the patient has no additional injury. This is a quick head-to-toe check to observe for any obvious bleeding or injury that may require immediate attention. It is necessary to stay with the patient until medical help arrives to ensure the ABCs. Oxygen and epinephrine should be available for administration on the physician's order. Usually 4 to 8 liters per minute of oxygen is administered by mask or nasal cannula, and 0.1 to 0.5 mg epinephrine 1:1000 is administered subcutaneously.

Constantly monitor the level of consciousness and vital signs and maintain an adequate airway and ventilation.

Positioning the patient is also very important. Often when a patient goes into anaphylaxis, a lying position cannot be tolerated. Usually the patient must be in a sitting or a semi-Fowler's position to expand the lungs and breathe more easily. Monitor the vital signs carefully, approximately every 2 or 3 minutes, note the skin color, and again monitor the airway. An oropharyngeal airway may be used at times to allow more air to enter the air passageways. When a reversal is not accomplished within a reasonable time, rapid transport to the hospital is necessary.

You should encourage patients with known allergies to wear a **Medic Alert bracelet** or **necklace** (see p. 771).

ASPHYXIA

Asphyxia may occur whenever there is an interference with the normal exchange of oxygen and carbon dioxide between the lungs and outside air. Obstruction of the airway is a common cause of asphyxia. This is commonly caused by foreign bodies, by the tongue, or by edema of the tissues, as seen in burns or inflammatory processes of the air passages. Drowning; electric shock; inhalation of smoke and poisonous gases; trauma to or disease of the lungs, bronchi, and trachea; or allergic reactions can all cause asphyxia. Basically the patient is apneic (not breathing). Immediate treatment is essential. **Follow the ABCs**—check for an open airway, breathing, and circulation. Open the airway if necessary and give artificial ventilation. Remove the underlying cause whenever possible. When both breathing and heartbeat are absent, give CPR immediately. Have oxygen available; it may be given when the patient is having difficulty breathing and also is often administered after breathing resumes to treat the resultant hypoxia (see Oxygen Administration in Chapter 7). Send for medical help or call the physician.

HUMAN, ANIMAL, SNAKE, AND INSECT BITES AND STINGS

Bites

Injuries resulting from animal or human bites may cause punctures, lacerations, or even avulsions, as the person attempts to pull away from the animal or human (see Chapter 6 for types of wounds). Human bites have a high potential for infection because of the high bacterial count in the human mouth. The danger of animal bites is rabies. Bites on the face, neck, or head are considered most serious and require immediate medical attention.

Human and animal bites.   The first aid care for human and animal bites is a thorough washing with soap and water for 5 minutes and copious rinsing under running water. An antibiotic ointment may be applied to the wound and then covered with a sterile or clean dressing. Keep the patient quiet and avoid movement of the affected part until attended by the physician. Report animal bites to the police or health department because the animal should be kept for observation for rabies. Collect information from the patient for the possibility of rabies. If the animal is not found and is believed to be rabid, treatment for rabies should be administered. Also, treatment against tetanus should be given.

Common insect bites.   Bites from ants, mosquitoes, and chiggers can be cared for by washing the affected parts with soap and water, applying a paste made from baking soda and a little water, or applying calamine lotion. Cover the site to keep it clean. When swelling is present, cover the area with a cloth saturated with ice water or a cold pack.

Tick bites.   Do not try to tear an embedded tick lose. Cover it with heavy oil (mineral or salad) or petroleum jelly to close the tick's breathing pores. Often this will disengage the tick at once; if not, allow the oil or jelly to remain in place for 30 minutes. If the tick does not disengage after this time, remove it with tweezers (close to the head of the tick), working slowly and gently and in a counterclockwise direction, so that all parts are removed. Wash the area with soap and water for 5 minutes. Apply an antibiotic ointment if one is available. Do not touch the tick with your hands because ticks can transmit several diseases. If the skin area becomes inflamed and swollen, if the patient develops a fever or flulike symptoms, or if you suspect or if symptoms are suggestive of Lyme disease, the physician must be notified.

Severe reactions to bites from spider, jellyfish, or insect or marine animal of unknown origin. Maintain an open airway; give CPR and treat for shock when necessary.

For jellyfish and other marine life, rub the affected area with sand and soak it in salt water. Apply a baking soda paste if available.

Keep the affected part immobile and below the individual's heart level. The victim should lie quietly and be covered with a blanket to maintain warmth. Wash the wound and apply ice wrapped in a towel or plastic bag or cold compresses to prevent spread of the poison and to prevent and reduce swelling. Summon the physician or have the victim taken to a hospital emergency room at once.

Antivenins can be given by professionals for black widow spider bites and for a scorpion sting.

Snakebites.   Much controversy has taken place in the past few years regarding the care of a victim of a snakebite. The current recommended care follows:

- Wash the wound with soap and water, blot dry, and apply a dressing (preferably sterile) and bandage.
- Immobilize the area.
- Keep the affected area lower than the victim's heart level.
- Get medical attention as soon as possible. Call the nearest physician or hospital to notify them to prepare antivenin.
- If possible, carry the victim who must be transported. If the victim must walk, have her or him walk slowly. Rapid movement must be avoided.
- If professional help cannot be obtained within 30 minutes, you should suction the wound using the suction cup from a snakebite kit.

Regardless of what you have heard, **DO NOT** apply ice, cut the wound, or apply a tourniquet.

Stings of bees, wasps, and hornets.   To care for a bee, wasp, or hornet sting, snap the barb off with your finger and then with tweezers try to remove the stinger. Run cold water over and around the sting or apply ice in a towel or plastic bag around it to relieve pain and slow the absorption of the venom. A victim of massive stings should be seen by a physician. If an allergic reaction develops, the victim must be immediately seen by the physician.

SEVERE BLEEDING (HEMORRHAGE)

Three types of bleeding can be observed from open wounds. Spurting of bright red blood from a wound indicates **arterial bleeding;** continuous flow of dark red blood indicates **venous bleeding;** and oozing of blood indicates **capillary bleeding.** Arterial bleeding is the most serious, requiring immediate control and medical intervention after the initial control to prevent severe shock or death. Generally, venous bleeding is easier to control than arterial bleeding because there is less pressure on the blood flow in the veins than in the arteries. However, venous bleeding may also be life threatening, especially if several large veins are involved. Capillary bleeding is easily controlled by first aid measures and the body's own clotting mechanisms.

Immediate action is imperative for any wound accompanied by severe bleeding because shock, loss of consciousness, and even death may occur from a rapid loss of blood in a short time.

Objectives of Wound Care
- To control the bleeding immediately
- To protect the wound from contamination and infection (as feasible; in emergency situations where sterile dressings are not available, you must use materials on hand, even if not sterile. It is more important to save the person's life by controlling the bleeding than to worry about preventing infection.)
- To treat for shock
- To obtain medical attention

Four Methods to Control Severe Bleeding
The following methods are listed in order of preference (Figure 17-20).

FIGURE 17-20 How to control severe bleeding. **A,** Apply direct pressure to the wound using a sterile gauze pad or clean cloth. **B,** Elevate the injured area above the level of the heart if there is no fracture. **C,** Apply a pressure bandage. The victim may be able to help you. **D,** If necessary, slow the flow of blood by applying pressure to the artery with your hand at the appropriate pressure point. (Courtesy The American National Red Cross.)

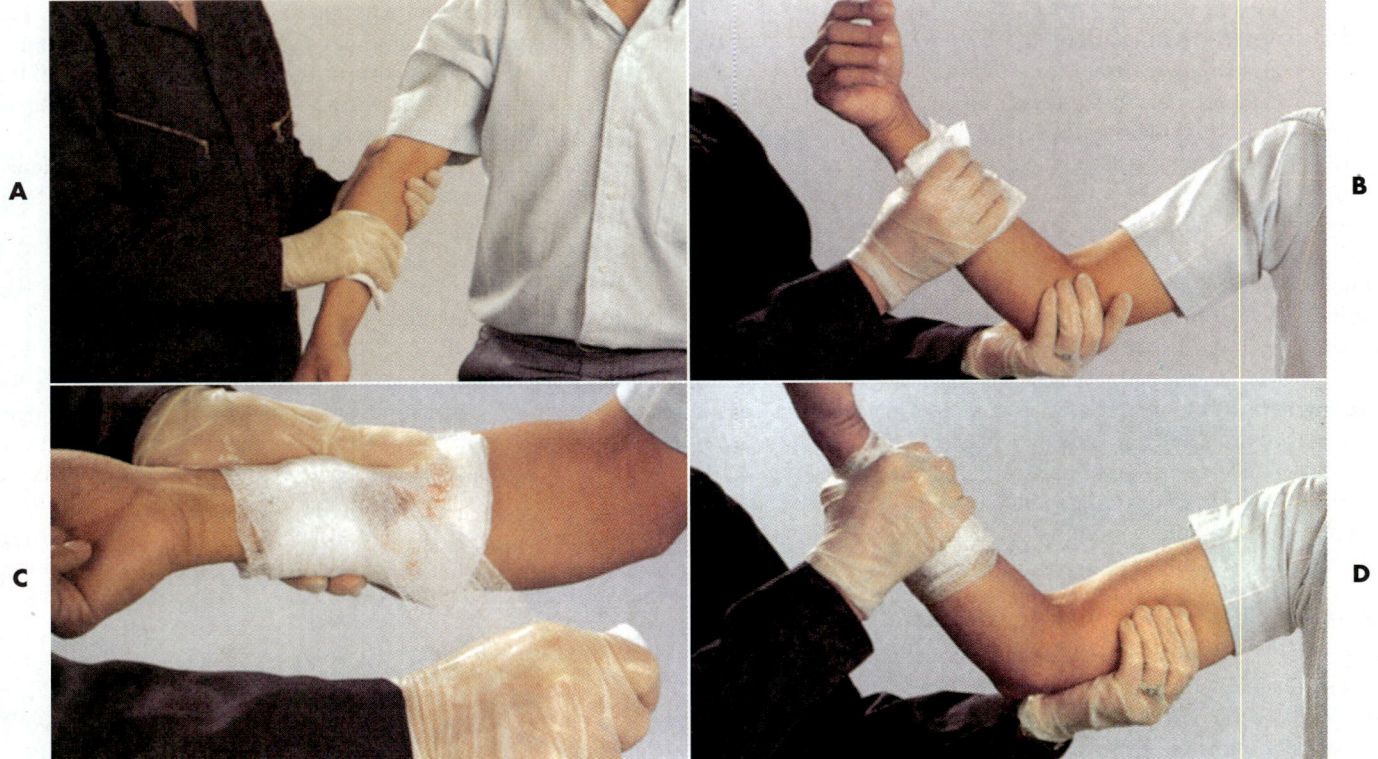

Direct pressure. Place a sterile dressing (or the cleanest cloth item on hand) over the wound site and apply hard, firm, direct pressure. This is usually effective in controlling severe bleeding. In the absence of dressing or cloth materials, apply direct pressure with the hand or fingers, but only until a compress is obtained. If a dressing becomes saturated with blood, do not remove it but place additional dressings directly over the saturated one and continue firm, direct pressure.

Elevation. Elevate a limb above the person's heart level in conjunction with direct pressure, unless a fracture is possible or if this action causes pain. Elevation helps reduce blood pressure within the limb, thus slowing down blood loss from the wound.

Pressure bandage. A bandage applied to control bleeding is called a pressure bandage. Cover the dressing that you have placed on the wound with a roller bandage using overlapping turns. Tie or tape the bandage in place. If blood soaks through, add more dressings and bandage over them.

Pressure points. When severe bleeding is not controlled with direct pressure, elevation of an affected limb, or a pressure bandage, the pressure point method can be applied in conjunction with the first three methods. The pressure point method compresses the blood vessel supplying blood to the wound against an underlying bone or muscle tissue in an effort to close it off and reduce the amount of blood flowing through the vessel to the wound site. This method can control bleeding in all but a few circumstances. The exact position of the pressure point must be known and located quickly; otherwise, significant blood loss will result. The **seven pressure points follow** (really 14, counting one on each side of the body) (Figure 17-21).

Temporal artery. Compression on the temporal artery may be used to control superficial wounds of the forehead or the frontal part of the scalp.

Facial artery. Upward and outward compression of the facial artery against the jawbone with two or more fingers may be used to control bleeding in the facial region.

Carotid artery. Compression of the carotid artery in the neck against underlying muscle tissue may be used to control only serious hemorrhaging in the head. When this pressure point is used, extreme care must be taken to avoid obstructing the person's airway. ***Do not*** apply pressure dressings around the neck.

Subclavian artery. Downward compression with the fingers on the subclavian artery just behind the collar bone (the

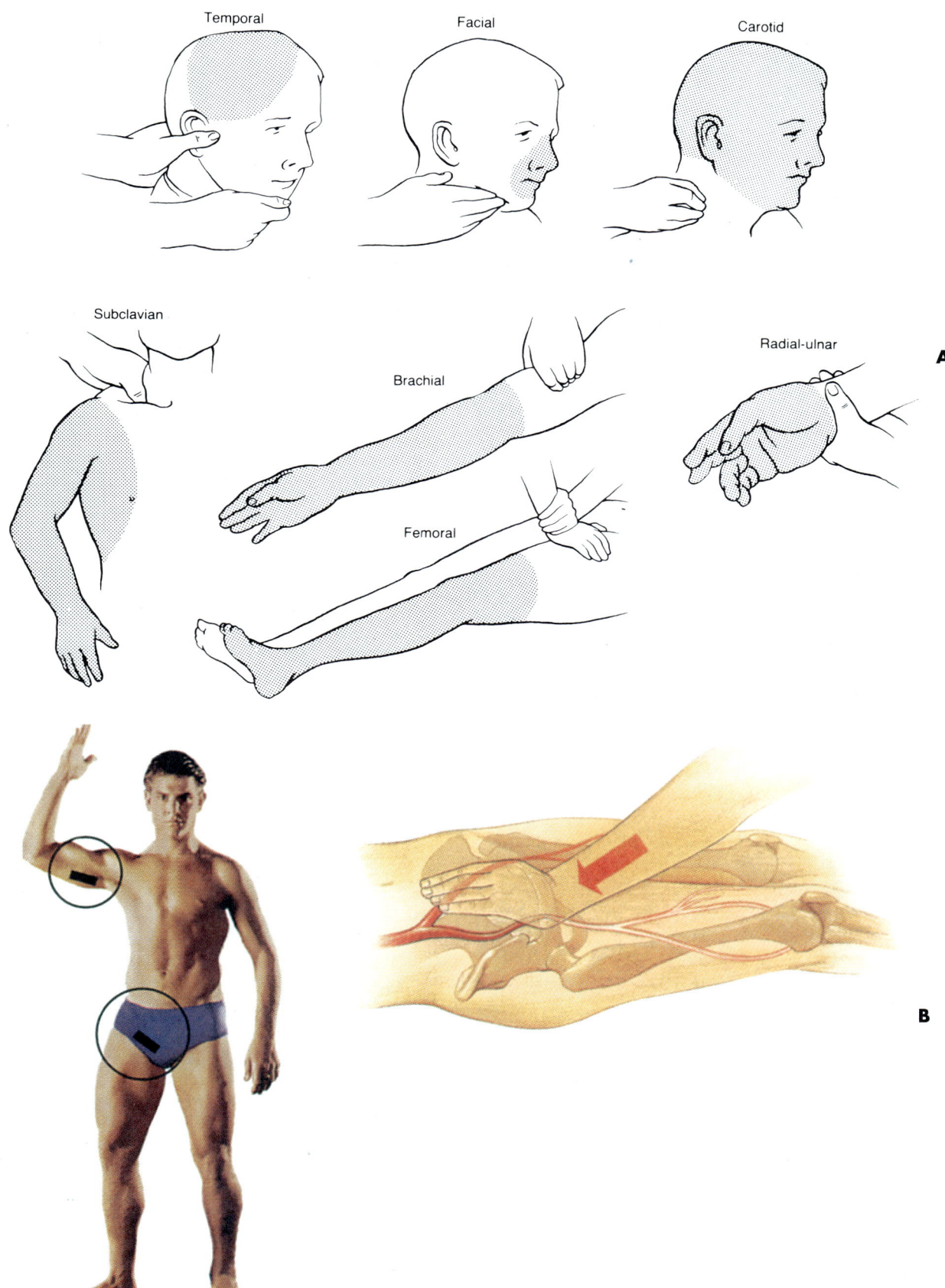

FIGURE 17-21 **A,** Location of pressure points. **B,** Pressure points are specific sites on the body where arteries lie close to the bone and the body's surface. Blood flow to an area can be controlled by applying pressure at one of these sites, compressing the artery against the bone. (**A** from Parcel G, Rinear C: *Basic emergency care of the sick and injured,* ed 4, St Louis, 1990, Mosby; **B** courtesy The American National Red Cross.)

Temporal

Facial

Carotid

Subclavian

Brachial

Radial-ulnar

Femoral

A

B

clavicle) may be used to control bleeding in the arm and upper shoulder regions.

Brachial artery. Compression of the brachial artery against the bone with the fingers applied midway between the shoulder and elbow on the inside of the arm may be used to control bleeding from the arm, hand, and fingers.

Femoral artery. Compression of the femoral artery (in the center of the groin area) against the pelvic bone with the heel of the hand may be used to control bleeding from the leg.

Radial artery. Compression of the radial artery on the anterior side of the wrist on the thumb side may be used to control severe bleeding from the hand or fingers.

Compression of the ulnar artery (on the little finger, anterior side of the wrist) should be used in conjunction with compression of the radial artery to control profuse hemorrhaging from the hand. If bleeding does not stop with compression on the radial and ulnar arteries, apply pressure to the brachial artery to control the bleeding.

Tourniquet

The use of a tourniquet is no longer recommended as standard first aid practice by the American Red Cross. The procedure is presented here to be used only in extreme cases that comply with medical practice in your locality.

The use of a tourniquet is dangerous and should be used only as a last resort to control severe, life-threatening hemorrhage when direct pressure, elevation, pressure bandage, and pressure point methods fail to control the bleeding. The dangers of nerve damage, blood vessel damage, and tissue damage exist when a tourniquet is applied; thus a **tourniquet must be avoided unless a life could be lost.** In essence, the decision to apply a tourniquet is a decision to risk the loss of the person's limb to save life. After the application of a tourniquet, it is imperative that the person be attended to by a physician. The following directions *must* be observed when a tourniquet is applied (Figure 17-22).

1. Use appropriate materials at least 2 inches wide, such as a stocking, a cloth, a folded triangular bandage, or a blood pressure cuff, if available.
2. Apply the tourniquet just above the wound, or just above a joint when the wound is in or below a joint area.
3. Wrap the tourniquet material around the limb twice, and secure it with a knot.
4. Insert a strong stick or similar object between the two loops and twist this object to tighten the tourniquet until bleeding stops. Tourniquets must be applied tightly enough to stop the bleeding; if applied too loosely, bleeding will increase.
5. Wrap the ends of the tourniquet material around the stick or similar object and tie it in place.
6. Make a written note of the time of application and the location of the tourniquet and attach this to the person's clothing, or mark this information on the person. Often

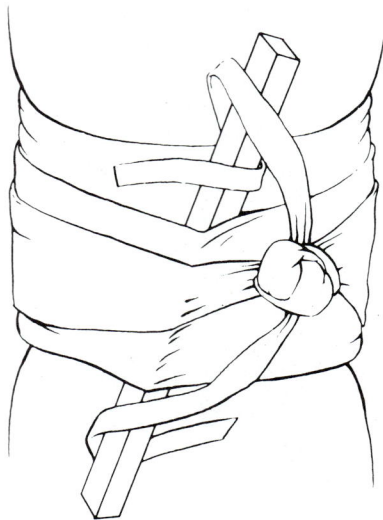

FIGURE 17-22 Procedure for application of tourniquet. (From Parcel G, Rinear C: *Basic emergency care of the sick and injured,* ed 4, St Louis, 1990, Mosby.)

people will mark a large *TK* (for tourniquet) on the injured person's forehead with lipstick when at the scene of the accident.

7. *Never* release a tourniquet once it has been applied. A tourniquet must be removed only by a physician, who can provide supportive treatment for shock.
8. Elevate the limb slightly if this does not cause further injury.
9. Treat for shock and give first aid for other injuries as required.
10. Transport the person immediately to receive medical attention.

Amputation

In cases of amputation, the amputated part should be kept cool and moist, if possible, and taken with the victim to the physician. With the advent of microsurgery, amputated limbs can often be reattached successfully, providing that damage to the surrounding tissues was minimal.

Further Wound Care

For capillary bleeding, direct pressure and the application of ice wrapped in a towel or plastic bag are useful. Remember that ice is not effective in controlling severe bleeding.

In all cases when caring for bleeding wounds, provide reassurance and emotional support to the victim and remain calm. If possible, estimate how much blood was lost because this will help the physician treat the person and determine if fluid replacement is necessary. However, remember that even an ounce of blood can discolor many dressings and that a cup of blood poured on the floor or ground covers a fairly large area; this is because blood that first comes from the vessels is thin, so a small amount looks like a lot. Also observe the actual bleeding—is it a minimal, moderate, or heavy flow? This information will aid the physician, in addition to guiding your decision for the use of a tourniquet.

When bleeding stops, bandage the dressings firmly in place. Do not remove the initial dressings because blood clots may be disturbed and bleeding may resume. Leave the cleaning and treatment of the wound to the physician.

Prevention of Contamination and Infection

To prevent infection, avoid touching the wound with an unsterilized dressing or your unscrubbed hands if possible. Do not disturb or remove the initial dressing placed over the wound.

BURNS

Burns are wounds caused by body contact with fire (dry heat), steam and scalding water (moist heat), electricity, chemicals, radiation (sun or nuclear rays), or lightning. Each year thousands of burns occur, many of which could have been prevented and many of which are fatal in both the young and old. Burns involving over one third to one half of the body are often fatal, especially in children. Theories on the treatment for burns have undergone many changes over the years; many remedies were advocated and later rejected. Current thought on the matter can best be summed up by following the three *B*'s and the three *C*'s.

B = *Burn*
  Stop the burning.
B = *Breathing*
  Check the breathing.
B = *Body examination*
  Examine where and how extensively the body has been burned and assess any associated injuries.

C = *Cool*
  Cool the burn.
C = *Cover*
  Cover the burn.
C = *Carry*
  Carry the burn patient to the nearest medical treatment facility.

In addition, current treatment practices condemn the application of greasy substances, ointments, powders, or antiseptics to a burned area.

Classification of Burns

Burns are classified as first, second, and third degree, depending on the depth of the wound; they are also classified according to the percentage of body surface involved (Figures 17-23 and 17-24).

Depth of wound. First-degree burns, also called superficial burns, involve only the outer layers of the skin. The skin is reddened without blister formation and is painful. The best example is a sunburn. **Second-degree burns, also referred to as partial-thickness burns,** involve deeper layers of the epidermis, are painful, and usually form blisters. **Third-degree burns, also called full-thickness burns,** are the most

serious, destroying all layers of the skin, including the hair follicles and the sebaceous and sweat glands. Nerves are destroyed; thus the wound is painless. Muscles, blood supply, and bones may also be destroyed in third-degree burns.

Body surface. The percentage of total body surface involved usually determines the severity of the burn. The body surface is divided into areas by the rule of nines. Each arm is 9%, each leg is 18%, the front or back of the trunk is 18%, and the head and neck are 9% of the total body surface.

A first-degree burn that involves more than 20% of total body surface, involves the face and airway, or impairs the person when walking or wearing clothes should receive medical attention. Any second- or third-degree burn involving more than 20% of the total body surface or the feet, hands, or genitalia is considered a serious burn in need of medical attention. When more than 40% of total body surface is burned, it is considered a *severe burn*.

First Aid Treatment for Burns
Objectives for care of first-degree (superficial) burns
- To relieve pain
- To prevent the formation of blisters

First-degree (superficial) burn care
1. Immediately submerge the burned part in cool water or place cold compresses directly on the burn.
2. Continue this treatment until pain has subsided when the cold is discontinued.
3. Apply a dry sterile dressing if the burn is in an area that will be irritated by clothing.
4. When running water is available, it is best to place the burned part under cold running water for 20 minutes. The reason is that, even though the top layers of the skin are cooled within a few minutes, the underlying tissue is still very heated, and the burn continues to cause tissue damage up to periods of 20 minutes after the initial burn.
5. For *small* superficial burns and burns with *small* open blisters that do not require medical attention, wash with soap and water, keep the area clean, and apply an antibiotic ointment to help prevent infection.

Objectives for treating second- and third-degree burns (partial- and full-thickness burns)
1. To treat the person for shock
2. To prevent infection
3. To relieve pain

Second-degree (partial-thickness) burn care
1. Immediately submerge the burned part in cold water for 1 to 2 hours *or* place under running water for 20 minutes.
2. **Do not** break blisters or remove tissue.
3. Cover with a dressing or clean cloth that has been wrung out in cool water.
4. Apply a dry dressing and loosely bandage in place.

FIGURE 17-23   **A,** Cross section showing structures of skin; **B,** classification of burns by degree. (From Parcel G, Rinear C: *Basic emergency care of the sick and injured,* ed 4, St Louis, 1990, Mosby.)

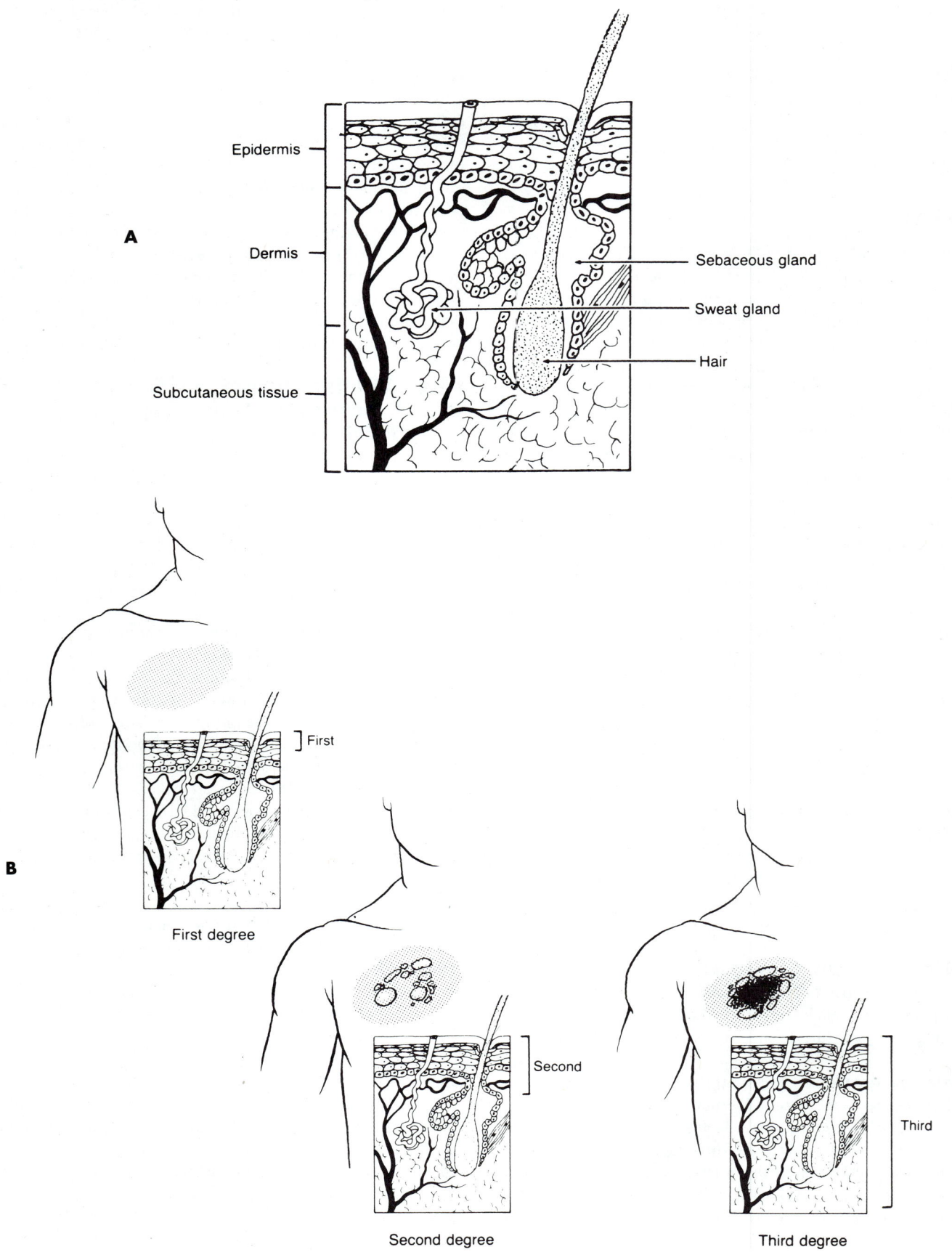

FIGURE 17-24   Classification of burns by body surface area. (From Parcel G, Rinear C: *Basic emergency care of the sick and injured,* ed 4, St Louis, 1990, Mosby.)

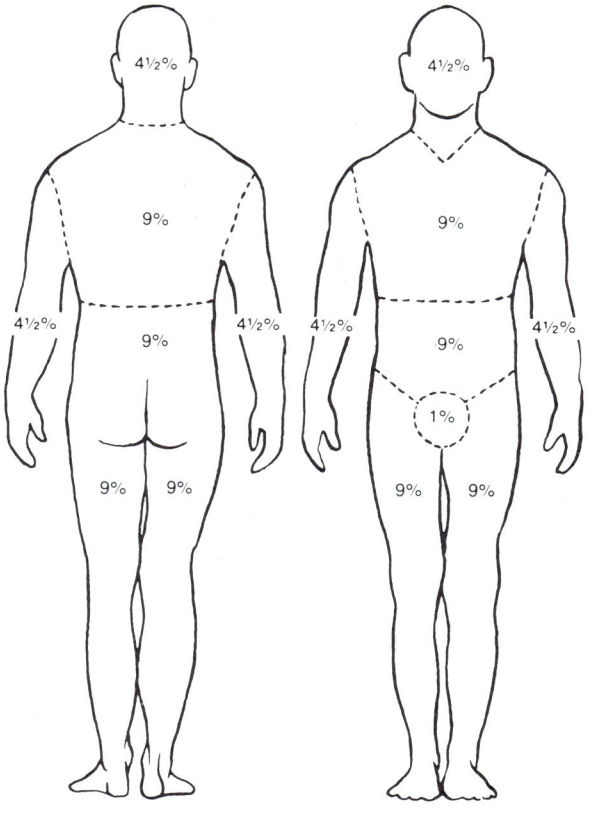

FIGURE 17-25   For chemical burns, wash immediately with copious amounts of cool running water for at least 5 minutes.

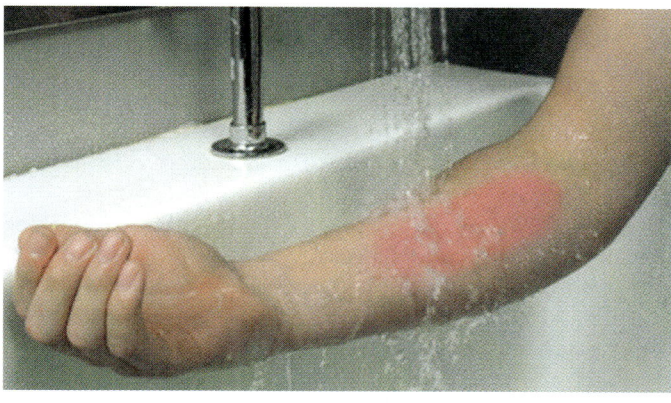

FIGURE 17-26   If chemical gets on face, flush face and eyes with a gentle flow of cool water.

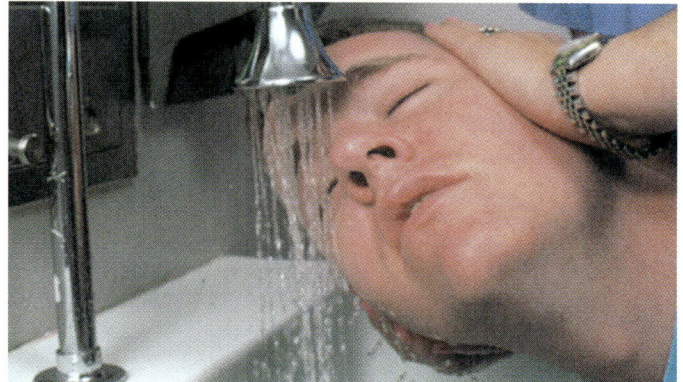

Third-degree (full-thickness) burn care

1. Stop the burning; check for breathing; remove the burning agent. Remove any smoldering clothing; certain synthetics retain heat. Remove any jewelry on the burned area. Clothing and jewelry retain heat and also can become constricting as edema develops. Do a quick body assessment to determine the extent and severity of the burn.
2. Keep the person lying down with the head a little lower than the legs and hips, unless the person has a chest or head injury or has difficulty breathing in this position.
3. Keep burned feet or legs elevated.
4. Keep burned hands above the level of the victim's heart.
5. Cool and cover the wound. Cover the burned areas with sterile dressings, if available, or a cloth or sheet. Pour copious amounts of cool water (**NOT** ice water) or saline, if available, onto the material covering the wound. Continue pouring cool water onto the material periodically because the burn continues to heat the water up to the material. If clean material is not available, water may be poured directly onto the wound. Do not use ice or ice water because this causes critical body heat loss. When the wound is cooled, wrap the person for transport to a medical facility. *Never open any blisters.* Covering the wound prevents moving air from reaching the wound, lessens pain, and reduces contamination, helping to prevent infection.
6. If adjoining surfaces of skin are burned, separate them with gauze or cloth to keep them from sticking together (such as between the toes or fingers, ears and head, arms and chest).
7. For **chemical burns,** wash immediately with *copious* amounts of cool running water for at least 5 minutes (Figure 17-25). Remove any clothing that was in contact with the chemical. If the chemical is on the face or eyes, flush the face and eyes with a gentle flow of cool water for at least 15 minutes (Figure 17-26). Remove contact lenses if the victim is wearing them. Try to find out what chemical caused the burn so that you can tell the personnel at the emergency department where the victim is taken. Also see the steps previously mentioned. **NOTE:** *Never* flush a phosphorus burn with any type of solution, including water, because this could cause tissue sloughing. Instead, *soak* the affected area in water.
8. For **facial burns,** prop the victim up and observe for signs of difficult breathing. Air passages could swell and cause breathing to be impaired or stopped. If you suspect a burned airway or burned lungs, continually monitor the victim's breathing.
9. If possible while awaiting transport for the person, take the pulse and respiration rates and blood pressure to assess impending shock.

10. Keep the patient warm and resting quietly. Chilling must be avoided to prevent additional discomfort and loss of energy.
11. Constantly provide emotional support for the patient.
12. Inform the patient before transfer is undertaken.

What *Not* to Do About Burns

* *Don't* pull clothing over the burned area—cut it away if necessary.
* *Don't* try to remove any pieces of cloth or bits of debris or dirt that are stuck to the burn.
* *Don't* try to clean the burn; *don't* use iodine or other antiseptics on it; and *don't* open any blisters that may form on the burn.
* *Don't* use grease, butter, ointment, salve, petroleum jelly, or any type of medication on any burn.
* *Don't* breathe on a burn and *don't* touch it with anything except a sterile or clean dressing.
* *Don't* apply ice directly to second-degree (partial-thickness) or third-degree (full-thickness) burns.
* *Don't* use absorbent cotton on burns.
* *Don't* change the dressings that were initially applied to the burn until directed to do so by a physician.

CEREBRAL VASCULAR ACCIDENT (STROKE)

A cerebral vascular accident (CVA), also called a stroke, is a disorder of the blood vessels of the brain that results in a lack of blood supply to parts of the brain. Main causes of a CVA include a cerebral thrombus or a cerebral embolus, a ruptured artery and a cerebral hemorrhage, compression of cerebral arteries (as from edema or tumors), and arterial spasms (Figure 17-27). The symptoms and effects of a CVA vary greatly. They can be slight or severe, temporary or permanent, depending on the cause, location, and extent of the damage in the brain. **Signs and symptoms of a CVA include the following:**

* Dizziness, mental confusion, headache, and poor coordination
* Difficulty in speaking or loss of speech
* Loss of bladder and bowel control
* Paralysis or weakness usually on only one side of the body
* Loss of vision, especially in one eye
* Difficulty in breathing and in swallowing
* Unequal size of the pupils
* Loss of consciousness

First Aid Measures for a Cerebral Vascular Accident

1. Loosen all constricting clothing, especially around the neck, to help improve breathing and circulation to the head.
2. Maintain an open airway.

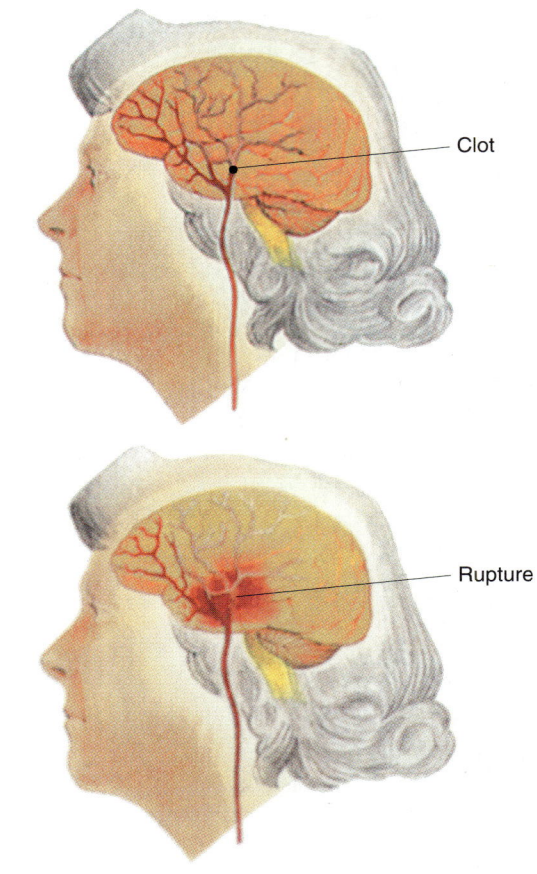

FIGURE 17-27   Cerebral vascular accident (CVA) can be caused by a cerebral thrombus or embolus, from a ruptured artery, and also from a cerebral hemorrhage. (From Ingalls AJ, Salerno MC: *Maternal and child health nursing,* ed 7, St Louis, 1991, Mosby.)

Clot

Rupture

3. Position the victim on the affected side so that secretions will drain from the mouth and thus prevent aspiration of saliva and mucus.
4. Keep the victim calm and provide reassurance that care is being provided.
5. If conscious, the victim may sit up or have the head elevated. This will help to lessen blood pressure in the head.
6. Do not give fluids unless the victim is able to swallow and is fully conscious. Discontinue all fluids if the victim vomits.
7. Seek medical attention as soon as possible. The victim usually needs to be hospitalized.
8. Be prepared to administer CPR if required.

CHEST PAIN

Chest pain can be associated with heart disease, lung disease, pain in the muscle fibers of the chest wall, and a few other conditions. It can be serious; therefore all patients with chest pain should be treated as if they are heart patients. First aid measures include the following:

HEALTH MATTERS

INFORMATION ABOUT STROKES

Approximately 400,000 first-ever strokes are reported each year in the United States. Over 4 million stroke survivors are alive today.

FOR MORE INFORMATION
The Stroke Connection "Warmline"
An information and referral service for stroke survivors, caregivers, and family members.
(800) 553-6321

The American Heart Association
(800) AHA-USA1
www.americanheart.org

National Stroke Association
Offers free screenings to inform people about their potential risk for stroke and what they can do to lower their risk.
(303) 649-9299, ext. 905

The American Academy of Physical Medication and Rehabilitation
(312) 464-9700

Stroke Caregiver Support
www.members.aol.com/scmmlm/nl.htm

HEALTH MATTERS

KEEPING YOUR PATIENTS INFORMED

STROKE IS A MEDICAL EMERGENCY! DIAL 911
KNOW THE WARNING SIGNS OF A STROKE
It is estimated that over 500,000 people in the United States suffer from a stroke each year. Stroke is the third-leading cause of death in the United States, following heart disease and cancer. In a stroke (cerebral vascular accident [CVA]), because blood supply is restricted or blocked to an area in the brain, the cells in that area are deprived of oxygen and nutrients. Brain cells deprived of oxygen can suffer from slight to severe and temporary to permanent damage and/or death. When brain cells don't function, the part of the body controlled by these cells cannot function either. For example, if the speech center in the brain is deprived of blood, the person will be unable to speak; if blood supply to areas in the brain that are in charge of motor coordination are obstructed, the person can be paralyzed. Blockage of blood to critical areas, such as the respiratory center or areas that affect heart function, could result in death.

Immediate attention to any of the warning signs may prevent a disabling or fatal stroke from occurring. See p. 764 for the signs and symptoms of a stroke. These will vary depending on the site and extent of brain damage.

Prevention and Risk Factors
Up to 80% of strokes are believed to be preventable by modifying key risk factors through either lifestyle changes and/or drugs. Therefore an awareness of the risk factors is important and information must be provided to patients.

Risk factors thought to increase a persons susceptibility to a stroke include the following:

Factors that cannot be changed or controlled:
- **Gender.** Studies have shown that men have a higher risk for stroke than women.
- **Age.** The risk of stroke more than doubles for a person every decade after age 55.
- **Race.** African Americans have a higher risk of strokes than whites; Hispanics are more likely to develop hemorrhagic strokes than whites.
- **Family history of strokes.** This increases a person's risk of having a stroke.

Factors that can be controlled, modified, or treated:
- **Hypertension.** Early detection and treatment of high blood pressure has significantly reduced the incidence of stroke. Treatment with medication for hypertension has been shown to reduce fatal and nonfatal strokes by 40%.
- **History of transient ischemic attacks (TIAs).** These are often referred to as "little strokes." TIAs cause minimal damage and serve as warning signs for potentially severe strokes in the future. About 10% of strokes are preceded by TIAs days, weeks, and even months before a major stroke. TIAs are temporary attacks that come on suddenly with short-lived and reversible symptoms. They last for only a few minutes to not more than 24 hours. Signs and symptoms include a numbness or weakness on one side of the body, slurred speech or inability to talk, visual disturbances ranging from blurred or double vision to blindness, and uncoordinated or staggered walking. Educating people about TIAs is extremely important because without treatment, the probability of having a serious stroke within the next 5 years is 25% to 35%.

Continued

- **Smoking.** Smokers have twice the risk of having a stroke than nonsmokers. If they quit smoking, their risk drops 50% in 2 years. Five years after quitting smoking, their risk for a stroke is nearly the same as nonsmokers.
- **Heart disease.** Heart disease can interfere with blood flow to the brain. Also, clots that develop in the heart can travel to the brain and obstruct blood flow to the brain cells.
- **Diabetes mellitus.** Diabetics have a higher risk and incidence of stroke than nondiabetics.
- **Blood fats.** Studies have shown that people with abnormally low amounts of high-density lipoproteins (HDLs) have more atherosclerosis in the walls of the carotid arteries that carry blood from the neck to the brain.
- **Physical inactivity.** Moderate amounts of exercise improve circulation and may increase HDLs, which in turn could lower the amount of cholesterol buildup in the blood vessels.
- **Obesity.** Being overweight puts an increased burden on the heart and blood vessels.

Dietary habits and exercise can help to reduce blood cholesterol and fat levels.

Treatment

Treatment for a stroke may include drugs, surgery, and rehabilitative therapy or any combination of these three treatments. The choice of medical treatment is determined by the condition that predisposes the person to a stroke or causes one or the potential benefit of the treatment after a stroke has occurred.

Common **drugs** used are anticoagulants and antihypertensives. Anticoagulants can reduce the blood's tendency to clot. They are used only when the potential or actual cause of decreased blood flow is clot formation. Antihypertensive drugs are used to decrease the pressure in the vessels and thereby reduce the risk of rupture. Newer thrombolytic drugs, commonly called "clot-busters" may also be used but *only* when the cause has been determined to be a clot (if given when the cause was a cerebral hemorrhage, they could worsen the patient's condition and possibly turn a serious stroke into a fatal one). These drugs *must* be given within the first 3 hours after

the onset of symptoms to halt the stroke process before lasting damage has occurred and usually only *after* a brain scan has been done to confirm that the stroke was *not* caused by bleeding. Thrombolytic drugs dissolve the clot and allow a return of blood flow and oxygen to the brain.

Surgical procedures used to prevent or lessen the severity of a stroke include the following:

- An endarterectomy. This surgery is now being used more often to prevent a stroke. In this procedure, atherosclerotic plaque is scraped from the inner lining of the carotid and/or vertebral arteries in the neck. The buildup of plaque in these vessels narrows and may totally obstruct the passageway for blood flow to the brain.
- A procedure involving patching or removing the section of an artery in which there is an aneurysm.
- A procedure involving removal of a blood clot in the artery.

Surgeons continue to study and develop ways to tie off tiny, bleeding cranial arteries with tiny clothespins and also ways to suction off blood that causes pressure on brain tissues.

Therapies

Rehabilitative therapies used to help patients regain physical function include the following:

- **Physical therapy.** Physical therapy employs the use of exercises and treatment with heat, water, or massage to restore function and movement.
- **Occupational therapy.** Occupational therapy teaches and helps patients with activities of daily living. It helps patients coordinate hand and eye movements to perform basic tasks, such as getting dressed and preparing food.
- **Speech therapy.** Speech therapy helps patients learn how to speak again.

All of these therapies are designed to help people return to independent living after suffering from a stroke.

1. Observe the symptoms.
2. Keep the patient quiet and warm. Allow the patient to rest. Often the patient finds it easier to breathe when in a semisitting or upright position. Do not have the patient walk any distance.
3. Loosen all tight clothing.
4. Administer 4 to 6 liters of oxygen (if you are in the office and have prior directions and permission from the physician).
5. Contact the physician. When the physician cannot be reached, call the EMS system in your community or an ambulance or the fire department.
6. Stay with the patient until medical help arrives.
7. If the patient is conscious, inquire if he or she has any medication on hand that is used for attacks of chest pain. The usual medication is nitroglycerin tablets, which are taken sublingually. You may give them to the patient with the patient's consent.
8. When feasible, obtain pertinent information from the patient. Use the PQRST method:
   P = Provoking
   What provoked the pain? Was the patient doing any physical activity, experiencing emotional upset or excitement, or just sitting quietly?
   Q = Quality of pain

Is it a sharp pain, prolonged oppressive pain, or unusual discomfort?

R = Radiation of pain

Where, if at all, does the pain radiate to? Is it in the center of the chest? Is it in the chest wall? Does it radiate to the abdomen or to the neck or to the left arm?

S = Severity

How severe is the pain—mild, moderate, or severe?

T = Time

When did the pain start? How long does it last? How frequently does it recur?

9. Keep an emesis basin handy in case the patient vomits.
10. At times, it may be necessary to start rescue breathing if breathing stops or CPR if there is no breathing and no pulse.
11. If in the physician's office, you may connect the patient to the electrocardiograph and record a few tracings for the physician to interpret. Leads II and V_1 are considered the monitoring leads.
12. Remain calm; offer emotional support and reassurance to the patient, because most patients will be anxious and frightened.

CONVULSIONS

Convulsions are the involuntary spasms or contractions of muscles caused by an abnormal stimulus to the brain or by changes in the chemical balance in the body. The primary effort in first aid for convulsions is to protect the patient from causing harm to the body during the convulsion.

1. Move items that may cause harm to the patient. Ask curious onlookers to remove themselves from the immediate area.
2. Loosen clothing around the neck and in any other area being constricted.
3. Place a padded bite block between the teeth to protect against biting of the tongue. *Do not* insert a bite block when force is required to get it in place. If an appropriate bite block is not available, one can be made by wrapping and taping a couple of pieces of gauze around two tongue blades. *Some suggest not to put anything between the patient's teeth. Check with the physician for his or her preference and policy.*
4. Do not restrain the patient's movements except to prevent injury. Protect the head at all times.
5. When movement has ceased, keep the patient lying down and allow him or her to rest.
6. Ensure an open airway.
7. If bleeding from a bitten tongue, excessive saliva, or vomit is present, turn the patient's head to one side to prevent aspiration of these excretions.
8. After all seizure activity has ceased, allow the patient to rest or sleep in a quiet, comfortable place until he or she is sufficiently oriented to time and place and capable of moving without weakness.

Anyone who has experienced a seizure (convulsion) should be seen by a physician, although the occurrence of one seizure is not considered an emergency. **If convulsive activity is repeated or occurs frequently, medical attention must be sought.**

If reporting the convulsion to the physician, providing a description of the convulsant activity is very important; that is, whether the convulsion was generalized or localized, how and where it started, how many convulsions there were, and how long they lasted. The *seizures* associated with epilepsy are a form of convulsion.

EPISTAXIS (NOSEBLEED)

Most nosebleeds are not serious and can be easily controlled. However, excessive bleeding requires medical attention and may require electrocauterization of the ruptured vessels causing the bleeding.

First aid for nosebleeds is relatively simple. Have the patient in a sitting position and pinch the lower portion of the nose between the thumb and index finger for 5 to 10 minutes. When this does not control the bleeding, apply ice packs to the nasal and facial areas. Place a moistened gauze pad gently into the bleeding nostril, leaving one end of the gauze outside so that it can be removed easily, and then pinch the nose between the thumb and index finger for 10 minutes. If this does not control the bleeding, medical attention should be obtained.

FAINTING (SYNCOPE)

Fainting is a partial or complete loss of consciousness of limited duration caused by a decreased amount of blood to the brain. A person may feel weak and dizzy, cold, or nauseated; appear pale; perspire; and have numbness or tingling in the hands and feet before fainting; or one may faint suddenly. **First aid** management for patients who faint is as follows:

1. Lay the person flat with the head lowered slightly.
2. Ensure an open airway.
3. Loosen tight clothing.
4. Apply cold cloths to the face. These are beneficial because of their stimulating effect.
5. Pass aromatic spirits of ammonia back and forth in front of the person's nose to allow inhalation. Avoid holding them too close to the person's nose.
6. Observe the person carefully, looking for anything unusual.
7. Observe for local weakness of the arms and legs and locate and count the pulse. These observations may be of great importance if the condition turns out to be something other than a fainting episode.
8. Keep the person resting quietly for at least 10 minutes after full consciousness has been regained.
9. Lower the head between the legs when the person is in a sitting position and begins to feel faint. Stay with the person and protect against falling should fainting occur.
10. When fainting lasts more than a minute or two, keep the person warm and resting quietly and summon the physician or transport to the hospital because the condition may not be a simple episode of fainting. It may, in fact, be a

symptom of diabetes, heart disease, epilepsy, stroke, or any one of many diseases.

FOREIGN BODIES IN THE EAR, EYE, AND NOSE

Ear

Foreign bodies lodged in the ear canal are often seen in children. *Do not* attempt to remove them. They must be removed by the physician because of the possibility of injury to the eardrum (tympanic membrane) and ear canal tissue.

If the foreign body in the ear is a live bug or insect, instill a few drops of sterile oil into the ear canal. This will asphyxiate and stop the movement of the intruder.

Eye

Foreign bodies in the eye are irritating and can be harmful because of the possibility of their scratching the eye surface or becoming embedded in the eye tissue.

Instruct the patient not to rub the affected eye. Wash your hands and examine the eye by pulling the lower lid down and turning the upper lid back. If the object is on either lid, take a moistened corner of a clean cloth and touch it lightly to try to remove it. Avoid applying any pressure on the eye. If the object is on the eye itself, do not attempt to remove it this way. At times, when the object is located under the upper eyelid or on the eye, it may be dislodged by pulling the upper eyelid forward and down over the lower lid; tears may dislodge the object. The eye then may be flushed with clean water (see also Eye Irrigation in Chapter 9.)

When the previous methods do not remove the object, it may be embedded. Cover the closed eye with a dressing and summon the physician.

Nose

When the object cannot be removed easily from the nose, a physician must be consulted. Instruct the patient to avoid violent nose blowing and probing the nose because these acts may only push the object deeper or injure the tissues of the nose.

FRACTURES

A fracture is a break in the continuity of a bone. Broad classifications of fractures are **open fracture**—one in which the bone penetrates the skin, producing an open wound, and **closed fracture**—one in which there is no break in the skin. Closed fractures are much more common than open fractures. Not all fractures prevent the patient from moving the injured part; therefore never ask the patient to move to determine the presence of broken bones. Movement of a fractured area may cause additional harm and, at times, permanent damage (Figure 17-28).

FIGURE 17-28   Types of fractures. (From Ingalls AJ, Salerno MC: *Maternal and child health nursing,* ed 7, St Louis, 1991, Mosby.)

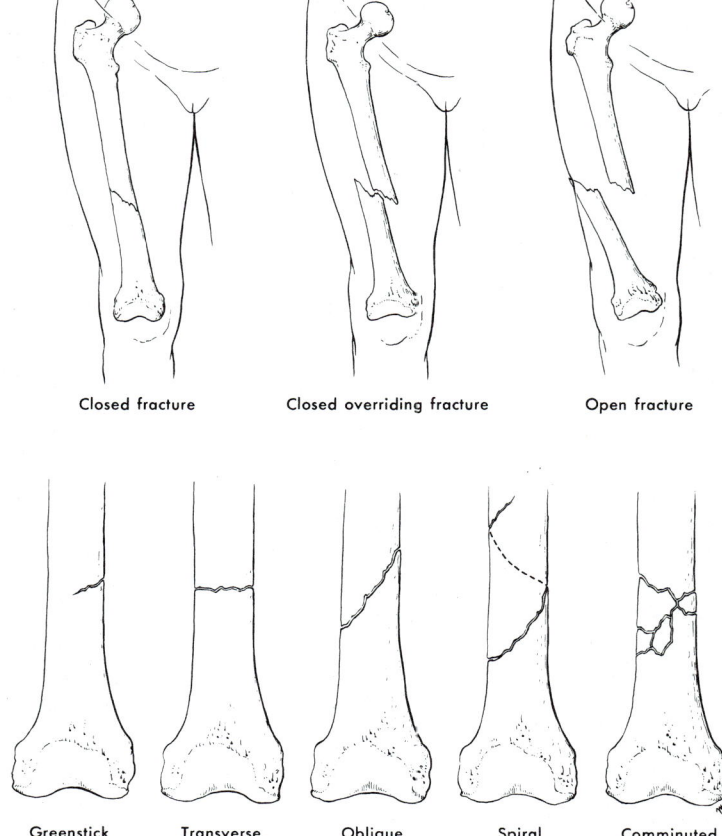

Closed fracture   Closed overriding fracture   Open fracture

Greenstick   Transverse   Oblique   Spiral   Comminuted

First Aid for Fractures

1. Treat for shock and give artificial respiration when necessary; keep the patient warm and quiet.
2. Prevent movement of the injured part and adjacent joints and do not move the injured part.
3. Elevate affected extremities when possible without disturbing the suspected fracture. This will help reduce hemorrhage, when present, and swelling.
4. Apply an ice bag to the painful area.
5. Never attempt to reduce (set) a fracture. This is the physician's responsibility.
6. Never attempt to push a protruding bone back into place.
7. For an open fracture, in addition to the preceding steps:
   a. Control any serious bleeding.
   b. Do not attempt to clean the wound.
   c. Avoid contaminating the wound; do not touch the wound.
   d. Do not replace bone fragments.
   e. Cover the wound with a sterile dressing or clean cloth material and secure in place with a bandage.
8. To prevent additional trauma when the patient has to be moved or transported, the injured part must be immobilized by applying splints or slings and bandages. Splints must be long enough to reach beyond the joint above and below the break on both sides. Pad improvised splints to prevent additional pressure or injury and tie them in place with bandages or strips of material. Make sure that the bandages or splints are not too tight. Normal circulation must not be hindered. Refer to a first aid textbook for additional information on the application of various types of splints.

Fractured Neck or Back

When a neck, back, pelvis, or skull fracture is suspected, *do not* attempt to move the patient. Trained medical or ambulance personnel are required. When the patient experiences a numbness or tingling around the shoulders and cannot move the fingers readily, a neck fracture is possible.

Symptoms suggestive of a back fracture are numbness or tingling in the legs or pain when trying to move the back or neck or inability to move the feet or toes.

In either of these cases, loosen the patient's clothing around the neck and waist. Do not move the patient and do not let the patient attempt to move because injury to the spinal cord may occur. Keep the patient warm and quiet and treat for shock, as indicated. Call for medical help immediately. The patient should be transported by ambulance to the nearest hospital.

Fractured Jaw

To treat a possible fractured jaw, tie a bandage around the chin and over the head to stop movement. Do not manipulate the jaw. Medical attention is required for treatment.

HEAD INJURIES

The severity of head injuries can vary greatly. The patient may appear normal, experience a headache, have a momentary loss of consciousness or lack of memory, be dazed, or be unconscious. Bleeding from the mouth, nose, ears, or scalp may be present; pulse may be rapid and weak; pupils of the eyes may be unequal in size; and pallor, vomiting, or double vision may be present. **In all cases, medical attention is imperative.** Even when the initial symptoms are minor, after a period of time, hours or days, the injured person may become drowsy, confused, or unconscious as a result of a head injury. A prompt recovery from a state of minor signs and symptoms may not be an indication of the seriousness of the injury. The following steps and precautions should be taken:

1. Assess the patient's physical and mental status. For physical assessment, check for signs as stated earlier and take the blood pressure if equipment is available. For mental assessment, when the patient is conscious, check for orientation as to time, place, name, and alertness and ask the patient to repeat a simple phrase. Talking with the patient is a good way to check the level of consciousness and alertness.
2. Keep the patient at rest in a supine position if the face is ashen and gray or raise the head and shoulders (together) if the face is flushed. **Never position the patient with the head lower than the rest of the body.**
3. Always ensure an open airway. Be prepared to give artificial respiration when necessary.
4. Control hemorrhage if present.
5. Do not give fluids by mouth.
6. Apply a dressing to a scalp wound and bandage it in place with a head bandage.
7. Take note of any period of unconsciousness and record it.
8. Observe and record any changes in the pupils of the eyes.
9. Take and record the blood pressure and the time of any changes (if the equipment is available). When the blood pressure begins to rise and if the pupils begin to dilate or the state of consciousness begins to decrease, this usually indicates an elevation of intracranial pressure.
10. If the patient is unconscious, gently turn the head to one side to prevent aspiration of any blood or mucus that may be present.
11. Keep the patient resting quietly until medical help arrives or the patient is transported to the hospital.

HYPERVENTILATION

Hyperventilation is a common complication of emotional upsets or hysterical situations. It usually affects persons who are anxious or high strung; have a history of job or home stress; are feeling anxiety from lack of sleep; have suddenly stopped taking prescribed drugs, such as diazepam (Valium); or have a history of drug usage that increases sensitivity of the respiratory centers, such as high concentrations of salicylate. These individuals usually unknowingly breathe too rapidly, which in turn disturbs the normal balance of carbon dioxide in the blood.

At the outset, individuals may feel a tightness in the chest and have a feeling of air hunger; they feel that they cannot fill the lungs because they can't get enough air. Often these individuals become apprehensive, which only leads to increased hyperventilation and at times to syncope (fainting). Palpitation of the heart, abdominal pain, and a feeling of fullness in the throat may also occur.

Immediate first aid treatment is to have the individual breathe into a paper bag held tightly over the mouth and nose for 10 minutes or more to replace the carbon dioxide that has been given off during hyperventilation. Removing the victim from the surroundings is helpful, because often people who are trying to help the victim become excited and anxious and unknowingly only promote the victim's anxiety and subsequent hyperventilation. In all cases, the first aid responder or medical assistant should be the calming influence and provide reassurance to the victim.

When frequent attacks of hyperventilation occur, the victim should seek medical attention for treatment of the underlying cause(s).

DIABETES EMERGENCIES: HYPOGLYCEMIA (INSULIN REACTION) AND HYPERGLYCEMIA (DIABETIC COMA)

Diabetes mellitus is a disorder of carbohydrate metabolism in which the ability to oxidize and use carbohydrates is lost and a subsequent derangement of protein and fat metabolism occurs. This results from disturbances in the normal insulin mechanism, a hormone secreted by the islets of Langerhans in the pancreas.

The problem is either an insufficiency of insulin or a resistance to the actions of insulin, or both. The main types of diabetes are **type I**, or insulin-dependent diabetes mellitus (IDDM), formerly called juvenile or childhood onset, in which the body does not produce insulin because of destruction of the insulin-producing beta cells of the pancreas. It is thought to be an autoimmune disease in which the pancreas destroys itself with its own antibodies. There appears to be a genetic tendency toward this type of diabetes (see Insulin Injections in Chapter 7). **Type II** or non–insulin-dependent diabetes, formerly called mature or adult-onset diabetes, is often diagnosed in people over 40 years old, although it can occur much earlier. In type II diabetes the person experiences a defect in insulin production *and* a tendency of the cells in the body to resist the action of insulin. It is estimated that in the United States alone, millions of people suffer from diabetes but are unaware of their condition. Therefore we should all be familiar with the most **common symptoms of diabetes,** which include the following:

- Thirst
- Frequent urination
- Fatigue and weakness
- Apathy
- Hunger

Further symptoms include the following:

- Blurred vision
- Irritability
- Numbness or tingling in the extremities
- Repeated infections of the urinary tract, skin, or gums
- Itchy skin

Sometimes there are no apparent symptoms, and the condition is only detected when a person has a complete physical examination. The presence of diabetes is confirmed by a fasting blood glucose level. If the blood glucose level is consistently elevated, the person has diabetes.

Adverse conditions can occur when a person with diabetes is undiagnosed or does not follow the therapy prescribed or when a disturbance occurs in the normal functions of the body. **Common complications of diabetes include the following:**

- Blindness
- Cardiovascular disease
- Cataract formation
- Congenital defects
- Dental caries
- Gangrene
- Glaucoma
- Impotence
- Kidney disease
- Stillbirths and miscarriages

Treatment should be obtained and followed diligently. The primary goal of treatment for both types of diabetes is the control of the person's blood glucose levels. Control of blood glucose levels can help to prevent complications and to maximize the individual's general health level.

All persons with diabetes, their immediate families, and persons in the health care professions should know the signs and symptoms and the treatment or immediate first aid for hypoglycemia (formerly called an insulin reaction, in which blood glucose levels fall and there is too much insulin or presence of insulin without food) and hyperglycemia (formerly called diabetic coma, a condition that may develop when there is lack of insulin and the blood glucose level is high in the diabetic patient's system) (Table 17-1). Diabetics should carry a card stating that they are diabetic, their daily insulin or oral hypoglycemic drug dosage, their address, and the name and address of their physician. Many diabetics wear Medic Alert bracelets or necklaces (Figure 17-29), which indicate their condition in case of emergency situations requiring treatment.

First Aid for Hypoglycemia (Insulin Reaction)

1. If the patient is conscious, give some form of simple sugar, such as hard candy, sugar, or sweetened orange juice. These are easily digested forms of sugar. Do not give candy bars for treatment of hypoglycemia. They contain many times the needed calories and also have proteins and fats that would slow down the absorption of glucose.
2. Seek medical attention if the patient does not respond readily to Step No. 1. The patient should respond within 15 to 20 minutes, if not sooner.

Text continued on p. 774

TABLE 17–1 **Signs and Symptoms of Hypoglycemia (Insulin Reaction) and Hyperglycemia (Diabetic Coma)**

	Insulin Reaction	Diabetic Coma
Onset	Sudden	Gradual
Skin	Perspiration, pallor, cold and damp skin (cool and clammy)	Flushed, warm, and dry skin, dry tongue
Behavior	Tremors, restlessness, fatigue, faint feeling, headache, confusion or strange behavior; may seem dazed or slow to respond; may appear irritable or grumpy	Weakness, drowsiness, lethargy
Gastrointestinal tract	Extreme hunger, nausea	Thirst, nausea, and vomiting
Vision	Double vision	Eyeball tension low
Respiration	Shallow	Difficulty in breathing or air hunger; rapid, deep, gulping respirations
Pulse	Rapid or normal	Rapid, weak
Speech	Slurred	
Breath	No acetone smell	Sweet or fruity odor; smell of acetone
Level of consciousness	May have loss of consciousness	Coma if unattended
		Apparent confusion and disorientation
Blood glucose	Low (40-70 mg/dl)	High (over 200 mg/dl)
Urine test	Sugar-absent, or a trace at most	Sugar-positive in high amounts
	Acetone-negative	Acetone-positive

FIGURE 17-29 **A,** Medic Alert bracelet and necklace. **B,** Diabetic medical identification card.

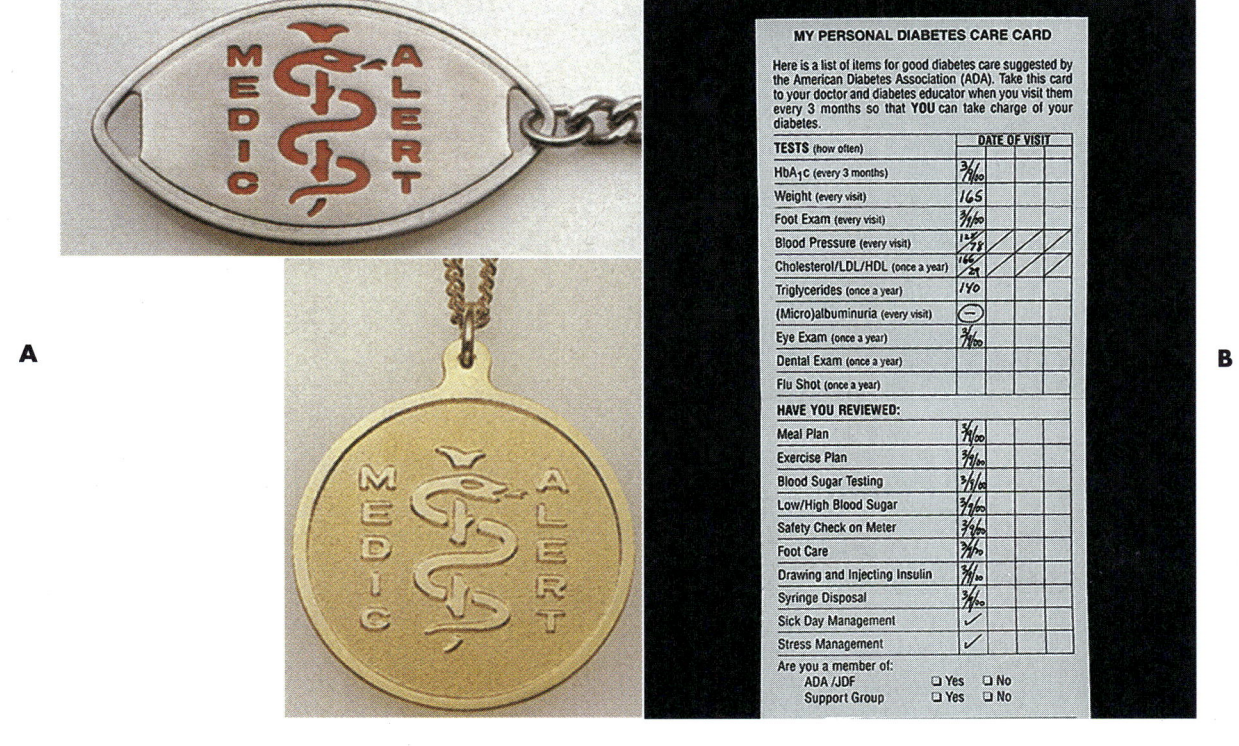

KEEPING YOUR PATIENTS INFORMED

MEDIC ALERT COULD SAVE YOUR LIFE*

1.   What is Medic Alert?

Medic Alert is the nation's leading emergency medical information service and is a nonprofit membership organization (under the 501[c][3] designation) headquartered in Turlock, California. It was founded in 1956 by Dr. Marion C. Collins and Mrs. Chrissie Collins to provide quickly accessible, vital personal medical information to protect its members and help save lives in emergency situations.

The trademarked Medic Alert emblem is worn as a bracelet or as a pendant on a neck chain and bears the internationally recognized insignia of the medical profession with the words "Medic Alert." The emblem provides special medical conditions of the wearer and the telephone number of the Emergency Response Center. Authorized emergency personnel can call this number collect from any phone around the world for the member's vital medical facts.

In 2001, Medic Alert celebrated its forty-fifth anniversary of service to its members.

2.   Why should people become members of Medic Alert?

People should become members for protection in emergency situations, for the resulting peace of mind that Medic Alert provides, and for identification when traveling. For those with medical conditions, membership in Medic Alert creates the confidence to travel domestically and internationally, knowing emergency medical personnel anywhere in the world can have almost immediate access to an individual's medical files if needed. Medic Alert members are active people of all ages striving to lead a full, satisfying life. The emblem they wear and the 24-hour computerized service behind it are an important contribution to their confidence in being able to participate fully in life's opportunities and adventures. Medic Alert serves people who enjoy life and, for example, go jogging, hiking, and take trips and vacations. Our society is mobile, and it makes sense for people to have a source of vital medical and family information that is readily available in a medical emergency.

"In a medical emergency, I need to know about your conditions and medications . . . and I need to know quickly. Having this information could help me save your life."

Stephan G. Lynn, MD, Director
Department of Emergency Medicine
St. Luke's–Roosevelt Hospital Center, New York

Medic Alert protection is especially important for emergency patients who are unconscious and cannot speak for themselves. However, even a conscious patient can be confused and apprehensive, if not frightened, in an emergency setting—he or she may give incorrect or incomplete medical information to the attending personnel. In addition, family members often cannot remember the details of their relative's condition, especially the exact medication being used; however, the Medic Alert computer system is able to report all such details almost immediately.

3.   Is this medical information held in confidence?

Yes! A medical file will not be provided over the phone or by fax unless the operator in the Medic Alert Emergency Response Center is assured that the caller is a legitimate emergency technician or physician or a person in a position to assist emergency medical personnel, who has the member's personal ID number (which is engraved on the bracelet) and is reacting to an urgent situation. Membership information is protected by Medic Alert and is not shared for any commercial purpose. Medic Alert is committed to the concept that medical information must be held in confidence and that members are entitled to the highest degree of privacy.

4.   What is an example of how Medic Alert has helped save a life?

In September 1995, Carmen G. suffered a severe gallstone attack that required emergency surgery. The attending nurse was preparing a syringe of penicillin until the surgeon-on-call pointed to the Medic Alert bracelet on her wrist and instructed her to look at it first. It read "Allergic to Penicillin," and a call to Medic Alert secured her entire medical record, including what antibiotic could be given without risk. That bracelet very probably saved Carmen's life.

5.   What does the emblem and jewelry look like?

The trademarked Medic Alert emblem is worn on a bracelet or necklace that bears the staff of Aesculapius, the internationally recognized insignia of the medical profession, with the words "Medic Alert." On the reverse side, the special medical conditions of the wearer are engraved, along with the member's identification number and the telephone number of the Emergency Response Center. Emergency personnel can call this number collect from any phone around the world. (Designer jewelry in gold or silver can also be purchased at additional cost.)

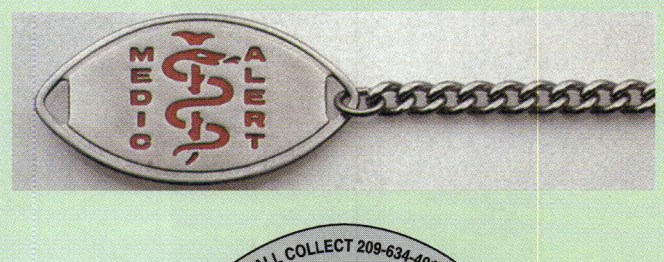

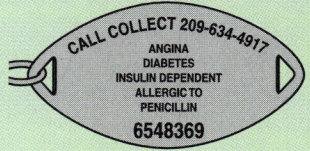

CALL 1-800-432-5378 FOR MEMBERSHIP INFORMATION

Over two and one-half million members worldwide feel better knowing they have the protection Medic Alert provides. You, too, can benefit from this medically approved emergency medical identification service. Join *now.* **Do it for life.**

"Medic Alert . . . can help protect patients' peace of mind, their ability to live independently and their lives"—American Hospital Association

*Courtesy Medic Alert, Turlock, CA 95382.

HEALTH MATTERS—cont'd

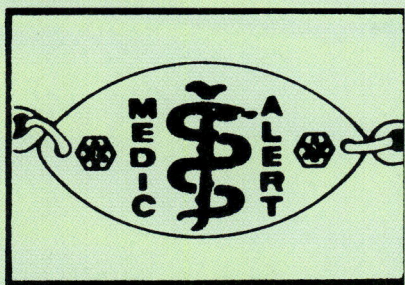

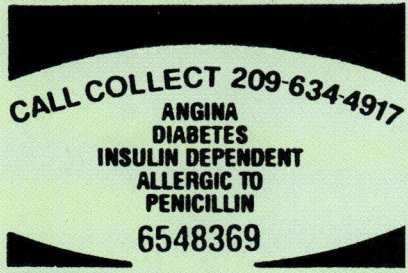

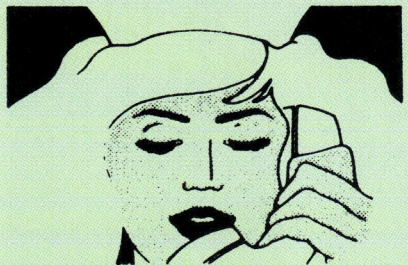

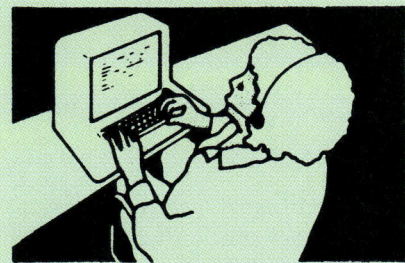

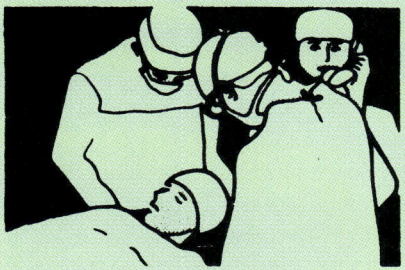

Here's How the Medic Alert System Works:

1. Your emblem, bearing the internationally recognized medical symbol, triggers Medic Alert, the world's only comprehensive emergency medical information system.

2. The emblem is engraved with your primary medical conditions, personal identification number, and Medic Alert's 24-hour hotline phone number.

3. A hotline call from a medical professional starts the information retrieval process.

4. Within seconds, Medic Alert's emergency operator responds with your computerized information.

5. Your vital data relayed back to emergency room staff helps medical personnel provide appropriate diagnosis and care and could save your life.

   As a backup to the Medic Alert System, you are provided with an annually updated wallet card.

- Medic Alert is the only internationally recognized emergency medical system that provides busy emergency personnel with vital patient information quickly, accurately, in one place, and on time.
- The international Medic Alert Foundation provides protection to members anywhere in the world 24 hours a day via the telephone emergency hotline.

Continued

HEALTH MATTERS—cont'd

Conditions, Allergies, and Medications Needing Medic Alert

Medical Conditions

- Abnormal ECG
- Adrenal insufficiency
- Alcoholism
- Alzheimer's
- Angina
- Asthma
- Bleeding disorder
- Cardiac dysrhythmia
- Cataracts
- Clotting disorder
- Coronary bypass graft
- Diabetes/insulin dependent
- Diabetes/non-insulin dependent
- Eye surgery
- Glaucoma
- Hearing impaired
- Heart valve prosthesis
- Hemodialysis

- Hemolytic anemia
- Hypertension
- Hypoglycemia
- Laryngectomy
- Leukemia
- Lymphomas
- Malignant hyperthermia
- Memory impaired
- Myasthenia gravis
- Pacemaker
- Renal failure
- Seizure disorder
- Sickle cell anemia
- Situs inversus
- Speech impaired
- Stroke
- Vision impaired
- No known medical conditions

Allergies

- Aspirin
- Barbiturates
- Codeine
- Demerol
- Horse serum
- Insect stings
- Latex
- Lidocaine

- Morphine
- Novocain
- Penicillin
- Sulfa
- Tetracycline
- X-ray dyes
- No known allergies

Medications

- Antianginal (specify)
- Antiarrhythmic (specify)
- Anticoagulant
- Anticonvulsant
- Antihistamine, regular use

- Beta blocker
- Steroid
- Chemotherapy agent
- Immunosuppressant
- Lipid-altering drugs

Special Needs

- Blood type (specify)
- Contact lenses
- Implants (specify manufacturer and model no.)

- Organ donor
- Advance directive for health care (see Chapter 4)
- Speaks (if other than English)

---

3. If the patient is unconscious, do not force fluids or food. Call the physician or take the patient to the hospital immediately.

First Aid for Hyperglycemia (Diabetic Coma)

There is *no adequate first aid* treatment for hyperglycemia or diabetic coma. *Immediate medical treatment is necessary.*

OPEN WOUNDS

Types of wounds include abrasions, avulsions, incisions, lacerations, and puncture wounds. See p. 327 and Figure 6-29.

First Aid for Minor Wounds

1. Wash your hands thoroughly before treating any wound to minimize the possibility of infection. Don disposable, single-use examination gloves.
2. Observe the wound to check for foreign objects, such as pieces of glass, wood, and dirt.
3. Control bleeding (see pp. 757-760).
4. Gently wash the skin around the wound with soap and water. Wash away from the wound, not toward it.
5. For minor cuts, scratches, and abrasions, wash the wound well with soap and water to remove foreign matter.

a. Lacerations and incisions may be irrigated with large amounts of water or normal saline. Do not apply an antiseptic unless instructed to do so by the physician.

b. For puncture wounds, gently squeeze the wound to encourage a small amount of bleeding to help wash out microorganisms. Then wash the wound with soap and water.

c. Wounds with severe bleeding should not be cleansed.

6. Cover the wound with a sterile dressing and bandage it in place. Use the cleanest material on hand when sterile dressings are not available.

7. Refer the person to the physician for follow-up care. Tetanus immunization may be required. Lacerations, incisions, and avulsions require medical attention because they may have to be sutured.

8. Advise the person to be alert for signs of infection and, if present, to seek medical attention. Signs to watch for are:

a. Swelling
b. Excessive redness
c. Heat and increasing tenderness
d. Drainage
e. Red streaks away from the wound
f. Fever
g. Excessive pain

POISONING

The symptoms of poisoning vary greatly and depend on the type and amount of substance taken. **All types of poisonings are considered emergencies that require immediate attention.** The following points should be considered when poisoning is suspected:

1. Look for any physical changes, such as an abrupt onset of pain or illness; burns or stains around the mouth or on the face, which would indicate poisoning with a caustic substance; breath odor, which may indicate the type of poison ingested; or depressed consciousness and irregular heartbeat.
2. Observe the surroundings for empty containers, spilled fluids, or containers of substances that would be poisonous if ingested.
3. Obtain information from the person or an observer when possible.

Objectives of First Aid Measures

1. To induce vomiting, **except** when the person has swallowed corrosive or petroleum products, when the person is unconscious, when the person is convulsing, or if the person ingested substances that could absorb rapidly and produce seizures (such as camphor or strychnine) or cause drowsiness, seizures, or coma (such as cyclic antidepressants)
2. To prevent absorption of the poison
3. To maintain an open airway, breathing, and vital functions
4. To obtain medical attention without delay

NOTE: The old thought that you should dilute or neutralize the poison is very controversial. Many experts believe that it may cause more harm than good, especially if it is done incorrectly. Therefore current recommendations are not to dilute or neutralize a poison without expert advice.

First aid.   *Speed is essential* to stop absorption of a poison. First aid for poisoning depends on the type of poison ingested. It is not possible for the person administering first aid or the medical assistant to know exactly what to do for all cases, but general guidelines must be followed:

1. In all cases, monitor the person's vital signs, maintain an open airway, and be prepared to administer CPR if necessary.
2. Make every effort to determine what, when, and how much was ingested.
3. Obtain specific information to follow. **Most specialists recommend that you should not carry out any specific first aid measures without expert advice (this may be analogous to not moving a trauma victim with a potential spine injury).**

   Call the physician, the poison control center that is in the nearest city, or the hospital emergency physician. Antidote labels may be on the product ingested, but *caution* must be taken because the label may be out-of-date and incorrect. Poison control centers are open 24 hours a day and maintain antidote information on several thousand available commercial products. Most states have a poison control center in the major cities. Keep this number on hand with other important telephone numbers.

4. Carry out the specific first aid instructions obtained.
5. When specific directions cannot be obtained, the following may be performed:
   a. If the person is awake and able to swallow, 1 glass of water may be given.
   b. **Do not induce vomiting** if the person (1) is unconscious or in a coma; (2) is having a convulsion; (3) has ingested a petroleum product such as kerosene, lighter fluid, or gasoline; or (4) has ingested a corrosive substance (for example, strong acids or alkalis). In these situations, if the person can swallow, give 1 glass of water.
6. Poison control centers **do not** advocate the use of syrup of ipecac without expert advice. They also suggest that activated charcoal be used only in the hospital.
   a. If the person has ingested a *noncorrosive* substance and is not unconscious or convulsing, the following may be suggested by the poison control center:
      (1) Give 1 tablespoon of syrup of ipecac, followed by 2 cups of water for children ages 1 to 12 years. For a person over 12 years of age, give 2 tablespoons of syrup of ipecac followed by 2 glasses of water. Keep children active. Repeat the same dose in 15 minutes if vomiting has not occurred. *Repeat only once.* The onset of vomiting will usually occur within 20 to 30 minutes.

      DO NOT give syrup of ipecac if the person has ingested anything that may cause seizures or drowsiness because by the time the person starts to vomit, he or she also could be having a seizure or be very drowsy, which increases the chance of the person aspirating the vomitus (studies have shown that aspiration happens approximately 50% of the times that vomiting is induced).
      (2) When retching and vomiting begin, place the person's head down with the head lower than the hips. This prevents vomitus from entering the lungs, causing further injury.
      (3) When the poison is unknown, save the vomitus and take it to the physician or hospital for analysis.
7. It is recommended **not** to dilute poisons taken in capsule or tablet form. The increased fluid in the stomach could speed the rate at which the capsule or tablet dissolves, thereby increasing the rate at which the poison would be absorbed into the bloodstream. NOTE: The universal antidote of 2 parts burned toast, 1 part milk of magnesia, and 1 part strong tea that was formerly recommended is now believed to be **useless.** Therefore do not waste time preparing this mixture for administration.
8. Arrange for transportation of the person to the physician or the hospital. **All cases of poisoning must receive medical attention.**
9. Remain calm at all times. Stay with the person and provide reassurance.

Many poisoning cases are related to drug abuse. To determine the proper first aid care to give in these cases, you should be aware of the characteristics of intoxication for drugs that are commonly abused. See Table 17-2 for selected effects of commonly abused drugs.

TABLE 17–2 Comparison of Selected Effects of Commonly Abused Drugs

Drug Category	Physical Dependence	Characteristics of Intoxication
Opiates	Marked	Analgesia with or without depressed sensorium; pinpoint pupils (tolerance does not develop to this action); patient may be alert and appear normal; respiratory depressions with overdose
Barbiturates	Marked	Patient may appear normal with usual dose, but narrow margin between doses needed to prevent withdrawal symptoms, and toxic dose is often exceeded and patient appears "drunk," with drowsiness, ataxia, slurred speech, and nystagmus on lateral gaze; pupil size and reaction normal; respiratory depression with overdose
Nonbarbiturate sedatives: glutethimide (Doriden)	Marked	Pupils dilated and reactive to light; coma and respiratory depression prolonged; sudden apnea and laryngeal spasm common
Antianxiety agents ("minor tranquilizers")	Marked	Progressive depression of sensorium as with barbiturates; pupil size and reaction normal; respiratory depression with overdose
Ethanol	Marked	Depressed sensorium, acute or chronic brain syndrome, odor on breath, pupil size and reaction normal
Amphetamines	Mild to absent	Agitation, with paranoid thought disturbance in high doses; acute organic brain syndrome after prolonged use; pupils dilated and reactive; tachycardia, elevated blood pressure, with possibility of hypertensive crisis and cerebral vascular accident; possibility of convulsive seizures
Cocaine	Marked	Paranoid thought disturbance in high doses, with dangerous delusions of persecution and omnipotence; tachycardia; respiratory depression with overdose
Marijuana	Absent	Milder preparations: drowsy, euphoric state with frequent inappropriate laughter and disturbance in perception of time or space (occasional acute psychotic reaction reported); stronger preparations such as hashish: frequent hallucinations or psychotic reaction; pupils normal, conjunctivas injected (marijuana preparations often adulterated with LSD, tryptamines, or heroin)
Psychotomimetics: LSD, STP, tryptamines, mescaline, morning glory seeds	Absent	Unpredictable disturbance in ego function, manifest by extreme lability of affect and chaotic disruption of thought, with danger of uncontrolled behavioral disturbance; pupils dilated and reactive to light
Phencyclidine	Unknown	Disinhibition, agitation, confusion, chaotic thought disturbance, unpredictable behavior, hypertension, meiosis, respiratory collapse, cardiovascular collapse, death
Anticholinergic agents	Absent	Nonpsychotropic effects such as tachycardia, decreased salivary secretion, urinary retention, and dilated, nonreactive pupils plus depressed sensorium, confusion, disorientation, hallucinations, and delusional thinking
Inhalants*	Unknown	Depressed sensorium, hallucinations, acute brain syndrome; odor on breath; often glassy-eyed appearance

*The term *inhalant* is used to designate a variety of gases and highly volatile organic liquids, including the aromatic glues, paint thinners, gasoline, some anesthetic agents, and amylnitrite. The term excludes liquids sprayed into the nasopharynx (droplet transport required) and substances that must be ignited before administration (such as marijuana).

POISON CONTROL CENTERS

Poison control centers have been established in many cities across the nation to provide quick and reliable information on possible poisonings or drug-related problems. They provide information on the appropriate first aid and clinical management to use for cases of suspected or known poisoning. Some centers also offer specialized poisoning treatment and consultant services, professional training, and poisoning prevention educa-

tion for consumers. Many centers are staffed by clinical pharmacists 24 hours a day, every day of the year.

Not all states have poison control centers; some rely on centers in nearby cities. Some states have state-designated centers that are located in two or three major cities in that state. Other states have poison control centers that are regional centers established by a particular city. These centers are usually financed locally and are usually located at major hospitals or ma-

Characteristics of Withdrawal	"Flashback" Symptoms	Masking of Symptoms of Illness or Injury During Intoxication
Rhinorrhea, lacrimation, and dilated, reactive pupils, followed by gastrointestinal disturbances, low back pain, and waves of gooseflesh; convulsions not a feature unless heroin samples were adulterated with barbiturates	Not reported	An important feature of opiate intoxication, caused by analgesic action, with or without depressed sensorium
Agitation, tremulousness, insomnia, gastrointestinal disturbances, hyperpyrexia, blepharoclonus (clonic blink reflex), acute brain syndrome, major convulsive seizures	Not reported	Only in presence of depressed sensorium or after onset of acute brain syndrome
Similar to barbiturate withdrawal syndrome, with agitation, gastrointestinal disturbances, hyperpyrexia, and major convulsive seizures	Not reported	Same as in barbiturate intoxication
Similar to barbiturate withdrawal syndrome, with danger of major convulsive seizures	Not reported	Same as in barbiturate intoxication
Similar to barbiturate withdrawal syndrome, but with less likelihood of convulsive seizures	Not reported	Same as in barbiturate intoxication
Lethargy, somnolence, dysphoria, and possibility of suicidal depression; brain syndrome may persist for many weeks	Infrequently reported	Drug-induced euphoria of acute brain syndrome may interfere with awareness of symptoms of illness or may remove incentive to report symptoms of illness
Similar to amphetamine withdrawal	Not reported	Same as in amphetamine intoxication
No specific withdrawal symptoms	Infrequently reported	Uncommon with milder preparations; stronger preparations may interfere in same manner as psychotomimetic agents
No specific withdrawal symptoms; symptoms may persist for indefinite period after discontinuation of drug	Commonly reported as late as 1 year after last dose	Affective response or psychotic thought disturbance may remove awareness of, or incentive to report symptoms of illness
No specific withdrawal symptoms	Occasionally reported	Same as in LSD intoxication
No specific withdrawal symptoms; mydriasis may persist for several days	Not reported	Pain may not be reported as a result of depression of sensorium, acute brain syndrome, or acute psychotic reaction
No specific withdrawal symptoms	Infrequently reported	Same as in anticholinergic intoxication

jor medical universities. You should post the telephone number of the nearest poison control center near your telephone both at work and at home so that you are able to obtain information as quickly as possible when the need arises.

More information on poison control centers can be obtained from:

The American Association of Poison Control Centers

National Capital Poison Center
Georgetown University Hospital
3800 Reservoir Rd. NW
Washington, DC 20007
Telephone: (202) 784-2088

For a list of poison control centers in the United States write to:

Publication Office of Veterinary and Human Toxicology
Comparative Toxicology Laboratories
Kansas State University
Manhattan, KS 66506
Telephone: (916) 532-5679

EMERGENCY TRAY/CRASH CART

See Chapter 7, p. 363.

FIRST AID KIT

Now is the time to check the first aid kit kept in the office, home, and family automobile. A properly equipped kit, with fresh supplies that are kept replenished after use, is a practical aid in relieving many minor injuries and ailments. It may even be lifesaving before medical help arrives. However, the best time to provide the office, home, or automobile first aid kit is *before* it is needed. The following first aid supplies are suggested:

1. Sterile gauze pads—2- and 4-inch squares
2. Sterile gauze roller bandages
3. Adhesive tape
4. Adhesive dressings in various sizes
5. Absorbent cotton—sterile
6. Triangular bandage
7. Elastic bandage
8. A mild antiseptic and antiseptic wipes
9. Syrup of ipecac
10. Analgesic, such as aspirin and acetaminophen
11. Petroleum jelly
12. Calamine lotion
13. Aromatic spirits of ammonia
14. Tweezers
15. A scissors with rounded ends
16. Clinical thermometer (digital thermometer may be used)
17. Flashlight with extra batteries
18. Safety pins
19. Sugar for diabetics
20. Ice bag and/or chemical ice pack
21. Disposable, single-use examination gloves
22. Airway or mouthpiece
23. Disposable face shields or resuscitation mask
24. First aid book

For automobiles, the American National Red Cross suggests a specially designed compact unit with standardized first aid materials fitted into a case, like blocks. The packet is readily stored, and the supplies do not become easily disarranged. Each packet is clearly labeled, and instructions for use are included. These kits can be obtained at auto supply stores and department stores with contents selected to meet the purchaser's particular needs. Ask your physician about other medications for such things as car sickness, upset stomach, and allergies. Take some road flares for car safety and a blanket in the car.

Regardless of how well equipped the first aid kit is, its effective use depends on individuals knowing how to give aid properly. A course in first aid, as well as training in CPR, can be an invaluable investment. For additional drugs and supplies that may be kept in the physician's office or clinic for emergency situations, see Table 7-3, Emergency Tray and Emergency Drugs.

CONCLUSION

In the event of a sudden illness or an accident that causes trauma to a person, the trained, competent medical assistant should be prepared to properly administer the appropriate first aid treatment and obtain medical assistance as needed. In time of emergencies, prompt action must be taken. Also, you must remain calm in all cases and provide care in a competent, orderly, and organized manner. Do not perform procedures that you have not been trained to do. To maintain your skills and knowledge in first aid and CPR, you should enroll in a refresher course every few years.

REVIEW OF VOCABULARY

The following are a hospital discharge summary received in the office on one of the physician's patients who had been in an accident, and a radiology report. After reading these, you should be able to discuss the contents with your instructor. Be prepared to define and explain any medical terms that are used. A medical dictionary, other reference books, and information given in preceding chapters of this book may be used as references for obtaining definitions or explanations of the contents of this report.

Discharge Summary

PATIENT: Will Nelson
ADMITTED: January 10, 20__
DISCHARGED: February 10, 20__
DISCHARGE DIAGNOSES

1. Multiple facial fractures, including fracture of the maxilla, mandible, nose, and right orbit.
2. Comminuted fracture, left patella.

HISTORY: This 22-year-old man was injured in a head-on motorcycle accident with another motorcycle at about 4:30 PM on January 10. The patient was brought to the emergency room of this hospital by ambulance.

PHYSICAL EXAMINATION: At the time of admission, the patient was conscious. He was alert and oriented and aware of his surroundings. Physical examination revealed gross bleeding from mouth and nose. There were multiple contusions and abrasions over the facial area. Blood pressure was 118/60, pulse was 74, respirations 16.

HEENT: The ears were clear. The eyes had marked ecchymotic areas present periorbitally, with diffuse edema in the periorbital area. The fundus on the left was clear. The fundus on the right was not seen. The nose was filled with blood clots, and there was some active bleeding in the nasal area. At the time of admission, this was not delineated clearly. There was a marked amount of blood in the right side of the mouth. The patient was unable to open his mouth because of deviation of the jaw. Neck was supple.

CARDIORESPIRATORY: Chest was clear to auscultation. There was a regular sinus rhythm with no murmurs.

GI: The abdomen was soft, without masses or organs palpable. Bowel sounds were active.

EXTREMITIES: There was ecchymosis and edema over the left knee.

NEUROLOGIC: The patient was conscious. The deep tendon reflexes were within normal limits, and there were no pathologic toe signs elicited.

DIAGNOSTIC DATA: X-ray studies at the time of admission revealed a fracture of the right patella, comminuted, and maxillary and mandibular fractures of the face. CBC at the time of admission revealed a hemoglobin of 12.6 g with a hematocrit of 38%. The hemoglobin on January 26 was down to 10.5 g with a hematocrit of 32% and WBC of 8300 with a normal differential. On February 2, hemoglobin was 11.7 g with hematocrit of 34%. Urinalysis on January 27 was normal. Serum electrolytes were normal on January 13. The chloride was 101 mEq/L. Pco_2 content 30 mEq/L. Potassium 3.5 mEq/L. Sodium 135 mEq/L. Serum osmolality ran from 276 to 282. On January 13, hemoglobin had dropped to 8.6 and 8.7 g, with a packed cell volume of 25% and mean proportional hemoglobin concentration of 34% and 35%. The patient was transfused with 2 units of blood at that time, and hemoglobin rose, on January 14, to 11.2 g, with a packed cell volume of 32%. X-ray examinations on January 10, at the time of admission, of skull, facial bones, left ribs, and left knee revealed multiple fractures of the facial bones, including the nasal bones and the mandible. There was a fracture of the left patella and, after surgery on January 12, a PA view of the chest (portable) revealed a hazy infiltration in the right upper lung field, resembling pneumonitis. A film of the right hand, on January 12, revealed a very small chip fracture of the palm as described. A portable chest x-ray film, on January 16, revealed the small patch of hazy infiltration in the upper right field, which was probably due to lung contusion. The chest otherwise was unremarkable. On January 14, stereo views of the pelvis revealed a gas pattern, heavy in the visible part of the abdomen. Bony structures were intact. There were no signs of dislocation of the hips. X-ray film of the left arm revealed the elbow and wrist to be intact. Cervical spine was negative, except for a fracture in the mandible as described. Lumbosacral spine showed anterior displacement of L5 on S1, and L1 was wedged very slightly anteriorly. It was not believed that this was a fracture. Waters' view of the sinuses revealed multiple facial bone fractures, evident with generalized haziness in the central part. On January 18, AP x-ray films of the facial bones revealed superior fractures of the nasal and maxillary bones, as well as the previously described fractured mandible. There were no specific changes.

HOSPITAL COURSE: On the night of admission, January 10, the patient was taken to the operating room where, under general anesthesia, he first had a tracheostomy by Dr. U.R. Belson. The patient then had a reduction of fracture of the mandible and maxilla with repair of facial lacerations and mucous membrane of the mouth and packing of the right antrum, reduction of nasal bones, and fixation of nasal packing. This was done by Drs. U.R. Belson, B. Beal, and I.B. Tucker. A simultaneous patellectomy was done on the left knee by Dr. P. Adamson. The patient did relatively well in the intensive care unit following surgery, maintained on antibiotics and tracheostomy care. On January 18, the patient was returned to the operating room where, under general anesthesia, Drs. U.R. Belson and I.B. Tucker performed open reduction of the fracture of the facial bones. The patient has continued to do well since that time on a general basis, requiring constant observation and very close and meticulous care of his tracheostomy site. He has been gradually ambulated from the bed to a wheelchair and ambulation in the room. The cast has been removed from the left leg. Sutures have been removed from his face. The patient was seen in consultation by Dr. I.B. Tucker, concerning the eyes, and he was found to have Berlin's edema from the fractures of the floor and rim of the right orbit. On January 11, the patient also was seen in consultation by Dr. P. Brown concerning advice for maintenance and following of his tracheostomy site and antibiotic therapy. The patient is being discharged today to his home, where he will be under observation by his father, Dr. W.F. Nelson, and will be followed by the physicians, as required, at general hospital.

Andrew Berger, MD

Diagnostic Radiology Consultation

EMERGENCY

DATE: January 4, 20__

PATIENT: David Lee

DATE: January 4, 20__

SOFT TISSUE—NECK:

COMPARISON: None available.

FINDINGS: Frontal and lateral views of the neck demonstrate abnormal retropharyngeal air, in keeping with most recent injury. The airway is open. The epiglottis is within normal limits.

IMPRESSION:

1. Abnormal retropharyngeal air, likely resulting from the recent injury.

Signed: M.S. Talbot, MD

THIS REPORT HAS BEEN ELECTRONICALLY AUTHENTICATED
BY THE DICTATING RADIOLOGIST

CRITICAL THINKING SKILLS REVIEW

1. List three factors that determine if a situation is an emergency.
2. As a medical assistant, you are responsible for rendering first aid when the need arises. Define first aid and state the contributions you can make for the physical and psychologic care of the victim in an emergency situation.
3. List four fundamental rules and procedures to follow in a medical emergency.
4. Mr. Bill Bailey has been experiencing uncomfortable pressure and pain in the center of the chest, shortness of breath, and slight nausea for the past 3 minutes. What medical condition do these symptoms suggest? What type of action should be taken for this condition?
5. While having lunch with a friend, a woman suddenly clutches her neck between her thumb and index finger. What should this indicate to you?
6. Define shock. List and explain the six types of shock. List eight outstanding symptoms of shock.
7. Dave Rubin has just had minor surgery in the physician's office. As you are assisting him after the procedure, you observe that he is very pale and his skin quite cold to the touch. You immediately take his vital signs and find that the pulse is weak and rapid, the blood pressure 92/70, and respirations 34 and shallow. What condition do you think he is experiencing? What must be your immediate actions?
8. Anna Westover is having a severe reaction to penicillin. Describe the first aid treatment that you could provide.
9. Ray Wood is cleaning the windows in your office. By accident, he breaks a window. He comes running to you at the desk. You observe that he is clutching his wrist and that bright red blood is spurting from his wrist, as well as from his hand and fingers. State the type of bleeding this would indicate, the vessel that may be cut, and the first aid treatment that you would administer.
10. List and locate the seven pressure points used to control severe bleeding.
11. State the difference between a first-, second-, and third-degree burn (superficial, partial-, and full-thickness burn).
12. After having blood drawn, Joanne Newman faints. State the first aid treatment that you would provide for this patient.
13. Ann O'Brien, a diabetic patient, is displaying the signs and symptoms of hypoglycemia or an insulin reaction. List six signs and symptoms of hypoglycemia (insulin reaction). State the immediate care that you could provide.
14. List six signs and symptoms of hyperglycemia (diabetic coma).
15. In the case of ingested poisoning, when should you not have the victim vomit?
16. When is the use of a tourniquet advisable?
17. List at least 15 items that you would include when compiling supplies for a first aid kit.

PERFORMANCE TEST

In a skills laboratory, with simulations of emergency situations, the medical assistant student will demonstrate skill in performing the following procedures without reference to source materials. The student needs a person to play the role of the patient. Time limits for the performance of each procedure are to be assigned by the instructor (see also p. 104.)

1. Demonstrate the proper first aid treatment to be administered to patients who have experienced all the emergency situations given in this chapter.
2. Demonstrate how to locate the seven pressure points to be used when controlling severe bleeding.
3. Demonstrate the proper method of applying a tourniquet to a patient's left arm; to a patient's right leg.

4. Demonstrate on the mannequin (if available) the correct method of administering CPR.

The student is to perform these activities with 100% accuracy before passing this chapter.

The successful completion of each procedure will demonstrate competency levels as required by the AAMA, AMT, and future employers.

INTERNET RESOURCES

Heartstream: ForeRunner (automatic external defibrillator [AED])
www.heartstream.com

American Heart Association
www.americanheart.org

American Heart Association
http://amhrt.org

Medic Alert
www.medicalert.org

American Red Cross
www.redcross.org

Poison Control Center
www.calpoison.org

North American Association for the Study of Obesity
www.naaso.org

American Diabetes Association
www.diabetes.org

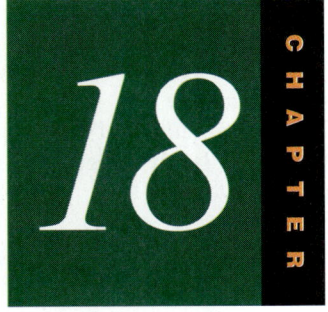
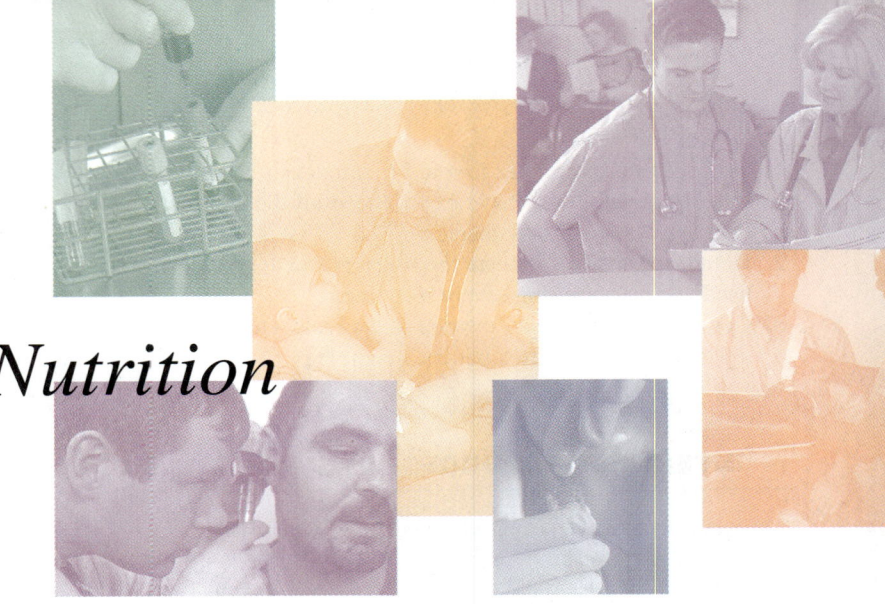

18 CHAPTER

Nutrition

■ Cognitive Objectives

On completion of Chapter 18, the medical assistant student should be able to:

1. Define, pronounce, and spell the vocabulary terms in this chapter.
2. List the six main nutrients required by the body to maintain health.
3. Summarize the functions of proteins, carbohydrates, fats, vitamins, minerals, water, and fiber in the body.
4. List four excellent sources of dietary protein.
5. Compare complete proteins and incomplete proteins and list one food source of each.
6. Distinguish between simple carbohydrates and complex carbohydrates, giving examples of each.
7. List at least four food sources each of saturated fats and unsaturated fats.
8. Explain the effects of saturated and unsaturated fats on cholesterol levels in the body.
9. Differentiate among and explain the functions of cholesterol, high-density lipoproteins (HDLs), and low-density lipoproteins (LDLs) in the body.
10. Define calorie and empty calorie. State six factors that determine a person's daily caloric requirement.
11. List three ways that you could incorporate more water into your daily diet.
12. Define vitamins and distinguish between the fat-soluble and the water-soluble vitamins.
13. List one function and one food source for each of the vitamins identified in No. 12.
14. Define minerals. Distinguish between the macrominerals and the microminerals.
15. Categorize foods according to the five basic food groups.
16. Discuss the relationship between overweight and disease risk.
17. Explain how good nutritional dietary habits can help to prevent cardiovascular disease and cancer.
18. Explain why it is important to lower the amount of fat and cholesterol in the average diet.
19. Explain the 10 dietary guidelines for Americans as recommended by the U. S. Department of Agriculture and the U. S. Department of Health and Human Services.
20. List 10 foods that are low in saturated fat and cholesterol.
21. List 10 foods that are high in saturated fats and cholesterol.
22. List 10 foods that are good sources of dietary fiber.
23. List the recommended number of daily servings from each of the five food groups, stating examples of food from each group.
24. Explain the benefits of increased fiber in the diet.
25. Discuss the reasons why it is important to use salt and sugar only in moderation. Discuss ways to limit the intake of salt and sugar.
26. List five groups of individuals who should *not* drink alcoholic beverages.
27. Discuss the 10 therapeutic diets discussed in this chapter, giving examples of foods that could be eaten in each.
28. State the average percentage of our daily caloric requirement that should be obtained from each of the following: proteins, fats, and carbohydrates.
29. Explain and list advantages of a vegetarian diet. Give examples of foods to eat and the recommended number of daily servings.

■ Terminal Performance Objectives

On completion of Chapter 18, the medical assistant student should be able to:

1. Demonstrate knowledge and understanding of healthful eating habits when discussing these with a patient.
2. Given a commercial food label, demonstrate and explain how to use the information to make healthy choices.
3. Given a commercial food label, demonstrate how to determine the percentage of calories in the food that are supplied from fat.
4. Using the Food Guide Pyramid recommendations, write out a sample menu for 7 days for a healthy adult.

5. Demonstrate knowledge in discussing the dietary goals and the recommended daily allowance of protein, fat, and carbohydrates.

6. Given a variety of foods, pick out those that would provide a good source of protein, saturated fats, unsaturated fats, fiber, carbohydrates, vitamins, and minerals.

7. Develop a personal plan for dietary habits and choices that promote health.

8. Provide instructions and patient education that are within the professional scope of a medical assistant's training and responsibilities as assigned.

VOCABULARY

digestion—The mechanical and chemical breakdown of food into substances small enough to be absorbed and used by body cells to maintain life.

food labeling—The nutritional information on a label of a food, including the serving size; the number of servings per container; the number of calories per serving; the number of calories from fat; and the amounts of protein, fat, saturated fat, carbohydrates, eight vitamins and minerals, cholesterol, sodium, dietary fiber, and sugars.

nutrient—A substance derived from food that provides the body with nourishment. Nutrients are essential for life. Each nutrient is responsible for particular body functions. Nutrients needed by the body include proteins, fats, carbohydrates, vitamins, minerals, and water.

nutrition—The science of the study of all of the processes involved with the taking in of food and drink and how they are used for proper body functioning and maintenance of health. The processes involved are the ingestion, digestion, and absorption of nutrients and the elimination of waste products.

obesity
- **mild obesity**—20% to 40% above one's ideal weight
- **moderate obesity**—41% to 100% above one's ideal weight
- **severely obese**—100% above one's ideal weight
  (see Chapter 3).

RDAs (recommended daily allowances)—The RDAs are defined as "the levels of intake of essential nutrients that, on the basis of current scientific knowledge, are judged by the Food and Nutrition Board to be adequate to meet the known nutrient needs of practically all healthy persons."

RDIs (reference daily intakes)—The RDIs are a set of dietary references based on the RDAs for essential vitamins, minerals, and, in selected groups, protein. The acronym *RDI* is replacing the term *U. S. RDA.*

uniform definitions—Nutrition language describing a food's nutrition content, such as "light," "low-fat," and "high-fiber" to ensure the same meaning for any product on which they appear.

The following terms are examples of uniform definitions, applying to their use on a food label:

low calorie—No more than 40 calories per serving in that food.

reduced calorie—The product has at least one-quarter fewer calories than the product it is replacing; for example, the reduced calories salad dressings in place of the regular salad dressings made by the same manufacturer.

sodium free—There are less than 5 milligrams (mg) of sodium in each serving of the food.

low sodium—There are 140 mg or less of sodium in each serving of the food.

very low sodium—There are 35 mg or less of sodium in each serving of the food.

unsalted—The product has been produced without any added salt. This product still contains the sodium that is a natural part of the food itself.

low fat—For each serving of the food, there are 3 grams (g) or less of fat.

low saturated fat—In each serving, there is 1 g or less of saturated fat in the food.

low cholesterol—In each serving of the food, there are 20 mg or less of cholesterol and 2 g or less of saturated fat.

lean—For each serving of the food, there are less than 10 g of fat, 4 g of saturated fat, and 95 mg of cholesterol.

extra lean—For each serving of the food, there are less than 5 g of fat, 2 g of saturated fat, and 95 mg of cholesterol.

reduced—The food contains 25% less fat, cholesterol, sodium, or calories than the regular product of the same food.

light *or* lite—For each serving, the food contains one-third fewer calories, 50% less fat, or 50% less sodium than the regular product of the same food.

free—Each serving of the food contains less than 5 calories, ½ g fat, 2 mg of cholesterol, 5 mg of sodium, or ½ g of sugar.

Additional terms are defined under their respective topics in this chapter.

NUTRITION AND YOUR HEALTH

The keys to healthful eating are moderation, balance, and variety. Nutrition scientists know that what you eat directly affects your long-term health. Dietary factors contribute substantially to premature death and preventable illnesses in the United States. For example, overweight to obesity, largely self-induced conditions, increase the risk for heart disease, various types of cancer, diabetes, stroke, and early death (Table 18-1).

Numerous scientific studies continually demonstrate that the typical American diet has:

TABLE 18–1 Relationship Between Overweight and Disease Risk

	Percentage of Increased Risk	
Disease	**(20%-30% Overweight)**	**(40% Overweight)**
Heart disease		
Male	32	95
Female	39	107
Cancer		
Male		
Prostate	37	39
Colon	26	73
Female		
Breast	16	53
Cervix	51	139
Endometrium	85	442
Ovary	0	63
Diabetes		
Male	156	419
Female	234	690
Stroke		
Male	17	127
Female	16	52
Other		
Chances of suffering from arthritis, gallstones, gout, and premature death also increase for both males and females.		
Obesity		
High percentage of body fat increases the low-density lipoproteins and increases total blood cholesterol.		

Courtesy American Cancer Society, San Francisco, Calif.

- Too many calories
- Too much cholesterol
- Too much fat, especially saturated fat
- Too much sodium and salt
- Too much sugar
- Not enough complex carbohydrates
- Not enough fiber

As a medical assistant, you may be involved in the **health education** of patients with special dietary needs. It is important to understand nutritional requirements, help patients from various cultures choose a variety of foods from each of the five food groups illustrated in the Food Guide Pyramid (Figure 18-1, *A* and *B*), and support patients in making behavioral changes to bring their diets into balance. Even small and simple changes in dietary habits can produce beneficial results.

THE FOOD GUIDE PYRAMID

The Food Guide Pyramid (see Figure 18-1, *A*) is an outline of what to eat each day. The idea of the pyramid is to show that everyone needs to eat more of the foods at the bottom of the

pyramid and lesser amounts of foods toward the top. No food is banned from this guide, but it does recommend fewer and smaller servings of some favorite foods such as those foods higher in fat, cholesterol, and sugar.

Patients should be reminded that overall good health requires a variety and different amounts of foods daily and to choose different foods from *each* of the five food groups to ensure a nutritious, as well as enjoyable, diet. Many foods are good sources of several nutrients. For example, vegetables and fruits are important for vitamins A and C, folic acid, minerals, and fiber. Breads and cereals supply B vitamins, iron, and protein; whole-grain types are also good sources of fiber. Milk provides protein, B vitamins, vitamins A and D, calcium, and phosphorus. Meat, poultry, and fish provide protein, B vitamins, iron, and zinc. No single food can supply all nutrients in the amounts needed. For example, milk provides calcium but little iron; meat provides iron but little calcium. A variety of foods must be eaten for a nutritious diet.

How Many Servings Are Needed

The Food Guide Pyramid shows a range of servings for each major food group. Most people should have at least the lower number of servings suggested from each food group. Some

FIGURE 18-1 **A,** Food Guide Pyramid: a guide to daily food choices. **B,** Serving sizes and suggested number of servings. (**A,** Courtesy U. S. Department of Agriculture/U. S. Department of Health and Human Services.)

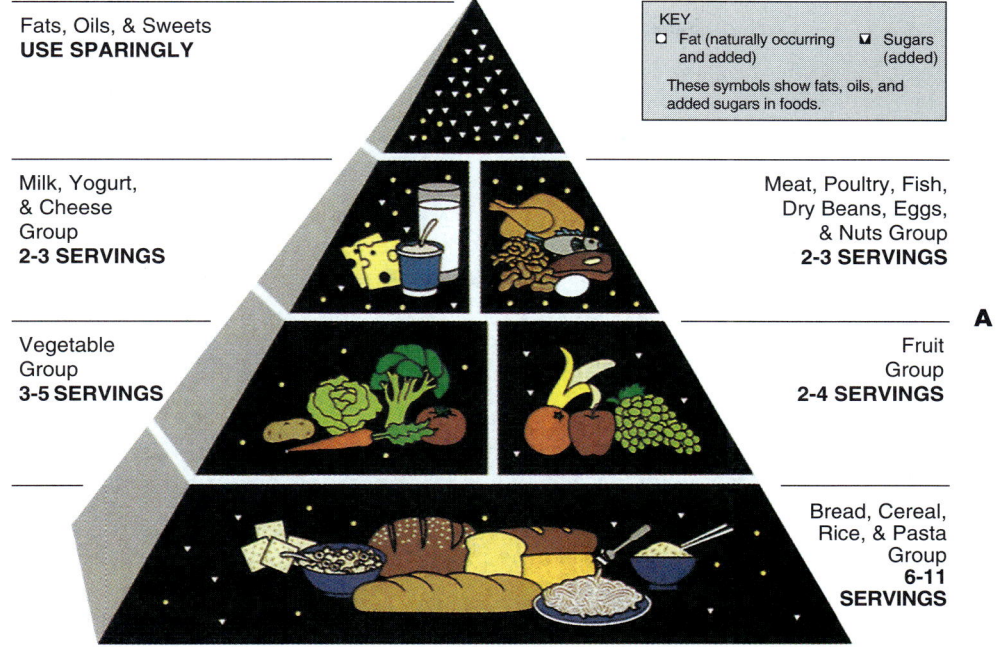

KEY
□ Fat (naturally occurring and added)   ☑ Sugars (added)
These symbols show fats, oils, and added sugars in foods.

Fats, Oils, & Sweets
USE SPARINGLY

Milk, Yogurt, & Cheese Group
2-3 SERVINGS

Meat, Poultry, Fish, Dry Beans, Eggs, & Nuts Group
2-3 SERVINGS

Vegetable Group
3-5 SERVINGS

Fruit Group
2-4 SERVINGS

Bread, Cereal, Rice, & Pasta Group
6-11 SERVINGS

A

B

WHAT COUNTS AS A SERVING?
Suggested daily servings and serving sizes in the Food Guide Pyramid food groups:

Grain Products Group (bread, cereal, rice, and pasta)
6-11 servings
1 slice of bread
1 ounce of ready-to-eat cereal
½ cup of cooked cereal, rice, or pasta*
½ bagel, bun, or English muffin
1 small tortilla
3 rice cakes
1 4-inch pancake

Vegetable Group 3-5 servings
1 cup of raw leafy vegetables
½ cup of other vegetables—cooked or chopped raw or dried*
¾ cup of vegetable juice
½ cup of cooked dry beans or peas **or** count this as
    1 ounce of the meat group

Fruit Group 2-4 servings
1 medium apple, banana, orange
1 melon wedge
1 cup berries
½ cup of chopped, cooked, or canned fruit
¼ cup of dried fruit
¾ cup of fruit juice (This **does not** include fruit drinks, fruit punch, or fruit-flavored sodas.)

Milk Group (milk, yogurt, and cheese) 2-3 servings
1 cup of milk or yogurt (8 ounces)
1½ ounces of natural cheese**
2 ounces of processed cheese**
1 cup custard pudding
½ cup ice cream

Meat and Beans Group (meat, poultry, fish, dry beans, eggs, and nuts) 2-3 servings
2-3 ounces of cooked lean meat, poultry, or fish (3 ounces is approximately the size of a deck of playing cards or the palm of your hand)
½ cup of cooked dry beans or 1 egg counts as 1 ounce of lean meat. Two tablespoons of peanut butter or ⅓ cup of nuts count as 1 ounce of meat.

* ½ cup of serving of fruits, vegetables, and cereals is approximately what could be held in the palm of an adult's medium-sized hand.
**1 ounce of cheese is approximately a 1 inch by 1 inch square.

people may need more because of their body size, activity level, and the number of calories needed.

Young children need the same variety as adults but may need fewer calories and smaller servings (see also Daily Caloric Requirements on p. 808).

Based on recommendations of the National Academy of Sciences and calorie intakes reported by people in national food consumption surveys, the following calorie levels are suggested for teens and adults:

- For many sedentary women and some older adults—*1600 calories*
- For most children, teenage girls, active women, and many sedentary men—*2200 calories*. Women who are pregnant or breastfeeding may need somewhat more.
- For teenage boys, many active men, and some very active women—*2800 calories*

TABLE 18–2   Sample Diets for a Day at Three Calorie Levels

	Lower (About 1600)	Moderate (About 2200)	Higher (About 2800)
Bread group servings	6	9	11
Vegetable group servings	3	4	5
Fruit group servings	2	3	4
Milk group servings	2-3*	2-3*	2-3*
Meat group† (ounces)	5	6	7
Total fat (grams)	53	73	93
Total added sugars (teaspoons)	6	12	18

*Women who are pregnant or breastfeeding, teenagers, and young adults to age 24 need 3 servings.

†Meat group amounts are in total ounces.

DIETARY GUIDELINES FOR AMERICANS 2000*

The *Dietary Guidelines* are designed to help healthy Americans age 2 years and older have diets that meet nutritional requirements, promote health, support active lives, and reduce chronic disease risks. Research often shows that diets high in fat, saturated fat, cholesterol, and salt and more calories than the body uses; and low in grain products, vegetables, fruits, and fiber raise the risk for serious chronic diseases.

The Food Guide Pyramid and the Nutrition Facts Label (see Figures 18-1 and 18-4) serve as educational tools to put the *Dietary Guidelines* into practice. The pyramid translates the recommended daily allowances (RDAs) and the *Dietary Guidelines* into the kinds and amounts of food to eat each day. The Nutrition Facts Label is designed to help you select foods for a diet that will meet the *Dietary Guidelines*.

The *Dietary Guidelines* include the following:

Aim, Build, Choose—for Good Health

Eating is one of life's greatest pleasures. Since there are many foods and many ways to build a healthy diet and lifestyle, there is lots of room for choice. Use this information to help you and your family find ways to enjoy food while taking action for good health.

The three basic messages—the ABCs for your health and that of your family are:

A = **A**im for fitness.
B = **B**uild a healthy base.
C = **C**hoose sensibly.

Ten guidelines point the way to good health. These guidelines are intended for healthy children (ages 2 years and older) and adults of any age.

Aim for Fitness
• Aim for a healthy weight.
• Be physically active each day.

Following these two guidelines will help keep you and your family healthy and fit. Healthy eating and regular physical activity enable people of all ages to work productively, enjoy life, and feel their best. They also help children grow, develop, and do well in school. Physical activity is a key component of weight management.

Build a Healthy Base
• Let the Pyramid guide your food choices.
• Choose a variety of grains daily, especially whole grains.
• Choose a variety of fruits and vegetables daily.
• Keep food safe to eat.

Following these four guidelines builds a base for healthy eating. Let the Food Guide Pyramid guide you so that you get the nutrients your body needs each day. Make grains, fruits, and vegetables the foundation of your meals. This forms a base for good nutrition and good health and may reduce your risk of certain chronic diseases.

These foods are emphasized because they provide vitamins, minerals, complex carbohydrates (starch and dietary fiber), and other substances that are important for good health. They are also generally low in fat, depending on how they are prepared and what is added to them before they are eaten. Be flexible and adventurous—try new choices from these three groups in place of some less nutritious or higher calorie foods you usually eat. Whatever you eat, always take steps to keep your food safe to eat.

Choose Sensibly
• Choose a diet that is low in saturated fat and cholesterol and moderate in total fat.
• Choose beverages and foods that limit your intake of sugars.
• Choose and prepare foods with less salt.
• If you drink alcoholic beverages, do so in moderation.

*U.S. Department of Agriculture and U. S. Department of Health and Human Services.

These four guidelines help you make sensible choices that promote health and reduce risk of certain chronic diseases. You can enjoy all foods as part of a healthy diet as long as you don't overdo on fat (especially saturated fat), sugars, salt, and alcohol. Read labels to identify foods that are high in saturated fats, sugars, and salt (sodium). The advice for children for fats and cholesterol is that after the age of 2 years, children should gradually adopt a diet that, by about 5 years of age, contains no more than 30% of calories from fat.

If your calorie needs are low, use sugars sparingly. The Nutrition Facts Label on foods gives the total carbohydrate and sugar content as well as total calories. Higher amounts of salt and sodium are found mainly in processed and prepared foods. Fresh fruits and vegetables have very little salt and sodium. Read the Nutrition Facts Label to identify foods lower in sodium. Numerous studies have shown that many people at risk for high blood pressure can reduce their risk of developing this condition by eating less salt and sodium. By eating more fruits and vegetables you increase the amount of potassium in your diet, which also may help to reduce high blood pressure.

If you drink alcoholic beverages, do so in moderation. Drink only moderate amounts, with meals, and when drinking does not put you or others at risk for any undesirable activity or consequence.

Aim, Build, Choose—for Good Health

By following these guidelines, you can promote your health and reduce your risk for chronic diseases such as heart disease, certain cancers, diabetes, stroke, and osteoporosis. These diseases are leading causes of death and disability among Americans. Your food choices, your lifestyle, your environment, and your genes all affect your well-being. If you are at risk for a chronic disease, it is especially important to follow the 10 Dietary Guidelines. So find out your family history for disease and your other risk factors for disease to make more informed decisions about how to improve your health.

These 10 guidelines will help you take action for good health. Find out some of the ways to aim for fitness, to build a healthy base, and to choose sensibly. Try combining familiar and unfamiliar foods for enjoyable, healthy eating. Become physically active. And keep your food safe to eat.

HEALTH MATTERS

KEEPING YOUR PATIENTS INFORMED

NUTRITION IN THE NEWS*

Nearly every day, research findings related to nutrition and health make the news. What should you do when today's report seems to contradict what you heard last week?

Your best bet is to use caution and common sense.

Use these tips for judging reports of food and nutrition research findings:

- Refrain from making changes in your food choices based on results from a single research study. The results of one study are just one piece of a bigger puzzle. Wait until more studies can confirm the results.
- Be wary of recommendations that promise a quick fix. Claims that sound too good to be true are usually just that.
- Remember to go beyond the headlines. Attention-grabbing headlines often oversimplify more complex findings. Bottom-line conclusions are usually reported at the end of a news story.
- Learn about the study methods. Longer studies, with more people, are more likely to produce valid results. However, be aware that the study results may not apply to you if the people studied are different in age, gender, health, or lifestyle.
- Check out the sources. Credible research is conducted by a respectable scientific or medical organization and is reported by a reputable newspaper, newsletter, magazine, or scientific journal.

*Courtesy *Food and Nutrition News*, 70(1):6, Winter 1998. Copyright by National Cattlemen's Beef Association, Chicago, Ill.

- Look for expert interpretation. Reports of research findings often include review and advice from nutrition and health professionals, such as a registered dietitian.

Advice for Today

Take the time to be well informed about diet and health, but use healthy skepticism when evaluating nutrition research findings. Until research findings are confirmed and consensus is reached, stick with the "tried and true" when it comes to diet and health recommendations.

- **Be realistic.** Set reasonable goals and make small changes over time—ones that you can stick with. Use the Food Guide Pyramid (see Figure 18-1, *A*) as your guide for choosing a variety of foods in healthy proportions.
- **Be flexible.** Balance your food choices over time. For example, savor your steak or pasta twice as much; eat half in the restaurant and take the rest home for tomorrow.
- **Be sensible.** Enjoy all foods; just don't overdo it. Steer clear of eating plans with rigid menus that limit your selection of foods or food groups.
- **Be adventurous.** Expose your taste buds to new flavors. Start by trying some foods you've never tasted—for example, fruits like mango, kumquat, or pomegranate; vegetables like jicama or kohlrabi; or an herb such as arugula.
- **Be active.** For overall fitness and health, include physical activity in your daily routine. The benefits are many—weight control, stress relief, muscle toning, increased energy, and feeling great!

NUTRIENTS

Six main classifications of nutrients required by the body to maintain health are proteins, fats, carbohydrates, vitamins, minerals, and water. These components are discussed according to composition, function, sources, and caloric requirements.

Proteins

Composition. Proteins are often thought of as the building blocks of our body. They are found in every living cell. Proteins are composed of chains of approximately 20 **amino acids, nine of which are called essential amino acids.** To function and survive, the body needs the nine essential amino acids contained in foods referred to as complete proteins. The remaining amino acids can be synthesized by the body.

Function. The main functions of protein include the following:

1. Promotes growth, repair, and maintenance of musculoskeletal and other body tissues.
2. Serves as a framework for bones, muscles, blood, hair, and fingernails.
3. Helps to regulate some body processes by serving as a component of hormones and enzymes.
4. Helps to maintain the acid-base balance in the body.
5. Serves as a source of energy (4 calories for every gram of protein consumed).

Sources. The essential amino acids must be obtained from the food we eat and are obtained from foods referred to as **complete proteins.** The best food sources of complete proteins are meat, poultry, milk, cheese, eggs, and fish. Foods that do not contain all of the essential amino acids are called **incomplete protein foods** and are of plant origin. Examples of these foods include legumes (dry beans and peas, soy bean curd [tofu]), grains, nuts, and seeds. A combination of various sources of incomplete protein foods provides an adequate amount of the amino acids needed for protein synthesis and are sometimes called **complementary proteins** (for example, peanut butter on wheat bread, macaroni and cheese, sesame seeds and chickpeas, rice and milk, rice-bean casserole, lentil curry on rice, and corn tortillas and beans).

Caloric requirements. Nutrition specialists recommend that 12% to 15% of our daily caloric requirement be derived from protein sources. Excess protein, like excess calories from any source, are stored as fat. Disease and injury affecting all body systems may require additional protein intake. Each gram of protein supplies the body with 4 calories.

To determine the average amount of protein to eat every day, based on the recommendation that **to maintain a healthy weight,** 12% of your daily required caloric intake should be obtained from protein, use the following formula:

Body weight in pounds (lb) × 0.36 grams (g)

For example:

- Desired weight = 120 lb
  120 × 0.36 = **43.2 g** of protein

- Desired weight = 160 lb
  160 × 0.36 = **57.6 g** of protein

Therefore these individuals should aim to have at least 43 or 57 g of protein per day. If your goal is to have a higher percentage of protein in your diet, you would adjust the number of grams accordingly. To help you to visualize grams, remember that 1 ounce of meat gives approximately 7 g of protein.

Fats

Composition. Fats (lipids) are composed of fatty acids in various combinations with glycerin. These fatty acids can be classified as either saturated or unsaturated. It is their chemical structure that makes them different.

Saturated fat. Saturated fat comes from animal sources (meats, lard, eggs, and dairy products) and plants (coconut oil, palm oil, and palm kernel oil). Products such as commercial cookies, nondairy whipped toppings and creamers, and commercial cake mixes contain hidden saturated fat (Figure 18-2). Saturated fat can increase the level of cholesterol in the blood. (For the amounts of both found in some common foods, see Table 18-3.) Too much cholesterol in the blood is associated with an increased risk of cardiovascular disease. No more than 10% of the required **daily caloric intake to maintain a healthy weight** should come from saturated fats. Reducing fat intake also reduces the risk for cancer of the breast, colon, and prostate and the occurrence of obesity.

Unsaturated fat. The two types of unsaturated fats are polyunsaturated and monounsaturated fats.

Polyunsaturated fat includes vegetable oils and fish oils (omega-3 fatty acids). Unsaturated fat is usually liquid at room temperature. The process of hydrogenation can convert some unsaturated fat into solid fat for cooking purposes. The production of margarine and shortenings are examples of hydrogenation.

Hydrogenation also causes some of the unsaturated fats to turn into **transfatty acids,** which also have a great effect on blood cholesterol levels (see Table 18-5).

Monounsaturated fat, the more beneficial unsaturated fat because it lowers cholesterol levels and low-density lipoproteins (LDLs), includes olive oil, canola oil, and peanut oil (Tables 18-4 and 18-5). Olive and canola oils are the oils that are recommended for use if you must use oil.

Function. The functions of fat in the body include the following:

1. Provides a concentrated source of energy (that is, every gram of fat provides 9 calories)
2. Helps to satisfy our appetite
3. Helps in making food taste good
4. Stores the fat-soluble vitamins
5. Aids in transporting the fat-soluble vitamins (A, D, E, and K)
6. Helps to keep our skin healthy
7. Is used for tissue building, but most of the fat is stored for future energy needs
8. Gives us stamina
9. Provides insulation for the body against low temperatures

Text continued on p. 792

FIGURE 18-2 Where's the fat? Hidden fat is found in products such as chocolate cake, nondairy whipped toppings, cookies, and milk. Visible fat is seen on meats, oils, and butter.

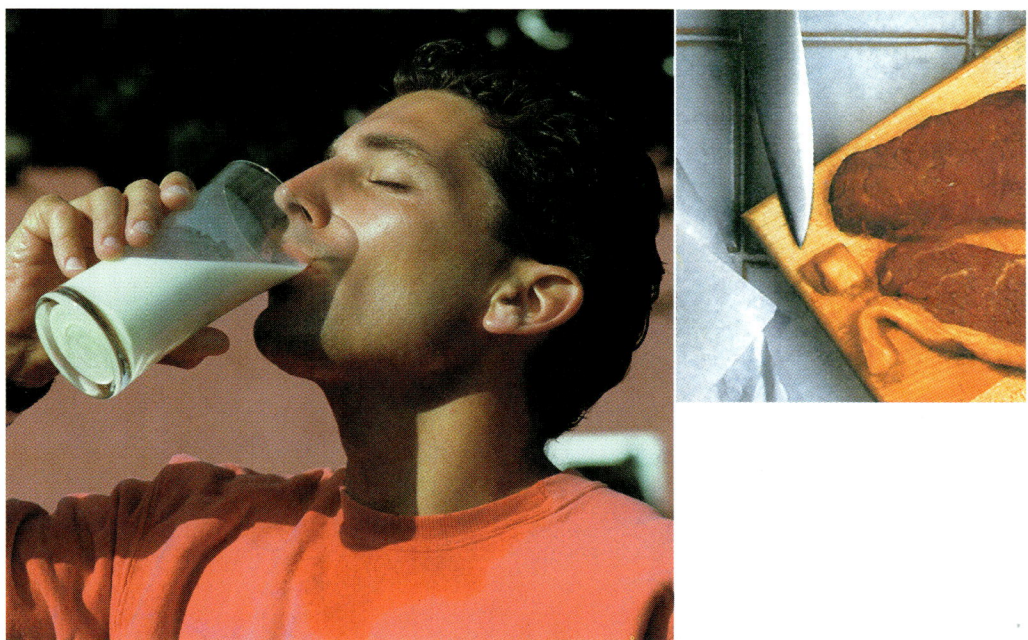

TABLE 18-3 Cholesterol and Saturated Fat Content of Selected Foods

Food (Amount)	Cholesterol (mg)	Saturated Fat (mg)
Lamb, 3 oz	85	3000-9000
Pork, 3 oz	55-75	3500-9200
Beef, 3 oz	55-75	2200-6000
Poultry (light meat), 3 oz	60	1000
Poultry (dark meat), 3 oz	85	4000
Liver, 3 oz	372	2500
Fish, 3 oz	40-60	1000-1700
Shrimp, 3 oz	90	400
Egg, 1 large	252	1700
Whole milk, 1 cup	34	4700
Lowfat milk, 1 cup	22	2700
Nonfat milk, 1 cup	5	—
Half and half, ½ cup	26	7800
Cottage cheese, ½ cup	15-23	1800-4900
Most cheeses, 1 oz.	16-30	4000-6000
Yogurt, 1 cup	5-20	500-4200
Ice cream ½ cup	30	6500
Ice milk, ½ cup	13	1900
Peanut butter, 1 Tbsp	—	1500
Butter, 1 Tbsp	34	6500
Margarine, 1 Tbsp	—	2100
Mayonnaise, 1 Tbsp	7	2000
Sour cream, 1 Tbsp	8	4600
Olive oil, 1 Tbsp	—	1500
Corn oil, 1 Tbsp	—	1400
Cottonseed oil, 1 Tbsp	—	3400
Salad dressing, (Italian), 1 Tbsp	—	1600
Chocolate, 1 oz	5	8400

TABLE 18–4   A Basic Primer on Fats in the Diet

On average, people in the United States eat about 42% of their total calories as fat. Many nutrition authorities have suggested it is best to restrict fat intake to no more than 30% of total calories, limiting saturated fatty acids to about a third of this amount. Limiting cholesterol is also important to your health. A basic definition of these terms and dietary suggestions follows.

Fat	Fat is the most concentrated source of food energy (calories). Each gram of fat supplies about 9 calories, compared with about 4 calories in a gram of protein or carbohydrates. In addition to providing energy, fat aids in the absorption of certain vitamins. Some fats provide linoleic acid, an essential fatty acid that is needed by everyone in small amounts. Butter, margarine, shortening, and oil are obvious sources of fat. Well-marbled meats, poultry skin, whole milk, cheese, ice cream, nuts, seeds, salad dressings, and some baked products also provide a good deal of fat.
Cholesterol	Cholesterol is not a fat, but a fatlike substance, found in the body cells of humans and animals. It is needed to form hormones, cell membranes, and other body substances. The body is able to make the cholesterol it needs for these functions. Cholesterol is not needed in the diet. Cholesterol is present in all meat, poultry and fish, in milk and milk products, and in egg yolks. It is **not** found in foods of plant origin, such as fruits, vegetables, nuts, grains, and seeds.
Fatty acids	Fatty acids are the basic chemical units in fat. They may be either saturated, monounsaturated, or polyunsaturated. All dietary fats are made up of mixtures of these fatty acid types. **Saturated fatty acids** are found largely in fats of animal origin, including whole milk, cream, cheese, butter, meat, and poultry. They are also found in large amounts in some vegetable oils, including coconut and palm. **Monounsaturated fatty acids** are found in fats of both plant and animal origin. Olive, canola, and peanut oil are the most common examples, along with most margarines and hydrogenated vegetable shortening. **Polyunsaturated fatty acids** are found largely in fats of plant origin, including sunflower, corn, soybean, cottonseed, and safflower oils. Some fish are also good sources.
To your health . . .	Eating a diet high in fat—especially saturated fatty acids—and cholesterol causes elevated blood cholesterol levels in many people. High blood cholesterol levels increase the risk of heart disease. Reducing fat is an especially good idea for those people who are limiting calories. Not only do fats provide more than twice the calories of proteins and carbohydrates, but they also contain few vitamins and minerals.
Moderation is the key	Eliminating all fats is not good for you either. For example, milk, meat, poultry, fish, and eggs all contribute fat, saturated fat, and cholesterol to our diet; but they also provide essential nutrients such as calcium, iron, and zinc. So the key is moderation. Focus on a balanced overall diet and avoid too much fat when possible by using lower-fat dairy products and lean meats and reducing the amount of fats added at the table.
How does your diet score?	Do the foods you eat provide more fat than is good for you? Answer the questions below, then see how your diet stacks up.

How often do you eat:	Seldom or never	1-2× per week	3-5× per week	Almost daily
Fried, deep-fat fried, or breaded foods?	❑	❑	❑	❑
Fatty meats such as bacon, sausage, luncheon meats, and heavily marbled steaks and roasts?	❑	❑	❑	❑
Whole milk, high-fat cheeses, and ice cream?	❑	❑	❑	❑
High-fat desserts such as pies, pastries, and rich cakes?	❑	❑	❑	❑
Rich sauces and gravies?	❑	❑	❑	❑
Oily salad dressings or mayonnaise?	❑	❑	❑	❑
Whipped cream, table cream, sour cream, and cream cheese?	❑	❑	❑	❑
Butter or margarine on vegetables, dinner rolls, and toast?	❑	❑	❑	❑

Take a look at your answers. Several responses in the last two columns mean you may have a high fat intake. Perhaps it's time to cut back.

Cutting back on fat	Here are 15 tips to help you avoid too much fat, saturated fat, and cholesterol in your diet: 1. Steam, boil, or bake vegetables; or for a change, stir fry in a small amount of vegetable oil. 2. Season vegetables with herbs and spices rather than with sauces, butter, or margarine.

TABLE 18–4 A Basic Primer on Fats in the Diet—cont'd

3. Try lemon juice on salads or use limited amounts of oil-based salad dressing.
4. To reduce saturated fat, use margarine instead of butter in baked products and, when possible, use oil instead of shortening.
5. Try whole-grain flours to enhance flavors of baked goods made with less fat and cholesterol-containing ingredients.
6. Replace whole milk with skim or lowfat milk in puddings, soups, and baked products.
7. Substitute plain lowfat yogurt, blender-whipped lowfat cottage cheese, or buttermilk in recipes that call for sour cream or mayonnaise.
8. Choose lean cuts of meat.
9. Trim fat from meat before and/or after cooking.
10. Roast, bake, broil, or simmer meat, poultry, or fish.
11. Remove skin from poultry before cooking.
12. Cook meat or poultry on a rack so the fat will drain off. Use a nonstick pan for cooking so added fat will be unnecessary.
13. Chill meat or poultry broth until the fat becomes solid. Spoon off the fat before using the broth.
14. Limit egg yolks to one per serving when making scrambled eggs. Use additional egg whites for larger servings.
15. Try substituting egg whites in recipes calling for whole eggs. For example, use two egg whites in place of each whole egg in muffins, cookies, and puddings.

For more information about fats and oils in your diet, contact:

The U.S. Department of Agriculture, Human Nutrition Information Service, Room 360, 6505 Belcrest Road, Hyattsville, MD 20782 and ask for a list of relevant publications.

The American Heart Association, National Center, 7320 Greenville Avenue, Dallas, TX 75231 or call your local American Heart Association office.

Your local county extension agent or public health nutritionist or dietitians in hospitals and other community agencies.

Courtesy the Worldview Quarterly, Nestle USA, Inc, Washington, D.C.

TABLE 18–5 Effects of Fats on Blood Lipids

Type of Fat	Effects on Blood Lipids	Sources
Saturated	Increases total cholesterol Increases low-density lipoproteins (LDLs)	Most red meats Lard Butter Hydrogenated shortenings Stick margarine Plant fats (tropical oils) • Coconut oil • Palm oil • Palm kernel oil Animal fats Milk products with high butterfat
Polyunsaturated (vegetable)	Decreases total cholesterol Decreases LDLs Decreases high-density lipoproteins (HDLs) May decrease the functions of the immune system Risks may outweigh the benefits	Safflower oil Sunflower oil Corn oil Soybean oil Cottonseed oil Sesame oil Soft margarine Nuts such as walnuts, pinenuts, brazil nuts, and chestnuts.

Continued

TABLE 18–5   Effects of Fats on Blood Lipids—cont'd

Type of Fat	Effects on Blood Lipids	Sources
Polyunsaturated (fish) (omega-3 fatty acids)	Decreases total cholesterol Decreases LDLs Increases HDLs Decreases triglycerides Retards plaque formation Reduces the body's tendency to form blood clots which can trigger a heart attack Aids the immune system	Cold-water fish • Mackerel • Salmon • Tuna • Trout • Anchovy • Herring
Monounsaturated	Decreases total cholesterol Decreases LDLs May reduce blood pressure May reduce blood sugar	Canola oil Peanut oil, peanuts Peanut butter Olives, olive oil Almonds Pecans Cashews Filberts Pistachios Avocados
Transfat (transfatty acids)	Increase total cholesterol Increase LDLs *May* decrease HDLs	Liquid oils that are partially hydrogenated to make them more solid and less greasy tasting Small amounts in meat and milk Vegetable shortening and foods made with vegetable shortenings, such as cookies, cakes, crackers, and other packaged foods; some peanut butters; and many but not all margarines

Sources.   Because currently there is so much talk about the disadvantages of fat (lipids) in the diet, some people are beginning to think that fat is not needed in their diet, but it is. Fat plays an important role in body functions and health. The problem is that most people eat too much fat. It is estimated that fat accounts for up to 42% of the daily calories in the average American diet. About 95% of the fat that is ingested is absorbed and used or stored in the body. Approximately 15% of the average person's body weight is fat. In addition to eating foods containing fat, the body converts some protein and carbohydrates that are eaten into fat.

Another area of concern is that about 50% of the fat that we eat is "hidden" fat. It is often not visible when we look at the food. For example, when you look at a piece of chocolate cake, you don't see little fat bubbles oozing out. What you do see is a nice, moist, crumbly texture of a product that may be very tasty to you. Other sources of hidden fats are snack foods, cookies, crackers, nondairy whipped toppings, nondairy creamers, and cereals. Many of these contain tropical oils (palm, coconut, and palm kernel oils), which are saturated fats. Many food items are labeled with the percentage of fat content. An example is 2% milk. Many people think that the whole gallon of milk has only 2% fat, which sounds like a low-fat food. They fail to realize that the 2% means the milk is 2% fat by weight not by volume;

thus in reality, in one serving of 2% milk containing 5 g of fat and 120 calories per serving, 37% of the total calories per serving come from fat. See p. 807 for the formula for determining the percentage of calories from fat in a food product.

Another example is a bran muffin. We often think muffins are a good source of fiber, and many times they may be; however, you must read the label because many packaged muffins are high in fat and sugar and low in fiber. In reading the label, you may see that the muffin contains eggs, palm oil (both containing fat), honey and sugar (both simple carbohydrates), and processed cake flour, which is low in fiber. That is not to say that you can never have another muffin in your life, but you should be aware of the contents of the food so that you can make more responsible choices, maintaining a diet of a *variety* of foods, even if you do indulge at times.

Caloric requirements.   We are advised to reduce our fat consumption so that fat makes up *only* 30% of our daily calorie requirement (Table 18-6). Many health experts recommend that 20% would be a better goal. These experts realize, however, that this suggestion is not very feasible, considering the dietary habits of Americans and the various foods available—unless the individual makes a very concerted effort. Each gram of fat provides the body with 9 calories.

TABLE 18–6 **Summary of Dietary Recommendations for Daily Caloric Intake**

Nutrient	Percentage of Total Diet	Recommendations Suggested by *Some* Nutrition Specialists
Protein	12%-15%	15%-20%
Fat	25%-30%	20%-30%
	• 10% Saturated	If 30% fat, then
	• 15%-20% Unsaturated; preferably more monounsaturated	• Less than 7%-8% polyunsaturated
		• Less than 7%-8% saturated
		• 10%-15% monounsaturated
Carbohydrates	58%-60%	60%-70%
	• 10% Simple	• Not more than 10% refined sugar
	• 48%-50% Complex	• Use mostly complex

Triglycerides. Most of the fats and oils that we eat are in the form of triglycerides. The triglycerides in foods are made up of mixtures of saturated, polyunsaturated, and monounsaturated fatty acids and glycerol. Before dietary fats are absorbed from the small intestine into the bloodstream, they are broken down into their smallest component parts—fatty acids. After absorption, the fatty acids regroup into bunches of three (tri) plus one molecule of glycerol. This chemical form/structure is called a **triglyceride.** For transportation purposes, triglycerides combine with proteins. These molecules are called lipo- (fat) proteins. Different types of lipoproteins have different functions. **Very-low-density lipoproteins (VLDLs)** transport triglycerides to the cells, where many are left to be used for energy, insulation, metabolism, and so on. The same lipoproteins travel on to the liver and pick up cholesterol. They are now **low-density-lipoproteins (LDPs)** and proceed to deliver cholesterol to the cells and blood vessels. **High-density lipoproteins (HDLs)** carry cholesterol away from the cells and arteries back to the liver to be broken down and excreted.

Blood tests are available to determine values for total cholesterol, HDLs, LDLs, VLDLs, and triglycerides. These measurements help in diagnosing a patient's risk for atherosclerosis. A high triglyceride level often accompanies a higher total cholesterol and LDL level and a lower HDL level. High levels of triglycerides in the blood also reduce HDLs and thus increase the risk of cardiovascular disease. Being overweight; having a diet high in calories, sugar, and refined starches; having diabetes; or drinking large amounts of alcohol can also cause high levels of blood triglycerides. Accepted triglyceride levels are 40 to 150 milligram/deciliter (mg/dl). Ranges of 250 to 500 mg/dl present an increased risk for heart disease.

Cholesterol

Composition. Cholesterol is an odorless, soft, waxy, fat-like substance found in body cells of animals and humans.

Function. Cholesterol is an important component for a healthy body because it is essential for the functioning of body systems such as the nervous system. It is also essential for the formation of cell membranes and many hormones, including the sex hormones, and other substances, such as bile salts and nerve fibers.

Sources. Cholesterol comes from two sources—from our own bodies and from food that comes from animal sources. **There is *no* cholesterol in foods from plant sources.** In addition, *saturated fats* found in animal fats and other sources are thought to contribute to the formation of cholesterol in the body, thereby increasing the body's normal supply and contributing to a high blood serum cholesterol level.

Cholesterol is transported to and from the body cells by compounds called **lipoproteins.** Of the several types of lipoproteins, which are classified according to their size and density, the main types are the HDLs and the LDLs. The HDLs are commonly referred to as the *"good guys"* or *"good cholesterol."* The LDLs are commonly referred to as the *"bad guys"* or *"bad cholesterol."* The LDLs are the major carrier of cholesterol in the bloodstream. They contain 60% to 70% of the serum cholesterol, whereas the HDLs contain 20% to 30% of the serum cholesterol. The *higher* the level of HDLs in the bloodstream, the *lower* the *risk* for cardiovascular disease. The LDLs carry cholesterol to blood vessels, where it is deposited. This leads to a narrowing of the blood vessels, thereby increasing the risk for cardiovascular disease. HDLs carry cholesterol away from the arteries and back to the liver for processing and removal, thereby helping to decrease the risk for cardiovascular disease.

Increased levels of serum cholesterol, associated with atherosclerosis, increase the risk for cardiovascular disease. On the other hand, it appears that *unsaturated* fats help to reduce the amount of cholesterol in the blood (see Table 18-5). When choosing foods, it is very important to look at the content of saturated fat present in addition to the amount, if any, of cholesterol (see Table 18-3) because even if the food is low in cholesterol but high in saturated fat, our bodies will turn the saturated fat into cholesterol. Some foods may contain no or low amounts of cholesterol but high levels of saturated fat. Chocolate is a good example. In 1 oz of chocolate, there is only 5 mg of cholesterol *but* 8400 mg (or 8.4 g) of saturated fat; thus even though the level of cholesterol is very low, the high amount of saturated fat will be changed into cholesterol and affect the cholesterol levels in the bloodstream.

Blood cholesterol is mainly influenced by total fat intake, especially saturated fat, and not by dietary cholesterol. Dietary cholesterol must not be confused with blood cholesterol.

Requirements. Our body produces all of the cholesterol needed for the functions it performs primarily in the liver and the small intestine; thus it isn't necessary to eat more. Most recommend that the daily intake of cholesterol be limited to 300 milligrams or less (Table 18-7; also see Table 18-3).

TABLE 18–7   The First Step in Eating Right Is Buying Right: A Guide to Choosing Low Saturated-Fat, Low-Cholesterol Foods

Following a low-saturated fat, low-cholesterol diet is a balancing act: getting the variety of foods necessary to supply the nutrients you need without too much saturated fat and cholesterol or excess calories. One way to ensure variety—and with it, a well-balanced diet—is to select foods each day from each of the following food groups. Select different foods from within groups, especially foods low in saturated fat (the left column). The amount and size of each portion should be adjusted to reach and maintain your desirable weight. As a guide, the recommended daily number of portions is listed for each food group.

	Choose	Go Easy On	Decrease
Meat, poultry, fish and shellfish (Up to 6 ounces a day)	*Lean cuts* of meat with fat trimmed; such as: • Beef Round, sirloin, chuck, loin • Lamb Leg, arm, loin, rib • Pork Tenderloin, leg (fresh), shoulder (arm or picnic) • Veal (all trimmed cuts except ground) Poultry without skin Fish Shellfish		"Prime" grade Fatty cuts of meat, such as: • Beef Corned beef brisket, regular ground, short ribs • Pork Spareribs, blade roll, fresh Goose, domestic Duck Organ meats Sausage, bacon Regular luncheon meats Frankfurters Caviar, roe
Dairy products (2-3 servings a day; 3 servings for women who are pregnant or breastfeeding)	Skim milk, 1% milk, low-fat buttermilk, low-fat evaporated or nonfat milk Low-fat yogurt Low-fat soft cheeses, like cottage, farmer, pot Cheeses labeled no more than 2 to 6 g of fat an ounce	2% milk Yogurt Part-skim ricotta Part-skim or imitation hard cheeses, like part-skim mozzarella "Light" cream cheese "Light" sour cream	Whole milk, such as regular, evaporated, condensed Cream, half and half, most nondairy creamers, imitation milk products, whipped cream Custard style yogurt Whole-milk ricotta Neufchatel Brie Hard cheeses, like swiss, American, mozzarella, feta, cheddar, muenster Cream cheese Sour cream
Eggs (No more than three egg yolks a week)	Egg whites Cholesterol-free egg substitutes		Egg yolks
Fats and oils (Use sparingly)	Unsaturated vegetable oils: corn, olive, peanut, rapeseed (canola oil), safflower; sesame, soybean Margarine; or shortening made from unsaturated fats listed above: liquid, tub, stick, diet	Nuts and seeds Avocados and olives	Butter, coconut oil, palm oil, palm kernel oil, lard, bacon fat Margarine or shortening made from saturated fats listed above

TABLE 18–7   **The First Step in Eating Right Is Buying Right: A Guide to Choosing Low Saturated-Fat, Low-Cholesterol Foods—cont'd**

	Choose	Go Easy On	Decrease
Breads, cereals, pasta, rice (6 to 11 servings a day)	Breads, like white, whole wheat, pumpernickel, and rye breads; pita; bagel; English muffin; sandwich buns; dinner rolls; rice cakes Low-fat crackers, like matzo, bread sticks, rye krisp, saltines, zwieback Hot cereals, most cold dry cereals Pasta, like plain noodles, spaghetti, macaroni Any grain rice	Store-bought pancakes, waffles, biscuits, muffins, cornbread	Croissant, butter rolls, sweet rolls, danish pastry, doughnuts Most snack crackers, such as cheese crackers, butter crackers, those made with saturated oils Granola-type cereals made with saturated oils Pasta and rice prepared with cream, butter or cheese sauces; egg noodles
Dried peas and beans (2 to 3 servings)	Dried peas and beans, like split peas, black-eyed peas, chick peas, kidney beans, navy beans, lentils, soybeans, soybean curd (tofu)		
Fruits and vegetables (2 to 4 servings of fruit and 3 to 5 servings of vegetables a day)	Fresh, frozen, canned or dried fruits and vegetables		Vegetables prepared in butter, cream, or sauce
Sweets and snacks (Use sparingly)	Low-fat frozen desserts, like sherbet, sorbet, Italian ice, frozen yogurt, popsicles Low-fat cakes, like angel food Low-fat cookies, like fig bars, gingersnaps Low-fat candy, like jelly beans, hard candy Low-fat snacks like plain popcorn, pretzels Nonfat beverages like carbonated drinks, juices, tea, coffee	Frozen desserts, like ice milk Homemade cakes, cookies, and pies using unsaturated oils sparingly Fruit crisps and cobblers	High-fat frozen desserts, such as ice cream, frozen tofu High-fat cakes, like most store-bought, pound, and frosted cakes Store-bought pies Most store-bought cookies Most candy, like chocolate bars High-fat snacks, such as chips, buttered popcorn High-fat beverages, like frappes, milkshakes, floats, and eggnogs

Label ingredients

Go easy on products that list any fat or oil first or that list many fat and oil ingredients. The following lists clue you in to names of saturated fat ingredients (decrease) and unsaturated ingredients (go easy on).

		Go Easy On	Decrease
		Carob, cocoa Oils, like corn, cottonseed, olive, safflower, sesame, soybean, or sunflower oil Nonfat dry milk, nonfat dry milk solids, skim milk	Cocoa butter Animal fat, like bacon, beef, chicken, ham, lamb, meat, pork or turkey fats, butter, lard Coconut, coconut oil, palm or palm kernel oil Cream Egg and egg-yolk solids Hardened fat or oil Hydrogenated vegetable oil Milk chocolate Shortening or vegetable shortening Vegetable oil (could be coconut, palm kernel or palm oil)

HEALTH MATTERS

KEEPING YOUR PATIENTS INFORMED

Being aware of your blood cholesterol levels is very important for the sake of a healthy heart and blood vessels and for reducing your risk for cardiovascular disease. Experts with the National Cholesterol Education Program advise healthy adults over age 19 to have a blood lipid panel done at least every 5 years and more frequently if deemed medically necessary. This blood test includes testing for total blood cholesterol, HDLs, and LDLs. The **cholesterol/HDL ratio** gives the physician the best indication of your present risk for cardiovascular disease. The test results below indicate if you are a low or high risk for cardiovascular disease.

Cholesterol Levels

	Desirable	Borderline	Danger
Total	Less than 200 mg/dl*	200-239 mg/dl	240 mg/dl or higher
HDL	35 mg/dl or higher	—	Less than 35 mg/dl
LDL	Less than 130 mg/dl	130-159 mg/dl	160 mg/dl or higher

*mg/dl means milligrams per deciliter (100 milliliters.)

Cholesterol/HDL Ratio

Risk Level for Heart Disease	Men	Women
Low	3.43	3.27
Average	4.97	4.44
Moderate	9.55	7.05
High	23.99	11.04

Source of these test values: *Mosby's patient teaching guides,* copyright 1997 by Mosby-Year Book.

HOW TO IMPROVE YOUR BLOOD VALUES

1. Eat smart. Change your diet to a low-saturated-fat and low-cholesterol diet.
2. Watch your weight. If overweight, reduce.
3. Move, be active—have regular physical activity. Even walking for 30 minutes at least three times a week will do. By losing extra weight and walking, it is possible to raise your HDLs by as much as 10% to 20%.
4. Don't smoke. Smoking can reduce HDLs significantly.
5. Take steps to reduce your blood pressure if it is too high.
6. Adopt ways to decrease and handle negative stress levels in your life.
7. Limit your intake of alcohol.
8. If these lifestyle changes mentioned do not control cholesterol levels, medication may be prescribed.

Is all this worth the effort? Absolutely and positively. Experts agree that "with exercise and diet, most women and men in this country who are headed for a heart attack could avoid it."

Carbohydrates

Composition. Carbohydrates are the most abundant and economical sources of energy. Carbohydrates are various combinations of sugar units. They are derived mainly from plants and are either simple (sugars) or complex (starches and fibers). When eaten, all carbohydrates except fiber break down into sugars.

Function. Carbohydrates provide the main source of energy for all body functions. There are 4 calories for every gram of carbohydrate. They are also necessary for the metabolism of other nutrients. In the body, carbohydrates are either absorbed for immediate use or stored in the form of glycogen. They can also be manufactured in the body from some components of fat and from some amino acids.

Sources. Carbohydrates are present, at least in small quantities, in most foods. The chief sources are the sugars (simple carbohydrates) and the starches (complex carbohydrates).

Sources of simple sugars include the following:

- *Refined sugars,* such as white and brown sugar, raw sugar, honey, and syrup
- *Naturally occurring sugars,* as found in milk, fruits, and vegetables

Some sugars are used as natural preservatives, thickeners, and baking aids in foods; they are often added to foods during processing and preparation or when they are eaten.

Like fats, much of the sugar consumed is hidden. Many fail to realize sugar is found in foods such as canned vegetables and fruits, ketchup, salad dressings, and cured meat products, as well as in many other food products.

On a food label, sugars include brown sugar, corn sweetener, corn syrup, fructose, fruit juice concentrate, glucose (dextrose), high-fructose corn syrup, honey, invert sugar, lactose, maltose, molasses, raw sugar, (table) sugar (sucrose), and syrup. A food would likely be high in sugar if one of the preceding terms appears first or second in the ingredients list or if several of them are listed.

Sources of complex carbohydrates or starches include the following:

- Vegetables such as broccoli, cabbage, cauliflower, carrots, yams, and potatoes
- Fruits such as citrus fruits and yellow fruits; for example, apricots, bananas, and cantaloupe
- Grains such as wheat, rice, oats, corn, breads, and pastas
- Cereals

Complex carbohydrates provide a good source for many vitamins and minerals. In addition, many provide a good source for dietary fiber. Generally, these foods are low in fat (Figure 18-3).

As with fats and proteins, if excessive amounts of carbohydrates are eaten, the body will change them into fats and store them as fat.

Caloric requirements.   The recommendation is that *less than 10%* of our total caloric requirements be obtained from refined sugars. *Complex carbohydrates should account for 50% to 60%* of our daily caloric requirement. The recommendation for most people is to decrease their intake of refined sugars and increase their intake of naturally occurring sugars and starches. Each gram of carbohydrate provides the body with 4 calories.

Vitamins (Table 18-8)

Composition.   Vitamins are organic compounds produced by plants and animals. Some vitamins are produced within our body, for example, vitamins D and K. However, the amounts produced by the body are not enough to meet the needs of the body. The best way to ensure that we get enough of all the vitamins is to eat a well-balanced *healthy* diet consisting of a variety of wholesome foods. Fruits and vegetables, whole grains, nuts and seeds, dairy products, meat, and seafood should provide all the vitamins needed. Vitamins are classified as either fat- or water-soluble. **Fat-soluble vitamins**—A, D, E, and K—dissolve in fat and are found in the fatty parts of food and body tissues. They are stored in the body until needed. **Water-soluble vitamins**—C and the B complexes—dissolve in water and are associated with the watery parts of food and body tissues. These vitamins *are not* stored in the body. Any excess

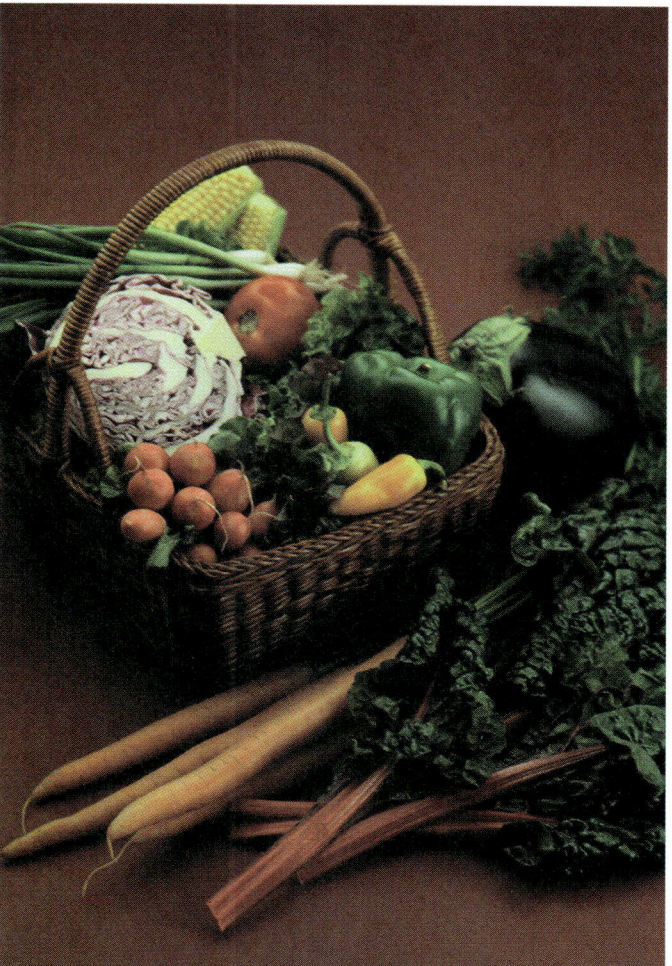

FIGURE 18-3   Fruits and vegetables in the diet **may help** prevent certain types of cancer, heart disease, and diabetes and reduce chances of hip fractures and dementia. (From Wardlaw GM: *Perspectives in nutrition,* ed 2, St Louis, 1993, Mosby.)

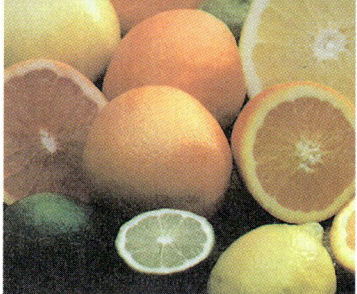

amounts of these vitamins not needed by the body are excreted in the urine. Therefore they must be eaten and replaced daily.

In the field of nutrition, more scientists now recommend increasing dietary intake of the **antioxidant vitamins**—*vitamin C, vitamin E, and beta-carotene (a form of vitamin A).* In addition to the functions outlined in Table 18-8, the antioxidants may also protect the body at the cellular level by preventing damage to body cells caused by *free radicals* (unstable oxygen molecules formed in the body during normal metabolic

TABLE 18–8   Vitamin Facts

Vitamin	U.S. RDA*	Functions	Best Dietary Sources
A (carotene)	5000 IU/day	Formation and maintenance of skin, hair, and mucous membranes; helps us see in dim light; bone and tooth growth; resistance to infection	Yellow or orange fruits and vegetables, green leafy vegetables, fortified oatmeal, liver, dairy products
B₁ (thiamine)	1.5 mg/day	Helps body release energy from carbohydrates during metabolism; growth and muscle tone	Fortified cereals and oatmeals, meats, rice and pasta, whole grains, liver
B₂ (riboflavin)	1.7 mg/day	Helps body release energy from protein, fat, and carbohydrates during metabolism	Whole grains, green leafy vegetables, organ meats, milk, and eggs
B₆ (pyridoxine)	2 mg/day	Helps build body tissue and aids in metabolism of protein	Fish, poultry, lean meats, bananas, prunes, dried beans, whole grains, avocados
B₁₂ (cobalamin)	6 μg/day (6 mcg)	Aids cell development, functioning of the nervous system, and the metabolism of protein and fat	Meats, milk products, seafood
Biotin	0.3 mg/day	Involved in metabolism of protein, fats, and carbohydrates	Cereal/grain products, yeast, legumes, liver
Folate (folacin, folic acid)	0.4 mg/day (400 mcg)	Aids in genetic material development and involved in red blood cell production	Green leafy vegetables, organ meats, dried peas, beans, and lentils
Niacin	20 mg/day	Involved in carbohydrate, protein, and fat metabolism	Meat, poultry, fish, enriched cereals, peanuts, potatoes, dairy products, eggs
Pantothenic acid	10 mg/day	Helps in the release of energy from fats and carbohydrates	Lean meats, whole grains, legumes, vegetables, fruits
C (ascorbic acid)	60 mg/day	Essential for structure of bones, cartilage, muscle, and blood vessels. Also helps maintain capillaries and gums and aids in absorption of iron, speeds healing, and helps prevent infection	Citrus fruits, berries, and vegetables—especially peppers
D	400 IU/day	Aids in bone and tooth formation; helps maintain heart action and nervous system	Fortified milk, sunlight, fish, eggs, butter, fortified margarine
E	30 IU/day	Protects blood cells, body tissue, and essential fatty acids from harmful destruction in the body; helps prevent heart disease, aids the immune system, and may help prevent Alzheimer's disease, cataracts, and some cancers	Fortified and multigrain cereals, nuts, wheat germ, vegetable oils, green leafy vegetables
K†		Essential for blood-clotting functions	Green leafy vegetables, fruit, dairy, and grain products

IU, International units; *mg*, milligrams; *μg and mcg*, micrograms.

*For adults and children over age 4.

†There is no U.S. RDA for vitamin K; however, the recommended dietary allowance is 1 μg/kg of body weight.

processes), tobacco smoke, air pollution, radiation, and other cancer-promoting chemicals. The antioxidants have the ability to neutralize free radicals. Many scientists believe that along with other factors, the resulting cellular damage could lead to the development of a number of *chronic diseases* including *heart disease, cancer,* and *cataracts.* Large-scale studies are being done to gain a better understanding of the potential benefits of taking antioxidant supplements. See Table 18-9 for foods rich in the antioxidants.

Function. Vitamins are required by every part of the body and are essential for growth, metabolism, health maintenance, and disease prevention. Vitamins work together and with other nutrients and in many energy-producing processes. They help to put protein, carbohydrates, and fat to use in the body. They serve as coenzymes working with enzymes to produce the right chemical actions at the right time. Vitamins are also needed by the body to produce hormones, blood cells, and other healthy tissues.

TABLE 18–8   Vitamin Facts—cont'd

Deficiency Symptoms*	Results of Toxicity	Processing Tips
Night blindness, dry and scaly skin, frequent fatigue	Toxic in high doses, but beta-carotene is nontoxic	Serve fruits and vegetables raw and keep covered and refrigerated. Steam veggies; broil, bake, or braise meats.
Heart irregularity, fatigue, nerve disorders, mental confusion	Nontoxic, as high doses are excreted by the kidneys	Don't rinse rice or pasta before and after cooking. Cook in minimal water.
Cracks in corners of mouth, skin rash, anemia	No toxic effects reported	Store foods in containers that light cannot enter; cook vegetables in minimal water; roast or broil meats.
Convulsions, dermatitis, muscular weakness, skin cracks, anemia	Long-term megadoses may cause nerve damage in hands and feet	Serve fruits raw or cook for shortest time in little water; roast or broil meats.
Anemia, nervousness, fatigue, and, in some cases, neuritis and brain degeneration	No toxic effects reported	Roast or broil meat and fish.
Nausea, vomiting, depression, hair loss, dry, scaly skin	No toxic effects reported	Storage, processing, and cooking do not appear to affect this vitamin.
Gastrointestinal disorders, anemia, cracks on lips	Some evidence of toxicity in large doses	Store vegetables in refrigerator and steam, boil, or simmer in minimal water.
Skin disorders, diarrhea, indigestion, general fatigue	Nicotinic acid form should be taken only under doctor's care	Roast or broil beef, veal, lamb, and poultry. Cook potatoes in minimal water.
Fatigue, vomiting, stomach stress, infections, muscle cramps	No toxic effects reported	Eat fruits and vegetables raw.
Swollen or bleeding gums, slow wound healing, fatigue/depression, poor digestion	Intakes of 1 g or more can cause nausea, cramps, and diarrhea	Do not store or soak fruits and vegetables in water. Refrigerate juices and store only 2-3 days.
In children: rickets and other bone deformities In adults: calcium loss from bones	High intakes may cause diarrhea and weight loss	Storage, processing, and cooking do not appear to affect this vitamin.
Muscular wasting, nerve damage, anemia/reproductive failure	Relatively nontoxic	Store in air-tight containers away from light.
Bleeding disorders in newborn infant and those on blood-thinning medications	Nontoxic as found in food	Store in air-tight containers away from light.

Courtesy the Food and Drug Administration, the American Institute for Cancer Research and the United States Department of Agriculture/Human Nutrition Information Service and Worldview Quarterly, Nestle USA, Inc, Washington, D.C. Vitamins A, D, E, and K are fat-soluble; all the rest are water-soluble.

***Many of the symptoms outlined under this heading can also be attributed to problems other than vitamin deficiency. If you have these symptoms and they persist, consult your doctor.**

Sources.   Sources of fat-soluble vitamins include:

- Vitamin A—Foods of animal origin, dark-green and deep-yellow vegetables
- Vitamin D—Milk, butter, and margarine (especially fortified), fish-liver oil, canned sardines and fish, egg yolks, and liver
- Vitamin E—Wheat germ, soybean, cottonseed, and corn oils
- Vitamin K—Green leafy vegetables, cauliflower, and pork liver

Sources of water-soluble vitamins include:

- Vitamin B_1 (thiamin)—Pork, liver, eggs, enriched cereals, wheat germ, nuts, and yeast
- Vitamin B_2 (riboflavin)—Liver, milk, wheat germ, wild rice, almonds, egg whites, and yeast

TABLE 18-9   Foods Rich in Antioxidant Vitamins

Foods Rich in Vitamin C	Amount	Milligrams
Broccoli	½ cup	58
Brussels sprouts	½ cup	35
Cantaloupe	¼ melon	56
Cauliflower	½ cup	34
Clams	1 pint	98
Currant, fresh	½ cup	101
Mango	1	53
Green pepper	1	89
Hot pepper	1	46
Kiwi	1	74
Papaya	1	187
Orange—California	1	80
Orange—Florida	1	68
Orange juice	6 oz	155
Grapefruit	½ fruit	120
Grapefruit juice	6 oz	185
Strawberries	1 cup	85

Foods Rich in Vitamin E	Amount	Milligrams
Dried apricots	1 cup	7
Mango	1	2
Olive oil	½ cup	12
Assorted nuts	1 cup	12
Pumpkin seeds	½ cup	2
Fortified cereals	1 cup	27
Sweet potato	1	5
Wheat germ	3½ cup	14
Sunflower seeds	3½ cup	44
Kale, raw	3½ cup	8

Foods Rich in Beta Carotene	Amount	International Units
Broccoli	½ cup	1,082
Carrots, cooked	½ cup	19,152
Carrots, raw	1	20,253
Sweet potatoes	1	21,822
Yellow squash	½ cup	3,628
Spinach, cooked	½ cup	7,371
Spinach, raw	½ cup	1,847
Tomato	1	766
Kale, cooked	½ cup	2,762
Cantaloupe	¼ melon	4,304

- Niacin—Liver, halibut, tuna, peanuts, poultry, enriched cereals, and yeast
- Vitamin B_6 (pyridoxine)—Molasses, wheat bran, wheat germ, soybeans, liver, corn, bananas, prunes, raisins, and yeast
- Vitamin B_{12} (cyanocobalamin)—Liver, beef, ham, shellfish, milk, and most cheeses
- Folacin (folic acid)—Green leafy vegetables, organ meats, and legumes
- Biotin—Organ meats, egg yolks, and legumes
- Pantothenic acid—Animal products, whole grains, and legumes
- Vitamin C—Citrus fruits, raw strawberries, liver, and raw vegetables (rutabaga, watercress, kale, parsley, turnip greens, broccoli, cauliflower, and peppers)

It is essential to store fresh food properly and use it within a minimum amount of time to preserve nutrients. Short processing techniques lessen the effect cooking has on foods rich in vitamins. The vitamins in food can be destroyed by pro-

TABLE 18–10A Recommended Calcium Intakes for Different Ages and Genders

Recommended calcium intakes*

Age/gender	mg/day
Children and Young Adults	
1-10 years	800-1200
11-24 years	1200-1500
Adult women	
Pregnant & Lactating	1200-1500
25-49 years (premenopausal)	1000
50-64 years (postmenopausal) taking estrogen	1000
50-64 years (postmenopausal) not taking estrogen	1500
65+ years	1500
Adult men	
25-64 years	1000
65+ years	1500

*Source: National Institutes of Health Consensus Panel, Optimal Calcium Intake, Revised Recommendations, 1994.

TABLE 18–10B Calcium Content of Foods

Food	Calcium (mg)
Skim milk, 1 cup	302
1% lowfat milk, 1 cup	300
2% lowfat milk, 1 cup	297
Whole milk, 1 cup	291
Buttermilk, 1 cup	285
Nonfat dry milk, 1 Tbsp	94
Milkshake, 10 oz.	457
Yogurt, plain, 1 cup	415
Yogurt, fruit flavored, 1 cup	345
Pudding, 1 cup	260
Frozen yogurt, 1 cup	200
Ice cream, 1 cup	170
Sherbet, 1 cup	100
Ricotta cheese, ½ cup	337
Cottage cheese, ½ cup	77
Swiss cheese, 1 oz	272
Cheese, most varieties, 1 oz	190
Cream cheese, 1 oz	23
Sour cream, 1 Tbsp	14
Half and half, 1 Tbsp	16
Whipped cream, 1 Tbsp	5
Sardines, with bones, 3 oz	372
Salmon, canned with bones, 3 oz	167
Tofu, processed with calcium sulfate, 3 oz	120
Oysters, raw, 7	113
Shrimp, canned, 3 oz	99
Legumes, dried, cooked, 1 cup	90
Almonds, ¼ cup	83
Brazil nuts, ¼ cup	65
Collard greens, ½ cup	179
Bokchoy, ½ cup	126
Turnip greens, from raw, ½ cup	126
Turnip greens, frozen, ½ cup	98
Rhubarb, ½ cup	106
Kale, ½ cup	103
Mustard greens, ½ cup	97
Broccoli, from raw, ½ cup	88
Broccoli, frozen, ½ cup	55
Spinach, ½ cup	84
Farina, cooked, 1 cup	147
Molasses, 1 Tbsp	137

longed heating or temperatures higher than boiling or can readily be destroyed by heat, especially slow cooking.

Caloric requirements. Vitamins *do not* supply any calories and thus no energy. For the daily minimum requirements of vitamins, see Table 18-8.

Minerals

Composition. Minerals are inorganic substances that make up nearly 5% of the body and are found in body tissues and fluids. The two major divisions of minerals are **macrominerals** (also called *major minerals*) and **microminerals** (known as *trace minerals*). On a daily basis, our body needs greater amounts of macrominerals than it does of microminerals. Macrominerals include calcium, phosphorus, magnesium, sodium, potassium, chloride, and sulfur. The trace minerals include iron, copper, iodine, manganese, cobalt, zinc, molybdenum, fluorine, selenium, chromium, nickel, tin, silicon, and vanadium.

Function. Minerals are needed for a variety of body functions, including the building of strong teeth and bones and the regulation of a number of body processes, including the metabolism of nutrients in foods, helping to maintain fluid balance among the body cells, heart function, muscle contraction, transmission of messages over the nerves, blood clotting, hormone production, and protein and red blood cell formation.

Sources. Minerals are essential in the metabolism of body cells. The best way to have the necessary minerals in your body is by eating a variety of foods in a balanced diet of carbohydrates, fat, and protein.

Growing children, teenage girls, and many women need to eat more **calcium-rich foods** to obtain the calcium needed for healthy bones throughout their lives. Adults with poor bone mass are more susceptible to osteoporosis. Postmenopausal women are most at risk for osteoporosis because of loss of the hormone estrogen, which has a protective effect on bones in the earlier years. Many physicians recommend dietary supplements and sometimes other medications (for older people) that can help to maintain healthy bones. See Table 18-10 for the current recommended calcium daily intake and foods rich in calcium.

Young children, teenage girls, and women of childbearing age must also eat enough **iron-rich foods.** During pregnancy and lactation, an iron supplement is usually recommended. Eating foods rich in vitamin C with iron-rich foods is suggested because they will help the body to absorb the iron. Cooking with iron pots can also add iron to the food. Some good sources of iron include the following*:

- Meats—beef, pork, lamb, and liver and other organ meats†
- Poultry—chicken, duck, and turkey, especially dark meat; liver†
- Fish—shellfish, like clams, mussels, and oysters; sardines; anchovies; and other fish†
- Leafy greens of the cabbage family, such as broccoli, kale, turnip greens, collards
- Legumes, such as lima beans and green peas; dry beans and peas, such as pinto beans, black-eyed peas, and canned baked beans
- Yeast-leavened whole-wheat bread and rolls
- Iron-enriched white bread, pasta, rice, and cereals. Read the labels.

Caloric requirements.   As with vitamins, minerals *do not* supply any calories and thus no energy. See Table 18-11 for more information on minerals.

Water
Composition.   Water is a vital nutrient needed for life and survival. Most of us could live for a few weeks without food, but all of us would survive for only a few days without water. The average healthy female is composed of 50% water, and the average healthy male is composed of 60% water. Men have more water because they have more muscle tissue, which holds more water. Women have more fat tissue, which holds less water than muscle tissue. The average adult contains 40 to 50 quarts of water. The body water is divided between two compartments called **intracellular** and **extracellular fluid compartments**. Water **inside** body cells is part of the intracellular fluid. This makes up about 63% of the total amount of body water. Water **outside** body cells is part of the extracellular fluid. It consists of the plasma in the blood, the interstitial fluid that surrounds body cells, the lymph, the cerebrospinal fluid, and specialized joint fluids. This makes up the other 37% of the total body water.

Function.   Every cell in the body needs water. It serves as a medium for all chemical reactions in the body. In addition, water does the following:

- Regulates the body temperature
- Carries oxygen and nutrients to all cells
- Removes wastes from all cells
- Lubricates the joints
- Protects tissues and organs

---

*Does not include complete list of examples. You can obtain additional information from "Good Sources of Nutrients," USDA, January 1990. Also read food labels for brand-specific information.
†Some foods in this group are high in fat, cholesterol, or both. Choose lean, lower-fat, lower-cholesterol foods most often. Read the labels.

- Prevents dehydration
- Replaces sweat losses during and after exercising or exposure to heat or elevated temperatures

Water is lost from our body daily through the processes of urination, respiration, and defecation and through the skin, whether perspiring or not.

Sources.   Water comes from three sources: beverages or other liquids; foods, especially vegetables and fruits; and water formed in the tissues as the result of metabolism.

Requirements.   Requirements for water vary with body size, metabolic rate, exercise, climate, type of diet, and other conditions such as pregnancy or illness. Individuals are advised to drink at least 6 to 8 cups of water daily although there is some water in foods such as fruits and vegetables and also in other beverages. Water is even found in foods such as chicken, cheese, eggs, hamburger, cookies, and crackers. Coffee, tea, and alcohol are *not* good fluids to use to replace water because the caffeine and alcohol act like a diuretic, causing water loss rather than replacement.

The simplest way to determine if you are drinking enough water is to check the color and amount of urine you excrete. If you are urinating only small amounts of urine and if it is dark in color, drink more water. If the urine is pale yellow or clear, it is an indication that normal water balance has occurred.

The Environmental Protection Agency (EPA) regulates the content of tap water. In many locations throughout the country, fluoride is added to the water supply to aid in preventing tooth decay in children. Most water is disinfected with chlorine. Water pipes lined with lead can contaminate the water from the tap. To avoid lead contamination, run the water until it is cold before using it because lead is more soluble in hot water.

To have your water supply checked and to obtain the location of a nearby certified laboratory, contact The Safe Drinking Water Hotline at 1-800-426-4791.

Bottled water may taste better to some people, but it may not be any healthier or safer than your tap water. Minimum standards for both are set by the Food and Drug Administration (FDA).

FIBER

Composition.   Fiber is an important element of our diet, although by definition it is not considered a nutrient. Dietary fiber is a complex mixture of cell walls of plants that are resistant to breakdown by the digestive tract. It is the indigestible part of a food.

The two major types of dietary fiber are as follows:

1. **Water-insoluble fiber** includes cellulose, hemicellulose, and lignin. They are not metabolized by intestinal bacteria and *do not* readily dissolve in water.
2. **Water-soluble fiber** includes gums, mucilages, and pectins. These substances readily swell or dissolve when put in water.

TABLE 18–11   **Summary of Water and the Major Minerals**

Name	RDA or Minimum Requirements	Major Functions	Best Dietary Sources	Deficiency Symptoms	Results of Toxicity	Most at Risk for Deficiency
Water	1 ml/kcal burned*	Medium for chemical reactions, removal of waste products, perspiration to cool the body	As such and in foods	Thirst, muscle weakness, poor endurance	Probably only in mental disorders, headache, blurred vision, convulsions	Infants with a fever, elderly in nursing homes
Sodium	500 mg	A major ion of the extracellular fluid, nerve transmission	Table salt, processed foods	Muscle cramps	High blood pressure in susceptible individuals	People severely restricting sodium to lower blood pressure (250-500 mg/day)
Potassium	2000 mg	A major ion of intracellular fluid, nerve transmission	Vegetables, fruits, milk	Irregular heartbeat, loss of appetite, muscle cramps	Slowing of the heartbeat, seen in kidney failure	Use of potassium-wasting diuretics, poor diets seen in poverty and alcoholism
Chloride	700 mg	A major ion of the extracellular fluid, acid production in stomach	Table salt, some vegetables	Convulsions in infants	High blood pressure in susceptible people when combined with sodium	No one, probably, if infant formula manufacturers control product quality adequately
Calcium†	800 mg (1200 mg ages 11-24)	Bones, teeth, blood clotting, nerve transmission, muscle contractions, cell regulation; reduces risks of osteoporosis and cancer of colon; seems to help prevent high BP and reduce symptoms of PMS	Dairy products, canned fish, leafy vegetables, tofu, fortified orange juice	Poor intake probably increased the risk for osteoporosis	Very high intakes may cause a form of kidney stones in susceptible people	Women in general, especially those who consume few dairy products
Phosphorus	Men: 350 mg	Bones, teeth, metabolic compounds such as ATP, ion of intracellular fluid	Dairy products, processed foods, soft drinks	Probably none; poor bone maintenance possible	Induces high levels of parathyroid hormone in kidney failure; poor bone mineralization if calcium intakes are low	Elderly consuming very nutrient-poor diets; total vegetarians? alcoholism?
Magnesium	Women: 280 mg	Bones, enzyme function, nerve and heart function	Wheat bran, green vegetables, nuts, chocolate	Weakness, muscle pain, poor heart function	Causes weakness in kidney failure	People taking thiazide diuretics
Sulfur	None	Part of vitamins and amino acids, drug detoxification, acid-base balance	Protein foods	None	None likely	No one who meets their protein needs

Adapted from Wardlaw I: *Perspectives in nutrition,* St Louis, 1993, Mosby.

*Just an approximation; best to keep urine volume greater than 1 L (4 cups).

†See Table 18-10.

Function.   Dietary fiber in the diet is required because of the important roles it plays in body functions. Some of the functions of fiber are as follows:

1. Fiber promotes increased chewing, which is good for the teeth.
2. Food sources of fiber are lower in fat than animal food sources, and most people need to decrease their intake of fat.
3. Fiber food sources increase a person's intake of vitamins.
4. Fiber food sources have less additives than processed foods.
5. Insoluble fiber promotes normal elimination by providing bulk for stool formation and thus hastening the passage of the stool through the colon.
6. Insoluble fiber helps to satisfy appetite by creating a feeling of fullness. It also aids weight control.
7. Fiber in the diet also helps to control weight because the foods *high* in fiber *generally* have fewer calories than other food sources.
8. Soluble fiber may play a role in reducing the level of cholesterol in the blood.
9. Soluble fiber is thought to slow down the release of carbohydrates from their source; it holds onto the sugar and releases it more slowly so that we derive the benefits of the sugar for a longer time.
10. Fiber is thought to be protective against heart disease, diabetes, breast and colon cancer, constipation, and diverticulosis because of some of the preceding functions. Only **some** nutrition experts have also associated fiber in the diet with a reduction of the number of cases of gallbladder disease, hiatal hernia, appendicitis, and varicose veins (Table 18-12).
11. Food sources rich in fiber are usually less expensive than foods from other sources.

Sources.   The main sources of dietary fiber come from grain products, fruits, and vegetables (Table 18-13). Dietary fiber is *not* found in animal products such as milk and meats.

Recommended amounts of fiber intake.   The National Cancer Institute recommends 20 to 30 g of fiber per day with an upper limit of 35 g. According to government surveys, average dietary intake of fiber varies from 12 to 17 g. Therefore for most people an increase in their fiber intake is recommended. Eating a variety of foods that contain dietary fiber is the best way to get an adequate amount. See Table 18-13 for a list of foods and the fiber content. The serving sizes used on the list are only estimates of the amounts of food you might eat. The amount of fiber in a serving depends on the weight of the serving. For example, ½ cup of a cooked vegetable contains more fiber than ½ cup of the same vegetable served raw because a serving of a cooked vegetable

TABLE 18–12   Type, Source, and Function of Fiber

	Source		
Water-Soluble Fiber	**Gums**	**Pectins**	**Function**
	Oatmeal	Apples	• Binds with cholesterol-containing bile acids in gut, preventing reabsorption
	Oat products	Squash	• Decreases blood cholesterol
	Dried beans	Citrus fruits	• Delays glucose absorption and gastric emptying
	Barley	Cauliflower	• Protects against heart disease and diabetes
		Green beans	
		Cabbage	
		Dried peas	
		Carrots	
		Strawberries	
		Potatoes	
Water-Insoluble Fiber	**Cellulose**	**Hemicellulose**	**Function**
	Whole wheat products	Bran	• Absorbs water
	Bran	Cereals	• Increases stool volume
	Cabbage	Whole grains	• Decreases stool transit time
	Green beans	Brussels sprouts	• Dilutes concentration of bile acids
	Broccoli	Mustard greens	• Protective against colon and breast cancer, constipation, and diverticulosis
	Brussels sprouts		
	Peppers		
	Apples		
	NOTE: Serving sizes:	½ cup beans, legumes, barley, rice	
		¾ cup cereals, oatmeal, oat bran	
		1 slice whole grain bread	
		1 medium fruit	

weighs more. Therefore the cooked vegetable may appear on the list, whereas the raw form does not. In this example, the raw vegetable provides dietary fiber—but just not enough in a ½ cup serving to be significant source of dietary fiber. A selected serving size in Table 18-13 contains at least 2 g of dietary fiber.

To retain dietary fiber in foods, serve fruits and vegetables with edible skins and seeds and use whole-grain flours. Cooking can reduce some of the dietary fiber in a food.

Increasing your dietary fiber intake should be done gradually to minimize potential side effects, such as gas, bloating, and cramps, which may occur if large amounts of fiber are

TABLE 18–13 Sources of Dietary Fiber

Food	Selected Serving Size*	Food	Selected Serving Size*
Breads, cereals, and other grain products		Dried, uncooked	¼ cup
Bagel, whole-wheat	1 medium	Raw	1 medium
Biscuit, whole-wheat	1 medium	Prunes, dried:	
Breads, multigrain, pumpernickel rye, white		Cooked, unsweetened	½ cup
and whole-wheat blend, whole wheat, or		Uncooked	¼ cup
whole-wheat with raisins	2 regular slices	Raisins	¼ cup
Bulgur, cooked or canned	⅔ cup	Raspberries, raw or frozen, unsweetened	½ cup
English muffin, whole-wheat	1	Strawberries, frozen, unsweetened	½ cup
Muffins, bran or whole-wheat	1 medium	Tangelo, raw	1 medium
Oatmeal:			
Instant, fortified, prepared	⅔ cup	**Vegetables**	
Regular or quick, cooked	⅔ cup	Artichoke, globe (french), cooked	1 medium
Pita bread, whole-wheat	1 small	Beans, green or lima, cooked	½ cup
Ready-to-eat bran cereals	1 ounce	Beets, cooked	½ cup
Rolls:		Broccoli, cooked	½ cup
Multigrain	1 large	Brussels sprouts, cooked	½ cup
Whole-wheat	1 medium	Cabbage, cooked	½ cup
		Carrots, cooked	½ cup
Fruits		Okra, cooked	½ cup
Apples:		Parsnips, cooked	½ cup
Dried, cooked, unsweetened	½ cup	Peas, green, cooked	½ cup
Raw	1 medium	Potato, boiled, with skin	1 medium
Applesauce, unsweetened	½ cup	Snow peas, raw or cooked	½ cup
Apricots, dried:		Spinach, cooked	½ cup
Cooked, unsweetened	½ cup	Squash, winter, cooked, mashed	½ cup
Uncooked	¼ cup	Sweet potato, baked or boiled	1 medium
Banana, raw	1 medium	Tomatoes, stewed	½ cup
Blackberries, raw or frozen, unsweetened	½ cup		
Blueberries, frozen, unsweetened	½ cup	**Meat, poultry, fish, and alternatives**	
Dates, chopped	¼ cup	***Dry beans, peas, and lentils***	
Fruit mixture, dried	¼ cup	Beans; black-eyed peas (cowpeas), calico,	
Guava, raw	1	chickpeas (garbanzo beans), lima, mexican,	
Kiwifruit, raw	1 medium	pinto, red kidney, or white; cooked	½ cup
Mango, raw	½ medium	Lentils, cooked	½ cup
Nectarine, raw	1 medium	Peas, split, green or yellow, cooked	½ cup
Orange, raw	1 medium		
Peaches, dried:		**Nuts and seeds**	
Cooked, unsweetened	½ cup	Almonds or chestnuts, roasted	2 Tbsp
Uncooked	¼ cup	Peanut butter	2 Tbsp
Pears:		Pine nuts (pignolias)	2 Tbsp
Canned, juice-pack	½ cup	Pumpkin or squash seeds, hulled, roasted	2 Tbsp
Dried, cooked, unsweetened	½ cup	Sesame seeds	2 Tbsp
		Sunflower seeds, hulled, unroasted	2 Tbsp

*A selected serving size contains at least 2 g of dietary fiber.

TABLE 18–14   Sodium Content of Foods

Food	Sodium (mg)	Food	Sodium (mg)
Fresh fruit, ½ cup or medium	2	Pretzels, 10 rings	336
Canned or frozen fruit	2	Hot cereal, ½ cup	1
Fresh vegetables, ½ cup	1-5	Instant hot cereal, ½ cup	280
Naturally high-sodium vegetables: carrots, celery,		Dry cereal, 1 cup	165-340
beets, spinach, kale, swiss chard	30-45	Rice, pasta, cooked with no salt	1
Canned vegetables, ½ cup	250-280	Seasoned rice and pasta mixes, ½ cup	600
Frozen vegetables, ½ cup (except naturally high)	5-15	Bread, 1 slice	170
Sauerkraut, ½ cup	750	Crackers, 4	120-200
Milk, yogurt, 1 cup	120	Vegetable oils	trace
Buttermilk, 1 cup	225	Butter or margarine, 1 tsp	50
Natural cheese, 1 oz	175	Bottled salad dressing, 1 Tbsp	200
Processed cheese, 1 oz	400	Canned soups, ½ can	600
Fresh meat, fish, poultry, 3 oz	75	Salt, sea salt, seasoned salt, 1 tsp	2300
Shellfish, 3 oz	150	MSG, 1 tsp	500
Ham, 3 oz	675	Baking soda, 1 tsp	820
Luncheon meats, 3 oz	1170	Baking powder, 1 tsp	330
Frankfurter, 1	540	Soy sauce, 1 tsp	365
Frozen dinners	1100	Worcestershire sauce, 1 Tbsp	315
Dried beans, ½ cup cooked	15	Catsup, 1 Tbsp	200
Canned baked beans, ½ cup	450	Bouillon cube, 1 cube	960
Unsalted nuts, ½ cup	1	Olive, 4 green	325
Salted nuts, ½ cup	230	4 ripe	130
Peanut butter, 2 Tbsp	200	Pickle, dill	903
Chips—10	220	Herbs and spices	trace

Sodium content of nonprescription drugs

Drug	Sodium Content per Dose
Alka-Seltzer (2 tablets)	935 mg
Bromo-Seltzer	717 mg
Fleet enema	250-300 absorbed
Metamucil instant mix	250 mg
Rolaids (2 tablets)	70 mg
Vicks' Formula 44 (2 tsp)	105 mg

eaten in a short time. When eating more dietary fiber, drink more fluids. Because fiber retains more fluid in the feces, more fluid is needed in the diet.

SALT AND SODIUM

Table salt contains sodium and chloride, both of which are essential in the diet. However, most Americans eat more salt and sodium than they need. Food and beverages containing salt provide most of the sodium in our diets, much of it added during processing and manufacturing.

In populations with diets low in salt, high blood pressure is less common than in populations with diets high in salt. Other factors that affect blood pressure are heredity, obesity, and excessive drinking of alcoholic beverages.

The recommended daily value for adults for sodium is 2400 mg or less or approximately 1 teaspoon. Most people are advised to eat less salt and sodium because they usually need much less than they eat and reduction will benefit those people whose blood pressure rises with salt intake. See Table 18-14 for the amount of sodium found in some foods and a few nonprescription drugs. Herbs and spices can be used to flavor food instead of salt.

ALCOHOL

Alcoholic beverages supply calories but little or no nutrients. Drinking them has no net health benefit, is linked with many health problems, is the cause of many accidents, and can lead to addiction. Their consumption is not recommended. If adults

If You Drink Alcoholic Beverages, Do So in Moderation

Some people should not drink alcoholic beverages:

- *Women who are pregnant or trying to conceive.* Major birth defects have been attributed to heavy drinking by the mother while pregnant. However, there is no conclusive evidence that an occasional drink is harmful, *but a safe level of alcohol intake during pregnancy* **has not** *been established.*
- *Individuals who plan to drive or engage in other activities that require attention or skill.* Most people retain some alcohol in the blood for 3 to 5 hours, after even moderate drinking.
- *Individuals using medicines, even over-the-counter kinds.* Alcohol may affect the benefits or toxicity of medicines. Also, some medicines may increase blood alcohol levels or increase the adverse effect of alcohol on the brain.
- *Individuals who cannot keep their drinking moderate.* This is a special concern for recovering alcoholics and people whose family members have alcohol problems.
- *Children and adolescents.* Use of alcoholic beverages by children and adolescents involves risks to health and other serious problems.

Heavy drinkers are often malnourished because of low food intake and poor absorption of nutrients by the body. Too much alcohol may cause cirrhosis of the liver, inflammation of the pancreas, damage to the brain and heart, and increased risk for many cancers.

Some studies have suggested that moderate drinking is linked to lower risk for heart attacks. However, drinking is also linked to higher risk for high blood pressure and hemorrhagic stroke.

Advice for today: If you drink alcoholic beverages, do so in moderation and don't drive.

If you don't drink, don't start.

What's Moderate Drinking?
Women: No more than 1 drink a day
Men: No more than 2 drinks a day

Count as a drink:

- 12 ounces of regular beer
- 5 ounces of wine
- 1½ ounces of distilled spirits (80 proof)

---

elect to drink alcoholic beverages, they should consume them in moderate amounts (see box).

CALORIES

Calories **are not** food, but rather the amount of energy that can be derived from protein, fat, and carbohydrate in food. Technically, a calorie is a unit of heat. One calorie is the amount of heat required to raise the temperature of 1 kg (kilogram) of water 1° Celsius.

The amount of energy that can be obtained from a food can be calculated from the amount of heat units or calories in that food using the following measurements.

- 1 g of protein provides 4 calories
- 1 g of carbohydrate provides 4 calories
- 1 g of fat provides 9 calories

NOTE: The fat in a food provides a little more than double the number of calories provided by protein and carbohydrates. This is important to keep in mind when trying to reduce or increase the number of total calories in a diet. When more calories are taken in than the body requires for its energy needs, the excess calories will be converted and stored as body fat. Also, the body is more efficient at converting fat (versus protein or carbohydrate) that is ingested into fat. **The following example demonstrates how the amount of calories consumed affects weight gain:**

1 pound of body weight = approximately 3500 calories
Daily caloric requirement for Mr. B. = 2000 calories
Daily caloric intake for Mr. B. = 3000 calories
Excess number of daily caloric intake = 1000 calories
Excess number of calories for 1 week = 1000 calories ×
7 days = 7000 calories

7000 extra calories ÷ 3500 calories/pound = 2 pounds

Therefore Mr. B. has just gained 2 pounds in 1 week.

The same formula can be applied to determine weight loss (that is, if you want to lose 2 pounds, you would have to eat 7000 calories less or burn off 7000 extra calories by increased activity).

A safe, healthy weight loss is 1 to 2 pounds per week. **Exercise along with dietary changes is the most effective way to lose weight and maintain the weight loss. Fad or crash diets should be avoided.**

To determine the number of calories in a cracker that is labeled as follows, use the following calculations:

1 cracker = 1 g of protein, 4 g of carbohydrate, and 3 g of fat
1 g of protein × 4 calories = 4 calories
4 g of carbohydrates × 4 calories = 16 calories
3 g of fat × 9 calories = 27 calories
TOTAL CALORIES = 4 + 16 + 27 = 47 calories

This means that in each cracker labeled in this way, there are 47 calories, the majority of which come from fat.

Formula for Determining the Percentage of Calories in a Food Supplied From Fat

1. Grams of fat × 9 = "Fat" calories
2. $\dfrac{\text{Fat calories}}{\text{Total calories} \times 100}$ = Percentage of calories from fat

Using the values given for the cracker, this equation would be:

1. 3 × 9 = 27
2. $\dfrac{27}{47}$ × 100 = 2700/47 = 57.4% of the calories in this cracker are supplied from fat.

Also see Table 18-15

TABLE 18-15 Fat in Foods

Low Fat (0%-20% of Calories)	High Fat (over 20% of Calories)
Fresh fruits and vegetables, fruit and vegetable juices, dried fruit	Olives, avocado, coconut, french fries, hash browns, potato chips
Most breads and cereals, noodles, pasta, matzoh, barley, bulgur, corn tortillas, popcorn (air popped), soda crackers, rye wafers, water crackers, Wasa and Ak Mak crackers, pretzels	Cornbread, biscuits, muffins, waffles, pancakes, granola, croissant, soft rolls, wheatgerm, flour tortillas, popcorn (oil popped), donuts, pastries, snack chips, snack crackers
Nonfat milk, nonfat dry milk, buttermilk, nonfat yogurt, low-fat yogurt, low-fat cottage cheese, sherbet, ice milk, frozen yogurt	Whole milk, low-fat milk, creamed cottage cheese, all cheeses, ice cream, whipping cream, half and half, nondairy creamer, lard, butter, margarine, oils, sour cream, cream cheese, tofu
Legumes, egg whites, cod, halibut, sole, flounder, red snapper, shrimp, scallops, squid, abalone, clams, crab, lobster, mussels, oyster, tuna in water, light meat of chicken and turkey (without skin), ham, Canadian bacon, veal, flank steak, round steak	Whole eggs, salmon, trout, swordfish, anchovies, sardines, mackerel, tuna in oil, dark meat of chicken and turkey, light meat of chicken and turkey (with skin), beef, pork, lamb, bacon, sausages, hot dogs, salami, cold cuts, organ meats, nuts, seeds, soybeans, commercial refried beans
Broths, bouillon, most soups, spices, herbs, sugar, jam, jellies, applesauce, apple butter, tomato sauces, mustard, ketchup, salsa, soy sauce, horseradish	Creamed soups, salad dressings, custard, mayonnaise, chocolate, candy bars, pies, cakes

To find the maximum amount of fat you can eat every day, according to the American Heart Association's recommendation that no more than 30% of your daily calorie intake should be obtained from fat, follow these recommended steps:

Step 1: Multiply your ideal weight by 15 if you are moderately active or by 20 if you are very active.

Step 2: From that total, subtract the following according to your age:
25 to 34, subtract 0
35 to 44, subtract 100
45 to 54, subtract 200
55 to 64, subtract 300
65 and older, subtract 400
This will give you your recommended daily calories. This is **only approximate**: ask your physician for guidance.

Step 3: Find your recommended calories intake on the chart that follows and read across to determine your daily fat allowance.

To visualize fat content in a food, be aware of the following*:

- One teaspoon (one pat) of butter or margarine has 4 g of fat.
- The fat content of one 8 oz glass of whole milk is equal to the fat in approximately 2 pats of butter (8 g of fat).
- Two french fries from a fast-food restaurant equal two whole baked potatoes ($\frac{1}{2}$ g of fat).
- One ounce of potato chips equals 20 oz of pretzels (10 g of fat).
- One peanut equals 2.86 cups of air-popped popcorn (0.86 g of fat).
- One corn chip equals 40 baby carrots (1 gram of fat).
- One chocolate donut equals 70 oranges (21 g of fat).

*Source: 1997 Illustrated Calendar of Fat by John Flaherty.

Daily Calories	Maximum Grams of Saturated Fat	Maximum Grams of Total Fat
1200	13	40
1400	16	47
1600	18	53
1800	20	60
2000	22	67
2200	24	73
2400	27	80
2600	29	37
2800	31	93
3000	33	100

Daily Caloric Requirements

Daily caloric requirements vary and depend on the following.

1. **Age:** Generally young people need more calories than older people.
2. **Sex:** Generally men need more calories than women.
3. **Body frame:** The larger the body frame, the more calories are needed to maintain the weight.
4. **Weight:** Heavier people need more calories than lighter people to maintain their weight.
5. **Percentage of body fat:** Women have more body fat (average 19% to 24%) than men (average 12% to 17%).
6. **Activity level:** The more active a person is, the more calories will be burned and needed to maintain body weight.
7. **Basal metabolic rate:** The basal metabolic rate is the amount of energy (calories) needed when the body is at rest to maintain basic body activities such as temperature, respiration, circulation, muscle tone, and peristalsis. This is a special test performed with the person at rest in a com-

FIGURE 18-4   Food label. Read food labels and note if the food has a high content of sugars or salt. (Courtesy Aetna Health Plans, San Bruno, Calif.)

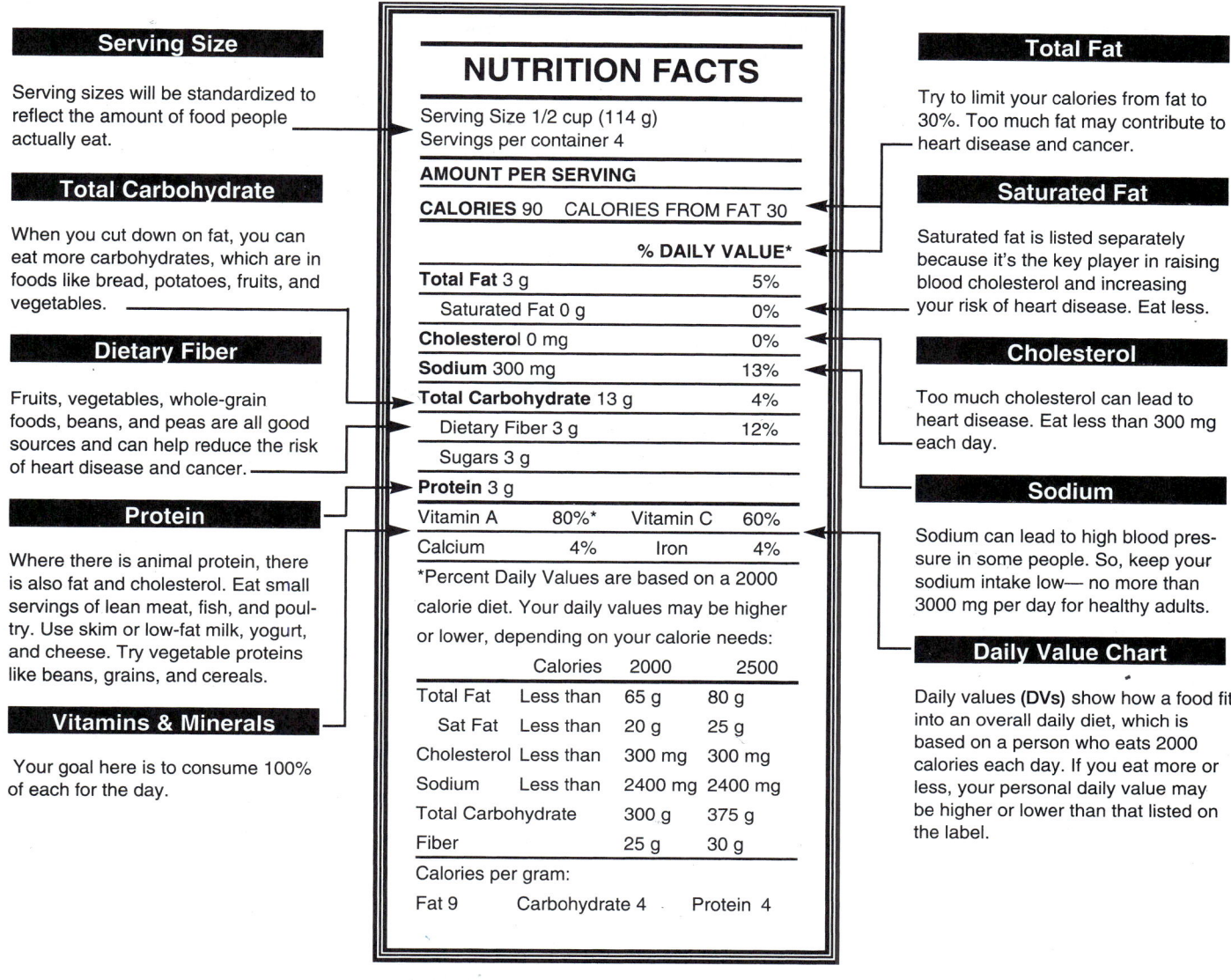

Serving Size

Serving sizes will be standardized to reflect the amount of food people actually eat.

Total Carbohydrate

When you cut down on fat, you can eat more carbohydrates, which are in foods like bread, potatoes, fruits, and vegetables.

Dietary Fiber

Fruits, vegetables, whole-grain foods, beans, and peas are all good sources and can help reduce the risk of heart disease and cancer.

Protein

Where there is animal protein, there is also fat and cholesterol. Eat small servings of lean meat, fish, and poultry. Use skim or low-fat milk, yogurt, and cheese. Try vegetable proteins like beans, grains, and cereals.

Vitamins & Minerals

Your goal here is to consume 100% of each for the day.

Total Fat

Try to limit your calories from fat to 30%. Too much fat may contribute to heart disease and cancer.

Saturated Fat

Saturated fat is listed separately because it's the key player in raising blood cholesterol and increasing your risk of heart disease. Eat less.

Cholesterol

Too much cholesterol can lead to heart disease. Eat less than 300 mg each day.

Sodium

Sodium can lead to high blood pressure in some people. So, keep your sodium intake low— no more than 3000 mg per day for healthy adults.

Daily Value Chart

Daily values (**DVs**) show how a food fit into an overall daily diet, which is based on a person who eats 2000 calories each day. If you eat more or less, your personal daily value may be higher or lower than that listed on the label.

NUTRITION FACTS

Serving Size 1/2 cup (114 g)
Servings per container 4

AMOUNT PER SERVING

CALORIES 90   CALORIES FROM FAT 30

		% DAILY VALUE*
Total Fat 3 g		5%
Saturated Fat 0 g		0%
Cholesterol 0 mg		0%
Sodium 300 mg		13%
Total Carbohydrate 13 g		4%
Dietary Fiber 3 g		12%
Sugars 3 g		
Protein 3 g		
Vitamin A	80%*	Vitamin C	60%
Calcium	4%	Iron	4%

*Percent Daily Values are based on a 2000 calorie diet. Your daily values may be higher or lower, depending on your calorie needs:

		Calories	2000	2500
Total Fat	Less than		65 g	80 g
Sat Fat	Less than		20 g	25 g
Cholesterol	Less than		300 mg	300 mg
Sodium	Less than		2400 mg	2400 mg
Total Carbohydrate			300 g	375 g
Fiber			25 g	30 g

Calories per gram:

Fat 9   Carbohydrate 4   Protein 4

No More False Claims

Now when you see words and health claims on food products, they will actually mean something. Here's a list of the most commonly used buzz words, along with their new government definitions:

Fat Free	Less than 0.5 g of fat per serving
Low Fat	3 g of fat (or less) per serving.
Lean	Less than 10 g of fat, 4 g or less of saturated fat, and 95 mg or less of cholesterol per serving.
Light (Lite)	1/3 less calories or no more than 1/2 the fat of the higher-calorie, higher fat-version; or no more than 1/2 the sodium of the higher-sodium version
Cholesterol Free	Less than 2 mg of cholesterol and 1/2 g (or less) of saturated fat per serving.

fortable environment 14 to 18 hours after the last meal was eaten.

The consumption of fat in the diet should be reduced so that fat makes up only 30% or less of a person's daily caloric requirement (also see Table 18-15).

Empty calorie is a term used to denote calories obtained from a food source that provides energy but very little other nutritional value. For example, the calories obtained from alcohol and refined sugars are thought of as being empty calories.

FIGURE 18-5 **A,** Vegetarian food pyramid. (Courtesy The Health Connection: [800] 548-8700.)

A

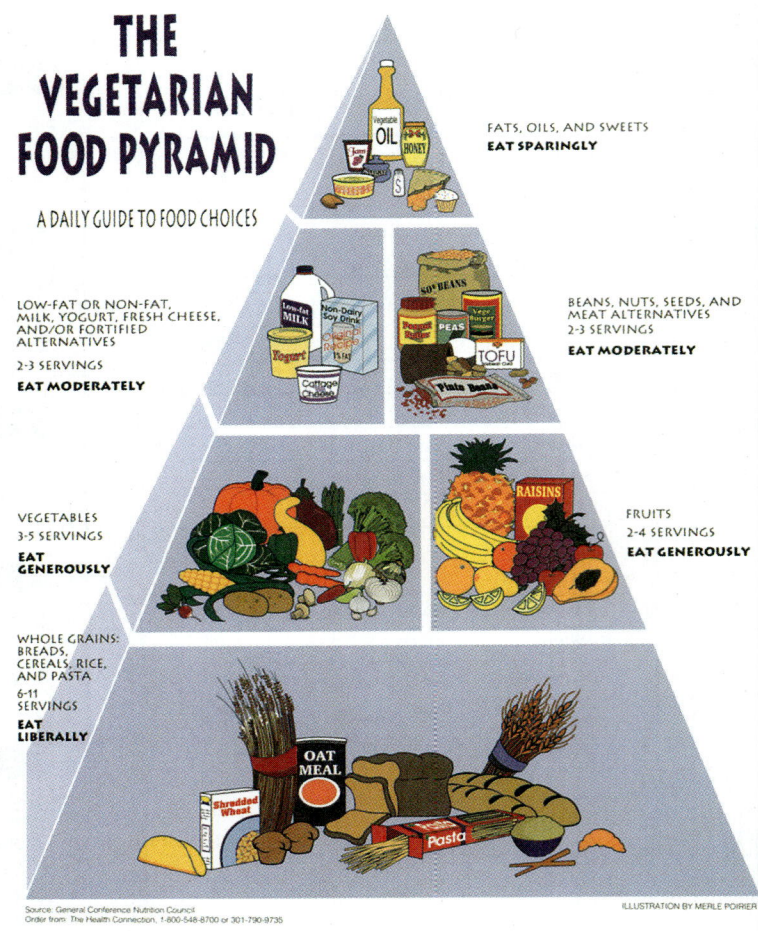

FOOD LABELING

Through the Department of Health and Human Services and the Food Safety and Inspection Service of the U. S. Department of Agriculture, the food industry is required to put a nutrition label on certain food products (Figure 18-4). The purpose of the label is "to help consumers choose more healthful diets and offer an incentive to food companies to improve the nutritional qualities of their products."

Food labels entitled "Nutrition Facts" must contain the following information:

Mandatory components
- Total calories
- Calories from fat
- Total fat
- Saturated fat
- Cholesterol
- Sodium
- Total carbohydrate
- Dietary fiber
- Sugars
- Protein
- Vitamin A
- Vitamin C
- Calcium
- Iron

Voluntary components
- Calories from saturated fat
- Polyunsaturated fat
- Monounsaturated fat
- Potassium
- Other carbohydrate
- Other essential vitamins and minerals
- Soluble fiber
- Insoluble fiber

The amount of grams or milligrams are listed to the right of each of the names of these nutrients, and the "% Daily Value" is also listed. This clarifies misinterpretations about foods with a high number. An example is a food with 140 mg of sodium, which represents less than 6% of the Daily Value for sodium, which is 2400 mg.

VEGETARIAN DIETS*

Some Americans adhere to vegetarian diets for reasons of culture, belief, or health. Most vegetarians eat milk products and eggs, and as a group, these **lacto-ovo-vegetarians** enjoy excellent health. Vegetarian diets are consistent with the *Dietary Guidelines for Americans* and can meet RDAs for nutrients. You can obtain enough protein from a vegetarian diet as long as the variety and amounts of foods consumed are adequate. Meat, fish, and poultry are major contributors of iron, zinc, and

Text continued on p. 813

*From "Dietary Guidelines for Americans," U. S. Department of Agriculture, U. S. Department of Health and Human Services.

FIGURE 18-5—cont'd B, Food groups with examples of foods and serving sizes. (Courtesy The Health Connection: [800] 548-8700.)

Limit foods high in fat, cholesterol, sugar, and salt.

Select relative portions to meet your caloric need.

Choose from a variety of whole grains, fruits, and vegetables.

Food Groups	One Serving Equals One Item	Nutrient Contributions		Sample Diet: Calories 1600	2200	2800	Food Choice Examples
Eat Liberally 6-11 Servings daily **Whole Grains and Legumes**	1 slice bread ½ cup hot cereal ¾ cup dry cereal ¼ cup granola ½ cup rice or pasta 1 tortilla 1 chapati ½ bagel or English Muffin 3-4 crackers ½ muffin ½ cup cooked beans	Complex CHO Fiber Protein Vitamin B_1 (Thiamine) Vitamin B_2 (Riboflavin) Vitamin B_6 and Niacin Iron Magnesium Calcium Trace minerals	Number of Servings	6	9	11	Grains: oats, brown rice, barley, millet, bulgar wheat, rye, corn, wheat, multi-grain, etc. Legumes: (see list below)
Eat Generously 3-5 Servings daily **Vegetables**	1 cup raw, leafy vegetable salad ½ cup cooked vegetables ½ cup chopped raw vegetables ¾ cup vegetable juice	Fiber Potassium Beta-Carotene Folate Vitamin C Calcium Magnesium	Number of Servings	3	4	5	Vegetables: broccoli, kale, cabbage, collards, spinach, pumpkin, carrots, winter squash, sweet potatoes, potatoes, parsnips, rutabagas, turnips, tomatoes, beets, eggplant, okra, summer squash, cauliflower
Eat Generously 2-4 Servings daily **Fruits**	1 medium, whole fruit ½ cup canned fruit ¼ cup dried fruit 1 cup berries ¾ cup fruit juice	Vitamin C Beta-Carotene Fiber Potassium Folate Magnesium	Number of Servings	2	3	4	Fruits: oranges, grapefruit, lemons, apricots, peaches, nectarines, plums, persimmons, apples, pears, kiwi, papaya, mango, pineapple, bananas, strawberries, raspberries, blueberries Dried Fruits: raisins, dates, pears, pineapple, prunes, peaches, figs
Eat Moderately 2-3 Servings daily **Legumes, Nuts, Seeds, Meat Alternatives**	½ cup cooked beans or peas 1/3 cup nuts (1 oz.) ½ cup tofu 2 Tbsp nut butter (1 oz.) ¼ cup seeds ¼ cup meat alternative 2 egg whites	Protein Zinc Iron Fiber Calcium Vitamin B_6 Vitamin E Niacin (B_3) Linoelic Acid	Number of Servings	2	2-3	3	Legumes: pinto, black, white, navy, soybeans, garbanzoes, lentils, blackeye, green pea, split pea, peanuts Nuts: almonds, walnuts, filberts, chestnuts, brazil, pecans, cashews Seed: pine nuts, sesame, sunflower, pumpkin Alternatives: tofu, meat alternatives
Eat Moderately 2-3 Servings daily **Dairy Products and/or Fortified Alternatives**	1 cup milk, nonfat or lowfat 1 cup soymilk (fortified) ¾ cup lowfat cottage cheese ½ cup soy cheese 1½ oz. fresh cheese 1 cup low-fat or non-fat yogurt	Calcium Protein Vitamins A and D Riboflavin (B_2) Vitamin B_{12}	Number of Servings	2	2-3	3	Dairy: milk, yogurt, cottage cheese, ricotta, other fresh cheeses Alternatives: soy or tofu milk, soy cheese

Eat Sparingly

Fats, Oils, Sugar, Salt

The small tip of the Pyramid shows fats, oils, salt, and sweets. These foods such as salad dressings and oils, cream, butter, margarine, sour cream, cream cheese, sugars, soft drinks, candies, and sweet desserts provide calories and are low in nutrients. Oils contain essential fatty acids. Most people should use these sparingly. For every tablespoon of fat added to a 2200 calorie diet, you increase the percentage of calories as fat by approximately five percent. Every tablespoon of sugar adds two percent calories as sugar.

- Use visible fats sparingly.
- Limit desserts to two or three per week.
- Use honey, jams, jelly, corn syrups, molasses, sugar sparingly
- Use soft drinks and candies very sparingly, if at all.
- Limit foods high in salt.

1 tsp salt (5 gm table salt) = 2000 mg sodium
1 T oil = 13.6 gm fat 120.0 calories
1 tsp oil = 4.5 gm fat 40.1 calories

1 T margarine	=	11.4 gm fat	102 calories
1 T mayonnaise	=	11.0 gm fat	99 calories
1 T sour cream	=	3.0 gm fat	30 calories
1 T cream cheese	=	5.0 gm fat	52 calories
1 T sugar	=	12 gm	48 calories
1 tsp sugar	=	4 gm	16 calories
1 T honey	=	21 gm	64 calories
1 tsp honey	=	7 gm	21calories

B

HEALTH **MATTERS**

KEEPING YOUR PATIENTS INFORMED

FOOD FACTS AND QUICK TIPS

- Read food labels to help you choose healthier foods—foods that are lower in fat, cholesterol, salt, and sugar.
- Food labels can help people avoid ingredients to which they are allergic.
- Hidden food allergies are often the cause of migraine headaches. Keep a food journal to see if certain foods are related to a headache on a consistent basis.
- When reading food labels, look for products that have 1 g or less of fat per ounce. In frozen meals, look for ones with less than 10 g of fat per serving.
- If you use margarine, look for brands that list "liquid" rather than "partially hydrogenated" oil as the first ingredient. Choose the liquid squeezeable, softer, or diet tub margarines. These are lower in transfatty acids.
- Look for the ingredient "whole wheat" on bread. Breads listed as "wheat bread" or with the ingredients "wheat flour," "enriched wheat flour," or "unbleached wheat flour" are made from *white flour* and *not* whole wheat.
- When buying juice, look for "100% juice" on the label. If the label contains the words "drink," "beverage," "ade," or "cocktail," you are getting something other than 100% juice. For example, Welch's Grape Juice Beverage or Dole Juice Cocktail. The four most nutritious juices are orange, grapefruit, prune, and pineapple.
- If you are susceptible to urinary tract infections, drink cranberry juice (also see Chapter 12, p. 554) (Cranberries and blueberries contain substances that prevent microbes from sticking to the wall of the urinary bladder, thus helping to prevent urinary tract infections.)
- Fruits and vegetables are low in fat and salt and high in vitamins, minerals, and fiber.
- Periodically try a vegetarian meal, using legumes such as beans, lentils, or peas. These foods are high in fiber, low in fat, and quite inexpensive.
- Vegetarians who *do not* eat dairy products can get their calcium from oranges, dried figs, legumes, collard or mustard greens, fortified tofu and soy milk, canned sardines with bones, and canned salmon with bones.
- Steam vegetables with herbs like rosemary and thyme for a great taste without any fat.
- Researchers estimate that plant-based diets with lots of fruits and vegetables combined with exercise and weight control could eventually reduce cancer incidence by 30% to 40%.
- If overweight, lose weight to reduce the risk of developing high blood pressure and heart disease.
- To determine if there is a lot of fat in a cracker, rub it with a paper napkin. If there is a grease mark on the napkin, there is a lot of oil (fat) in that cracker.
- To help determine if you are getting the right balance of nutrients in your diet, fill two-thirds of your meal plate with carbohydrate-rich foods, such as fruits, vegetables, grains, beans, pasta, and bread. Think of foods that grow. Think color—"*colorize your diet*"—have a great variety of yellow, red, bright dark green, purple, orange. Examples include carrots, tomatoes, broccoli, spinach and other greens, scallions and other members of the onion family, green beans, yellow squash, pineapple, papaya, watermelon, peaches, plums, blueberries, strawberries, and raspberries. The remaining one-third of your plate should have protein-rich foods such as lean, trimmed and skinned chicken and turkey, other lean meats, fish, peas and lentils, dried beans, and low-fat or fat-free dairy products.
- For yourself or a party, create a color wheel—a plate with various fresh fruits and vegetables of bright colors. This will look and taste great.
- Nutrition's **top 10 fruits and vegetables:** broccoli, cantaloupe, carrots, kale, mango, pumpkin, red bell pepper, spinach, strawberries, and sweet potato.
- To help you increase your fiber intake, start the day with a high-fiber cereal that provides at least 5 g per serving; eat at least five or more servings of fruits and vegetables each day; use whole-grain breads with 2 or 3 g of fiber per slice; and add beans to salads, soups, or casseroles and other dishes.
- Retain dietary fiber in foods by serving fruits and vegetables with edible skins and seeds and use whole grain flours. (Cooking can reduce *some* of the dietary fiber in a food.)
- Reduce or avoid the use of regular soft drinks. A 12-ounce can contains 9 teaspoons of sugar.
- Taste and eat food *without* adding additional salt. Reduce the amount of salt used when cooking. Try using other herbs and spices to season food.
- Research shows that calcium, vitamin D, potassium, and magnesium all contribute to strong bones by maintaining bone mineral density and therefore help to prevent osteoporosis.
- Calcium is the foundation of strong bones. If you are unable to get enough calcium from food, consider taking calcium supplements—preferably calcium carbonate or calcium citrate. Calcium citrate seems to absorb better in the elderly because they have less acid in their stomach.
- Bone density begins to decline when people reach their late 30s and early 40s. Bone loss accelerates *after* menopause in women.
- Physical activity during childhood promotes healthy bone development. Bone density is also established during adolescence and early adulthood. This is why adequate calcium intake is so important during these periods. Throughout life, weight-bearing exercises, such as walking, dancing, running, jumping rope, stair climbing, tennis, basketball, strength training, and aerobics, can help to increase bone mass and protect against bone loss.
- **Osteoporosis** is a disease in which excessive bone loss leaves the skeletal system abnormally vulnerable to fractures, especially in the forearms (near the wrists), hips, and spine. The bones affected become very brittle and porous and therefore

break easily. Loss of bone mass and/or fractures of the vertebrae produce characteristic changes in the curvature of the spine. Osteoporosis usually affects people between the ages of 50 and 70 years. As people age, as much as 6 to 9 inches in height can be lost, and a humpback can develop in the thoracic vertebral area. The ideal time to prevent osteoporosis is during the younger years, but it is never too late to begin a preventive program. Start with a calcium-rich diet and regular weight-bearing exercises. These are important defenses against accelerated bone loss and osteoporosis. Also, avoid smoking and excessive use of alcohol. Postmenopausal women should also discuss hormone replacement therapy (HRT) with their physician.

Risk factors for osteoporosis include the following:

- Small, petite female frame
- Thin body type
- Caucasian or Asian ancestry
- Family history of osteoporosis
- Sedentary lifestyle
- Excessive use of alcohol
- Smoking
- Diet high in protein or caffeine or sodium or sugar
- Low calcium intake
- Early menopause
- Certain medications (such as large doses of thyroid preparations or cortisone-like drugs used for asthma, arthritis, or cancer).
- Mature (older) adults who are less active generally need fewer calories, so it is very important that the calories they eat be nutrient rich and include portions from all of the food groups.

Good nutrition can help people prevent disability. Those who find it difficult to eat enough food to include all the recommended daily nutrients could take a basic multivitamin. Women should also discuss calcium supplements with their physician to reduce the risk of osteoporosis.

- Mature (older) adults can help preserve cognitive function by getting adequate amounts of vitamins B_6, B_{12}, and folic acid. These vitamins may also play a complex but very important role in preventing heart attacks. Good sources of these vitamins include fish, poultry, lean meats, whole grains, low-fat and/or nonfat dairy products, green leafy vegetables, and dried beans.
- Dietary supplements (vitamin, mineral, herbs, and amino acid tablets or solutions) are classified as food, not drugs; therefore they are not regulated by the Food and Drug Administration. They cannot claim to treat, cure, or prevent disease. They can only claim to improve health. If using supplements, you must know what you want to take and *why*.
- People who are pregnant or breastfeeding, chronically ill, elderly, under age 18, or taking prescription or over-the-counter drugs should check with their physician before starting a dietary supplement. Certain supplements can boost blood levels of certain drugs to dangerous levels. Some herbs could have strong or stronger side effects than prescription drugs.

Studies show that healthy habits not only add more years to your life, they add more life to your years. **Promotion of healthy living habits is an essential part of everyone's responsibilities.**

As Thomas Edison once said, "The doctor of the future will give no medicine, but will interest the patients in the care of the human frame, in diet, and in the cause and prevention of disease."

B vitamins in most American diets, and vegetarians should pay special attention to these nutrients.

Lactovegetarians include dairy products in their diet but no other animal products, such as eggs.

Vegans eat only food of plant origin. Because animal products are the only food sources of vitamin B_{12}, vegans must supplement their diets with a source of this vitamin. In addition, vegan diets, particularly those of children, require care to ensure adequacy of vitamin D and calcium, which most Americans obtain from milk products (Figure 18-5).

CULTURAL AND ETHNIC GUIDE TO GOOD EATING

Food preferences may vary within a culture or ethnic group. The socioeconomic situation of people also greatly influences their food selections and preparation. A healthy diet in any culture is one that provides the key nutrients essential for good health, incorporating current guidelines as presented in this chapter. *All foods in moderation* can fit into a healthy diet. It is a matter of balancing choices. Each food

group has key nutrients essential for body functions, growth, and repair.

See Table 18-16 and Table 18-17 for similarities and differences in food choices that are common in a few of the many cultures in the United States. These tables can be used as **teaching tools when explaining to patients** that they can still be eating their traditional foods while following the guidelines that promote health and prevent disease. These tables can also broaden your own awareness and choices as you learn of foods and customs from cultures other than your own. The emphasis for healthy eating habits remains the same, that is, eat a wide variety of foods, more low-fat and less high-fat foods, more fruits and vegetables, and much more (low-fat) foods from the whole grains, bread, cereals, rice, and pasta group.

Understand that food choices can be different and nutritionally sound.

THERAPEUTIC DIETS

Modification in the amount and type of food ingested may be needed for some medical conditions to aid in the treatment

Text continued on p. 816

TABLE 18–16   Cultural and Ethnic Guide to Good Eating

Culture	Cereal, Rice, Pasta, Bread Group	Fruit Group	Vegetable Group	Meat and Alternatives	Dairy Group* (Additional Sources of Calcium)
African American	Refined breads Hot yeast breads Cornbread Biscuits, pancakes Cream of wheat Oats, grits, rice Cornmeal, flour Corn flakes Macaroni, spaghetti	Oranges Melons Lemons Strawberries Grapes Bananas Peaches Fruit cocktail Pineapples Apples	Leafy greens Tomatoes Sweet potato Carrots Pumpkin Green pepper Collard Chard Turnip greens Cabbage Radishes String beans Beets, onions Green peas, corn	Pork organs Chitterlings Beef, lamb, tripe Chicken, turkey, duck, goose Fish, tuna, salmon Eggs, nuts, Cow peas, beans Peanut butter	Homogenized milk, buttermilk Ice cream Puddings Cheese
Hispanic	Rice, oats Corn meal Corn flakes Thin spaghetti Noodles, macaroni Sweet breads, Flour and corn Tortillas Biscuits Tamales Enchiladas	Pumpkins Peaches Guava fruit Oranges Lemons, limes Papaya Cactus fruit Zapote, apples Bananas Mangos	Spinach Wild greens Tomatoes Carrots, corn Green pepper Cactus leaves Potatoes Cabbage Summer squash Green peas Green beans Hominy, beets Celery, onions	Pork, beef Lamb, tripe Chicken Hot sausage Beef intestines Fish, bologna Frankfurters Eggs, nuts Dry beans Chick peas	Milk, cheese (Monterey Jack, parmesan, Mexican, and cottage cheeses) Flan Ice cream
American Indian	Refined bread Whole wheat Bread, biscuits Cornbread Pancakes Cream of wheat Oatmeal, rice Dry cereal Flour tortillas Hominy	Pumpkin Oranges Grapefruit Melon, lemon Strawberries Grapes, pears Bananas Fruit cocktail Peaches Apples Pineapple	Tomatoes, carrots Yellow squash Leafy greens Watercress Turnips, cabbage Mustard greens Green peas Green beans Beets, onions Cucumbers Potatoes Corn Eggplant Lettuce	Pork, beef Lamb, duck Turkey, goose Rabbit Fish, shell fish Eggs, legumes Blackeyed peas Sunflower seeds California walnuts Acorns Pine nuts Peanut butter	Fresh milk Goat milk Sheep milk Ice cream Cream pies
Vietnamese	Thin rice noodles Thick rice noodles Rice paper Rice cracker Rice	Mango Papaya Persimmon Pineapple	Ong choy Bamboo Pumpkin Taro	Green beans Black beans Black eye peas Mung beans	Tofu Small dried fish with bones

Source of Asian Foods: California Milk Advisory Board.

*Dairy foods are generally not part of the traditional diets of Asia (with the exception of India). The Asian diet is distinguished for its emphasis on a plant-based diet. When dairy foods are consumed on a daily basis, low-fat foods should be used. Products that could be used include milk, cheese, ice cream, tofu, calcium-fortified soy milk, yogurt, and condensed milk. Calcium-fortified juices can also be used for a good source of calcium otherwise supplied by dairy products.

TABLE 18–16 **Cultural and Ethnic Guide to Good Eating—cont'd**

Culture	Cereal, Rice, Pasta, Bread Group	Fruit Group	Vegetable Group	Meat and Alternatives	Dairy Group* (Additional Sources of Calcium)
Filipino (Tagalog)	Spaghetti	Mango	Bitter melon	Pork or beef	Sardines
	Toasted bread (bitkotso)	Strawberries	Chayote	Crab	Small dried fish with bones
	Wheat noodle (misuwa)	Papaya	Long beans	Dried fish	Seaweed
	Rice	Guava	Spinach	Peanuts (mani binusa)	
Korean	Rice cake	Grapes	Spinach	Pork or beef	Tofu
	Ramen	Strawberries	Chrysanthemum	Pureed soy	Small dried fish with bones
	Porridge	Pear	Squash	Bean	Seaweed
	Barley	Persimmon	Bean sprouts	Fish cake	Soup bones
	Rice			Crab	
Japanese	Ramen	Tangerines	Spinach	Fish cake	Tofu
	Steamed buns	Peach	Broccoli	Octopus	Small dried fish with bones
	Buckwheat noodles	Grapes	Sweet potato	Squid	Seaweed
	Soba	Melons	Snow peas	Pork or beef	Leafy green vegetables
	Rice			Most fish and seafood	
Chinese	Rice noodles	Mango	Bitter melon	Crab	Tobu
	Bun (bow)	Orange	Bean sprouts	Duck	Small dried fish with bones
	Porridge	Cantaloupe	Taro	Peanuts	Leafy green vegetables
	Oatmeal	Grapes	Chinese broccoli	Almonds	
	Rice				

TABLE 18–17 **Do's and Don'ts of Ethnic Foods: What to Serve—What to Avoid**

Culture	Serve Low-Fat Foods	Avoid High-Fat Foods
Hispanic	Ceviche (marinated seafood)	Fried tortilla chips/nachos
	Gazpacho (cold tomato soup)	Refried beans (made with lard)
	Soft flour tortillas (no lard)	Chorizo (sausage)
	Black bean soup	Beef, cheese, chimichanga
	Yellow or plain rice	Fried, stuffed dough; taco (fried shell); tostado
	Chili with beans (no meat)	Sour cream/guacamole (avocado dip)
	Bean, chicken, or seafood fajitas, enchiladas, or burritos	Flan (custard)
	Salsa (spicy, red sauce)	Sopapillas (fried pastry)
	Red beans with rice	
	Arroz con pollo (rice with chicken)	
	Taco salad (no fried shell)	
American Indian	Dried peas and beans	Fried bread
	Corn	Fried mutton
	Mutton (roasting, boiling, baking, underground steaming, trim off fat)	Fried potatoes
	Turkey	Potato chips
	Wild vegetables (celery, onion, spinach, potatoes)	Lard
	Green beans, corn, tomatoes	High fat lunch meats, sausage, bacon
	Apples, oranges, peaches, fruit cocktail	
	Cornmeal mush	
	Watermelons, wild sumac berries	
	Kneel down bread	
	Hominy	

Data from: The State CASBO Child Nutrition Research and Development Committee, Sacramento, Calif.

Continued

TABLE 18–17   **Do's and Dont's of Ethnic Foods: What to Serve—What to Avoid—cont'd**

Culture	Serve Low-Fat Foods	Avoid High-Fat Foods
Asian-Pacific Islander	Stir fried vegetables	Tempura battered vegetables
	Steamed rice	Fried rice
	Stir fried meats, fish, poultry	Eggrolls
	Tofu	Deep fried meats
	Cabbage, tomatoes, mustard greens in salads, squash, broccoli	Peking duck
	Fresh fruits	
African-American	Chicken, baked or broiled	Fried chicken
	Steamed or stir fried greens	Pork, hot dogs, lunch meats
	Broiled catfish	Boiled greens with pork fat
	Black-eyed peas with turkey ham	Fried catfish
	Legumes (kidney beans, pinto beans, red beans)	Black-eyed peas with ham hocks
	Corn, okra, rice, sweet potatoes	Fried pork rinds
	Pasta	Fruit pies
	Fresh fruits and vegetables	
	Chitlins (chitterlings)	

process. The following are examples of special diets that may be used.

Clear Liquid Diet

A clear liquid diet may be required before the patient has certain laboratory tests or other examinations. It may also be recommended after episodes of diarrhea or vomiting. It generally provides little nutritional value but does provide needed fluids and relieves thirst.

Foods recommended
- Clear soups such as broth or bouillon
- Clear coffee, tea, or carbonated beverages, such as ginger ale, 7-Up, and Sprite (as allowed and tolerated)
- Clear fruit juices (without pulp), such as apple, cranberry, or white grape juice
- Plain, flavored gelatin and popsicles
- Hard, clear candies

Full Liquid Diet

A full liquid diet may be used for a patient who cannot tolerate or chew solid foods, for someone who has acute gastritis and infections, or for patients before and after surgery.

Foods recommended
- All liquids allowed on the clear liquid diet
- Milk, milkshakes
- Strained fruit and vegetable juices
- Creamed soups, strained soups
- Ice creams, custards, puddings

Mechanical Soft Diet/Dental Soft Diet

A mechanical or dental soft diet may be required for patients who have difficulty chewing because of sore gums or lack of teeth and for those who have difficulty in swallowing.

Foods recommended
- Chopped or ground meats and vegetables
- Soups
- All liquids
- Casseroles
- Canned fruits
- Well-cooked vegetables
- Tender meats such as baked chicken or turkey

High-Fiber Diet

A high-fiber diet may be beneficial for a patient who has constipation, diverticulosis, diabetes, or irritable bowel syndrome and for everyone as protection against these conditions. In addition, it may aid in the prevention of cardiovascular disease and breast and colon cancer (also see the previous section on fiber, pp. 802-805). Processing and cooking foods reduce the fiber content in foods.

Foods recommended
- All foods with increased emphasis on fiber-rich foods, which include vegetables and fruits, especially raw fruits and vegetables, legumes, whole-grain breads, and cereals (see Tables 18-12 and 18-13).

Low-Residue or Low-Fiber Diet

A low-residue diet, also called a low-fiber diet, is recommended for patients with indigestion, diarrhea, colitis, and ileitis, as well as for patients who have had a colostomy and for those having radiation therapy.

Foods Recommended
- Eggs
- Lean beef, chicken, turkey, veal, lamb
- Refined flour, breads and rolls, rice, noodles, spaghetti
- Cooked cereals

- Cooked vegetables
- Fruit juices
- Canned or stewed fruits; bananas are allowed
- Soups BUT NO creamed soups or any milk products
- Desserts *without* milk, milk products, nuts, or seeds

These foods must **NOT** be fried or cooked with milk or milk products and must **NOT** be highly seasoned.

Low-Fat Diet

A low-fat diet is generally recommended for a patient who has liver, gallbladder, or pancreatic disease. It is also highly recommended for everyone to reduce the risk of cardiovascular disease and cancer of the colon, prostate, and breast, as well as obesity. Adult patients for whom a low-fat diet is prescribed are allowed between 30 to 50 g of fat per day. Amounts vary for children.

Foods recommended (Figure 18-6)

- Up to 5 oz of meat per day—baked, broiled, roasted, or steamed. It must *not* be fried or served with gravy. All visible fat must be removed before cooking.
- Fruits
- Vegetables—but no fried vegetables
- Skim milk, low-fat or nonfat yogurt, and low-fat cheeses
- Ice milk—chocolate, strawberry, vanilla
- Whole grain breads (nonfat)
- Cold cereals, cooked cereals, soda crackers
- Unbuttered popcorn
- Plain angel food cake, vanilla wafers, ladyfingers, graham crackers, arrowroot cookies
- Pudding made with skim milk, as well as rice pudding and tapioca
- Fruit whips made with gelatin or egg whites
- Fats (strictly limited)—measured amounts of margarine, salad dressings, vegetable oils. Generally only 3 servings per day of either 1 teaspoon or 1 tablespoon depending on the fat.

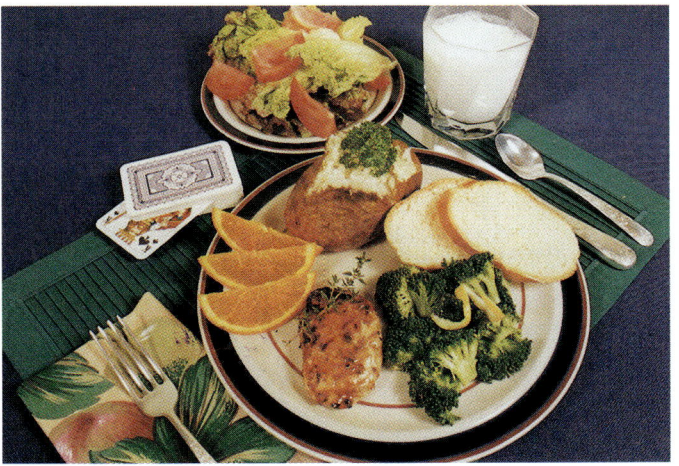

FIGURE 18-6   Low-fat dinner. (From Wardlaw GM: *Perspectives in nutrition,* ed 2, St Louis, 1993, Mosby.)

Sodium Restricted/Low Sodium/Salt-Free/No Added Salt/Low-Salt Diets

A diet with varied amounts of sodium or salt is used for patients with high blood pressure, congestive heart failure (CHF), fluid retention, renal disease, and cirrhosis.

The amount of sodium should be specified. Sodium is found in most foods naturally, so a salt-free or no-salt diet is technically impossible (see Table 18-14).

Mild restriction.   4000 to 5000 mg of sodium per day (174 to 217 mEq)

- Limited use of foods high in sodium
- 1/2 teaspoon of table salt is allowed each day

Moderate restriction.   2000 mg of sodium per day (87 mEq)

- Omit foods with a high sodium content
- 1/2 teaspoon of table salt is allowed each day or the equivalent in prepared foods
  1000 mg of sodium per day (45 mEq)
- Omit canned or processed foods containing salt
- No salt is allowed in preparation of food or at the table

Strict restriction.   500 mg of sodium per day (22 mEq)

- Omit canned or processed foods containing salt
- No salt is allowed in preparation of food or at the table
- Low-sodium bread must be used rather than regular bread
- Omit vegetables containing high amounts of natural sodium, such as sauerkraut, pickles, celery, frozen corn, frozen mixed vegetables, frozen vegetables in sauce, frozen peas, frozen lima beans

Severe restriction.   250 mg of sodium per day

- THIS DIET IS NOT RECOMMENDED, BUT IT COULD BE USED FOR SHORT TERM OR TESTS ONLY.
- The same restrictions as outlined for the 500 mg/day are to be followed. In addition, limit protein foods and use low-sodium milk in place of regular milk.

When a patient is placed on a sodium-restricted diet, instructions must be given to read *all* the labels on a food for the sodium content even if the product states "low sodium." This could mean that it is low sodium, only in comparison with the regular product from that manufacturer and still contains more sodium than the patient should have. (Low sodium is 140 mg or less per serving.)

Food recommended for a 1000-mg (1-g) sodium diet

- Plain, unprocessed foods, including fresh fruits and vegetables or those processed without added sodium
- Whole or skim milk

- Unsalted cheddar cheese and cottage cheese
- Unsalted breads, crackers, cooked cereals, dry cereals, rice, noodles
- Unsalted popcorn
- Flour (but not if self-rising flour)
- Unsalted nuts
- Unsalted margarine, oils, and butter
- Fresh or frozen meats
- Fresh fish (no shellfish or canned fish)

Reduced-Calorie Diet

A reduced-calorie diet is used for patients needing to lose weight or to aid in maintaining a desirable weight.

Foods recommended. In general, all of the basic five food groups should be included with smaller servings. Low-fat foods are often encouraged.

Peptic Ulcer (Gastric and Duodenal) Diet

The pain experienced with a gastric ulcer is increased with eating. The pain experienced with a duodenal ulcer is often relieved by eating. Diets used for patients with ulcers have changed significantly in the past decade. The bland, low-fat, low-fiber diets with frequent small feedings of milk or cream had no scientific basis and thus have been *discontinued.* Also, it is now known that milk protein stimulates acid secretion, thereby interfering with ulcer healing and related pain. Currently an ulcer diet restricts only those foods that have been shown to interfere with the healing process.

Recommendations

- Eat small-to-moderate servings at mealtime to avoid gastric distention.
- Avoid caffeine-containing foods (coffee, tea, colas, chocolate), decaffeinated coffee, all alcohol, and black or red pepper. These foods are known to increase gastric acid secretion.
- Some individuals must avoid gas-producing foods because they have a tendency to cause distress. Examples include

carbonated beverages, onions, brussel sprouts, cauliflower, and cabbage.

BRAT

The acronym *BRAT* stands for a special diet comprising *bananas, rice, applesauce,* and *toast.* It is often prescribed for patients recuperating from gastrointestinal problems with symptoms of nausea, vomiting, and diarrhea.

Diabetic Diet

A diabetic diet is ordered as part of the treatment program for a patient who has diabetes mellitus. Many factors, including the patient's activity level and insulin dosage or other diabetic medication have to be considered. The physician works with a dietitian and provides the patient with a diet to include a set amount of grams of protein, fat, and carbohydrates. Food exchange lists are provided for patients so that they can select various foods and the correct amount from the basic five food groups.

For years, diabetics were not allowed to have sugary foods such as cake, cookies, salad dressings containing sugar, and so on. Newer guidelines state that diabetics can have limited amounts of sugar, honey, and other sweeteners (simple carbohydrates) occasionally. When eating these foods, diabetics must substitute them for other carbohydrates, such as breads and cereals (complex carbohydrates), that they would normally eat. What was learned was that the **critical factor affecting blood sugar** was the *total* amount of carbohydrate in the diet rather than its source. This means that a cookie and a slice of bread, which both contain 15 g of carbohydrate, have the same effect on blood glucose levels. However, high sugar foods are often high in fat and often lack other needed nutrients. What must be considered is that when total calories and nutrients are determined, sugar can be eaten in *modest amounts as part of a balanced meal.* Diabetics must be taught by a physician, a registered dietitian, or a certified diabetic educator how to calculate the nutritional makeup of their meals and how to substitute sugar for other carbohydrates.

Also see Insulin Injections in Chapter 7, p. 402, and Diabetes Emergencies—Hypoglycemia and Hyperglycemia in Chapter 17, p. 770.

TABLE 18-18 The DASH Diet

The "combination diet" is rich in fruits, vegetables, and low-fat dairy food and low in saturated and total fat. It also is low in cholesterol; high in dietary fiber, potassium, calcium, and magnesium; and moderately high in protein.

The DASH eating plan shown below is based on 2000 calories a day. Depending on caloric needs, the number of daily servings in a food group may vary from those listed.

Food Group	Daily Servings	Serving Sizes	Examples and Notes	Significance of Each Food Group to the DASH Diet Pattern
Grains and grain products	7-8	1 slice bread ½ cup dry cereal ½ cooked rice, pasta, or cereal	Whole wheat bread, English muffin, pita bread, bagel, cereals, grits, oatmeal	Major sources of energy and fiber

To learn more about high blood pressure, call 1-800-575-WELL or visit the NHLBI website at http://www.nhlbi.nih.gov/nhlbi/nhlbi.htm. DASH is also online at http://dash.bwh.harvard.edu.

TABLE 18-18 **The DASH Diet—cont'd**

Food Group	Daily Servings	Serving Sizes	Examples and Notes	Significance of Each Food Group to the DASH Diet Pattern
Vegetables	4-5	1 cup raw leafy vegetable ½ cup cooked vegetable 6 oz vegetable juice	Tomatoes, potatoes, carrots, peas, squash, broccoli, turnip greens, collards, kale, spinach, artichokes, beans, sweet potatoes	Rich sources of potassium, magnesium, and fiber
Fruits	4-5	6 oz fruit juice 1 medium fruit ¼ cup dried fruit ¼ cup fresh, frozen, or canned fruit	Apricots, bananas, dates, grapes, oranges, orange juice, grapefruit, grapefruit juice, mangoes, melons, peaches, pineapples, prunes, raisins, strawberries, tangerines	Important sources of potassium, magnesium, and fiber
Low-fat or nonfat dairy foods	2-3	8 oz milk 1 cup yogurt 1.5 oz cheese	Skim or 1% milk, skim or low-fat buttermilk, nonfat or low-fat yogurt, part-skim mozzarella cheese, nonfat cheese	Major sources of calcium and protein
Meats, poultry, and fish	2 or less	3 oz cooked meats, poultry, or fish	Select only lean; trim away visible fats; broil, roast, or boil, instead of frying; remove skin from poultry	Rich sources of protein and magnesium
Nuts, seeds, and legumes	4-5 per week	1.5 oz or ⅓ cup nuts ½ oz or 2 Tbsp seeds ½ cup cooked legumes	Almonds, filberts, mixed nuts, peanuts, walnuts, sunflower seeds, kidney beans, lentils	Rich sources of energy, magnesium, potassium, protein, and fiber

HEALTH MATTERS

KEEPING YOUR PATIENTS INFORMED

TIPS ON EATING THE DASH WAY
- Start small. Make gradual changes in your eating habits.
- Center your meal around carbohydrates, such as pasta, rice, beans, or vegetables.
- Treat meat as one part of the whole meal, instead of the focus.

- Use fruits or low-fat, low-calorie foods, such as sugar-free gelatin, for desserts and snacks.

REMEMBER: If you use the DASH diet to help prevent or control high blood pressure, make it part of a lifestyle that includes choosing foods lower in salt and sodium, keeping a healthy weight, being physically active, and if you drink alcohol, doing so in moderation.

Source: National Institute of Health

The DASH Diet

This eating plan is from the "Dietary Approaches to Stop Hypertension" (DASH) clinical study funded by units of the National Institutes of Health. The final results of the DASH "combination diet" showed that it lowered blood pressure and so may help prevent and control high blood pressure (Table 18-18). (See also Prevention, Detection, and Evaluation of High Blood Pressure in Chapter 3.)

PATIENT TEACHING

The physician, dietitian, or the medical assistant must work with the patient and possibly the family to individualize any diet recommended for therapy. Nutritional assessments should be done to find out what the patient usually eats and likes and then to see how small changes can be made to fit his or her needs. The patient needs to know how to select the right foods, incorporating as many family and cultural favorites as possible. The patient may need instruction in reading a food label so that informed decisions can be made regarding food choices. Standard diet forms are not generally used anymore because they often confused the patient with too much information, and thus the patient did not pay attention to any of the recommendations.

Always provide patient education verbally and have available educationally appropriate and culturally sensitive printed materials to give to patients. Printed materials may also be left in the waiting room for the patient to read and take home.

CONCLUSION

You have now completed the chapter on nutrition. Given your knowledge of dietary guidelines and therapeutic diets, you should be able to identify an appropriate food plan for patients requiring a standard diet and for patients requiring any one of the special therapeutic diets.

Use this information to make informed decisions for yourself when selecting the foods you eat. Science has proven that dietary habits have a direct connection to major diseases, such as cardiovascular disease and cancer. Become more familiar with the varied choices of food that can provide the essential nutrients needed to promote health and prevent illness. Evaluate your own eating habits and start to make any needed changes slowly so that in time you will be eating healthier and tasty foods and experiencing the long-term benefits of doing so. Encourage your family and friends to do the same. **Habits do affect health, and health does affect habits and lifestyles.** *Remember* "Health is your biggest asset."

> **"If we could give every individual the right amount of nourishment and exercise, not too little and not too much, we would have found the safest way to health."**
> **HIPPOCRATES, 431 BC**

REVIEW OF VOCABULARY

Rather than a review of the vocabulary for this chapter, a psychiatric case history on *bulimia nervosa* is presented. Bulimia is one of the very serious and potentially dangerous eating disorders. Research shows that 4 of 100 and possibly more young female college students in the United States are bulimic. Bulimia also affects males but in much smaller numbers. However, with the media's increased focus on the "lean look," incidences of bulimia are increasing in both sexes.

Bulimics consume large amounts of food rapidly (as much as *10,000 calories* at a time), and then, so that they will not gain weight, they purge through self-induced vomiting, use of laxatives and diuretics, fasting, vigorous exercise, strict dieting, or any combination of these behaviors. This addictive binge-purge behavior is usually done in secret and occurs once or twice a week up to many times in 1 day. Without stopping this behavior and getting treatment, bulimia can be *fatal* due to cardiac arrest or kidney failure.

Case Example of a Patient With Bulimia

Patient self-presented at an outpatient facility within the community mental health system.

Patient was a 22-year-old Caucasian woman, by the name of P. P presented well dressed and was soft spoken; she was of small stature and slight build. Her affect was appropriate, her thought processes linear, and thought content rational. She exhibited no signs of psychosis and reported no substance use besides an occasional alcoholic drink, about every 2 weeks.

Presenting Complaint: P's presenting complaint was that she had been bingeing and throwing up for about a year. P described the following behaviors: She would fast for periods of time and then overeat, eating to a point beyond fullness. She would then purge by throwing up. The binge-purge behavior occurred anywhere from 4 to 5 times a week. P reported that she had been wanting to stop this behavior but had been unable to do so on her own.

P had never been in therapy before and upon questioning reported no past or current medical problems. Because of the physical nature of her illness, a thorough physical examination was recommended by the clinician. P did not exhibit any outward physical signs of bulimia. There were no scars on her fingers, nor did she have dental problems. The physical she underwent revealed no health problems.

Family History: P had two older sisters, one of which was still living at home with the parents. P reported that she felt very close to her family and that nothing had really bothered her while growing up. She reported a "happy childhood." P excelled in school, always having a high GPA, and at the time she was seen, was currently enrolled in school. She also worked part-time, doing clerical work.

P had recently moved to California from her home state, to fulfill her profession's training and school requirements. P was in close contact with her parents, who were living in another state. She would call them three to four times a week, or her mother would call her. P reported that she had very few friends and that she desperately wanted to have a pet, to "love me unconditionally."

Therapy Focus: As the theme of unconditional love and P's craving for it were further explored, P started talking about the pressures she had always felt to achieve and to work hard, which had always been most important to her mother. P reported that her mother had never told her that she loved her but always encouraged her to work hard and "tough it out." Initially P declared that that was fine with her. As the work continued, P started talking more about her need for unconditional love.

Tying old experiences to her present behavior, P explored some of her feelings around her bulimic behavior. She was asked to keep a journal of her behaviors, thoughts, feelings, and events preceding her behavior and after the behavior. This exercise made P more aware of her emotions and patterns tied to her bulimic behavior. P noticed that she would overeat when she wanted to reward

Case Example of a Patient With Bulimia—cont'd

herself or at times when she was angry. After eating a lot of food she would feel guilty because she was afraid she would gain weight, so she would throw up. P described the purging behavior as a "high." It fulfilled the function of ridding herself of unwanted food, and it had turned into a self-reinforcing behavior in itself.

P had never learned how to self-soothe, to feel good about herself without achieving something that would draw praise from her mother. The eating disorder was an attempt on her part to both soothe herself and reward herself. It also stood for a lot of anger that she held toward her mother and provided a way for her to "stuff her feelings." She needed to learn about healthier ways to cope and to express her feelings. By identifying the pattern of her disorder and exploring its purpose in therapy, P was gradually able to change some of her eating disordered behaviors.

One of the aims of therapy was for P to engage in other behaviors (besides eating and throwing up) that made her feel good. Initially this was difficult because P was very out of touch with her own needs and feelings. She had spent most of her life trying to please her mother. P was scared of her own needs and discovered that she had unconsciously held the belief that the expression of her own needs would ultimately lead to the wrath and then loss of her mother. The task of identifying needs and feelings for herself was an important task in P's development.

As P became more clear about her own experiences and needs, she was able to incorporate other coping behaviors, instead of unconsciously trying to soothe herself by overeating. P took part in an assertiveness class and made a few friends who she would talk to at times, instead of reaching for food. By the end of therapy, which had to be terminated because of the session limit imposed by the institution, P was bingeing a lot less and would only occasionally engage in purging behaviors. She was interested in further therapy and thus was given three referrals of therapists who have experience in the area of eating disorders. P followed up on the referrals and chose one of the therapists to work with.

Diagnosis on Axis 1: 307.51 Bulimia Nervosa, Purging Type.

CRITICAL THINKING SKILLS REVIEW

1. Using the dietary guidelines and the Food Guide Pyramid, write a sample menu/food plan for the next 3 days.
2. List the five main nutrients (excluding water) and give three food examples for each.
3. Explain the difference between HDL and LDL.
4. List the fat-soluble vitamins and the water-soluble vitamins, stating foods that are a good source of these vitamins.
5. Explain the difference between a full liquid diet and a clear liquid diet.
6. List five benefits of increasing the fiber in your diet.
7. Explain why water is so important to the body.

For food and nutrition information and a referral to a registered dietitian in your area, call the Consumer Nutrition Hot Line at (800) 366-1655. For customized answers to your nutrition questions, call (900) CALL-AN-RD ([900] 225-5267). Visit ADA on World Wide Web at http://www.eatright.org

INTERNET RESOURCES

The American Anorexia/Bulimia Association, Inc.
www.aabainc.org

FDA Center for Food Safety and Nutrition
http://vm/cfsan.fda/gov

Fast Food Facts
www.olen.com/food

National Dietetic Association
www.eatright.org

Fitness Resources
http://rampages.onramp.net/~chaz

Screening for Postmenopausal Osteoporosis
http://cait.cpmc.columbia.edu/texts/gcps/gcps0056.html

Diet & Nutrition Resource Center
www.mayo.ivi.com/mayo/common/htm/dietpage.htm

Weight Watchers Interactive
www.wwgroup.com

Doctors Guide to Osteoporosis
www.pslgroup.com/OSTEOPOROSIS.HTM

Optimum Calcium Intake
www.nih.gov/niams/news/calsum/htm

American Dietetic Association
www.eatright.org

North American Association for the Study of Obesity
www.naaso.org

abdominal pulse Abdominal aorta pulse.

abdominal respirations The inspiration and expiration of air by the lungs accomplished primarily by the abdominal muscles and diaphragm.

accelerated respirations More than 25 respirations per minute, after 15 years of age.

acetonuria (as″e-to-nu′re-ah) or **ketonuria** (ke″to-nu′re-ah) The presence of acetone or ketone in the urine.

acrotism (ak′ro-tizm) Apparent absence of pulse.

addiction (ah-dik′shun) An acquired physiologic and/or psychologic dependence on a drug with tendencies to increase its use.

agglutination (ah-gloo″tin-na′shun) A clumping together of cells, as of blood cells or bacteria. An example is when red blood cells (RBCs) clump together as a result of an incompatible blood transfusion.

agranulocyte (a-gran′u-lo-sit″) A white blood cell (WBC) with a clear or nongranular cytoplasm. There are two types, monocytes and lymphocytes.

albuminuria (al-bu″mi-nu′re-ah) The presence of serum albumin in urine.

allergen (al′er-jen) Any substance that induces hypersensitivity.

allergy (al′er-je) An unusual and increased sensitivity (hypersensitivity) to specific substances that are ordinarily harmless.

alternating pulse Alternating weak and strong pulsations.

AMA American Medical Association.

amplify (am′pli-fi) To enlarge, to extend.

Anaerobic Culturette culture collection system This system offers the same basic properties of the Culturette, plus a standardized and dependable anaerobic environment for transport of anaerobic bacteria. The transport medium once released maintains an anaerobic environment for up to 48 hours. Many laboratories request that the anaerobic culture system be used when taking a wound culture. (*See also* Culturette.)

anaphylactic (an″ah-fi-lak′tik) **shock** An intense state of shock brought on by hypersensitivity to a drug, foreign toxin, or protein. Early symptoms resemble an allergic reaction, then increase in severity rapidly to dyspnea, cyanosis, and shock. This can be fatal if emergency measures are not taken immediately (see also Chapter 17, Allergic Reactions to Drugs).

anaphylaxis (an′ah-fi-lak′sis) An unusual or hypersensitive reaction of the body to foreign protein and other substances; often caused by drugs, foreign serum (for example, tetanus), and insect stings and bites.

anemia (ah-ne′me-ah) There is a variety of forms of anemia, but broadly speaking, it is a lack of red blood cells in the circulating blood or a reduction of hemoglobin, or both. Anemia is thought of as a symptom of a disease or disorder; it is not a disease.

anesthesia (an″es-the′ze-ah) The loss of sensation or feeling.

anisocytosis (an-i″-so-si-to′sis) A state of abnormal variations in the size of red blood cells in the blood.

anoscope (an′no-skop) A speculum or endoscope inserted into the anal canal for direct visual examination.

antidote (an′ti-dot) An agent used to counteract a poison.

antiseptic (an′ti-sep′tik) A substance capable of inhibiting the growth or action of microorganisms, without necessarily killing them; generally safe for use on body tissues.

anuria (ah-nu′re-ah) The absence of urine.

apnea (ap-ne′ah) Cessation or absence of breathing.

applicator A slender rod of glass or wood with a pledget of cotton on one end used to apply medicine or to take a culture from the body.

arrhythmia (ah-rith′me-ah) A variation from the normal or an irregular rhythm of the heartbeat.

arthritis (ar-thri′tis) Inflammation of a joint.

artificial respiration Artificial methods to restore respiration in cases of suspended breathing.

asepsis (a-sep′sis) The absence of all microorganisms causing disease; absence of contaminated matter.

aspiration/needle biopsy Removal of material from an internal organ by means of a hollow needle inserted through the body wall and into the affected tissue.

atopy (at″o-pe) A hypersensitive state that is subject to hereditary influences, such as hay fever, asthma, and eczema.

atrium (a′tre-um) One of the upper chambers of the heart. The right atrium receives deoxygenated blood from the body, whereas the left atrium receives oxygenated blood from the lungs. (The plural is **atria**.)

auricle (aw′ri-kl) The outer projection of the ear; also known as the pinna (pin′nah).

bactericide (bak-ter′i-sid) A substance capable of destroying bacteria but not spores.

bacteriology (bak-te″re-ol′o-je) The study of bacteria.

bacteriolysis (bak-te″re-ol′i-sis) The destruction of bacteria.

bacteriostatic (bak-te″re-o-stat′ik) A substance that inhibits the growth of bacteria.

bacteriuria (bak-te″re-u′re-ah) The presence of bacteria in urine.

band-form granulocyte A granular WBC in a stage of development.

benign (be-nin) **hypertension** Hypertension of slow onset that is usually without symptoms.

bigeminal (bi-jem′in-al) **pulse** Two regular beats followed by a longer pause. It has the same significance as an irregular pulse.

bimanual (bi-man′u-al) With both hands, as bimanual palpation.

biochemistry (bi″o-kem′s-tre) The study of chemical changes occurring in living organisms.

biologic death The condition that results when the brain has been deprived of oxygenated blood for a period of 6 minutes or more and irreversible damage has probably occurred.

biopsy (bi′op-se) Removal of tissue from the body for examination.

biopsy forceps Two-pronged instruments of varying sizes and shapes used to remove tissue from the body for examination.

Biot respiration   Irregularly alternating periods of apnea and hyperpnea; occurs in meningitis and disorders of the brain.

blood culture   Used in the diagnosis of specific infectious diseases. Blood is withdrawn from a vein and placed in or on suitable culture media; then it is determined whether or not pathogens grow in the media. If organisms do grow, they are identified by bacteriologic methods.

blood dyscrasia (dis-kra′ze-ah)   An abnormal or diseased condition of the blood.

BNDD   Bureau of Narcotics and Dangerous Drugs (a federal government agency of the DEA).

bowel movement   The elimination/excretion of fecal material from the intestinal tract.

bradycardia (brad-i-kar′di-a)   Slow heart action; extremely slow pulse, generally below 60 beats per minute.

bronchoscope (brong′ko-skop)   An endoscope designed specifically for passage through the trachea to allow visual examination of the interior of the tracheobronchial tree.

bronchoscopy (bron-kos′ko-pi)   Internal inspection of the tracheobronchial tree with the use of a bronchoscope; used for diagnostic or treatment purposes. For diagnosis, the physician will inspect the interior of the bronchi and may obtain a sample of secretions or a biopsy of tissue; for treatment, foreign bodies or mucous plugs that may be causing an obstruction to the air passages can be located and removed.

bursitis (bur-si′tis)   Inflammation of a bursa. The most commonly affected is the bursa of the shoulder.

canthus (kan′thus)   The inner canthus is the angle of the eyelids near the nose; the outer canthus is the angle of the eyelids at the outside corner of the eyes.

cardiac (kar′de-ak) **arrest**   Sudden and often unexpected cessation of the heartbeat. Permanent damage of vital organs and death are probable if treatment is not given immediately.

cassette (kah-set′)   A lightproof aluminum or Bakelite container with front and back intensifying screens, between which x-ray film is placed when used for x-ray examinations.

cautery (kaw′ter-e)   A hot instrument used to cut or destroy tissue, causing hemostasis at the time.

cerumen (se-roo-men)   Ear wax secreted by the glands of the external auditory meatus.

chemotherapy (ke″mo-ther′ah-pe)   The use of drugs (chemicals) to treat disease; a type of therapy used for cancer patients in which powerful drugs are used to interfere with the reproduction of the fast-multiplying cancer cells.

Cheyne-Stokes (chan-stoks) **respirations**   Respirations gradually increasing in rapidity and volume, until they reach a climax, then gradually subsiding and ceasing entirely for from 5 to 50 seconds, when they begin again. These are often a sign of impending death. Cheyne-Stokes respirations may be observed in normal persons (especially the aged) during sleep or during visits to higher altitudes.

clinical death   The state that results when breathing and circulation have stopped.

colicky   Acute intermittent abdominal pain usually caused by spasmodic contractions.

concussion (kon-kush′un)   The injury that results from a violent blow or shock.

concussion of the brain   A violent disturbance of the brain caused by a blow or fall.

conduction (kon-duk′shun)   The passage or conveyance of energy, as of electricity, heat, or sound.

conjunctiva (kon″junk-ti′vah)   The delicate membrane lining the eyelids and reflected onto the front of the eyeball.

constant fever   High fever with a variation not exceeding 1 or 2 degrees F (0.06° or 1.2° C) between morning and evening temperatures.

constipation (kon-sti-pa′shun)   A condition in which the waste material in the intestine is too hard to pass easily or in which bowel movements are so infrequent that discomfort results.

contact dermatitis   Dermatitis caused by an allergic reaction resulting from contact of the skin with various substances, such as poison ivy, or chemical, physical, and mechanical agents.

contaminated, contamination (kon-tam″i-na′shun)   The act of making unclean, soiling, or staining, especially the introduction of disease germs or infectious material into or on normally sterile objects.

contraindication (kon″tra-in″di-ka′shun)   Condition in which the use of certain drugs or treatments should be withheld or limited.

contusion (kon-too′zhun)   A bruise, indicating injury to tissues without breakage in the skin. Discoloration appears because of blood seepage under the surface of the skin.

cornea (kor′ne-ah)   The transparent section of the eyeball that permits light to enter the eye. It is part of the focusing system of the eye.

cross-tolerance   Cross-tolerance can develop when tolerance to one drug increases the body's tolerance to drugs in the same category. For example, a tolerance to one depressant drug leads to a tolerance of other depressant drugs.

crude drug   An unrefined drug.

culture (kul′tur)   The reproduction or growth of microorganisms or of living tissue cells in special laboratory media (the material on which the organisms grow) conducive to their growth. Various types of cultures follow.

culture medium   A commercial preparation used for the growth of microorganisms or other cells. (Types of culture media are described in Chapter 11.)

Culturette   A commercially prepared bacterial culture collection/transport system, consisting of a sterile plastic tube with applicator. Modified Stuart's transport medium is held in a glass ampule at the bottom end, to ensure stability of medium at the time of use. Transport medium is released only after the sample is taken, by crushing the ampule. A moist environment (not immersion) is maintained up to 72 hours to preserve the specimen.

Culturette II culture collection system   This is identical to the Culturette, with the exception that the plastic tube contains two applicators and the ampule contains twice the medium (1 ml).

cumulative action of a drug   A drug accumulates in the body; it is eliminated more slowly than it is absorbed.

cystoscope (sist′o-skop)   A hollow metal tube instrument (endoscope) designed specifically for passing through the urethra into the urinary bladder to permit internal inspection. The bladder interior is illuminatd by an electric bulb at the end of the cystoscope. Special lenses and mirrors allow the bladder mucosa to be examined for calculi (stones), inflammation, or tumors.

cystoscopy (sis-tos′kop-i)   Internal examination of the bladder with a cystoscope. Samples of urine for diagnostic purposes can be obtained by passing a catheter through the cystoscope into the bladder or beyond, up into the ureters and kidneys. Also, radiopaque dyes may be injected through the cystoscope into the bladder or up into the ureters when taking x-ray films of the urinary tract.

cytology (si-tol′o-je)   The study of the structure and function of cells.

DEA   Drug Enforcement Administration. This is the federal law enforcement agency charged with the responsibility of combating drug diversion.

debridement (da-bred-ment′)   The process of removing foreign material and devitalized tissue.

defibrillation (de-fi″bri-la′shun)   The application of electrical impulses to the heart to stop heart fibrillation.

density   The quality of being dense or impenetrable.

dermatitis (der″mah-ti′tis)   Inflammation of the skin.

detail   The sharpness of the radiograph image.

diaphragmatic respiration   Performed mainly by the diaphragm.

diarrhea (di-a-re′a)   Rapid movement of fecal material through the intestine, resulting in poor absorption, producing frequent, watery stools.

digital (dij′i-tal)   The use of a finger to insert into a body cavity, such as the rectum, for palpating the tissue.

dilute   To weaken the strength of a substance by adding something else.

disinfectant (dis″in-fek′tant)   A substance capable of destroying pathogens, but usually not spores; generally not intended for use on body tissue, because it is too strong.

diuresis (di″u-re-′sis)   An abnormal, increased secretion of urine as seen in diabetes mellitus or diabetes insipidus or when drinking large amounts of fluid; this can be artificially produced by drugs with diuretic properties.

don   To put an article on, such as gloves or a gown.

drug idiosyncrasy (id″e-o-sing′krah-se)   An unusual or abnormal response or susceptibility to a drug that is peculiar to the individual.

drug tolerance   The decreased susceptibility to the effects of a drug after continued use. In this case an increased dosage would be required to produce the desired effects because the initial dose would be ineffective.

dysplasia (dis-pla′ze-ah)   An abnormal development of tissue.

dyspnea (disp-ne′ah)   Labored or difficult breathing.

dysuria (dis-u′re-ah)   Painful or difficult urination.

electrocardiograph (e-lek″tro-kar′de-o-graf″)   The instrument used in electrocardiography.

electrolyte (e-lek′tro-lit)   Substances that separate into their component atoms when dissolved in water. They play an important part in maintaining fluid balance and a normal acid-base balance and in the functions of cells in the body. EXAMPLES: sodium, potassium, calcium, magnesium, chloride, and bicarbonate.

electrophoresis (e-lek″tro-fo-re′sis)   A laboratory method used to diagnose certain diseases by analyzing the plasma protein content.

endoscope (en′do-skop)   A specially designed instrument made of metal, rubber, or glass that is used for direct visual examination of hollow organs or body cavities. All endoscopes have similar working elements, even though the design will vary according to its specific use. The viewing part (scope) is a hollow tube fitted with a lens system that allows viewing in a variety of directions. Each endoscope has a light source, power cord, and power source; examples include bronchoscope, cystoscope, proctoscope, and sigmoidoscope.

endoscopy (en-dos′ko-pi)   Visual examination of internal cavities of the body with an endoscope (for example, a proctoscope, bronchoscope, cystoscope, gastroscope, and laryngoscope).

enema (en′e-mah)   The introduction of a solution into the rectum; for an x-ray examination of the colon, a radiopaque solution is administered by enema.

enuresis (en″u-re′sis)   The involuntary excretion of urine, especially at night during sleep; bedwetting; most commonly seen in children with either physical or emotional problems.

epinephrine (ep″i-nef′rin)   A hormone produced by the adrenal glands. Epinephrine can be administered parenterally, topically, or by inhalation. It is used as an emergency heart stimulant, to relieve symptoms in allergic conditions, and to counteract the lethal effects of anaphylactic shock.

erythrocytosis (e-rith″ro-si-to′sis)   Increased numbers of red blood cells (erythrocytes).

essential hypertension (idiopathic or primary hypertension)   Hypertension that develops in the absence of kidney disease. Its cause is unknown. About 85% to 90% of the cases of hypertension are in this category.

eupnea (up-ne′ah)   Easy or normal respiration.

excisional biopsy   Removal of an entire small lesion.

excreta (ek-skre′tah)   Waste material excreted or eliminated from the body. Feces, urine, perspiration, and also mucus and carbon dioxide (CO_2) can be considered excreta.

excrete   To eliminate useless matter, such as feces and urine.

excretion (ek-skre′shun)   The elimination of waste materials from the body. Ordinarily, what is meant by excretion is the elimination of feces, but it can refer to the material eliminated from any part of the body.

excruciating pain   Torturing, extreme pain, often intractable.

exfoliative cytology   Microscopic examination of cells desquamated (shedding) from a body surface as a means of detecting malignant change.

expectorate   The ejection of sputum and other materials from the air passages.

exquisite pain   Intense pain to which an individual is extremely sensitive.

external auditory meatus (me-a′-tus)   The canal or passage leading from the outside opening of the ear to the eardrum. Also called the external acoustic meatus.

external ear   Includes the auricle, or pinna, and the external auditory meatus.

FDA   Food and Drug Administration (a federal government agency).

febrile (feb′rile) **pulse**   A full, bounding pulse at the onset of a fever, becoming feeble and weak when the fever subsides.

feces (fe′sez)   Body waste excreted from the intestine; also called stool, excreta, or excrement.

fever   Pyrexia, or elevation of body temperature above normal, 98.6° F (Fahrenheit) or 37° C (centigrade or Celsius) registered orally. Some classify it as:

Low	99° to 101° F
	(37.2° to 38.3° C)
Moderate	101° to 103° F
	(38.3° to 39.5° C)
High	103° to 105° F
	(39.5° to 40.6° C)

- **crisis** Sudden drop of a high temperature to normal or below; generally occurs within 24 hours.
- **intermittent fever** Variations with alternate rises and falls, with the lowest often dropping below 98.6° F. An intermittent fever reaches the normal line at intervals during the course of an illness (for example, AM 98° F, PM 101° F).
- **onset** Beginning of a fever.
- **remittent fever** Variations in temperature but always above 98.6° F (37° C), a persistent fever that has a daytime variation of 2° F (1.2° C) or more (for example, AM 100° F, PM 103° F; AM 99° F, PM 102.4° F).

fibrillation (fi″bri-la′shun) A cardiac arrhythmia characterized by rapid, irregular, and ineffective electrical activity in the heart. Ventricular fibrillation is a common cause of cardiac arrest.

fixation of a smear Spraying with or immersing a slide into a special solution, drying the slide over a flame, or air-drying to harden and preserve the bacteria for future microscopic examination.

flatulence (flat′u-lens) Excessive formation of gases in the stomach or intestine.

flatus (fla′tus) Air or gas in the stomach or intestine.

fluoroscope (floo′ro-skop″) An instrument that is used during x-ray examinations for visual observation of the internal body structures by means of x-rays. The body part that is to be viewed is placed between the x-ray tube and a fluorescent screen. As x-rays pass through the body, shadowy images of the internal organs are projected on the screen.

fluoroscopy (floo″or-os′ko-pe) Visual examination by means of a fluoroscope.

forced respiration Voluntary hyperpnea.

formicant (for′mi-kant′) **pulse** A small, feeble pulse.

frequency The need to urinate frequently.

fungicide (fun′ji-sid) A substance that destroys fungi.

gastroscopy (gas′tros′ko-pi) Internal inspection of the stomach with a gastroscope.

gelatin culture A culture of bacteria on gelatin.

germicide (jer′mi-sid) A substance that is capable of destroying pathogens.

glucosuria (gloo″ko-su′re-ah) or **glycosuria** (gli″ko-su′re-ah) Abnormally high sugar content in urine.

granulocyte (gran′u-lo-sit″) A white blood cell (WBC) having granules in its cytoplasm. These types of WBCs are neutrophils, basophils, and eosinophils.

guaiac (gwi′ak) **test** The preferred chemical test to determine the presence of occult blood in feces.

guarding A reflex usually related to abdominal pain; the action of muscles tensing, knees drawn up and/or hand placed over a part to prevent examination and/or protect against increasing pain.

habituation Emotional dependence on a drug because of repeated use but without tendencies to increase the amount of the drug.

hanging drop culture A culture in which the bacteria are inoculated into a drop of fluid on a coverglass and then mounted into the depression on a concave slide.

health The state of mental, physical, and social well-being of an individual, and not merely the absence of disease.

hematuria (hem″ah-tu″re-ah) The presence of blood in urine.

hemoglobin (he″mo-glo′bin) A protein in a red blood cell that carries oxygen and carbon dioxide. The pigment in hemoglobin is what gives the blood its red color. The protein in hemoglobin is globin; the red pigment is heme. For the body to make hemoglobin, it must have iron, which is derived from the food we eat.

hemolysis (he-mol′i-sis) The destruction of red blood cells with the release of hemoglobin into the plasma.

hemoptysis (he-mop′-ti-sis) Coughing up blood as a result of bleeding from any part of the respiratory tract. The appearance of the secretion in true hemoptysis is bright red and frothy with air bubbles.

HHS Health and Human Services (a federal government agency).

histology (his-tol′o-je) The study of the microscopic form and structure of tissue.

hyperbilirubinemia (hi″per-bil″i-roo″bi-ne′me-ah) Increased or excessive levels of bilirubin in the blood.

hypercalcemia (hi″per-kal-se′me-ah) Increased or excessive levels of calcium in the blood.

hypercholesterolemia (hi′per-ko-les″ter-ol-e′me-ah) Excessive levels of cholesterol in the blood.

hyperchromia (hi′per-kro′me-ah) An abnormal increase of the hemoglobin levels in red blood cells.

hypercythemia (hy′per-si-the′me-ah) An excessive number of red blood cells in the circulating blood.

hyperemia (hi′per-e′me-ah) An excessive amount of blood in a part.

hyperglycemia (hi″per-gli-se′me-ah) Excessive amounts of glucose in the blood.

hyperkalemia (hi″per-kah-le′me-ah) An excessive level of potassium in the blood.

hypernatremia (hi′per-na-tre′me-ah) An excessive amount of sodium in the blood.

hyperoxemia (hi″per-ok-se′me-ah) A condition in which the blood is excessively acidic.

hyperpnea (hi″perp-ne′ah) Increase in rate and depth of breathing.

hyperproteinemia (hi″per-pro″te-i-ne′me-ah) An excessive amount of protein in the blood.

hypertension (hi′per-ten′shun) High blood pressure; a condition in which the patient has higher blood pressure than normal for his or her age; (for example, systolic pressure consistently above 160 mm Hg and a diastolic pressure above 90 mm Hg).

hyperventilation Increase of air in the lungs above the normal amount; abnormally prolonged and deep breathing, usually associated with acute anxiety or emotional tensions.

hypo (hi′po) A word part meaning an abnormal decrease or deficient amounts. If you replace this word element and definition for the word element "hyper" in all of the preceding terms (except in hyperemia and hyperoxemia), the correct meaning will be defined.

hypotension (hi′po-ten′shun) A decrease of systolic and diastolic blood pressure to below normal; for example, below 90/50 is considered low blood pressure.

hypothermia (hi′po-ther′me-ah)   Low body temperature.

hypoxemia (hi′ pok-se′me-ah)   A deficient amount of oxygen (O_2) in the blood.

hypoxia (hi-pok′se-ah)   Reduced amounts of oxygen to the body tissues.

immunization (im″u-ni-za′shun)   The process of rendering a person immune (protected from or not susceptible to a disease) or of becoming immune; often called vaccination or inoculation. A process by which a person is artifically prepared to resist infection by a specific pathogen.

immunosuppressive agents   Drugs that inhibit the formation of antibodies to antigens that may be present.

incisional biopsy   Incision into and removal of part of a lesion.

incontinence (in-kon′ti-nens)   The inability to refrain from the urge to urinate. This may occur in times of stress, anxiety, anger, postoperatively, or from obstructions that prevent the normal emptying of the urinary bladder, spasms of the bladder, irritation caused by injury or inflammation of the urinary tract, damage to the spinal cord or brain, or development of a fistula (an abnormal tubelike passage) between the bladder and the vagina or urethra.

incubation (in″ku-ba′shun) **period**   The interval of time between the invasion of a pathogen into the body and the appearance of the first symptoms of disease.

incubation (in″ku-ba′shun)   When pertaining to bacteriology, this term refers to the period of culture development.

induration (in″du-ra′shun)   An abnormally hard spot; a process of hardening.

infection (in-fek′shun)   A condition caused by the multiplication of pathogenic microorganisms that have invaded the body of a susceptible host.

- **acute**   Rapid onset, severe symptoms; usually subside within a relatively short period.
- **chronic**   Develops slowly, milder symptoms; lasts for a long time.
- **latent**   Dormant or concealed; pathogen is everpresent in the host, but symptoms are present only intermittently, often in response to a stimulus. At other times the pathogen is dormant.
- **localized**   Retricted to a certain area.
- **generalized**   Systemic; involving the whole body.

infectious mononucleosis   Also called glandular fever, it is an acute infectious disease, caused by the Epstein-Barr virus.

inoculate (i-nok″u-lat)   In microbiology, this refers to introducing infectious matter into a culture medium in an effort to produce growth of the causative organism.

insufflator (in′suf-fla-tor)   An instrument, device, or bag used for blowing air, powder, or gas into a cavity.

intermittent pulse   A pulse in which occasional beats are skipped.

intractable   Unmanageable; not controllable with conventional means, that is, rest, heat, or medication.

ionizing (i″on-i-zing)   Radiant energy given off by radioactive atoms and x-rays.

irradiate (i-ra″de-at)   To treat with radiant energy.

irradiation (i-ra″de-a′shun)   Exposure to radiation; the passage of penetrating rays through a substance or object.

irregular pulse   A pulse with variation in force and frequency; an excess of tea, coffee, tobacco, or exercise may cause this.

ischemia (is-ke′me-ah)   A deficient amount of blood in a body part caused by an obstruction or a functional constriction of a blood vessel.

isocytosis (i″so-si-to′sis)   A state in which cells are equal in size, especially equality of size of red blood cells.

labored breathing   Dyspnea or difficult breathing; respiration that involves active participation of accessory inspiratory and expiratory muscles.

laryngeal (lar-in′je-al) **mirror**   An instrument used to view the pharynx and larynx consisting of a small rounded mirror attached to the end of a slender (metal or chrome plate) handle.

laryngoscope (lar-in′go-skop)   An endoscope used to examine the larynx. It is equipped with mirrors and a light for illumination of the larynx.

leukemia (lu-ke′me-ah)   A malignant disease of various types that is classified clinically as acute or chronic, depending on the character and duration of the disease; myeloid, lymphoid, or monocytic, depending on the cells involved. This disease affects the tissues of the lymph nodes, spleen, and/or bone marrow. Symptoms include an uncontrolled increase of white blood cells, accompanied by a decrease in red blood cells and platelets. This results in anemia and an increased tendency to infection and hemorrhage. Other classical symptoms include pain in bones and joints; fever; and swelling of the liver, spleen, and lymph nodes. The precise cause is unknown.

leukocytosis (lu″ko-si-to′sis)   An increased number of circulating white blood cells.

leukopenia (lu″ko-pe′ne-ah)   A deficient number of circulating white blood cells.

lienteric stool   Feces containing much undigested food.

ligate (li′gat)   To apply a ligature.

ligature (lig′ah-tur)   A suture; material used to tie off blood vessels to prevent bleeding or to constrict tissues.

light therapy or phototherapy (fo′to-ther′ah-pe)   The use of light rays in the treatment of disease processes. By custom, this includes the use of ultraviolet and infrared or heat rays (radiation).

lysis   Gradual decline of a fever.

macrocyte (mak′ro-sit)   The largest type of red blood cell; seen in cases of pernicious anemia (vitamin B_{12} deficiency) and folic acid deficiency.

macroscopic (mak-ro-skop′ik) **examination**   An examination in which the specimen is large enough to be seen by the naked eye.

malignant (mah-lig′nant) **hypertension**   Hypertension that differs from other types in that it is a rapidly developing and may prove fatal if not treated immediately after symptoms develop, before damage is done to the blood vessels. This type occurs most often in persons in their twenties or thirties.

Mayo (ma′o) **stand**   A stand with a flat metal tray used to hold sterile supplies during an aseptic procedure.

medical microbiology   The study and identification of pathogens and the development of effective methods for their control or elimination.

melena (me-le′nah)   Darkening of stool by blood pigments.

microcyte (mik′ro-sit)   An abnormally small red blood cell, found in cases of iron deficiency anemia and thalassemia.

microorganism (mi-kro-or′gan-ism)   A minute living body not perceptible to the naked eye, especially a bacterium or protozoon; these are viewed with a microscope.

microscopic (mi-kro-skop′ik) **examination** An examination in which the specimen is visible only with the aid of a microscope.

miotic (mi-ot′ik) A medication that causes the pupil of the eye to contract.

modality (mo-dal′i-te) Therapeutic agents used in physical medicine and physical therapy.

mononucleosis (mon′o-nu″kle-o′sis) An abnormal increase of the mononuclear white blood cells in the blood.

mydriatic (mid″re-at′ik) A medication that causes the pupil of the eye to dilate.

myocardial infarction (mi″o-kar′de-al in-fark′shun) **(MI)** The formation of ischemic necrosis in the heart muscle caused by an interference of blood supply to the area.

myocardium (mi″o-kar′de-um) The heart muscle.

nasal speculum (na′zl spek′u-lum) A short, funnel-like instrument used to examine the nasal cavity.

necrosis (ne-kro′-sis) The death of a cell or a group of cells because of injury or disease.

negative culture A culture made from suspected material that fails to reveal the suspected microorganism.

normal flora Microorganisms that normally reside in various body locations, such as in the vagina, intestine, urethra, and upper respiratory tract and on the skin. These microorganisms are non-pathogenic and do not cause any harm (they may become pathogenic and cause harm if they are introduced into a body area in which they do not normally reside).

objective symptom A symptom that is apparent to the observer; also called a sign, for example, rash, swelling.

obstipation (ob′sti-pa′shun) Extreme constipation caused by an obstruction.

occult blood Obscure or hidden from view.

occult blood test A microscopic or a chemical test performed on a specimen to determine the presence of blood not otherwise detectable. Stool is tested when intestinal bleeding is suspected, but there is no visible evidence of blood in the stool.

ocular (ok′u-lar) Pertaining to the eye.

oliguria (o″i-gu′re-ah) Scanty amounts of urine.

ophthalmic (of-thal′mik) Pertaining to the eye.

ophthalmology (of″thal-mol′o-je) The study and science of the eye and its diseases.

ophthalmoscope (of-thal′mo-skop) An instrument used for examining the interior parts of the eye. It contains a perforated mirror and lens. When the ophthalmoscope is turned on and brought close to the eye, it sends a narrow, bright beam of light through the lens of the eye. By looking through the lens of the instrument, the physician is then able to examine the interior parts of the eye, including the lens, anterior chamber, retinal structures, and blood vessels, to detect any possible disorders. Many ophthalmoscopes come with an interchangeable otoscope, throat illuminator head, or nasal illuminator head.

oral examination Examination pertaining to the mouth.

orthopnea (or″thop-ne′ah) Severe dyspnea in which breathing is possible only when the patient sits or stands in an erect positon.

orthostatic (or″tho-stat′ik) **hypotension** Hypotension occurring when a patient assumes an erect position.

oscilloscope (o-sil′o-skop) An instrument for visualizing the shape or wave form of sound waves, as in ultrasonography, or of electric currents, as when monitoring heart action and other body functions.

otic (o′tik) Pertaining to the ear.

otology (o-tol′o-je) The study and science of the ear and its diseases.

otoscope (o′to-skop) An instrument used for visual examination of the external ear canal and eardrum.

pacemaker (pas′mak-er) The pacemaker of the heart is the sinoatrial node located in the right atrium.

Papanicolaou (pap″ah-nik″o-la′oo) **smear or test** A smear examined microscopically to detect cancer cells from body excretions (urine and feces), secretions (vaginal fluids, sputum or prostatic fluid), or tissue scrapings (as obtained from the stomach or uterus); most commonly done on a cervical scraping to detect abnormal or cancerous cells in the mucus of the cervix. This test is often referred to as a Pap smear or test.

parasite (par′ah-sit) An organism that lives on or in another organism, known as the host, from which it gains its nourishment (for example, fungi, bacteria, and single-celled, and multicelled animals).

pathogen (path′o-jen) A disease-producing substance or microorganism.

pathogenic (path′o-jen′ic) Pertaining to a disease-producing microorganism or substance.

pathogenic microorganism One that produces disease in the body.

PDR *Physicians' Desk Reference,* a book on drugs.

pelvic examination Examination of the external and internal female reproductive organs.

percussion (per-kush′un) **hammer** A small hammer with a triangular-shaped rubber head used for percussion.

pericarditis (per″i-kar-di′tis) Inflammation of the pericardium, the fibroserous sac enveloping the heart.

phagocytosis (fag″o-si-to′sis) The process by which white blood cells destroy and engulf or ingest harmful microorganisms.

physical signs Objective manifestations of disease that are apparent on a physical examination; observable changes representing alterations resulting from a disease or dysfunction in the body (*see also* Sign).

placebo (plah-se′bo) An inactive substance resembling and given in place of a medication for its psychologic effects to satisfy the patient's need for the drug; it hopefully will produce the same effect as the real medication through psychologic means. A placebo may be used experimentally.

poikilocytosis (poi″ki-lo-si-to′sis) The presence of red blood cells in the blood that show abnormal variations in their shape.

polycythemia (pol″e-si-the′me-ah) An abnormal increased amount of red blood cells or hemoglobin.

polyuria (pol″e-u′re′ah) Excessive excretion of urine.

positive culture A culture that reveals the suspected microorganism.

positive findings Evidence of disease or body dysfunction.

postoperative (post-op′er-ah-tiv) Pertaining to the period following surgery.

postural hypotension Hypotension occurring on suddenly arising from a recumbent position or when standing still for a long time.

preoperative (pre-op′er-ah-tiv) Pertaining to the time preceding surgery.

proctoscope (prok′to-skop) A specially designed tubular endoscope that is passed through the anus to permit internal inspection of the lower part of the large intestine.

prodrome   An early symptom, indicating the onset of a disease, such as an achy feeling before having the flu.

prognosis   A statement made by the physician indicating the probable or anticipated outcome of the disease process in a patient; usually stated simply as good, fair, poor, or guarded.

prophylaxis (pro″fi-lak′sis)   Prevention of disease.

proteinura (pro″te-in-u′re-ah)   An abnormal increase of protein in urine.

psoriasis (so-ri′ah-sis)   A chronic inflammatory recurrent skin disease characterized by scaly red patches on the body surfaces. The lesions are seen most often on knees, elbows, scalp, and fingernails. Other areas often affected are the chest, abdomen, palms of the hands, soles of the feet, and backs of the arms and legs. The cause is unknown, although a hereditary factor is suggested.

pulse deficit   The apical rate is greater than the radial pulse rate.

pulse pressure   The difference between the systolic and the diastolic blood pressure.

EXAMPLE: If BP is 120/80,

$$
\begin{array}{r}
120 = \text{systolic pressure} \\
-\,80 = \text{diastolic pressure} \\
\hline
40 = \text{pulse pressure}
\end{array}
$$

A pulse pressure consistently over 50 points or under 30 points is considered abnormal.

pure culture   A culture of a single microorganism.

pure drug   A refined drug; one that has been processed to remove all impurities.

pyuria (pi-u′re-ah)   The presence of pus in the urine.

qualitative tests   Used for screening purposes. These tests provide an indication as to whether or not a substance is present in a specimen in abnormal quantities. A qualitative test does not determine the exact amount of a substance present in a specimen. Color charts are usually used to interpret qualitative tests. Sometimes they are called semiquantitative tests. Results are reported in terms such as trace, small amount, moderate, large amount, or 1+, 2+, 3+ or simply as positive or negative.

quantitative tests   More precise tests. They determine accurately the amount of a specific substance that is present in a specimen. A high level of skill is required to perform these tests on sophisticated equipment. Results are reported in units such as grams (g) per 100 milliliters (ml), or milligrams (mg) percent, or milligrams per deciliter (dl).

radiating   Diverting from a common central point; for example, gallbladder pain begins in the right upper quadrant of the abdomen, and it is diverted from that central point to the right flank and right scapular area.

radiation (ra″de-a′shun)   Electromagnetic waves of streams of atomic particles capable of penetrating and being absorbed into matter. Examples of electromagnetic waves are x-rays, gamma rays, ultraviolet rays, infrared rays, and rays of visible light. Atomic particles are alpha and beta particles.

radiogram (ra′de-o-gram″)   A picture of internal body structures produced by the action of gamma rays or x-rays on a special film.

radiograph (ra′de-o-graf″) or **roentgenograph** (rent′gen-o-graf) or **roentgenogram** (rent′gen-o-gram″)   The film or photographic record produced by radiography.

radiography (ra″de-og′rah-fe)   The taking of radiograms.

radioisotope (ra″de-o-i′so-top)   A radioactive form of an element consisting of unstable atoms that emit rays of energy or streams of atomic particles. Radioisotopes occur naturally, as in the case of radium, or can be created artificially, as in the case of cobalt.

radiologist (ra″de-ol′o-jist)   A physician specialist in the study of radiology.

radiolucent (ra″de-o-lu-sent)   That which permits the partial or complete passage of radiant energy such as x-rays. Dense objects appear white on the x-ray film because they absorb the radiation. An example of this is bone.

radionuclide (ra″de-o-nu′klid)   A radioactive substance.

radiopaque (ra-de-o-pak′)   That which is impenetrable by x-rays and other forms of radiant energy; matter that obstructs the passage of radiant energy, such as lead, which is commonly used as a protective device.

rales (rahls)   An abnormal bubbling sound heard on auscultation of the chest; often classified as either moist or crackling and dry.

rebound tenderness   A sensation of pain felt when pressure applied on a body part is released.

regular pulse   The rhythm of the pulse rate is regular.

renal hypertension   Hypertension resulting from kidney disease.

reservoir (rez′er-vwrar)   The source in which pathogenic microorganisms grow and from which they leave to spread and cause disease.

resistance (re-zis′tans)   The ability of the body to resist disease or infection because of its own defense mechanisms.

reticulocyte (re-tik′u-lo-sit)   A nonnucleated immature red blood cell. Generally, of all the red blood cells in the circulating blood, less than 2% are reticulocytes.

rhythm strip   A rhythm strip is an ECG (or EKG) recording of a single lead that is used to determine the rhythm of the heartbeat, such as a fast, slow, regular, or irregular rhythm, and certain types of ventricular fibrillation. It is also used to determine if the patient is in any type of heart block, such as third-degree heart block. The rhythm strip gives a one-dimensional picture of the beating of the heart, which determines only the rhythm of the heartbeat in contrast to the 12-lead ECG, which can slow damage to the heart and other conditions. Data from the rhythm strip can be a useful "screening" tool because frequent runs of arrhythmias can be more easily observed. The rhythm strip can also be used to confirm the basic assessment made on the 12-lead ECG. Currently for the rhythm strip, most practitioners will record lead V_1, and possibly Leads V_2 and V_5, although one could record any lead that is desired. Rhythm strips are frequently recorded from a continuous cardiac monitor in intensive care units in the hospital and by paramedics when they are in the field in emergency situations.

roentgenologic (rent-gen-ol′oj-ik)   Pertaining to an examination with the use of x-ray film (radiographs).

saliva (sah-li′vah)   The enzyme-containing secretion of the salivary glands in the mouth.

sclera (skler′ah)   The white outer layer of the eyeball. It is touch sensitive and is transparent over the front of the eyeball.

secondary hypertension   Hypertension that is traceable to known causes, such as a pheochromocytoma (tumor of the adrenal gland), hardening of the arteries, kidney disease, or obstructions to kidney blood flow. Approximately 10% to 15% of the cases of hypertension are secondary. Patients with secondary hypertension can often be cured if the underlying cause can be eliminated.

sepsis (sep′sis)   A morbid state or condition resulting from the presence of pathogenic microorganisms.

septicemia (sep″ti-se′me-ah)   A condition in which bacteria or toxins are in the blood.

serologic (se-ro-loj′ik) test   A laboratory test involving the examination and study of blood serum.

serum (se′rum)   The clear, straw-colored liquid portion obtained after blood clots; it consists of plasma minus fibrinogen, which is removed in the process of clotting.

side effect   A response in addition to that for which the drug was used, especially an undesirable result.

untoward effect   An undesirable side effect.

sigmoidoscope (sig-moy′do-skop)   A tubular endoscope used to examine the interior of the sigmoid colon.

sign   Sometimes called a physical sign; any objective evidence (apparent to the observer) representing disease or body dysfunction. Signs may be observed by others or revealed when the physician performs a physical examination; examples include swollen ankles, a distended rigid abdomen, elevated blood pressure, and decreased sensation.

Sims' vaginal speculum   A form of bivalve speculum used in the examination of the vagina and cervix.

slow pulse   A pulse between 40 and 60 beats per minute, often found among the elderly and among athletes at rest.

smear (smer)   Material spread thinly across a slide or culture medium with a swab, loop, or another slide in preparation for microscopic study.

smear culture   A culture prepared by smearing the specimen across the surface of the culture medium.

specimen (spec′i-men)   A small part or sample taken to show kind and quality of the whole, as a specimen of urine, blood, or other body excretions, or a small piece of tissue for macroscopic and microscopic examination.

speculum (spek′u-lum)   An instrument used for distending or opening a body cavity or orifice to allow visual inspection; a bivalve speculum is one having two parts or valves.

spore (spor)   A reproductive cell, usually unicellular, produced by plants and some protozoa and possessing thick walls to withstand unfavorable environmental conditions. Bacterial spores are resistant to heat and must undergo a prolonged exposure to extremely high temperatures to be destroyed.

sprain (spran)   A joint injury in which some fibers of a supporting ligament are ruptured, but continuity of the ligament remains intact. There may also be damage to the associated muscles, tendons, nerves, and blood vessels.

sputum (spu′-tum)   A mucous secretion from the trachea, bronchi, and lungs, ejected through the mouth, in contrast to saliva, which is the secretion of the salivary glands.

stab culture   A bacterial culture made by thrusting a needle inoculated with the microorganisms under examination deep into the culture medium.

stabbing pain   Deep, sharp, intermittent pain.

sterile (ster′il)   Free from all microorganisms.

sterile field   A work area prepared with sterile drapes (coverings) to hold sterile supplies during a sterile procedure.

sterile setup   Specific sterile supplies used in a specific sterile procedure.

stertorous (ster′to-rus) **respirations**   Characterized by a deep snoring sound with each inspiration.

stethoscope   An instrument used in auscultation to amplify the sounds produced by the lungs, heart, intestines, and other internal organs; also used when taking a blood pressure reading.

stock supply   A large supply of medications kept in the physician's office or pharmacy.

stool (stool)   Body waste material discharged from the large intestine; also called feces or bowel movement.

strain (stran)   An overexertion or overstretching of some part of a muscle.

streak culture   A bacterial culture in which the infectious material is implanted in streaks across the culture media.

subjective symptoms   Symptoms of internal origin that are apparent or perceptible only to the patient; examples include pain, dizziness (vertigo).

suture (soo′cher)   Various types and sizes of absorbable and nonabsorbable materials used to close a wound with stitches.

swab (swob)   A small piece of cotton or gauze wrapped around the end of a slender stick used for applying medications, cleansing cavities, or obtaining a piece of tissue or body secretion for bacteriologic examination; also known as a cotton-tipped applicator.

symmetry (sim′et-ri)   Correspondence in form, size, and arrangement of parts on opposite sides of the body.

symptom   Any subjective evidence of disease or body dysfunction; a change in the physical or mental state of the body that is perceptible or apparent only to the individual; examples include anorexia, nausea, headache, pain, itching.

syndrome   A combination of symptoms resulting from one cause or commonly occurring together to present a distinct clinical picture; an example is the dumping syndrome, which consists of nausea, weakness, varying degrees of syncope, sweating, palpitation, and sometimes diarrhea and a feeling of warmth. This may occur immediatley after eating in patients who have had a partial gastrectomy.

tachycardia (tak″y-kar′di-a)   A pulse of 170 or more beats per minute; abnormal rapidity of heart action.

tear (lacrimal) glands   The glands on the underside of the upper lids that secrete a fluid to keep the eyes moist.

tendinitis (ten′di-ni′tis)   Inflammation of a tendon; one of the most common causes of acute pain in the shoulder.

thready pulse   A pulse that is very fine and scarely perceptible, as seen in syncope (fainting).

threshold   The level that must be exceeded for an effect to be produced; the level of pain that an individual can tolerate without external intervention. Threshold is unique to each individual, and the overall physiopsychologic makeup of an individual must be considered when evaluating pain.

thrombocyte (throm′bo-sit)   A blood platelet.

thrombocythemia (throm″bo-si-the′me-ah)   An increased number of platelets in the circulating blood.

thrombocytopenia (throm″bo-si″to-pe′ne-ah)   A decreased number of platelets in the circulating blood.

tissue culture   The growing of tissue cells in artifical nutrient media.

tongue blade   A flat, thin, smooth piece of wood or metal with rounded ends approximately 6 inches long; also called a tongue depressor. It is used for pressing tissue down to permit a better view when examining the mouth and throat. In addition, it may be used for application of ointments to the skin.

tonometer (to-nom′e-ter)   An instrument used to measure tension or pressure, especially intraocular pressure.

tourniquet (toor′ni-ket)   A constricting device used to compress an artery or vein to stop excessive bleeding or to prevent the spread of snake venom.

toxicity (tok-sis′i-te)   The nature of exerting harmful effects on a tissue or organism. The level at which a drug becomes toxic to the body. Minor or major damage may result.

toxin (tok′sin)   A poisonous substance produced by pathogenic bacteria and some animals and plants. The toxins produced by bacteria include toxic enzymes, exotoxins, and endotoxins. Toxins in the body cause antitoxins to form, which provide a means for establishing immunity to certain diseases.

transfer forceps   A type of instrument (forcep) that is kept in a chemical disinfectant or germicide and used for transferring or handling sterile supplies and equipment.

transient   Fleeting, brief, passing, coming and going.

tuning fork   A steel, two-pronged, forklike instrument used for testing hearing; the prongs give off a musical note when struck.

tympanic (tim-pan′ik) **membrane** (TM)   The eardrum; it serves as the membrane that separates the external auditory meatus from the middle ear cavity.

type culture   A culture that is generally agreed to represent microorganisms of a particular species.

unequal pulse   A pulse in which some beats are strong and others are weak; pulse in which rates are different in symmetrical arteries.

unit-dose   A system that supplies prepackaged, premeasured, prelabeled, individual portions of a medication for patient use.

uremia (u-re′me-ah)   A toxic condition in which there are substances in the blood that should normally be eliminated in the urine.

urgency   The need to urinate immediately.

urination (u″ri-na′shun), **voiding, micturition** (mik″tu-rish′un)   The act of passing urine from the body.

urine (u′rine)   The fluid containing certain waste products and water that is secreted by the kidneys, stored in the bladder, and excreted through the urethra.

urobilinogen   A colorless compound formed in the intestines by the reduction of bilirubin.

USP-NF   *United States Pharmacopeia-National Formulary,* a drug book listing all official drugs authorized for use in the United States.

vaccination (vak″si-na′shun)   The introduction of weakened or dead microorganisms (inoculation) into the body to stimulate the production of antibodies and immunity to a specific disease.

venipuncture (ven″i-pungk′tur)   Puncturing a vein to collect a blood specimen or to administer a medication.

venous pulse   A pulse in a vein, especially one of the large veins near the heart such as the internal and external jugular. Venous pulse is undulating and scarcely palpable.

ventricle (ven′tri-kl)   One of the lower chambers of the heart. The right ventricle receives deoxygenated blood from the right atrium and pumps this blood through the pulmonary arteries to the lungs; the left ventricle receives oxygenated blood from the left atrium and pumps this blood out through the aorta to all body tissues.

vesicle (ves′i-kl)   A circular, blisterlike elevation on the skin containing fluid.

viable (vi′ah-bl)   Able to maintain an independent existence.

virulence (vir′u-lens)   The degree of ability of a pathogen to produce disease.

vitamin K   A vitamin that is essential for the formation of prothrombin and the normal clotting of blood. A deficiency may result in hemorrhage because of a prolonged prothrombin time.

voltage (vol-tij)   The electromotive force measured in volts (the units of force for electricity to flow).

wheal (hwel)   A temporary, more or less round, elevation on the skin that is white in the center and often accompanied by itching.

Special Vocabulary

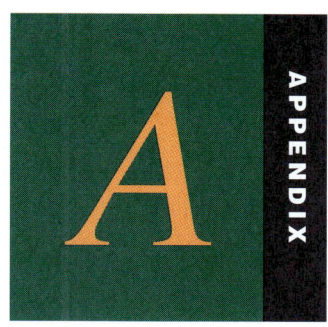

Part 1: Vocabulary Used When Recording Information Obtained From the Review of Systems

The following vocabulary lists **some** of the terms that an examiner may use when recording the *subjective* **findings** of the review of systems (ROS) of a patient. Terms are presented in the order in which they appear in the patient's ROS and under the body part or system for which they are used in describing ROS findings (see also Chapter 4).

Eyes

photophobia (fo″to-fo′be-ah) An abnormal visual intolerance to light.

Ears

tinnitus (ti-ni′tus) A ringing or buzzing noise in the ears.

Nose

coryza (ko-ri′zah) A head cold; an acute inflammation of the nasal mucous membrane with a profuse discharge.

epistaxis (ep″i-stak′sis) A nosebleed; hemorrhage from the nose. Many episodes of epistaxis are caused by the rupture of the small vessels over the anterior part of the cartilaginous nasal septum.

Respiratory

asthma (az′mah) Recurrent attacks of difficulty in breathing (dyspnea) with wheezing that is caused by spasms in the bronchial tubes.

expectoration (ek-spek″to-ra′shun) The coughing up, expulsion, or spitting out of material (mucus, sputum, or phlegm) from the throat, trachea, bronchi, or lungs.

hemoptysis (he-mop′ti-sis) The spitting and/or coughing up of blood from the respiratory tract caused by bleeding in any part of the respiratory tract. In true hemoptysis, sputum is frothy with air bubbles and bright red. (Hemoptysis must not be confused with *hematemesis,* in which a dark red or black substance is ejected from the gastrointestinal tract.)

hyperventilation (hi′per-ven″ti-la′shun) Abnormal deep and prolonged breathing; increase in the inspiration and expiration of air resulting from an increase in the depth or rate of respirations or both. This results especially with depletion of carbon dioxide. This condition is often associated with emotional tension or acute anxiety situations.

Cardiovascular (CV)

palpitation (pal″pi-ta′shun) An unusually strong, rapid, or irregular heartbeat, usually over 120 beats per minute (normal heart rate varies between 60 to 100 beats per minute). Palpitation is often the result of strong exertion, nervousness, excitement, or the taking of certain medications. Palpitations may also result from a variety of heart disorders.

peripheral (pe-rif′er-al) **edema** Pertaining to the periphery, which means the surface or outward structures; *edema* (e-de′mah) An abnormal accumulation of fluid in the intercellular spaces of the body.

varicosity (var″i-kos′i-te) Pertaining to a varicose condition; distended, swollen veins.

Gastrointestinal

anorexia (an″o-rek′se-ah) Loss of appetite. Anorexia can be caused by illness, emotional upsets, or unattractive food.

colic (kol′ik) Pertaining to the colon; abdominal pain caused by spasmodic contractions of the intestinal tract.

constipation (kon″sti-pa-shun) Difficult elimination of fecal material from the intestinal tract; often the infrequent passage of waste material that is hard to eliminate easily results in the passage of unduly dry and hard fecal material.

diarrhea (di″ah-re′ah) The rapid movement of fecal material through the intestine, the feces having more or less fluid consistency; primarily a result of increased peristalsis in the intestinal tract.

distention (dis-ten′shun) The state of being stretched out, or distended.

dysphagia (dis-fa′je-ah) Difficulty in swallowing.

flatus (fla′tus) Air or gas in the gastrointestinal tract.

hemorrhoid (hem′o-roid); also called *piles* A dilated blood vessel in the anus that may bleed, cause discomfort or pain, and itch.

jaundice (jawn′dis); also called *icterus* (ik′ter-us) A symptom of different disorders of the gallbladder, liver, and blood characterized by yellowness of the skin, mucous membranes, and whites of the eyes caused by excessive bilirubin in the blood and deposition of bile pigments.

melena (me-le′nah) Black fecal material; blood pigments darken the feces.

Genitourinary (GU)

enuresis (en″u-re′sis) The involuntary excretion of urine, especially at night during sleep; bedwetting; most commonly seen in children with physical or emotional problems.

frequency (fre′kwen-se) The need to urinate frequently.

hesitancy Dysuria caused by nervous inhibition or obstruction in the vesical outlet.

incontinence (in-kon′ti-nens) The inability to refrain from the urge to urinate. This may occur in times of stress, anxiety, or anger; after surgery; or because of obstructions that prevent the normal emptying of the urinary bladder, spasms of the bladder, irritation caused by injury or inflammation of the urinary tract, damage to the spinal cord or brain, or the development of a fistula (an abnormal tubelike passage) between the bladder and the vagina or urethra. The word also may refer to fecal incontinence caused by nervous disorders or weakening of the anal sphincter.

nocturia (nok-tu′re-ah) Excessive urination at night.

potency (po′ten-se) The ability of a male to have sexual intercourse.

renal colic (re′nal kol′ik) Spasms accompanied by pain that radiates from the kidney region around to the abdomen and into the groin. Renal colic is experienced during movement of a stone in the ureter.

retention (re-ten′shun) The process of urine accumulating in the bladder because of the individual's inability to urinate.

urgency The immediate need to urinate.

urination (u″ri-na′shun); also called *micturition* (mik ″tu-rish′un) Voiding; the act of passing urine from the body.

venereal (ve-ne′re-al) **disease** A disease that is transmitted by sexual contact and intercourse. Venereal disease is now more commonly referred to as *sexually transmitted disease.* Abbreviations used are VD and STD.

Female reproductive

abortion (ah-bor′shun) The termination of a pregnancy before the fetus is capable of surviving outside of the uterus. In lay terminology, *abortion* refers to a deliberate interruption of pregnancy by various methods, and *miscarriage* refers to the natural loss of the fetus (*spontaneous abortion*).

dyspareunia (dis″pah-ru′ne-ah) Difficult or painful genital sexual intercourse in women.

gravida (grav′i-dah) A pregnant woman. During the first pregnancy the woman would be referred to as gravida I (*primigravida*), and so on, with each succeeding pregnancy.

leukorrhea (loo″ko-re′ ah) An abnormal yellow or white mucous discharge from the cervix or vaginal canal. Leukorrhea may be a symptom of pathologic changes in the vagina and endocervix.

menarche (me-nar′ke) The beginning of the menstrual functions in a woman.

menopause (men′o-pawz) The period in a woman's life at which the menstrual cycles decrease and gradually stop; the period when menstruation and the ability to have a child cease because the ovaries stop functioning. Menopause is often referred to as *the change of life* and also called the *climacteric.*

parous (pa′rus) Having borne at least one child. For example, if a woman has one live child and is now pregnant for the second time, she would be referred to as gravida II, para I (*see* Gravida).

Endocrine

goiter (goi′ter) An enlargement of the thyroid gland.

Skin

allergy (al′er-je) An abnormal condition of individual hypersensitivity to substances (*allergens*) that are usually harmless. Allergens, substances capable of inducing hypersensitivity, can be almost any substance in the environment. Examples of allergens to which people become sensitive include dust, animal hairs, plant and tree pollens, mold spores, soaps, detergents, cosmetics, dyes, foods, feathers, plastics, and even some valuable medicines. When the allergen is in contact with or enters the body, it sets off a chain of events that brings about the allergic reaction. The allergen itself is not directly responsible for the allergic reaction. An allergy does not develop on the first contact with the allergen but can develop on the second contact or even years later, after repeated contact with the allergen. Signs and symptoms of allergies include sneezing, stuffed up and running nose, watery eyes, itching, coughing, shortness of breath, wheezing, rashes, skin eruptions, slight local edema, and mild to severe anaphylactic shock, which can be fatal unless treated.

mole (mol) A discolored blemish or growth on the skin; also called a *nevus.*

ulcer (ul′ser) An open sore or lesion on the surface of the skin or mucous membranes of the body, produced by the sloughing of dead inflammatory tissues.

Musculoskeletal

atrophy (at′ro-fe) A wasting away and decrease in size of a normal tissue or organ.

dislocation (dis″lo-ka′shun) The displacement of a bone from its normal position in a joint.

fracture (frak′chur) A break in the continuity of a bone. Broad classifications of fractures are *open fracture,* in which the bone penetrates the skin, producing an open wound; and *closed fracture,* in which there is no break in the skin.

spasm (spazm) An involuntary sudden movement or contraction of a muscle or group of muscles, commonly accompanied by pain and varying from mild twitches to severe convulsions. Spasms may be **clonic,** in which muscles alternate between contacting and relaxing; or **tonic,** in which the contraction of the muscle is sustained. Tonic spasms are the more severe type, because they are caused by diseases that affect the brain or central nervous system, such as rabies or tetanus.

tetany (tet'ah-ne)   A continuous tonic spasm of a muscle without distinct twitching. The spasms are usually sudden, periodic, or recurrent; and they involve the extremities.

Neurologic

convulsion (kun-vul'shun)   Involuntary spasms or contractions of muscles caused by an abnormal stimulus to the brain or by changes in the chemical balance of the body.

paralysis (pah-ral'i-sis)   A state caused by damage to parts of the nervous system, resulting in impairment or loss of motor function in a part or parts of the body.

paresthesia (par"es-the'ze-ah)   An abnormal sensation experienced without an objective cause. Examples include a burning, tingling, or numb feeling.

tremor (trem'or)   An involuntary quivering or trembling movement of the body or limbs caused by alternate contractions of opposing muscles. Tremors may have a psychologic or a physical cause or both.

vertigo (ver'ti-go)   A sensation of dizziness (that is, rotation of oneself or of external objects in one's surroundings).

Part 2: Vocabulary Used in Recording Physical Findings

The following vocabulary lists **some** of the terms that an examiner may use in recording the **objective findings** of the physical examination of a patient. Each term is presented under the body part or system for which it is used when describing the findings of the physical examination. The order in which the body part or system is presented follows the usual sequence that examiners follow in performing a physical examination.

Skin

abrasion (ah-bra'zhun)   A scrape on the surface of the skin or on a mucous membrane (for example, a skinned knee).

avulsion (a-vul'shun)   A piece of soft tissue that is torn loose or left hanging as a flap.

contusion (kon-too'zhun)   A bruise; an injury to the tissues without skin breakage. In a contusion, blood seeps into the surrounding tissues from the injured and broken blood vessels, causing pain, tenderness, swelling, and discoloration of the surface skin.

cyanosis (si"ah-no'sis)   A bluish discoloration of mucous membranes and skin.

ecchymosis (ek"i-mo'sis)   A round or irregular nonelevated hemorrhagic spot on mucous membranes or skin. The appearance is that of a blue-black or purplish patch changing to yellow or greenish brown. An ecchymosis is *larger* than a patechia.

erythema (er"i-the'mah)   A redness of the skin caused by capillary congestion in the lower layers of the skin. Ery-

thema is present in any inflammatory process, infection, or injury of the skin.

jaundice (jawn'dis)   See ROS vocabulary under Gastrointestinal.

laceration (las"e-ra'shun)   A tear or jagged-edged wound of body tissue.

petechia (pe-te'ke-ah)   A tiny, round, nonraised, purplish-red spot caused by submucous or intradermal hemorrhage. Later a petechia will turn blue or yellow. Small red patches.

purpura (per'pu-rah)   Purpura is a hemorrhagic disease of obscure cause. It is characterized by the escape or discharge of blood from vessels into tissues under the skin and through mucous membranes, producing small red patches and bruises on the skin.

turgor (tur'gor)   The condition of normal tension or fullness in a cell.

ulcer (ul'ser)   See in ROS vocabulary under Skin.

urticaria (ur"ti-ka're-ah)   Also called *hives.* An inflammatory reaction of the skin characterized by the appearance of slightly elevated red or pale patches that are often itchy.

Eyes

acuity (ah-ku'i-te)   Clearness, sharpness, or acuteness of vision.

adnexa (ad-nek'sah)   Accessory organs of the eye.

arcus senilis (ar'kus seni-lis)   An opaque white ring partially surrounding the margin of the cornea, usually seen in people 50 years old or older. This condition often occurs bilaterally and is a result of fat granules depositing in the cornea or lipoid degeneration.

fundus (fun'dus) **(of the eye)**   The back portion of the interior of the eye. The physician can observe this part of the eye by looking into or through the pupil of the eye with an ophthalmoscope.

nystagmus (nis-tag'mus)   The constant, involuntary, rhythmic movement of the eyeball in any direction.

papilledema (pap"il-e-de'mah)   Edema and inflammation of the optic nerve, usually caused by intracranial pressure as a result of a brain tumor pressing on the optic nerve.

ptosis (to'sis)   A drooping of the upper eyelids caused by paralysis.

Ears

cerumen (se-roo'men)   Earwax.

tympanic (tim-pan'ik) membrane; also called *eardrum*   A thin membrane that separates the middle ear from the outer ear.

Nose

nares (na'rez)   The external openings into the nasal cavity; the nostrils.

nasal septal defect   A deviation of the bone and cartilage that divides the nasal cavity so that one part of the nasal cavity is larger than the other. On occasion this may produce difficulty in normal breathing, prevent normal drainage from infected sinuses, and interfere with the normal flow of mucus from the sinuses when one has a cold.

Neck

supple (sup′l)   Easily movable.

Respiratory system

fremitus (frem′i-tus)   A vibration or tremor felt through the chest wall, usually during palpation.

tactile fremitus   A vibration felt when a person speaks.

tussive fremitus   A vibration felt when a person coughs.

vocal fremitus   A vibration heard during auscultation of the chest wall when a person speaks.

friction rub; also called *rub*   A sound heard during auscultation that is produced when two serous membrane surfaces rub together.

rale (rahl)   An abnormal respiratory sound heard when the physician auscultates the chest. A rale indicates a pathologic condition. There are many types of rales. Examples include a *dry rale,* which is a whistling or squeaky sound as heard in a person who has bronchitis or asthma; a *moist rale,* which is produced by fluid in the bronchial tubes; and a *crepitant rale,* which is a dry, crackling sound heard in the early stages of pneumonia when the person completes an inspiration.

resonance (rez′o-nans)   The quality of sound heard when the physician is examining the chest wall by percussion.

rhonchus (rong′kus) (pl. *rhonchi*)   A dry rale in the bronchus or a rattling in the throat.

rub   *See* Friction rub.

sputum (spu′tum)   The mucous secretion that comes from the lungs, bronchi, and trachea and that is ejected from the mouth. *Saliva* is not the same as sputum; saliva is secreted from the salivary glands in the mouth.

stridor (stri′dor)   A harsh, shrill respiratory sound heard during inspirations in individuals who have laryngeal obstruction.

Cardiovascular system (CVS)

bruit (bru′e)   A blowing sound heard over an aneurysm during auscultation of the cardiovascular system.

congestion (kon-jes′chun)   An abnormal accumulation of blood in a body part.

ecchymosis   See under Skin.

engorgement (en-gorj′ment)   A distention of a body part with blood.

erythema   See under Skin.

gallop (gal′op)   A disordered rhythm of the heart heard during auscultation. In a gallop rhythm, three or four extra sounds are heard during the diastolic phase; the sounds are related to atrial contraction.

infarction (in-fark′shun)   A localized area of deficiency of blood in a part causing death to the cells. This is caused by blockage of arterial blood supply to the area. With reference to the heart, the term *myocardial infarction* is used. This pertains to the death of the cells in the myocardial layer of the heart caused by the lack of blood supply to the area.

ischemia (is-ke′me-ah)   The deficiency of blood in a body part. Ischemia may be caused by an obstruction in a blood vessel such as from a clot or cholesterol deposits, or by a functional constriction.

murmur (mer′mer)   A sound heard during auscultation that is cardiac or vascular in origin, especially a periodic sound of short duration. This sound may be heard over the aortic valve, over the apex of the heart, or over an artery; all of these indicate possible disease in the particular area.

petechia   See under Skin.

purpura   See under Skin.

resuscitation (re-sus″i-ta′shun)   The act of restoring life or consciousness to a person whose respirations have stopped and who is thought to be dead.

rub; also called *friction rub*   See under Respiratory System.

pericardial rub   A rub associated with inflammation of the pericardium. When this condition is present during auscultation, the physician will hear a grating or scraping sound with the heartbeat.

thrill (thril)   A vibration that is felt by the physician when palpating the area over the heart, either during diastole or systole.

Abdomen

ascites (ah-si′tez)   An abnormal excessive accumulation of serous fluid in the peritoneal cavity that may cause abdominal distention. Ascites can be caused by a variety of conditions, some of which are tumors, kidney and heart disease, inflammation of the abdominal cavity, and cirrhosis of the liver.

contour (kon′toor)   The outline or shape, as of the abdomen.

distention   See under ROS vocabulary.

flaccid   Relaxed, soft, weak, flabby; applied especially to muscles that lack muscular tone.

hernia (her′ne-ah)   An abnormal projection or protrusion of an organ or tissue or part of an organ through the wall of the cavity in which it is normally contained.

protuberant (pro-tu′ber-ant)   With reference to the abdomen, an area that projects out or is prominent beyond the usual surface abdominal area.

scaphoid (skaf′oid)   In reference to the abdomen, appearing as having a hallowed anterior wall; boat-shaped.

rigidity (ri-jid′i-te)   A state of being stiff or inflexible.

Gastrointestinal system

caries (ka′re-ez, kar′ez)   The decay of teeth or bone.

distention (dis-ten′shun)   See under ROS vocabulary.

fissure (fish′er)   A slit or cracklike sore. For example, an anal fissure is a lineal ulcer at the border of the anus.

fistula (fis′tu-lah)   An abnormal tubelike passage from a tube, organ, or cavity to another cavity or organ or from an internal organ to a free body surface.

hemorrhoid (hem′or-roid)   A varicose (enlarged) vein in the mucous membrane just outside (external hemorrhoid) or inside (internal hemorrhoid) the rectum. Also called *piles,* these enlarged veins may be painful and itchy and may bleed.

peristalsis (per″i-stal′sis)   A wavelike movement by which tubular organs and the alimentary canal propel their contents. Peristalsis is an involuntary movement seen in tubes that have both circular and longitudinal layers of smooth muscle fibers.

Reproductive system

adnexa (ad-nek′sah)   Accessory organs of the uterus (ovaries, uterine tubes, and ligaments).

atrophy (at′roo-fe)   A decrease in size of organs or tissues after having reached full functional development. Atrophy is seen in the female reproductive organs after menopause.

gravida   See under ROS vocabulary.

introitus (in-tro′itus)   The opening into a body cavity or canal, as the opening into the vagina.

involution (in″vol-lu′shun)   The retrogressive change in the size and the vital processes of organs and tissues after they have fulfilled their functions, such as seen after menopause or in the reduction in size of the uterus after birth.

parous   See under ROS vocabulary.

Musculoskeletal (MS) system

crepitation (krep″i-ta′shun)   A crackling, grating sound produced by movement of the ends of a fractured bone.

exostosis (ek″sos-to′sis)   A new bony growth arising and projecting from the surface of a bone, characteristically capped by cartilage.

flaccid   See under Abdomen.

gait (gat)   The style or manner in which a person walks.

kyphosis (ki-fo′sis); also called *hunchback*   When viewing a person from the side, the examiner sees an abnormal convexity in the curvature of the thoracic spine.

lordosis (lor-do′dis)   An abnormal forward curvature of the lumbar spine.

protuberance (pro-tu′ber-ans)   A part that projects or is prominent beyond the usual surface area.

rigidity   See under Abdomen

scoliosis (sko″le-o′sis)   A lateral curvature of the vertebral column that usually consists of two curves, one in the opposite direction from the first.

supple (sup′l)   Flexible, limber, or easily bent.

Extremities

claudication (klaw″di-ka′shun)   Limping, lameness.

intermittent claudication   A severe pain, tension, and weakness in the calf muscles that occurs after walking has begun and that subsides when walking stops and the limb has been resting. This condition is seen in patients with occlusive arterial disease in the limbs.

clubbing (klub′ing)   A process or result of rapid reproduction of the soft tissue on the ends of the fingers and toes, as seen in adults with long-standing pulmonary disease.

edema (e-de′mah)   An abnormal accumulation of fluid in the body's intercellular spaces. It can be local or general.

passive congestion (kon-jes′chun)   An abnormal accumulation of blood in an area on the body.

ulcer (ul′ser)   See under ROS vocabulary.

varicosity (var′i-kos′i-te) (pl. *varicosities*)   The condition of being varicose; a swollen, distended, enlarged, and twisted vein.

General

cachexia (kah-kek′se-ah)   A general state of ill health, wasting away, and malnutrition, as seen in many chronic diseases.

dehydration (de″hi-dra′shun)   The condition that results when water output exceeds water intake; the excessive loss of water from the tissues or body.

diaphoresis (di″ah-fo-re′sis)   Perspiration.

emaciation (e-ma″se-a′shun)   A condition in which the body is extremely thin and wasting away. Emaciation is generally caused by extreme malnutrition or diseases of the gastrointestinal tract.

fingerbreadth (fin′ger-bredth)   The width of the finger from side to side, used when measuring the width of something, such as a lesion, or when measuring the distance between two areas (for example, "two fingerbreadths from the umbilicus").

lethargic (leth″ar′gic)   The state of being indifferent, drowsy, or sluggish.

patulous (pat′u-lus)   The state of being open, spread apart widely, or distended.

tenderness (ten′der-nes)   A sensitivity to touch or pressure.

Small Business
An Entrepreneur's Plan

Small Business
An Entrepreneur's Plan

Lee A. Eckert
Saddleback Community College

J. D. Ryan
Saddleback Community College

Robert J. Ray

Harcourt Brace Jovanovich, Publishers
San Diego   New York   Chicago   Atlanta   Washington, D.C.
London   Sydney   Toronto

This book is for entrepreneurs everywhere:

May you prosper and grow rich.

May you be forever strong.

May you always ace the Big Guys.

A number of the case studies in this book are adapted from the authors' column, "Owning the Store," a weekly feature of the *Register* of Orange County, California. The authors gratefully acknowledge the publishers of the *Register* for permission to adapt this material.

Illustrations
Jennifer Hewiston, *Kull/Breidenthal Design*

ISBN: 0-15-581220-3

Printed in the United States of America

To the Instructor

The purpose of *Small Business: An Entrepreneur's Plan* is to make students "street smart" about creating, managing, and gaining profit from a business of their own. The book has gone through three tough semesters of prepublication testing, and over 2,000 of our students have succeeded in business by using the tools presented in this textbook.

You have undoubtedly looked at other small business texts. On page one, they begin, slowly, painfully, and steeped in gloom. On page two, they quote dark failure statistics, almost proudly, from the Small Business Administration. By page three, the student is feeling awful for even daring to think about small business.

This book is different.

We begin with hopes, dreams, and the sweet thrill of adventure. Then we carry the student, step by step, to the creation of a winning Business Plan.

A Business Plan is the key to success in small business.

What Is a Business Plan?

A Business Plan is a written document that provides goals and directions for a business. The business may be already up and running, or it may be still in the conceptual phase. A Business Plan works either way. Plans are flexible enough to meet any challenge. A plan for a retail store in a huge shopping mall will obviously differ from a plan for a computer repair facility run from the home, but all plans have four qualities in common: First, a Business Plan keeps those entrepreneurial energies on track; second, it provides a means of filtering out random business ideas that would otherwise waste time and soak up energy; third, it provides a logical pathway to success; and finally, it can act as a showcase that tells the world about your business.

Why is this planning concept so valuable to you and your students? Because a Business Plan is a natural teaching tool. It motivates. It monitors. It controls direction, screens data, deepens learning, and builds confidence. Best of all, it eases your judgmental burden as an instructor by providing an objective proving ground for glittery, half-baked ideas that may light the room with surface dazzle, but which, under scrutiny, are unsound.

The act of creating a Business Plan will of itself educate your students.

Organization of the Text

Each chapter of *Small Business* is linked to a specific section of the Business Plan. Some chapters serve as building blocks to help the student create the business section of the plan. Other chapters provide the student with the background necessary to understand and create the financial section (where three important financial statements create a moving picture of your business finances). A simple pie chart at the beginning of each chapter tells the student how that chapter relates to the finished plan.

We also include a chapter on the "why" and "how" of using a microcomputer in small business. We think no more useful tool exists for the busy entrepreneur. (The manuscript for this book was written on an IBM-PC using Easy Writer II.)

Action Steps

One of the keys to success in any adventure (whether going on safari, hunting for a job, or attending college) is to have the right motivation. To help motivate your students in the adventure of small business, we've provided a series of Action Steps that begin in a familiar realm—the student's concepts, dreams, and high hopes—and then move out into the marketplace, where the student learns through research how best to turn those dreams into reality.

The Action Steps cover all phases of business learning—industry analysis, the art of customer profiling, testing the competition, designing a promotional campaign, projecting finances, creating business opportunities, and so on—and they are expanded by over forty case studies that discuss business concepts in human terms.

By themselves, the Action Steps make quick reading, and all you have to do is choose the steps and make the assignments. The steps are previewed at the beginning of each chapter, reviewed at the end of each chapter, and indexed at the back of the book.

Additional Aids

Aside from the Action Steps, there are other aids to provide painless semesters:

Running Glossary. Key terms (positioning, product innovation, core market, Third Wave, pyramid hierarchy, and so on) are defined in the margin as they appear in the text. This simplifies the learning of key words, which is at the heart of any educational task.

Graphics. Complex step sequences like Power Marketing have been bolstered by illustrations, so as not to slow momentum. We are grateful to our publisher, who has made every attempt to keep the book accessible to your students.

Study Guide. Located at the back of the book, this guide provides enough ideas and projects to keep students involved and on track.

Instructor's Manual with Test Bank. It includes tests, teaching tips, ideas for discussion, suggestions for guest speakers, book reports, and projects in the marketplace.

In short, this package was designed with both the professor and the student in mind.

Our Wish

We hope you enjoy using *Small Business: An Entrepreneur's Plan* as much as we enjoyed writing it. We think small business is the wave of the future, the backbone of the country, and an especially promising opportunity that is often overlooked by women, minorities, and immigrants. We think small business is where the country is headed and how it will continue to grow economically. As small business educators, we want to ride the cutting edge of entrepreneurship—right out to the stars.

Along those lines, we'd like to hear from you. If you develop something for teaching small business that you'd be willing to share, please write us in care of the publisher.

Good luck with the book.

Acknowledgments

We couldn't have written this book without a lot of help from a lot of people. The book is built on a foundation of case studies, with Action Steps taken from real life tactics in the marketplace.

Someone has tried to do it out there in the real world. We just wrote it down.

Our thanks go to: Spike Atkinson, owner-operator, Clavo's Cantina; Ron Barley, president, B/T Western Corporation; Greg Beck, of Beck, Wilson and Nolan, a law corporation; Robert Bulmahn and Pam Bulmahn, microcomputer consultants; Lynn Dick, owner-operator, Travel Country of Irvine; Jean Femling, freelance writer, Costa Mesa; Jim Grammer, president, Gramco Manufacturing; Jim Hodgson, president, Syllabus, Inc.; Murry Katzen, group operations manager, Levitz Furniture Corporation; Michael M. Kolbenschlag, business editor, the *Register* of Orange County; Jean Lowe and Ron Lowe, owner-operators, Swedish AutoService; Marjorie Luesebrink, professor, Saddleback Community College; Mort Meiers, instructor in small business, Lake Tahoe Community College; Ginny Metz, co-owner/operator, Shoppers' Shuttle; Cheryl Moore, owner-operator, Broek-Moore Store for Cooks; Barbara Moss and Tom Moss, co-owners, The Pleasure Company, Inc.; Howard Snyder and Nancy Snyder, owner-operators, Totem Book Store; Terry Thorpe, Saddleback Community College; Steve Waddell, U.S. Small Business Administration; and Jim Weaver, owner-operator, Toy Junction.

We are also grateful to our reviewers, who gave us suggestions for revision that made the book smoother and better: Colleen Demaris, Bellevue Community College; Carol Eliason, director, National Small Business Training Network of the American Association of Community and Junior Colleges; Evelyn Fine, Daytona Beach Community College; Dale E. Kerby, Albuquerque Technical-Vocational Institute; Judy Nye, associate director, National Small Business Training Network, and director, Women's Business Programs, of the American Association of Community and Junior Colleges; Norman Pacula, College of Marin; Harry J. Swanson, coordinator, Small Business Development Center, Southern Utah State College; and Raymond S. Weisler, professor of business administration, California State University, Dominguez Hills. And we are grateful to Charles McCormick and Bill Teague of Harcourt Brace Jovanovich for their willingness to work with us when the going got tough.

LEE A. ECKERT

J. D. RYAN

ROBERT J. RAY

Contents

Owning the store is the Great American Dream. Henry Ford started small; so did Apple Computers. Small business is going to be even more dynamic in the Information Society. Market gaps will open, and entrepreneurs with dreams and fast foot-work will fill the gaps before big business, with its layers of bureaucracy, can begin to move. There are two tricks to success: (1) Study the market with New Eyes; and (2) write a Business Plan that keeps your creativity on track.

How to understand the large trends at work in our society, and how to recognize business opportunities as they develop—these are skills any entrepreneur needs. We show you these skills and more: How to apply the life-cycle yardstick to any industry, how to read a customer's life-style from a shopping cart or from a walk through the customer's neighborhood, and how to analyze any industry to discover market gaps.

The secret of market research in small business is a tool called Power Marketing, represented by a funnel that allows you to take in everything—your own hopes and dreams, business objectives, industry research, problems and opportunities, and mad solutions—and organize it along a matrix for your consideration. As if by magic, your options become clear, and you can choose a solid business idea that will suit your needs.

The Target Customer is the key to your survival in small business. Know the buying habits of your Target Customer, and you can't fail. By profiling your Target Customer, you can refocus your product or service. Profiling should be a continuous process in any business. This chapter gives you techniques to make profiling fun as well.

corporations. Included in this chapter are probing questions you can ask a lawyer to determine which form of ownership—and which lawyer—is right for you.

Entrepreneurs have lots of energy, much foresight, and big egos. We encourage you to find out where you are strong and where you are weak. Then we give you techniques to help you build a balanced team that will complement your strengths. We also suggest sources for finding good people and ways to make the most of your people resources once you have assembled them.

This chapter offers special help for people interested in buying or franchising an existing business. Every business in the country is for sale sooner or later—including a lot of losers. The losers are usually easy to spot, because they're listed in the newspaper ads. Better deals are often found elsewhere. If you play detective, really investigate, know your industry, and luck onto a hungry seller, you can get a deal on everything from terms to used equipment.

The computer works for small business both as a tool and as a symbol. As a tool, it helps you become more effective wherever highly repetitive tasks are involved. As a symbol, it points to the future. In this chapter we discuss the right way to shop for a computer system, and we include a list of do's and don'ts for the first-time computer buyer.

Your Business Plan is your road map to riches in small business. It will keep you on track when your creativity threatens to derail you. It will tell the world what business you're in. And it's portable enough to be sent anywhere. This final chapter rounds out your entrepreneurial journey by bringing all the data home—and by helping you organize a winning Business Plan.

How to Use This Book

This book tells you how to create a tool that could save your life and make you rich. The tool is called a Business Plan. And the great thing is that you build the plan yourself—around your personality, around your own dreams, around your own small business.

Your Business Plan is a document that provides goals and directions for your business. It's very personal, very private; yet it is also a show-case. When it's finished—typed, enclosed in a snappy folder, supported by numbers, photographs, letters of reference, and diagrams—your Business Plan tells the world (bankers, vendors and lenders, venture capital-ists, credit managers, key employees, family, friends, and so on) what business you're in.

Your finished plan is a blueprint for your business. It provides a walk-through of your industry, excites potential lenders, shows what a great planner you are, and underlines the reasons customers are going to clamor for your product or service. When customers clamor, you get rich.

Having a showcase is important. But the plan in process has a second function—channeling your creative energies. One reason you're reading this book is because you're creative. You like to build, to pull things together, to plant seeds and watch things grow, to develop projects, and to produce results. When your mind is cooking, you probably have the feeling you could start a new business venture every four hours.

That's when you need a plan—to keep your entrepreneurial energies on track while the creative steam rises. A Business Plan keeps your creativity grooved.

You've always had this dream of working for yourself, of being your own boss, of owning the store. Don't destroy your dream by entering the grand arena unprepared. Read the book. Put yourself through the paces. Exercise those winning muscles. And *Small Business: An Entrepreneur's Plan* will help you get where you want to go by giving you a personalized road map.

You start with your own dreams of success. You work through 68 Action Steps. You wind up at the end with a street-smart Business Plan. And when you take a breather and look back, you'll have some exciting memories.

If at this stage you feel overwhelmed, don't worry. Other entrepreneurs have started out just where you are now. You can read about them in the case studies in this book—studies based on people in real life—friends, associates, fellow entrepreneurs, students—although the names have been changed. And the lessons they've learned, we're passing on to you.

We'll also help you focus your energies by showing you—with a pie chart at the beginning of each chapter—how far you have progressed toward completing your Business Plan. There are two sections to the finished plan, as shown in Figure A. Section I, The Business, is made up of seven building blocks (see Figure B). Here you describe the important aspects of your business idea. Section II, Financial Statements, consists of three financial statements (see Figure C). Here, thanks to a lot of careful research and computation, you prove that your dream can be made a reality.

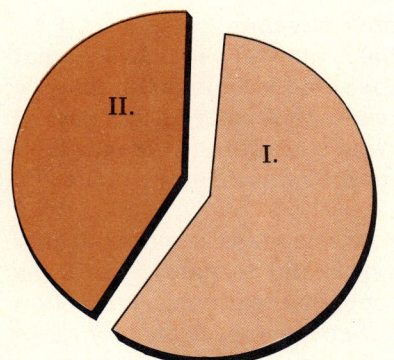

I. The Business

II. Financial Statements

FIGURE A
Your finished Business Plan will back up a complete description of your business with detailed financial statements.

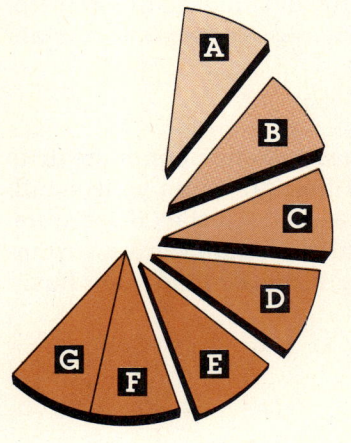

A Description of Product or Service

B The Market and the Target Customer

C Competition

D Marketing Strategy

E Location

F Management

G Personnel

FIGURE B
The business section is made of seven building blocks as shown.

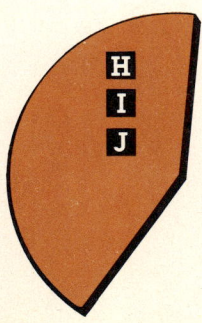

H Projected Income Statement (Profit and Loss)

I Projected Cash Flow

J Projected Balance Sheet

FIGURE C
The final result of all your work on finances will be three financial statements.

Study Guide

Another aid to help you understand the text and to help you create a plan for your business is the Study Guide at the back of the book. Objective questions test your knowledge of basic concepts; short-answer questions serve as worksheets that will help you complete various Action Steps—just as the short-answer questions that follow will help you with Action Step 1. The Study Guide is perforated, so you can take relevant pages with you out into the arena of the marketplace, and so you can hand in pages for review as requested by your instructor. Completed sections of the Study Guide can be removed to serve as rough notes for the completion of your Business Plan.

The Fast-Track Entrepreneur and the Creative Dreamer

Your instructor will set the pace for your class, but you should know that you can read this book on at least two levels. One level is fast-track. It's for the action-oriented entrepreneur, who wants to get started right away. The other level is for the creative dreamer, who can afford to take the time to savor the atmosphere in the arena of small business, and who enjoys taking things as they come.

On the fast track, you can read the 68 Action Steps throughout this book to lock in your own personal overview and to gain a compass reading of where you are heading. (For people in a real hurry, the Action Steps are indexed at the end of this book.) Then come back and complete each step. (If you're already in business, you may want to be even more selective. You can turn directly to the chapter that most interests you—Chapter 10, Shaking the Money Tree, or Chapter 12, Fun-Time: Building Your Winning Team.) On the other track, you are given the background for each Action Step as it appears. The text provides information to help you act, while numerous case studies show business concepts in human terms.

Your First Action Step

If you're unsure which category (action-oriented entrepreneur or creative dreamer) applies to you, Action Step 1 will help. It starts your small business adventure by asking you to profile yourself—just as if you were a Target Customer. Use the spaces provided to make sure you know your dreams and your personality—the first step in developing your Business Plan.

How would your best friend describe you?

_____

_____

How would your worst enemy describe you?

_____

_____

How would you describe yourself?

_____

How much money do you need to survive?

_____

How much money do you need to do everything you wish to do?

_____

What's your education level?

_____

What's your occupation?

_____

Where do you live now? (Describe home, residential area, geographical area, amenities, and so on.)

_____

_____

_____

_____

Where would you like to live?

_____

_____

_____

Profile Yourself as if You Were a Target Customer

Who are you? What do you want out of life? To find out, we're going to introduce you to a concept that we'll discuss more fully in Chapter 4. It's called profiling your Target Customer. Only this time, *you* are the one being profiled.

Answer the questions that appear in the text. Write your answers in the spaces provided—this is *your* book to use as *you* want—and by the time you are finished, you'll have completed your first profile. Then take a look at the person you've just described. That person is the budding entrepreneur.

What's the ideal small business for that person to get into? The answer to that question is found in the rest of this book.

Before you continue, mark the space provided to show that you've completed the Action Step.

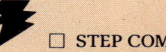 ☐ STEP COMPLETED

What is your current net worth?

_____

What do you spend the most money on each month?

_____

_____

How long is your vacation?

_____

How long would you like it to be?

_____

Look around your house and begin to list products you have bought from firms that see you in their sights as their Target Customer.

_____

_____

_____

_____

_____

_____

Small Business
An Entrepreneur's Plan

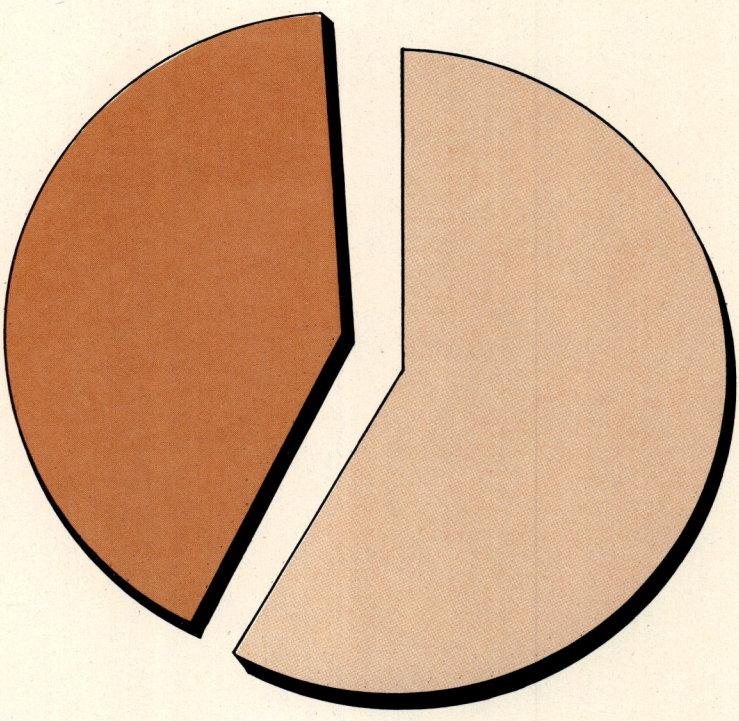

FIGURE 1.1 Before you begin your Business Plan, investigate doorways to the Information Society.

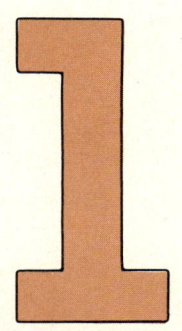

Doorways to the Information Society — Your Great Adventure

To understand where business is headed in the next 5–10 years.

To learn how you fit in and how you can survive, prosper, and get rich.

To brainstorm your way to a clear picture of success in small business.

To identify successful (and unsuccessful) businesses in your community, so you can use them as guidelines.

To discover your personal strengths for developing an accomplishment-oriented skills picture.

To hone your information-gathering skills so that you can experience the excitement of doing effective research.

To expand your knowledge of small business by going out into the marketplace and interviewing small business owners.

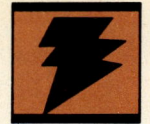 Welcome to the Information Society.

Briefly, the Information Society is a massive movement of an entire civilization away from industry and smokestacks and assembly lines — and toward the computer and every business that is remotely computer-connected. The Information Society is an outgrowth of the nation's move towards a service economy, which began in earnest in 1945, at the end of World War II.

If you're an intrepid entrepreneur — ready to start the great adventure of small business — this could be your golden moment.

THE AGE OF INFORMATION

Alvin Toffler writes about the coming Age of Information in *The Third Wave* and also in *Previews and Premises.* John Naisbitt writes about the Information Society/Economy in *Megatrends*, a crystal ball in book form which forecasts the next 10–15 years. For the busy entrepreneur, *Megatrends* is a must read.

Writing early in the 1980s Naisbitt predicted that by the mid eighties 75% of all jobs will "involve" computers. His prediction has come true. Our latest statistics place the total revenue of the Information Industry at $800 billion, which means that Information will soon be half of the Gross National Product.

What that means for small business is opportunity. Because if you can produce information, or copy it, or transmit it, or speed it up, or float it in like money from London to Singapore, or educate people about it, or service the machinery that produces it, or feed and clothe and entertain the people who specialize in information — Toffler calls them **mind workers** — you can prosper in small business.

Entrepreneurial Opportunities in Mind Work

To get a handle on information, you may have to **reposition** yourself. You'll probably have to learn a new skill or two. But you can do it. And you can win at it. And you can have fun doing it.

If the Information Society seems remote, take a look at this list of jobs that directly involve mind work:

teacher	engineer
stock broker	bureaucrat
librarian	politician
architect	writer
social worker	newspaper reporter
personnel analyst	editor
banker	clergy

mind workers
information specialists in
the Information Society

reposition
strategic adjustments to
the fluid state of the market

secretary	lawyer
health professional	insurance person
researcher	clerk
accountant	advertising executive
artist	salesperson

People in these jobs deal in information.

Tom Jackson, in his terrific book *Guerrilla Tactics in the Job Market,* predicts two things about your working life:

1. You will change jobs 10 times during your lifetime.
2. You will change career paths 3 – 4 times!

One of those career paths could very well be in the arena of small business — owning the store, working for yourself, not taking orders, being your own boss for a change. All you have to do is locate the right doorway and be prepared to step through it when the gong sounds.

Toffler's Waves

As you read these words, we are poised between the Second and Third waves, between the smoky remnants of the Industrial Age and the oncoming computer beeps that herald the Age of Information.

Industrial Age machinery still exists, but the Industrial Age yardsticks (depression, recession, industrial averages, and GNP) have lost much of their meaning. Furthermore, the new buzzwords — cognitariat, mind map, high touch/high tech, decision load, megabyte, mind worker, networking, and role diversity — don't seem to measure our progress with much precision.

THE NEW MARKETPLACE

When the old yardsticks don't work, society gets the shakes. When society gets the shakes, cracks open in the corporate floor, tastes get more specialized, and new market **gaps** appear.

That's good news for the alert **entrepreneur.** Entrepreneurs have a keen sense of trends, of change, of which way the wind is blowing in the marketplace. Entrepreneurs are insatiably curious. They read. They listen.

Derek Campbell was like that:

"After five years of faithful service as a pilot, I was furloughed by the airline that employed me, so I had time to look around and think about my future. One of the books I read was *Megatrends*. It was like seeing a lighthouse beacon after a long and dark sea-voyage."

gap
an area in the market where emerging demands are not being met

entrepreneur
a visionary self-starter who loves the adventure of the new enterprise

Derek Campbell — Information Engineer

When Derek Campbell was furloughed the third time from his pilot's job with a major airline, he was frustrated and angry at the world. Derek had done his work, and he'd loved flying the big planes, but the airline industry was in chaos. Size didn't make any difference. Even the giants were in trouble.

''Three furloughs and you're out,'' Derek said. ''For me, that was the handwriting on the wall. I was fed up with working for someone else, tired of being a puppet on someone else's string. It was time to call a few tunes of my own.''

Like a lot of entrepreneurs, Derek was a workaholic. His first move was to make a list of his past accomplishments, his strengths, his skills. He had a bachelor's degree in engineering, an M.B.A., and several years of experience as an instructor in the Marines.

And — he'd always been interested in computers.

Derek hired himself out as a computer consultant. His work was largely on the phone, making contacts, locating prospects. Then he'd go out for a location visit and size up the problems.

''Literally everyone on my list could have used some kind of computer,'' Derek recalls. ''And that's what gave me the idea to start an educational facility. There was, on the one hand, a crying need for more efficiency. And on the other hand, there was a lot of fear and misunderstanding about computers in general and about small computers in particular.''

So Derek kept his consulting business going while he organized a founder's team to help him brainstorm strategies for a computer school. It was an interesting mix of men and women: two lawyers, another ex-pilot, a banker, a marketeer from big business, a numbers wizard, and an expert in corporate mergers.

Derek used his microcomputer to create a stunning 85-page **Business Plan.** The plan helped him get a line of credit from a local bank for $40,000. And nine months after the idea had first hit him, Derek and his team ran their first class — Computer Fundamentals.

''Planning makes all the difference,'' Derek says. ''The minute we opened the doors, we had business. That told us we had targeted our industry, and our particular segment, accurately. Of course, if you don't stay in there punching, don't keep your image right out there, trade tends to fall off. But **gap analysis** helped us find our foothold in the marketplace — computer education — and it's paying off fast. We're in the information business to stay. We're not pushing hardware. We're not pushing software. We're here to teach people how to help themselves by learning the vast capabilities of the microcomputer.''

Derek leans back, clasps his hands behind his head, and smiles.

''And the best part of all is — it's great fun!''

Business Plan
a blueprint for your business expansion or start-up

gap analysis
a sophisticated tool for locating and measuring market potential

What can we learn from Derek Campbell?

1. He was able to turn adversity into opportunity.
2. He knew his strengths: engineering, teaching, computers.
3. He saw a gap in the marketplace.
4. He knew where to go for information to develop a terrific

Business Plan. (The plan proved on paper that his computer school would earn him a handsome return on his investment.)

5. He was ready for self-employment.

Derek Campbell became a beneficiary of the Information Age.

The First Wave was Agriculture. Most workers were farmers or farm workers. The *Second Wave* was Industry. Most workers were laborers. If you look back over your shoulder at the seventies, you can see the crumbling structures of our Industrial Age — GM, Exxon, Ford, Texaco, TWA, and so on. They dominated the world. As the Information Society approaches, we can ask — how effective were those huge organizations? In what areas are they now vulnerable?

Second Wave
the Industrial Age, which began with the Industrial Revolution

MAJOR CORPORATE GIANTS SHRINK AS AGE OF INDUSTRY FADES

Each year, *Fortune* magazine publishes a list of the 500 largest firms in the nation. In April, 1984, *Fortune* came to Naisbitt's conclusion — the giants no longer create new jobs. In fact, during the decade of the seventies, the word among the *Fortune* 500 was "retrenchment" or cutting back, and that's what they did.

They cut employment 10%, from 15.5 million to 14 million jobs. At the same time, sales per employee rose 11.5% during the seventies.

Impressive? Yes. Survival always is. But at the same time, the nation's small businesses created 6 million new jobs.

Let's hear it for small business.

There are now more than 16 million small businesses in the United States, which make up 97% of all nonfarm businesses. Sixty-six percent of all new jobs were created by small businesses between 1970 and 1980. The *only* new jobs created, nearly a million, between 1980 and 1982 were created by small businesses.

Why do these new firms survive? Because they are founded by people who are not afraid of risk. Because they can effect changes quickly, without going through umpteen layers of managers and vice-presidents. Because they are in touch with their customers. Because — they are not huge.

THE MYTH OF SMALL BUSINESS FAILURE

You can't talk to anyone on the street about small business without having the subject of failure come up. Indeed, the Small Business Administration (SBA) tells us that 55% of all small businesses fail in their first five years. That's not true! The SBA bases its conclusions on the U.S. Census of Business, which is taken in every year that ends in a 2 or a 7.

So, if you start a business in 1987, and you aren't at the same address when 1992 rolls around, you go down on the charts as another failure.

Or, if you start out as a sole proprietor and then take on a partner and change your business name and then merge with a corporation and move into the corporate GHQ, you go down on the charts as a failure.

Or, if you latch onto a trendy fad, ride it for a year or 18 months, then take your profits and go on vacation, you're classified as a failure. We know for a fact that's what happened to Mr. Dahl, the man who created the Pet Rock back in the seventies. He found a fad. He produced a product to take advantage of the fad. When the fad wound down, Mr. Dahl took his profits and left the marketplace.

That's not failure. That's smart marketing.

What is a Small Business?

For the past three decades, businesses have been classified by a coding system known as Standard Industrial Classification Codes. You've probably heard the abbreviation, SIC. (We deal with SIC codes in depth in the next chapter.) When you go to the SBA to borrow money, they use three criteria, linked to SIC codes, to determine how small is small. They say a business is a small business if:

1. It does not dominate the industry.
2. It has less than $10 million in annual sales.
3. It has less than 1,000 employees.

There are exceptions to all of these.

For the purposes of this book, a small business is any venture with spirit, any business you want to start, any idea you want to chase into the marketplace. It could be part-time, something you do at home, something you try alone, something you need a team for.

If you prove it out on paper first, there's a good chance you'll be successful.

If you plan to win, there's a good chance you'll win.

If You Fail to Plan, You're Planning to Fail!

To get the maximum benefit from this book, you'll need to go beyond its pages and experience the risk and joy and thrust of entrepreneurship. You'll read a lot, of course. You'll construct your own Plan.

The Action Steps will help you plan. They'll also give you energy boosts, and that helps your momentum. You've already taken a crack at profiling yourself as a consumer in Action Step 1. In the next Action Step, you'll focus on some of your past accomplishments. The purpose here is to give you confidence. After all, you've come this far, right?

Action Step 2 is designed to trigger your imagination and get you rolling. Small business is your dream, it reflects your personality, and when you start planning, you'll learn more about yourself than you'd ever learn from group therapy or from years with a psychiatrist.

ACTION ⚡ STEP 2

Explore Your Past Accomplishments

Begin by listing all the things in your life that you're proud of. What, for example, gave you the most satisfaction? What is your sweetest memory? How old were you? What were you doing at the time? Were you alone or with someone? How did it feel to be victorious? How did it feel to be in control?

Then move to the present. Where are you now? What about the future? Where do you want to be in three years? In five years? In 10? In 20?

Spend some time on this list. Share it with friends. Ask for their input. And don't ever finish compiling.

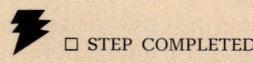
⬜ STEP COMPLETED

Remember, you're an entrepreneur. You can adapt to the changes in the marketplace quickly, while large firms are locked in by their corporate hierarchy. This Action Step gives you the confidence to get rolling.

The same thing happened to Joe Talmadge. He inventoried his skills and interests. He'd already known the thrill of bringing a new product into the marketplace. But he was frustrated working for someone else.

Frustration can be a creative force, especially when it's experienced by the right individual.

Frustration made Joe Talmadge even more inventive.

Case Study

Joe Talmadge — Liqueur Expert

The autumn that Bailey's Irish Cream hit the marketplace, Joe Talmadge was working as a specialty liqueur marketing expert for a major distillery.

The figures for that fall speak for themselves. The suppliers had 100,000 cases of Bailey's in the marketplace. They thought it would last through Christmas — which was two months away. The market surprised everyone. The Bailey's sold out in four days. And Joe Talmadge saw an opportunity — a gap in cream-based liqueurs.

In his kitchen at home, Joe and his wife got creative with different old family recipes until they came up with a smooth taste. He wanted to **position** his product against Ireland, the home of Bailey's, so he found a family of winemakers in Italy. They'd been in business for 300 years, which gave Joe the sense of history he wanted, and they had a fantastic supply of old bottle molds — embossed with their regal family crest — and that gave Joe the image he was after.

Gambling a little, Joe named his liqueur Creme de Napoli.

There were problems — manufacturing, distribution, the basic instability of cream, the Italian government and its endless red tape — but Joe persevered and selectively spent money in his test market. It took several months, but he gradually expanded his market area, proving he had a winner. And two years after he had concocted the recipe for Creme de Napoli at his kitchen table, Joe Talmadge sold the product to a major international liquor maker.

How much did he get? Creme de Napoli sold for just under seven figures. That's almost $1 million. As part of the deal, he was hired by the purchasers for one year at a very good salary.

But Joe Talmadge is an entrepreneur. He loves risk. He likes being in control. Working for someone else frustrates him. And six months after selling Creme de Napoli, he had left the international liquor giant and started his own independent marketing and consulting business.

Joe understands the market. He solves problems. He travels. He loves his work. And he is financially secure so that he doesn't have to work unless he chooses to.

When Joe Talmadge thinks back, he remembers how it all started at his kitchen table, being creative, working with his wife, taste-testing, trying to come up with a product to position against Bailey's.

position
your niche in the eyes of
your Target Customer

GETTING ORGANIZED

How can you operate like Joe Talmadge? First, you need to get organized — which brings us to Action Step 3. After all, you can't join the Information Society until you get your own information organized.

What's keeping you from getting organized?

Some people resist the advice given in Action Step 3 because they have the feeling that getting organized will stifle their creativity. Travel Agent Marci Reid was like that. Then she learned the value of starting her own Adventure Notebook.

Case Study

Marci Reid — Travel Agent

Marci Reid loved to travel, so when she graduated from high school, she went right out and got herself a job with a travel agency. For 14 months, she was a secretary, until she learned the business. From her first week, Marci kept a diary form of notebook, listing what seemed to be important elements of the travel business.

For the next dozen years, Marci worked for three different agencies. The notebook grew. She spent four years in Europe — France, the Greek islands, Spain — and when she returned home she knew it was time to strike out on her own. Her notebook now filled four volumes.

"I can do this better," Marci said to a friend. "I know the business. All I need are a few more business skills. Then I can have my own agency." So, Marci talked with a friend she'd been considering for a partner. Then Marci enrolled in a course in entrepreneurship. She wanted help in refining her voluminous notes into a workable Business Plan.

Here's what Marci said about it all in retrospect:

"That first night in class, it was made really clear that you've got to plan every move. I admit I fought the idea at first, mostly because I was so eager to get started, but also because I was worried that too much planning would throttle my creativity. But then as I went through each step of building the business plan, the patterns began to appear and I got a glimpse of how things would work out in the long run and I didn't feel cramped at all. My travel industry diary turned into an **Adventure Notebook.**

"It was high anxiety there at first. Our contractor was four months behind, so we were forced to rent space that was almost ten miles away from our **Target Customers.** When we couldn't get our location right away, our banker chopped our line of credit in half. Luckily, we had followed the advice of our teachers and we had a **backup bank.** Then an airline strike forced us to stay up three nights rerouting customers. Without a plan, we'd have gone under.

"Now that Adventures in Travel is three years old, my partner and I are thinking about another start-up. The other evening, I brought out my Adventure Notebook — the one I'd used to plan our travel agency — and read it through. I was amazed at its accuracy, and what it proves is that you can do a lot in life if you get organized."

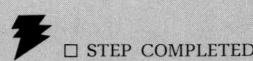

ACTION STEP 3

Organize Your Information

If you're the typical entrepreneur, you probably put 90% of your important data on the back of an envelope.

Good work. Now that you're doing this for real, get yourself an organizer, some kind of container (a shoebox, a briefcase, a folder) to put those old envelopes in.

Or treat yourself to an Adventure Notebook — spiral-bound, three-ring — something with pockets so you can keep track of small items like ticket stubs.

Give this organizer a name. Name it something creative, so that it reflects the mood of your adventure.

Write everything down.

Make lists.

And while you're at it, remember to keep written records of your expenses for the IRS.

☐ STEP COMPLETED

Adventure Notebook
storage place for valuable
business information

Target Customer
a customer with the
highest probability of
buying your product or
service

backup bank
a bank which offers
alternative financial
resources

Most people begin a new business with less planning than they give the family vacation.

Marci's Adventure Notebook was the incubator for ideas that became the Business Plan that proved, on paper, that she could be successful. As they continue in business, Marci and her partner continue to up-date their plan. In the next chapter, we'll show you how to select a business idea and how to start planning for its success.

WHAT IS SUCCESS?

Success is how you define it.

Action Step 4 is optional, but fun. Thinking about success can be stimulating and enlightening. What makes a business successful? Unsuccessful? How do you measure success? How do your friends measure it?

Action Step 4 relies on guesswork as to what businesses are doing well. Only a detailed examination of their books would provide total accuracy. But we still urge you to exercise your marketplace intuition. Personal observation is a good way to open your awareness to what might be happening to small firms in your community.

For example, next time you eat out, try this:

Estimate the number of customers while you're there.

Estimate the total number of customers for the day.

Estimate the average cost per meal.

Multiply average cost times total number of customers.

Pretty soon, you'll begin to get the feel for who is not winning. Observe the small businesses you patronize with **New Eyes** and success factors will begin to emerge.

Success is something only you can judge. Income is measurable. So is Return-on-Investment (ROI). But success wears many faces, and you need to think about that as you start your adventure.

Try the following checklist on success. At the end, add other items that might be special to you?

Is success measured for you in dollars? How many?

_____$25K a year.

_____$50K.

_____$100K.

_____$250K.

_____$1,000,000.

_____Return-on-Investment. How much?

Or is success measured in other ways?

_____Being able to enjoy a certain lifestyle.

_____Friendly customers who appreciate the service.

 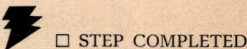
New Eyes

Every day you are exposed to the secrets of business success, and also of business failure. Just by taking the blinders off and looking around, you can teach yourself a lot about how to succeed in small business. We call this process, ''Seeing with New Eyes.''

Henry Ford used New Eyes when he observed the assembly method of dressing beef in the Chicago stockyards. He borrowed the concept for auto assembly and the rest is history.

Seeing with New Eyes is a concept we'll return to again and again as we go through this book.

_____Power.

_____Being able to live where you want.

_____Providing employment for others.

_____Being the best business for your area.

_____Looking out the door and seeing long lines waiting for your service.

_____Time to do what you want.

_____Teamwork — a smooth operation, with lots of key employees reporting to you.

_____Fame — your face on TV, your name a household word.

_____Control — things always done your way.

Or is success measured by concrete achievements, like the car you drive or the location of your dream house? Where would you rather live?

_____ In the heart of a lavish upscale residential area.

_____ A penthouse, atop a tall building, in the poshest metropolitan area of your choice.

_____ Anywhere that's safe.

_____ A place where your kids can play.

_____ A quiet cabin on a quiet lake looking out across clear blue water.

_____ A fancy city apartment, beautifully decorated.

_____ A tropical island, isolated, quiet.

What special items measure success for you?

_____

_____

_____

INFORMATION AND YOU

Self-Knowledge as Information

The people who thrive in the Information Society know how to organize information so that it becomes effective — and therefore valuable. As we describe the new Information Society, we're also introducing you to a new source of information — yourself. If you can gather self-knowledge and then organize it to make it effective, you'll have a valuable base of information to use in determining the best entrepreneurial path for you.

You already have an idea of how you view success. Now complete Action Step 5 to see how equipped you are to get it. Action Step 5 asks you to examine **personal skills** — and the result will greatly add to your store of information.

Once you have a better picture of your own skills, you will be better equipped to see correspondences between what you can do and what

personal skills
your strengths, where you shine, the tools that help you grow

needs to be done around you. Does it seem strange to inventory your own skills like this? It shouldn't.

It is not too late to get to know yourself, especially if you're going to change career paths three to four times in one lifetime.

English major Nancy Tremaine learned in her career that she possessed highly developed communication skills. As writers go, Nancy was moderately successful. But she wanted more. She learned to look at herself and at the marketplace with New Eyes. That defrosted her frozen mind-set. When Nancy's perceptions thawed, she became a more successful person by her own individual standards.

Case Study

Nancy Tremaine — English Major

Nancy grew up reading books and keeping a diary, so when she went to college, she decided to major in English literature. When her parents asked her what she would do when she got out of school, Nancy always told them she would teach.

Well, the economy sagged and things didn't turn out that way.

When Nancy graduated, there were no jobs in teaching. She worked as a secretary for a while, then tried sales, then did a long stint as a copy editor for a couple of magazines.

She was thirty before she began to write.

She wrote novels. She got encouragement from her friends. She was disappointed when nothing sold. She kept on writing. She wrote all night long. In the morning, she would drag herself to work. Her job suffered. When circulation figures dropped, the magazine had to make cutbacks. Nancy lost her job.

Now she was scared.

She had a little money saved. She would write all morning, then hunt for a job in the afternoon. She sold two articles. The money kept her going for a while. Then a friend told her about a marketing class at the local college. At first, Nancy wasn't interested. Art was her life. Marketing was for the masses.

The friend dragged Nancy to the course.

Surprise: Nancy found herself more interested than she could ever have imagined. That next term, she registered for Marketing I.

Three things struck her right away:

1. "We live in a **marketing lab,**" the teacher said. "And someone is always testing to see what our consumption patterns are. When you market, do the same."
2. "It doesn't take all that much to be better than your competition," the teacher said. "All you really have to do is look around with New Eyes."
3. "Henry Ford has a great saying," the teacher said. "He'd call up Production and say: 'Color? They want color? Give them any color so long as it's black.'"

Nancy liked that image — rows and rows of black Model T Fords on an endless production line. The image of Henry Ford's black cars re-

Continued

 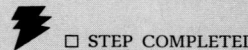

Inventory Your Personal Skills

What's in your skills repertoire that will launch you into the hot growth industries?

Now that you've had your fling at dreaming, interact with reality by listing all the things you can do and are good at.

What kind of work do you do?

What kind do you really enjoy?

What are your hobbies?

What really excites you?

Do you like to work alone?

Are you a self-starter?

If you were to ask three people who really know you to list your three major skills, what would they say?

Circle your skills — sell, write, negotiate, soothe, counsel, synthesize, coordinate, create, analyze, compile, teach, persuade, tend, plant, nurture, supervise, help out, copy, add and subtract, follow instructions, delegate, lead.

Make a list of your top five. Make a list of the five that are impossible for you.

□ STEP COMPLETED

marketing lab
a slice of the real world
made manageable so you
can test, test, test

minded her of a writer who writes without thinking of the reader. Both were trapped in a production mind-set.

She chose K-mart as her marketing lab. She went in to look around with New Eyes. She was standing at the book racks, thinking of Henry Ford, when it hit her.

Here's Nancy:

"Suddenly, I remembered what the marketing teacher had been saying. '*Look Around.* Where are the lines? The crowds? What's turning people on?' To humor him, I looked around.

"Off to the left, there were 37 kids playing arcade games. Behind me, about 20 people were watching Monday night football. Off to my right, a line of people stood at the credit window.

"I was about to give it up when it hit me. Games. Escape. Amusement. Money. Was I excited! I went through the store, taking notes, and when I finished I had 72 ideas I knew would make me rich. I could have kicked myself for not noticing any of this before.

"The next day, I made an appointment with my marketing prof and he helped me narrow down my choices with something he called a decision filter. [Decision filters are discussed in Chapter 3.] I realized I'd had my head buried in the sand for more than a dozen years."

On the advice of the marketing teacher, Nancy did a thorough skills analysis. She discovered in herself qualities of nurturing, tending, creating, negotiating, and exploring. She was always a good writer, and now she developed marketing tools to help her aim words at specific audiences.

Her new novel, aimed at the shoppers she'd observed that night in K-mart, sold. When she had sold three more, Nancy gathered a core group of three writing friends, taught them her techniques, and started a seminar business for writers.

She now employs 17 people in her seminar business. Nancy has joined the Information Society. And her discovery of her skills has allowed her to do what she wanted to do in the first place — teach.

The Importance of Research

Research opens doors to the Information Society. There are three approaches to research. You'll need a combination of all three to make it big in small business.

1. Primary Research.   That's interacting with the world. Talking to people. Interviewing. Asking small business owners where they were when the entrepreneurial bug bit, who they bank with, what luck they've had with lawyers and accountants, what they'd change the second time around.

primary research
direct interaction with the world through interviews and observation

2. Secondary Research.   That's when you read, secondhand, what someone else has discovered. You go to the *Business Index* in the library. You look up "Small Business." You locate magazines or newspapers which contain information you think will be helpful.

Or you write off to trade associations in your industry. You find data on sales that will help you project how much money you can make in small business. Good techniques here will save you lots of footwork.

3. New Eyes Research.   You play detective. You become the Mystery Shopper as you check out your competition. You sit in your car and take telephoto pictures of a business you're thinking of buying. When Target Customers appear, you photograph them so you can profile them later. You stand in a supermarket, trying not to look nosy, and observe what's in the shopping carts.

Steak + Scotch + Cigarettes + 17 bottles of 7-Up = Party time

Cereal + Dog food + Diapers + Baby food = Family with children

New Eyes research is when you creatively use the techniques of **psychographics** to generate **profiles** of your Target Customers. (Remember Action Step 1?) See Figure 1.2 for how psychographics works.

New Eyes research is fun. Combined with books and publications like the *Wall Street Journal* — one of the best sources of up-to-date business news information — and talking to people, it will get you all the way to the Business Plan.

And the Business Plan will either make you a success or prove that the idea won't be worth any more of your time.

psychographics
analyses of life-styles

profiles
descriptive features of your Target Customer

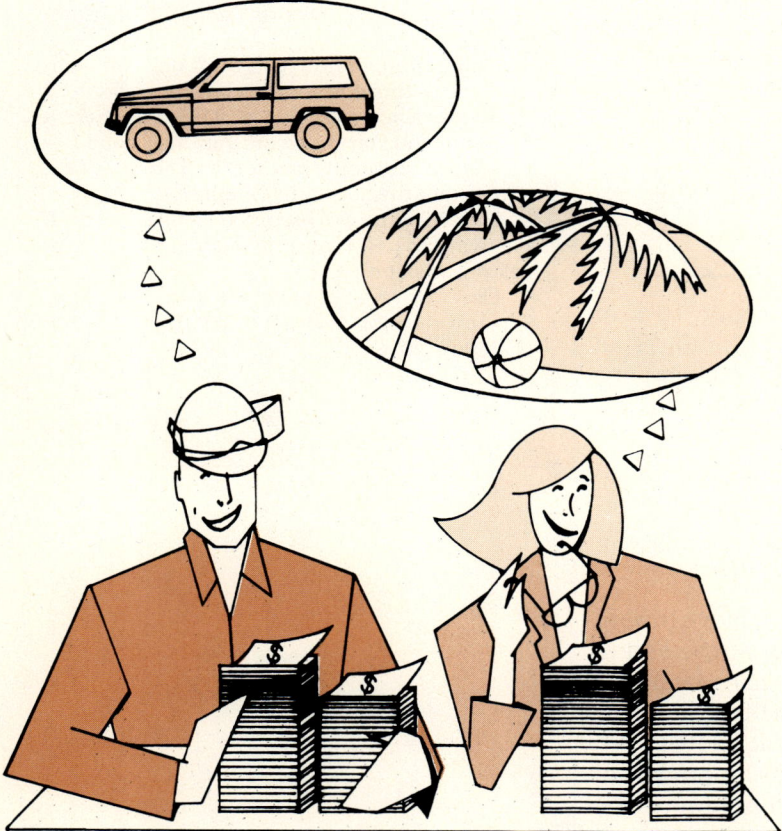

FIGURE 1.2 To use psychographics, think about patterns of consumption and life-style. For example, any two people, each with $20,000 to spend, would make different choices.

Now it's time to start filling your Adventure Notebook with bits of survival information. And how do you do that? You get started on Action Step 6. You interview owners of small businesses.

A fun exercise when you're interviewing business owners is to develop a Secret Profit Profile. Use this example as a model for your own work.

In the course of your interview, find out a few key numbers. You'll need to know gross sales, cost of goods sold, rent, salaries (owner, management), and how much they spend on marketing (advertising, commissions, promotions, and so on). You can estimate the other expenses and come up with a range that will help you when it comes time to work with your own numbers.

For example, let's take a business with $500,000 in sales. The CofGS (cost of goods sold) averages 53%. Rent is $2,000. Total salaries are 15% of gross sales. They spend 6% of their gross on marketing.

That much you know from your interview. You can estimate benefits, including FICA costs, at 20–30% of salaries. Other expenses (supplies, utilities, phone, accounting, legal, auto, entertainment, and so on) will be from 8–12%.

Here's how you get to your Profit Profile:

	High Side	Low Side
Sales	$500,000	$500,000
CofGS (53%)	265,000	265,000
Gross Profit	235,000	235,000
Marketing	30,000	30,000
Salaries	75,000	75,000
FICA/Benefits	15,000	22,500
Rent	24,000	24,000
Other Expenses	40,000	60,000
Net Profit	$ 51,000	$ 23,500

On the high side, the Profit Profile is slightly better than 10%, or $51,000. On the low side, it's slightly below 5%, or $23,500. (That $23,500 is not as low as it looks; the owner has already taken out a salary and most likely auto and entertainment expenses.)

SUMMARY

The Information Society is an outgrowth of the nation's move toward a service economy, which began in earnest in 1945, at the end of World War II. By the early 1980s, less than four decades later, the information industry was doing $800 billion a year, which was close to 50% of the Gross National Product. Looking back, we can see changes in the seventies that are directly related to the growth of information as a business. Big Business, a product of the Industrial Age, began to retrench, cutting its labor force. At the same time, small business created 6 million new jobs.

ACTION ⚡ STEP 6

Take your New Eyes out into the Arena of the Marketplace

Interview at least three people who are self-employed as small business owners. One of them should be in your own area of interest. (If you're a potential competitor, you may need to travel 50 miles or more to get real help.)

Successful entrepreneurs love to tell the story of how they made it. Make an appointment and be up front with why you want the information.

Find a time when a small business owner isn't busy, and you'll be amazed at how much help you can get.

Open-ended questions are best, because they leave room for embellishment. Here are some samples to start you off:

When did you first decide to start your own business?

What was your first step?

What were your feelings then?

If you had it to do all over again, what would you do that's different?

What were the pivotal moments when you felt events were changing with great drama?

How large a part does creativity play in your particular business?

What are your rewards (tangible or intangible)?

Depending on how you hit it off, you want to think of these first interviewees as sources of marketplace experience. They can help a lot when you start to locate your taxi squad — lawyer, accountant, banker, and so on. (Taxi squads are discussed in Chapter 12.)

Helpful hint: Be prepared to take notes. If you want to use a cassette recorder, be sure to ask permission.

Don't worry about evaluation at this stage. The information will fall into patterns sooner than you think.

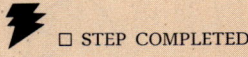
□ STEP COMPLETED

Three of our four case studies are connected to the information business. The computer school trains people to use the tools of the future. The travel agency is an information conduit between travelers and the machinery of travel. The writing consultant didn't get anywhere with her life until she realized she was dealing in pure information.

THINK POINTS

⚡ The Information Society is the big event of the next 15 years.

⚡ To find a door into that society, try looking around with New Eyes. One door may lead to broader thoroughfares.

⚡ Get reckless on paper. Prove your venture with numbers and words before you enter the arena.

⚡ Even though you may not be in business yet, you can intensify your focus by writing down what business you think you want to try. Stay flexible.

REFERENCES

Buzan, Tony. *Use Both Sides of Your Brain.* New York: E. P. Dutton, 1976. Teaches the fine art of mind mapping (which helps the fine art of brainstorming).

Jackson, Tom. *Guerilla Tactics in the Job Market.* New York: Bantam Books, 1978.

Naisbitt, John. *Megatrends: Ten New Directions Transforming Our Lives.* New York: Warner Books, 1982. A must read for entrepreneurs.

Nulty, Peter. "The Princes of Productivity." *Fortune*, April 30, 1984, 253–56. Nulty backs up—with numbers that define the retrenchment of the *Fortune* 500—what Naisbitt (see previous entry) is saying.

O'Boyle, Thomas F. "Other Steel Firms Consider Merging in Wake of LTV Offer for Republic." *Wall Street Journal*, November 9, 1983, Sec. 2, 1. A story from the Industrial Age, with mergers compared to marriages. Good picture of a smokestack industry.

Ries, Al, and Jack Trout. *Positioning: The Battle for Your Mind.* New York: Warner Books, 1982. Two New York City ad executives offer advice on how you can position yourself in the marketplace.

Rico, Gabriele. *Writing the Natural Way: Using Right-Brain Techniques to Release Your Expressive Powers.* Los Angeles: J. P. Tarcher, 1982. Introduces a form of mind mapping called "clustering." Good for the entrepreneur in a hurry.

Toffler, Alvin. *Previews and Premises.* New York: William Morrow & Co., 1983.

————.*The Third Wave.* New York: William Morrow & Co., 1981.

ACTION ⚡ STEP
REVIEW

The keys to success in small business are planning and momentum. In this chapter, five action steps help you focus on both.

2 Boost your confidence by looking back on your past achievements. What stepping-stones got you here? How did victory taste?

3 Get organized. It's the first step in planning. Entrepreneurs typically move so fast they don't take the time to plan. If you fail to plan, you're planning to fail.

4 Now focus on success. What does the world mean by success? What do you mean?

5 Develop your skills picture. What can you do? What do you hate doing? What do you need to learn to survive in the marketplace?

6 Now it's out of the classroom into the real world, where you interview small business owners who are doing something close to what you'll do with your own business.

A Description
of Product
or Service

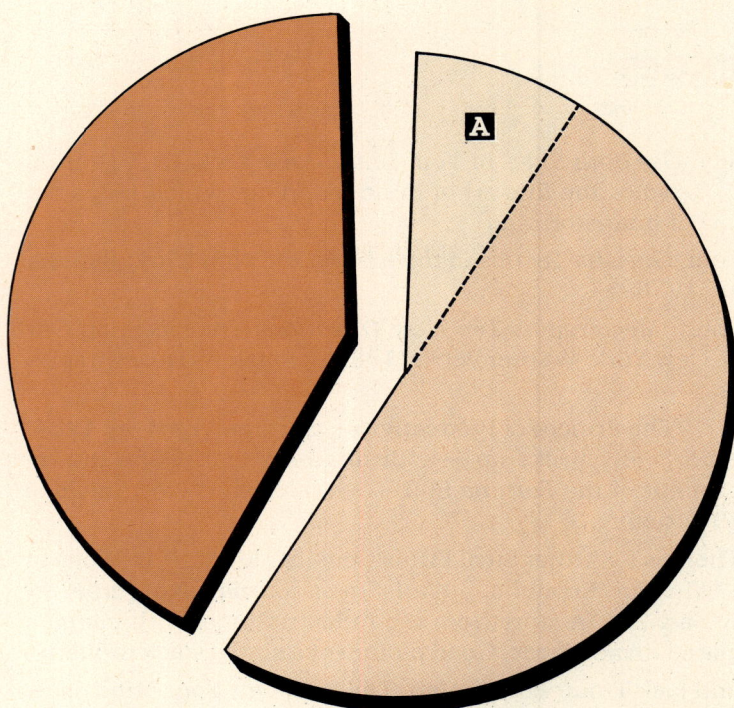

FIGURE 2.1 Chapter 2 starts you building your Business Plan by getting you to see the Big Picture and to define your own product or service.

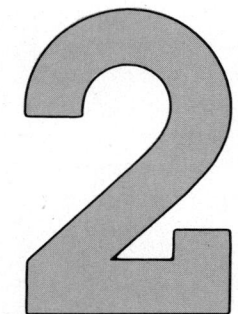

The Big Picture: Charting Trends for Your Small Business

To understand how to analyze the potential for small business success by applying the life-cycle yardstick to industries, products, services, and even locations.

To know what business you're really in.

To experience the techniques of creative brainstorming.

To use diagrams and mind maps to explore the force of market segmentation.

To discover market signals as one key to the ups and downs of trends.

To probe for market forces that lie beneath the trends.

To use your New Eyes to deduce a life-style from the contents of a shopping cart.

To select information sources that will provide the most efficient help, thereby saving you time.

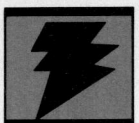

A good Business Plan begins with a Big Picture or industry overview. There are good reasons why you should build your own window to look at the Big Picture and where your small business fits in. One good reason is that the Big Picture is changing all the time. By charting the larger trends in society and in business, you—as a flexible entrepreneur—will be able to make sure you're in the right business at the right time. After all, entire industries go through life cycles, segments within industries go through different life cycles, and individual products and services also pass through cycles of birth, growth, maturity, and decline. We've already established one general trend—the move from an Industrial Society to an Information Society. Chapter 2 gives you the tools you need to examine the Big Picture in more detail.

LIFE CYCLES AND YOUR BUSINESS SUCCESS

Because it is so much easier to succeed in a **growth segment** of a growth industry, you can help yourself by identifying where you are in the **life cycle.**

If you'll look at the life-cycle diagram in Figure 2.2, you can see the auto industry as a whole is very mature. Yet some segments of that industry are promising—mini vans, sports models, and upscale foreign imports. Despite traffic jams, people are still driving. But the cars they drive show they are making choices that reflect changing lifestyles.

The growth segments of the auto industry are ''after-market'' products that are sold to people who are keeping their cars longer. Examples are paint, detailing, electronic accessories, and engine rebuilding. If you're interested in the auto industry, try the after-market!

A well-developed industry overview helps you identify gaps and needs in every market. (In Figure 2.2 we've left some spaces for you to write in industries that have a special interest for you.)

KNOW YOUR BUSINESS

What Happened to the Railroads Can Happen to You

Trains were once a major national force, too. For one explanation of how a huge (and highly dominant) industry can enter the decline stage, let's look back at what happened to the American railroads. Half a century ago, rail lines crisscrossed the continent. You could step aboard a train in New York City and ride in safety, ease, and splendor all the way to California. Trains were the great movers of products and people. The railroad companies owned timber, grazing land, and mineral rights. The train names (Chief, Super Chief, California Zephyr, Commodore Vanderbilt, New York Express, Texas

growth segment
an identifiable slice of an industry that is expanding more rapidly than the industry as a whole

life cycle
four stages, from birth to death, of a product, business, service, industry, or location

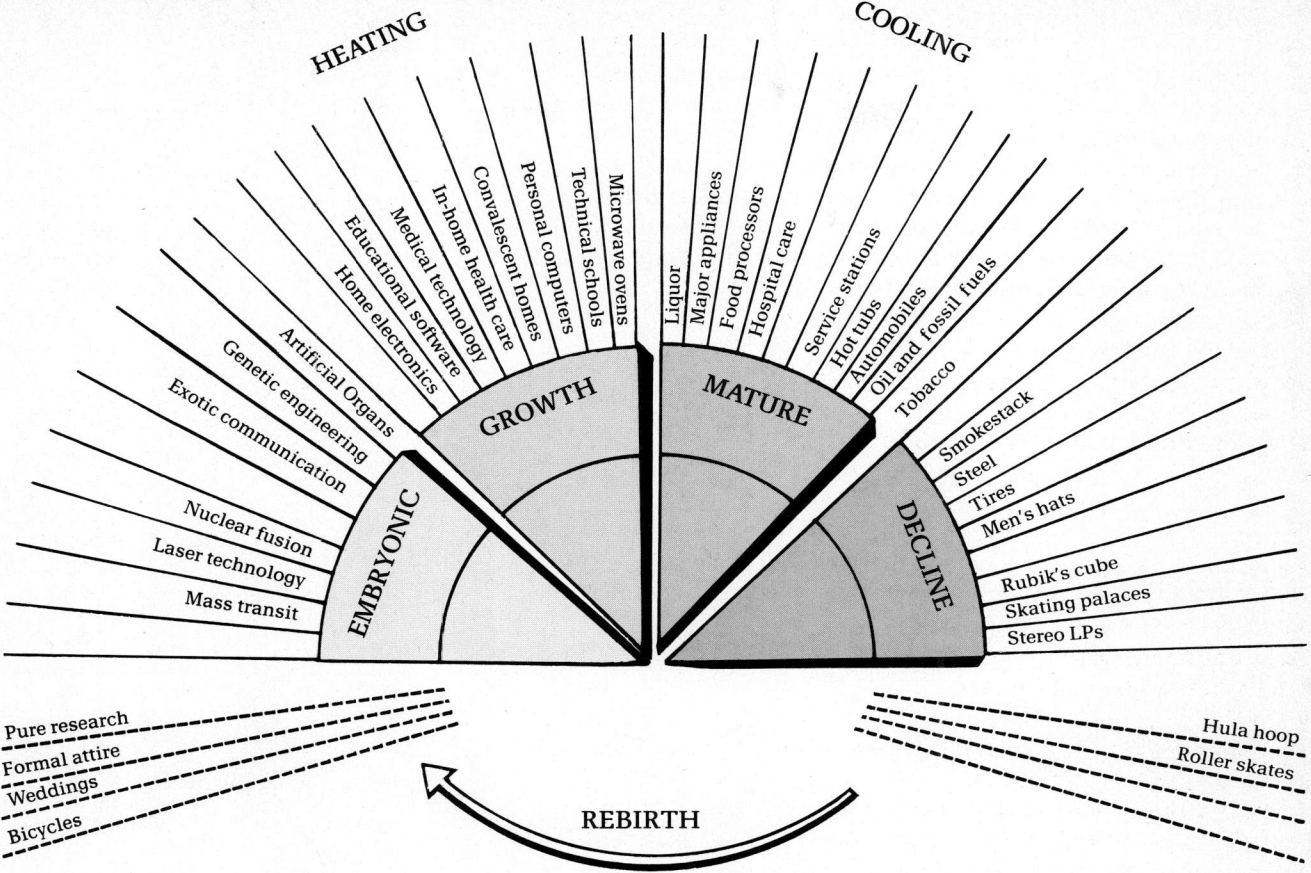

HEATING

COOLING

Mass transit
Laser technology
Nuclear fusion
Exotic communication
Genetic engineering
Artificial Organs
Home electronics
Educational software
Medical technology
In-home health care
Convalescent homes
Personal computers
Technical schools
Microwave ovens
Liquor
Major appliances
Food processors
Hospital care
Service stations
Hot tubs
Automobiles
Oil and fossil fuels
Tobacco
Smokestack
Steel
Tires
Men's hats
Rubik's cube
Skating palaces
Stereo LPs

EMBRYONIC

GROWTH

MATURE

DECLINE

Pure research
Formal attire
Weddings
Bicycles

Hula hoop
Roller skates

REBIRTH

Special) spoke of American confidence, empire-building, power, and the grand strategy of efficient transportation.

It was a magnificent era.

Yet, somewhere along the line, railroad magnates made a simple error — they forgot what business they were in. And that, coupled with jumbo jets, the automobile, the interstate highway system, and the general fickleness of consumers, was the beginning of the end.

Railroads entered the decline stage. Can they come back? Major cities are asking the government for billions to build light rail people-movers. Amtrak still runs a few trains here and there. There is talk of bullet trains, with designs borrowed from the French or the Japanese. Is railroad rebirth idle talk? Was what happened to those huge companies inevitable? Let's see.

FIGURE 2.2 Every industry goes through this life cycle. You need to know where your business fits in the cycle, too.

Here's What the RRs Said	Here's What the RRs Might Have Said
"We're in the railroad business."	"We're in the transportation business."

Did the same lack of vision move the auto industry into decline?

Keep Defining Your Business

To make use of this lesson, keep **defining your business.** Once a month is not too often, especially before the start-up. After you define your business, check signals with potential Target Customers, who may perceive your business differently. You may have to print up new letterhead stationery after you talk to them, but as business expenses go, that's a small price to pay to overcome customer confusion.

Here is a small-scale example demonstrating the importance of understanding what business you are really in.

defining your business
developing a clear picture of what business you are really in

---

Case Study

Mary Clark

Mary Clark was a 40-year-old school teacher who was always more interested in riding her prize-winning saddle horses than she was in teaching. When Mary's grandmother died, leaving her $200,000, Mary made a down payment on a boarding stable and retired from teaching forever, she thought.

The boarding stable was run down. It had stalls for 100 horses. Only 40 were occupied. Mary did everything she could think of to make the place better for horses. She spent $57,000 rebuilding, painting, grading. She made Clark's Stables a very attractive place. She bought the highest quality of feed. She gave the horses the best care money could buy.

When horse owners took their horses to other stables, Mary couldn't understand. She had not increased fees. She treated the horses like friends. In six months, 37 of her 40 customers were gone. In nine months, she was behind on her mortgage payment. Her tenth month, Mary sold Clark's Stables.

What business was Mary in? Write your answer here:

_____

_____

_____

Mary made the simple mistake of thinking horses were Target Customers. They weren't. But young girls between the ages of 7 and 14 were.

The business Mary thought she was in was stabling horses. The business she was really in was providing services for girls who rode horses. They wanted recreation, training, social activities. Mary's customers left because the other stables were providing lessons, trail rides, fun barbeques, pony and horse shows.

Today, Mary is back in the classroom wondering why people don't care more about their horses.

Before you make Mary's mistake, complete the following Action Step. Action Step 7 makes sure you know what business you're really in.

ACTION ⚡ STEP 7

Define Your Business

Then test your definition by reaching out, beyond the classroom.

1. Brainstorm what business you're really in. Let your mind play at this. Try to keep negative statements to a minimum.

2. Once you know what business you're in, visit your printer and order some one-color business letterhead stationery. (One-color is cheaper. Saves you money up front.)

3. Next, visit your library and look for a thick publication called *Encyclopedia of Associations* and locate the name of a trade association your business would be a part of. Make a note of the address, city, phone, and contact person.

4. While in the library, also check *The IMS Ayer Directory of Publications* for a trade journal that covers your industry. Try to find one that's not connected to the association you found in item 3, above. Note the publication name, publisher's name, address, city, phone, and cost (if any).

5. Finally, look in the *Thomas Register of American Manufacturers* for the name of a company that manufactures a part or a product that will be needed in your business. Note the name of part or product, manufacturer, address, city, and phone.

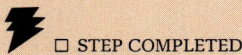 ☐ STEP COMPLETED

Your Real Business

What business are you really in? What business do you want to be in? Naming anything is a game of words, and a small business is no exception. Run through the chart below. It will help you define your own business. If you're hesitant about defining at this early stage, remember what happened to the railroads—and to Mary Clark's stable.

If You're In	Try Saying This
Software sales	"I'm in the problem-solving business."
Pie-baking	"I'm in the taste satisfaction business."
Medical manufacturing	"I'm in the $6 million man business."
College teaching	"I'm in the Information Business."
Medicine	"I'm in the healing business."
Auto sales	"I'm in the ego-gratification business."
Mattresses	"I'm in the sound sleep business."
Cameras	"I'm in the happy memory business."
Gourmet cookware	"I bring fun back into the kitchen."
Locksmith	"I'm in the security business."
Badge manufacturer	"I'm in the recognition business."

KNOW YOUR MARKET

When you know what business you're in, you can develop an effective **marketing strategy.** So let's get started. Define your business here:

_____

_____

Explain why you chose this definition and how it relates to the Target Customer:

_____

_____

_____

_____

Action Step 8 will help you learn more about your local marketplace. New Eyes research, combined with your secondary research efforts, will help you prove that your Business Plan will work. Action Step 8 should be more than a one-time exercise. It should be the start of an entrepreneurial habit. Keep moving. Keep looking for market signals. (And see "Life in a Marketing Lab" on page 22.)

ACTION ⚡ STEP 8

What's New? What's Hot? What's Cooling Fast?

Find out!

1. Take your New Eyes out into the marketplace and observe what's happening at the local or regional level. Prowl around a supermarket and analyze what's going on. A locally owned store will give you a clearer picture than a chain, because it is meeting needs in your area.

   What's on sale? What's dusty? What's new? What's not here? What is the store promoting and what conclusions can you draw about the store's marketing strategy? Which department has the most space? The longest lines? The most workers? The highest prices? Guesstimate the shelf velocity of certain products. (See sidebar on shelf velocity, page 35.)

   Move on to other locally owned stores —hardware, drugstores, restaurants, gift shops, and so on. And keep analyzing.

2. Give your New Eyes research a data base by checking with your local newspaper. Visit the marketing department and ask to see research they've compiled on the area.

3. Visit your library and study a copy of *Annual Survey of Buying Power*, published by *S & MM* magazine. For your city or county, note:
   a) Total dollars spent on autos and related products.
   b) Percentage of households earning more than the national average.
   c) Total city/county population.

   How does your New Eyes research correlate with what you found in the secondary sources?

⚡ ☐ STEP COMPLETED

marketing strategy
an action plan for winning
in the marketplace

Market Signals

Market signals are everywhere—in the newspaper (classified ads, display ads), in the lines at the theater, in the price-slashing after Christmas, in discount coupons, rebates, closings, and Grand Openings. With practice, you can follow a product right through the life cycle.

For example, take designer jeans. In the early 1980s, a massive ad campaign convinced otherwise sane Americans they should pay $40 and up for jeans carrying designer labels. The jeans were available only in the posher stores. A year or so later, designer jeans had reached the discount stores. Jeans that had sold for $55 were now selling at **Deep Discount**—$9.99.

A bargain? Yes. And also a trend.

What items have you noticed going through a life cycle, from upscale out of sight to Deep Discount?

_____

_____

_____

_____

Now go back to the industry life-cycle wheel and see if you can fill in more spaces.

Warning Signals

When merchandise slides into Deep Discount, the marketing party is over. The air is chilly. The market is flooded. Sinking is likely. Drowning is now possible. If that's happened to your job—or to your business—it's time to find a growth segment of a growth industry.

OPPORTUNITIES FOR GROWTH

The average American will have at least four different kinds of jobs in one lifetime. No one has a completely secure job. Rhonda Van Warden thought she did—but when she learned that her position was being eliminated, she started to look at the trends in her community, in the nation. Rhonda had some great assets. She was intelligent. She was a good listener. And she was flexible enough to see herself in a totally new role if opportunity knocked.

Case Study

Rhonda Van Warden — Private Screenings

Rhonda was a great teacher. She had a warm personality, a terrific smile, and an intuitive understanding of what kids needed from the world of adults. When she was offered a job as a counselor for the school

Continued

Deep Discount
cutting the price to near cost, cost, or below cost

Life in a Marketing Lab

We live in a marketing lab. To discover the truth of this, go out into the arena of the marketplace (as in Action Step 8) and see how other businesses succeed—or fail—in their marketing efforts.

Locally owned stores present a good picture of marketing on a local level. National chain stores will show you what the country is buying. Department stores and mass merchandisers adjust very quickly to changes in the market. Every square foot is expected to make a contribution to sales and profit. The next time you're in a store, ask yourself these questions:

How are areas expanded or contracted to adjust to market demand?

How are special displays placed during demand periods?

What is the location of products with the highest gross margin?

Did you ever notice how cafeterias display soups, salad, and desserts first? They are high-margin goods. Management wants you to build your meal around them.

Can you remember the last time you bought film and they tried to sell you fresh batteries for your flash? Or the time they tried to sell you a scarf to match a purse? Or a shoe tree to keep your shoes new?

Now that you know we live in a marketing lab, how can you turn this knowledge into power for yourself?

where she'd worked as a teacher, Rhonda didn't hesitate. As a counselor, she knew she could reach more kids.

Then the district cutbacks started. Due to forces beyond her control, Rhonda was furloughed. Naturally, she was very upset. Here she'd been working overtime, supporting the system, counseling her heart out, and what did she have to show for it?

Not much.

But Rhonda's a fighter who doesn't give up easily. She took seminars. She read books about job-hunting. She networked her friends for leads.

One day she was talking to a couple of friends, and the talk turned to ladies' intimate lingerie.

"What I wish," one friend said, "is that a girl could own some of that semi-sexy stuff without having to be seen going into Le Sex Shoppe to buy it."

"There's always the catalogs, dear," the other friend said. "There are ads in the back of every magazine I subscribe to."

"I don't trust those catalogs," the first friend said. "When I pay hard-earned money for frilly underwear, I want to see what I'm buying."

They turned to Rhonda. "You're sitting there not saying a word, Rhonda. What's your view on this?"

"I think," Rhonda said, smiling, "I've just discovered the business I want to be in."

Rhonda's idea was to network her women-friends for potential target customers who would be interested in attending a private showing of ladies' intimate undergarments. Rhonda came up with the name for her business, Private Screenings. She had letterhead stationery printed. And she began to contact suppliers and manufacturer's reps. They were interested in her idea.

Her first "private screening" was well attended. There were only ladies present. As a group, the ladies spent just under $1,000 that first night. They felt safe, private. Ten years ago, they'd never have considered buying intimate underwear. But times change.

Rhonda went on from the first success to develop a line of products, which she sells through her own catalog. Her husband has joined her in the business, and she has hired someone else to present her intimate merchandise through seminars (the seminars are still held in private homes). Rhonda spends most of her time recruiting personnel and developing new products.

"When I started into this business," Rhonda admits, "I thought it might help supplement my husband's income. But it's expanded so much we have to scramble to keep up with orders. We travel a lot, talking to manufacturers abut the next trend, picking up ideas. Now my husband works full-time in the business."

Recognizing Trends

Rhonda was a sharp reader of market signals — the major **trends** that were changing the way people think and act. (See "An Overview of *Megatrends*" on page 24.) What trends are at work in Rhonda's success?

trends
pathways to your future

1. **Specialized Consumer Tastes.** Rhonda's target customers are middle-class women in their forties and fifties. They like

An Overview of *Megatrends*

You can't talk about trends without referring to John Naisbitt's best-seller, *Megatrends.* Naisbitt provides us with 10 major movements (he calls them *transformations* or *megashifts*). If you want to know the way things are moving, read *Megatrends,* which grew out of a data base of 6,000 local newspapers monitored for a dozen years. If you want to verify Naisbitt's overview (the book was published in 1982, and needs updating), just glance at the front page of the *Wall Street Journal,* on almost any day of the week.

Here's a quick overview of Naisbitt's overview. We are moving

1. From an industrial society to an information society.
2. From forced technology to a balance between high tech and high touch.
3. From a national economy to a world economy (see mergers and joint ventures between U.S. car makers, Europe, Japan).
4. From short-term cover-ups to long-term planning.
5. From centralized structures to more local control by states, counties, cities, neighborhoods, and private associations.
6. From institutional help to self-help (health, wellness, education, the entrepreneurial explosion in business, and so on).
7. From representative democracy to participatory democracy (independent voters, new political parties, tax initiatives, referenda, consumerism as marketplace control).
8. From hierarchies (corporate and government pyramids crumble) to networking (clustering together, sharing, the horizontal link).
9. From North (Frost Belt) to South (Sunbelt—especially to the West, Southwest, Florida). [See the *Wall Street Journal's* weekly Section II columns on Regions and Real Estate for updates and refinements in the North-South Megashift.]
10. From Either/Or to Multiple Option—doing your own thing is now not only possible, but also feasible and profitable. [Nineteen million singles, more than 750 models of cars and trucks sold in the U.S., rise in birth rate in women over 30, explosions in art, religion, designer fruit and vegetables—all spell opportunity for the eager entrepreneur].

Naisbitt's advice on what to do with a trend once you see it: "Trends, like horses, are easier to ride in the direction they are going."

SOURCE: Adapted from John Naisbitt; *Megatrends: Ten New Directions Transforming Our Lives* (New York: Warner Books, 1982), by permission of Warner Books, Inc.

their privacy. Most of them would be uncomfortable walking off the street into a store to ask to see some intimate apparel. When Rhonda brings the merchandise to them, they feel both safe and special. Their sense of adventure is free to soar.

2. **High Tech/High Touch.** You can't stop the approach of computers and the Information Age. But we all try to balance the electronic effects of whirring machinery by an occasional

human response — Rolfing, EST, dance, the arts, feeding our fantasies. Private Screenings capitalizes on our urge for softness, and as such, it is part of the trend that *Megatrends* calls high touch.

3. **Relaxing National Attitudes About Sex.** Private Screenings was founded in the early eighties, and reflects a more exploratory attitude in the area of sex.

What trends do you see operating in Private Screenings?

_____

_____

_____

_____

The Right Place at the Right Time

There is another kind of opportunity for growth that you should be aware of. Not only is it easier to penetrate a growth industry with a new product or service, it is also wise to consider a growth geographic area. Table 2.1 (page 26) lists areas where population shifts will be felt most dramatically. For many businesses, it pays to be where the customers are. Is your area listed in Table 2.1? (Later, in Chapter 7, we'll go into the fine points of choosing the right location for your business.) It's interesting to note that of the 25 fastest-growing markets listed in Table 2.1, eight — or nearly a third — are in Florida. In *Megatrends,* Naisbitt identifies Florida as a ''bellwether'' state.

LOOKING BEFORE YOU LEAP

One good reason to get the Big Picture and to see how your small business fits in with changing trends is that by doing a little preliminary research, you can save yourself a tremendous amount of grief down the road. In fact, one reason to engage in research is to see just where that road will lead you. In Action Step 9 we ask you to literally walk down a road — the one you'll use for **walking the neighborhood** of your target customer. By using your New Eyes — and employing a little primary research — you will be able to probe the lifestyle of your potential Target Customer. What does this view of your Target Customer tell you? Does it confirm your hunches? Does it inspire you to modify the way you define your business? Complete Action Step 9 and find out how to hunt for **clues to life-style.**

Deep Research

Depending on your business, and depending on the kind of person you are, you may want to engage in deep research. Granted, it takes longer than a stroll through your target neighborhood, but for entrepreneurs with a complex dream to realize — or for entrepreneurs who are very careful about the business they want to go into — it makes

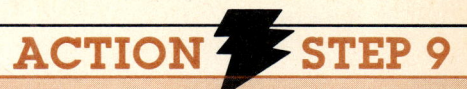

ACTION STEP 9

Probe the Life-style of Your Potential Target Customer Before You Plunge into a New Venture

Walk the neighborhood that is your Target Customer's habitat.

The best time to walk a target neighborhood is on the weekends, when the garage doors are open.

You're looking for clues to life-styles.

How many cars? What makes and models? How old? What condition? (Sports cars or low-slung two-door hatchbacks indicate the owners are young, or trying to be. Station wagons suggest families. A fleet of Mercedes or Jags means you're upscale.)

Any sports or recreation equipment? Any tools? Any pets, doghouses, stables?

What's the maintenance level of the homes? Are they patio homes? Condos? Townhouses? Single-family? Estimate the number of bedrooms, baths, square feet, and so on. Then pay a visit to your local real estate office and get an estimate on local housing costs. Use these costs to estimate household income. (If the average price for a home in your target neighborhood is $125,000, and buyers can finance $100,000, the household income will probably be around $50,000–$60,000.)

If you don't have time to walk the neighborhood, bike it or drive it.

Study your Target Customer — from all angles. You can't afford to make any blind guesses.

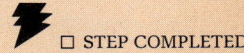 ☐ STEP COMPLETED

walking the neighborhood
tramping through the dust and gold of the marketplace

clues to life-style
reading your Target Customers by observing what's important to them

TABLE 2.1 Biggest Markets of 1986 and Fastest and Slowest-Growing Markets

Biggest markets in 1986

Rank 1981	Rank 1986	Metropolitan Market	1986 Pop. (Thous.)	% Change 1981–86
1	1	New York	8,726.2	− 2.9%
2	2	Los Angeles – Long Beach	7,753.3	+ 2.6
3	3	Chicago	7,232.0	+ 1.4
4	4	Philadelphia	4,664.7	− 0.7
5	5	Detroit	4,301.0	− 0.6
6	6	Boston	3,654.0	− 0.1
10	7	Houston	3,597.6	+17.1
9	8	Dallas – Fort Worth	3,433.3	+11.4
7	9	San Francisco – Oakland	3,363.2	+ 2.5
8	10	Washington, DC	3,170.4	+ 2.8
11	11	Nassau – Suffolk, NY	2,680.5	+ 2.5
12	12	St. Louis	2,401.9	+ 2.1
16	13	Atlanta	2,355.6	+11.7
17	14	Anaheim-Santa Ana-Garden Grove, CA	2,298.2	+13.5
14	15	Baltimore	2,253.7	+ 2.8
15	16	Minneapolis – St. Paul	2,243.1	+ 4.5
18	17	San Diego	2,217.7	+13.4
13	18	Pittsburgh	2,173.3	− 3.0
21	19	Miami	1,933.8	+10.4
22	20	Denver-Boulder	1,916.0	+13.1
24	21	Riverside-San Bernardino-Ontario, CA	1,907.8	+16.0
26	22	Phoenix	1,894.1	+17.0
23	23	Tampa – St. Petersburg, FL	1,893.3	+14.5
19	24	Newark, NJ	1,892.9	− 2.8
20	25	Cleveland	1,857.0	− 0.7
25	26	Seattle-Everett	1,745.8	+ 6.2
29	27	San Jose, CA	1,479.5	+10.4
27	28	Cincinnati	1,420.0	+ 1.0
31	29	Portland, OR	1,402.9	+ 9.8
28	30	Milwaukee	1,401.8	+ 0.2
30	31	Kansas City, MO	1,374.1	+ 2.6
33	32	New Orleans	1,286.8	+ 6.0
37	33	Fort Lauderdale – Hollywood, FL	1,280.1	+18.3
36	34	San Antonio	1,204.0	+ 9.2
34	35	Indianapolis	1,202.1	+ 2.3
38	36	Sacramento	1,184.3	+12.2
32	37	Buffalo, NY	1,170.0	− 4.3
35	38	Columbus, OH	1,148.4	+ 3.7
40	39	Salt Lake City – Ogden	1,125.1	+14.5
39	40	Hartford-New Britain-Bristol, CT	1,055.7	+ 0.4
		Total	101,295.2	+ 4.3%

Tomorrow's fastest-growing markets

Rank	Metropolitan Market	% Growth 1981–86	1986 Pop. (Thous.)
1.	Fort Myers – Cape Coral, FL	22.9%	274.0
2.	Provo-Orem, UT	21.7	286.5
2.	Olympia, WA	21.7	162.9
4.	Ocala, FL	20.6	159.0
5.	Las Vegas	20.5	594.3
6.	Fort Collins, CO	19.9	192.4
7.	McAllen-Pharr-Edinburg, TX	19.7	363.2
8.	Boise, ID	19.6	221.2
9.	Reno	19.3	246.8
10.	Bryan-College Station, TX	19.2	119.3
11.	Richland-Kennewick-Pasco, WA	19.1	184.5
12.	Casper, WY	18.7	90.6
13.	Redding, CA	18.5	146.1
14.	Sarasota, FL	18.4	256.0
14.	Santa Cruz, CA	18.4	237.5
16.	Fort Lauderdale-Hollywood, FL	18.3	1,280.1
17.	Orlando, FL	18.0	881.8
18.	Santa Rosa, CA	17.7	374.6
18.	Brownsville-Harlingen-San Benito, TX	17.7	261.4
20.	West Palm Beach – Boca Raton, FL	17.5	727.9
21.	Houston	17.1	3,597.6
21.	Bradenton, FL	17.1	184.6
23.	Phoenix	17.0	1,894.1
24.	Tucson, AZ	16.8	663.6
25.	Tallahassee, FL	16.6	197.0

Tomorrow's market losers

Rank	Metropolitan Market	% Loss 1981–86	1986 Pop. (Thous.)
1.	Jersey City, NJ	−4.9%	522.7
2.	Buffalo, NY	−4.3	1,170.0
3.	Pittsburgh	−3.0	2,173.3
3.	Utica-Rome, NY	−3.0	307.1
5.	New York	−2.9	8,726.2
6.	Newark, NJ	−2.8	1,892.9
7.	Paterson-Clifton-Passaic, NJ	−2.0	435.5
8.	Muncie, IN	−1.6	125.9
9.	Akron, OH	−1.5	646.9
10.	Dayton, OH	−1.4	814.2
10.	Elmira, NY	−1.4	95.7
12.	Steubenville-Weirton, OH-WV	−1.2	160.3
13.	Springfield, OH	−1.1	181.0
14.	Pittsfield, MA	−0.8	143.0
15.	Philadelphia	−0.7	4,664.7
15.	Cleveland	−0.7	1,857.0
15.	Great Falls, MT	−0.7	79.9
18.	Detroit	−0.6	4,301.0
19.	Youngstown-Warren, OH	−0.5	527.5
19.	Anderson, IN	−0.5	138.4
19.	Burlington, NC	−0.5	98.7
22.	Binghamton, NY	−0.3	299.9
23.	Boston	−0.1	3,654.0

SOURCE: "Biggest Markets of 1986 and Fastest and Slowest-Growing Markets." *Sales & Marketing Management's 1982 Survey of Buying Power—Part II, 10.* Sales & Marketing Management.

sense to be thorough. Deep research is at the opposite end of the spectrum from Action Step 9. Later in this chapter we give you more tools for completing the right amount of research for you.

Two years of deep research is not for everyone who goes into small business. But Rich Cameron was a very precise and careful person.

If you are considering a venture you know very little about, then you should work in that kind of business to get experience.

If you can't work in it, then do what Rich Cameron did.

Case Study

Rich Cameron — Seminar Junkie

When Rich Cameron celebrated his 35th birthday, he was in the marketing end of the computer industry. The industry was doing all right, but Rich was frustrated with his job.

"I was your typical workaholic," Rich said. "I'd do overtime at the office, put out a lot of energy for the company, and then wonder why I didn't feel terrific. If someone had told me I was experiencing Corporate Burnout, I'd have laughed in his face."

Rich had been in the habit of changing jobs when he got frustrated. He'd started working as a grocery boy when he was 12, and since then he'd worked in sales, management, real estate, insurance, finance, research, and programming. Now he started to look around for something else to do. He arranged a four-day work schedule, ten hours a day, and he spent the three other days exploring.

"When I was a kid in high school, my dad took me aside and gave me some valuable advice. 'Son,' he said. 'Remember this. You are your greatest resource.' So one of the first things I did, before I checked out the marketplace, was to take some aptitude tests. They told me three things: 1) I was good with spatial problems; 2) I liked being creative; 3) I liked to play. The last one — play — was the one that threw me. I'd grown up in a family where we learned to work hard, and play was a word I didn't use much. It took me more than a year to accept the fact that I liked to play."

While he was digesting this news about himself, Rich took seminars, mostly in small business, and he also kept to his schedule — 4 days for the boss, 3 for adventure. He walked over a hundred neighborhoods. He interviewed over a hundred small business owners. He studied **traffic patterns,** shopping habits, trends. At the end of the first year, he knew he wanted to combine work and play by opening a toy store. He was about to settle on a location in a major shopping center when he happened to interview the owner of an antique store.

Rich asked the antique store owner why he'd chosen this location.

"We did research," the man said. "My wife is the mathematician of the family. She worked the whole thing out on paper."

"Great," Rich said. "I've been at it for more than a year, myself. What kinds of things did she do?"

"We counted the cars in the parking lot," the owner said. "We counted them every day for two weeks. This lot was packed solid from dawn to dark."

Rich looked out. Today, the parking lot was packed. "What about weekends?" he asked.

Continued

traffic patterns
pathways and frequency
of travel

The antique owner looked at the floor. ''Now there,'' he admitted, ''we've been having problems — ever since we lost our anchor tenant.''

''How long ago was that?'' Rich asked.

''Six months ago tomorrow,'' the man said.

Rich thanked the owner and kept on exploring. He had liked this center. It was nearly a perfect target neighborhood. Yet, something was wrong. He could feel it.

Rich was still talking to store owners when evening rolled around and the parking lot began to empty, fast. Rich stopped his interviews to do some New Eyes observing. A car full of people would pull into the lot, stop. Everyone except the driver would leave the car and proceed to other cars. The drivers did not go into any of the stores to shop. Rich quickly saw a pattern: This particular center was a drop-off area for car-poolers on their way to jobs in the city.

''I'd been interviewing store owners all afternoon,'' Rich says, ''and not one of them told me about the car-pooling situation. Maybe they didn't know. Maybe they were hiding something. Either way, it was a signal for me to keep on looking.''

It took Rich Cameron two years to find what he was looking for — a location close to a target neighborhood packed with kids and young parents and station wagons and toys.

He named his store Toys from Middle Earth. Now he works 70 hours a week until the Christmas Season, when he works 100. He's not frustrated any more.

''The only thing you've got to watch in the toy business,'' Rich says, ''is how fast a trend can end. One week, you're selling hula hoops like crazy. The next week, the hula hoops wouldn't move at half price, and the kids are coming in the store asking for gear they've seen on a new TV show or adventure movie. To make it in toys these days, you need to keep one eye on the kids, the other on the future.'' He grins. ''If you'd told me that a couple of years back, I wouldn't have believed you. But you learn to read the customers in this business. Or you go under.''

Rich Cameron won't go under. He likes to win too much.

Quest for Hard Data

Rich Cameron spent two years researching the toy industry. Today, his toy business is growing steadily because he planned well.

Rich is a researcher to model yourself after. He integrated New Eyes research with hard data from secondary sources.

In the list that follows, we have indicated some valuable secondary sources that you can use to begin gathering hard data:

Newspapers. John Naisbitt's Trend staff monitors 6,000 regional and daily newspapers. *Megatrends* grew in part out of that research. Study your local newspaper, starting with the classifieds and display ads. For a bigger picture, we recommend the *Wall Street Journal.*

Magazines. The ads tell you what's hot and where the money is flowing. The articles keep you current. If you haven't looked at it already, check out *S & MM* (the new name for *Sales and Marketing Management Magazine*) which publishes two supplements of interest to small business pioneers: the *Survey of Buying Power* (listed by counties all across the U.S.) and an annual *Survey of Industrial and Commercial Buying Power* (which gives you a dramatic, Big Picture look at regions, counties, industries, and metro areas). *S & MM* supplements are definitely must-read materials.

Trade Journals.   A valuable source once you know what industry you're in. Use your new business letterhead to write trade associations. A brief list is included in Appendix C of this book. You can find detailed addresses in the *Encyclopedia of Associations* and in *The IMS Ayer Directory of Publications.*

Banks.   Banks are in the business of renting money, and any bank above medium size will have a research staff (economists, marketing experts, and so on) who write forecasts and reports of economic trends. Ask to see those reports.

Planning Offices.   Cities and counties employ planners to chart the future and plan for growth. Most phone directories have an information number you can call to find out where these offices are. For the best service, however, you'll need to pay the office a visit, make friends, be pleasant and patient. Many counties use federal data to develop annual Progress Reports.

Reports from Colleges and Universities.   State universities publish annual and semiannual reports on economic conditions, which you can usually get by writing to the public relations office. Reports are also published by private institutions of higher learning with special interests in business. Inquire in your area.

Real Estate Firms.   The larger commercial and industrial firms have access to developer's site research. The more specific you can be on your requirement, the easier it will be for them to help you. Familiarize yourself with the dynamics of the area. What firms are going into business? What firms are leaving business? For more details on this, see Chapter 7, on Location.

The SBA.   The Small Business Administration of the U.S. government has many booklets. Call the nearest office or write to U.S. Small Business Administration, P.O. Box 15434, Fort Worth, Texas 76119. Put tax dollars to work for you.

Federal Depositories.   Scattered across the land are special libraries which contain various sources of census information: CMSAs (Consolidated Metropolitan Statistical Areas), such as New York–Long Island–Southwestern Connecticut–Northern New Jersey, 17 million people; PMSAs (Primary Metropolitan Statistical Areas), such as New York City; and MSAs (Metropolitan Statistical Areas), such as Peoria, Fresno, and so on. These three categories used to be grouped under SMSA—Standard Metropolitan Statistical Area—a category that will linger in the minds of marketeers for another decade or so. No matter what you call it, you can find census information in these Federal Depositories, where the 1980 SMSA for your area is probably still intact. Also check a booklet called *County Business Patterns.* For the whereabouts of the nearest depository, see our list in Appendix C, or check with your friendly reference librarian.

trade journals
publications directed to the specific needs of an industry

SIC Codes

While you're scanning the Big Picture for trends, you might want to develop a feel for what you can do with SIC Codes. Start with your code first. It will help you define your industry. It will orient you in the Big Picture.

SIC means Standard Industrial Classification. It's a numerical system that assigns a number to almost any identifiable industry. SIC numbers come in three groups:

2-digit — Major Group (36)
3-digit — Industry Group (366)
4-digit — Specific Industry Group (3662)

SIC codes are contained in a government publication, available at most libraries, called *The Standard Industrial Classification Manual.* The simplest way to use it is to go right to the alphabetical index, find the industry you think you're in. Then go to Major Group, Industry Group, and Specific Industry.

For example, let's say you're a creative entrepreneur who's just invented a device that will make radio transmission easier. Your primary market will be manufacturers of radio equipment. You could have a secondary market among telephone equipment makers. You can manufacture the device for $4.22 per unit. But before you start production, you want to assess the size of the market.

So you find your SIC classification in the alphabetical index, under number 3662, Radio & TV Communication Equipment. That's you, all right. You turn to Major Group 36, Electrical, Electronics, then to Specific Industries under 3662. You notice that 3661 is Telephone & Telegraph Supplies, which is another industry category you need to explore.

You also notice that the SIC codes have led you so far and no further. That's because the government does not release *sources* for its data. A good thing for the government, perhaps. But not for you.

Q. Where do you go from here?
A. Private enterprise.

In Figure 2.3, we suggest three different tracks you can follow with your SIC code, depending on the nature of your quest.

Track I. Track I leads to S & MM's *Survey of Industrial and Commercial Buying Power,* an annual study of markets. The *Survey,* which is available at most libraries, gives you a Big Picture look at business trends at the national level:

Major industry groups.
Top 50 counties by manufacturing activity.
50 leading industrial metropolitan markets.

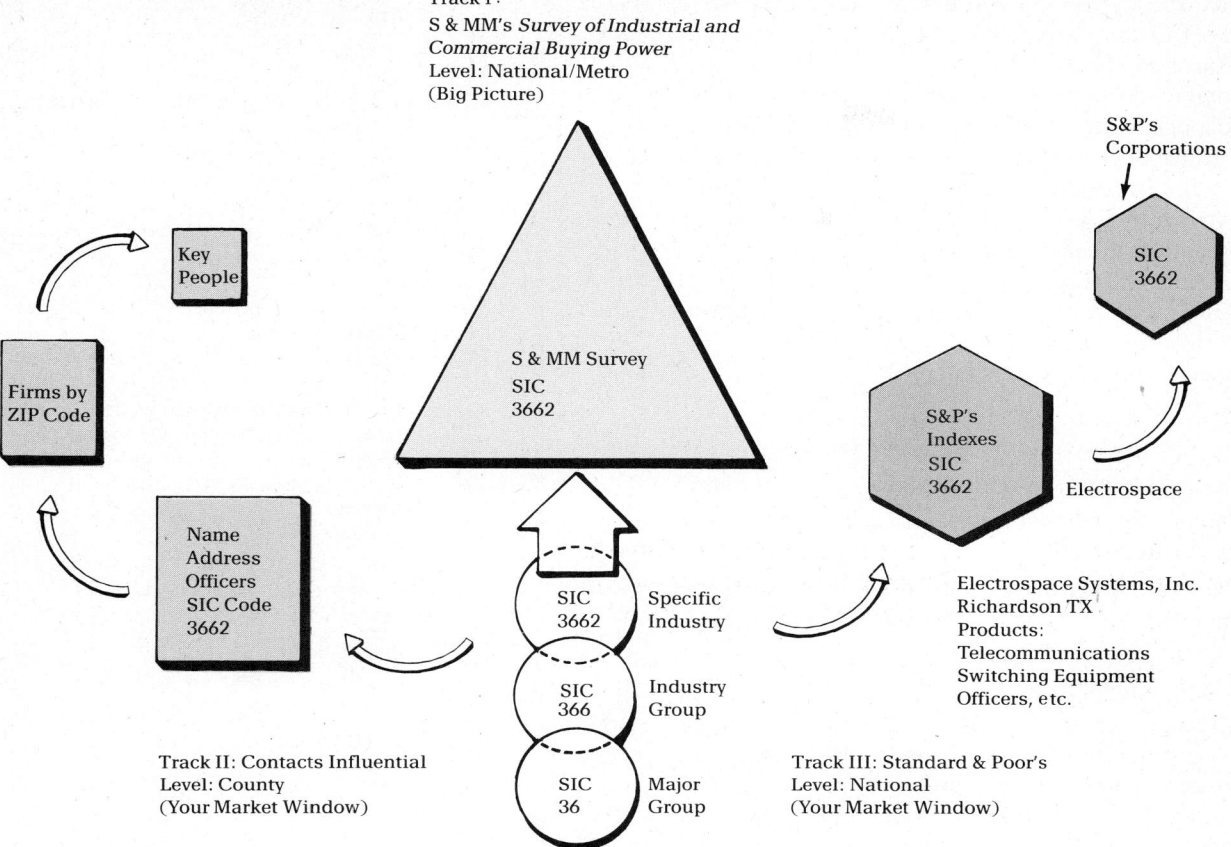

Track I:
S & MM's *Survey of Industrial and Commercial Buying Power*
Level: National/Metro
(Big Picture)

S&P's Corporations

SIC 3662

Key People

Firms by ZIP Code

S & MM Survey SIC 3662

S&P's Indexes SIC 3662

Electrospace

Name Address Officers SIC Code 3662

SIC 3662   Specific Industry

SIC 366   Industry Group

SIC 36   Major Group

Electrospace Systems, Inc.
Richardson TX
Products:
Telecommunications Switching Equipment
Officers, etc.

Track II: Contacts Influential
Level: County
(Your Market Window)

Track III: Standard & Poor's
Level: National
(Your Market Window)

Regional and state summaries of manufacturing markets.

Profiles of the 50 biggest manufacturing industries.

And, if you're still following that SIC number 3662, you get a breakdown, by employment totals, total shipments, percentages of SIC classifications, and so on, of the top 71 counties in the country. You know that Los Angeles County, for example, has 83 plants that make radio and TV equipment. Up above, in 3661, Cook County, Illinois, has 8 companies that make telephone/telegraph gear.

Now, depending on your business and how wide you want to fling your marketing net, you take either one of two tracks.

Track II leads to *Contacts Influential.*

Track III leads to Standard & Poor's *Register of Corporations, Directors, and Executives.*

Track II. *Contacts Influential* operates at the county level. You follow your SIC 3662 to the first Contacts book, which gives you the name of the corporation, the address, the phone, the key officers. Then you double-check your data in the section where the 3662 firms are listed by zip code. Finally, you look up your list of key officers, in their own section.

SIC 3662 has led you to some possible contacts at the county level. If you feel that your device would be easy to market at the national level, go on to Track III.

FIGURE 2.3 Working from the SIC codes, you can follow three different tracks to see how your business relates to national and local markets.

Track III.   SIC 3662 will lead you first to Standard & Poor's *Index,* where you locate the company you want, Electrospace Systems, Inc., located in Richardson, Texas.

Now you move to a second S & P volume, *Corporations,* where you look up Electrospace Systems. Here you'll find the address, phone, a list of officers, number of employees, regional contacts, sales for the previous year, a list of products, and your friend, SIC 3662.

Since the listings in S & P's *Corporations* are alphabetical, you'll find other interesting corporations beginning with *electro* — Electronics Corp. of America, Electronics Corporation of Texas, Electronics Research, Inc. (which makes FM broadcasting antennas, which might give you another market tie-in), and so on.

Let's summarize how SIC codes can help you:

1. They help you discover what industry you're in.
2. They help you define the boundaries of that industry.
3. They help you locate customers and suppliers within that industry.
4. They help you reach out to other industries, thoughtfully and systematically.

So have fun with SIC codes!

Figure 2.3 gives you a schematic of the three tracks you can follow, using the SIC codes. Once you're looking at SIC codes, use the same idea for a schematic to track your own industry.

Now that you know how to use SIC codes, relax and try a creative exercise. Action Step 10 sends you back to consult with your friends on a very weighty topic: segmentation and gap analysis.

USING THE BIG PICTURE TO FIND MARKET GAPS

Working from Mind Maps

By using mind maps and diagrams to create a Big Picture for a particular industry, you will begin to get a feel for locating gaps in the market. The diagram in Figure 2.4 was derived from an informal mind map several entrepreneurs drew as they discussed various **segments** of the health-care industry. You'd be surprised at how a simple sketch can trigger a meaningful discussion of an industry and its segments.

First the entrepreneurs drew a circle to represent the entire health-care industry. Then, as they talked, they listed segments of the industry. Once they had a fairly complete list of segments, they roughly allocated portions of the circle — or, if you prefer, slices of the pie — to each segment. Note that most segments of this industry are still in the growth stage — a number are listed on our life-cycle diagram at Figure 2.2. Our entrepreneurs decided to focus on in-home health care. They felt that this particular segment had a great deal of potential — for a number of reasons. One big reason is that other segments of the industry emphasized hardware and institutions.

 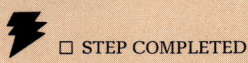
segments
identifiable slices of an
industry

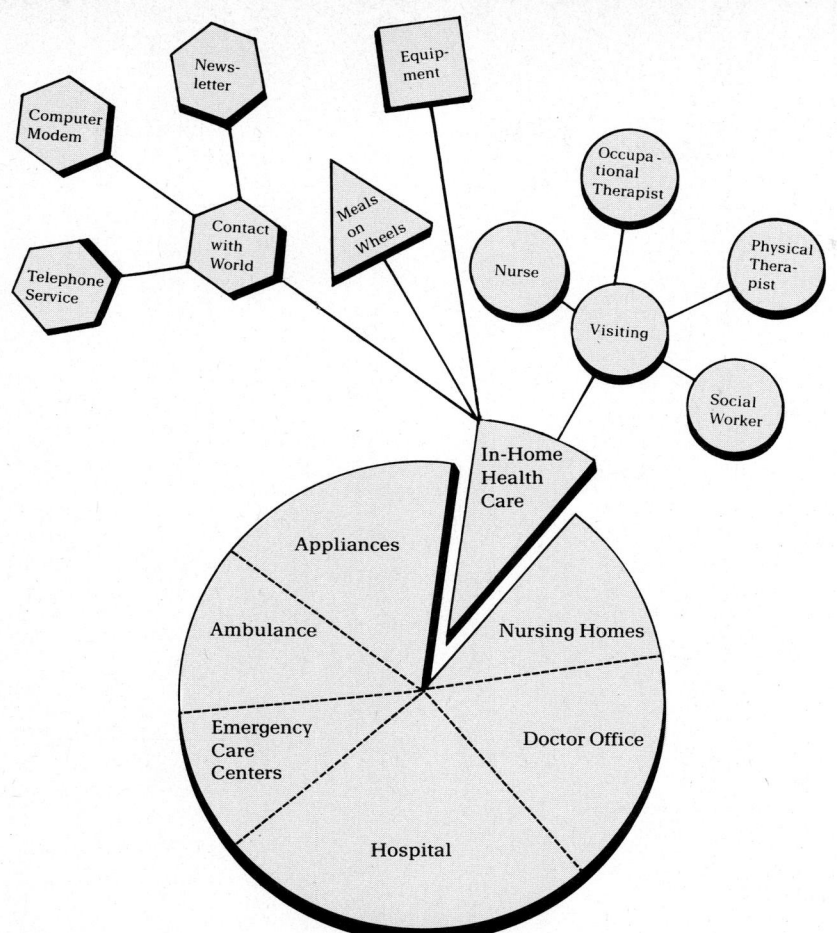

FIGURE 2.4 This diagram is derived from a mind-map analysis of just one segment of the health care industry. You can use mind maps to explore *your* industry.

Other businesses had no problem in seeing the potential of selling expensive, specialized machinery or other products to highly visible institutions. In-home health care appealed to our entrepreneurs because it took a certain amount of creative initiative just to conceive of this segment as an existing, opportunity-filled market.

As they brainstormed, the entrepreneurs discovered additional components of their chosen segment. Each new idea went into the mind map. Later, they recognized specific clusters of components, and quickly revised their map to visualize their new ideas. When they were done, they discovered four sections of the segment that looked promising. In addition to the obvious requirements for services like Meals on Wheels, and the highly visible market for specialized equipment, the entrepreneurs saw that the two major needs of most outpatients are contact with the outside world and visits from a battery of qualified service personnel. Of the four sections, they decided that the biggest market gap occurred in the area of contact with the outer world. Customized newsletters, specialized telephone services, and a new market for computer modems were three ideas that looked especially appealing—all because they had been ignored by others.

Maybe other entrepreneurs had overlooked these gaps because they lacked experience using mind maps.

The real mind map our entrepreneurs created was messier than the one reconstructed in Figure 2.4. What's important is that their map allowed the entrepreneurs to visually express what had been a hidden market opportunity. In other words, they used a mind map to give them the Big Picture, and then they located the market gaps.

Working from Major Trends

In the case study that follows, entrepreneur Fred Hayes shows us how to search for gaps and opportunities by taking a long look at a major trend — the **Baby Boom.**

"I got into baby bedding by studying the home," Fred said. "What did it need? What would it be like five years from now? Then I targeted the last wave of Baby Boomers — they were in their late 20s when I founded Sweet Dreams Bedding — and my **market research** told me they were having fewer kids, but spending more money on them. So I positioned my products in what we call the New Nursery. My first year, sales were spotty. My second year, I grossed over $1 million. I listen to my customers, and they tell me what I should produce. That New Nursery is my marketplace."

Baby Boom
an increase in the national birth rate between 1946–1963

market research
data collection and analysis on your current or potential market areas

Case Study

Fred Hayes — Super Seamster

Fred Hayes is a big man, six two, weighing 210 pounds. He served in the Air Force, where he learned to sew, on industrial machines, and to do construction work. When he left the service he made good money in commercial construction.

An on-the-job accident put an end to that career.

Fred was in the hospital three weeks, recuperating, and when he got out, the pain in his back told him he wouldn't be able to continue the construction work.

Fred was bitter, but willing to shift careers:

"Okay, I was 41 years old. I had two great kids and a good marriage. My workmen's comp kept me going long enough for me to look around for a job, and it was clear that no one wanted to hire me.

"That meant I was going to have to work for myself.

"I signed up for a seminar in small business. I was a stand-up student, because it hurt to sit for more than 20 minutes at a stretch. But I got the message of small business loud and clear:

"'Know what business you're in,' the prof said. 'Scrounge up some customers who agree with you. Ask them what products they need and want. Find out what they can pay. Make the product. Ship it. Always pay your bills. And make sure you're pals with your banker before you run short of cash.'"

It was good advice, and Fred took it. Market research told him there was room in the baby bedding business, and he found a job sewing for a mattress manufacturer, to learn the business from the inside. In his spare time, he designed a nursery set for his neighbors, who had a new

Continued

ACTION ⚡ STEP 11

Decode the Secrets of the Shopping Cart

Use your New Eyes to uncover the life-style of your Target Customer by analyzing the contents of a supermarket shopping cart.

The next time you're in a supermarket, deduce the life-styles of the shoppers by observing their behaviors. Give each subject a fantasy name, perhaps associated with a product (Susan Cereal, Steve Steak, Eloise Sugar) so that you can remember your insights. What can you deduce from the contents of each subject's shopping cart? What do their shoes say? Their clothes? What does their jewelry tell you? Or their hairstyle? Put these deductions together with a demographic checklist (sex, age, income, occupation, socio-economic level), and then decide how many of these shoppers are potential Target Customers for your business.

Trained marketeers look for a category of buyer known as Heavy User. A Heavy User of beer would drink 24 cans a day. A Heavy User of apples would eat 20–30 a day. A Heavy User of cigarettes would smoke at least two packs a day.

Who are the Heavy Users in your business? The *potential* Heavy Users?

Got the Big Picture?

 ☐ STEP COMPLETED

baby. They were impressed. And that's how Sweet Dreams Bedding began.

That first year, Fred worked out of his home. When orders came in, he hired some help and moved into a small warehouse. As someone else took over the sewing, Fred went into sales. He kept an accurate customer file, and always was careful to ask what customers liked about the product.

"When you're in the baby business," Fred says, "and especially in the bedding segment, you study birth rates. I spent half my life in the library, looking at SIC codes and census tracts. I knew the Baby Boomers wouldn't have babies forever."

But business is funny, and that second year Fred made a discovery — the young families that were spending more money on their children were concerned with the total look of their nurseries. That gave Fred the clue to move into coordinated nursery items — pillow slips, dust ruffles, coverlets — all with the same design.

"'Trends are like customers,' my small business prof used to say. 'You can spot some of them by standing outside and staring through the window. But others won't show themselves until you're in business, working and sweating away, wondering whether or not you'll make it.'"

Working from the Heavy User

Before we turn from the subject of using the Big Picture to find market gaps, we'd like to suggest one more way to open a window on the Big Picture. In this method you work up a Big Picture by looking at your Target Customers, by determining their life-styles, and then by looking to see if you find any Heavy Users — or potential Heavy Users — for your particular product or service. Action Step 9 provided one technique for learning more about your Target Customer, and now Action Step 11 (opposite) provides another. This time you use the shopping cart as the window through which you view the Big Picture.

Action Step 11 can help you make some informal judgments about the marketplace that will bring you closer to discovering market gaps. It asks you to practice **shopping-cart analysis.**

BEYOND THE BIG PICTURE

The Big Picture of today may not be the Big Picture of tomorrow. In closing this chapter, we want to let you know of a development that may someday become a Fourth Wave that carries civilization beyond the Age of Information — or Third Wave — that was discussed in Chapter 1. This development is bio-technology, or Bio-Tech for short. And as you will see in our boxed insert on Bio-Tech (see page 36), some of the things that can be accomplished are truly amazing.

At the very least you should be aware of Bio-Tech as a possible future that's waiting to happen. Or it could be that the Bio-Tech of today will provide the missing solution to a market gap that has

Shelf Velocity at Work

Shelf velocity is the speed at which a product moves from storage to shelf to customer. If you are selling an item with a small profit margin, you need tremendous shelf velocity to survive. If you are selling items with huge margins, your focus is elsewhere.

Estimate the shelf velocity for each of the items below:

Iceberg lettuce.

Ski boots.

Bikini bathing suit.

Bricks in a brickyard.

Paperback books.

Cosmopolitan magazine.

Potato chips.

Diamonds.

Ice cream.

Yesterday's newspaper.

You can learn about shelf velocity and turn ratios by making contact with trade associations in your industry. You can take a New Eyes look at shelf velocity the next time you walk into a store.

The high velocity items are usually in the back of the store. That forces you to walk past slow-moving items. In a supermarket, milk and bread are on the back wall. In a liquor store, beer is a long way from the door.

Also — high velocity items occupy a higher percentage of shelf space. Compare the shelf space for potato chips to the shelf space for peanuts or corn nuts.

How fast will your products need to move?

shopping-cart analysis
a process of primary research in which you observe purchases in a supermarket, drug store, or other mass market arena

otherwise resisted successful exploration. At the most it should remind you that part of knowing the Big Picture is advance knowledge of coming trends.

In such momentous times it's exciting to be in small business.

And that's probably why you're an entrepreneur.

Bio-Tech — The Fourth Wave?

Their names are tied to the word *genetics* — Amgen, Genentech, Biogen NV, Gentest, Calgene, Genex, Agrigenetics — and they may be headed for a $40 billion industry by the year 2000. Their labors range from creating tiny bugs that eat rocks to let the oil through, to producing an interferon nasal spray to fight the common cold, to searching for the Holy Grail — a chemical marker to help diagnose cancer.

They are the bio-technicians. Their tools are chemicals, enzymes, monoclonal antibodies, vaccines, recombinant plasmids. They are trying to make pork chops grow on trees.

What does Bio-Tech mean for small business?

1. The possibility of getting in on the ground floor of a revolution — if you know your plasmids (one company, International Plant Research Institute of San Carlos, California, was founded on $10,000).
2. A chance for rapid growth (by the year 2000, projected sales are invariably in the billions of dollars).
3. A handhold on shaping the future (rot-resistant potatoes to grow in the tropics; frost-resistant wheat to grow in cold climes).

Bio-Tech, like Information, is not for everyone. If you're inclined toward re-shaping life through genetic engineering, you'll need training and vision and a friendly banker for your R & D.

A pioneer in Texas points the way for adventurers. His name is Al Swan. He's developed three kinds of bugs to extract the last drop of oil from a well. After the drillers leave, Al Swan moves in with his gear — one dump truck filled with water, 25 barrels of molasses, and several million bacteria. Swan pumps his mixture into the dried-up well. It takes about a month, as

1. Bug-strain one eats the rock, freeing trapped oil.
2. Bug-strain two thins the oil so it flows.
3. Bug-strain three creates gas to move the oil topside.

As they finish off the molasses, the bugs die. But Swan's working on a strain that eats oil instead of sugar.

Is Bio-Tech the small business for you?

SOURCE: Adapted from Jim Mintz, "Special Report on Biotechnology," *Venture* (February 1984). Reprinted from the February 1984 issue of *Venture, the Magazine for Entrepreneurs,* by special permission. © 1984 by Venture Magazine, Inc., 35 West 45th St., New York, N.Y., 10036.

SUMMARY

The trend of our civilization is *away* from the smokestacks of heavy industry and *toward* information, computers, and data-processing. Within this general trend, individual products and services go through a four-phase cycle — birth, growth, maturity, decline. Before you open the doors of your small business, you need to know what phase you're in. For example, if you think there's easy money in selling microcomputers, you need to know that this industry has passed its growth stage and is now maturing. If you want to install solar products, you need to know that this industry has left the birth stage and is now entering an area of growth. If you're thinking about opening a toy store, you need to know that this industry is mature, and that you'll have to steal customers from other people.

Remember what happened to the American railroads. Less than a hundred years ago, railroads were a powerful industry. They forgot what business they were in and they are no longer powerful. (Is the same thing happening to some of the smaller firms you know?)

By being alert to market signals — and by combining New Eyes research with research of secondary sources — you will be able to chart large trends and to place specific products in the life cycle.

Various sources of hard data are recommended: newspapers, magazines, trade journals, banks, planning offices, reports from colleges and universities, real estate firms, the SBA, and federal depositories. SIC (Standard Industrial Classification) codes will help you formally identify your industry, define its boundaries, locate customers and supplies, and reach out to other industries.

ACTION ⚡ STEP
——— REVIEW ———

Action Steps in Chapter 2 help you organize the construction of your own window into the Big Picture.

7 You define your business by deciding what business you're really in. Then you have fun designing your own business letterhead. Locate your trade associations in the *Encyclopedia of Associations*, start writing off for industry information, and you're on your way.

8 When you look at trends in the local marketplace, you'll see what's new, what's hot — and what's dusty.

9 There is no better way to analyze your Target Customers than to walk their neighborhood during the weekend when the garage doors are open.

10 By getting together with your friends on the weighty topics of segmentation and gap analysis, you can brainstorm your way to a clear view of unexplored opportunities in the Big Picture.

11 This Action Step helps you uncover the life-style of your Target Customer by analyzing the contents of a shopping cart. This one can be fun.

THINK POINTS

⚡ The most valuable tool you can have for charting trends is the four-stage life-cycle yardstick. The life-cycle yardstick helps you plant yourself in a growth industry; it helps you decide what business you're really in; and it leads you to gaps and segments that look promising.

⚡ Once you know what segment you're in, you can focus on your market research with New Eyes.

⚡ While the major corporations are floundering around in Toffler's Trough, between the Second and Third Waves, you can latch onto a trend that will help you survive (in style) for the next 10 – 15 years.

⚡ Even Big Pictures change. By staying alert to trends, and by looking around you with New Eyes, you can be prepared for the changes before they happen.

⚡ What new markets have been created by the Baby Boom of the Baby Boomers?

REFERENCES

Akey, Denise, ed. *Encyclopedia of Associations.* Vol. 1, *National Organizations of the U.S.;* Vol. 2, *Geographic and Executive Index;* Vol. 3, *New Associations and Projects.* 17th ed. Detroit: Gale Research Co., 1982.

Buss, Dale D. "GM Weighing More Big Cuts in Work Force. *Wall Street Journal,* February 21, 1984. Predicts a cut in the GM work force up to 120,000 people by mid-1986. An internal company document talks about wage increases based on corporate performance, robotics, and "aggressive productivity."

"Chrysler, Having Cut Muscle as Well as Fat, Is Still in a Weak State." *Wall Street Journal,* July 15, 1983. Summarizes the Chrysler saga from bail out to repayment of the first $400 million to U.S. government. Excellent piece on a segment of the auto industry.

Contacts Influential. Cleveland, Ohio: Contacts Influential International, 1984. A comprehensive body of business information on the county level that takes off from SIC codes and goes through firms by zip code, key individuals, all the way to a business telephone index. If your library doesn't have this reference, it's because a subscription costs $1,000 a year. For more information, write Contacts Influential Marketing Information Services, 20950 Center Ridge Road, Suite 106, Cleveland, OH 41116.

Engelmayer, Paul A. "Worker Owned and Operated Supermarket Yields Financial Success, Personal Rewards." *Wall Street Journal,* August 18, 1983. Heartwarming piece about the union and union-member purchase of a going-out-of-business A & P supermarket in Philadelphia. The story reads like a page from Naisbitt's book — the end of the pyramid, the demise of the large corporation, the move to local control and local ownership. Along with *Megatrends,* the Journal can keep you current with what's happening in the world and in business.

The IMS Ayer Directory of Publications. Fort Washington, Pa.: IMS Press, 1984. Good starting point for running down trade associations and trade publications. Note that we have a brief list of major associations in Appendix C.

Naisbitt, John. *Megatrends: Ten New Directions Transforming Our Lives.* New York: Warner Books, 1982. Naisbitt's book makes trend-charting easy. The book is well-written, positive, and farsighted. We've said it before — *Megatrends* is a must read for entrepreneurs.

Rifkin, Jeremy. *Algeny: A New Word — A New World.* New York: Penguin Books, 1984. A negative view of genetic engineering. Rifkin likens Bio-Tech to a tougher version of the Dutch Elm disease that ravaged trees in the Midwest.

Standard & Poor's Register of Corporations, Directors and Executives. New York: Standard & Poor's Corporation, 1984. The S & P directories are in most libraries.

Survey of Buying Power. New York: Sales & Marketing Management Magazine, 1983. S & MM publishes annual supplements to its magazine that are extremely helpful to the small business owner. We also like their *Survey of Commercial and Industrial Buying Power.* If your library doesn't have these volumes, you can write for more information to the S & MM office at 633 Third Avenue, New York, NY 10164-0563.

Tepper, Terri, and Nona Dawe Tepper. *The New Entrepreneurs: Women Working from Home.* New York: Universe Books, 1980.

Thomas Register of American Manufacturers and Thomas Register Catalog File. New York: Thomas Publishing Co., 1984. If you're wondering whether your invention has already been invented, check the Thomas' catalogs of manufacturers—complete with product descriptions, photos, and so on.

A Description
of Product
or Service

B The Market
and the
Target
Customer

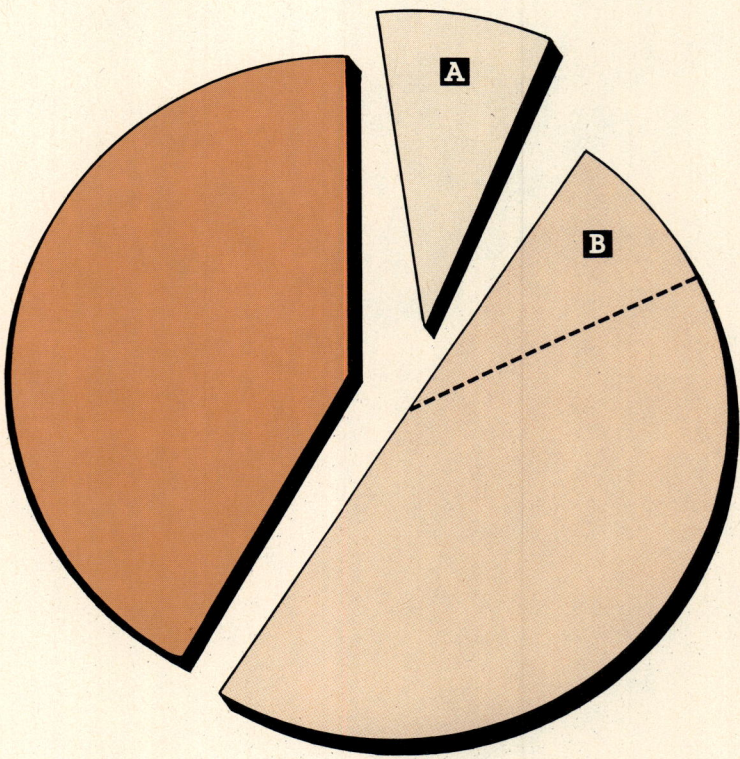

FIGURE 3.1 Chapter 3 furthers your Business Plan by introducing the concept of "Power Marketing."

3

Power Marketing

LEARNING OBJECTIVES

To mesh your personal business objectives with the vast opportunities in the marketplace.

To learn to accept your business objectives as a force which can give a positive and unique thrust to your business.

To narrow your industry research down until viable gaps begin to appear.

To use an industry chronology to gain insight into hidden pockets of the life cycle.

To expand your New Eyes approach into a whole-brain approach, so that you are using your intuition (it imagines the future) as well as your analytic ability (it interprets the past).

To turn problems into opportunities.

To combine demographic (population) data and psychographic (picture of a life-style) data into your first customer profile.

To begin to watch for Heavy Users for your product or service.

To brainstorm creatively.

To use a matrix grid to blend your objectives and your research findings into a portrait of a business.

 **L**ife in the Information Age is exciting. Opportunities exist that were unheard of five years ago. The speed is exhilarating. If you've done only a fraction of the research suggested in Chapter 2, you're now experiencing information overload. That's understandable. You're creative. You're wound up. Unless you live 200 years, you've packed in more ideas than you can follow up.

What you need is a filter system, something like a wine press or a *moulin* (a French kitchen machine that makes applesauce). You have all this information and all these ideas. You need a sifter.

WELCOME TO POWER MARKETING

Power Marketing is a tool that will help you exploit gaps in the marketplace. It connects your skills to your research. It tells you what new skills you'll need to develop. It aims the power of your mind at a particular segment of small business.

If you'll look at Figure 3.2, you'll see that Power Marketing requires seven moves. If you've been doing each Action Step as you move through the book, you'll be ahead of the game now. Here's a quick preview of what Power Marketing can help you do:

1. Identify your business (and personal) objectives.
2. Dig deeper into your favorite industry.
3. Identify 3–5 industry segments.
4. Turn problems into opportunities.
5. Brainstorm "mad" solutions.
6. Sift your objectives and solutions.
7. Concentrate on your particular segment.

A lot of entrepreneurs are using Power Marketing and don't know it. This chapter streamlines the process so that you can use it too — consciously and effectively.

At this point, you have just begun to plan. The marketplace lies open in all its excitement and confusion. The most important thing is not to lose your momentum. Momentum is confidence. Confidence helps you to win. The beauty of Power Marketing is that you start out by *using* your excitement to generate the "raw material"; the later stages of the process will help you come up with something even more valuable: a winning business concept.

Power Marketing is like a huge funnel, equipped with a series of idea filters. (See Figure 3.3 on page 44.) You throw in everything — goals, personality, industry data, problems, hopes, fears — and you come out at the end with a solid business idea. You'll know where you're going.

And that is power.

To illustrate how Power Marketing works, we've developed a case study that leads you through all seven steps. At this point, we're also introducing an important concept — teamwork.

ACTION  STEP
PREVIEW

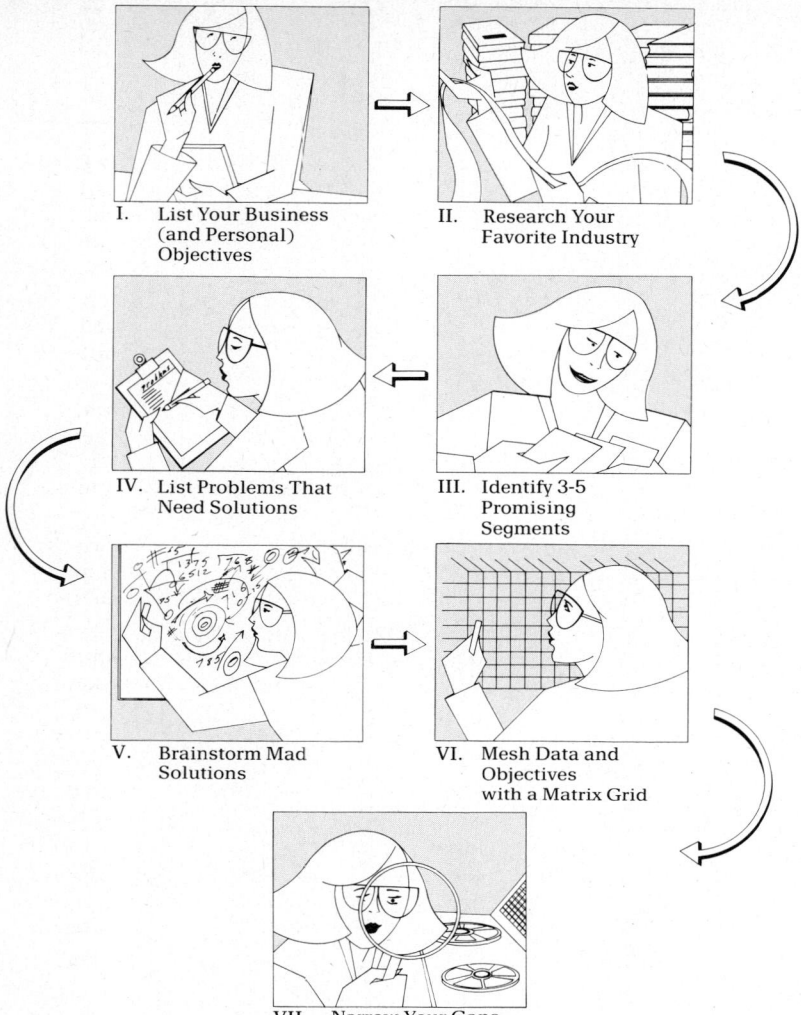

I. List Your Business (and Personal) Objectives

II. Research Your Favorite Industry

III. Identify 3-5 Promising Segments

IV. List Problems That Need Solutions

V. Brainstorm Mad Solutions

VI. Mesh Data and Objectives with a Matrix Grid

VII. Narrow Your Gaps

FIGURE 3.2 The seven secret moves of Power Marketing.

Case Study

Introducing the Info Team

Five principals teamed together to explore opportunities in some segment of the Information Industry. They chose Information because they saw it was the wave of the future, and that it accounted for at least 50% of the Gross National Product (GNP).

The opportunity was certainly there. But anything that huge would be hard to define. So the team needed a systematic process to help them explore gaps.

Before we get into the process, here are brief profiles of each principal:

Principal A — an organizer with experience in small business consulting. His background was in engineering and commercial flying. He had a strong feeling about the power of computers long before they became popular.   *Continued*

Principal B—a manager, marketeer, and teacher. Her background was in big business and psychology.

Principal C—an attorney.

Principal D—a teacher, seminar leader, and consultant to small business. His background was corporate. His expertise was in marketing of industrial products.

Principal E—a teacher, seminar leader, inventor, engineer, and programmer. He had worked with the mass transit industry in Japan where he had first encountered robotics. His expertise was in the creation of products.

All five members had extensive experience in owning and operating small businesses.

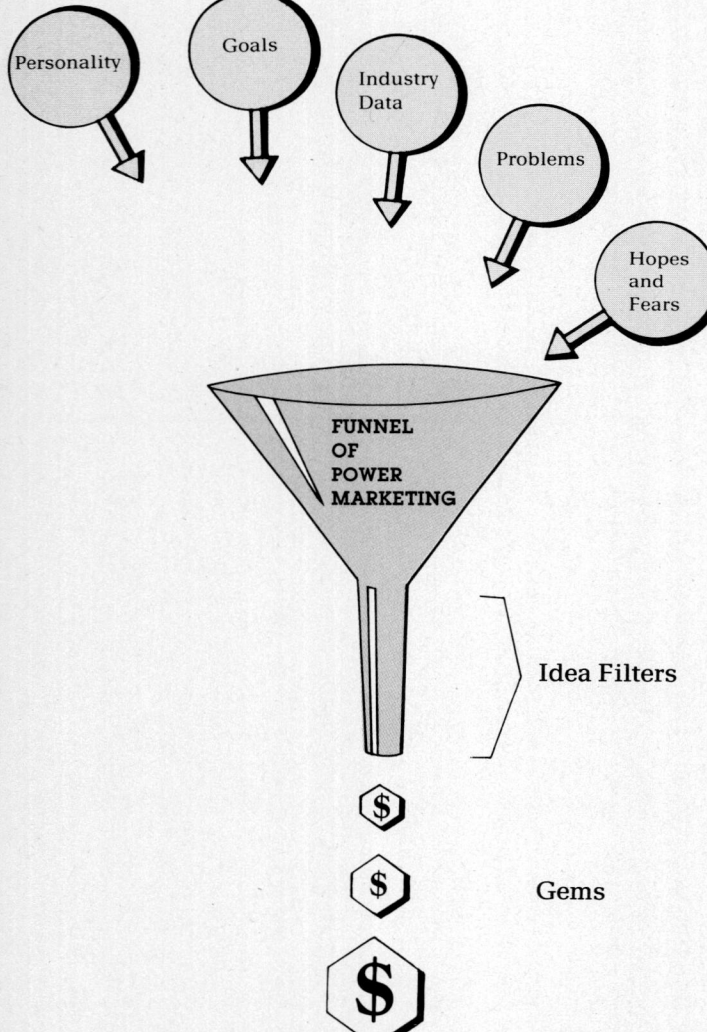

FIGURE 3.3 One way to look at Power Marketing is as though it were a huge funnel, equipped with a series of idea filters.

KNOW YOUR OBJECTIVES

Now you know the background of each of the principals — but why are they gathered for this particular project? No doubt they each have various **business objectives,** but what are they? You could just as well ask yourself why you are now in, or about to start, a small business. And that is what Action Step 12 asks you to do — to list your business (and personal) objectives. (In small business, business objectives are often the same as personal objectives!) Action Step 12 will help you express your goals in a nonjudgmental way. Don't limit the range of your imagination in this Action Step. If your business desires are a confused jumble, imagine what it was like when all five team members started in!

They started by listing their individual business objectives, and then they tried to boil the list down to objectives everyone could agree on.

Agreement wasn't easy.

Case Study

Brainstorming Business Objectives

They argued a long time, but they came up with nine objectives that sounded like heaven.

1. **Psychic Rewards.** They wanted to build something, to plant a seed and watch it grow.
2. **Teamwork.** They wanted to be a part of something bigger than themselves. Each member of the team had strengths and weaknesses. With luck, blending, and balancing, the team could be greater than the sum of its parts.
3. **Financial Returns.** They wanted to see a respectable ROI (Return on Investment) — 25% at a minimum.
4. **Safety.** They did not want to lose money.
5. **Growth Industry.** The members of the team had a combined business experience of 163 years. They had known failure. They had known success. They wanted a booming segment of a **growth industry.**
6. **Time.** Getting a business up and running takes a year at least. Sometimes, it takes longer. They wanted a business that would last at least three years.
7. **No Competition.** They wanted no viable **competition** for the opening phase of their operation.
8. **Key People.** They wanted to attract the best people in the field.
9. **Fun, Adventure, Excitement.** From experience, they knew that starting a small business, even in a growth or glamour industry, would involve hassles, problems, expensive surprises. So they wanted to make sure they'd be in a business where they would be having fun.

Continued

---

business objectives
measurable goals a
business is trying to reach

ACTION 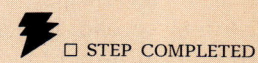 STEP 12

List Your Personal and Business Objectives

What do you want from small business? Money? Fame? Job security? To be your own boss? Freedom to explore the marketplace? Control of your own professional destiny?

Or maybe you just want to be President of the company.

Think back to the forces that made you consider small business in the first place. What were those forces? Where were you when you first thought about owning the store? How have circumstances changed your goals?

You probably will not have trouble writing down objectives, but if you do, flip back to your notes on your dream year (Action Step 3) and to your skills analysis (Action Step 5).

List anything, whether within reason or not, whether embarrassing or not. The matrix grid will sift it for you later.

In the case study that follows, you can see the team wanted the moon.

□ STEP COMPLETED

---

growth industry
an industry with an annual
sales growth that is
considerably higher than
the national average

competition
the contestants in your
arena who are fighting
you for business

That's quite a list of objectives, but they were convinced that they still had made the right choice with the Information Industry. What industry would you choose?

RESEARCH

Organizing Your Information

We all have a favorite industry, and Action Step 13 gets you started researching your favorite. An industry is a broad classification, and what you're aiming for in this Action Step is a similarly broad overview. Your favorite industry could be transportation, entertainment, food service, travel, education, publishing, retailing, construction, small manufacturing, information, or anything that looks interesting. But get started on whichever industry you choose — and get started on Action Step 13 — now.

Look for information from your previous Action Steps. Pay a visit to your local library for a look at periodicals like the *Wall Street Journal, Venture,* or other general business or news sources. The *Reader's Guide to Periodical Literature* will point you to dozens of helpful articles in your field. Or ask your local librarian for help. What you hope to come up with is a good picture of how the trends are breaking in your favorite industry. Later you can determine how best to take advantage of those trends — right now the important goal is information.

To focus on any industry, you'll want to organize the information you gather. Action Step 13 recommends that you organize your research into categories like life cycle, speed of change, history, competition, recent industry breakthroughs, costs of positioning yourself, customer spread, and so on. (Often the very nature of your industry will determine which categories you choose.) One important function of these categories is that you can later use them as idea filters — when it comes time for you to sift your ideas through the funnel of Power Marketing. For example, one category which is usually helpful as a filter is the life-cycle yardstick. (Learn to use it fast, like a reflex. When you see a business, label it with one of the four phases.) A mature segment of a mature industry is not going to leave much room for a creative entrepreneur.

A second helpful category is competition, which we'll be discussing in detail in Chapter 5. Competition varies with each stage of the life cycle, and you can imagine how useful competition is as an idea filter.

A third category that might be helpful is the concept of industry **breakthrough.** What is there in your industry that really hums? It could be technological, like the microchip. It could be theoretical, like Theory Z, a management theory which was imported from Japan. Using this category as a filter, you could ask yourself if your business idea is taking advantage of the current breakthrough.

We may be getting ahead of ourselves by talking about idea filters now. Let's get back to categories as a useful way to organize your

 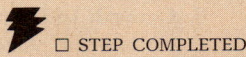
breakthrough
finding a way through, over, under, or around the wall

information. First, let's see how our Info Team used some of the categories to organize—and to analyze—their research. Use their brief analyses as models for your own exploration.

Industry Research

With all of the research they gathered, the team decided to concentrate on the role of the microcomputer within the Information Industry. Their findings:

Life Cycle.   Hardware seems to be maturing. The life cycle of a particular machine can be as short as 18 months (*Wall Street Journal*, August 19, 1983). The life cycle of a piece of software can be longer. Wordstar, a complex but powerful word-processing program, stayed on the software bestseller list for months. But the early electronic spreadsheet programs (Visicalc, Supercalc) are being challenged by new integrated systems like Lotus 1-2-3 or Symphony.

(*Problem:* Finding a gap that has a longer life cycle.)

Competition.   Heaviest competition is in manufacturing and retailing of hardware. Next heaviest is in creating and retailing of software. From a distance, this seems like holdover behavior from the Industrial Age, but that doesn't make it any less fierce.

(*Problem:* Finding a duck pond that's not crowded with hungry hunters.)

Industry Breakthrough.   Printed circuits, microcircuits, and so on. From the consumer point of view, the major breakthrough might have been with components—the computer system (computer, display terminal, detachable keyboard, printer, and other add-ons) now bore some resemblance to a home stereo system (stereo, turntable, tape deck, speakers, and other components). Hooking up a system, if it worked, was fun. Detachable parts are easier to move and easier to haul in for repair. Another major breakthrough could have been with the portables, introduced by Osborne in July, 1981, and with the lap models, which came in 1982.

(*Problem:* if you get into the Information Age, which hardware do you aim at? Which software do you use?)

Quick Conclusion.   You can't get enough data fast enough. The speed of the field is overwhelming, breathless, and exciting. You can't stop long enough to make a decision. Yet you must stop to breathe.

Well, the Info Team isn't anywhere near a final decision yet, but that's exactly the point. At this stage of Power Marketing, the team is still making the most of its research to understand its chosen industry—the decision-making stage comes later. Right now we want to share with you one other category the Info Team used to organize and analyze its research—a selective **industry chronology.** A selective chronology is useful—especially in a fast-breaking industry like information—because it gives you a feel for the rhythm of the important trends at work. A selective chronology could be just

industry chronology
the time sequence of major developments in an industry

the thing to let you position your business venture to be at the right place at the right time. The chronology can also help you take the long view of your chosen industry. Here's what the Info Team came up with.

Case Study

Selective Chronology

1977. Apple introduces the micro.

1981. 1 million computer systems shipped by U.S. manufacturers.

1982. Adam Osborne launches new sewing-machine size portable. IBM sells 2 million computers. Apple still in first place with 33% of market. According to Naisbitt's *Trend Letter* (July 27, 1983), personal computers in homes increase from 340,000 to 2.4 million. At Comdex, the microcomputer industry's giant show in Las Vegas, the new "wrinkle" is that more people are developing more software for the IBM-PC than for any other 16-bit machine. (*Inc.*, March 1983.)

February 1983. Pacific Stereo decides to explore computer retailing. (*CRN*, February 7, 1983)

August 1983. Computerland of Connecticut drops its six-year-old Apple contract, and Softmart, Inc., launches a network of stores devoted entirely to IBM-PC software (*CRN*, August 22, 1983). Kaypro, the other portable, goes public; six-month sales were $26.1 million, up from previous $1.9 million; to date, Kaypro has sold 47,500 units; analysts think Kaypro may survive (*Wall Street Journal*, August 26, 1983).

September 1983. Osborne, the creator of the first portable computer, seeks bankruptcy protection.

December 1983. Suffering from low sales for Lisa, Apple computer counts heavily on Macintosh to keep company afloat.

August 1984. IBM drops prices and adds features to PC Junior.

August 1984. Apple introduces portable PC.

Case Study

Random Predictions

Future Computing. Future Computing, a market research firm, predicted that software sales volume would reach $2 billion in 1983. By 1988, says the research firm, volume will be six times greater (*Wall Street Journal*, August 26, 1983).

Dataquest. According to Dataquest of Cupertino, California, the business in simplified, fault-tolerant computer processing systems (for airline reservations or banking transactions, for example) was $3.6 billion in 1980 and will grow to $19.5 billion by 1985 (*Venture*, November 1982).

Nation's Business. By 1986, the number of computers will be 5.9 million. The number of desktop computers will be "staggering" (*Nation's Business*, December 1982).

Note how the team made use of existing predictions to get a feel for the future of their industry as well as its recent past. The result is a brief, selective chronology that sums up their industry's past, present, and future. What did the team do next, now that the research was in? The same thing you'll have to do: Look for market gaps (unmet needs in the marketplace) and promising industry segments.

MARKET GAPS AND INDUSTRY SEGMENTS

When you write your Business Plan, you'll need to explain why you chose a particular market segment. If you choose the right segment — and you communicate your excitement — you'll have developed a hook for the banker or venture capitalist who's reading your plan. Action Step 14 sets the stage for writing that section of the Plan. It helps you focus on gaps in the marketplace.

There's a secret to focusing on market segments or gaps, and Action Step 14 just gave you that secret. Once you've chosen a few promising segments, you consider who your Target Customer is. Very often, the Target Customer helps you define your true market. That's why it pays to profile your Target Customer. (The Target-Customer profile can act as one more idea filter in the funnel of Power Marketing.)

The minute you get to people, you've found your segment.

In the following scenario, we see how our team made a few quick decisions to focus on a particular segment of the industry. "After that, we started to look at people," Principal A says. "The minute you get to people, you've found your segment." Let's see how the Info Team developed their first profile and how it led to a different market.

 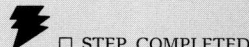
Case Study

Identifying Segments, Gaps, and Target Customers

After looking hard at the Information Industry and after analyzing their research, the team quickly segmented the industry. They used a pie chart, as reproduced in Figure 3.4 on page 51. [Pie charts are great because they're easy to use. Try using a pie chart to segment your industry.] The team made some fast conclusions:

1. Hardware production was out.
2. Software writing or creation was possible.
3. The main gap seemed to be in education and training.

As soon as they identified this gap, team members began to think of the people who use microcomputers. The words flew about the room as team members thought of various users: "Business people!" "Hobbyists!" "Students!" "How about engineers?" "Don't forget word processors!" "And educators!"

Continued

"We started off discovering two things all these potential users had in common," Principal A says, "and they were **computerphobia** and a lack of education in how to use computers. We followed these needs all the way through the Information Society to a successful business." By now, there was no doubt. The main gap was in computer training.

The team quickly realized they needed to define their market further. One way they did this was to profile their Target Customers. They identified two kinds of customers—personal and industrial. The profiles that emerged from the group discussion were interesting indeed.

Primary Target Customer

The main potential recipients of this training looked like this:

Sex: predominantly male

Age: 18–35

Education: Some college

Owns PC: 30%

Access to computer at work: 52%

Lives near computer store: 73%

Income: $35,000 and up a year

This customer was the primary target, and quickly led to a more obvious target—the customer's employer.

Secondary Target Customer

Size of business: 1–30 employees

Annual income: $250,000–$5 million

Major output: Paper, reports (a few firms in small manufacturing)

Location: 15 mile radius of the team's 100% location

Figure 3.5 on page 52 reproduces the mind map that the Info Team used to help define their business. They started with a total market (in this case, computer education) and were soon discussing hardware, location, and Target Customers. In an hour or so they had gone from an industry overview to a detailed picture of a very promising market gap!

PROBLEMS

Once you have identified at least two major target markets, you are in a position to take a closer look. One way to do this is to search for **problems** in the industry.

Action Step 15 gets you started on this list. And for good measure, we'll show you how the Info Team listed problems in their industry.

ACTION ⚡ STEP 15

List Problems in the Industry that Need Solutions

When you surveyed your friends in Action Step 10, you were approaching the list of problems you need to develop now.

The difference is, now you want to list problems that are unique to the industry you've been exploring.

Follow your success with Action Step 10 and get together with some people who know something about your industry. Ask them for input. Write everything down.

Then develop your list of problems.

The more problems you can find, the wider will be your opportunities to prosper in your segment.

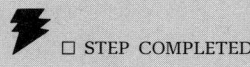

☐ STEP COMPLETED

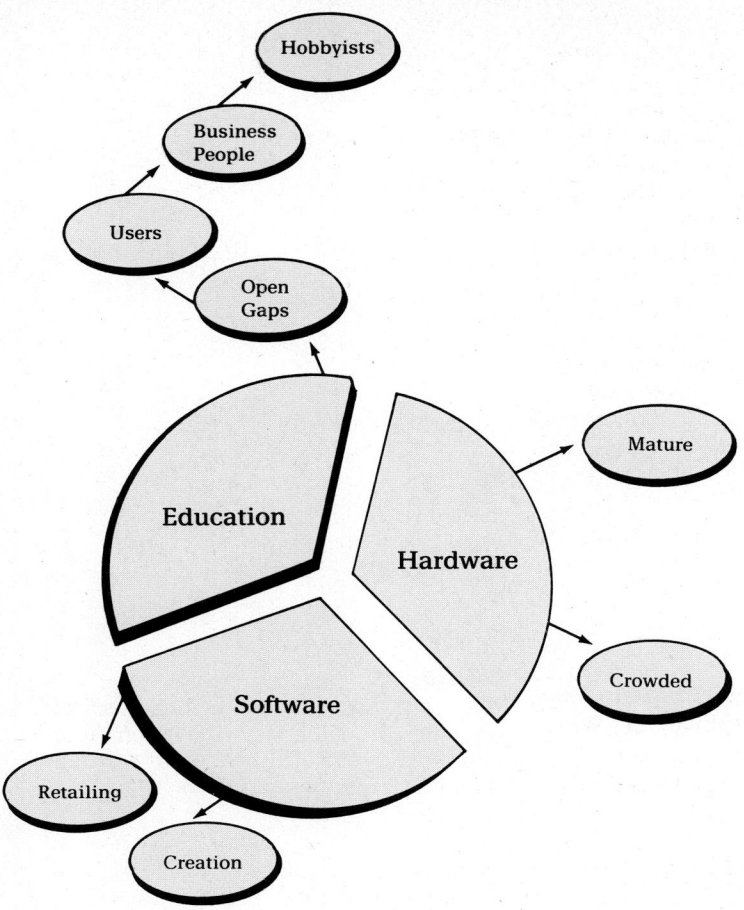

FIGURE 3.4 By segmenting the Information Industry, the team was able to identify the biggest gap with the greatest growth potential.

Follow this list carefully, and then **extrapolate** to your own. (You may find that some problems carry over.)

extrapolate
to project known data into an area that is as yet unknown

Case Study

Listing Problems in the Computer Industry

    1. User Frustration. The most obvious problem in the microcomputer segment of the Information Industry was user frustration. In their haste to join the Information Society, buyers had raced out to purchase sophisticated hardware. Hardware won't do anything without **software**—except drink up electricity. Software creators, sensing a tremendous market gap, flooded the market with software, not all of it good, and most of it plagued with Problem 2.

    2. Poor Documentation. The printed matter that was supposed to explain the software was disorganized and clumsily written, thus making the entire system user-unfriendly and even user-hostile.

    3. Minimal Support from Manufacturers. Because of the **short life cycle** of their product, computer makers were putting the bulk of their energies into creating new products so they could compete in the marketplace. A few software makers had established toll-free, 800-

Continued

software
the information base that tells the hardware what to do

short life cycle
a very rapid movement from birth to death of a product or service

number hotlines to answer questions from frustrated users. But toll-free numbers do not solve this real problem.

4. Minimal Support from Retailers. Retail merchants who sold hardware and software had little time to provide service after the sale. Salespeople, trained to sell and close deals with all the energy of the fast-track, were unavailable following the sale. Increased price-cutting by dealers led to an even lower level of service and training.

5. Mounting Buyer Exasperation. After the computer purchase, the average buyer made ten trips back to the retailer for information, help, troubleshooting, explanations, and hand-holding.

6. Clumsiness in the Marketplace. The rare retailer that did attempt training used conventional classroom techniques, and used them poorly. The student—the new computer user—would suffer through dull lectures, rote drill, and the exasperation of an instructor trying to teach people about computers with a blackboard and a piece of chalk.

SOLUTIONS

The Info Team recognized that here was a clear case of failure to meet human needs. The gap was widening in the marketplace, and when that happens, you have a clear signal for transforming problems into opportunities. Before we follow our team through this process, follow

FIGURE 3.5 The Info Team used a mind map to help them define their business. They started with a total market—computer education—and finished with a detailed picture of a promising market gap.

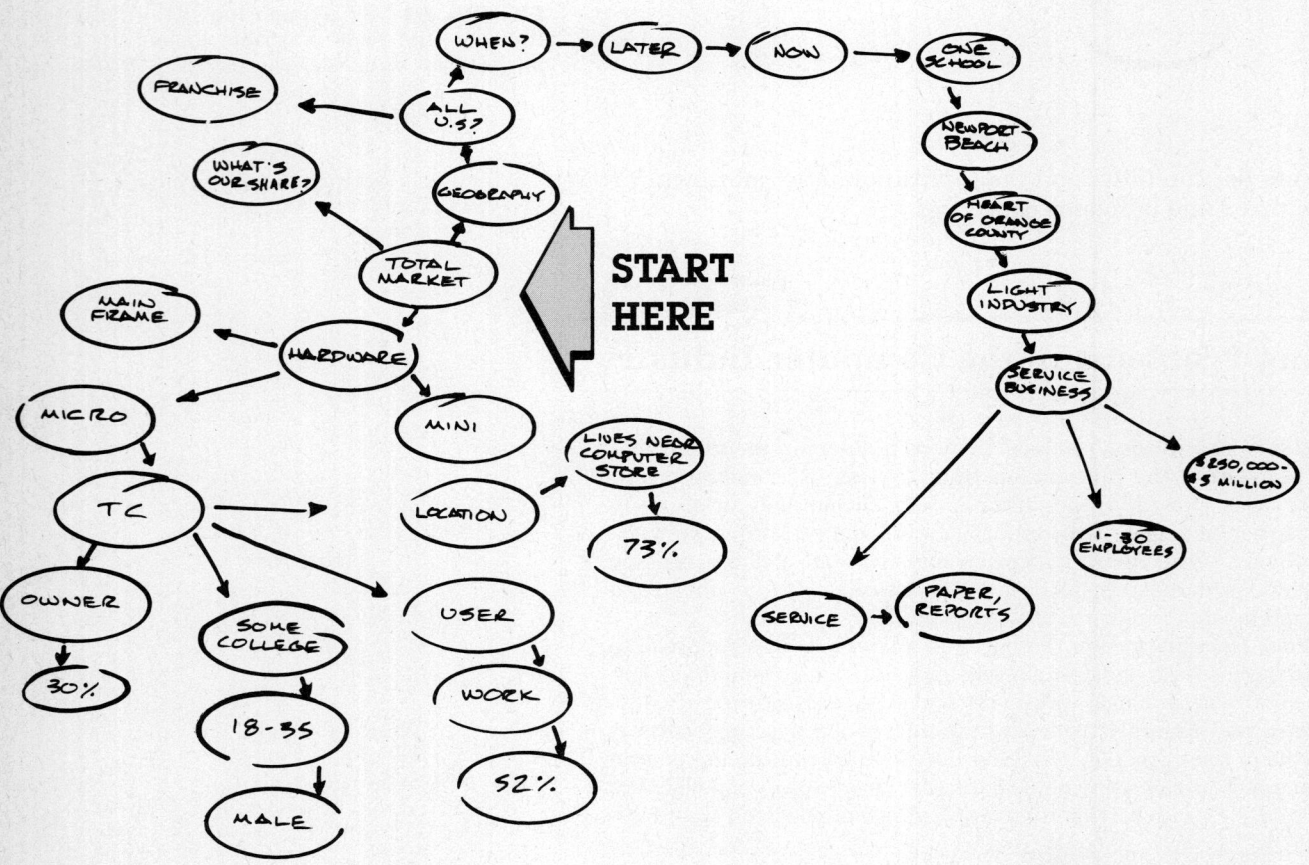

your own list of problems. Every problem can be turned into an opportunity, and Action Step 16 gets you started on that process. We don't expect you to go through this calmly and logically. We expect you to brainstorm mad solutions. (You can filter your ideas through the funnel of Power Marketing later. Right now you need the raw material!)

When human needs aren't being met, you have a widening gap in the marketplace, and a clear signal for transforming problems into opportunities.

Brainstorming is a subtle art used by many large corporations to probe the unconscious mind for ideas. You begin small, with ideas that could seem erroneous, and then, as you gain momentum, your concepts develop. The key to brainstorming is to keep the negative ideas to a minimum so that creativity gets all of the energy.

What follows is a recap of a brainstorming session held by the Info Team as they began to turn problems into opportunities. You can see at this stage how personality and motivation meshes with business objectives.

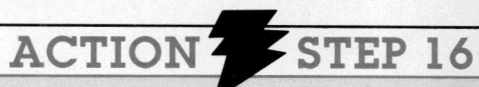

ACTION STEP 16

Brainstorm Mad Solutions

Okay, here's where you get creative. You've just listed problems in your industry. Now figure out how to solve them.

There's a good chance you'll come up with better ideas in the long run if you just let your imagination run fast and free.

Don't stop yourself with a lot of logic and reason — not at this stage — but just let your mind work at top speed.

You might begin with a quick overview of what you know so far, then slide over into solutions.

A cassette recorder will be useful if you do your best thinking "out loud."

Have fun.

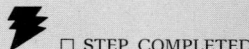
☐ STEP COMPLETED

Case Study

Brainstorming Mad Solutions

To start with a quick overview of problems they had discovered, Principal A took the lead.

"All right," Principal A said. "What we've got here are unhappy micro owners. They've just spent anywhere from $1,000 to $15,000 on a system that was supposed to streamline business operations. Only the system won't perform as specified."

"So," D asked. "What's their first move?"

"Easy," E said. "They go to the documentation. But it was written by an engineer in something that only looks like English, and they can see it would take a couple of months to translate the manual and apply it to their business."

"Yes," B said. "Only they don't have two months. The reason they bought this system in the first place was to save time and upgrade production. Now the poor users have this expensive hardware just sitting there, soaking up electricity and humming at them."

"That's exactly right," C said. "And they are *still* doing their books caveman style."

They had defined the problem. Now was the moment for brainstorming.

"So what do we do about it?" A asked.

"I've got it," D says. "Let's rent a jet, fly to Armonk, and take over IBM."

(Laughter)

"I have a better one," D said. "Let's retool the Business Plan, take it to some venture capital people I know, set up a software company. I know a venture capitalist in L.A. who'd love to get his hands on a hot software company. He could sell it before we got it put together."

"I'm beat," C said, yawning. "When's the next boat for Tahiti?"

"I feel silly, saying this," B said, "but why couldn't we invent a robot? The robot could take the place of the office staff. We could

Continued

program him to run the computer. Once a month we'd drop by, give him some DW-40, and replace his battery."

"I know this guy in Hong Kong," D says, grinning. "He'd love to have a contract for a robot that does word processing. And he's got the Japanese contacts to make it fly."

"Let's run seminars," E said. "We could train people to care for their computerized robots."

"Let's push that seminar idea," A said.

"Yes," B said. "Seminars."

"Push it all the way to Tahiti?" C asked. "Or Armonk?" C was tired.

"What about a school?" A asked.

"School? What kind of school?" E asked.

"A computer school. One that teaches software."

"My Uncle Charley's a farmer, back in Dubuque," D said. "He just bought a micro. Uncle Charley could be our first student."

"It's not a bad idea, you know," B said. "Our school would have to be fast. No quarters or semesters. And it would have to be well organized."

"She's right," D said. "Business people are busy."

"And it would have to be user-friendly," A said, beginning to write on the board. "That would solve one huge problem."

"It would have to be comfortable," E said. "I always learn faster when I'm comfortable."

B smiled, warming to the idea. "We could guarantee learning."

"How?" C asked.

"There won't be grades in our school. So if customers don't get it the first time through, they can come back for a second try."

"Like mail order," E said. "We give them a guarantee."

"Right," B said.

"I like it," A said.

"So do I," E said.

"I hate to admit it, guys," C said, "but I kind of like it, too."

[That wasn't a bad idea D had, about his Uncle Charley becoming the first student at the software school. See the boxed article, "Marketing Micros down on the Farm," on page 58.]

Let's try to summarize:

1. The school would have to be near computer stores.
2. The school would have to be in the heart of a solid market of micro-users.
3. The school would have to be comfortable, priced right.
4. The school would have to look like an executive board room, not a classroom. For their Target Customers, atmosphere was a big selling point.

It's helpful to summarize after a brainstorming session, so that you identify the most useful ideas. After you summarize, do a quick mind map. Then you'll have most of your experience down on paper. Figure 3.6 shows the mind map that the Info Team drew up.

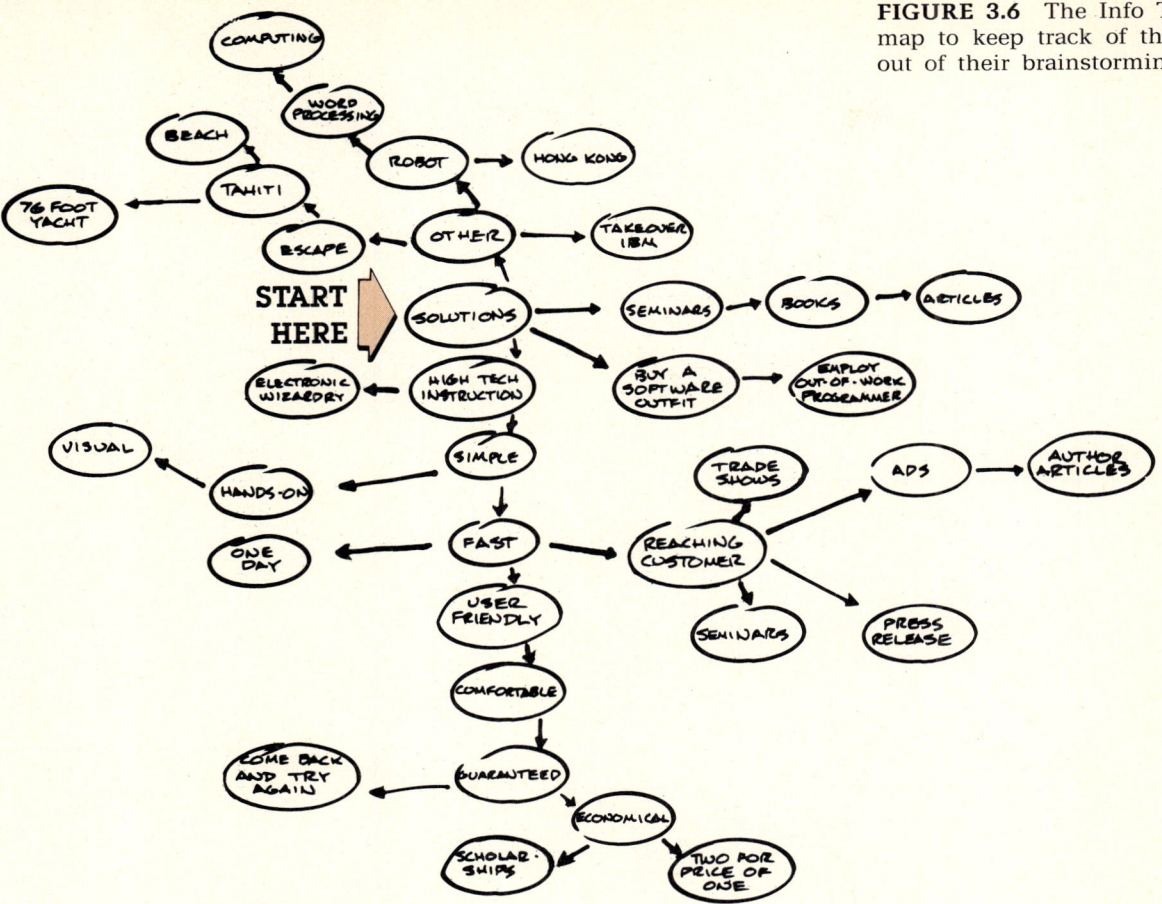

FIGURE 3.6 The Info Team drew a mind map to keep track of the solutions to come out of their brainstorming session.

MATRIX ANALYSIS

Some people really like mind maps. Others prefer a more methodical system for arriving at conclusions. A **matrix grid** is one such system. After you have brainstormed your way through a series of solutions, use a matrix grid to get even more focus. On page 56, Action Step 17 walks you through the process. We've also included a sample matrix grid at Table 3.1. This particular matrix is the one used by our Info Team—*before* they started assigning values.

As the team members worked through the matrix, the pattern of the software school became more defined, and new problems surfaced. Let's join them now.

It should be obvious that the matrix analysis is one of the most powerful idea filters available to you as you funnel your hopes and plans through the Power Marketing process. The beauty of the matrix analysis is that it allows you to consider crazy and creative solutions, and it keeps you true to your personal and business objectives. And it makes you a very effective entrepreneur.

matrix grid
a screen or filter through which ideas are passed in order to form solutions

TABLE 3.1 Matrix Grid for Proposed Information Business

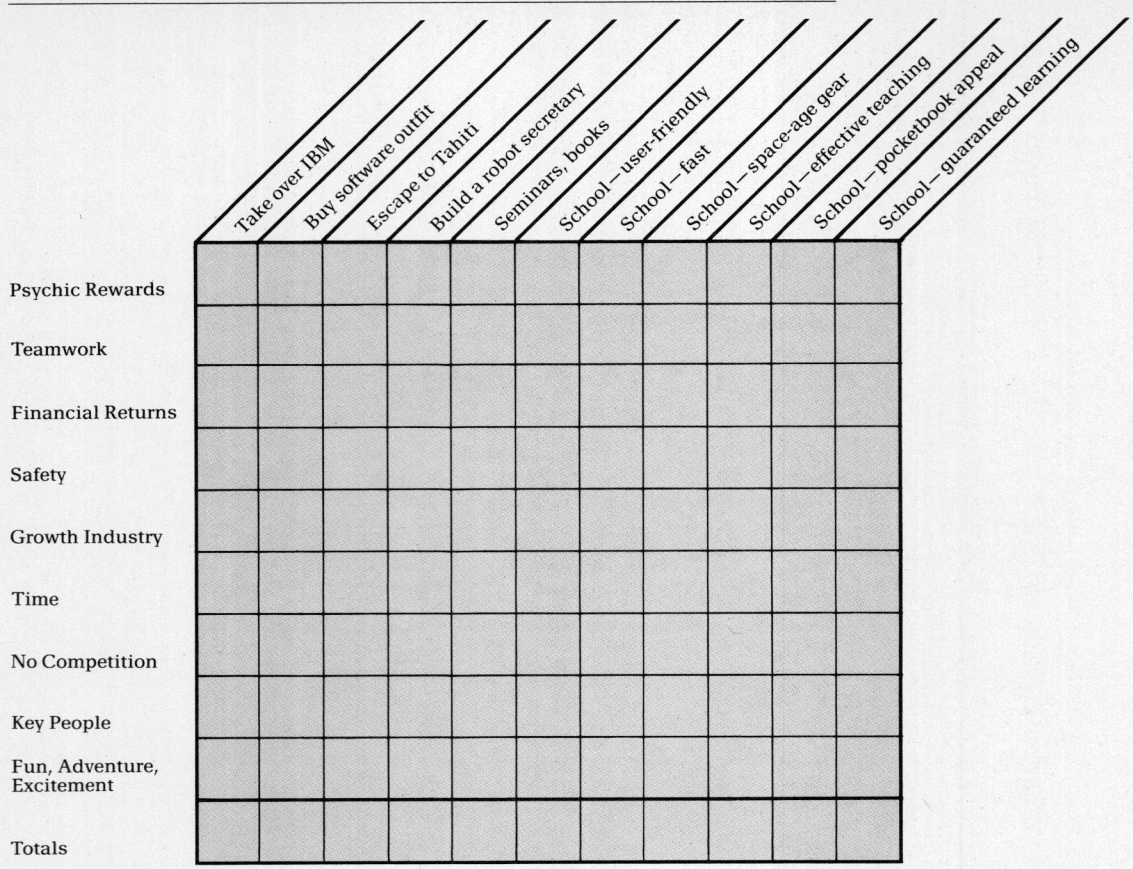

Continued

Working the Matrix Grid

Case Study

When the numbers were tallied, here's what the team saw:

Four out of five of the team members wanted to take over IBM. It would be great fun, they said. They could move the GHQ from Armonk to Orlando. IBM was overconfident, they believed, and a takeover would provide them with psychic rewards equaled only by the conquest of the Holy Land by medieval crusaders.

The dissenting team member wanted to escape to Tahiti. Tahiti was his psychic reward, and he had a friend at the Bank of Tahiti who had guaranteed him 15% on his money. This team member had always been fascinated by offshore banking.

Three team members thought the Hong Kong robot was a great idea. When the robot wasn't programming with dBase II, it could sub as a janitor or maid in the homes of the founders.

Two team members knew of software companies for sale. They urged the others to pool their money for a buyout. Buying companies gave both great pleasure.

Continued

ACTION ⚡ STEP 17

Mesh Solutions and Objectives in a Matrix Grid

A matrix analysis will help you focus, especially if you're working with a group and you have diverse objectives to satisfy. If you put the grid up on the wall, all members of the team can participate.

Along the far left side, make a vertical list of the objectives you brainstormed in Action Step 12.

Along the top, list the solutions you came up with in Action Step 16.

To score, you can use a ten-point scale, or you can use +, 0, and −.

Plus (+) = 3.
Zero (0) = 2.
Minus (−) = 1.

When you've filled in the boxes, you add up each column. That tells you where your intensities are. The rest is up to you.

A sample matrix is shown in Table 3.1.

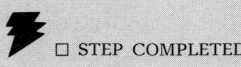 ☐ STEP COMPLETED

The school to teach software emerged as the really viable option. Here's what the school would do:

Solve problems. Business people have business problems to solve, tasks to perform. The school would teach them how the computer can reduce their work load. All you would need is an open mind and the right software.

Provide clarity. Software documentation is confusing. The school would devise a teaching system that was streamlined and clear.

Offer speed. Business people are in a hurry. Time is money. Could the school teach software in a month? A week? A day?

Build a **psychological cushion**. The founders would start a club. Once a student took a course, that student would become a club member for life and could retake any course.

Ask a reasonable price. Studies showed that business people would pay $100 a day to learn software, and the school would offer courses that were competitively priced.

Make it fun. If clients have fun learning, they'll relax and learn more. If they learn more, they'll spread the word about the school.

As a result of meshing their previous objectives with the mad solutions they generated, the Info Team identified which of their solutions best fit their objectives. They ended up with a fairly reasonable picture of a red-hot business opportunity. And they had great fun along the way.

Did the team rest on its laurels? Sure — for a few minutes. Then they started in again to get an even better picture of their Target Customer. First they reviewed what they had discovered so far, and then they began to dig in deeper and to narrow their market gap further. We'll leave them in the middle of their discussion now, energized and excited by the possibilities opened up to them by Power Marketing.

psychological cushion
a unique, untouchable rung on the ladder in your Target Customer's mind

NARROWING THE GAP

Now you're ready for the final move of Power Marketing. Action Step 18 will take you through this last stage. It is extremely important, because it gives you the chance for a final focus on your main business idea.

Write the name of your industry here:

_____

Write the name of your segment here:

_____

Now, before you lose the feel for the process of Power Marketing, try sketching out a rough picture of your journey through your favorite industry. You should know the route pretty well by now. Action Step 18 will be your guide.

ACTION ⚡ STEP 18

Narrow Your Gaps

All right, you've found your segment. You've tested parts of it. The trick now is to stay with this segment until you know whether or not it will work for you.

One way to keep concentrating is to do a simple sketch or diagram that reminds you how far you've already come. Use Figure 3.2 to help you recap the seven moves of Power Marketing.

Get yourself a large sheet of paper. Begin with your objectives and move through a review of what has happened.

At the end of your sketch, identify the main gap in your industry that really looks promising.

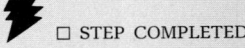
☐ STEP COMPLETED

Marketing Micros down on the Farm

• At a tent show in Iowa, farmers are met with a banner that reads: "Digital: The World's Second-Largest Computer Company." They ask the obvious question: "So who's number one?" [Illustrates a clear case of positioning by DEC, Digital Equipment Corporation, which also promotes its name by handing out baseball caps emblazoned with DEC.]

• At the same show, number one IBM promotes with this slogan: "The little computer with the high yield."

• *Agricomp*, a computer magazine targeted at farmers, puts out these ownership percentages:

　　Apple: 47%
　　Radio Shack: 22%
　　IBM: 15%
　　DEC: Less than 1%

• IBM began analyzing the farm computer market in 1981. One distribution channel is Valmont Industries (Omaha), a manufacturer of irrigation equipment. In 1983, there were 100 ValCom Computer Centers in the Farm Belt.

• Much of the early farm software came from kitchen-table (small business) operations run by farmer-programmers who saw an empty niche in the marketplace.

• Is farming an Information Business? A program called "Complete Crop Model" contains 2,500 mathematical formulas. The Info-Farmer enters acreage, marketing plan, cash flow, grain prices. The computer gives him back an income statement, a balance sheet, and a projection based on what-ifs that are real — what if he planted more, what if he bought a tractor, etc?

SOURCE: Adapted from Meg Cox, "Farmers' Growing Demand for Computers Draws Many High-Tech Firms into Market," *Wall Street Journal*, December 22, 1983. Reprinted by permission of *Wall Street Journal*, © Dow Jones & Company, Inc., 1983. All rights reserved.

As you bring your target market in better focus, your Target Customer will also become better defined, and you can work back and forth from one to the other. And you can use the techniques of Power Marketing at any time you think they will help you define your dream.

SUMMARY

Power Marketing — which we have likened to a funnel of power that filters your goals and plans so that you end up with a solid business idea — gives you a new confidence in your approach to the marketplace. It works with teams, small corporations, partners, and sole proprietors.

To illustrate the power of Power Marketing, we've explored a case study for a five-person team who began exploring the Information

Industry and wound up with a winning business concept: a software school — a training facility to teach people how to use complex computer programs in one day.

1. The team began in a group brainstorming session, listing business (and personal) objectives.
2. Using the life-cycle yardstick for an overview and an industry chronology to give them historical depth, the team researched the Information Industry. They focused on that segment forming around the microcomputer.
3. Despite the apparent chaos, promising segments began to emerge. Hardware (both production and retailing) was eliminated (too much competition). Software creation was a possibility. The real gap was in software education.
4. The team listed problems: user frustration, poor documentation, minimal support from manufacturers, minimal support from retailers, and so on.
5. The team brainstormed solutions to the list of problems.
6. The team built a matrix grid. They listed objectives along one side, solutions along the top. By matching, they discovered which solutions would satisfy which objectives. A software school would satisfy the most objectives.
7. With the project firmly in mind, they began to dig deeper into their chief survival mechanism — the Target Customer.

THINK POINTS

⚡ Be bold about brainstorming your business objectives. Who knows — some of them may take you through a doorway you didn't know was there.

⚡ Build your dream business around *your* likes and strengths.

⚡ The customer is always right, so make sure you have the right business. The Target Customer can always be profiled.

REFERENCES

White, Richard M. *The Entrepreneur's Manual.* Radnor, Pa.: Chilton Book Co., 1974. Excellent discussion of gap analysis, which is a larger, corporate version of Power Marketing.

ACTION ⚡ STEP
REVIEW

In Chapter 3, seven Action Steps take you through the seven secret moves of Power Marketing.

12 You start out by listing your business objectives — fame, money, being your own boss, planting yourself in a growth industry, no competition, and so on.

13 Then you dig more deeply into your favorite industry through research. (Two very helpful tools here are the life-cycle yardstick and an industry chronology.)

14 Your research allows you to identify promising gaps or segments in the industry. You are hunting for your own market niche.

15 Now that you have focused on the most promising segments, you list problems in need of solutions.

16 Those problems represent opportunities. Now you let yourself be creative and brainstorm wild solutions.

17 You use a matrix grid to mesh your solutions with your business objectives. This process leads naturally to the next Action Step.

18 By reviewing the process thus far, you watch your Target Customer surfacing, and at the same time you see the gaps narrow down into a solid business idea.

A Description
of Product
or Service

B The Market
and the
Target
Customer

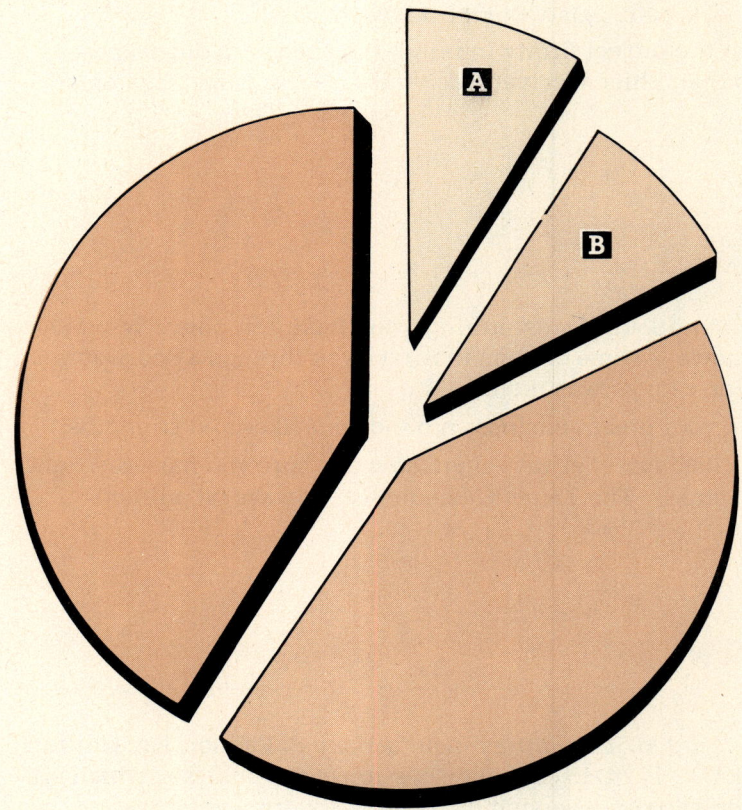

FIGURE 4.1 Chapter 4 completes your investigation of markets and Target Customers by taking you through a profile of your Target Customer.

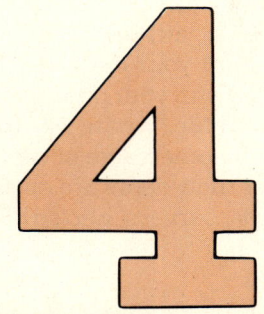

Profiling Your Target Customer

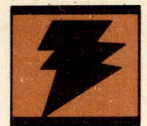

Your Target Customer is your key to survival in small business. A *customer profile* is the tool that draws a circle around that customer. To generate that profile, you will need to use a combination of demographic data—the statistical analysis of age, sex, income, education, residence, size of business or industry, and the like—and psychographics—the firsthand, intuitive insight into life-style, buying habits, patterns of consumption, attitudes, and so forth. The importance of drawing a circle around your customer is that you can turn the circle into a target, and then aim your product or service effectively—if you have an accurate profile. Small wonder that many entrepreneurs profile their Target Customers five or more times before they open their doors—and, after their doors are open, they continue to gather new data (from file cards, surveys, and so on) and draw new profiles every month.

AN EMPIRE BUILT ON THE TARGET CUSTOMER

Flashback

We are back in the fifties. Boys are in crewcuts and girls are wearing their hair in ponytails. Their parents are listening to a Senator named Joe McCarthy. Ike is in the White House. A woman named Monroe is about to become America's chief sex symbol. At the movies we're watching newsreels of a costly ''police action'' on a remote Asian peninsula called Korea. The Russians are getting ready to launch Sputnik. Color TV is only a rumor at R.C.A.

And in snowy Chicago, a visionary named Hugh Hefner is sitting at his kitchen table, probing the future with **New Eyes.**

Hefner sights his Target Customer and builds the vast *Playboy* empire.

Hefner isn't rich yet. He's a long way from being a success. And Playboy West—the legendary mansion in sunny Los Angeles with the fantasies, the bunnies, the bodyguards, and the celebrity parties—is still a faraway dream.

Later, historians looking back would call this the Silent Generation.

What Did Hefner See?

So what did entrepreneur Hefner see when he looked out from his Chicago flat?

He saw his **Target Customer.** (See Figure 4.2.)

He saw his Target Customer, and his Target Customer made him rich, famous, and envied around the world.

Hefner's Target Customer gave him an empire. You could almost call it an Information Empire.

New Eyes
playing Marketplace Detective, taking the blinders off, targeting opportunities with your intuition

Target Customer
a person who has the highest probability of buying your product or service

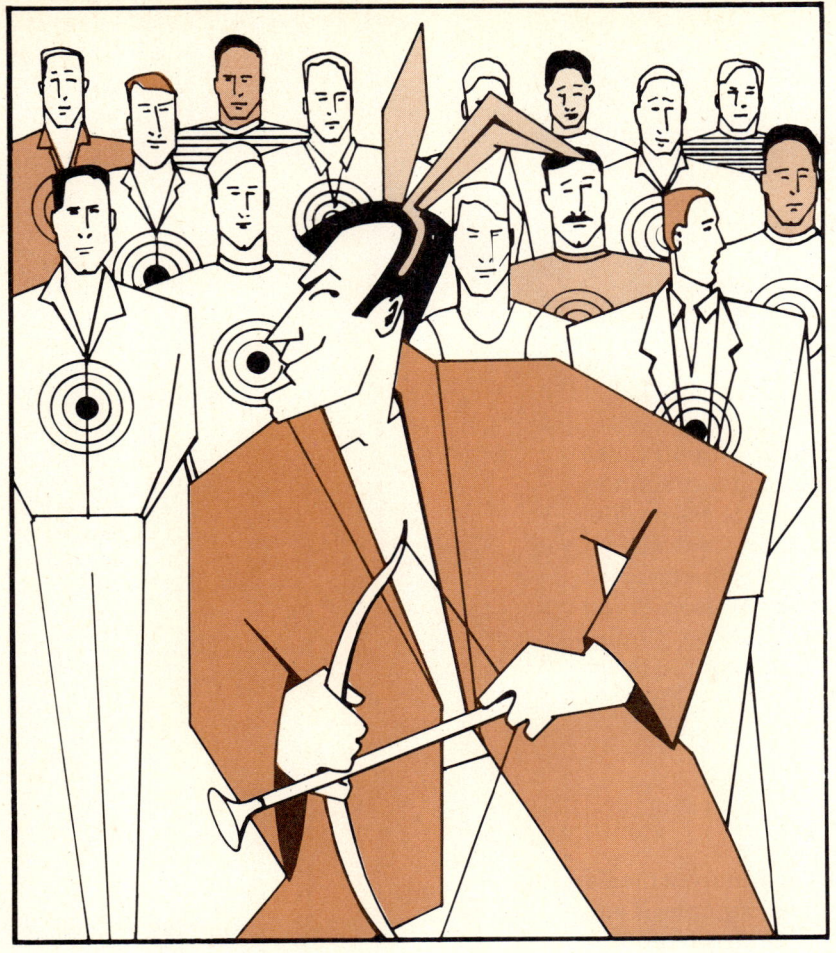

FIGURE 4.2 Entrepreneurs have built empires by aiming their messages at the right Target Customers.

The entrepreneur with a dream can learn a lesson here. Study Hefner. Find out what he learned about his Target Customer. Use that knowledge to help you own the store.

We weren't being facetious about the *Playboy* empire being one of information. *Playboy* is meant to communicate, and Hefner's message hasn't changed in the last quarter of a century. Play, he said. Play your ears off. You owe it to yourself to play. Play hard and never grow old and find a playmate to keep you young.

Of course, anyone could say that. But Hefner was careful to aim his message at a target audience that was super receptive. Here's a quick profile of his Target Customer:

Hefner's Target Customer

Sex: Male
Age: 18–34 (75%)
Education: Some college (52%)
Background: Upper middle class
Income: $35,000 annually (current dollars—25 years ago, income was $4,500)

Married: 50%

Residence: urban/suburban (64%)

Purchasing habits:

Consume more than 7 drinks per week: 25%

Consume more than 10 drinks per week: 18%

Consume more than 15 drinks per week: 12%

Own 3 or more cars: 17%

Heavy smokers: 21%

Purchased car new: 54%

Purchased 7 or more dress shirts per year: 17%

Purchased 4 or more pairs of shoes per year: 16%

The important thing to remember is that Hefner didn't pull those **demographics** out of thin air. He knew how to use secondary sources like newspapers and radio stations to help him complete his profile. You can do the same thing with your Target Customer. (Material on the *Playboy* target reader is adapted from *Subliminal Seduction: Ad Media's Seduction of a Not-So-Innocent America,* by Wilson Bryan Key, pages 118–119, and is used by permission. See the "References" section at the end of this chapter for full bibliographic information.)

demographics
key characteristics—age, sex, income, education, occupation, etc.—of the nation's consumers

THE POWER OF PROFILING

One easy way to understand the power of profiling is to analyze media sources that are aimed at different Target Markets. For example, if you know what your Target Customer reads, you can get in-depth profiles from magazines and newspapers, because they need to know such information for advertising. Although in this chapter we will focus primarily on magazines, you can take advantage of almost any of the media—especially the commercial ones, because of the useful information contained in ads. We could just as easily expand our discussion to include TV programs and radio stations, and to a lesser extent, books and movies. For an idea of the difference between the target readers of one magazine and another, think what you would find if you contrasted *McCall's* with *Playboy.*

In a minute we're going to do just that.

WHAT CAN WE LEARN FROM MAGAZINES?

Often, we move past magazines without a sideways glance. That's unfortunate, because magazines hold the key to many questions about marketing. Most people see a magazine as a glossy cover wrapped around ads and editorial copy. With New Eyes, however, you can see that a mass-market magazine exists because it is a channel to the subconscious of a certain type of reader.

This knowledge about the way a reader thinks and feels gives you power.

If you stand in the center of the marketing lab and study the advertisements in a magazine, you can learn about target markets, consumption patterns, and buying power. Put yourself in an analytical frame of mind by counting the ads. Then look for products that dominate the ads — these products are probably aimed at Heavy Users. Next, study the models. They are fantasy images for the Target Customer to identify with, connect with, and pursue. The activities pictured in the ads enlarge the fantasy and link it to real life through narrative.

A good ad is a slice of idealized life, a picture that beckons the customer toward the product.

We took one issue of *Playboy* (it has a carefully profiled reader) and one of *McCall's* (an obviously different target market) and did a New Eyes analysis. After looking at the data, we drew a few conclusions. We developed categories as we went along, because the magazines and the kinds of ads in them suggested such categories. (That's one of the nice things about New Eyes Research — you can expand the model fast.) Our categories were as follows:

Total number of ads one-third page or more

Ads aimed at Heavy Users (products advertised the most)

Huge ads (ads of 2 pages or more)

Demographics of models (age, income, occupation, race, gender)

Main activities depicted

Objects depicted (include mail order, if any)

An Analysis of *McCall's*

The total number of ads of one-third page or more was 80. Thirty-six ads were devoted to food, dieting, or eating, which suggests that the Heavy Users who read *McCall's* not only enjoy their foods, but also cook and probably feel that cooking is a great way to express themselves creatively. Dieting is the escape hatch that attempts to balance any indiscretionary overindulgence in food.

Five of the diet or food ads ran two pages. Twenty-one ran a full page. The next major product grouping was clothes — two double-page ads, eight full page. After clothes come cigarettes, with three double-page ads and five full pagers. There were six ads for beauty, skin, or hair care, three for intimate accessories (bras or pantyliners), five for children (shoes, cereal, baby food, toothpaste), and two for headache pills. A two-page ad for Kools cigarettes was dominated by a Porsche 928-S equipped with a Blaupunkt audio system.

Liquor was not advertised in this issue. Nor were cars.

Female models ranged in age from late-teen Brooke Shields to a couple of women in their late forties or early fifties. All models seemed comfortably well off, but not ostentatiously wealthy. All were white.

See Figure 4.3 on page 66 for a visual representation of our analysis of the advertising data.

The major activity depicted was smiling into the camera. One ad showed the lower three-fourths of a woman talking on the phone in an office as she advertised L'eggs, a brand of panty hose. Another showed a slender, slightly perspiring woman drinking Sprite with a background of weights and chrome barbells. In general, the ads with

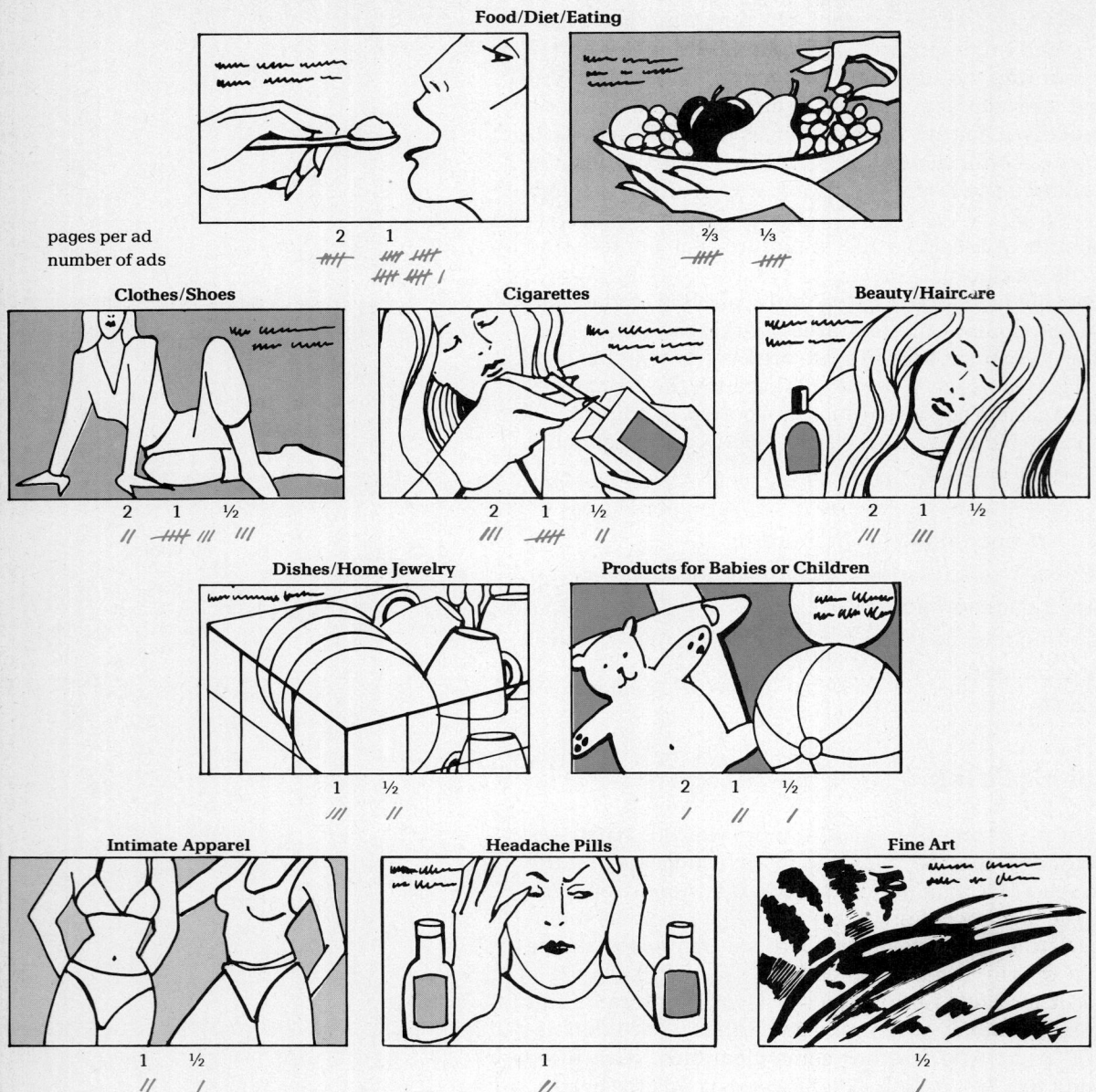

Food/Diet/Eating

pages per ad
number of ads

Clothes/Shoes   **Cigarettes**   **Beauty/Haircare**

Dishes/Home Jewelry   **Products for Babies or Children**

Intimate Apparel   **Headache Pills**   **Fine Art**

models pictured a world of charm and order, of women in control of themselves. Models were either young and famous, like Brooke Shields and Christie Brinkley, or they were aging gracefully.

Eight men, including Superman, made it into the *McCall's* ad stable: the Marlboro man, the Barclay's man, a Mazola man, three musicians touting Kools, and Bill Cosby, advertising Jello. The median age was between 35–50. The Marlboro man rides a spirited horse across an autumn landscape. The Barclay's man lights his own cigarette while he turns his eyes to the left, where an elegant female hand holds a glass of bubbly. The Mazola man—a husband archetype—is pictured with some apparatus to test blood pressure, suggesting the connection between eating Mazola and living longer. Bill Cosby, the only non-white adult, is surrounded by children munching jello. (One of the six children is black.)

FIGURE 4.3 By keeping track of the amount of space given to various categories of ads, you can determine what Target Customer a magazine is aimed at.

Aiming the Product

The objects depicted in these *McCall's* ads aim at the home, the hearth, the happy homemaker. A clean floor tied with a huge red ribbon extols the virtues of Brite. Food is celebrated with a plate of fancy spaghetti, cake mix, instant pie dough, a set of china, or a chocolate cream pie. Mail-order items are scarce. Most come from the magazine itself: a *McCall's* pastry cloth set and a *McCall's* tart pan.

McCall's Target Readers

What does this data tell us about *McCall's* readers?

1. They are predominantly female, ages 19 – 55, with a household income in the upper middle range. They live in metro-suburban areas. A high percentage are married, with children under 18. A high percentage are employed. The percentage of white readers outweighs any minority group.
2. They focus on the home. Their adventures occur in the kitchen, when they create with food.
3. They make buying decisions on lots of small purchases like moisture-whip Maybelline, Shaklee's instant protein, cigarettes, or Sizzlean.
4. They are object-centered, private about bedrooms and intimate wear. If they dream about escape, they do so briefly, with lots of control. If they use alcohol, they use it sparingly, or in private.

(This data checks out with the material we requested from *McCall's* **Display Ad Department.** The point of New Eyes analysis is that you can arrive at some exciting conclusions on your own. Let's try the same analysis on *Playboy*.)

Display Ad Department
a department of a magazine or newspaper which might provide market data

An Analysis of *Playboy*

The issue of *Playboy* contained 292 pages (*McCall's* had 158), with 79 ads that were one-third of a page or over. Thirty-three of these ads were for hard liquor (Scotch, gin, brandy), which corroborates the findings in *Subliminal Seduction* about *Playboy* readers also being Heavy Users of alcohol. Twenty-six of the liquor ads were full page, two covered two pages, and five were half-pagers. The next cluster came with 22 ads for electronic entertainment gear — video/audio/camera/stereo/phones/fuzzbusters. There were eight ads for cigarettes, which ties the *Playboy* smoker with the smokers for *McCall's.* Eight were for clothes, four for perfume, cologne, or diamonds. The largest ad was a five-page superspread for the new Nissan 300ZX, a hummer of a car, guaranteed to prolong your playing life, and suggesting that enough *Playboy* readers have the income to afford a sports car to make advertising worthwhile.

In contrast to *McCall's, Playboy* had no food ads. The center of the *Playboy* reader's attention is on a world beyond hearth and family.

Except for a wry and satiric Santa Claus (advertising Crown Royal), the male models ranged in age from 25 to 45. Several were indoorsy muscle-types working out on expensive exercise equipment. Most of the outdoorsy types wore work clothes, uniforms, heavy boots, and mustaches. The female models ranged in age from 21 to 30, from girlish flirts to elegant women in control. In several of the ads, one man would be sandwiched in between two women, suggesting that the reader will have an abundance of female companionship if he only plays his cards with *elan*.

Product Crossover

The only product strong enough to cross over from *McCall's* to *Playboy* was Marlboro. In the pages of *Playboy*, the Marlboro Man is closer to us, less romantic, more rugged. He has replaced his *McCall's* horse with the macho roping of a calf, symbol of dexterity and control.

Playboy ads have more action than *McCall's* ads, with romantic settings at the top of the world (Hennessy cognac), adventure settings in the wilds (Camel), and rescue settings on isolated Arctic ice (Winston). The Gordon's gin ad shows two black models (male pianist, female dancer in white tights) in a tastefully austere, mirrored studio.

Aiming the Product

The objects depicted in the ads are machines for grown-up play, such as Toyota trucks, fire-red Nissan sports cars, radar detectors, videos, stereos, and cameras. The Good Life indoors at night balances the Rugged Life outdoors in the daytime. Night and day. For the *Playboy* reader who can afford it, it's the best of all possible worlds.

This issue contained one mail-order ad (with toll-free number included) for Karess sheets. The other mail-order ads offered products from Playboy: the magazine itself, the Playmate calendar, and various Playmate and adventure videos.

Playboy's Target Readers

We already have demographic data on *Playboy* readers. What does our New Eyes research tell us about them?

1. The Good Life costs, but it's worth every penny. Female companionship is available if the *Playboy* readers have the bucks. If they can't handle the fire-red Nissan right now, they can settle for the tony grey VW Quantum.
2. They make big-purchase decisions: cars, stereos, phone systems, cameras, and video. They're Heavy Users of hard liquor.
3. They spend a hefty percentage of their income on entertainment — some to set the stage in their apartments, a lot more out in the playgrounds of the world. (In this issue, snow-covered mountains called to the winter sports enthusiast, ''Come and ski.'')
4. They are filled with hopes of achieving the Good Life permanently. Until that time, *Playboy* will line their dreams with products from the Playboy Information Empire.

Play is serious business, requiring a hefty investment. If an advertiser in *Playboy* spends $50,000 for a full-page ad, that ad has to bring him $1 million in gross sales — 20 times the cost of the ad — before he breaks even. What that means for you is that expensive ads are highly targeted. They must hit the target or the advertiser withdraws business.

MAGAZINES AND PROFILING YOUR TARGET CUSTOMER

To help you get a handle on profiling, in Action Step 19 we have designed an interesting exercise — analyzing the advertising in a magazine which is read by your Target Customer.

As usual, you begin with yourself, with what you read, and then you widen your search to include potential customers. Have fun with this one.

You should get into the habit of profiling. It's the key to success in small business. To help you get a handle on profiling target readers of magazines, take a look at the boxed article on page 70. (Information for customer profiles is also available from local newspapers and radio and TV stations. For other specific data, you can contact trade associations through the *The IMS Ayer Directory of Publications* or the *Encyclopedia of Associations,* which are discussed in Chapter 2.)

In the Age of Information, how much data do you need to gather before you arrive at knowledge? In an age of highly specialized customer tastes, who survives?

How many **general interest magazines** did you spot on the racks? How many do you read? How many do you subscribe to?

Life. Look. Colliers. Coronet. Saturday Evening Post. They were all general interest magazines, all aimed at the "general" reader.

Did you spot them in your research quest? Or have they gone the way of the railroads?

Who's surviving in the magazine game these days?

Magazine	Target Reader	Circulation
D & B Reports	Owners or top managers of small businesses; $9 million annual sales.	71,630
EasyRiders	Rugged guys; enjoy choppers, good times.	488,000
Money	Middle-upper income, sophisticated reader.	1.1 million
Penthouse	Male; 18–34; upper-income; college.	5.3 million
Cosmopolitan	Female; 18–34; middle-income; career-minded	2.5 million

Is the phenomenon of the highly specialized audience here to stay? Good question. *Saturday Evening Post* and *Life* have been revived — as monthlies. The *Post*'s circulation is around 500,000, slightly more

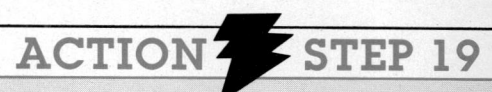

ACTION STEP 19

Analyze the Tactics of Mass-Market Magazines

Combine primary, secondary, and New Eyes research to study the magazines and their target readers; then apply what you learn to your own business.

Part A. New Eyes and Primary Research. Find a magazine rack in any store. Glance quickly at the covers. List five that reach out and grab your mind. They are aimed at you. Do you buy any of them? Are you a subscriber? What do you get from them?

Now, step back from the rack and observe other shoppers. Make notes on what magazines they are buying. How many purchases could you have predicted?

If you have a chance, interview a couple of these magazine buyers. Ask them why they bought what they bought. While they are answering, build reader profiles in your mind. Without being too obvious, collect as much demographic data as you can on these shoppers. Could any of them be your TC?

Part B. Secondary Research. Choose five magazines that you think your TC would read. Using your business letterhead, write the magazines and ask for media kits and reader profiles.

Tell them that you're in business or in the planning stage for a new business; that you're looking around for places to advertise; and that you'd like some information on subscribers, readers, and ad rates.

Address your letter to the Display Advertising Department.

Part C. Comparative Analysis. When the magazine demographic data arrives, compare it with what you learned and surmised on your own.

How close were your New Eyes Profiles?

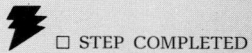 ☐ STEP COMPLETED

general interest magazines
publications directed at a mass audience, across demographic lines

---

Getting a Handle on Profiling

To help you get a handle on profiling your Target Customer using magazines, we're giving you a model to follow. This incredible wealth of information comes from an analysis of *Vogue* magazine in *Subliminal Seduction* by Wilson Bryan Key.

- The average age of *Vogue* readers is in the early thirties and 72 percent are married—if not happily at least comfortably. Some, the younger ones with high upward-mobility husbands, work. The majority, however, are married to men with managerial or executive responsibilities who are quite likely to be older than their wives. Men usually hit their high earning peak in the mid to late forties.
- A significant portion of *Vogue* readers will be in their second marriage, their husbands in their second, third, or fourth marriage.
- The place of children in the life of the *Vogue* reader is curious. Two-thirds of *Vogue* families have no children under 18. This can mean two things: Most of the readers are well over 40 (which does not seem to be the case), or they live in a marriage in which children do not play an important role.
- The *Vogue* reader is well-educated — 78 percent attended college, 41 percent graduated. Of their husbands, 83 percent attended college, 64 percent graduated; in their occupations (which really determine lifestyle, fashions, clubs, travel, sport, and amusements) 35 percent are professionals and 32 percent are executives, proprietors, managers, or officials.
- Ninety-seven percent of *Vogue* readers belong to one or more clubs. They entertain frequently with dinner parties, buffets, and luncheons, and they are entertained equally as often with a total average of 6.4 engagements monthly.

SOURCE: From the book *Subliminal Seduction: Ad Media's Seduction of a Not-So-Innocent America,* pp. 149–152, by Wilson Bryan Key. © 1973 by Wilson Bryan Key. Published by Prentice-Hall, Inc., Englewood Cliffs, NJ 07632.

---

than *EasyRiders'*, and *Life's* is 1.3 million. What does this tell you about surviving in the marketplace? Tastes are more specialized. Will riches ever return to the mass market?

A DIFFERENT KIND OF TARGET READER

"Our readers," a publisher of romance novels wrote, "are starved for the Good Life. Most of them will never see Europe, never eat in an elegant restaurant, never meet anyone famous or important. Their days are spent scrimping, watching the budget, doing dishes and the laundry. Their husbands are indifferent. If our readers work, they hold down jobs that are dull. They are going nowhere, and they want to read about women who have it made, who never think twice about what something will cost. Our readers live vicariously — they want to have the confidence of someone who has everything!"

Sarah Routledge thought that she had trouble conceiving of markets and customers. But once she found a way to profile readers, she discovered that markets and customers were easy to understand. She also discovered a larger target market.

Case Study

Sarah Routledge — Cook, Writer, Entrepreneur

Sarah Routledge was 52 when her husband died. She'd been married 31 years. She missed him terribly. Her two children lived 3,000 miles away, in California. They flew in for the funeral, looking fit, tanned, rushed. They both smiled a lot. After the ceremony, they both invited their mother to come out for a visit. Three days in her son's house — in a smoggy southern California suburb — and Sarah went back home.

New England — she belonged there.

Sarah grieved for her husband. To stay busy, she began to bake fine home-made pies for the Old New England Restaurant down the road. The money coming in every week helped pay the bills, which were scary. Her busband had always handled the money, and there had always been enough, even with the children, but now it seemed as if the insurance checks wouldn't quite stretch from month to month.

Sarah baked more pies.

In the tourist season, business was brisk, so Sarah hired a local girl to help out. In a year, her small business had made enough money to pay the bills, expand her kitchen, and hire another girl. Sarah had some time now, so she went back to college. She'd always loved to read. The course she took was How to Write a Mystery Novel.

Sarah's stories were set locally — with old houses, dense forests, and small New England towns — and she did eight revisions before her teacher was satisfied. When she was almost ready to give up, her teacher said he'd send it to New York, to a friend of his in the publishing business.

Sarah was nervous. She'd always held publishers in high esteem. She didn't want to be hurt or disappointed.

Surprise — the publisher liked her story, wanted to publish it, and wanted to see more.

In the next three years, Sarah sold five mysteries. She turned out to be a superior story teller, and she enjoyed sitting in a corner of the house with a fire going, spinning out mysteries. She made an average of $3,000 on each book — not much, unless you were thrifty. Sarah was.

Then, one wintry November morning, Sarah's New York publisher broke her heart by turning down her sixth novel. "The **market** is terrible for mysteries," he wrote. "Try me again when this has blown over."

Sarah was confused. She didn't understand. Market? What market? The only market she knew was Eldredge's, down the road, where she sold extra pies. Of course, she remembered her husband when he used to grouse about the stock market. She also remembered not paying much attention. No, markets were not Sarah's cup of tea.

A year passed. Sarah kept on writing. Two more mysteries were turned down, for the same vague reasons. Now Sarah was nervous. Her expenses in the pie business had increased, and a new person, a young woman who had just moved out from Boston, had set up in competition. She'd been counting on the money from her books, which was now drying up.

Fighting back the tears, Sarah began to study what went on in the
Continued

market
where you meet your
customers for the purpose
of doing business

world of publishing. She read *Publisher's Weekly,* a trade journal. She read biographies, books by agents, books by publishers. She did not unearth any secrets.

Then one day, Sarah ran into a woman in the library. She was younger than Sarah, and she was carrying a stack of paperback romances. With gentle probing, Sarah learned that the woman read as many as ten romances a week. She belonged to two romance book clubs and a romance reader's group.

"What organization," Sarah thought. And then she began to wonder how many romance readers there were in New England. How many on the East Coast? How many across the country?

That question carried her through a secret doorway — right to a new set of Target Readers.

Working with her New England diligence, Sarah did some research on the leisure-time activities of the American housewife. In an obscure marketing journal, she found a 1970 study that said housewives spend almost 70% of their leisure time reading. Not mysteries, Sarah thought. A study in *Publisher's Weekly* said that 37% of the fiction sold was romance fiction.

That explained some of what her publisher had been talking about. A market meant people. In publishing, a market meant readers. Now why hadn't he said that in the first place?

To follow up, Sarah wrote to romance publishers, requesting information on the mechanics of writing romance fiction. She got back detailed reader profiles, plot suggestions, length of each type of romance — a blueprint for writing a book.

"Our readers," one publisher wrote, "are starved for the Good Life. Most of them will never see Europe, never eat in an elegant restaurant, never meet anyone famous or important. . . ."

Sarah read through all the material carefully. None of her friends read romances, but if she used a pen name no one would know what she was up to. Two days later, Sarah sat down to write her first romance novel, *Amelia Thorn.* It was snapped up by the publishers. It sold 300,000 copies and made more money in its first print run than all of Sarah's mysteries combined. Her second romance, *Rachel Duncan,* outsold *Amelia Thorn,* and forced Sarah to find an honest lawyer who helped her to incorporate.

She has been a **corporation** for two years now. Six young women work for her, baking pies, and she is planning to start her own publishing operation — to do a cookbook called *Sarah's Pies.* One of the things she discovered doing research on publishing was that the bigger publishers didn't like to do small print runs because they didn't make any money. That left a market gap for Sarah.

Before she finished the pie book, she hired a young man from one of the business schools to do some market research for her. He seemed to think there would be 25,000 readers for her book.

Sarah Routledge had discovered the key to small business.

"I think what helped me the most," she says, "is when I discovered I was in business. Because when you're in business, then you think about your customers. Before, all I'd thought about was pies and books. Customers are the key.

"Finding the right customers is like slicing a pie," Sarah goes on. "You take out only what you need for yourself. You leave the rest for somebody else. If someone comes along and wants the whole pie, then you have a choice — either you move on or you dig in your heels and fight. The key to business, whether it's baking pies or writing books, is to know who's going to eat 'em or read 'em."

(We'll continue with Sarah's thought about digging in and fighting in the next chapter, on Competition.)

corporation
a legal entity that stands separate from its owners

MAKE PROFILING A REFLEX

We're trying to help you make customer profiling a reflex. If you keep after it, profiling is the tool that helps you intensify your focus on the all-important marketplace.

In the box below is a pair of contrasting profiles from *Nine American Lifestyles* — Arnold Mitchell's book about psychographics in

---

Contrasting TCs: One Trick to Profiling

While you are training your New Eyes to zoom in on the marketplace, it's sometimes helpful to profile two very different Target Customers. Below, you'll see material adapted from *Nine American Lifestyles* by Arnold Mitchell analyzing the consumption patterns of two distinctive customer groups.

Belongers. Belonger households are major buyers of both large and compact American-made autos. Important current purchase considerations to them are convenient dealer locations, cost of repairs and servicing, and safety features, the last probably reflecting concerns for the family. Exterior styling is relatively unimportant. They prefer American-made cars to imports.

In appliances, Belongers show a higher-than-average level of ownership of freezers and lower ownership levels for dishwashers, garbage disposals, food processors, and microwave ovens. These patterns possibly reflect their preference for doing things in the traditional way, as well as their older homes and rural living habits.

In clothing Belonger women are particularly frequent wearers of slacks. Slacks appear to be sufficiently ingrained in their life-styles that employment status has little effect.

Belongers are substantially below average in consumption of all types of alcoholic beverages and regular carbonated soft drinks. A higher-than average percentage consume fruit juices as well as regular and decaffeinated coffee.

Experientials. Experiential households have among the highest incidence of ownership of compact, subcompact, and small specialty cars. They are the highest in ownership of, and preference for, foreign cars, and they show the highest ownership of European cars of any VALS type.

Ownership of dishwashers and garbage disposals is among the highest in the typology. Ownership of recreational equipment is also high: Experiential households are substantially above average in owning camping or backpacking equipment and racing bicycles. In home electronic products higher-than-average ownership levels prevail for photo games and prerecorded and blank recording tapes.

Experiential women show an interesting pattern in their clothing preferences. Disproportionately more wear jeans, skirts, and dresses. They wear bras less frequently than any of the other VALS types, perhaps reflecting their "free spirits." Experiential men are among the most frequent wearers of jeans and sport and casual shirts, but they also wear suits more often than average.

Wines, including champagnes, and domestic and imported beers are the favored alcoholic beverages.

SOURCE: Reprinted (with slight changes) by permission of Macmillan Publishing Company from *Nine American Lifestyles: Who We Are and Where We Are Going* by Arnold Mitchell, pp. 91–92, 132–133. Copyright © 1983 by Arnold Mitchell.

America. We've selected Belongers and Experientials. Belongers are outer-directed while Experientials are inner-directed. It might help to do a a comparative chart, just to make the differences in consumption patterns stand out. Read through these profiles and then complete Action Step 20 on your own Target Customer. (We'll return to Mitchell and *Nine American Lifestyles* in a minute.)

THE TARGET CUSTOMERS YOU CANNOT SEE

One reason people go into business for themselves is because they can't work for someone else. Maybe they're mavericks who don't like to take orders from a boss. Maybe they're dreamers who love their own ideas. Or maybe they've had an accident that prevents them from holding down a job with a large firm.

That's what happened to Fred Bowers.

Here's what Fred says of his start-up.

"When I went into the soccer segment of the retail sporting goods business, I had mostly kids in mind. Then, after I'd been in business awhile, these adults started coming in — guys from Britain, Mexico, Germany — and I kicked myself for not having seen them before. I couldn't, I guess, because they were invisible."

Case Study

Fred Bowers — Segmenting Retail Sporting Goods

Fred Bowers was planning on being a career Marine when he fell out of a training helicopter. He could still walk, painfully, but his military career was over. With a medical discharge in his pocket, Fred looked around for work.

"I'd always loved soccer," Fred said. "I'd been a pretty fair player and I'd had two stints of coaching, so that gave me a good angle on the kids. I thought there might be a place for a soccer specialty shop, but before I went around asking my friends for money, I spent a year checking it out."

Fred found 18 sporting good shops in the area he was interested in. None of them really dealt with soccer in depth. When he began profiling his Target Customers, Fred came up with two easy targets:

Primary target: boys, age 6–17
Secondary target: girls, age 6–12
Household income (both targets): $28,000–$32,000
Socio/Econ: middle, upper middle
Interest: sports

Then Fred segmented the youngsters into two groups:

1. School teams.
2. Teams in the AYSO, American Youth Soccer Organization.

Continued

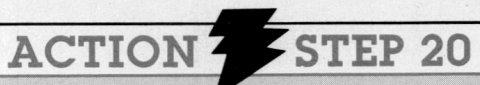

ACTION STEP 20

Profile Your Target Customer

Use demographics and psychographics to draw a circle around your Target Customer. You may find it useful to list your own categories as developed in Action Step 19 or in earlier research.

Clues: What does your TC read? What is in his or her shopping cart? What kind of car does your TC drive? What does that car tell you about the TC's self-image? What does the TC drink? What does the TC do for leisure, for recreation, for entertainment?

Now that you're deeper into your adventure, you will have more information about the kinds of TCs you should aim your product or your service at. (See the sidebar below, "Three Kinds of Target Customers.") Think —and dream—about your TC often. Your Target Customer is your key to survival in small business. The better you can draw a circle around your customer, the better you can aim your product or service. And you can't do too many of these profiles.

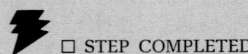 ☐ STEP COMPLETED

Three Kinds of Target Customers

Entrepreneurs we have known tell us you should be watching for at least three TC groups:

1. **Primary.** This TC is perfect for your business, and could be a Heavy User.
2. **Secondary.** This one almost slips away before you can focus the camera. (The word processors in the Team Case Study in Chapter 3 were secondary TCs.) Sometimes your secondary TC will lead you to the third customer—who is invisible at first.
3. **Invisible.** This customer appears after you open the doors, after you have the courage to go ahead and start up.

He'd done such close work on his Target Customers that when he showed his 52-page Business Plan to a couple of investors, they put up all the money for the start-up of Soccer City. Because of Fred's knowledge of the game, his store prospered. Schools counted on him for an honest deal. Parents of players counted on him for advice on equipment.

"I thought I'd just be selling," Fred said. "What I was really doing was providing a **service.**"

After he'd been in business a year, a third market began to emerge. The customers in this third group were adults, mostly foreign-born, from places like Britain, Germany, Mexico, South America. They had grown up playing soccer. To them, the game was a fiercely national sport, full of deep memories. To keep those memories strong, these heretofore invisible customers would drive 50–75 miles to Fred's shop for that special piece of equipment they couldn't find anywhere else.

"They didn't show up in my research," Fred said. "If I hadn't opened up, they would never have appeared. Now they make up at least 30% of my business. One day they weren't there. The next day, they had surfaced. I like that. I like it a lot. It makes the whole adventure more interesting."

WHERE DO YOUR TARGET CUSTOMERS FIT ON THE VALS ONION?

VALS is an acronym for a profiling system developed at SRI International, a Menlo Park firm that specializes in market research. VALS means Values and Lifestyles, and Arnold Mitchell, the author of *Nine American Lifestyles,* has developed an onion diagram that places nine life-styles (described on page 76) in relation to each other.

The VALS Onion is one more tool available to you to help you profile your Target Customer. As shown in Figure 4.4 (on page 77), Survivors are at the bottom, Integrateds at the top. Where are Fred's soccer players?

For an answer, study Figure 4.4 for a moment, referring to the boxed article on page 76 as needed.

After you find Fred's Target Customers, look for your own. Who on the great VALS onion will buy your product or service?

List 3 VALS groups here:

_____

_____

_____

You don't have to be a romance writer or a soccer coach to find Target Customers. One good way to pinpoint your target is to **interview.**

Action Step 21 sets you out to interview your potential TCs. And now is the time. You know where your TC hangs out. You know its habits, income, sex, personality, type of business, and buying patterns. You can guess at its dreams and aspirations. You've identified the Heavy Users of your product or service. Now is the time to go out there and start interviewing.

service
a perishable commodity that must be used as it becomes available

ACTION ⚡ STEP 21

Interview Prospective Target Customers in Your Business Segment

After you have profiled several TCs, it's time to take a big step. You move from the tidy world inside your head to the noisy arena of the market place. You discover how accurate your concepts are by rubbing elbows with the people who'll be buying your product or service.

Prepare your questions in advance. Then go find your TC. Consider questions like the following:

How do you like the business?
What products did you buy?
Were the people helpful and courteous?
How did you learn about the business?
Is this your first visit? How often do you shop here?
What are you looking for that you didn't find?
Where do you live?
What do you read?

Remember, no one is totally satisfied, and your questions may unearth some gaps that you never knew of before.

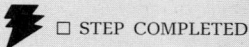 ⚡ ☐ STEP COMPLETED

interview
a planned conversation with another person or group of persons designed to elicit specific information

A lot of people go into small business because they don't have much choice. They find they have to learn new skills.

Using Secondary Data to Segment Your Markets

Nine American Lifestyles is almost as helpful to the eager entrepreneur as *Megatrends*. Author Arnold Mitchell, director of the VALS (Values and Lifestyles) Program at SRI International, gathered data for 20 years before coming out with the book. Find your Target Customer in Mitchell's nine classifications.

Survivors. Old; intensely poor; fearful; depressed; despairing; far removed from the cultural mainstream; misfits. There are 6 million Survivors. Most are over 65. 77% are female, with incomes under $7,500 and education median of 8th–9th grade.

Sustainers. Living on the edge of poverty; angry and resentful; streetwise; involved in underground economy. There are 11 million Sustainers. 58% are under 35. 55% are female, with median income of $11,000, median education of 11th grade.

Belongers. Aging; traditional and conventional; contented; intensely patriotic; sentimental; deeply stable. There are 54 million Belongers. Median age is 52. 65% are female, with median income of $17,500. About 50% graduated high school.

Emulators. Youthful and ambitious; macho; show-off; trying to break into the system, to make it big. There are 16 million Emulators. Median age is 27. 53% are male, with median income of $18,000 and more education than high school.

Achievers. Middle-aged and prosperous; able leaders; self-assured; materialistic; builders of the "American Dream." There are 37 million Achievers. Median age is 37. 60% are male, with median income of $31,400. 32% are college graduates or more.

I-Am-Me. Transition state; exhibitionistic and narcissistic; young; impulsive; experimental; active; inventive. There are 8 million I-Am-Mes. 91% are under 25. 64% are male. Median income is $8,800. Some college.

Experiential. Youthful; seek direct experience; person-centered; artistic; intensely oriented toward inner growth. There are 11 million Experientials. Median age is 27. 55% are female. Median income is $23,800. 38% are college grads or more.

Societally Conscious. Mission-oriented; leaders of single-issue groups; mature; successful; some live lives of voluntary simplicity. There are 14 million SCs. Median age is 39. 52% are male. Median income is $27,200. 58% are college graduates. 39% have some graduate school.

Integrated. Psychologically mature; large field of vision; tolerant and understanding; sense of fittingness. There are 3.2 million Integrateds.

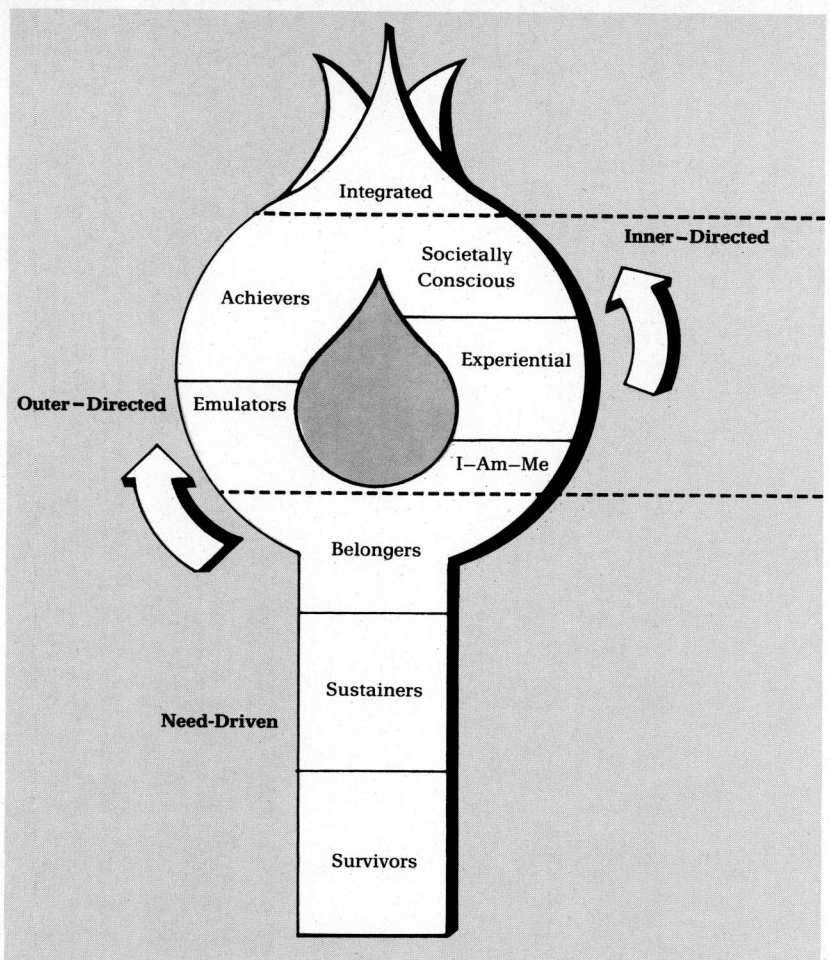

SOURCE: Reprinted (with slight changes) by permission of Macmillan Publishing Company from *Nine American Lifestyles: Who We Are and Where We Are Going* by Arnold Mitchell. Copyright © 1983 by Arnold Mitchell.

FIGURE 4.4   Where are you on the VALS onion? Where is your Target Customer?

Fortunately, entrepreneurs are a bright lot. They learn fast.

And they know how to hang on.

In the case study that follows, we see how Action Step 21 could be applied. When Julia Gonzales found herself about to go into her own small business, the first thing she did was to start interviewing.

Case Study

Julia Gonzales — Entrepreneur by Default

I didn't plan to become an entrepreneur. It just happened. It's no secret. I was distressed when my husband was transferred to another city. I couldn't blame him wanting the transfer, of course, but I had a terrific job, too — manager of a full-line baby furniture and bedding store —

Continued

and to keep both job and husband I'd have had to commute over a hundred miles a day five days a week.

I made the choice and quit my job.

But I wasn't happy, and it was hard getting by on one salary when we had been bringing in two. I decided to look for work, and that's when I found that my reputation had preceded me. Store owners knew where I'd worked, and they were afraid that all I wanted to do was get a feel for the area and set up in competition with them.

They inspired me: When I couldn't find work, I decided to compete with them. Anybody that afraid gave me hope.

One thing I had learned on my way up from stock clerk to store manager was that it pays to know your customer. So in the mornings I'd get the kids off to school and then I'd park my car a block away from a baby store and I'd strike up conversations with customers as they came out.

"Hi," I'd say. "My name's Julia Gonzales, and I'm doing market research for a major manufacturer who's interested in this area, and I was wondering if you could answer a few questions about babies."

The winning smile must have helped. I like people. I guess it shows. Having two kids helps me understand mothers, too.

I always dressed nicely. I had a clipboard. I'd ask the obvious questions:

"How do you like the store?"

"What products did you buy?"

"Were the people helpful and courteous?"

And so on.

Sometimes, I parked in the alley to research the delivery trucks. Other times, on the beach or in the shopping malls, I would stop every pregnant lady I saw. I developed my own list of questions for pregnant gals:

"Did you have a baby shower?"

"What gifts did you like best?"

"What seemed most useful?"

"What are you buying now?"

"What are you delaying buying?"

"What plans are you making for nursery redecoration?"

"What do you really need most?"

The research was time-consuming, but after I'd talked with 30 young women, I had enough information to help me make some sound judgments. I also knew my competition and where their weaknesses were. And when I located my new store, I plopped it down in the middle of a coming baby boom.

How Can This Case Study Help You?

When Julia discovered she had to work for herself, she quickly began to research her Target Customers. The method she chose was interviewing. You can do the same thing for your business. Work out your questions in advance. Leave some of them open-ended, so that your potential customer will have more to say than "yes" or "no."

You can begin with Julia's questions. (How did you like the store? Did you find everything you wanted?) More will come to you after you've done a couple of interviews.

So get out there and try a few!

WHY YOU SHOULD PROFILE YOUR TARGET CUSTOMER

Profiling your TC is all important, for these reasons:

1. You'll know how to communicate your message with a minimum of confusion when you know who your customer really is. You'll be better able to decide how to market your product or service — whether it's through direct mail, newspapers, radio, direct sales, etc.
2. You'll know what additional service your TC will want, such as delivery, credit, gift wrapping, installation, post-sale service, and so on.
3. You'll know how much the TC can pay. That will give you a firm sense of pricing.
4. You'll know what the TC wants in quality.
5. You'll know where large groups of TCs are located, so you can market directly to them.
6. You'll know who else is after your TC.

Knowing who else is after your TC may be the most important thing.

When Hugh Hefner had the vision about *Playboy,* he was alone in that market. His Target Customers were between the ages of 17 – 34. That was over 30 years ago. Those same customers are now between the ages of 47 – 64, and recent surveys have suggested that *Playboy's* readership is getting smaller. Part of any product's life cycle depends on the age of the customers. What is the life cycle of a magazine?

In autumn of 1982, *Penthouse* magazine started running ads in major newspapers claiming that it would run *Playboy* out of the arena.

There is a word that covers this phenomenon when someone is after your Target Customers.

The word is competition.

And that's what we're covering in the next chapter.

SUMMARY

There are a number of ways to profile your Target Customer. One powerful approach is to take advantage of the information provided directly and indirectly by the advertising in popular magazines (or other commercial media). If the magazine's target reader is also your Target Customer, it's almost as if the magazine did your profile for you. Another approach is to take advantage of categories defined by researchers in the field, as with Mitchell's *Nine American Lifestyles.* These categories will provide fully thought-out descriptions of types you already recognize. If one of your Target Customers fits one of the categories, once again you have received a tremendous boost towards completing your profile.

This preparation in itself may be enough to allow you to profile your Target Customer. But you need to test your profile against reality. That's why we also have you interview potential Target Customers directly. No doubt you will need to refine or rework your profile once you compare it against the real thing. Remember: Profiling should be an ongoing process. Your Target Customer will change over time and you will uncover additional Target Customers only after you have been in business awhile. Revise your profile as you go.

If you are a true entrepreneur, you will find your contacts with Target Customers—and the challenge of keeping the Target Customer properly in focus—stimulating and fun.

THINK POINTS

⚡ Psychographics comes from *psyche*, a Greek word meaning soul or spirit, and from three other Greek words (*gramme, gramma, graphein*). Put them all together and you come up with a fancy definition for psychographics—charting the customer's mind, soul, or spirit. Psychographics makes your Target Customer a sitting duck.

⚡ Profiling draws a magic circle around your Target Customer. Moving the customer to the center of that circle transforms the whole arena into a bull's-eye.

⚡ Segmenting is like slicing a pie into pieces.

⚡ You can save yourself a lot of steps by *using market research done by others.* Contact magazines and newspapers. They employ market researchers.

REFERENCES

Barnhart, Helene Schellenberg. *Writing Romance Fiction for Love and Money.* Cincinnati, Ohio: Writers Digest Books, 1983.

Bernstein, Peter W. "Psychographics Still an Issue on Madison Avenue." *Fortune,* January 1978. Early Pinto advertisements linked the car with a frisky pony. Market probes by a major research firm indicated that buyers wanted a dependable car. The next run of ads showed the Pinto on a split screen with the Ford Model A—symbol of a reliability that was legendary. Good example of response to the wishes, dreams, and mythic desires of the market.

Brady, Frank. *Hefner.* New York: Macmillan, 1974. Easy-to-read book about the man who founded an empire on an image—the bunny rabbit, playboy of the animal world.

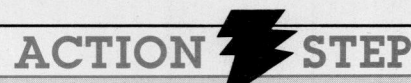

ACTION ⚡ STEP
REVIEW

Three Action Steps in Chapter 4 help you zero in on Target Customers:

19 In this Action Step you get inside the covers of mass-market magazines, where you develop your profiling reflexes. You can use this tool on your own market.

20 Moving logically from Action Step 19, here you are given a chance to profile your own potential customers. This is fun and it draws you closer to the key to your business survival—your Target Customer.

21 We introduce you here to the concept of interviewing to gather primary data on your Target Customers. And better than conceptualization, you actually go out and interview. (Your first taste of interviewing was in Action Step 6, when you interviewed small business owners.)

Byer, Stephen. *Hefner's Gonna Kill Me When He Reads This. . . .* Chicago: Allen-Bennett, 1972.

Hawkins, Delbert I., Kenneth Coney, and Roger Best. *Consumer Behavior: Implications for Marketing Strategy.* Dallas: Business Publications, 1980.

Key, Bryan Wilson. *Subliminal Seduction: Ad Media's Seduction of a Not-So-Innocent America.* Englewood Cliffs, N.J.: Prentice-Hall, 1973. Fascinating study of methods used by the media to persuade us to buy things. Chapter 7, on *Playboy,* and Chapter 8, on *Cosmo* and *Vogue,* are especially valuable for helping you *zero in* on target markets.

Mitchell, Arnold. *Nine American Lifestyles: Who We Are and Where We Are Going.* New York: Macmillan Publishing Co., 1983. A comprehensive data-based study on psychographic patterns in America. Contains an illuminating chapter on Europe. Because it projects the future, it is an excellent companion to *Megatrends.*

Publishers Weekly Yearbook: News, Analyses, and Trends in the Book Industry. New York: R. R. Bowker Publishing Co., 1983.

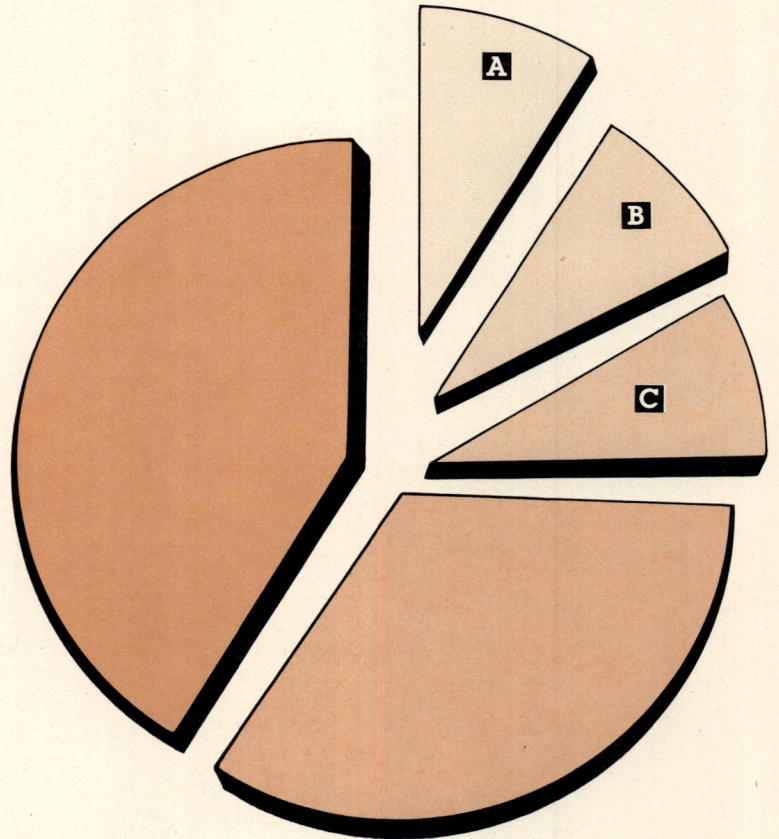

A Description of Product or Service

B The Market and the Target Customer

C Reading the Competition

FIGURE 5.1 Chapter 5 adds to your Business Plan with information on how to outsmart the competition.

5

Reading the Competition

LEARNING OBJECTIVES

To expand the concept of the four-phase life cycle to illuminate the changing force of competition in each phase.

To define the competitive arena in terms of size, growth, profitability, innovation, market leaders, market losers, and potential competitors.

To understand the value of positive positioning.

To conceptualize competition as a struggle or climb up a ladder inside the mind of the Target Customer.

To evaluate competitors by using all three dimensions of research (primary, secondary, and New Eyes).

To develop your skills at playing Marketplace Detective as you set up surveillance on your competitors.

To develop a competitor test matrix which will allow you to compare intensities of competition.

To learn imaginative ways to disarm competitors.

To think about ways to change the arena.

Like everything else in life and in business, competition goes through a cycle of four stages: embryo, growth, maturity, decline. In this chapter we examine all four stages in general; then we look at ways you can meet and beat your competition. Briefly, we can describe the four stages as follows:

1. In the *embryonic* stage, the arena's empty. There's just you and your idea for a product or service and a tiny core market.
2. As your industry *grows*, competitors smell money and attempt to **penetrate the arena** to take up positions they hope will turn to profit. Curious target customers come from all directions. You have visions of being rich forever.
3. As the industry *matures*, competition gets fierce and you are forced to steal customers to survive. Shelf velocity slows. Production runs get longer. Prices start to slide down.
4. As the industry goes into *decline*, competition becomes desperate. Many fail; other weary competitors leave the arena, which is now silent except for the echoes of battle.

A LIFE–CYCLE SCENARIO

The following scenario will deepen your understanding of the life cycle of a product. As a product travels the cycle, business people adopt different strategies to meet changing circumstances in the marketplace. In this scenario, we again emphasize the importance of teamwork in small business. In Chapter 3, we saw the Info Team at work. In Chapter 5, we have a manufacturing team which brainstorms its way to a brilliant success.

As you read "Skates for Ducks," try to visualize other goods and services as they travel the life cycle.

penetrate the arena
a calculated thrust into the marketplace

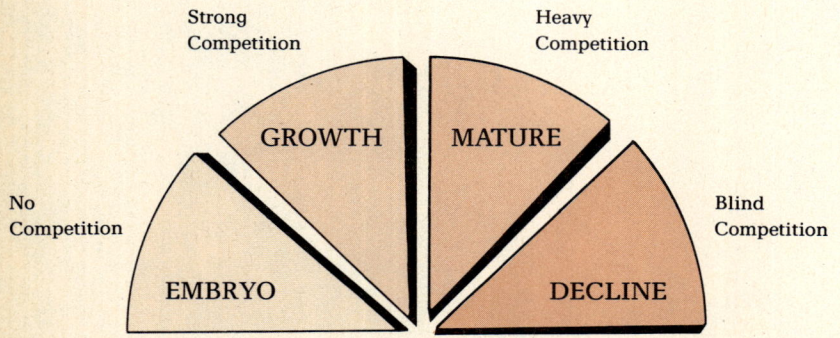

FIGURE 5.2 The competition life cycle defines four stages in the intensity of competition that every product or service must face.

Case Study

Scenario — Skates for Ducks

Over lunch one Friday, four friends who worked for XRD, the giant telecommunications **conglomerate,** began talking about founding their own company.

Betty, an energetic woman with an M.B.A. from Wharton, was in marketing and sales. Before coming on board at XRD, Betty had worked for Exxon, IBM, and TRW. Even though she had just received a promotion and a good raise, Betty was getting tired of having her marketing strategies shot down. She was ready to try entrepreneurship on her own.

Bruce was a junior vice-president. His favorite saying was "Let's have the bottom line, here." Bruce's dream was to be president of XRD, then Chairman of the Board, then U.S. Senator, then President of the United States. His hero was John DeLorean. "John was framed on the drug thing," Bruce was fond of saying. "It was an obvious case of entrapment. The company was his family. He was just trying to save his family." Bruce's desk was a paper jungle. He was impatient with subordinates. He was barely 35, yet his hair was turning grey. He suffered from a stomach ulcer.

Hugh was in Design. He worked a flex-time schedule in the XRD Creative Dungeon, and came to work in jeans and blue work shirts and running shoes. Hugh could program a computer in his sleep. Because shaving took him away from his creativity, Hugh wore a beard. You could drive by his home any night or on the weekends and find him tinkering away. Hugh devoured books on art, computers, architecture, self-hypnosis, investing, and right-hemisphere power.

Dan was in Public Relations. He had a B.A. in journalism from Columbia University, and he'd worked for an ad agency for 10 years before coming to XRD. Dan dressed in three-piece suits from Savile Row. He drove a red convertible. He was always looking for a party, and if someone wasn't throwing one, Dan would offer.

Act One

"Listen, fellow inmates," Hugh said, finishing the last of his cola. "Last night, I came up with an idea that will make us all rich."

Bruce's ulcer was bothering him. He glared at Hugh. "Spare us the details, Hughie. Let's just have the bottom line, okay?"

"Skates for ducks," Hugh said, smiling like a mad inventor.

Betty's marketing intuition told her some exciting changes were about to take place. "Don't jump on him, Bruce," Betty said. "Go ahead, Hugh."

"Ice skates?" Dan asked. "Or roller?" Dan was already thinking of promotional angles.

"You're off the deep end, Hugh-Boy," Bruce said, staring around the table. "Why ruin a good lunch with your usual holistic nightmares?"

"Take the afternoon off, Bruce," Betty said. "Play some racquetball. They're working you too hard up there in the Executive Tower."

"I've got tennis elbow," Bruce said. "Or I'd be on the court now."

"You ever watch a duck?" Hugh asked. "They can stand on one foot. Their leg muscles are rock solid. And they have all these feathers that would keep them from getting cold on the ice."

"The **core market** is pretty thin," Betty said. "But I like the idea. It has an innovative touch that's almost sexy. Can we have something for the December Show?"

Continued

conglomerate
an organization involved in several diverse businesses

The Embryonic Stage

The embryonic stage is marked by excitement, naive euphoric thrust, clumsiness, a high failure rate, and much brainstorming. Pricing is experimental. Sales volume is low, and production and marketing costs are high. At this stage, it's difficult to find distributors and resellers demand huge gross margins. Profit is chancy and speculative. Shrewd entrepreneurs, however, can close their eyes and divine the presence of a core market. Competition has not yet appeared.

core market
customers whose perceived needs best fit a product's characteristics

"I'm testing the prototype Saturday. At Dorman's Pond. It's a tame duck, of course, but you're all welcome to observe."

"The real market's in wild ducks," Betty said.

"The real promo angle, too," Dan said.

"You're all crazy," Bruce said, and walked away from the table.

So on Saturday, only Dan and Betty showed up for the test. They were amazed. Hugh's duck skated across the ice of Dorman's Pond serenely, like a creation out of a Walt Disney film. A gaggle of Mallards gathered to watch the performance, and one younger Mallard came up afterward to try on the skates.

The Mallard was a natural. He swirled out onto the ice, doing ripostes and pirouettes. Watching, Betty was thrilled. The ducks on the sidelines applauded. Betty sensed widespread customer interest.

"This is exciting," Betty said.

"The PR possibilities are endless," Dan said. "We'll start with an autograph party this spring, as they fly north, out of Mexico and South America."

The three friends had been in business before, so they started on a small scale. Hugh found a manufacturer in the next town who would make a hundred pairs of duck skates. They promoted the skates with a direct mail piece to duck owners in the local area. "Win a free pair of skates for your duck," the promo said. "Enter your duck in the Dorman's Pond Regional."

They developed an essay contest at the local high school. The topic was "Should American Ducks Have Access to Jet-Powered Ice Skates?" (The jet-powered models were still on Hugh's drawing board, but this was the moment to test the market for **product innovation.**)

The response from the students was an overwhelming *yes*.

Their skate manufacturer thought he had enough inventory to last until Christmas. Surprise. All 100 pairs were sold within a week. Catalog houses were calling, wanting the skates. The core market had emerged.

The three friends were excited. They hadn't lost money. There was still no competition in sight.

One problem surfaced. At the duck races in West Ossipee, New Hampshire, three Fleet Mallards sustained severe injuries when they achieved ice speeds in excess of 237 m.p.h. and their skates flew off.

Act Two

Hugh, working late one night in his garage, developed a product innovation: a velcro heel strap that solved the flying skate problem. Endorsements by famous ducks quickly followed. Television networks began selling time for events featuring ducks on skates. As soon as Betty and Dan created a suitable company name—The Fire and Ice Skate Company—Bruce resigned from XRD and came on board as president.

There was an ugly occurrence during **distribution.** A railroad car loaded with the all-new Luke Skywalker rocket-powered skates was hijacked by a gang of masked coots. Several coots were blown away when the skates they were wearing exploded. Editorials across the land carried the same message: "Technology kills."

In Hollywood, celebrities who had never given a thought to ducks on skates were now sponsoring duck races, skate regattas, and skate ballets.

On New York's Publishers Row, major publishing houses entered a race to see who could bring out the definitive study of duck behavior. Would skating change the face of duckhood over the planet?

In Texas, an entrepreneur at A & M in College Station developed an

Continued

product innovation
improvement in the utility
or design of a product

The Growth Stage

The growth stage is marked by product innovation, strong product acceptance, the beginnings of brand loyalty, promotion by media sizzle, and a nailing down of ballpark pricing. Product innovation occurs. Distribution becomes all important. Resellers who laughed during the embryonic stage now clamor to distribute the product. Strong competitors, excited by the smell of money, enter the arena of the marketplace. Profit shows signs of peaking.

distribution
the physical movement of
the product from
manufacturer to ultimate
consumer

Arctic Refractor that would freeze over a medium-sized lake in three hours flat. DuPont and GE put their plants into 24-hour R & D to show the world who would build the first Arctic Refractor. Meanwhile the U.S. Government hired biologists to train ducks to stop migrating.

"We don't want them skating in Mexico," said one government spokesman. "That would be unpatriotic. We need them up here — at home on America's glorious lakes — to boost the national morale." All over the duck world, ducks were entering the work force. Parallax, Inc., the noted motivation research firm, stated that the major reason for this influx was to increase discretionary duck income to buy upgraded skates.

Wary of being exploited, ducks began to demand higher wages. They wanted their own show. In Pittsburgh, duck skater's unions began, then spread south and west.

Fire and Ice Skate Company had been in business only a short 18 months when it declared an astronomical dividend. Hugh's new developments, coupled with aggressive management from Bruce, marketing expertise from Betty, and superpromotions from Dan, enabled the four friends to pay themselves $2 million apiece (combined salary and executive perks). Bruce decided to fire their small accounting firm and sign with one of the Big Eight. Dan decided to throw a party.

With three Scotches in him, Bruce slapped Hugh on the back and admitted he had been hasty for calling him crazy.

"*Time* wants me for their cover," Bruce said. "What's on the drawing board, anyway? Anything cooking?"

"Yes," Hugh said. "I'm off to Tibet."

"Tibet?" Bruce was shocked. "What for?"

"Ideas," Hugh said, pointing to his right brain. "Ideas."

Act Three

Price wars plagued the industry. Mallard Eski-Skates made cuts of 25%. Canadian Goose Ltd., the makers of the Luxury Ugly-Duckling Model, slashed prices by 40%. At Fire and Ice GHQ in Manhattan, Bruce took a look at the balance sheet and called down to Design with orders for 17 new variations of the Fire and Ice Turbo Skate.

Betty came up with a creative idea to save the firm — the Duck Skate Palace in Armonk, New York — but her bank said Fire and Ice was overextended on lines of credit as it was. Up in PR, Dan hadn't had an idea for media sizzle in days. The Fire and Ice computer told the story — the end was near.

"Where is Hugh when we need him?" Bruce asked, at the meeting of Executive Group on Friday. "We're in a trough. He could bail us out."

"Our marketing data says we've peaked, dear," Betty said. "The Armonk Skate Palace was our last stand for this product."

"Show me that on the bottom line," Bruce said, aggressively.

"I'm thinking about moving to Florida," Dan said. "According to this guy Naisbitt, that's where the action is."

That day, the Executive Group meeting disintegrated into wild schemes and bickering. After the meeting broke up, Bruce kept his accounting department working through the night. "You people will stay here," Bruce said, "until you produce me a spreadsheet that does not forecast the end of my world."

But the numbers would not lie.

Act Four

That year, Fire and Ice Skate Company tripled production — over 17 million skates for ducks. Prices were slashed. New colors were added.

Continued

The Mature Stage

The mature stage is marked by zero modifications. Design concentrates on product differentiation instead of product improvement. Competitors are going at it blindly now, running on momentum even as shelf velocity slows. Production runs get longer, so firms can take full advantage of capital equipment and experienced management. Resellers, sensing doom, are cool on the product. Advertising investments increase, in step with competition. Some firms go out of business. Prices are on a swift slide down. Any competitor who enters the production segment of the skate market now is either dumb or over-confident or both. In the once-hot marketplace, there is a pervasive air of depression.

Velcro straps were striped with silver and gold. Five million pairs had to be sold at Deep Discount.

On December 26, Mallard Eski-Skates, the major competition, filed for Chapter Eleven.

Bankruptcy.

Fire and Ice closed plants in California, Texas, Alabama, and southern New Hampshire.

On location at a lake site in Louisiana, DuPont's Prototype Arctic Refractor blew up, killing several hundred ducks and splattering over a million fish across northern New Orleans.

Ducks reacted by dropping their skates onto city streets at rush hour. The knife-sharp blades cut into the very heart of city traffic.

"How awful," Betty said.

"I'm off to Florida," Dan said. "What will you give me for my stock?"

"Great news, men," Bruce said. "We just killed Canadian Goose, Ltd. They closed all their plants."

"We must do something," Betty said.

"I'm selling my car," Dan said. "Any takers?"

In the midst of chaos and depression, Hugh arrived from Tibet with an idea—a 10-speed Turbo Skate for people on the go.

As he was leaving, Dan met Hugh in the hall outside Executive Tower. Hugh had the sketches for the new Turbo Skate in his shirt pocket. Dan noticed that Hugh's beard could use some immediate barbering.

"Great idea, Hugh!" Dan said. "Why didn't you think of this before?"

"It came to me on a mountaintop in Tibet," Hugh said, smiling peacefully. "How is everything in the corporate universe?"

"I think," Dan said, "that we are back in business."

Dan promoted the new Turbo Skate with an ad showing a young man in sweater and scarf, sitting at the edge of a frozen pond. The ad copy read as follows:

Romance fading? Dazzle her with the new F & I Turbo. With ten speeds, you can skate uphill, skate to work, or write her name in ice!

Production geared up to make the Turbo. Bruce became F & I CEO and brought in a new man—a hotshot manager from the soft-drink industry—as president. Dan got busy making a documentary on the history of the skating duck movement. It would make great PR, he said, and enhance the company image. The documentary was set to air on network TV. Betty spent most of her time at trade shows, promoting the new 10-speed skates. She got an endorsement from a retired Olympic figure skater, and that led to the idea to have a Turbo Skate Power Championship at the next Winter Olympics. Bruce the competitor fell in love with that idea and joined Betty on the road as they networked their way into the highest skating circles in the land. On their last joint report to Executive Group, Betty and Bruce announced their engagement.

When last seen, a bearded, glassy-eyed Hugh was locked in the lab at Fire and Ice, working on an idea for two computer games—Skates in Space and The Duck in the Dungeon—while he made final sketches for his Hobby Skate model kit, to be sold in toy stores at Christmas.

The Decline Stage

The decline stage is marked by extreme depression in the marketplace. A few firms still hang on. R & D ceases. Promotion vanishes. Price wars continue. Opportunities emerge for entrepreneurs in service and repair. Diehards fight for what remains of the core market. Resellers laugh at sales people.

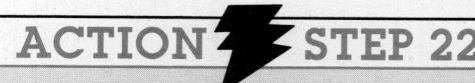

ACTION STEP 22

Position Yourself in the Grand Arena of the Marketplace

Competition is a kind of mind-game. To find out what that means in business, read a book called *Positioning: The Battle for the Mind,* by Al Ries and Jack Trout. *Positioning* sharpens the process of competition by helping you focus on the mind of the prospect, or Target Customer.

Inside your Target Customer's mind are many ladders—ladders for products, ladders for services, ladders for sports figures and TV programs and banks and wine and rent-a-cars.

To compete, you have to get a foothold on your industry ladder inside the Target Customer's mind.

Or build a new ladder.

But before you try anything that fancy, why not locate a couple of ladders and give them a try?

1. See which firm is at the top. That one is your major competition. Studying the Top Position will trigger ideas on how you can compete.

2. Try a short climb. When you run into a competitor, make some notes. What is good? What is bad? What is formidable? What can you learn?

3. When you are about halfway to the top, look around and reprofile your Target Customer. Is the profile the same as the one you did from the floor of the arena? Or has climbing changed your perspective?

4. Before you get to the top, ask yourself two questions:

Do I really want to be here?

What business am I really in?

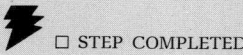

☐ STEP COMPLETED

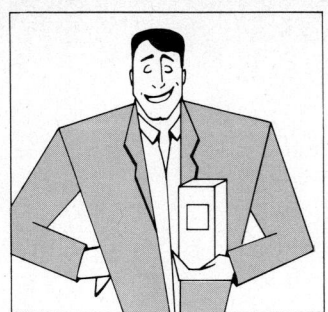 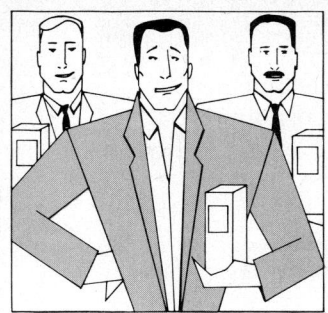 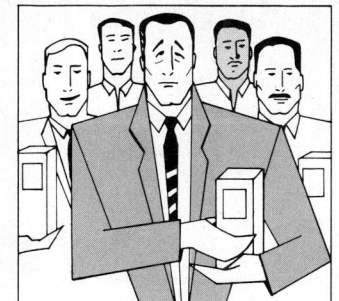 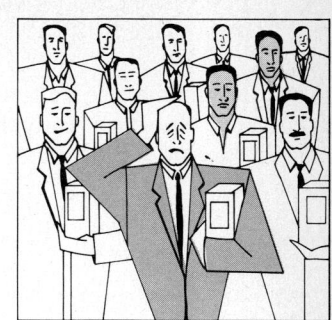

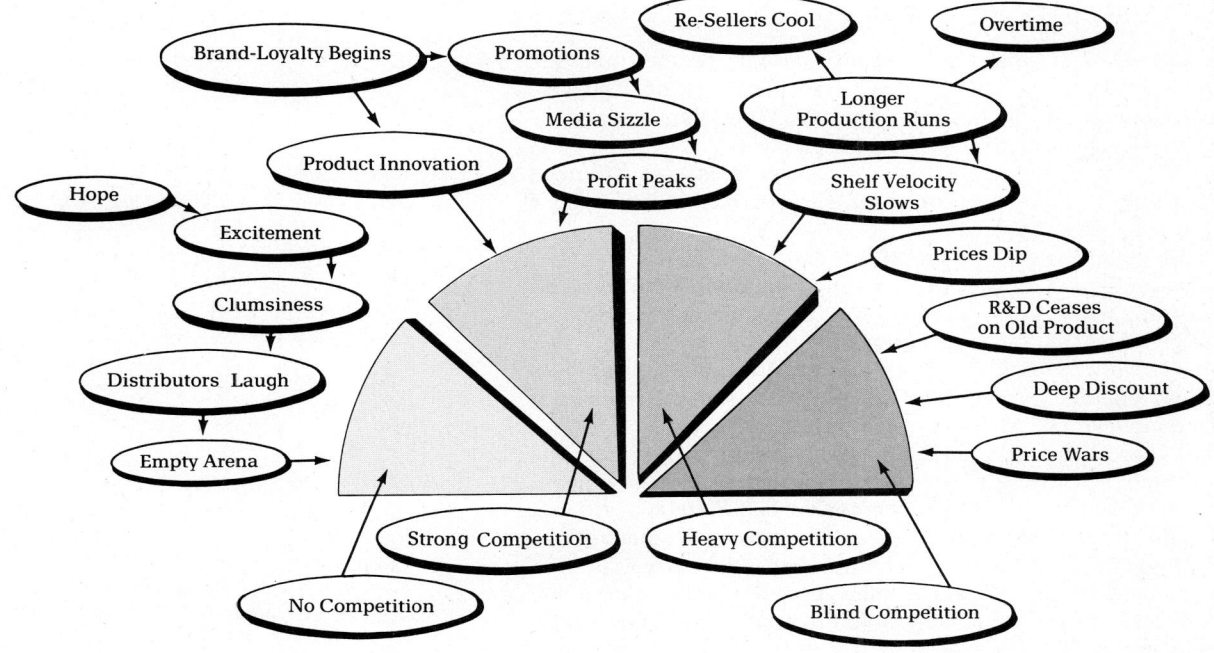

FIGURE 5.3 Different competitive strategies are needed in each stage of the competition life cycle.

Our life-cycle scenario is only partly facetious. The facts are that to survive, you must know what stage of the life cycle you are in and plan your competitive strategies accordingly. See Figure 5.3 for a visual reminder of these facts.

Where is your industry on the great arc of the life cycle? What does that mean for you at start-up time? What does that mean for your survival? When your industry starts into maturity and decline, will you be ready with Plan B?

COMPETITION AND POSITIONING

Competition in business is no mystery. It takes place on a ladder in an arena inside the Target Customer's mind. The winners of this competition find the ladder and wrestle for positions at the top. Action Step 22 could give you a winning advantage in this process.

Competition in a Mature Industry

If you're in a mature industry, you're going to have to steal customers to survive. The case study that follows will show you one way of doing it — by giving better service.

Case Study

Roy Modell

Roy Modell grew up in Arkansas. When he was 18, he decided to see the world. He wound up in Detroit. He was an independent kind of guy. He worked for someone else awhile, found he didn't like it, and opened his own business — a gas station.

"I did like a lot of guys in Motown," Roy says. "I just sort of jumped into something. It went along okay for a while, but then one day I realized the business was broke."

Roy worked for five years to pay off his debts.

The five years paid off. Roy built a solid reputation with three oil companies, and when he moved to the West Coast, oil reps would come to him to give him first bid on a station site.

He was down in Orange County, running two stations. There was one of those planned communities going in, and the oil rep said it would be a money-maker. Here's how Roy checked it out.

Around 7:30 in the morning, he parked across the street from the only other station within three miles. He counted the cars buying gas for an hour. He developed his own **competitor test matrix,** a grid that he used to rate the competition. For example, he noted the make of car, then correlated that with time at the pump. He had industry figures on tank capacity for all vehicles, and he knew, from long experience in the service station business, the average amount of gas for each type of car.

Roy had an insider's knowledge.

He came back around noon, and then again during the rush hour. He compared weekday business with business on the weekends, just before people went out for some distance driving.

In the employee sector, Roy saw a lot of opportunity for competition. "They were pump jockeys," Roy says. "They could have been more courteous. They made five moves where one should have done. And there wasn't much attempt at selling TAB [tires, accessories, batteries]. That could have been because the owner wasn't around much."

In any **mature industry,** Roy knew, you have to be ready to steal customers from your competition. The way he did it was with service.

Roy put in his bid and his station opened up — at a great **location.** He had a busy corner in a medium-sized shopping center. And it was a good **layout.** There were three service bays, always full, with two cars parked on the driveway outside, waiting to get in. After a good long look at the tire dealers in his area, Roy began running ads in the Sunday paper.

In less than a year, he outsold most of the tire stores.

competitor test matrix
a grid used to get a clear picture of the strengths, weaknesses, and sales volume of your competitors

mature industry
growth has slowed here, few new competitors, strong competition, little real new product innovation

location
physical place of a business

layout
physical arrangement of a business which attempts to maximize productivity

Roy succeeded because he made a game out of his business. He knew what business he was in. He knew where his business was in the Great Industry Life Cycle. He knew how to compete.

Scouting the Competition

Your next step is to follow Roy Modell's lead and study your competition. Action Step 23 will help you. Remember — work from your strengths. Strength is built on knowledge. Knowing your competitors will increase your confidence. Only then can you win.

With a competitor checklist, you can keep track of all your competitors.

As you study your competitors, organize your observations into a list of categories. Then rank each competitor on a scale of 1 to 10 for each category. By the time you are finished, you will have completed a competitor test matrix that will give you an instant overview of your competition — and your opportunities.

Plan A and Plan B

The two case studies that follow illustrate two tactics for disarming your competition. In the first case, Ben Jones grabs an exclusive rung on his Target Customer's ladder by being unique. In the second case, Ford Johnson is always one step ahead of the competition because he is ready with a **Plan B.**

Plan A: How to keep your image in the mind of the prospect.

Case Study

Ben Jones

Ben Jones believes in keeping his **image** right up there. When he ships expensive camera lenses (some wholesale for $2,000), he always makes sure they remember him in the shipping room — he has the lenses packed in popcorn, or in courtesy bags of Virginia peanuts.

The bags are stamped with Ben's company logo.

The people who work in the shipping room are Ben's Target Customers.

In addition, Ben sends out cards on April Fool's day (instead of at Christmas), and when he visits clients he wears a Superman suit. He definitely maintains a **presence.**

His clients always remember Ben Jones.

Plan B: How to compete with your own products.

Case Study

Ford J. Johnson

Ford J. Johnson has been in mail order for a dozen years now. He says it gives him more freedom to be creative. Ford was trained as an electri-
Continued

ACTION STEP 23

Disguise Yourself as the Mystery Shopper

Probe your competitors. Then build your own competitor checklist.

Part A. Study your competitors from the outside. Analyze their layout, location, parking, advertising, image. How is the business perceived by the Target Customers? By the neighbors? By passersby? How long are the lines? Are people walking out loaded or empty?

If this were your business, and you had unlimited funds, what would you do differently in the area of image and atmosphere?

Part B. Now move inside. What's the layout like? Is the service swift and pleasant and efficient? How are you greeted? How would you score the quality of merchandise? Is there music? How would you characterize the atmosphere? Is the place clean?

If you can't move inside without blowing your Mystery Shopper Disguise, do some cagey telephone shopping. You can tell a lot from a phone call survey that's prepared in advance.

Where are your competitors vulnerable? What gaps aren't they filling? How can you be better?

☐ STEP COMPLETED

Plan B
the counter-attack blueprint that you have ready to implement depending on fluid shifts in the marketplace

image
the way a business is perceived

presence
a heightened awareness in the mind of your Target Customer

cal engineer, and he spent a good 20 years in the aerospace industry before breaking free.

In a dozen years, Ford has developed and marketed over two hundred products — from a Mylar heat sheet (for pets) to Engine Coat (a motor lubricant using Teflon) to Space Monkeys (dried shrimp eggs that hatch when dropped into water).

Ford has a hundred strategies for handling his competitors. The best one is how he competes with himself.

Here's the way it works:

He hits the marketplace with a quality product. It retails for $12, and his price nets him a reasonable profit after overhead. Because he deals with established mail order houses (they ship to thousands and thousands of customers), Ford knows someone out there will copy his idea and try to ace him by bringing out a lower quality product for less.

So for the first couple of runs, Ford manufactures a quality product, using the best materials available. It sells for full price, and Ford is waiting for the phone to ring. When it does, he knows it's the buyer from the catalog house, telling him there's a competitor waiting in the wings with an **inferior product** that will retail for $6 — half of what Ford's costs.

Ford has a cheaper one ready to roll.

"When do you need them and how many can you handle?" Ford asks.

"Wait," the buyer says. "What kind of numbers are we looking at?"

"Mine will retail for $5.75," Ford says. "And I can have 10,000 on your loading dock by two weeks from tomorrow."

"You're kidding," the buyer says. (He's new on the block. Other buyers have watched Ford work before.)

"Can you move 20,000?" Ford asks.

"Ten for sure," the buyer says. "And if we need more I'll get back to you in two weeks."

"Over and out," Ford says. "It's great doing business with you."

Now, let's really get an in-depth understanding of your competitors. The more you understand your competitors, the easier it will be to visualize the position of your new company in the grand arena of the marketplace. Action Step 24 will help you dig.

If you're a potential buyer, everybody will compete for your dollar. If you change positions and become the store owner, you'll want to move fast to locate the ladder inside your TC's mind. If you can't locate the ladder, or if all else fails, change the arena where the ladder rests.

CHANGING THE ARENA

The following two cases illustrate how two large companies successfully changed the arena and won a huge slice of the market.

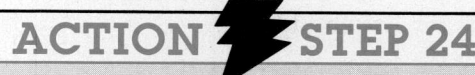

inferior product
lower in utility than the product it's being compared to

ACTION STEP 24

Using Every Network Connection You Can Find, Dig Beneath the Surface of Your Competitors

Leave your Mystery Shopper Disguise at home and really dig into this competitor research. Some of it will be easy: yellow pages, newspapers, trade advertising, signs, former and present customers.

Interview everyone who will talk to you.

If your competitors have stock that is publicly traded, call your stock broker or look up your competitors in Moody's or Standard and Poor's.

Another neat trick is to ask your librarian to get you a 10K corporate report. (A 10K is required of public companies by the IRS.) In addition, most firms are listed and rated by Dun and Bradstreet. Ask your friendly banker for a peek at the D & B reports.

Keep expanding your own competitor test matrix. Use a 1 – 10 scale on everything you can see, hear about, touch (image, location, advertising, the sign outside, the way the employees dress, parking, Target Customers, product mix, pricing, hours of service, and so on).

Whenever you unearth some hard data, compare it with industry averages.

Keep looking until you find some areas of vulnerability.

□ STEP COMPLETED

Case Study

A Major TV Network

Several years back, ABC had only college football. The other major networks, NBC and CBS, had pro football covered, and pro football had captured most of the viewers, and that spelled advertising dollars.

What did ABC do?

It **changed the arena** and started Monday Night Football.

ABC could change the arena because it was sure what business it was in—the entertainment business. And a larger market was prepared to be entertained on Monday night than on Sunday afternoon.

changing the arena
transforming a product or service by adding a simple benefit that has immediate customer appeal

Case Study

A Major Electrical Manufacturer

Manufacturer B, a very large electrical manufacturer, wanted to penetrate the market for movie projector lamps. The problem was that Manufacturer A had the market sewed up.

Manufacturer B's creative, entrepreneurial-type people went to work on the problem and discovered an **area of vulnerability:** They designed a new bulb with a four-prong locking flange pin. The new bulb was easy to install, it was safe, and the new design provided better focusing.

To promote the new bulb, Manufacturer B gave away sockets that were fitted to it, and bases to set the sockets into.

It was the system approach.

Because the whole new system from Manufacturer B worked better and more smoothly than the piecemeal approach provided by Manufacturer A, the customers (Kodak, Bell and Howell, and other big companies) went for it.

By the time Manufacturer A woke up to the change in the arena, it was almost too late, and when they started making bulbs with locking flange pins, they had to pay Manufacturer B, who owned the patent.

area of vulnerability
your competitor's soft underbelly, Achilles' Heel — weaknesses ready for you to exploit

There's something we can learn from this last case study.

This story has a moral—the arena that shifted this multimillion-dollar market was the size of a quarter. Because that was the size of the new socket.

Now is the time to formulate your own plan for dealing with the competition. Action Step 25 shows you how. Don't forget that your competitor's area of vulnerability may be no bigger than a quarter.

ACTION ⚡ STEP 25

Formulate Your Plan for Disarming Your Competitors

Make this a brainstorming session. Start with a crazy idea (packing expensive gear in popcorn and competing with yourself are two examples) and really let go with the wild ideas.

Keep your mind on the industry ladder as you brainstorm. What's unique about your product or service? Are you supplying something your Target Customer wants and/or needs? What tactics, of your competitors, can you utilize? If you start out in an embryonic industry and suddenly the arena is filled with competitors, do you have Plan B?

(For some ideas on how one firm dealt with competitors, see Chapter 15, "Showcase: Pulling Your Plan Together.")

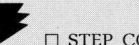 ☐ STEP COMPLETED

SUMMARY

One way to get an overview of competitive forces at work is to use the life-cycle yardstick.

In the *embryonic stage,* the arena is empty. Competitors are invisible. Your Target Customer is a dim profile on yellow paper. Potential customers ignore you. Suppliers and distributors laugh at you.

In the *growth stage,* competitors enter the arena and Target Customers surface. They have been waiting for your product for years! Smart distributors sign you up.

In the *mature stage,* competition makes shelf space scarce and you are forced to steal customers to survive.

In the *decline stage,* a few competitors hang on, tenaciously. By now, you have shifted your energies to a new arena, where you will quickly re-position yourself for another new enterprise.

Competition is a mind game, because that is where buying decisions are made. To explore this idea, read a terrific book called *Positioning: The Battle for the Mind,* by Al Ries and Jack Trout.

A number of case studies in the chapter show how successful entrepreneurs have disarmed the competition — by stealing customers, by scouting the competition for strengths and weaknesses, by maintaining a highly visible presence, by being ready with a Plan B, or by changing the arena of competition.

THINK POINTS

- Do it smarter.
- Do it classier.
- Do it with more style.
- Do it with more features.
- Provide more service.
- Do it faster.
- Treat your Target Customers like people. Consider their needs first.
- Be unique.
- Buy your competition out in a midnight stock takeover.
- Change the arena.
- Keep your image in the mind of the prospect.
- Become your own competition.
- Change the arena where the competition takes place.
- Beat your competition by being better, faster, safer, and easier to use.
- A new firm will never win a price war.
- Old habits are tough to break. Give your TC *several* strong reasons to switch over to you.

ACTION STEP REVIEW

22 Competition in business takes place inside the mind of the Target Customer. If you are going to win, you have to find your industry ladder inside your TC's mind. Then make sure you've got a foothold on the ladder before you begin to climb.

As you climb, keep profiling your Target Customer. As you encounter competitors, keep asking yourself this question — what business am I really in?

23 Build your own Competitor Checklist. Who are your main competitors? What are they doing that's strong? What are they doing that is weak? What can you learn from studying them in detail?

24 Study your competitors through customer interviews, corporate reports, and kinds of advertising they do. How tough is it going to be to disarm these competitors? What do you think will be your market share?

25 Now that you know your competitors, brainstorm ways you can win. What is unique about your product or service? Are you filling a need? If you started out in an industry segment that was embryonic, and suddenly it is overflowing with competitors, do you have Plan B? What can you do to change the arena?

REFERENCES

Baty, Gordon B. *Entrepreneurship: Playing to Win.* Reston, Va.: Reston Publishing Co., 1974.

"European Luxury Cars Capturing a Growing Share of the U.S. Market." *Wall Street Journal,* May 6, 1983.

Kahn, Joseph P. "800-356-9377." *Inc.,* July 1983, 51–62. Someone is after your 800 number, which is your key to telemarketing in the Age of Information. Across the nation, dialers can reach 356-9377 by spelling F-L-O-W-E-R-S. Who got the number? A trucking firm.

Ries, Al, and Jack Trout. *Positioning: The Battle for Your Mind.* New York: Warner Books, 1982. The best book around on the power of positive positioning.

Schwartz, David J. *Marketing Today: A Basic Approach.* New York: Harcourt Brace Jovanovich, 1977.

A Description
of Product
or Service

B The Market
and the
Target
Customer

C Reading the
Competition

D Marketing
Strategy

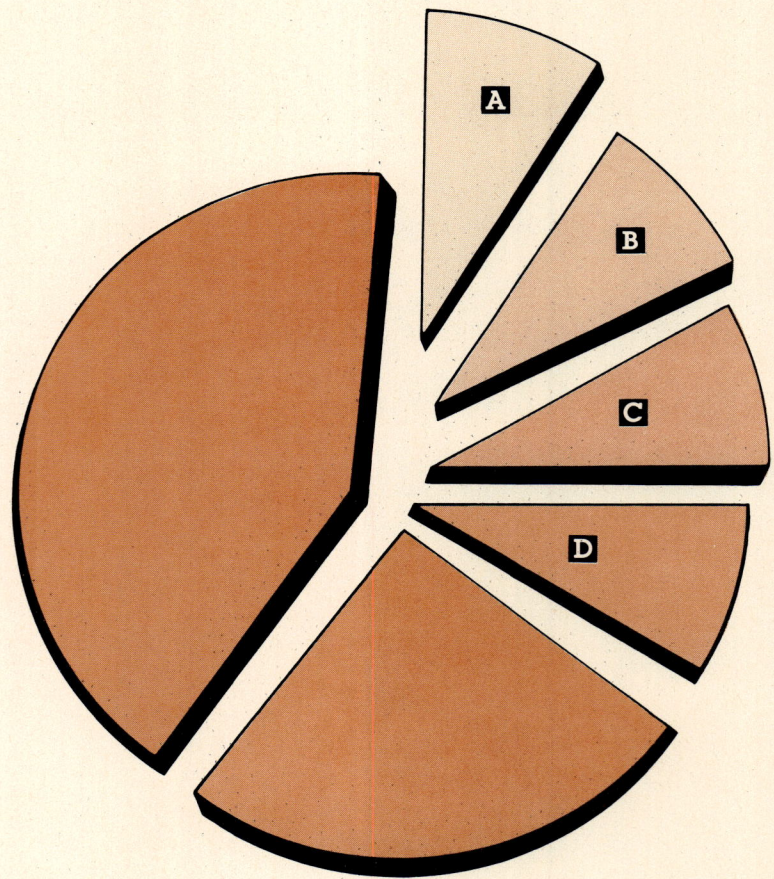

FIGURE 6.1 Chapter 6 will help you put together the Marketing
Strategy section of your Plan by giving you the tools you need to
reach your customer.

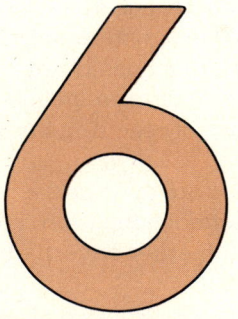

Promotion: Making That Customer Connection

LEARNING OBJECTIVES

To learn how to communicate to Target Customers using both conventional and creative promotional methods.

To develop an overview of promotional tools.

To decide, through research and testing, which tools form the central core of your promotional strategy.

To get free publicity, so you can tell your customers what you are selling without having to spend money on advertising.

To maximize the power of a small advertising budget.

To learn the value of personal selling for the smaller firm.

To try brainstorming techniques to help you arrive at the right promotional mix for your small business.

To develop a customer list.

To target customers with maximum effectiveness for the dollar.

To learn the magic of networking, so that you can have dozens of unpaid professionals promoting for you.

To locate networks.

To build your own network.

 **N**ow that you have profiled your Target Customer and have gained a sense of competition and market niche, it's time to plan a promotional strategy. But each business is unique, and you don't want to throw away money on promotional schemes that don't work.

For example, if your Target Customer is female, age 45–55, with an income of $100,000 and up, college educated, with a suburban residence, owns three cars (one of which is a Mercedes limousine), rides horseback 10 hours a week, reads *Practical Horseman* and *Performance Horseman,* you'll have a good chance of reaching her with direct mail.

If, on the other hand, your Target Customers are male and female, age 24–57, income of $17,000, with a high school education, you're going to have to resort to some form of mass market advertising or rethink your target market.

Market research is your strategy for locating your Target Customers and finding out where they itch. Promotion is letting them know your business can scratch their itch and make them happy in the process.

Promotion is the art or science of moving the image of your business into the prospect's mind. *Promotion* comes from the Latin verb, *movere,* which means ''to advance,'' ''to move forward.'' (It's an aggressive word, so learn to say it with a smile!)

PROMOTIONAL STRATEGIES

The Right Promotional Mix

The key to finding the right promotional strategy for your small business is to consider a wide variety of promotional approaches and then to pick the right **promotional mix.** Let's look at some of the potential elements of that mix:

Paid media advertising.
Point-of-purchase displays.
Catalog sales.
Direct mail.
Money-back guarantee.
Free ink/free air.
Personal selling.
Trade shows.
Industry literature.
Working visibility.

All of these elements together make for a rich promotional mix. Check the elements *you* feel comfortable with. For a closer look at these strategies, read on.

promotional mix
all the elements that you blend to maximize effective communication with your TC

Potential Strategies

Paid Media Advertising. A surefire way to reach out is by ads in radio, newspaper, television, magazines, and trade journals. Advertising tickles the Target Customer's mind. With a good ad, you can gain the attention and interest of your Target Customer. You can reach right into your TC's mind and create the desire to buy from you.

Advertising has some obvious drawbacks: 1) it can cost plenty to create; 2) if you don't spend even more money, your ad won't get exposure; and 3) **preferred placements** go to big spenders.

Advice:

Your best ad is yourself. Stay visible.

Check with vendors. Ask for tear sheets, copy, cooperative advertising money, and help on layouts.

Check with marketing departments of newspapers. Ask for help, advice, information.

Newspapers often offer special supplements at reduced cost. The offer often includes free editorial copy.

Explore creative **co-op advertising.**

Don't be afraid to **piggyback.** Let Madison Avenue build the market. Then use your promotional mix to tell the TC where to buy: *at your place.*

Start small, and test, test, test.

Point-of-Purchase Displays. This is a great gimmick for impulse buys. Good for last-minute stuff like paperbacks, L'eggs, candy, magazines, and gum. A sharp **P-O-P** improves your image by making your underfinanced start-up look like a million dollars. A good P-O-P is like a tireless silent salesperson, always on duty.

There are problems with these displays: 1) you can't sell large items because they crowd customers at the cash register, and 2) the display must sell itself as well as the product. (A tacky P-O-P will turn prospective customers *off* instead of *on.*)

Advice:

Do weekly evaluations of all P-O-Ps. Make sure your silent salespeople are doing their work.

Catalogs. This sales tool is just right for isolated shoppers — or shoppers in a hurry — who want specialty items like camping gear, jewelry, rare books, or Star Pets. Some shoppers just want privacy. **Catalog houses** like Sunset House, Spiegel, and L. L. Bean don't usually manufacture anything, so they are always looking for good products. Use catalogs as another kind of silent salesperson to reach smaller customers.

If you try printing your own catalogs, you'll run into at least two problems: 1) cost (they are expensive to print, expensive to mail); 2) size limitations (it's tough to sell anything by catalog that's big, bulky, or inconvenient to ship).

---

preferred placements
best locations within a publication, in a store, in a business area; or the best time-slots on TV or radio

co-op advertising
when manufacturers co-sponsor or contribute to the retailer's cost of advertising

piggyback
a technique that allows you to tie in your local ad campaign to capitalize on the hoopla generated by national advertising

P-O-P (point-of-purchase)
a display which acts as a silent sales clerk, for a specific product

catalog houses
businesses that specialize in buying products that are in turn resold via catalogs

Advice:

Let major catalog houses do your promotion.

Make sure you can deliver. Their principal concern will be your ability to keep them supplied if your product takes off.

Before you get in too deep, try a few major houses with a **product description** plus photographs. If they don't like your product, they may help you locate a catalog house that will. The feedback will be invaluable.

Direct Mail.   This promotional tool lets you aim your brochures and flyers where they will do the most good. **Direct mail** is very important for small business, because it can go to the heart of your target market.

The success of direct mail depends on your ability to *define* the target market. If the market is too fragmented to get your arms around, direct mail is not for you.

Advice:

Stay up nights if you have to, but define that target market.

Develop customer lists. (See Action Step 28.)

Money-Back Guarantees.   You may not have thought of a guarantee as a form of promotion, but it is. You can reach security-minded customers by emphasizing the no-risk features of your product.

The problem is that you have to back up your guarantee with your own time and your own money.

Advice:

Figure 5% into your pricing to cover returned goods. If the product is fragile or easily misused — and people have been known to misuse just about anything — build in a higher figure.

Free Ink/Free Air.   Reviews, features, interview shows, press releases, and newspaper columns cost you nothing, and they are tremendously effective. **Free ink/free air** are among the best ways a small business can promote because they establish your company in a believable way. The average Target Customer is likely to attach more credence to words that are not paid advertising.

The obstacle here is getting media people to think your business is newsworthy.

Advice:

Every business is newsworthy. Dig until you find something.

Know your media people. Aim your release at *their* Target Readers.

Make your press kit visual. Send accompanying photos of your principals, the facility, and the product or service in use.

Present your press kit in an attractive folder to influential representatives of the media.

product description
a list of the features and benefits of a product

direct mail
advertisement or sales pitch that is mailed directly to your TC

free ink/free air
information concerning your business published or broadcasted free of charge

Personal Selling.   It doesn't matter that you've never sold before. No one is a better salesperson than you are. You are the business. If you listen carefully, your Target Customers will *tell* you how to sell them your product or service. That's why a good salesperson is a creative listener, not a fast talker.

Unfortunately, **personal selling** is expensive, especially if you have to pay others to do it, and it will boost your overhead (unless you pay your sales people only by earned commission). And if you try to do it all yourself, often you can't be everywhere you're needed.
Advice:

> Make everyone in your business a salesperson. It's security for them, because if they don't help and nothing sells then they don't have a job. Remind them your TC needs a lot of TLC.
>
> Consider developing a **network of sales reps** who will work on a percentage of sales. Keep cheerleading. Reps need encouragement, too.
>
> Increase your personal visibility. Join **Lead Clubs** in your area. Join service clubs and trade associations. Write a newspaper column. Be bold. (And see the sidebar on page 103, ''Bite a Lion on the Tail.'')

Trade Shows.   These shows display your product or service in a high-intensity way. Trade shows develop that carnival, county fair atmosphere which can be so necessary in business. Besides, your appearance at a trade show asserts your position in your industry.

However, if the show is not in your area, you'll have transportation costs. And the booths are expensive. And unless you're careful and you really make a study of the layout, you can buy a space that is thin on **traffic.**
Advice:

> Piggyback spare booth space from another small business owner.
>
> Combine functions by doing some market research while you're promoting (see the case study on Frank Williams later in this chapter.)
>
> Study the floor plan. Position yourself in a high traffic area like the pathways to the entrances, exits, restaurants, rest rooms, and giant exhibitors. (See Figure 6.2 for an idea of how the traffic flows at a trade show.)

Industry Literature   Become a source of information in your industry by producing brochures, newsletters, handbooks, product documentation, annual reports, newspaper columns for the layman, or even the Bible for your Industry. (How would you like to be recognized as an expert in your field?) We think this is one of the best promotional devices around.

You may balk if you're not handy with words.
Advice:

> Hire yourself a writer.

---

personal selling
selling and taking orders by an individual salesperson

network of sales reps
independent business people who normally operate in a specific geographic area, and who sell a number of noncompeting products and services

Lead Clubs
a group of business and professional people who meet regularly to exchange sales prospects and tips

traffic
movement of vehicles and pedestrians

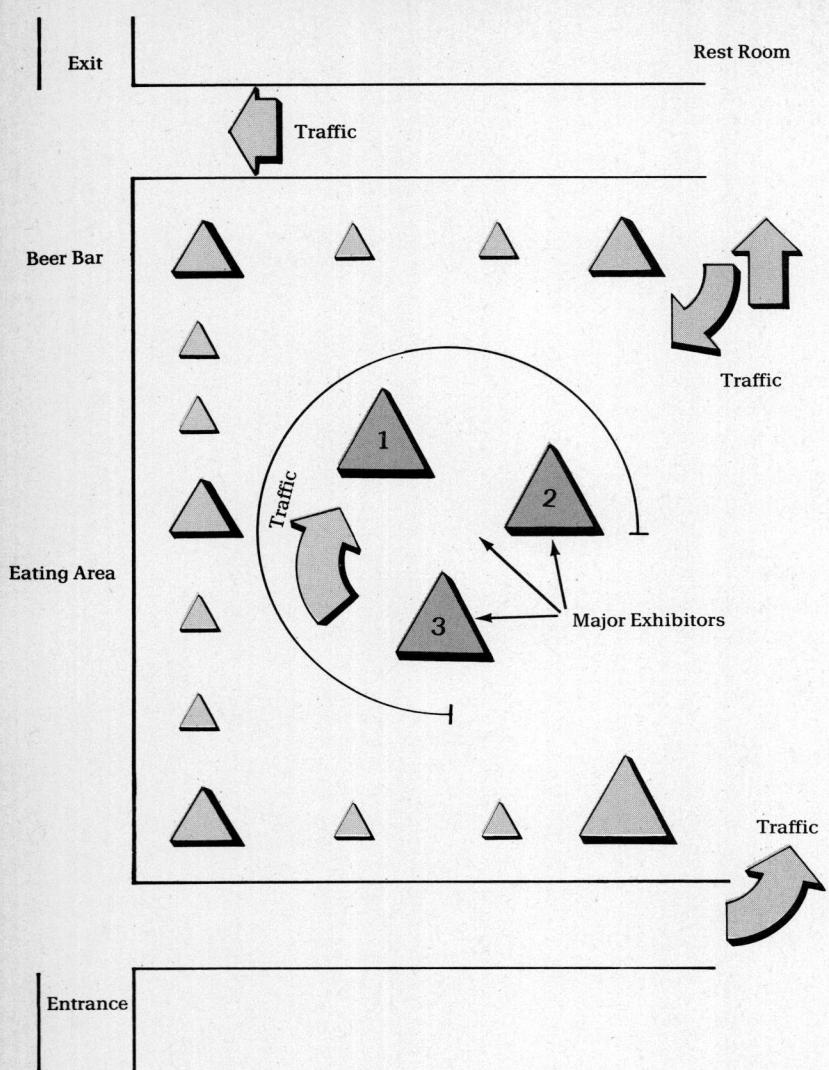

FIGURE 6.2 If you learn to read the layout of a trade show for where the largest traffic flows will be, you can position your booth to take advantage of that traffic.

Talk is cheap. If you get your thoughts down on paper, you're two steps ahead of the talkers.

Don't be afraid of audacity. It stirs the blood.

Working Visibility.   In Chapter 5, our case study on Ben Jones painted a picture of an entrepreneur who knew how to maintain a presence. You can do the same thing even on a small budget. Most service firms display their presence as they work. In other words, they put signs on everything: on their business, on their trucks, and on the sites where they go out and work. Wherever they're busy, they let people know it. They stay visible.

The drawback here is similar to one of the drawbacks with P-O-P displays. If the presence you maintain doesn't sell itself—if it is unattractive, of if it calls attention to an unsavory part of your business—you are losing potential customers, not gaining them.

Advice:

Exploit your public activities with signs that tell people who you are.

Review your displays weekly. Make sure the message works.

The Right Decision

Any promotion or promotional mix that advances the image of your business is worth considering. You've just surveyed some of the most common and traditional means of promotion. Before you decide on your promotional strategy, you want to make sure you're open to all options. That's why we're going to ask you to keep an open mind, as you brainstorm your *ideal* mix of strategies, as you examine further creative promotion campaigns, and as you learn to understand the importance of planning ahead. Then you will truly be able to make the right decision.

PLANNING AHEAD

You need to make a lot of intelligent noise before you open your doors. When you open, open with a bang. Start-ups are ironic — you need to spend bushels of money to overcome buyer inertia, yet you don't have those dollars to spend. What's an entrepreneur to do?

When promoting, use your head instead of your checkbook.

Plan for your opening now. Few businesses are profitable right away. Many of the promotional tools we've just discussed cost very little. You must lure customers. You must build confidence that you are in this game to win. When promoting, use your head instead of your checkbook. And keep your Target Customer clearly in mind. How will your product or service benefit your TC?

Don't Keep Your Business a Secret

Elsewhere in this book, we stressed that if you fail to plan, you're planning to fail. When it comes to promotions, if you fail to plan promotions, you're planning to keep your business a secret.

Brainstorm Your Ideal Promotional Campaign. One way to stop from keeping your business a secret is to brainstorm an ideal **promotional campaign** with no holds barred and with no worries about costs. Action Step 26, on page 104, makes sure you consider all of your creative ideas before you discard them because you think they are unrealistic. Try getting crazy with this Action Step. Creative solutions often come from bizarre mental activity!

Look at Other Creative Promotion Ideas. You'll want to save the ideas you come up with in Action Step 26 — we'll make good use of them later. Now to add to your list, take a look at how other entrepreneurs have applied ingenious — and cost-effective — solutions to

Bite A Lion on the Tail

For whatever reason, many people are afraid of personal selling. You can make that fear your challenge. Ever hear of the surefire cure for fear of lions? You just bite a lion on the tail.

It's the same way with fear of elevators. The best cure is to ride in lots of elevators.

If you're afraid of selling, go out and become your own best salesperson. *You can do it* — not only because you know the business better than anyone else, but because your very hesitancy indicates that you will be truly sensitive to your customer's needs. But don't just go out there and be sensitive.

Go out and bite a lion on the tail.

promotional campaign
a sales program designed to sell a specific product or service, or to establish an image/benefit/point

their promotional needs. See the boxed article, "Creative Borrowings from *Streetfighter*," on the following page. (Later in the chapter we'll also consider four quick case studies from our own file on creative promotions.) As you'll see throughout this chapter, the entrepreneurs who succeed in their efforts are the entrepreneurs who have the best fix on their Target Customers. They are also the entrepreneurs who understand the full importance of market research.

PROMOTIONS AND MARKET RESEARCH

As you gain experience in promoting your small business, you'll find out for yourself just how much promotional strategy and your Target Customer are interlocked. That's why you can't plan your promotional mix without dipping back into market research. The pros manage to do both at the same time. But don't take our word for it — ask the entrepreneur in the case study that follows.

Many Roads to the Marketplace

"Market Research" may sound like something only a large organization can do. Here is one example of market research made simple. Entrepreneur Frank Williams saw a need, then combined his research with promotion — a smart recipe. And — he used a freebie for a come-on.

Case Study

Frank Williams — Trade Show Research and Promotion

Frank Williams was really happy with his microcomputer until the switch went out two days after the 90-day warranty was up. Frank put the micro into his car and drove to the repair shop.

"You turn it on and off a lot?" the repairman asked.

"Of course," Frank said. "Several times a day. Why?"

"That's what wore it out," the repairman said. "The switch is the only moving part. The rest of this baby will last ten years, at least."

The repair bill was $150, and when Frank got back home he gave the situation some thought. The reason he had to keep turning the machine off was so his youngest child wouldn't mess up his files. The easiest way to handle it was to turn the machine off.

The lock box came to Frank as he was dropping off to sleep. That next weekend, he designed a prototype of wood. His model had a hinged lid and a brass lock, and a space-age look. Frank took it to a friend of his who was a manufacturer. The friend thought it would fly. They consulted their wives on colors and the group came up with eight — red, orange, yellow, black, beige, blue, white, and avocado.

"That's a lot of paint," the manufacturer said. "How can we narrow it down?"

"Market research," Frank said.

continued on page 106.

Brainstorm the Perfect Winning Promotional Campaign for Your Business

Disregard all budgetary restraints. Pretend that money is no object. Close your eyes. Sit back. And develop the ideal campaign for connecting with your Target Customers.

If your product or service needs a multi-million-dollar advertising promotion, with endorsements by your favorite movie star, fantasize that it's happening now.

If you need a customer list created in marketing heaven, specify exactly what you need and it is yours.

If you are looking for the services of a first class catalog house, just whisper the name three times and you are in business.

If your business at its peak could use a thousand delivery trucks with smiling delivery people who make your TC feel terrific, write down "1,000 smiling delivery people."

If your product is small, brainstorm the perfect Point-of-Purchase device, one that is equipped with slot machines with money-tubes that are connected to your private bank vault.

Watch the money roll in.

This chance to ignore costs won't come around again. (Reality is right around the corner.) But for now, have fun.

☐ STEP COMPLETED

Creative Borrowings from *Streetfighter*

The Streetfighter is a newsletter created by a midwest entrepreneur who believes in "duking it out" to attract business. His name is Jeff Slutsky. His business is RMI, a retail marketing institute. Jeff Slutsky not only gets PR for other businesses, he's the Wizard of Free Ink for RMI, and has been written up in *Entrepreneur, Nation's Business, The Chicago Sun-Times, Inc.*, and the *Wall Street Journal*. He has been the subject of a Cable News Network feature. Entrepreneurs could do worse than study Slutsky's style.

Trends. What's hot? What's cool? What's melting in your arms?

Sales people at Wisman's Trusted Appliances & TV, Inc., felt they were losing business when customers left the store to comparison shop. Slutsky's Streetfighter solution — he packed a freezer with ice cream. Every customer who looked at a Wisman freezer got a half-gallon carton, free. Instead of comparison shopping, the customer raced home to refrigerate. That gimmick kept Wisman's in the mind of the prospect and helped increase sales by 11%.

Contest? Fat prize? Insure yourself with Lloyd's.

A print-shop owner was tapped for $750 by the organizers of a charity golf tournament. Slutsky's client could have been lost among the donors, so he offered a hole-in-one contest prize of $10,000, to be split between the first golfer to ace the ninth hole and the charity. The owner's picture was taken with an oversize check, and the media kept cameras trained on the ninth hole. And if the golfer had sunk one? No problem. Slutsky's client was insured with Lloyd's of London against business loss with a premium of $450 — $300 less than his line on the donors board.

Upscale restaurant? Keep 'em standing in line.

A restaurant in a large metro area ran small ads announcing its opening, saying reservations were a must. People calling to make reservations were told by a *maitre d'* that the place was busy for the next three months and couldn't accept reservations. The reason was that they were under construction for those first three months. By opening day, diners stood in line for tables. The business didn't spend much money, but got a lot of impact through word-of-mouth.

Cross promotion keeps anger cooled.

An apartment house, partially occupied, needed to fill vacant units. Slutsky guided management to bypass the collective ire of tenants by offering 5,000 certificates to local colleges and credit unions. The certificates guaranteed one month's free rent on a 12-month lease to members or students only.

SOURCE: Adapted by permission from *Streetfighter*, a newsletter published by RMI, P.O. Box 15719, Fort Wayne, IN 46885. Telephone (219) 485-7037. The *Streetfighter* motto is "Don't outspend the competition. Out-think 'em."

Frank took a prototype Lock Box to a computer trade show. He put up a large sign that said: **Register here for your free Micro Lock Box.**

People crowded into Frank's booth to sign up. The card had a place for their name, address, phone number, type of computer, and — what color they would like.

It worked. Frank's market research was cheap and fast. In a day and a half, Frank got 1,400 people to tell him what color Lock Box they wanted.

The overwhelming favorite was beige.

And he had a good start on a customer mailing list.

By being curious and thorough, Frank Williams had discovered one of the secrets of the marketplace: You can promote and do market research at the same time.

And the other secret he learned was just as good: If you don't know what your Target Customers want, all you have to do is ask them.

Ask Your Customers

When you're trying to brainstorm your promotional campaign, ask your customers how they perceive your business. Then ask them questions:

What do they want?
Where are they from?
How did they find you?

If you have trouble getting their attention, offer them something free.

THE PROPER USE OF FREEBIES

Freebies in General

Freebies are a tremendously effective promotional gimmick. You can use them to get your customer's attention, to create interest in a new product, or (like Frank Williams) to gather market research. Freebies don't have to be extravagantly expensive; they do have to help you connect with customers. See the boxed article on the following page for a number of inexpensive freebies that entrepreneurs have used to grab the mind of the Target Customer. (Note that many of the freebies are purely informational. Could you boost sales by offering free advice?)

Discount Coupons

Discount coupons are a special form of freebie. Coupons give you positive feedback on your promotion. They should have an expiration date and multiple-use disclaimers (as, for example, a disclaimer that the coupon cannot be used in conjunction with other promotions or

How Street-Smart Are Your Freebies?

Every business has a "freebie" that will help grab the mind of its Target Customer. This book is full of examples: the toy store retailer who gave away a large jar of pennies in exchange for a start on a customer mailing list; the appliance store that gave away ice cream so that potential customers wouldn't have time to price freezers elsewhere; the inventor who gave away one computer lock-box in exchange for a mailing list of 1,400 names. To trigger your imagination, we've listed more examples of effective, street-smart freebies below.

Free Orange Juice.   A manufacturer of a new juice squeezer gave away free orange juice at a trade show.

Hot Dogs.   A retailer obtained hot dogs and buns from a local hot dog maker, then advertised with promotions that read "Bring Your Buns to Hastings August Sale At Noon." Retailer's cost was $66. At noon, the line of hot dog lovers stretched around the block. Curious customers, lured by free food and the carnival atmosphere, walked into the store to check out the sale.

Health Drink.   A distributor of an expensive food blender gave away cups of a health drink at a trade show. A booklet of recipes followed, free. Salespeople were on hand to take orders for the blender.

Advice.   A men's clothing store hired a woman fashion consultant at Christmas to give advice to women who came in to shop for presents for men.

A flower shop passed out "Green Thumb" information leaflets on plant care.

A hardware store took over the parking lot for a "home improvement weekend." Professionals were on hand to give tips and instruction on laying tile, repairing garden hoses, fixing leaky faucets, and installing dead-bolt locks.

SOURCE: Adapted in part from *How to Get Free Press* by Toni Delacorte, Judy Kimsey, and Susan Halas (San Francisco: Harbor Publishing, 1981) pp. 120–121, 125, 127, 131–132.

discounts). They should be coded to identify the source (so you can find out where your advertising is paying off), and they should be tested in small quantities before major use.

MAKING DECISIONS

By now you should be ready to make a few decisions about your promotional mix. Let's begin with price.

Price Tags

Freebies, like other promotional strategies, come with definite price tags. We want you to take your ideal promotional strategies from Action Step 26 and pick the top four or five elements. Then determine the price tag for each. (For example consider the difference in costs between a **magazine ad** and a **press release.**) Action Step 27 walks you through the process.

Don't be discouraged if price knocks out part of your ideal promotional mix. That's why we've filled this chapter with so many inexpensive promotional ideas. And in the meantime, you have used the powers of your imagination to brainstorm the best possible promotional effort for your business.

Even as you make decisions, keep thinking of that best possible effort — and of your Target Customer — and you can't go wrong.

Concentrating Your Efforts

Often just one element proves to be the secret ingredient that lets a business grab customers. In the examples that follow, each entrepreneur, often in desperation, discovered that magical missing ingredient. Maybe by reading what they have to say, you'll discover what promotional element you'll want to concentrate on.

Our friends in small business have shared some promotional secrets with us. They worked. Now we're sharing them with you.

Case Study

Four Quick Case Studies from Our Promotions File

Earth-to-Air Travel, Inc. — Newsletter

The travel agency missed out on one advertising opportunity, but with fast footwork they found a better technique.

We missed out on the one and only yearly ironclad deadline for getting our ad into the Yellow Pages, so we made up for that by placing fun-type ads in community newsletters within a two-mile radius of our agency. Our best response came from a mobile home park less than a mile away, and we discovered a gold mine of retirees with steady incomes.

Those folks dearly love to travel.

The ads didn't cost much, and we used them to keep our visibility high.

By studying the community newsletters, we came up with our own format, and now we send out our own agency newsletter every couple of months. On the front page we feature a catchy travel theme, along with a picture of our employees. The picture helps us connect, especially with first-time customers. They see our smiling faces, and when they walk through that door, most of them feel they know us.

We're already on the way to being friends.

Continued

ACTION ⚡ STEP 27

Return to Reality by Adding Price Tags to Each Magic Ingredient of Your Promotional Mix

What will your Customer Connection cost?

Go back to Action Step 26 and list the top four or five connections you want with your customers. Then research what each will cost.

Say you have chosen magazine advertising, direct mail, press releases in the local newspapers, and personal selling.

1. Magazine Ads. This choice assumes you know what your TC reads. Good. Contact the display ad department of the magazines. Ask for their media kit and a reader profile. At the same time, ask for rates on mailing lists for geographic areas you want to reach.

2. Direct Mail. Locate Mailing List Brokers in the Yellow Pages under Direct Mail. Tell them what business you are in and ask for information and strategy tips. Ask for sample names so you can check mailing list accuracy against your TC profiles. Compare the costs of lists from brokers with lists from magazines.

3. Press Releases. Visit the marketing department of your local newspaper for information on targeting its readers. Use this information to angle your release. In the release, double-space your copy. Make sure you catch the reader's attention. Keep the message simple. Be sure to wield the five W's (who, what, where, when, why) and the noble H (how) of journalism.

4. Personal Selling. If you cannot reach customers this way yourself, you will need to budget for someone who can. If you are planning on selling yourself, locate Lead Clubs in your area and start building your own network. Figure your salary and expenses as a promotional cost. (For tips on how to profile your personality and how it can be balanced by others, see Chapter 13, Team Building.)

Once you know what each ingredient of your promotional mix will cost, you can decide what you can afford.

 □ STEP COMPLETED

The Software School — Direct Mail

It helps to know where your customers are before you start to promote — The Software School found out in an alternative to newspaper ads.

When we started The Software School, we quickly discovered that the major local newspaper covered the northern half of the county, while the market we'd targeted — executives and small business microcomputer owners — lived in the southern half. The one sure way to reach the center of the market was with a direct mail piece. Our strategy was to buy a list from a magazine whose readers matched our customer profile — in this case, *Personal Computing* — and then we sent out our brochure.

The response was terrific. We generated enough business for a healthy start-up, and satisfied customers sold for us after that by talking up our one-day teaching system.

Direct mail allowed us to fire a rifle shot into the heart of our market. And when you're just starting out in a new venture, you're so busy and overworked that you're grateful for accuracy.

Argosy Auto Parts — A Sign on Your Car

Sometimes your customer may need help finding you.

The main reason we chose Argosy was because we thought it was a good name. My husband had 32 years of experience in the auto parts trade — in retailing and also in distribution — and when we opened our store in South Coast we felt it was a guaranteed money-maker.

We opened our new store in midsummer, but by September we were ready to call it quits. Sales had averaged only $2,000 a month, and that wasn't enough to pay the rent.

Fortunately, we got help from a small business seminar. It was made clear to us that although everyone was familiar with the name, Argosy, very few people knew we were Argosy in South Coast.

Our first step was simple — we parked the car on the main street near our store. On the back was a large sign, with an arrow pointing to our store. The sign read

ARGOSY AUTO PARTS

Business began picking up right away, and that gave us the confidence to make contact with service stations in the area.

Gradually, we built up our own network. I joined some local service clubs, and that led me to a sales lead club. We meet once a week, for breakfast, and if you don't bring someone a lead, you have to pay a dollar into the kitty.

Things are all right now, but when I look back, I know that without that sign on the car we'd be out of business.

Garment Guide — Free Ink

Here's how to use free ink.

When my partner and I got the idea for guiding shoppers through the L.A. garment district, we thought it would be so exciting we wouldn't have to do much except stop off once a week to make bank deposits.

Were we ever wrong.

sign on car
a simple promotional technique — you park your car or truck in a high-traffic area — the sign points the way to your business

Continued

We ran a good-sized ad in the local paper. It filled a couple of buses, but then our market ran out, because those customers didn't need a return trip on the bus. We had some flyers printed up and we covered every car in every local parking lot.

Two thousand flyers netted us half a bus.

Then I just happened to read a feature story in the View section of the *L.A. Times* — about a tour to Hollywood and Universal Studios — and on an impulse I called the reporter up and told her about Garment Guide.

It worked.

On the next trip, the reporter came along, and brought a staff photographer. Two weeks later, we had a story on the front page of the View Section — a beautiful third of a page — and customers began calling us! Our local papers followed a month or so later with features about the service, and after we got bigger, a TV reporter profiled us for one of the evening news magazines on television.

Now business is great. We haven't had to advertise for 18 months.

Ask me what kind of promotion I believe in, I'll tell you.

Free ink.

We hope you found inspiration in these stories of entrepreneurs who, through planning or perseverance, found the secret ingredient for a successful promotional mix. And if you're still looking, that's all right too. We've saved a detailed discussion of two of the most useful promotional tools — for *every* small business — for last. Those tools are mailing lists and networking.

MAILING LISTS

Sometimes the secret ingredient in a promotional mix is the careful use of a **mailing list.** You need more than a mere list of names and addresses. What you need is a list that goes to the heart of your target market.

> **mailing list**
> names and addresses of potential customers

One of the most important tools for small business survival is an accurate and up-to-date mailing list. To explore the angles of the mailing list, study your Target Customer with New Eyes.

Entrepreneur Mel Cartwright developed a database on his Target Customers in a fun and painless manner — in the midst of his Christmas promotion. His story starts on the opposite page.

You may not need a Rent-a-Santa, but you do need well-organized information. Action Step 28 (see opposite) asks you to shape up the information you already have. See how the concept of a mailing list may begin with a **customer file,** but expands to include your other contacts as well. You can't help but gather information as you operate your small business. With good files, that information becomes useful. With organization, information becomes a source of power. Action Step 28 shows you how to tap that source.

> **customer file**
> a list of persons or firms that have purchased from you

Case Study

Mel Cartwright

Mel Cartwright had worked for three large corporations before he decided to vote for freedom and start a small business. He used some money of his own and founded Mel's Toys on the East Coast. For the first six months, business was fair, and Mel broke even. Sales picked up dramatically the day after Thanksgiving. The parking lot in the shopping center was crammed with cars. And Christmas-conscious people came in hunting for gifts for their children.

On that Friday after Thanksgiving, Mel made more money than he had all of September.

"The toy business is seasonal," Mel said. "And with all those people coming through the door, I wanted to make sure I developed a solid customer base."

So for three weeks, Mel hired a Rent-a-Santa and a professional photographer. Every child that came into Mel's Toys was photographed, free, on Santa's knee. While the children were being photographed, the parents filled out information cards.

Name. Age. Toy preferences. And date of birth.

At the end of the three weeks, Mel had developed a fine customer list. He also had one valuable piece of information — the date of birth of every child who had been photographed.

So, every time a birthday rolled around, Mel mailed a small inexpensive toy along with some copies of the Santa photograph. As an added bonus, he made the negatives available to parents, many of whom ordered Christmas cards picturing their child talking to Santa.

As his mailing list grew, Mel came up with another idea.

"I was at the cash register one day when one of my employees was sick with the flu, and I noticed five customers in a row who spent more than $50. I kept those checks and credit card slips separate, and at the end of the day I xeroxed them off and started a Big Spender List. Today, my Big Spender List has grown to several hundred customers, and I've developed a special mailer aimed just at them."

I wish someone would have told me how important a mailing list would be in this business before I got into it. With what I know now, I think I could branch off into at least a dozen industries and do very well."

Cartwright smiles. "And to think it all began with a Rent-a-Santa."

ACTION STEP 28

Shape Up Your Files on Your Target Customers, Your Competitors, the Media, and Your Vendors

Begin with a study of what your TC reads. Move from there to a reader profile and a mailing list, to find out where your TC's are concentrated.

For every customer you contact, make up a file card. Use your handy demographic set-up (sex, age, income, education, and residence — or size of company, type of industry, what department did the buying, and so forth) and launch yourself early into analyses of life-style or business-style.

If you have a microcomputer, now is a great time to use it.

Try to segment the Big Spenders and develop a special strategy for them. (Every industry has its Heavy Users. Who are the Heavies in your industry?)

Start a media file by contacting all potential advertising media in your area. Ask for rate cards and demographics.

If you did not do it in Chapter 5, start a file on your competitors, and how they promote. Try to learn what is working. What ideas can you borrow? Or steal?

Start a How-Can-They-Help-Me File on your vendors and suppliers. See Action Step 42 in Chapter 10 for suggestions on creating your own vendor statement. Most vendors have been in the industry awhile. Show them your Business Plan, ask for advice, listen carefully. You may not buy from them, but the information you obtain could save your neck.

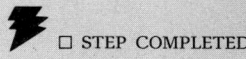 ☐ STEP COMPLETED

NETWORKING

Another source of promotional power is the technique of **networking.** In Figure 6.3 (page 112), we see the technique in action.

Networking floats the image of your business out across a lattice-work of noncompetitive helpers. It is the wave of the future in small business.

networking
communicating through person-to-person channels in an attempt to sell or gain information

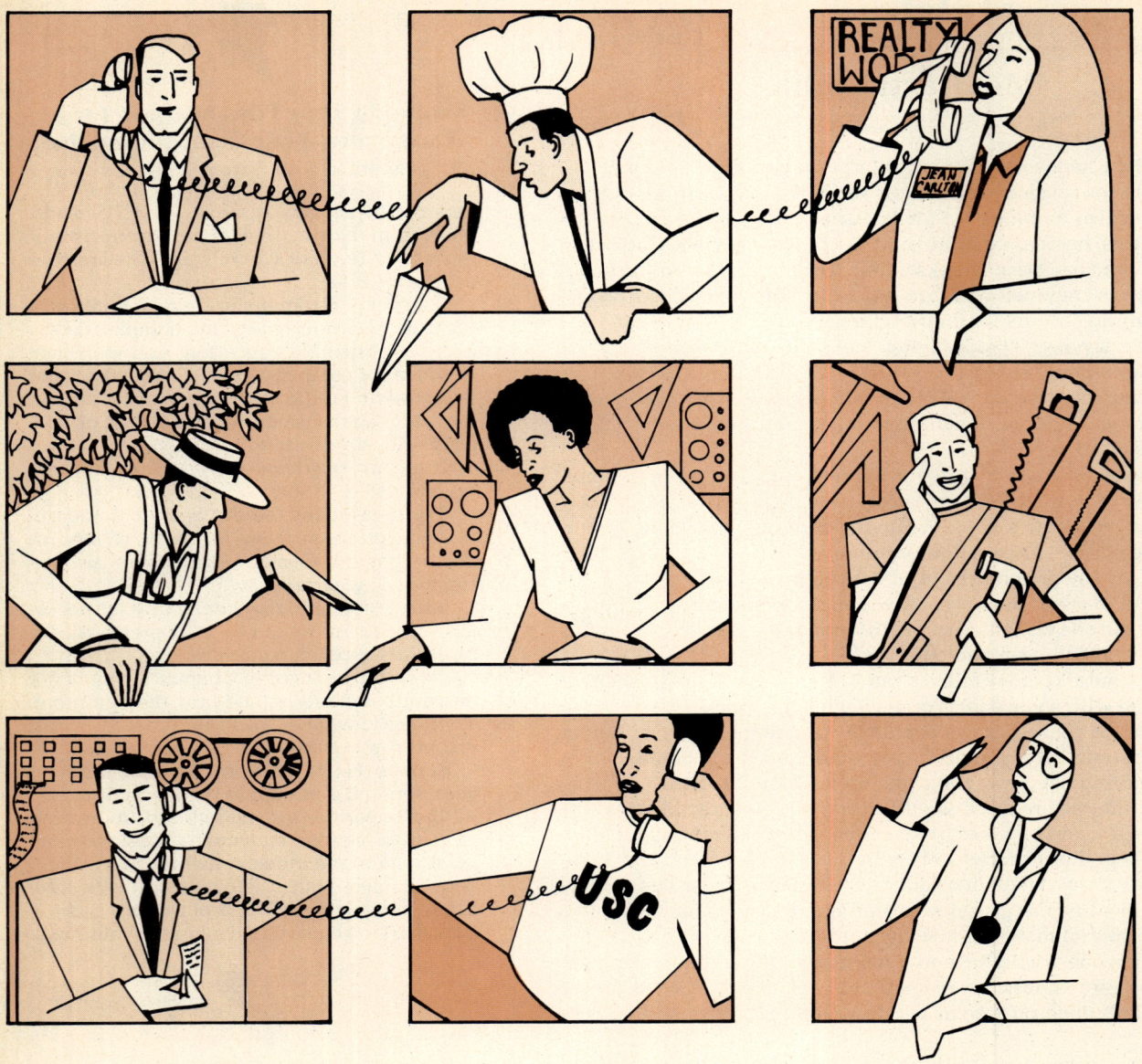

Listen to Gena D'Angelo explain why she likes networking.

FIGURE 6.3 Networking friends and acquaintances can produce a creative, vital flow of information; it can be used to gather sales leads and to float the image of your business out into your community.

Case Study

Gena D'Angelo

When Rob and I decided to go into business for ourselves, we looked around for more than a year. I had some training in graphics and Rob's good with numbers, and what we finally decided on was a franchised mail-box operation. We paid the franchisor a flat fee and a percentage of our gross. They gave us aid and assistance and a well-developed business plan.

What they didn't tell us about was networking.

When you're in the mail-box business, good service is how you forge ahead. We knew we had to promote our image and we tried everything

Continued

—brochures, leaflets, flyers, and full-page display ads in the local newspapers.

But the business didn't start rolling in until I joined my first network.

It was called a Sales Lead Club. The membership was varied. We had a real estate broker, an insurance agent, the president of a small bank, the owner of a coffee service, a printer, a sign manufacturer, a man who had a chain of service stations, a sporting goods store owner, a travel agent, two small manufacturers, and a local contractor. The way our club works is that we meet once a week for breakfast. If you don't bring at least one sales lead for another club member, you have to put a dollar into the kitty.

I got more business from that club than from all my other promotional efforts.

So I joined one more, and then I used the contacts I made to build my own network.

Business has been good ever since. We opened our second shop last April, put in a word processor to keep up with the typing, and added an answering service. That first year, we networked our way to even more business, and we're planning a third shop ten miles south of here by this time next year.

Networking gives you confidence, while at the same time it allows you to pass on helpful information to people who aren't competing with you.

Why You Should Network

Look around: The days of the **pyramid hierarchy** are drawing to a close, and it is now sunset in the industrial desert. Church, State, Family, Corporation, and Neighborhood—the old structures are crumbling, wheezing, and breaking apart.

One reason is Toffler's Trough. The old structures are wallowing in the cultural trough between Toffler's Second Wave (the Industrial Age) and the Third (the Age of Information).

A network can make a cozy place for your business even in Toffler's Trough.

As the engines of society slow down and break apart, they lose their efficiency. When that happens, people begin to ask questions, and they begin to cluster together.

They cluster for all kinds of reasons—to trade information, to solve problems, to nurture each other, or to help out in the survival game.

This clustering is called networking.

Networking Is Not New

You've probably been doing it all your life. In school, you networked for information about teachers and courses. When you moved into a new community, you networked for information about doctors, dentists, car service, babysitters, and bargains—all the life-supporting details that make up existence. On the job, you networked your way to sales leads, or brainstormed your way to better designs, or got in a huddle with some fellow managers or coworkers to solve problems.

As a small business entrepreneur, you can network your way to a

---

ACTION ⚡ STEP 29

Build Your Own Network of Pathways into the Information Society

Start at the center of the web, because that's where you are, and make a list of the people you know.

Put circles around each person, and then draw spokes from each name, and write down what you know about them—business, hobbies, residence, children, interests, and who they might know.

Now recall where you met each person. Does the meeting place tell you anything helpful? Are you members of the same group or club? What interests do you share? What, after all, is the connection here?

Now, from all these people, build a couple of core groups. Start with two or three people. Are they interested? Are they diverse enough? (You'll need doers, stars, leaders, technicians, an organizer or two—depending on your own talents. See Chapter 12, on Team Building.)

Make sure the people you are contacting are not competing for the same Target Customers.

Set up a meeting. If you are working, breakfast usually works best. If the core group catches on, you can share phone duties and arrange further meetings.

Before you know it, you will be networking your way through the channels of the Big Picture, business to business.

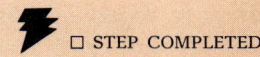 ☐ STEP COMPLETED

---

pyramid hierarchy
a form of bureaucratic organization with the Pharoah, Chief, King, President, Chairman, Chancellor, CEO, or Boss at the top, all others below

surprising number of new customer connections. And customers spell success.

If you don't have a network, use Action Step 29 to build your own.

Networking Is for You

Networking is a very powerful tool for small business. And it's just waiting for you to start. Our last Action Step helps you develop your own network and to build your own **core groups** of people within it. Because a network grows naturally from the loose association of people you already know, and because you are at the center of the net, networking is for you.

core groups
clusters of influential, key individuals that share a common area of interest

SUMMARY

Promotion is the art or science of moving the image of your business into the prospect's mind. Anything that advances that image is a good tactic to consider. We recommend that you survey the range of promotional strategies available to you and then choose the promotional mix that will work best for your unique business. Potential strategies include paid media advertising, point-of-purchase displays, catalog sales, direct mail, money-back guarantees, free ink and free air, personal selling, trade shows, industry literature, and working visibility.

We also recommend that you be open to creative solutions to the problem of promoting while on a budget, and we give examples of how other entrepreneurs responded to that challenge. Other topics covered include the proper place of freebies, the reasons why an accurate and up-to-date mailing list is a must for survival, and the importance of networking for sales leads and other information.

Throughout the chapter, we stress the interlocking relationship of market research — your strategy for locating your Target Customers and finding out where they itch — and promotion — letting your customers know your business can scratch their itch and make them happy in the process.

If there is one overall message to the chapter, it is that when promoting, you should use your head instead of your checkbook.

THINK POINTS

- Be unique with your promotions. Instead of Christmas cards, send Thanksgiving cards or April Fool cards.
- Stand in your Target Customer's shoes. Think like your TC. Find that need. Find that ladder in the TC's mind.
- Stay visible. Keep sending up colorful balloons.
- A world in transition means more opportunities for your small business. Fast footwork keeps you in the game.
- To start your own mailing list, give away something for free. In return, potential customers will give you their names.
- Rent a Santa. Rent a robot. Rent a big, hot-air balloon. Rent a talking dolphin. You want to create excitement. Excitement sells.

ACTION ⚡ STEP
REVIEW

26 A very good warm-up exercise is to close your eyes and design the perfect promotional mix for your small business. For a moment, forget about budgetary restraints and go all out. Need a media blitz? You've got it. Need a thousand salespersons? You've got them. At the same time, you visualize the profits rolling in.

27 The next step is to add price tags to each ingredient of your promotional mix. You can do this by contacting display ad departments for magazines and newspapers, direct mail brokers, trade show organizers, and catalog houses.

28 Create a file for every contact you make in the promotional business. While you are creating these files, expand your efforts to a customer file, a vendor file, and (if you did not do it in the last chapter), a competitor file.

29 One of the best tools for making contacts with customers is a network. A network can be informal (friends, family, coworkers or people who share the same interests) or formal (service clubs and sales leads clubs).

When you think you have it made, keep making that customer connection anyway. You will never be so big that you can disconnect. Remember that and you will be famous.

REFERENCES

Blake, Gary, and Robert W. Bly. *How to Promote Your Own Business.* New York: New American Library, Plume Books, 1983. A nicely written paperback. Good tips on trade shows, press releases, and writing copy.

Delacorte, Toni, Judy Kimsey, and Susan Halas. *How to Get Free Press: A Do It Yourself Guide to Promote Your Interests, Organization, or Business.* San Francisco: Harbor Publishing, 1981. Contains an excellent chapter called "PR for Small Businesses," which has many ideas for solid promotions.

Delano, Sara. "How to Get a Fix on Free Ad Dollars." *Inc.,* July 1983, 94–96. Cooperation among noncompeting retailers—a clothing store, a computer store, and a car dealership—creates snappy ads and allows the costs to be split.

Eckert, Lee, Joe Ryan, and Bob Ray. *Leads Clubs/Orange County Networks.* Laguna Hills, Calif.: Owning the Store, 1984. A listing of local county and metro leads clubs that began in *The Register,* Orange County's largest newspaper (circ. 270,000), but grew too large for the newspaper to support. It is now published and distributed, at a nominal cost, to the networking public. For information, write Owning the Store, P.O. Box 3426, Laguna Hills, CA 92654-3426.

Jacobs, Sanford L. "Split Yellow Pages Highlights Problems in Phone-Book Ads." *Wall Street Journal,* December 8, 1983. You've probably seen those business-to-business yellow pages floating around. Straight talk in this essay about what you get when you buy any kind of ad in any of the yellow pages.

Kleiman, Carol. *Women's Networks: The Great New Way for Women to Support, Advise, and Help Each Other Get Ahead.* New York: Ballantine Books, 1980.

Naisbitt, John. *Megatrends: Ten New Directions Transforming Our Lives.* New York: Warner Books, 1982. Naisbitt devotes most of his Chapter 8 to networking for the future.

Ouchi, William. *Theory Z: How American Business Can Meet the Japanese Challenge.* New York: Addison-Wesley Publishing Co., 1981.

Slutsky, Jeffrey, and Woody Woodruff. *Streetfighting.* Englewood Cliffs, N.J.: Prentice-Hall, 1984. Slutsky is the owner and founder of the Retail Marketing Institute. He publishes an entertaining newsletter, tailored for small businesses, which you can subscribe to. The address is RMI, P.O. Box 15719, Fort Wayne, IN 46885.

Welch, Mary S. *Networking: The Great New Way for Women to Get Ahead.* New York: Harcourt Brace Jovanovich, 1980. Contains lists of networks already in progress.

A Description of Product or Service

B The Market and the Target Customer

C Competition

D Marketing Strategy

E Location

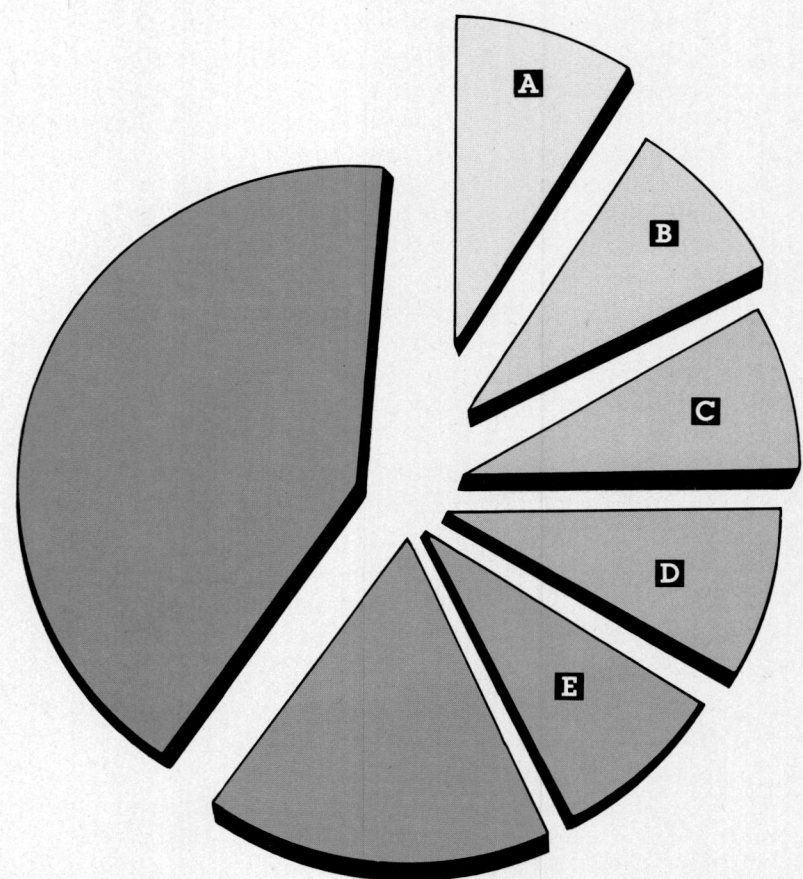

FIGURE 7.1 Chapter 7 helps you put together the Location section of your Plan by giving you a complete understanding of the dynamics of location.

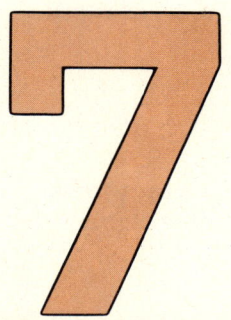

Location

LEARNING OBJECTIVES

To understand the importance of location.

To understand that each business has its own 100% location.

To brainstorm until you have a mental picture of that 100% location to guide you in your search.

To increase your awareness of location dynamics.

To develop your *own* checklist for finding your best location.

To use professional help, like commercial real estate brokers, when you are searching out a location.

To develop your own checklist for negotiating the best possible lease contract with your landlord.

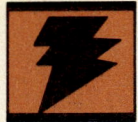

One of the most important decisions for a business to make is location. In retail, a location is very important, and the retail lease reflects this importance by being long and complex — often running 30 – 50 pages. It's important to remember that lease documents are drawn up by lawyers who work for the landlord. Language is malleable and is meant to be changed.

ENTREPRENEURS — READ YOUR LEASE

In the case study that follows, entrepreneur Mick Beatty forgot to read the terms of his lease. He thought he had a "gentleman's agreement" with his lessor. Mick was wrong.

Case Study

Mick Beatty — Controlled by the Lease

I was on vacation from the East Coast when I discovered the **perfect location.** It was in the sleepy tourist town of Laguna Beach, on the edge of the world in a fabulous part of Southern California.

It was late summer, I remember, and I'd just spent a week driving down the coast from Washington State, and when I reached Laguna I thought I was home.

I discovered Eddie's Pub my first evening in town. It faced the beach, and sitting there sipping a cool one you could watch the sun reflect off the water. From time to time, people would drift in for a casual drink, and while I was sitting there, feeling like a million, I must have talked to 20 different folks.

They loved the place, too. And most of them looked upscale.

Vacations don't last forever and when I got back home I kept thinking about Eddie's in Laguna. I was working then for one of the giant **megacorporations,** making good money in a pressure cooker of a job, and even though I was enough of a culture freak to appreciate New York City, the winters were rough and I wanted more out of life. The first day it snowed, I sat in my office, staring out the window, thinking about those three days I'd spent in Laguna, on the beach.

A business trip took me to Los Angeles that next spring, and I managed to haggle for an extra day so I could stay overnight in Laguna and stop in for a drink at Eddie's.

Double surprise.

The sun was shining. Eddie's Pub was for sale.

I called my banker back East. He said I was crazy. I phoned two buddies, one from college, one from the Army. They thought it would be fun to be part of a new venture and were ready to invest. I talked to Eddie, the owner, made a deal to pay him so much down and the rest out of profits, and suddenly I owned a small business.

When I phoned my boss back East, he said I was crazy, too. "That whole beach is a dream," he said. "I was stationed there during the war, and I know. One day you'll wake up and it won't be there any more." My boss paused, and what he said next saved my life. "Tell you what, Mick. Don't pull the plug until you're absolutely sure. We'll give you six

Continued

perfect location
the optimum physical site
for a business firm

megacorporations
huge corporations

months. If you're still out there dreaming, send in your resignation. Meanwhile, have fun. Every man needs a fling before he settles down."

I said okay, and thanks. And that was that.

The location at Eddie's is only 450 square feet. The layout is long and narrow, and we use mirrors from the Gay Nineties to give the place atmosphere. The traffic is mostly walk-in—beach people, stray tourists—and the only promotion I had to do was to put up a sign that said HAPPY HOUR 4 – 6:30. I shook hands with my customers, passed out complimentary drinks, served the best expresso south of Los Angeles, and started making money my first day.

Then trouble showed up.

I hadn't been open a week when I got a call from my **landlady.** She was a crusty voiced lady who I'd barely talked to, and she said over the phone that there had been some complaints about the music.

"Hey," I said. "I'm sorry. Who's complaining?"

"Your neighbors," she said. "They have rights, too, you know."

"Is it too loud?"

"No," she said. "It's not the volume. It's that rock stuff that's causing the trouble. It irritates the other customers."

"Rock?" I said. "It's not rock, it's more like—"

"I don't know what you call it," my landlady said. "But it's got to stop. And right now."

"My customers like it," I argued. "The music is part of my atmosphere."

"Young man," she said, "what your customers like is neither here nor there. I own that property, and I have other tenants to think about. And if you have any questions, I'd advise you to read your **lease.**"

She hung up.

Well, I read the lease, carefully. And then I saw a lawyer. He confirmed what I'd read—according to the terms of the lease, my landlady had the power to tell me what kind of music I could play in my own small business.

Incredible, but true.

I tried turning off the music. Right away, my customers missed it. Drink orders fell off. I surveyed my neighbors and made a list of songs they didn't find offensive, but when I played that junk in the bar, my steady customers (who were becoming less steady) asked me to turn it off. As a last resort, I even visited my landlady and tried to **renegotiate the lease.** But she wouldn't budge.

There was only one thing to do. I sold the business. I went back to my job on the East Coast. I still owe some money to my partners, and when it snows I aways think of the sun on the water at Laguna. Oh, I'll go back sometime. But right now I'm a little soured on the place. It's too bad. They've got a great beach. And a great little bar where you can sit and watch the sun go down. My advice?

Read the small print.

landlord/landlady
a person/business you pay rent or lease payments to

lease
contract for occupancy

renegotiate the lease
obtaining a new or modified contract for occupancy

WHEN DO YOU NEED A GREAT LOCATION?

A good location can make everything easier for a new business. A highly visible building will save you advertising dollars. Once you've been discovered and have your customers coming in regularly, location becomes less important.

For retail, location is absolutely essential.

What kind of business could you open where location is secondary?

While you're thinking about that one, work through Action Step 30, which should help you to analyze the effect location has on your shopping habits. Use New Eyes to examine your own consumer behavior.

You could expand this Action Step by interviewing purchasing agents and buyers of commercial and industrial goods. Ask them what impact location has on their choice of vendors or on their employees. Once you understand how location affects spending habits, you will be better equipped to make your own **site analysis.** But you'll need more than understanding. You'll also need some hard information.

CENSUS INFORMATION IS YOURS FOR THE ASKING

Census Tracts and SMSAs

You stay in a location for a while because it's expensive to pack up and move. Selection is important and you need reliable information to make sure you're in the heart of your target market.

> **Through its data from the U.S. Census, the federal government has supplied you with that information. All you have to do is gather it and then read it right.**

Every ten years, the government pulls together some valuable data. Up until 1982, it was compiled for large population blocs known as SMSAs (Standard Metropolitan Statistical Areas) in statistical form broken down by tract (a smaller geographic area within the SMSA) and by demographic categories like age, income, and so on. Following 1982 (the next census will be in 1990), data will fall into one of three subdivisions: CMSAs (Consolidated Metropolitan Statistical Areas), PMSAs (Primary Metropolitan Statistical Areas), and MSAs (Metropolitan Statistical Areas). See Chapter 2 for a more detailed explanation of the reorganization of census information. Fortunately, the data for the 1980 Census is still organized by SMSAs.

Your first step is to locate a Federal Depository. Check our list in Appendix D, or see your friendly reference librarian.

Tract Data for Small Business

Your second step is to find your general area (SMSA), then find your tract by number on a map. Census information comes in different sizes. Data organized by tract provides the kind of information most needed by small business. Once you find your tract number, you dig in and begin to probe. By checking various tables, you will be able to find such information as income (Table P-11, Income and Poverty Status in 1979), occupation (Table P-10, Labor Force and Disability Characteristics of Persons), and education (Table P-9, Social Characteristics of Persons).

A fourth helpful table compiles values of houses in your tract, tells

---

site analysis
a detailed study of the pros and cons of different possible locations for your business

ACTION ⚡ STEP 30

Use New Eyes to See How Consumers Respond to Location

Take a couple of minutes to analyze how location affects your own personal spending habits.

For example, where do you buy gas for your car? Do you buy it on your way to work or school? Or on your way home? Why?

Now, with your planning notebook in hand, look through your home. How much did location affect your decision to purchase what you see around you? Here's a list to start you off:

1. Cigarettes or candy.
2. Washing machine.
3. Art work on the walls.
4. Carpeting.
5. Dry cleaning service.
6. Mail order (seeds, books, magazines, or other products).
7. Custom crafted golf clubs.
8. Eyeglasses.
9. Wig, toupee, or artificial dentures.
10. Designer clothes.
11. Wrist watch.
12. Power tools.
13. Packaged food.
14. TV set.

Feel free to add to this list.

How far did you travel, for example, for your last good meal with a friend?

Or, at another level, how far would you travel to find a brain surgeon if you knew you needed that particular service?

What kind of conclusions can you draw about the power of location when you make a purchase?

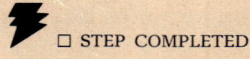 ☐ STEP COMPLETED

SMSA Index Map

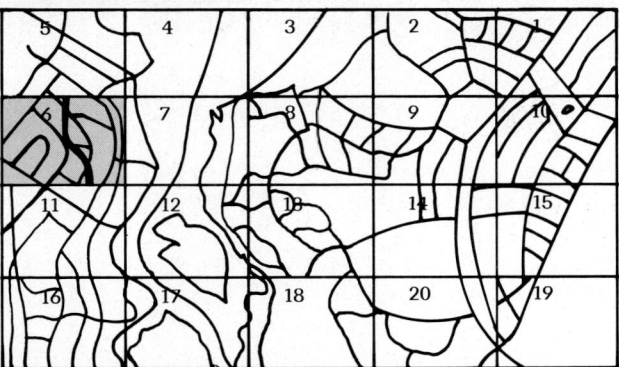

1. Use the index map to locate the detailed sheet map showing the area you want to investigate.

Detailed Sheet Map

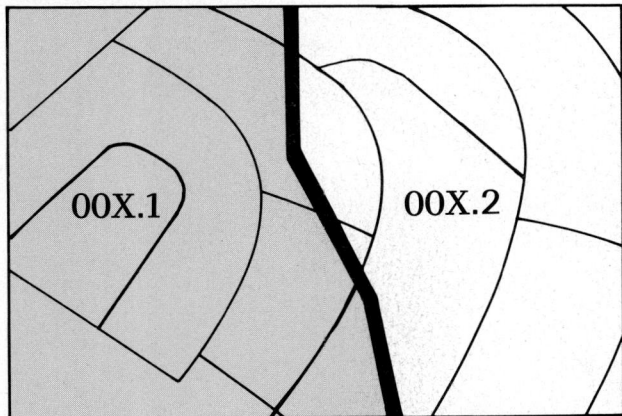

2. Use the detailed sheet map to determine the number of the tract you want to research.

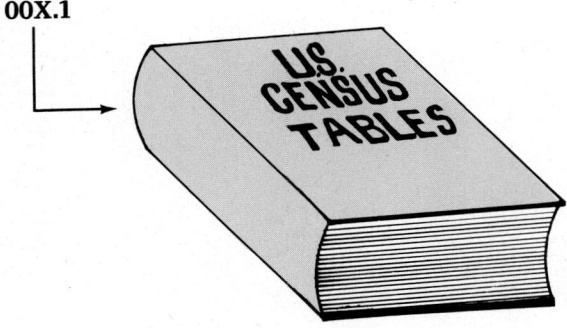

3. Use the tract number to unlock information from the U.S. Census Tables.

FIGURE 7.2   Unlock the information in the Census Tables by following three steps.

you the median rents charged, tells you how many homes are rented, and breaks down renters by race and origin (Table H-1, Occupancy, Utilization, and Financial Characteristics of Housing Units).

(When you're working with government documents, your first task is to learn how to interpret bureaucratic language. Government prose has a high fog index. Don't let the fog get in the way of your research.)

This information is of tremendous value to the entrepreneur. To help you learn how to use this census data, let's take a statistical stroll through two tracts in the same SMSA.

A WALK THROUGH TWO CENSUS TRACTS

For the following exercise in census data analysis, we chose two tracts from the 1980 Census for the Anaheim – Santa Ana – Garden Grove SMSA (an area in the heart of Orange County, California, and on the western edge of the Sun Belt). Both tracts have between 2,700 and 3,000 persons, which aren't bad numbers for a target market. Tract 740.06 is from the city of Santa Ana. We'll call it Tract SA. Tract 630.07 is from the city of Newport Beach. We'll call it Tract NB.

Finding Your Tract Number

To locate our tract numbers, we referred to the large index maps which accompany the census data. We located Newport Beach on the index map for our SMSA, for example, and we could tell that the specific area we wanted would be shown in more detail on sheets 21 and 28. Turning to sheets 21 and 28 we found that the small area we were interested in was Tract 630.07. Our procedure for the tract in Santa Ana was the same. Figure 7.2 (on page 121) illustrates the process in a simplified manner.

Once you have your tract number, you're ready to unlock the information from the census tables.

Using the Census Tables

Actual census tables look formidable — with 13 or 14 long columns per page listing statistical data in fine print — but they can be easy to use if you know what to look for. As we continue our walk through two census tracts, we'll highlight the key numbers from each table. Also, to make this exercise a little easier to handle, we've only reproduced portions of the tables, and we show only the columns for our Tract NB and Tract SA. (We've also used larger type!)

Now let's take a look at how to find the kinds of information about your target market that you want to know.

Income.   Small business depends on accurate targeting, so one clue you're looking for is discretionary income. If two households have incomes of $20,000 each, but household A must support seven people on that income and household B has to support only one, there's a good chance household B will have more discretionary dollars.

The census lists that information under its Table P-11, which we show in our Table 7.1(a). The median income for Tract SA was

TABLE 7.1(a)   Census Table P-11, Income and Poverty Status in 1979, can be useful for determining the income of various census tracts.

Census Tracts	[Tract NB] (0630.07)	[Tract SA] (0740.06)
INCOME IN 1979		
Households	**1 057**	**1 384**
Less than $5,000	38	88
$5,000 to $7,499	19	99
$7,500 to $9,999	—	83
$10,000 to $14,999	52	279
$15,000 to $19,999	63	227
$20,000 to $24,999	81	218
$25,000 to $34,999	107	258
$35,000 to $49,999	152	107
$50,000 or more	545	25
Median	$51 061	$18 264
Mean	$69 568	$19 319
Owner-occupied households	**912**	**335**
Median income	$53 545	$22 476
Mean income	$72 180	$24 748
Renter-occupied households	**145**	**1 049**
Median income	$30 494	$16 696
Mean income	$53 137	$17 585
Families	**888**	**563**
Median income	$55 965	$21 696
Mean income	$77 461	$22 170
Unrelated individuals 15 years and over	**197**	**1 291**
Median income	$19 712	$10 861
Mean income	$23 815	$11 242
Per capita income	**$24 373**	**$9 667**
INCOME TYPE IN 1979		
Households	**1 057**	**1 384**
With earnings	925	1 337
Mean earnings	$60 068	$19 019
With Social Security income	117	75
Mean Social Security income	$4 662	$2 686
With public assistance income	—	7
Mean public assistance income	—	$1 405
MEAN FAMILY INCOME IN 1979 BY FAMILY TYPE		
Families	**$77 461**	**$22 170**
With own children under 18 years	$68 252	$22 657
Without own children under 18 years	$85 652	$21 799
Married-couple families	**$82 604**	**$23 944**
With own children under 18 years	$74 619	$28 104
Without own children under 18 years	$89 433	$21 647
Female householder, no husband present	**$23 569**	**$17 120**
With own children under 18 years	$18 957	$13 613
Without own children under 18 years	$31 374	$23 625

(Note: Data are estimates based on a sample.)
SOURCE: Adapted from 1980 U.S. Census.

TABLE 7.1(b) Census Table P-10, Labor Force and Disability Characteristics of Persons, helps you determine what occupations are represented in each census tract.

Census Tracts	[Tract NB] (0630.07)	[Tract SA] (0740.06)
LABOR FORCE STATUS		
Persons 16 years and over	**2 361**	**2 426**
Labor force	1 494	2 134
Percent of persons 16 years and over	63.3	88.0
Civilian labor force	1 485	2 125
Employed	1 433	2 081
Unemployed	52	44
Percent of civilian labor force	3.5	2.1
Female, 16 years and over	**1 208**	**1 253**
Labor force	554	1 043
Percent of female, 16 years and over	45.9	83.2
Civilian labor force	554	1 043
Employed	542	1 037
Unemployed	12	6
Percent of civilian labor force	2.2	0.6
With own children under 6 years	60	131
In labor force	24	58
Married, husband present	775	384
In labor force	285	254
Civilian persons 16 to 19 years	**289**	**126**
Not enrolled in school	25	69
Not high school graduate	18	7
Employed	12	7
Unemployed	—	—
Not in labor force	6	—

$18,264. For Tract NB, it was $51,061. The mean income for Tract SA was $19,319, while for Tract NB it was $69,568.

The mean household income for families in Tract SA is just over $22,000. For Tract NB, it's over $77,000. Mean family income for married couples in Tract SA rises to just under $24,000, while in Tract NB it rises to more than $82,000. The highest mean family income in Tract NB is recorded for married couples with no children under 18 years: over $89,000. In Tract SA, that same category is less than $22,000.

Income never tells the whole story in site analysis. But it's a very good starting point, and Tract NB has households with at least three times the income of households in Tract SA.

Occupation. A look at Census Table P-10 — our Table 7.1(b) — shows more people working from Tract SA, where the highest percentage of employed workers (850, almost 41%) are in technical, sales, and administrative support.

TABLE 7.1(b) Continued

Census Tracts	[Tract NB] (0630.07)	[Tract SA] (0740.06)
OCCUPATION AND SELECTED INDUSTRIES		
Employed persons 16 years and over	**1 433**	**2 081**
Managerial and professional specialty occupations	632	781
Executive, administrative, and managerial occupations	384	413
Professional specialty occupations	248	368
Technical sales, and administrative support occupations	592	850
Technicians and related support occupations	36	118
Sales occupations	360	250
Administrative support occupations, including clerical	196	482
Service occupations	69	162
Private household occupations	6	7
Protective service occupations	13	4
Service occupations, except protective and household	50	151
Farming, forestry, and fishing occupations	7	—
Precision production, craft, and repair occupations	97	122
Operators, fabricators, and laborers	36	166
Machine operators, assemblers, and inspectors	14	93
Transportation and material moving occupations	—	23
Handlers, equipment cleaners, helpers, and laborers	22	50
Manufacturing	243	589
Wholesale and retail trade	348	480
Professional and related services	315	390

(Note: Data are estimates based on a sample.)
SOURCE: Adapted from 1980 U.S. Census.

In Tract NB, the highest percentage of workers (632, a bit over 44%) are either managerial or professional. Tract NB also has a higher percentage of people in plain old sales occupations — 360, or a little over 25%, while Tract SA has only 250, or 12%.

Salespeople make good money.

If you want a deeper contrast, one tract in Newport Beach (Tract 645.01, not shown) lists 2,451 persons working, with only 95, or 3.8%, in managerial or professional occupations.

Education.   This data will be more important if you're in a business like entertainment, the arts, publishing, travel, recreation, or leisure-time activities.

TABLE 7.1(c)   Census Table P-9, Social Characteristics of Persons, gives you information on the level of education in each census tract.

Census Tracts	[Tract NB] (0630.07)	[Tract SA] (0740.06)
NATIVITY AND PLACE OF BIRTH		
Total persons	**3 001**	**2 784**
Native	2 831	2 504
Born in State of residence	1 416	1 098
Born in different State	1 400	1 386
Born abroad, at sea, etc.	15	20
Foreign born	170	280
LANGUAGE SPOKEN AT HOME AND ABILITY TO SPEAK ENGLISH		
Persons 5 to 17 years	**719**	**260**
Speak a language other than English at home	59	15
Percent who speak English not well or not at all	13.6	—
Persons 18 years and over	**2 189**	**2 390**
Speak a language other than English at home	233	323
Percent who speak English not well or not at all	2.6	10.2
SCHOOL ENROLLMENT AND TYPE OF SCHOOL		
Persons 3 years old and over enrolled in school	**1 070**	**751**
Nursery school	25	12
Private	18	12
Kindergarten	22	13
Private	7	5
Elementary (1 to 8 years)	367	185
Private	107	8
High school (1 to 4 years)	355	32
Private	35	—
College	301	509
YEARS OF SCHOOL COMPLETED		
Persons 25 years old and over	**1 921**	**1 575**
Elementary: 0 to 4 years	—	5
5 to 7 years	16	6
8 years	6	24
High school: 1 to 3 years	68	107
4 years	371	330
College: 1 to 3 years	549	587
4 or more years	911	516
Percent high school graduates	95.3	91.0

(Note: Data are estimates based on a sample.)
SOURCE: Adapted from 1980 U.S. Census.

TABLE 7.1(d)   Census Table H-1, Occupancy, Utilization, and Financial Characteristics of Housing Units, is useful for learning about the number of owner-occupied housing units, the number of rentals, and the value of real estate.

Census Tracts	[Tract NB] (0630.07)	[Tract SA] (0740.06)
Total housing units	**1 138**	**1 988**
Vacant seasonal and migratory	8	3
Year-round housing units	1 130	1 985
YEAR-ROUND HOUSING UNITS		
Tenure by Race and Spanish Origin of Householder		
Owner-occupied housing units	911	302
Percent of occupied housing units	86.0	21.8
White	892	267
Black	. . .	9
American Indian, Eskimo, and Aleut	. . .	3
Asian and Pacific Islander	10	14
Spanish origin	11	12
Renter-occupied housing units	148	1 082
White	142	939
Black	. . .	39
American Indian, Eskimo, and Aleut	. . .	8
Asian and Pacific Islander	3	66
Spanish origin	3	74
Rooms		
Year-round housing units	**1 130**	**1 985**
1 room	—	68
2 rooms	4	220
3 rooms	12	471
4 rooms	57	739
5 rooms	154	348
6 rooms	203	74
7 rooms	257	43
8 or more rooms	443	22
Median, year-round housing units	7.0	3.8
Median, occupied housing units	7.0	3.9
Median, owner-occupied housing units	7.2	4.8
Median, renter-occupied housing units	5.1	3.7

[Continued]

Census Table P-9, which we show in Table 7.1(c), tells us there are 91% high school graduates in Tract SA, and a little over 95% in Tract NB—not much difference. When you reach years of college completed, the picture sharpens. Tract NB has 911 people who finished 4 or more years of college. That's over 47% of the people surveyed. Tract SA has 516, or less than 32% of the people surveyed.

TABLE 7.1(d)   Continued

Census Tracts	[Tract NB] (0630.07)	[Tract SA] (0740.06)
VALUE		
Specified owner-occupied housing units	636	89
$50,000 to $59,999	—	1
$60,000 to $79,999	3	7
$80,000 to $99,999	4	34
$100,000 to $149,999	23	46
$150,000 to $199,999	125	—
$200,000 or more	481	1
Median	$200000+	$101 700
CONTRACT RENT		
Specified renter-occupied housing units	136	1 038
Median	$500+	$340

(Note: Data are estimates based on a sample.)
SOURCE: Adapted from 1980 U.S. Census.

If you match up this census data with some of the consumption patterns from the VALS lifestyles from Chapter 4, (Emulators, Achievers, Experientials, and so on), you can find out what they buy and what their dreams are.

All of that helps with site selection.

Who Lives Where.   Another helpful category is Census Table H-1, Occupancy, Utilization, and Financial Characteristics of Housing Units. See our Table 7.1(d). Here you can learn the number of owner-occupied units, the number of rentals, the value of real estate, and so on.

In Tract SA, for example, there are over 1,000 renter-occupied housing units out of a total of almost 2,000 housing units. In Tract NB, there are 148 renter-occupied housing units out of a 1,138 total. This works out to over 54% renter-occupied units for Tract SA, and 13% for Tract NB.

Tract NB also has larger housing units—443 with eight or more rooms. The median values are higher in Tract NB—more than $200,000 versus $101,700 in Tract SA. And the rents in Tract NB are higher—over $500 versus $340 in Tract SA.

Think about it this way. What do renters need? What do home-owners need? Renters generally live in multiple dwellings (apartments or condos) where space is limited. Renters will be in the market for portable things, smaller appliances they can carry with them when they move on. Limited space means renters will buy space savers.

Homeowners, on the other hand, will be a market for larger appliances, furniture, big ticket items that don't need moving around.

TABLE 7.2   Census Table H-7, Structural, Equipment, and Household Characteristics of Housing Units, is just one example of the kinds of specialized information waiting for you in various census tables.

Census Tracts	Greenfield City, Milwaukee County		
	Tract 1201	Tract 1202	Tract 1203
Year-round housing units	**1 586**	**4 525**	**884**
SELECTED CHARACTERISTICS			
Complete kitchen facilities	1 586	4 491	877
1 complete bathroom plus half bath(s)	473	1 355	399
2 or more complete bathrooms	356	497	70
Air conditioning	1 057	3 461	565
Central system	385	1 092	267
Source of water, public system or private company	1 276	4 475	856
Sewage disposal, public sewer	1 288	4 520	884
UNITS IN STRUCTURE			
1, detached or attached	1 071	2 147	668
2	45	175	141
3 and 4	—	100	—
5 to 9	10	604	40
10 to 49	440	1 161	35
50 or more	20	333	—
Mobile home or trailer, etc.	—	5	—
HEATING EQUIPMENT			
Steam or hot water system	316	1 667	92
Central warm-air furnace	1 058	2 605	782
Electric heat pump	35	39	—
Other built-in electric units	138	145	6
Other means	39	69	4
None	—	—	—
Occupied housing units	**1 543**	**4 443**	**874**
HOUSE HEATING FUEL			
Utility gas	946	3 597	728
Bottled, tank, or LP gas	24	13	—
Electricity	203	241	6
Fuel oil, kerosene, etc.	313	579	133
Other	57	13	7
No fuel used	—	—	—

(Note: Data are estimates based on a sample.)
SOURCE: Adapted from 1980 U.S. Census.

Other Census Information

This quick analysis has only scratched the surface of the vast census data bank. We have tried to show you what to look for first, and where it might lead. For example, to save space we left out a number of categories from our sample tables in Table 7.1. In the complete Census Table P-9, which we excerpted for our Table 7.1(c), you can learn what form of transportation people in each tract use to go to work, and where their place of work is.

If you have a specific business in mind, there are probably tables that will apply. For example, say you just inherited seven oil-delivery trucks, and you have a chance to get into a partnership selling utility gas or heating oil. One of your problems is finding out where the customers are, so you can locate your holding tanks and your general headquarters close to their center. You live near a lake in the Midwest, in Greenfield, Wisconsin, but your spouse says Greenfield is no place for oil tanks. You go to your nearest Government Depository, on the campus of the University of Wisconsin. You find the Milwaukee SMSA and you look up Table H-7, Structural, Equipment, and House-hold Characteristics of Housing Units. This table is reproduced in Table 7.2 on page 129. You are a nuts-and-bolts person, so you start with Tract 1201 in the city of Greenfield. (Tract 1202 is where you live.) Under Tract 1201 you find a section called House Heating Fuel, where you learn that of 1,586 total housing units, 946 units use utility gas, 313 units use fuel oil or kerosene, and the other units use other heating fuels to lesser degrees.

That doesn't give you a lot of hope. But right next to Tract 1201 is Tract 1202, where the numbers for utility gas are higher — 3,597. You feel a surge of hope. You don't have the total picture yet, but at least you're on the way.

And all with the help of government statistics.

The Problem with Census Data

The government takes a population census every 10 years. A location could have changed dramatically between censuses. We think the census works best for mature geographic areas like the Midwest and mature industries like automobiles, service stations, or heating oil. The census is a good starting place. Then, if you match what you found from tract analysis with information from other sources, you should begin homing in on your location.

HOMING IN ON YOUR BEST LOCATION

To help you determine that best location, the list of categories that follows will allow you to generate your own **location checklist**.

Assigning Values

Using a scale of 1 to 10, assign a numerical importance to each of the following categories in the blanks provided, with 1 indicating the least important and 10 the most important. When you finish scoring, go back and note the categories with the higher numbers — say anything above a 5. Then read the rest of the chapter and come back to review the values you put down. Change whatever numbers you have

location checklist
a detailed list of important
factors to consider when
selecting a business site

to. When you are completely done, transfer the most important categories onto a piece of paper. This list then becomes your personal checklist for selecting your best location.

Creating a Location Checklist

____ **Target Market.** How far will your customers have to travel to get to you? (*Hint:* Information on the traffic count for your area may be available from the department of highways or independent research firms.) Are you in a business (flowers, dry cleaning, plumbing, or pizza carry-out) that can travel to the customers? If you're traveling, how far can you travel and still make a profit?

____ **Transportation Lines.** How much will your business depend on trucks, rail, buses, airports, shipping by water? If you're in manufacturing or distribution, you'll need to do some careful analysis of your major transportation channel. It's also a good idea to have a **backup transport system.** A good technique here is to diagram your site, then diagram all the lines of transportation your business will be using.

____ **Neighbor Mix.** Who is next door? Who is across the way? Consider your **neighbor mix.** Who is going to help you pull target customers? In your immediate area, which business pulls the most customers? If you're considering a shopping center, who is your anchor tenant (the big department store or supermarket that will act as the magnet for the center)?

____ **Competition.** Do you want competitors miles away or right next door? Think about this one. If you're in the restaurant business, you may want to set up along a Restaurant Row. (A good example of a workable Competitor Cluster is San Diego's famous Mile of Cars—Chevrolets, Datsuns, Dodges, Toyotas, VWs, and so on—which cuts down customer driving time and allows for easy comparison shopping.)

____ **Security, Safety.** How safe is it? Are you in a high crime area that looks safe as a nursery at high noon but turns into an urban jungle near midnight? Is there anything you can do beside sleeping on the premises to increase your security?

____ **Labor Pool.** Who will be working for you, and how far will they have to commute? Does your business require a bigger **labor pool** at certain peak periods of the year? How easily will you be able to find that kind of help? Will you need skilled labor? Where's the nearest pool? Train stop? Bus stop? Subway? Will you need technical people? How far will they travel?

____ **Ordinances.** What state, county, or city rules will affect your location? For example, are there sign **ordinances,** or can you put up whatever sign you need to attract customers? Signage— sign requirements that could affect both the size of signs and where they could be placed—will affect your visability.

   Local ordinances are often included in zoning regulations. How is your location zoned?

____ **Services.** Police, fire, security, trash pickup: What do you get for your taxes, and who pays for the rest?

____ **Costs.** Purchase price if you're buying. Rent or lease if you are

backup transport system
a secondary means of delivery or shipment to use when your primary system can't deliver

neighbor mix
the industrial/commercial make-up of businesses in close proximity to yours

labor pool
qualified people who are available for employment near your business location

ordinances
city/county laws governing business locations

not. (We advise against buying property and starting a business at the same time. It diverts your precious energies. It diverts capital you will need for the business.) Other costs include taxes, insurance, utilities, improvements, association dues, and routine maintenance. You want to know who pays for what. For example, there's a big difference between a gross lease — where your costs are fixed and there are no additional assessments — and a triple net lease — where you are charged for taxes, insurance, and improvements in addition to a base rental fee. See the section in this chapter on how to rewrite a lease, and see the case study on Charlene Webb, also in this chapter.

_____ **Ownership.** If you're still planning to buy the property, whom will you get to advise you on real estate? Consider a lease, with option to buy.

_____ **Accessibility.** Will your Target Customers, lured by your creative promotions, find you easily and have a place to park when they get there? Or will they have to climb over ugly obstacles that spoil the mood you're trying so hard to create?

_____ **Space.** If you need to expand, can you knock out a wall or will you have to move to a new site? Take a good look at the footprint of the building — the configuration of the building and the space it takes up on its lot.

_____ **History of Property, Stability of Landlord.** How long has the landlord owned this property? Is it likely to be sold while you're a tenant? If the property is sold, what will happen to your business? What will happen to your tax obligations? If the property goes up for sale, do you want the first crack at making an offer?

_____ **Physical Visibility.** Does your business need to be seen? If so, how does your location enhance its visibility? Can you make alterations in your location such as building or area to increase your visibility?

_____ **Life Cycle of the Area.** Consider the **location life cycle.** Is your location in an area that is _embryonic_ (vacant lots, open space, emptiness), _growing_ (high rises, new schools, lots of construction), _mature_ (building conversions, cracked streets, sluggish traffic), or _declining_ (graveyards, emptiness)? If you locate here, where will the area be in five years? What will that do to your business?

_____ **Image.** How important is image in your business? How will location affect your image? Can you get the image you want in this location? How far would you have to travel to find your 100% location?

_____ **Parking.** Is there enough parking for peak periods of demand?

WHAT IS THE PERFECT LOCATION?

The perfect location is different for every enterprise. If you're in the house-cleaning business, you can work out of your station wagon and your telephone. If you're in mail order, you can work out of a P.O. box. Action Step 31 allows you to brainstorm your **100% location.** (Use a mind map to help you get going.)

ACTION 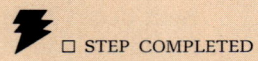 STEP 31

Fantasize Your 100% Location

Sit down where you will not be disturbed and brainstorm the 100% location for your small business.

For example, if you were going to open a candy, cigarette, and cigar stand, you might want to locate in the center of New York's Grand Central Station, where 10,000 people pass by every hour.

Or if you want to open an upscale boutique, you might want to visualize a short but profitable street in Beverly Hills called Rodeo Drive.

Once you have the general area in mind, write down what else is terrific about this location.

Writing everything down will give you guidelines to work from as you move out to explore actual sites in the real world.

☐ STEP COMPLETED

---

location life cycle
stages from birth to death of a commercial or industrial area

100% location
mythical perfect location — a useful benchmark for your site-search

Case Study

Marcia Meadows — Site Analysis

Michael, my husband, had worked in the automotive industry for 17 years — the last dozen in California — when his company decided to transfer him back East.

The new job would give him a nice promotion, and for a while we were happily making plans. Then one day, coming back from the beach with the kids asleep in the back seat, I suddenly knew I didn't want to leave California. We had a lovely home. The children had their friends. And Michael and I both dreaded the East's long bleak winters.

So we decided to start our own small business. Michael knew about cars — Saabs and Volvos mostly — and I got busy and took a course in small business at the local community college.

The first thing we did was locate our competitors. The largest was in the north part of the county. The next largest was west, a couple of miles from the beach. One was to the south.

If you drew connecting lines on an area map, our three competitors each formed one point of a wide-spread triangle.

There was no one in the middle, and Michael knew from experience they couldn't handle all the repair business.

Our next step was to get a list of all the Volvo owners in the area. We contacted the Department of Motor Vehicles, and they were very helpful.

For several days, we stuck little colored pins into our area map — one pin for each Volvo owner — and as the number of pins grew we noticed a steadily growing cluster right in the middle of our three competitors, and that's where we located our repair business.

Our research and planning worked. We're very glad we did not leave our home to move back into winter.

MORE SITE DATA FROM THE FEDERAL GOVERNMENT

In the preceding case study, location was important for a couple of reasons:

1. Convenience. Customers will only drive so many miles to have their cars repaired.
2. Equipment. A major expense in car repair service is equipment, and you don't want to be moving that from one location to another.

As you prepare to find the best location for your business, there is another source of data from the federal government that you should consider. It's a book called *Starting and Managing a Small Business of Your Own*. Table 7.3 (page 134) is from the 1982 edition, and it shows the number of inhabitants per kind of retail establishment on a national average. Is your future business listed there too? If so, you have one more tool for determining where you should locate. For example, if you're going to open a shoe store, you don't want to locate

TABLE 7.3   Number of Inhabitants per Store by Selected Kinds of Business (National Average for 1977)

Kind of Business	Number of Inhabitants per Establishment	Kind of Business	Number of Inhabitants per Establishment
Food Stores		**Building Material & Hardware Dealers**	
Grocery stores	1,191	Lumber & other building material dealers	7,366
Meat or fish (sea food) markets	12,647	Paint, glass & wallpaper stores	18,266
Fruit stores & vegetable markets	27,139	Hardware stores	8,067
Candy, nut & confectionary stores	23,752	**Automotive Dealers**	
Retail bakeries	10,706	Motor vehicle dealers, new and used	6,921
Dairy products stores	25,712	Motor vehicle dealers, used cars only	5,757
Eating, Drinking Places		Tire, battery & accessory dealers	4,538
Restaurants, lunchrooms, caterers	776	Boat dealers	32,509
Cafeterias	776	Gasoline service stations	1,207
Refreshment places	776	**Miscellaneous**	
Drinking places (alcoholic beverages)	2,273	Used merchandise stores	1,294
General Merchandise		Book stores	16,758
Variety stores	12,265	Stationery stores	33,206
General merchandise stores	9,377	Drug stores	4,299
Apparel & Accessory Stores		Florists	7,255
Women's ready-to-wear	4,747	Fuel Oil dealers	19,976
Women's accessory & specialty stores	31,304	Gift, novelty & souvenir shops	6,260
Men's & boys' cothing and furnishing stores	9,396	Hobby, toy & game shops	11,493
Family clothing stores	9,888	Jewelry stores	6,249
Shoe stores	7,641	Liquified petroleum gas (bottled gas dealers)	29,171
Furniture, Home Furnishings and Equipment Stores		Mail order houses	19,449
Furniture stores	5,223	Merchandising Machine operators	15,799
Floor covering stores	12,391	Optical goods stores	2,144
Drapery, curtain and upholstery stores	18,669	Sporting goods stores & bicycle shops	6,782
Household appliance stores	12,148		
Radio & television stores	8,610		
Record shops	15,517		
Musical instrument stores	15,517		

SOURCE: Wendell O. Metcalf, *Starting and Managing a Small Business of Your Own* (Washington, D.C.: Small Business Administration, 1982), 23. This table is based on information from the Bureau of the Census, U.S. Department of Commerce. Number of establishments with payroll based on July 1, 1976 population estimates prepared by the Census Bureau for the Office of Revenue Sharing from the 1977 *Census of Retail Trade*.

where there are already more shoe stores than inhabitants to support them — not unless you have good reason to believe you can steal customers right and left.

Note that the SBA's 1982 table is based on the 1977 *Census of Retail Trade*. These figures are not current, but they're still useful. When we compare them to information taken from the 1973 edition of the same book (based on the 1972 *Census of Retail Trade*), we discover an important trend at work: The number of people needed to support every establishment listed dropped from one census to the other. Why? Reasons on the consumer side include more specialized tastes and increased discretionary income. On the retail side, some retailers have increased the variety of products they offer. Selected examples of these decreases are shown as follows:

Number of Inhabitants Needed to Support a Retail Business

	1972	1977
Retail bakeries	12,563	10,706
Boat dealers	61,526	32,509
Men's & boy's clothing	11,832	9,396
Record shops	112,144	15,517
Hardware	10,206	8,067
Hobby, toy, game	61,430	11,493
Jewelry stores	13,495	6,249
Florists	13,531	7,225
Paint, glass, wallpaper	22,454	18,266

The government takes an economic census every five years. We were unable to locate an SBA analysis based on data from the 1982 *Census of Retail Trade*, although one will no doubt be available.

These numbers are not the total picture, of course, and they'll need to be supplemented and sharpened by other demographic data like age, income, household size, and marital status. But they do give you another way of looking at site selection.

When you start looking for your location, keep these numbers in mind.

SUGGESTIONS FOR LEASING

Commercial Realtors and Other Professional Help

We strongly urge you to get professional help when it comes time to start looking seriously for your new location.

A **commercial real estate office** — especially one for a large national firm — will be a source of information about growth in the community and, of course, about available sites. A lawyer can review the lease offered by your prospective landlord and offer suggestions about how you can protect yourself. Action Step 32 gives you even more reasons to follow through on our advice.

ACTION STEP 32

Seek Professional Help in Choosing a Location

When you really start to look, pay a visit to a commercial real estate office.

Perhaps the simplest way to begin is with a large firm, like Coldwell Banker. They're nationwide, and they have extensive information on commercial properties. A large firm will also have enough people on the staff to show you around.

A commercial real estate firm should have access to planning reports and demographic information that will tell you about growth in the community.

These reports are free. Have your plan well in mind. Make an appointment. Dress conservatively.

And leave your checkbook at home!

P.S. Once you choose a site, a lawyer can be a big help in interpreting your lease.

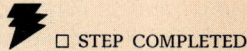 □ STEP COMPLETED

commercial real estate office
a real estate firm that specializes in selling and leasing business properties

Have Plan B Ready if Your Anchor Tenant Sinks

Bette Lindsay had a soft spot for books, so when she finally chose a business, it was a bookstore. She researched everything—trends, census data, newspapers, reports from real estate firms, the major suppliers—but she neglected to analyze her dependency on an **anchor tenant.**

Would you have made the same mistake?
Or will you have Plan B ready?

anchor tenant
a business firm in a commercial area that attracts customers

Case Study

Bette Lindsay—A Costly Surprise

My husband and I researched the small business field for almost two years before we took the plunge.

My heart kept bringing me back to books.

I've been reading since I was seven, and I'll always have a soft spot for a well-written story, so when this new shopping center opened up a mile from our home, I told my husband, "This is it."

Everything looked perfect. There was a new anchor tenant coming in, a food store that would draw in lots of customers. And our real estate agent, the one we'd been working with during most of our search, showed us a report on the demographics of the area that showed we were smack in the middle of a well-educated market. According to statistics put out by the federal government, a bookstore needs a population of 28,000 people to survive.

Our area had 62,000 people in it, and the closest bookstore was over five miles away.

Everything else looked good, too. We had lots of parking. The neighbors that had moved in (there were only three hardy pioneers like ourselves) were serious about their business, yet pleasant to work with.

We wanted to get in for Christmas, because December is the peak season for bookstores, so we set a target date of mid-October. The contractor was still working when we opened a month later.

We started off with an autograph party. We advertised some bestseller specials. And even though construction work from our anchor tenant blocked access, we had a very good Christmas that year.

My mother always told me, "Never count your chickens before they're hatched."

In mid-January, all construction work stopped on our anchor tenant's new building. The next day, we read in the paper that his company had gone bankrupt.

Well, the first thing I did was to call the landlord. He was out of town, and my call was referred to a property management company. All they did was collect the rent.

January was slow. So was February. So was March. In April, two of our neighbors closed up. The construction debris was blocking customer access. And it was a mess.

In May, I finally succeeded in getting ahold of the landlord, to try to re-negotiate the lease, but his story was sadder than mine.

It was 14 months from the day we moved in that we finally got our anchor tenant. If I'd suspected any problems like that, I could have built protections against them into our lease.

That was one expensive mistake that does not bear repeating.

Most small businesses are not destination locations and must count on anchor tenants to draw traffic. Bette made an assumption that the anchor tenant in her center would be there forever.

Rewriting the Lease

You live with a lease (and a landlord) for a long time. If you're successful in a retail business, most landlords will want a percentage of your success based on your **gross.** If you're not successful, you're going to want a bevy of Plan Bs and a **location escape hatch.**

The big word here is *if*.

If the furnace breaks down.

If the parking lot needs sweeping.

If the anchor tenant goes under.

If the building gets sold.

Your mission is to peer into the future and handle all these gut-busting possibilities with precise words and precise numbers.

Before signing on the dotted line, take some time to rewrite your lease.

Read the lease. When you see something you don't understand or don't like, strike through it. Rewrite the sentences if you have to. It's your lease, and you're not bound by the legalese. If you need help from a lawyer, get a lawyer. And make sure that your landlord (or the leasing agent) agrees with your changes by initialing every one.

Here's a list of reminders to start you on your rewrite.

1. **Escape Clause.** If the building doesn't shape up or the area goes into eclipse, you want out fast. Be specific. Write something like this into your lease: "If three or more vacancies occur in the center, tenant can terminate lease."

2. **Option to Renew.** Most businesses need a year or at least 6 months to get going. It your business does well, you want to stay put. If it doesn't, you don't want to be saddled with a heavy lease payment every month. Get a lease for one year, with an **option to renew** for the next two or three.

3. **Transferring Your Lease.** Circumstances might force you to sublet. In the trade, this is called "assigning." If these circumstances arise, make sure you can transfer your lease without a heap of hassle.

4. **Cost-of-Living Cap.** Most leases allow the owner to increase rents with the inflation rate. To protect yourself, insist on a **cost-of-living cap** so that your base rate won't increase faster than your landlord's cost. Try for half of the amount of the Consumer Price Index (CPI), a standard measure. If the CPI goes up 10%, your rate only goes up 5%. It's fair, because your landlord's costs don't change much. Major tenants in your center will insist on a cap. Act like a pro when negotiating your lease and you will be treated like one.

---

rewriting your lease
a protective tactic to put language in the lease that protects you as well as the landlord

gross
total amount

location escape hatch
a way to cancel or modify your lease if the landlord fails to meet certain specified terms

option to renew
a guaranteed opportunity at the end of your lease to extend for another specific period of time

cost-of-living cap
an agreement which states that the rent from one year to another cannot be increased by more than the CPI for the same period

5. **Percentage Lease.** A percentage lease is common in the larger retail centers. The tenant pays a base rate plus a percentage of gross sales. Inflation can hurt you unless the owner agrees to raise the base-rate minimum along with the inflation rate.

6. **Floating Lease Scale.** If you're a pioneer tenant, the first in a center, and you're surrounded by symbolic rocks and dirt and construction machinery, you should negotiate a payment scale based on occupancy. For example, you specify that you'll pay 50% of your lease payment when the center is 50% occupied, 70% when its 70% occupied, and 100% when it's full. You can't build traffic alone, and motivation is healthy for everyone, including landlords.

7. **Start-up Buffer.** There's a good chance you will be on location fixing up or remodeling long before your first customer gives you your first sale. Tell your landlord of this problem and negotiate two to three months of free rent. The argument: If your business is a success, the landlord, who is taking a percentage, will make more money. If your business is slow, or if it fails, the landlord will have to find a new tenant. You need breathing space. You have signed on for the long haul. By not squeezing you to death for cash, the landlord allows you to put more money into inventory, equipment, service, and atmosphere — the things that make a business go.

8. **Improvements.** Unless you're a super fixer-upper, you don't want to lease a location equipped with nothing but a dirt floor and a capped-off cold water pipe. You want the right atmosphere for your business, but you don't want to use all your cash to pay for it before you open. Negotiate with the landlord to make improvements and spread the total payments out over the total time of the lease. Or find an existing space that doesn't require heavy remodeling.

9. **Restrictive Covenants.** If you're running a camera store and part of your income derives from developing film, you don't want a film developing booth springing up in your center. If you're running a hearing aid store, you don't want a stereo store to move in next door. Build all the protection you can into your lease. And make sure you fully understand what existing CC & Rs (conditions, covenants, and restrictions) you will be subject to. Sometimes these CC & Rs are in a separate document. Get a copy and read it, because it is nearly impossible to change these pre-existing restrictions.

restrictive covenants
a list of things you can't do

10. **Maintaining the Location.** If the parking lot needs sweeping, who takes care of it? If the air conditioner goes out, who pays for service? If the sewer stops up, who handles the repairs? Get all this written down in simple language. Your diligence with words and numbers will pay off.

Let's watch one entrepreneur protect her small business by thinking and rewriting before she signs.

Case Study

Charlene Webb — How to Rewrite a Lease

My partner and I were both in education, so doing research for our gourmet cookware store didn't seem unnatural. Our target **grand opening** date was October, because we wanted to catch the holiday cycle as it started up, so during Easter we spent a week in the Los Angeles area talking to owners of gourmet cookware shops.

There's one on every corner.

We spent five days, Monday to Friday, and we saw an average of 15 shops a day. The owners we talked to were helpful — because they knew we were going to open up 60 miles away.

When Easter vacation was over, we went back to our jobs at school, minds loaded with information, hearts full of hope. Time pressures were heavy. For an October opening, we knew we had to spend the summer on layout, image, and atmosphere.

We had to find a dream location.

Three days before the end of spring term, we found a site — in a very safe and secure center near a convenient freeway off-ramp. Our nearest competition was six miles away, and some figures from a population study told us we had about 55,000 people from the surrounding area to support us.

The next step was to negotiate the lease.

Perhaps it was because I'd been an English teacher. Perhaps it was because my father was a lawyer. But whenever I came across a passage in the lease document I didn't like or didn't think was fair to us, I crossed it out. Several times I rewrote passages in the lease, and when it was all over — my changes discussed with the landlord and then initialed by both of us — I had made four changes that really gave our business some flexibility and breathing space.

1. We got a one-year lease with option to renew for the next two. I knew if I was going under, it would be that first year, and I didn't want to be responsible for paying a lease if our shop went under.

2. We got three months free rent. I was very straightforward with the landlord on this. I said, "Look here, I can pay you three months rent out of what cash I have left after fixing up the interior, or I can put that money into inventory that will help my start-up. I think it would be a benefit to both of us if I were to put that money into inventory." The landlord agreed with me.

3. We got what's called a cost-of-living cap on the percentage the landlord raises our rent each year. Our cap is 10%. If I ever do another lease negotiation, I'm planning to go for 5%.

4. We would not let the landlord or any of his representatives look at our books.

grand opening
a splashy celebration announcing your entry into the market arena

More Survival Tips from Charlene Webb

Charlene's shop started off nicely, with a grand opening party spiked by invitations to 500 friends, and friends of friends. To bring in business, she started a cooking school, and her students have become good customers. Once a week, she runs a special treat called Lunch and Learn.

For $5.75 and 50 minutes of their time, customers get a glass of wine, a quick cooking lesson, and the lunch they cooked themselves. The Heavy Users in Charlene's business are women. Lunch and Learn targets men and brings them into the store. Then they come back to buy gifts.

Charlene has developed her own customer list, which now numbers 2,500 names. She mails a quarterly newsletter to her customers informing them of upcoming classes and product promotions. She stays visible in the community by being actively involved in music, the chamber of commerce, and the bank (she's now on the board of directors).

When people ask her to look back over the last couple of years, from start-up to where she is now, Charlene says there is one thing she would do differently.

> I'd buy a cash register. It's marvelous. It keeps track of everything. When you're a customer, you don't realize, because all you see is the total that some faceless salesperson puts down on your charge card. But when you become a merchant retailer, you're on the business end of a cash register, which is sort of like the economic turnstile of your whole business. On normal days, you'll work 10–12 hours. At Christmas, you'll work 18 hours a day, and you'll need to multiply yourself into three different people to get everything done, and that's when you'll think Heaven, after all, is a cash register.

SUMMARY

For many small businesses, the importance of location cannot be overstated. A good location can make everything easier for a new business. A highly visible building will save you advertising dollars. Of course, for retail businesses, location is essential.

We encourage you to develop your own understanding of the relationship between location and consumer response. We show you how to use census information to research potential target markets. We provide you with a list from which you can create your own checklist for analyzing sites. And we refer you to the SBA booklet, *Starting and Managing a Small Business of Your Own,* which contains estimates of how many people it takes to support certain businesses. (How many people does *your* business need to support an adequate number of target customers?) All of these tools should help you home in on your best location. Throughout the chapter, we stress that the perfect location is different for every enterprise; we also encourage you to brainstorm the 100% location for your business.

Because most entrepreneurs will be leasing their business sites, in the case studies and in the text we repeatedly underscore the importance of reading and even rewriting your lease *before* you sign. Leases

ACTION STEP REVIEW

30 To get a sense of the power of location, focus for a moment on your own buying habits. How far do you travel for candy, cigarettes, beer, a movie, car repairs, eyeglasses, a doctor, a dentist, a new car, a microcomputer? How far did you travel the last time you had dinner with an old friend? If you needed brain surgery, how far would you travel?

31 After you assess the power of location, brainstorm your 100% location. Leave all geographic and budgetary restraints behind and have some fun developing the perfect site for your small business. This exercise will whet your appetite and make you think of things you really need in your location.

32 If you need help, get it. A commercial real estate broker can help you check out locations. A lawyer is invaluable for reading your lease.

supplied by the lessor (your landlord or landlady) are written to favor the lessor, and you (as lessee) have every right to protect your own interests.

THINK POINTS

⚡ Leases are written *for* landlords by attorneys employed *by* landlords. Every word in a lease is put there to protect the landlord.

⚡ Have *your* attorney read the lease and offer suggestions about how you can protect yourself.

⚡ The irony of the location quest is that you need the best site when you can least afford it.

⚡ Take your time with location choices. If you lose out on a hot site, don't worry. Another one will appear shortly.

⚡ Have your landlord pay for site improvements and spread the payments out over the term of the lease.

⚡ You may have heard about lease-breaking parties. Take it from us. There's no such thing. They don't work.

⚡ If your business is drive-up, make sure you've got ample parking.

REFERENCES

Burstiner, Irving. *The Small Business Handbook: A Comprehensive Guide to Starting and Running Your Own Business.* Englewood Cliffs, N.J.: Prentice-Hall, 1979. Good, solid chapter on location.

Metcalf, Wendell O. *Starting and Managing a Small Business of Your Own.* Washington, D.C.: Small Business Administration, 1982. Statistics always lag behind reality. There is good information here, but you will need to update these figures by contacting trade associations in your industry.

Sullivan, Daniel J., and Joseph F. Lane. *Small Business Management: A Practical Approach.* 2nd ed. Dubuque, Iowa: William C. Brown Co., Publishers; 1983. The chapter on location contains a model study of the southern San Mateo County market. The study was prepared by the *Redwood City Tribune,* and it is a good example of the kind of help you can get from your local newspapers.

A Description of Product or Service

B The Market and the Target Customer

C Competition

D Marketing Strategy

E Location

H Projected Income Statement

I Projected Cash Flow

J Projected Balance Sheet

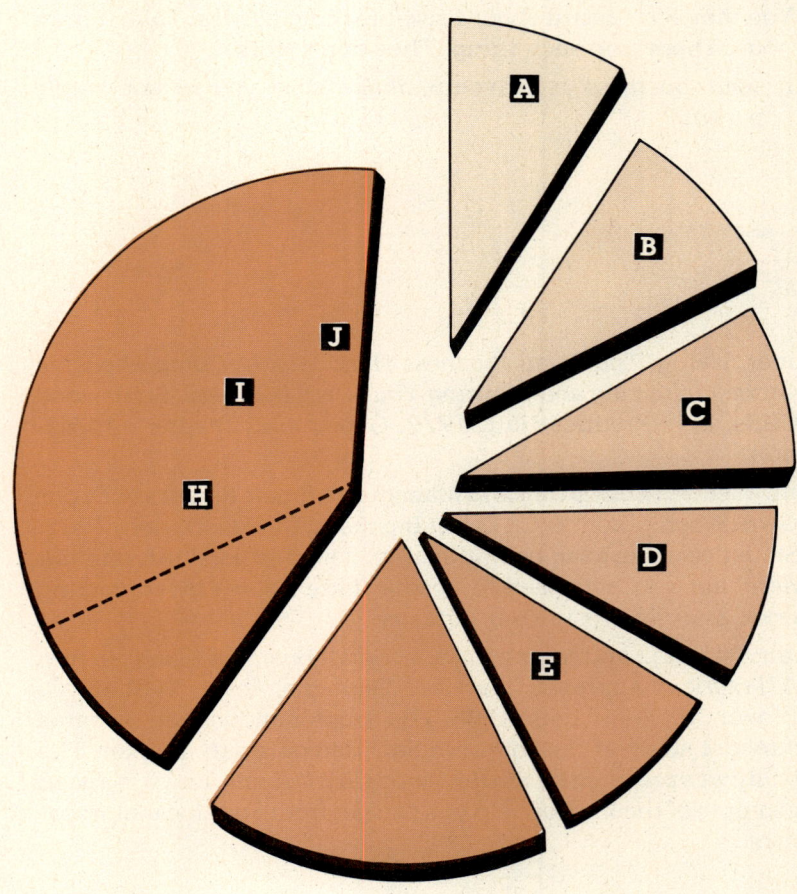

FIGURE 8.1 Chapter 8 prepares you for computing the financial section of your Plan by anticipating surprises you can't afford.

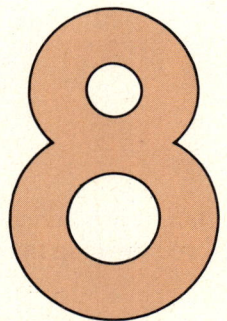

Surprises You Can't Afford

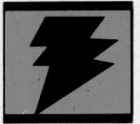 **I**n earlier chapters, we've talked about the need for Plan B—an alternate strategy for bailing your business out of a tight spot in the marketplace. In Chapter 8 we deal with that necessity in more detail. You're a budding entrepreneur. You have lots of energy. You get ideas fast. You pride yourself on being results-oriented.

ARE YOU READY WITH PLAN B?

For you, Plan B is a must. You can start on your Plan B with a checklist for problems and solutions, which we will help you develop later on in the chapter.

The Inspector Cometh

For now, focus on the following case study—about a creative guy who took care of everything for his business except a city ordinance.

Case Study

Tommy Mankiewicz — The Sandwich King

Tommy Mankiewicz was in a poker game with a couple of old Army buddies when the idea came up for a small business.

"Dry cleaning," Rick said. "You can work out of the garage. All you need's a panel truck and a customer list. It's like coining money, right from the start."

"Sandwiches," George said. "And I know just the place. Traffic 25 hours a day. Beach traffic, commercial, commuters, blue collar, kids on their way from school. Gimme two cards."

George had been in sandwiches down in Florida. After a couple of beers, Rick and Tommy would call George the Sandwich King. It was assumed George knew a lot about making it big in business.

"How much would it cost?" Tommy asked.

George whipped out pencil and paper, and pushed a few numbers around on paper. "Figure twenty grand apiece, tops," he said. "Figure to double your twenty in 18 months, easy."

"Those are nice numbers at the end," Tommy said. "But which one of you big spenders can loan me the twenty at the beginning?"

"Hey," George said. "No problem. They don't call me the Sandwich King of Pompano Beach for nothing. You give me a **handshake** now and your name on a paper later and we're in business."

Tommy thought about it. He was working for the state, making okay money, but next year his oldest kid would start to college, and the house could use some refurbishing, and his wife was after him to buy some new living room furniture.

Besides, he'd always wanted to own his own business.

Continued

handshake
a way to form a
partnership that is only as
good as the character
and memory of the
shakees

So Tommy and Rick shook hands with George.

George was between jobs, so he handled most of the details. He found the location, negotiated with the landlord, talked to the equipment **vendors,** and bought a great-looking sign. Tommy and Rick each prepared a **financial statement,** to hand over to the banker George knew, and Tommy made several long distance calls to relatives and friends, asking for **start-up money.**

On weekends, Tommy and Rick and their wives spent all day at the site, fixing the place up. Tommy worked hard. He was good with tools, and he could build cabinets and shelves. But what really got him going was making fancy sandwiches.

''Hey!'' Rick said. ''This tastes great! Serve enough of these and we'll be famous!''

''Yes,'' Rick's wife said. ''And they have eye appeal, too.''

Everyone agreed. Tommy made the best sandwiches in the world. His stylish creations would add quality to the shop.

Tommy was pleased. He'd always had a touch of **creativity,** way down deep, and now it had a chance to come out and take its place in the world. He was in the middle of one of his creations when the city **inspector** arrived. (See Figure 8.2.)

The inspector was a heavy-set man with beady eyes and a clip board. He walked around the inside of the store, frowning, making notes. The inspector distracted Tommy, took his mind off what he was doing. Tommy was at the counter, working the big French chef's knife. He could hear the inspector in the next room, walking around. Tommy wished that his partner George was here, to handle this end of the business.

Then the inspector appeared in the doorway.

''Where's the restroom for the disabled?'' he asked.

''What?'' Tommy said, feeling a chill on the back of his neck.

''The disabled restroom. You know, wide enough for a wheelchair, regulation railing along the wall, special raised toilet facility. You gotta have one.''

''Can you wait for my partner?'' Tommy asked. ''He just stepped out. If you'll talk to him, I'm sure he —''

But the inspector just stood there, shaking his head. And Tommy knew that George hadn't taken care of it, and even when George did get there, all the inspector did was read them chapter and verse of the **municipal code,** and there it was, right there, in language even a lawyer couldn't understand.

Every public place had to have a restroom for the disabled. There was only one place for it in the shop. And that meant they had to tear out a wall and put in a drain and move some machinery around in the kitchen and replumb everything.

The surprise cost just under $12,000.

And when the inspector came by to check out the work, he sat at the counter working on a plate of Tommy's freshest creations and told Tommy they were lucky not to be fined right off the bat.

''I knew you were an honest guy,'' the inspector said, ''who just got his tail caught in the wringer. I meet all kinds in my work, but I could tell from the way you handled those sandwiches you didn't mean anybody any harm. That's why I didn't drop it on you from the start.'' The inspector selected a special sandwich. ''These are great. Once you guys get going, these sandwiches will make you famous.''

The work on the new bathroom delayed the opening of Tommy's shop more than a month.

vendors
suppliers of goods or services to business

financial statement
a list of assets and liabilities that will show your net worth

start-up money
all funds necessary to open the doors and to keep them open until you reach positive cash flow

creativity
the ability to create

inspector
a local government employee whose task is to ensure that codes and ordinances are adhered to

municipal code
provisions to ensure the safety and health of a political jurisdiction

Planning Ahead

Reading about Tommy Mankiewicz and the Inspector, it's easy to say "I told you so." It's easy to second guess the situation and say to yourself, "The guy should have thought about the handicapped."

Easy to say.

But Tommy had just discovered he was an entrepreneur. He was having fun being creative. He got busy, lost himself, and suddenly the world appeared at his door, holding a clipboard and reading off regulations (as shown in Figure 8.2).

The same thing can happen to you.

And that's why you've got to plan for everything, even surprises.

If you get into the habit of making lists, doing mind maps, and writing everything down, you'll have a better chance at surviving in small business. Putting your ideas down in words lets you look at them with a certain amount of objectivity. It also helps you focus if you connect your ideas to specific dollar amounts, which is what we ask you to do in Action Step 33.

(Near the end of this chapter there's a list of surprises that have

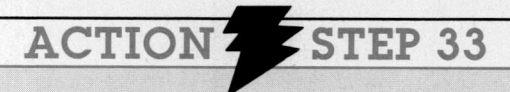

Plan Ahead for Expensive Business Surprises

Now that you've got your business well in mind, take a few minutes to brainstorm your way through a list of expensive surprises that could hurt your business or threaten its survival.

You can either use a time frame (start-up surprises, first year surprises, and so on) or just move through your list by free association.

When you finish your list, go back through and circle all the surprises that have any connection at all with money.

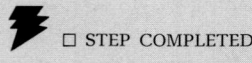 ☐ STEP COMPLETED

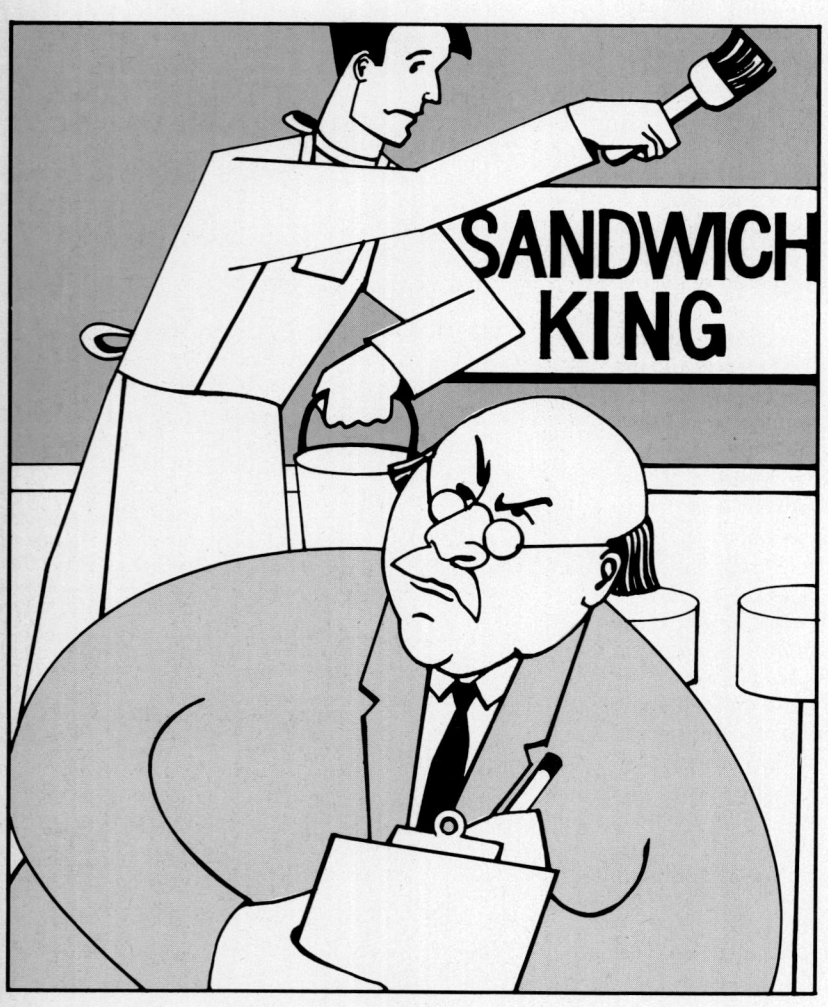

FIGURE 8.2 Many an entrepreneur has been surprised by an inspector with beady eyes and a clipboard.

happened to entrepreneurs and business owners, and we've included a checklist on what they might have done to slice the surprises to a fraction of what they were.)

PAYING THE PIPER WHEN THE PURSE IS THIN

If Ginny Henshaw had made a list of possible surprises, she would have been better prepared for what happened.

Case Study

Ginny Henshaw — Day-care Center

The reason I decided to start a preschool day-care center was because I really like kids. I'm a person with a lot of extra warmth, and so I talked it over with my husband, who said he'd help out if I got in over my head.

I think we planned things pretty well. We searched out a good location — smack in the middle of a housing area of new families with an average of 2.3 children apiece — and then we spent weekends painting and fixing up. It was fun. We worked hard. Putting our labor into the place that way made us feel a part of something warm and cozy.

Well, about three weeks before opening, we called the light and power people to ask them to turn on some lights.

"Sure thing," they said. "Just send us a check for $700 as a **utility deposit** and the lights will be on in a jiffy."

"What?" I asked. "Did you say $700?" I knew we had around $800 in the kitty. But that was for emergencies.

"That's right. You're a new commercial customer with a good credit rating. That's why the figure's so low."

"You think $700 is low?" I asked. I was shocked.

"For your tonnage," they said, "it's right on the money."

"Tonnage? What tonnage?"

"Your air conditioner," they said. "That's a five-ton unit on your roof. Figure you run it for a month, that's $310. The other $40 is for lights."

"But we're not planning to run it!" I said. "The breeze here is terrific. We don't need the air conditioner."

"Sorry, Ma'am. Our policy is pretty clear. As I said, sometimes we get three months deposit. But from your business, we'll only require the two. Would there be anything else I can help you with today?"

"No," I said. "Nothing."

How much will it cost you to open the doors of your business?

Action Step 34 helps you develop a list of tangible and intangible costs before you start out, to protect you against surprises. The Action Step also leads you to an SBA worksheet so that you can calculate exactly how much money you'll need to start out. The SBA has divided the costs into ongoing costs and costs you have to pay only once — which is an easy way to think about the costs of opening the doors to your business.

utility deposit
a cash reserve required of a new business by public utility companies

ACTION ⚡ STEP 34

Attach Price Tags to Your Business

Sit at your desk and look around with New Eyes.

Part A. List the items on the desk. Pencils, paper, telephone, typewriter, microcomputer, business cards, calendar, and so on.

List the desk, lamp, chair, bookcase, filing cabinet, and coffee machine. Now go through the drawers, listing every item you use to make your work run easier and smoother.

When you finish the first list, start another one for those large invisible costs, some of which you might take for granted. Think about things like insurance protection, rent, utilities, deposits, taxes, legal services, or accounting services.

Part B. When you finish your lists, add prices to each item.

If you don't know precise amounts jot down a ballpark figure and move on. You can get the exact amount later.

Part C. Move all your items to the handy SBA worksheet in Figure 8.3 on page 148.

As you gather more information, add in the numbers on this sheet.

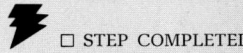 ☐ STEP COMPLETED

FIGURE 8.3 This SBA worksheet will help you estimate how much cash you need to open your business.

ESTIMATED MONTHLY EXPENSES	Your estimate of monthly expenses based on sales of $ _____ per year	Your estimate of how much cash you need to start your business (See column 3.)	What to put in column 2 (These figures are typical for one kind of business. you will have to decide how many months to allow for in your business.)
Item	Column 1	Column 2	Column 3
Salary of owner-manager	$	$	2 times column 1
All other salaries and wages			3 times column 1
Rent			3 times column 1
Advertising			3 times column 1
Delivery expense			3 times column 1
Supplies			3 times column 1
Telephone and telegraph			3 times column 1
Other utilities			3 times column 1
Insurance			Payment required by insurance company
Taxes, including Social Security			4 times column 1
Interest			3 times column 1
Maintenance			3 times column 1
Legal and other professional fees			3 times column 1
Miscellaneous			3 times column 1
STARTING COSTS YOU ONLY HAVE TO PAY ONCE			Leave column 2 blank
Fixtures and equipment			Fill in worksheet 3 on page 12 and put the total here
Decorating and remodeling			Talk it over with a contractor
Installation of fixtures and equipment			Talk to suppliers from who you buy these
Starting inventory			Suppliers will probably help you estimate this
Deposits with public utilities			Find out from utilities companies
Legal and other professional fees			Lawyer, accountant, and so on
Licenses and permits			Find out from city offices what you have to have
Advertising and promotion for opening			Estimate what you'll use
Accounts receivable			What you need to buy more stock until credit customers pay
Cash			For unexpected expenses or losses, special purchases, etc.
Other			Make a separate list and enter total
TOTAL ESTIMATED CASH YOU NEED TO START WITH	$		Add up all the numbers in column 2

SOURCE: Small Business Administration, *Business Plan for Retailers,* SBA Marketers Aid 71 (Washington, D.C.: Small Business Administration, 1981).

Don't Run out of Money

Failure to identify all possible costs may cause you to run short of money before you open your doors. If your estimates are not well developed, you might double them or triple them to stay safely within your budget. This is no time for wishful thinking. You want to run lean and mean.

How Much Money Do You Have Now?

The next question to ask is — do you have enough money for a start-up? You can keep this simple by getting a total **cash value** for your assets (what you own), a total for your **liabilities** (what you owe), and doing some easy arithmetic to calculate your net worth.

Get some practice by doing Action Step 35.

Personal Financial Statement

Action Step 35 was just a warmup. You should begin to work up a formal statement of your worth. Figure 8.4, on page 150, is a bank form for a personal financial statement. (Banks provide these forms to loan applicants.) Use this form (or get one from your bank) to develop your own, more presentable, personal financial statement. As you fill the form out, plan on supporting your numbers with documents — bank statements, photostats of stock certificates, your savings passbook, and so on. Think of this statement as your personal balance sheet.

Pulling together a personal financial statement is important for two reasons:

1. It tells you how much money you have now.
2. It forces you to get organized.

(And if later you discover you do need to apply for a loan — which we discuss in Chapter 10, "Shaking the Money Tree" — you'll be that much more prepared.).

Time Lags Are Harsh Reality

We've said before that it's going to be a while before your business starts making lots of money. In small business, you don't just rent a location and throw open the doors and get rich quick the same day.

You want to be aware of every time lag. And what does awareness mean?

Awareness means you've planned everything down to the last doorknob. Awareness means you don't quit your job until you've finished you business plan and checked with your banker (and your backup banker) and know you have enough money to make it through whatever surprises await in the grand arena of the marketplace. Awareness means you're not surprised when your business does not support you (right away) in the manner to which you've become accustomed.

A business is a living, breathing entity.

But it takes time before it lays the golden egg.

Be prepared to wait awhile.

---

cash value
worth of tangible and intangible possessions when converted to cash

liabilities
a sum total of what you owe

ACTION ⚡ STEP 35

Develop Personal Financial Statement

Part A. List everything you own with cash value: cash, securities, life insurance, accounts receivable, notes receivable, rebates, refunds, autos, other vehicles, real estate, vested pension, Keogh or IRA.

Don't stop now.

List home furnishings, household goods, big appliances, sports equipment, collectibles, jewelry, tools, livestock, trusts, patents, memberships, business interests, investment clubs. . . .

Add it up for total assets.

Part B. List every dime you owe to someone or something: accounts payable, contracts payable, notes payable (car loans, etc.), taxes, insurance (life, health, car, liability, etc.), mortgages, real estate loans, and anything else you owe. Add it up for total liabilities.

Part C. Subtract your liabilities from your assets. That gives you a net worth. Now you know how much you have. That will give you a better idea of how much you need to raise to start your business.

Good luck.

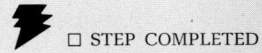 ☐ STEP COMPLETED

FIGURE 8.4 A personal financial statement form—available at any bank—will help you construct an accurate picture of your net worth.

ASSETS		LIABILITIES	
Cash in Wells Fargo	$	Notes Payable Banks—Schedule I	$
Cash in other—identify		Secured	
Stocks and Bonds—Schedule II		Unsecured	
Accounts Receivable		Accounts/Bills Payable—Schedule I	
Cash Surrender Value Life Insurance			
Face Value $			
Real Estate—Schedule III		Mortgages Payable on Real Estate—Schedule III	
Automobiles		Other debts—itemize	
Other Assets—Itemize			
		Total Liabilities	
		Net worth (total assets less total liabilities)	
TOTAL ASSETS	$	**TOTAL LIABILITIES PLUS NET WORTH**	$

SOURCES OF INCOME		SCHEDULE I—DEBTS AND CREDIT REFERENCES		
Salary	$	Notes Payable, Banks, Credit Cards, Dept. Stores, etc. itemized. (All debts are listed ☐ Yes ☐ No)		
Spouse's Salary—(if applicable)				
Bonus and Commissions		NAME AND ADDRESS OF CREDITOR	BALANCE	MO. PMT.
Real Estate Income—Net				
Dividends				
Other Source (**Note:** you need not list income from alimony, child support or maintenance unless you wish it to be considered.)				
		Alimony, Child Support, Maintenance		
Total	$	Totals	$	$

SCHEDULE II—STOCKS AND BONDS

DESCRIPTION	WHERE QUOTED	COST OR MARKET	TITLE IN NAME OF	QUANTITY	VALUE

SCHEDULE III—REAL ESTATE

DESCRIPTION/ADDRESS	DATE ACQUIRED	TITLE IN NAME OF	COST	MARKET VALUE	MORTGAGE DUE TO	AMOUNT	MO. PMT.

SCHEDULE IV—SEPARATE PROPERTY

Complete if married, and any assets listed above are separate property.

DESCRIPTION	TITLE IN NAME OF	VALUE

GENERAL INFORMATION—CONTINGENT LIABILITIES

Have you ever had a repossession? ☐ Yes ☐ No   Have you ever declared bankruptcy? ☐ Yes ☐ No

Are you an Endorser, Guarantor, Co-maker? ☐ Yes ☐ No

Are you a party to any Claims, or Suits? ☐ Yes ☐ No

Do you owe any taxes for years prior to the current year? ☐ YES ☐ NO   AMOUNT: $ _____

SOURCE: "Statement of Financial Condition," from Application for Loan— Individual(s), Wells Fargo Bank, N.A. Reproduced by permission of Wells Fargo Bank, N.A.

OPPORTUNITY COSTS

Before You Take the Plunge

Before you jump into your own venture, make sure that you are honest with yourself. What are the opportunity costs? What would happen to your finances if you chose to keep working for someone else and did not go into business? Action Step 36 allows you to find out, and the dollar **projection** you come up with should let you know precisely what you're getting into. If it hurts you to think about what you'd be giving up to go into business, maybe you're not ready for the plunge.

What Does Success Mean to You?

Money isn't the only measure of success. You need to open your New Eyes wide and search the marketplace for what you really want. Make a list. Do a mind map. Dig deep into yourself and what makes you tick.

projection
an intelligent forecast into the future

Projecting Opportunity Cost

A. Project your salary (next 12 months) _____

B. Add in benefits from your employer
   Life insurance _____
   Disability insurance _____
   Health insurance _____
   Pension plan _____
   Company car _____
   Social Security (employer's contribution) _____
   Expense account _____
   Bonuses _____
   Other _____
   Total benefits _____

C. Figure in potential income on the capital
   you're planning to invest in your small
   business.
   (Example: $25,000 × 7.75%
   = $1,937.50 for one year) _____

D. Add in your time. How many hours per week
   are you planning to work in your new
   business? _____
   Subtract the number of hours you now work _____
   Leaves hours available for moonlighting _____
   Multiply moonlighting hours times hourly
   rate times 50 weeks _____

E. **Total opportunity cost** (current potential
   income for one year) _____

AN OUNCE OF PREVENTION

When survivors from any field or profession get together, they like to tell horror stories.

We have collected a few of these in the surprise area and come up with some **preventive action.**

You can probably think of more.

ACTION ⚡ STEP 36

How Much Could You Make if You Did Not Go Into Business?

Now that you know what you're worth, take a couple of hours out and calculate what would happen, money-wise, if you kept on with what you were doing and then added in the extra time you're going to have to spend in your new business.

Use the box "Projecting Opportunity Cost" for your calculations.

Part A. Project your salary for the next 12 months.

Part B. Add in benefits from your employer, as shown. Make sure you include anything else you don't have to pay for (parking, Xerox, paper clips, etc.).

Part C. Now figure in the potential income on the capital you're planning to invest in small business. You would be earning interest on this money if you invested it elsewhere.)

Part D. Add in your time. For example, if you're planning to work 60 hours a week in your new business (entrepreneurs report up to 100 hours a week during peak seasons), subtract 40 (your normal work week) from 60 and figure how much you could earn per hour moonlighting, times 20 hours a week, times 50 weeks a year.

Part E. Total up your potential income for one year if you did not go into small business.

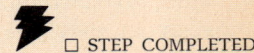 ☐ STEP COMPLETED

preventive action
positive steps taken to minimize risk of potential adversities

Surprise	Prevention
Your landlord decides to evict you and your business.	Get a lease. Rewrite the lease to favor your business. Keep in contact with the landlord. Make sure you have a renewal clause.
The local newspaper does not run ad for your Grand Opening.	Make connections with all media. Develop a **tickler file.** Make sure you see proof sheets. Withhold payment until they do it right.
An hour after you sign your name to guarantee the lease, your best friend and partner gets cold feet and pulls out. You do not have a thing in writing to protect you against **partner's remorse.**	Line up partnership commitments before the big day. Open a special **escrow account.** Everybody deposits. Everybody signs.
For eight weeks, during your peak season, the city keeps the sidewalk in front of your store torn up. The noise is deafening.	Network your way into **city hall.** Make sure you know your representative. Try to rally media sympathy. Use the underdog angle.
Your general contractor goes bankrupt.	Get a **completion bond.** Ask the bonding agency to expedite.
Your bookkeeper disappears with $100,000, your books, two trade secrets from the company safe, and your spouse.	A fidelity bond would have protected you against financial loss. Small businesses are more likely to be embezzled than larger firms.
Your **key employee,** the best sales person in your small firm, is hired away by the competition.	Woo key employees. Keep them involved and informed. Do not take them for granted. Think about giving them a piece of the business. Check the horizon for pirates.
Due to an administrative error, the bank calls your loan. It is payable in 30 days. If you would like to cash out, they will give you 25 cents on the dollar.	Take a banker to lunch. Take a **backup banker** to lunch. Back up the backup banker with a backup.
A new customer pays you by check, takes delivery of the goods, then stops payment on the check before you make it to the bank. You were too busy to double-check.	No matter how creative you are, take time out for important survival tasks.

tickler file
a calendar-based reminder system

escrow account
funds held by a neutral state-regulated third party until certain prestated conditions are met

partner's remorse
backing out of a deal before the business gets rolling

city hall
local government of the nearest bastion of municipal authority

completion bond
an insurance policy that will pay for finishing a project

key employee
a worker whose loss would seriously affect the future of your business

backup banker
another banker who would like your business and is ready to help

Surprise	Prevention
Your largest customer declares bankruptcy. The money owed you in receivables is 77% of your gross annual sales.	Do not keep all your eggs in one basket.
The bank where you have your checking account refuses to extend you a $3,300 line of credit to buy a piece of equipment that will double your business. The bank has a policy of not lending money to small firms.	Keep your banker in your information loop. Make sure you give your banker updates on your Business Plan. Get a backup bank. Discuss money long before you need it.
A new energy crisis makes 1974 look like child's play. Cars line up, hungry for gas, blocking the traffic to your store.	See the following case study.

At some time in your business life, you're going to have to turn a lemon into lemonade.

Case Study

Terry Adkins—Turning a Lemon into Lemonade

Terry's Donut Place got off to a slow start—$275 a day for the first month, when what they needed was closer to $700—but then things started picking up, $310, $380, $475, and both Terry and his wife knew they were going to make it, after all.

By Easter of the second year, they were pulling in $850 on the weekdays and close to $600 on weekends, when the trade naturally slowed down, and they were just beginning to plan their first summer vacation in six years when the Energy Crisis hit.

It didn't get as nasty in Terry's city as it did in the big cities, but it was bad enough.

Cars lined up for blocks to wait for available gas. Terry noticed the effect in his center because there was a major oil company station on the corner. The oil crisis hurt Terry's business. Terry's customers were either waiting in line for gas, or they couldn't drive in for their morning donuts without crashing through the lines of waiting cars.

Sales dropped. If the shop pulled in $200 a day, Terry called it profit. It wasn't, of course. And it wouldn't come anywhere near paying the bills.

Terry was in despair.

After a week of no business, Terry had an idea. He borrowed a shopping cart from the super market. He bought a 50-cup coffee urn. He

Continued

brewed coffee. He loaded the urn onto the grocery cart. He stacked boxes of donuts around the urn. And then he moved down the line of cars, selling his wares.

While he sold donuts, Terry got to know the people in the cars. The second day he went out with his grocery cart, he took along a paper and pencil, to write down folks' names. Beside the names he wrote what kinds of donuts they liked. He didn't know it was called "market research." It just seemed like the smart thing to do.

Terry didn't make as much money as he had before the Energy Crisis, but he made enough to keep going while things got sorted out over in the Persian Gulf. And when the Energy Crisis was over, Terry had more than a hundred new customers.

And because of the careful market research he'd done, he knew what kind of donuts they liked.

WHERE TO GO AFTER PLAN B

One of the reasons you can succeed in small business is fast footwork. You can move more quickly than the Big Guys. After you develop Plan B, work on Plans C and D.

And repeat this over, to yourself: "We are entrepreneurs. We never sleep."

SUMMARY

Start-up time needs to be smooth. What you do not need are expensive surprises that knock you and your business for a loop. So before you open your doors, you want to have anticipated as many unexpected and unpleasant surprises as possible.

You need to have a plan of action—a Plan B—laid out for every surprise you anticipate.

One way you can be prepared is to know how much it will cost you to open the doors of your business. You can also develop a personal financial statement and determine the opportunity cost of going into your new business to complete the picture of your financial preparedness. (Being caught short of cash can be a fatal surprise.)

To further prepare you for surprises, we list a number of common horror stories and the preventive measures you can take to protect yourself from similar calamities. We end the chapter by reminding you that a good entrepreneur has the drive to make the best of a bad situation. That same drive will help you go beyond being prepared with a Plan B—you will develop a Plan C and a Plan D as well.

There are two things to remember about surprises: First, you need to anticipate everything you can (and plan, plan, plan); second, when you can't anticipate, be sure you see the new problem quickly (New Eyes) and handle it with creativity and zest (Whole Brain). For a boost in this direction, reread the Terry Adkins case study on turning a lemon into lemonade.

ACTION ⚡ STEP
REVIEW

Four Action Steps help you anticipate surprises:

33 You can plan ahead. You can use your New Eyes to peer into the future and develop strategies for dealing with unforeseen events that could cripple you. You don't need to be paranoid. You just need to be alert.

34 Add price tags to your dream business. A helpful exercise before you open the doors is to make lists of all equipment needs, and then pencil in costs. List everything you can see first: telephone, desk, chair, pencils, computer, computer paper, printer, Xerox machine, lamp, filing cabinet, and so on. As you give each item a price, check classifieds for used equipment prices. When you finish pricing the things you can see, list costs for those important intangibles like insurance, electricity, utilities, taxes, and legal service.

35 Develop a personal financial statement to find out your net worth. This is good practice. It organizes you. In many cases, it builds confidence because it tells you that you're worth more than you thought. Setting down your assets and liabilities on paper is a good beginning for tackling the numbers in business.

36 By now, you probably have some idea of how much money you're going to need for a start-up, how long it will take to break even, and when you'll begin making a profit. Most small businesses don't make money for the first year, and if that's true for your business, you want to face facts now. One way to face facts is to determine how much you'd make in that first year if you *didn't* go into business.

THINK POINTS

- Be prepared for your competition to counter-attack.
- Be aware of closing dates for Yellow Page advertising, and other key media.
- Keep a time log that tells everyone (you, your founders, your key employees) where you are on the Plan.
- Make sure your partners are as committed as you are.
- Develop a checklist of unforeseen circumstances that can hurt your business.
- Always have Plan B.

REFERENCES

Donoghue, William E., with Thomas Trilling. *No-Load Mutual Fund Guide: How to Take Advantage of the Investment Opportunity of the Eighties.* New York: Harper & Row Publishers, 1983. An investment guide which can save your money from a lot of surprises. Donoghue's SLYC system (Safety, Liquidity, Yield, Catastrophe-Proofing) is one smart alternative to small business start-ups. He predicts bank swallow-ups—two dozen superbanks by the end of the eighties. A thought-provoking book.

A Description of Product or Service

B The Market and the Target Customer

C Competition

D Market Strategy

E Location

H Projected Income Statement

I Projected Cash Flow

J Projected Balance Sheet

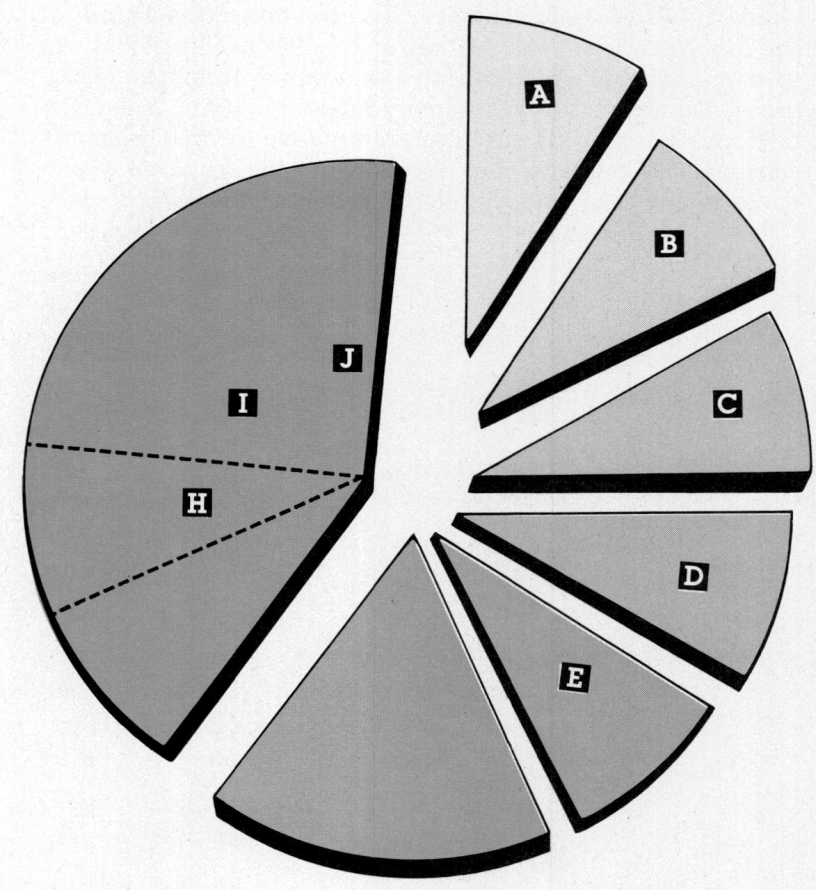

FIGURE 9.1   Chapter 9 helps you generate the financial section of your Plan by bestowing on you the powers of numerical projection.

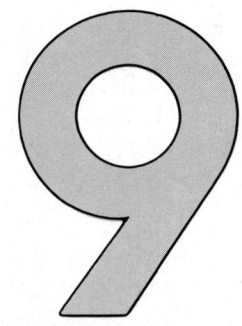

The Powers of Numerical Projection

LEARNING OBJECTIVES

To develop the ability to use numbers to project your business future.

To develop your own strategies for cash management.

To project sales on a monthly basis.

To search your own financial history for creative ideas on how you dealt with shortfalls in the past.

To understand that you pay your bills with cash, not profit.

To understand that the government taxes you on paper profit, whether you have any cash or not.

To learn the power of ratios as a cash management tool.

To create an income statement.

To create a cash flow projection.

To use the powers of numerical projection to help you decide what legal form you will choose for your business.

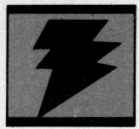

In this chapter, we're going to urge you to launch yourself out across the unknown. We're going to ask you to move past your start-up plans and cantilever your adventure out over an obscure and shapeless future. We're going to ask you to peer into the future with New Eyes and make a brave attempt to forecast what will happen to your business in your first year of operation.

CHART YOUR BUSINESS FUTURE WITH NUMBERS

For example, which months will be strong in your particular business? Which will be weak? What will your sales total be for that first year? For the second? For the third?

How much profit will you make? Or will you be forced to take a loss? How will your projected profit or loss affect the legal form such as partnership or corporation you choose for your business?

Running out of money in business is the end. To avoid running out of money, chart your business future across some numbers and plan, plan, plan.

What will your cash picture look like when you spread those start-up dollars out across a full year? How fast will your business grow? What would rapid growth do to your cash picture?

Has anything in your life prepared you for handling money in business?

Starting with the Past

One easy way to chart your business future is to face your past.

Civilization runs on money, and everyone has ups and downs. What were some of yours? Let Action Step 37 help you face your financial past so you can chart your financial future. You never know when a **Plan B for meeting expenses** will come in handy.

Pulling Together Survival Information

In the previous chapter, you worked out a personal financial statement. In the previous Action Step, you recalled personal survival tactics — how you dealt with money problems in the past. Your next step is to begin building a business budget, which is similar to a **personal budget.** Down below, we've listed four ideas for you to think about, generally, before you plunge into details. They are: sales forecast, seasonality, cash management, and profit and loss.

We'll discuss them briefly before moving on. And remember, your expenses are someone else's sales.

Plan B for meeting expenses
an alternative course of action for paying the bills in emergencies

personal budget
your own financial picture that allows you to meet prioritized dollar needs

1. **Sales Forecast.** Before you jump into a business, you need to figure out how many sales dollars you can produce in a given period of time. You can pull a first-year forecast together by combining information on sales from business owners, trade associations and your own marketing plans.

2. **Seasonality Scenario.** Almost every business will have its peaks and valleys during the year. You need to write a brief **seasonality** scenario for the first year of your particular business.

3. **Cash Management.** Because of time lags (checks clearing, dating, credit sales, credit cards, bad risks, human factors, paperwork, weekends, and so on), you may not get paid the same day you make a sale. Meanwhile, you have to pay cash out for labor, taxes, rent, utilities, and inventory. If your business is going to stay afloat in this turbulent trough between credit and creditors, you have to know where every nickel is. Long before the nickels stop trickling in, you have to make arrangements for help.

   Cash management means knowing where the nickels are every month and maximizing the benefits of the money you are holding.

4. **Profit and Loss.** Unless you are the exception to the rule, you are not going to make lots of money your first week in business, and if you get rich, you will get rich slowly. A projected profit and loss statement will tell you when you are going to start making a profit, which has to come before you start to get rich. And if you're not going to make a profit for a while, you might want to structure your business so that your losses can be deducted from personal taxable income.

HOW TO CHART INCOME BEFORE YOU OPEN YOUR DOORS

Forecasting Sales

The following case study illustrates the value of planning. The case is about a bookstore operation, and it is valuable because the owners went through three important steps:

1. They developed a seasonal scenario so that they were not surprised by the Christmas Crush and the February Blues.
2. They gathered data from their trade association, which gave them ballpark numbers.
3. They developed their own method of projecting sales by using ratios.

In any retail operation, you want to separate your product mix according to how fast it moves. The term for this is "shelf velocity." In the bookstore case, industry data told the owners to separate paperbacks from hardbacks because the shelf velocity for each category was different.

seasonality
the recognition that business, like life, flows in cycles connected to the four seasons

cash management
the tightrope balancing of liquid money resources to obtain maximum benefit from each dollar

ACTION ⚡ STEP 37

Recall Hard Times to Plan for the Future

List the times in your life when you ran out of money; then look ahead.

Part A. Your Personal Money Past. Look back over your life to the days when you were not so street smart, and try to remember hard times.

Where were you and what were you doing? What was your age at the time? How much training did you have? Who was there with you? How many people did you have depending on you? How did you feel about running out of money? Angry? Sick? Depressed? Victimized?

How did you solve the problem? Did you moonlight? Did you get a loan? Did you take out another mortgage? Did you try to tighten your belt and run leaner?

Part B. Your Personal Money Future. Look ahead into the next year, and list your expenses, such as shelter, food, medical expenses, transportation, insurance, phone, school, clothes, and utilities—and then add in 10% for a contingency fund. (If you need a form with blanks to fill in, ask your banker. Banks usually carry personal budget forms for their customers.)

Next, list the tactics you have developed to handle these expenses. If it looks as though you are not going to have enough money, what is your Plan B?

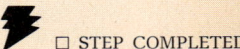 ☐ STEP COMPLETED

Patricia French — Retail Bookstore

We planned every phase of our bookstore operation. My husband, Don, has always been a great reader, and my friends in college used to accuse me of being a bibliophile — but we quickly discovered when we did our research that a bookstore is a business. In business, you either grow fast or you don't survive, so we found ourselves mastering a lot of new skills, fast.

Running a bookstore is not the same as being a happy-go-lucky English major in college.

We worked and saved for several years — bookstores, teaching, advertising — so when we started our business we had over $30,000. In addition, we got our friends interested, and they contributed over $50,000 more. With that in hand, we wrote up an 80-page business plan and went to our banker, who extended us a line of credit for $25,000.

The location we found had about 2,500 square feet of floor space, and data from the ABA (American Bookseller's Association, the major trade association) indicated that sales for that size store in this demographic area would be around $130,000 annually. (Our major competitor had done $150,000.)

The first question was how much to spend on inventory. To answer that, Don used a ratio method of inventory projection.

First, we found the annual **turn ratio** for hardbacks, which was 3. Then we found the annual turn ratio for paperbacks, which sell faster. That was 5.

To find the amount we needed for initial inventory, we first multiplied the percentage for gross sales times the annual sales figure.

Industry figures told us hardbacks would account for 60% of sales (that meant paperbacks would equal 40% of sales):

$$60\% \times \$130,000 = \$78,000 \text{ annual hardback sales}$$

Next, we figured cost of sales, which has gone up. It's now 65%. We multiplied 65% times $78,000. That came to $50,700, which was the annual cost of (hardback) goods sold.

In order to develop the start-up hardback inventory, we divided the cost of goods sold by the annual turn ratio, which for hardbacks was 3.

$$\frac{\$50,700}{3} = \$16,900$$

So we knew our estimated cost for the initial hardback inventory would be $16,900.

We went through the same procedure for paperbacks, multiplying annual sales by percentage of sales and by cost of sales, and then dividing by the turn ratio:

$$\frac{\$130,000 \times 40\% \times 65\%}{5}$$

$$\frac{\$52,000 \times 65\%}{5} = \frac{\$33,800}{5} = \$6,760$$

Continued

Finally, when we added the two figures, we came up with $23,660, or almost $24,000, needed for initial inventory.

It was a lot of money. It was also a relief — to know where we were going.

After we'd been in business for a year, we did an exercise which we should have done before. We plotted out a **scenario for a year,** and we assigned percentages of sales for each month.

A scenario gives you a feel for the future, based on the past.

When we first went into the bookstore, we knew that Christmas would be our **peak time.** But we didn't realize the extent of the peak. That holiday season accounts for at least a third of our business. When you realize that, you can be better prepared. Here's our scenario:

January (6.5%). January is an anticlimax to Christmas, but it's still busy because of gift certificates and exchanges. Don and I run some good specials at the end of January, prior to taking our yearly inventory. Even though sales are slowing down, we have to order new titles, because publishers (our suppliers) are giving us advance notice on their lists for spring.

February (4.5%). Very quiet. We take inventory, weed out stuff that didn't sell, send it back. We meet a lot of publisher's reps, who are out on the road pushing new titles.

March (5%). On March 15th, we have an Ides of March sale. Next year, we're planning a St. Patrick's Day tie-in.

April (5%). Still slow. We get a slight jump in sales after the 15th, mostly because Spring vacation gives some people time to read.

May (8%) and June (8%). Two holidays — Mother's Day, Father's Day — plus weddings and graduation, give us our second busiest season. Art books and gift editions do well. Also encyclopedias and how-tos.

July (6%) and August (7%). We're not in a tourist area, and summers for us are slow. We sell mostly easy-to-read paperbacks and our minds are on ordering books for Christmas.

September (9%). Saved by back-to-school purchases. We're interviewing people for Christmas jobs and making last-minute purchases on gift items.

October (10%) and November (12%). The start of the busy season. Customers sense it, and we can feel the momentum. The rush is just around the corner. We usually hire more sales help at this time.

December (19%). The crush. I work the front while Don stations himself in back, inputting our sales into the computer. We gather information daily so we can spot the direction holiday sales will take. It's different every year, but with two years of data gathering and **charting sales** behind us, Don knows he's getting a feel for what really happens. And that helps us plan ahead for next year.

scenario for a year
combining seasonality with sales percentages to produce a picture of the peaks and valleys of the business cycle

peak time
a high-volume period when maximum inventory and resources are needed

charting sales
a graphic presentation of historical sales data

After the first year of business, sales forecasting will become easier. Keep records that first year, so you'll know how your own peaks and valleys correlate with the seasonality of your industry.

Most businesses are seasonal, and you'll need to develop strong control systems to manage your financial resources. Start now to identify alternate sources of credit and also ways to collect cash from customers before all of your products or services are delivered.

Forecasting Collections

What businesses are seasonal? When can you collect ahead of time?

If you're in the ice cream business, sales will heat up in summer. The same is true of hardware (especially home improvement supplies) and auto parts, when everyone is getting the travel bug.

If you run a ski shop, you might have to order your skis at a summer trade show, pay for them when they arrive in September, and wait until late March to make the final sale.

If, on the other hand, you're in the bed-and-breakfast business, you can collect your money ahead of time — sometimes as far ahead as six months — and have it spent or invested long before you have to deliver the bed and breakfast.

The same is true for airlines, insurance companies, magazines, newspapers, advertising agencies, travel agents, universities that charge tuition, printers, and caterers.

If you're on the receiving end, it's nice to know there are businesses which collect the dollars up front.

What's it like for your business?

Charting Your Income Scenario

Now it's your turn to project an income scenario. Action Step 38 takes you through the process. Note that more than just sales are involved — you will also need to project times of collection and other time lags so you can get a feel for the way cash will flow through your business. The Action Step winds up by asking you a pointed question: Now that you have seen your sales percentages, what **management strategies** will you develop to get more control of your business?

It's better to tackle that question *before* you open your doors. Think about that as you read the following case study. It tells the story of how Laserian, Ltd., a flashy company in a glamorous growth industry, got into money trouble because its CEO didn't bother with cash management.

He was a creative kind of guy.

Case Study

Gerald R. Fiske — Laser Optics

Jerry Fiske's Laserian, Ltd., a manufacturer of laser optics, had just started its second year of operation when it started to run out of money.

Jerry was an engineer and an inventor, and he had been fooling around with lasers for 20 years before he got some backers together to found Laserian, Ltd. He knew lasers, and every instinct told him it was the hottest growth industry going, and when Jerry solved one of the tricky problems in the industry, he knew he was going to be rich and famous.

The problem that Jerry solved was light leakage. Big communications companies were experimenting with sending messages through glass fiber tubes, which were a lot more efficient for carrying information than plain old wires. The messages traveled without a hitch as long

Continued

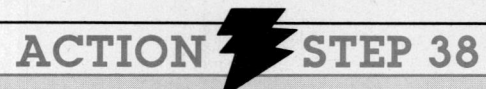

ACTION STEP 38

Spread out the Year in an Income Scenario

Write out a typical scenario for one hypothetical year in your business.

You can do part of the scenario with New Eyes — just look around at obvious forces such as weather, heat, cold, time, and expense — and mix carefully with life cycle, location, and competition as they relate to your business.

You will have to do the rest of the scenario with information gleaned from other small business owners and from trade associations.

When does your industry collect money? Before the sale? During the sale? After the sale? Long after the sale?

When will you have to pay for your inventory?

What is the shortest time lag you could see between the time you pay for inventory and the time you receive money (payment, hard dollars) for the sale of that same inventory?

What is the longest time lag? When will you declare a lag a bad debt?

If you are in manufacturing, and you have to alter or reshape or rebuild the raw materials into a product, what kind of time lag will there be?

Now that you have seen your sales percentages for a year, what management strategies do you need to develop to get more control of your business?

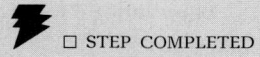 ☐ STEP COMPLETED

management strategies
making directional decisions

as the tubes were straight, but whenever there was a bend in the tube, some of the light would continue on in a straight line.

Result: light leakage and a garbled message.

Jerry solved the problem with a special coating inside the tube which would bounce the light into a graceful curve, and thus help it to glide around corners.

At the moment he ran short of cash, Jerry was working in the lab on no less than a dozen different applications of his discovery. At the same time, other Laserian engineer-inventors were designing a new scanner that would read labels for the food industry.

At Laserian, Ltd., the research and development people, who ran the place, came to Jerry to tell him the company needed a **cash injection.**

"We're out of money, Jerry. What's the story?"

Jerry didn't know. So he put on his coat and tie and went off to see Phil Brill, his banker.

First Visit

"Jerry," Phil said, shaking hands. "Glad you called. Long time, no see."

Jerry handed Phil a roughed-out profit and loss statement on the back of an envelope. Phil took the envelope, glanced at the figures, then looked at Jerry.

"How's the laser business, anyway?"

"Booming," Jerry said. "We've got orders pouring in for this new scanner. Every food chain in the country wants one the day before yesterday. We're starting up production of a new holographic camera — one that will take pictures of automobile tires to check for defects. The Air Force has sent six guys around because they want us to sign a contract to work on a new cryptographic device. The numbers speak for themselves, Phil. We did $300,000 in sales this month and had a profit of $52,000 plus."

The banker looked at the numbers on the envelope:

Sales $300k

Cost of Goods Sold $172k

Gross Profit $108k

Expenses $76k

Profit $52k plus

"How much do you need?"

"Thirty thou should do it, Phil. Just for odds and ends until our receivables start pouring in."

Jerry was one of those guys who could pick up key words and use them right away. "Receivables" was one of those words.

"From the look of these numbers," Phil said. "I'd say you'd be good for it."

Jerry smiled. This was easy street. "I never argue about money," he said.

Later that week, he had a check for $30,000. He turned the check over to his manager and got back into the lab, where he was happy.

One month later, Laserian ran short of cash again.

Second Visit

"Sorry to bother you again, Phil," Jerry said. "But we need another short green transfusion." Jerry was smiling. He had received money before, and he knew this was a piece of cake.

Continued

cash injection
infusion of dollars into a business, usually at a critical point in history of the business

"How much this time?" the banker said.

"What about ninety grand?" Jerry asked.

"Sounds steep," Phil said. "What's your cash picture?"

Jerry smiled. "We're in terrific shape, Phil." Jerry handed the banker a sheet of graph paper that contained a short column of numbers. "Take a look at this month."

	Feb.
Sales	$320,000
Cost of Goods Sold	184,000
Gross Profit	136,000
Expenses	87,000
Profit	49,000

The banker studied the figures without saying anything.

"Feast your eyes, Phil. Sales are up over last month. The total profit for the last two months is over a hundred grand. If things keep up at this rate, we'll have $5 million in sales by the end of the year. And that means a million in profits."

The banker looked up at Jerry. "What's the money for?" he asked.

"Plastic," Jerry said. "Everything we build is housed in plastic, and my purchasing guy found a real deal. That stuff's made with oil, you know, and if the world runs short of oil, we've got to have enough plastic to get us through."

"A sound point," Phil said.

"I'm in kind of a hurry, Phil. When can I get the check?"

"Can you have your accountant get me a completed profit and loss statement?" Phil asked. "And do something on **cash flow**?"

"Can do," Jerry said. "I'll get my people right on it."

"Let us see the numbers," Phil said. "I'll get back to you."

Walking out of the bank, Jerry was disappointed in the banker's conservative attitude. He thought briefly of changing banks, then swung his mind back to the excitement of lasers.

Back at the plant, he told his manager to do up a profit and loss statement and a cash flow projection, and then he got back to his inventing.

This time, it took the bank almost three weeks to approve the loan. And two loan officers came out to have a look at Laserian, Ltd.

Apparently, they liked what they saw, because the check came through just in time.

The $90,000 lasted only a couple of months, so Fiske went to see his banker for a third time.

Third Visit

"I'll bet you know why I'm here," Jerry said.

"You'd better tell me, just the same," Phil said.

This time, Jerry was ready with some computerized **spreadsheets.** He unrolled them in front of the banker. "Look at those numbers, Phil. Feast your eyes. That's over a million in sales you're looking at. It's also over $220,000 in profits, counting next month. The sales are already on the books, and we're showing a backlog that will carry us for two more months."

The banker studied the **spreadsheets.** (See Table 9.1) He noticed they covered only the first four months.

Continued

cash flow
the lifeblood of any
business

spreadsheets
displays of critical
accounting data

Phil was a banker. Numbers were his business. He'd seen thousands of spreadsheets come across his desk. He knew that fast growth could kill a company that wasn't ready for it.

"How much do you need this time, Jerry?"

Jerry smiled. He thought he'd found a money tree.

"Thirteen thousand looks like what we need, but I thought we could double that, just to be on the safe side." Jerry paused. "Let's say $30,000."

"You're already into us for $120,000," the banker said. "Before you get any more, I'd like to discuss how we're getting the one-twenty back."

"Hey," Jerry said. "I'm good for it. Look at those numbers!"

The room was silent. For a long time, the banker didn't say anything. When he finally said something, it was no.

TABLE 9.1   The Laserian, Ltd., Income Statement

	Jan.	Feb.	Mar.	Apr.	Totals (four months)
Sales	300,000	320,000	360,000	380,000	1,360,000
Cost of Goods Sold	172,500	184,000	207,000	218,500	782,000
Gross Profit	127,500	136,000	153,000	161,500	578,000
Expenses					
Sales — Commissions	27,000	28,800	32,400	34,100	
Advertising/Promotional	1,500	1,600	1,800	1,900	
Travel	500	5,000	2,000	5,000	
Equipment Rental	800	800	800	800	
Auto/Truck	1,300	1,300	1,300	1,300	
Repair/Maintenance	800	800	900	900	
Rent	12,000	12,000	12,000	12,000	
Supplies	1,500	1,600	1,800	1,900	
Telephone	4,000	4,400	4,900	5,300	
Utilities	1,200	1,200	1,200	1,200	
Insurance	1,700	1,700	1,700	1,700	
Legal/Accounting	2,500	2,500	2,500	2,500	
Dues/Subscriptions	250	400	400	400	
Salary — Management	15,000	16,000	17,000	18,000	
Salary — Staff	3,000	5,000	7,000	9,000	
Miscellaneous	1,000	1,100	1,100	1,200	
Interest on Bank Loan		1,900	1,900	1,900	
Payroll Taxes	1,300	1,500	1,700	1,900	
Total Expenses	75,350	87,600	92,400	101,000	356,350
Net Before Taxes	52,150	48,400	60,600	60,500	221,650
Tax Reserve	23,450	21,800	27,300	27,300	99,850
Net Profit After Taxes	28,700	26,600	33,300	33,200	121,800

What Went Wrong?

Bankers don't like surprises. The banker's job is to protect bank depositors, and bankers all over the world worry about small firms that don't plan in advance. Jerry Fiske's banker did not feel that the bank could afford to underwrite Laserian's prosperity, which was based on uncontrolled growth, regardless of Laserian's **gross profit.**

Therefore, Jerry Fiske did not get the money he needed to sustain the rapid growth of his company. The company was out of control, and Jerry didn't see it even when the numbers were down on paper.

What could Jerry have done differently? If he had prepared a cash flow projection ahead of time, his shortfall would have been predicted, and he could have applied for one big loan instead of a series of smaller, haphazard loans. Table 9.2 shows what that ideal cash flow

gross profit | net sales minus cost of goods sold

TABLE 9.2   Jerry Fiske wishes that the Laserian, Ltd., Statement of Cash Flow looked like this.

	Jan.	Feb.	Mar.	Apr.
Cash-on-Hand/Start of Month	10,000	170,800	74,900	52,100
Cash Received/Accounts Receivable	210,000	280,000	316,000	352,000
Three-Year Bank Loan	200,000			
Total Cash Available	420,000	450,800	390,900	404,100
Cash Disbursements				
Manufacturing Disbursements				
Packing, etc.	18,000	19,000	21,000	23,000
Material	123,000	224,000	172,000	198,000
Outside Labor	44,000	49,000	53,000	57,800
Other Disbursements				
Sales — Commissions	14,000	27,000	28,800	32,400
Salary — Management	12,000	12,800	13,600	14,400
Salary — Staff	2,700	4,500	6,000	7,600
Payroll Taxes	4,500	4,500	5,300	6,000
Advertising/Promotional	1,400	1,500	1,600	1,800
Travel	500	500	5,000	2,000
Auto/Truck	1,300	1,300	1,300	1,300
Equipment Rental	2,400			2,400
Repair/Maintenance	800	800	900	900
Rent	12,000	12,000	12,000	12,000
Supplies	1,400	1,500	1,600	1,800
Telephone	2,500	4,000	4,400	4,900
Utilities	1,200	1,200	1,200	1,200
Insurance	4,000			
Legal/Accounting	2,500	2,500	2,500	2,500
Dues/Subscriptions		1,200		
Miscellaneous	1,000	1,100	1,100	1,200
Loan		7,500	7,500	7,500
Total Disbursements	249,200	375,900	338,800	378,700
Cash Flow for Month	170,800	74,900	52,100	25,400

would look like with an adequate loan of $200,000 in place. The bottom line in Table 9.2 is "Cash Flow for Month."

What you aim for — over and above paper profits — is positive cash flow. You want enough money available so that you can buy what you need to stay in business.

Now let's revise Table 9.2 by taking away Jerry's one-time loan of $200,000 and watch why Jerry had to run to the banker so often. January's cash flow becomes negative ($170,800 − $200,000 = − $29,200). No wonder Jerry needed to borrow $30,000 in a hurry! This negative cash flow carries on through. If we assume that Jerry wasn't able to borrow any money at all, our revised cash flows for each month would be

	Jan.	Feb.	Mar.	Apr.
Cash-on-Hand/Start of Month	$ 10,000	$(29,200)	$(117,600)	$(132,900)
Cash Received/Accounts Receivable	210,000	280,000	316,000	352,000
Bank Loans	—	—	—	—
Total Cash Available	220,000	250,800	198,400	219,100
Total Disbursements	249,200	368,400	331,300	371,200
Cash Flow for Month	$(29,200)	$(117,600)	$(132,900)	$(152,100)

If you're figuring along, you'll notice that Total Disbursements now differ from the Total Disbursements in Table 9.2. This is because if there is no loan, there won't be any loan payments of $7,500 in February, March, and April. Note also that in spreadsheets, a negative amount like − $29,000 is often shown in parentheses, as $(29,000).

Fortunately, Jerry bagged a few loans, but another quick revision of the cash flow shows that $30,000 in January and $90,000 in February weren't enough:

	Jan.	Feb.	Mar.	Apr.
Cash-on-Hand/Start of Month	$ 10,000	$ 800	$ 2,400	$(12,900)
Cash Received/Accounts Receivable	210,000	280,000	316,000	352,000
Bank Loans	30,000	90,000	—	—
Total Cash Available	250,000	370,800	318,400	339,100
Total Disbursements	249,200	368,400	331,300	371,200
Cash Flow for Month	$ 800	$ 2,400	$(12,900)	$(32,100)

And remember, for these same four months, Laserian, Ltd., showed $121,800 of net profit after taxes.

What's the Moral?

Although Laserian was profitable on paper (see Table 9.1), every month that sales increased saw an increase as well in accounts receivable (money owed the company but not yet paid). Because the company was expanding, money had to flow into inventory. Past sales could not generate enough cash to support the growth. Without outside sources of cash, the company could not keep up.

> **Project your income and cash flow ahead of time.**

Project your income and cash flow *before* you open your doors — for at least a year in advance. If your numerical projections are sound, your banker will be likely to loan you a large amount for start-up costs. If your projections are haphazard, you may get the same answer that Jerry Fiske got when asking for a lesser amount: *No.*

INCOME STATEMENT AND CASH FLOW: IMPORTANT PROJECTIONS

A projected income statement tells you when you're going to make a profit on paper. A cash flow projection tells you whether or not you can pay the bills and when you'll have to visit the banker. Both the income statement and the cash flow projection are necessary for the survival of your business.

Projected Income Statement

When you project your income statement, it's like projecting a moving picture of your business. If you're careful in how you prepare your numbers, that movie can be reasonably accurate. Action Step 39 leads you through this projection step by step. (*Note:* You already have a head start because you forecast sales in Action Step 38.) We also supply you with a worksheet from the SBA (see Figure 9.2).

If you discover you won't be making a profit for the first two years, you're going to need a very good plan, a team of terrific investors, and an understanding banker.(See the case study on Herman, Terry, and Mitch for what to do when your Business Plan forecasts losses for the first year or so of operation.)

Cash Flow Projection

As we learned in the preceding case study on Jerry Fiske, an income statement doesn't tell you the whole story — even a documentary movie is shot from only one angle at a time. It's nice to watch paper profits, but you also need to see what is happening to real cash. Figure 9.3, on page 170, shows the typical pattern of cash flow: a lot of worry until real profits appear.

ACTION ⚡ STEP 39

Project an Income Statement — A Moving Picture of Your Business

You may want to adapt the SBA worksheet "Projected Statement of Sales and Expenses for One year," reproduced on the opposite page, for use in this Action Step.

Part A. First generate your numbers for the year as follows:

1. Using data from trade associations and small business owners, forecast your sales for the year.

2. Figure your cost of goods sold, subtract that from sales, and you have gross profit.

3. Add up all expenses and subtract those from gross profit. That gives you the net before taxes.

4. Subtract taxes. (Uncle Sam, who uses what we might call Old Eyes, will tax you on paper profit, so you have to build this figure in.)

The figure at the bottom is net profit after taxes for the year.

Part B. Now spread these figures out month by month to create a kind of moving picture of your business. Your net profit, after taxes, may be negative for a number of months during your start-up.

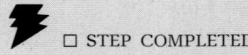
⚡ □ STEP COMPLETED

Projected Statement of Sales and Expenses for One Year

	Total	Jan	Feb	Mar	Apr	May	Jun	Jul	Aug	Sep	Oct	Nov	Dec
A. Net Sales													
B. Cost of Goods Sold													
1. Raw Materials													
2. Direct Labor													
3. Manufacturing Overhead													
Indirect Labor													
Factory Heat, Light, and Power													
Insurance and Taxes													
Depreciation													
C. Gross Margin (Subtract B from A)													
D. Selling and Administrative Expenses													
4. Salaries and Commissions													
5. Advertising Expenses													
6. Miscellaneous Expenses													
E. Net Operating Profit (Subtract D from C)													
F. Interest Expense													
G. Net Profit before Taxes (Subtract F from E)													
H. Estimated Income Tax													
I. Net Profit after Income Tax (Subtract H from G)													

SOURCE: Small Business Administration, *Business Plan for Small Manufacturers*, SBA Management Aid 2.007 (Small Business Administration: Washington, D.C., 1981), 8.

Cash flow projection is a tool to help you control money.

Now that you understand the need for not running out of cash, here's a tool to help you control its flow. Action Step 40 (see page 172) leads you through a monthly cash flow projection. We also supply an SBA worksheet you can use to prepare your projection (see Figure 9.4 on page 171).

When you're through with Action Step 40, show the results to an expert. Does the picture look accurate? It's better to know the truth now, while you're working on paper. Paper truth is a lot easier on the pocketbook than real truth.

FIGURE 9.2 This worksheet from the SBA will allow you to project a yearly income statement— and to spread your projections out month by month.

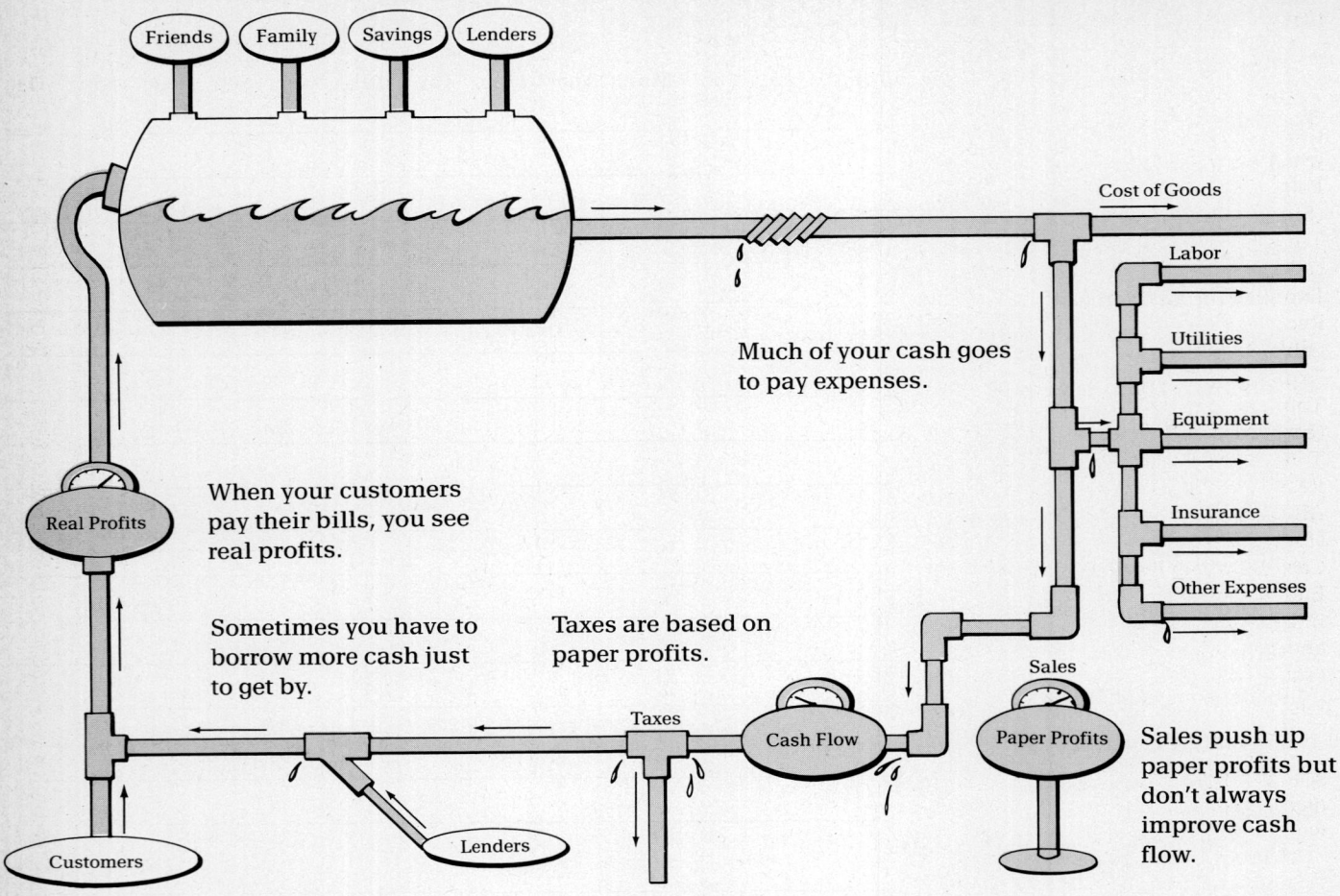

When your customers pay their bills, you see real profits.

Sometimes you have to borrow more cash just to get by.

Taxes are based on paper profits.

Much of your cash goes to pay expenses.

Sales push up paper profits but don't always improve cash flow.

WHAT ARE THE KEY NUMBERS IN YOUR BUSINESS?

Knowing a few key numbers can help you avoid painful surprises. If you know your costs (variable and fixed) and your gross sales, you can use a couple of break-even formulas to tell you when you will start making money. Break-even is handy at start-up time, after you have completed your cash flow projections, and also anytime you are ready to launch a new product or service.

FIGURE 9.3 This simple cash flow diagram shows the typical time lag between the dry rattle of paper profits and the thundering gush of real profits. Unless you plan ahead for that lag, you could find yourself high and dry.

Case Study

Break-Even Analysis

A small manufacturing company was completing a plan for its second year of operation. Their first year sales were $177,000. Their fiscal year ended in December. A sales breakdown for the last three months of their first year looked like this:

Continued

Estimated Cash Forecast

	Jan	Feb	Mar	Apr	May	Jun	Jul	Aug	Sep	Oct	Nov	Dec
1. Cash in Bank (Start of Month)												
2. Petty Cash (Start of Month)												
3. Total Cash (add 1 and 2)												
4. Expected Accounts Receivable												
5. Other Money Expected												
6. Total Receipts (add 4 and 5)												
7. Total Cash and Receipts (add 3 and 6)												
8. All Disbursements (for month)												
9. Cash Balance at End of Month in Bank Account and Petty Cash (subtract 8 from 7)*												

* This balance is your starting cash balance for the next month.

SOURCE: Small Business Administration, *Business Plan for Small Manufacturers*, SBA Management Aid 2.007 (Small Business Administration: Washington, D.C., 1981), 9.

FIGURE 9.4 A second worksheet from the SBA allows you to project monthly cash flow.

October	$24,000
November	29,000
December	15,000
	$68,000

The owners took a look at the numbers and called in a consultant to help. The consultant gathered information from sales reps, owners, and customers and projects sales for the second year at a whopping $562,000. The owners reacted with disbelief.

"You're crazy," they said. "That's over three times what we did last year."

The consultant smiled. " Didn't you tell me you were going to add three new products?"

"Yes."

"And new reps in March, June, and September?"

"Yes, but—"

"And what about those big promotions you've got planned?"

"Well, sure. We've planned some promotion. But that doesn't get us anywhere near three times last year.

"All right," the accountant said. "Can you do $275,000?"

The owners got into a huddle. Based on the fourth quarter, they were sure they could stay even, and 4 times $68,000 (4th quarter sales) was $272,000. They knew they had to do better than last year.

"Sure. No problem. We can do $272,000."

"All right." said the consultant, rolling out his break-even chart.

Continued

"I've just projected $562,000 in sales for the year. To break even, you only need $275,000."

"Hey," the owners said. "We're projecting $90,000 the first quarter."

"I'm glad you're thinking my way," the consultant said. "Because if you don't believe you can reach a goal, you'll never get there." He paused, then said: "By the way, that $90,000 is three times what you did your first quarter last year!"

"Just tell us what to do," the owners said.

Based on a careful cash-flow analysis, the consultant determined that the company would need to borrow money. They knew their business—industry trends, product line, competitors, sales and promotion plans—but there was no way the bankers would believe a tripling of growth. The key to getting the loan was to convince the bankers the company could do better than the break-even, at $275,000. The break-even chart (see Figure 9.5) was built on the $562,000 sales figure.

Footnote: The banker granted the loan because he realized the company could pass the break-even point, and then some. The key, as usual in business, was a combination of numbers and human confidence.

In Figure 9.5, note that after $280,000 in sales the firm has passed its break-even point and is making a profit.

PROJECTIONS HELP DECIDE YOUR BUSINESS FORM

Working with numbers (sales projections and cash flow) can help you decide the legal form your business takes. The three partners in the next case were smart. Numerical projections told them they would not make a profit for several months after they opened the doors. So they held onto their jobs and used the losses to offset their regular income.

Once they understood that the break-even point would not occur until the end of the first eight months, they chose a Subchapter S corporation—a legal form which gives you some protection while at the same time it allows you to write losses off on your personal income tax.

Case Study

Herman, Terry, and Mitch — The Numbers Talk

Three bowling buddies got together over beers one night after a big win over the best team in their league, and they started griping about their jobs.

"My boss hates my guts," Herman said. "I feed him great ideas and he just shoots them down. Boom!"

"Yeah," Terry said. "I came up with a boiler plate that would save
Continued

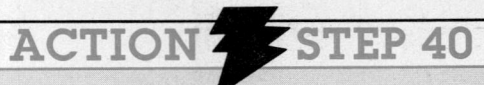

ACTION STEP 40

Project Your Cash Flow — Spreading out the Green

If you don't have access to a computer and an electronic spreadsheet program, get yourself a spreadsheet from your bank or adapt the worksheet from the SBA on page 171 and begin projecting your cash across the first year of your business.

1. Write down all the cash you'll start the year with.

2. For each month, enter the amount of cash you'll receive from sales or accounts receivable.

3. Enter any loans in the month you receive the cash from the lender.

4. Total the above, which will give you the cash available for each month.

5. Now list all disbursements (cash going out). Spread these out, too.

6. Then subtract disbursements from cash available which gives you a monthly cash flow. Carry this figure forward (to point one for each succeeding month).

7. Now examine your work. Have you explored the quirks of seasonality? Have you discovered the minimum and maximum time lags between when you make a sale and when the business gets paid in cash for that sale? Does the picture look accurate? Have you checked with an expert?

8. Try the What-If Test:

If your cash-flow picture looks good, you can test your money management skills by dropping in a couple of what-ifs.

What surprise expenses could throw a monkey wrench into your new business?

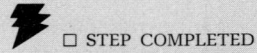 ☐ STEP COMPLETED

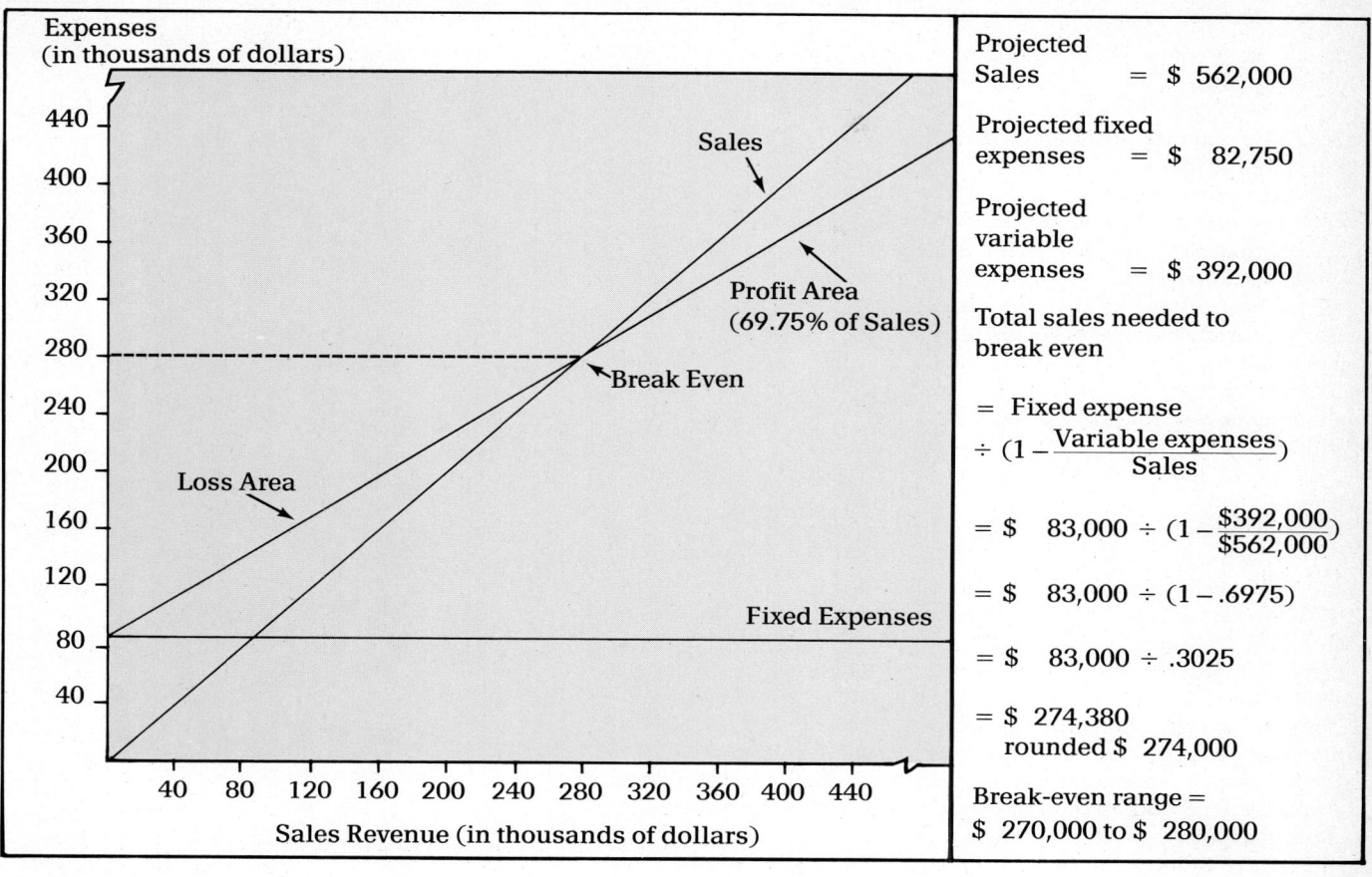

Expenses (in thousands of dollars) [y-axis: 40, 80, 120, 160, 200, 240, 280, 320, 360, 400, 440]

Sales

Profit Area (69.75% of Sales)

Break Even

Loss Area

Fixed Expenses

Sales Revenue (in thousands of dollars) [x-axis: 40, 80, 120, 160, 200, 240, 280, 320, 360, 400, 440]

Projected Sales = $ 562,000

Projected fixed expenses = $ 82,750

Projected variable expenses = $ 392,000

Total sales needed to break even

= Fixed expense

$\div (1 - \dfrac{\text{Variable expenses}}{\text{Sales}})$

= $ 83,000 $\div (1 - \dfrac{\$392,000}{\$562,000})$

= $ 83,000 $\div$ (1 − .6975)

= $ 83,000 $\div$ .3025

= $ 274,380 rounded $ 274,000

Break-even range = $ 270,000 to $ 280,000

FIGURE 9.5 A simple break-even chart like this may be all it takes to convince your banker that a small loan now means big profits later.

my company upwards of $50k per annum, and they just smiled me out the door.''

"Both of you should quit," Mitch said, "and go into the pizza business with me."

"Too risky," Terry said. "Statistics show you can lose your house and everything when you start too small."

"I worked in a restaurant once," Herman said. "Back in high school. For the people who owned it, it was like coining money. Especially during the season."

"Does that mean you're interested?" Mitch asked. "Or just being your old late-fifties self?"

"I'm interested," Herman said, draining his beer glass. "And so is Terry the Numbers Man."

Terry worked in his company's accounting department. He knew the ins and outs of pro forma statements and cash flow management.

"I think there's room in this town for an innovative pizza parlor," Terry said. "My brother-in-law's into one in Duluth, and I've seen the books for his second year. He's making a profit just on the write-off."

"I like it," Herman said. "I like the sound of being my own boss."

"Herman Smith," Mitch said. "The Great Entrepreneur."

"My advice," Terry said, "is to hang on to your jobs while I pull some numbers together. They'll tell us a lot."

"Well, hurry it up," Herman said. "My boss is on my nerves."

Terry worked four solid weeks on the numbers. Herman and Mitch couldn't believe it took so long. They had both drawn up personal

Continued

financial statements. They were both ready to put $20,000 each into Three-Way Pizza—the name they'd settled on.

Then Terry came back with the bad news. He showed it to them on pale green computer printouts. All Herman and Mitch could understand were the totals.

All three partners were putting in $20,000 apiece. That was a total of $60,000 to start a business. Just the sound made them feel rich.

In addition, they were borrowing $30,000 from family and friends. Total start-up capital—$90,000. A king's ransom.

"Expenses will eat us alive the first year," Terry explained. "Even with the leased equipment. As you can see, the big expenses are for salaries and supplies. We've got to have a first-rate hostess, and they don't come cheap. And if we go into the pizza delivery business, where the money is, we won't reach the break-even point for at least eight months."

"Lucky for me I didn't kiss off my boss," Herman said. He felt depressed.

"Ninety grand," Mitch said, "is just a drop in the bucket."

"There is a way," Terry said. "Let me talk to my buddy, John, the tax lawyer. He specializes in small businesses."

"All lawyers are crooks," Herman said. "Why, I remember, back in Oshkosh, there was this lawyer who. . . ."

Terry and Mitch met with John, the tax lawyer, while Herman went bowling alone. The lawyer came up with the following solution:

Three-Way Pizza should be chartered as a **Subchapter S Corporation.** (The S stands for *small.*) All three partners were in a 40% tax bracket. Except for their families, they had few deductions. As founders of a Subchapter S Corporation, they could deduct early business losses on their personal income tax returns.

"Hey." Herman said, when he heard. "This is better than my crummy tax shelter plan at work. Why didn't you guys think of this in the first place?"

Three-Way Pizza opened in February, three months before the start of the summer season. It lost money for seven and a half months, but then began making a small profit. The partners were better off at tax time. And by the second year, they were realizing a nice profit.

At that time, they converted to a regular corporation.

Subchapter S Corporation
a small, closely held corporation that is taxed like a sole proprietorship

SUMMARY

Entrepreneurs have problems with charting business numbers for a couple of reasons: 1) they're typically in a hurry and do not take the time to sit down and do the figuring, and 2) they're creative and highly visual with their information intake—numbers turn them off or make them nervous.

The trick when working with numbers is to make them realistic and not hypothetical. That means you relate every projected number to your business and to industry standards, and you document your projections in your Business Plan.

When you read a case study about a crazy inventor who keeps his numbers on the back of an envelope and who keeps asking for money because he cannot track cash flow, your immediate response will likely be to close the book and say, ''That fellow should have been more businesslike and stayed on top of his finances.''

But if you were in the ice cream business and you knew you could double your sales with a new $5,000 freezer, and you went to your banker and asked for money and he looked at your envelope with your scrawled numbers and shook his head—well, you would have a different feeling about *that* situation.

Because the numbers were *your* numbers.

And that is the secret. You need to make *your* numbers believable by keeping them realistic and by documenting them properly. Your numbers will always speak to you. You have to make sure they speak to others.

THINK POINTS

⚡ It's cheaper to make your errors on a spreadsheet, before you go into business.

⚡ An income projection can help tell you what legal form is best for your business. It you're going to make lots of money early, think about incorporating. (For tips, see Chapter 12.)

⚡ When you work out numbers for your Business Plan, hit the return-on-investment section with underlines.

⚡ When you visit your banker to ask for money, make sure you know how much you're going to need way out there in the future.

⚡ Projecting will help you control the variables of your business — numbers, employees, promotion mix, product mix, and the peaks and valleys of seasonality.

REFERENCES

Bank of America Marketing Publications Department. *Bookstores.* Small Business Reporter Series. San Francisco: Bank of America, 1979. The B of A SBR series has several excellent booklets that contain information on ratios and other hard-to-find items. Most B of A branches have booklets on hand, or you can write SBR Series, Bank of America, Department 3120, P.O. Box 37000, San Francisco, CA 94137.

Business Plan for Retailers. Washington, D.C.: Small Business Administration, 1981.

Business Plan for Small Manufacturers. Washington, D.C.: Small Business Administration, 1981.

Milling, Bryan E. *Cash-Flow Problem-Solver.* Radnor, Pa.: Chilton Book Co., 1981.

Purcell, W. R. *Understanding a Company's Finances: A Graphic Approach.* Boston: Houghton Mifflin, Co., 1981.

ACTION ⚡ STEP
REVIEW

Four Action Steps help you bring your numbers into focus:

37 Close your eyes and recall a couple of times in your life when you ran out of money, or when you had to scratch for money. Where were you? How old were you? Did it affect you alone? Did it affect others? Could it have been avoided? Did you feel victimized? Trapped? Angry? Depressed? Hopeless? Ready to fight?

How much money did you need to lift you out of your tight spot?

38 The next thing to do is to develop a typical sales scenario for your business for one year. This is very important! Every business has peaks, when sales are hot, when you will have to hire extra people. Using industry data, you should plot out percentages of sales for each month of the year.

39 Once you have projected sales for a year, you can develop your income statement. The income statement shows you when you are going to start making a profit. Take this in small bites, as outlined in the Action Step. As you follow that outline, remember that these are *your* numbers. They affect the survival of *your* business.

40 A cash flow projection tells you whether or not you can pay the bills. If you are going to run out of money seven months after you open the doors, and you know about it early, you have the breathing room to plan. Again take the cash flow projection in small bites, as outlined. When you have finished, check your work. Add an emergency fund for unforeseen surprises. Then have your work checked by an expert.

A Description of Product or Service

B The Market and the Target Customer

C Competition

D Marketing Strategy

E Location

H Projected Income Statement

I Projected Cash Flow

J Projected Balance Sheet

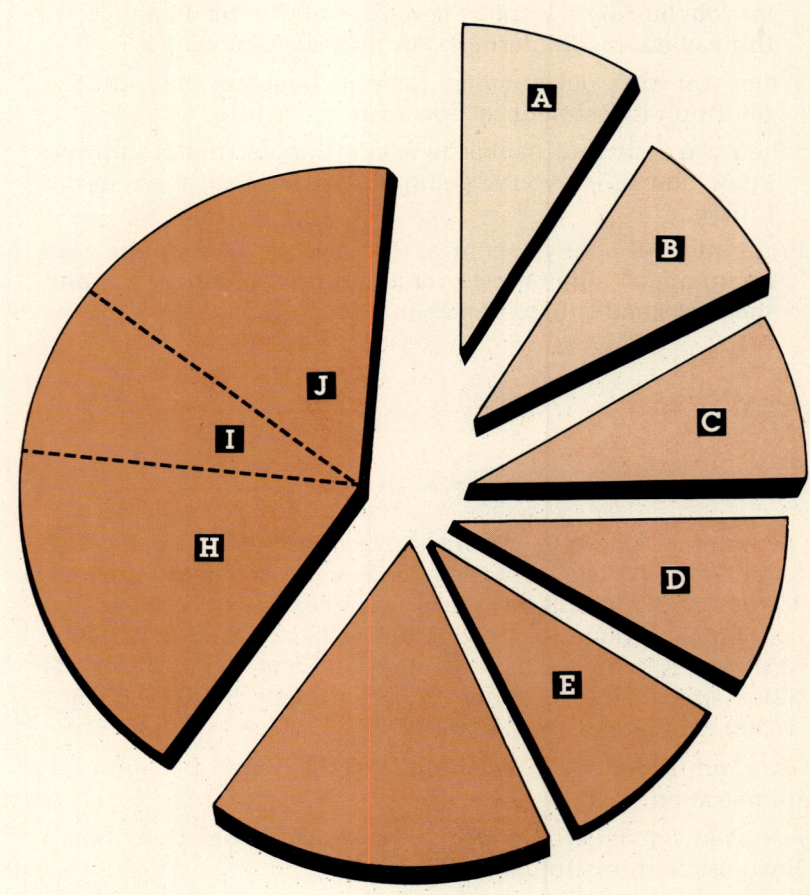

FIGURE 10.1 Chapter 10 prepares you for dealing with the financial section of your plan by taking you through the world of money.

10

Shaking the Money Tree

LEARNING OBJECTIVES

To understand that you need to establish connections in the world of money.

To understand that your banker can be one gateway to the world of money.

To develop strategies for working with your banker.

To develop more sophistication when you conceptualize money and its power.

To develop confidence and street survival skills in the worlds of high and low finance.

To learn how to seek out potential lenders.

To learn how to generate cash from customers.

To develop a vendor application that will allow you to make intelligent purchasing decisions quickly.

To scour the lending arena for dollars to fund your new business.

To probe the highest offices of government to request help with this enterprise and with future enterprises.

 **D**oes it sound too easy if we tell you simply to go out and shake a money tree to find financing for your small business? It may not be quite that easy. First you must become familiar with the world of money. Then you must be able to tell the forest from the trees. And then you must find the right tree. On the other hand, you might be surprised at how money turns up if you start looking for it.

LOOKING FOR MONEY

Before we get to specifics, let's follow one man as he makes discoveries about the world of money.

Case Study

The Organization Man Who Needed to Escape or Go Mad

Once upon a time, there was a man who hated his job.

His name was Alexander Adams. He was employed by HAL Corporation, a giant telecommunications conglomerate, headquartered in upstate New York. The year he decided to escape, Alex's title was Assistant to the Associate Vice President for Region X, Subsection C, Department of Marketing and Market Research.

At HAL, Alex's forte was product development. His territory was the East Coast, from New England to South Carolina. He worked 50–70 hours a week and traveled away from home at least two weeks out of three. Alex was married to the former Jayne M. Barrows, of Grosse Pointe, Michigan. They had two children, Donna, 13, and George Roy, 11. Donna was the scholar of the family. Her dream was to live in Paris, attend the Cordon Bleu School, and paint street scenes from the 19th century. George Roy's dream was to drop out of school, join the CIA, and fight international terrorism.

Alex Adams was creative. He was valuable to HAL because his innovative ideas allowed his employer to change the competitive arena. For example, when the company brought out its famous HAL-PC, Alex had the idea, late at night, to follow the PC up with HAL-XT (a PC loaded with a Winchester hard disk), and then with HAL-JR, a pint-sized teenage HAL with muscle and the capability to run most of HAL's software.

Down deep, Alex knew that the computer was a toy and that the great international electronic networking apparatus was just so much gossip at light-speed. But money was money, and his experience told him it did not grow on trees, so he kept working on new ideas. He used his kids as a Capability Lab. If Donna (and especially the restless George Roy) could stay with something 30 minutes and not get bored, Alex would take the idea upstairs, to the boys higher in the HAL pyramid.

The problem was that the boys upstairs shot 78% of his ideas down. And it always hurt.

Continued

One day in May, after he had gone in with a really terrific idea and watched them take their crazy potshots, Alex made a decision. He told his wife about it at dinner.

"I'm getting out," he said. "I've had enough."

"Have some more meat, dear," Jayne said. She had seen her husband in these moods before. Eventually, he got back into the company harness.

"Remember the idea I had last night? The one about the double mini-disks in one slot and the Winchester in the other?"

"Of course," Jayne lied. "I remember all your ideas, dear."

"Well, they shot it down. Bang-bang. Just like that."

"Who did, dear?"

"The whole gang. Armstrong, White, Baxter, Angeleno, even my pal, Fred Samson. This is the fifth time in two months. I feel strangled. I feel caged. If I don't get out, I'll go crazy."

"Don't talk foolishness, dear. We have a lovely life." Jayne indicated the house, the china, and the fancy wedding crystal in the glass cabinet, but Alex knew she was talking also about the country club, the parties, and her women friends. Just last week, Jayne had been invited to lunch by Mrs. William H. Thorngill, wife of HAL's CEO. Letitia Thorngill (*née* Atwater) was the Queen of Armonk society, and Jayne Barrows Adams wanted in.

"Yes," he said. "And I'm paying for the whole shebang with pounds of my flesh."

"It scares me to hear you talk that way, dear."

"It scares me not to." he said, and left the table.

Alex got most of his good ideas in dreams. That night, he dreamed about a man on a shady park bench. The man wore a Palm Beach suit. A straw boater rested on the bench beside him, on top of a folded copy of the *Wall Street Journal.*

The man was feeding the pigeons. One of the pigeons was Alex Adams. When Alex recognized his own face above the plump body of a pigeon eating corn nuts, he woke, sweating.

On his next business trip, Alex found himself in New York. He had twenty minutes between meetings, so he took a walk in Central Park. It was a lovely day, soft air, the smell of blossoms. As he came around a bend in the walk, he saw the man in the Palm Beach suit. He was feeding pigeons. As Alex came up, the man smiled, said hello, held out his hand. Alex took it. The hand was rough with age, strong, steady. For some reason — the sharp blue eyes, probably — the man reminded Alex of his grandfather on the farm back in Missouri. They talked. The man in the Palm Beach suit seemed to know a lot about finance. He hinted that he had been an unofficial adviser to three U.S. Presidents and one successful Balkan Prince! Alex told the man about his job, his feeling of being caged, and his desire to escape. The man offered Alex some free advice.

"I felt that way once," the man said. "When they wanted me to go into the family business, up Armonk way. I was afraid to go out on my own. And yet I heard the call of adventure. If I'd worked in the family business, I'd have gone crazy early. It should be easier now, because the financial market is so splintered, and there are a ton of opportunities out there. Here's what I'd do if I were your age — first, hang on to your job while you build up some personal credit. Do you get those offers in the mail — just sign your name here for credit?"

"Sure. I throw them away."

"Well, start gathering them together."

Continued

Alex could get a hundred thousand in credit, the man said, just by signing his John Henry.

"You own your house?" the old man asked.

"Yes," Alex smiled. "And so does the bank."

"Use your house as collateral to open another line of personal credit. Where do you bank?"

"One of the big interstates."

"All right. Find out whether or not they lend money to small operators. If they don't, you find yourself a smaller bank — one where you can shake hands with the president when you go in to do business. What's your cash position?"

"Eleven thousand," Alex said. "In CDs. It's our emergency fund."

"How much can you borrow, short term?"

"I don't know. Why should I?"

"Because you want to open your new account with a big bankroll. Try to open with a minimum of $10,000. Then when potential creditors ask your bank about your credit, the bank will only say that you opened with a five-figure amount. You want to make their eyes pop. Get ahold of your friends and relatives. Offer them a half percent over what they're making, for just long enough to open the account. You pay them back fast, once you get the account opened."

"That's a great idea!" Alex said.

The man talked for several more minutes, giving Alex more good ideas. Then he asked: "How will you make money, once you've escaped from HAL Corporation?"

"I'm good at marketing," Alex said. "I won't have any problem finding something else."

"That's just another cage, isn't it?"

"No." Alex said. But he knew it was, and the idea made him sad.

A pigeon waddled up for some corn nuts. The old man reached into his candy-striped sack and brought out a handful of corn nuts. As he dropped them one at a time, he said something to Alex that struck home:

"Life's pretty simple. There are the pigeons, waiting to get fed. And there are the feeders. It's all in deciding what end of the corn nut you want to be on."

Alex said nothing. He thought of his dream, when his face had been attached to the body of a feeding pigeon. He was overwhelmed with insight. He was also late for his next appointment. As the two men shook hands, the old man handed Alex a package. Alex hurried off. There were things he had to do for HAL, so Alex didn't open the package until two days later to find two books, a clipping from the *Wall Street Journal,* and a business card from the man on the park bench. One book was *Megatrends.* The other was *Nine American Lifestyles.* Reading them blew Alex's mind. The information was so relevant, so timely, so easy to absorb.

The *Journal* clipping was about our aging population. Today, it said, there are 27 million people 65 years or older, and by the year 2030 — when Alex would be 81 and retired in Florida — there would be 64 million Americans over 65. *Megatrends* said Florida was a bellwether state and a forecaster of patterns to come, with lots of young people, lots of old people, and a huge age gap in between. *Nine American Lifestyles* said households would increase from 89 million now to 97 million by 1990, and household size would decrease from 2.59 persons in 1985 to 2.50 in 1990.

Continued

Alex was not creative for nothing. He put the facts together: Florida, population over 65 increasing, and household size decreasing. He linked them to some personal considerations — his need for escape, his plan to retire in Florida, his need for a job, his creativity. Then he thought of people he knew. His father had just been mugged two blocks from his front door in a St. Louis suburb. His mother hated the Midwest cold. Some of their friends had already retired to Orlando.

His excitement kept him awake that night. He called his parents early the next day.

Alex explained his idea: Emerson Landing, a specially designed condo complex for seniors. It would contain medium-priced living quarters, various social areas, easy access to markets, a convalescent recuperation area (post-hospital care at modest prices), and a wellness clinic (to keep the elderly out of nursing homes).

Alex's parents weren't wealthy, but they offered him $47,000 up front and $90,000 more when their house was sold. Furthermore, the idea of getting out of the ice and snow and danger was so exciting, they volunteered to help him raise funds among their friends, in return for a small percentage off the top.

Alex Adams' escape machine was in motion.

He retured to Armonk and spoke with his banker, who liked the idea and offered to help Alex develop a Business Plan. His interstate bank was interested in Florida developments, he said. And they loved real estate projects that were created by innovative people who had their numbers together.

There was only one stumbling block ahead — Jayne Barrows Adams, Alex's wife.

Consequently, he was surprised at her response. His wife was both afraid and excited by Alex's plan. When he laid the numbers out for her, Jayne frowned, pursed her lips, said she'd have to think about it. Later that evening, when the couple were preparing for bed, Jayne asked if there might not be something she could do once Emerson Landing got going.

"Like what?" Except for volunteering a few hours for the church fund-raisers, Jayne had never worked.

"Oh, I don't know," she said. "Perhaps a boutique. Women that age have lots of money to spend. Their children are gone. They need amusement. My mother has ideas. I could ask her."

"I think that's a great idea, dear," Alex said. "I think that's terrific."

Alex made one phone call before retiring. He called the old man he'd met on the park bench, to thank him.

"Is there room for another investor?" the old man asked. "This city's too cold, and I've been needing to get my teeth into a project."

"You don't mean —?" Alex cried.

"Why don't we have lunch and talk about it. I can free up some capital. How does $17 million sound?"

"Ulp," Alex said. "I mean, it sounds terrific."

"Let's get rolling," the old man said. "These old fires have been banked too long."

"Yes, sir," Alex said.

And that night, Alex Adams had an entire set of beautiful entrepreneurial dreams — in technicolor.

What Can You Learn from Alex Adams?

When Alex Adams needed to escape from the golden handcuffs of HAL Corporation, what did he do? Did he insult his boss? No. Did he march into his bank and demand $100,000 in seed capital? No.

What Alex did was to plan:

1. He located someone who knew more about money than he did. He learned from this person.
2. He eyeballed trends in the marketplace. He read. He used his New Eyes to analyze and sense what was going on around him. He explored new territory.
3. He lined up banking connections and lines of credit before quitting his job with HAL.
4. He started looking for money close to home — his parents, friends of his parents. A good idea surfaced, and people were eager to invest.
5. He opened his business bank account with an impressive dollar figure. Later, when he went to the bank for a credit line, he had smooth sailing.

Preparing for the Search

Before hunting the great money tree, prepare, prepare, prepare.

Research the World of Money. Money creates its own world, with its own customs, myths, and rules. Before you go around begging with your hand out asking for money, spend three or four months studying the **world of money.** If you are new at this, a good place to start is *Money* magazine (see the great piece on money for the small business in December, 1982). Then go on to books like *The Small Business Guide to Borrowing Money, The Seven Laws of Money, How to Buy Money,* and the other sources listed in our reference section.

Sit at the Feet of a Money Guru. Make a secret list of three people who know more about money than you do. Seek one out. Begin to build a money network.

Buy Some Stock. Invest a small amount of money in a few shares of **common stock** of a business you want to know about. When you read those financial reports, monitor your emotions. Write down how you feel as you open up the *Wall Street Journal* to check the roller-coaster of your ups and downs. When it comes time to ask people to invest in your business, read over what you wrote.

Know the Litany of the Four Cs.

Capital. How much liquid cash (savings and checking accounts) do you have?

Character. Do you pay your bills on time?

Capacity. Do you have the ability to repay the loan out of the profits of the business?

Collateral. Which of your tangible assets, such as your infant child, Porsche, securities, beach condo, life insurance, can you use to secure a loan?

world of money
a strange and mysterious place where all sign-posts are written in $ signs

common stock
a certificate of equity ownership representing a certain number of shares

Four Cs
a classical series of questions lenders use to screen potential borrowers

Sketch out Your Business Plan Now. The Business Plan is your showcase for displaying all the ideas and information you've gathered in your venture adventure. A suggested format for the plan appears in Chapter 15. If you start thinking about your plan early and test it out on family, friends, and bankers, your chances of success in small business will increase in quantum leaps.

Befriend a Banker; Befriend a Backup Banker. Banks are conservative, and they probably will not want to lend you start-up money unless you pledge real property or securities. But **bankers** can lead you to money sources you hadn't considered. One useful tactic is to seek your banker's advice on pulling your Business Plan together. If you get your banker's input, he will have a hard time refusing help later on. Your banker is one gateway to the world of money.

You will want to know more than one banker.

YOUR BANKER

Befriending the Guardian

Action Step 41 gets you started on our last piece of advice—befriending a banker. We ask you to begin with your current banker.

> **To make friends with the Guardian at the Gate, start from where you are.**

You want to bring your banker into your **information loop** and involve your banker in your business idea. People lend money to people, and bankers are people. They get excited about good ideas.

It will help your trek through the money world to stop thinking about a banker as someone who will lend you an umbrella only on a sunny day. You would not lend money to a stranger, and when you walk in off the street, you want to make sure your banker knows what you are up to. More suggestions for dealing with your banker follow.

How to Deal with a Banker

Bankers are people, and people like to give advice. Here are some strategies for dealing with bankers.

1. Never ask a banker for money. Always ask for advice and information.
2. A **bank** is like a formidable medieval fortress or a great modern cathedral. It is designed to intimidate, and to give the lender a psychological edge. Cut through this obvious web of symbolism and money mythology with New Eyes. If you choose to see a banker on his or her own turf, always: 1) make an appointment (it's polite; it also makes the banker feel worthwhile); 2) dress conservatively (nothing impresses a banker like order and neatness); 3) act as if you don't need any money.
3. Think about luring a banker to **your turf.** Say: "I can't tell you exactly what my shop is like. Why not come out for a

bankers
gateways to the world of money

information loop
a network of people who need to be kept informed with updates of your business successes

bank
a place where some people park their money

your turf
a place you invite your banker to when you want advice and information

look-see? We could have lunch. How's Thursday around noon?'' On your own turf, you will be in a stronger position. You should feel more at ease and communication will flow more easily for both parties.

4. Once you have your loan or line of credit, stay in touch with your banker. Keep your Business Plan up to date and keep your banker friend informed about how things are going in your business. Keep positioning yourself on the ladder in your banker's mind.

5. While you're negotiating with one bank, get yourself a backup bank. You can use information from one bank to cross-check the other bank. Shop for money like you would shop for any major purchase. The deals could surprise you.

6. Negotiate for your line of credit or loan while you are still employed. A personal line of credit is often reviewed annually. You may have to prove that you are still a good credit risk after you are in your own business. But if you keep up a good credit rating, chances are good you will be able to keep the personal lines of credit.

7. Some questions to ask your prospective banker:
What are your lending limits?
Who makes the decisions on loans?
What are your views on my industry?
What experience do you have in working with businesses like mine?
Could you recommend a highly qualified lawyer? Bookkeeper? Accountant?
Are you interested in writing **equipment leases**?
What kind of terms do you give on **accounts receivable** financing?
Does your bank offer VISA and Mastercards for business? What credit limit could I expect for my business credit cards?
What kind of handling charge will I have to pay on credit card receipts?
What kind of interest can I earn on my business checking account?
Do you have a merchant's or commercial window?
Do you have a night depository?
If you can't lend me money, can you direct me to people who might be interested?
Do you make **SBA guaranteed loans**?
If I open up a business checking account here, what else can you do for me in the community?

Your Banker Is a Member of the Team

A helpful banker can be an entrepreneur's best friend and a member of your auxiliary management team.

Business growth demands money from external sources. The more successful you become, the more likely you will need a close bank relationship to help you finance prosperity. If you grow at more than 25% a year, you'll need lots of help from the bank. Manufacturers get into trouble fast, but even service firms have to wait for their customers to make payments.

equipment leases
long-term arrangements from a bank or leasing company which allow you to rent capital equipment

accounts receivable
what is owed to a firm

SBA guaranteed loans
loans where up to 90% of loaned funds are insured by the federal government

Meanwhile, your creditors and employees want their money now.

Advice: Keep your banker in your information loop. Bankers are more willing to help if they understand your needs.

In the next case study, you can see how one young man handled his problems with cash flow by allowing a banker to understand the business he was in.

Case Study

Steve McWhorter — Inventor

Things went really well that first year. My third invention — a battery-operated fuel monitor for the new diesel turbos being made in Germany — was selling like hotcakes, and I'd found a great production manager to keep things going down on the line.

Then we had cash flow troubles.

It happened in February of our second year when a couple of the big car makers — customers that purchased at least 50% of our product — slowed down on their payments. Some payments were more than ninety days past due.

I stay pretty much in the lab and the shop, because that's the fun part of the business for me, so I didn't find out about the cash problems for almost three weeks. When I did find out, we invoiced the customers again. Still no money. The first week in March, I had trouble meeting the payroll. The second week I had to pay a couple of crucial supplier accounts. The third week, except for petty cash, the company was almost out of money.

I gave my banker a call. We were on good terms, and I had four accounts at her bank, and when I told her my problem, she said: "How much do you need? And for how long?"

Instant **line of credit.** What a relief.

Well, we got that squared away, and after things were rolling smoothly again, my banker sat down with me and the company books, and we worked out a strategy for bridging the gap between billing and customer payment.

The thing I remember from those sessions was that the whole subject bored me, so that very afternoon I started looking around for someone to help out on the numbers.

My banker helped here, too, with advice and recommendations about what kind of person would be best at keeping track of money.

When I worked for someone else, I never thought of a banker at all. Since I've been in business, I've come to realize a banker can be a businessperson's best friend.

line of credit
an unsecured lending limit

SECRETS OF SMALL BUSINESS SURVIVAL

Make Those Dollars Work Overtime

Steve McWhorter discovered the art of managing money in the eleventh hour. It's no secret that start-ups are expensive, and those first few months can be a make-or-break time for the entrepreneur. You want to make your dollars work efficiently.

1. Find out who you have to pay right now.
2. Find out who can wait awhile.
3. Keep asking what you're getting for your money.

If you work the dollars you do have, you won't have to shake the money tree so hard.

Tips on Saving Money

Read through the list below. How many of these ideas have you thought of? How many are new to you?

1. Persuade your customers to give you **cash deposits** when they place their orders.
2. Persuade your vendors to give you more **trade credit** or **dating** and more time to pay. (See Action Step 42.)
3. Lease your equipment.
4. Run a lean operation. No waste.
5. Work out of your home.
6. Get your business landlord to make **on-site improvements** and finance the cost over the term of the lease.
7. Stay on top of your receivables. Be aggressive.
8. Keep track of everything. Try to resell whatever waste or by-products you have in your particular business.
9. Return goods that aren't selling.
10. Take markdowns quickly on **dead goods.**
11. Use as little commercial space as you can.
12. If your customers do not visit your business facility, it does not have to be highly visible or attractive.
13. When you have to borrow money, shop around.
14. Make sure your **liquid cash** is earning interest.
15. Shop **nonbank lenders** like commercial credit firms.
16. Do not collateralize your loans — unless you have no choice.
17. Survey your friends and relatives — they might lend you money at higher rates than they could get in the money markets, but for less than you would pay institutional lenders.
18. Look into **R & D partnerships** for product development funds.
19. Befriend a venture capitalist who funds your type of firm.
20. Consider selling limited partnerships. You become the general partner with little or none of your own capital invested.

Vendor Applications

An often overlooked technique for reducing your capital requirement is to probe your vendors (major suppliers) for the best prices and terms available. Professional buyers and purchasing agents ask their vendors to fill out an information sheet that forces them to write down all the terms and conditions of their sales plans.

This is a good idea for you.

A small business must buy professionally and a **vendor application** will help you do just that. With a vendor application, your ven-

---

cash deposits
funds paid in advance of delivery

trade credit or **dating**
an extension of the payment term by the vendors into the near future

on-site improvements
modifications to real estate to meet special needs of the business

dead goods
merchandise no longer in demand

liquid cash
funds that you can use immediately, usually held in checking or other accounts

nonbank lenders
institutional lenders other than banks

R & D partnerships
a separately funded venture partnership that has certain tax advantages for investors

vendor application
a personally designed form which allows you to negotiate with each vendor from a position of informed strength

dor's verbal promises become written promises. How well you buy is as important as how well you sell. To compete in your arena, you need the best terms and prices available.

Action Step 42 will help you concentrate on a vendor application.

Vendor Application Starter Kit

Action Step 42 asks you to design your own vendor application. Here's a kit to get you started. The following list of questions gives you the basics. You'll probably add more questions as you gain experience.

1. Source (vendor's name).
2. Address/Phone.
3. Sales rep's name.
4. Business phone. (Will vendor accept collect calls?)
5. Home phone (for emergencies).
6. Amount of minimum purchase.
7. Quantity discounts? How much? What must you do to earn?
8. Are dating or extended payment terms available?
9. What are the advertising/promotion allowances?
10. Policies on returns for defective goods. (Who pays the freight?)
11. Delivery times.
12. Assistance (technical, sales, and so on).
13. Product literature available.
14. Point-of-Purchase material.
15. Support for Grand Opening. (Will supplier donate prize or other support?)
16. Nearest other dealer handling line.
17. What special services can the sales rep provide?
18. Will vendor give you a **tax-credit pass-through** on lease equipment?
19. Get your supplier's signature, the date, and some kind of agreement that you will be notified of any changes.

Remember the application is the starting point for further negotiations. Revise the master of your application form as you learn from experience how vendors can help you in your particular business.

ACTION ⚡ STEP 42

Design Your Own Vendor Application

One of the best ways to save money is to get help from your vendor/supplier. To do that, you will need to create your own special form which specifies, in writing, terms to be negotiated.

Be tough. Be firm. Be pleasant.

You will want to personalize this form with the name of your business at the top. We give you a starter kit for developing your own vendor application on this page.

The vendor form will give you talking points. Most vendors hold something back, and it is up to you to be a barracuda and get the best deal for your business.

When negotiating, use a lot of open-ended questions like: "What else can you do for me?"

You do not have to be nasty. Just keep negotiating.

⚡ ☐ STEP COMPLETED

---

tax-credit pass-through
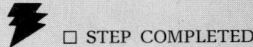
an agreement from the provider of a leased product which allows you to take the investment tax credit

---

Case Study

Rich Cameron — Toys from Middle Earth

You have met Rich Cameron before in these pages. He was in marketing, working for a large firm, when he decided to go into business for himself. He attended seminars, interviewed owners, walked neighborhoods, read trade journals.

Rich wound up opening a toy store in a shopping center where a Safeway supermarket was the anchor tenant. The store opened in May,

Continued

but Rich knew from doing industry research that he would have to start placing orders for the Christmas season right away.

The problem was that his store would hold $100,000 worth of toys, but Rich had only $30,000 to use for his inventory. He knew he would have to be well-stocked by Thanksgiving or miss out on the profitable holiday rush.

The unwritten rule in a new business is that suppliers want you to pay cash up front — for everything. You are a new account, unproven in the grand arena of trade and commerce, and they want to wait and see how you do before extending credit.

Rich Cameron found a way to get around that unwritten rule.

He showed his Business Plan to the credit managers of his suppliers. What happened?

"They were amazed," Rich says. "They'd been dealing with toy store owners for years, and mine was the first Business Plan they'd seen from a toy store owner. I showed them everything in black and white — industry trends, projections, marketing plan, management-team statistics, promotion strategy, everything — and when they finished reading, I had my extended dating terms."

The Business Plan didn't do all Rich's work for him. He also developed his own personalized Vendor Application, to use when he spoke to salespeople.

"A Vendor Application will really help you," Rich says, "because the survival items are written down. It's got the information organized and it puts sales reps on the spot. If they want your business to succeed, they have to deal with the questions.

"I got some strong resistance when I brought out my Vendor App. One guy spent 30 minutes on long distance, telling me why he wouldn't sign it. He wanted all cash up front for the first sale, 75% cash for the second, 50% for the third, and 30% of net after that. But using the App, backed by my Business Plan, I was able to negotiate him into dating, which means I bought toys in early summer and didn't have to pay for them until December 10. Dating saved my business."

Rich smiles as he recalls those early days. "The interesting thing about negotiating is that it gets you in close enough so you can ask for other assistance. A lot of my advertising and promotion comes free through the vendors because they want my store to be a success. If I hadn't gone in to deal, they wouldn't have known I was going to be a major customer for the long run. And I couldn't have moved confidently without that Vendor Form."

If you're a new account, flash 'em your Business Plan. Then flash 'em your vendor application. Tell vendors you're going to be a very important customer, very soon. And remember those who helped you out.

SCOUTING THE FOREST

By now you've befriended a banker, you've increased your money savvy, and you have prepared a vendor application. Now is the time to zero in on your **lenders.** Action Step 43 asks you to prepare yourself on paper first by listing potential lenders and investors (the next section discusses sources of capital) and second by developing your persuasive tactics ahead of time. Without persuasive **inducements to lenders,** they have no reason to invest in your business. If you need

lenders
persons or firms who advance money

inducements to lenders
an extra benefit offered to lenders — including stock warrant, discount, or control of company

help in listing your reasons, you might begin by profiling your Target Customer, the one who's out there waiting for your product or service. You might list industry trends, and dovetail them with a scenario of where your product or service fits. Move from there to marketing strategy, selling, the profit picture, and return on investment (ROI).

The final part of Action Step 43 asks you to test your tactics out on friends. Ask your friends to respond as potential investors. Here you *want* to hear their objections so you can answer their objections on paper. When you are through with this Action Step, you will be truly prepared to meet your lender.

SHAKING THE MONEY TREE

In Action Step 36 you prepared a personal financial statement that gave you an idea of your net worth. You can use that information here, as you start to shake the money tree.

You are going to have to put cash of your own on the line, but the pain will be translated into excitement once your business gets going.

Face it. It is your business, and you are going to have to use some money of your own. That's only fair. But you might be surprised at how money turns up if you start looking around with New Eyes.

Sources of Capital

Start with the list below, adding to it when you think of a new source we haven't thought of.

1. Savings.
2. Borrow on your life insurance.
3. Refinance your car, boat, camper.
4. Take out a **second mortgage.** A third? A fourth?
5. Get a line of unsecured personal credit from your bank, credit union, or other financial institution (see item 10 following).
6. Research your assets (coin collections, old baseball cards, or whatever).
7. Sell that crummy stock you have been holding. Take a loss. Write it off. Or get a loan on the securities you want to retain.
8. Get a part-time job. Moonlight your way to more money.
9. Network your friends and family. You will be surprised at the nest eggs lying there.
10. Look at nonbank sources (see Figure 10.2 on page 190):
    a. Savings and loan associations
    b. Credit unions
    c. Insurance companies. They prefer to make big loans — starting at $1 million.
    d. Commercial credit corporations. For example, Control Data and the Money Store make SBA guaranteed loans.

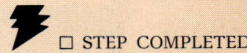

ACTION STEP 43

Prepare Yourself to Meet Your Lenders

Know who your potential lenders are and know why they should want to help you.

Part A. List potential lenders and investors. Begin with family and friends and move out to business acquaintances and colleagues. Don't forget institutional lenders.

Part B. Now quickly list reasons why lenders should invest in your business. What inducements are you offering potential investors? If you're offering them a very small ROI, what have you got to offset that?

Think about the legal form of your business. Would you attract more investors if you formed a corporation?

Part C. Test your tactics out by talking to a few friends. Tell them: "This is just a test, and I'd like your reactions to my new business venture." Watch their reactions.

Now list all the objections they gave you — reasons why they couldn't loan you any money.

Answer all objections on paper first. Are there objections you cannot answer? What does this mean for your business?

□ STEP COMPLETED

second mortgage
a second lien or note on real property that is subordinated to the first mortgage

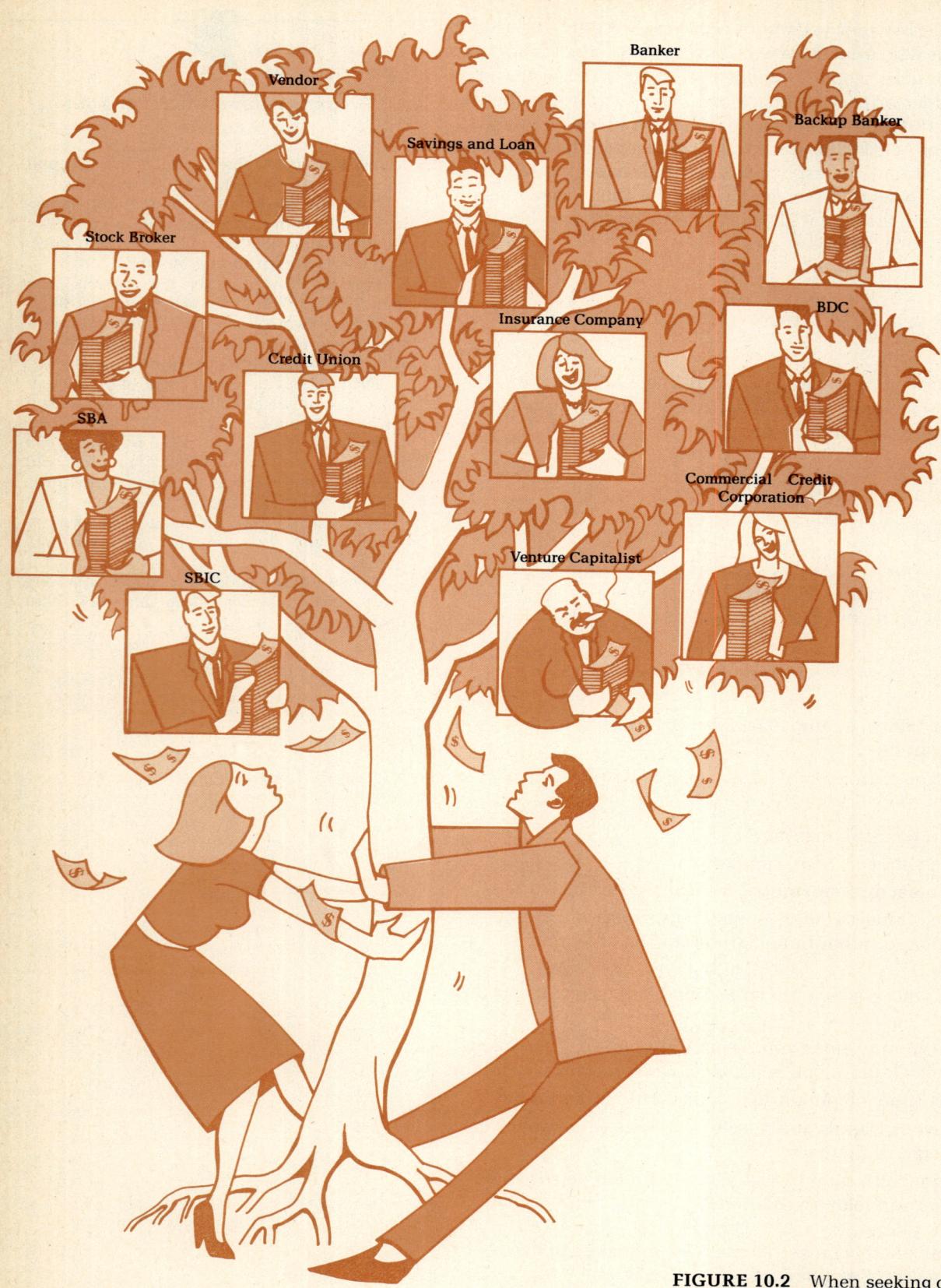

FIGURE 10.2 When seeking out institutional lenders, don't stop with just one bank. Lenders come in many shapes and forms.

e. **Cooperative venture with customers.**
f. Stock brokerage houses.
g. SBA (discussed in the following).
h. SBICs (discussed in the following).
i. Venture capitalists (discussed in the following).
j. BDCs (discussed in the following).

We discuss several potential money trees as follows.

Small Business Administration

The Small Business Administration **(SBA)** of the U.S. government has two major categories of loans, guaranteed and direct. The guaranteed loans are from your bank or nonbank lender. The direct loans go from the federal government right to your business. Direct loans are scarce. Guaranteed loans are changing.

The guarantee is between the SBA, an arm of Congress, and the bank. If your business goes under, up to 90% of your loan is insured by the federal government. (This figure is dropping, perhaps to 75%, and you need to check the latest information at your nearest SBA office.)

In 1981 (statistics are slow to catch up to reality), the SBA made just over 22,000 guaranteed loans, and about 3,600 direct loans.

That's not very many loans, especially when compared to the number of new business corporations for 1983: 600,000.

The numbers seem to be stacked against small business. Six hundred thousand new corporations (partnerships and sole proprietorships are not counted), yet only 25,000 loans. Those numbers give every small business person a reason to write Washington. (See Action Step 46.) If you want to challenge those odds, you can apply for an SBA loan, but only after you have been turned down by a bank (not a process that builds confidence). If you live in a huge metro area (like one of the SMSAs or CMSAs of the Census Bureau — see Chapter 7), you have to be turned down by two banks.

In December of 1981, according to *Money* magazine, the SBA began a new program to award grants to high-tech firms for research. The first-year grants have a ceiling of $50,000. If your company makes it to the second year, you can apply for as much as half a million.

Information about this program, which is called Small Business Innovation Research (SBIR), can be had by writing SBA, 1141 L St. NW, Washington, D.C. 20416.

Small Business Investment Companies

Small Business Investment Companies **(SBICs)** are privately operated companies that are licensed by the SBA to provide money to small firms.

Most SBICs are owned by banks or groups of private individuals. The money for loans comes from the SBA, which gets it from the U.S. Treasury, which gets it from you.

In 1982, there were about 360 SBICs in the United States. According to Thomas Martin, in *Financing the Growing Business*, SBICs are all over the place with their money: two hundred thousand dollars of

---

cooperative venture with customers
a lucky break where you find a major user who will finance your business

SBA
federal agency whose prime mission is to help small business

SBICs
nonbank lending institutions licensed by the SBA to provide money to small business

start-up money for a telephone equipment company, $200k for town-house construction, $650K three-way team purchase of convertible debentures, $250K four-way team financing for an already existing business, and $150K second-stage money for a sportswear distributor.

To get money from an SBIC, you need a Business Plan. (See Chapter 15 for an outline and sample plan.)

About 60% of the SBICs are members of NASBIC (National Association of Small Business Investment Companies), which has a directory listing its loan policies. The directory is free. Write NASBIC, 618 Washington Building, Washington D.C., 20005. Telephone (202) 638-3411. Try to call collect.

There are about 130 special SBICs that lend money only to firms that are owned by the disadvantaged. "Disadvantaged" here includes Vietnam veterans. For information, contact American Association of Minority Enterprise Small Business Investment Companies (MESBIC) 915 15th St., Washington, D.C., 20005.

Venture Capital Firms

With venture capital firms we enter an area of myth, the world of high rollers and higher flyers.

Banks lend money that is secured, usually by real estate. Venture capitalists don't lend money; they buy a piece of your business. The reason they'll buy a piece is that they are gambling on rapid growth so they can reap a 300%–500% return on their investment (ROI). The payoff for most venture capital firms occurs when your company is large enough to interest enough investors for a public issue of common stock. When you "go public," the venture capital people can take their money out.

Venture capital people prefer to enter the financial picture at the second stage of a firm's development, when the business has proven its potential and now needs a large infusion of cash to support growth.

When they invest money, venture capital firms like high-tech concepts in embryonic industries with high growth potential. As we move toward the year 2000, venture capital companies will grow in number and become more significant in the financing of entrepreneurial America.

Venture capitalists come in lots of shapes — family firms (Rockefeller), industrial arms (GE), bank arms (B of A), and other arms (insurance companies, finance companies). The names smack of adventure — Bay Venture Group (San Francisco), Zero Stage Capital Equity (Cambridge), Nautilus (Boston).

And some of the myths are real. Venrock, the Rockefeller arm, was in on the birth and dynamic growth of Apple.

Venture capitalists will let you run the show if you give them a healthy ROI.

There's a good list of names and addresses in *The Guide to Venture Capital Sources*, listed in our reference section. Names of local and regional venture capital firms are sometimes compiled by business editors of newspapers. *Inc.* magazine publishes an updated list in December, and *Venture* magazine publishes a yearly list called "The Venture Capital 100" in its June issue.

According to *Venture*, such firms invested $1.38 billion in 1982, a 12% increase over 1981.

Business Development Corporations

Business Development Corporations (BDCs) are private outfits operating inside states. Their goal is to increase employment within their specific state. New York has the largest BDC in the country.

You can locate your state's BDC by contacting your state economic development agency. Try the government information number in your white pages.

POLITICAL ACTION

Action Step 44 is optional and will not become a part of your Business Plan. It might, however, become a part of your strategy for contacting and educating the federal government.

As a private citizen who is interested in the growth of our economy, you should consider taking a more active role in the political system. You pay taxes. You have rights. Learn to express them logically,

ACTION STEP 44

Write an Angry Letter

This Action Step is optional, but you might find it very satisfying! Write to your Congressman and Senator about the state of small business in your area and tell them what kind of help you need.

1. Tell them why you think the tiny trickle of money for small business is disgraceful.
2. Tell them about the times when a small business could use a break on taxes.
3. Beg them to decrease the mountain of paperwork required when you try to get help from Uncle Sam.
4. Somewhere in your letter, remind your representative that small business is the backbone of America.

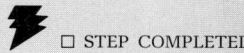

☐ STEP COMPLETED

Letter from a Small Business Owner

The Honorable ———
Capitol Office Building
Washington, D.C.

Dear Senator [or Congressman]:

I'm writing to you because, as a small business person, I feel both neglected and harassed by Uncle Sam.

Let me be specific. My computer software business is two years old. This year, I went to the SBA for a loan. My business is growing, and as I'm sure you know, it takes capital to expand. The paperwork for the SBA loan took two weeks, with three people on my staff working on it almost full-time. Today, I learned that the SBA was out of money, and I was informed that I'll have to go elsewhere for my expansion capital.

Why are small businesses, which are producing jobs and goods, forced to beg for help, while Big Business, which is a declining force in the economy, is given tax breaks and bail-outs?

My point is this: Small businesses typically need help in the first three to five years. During this period they are cash poor, despite profit statements and taxable income. Therefore, we need more SBA loans, and at a decent rate. We need to delay or defray taxes until cash flow catches up with paper profits. And we need to simplify the paperwork needed to apply for the loans.

When small business fails, everyone loses — the owners, the banks, the customers, all levels of government (no taxes coming in), the suppliers, and the employees. When small business succeeds, everyone wins. In a free economy, business creates new jobs, more innovation, more tax revenue, and a larger number of positive, energetic, free-spirited people.

Let's get together, Senator, and make sure small business succeeds. The success of the country — yours and mine — depends on it.

Cordially,

———

coherently, systematically. Writing to your representative is a good place to start.

And remember, in the Information Society, the world runs on words — whether on paper or by electronic communications.

We don't think small businesses are getting enough help from the federal government. What do you think?

We provide a sample letter on page 193. But write your own letter, listing your own problems, in your own words. Compare your letter to ours. Try to make yours better.

Beyond writing letters, talk your problems and needs up among small business owners. Try to get a group effort going. Politics is a numbers game, and groups carry a bigger stick than individuals. (According to *Inc.*, June 1983, the Democrats are starting a Small Business Council — a road show sponsoring town meetings for small business across the country. It's up to you to find out which politicians are doing the most for small business.)

SUMMARY

Money creates its own world, with its own customs, rituals, and rules. Before you start asking people for money for your small business, spend three to four months researching the world of money. Here are some paths to streamline your research:

1. Read back issues of *Money* magazine.
2. Read books like *The Small Business Guide to Borrowing Money, Up Front Financing*, and *The Seven Laws of Money*.
3. Find someone who knows more about money than you do. Ask questions.
4. Invest a little money in a few shares of stock in a business you want to know about. Read the stockholders reports.
5. Know that loans are made on the basis of the Four Cs — Capital, Character, Capacity (to repay), and Collateral.
6. Take an hour out to outline your Business Plan. You will need the plan to show to bankers, vendors, and lenders. For now, an outline is good enough. (See Chapter 15 for a model plan.)
7. Begin thinking of a banker as your gateway to the world of money.

THINK POINTS

- Your banker can be a doorway to the world of money. Use that door.
- How well you buy is as important as how well you sell.

ACTION STEP REVIEW

Four Action Steps help you focus on the world of money and what it means to you:

41 Use your banker as a resource to help you design your Business Plan. Strategies for dealing with bankers are listed in the text, but perhaps most important is always to ask for advice; never ask for money.

42 Save money by getting help from your vendors and suppliers. The key here is to develop your own Vendor Application, a form that allows you to negotiate important survival assistance and to get it in writing.

43 Focus on what money means to others by listing reasons why lenders would give you money for your business. You may want to begin by listing potential lenders. Then develop persuasive tactics. You can test your persuasive powers on your friends. Watch their reactions, and list objections. Then work out answers to the objections.

44 After you have explored the various sources of money (SBA loans, SBICs, Venture Capital firms, BDCs, and so on), you might feel like writing a letter to Washington about the state of small business financing.

- Business is a game. Vendors enjoy having secrets. It is up to you to make your best deal.
- Whether you are dealing with bankers or vendors, use lots of open-ended questions like, ''What else can you do for me?''

REFERENCES

Burlingham, Bo. ''Let Them Make Mudpies.'' *Inc.,* July 1983, 65–74. Inside look at the way one loan application was turned down by the SBA.

''The Democrats Are Coming!'' *Inc.,* June 1983, 38, 43.

Eisenberg, Richard, ''Financing Your Venture.'' *Money,* December 1982, 75–82.

Goldberg, Philip, and Richard Rubin. *The Small Business Guide to Borrowing Money.* New York: McGraw-Hill, 1980.

Gumpert, David E., and Jeffrey Timmons. *The Insider's Guide to Small Business Resources.* New York: Doubleday & Co., 1982.

Klugman, Ellen. ''How to Attract Money.'' *Working Woman,* October 1980, 83–86, 112.

Martin, Thomas J. *Financing the Growing Business.* New York: Holt, Rinehart & Winston, 1980.

Nelson, Wayne E. *How to Buy Money: Investing Wisely for Maximum Return.* New York: McGraw-Hill, 1981.

Nicholas, Ted. *Where the Money Is and How to Get It.* Wilmington, Del.: Enterprise Publishing, 1976.

''Open a Boutique—Risks to Riches in the Rag Trade.'' *Working Woman,* January 1979, 59–60.

Phillips, Michael, et al. *The Seven Laws of Money.* New York: Random House, 1974.

Posner, Bruce G. ''How S & L's Stalk the Business Market.'' *Inc.,* July 1983, 99–102. New 1982 regulations allow S & L's and savings banks to invest specified percentages of their assets in commercial loans. See your neighborhood thrift officer.

———. ''A Rare Case of Bourgeois Values.'' *Inc.,* June 1983, 71–76. Interesting piece about Bourgeois Fils, an investment banking firm in New Hampshire, which puts together money packages for venturers.

Pratt, Stanley E., ed. *The Guide to Venture Capital Sources.* 7th ed. Wellesley Hills, Mass.: Capital Publishing, 1984. This guide costs $90, so try your library first. You can contact the publisher at P.O. Box 348, Wellesley Hills, MA 02181.

Zonana, Victor F. ''Despite Greater Risks, More Banks Turn to Venture Capital Business.'' *Wall Street Journal,* November 28, 1983. Seventy banks now have venture-capital subsidiaries, and they include Bank of America, Continental Illinois, and First Chicago. Ask your banker about it.

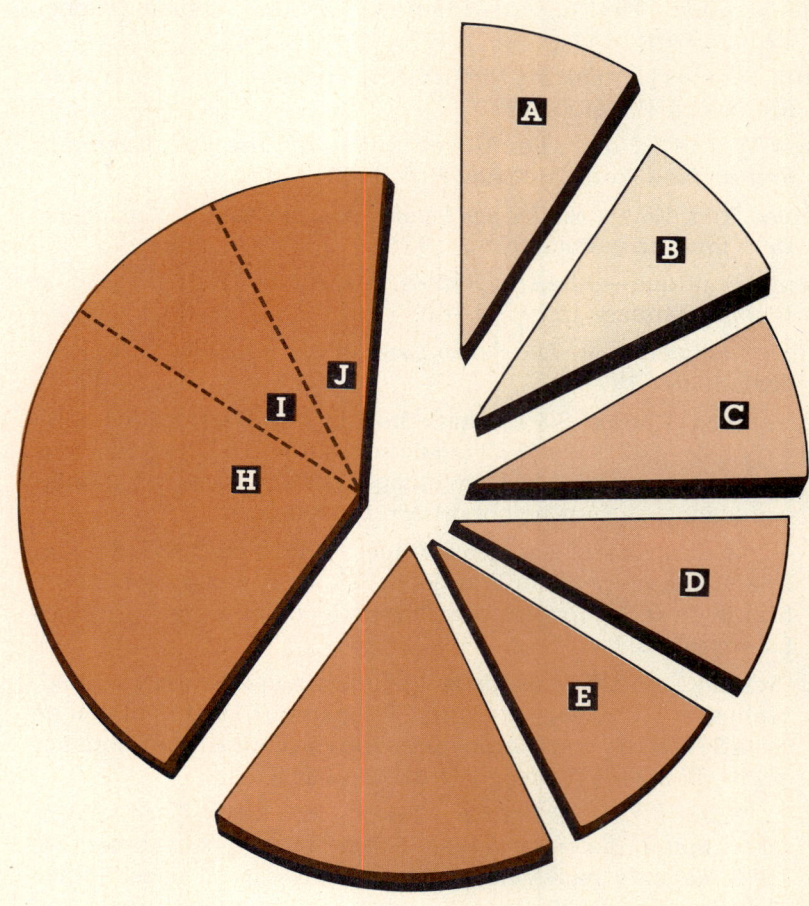

A Description of Product or Service

B The Market and the Target Customer

C Reading the Competition

D Marketing Strategy

E Location

H Projected Income Statement

I Projected Cash Flow

J Projected Balance Sheet

FIGURE 11.1 Chapter 11 adds to your financial expertise by explaining why and when you should consider incorporation.

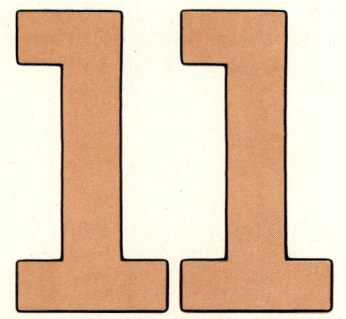

When Should You Incorporate?

To decide which of the three legal forms (sole proprietorship, partnership, corporation) is best for your business.

To understand why you need to get everything in writing even if it is not required by law.

To use your imagination to think ahead when you are going into business with anyone but yourself.

To understand the power of psychological forces, and to build appropriate escape routes for yourself when you bring those forces into your business.

To understand that all escape routes must be in writing, usually from the hand of an attorney.

To develop tactics for finding the right attorney.

To develop questions for probing the mind of that attorney.

To explore the reasons for thinking about incorporating.

To recognize the signals for your own incorporation.

To discourage yourself from considering the romance of ''offshore'' incorporation.

 **Y**ou may run your small business as a sole proprietorship or in partnership with another entrepreneur, and as far as you're concerned, your business is already in the best possible legal form. Are you sure? Or you may be in the planning stages of your new business, but you don't know what legal form (sole proprietorship, partnership, or corporation) is best. In this chapter we will look at clear financial signals and hidden business liabilities that should help you look ahead and decide which legal form will work for you.

IT PAYS TO LOOK AHEAD

Don't learn your lessons the hard way — that's what happened to Phil Johnson.

Q. You are in a great business, with a partner you trust and respect. When should you *incorporate*?
A. Sooner than you think.

Case Study

Phil Johnson in ''My Partner, My Pal''

The power sailer was my idea. My partner, Steve Savitch, said it would break us, and I should have listened to him. Steve's an engineer and inventor. He's great with numbers and computers, but he doesn't know much about people, which is my department. We'd been friends for a dozen years, at least, and we'd been partners — Savitch and Johnson, Business Consultants — for the last three.

This was the first year we were going to clear over $60K apiece.

Steve's tight with a nickel. I knew he'd sock his money away in a **money market fund** at a conservative rate. But I had this idea that we could buy a boat for the partnership, write off the down payment as expense, and do our company image a world of good.

Selling is 50% sweat, 40% image and 10% product. I've been in sales all my life. I know.

''I don't know, Phil,'' Steve said when he saw the boat. Her name was *The Ninja*. She was 46 feet long, with polished brass fittings and wood that gleamed back at you when you smiled. ''What does a fancy rig like that have to do with anything?''

''Image, Steve,'' I said. ''Image.''

''Uh-oh,'' Steve said. ''Here we go with the unmeasurable intangibles.''

''It's not intangible when you think about those prospects coming out from Chicago a week from tomorrow,'' I said. ''A cruise to Catalina should soften them up, don't you think?''

''Maybe,'' Steve sighed. He gave me his engineer's thin smile. ''I trust you, Phil. You're the people person.''

Steve's reluctance faded some when he saw the numbers. The power sailer was listed at 25% below market and the owner was eager to carry back some paper. We took our banker for a sail that weekend, and by Monday at noon, we had a check for the difference. The first payment wasn't due for a month, and when Steve and I went out with our wives, I tell you, I felt like a prince of the sea. I have to admit we'd pulled off a

Continued

incorporate
the process of choosing to become an artificial and/or immortal business entity

money market fund
a pool of managed money that is secured by short-term corporate IOUs

smooth deal, and I kept patting myself on the back every time I thought about the **write-offs.**

The Ninja boosted business, just like I'd thought. We closed the Chicago deal and we were busy on a couple of others that looked promising. We made the first payment with no trouble, and when Steve **counter-signed** the check, he even admitted he was beginning to like the boat.

"If it's okay with you, Phil, I'm going to sleep there a couple nights this week. My house is full of in-laws, and I've got to get my projections done for those guys from St. Louis.

"Be my guest," I said.

So for a couple of weeks, Steve took his portable computer and slept on *The Ninja.* We took her out that weekend, with four prospects from St. Louis, and Steve seemed a little preoccupied. I closed the deal with them Sunday, 15 minutes before putting them on the plane for home, but when I called Steve's house to tell him the good news, his wife, Mary, told me he was still at the boat.

Thinking back, later, I remembered hearing something funny in Mary's voice. At the time, I was so excited I didn't think anything about it.

Monday, Steve didn't come to work until almost noon. He looked hung over, but he handed me his projections and we got on with planning our strategy for the next couple of weeks.

"Anything wrong, partner?" I asked. "You seem a little far-off today."

"Sorry," Steve said. He was never one to admit to having emotions. "My mind wandered a bit there. Where were we?"

I should have gotten suspicious right then. But I'm not one to pry, so I didn't. We all like our privacy.

On Tuesday and Wednesday, Steve was at the office when I got there, working away at his computer. On Thursday, the first thing I saw when I got to work was a stack of computer printouts two inches high. It was Steve's half of the next three jobs.

By noon, Steve still hadn't made it to work. I called his house. No answer. I thought of driving down to the dock, to check the boat, but I had to pick up a couple of clients at the airport. They were flying out from Minneapolis. We were scheduled for an evening aboard *The Ninja.* When we arrived at our dock, around 4:30 that afternoon, there was no sign of *The Ninja.* Someone from the boat next door said Steve had taken off early this morning. With a woman on board.

I was in shock. There I stood, with two pale clients dressed in deck shoes and Bermuda shorts, and my partner was off somewhere with our power sailer.

Then Joey, the guy who pumps gas, came up waving a gas bill for $800 — one I'd thought Steve had paid. And the bad news didn't end there.

The next day, I got a call from a fellow who sells radar equipment. Seems Steve had bought $2,000 worth of radar, and this fellow was wondering when he would be paid.

As I hung up the phone, my secretary buzzed me. It was Mary Savitch, Steve's wife, and she wanted to know where Steve was.

Now my stomach was really hurting.

My partner Steve was gone — no one knew where — and I was liable for all his business debts. That included payments on *The Ninja.* Terrific.

The problem was that Steve and I had never seen the need for having anything in writing. We were both men of good faith. We had both pulled our weight in the business. And we had balanced each other with our various skills.

Continued

write-offs
legitimate business deductions you can report to the IRS

counter-signing
a situation in which two or more signatures are required before action can occur

Now that Steve was gone, I guess I felt pretty lost for quite a while. And I also felt angry. And betrayed.

For the first time in 22 years of business, I made an appointment to talk to a lawyer. He just shook his head.

''You should have come to me sooner, Phil,'' he said. ''A lot sooner.''

While I was paying off Steve's bills and trying to keep the business going by myself, I heard some gossip from the dock. It seems Steve had met a woman down there and had decided to run off with her without telling anyone, including me.

And there I was, holding the bag.

Just last week, when I was closing the place down and getting ready to go back to work for my old boss, I got this postcard from Steve, from Tahiti. It was Steve's handwriting, all right. So precise it could have been set on a typesetter.

''Sorry, Phil,'' it read. ''Didn't mean to run out on you, pal. It was the only way I could handle it. These things happen. Wanda says hi. Your pal, Steve.''

You can form a partnership with a handshake. You can dissolve a *partnership* by dying or destroy it by sailing out of town on your power sailer.

A partnership, as lots of people find out too late, is only an accounting entity. It's not a shield between you and your trouble. It won't make your business immortal or continuous. It's taxed at the same rate you are.

That's something you want to find out long before income tax time.

The Good and Bad of Partnerships

The great thing about partnerships is that they're warm, easy to form, and feel good, right from the start. You can form a partnership with a handshake, or dissolve it without one. (Several case studies in this chapter show the unforeseen problems that can arise from **dissolving a partnership.**) The best reason to form a partnership is that it makes you feel warm and cozy with people you get along with.

When you form a partnership, you have to deal with a paradox. As a business form, the partnership doesn't do much for you. In fact, only 8% of the small businesses in the country are partnerships. Yet, as many partners admit, there are sound psychological reasons for wanting to go into business with someone else.

What are some of those reasons?

Maybe you've done your personal skills analysis, and you realize you need to **balance skills** in a couple of critical areas. (Example: You're an engineer with 20 creative ideas a day, but you couldn't sell canned heat in an Arctic snowstorm.) Or maybe you don't have quite enough money and you meet someone who can help your new business out with capital. Or maybe you get along with people and love to sell and need to team up with an inventor/producer who can fill your life with products.

These feelings are real, and can't be ignored. You aren't alone and all of us need help.

But before you enmesh yourself in a partnership, read on and consider the alternatives.

partnership
an enterprise in which two or more people are engaged as owners or owner/operators

dissolving a partnership
the separation of the partners, an eventuality that needs to be prepared for with intricate planning and much thought

balancing skills
choosing coworkers with abilities that complement your own

THE THREE LEGAL FORMS FOR SMALL BUSINESS

Your small business can exist in one of three legal forms: a sole proprietorship, a partnership, or a corporation. Beyond the mental images we have of these forms of business ownership (see Figure 11.2), there are business realities—and various amounts of paperwork—that you should know about.

1. Sole Proprietorship

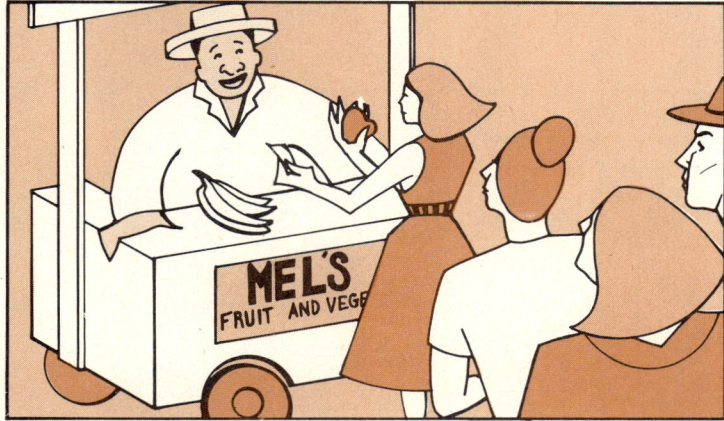

2. Partnership

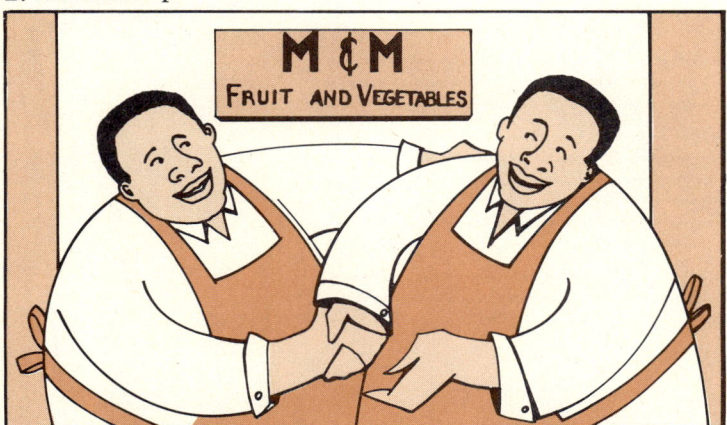

3. Corporation

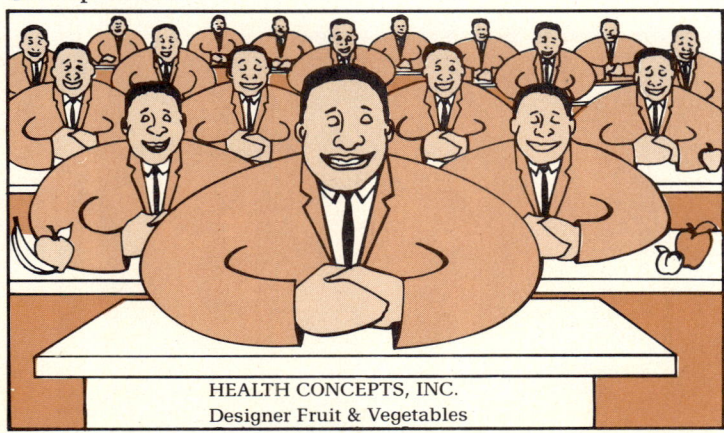

FIGURE 11.2 Shown are common mental images of the three legal forms of business ownership. Beyond these images there are business realities that you should investigate before you decide which form is right for you.

Sole Proprietorships

Most small businesses start as sole proprietorships. Once you start a business on your own — without partners — you are a sole proprietor. (See the case study on Rich Cameron in Chapter 2, beginning on page 27.) After all, when you run your business as a sole proprietorship, the paperwork is easy. You might get by with a city business license, a resale license, and a doing-business-as or fictitious business statement (DBA). And if you use your own name, you won't even need the DBA. But you may also discover that your business is sending you signals that another form will better suit your needs.

FIGURE 11.3 A sample partnership agreement between R. D. Bacon and W. L. Shakespeare, both of Radar, Iowa.

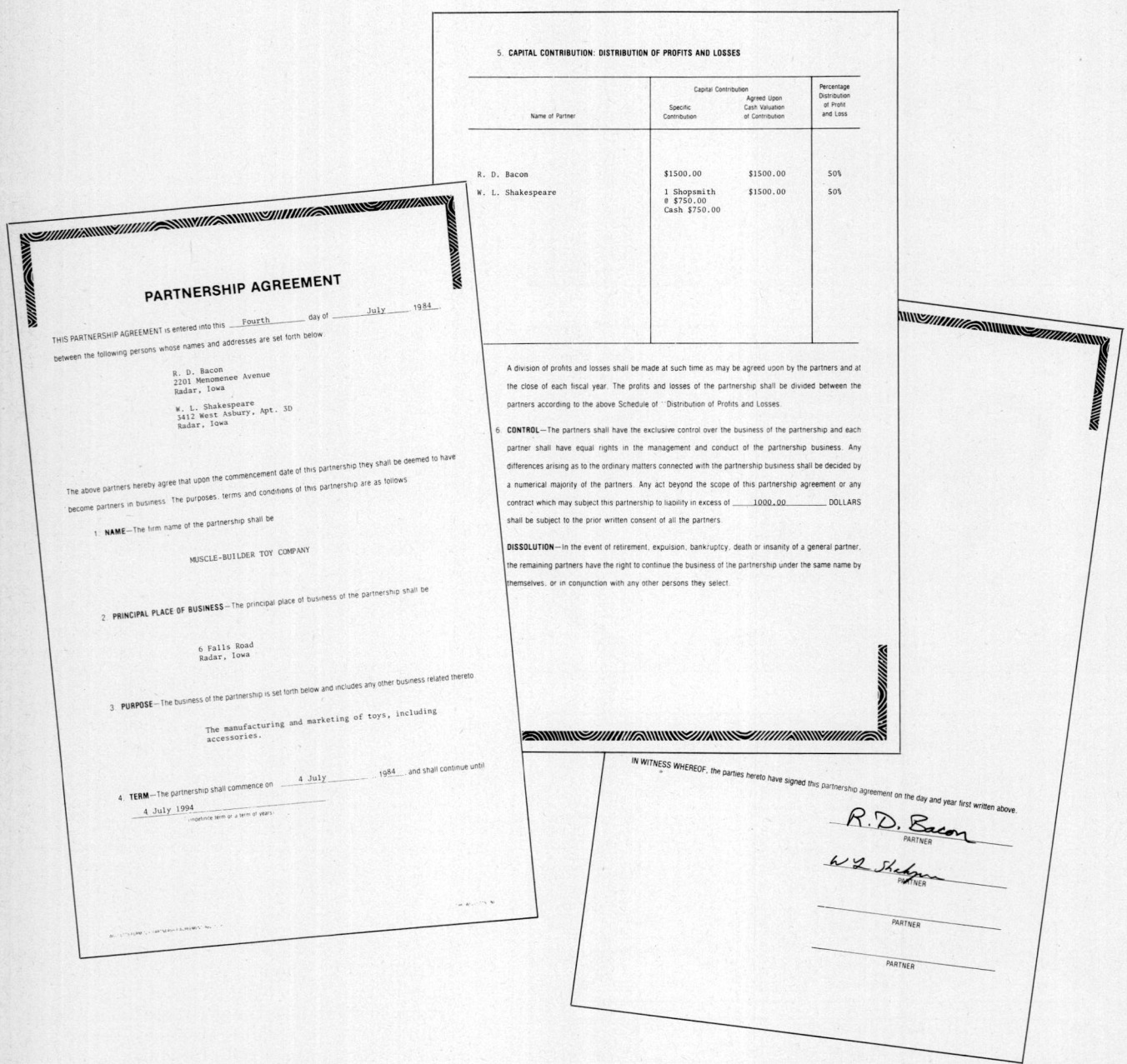

Partnerships

Other times, a small business starts as a partnership, and it can work great. The paperwork to start up is almost as easy as for a small proprietorship—although you would want a good lawyer to put together the right partnership agreement for you, it is possible to form a valid partnership with a handshake. But don't. Sign a partnership agreement; you'll be glad you did in the long run. (See Figure 11.3 for a sample partnership agreement.)

Corporations

Throughout this chapter we will continue to give you good reasons to at least think about incorporating your small business. But of the three legal entities to choose from, a corporation requires the most—and the most careful—paperwork. That's right, you'll need a lawyer. In just a minute, we'll give you tools for locating the right lawyer for you—plus magic words to show your lawyer you know more than the lawyer thinks you do.

Choosing the Best Legal Form for You

Before you decide, finish reading this chapter. At least study Table 11.1 on this page. Then do a projected cash flow and a projected P and L, to get a ballpark look at your first couple of years. Decide, on the

TABLE 11.1 Comparison Chart on Legal Forms

	Control	Need for Written Agreements	Raising Money	Taxes	Liability	Continuity
Sole proprietorship	absolute	none	one-person show save, save, save	$ or ($) go with personal income	personally liable for everything	It's on your back
Partnership (limited)	total control by general partner	overwhelming	lots of laws	$ or ($) passed onto ltd. partners	ltd. partners are liable only for $ invested	death cancels parnership
Partnership (general)	divided	locate super lawyer	easier if more parties sign	$ or ($) passed on to partners	personal liability for debts or misdeeds of partners	depends on buy-sell agreement
Corporation	shared (could be absolute)	locate super lawyer	market your snob appeal	taxed in tiers of $25K (tax year can be changed)	shield between you & world	potential for immortality
Subchapter S	shared (could be absolute)	much red tape (get a lawyer)	limit on number of stockholders	a good deal if you're losing $$$$$	corporate protection	potential for immortality

basis of a really accurate business analysis, what the best legal form for your business is.

Because that's all it is—a form, a shape. To the consumer, legal forms are invisible. To you, the right shape is absolutely essential. You want it to be rock solid, stable, protective—yet you want to be able to change the shape if it's not working.

WHY YOU NEED A LAWYER

Because businesses are built on people, you need a business structure that gives you flexibility when the people in your business want a change. Don't underestimate the power of psychological forces. The case studies and the six questions to ask your lawyer provided in this chapter are all designed to help you anticipate those internal forces at work that can make you wish you had planned escape routes ahead of time.

Only a good **small business attorney** can help you create the right business structure for a partnership or a corporation—a structure that gives you the flexibility you'll need. Action Step 45 tells you how to shop for the right lawyer. Read it—and the rest of the chapter—and then act.

After you read this chapter, continue your exploration of legal forms by taking a lawyer to lunch.

Magic Words: Six Questions to Ask Your Prospective Lawyer

The following warm-up questions will let you find out just how sharp your prospective lawyer is. And they'll get the discussion started in the right direction. The questions will also let the attorney know the caliber of the client he or she might be getting. Don't be shy about asking tough questions: Remember, you're buying lunch.

Question 1. What kind of signals suggest that I should designate my company stock as IRS Section 1244?

Section 1244 of the **IRS Codes** could save you a lot of money. For example, if you form a company and the stock becomes worthless (or if you're forced to sell it at a loss), Section 1244 allows you to deduct up to $50,000 per year as ordinary income. You must write the magic words "Section 1244 Stock" into your corporation's by-laws, and you'll need a lawyer or tax adviser to write it correctly. If you don't have the 1244 privilege, you'll be allowed only a capital loss, which is a lot less. If you win, you want to win big. If you lose, you want to have the loss work for you, not against. Section 1244 gives you credit for trying.

Question 2. Can you give me a concrete example of how IRS Section 368(a)(1)(B) works?

After you've gotten rich slowly in your small business, you may want to liquidate, take your profits, and retire to a beach in magical Tahiti. If you do a simple sale, you create tax problems. Section

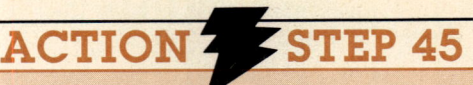

ACTION STEP 45

Take a Lawyer to Lunch

Network your business contacts until you get the names of 3–5 attorneys who know something about forming small business corporations and partnerships.

Concentrate on those who have worked in your industry.

Call up. Check them out on the phone. Take the most promising candidates to lunch. (*Remember:* This is a write-off.)

What you're looking for first is someone you can get along with.

Then look for experience in the world of small business. A hot trial lawyer may have a lot of charisma on television, but you want a nuts-and-bolts small business specialist who can save you time, pain, and money.

During lunch, find out about fees and costs. Compare the cost, for example, of having your lawyer write up a complex partnership buy-out agreement with the cost of setting up a corporation.

Following this Action Step, you'll find some questions to start you off in your discussions with your prospective attorney.

A good lawyer has a different perspective that will be helpful to the formation of your business. You may have to look awhile. It may cost you some dollars up front. But there's no substitute for good legal help.

P.S. Lunch is optional—but your inquiries are vital.

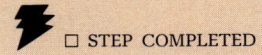 ☐ STEP COMPLETED

small business attorney
an attorney who specializes in small business

IRS Codes
federal government tax regulations

368(a)(1)(B) allows you to exchange your corporate stock (and control of the company you've built over the years) solely for stock in another — probably larger — corporation. Later, when you need money, you wait for the stock market to soar and then you peel off those larger certificates.

Question 3.   How does my corporation handle the **depreciation** recapture rule?

If your business doesn't have equipment, skip this one. One of your big tax write-offs is equipment depreciation. If the sale of your corporation includes equipment, you drop into a trap called IRS Section 1245, which means you take back those earlier write-offs as **ordinary income.** This one question should provide a nice test for your lawyer.

Question 4.   What strategies should we use to avoid "disposition of installment income" upon the sale of my corporation?

If you get paid in installments when you sell your corporation, logic dictates you should get taxed in installments. Wrong. The word "disposition" means you've just done away with tax installments. Unless you protect yourself before the sale, you'll be paying all those taxes in the year of the sale while you get the money from your buyer in droplets over the years.

Question 5.   How do I make sure I get my tax deduction when I pay the owner for a **noncompetition covenant**?

Answer: You've got to earmark it and put it in writing. Say you pay $200,000 for a business. Make sure that a specified portion is labeled — for example: "This $50,000 is specifically paid to the owner as a covenant not to compete for the next 5 years."

Question 6.   I want to make a business loan to a semi-bad risk (a family member, a worrisome in-law, or the like) without crippling my bank account and killing my business reputation. How do I make that loan and still protect myself?

Answer: Co-sign. 1) You're not out money right away, and 2) if the bad risk you co-signed for defaults on the loan, you can refer yourself to IRS Section 166(5), which allows you to write off bad debts made from guaranteeing someone's business loan.

If you borrowed the money and lost through the same default, that would amount to a mere capital loss — with a limit of $1,000 a year in deductions.

Network your contacts for a lawyer with experience in your industry. You're out there on the field, playing to win. Your lawyer is part of your *taxi squad*.

WHAT HAPPENS WHEN YOU DON'T LOOK AHEAD

If you don't use a good lawyer to help you structure your business, you probably won't have a plan to handle contingencies, and unforeseen events can take you by surprise. If Paul Webber had used his imagination to look ahead, his story might have turned out differently.

---

depreciation
a clever method of deducting the expense now of the future replacement of a capital good

ordinary income
the earnings of the individual taxpayer

noncompetition covenant
an agreement by the seller of a business not to engage in a similar business for a specified period of time

taxi squad
human resources outside your business whom you can call on as needed

Case Study

Paul Webber — Programmer Entrepreneur

Paul was a computer programmer when he met Jerry Dominic. Jerry was a likeable guy and a dynamite salesman, and after he'd read *Megatrends* he knew there was money to be made in the information business, so he got together with Paul and they formed a software consulting business. They specialized in microcomputers, because that's where the action was. Their first year was okay—they netted over $40,000 apiece—but their second year was looking even better.

By May of their second year, their projections told them they might make something like a hundred thousand each before the end of summer.

It felt great to be rich.

To celebrate, they went to a neighborhood bar for a couple of drinks. Jerry got into an argument with a bald-headed guy about politics. There was a quick fistfight and Jerry ended up on the floor. As Paul stooped down to help Jerry up, he noticed his partner felt heavy, like dead weight.

At 49 years old, Jerry Dominic was dead of a heart attack.

Two days after the funeral, Paul was on the phone to a customer when Jerry's widow walked in. She was dressed in dark clothes. Her name was Mildred. And she had just inherited Jerry's half of the business.

Paul didn't like it, but there was nothing he could do. He knew how Mildred Dominic felt. He also knew he would have to break his back to teach her the business. Computer software was fast-track and super-competitive—it changed before you could take a breath—and Mildred would have to learn an awful lot in a very short time.

Paul was a good guy, so he tried. The first week, he was extra tired because he was handling his own customers while he spent long hours with Jerry's widow, trying to phase her into the business. The second week, two of Paul's customers on hold defected to a competitor. Paul heard about it on the grapevine. The third week, the company almost ran out of cash and Paul had to dump in $5,000 from his personal account to keep suppliers happy.

The other problem was that Mildred, Jerry's widow, wasn't learning the business. She was getting in Paul's hair, and she was spending money. But she wasn't able to hold up her end, and there was no improvement in sight.

Paul hung on for a couple more weeks. Then he did the only thing he could do for his own survival: He took what customers he had left and rented an office six blocks away and tried to keep going. He figured he had paid his dues to Jerry. He hoped Jerry understood, wherever he was.

Sometimes, Paul wishes he and Jerry had had something in writing to cover **contingencies.** In business, you always need a Plan B.

contingencies
unforeseen events in the future which alert you to develop Plan B early

partnership agreement
a written agreement between two or more partners that should specifiy profit sharing, capital gains distribution, and tactics for painless dissolution

Advice: If you still want to form a partnership, get a lawyer to draw up a *partnership agreement* and consult your insurance agent about taking on some protective insurance.

If you're able to look ahead, you'll avoid problems regardless of the legal form of your business. Next, we'll help you look ahead at incorporation.

CORPORATIONS AND SMALL BUSINESS

In the section that follows, we give you eight good reasons for thinking about incorporation before you take the plunge. In general, we think most owners of small businesses fail to incorporate because they don't see the clear signals their businesses are giving. If you don't see the signals, don't incorporate. If you do, check out an attorney. (See the sidebar, "Three Clear Signals That You Should Consider Incorporation.")

Eight Reasons to Think About Incorporating

1. You Limit Your Liability. A corporation acts like a shield between you and the world. If your business fails, your creditors can't come after your house, your beach-condo, your Porsche, your first-born, your hard-won collectibles — provided you've done it right.

To keep your corporate shield up, make sure you: 1) hold scheduled meetings; 2) keep up the minute book; and 3) act as if you are an employee of the corporation.

Here's an everyday example of the corporate shield at work: your secretary gets into a fender-bender while driving on company business; if you're a corporation, the injured parties will come after your corporation and not you.

(If your employees use *their* cars on company business, make sure they're insured for a minimum of $1 million.)

2. You Change Your Tax Picture. The income from corporations is taxed in **tax tiers.**

	Pre-1982	1982	1983 and beyond*
First $25K	20%	16%	15%
Second $25K	22%	19%	18%
Third $25K	30%	30%	30%
Fourth $25K	40%	40%	40%
Over $100K	46%	46%	46%

* Tax laws change. Check with the IRS.

Now, what does this mean to you as a small business person? Let's say you're a sole proprietor and you make $60,000 in 1984. The tax table for 1984 says you'll pay 38% tax on that $60,000, or $22,800. Ouch.

Now let's say you're in the same business, only you're the founder and key employee of a corporation. You take a salary of $35,000, which is taxable at around 28%, or about $10,000. In both ownership examples, you want to keep $21,000 in the business to support next year's growth.

What does the tax picture look like?

Three Clear Signals That You Should Consider Incorporation

If you are in business now and are thinking about incorporation, answer these three questions first. Your business may already be giving you signals that you should incorporate soon.

1. Could you be sued? If you are vulnerable to litigation, then incorporate or buy lots of protective insurance.
2. Are your profits more than $50,000 a year? If the answer is yes, then incorporate for tax reasons.
3. Do you want a different, more prestigious image? Again, if the answer is yes, incorporate.

tax tiers
a graduated series of tax obligations

	No Corporation	Corporation	
		Corporation	You
Profits	$60,000	$60,000	
Salary (expense)	–0–	35,000	$35,000
Taxable income	60,000	25,000	35,000
		×15%	
Income tax	22,800	3,750	10,000
After tax	37,200	21,250	25,000
Money for next year's growth	21,000	21,000	–0–
Personal spendable	16,200		25,000

If you incorporated with this tax picture, you would end up paying $9,050 less in taxes. That's over 50% more personal spendable income. It pays to check into what a corporate structure can do for you.

3. You Control Your Fiscal Year.   As a sole proprietor or partnership, your fiscal (tax) year ends on December 31, whether you like it or not. As a corporation, you can decide where you want your **fiscal year** to end. You might actually save money, because you can plan for the best action (buy, invest, sell, and so on).

4. You Upgrade Your Image.   What does the word, *corporation*, mean to you? IBM? Exxon? TRW? Texaco? TWA? GM?

Heavy hitters, right?

Let's look at the word with New Eyes.

Corporation comes from the Latin, *corpus,* which means ''body.'' *To incorporate* means to make or form or shape into a body. Looked at from that angle, ''incorporating'' starts to sound creative.

It will sound that way to lots of your Target Customers, too.

As a corporation, you can:

1) Have more clout and solidity in the world.
2) Attract better employees.
3) Enjoy more prestige.

5. You Have the Opportunity of Channeling Some Heavy Expenses.   With some legal help, you can write a medical assistance clause into your by-laws. Here's the way it works:

1. Your corporation pays the **insurance premium** on your health insurance.
2. Your corporation reimburses you for the deductible
   a. Your corporation writes off the money paid to you as a business expense
   b. You aren't liable for taxes on the reimbursement

6. You Simplify the Division of Multiple Ownership.   As an example, say you're going into the printing and graphics business with two very good friends.

fiscal year
a flexible date set by a corporation which gives the owners partial control over the timing of taxes

insurance premium
a rated payment on insurance coverage

The business needs $110,000 to get started.
You can put your hands on $60,000.
Friend A delivers $25,000.
Friend B delivers $15,000.
You borrow the other $10,000 from your friendly banker.
The way to handle the ownership is with stock. You get 60%. Friend A gets 25%. Friend B gets 15%.

7. You Guarantee Continuity.   If one of your stockholder/founders departs by power sailer or other means, the corporation keeps on chugging. That's because you've gone through a lot of red tape and planning to set it up that way.

It's one of the few justifications for red tape we know of.

8. You Can Offer Internal Incentives.   When you want to reward a special employee, you can offer some stock or a promotion (for example, a Vice Presidential title) in addition to (and sometimes in place of) pay raises. Becoming a corporate officer carries its own special excitement, and this gives you flexibility.

What a Corporation Will Not Do

Becoming a corporation won't solve all your problems. For example, a corporation will not do any of the following:

Immunize you against creditors (the bankers and creditors will
   still want a personal guarantee — which could mean your house.)
Make you immortal.
Eliminate taxes altogether.
Do your market research for you.
Make those cold calls when you need business.
Save a marriage that's already on the rocks.

In this chapter we've made a strong case for incorporation. For an alternate view, see the boxed article on page 210.

DO RESEARCH ON CORPORATIONS NOW

We've told you a lot of what you need to know, but don't stop yet. Action Step 46 gets you started on secondary research now. It takes time to incorporate properly, so it pays to get started early.

A Word About Subchapter S

Subchapter S corporations are semicorporate bodies that attempt to limit the owner's liability while still allowing a pass-through of busi-

---

ACTION ⚡ STEP 46

Do Some Secondary Research on Corporations

Before you take any action about legal forms, you need a lot of information.

Read books like *Inc. Yourself* by Judith McQuown, *How to Form Your Own Corporation Without a Lawyer for Under $50* by Ted Nicholas, and *Incorporating Your Business* by John Kirk.

Once you get familiar with the broad concepts, do some research on specific corporations (start with your incorporated competitors) in your industry. You can get information from the library, from a stock broker, or by writing the corporation.

While you're doing this research, keep looking around with New Eyes.

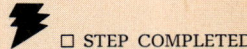 ☐ STEP COMPLETED

Don't Incorporate for the Big "Inc." or the Pension Plan Alone.

If you're thinking about incorporating just to get the "Inc." after your name or because you think it's the "in" thing to do, stop and give the matter a re-think. In 1982, Congress changed the rules to discourage incorporation by professionals — doctors, lawyers, consultants, big-time athletes, entertainers, enginers, architects, et al. — and small business owners, as usual, take the legislative fallout. Prior to 1982, a small business owner was forced to incorporate to put money away for retirement. Because of the 1982 ruling, you've got three choices on your pension plans if you'd still like to be a sole proprietor.

1. A "Keogh" for 15% of earnings up to $30,000.
2. A "money-purchase" plan for 25% of earnings up to $30,000.
3. A "defined-benefit plan" which allows you to fund a pension plan as large as $90,000 per year.

So if you're in business to feather your nest for those retirement years, network your way to a lawyer and give the legal form of your business some thought. A good insurance plan might handle your liability problems — and allow you to handle the business helm as sole proprietor.

Warning: You'll still need legal help setting up your pension plan. Lawyers and accountants are two valiant mainstays of the Information Society.

SOURCE: Adapted from Janet Bryant Quinn, "To Inc. or Not To Inc." *Newsweek* (January 9, 1984). Copyright 1984, by Newsweek, Inc. All rights reserved, reprinted by permission.

ness losses to the personal income statement of the owners, founders, and others.

The name Sub S comes from a 1958 section of the IRS code, where it leaped from the pages of an IRS document to the world. Now it's a buzzword.

There were some changes made in Sub S corporation rules in late 1982 (higher owner retirement ceilings, 35 shareholders instead of 25, two classes of stock instead of one, a broadening of allowable income from passive sources such as rents, and so on).

But most tax authorities still hold that you want to form a Sub S only if your company is going to be losing money for the first year or so.

Most states have specific time requirements for filing.

Not all states recognize the tax aspects of the Sub S category.

It takes time to incorporate. Do it early, if the signs point that way, and save yourself some grief.

Look at how the corporate shield protected the entrepreneur in our next case study.

Easy-Cup Coffee Service — The Corporate Shield

Henry Bemis was going great guns with his coffee service when a piece of his equipment spewed boiling water all over the hands of Jody Dawn, a professional model.

Miss Dawn's hands earned her just over $200,000 a year. The day her hands were burnt, she was at a branch of a major bank, doing a DeBeers-sponsored commercial for diamond rings and safety-deposit boxes.

Her model's hands were her living and her future. On the advice of her attorney, Miss Dawn sued Henry Bemis and his Easy-Cup Coffee Service.

Henry had insurance, of course. But it stopped at $350,000, and the courts were about to award Miss Dawn two million dollars.

Here's the way they figured it:

She made $200,000 a year.
She could figure on an active career of at least ten years.
Ten years × $200,000 = $2,000,000.

Luckily, Henry had the good sense to incorporate when he first went into business. So while the courts went after Easy-Cup Coffee Service, Inc., Henry's house and car and personal properties were safe.

Also, because he'd gotten into a couple of networks, Henry was able to start another business right away.

This time, he didn't go into coffee.

SUMMARY

There are three legal forms for your small business: sole proprietorship, partnership, corporation.

You can run a business as a sole proprietorship with a minimum of hassle — you might only need a city license, a resale license, and a DBA, or fictitious name statement. (If you use your own name, you won't even need a DBA.)

The legal paperwork for a partnership is almost as hassle-free. You can form a partnership with a handshake and disssolve it without one. There are good psychological reasons for forming a partnership. Let's say you're an inventor; you need a partner who can manage and sell. Let's say you're good at marketing; you need a partner who can run the office and keep the books.

Only 8% of the small businesses in the country are partnerships. If you decide a partnership is right for you, get a lawyer to pull together a partnership agreement to protect you against trouble.

ACTION STEP REVIEW

Two Action Steps teach you more about legal forms.

45 When you take a lawyer to lunch, use the time to determine the lawyer's personality. Can you get along with this lawyer? Does this lawyer understand your small business? Once you've decided you can work with a lawyer, ask some of the questions provided in this chapter.

46 In this Action Step, you read some books on corporations and the art of incorporating. A list of books is included in the Reference section. You can also contact your librarian and your stock broker for information on corporations.

Forming a corporation will take the most paperwork, but it gives you more flexibility, as well as a shield to protect you in case your business hurts someone. With a corporation:

1. You limit your liability.
2. You change your tax picture.
3. You control your fiscal year.
4. You upgrade your company image.
5. You can rechannel some expenses (like medical).
6. Your company stock can simplify multiple ownership.
7. You can guarantee continuity.
8. You can offer internal incentives to key employees.

One green light for incorporating is when you make $50,000 or more in your business.

THINK POINTS

- We only remember what we want to. Get everything in writing.
- A green light for incorporating is when you make $50,000 or more per year.
- If your business is small and you like it that way, keep it simple like your hobby.
- Most growth businesses need outside infusions of cash. Don't pay Uncle Sam more than you have to.
- When you create corporate stock in your by-laws, think about creating at least 10 times more than you intend to sell at start-up.
- Even when you incorporate, a banker will still want a personal guarantee for loans.
- Forget about incorporating in Nevada or Delaware (unless you live there), or in exotic offshore locations. You'll be a foreign corporation (out-of-state) and you'll have to pay extra to do business at home.

REFERENCES

Ames, Michael D., and Norval L. Wellsfry. *Small Business Management.* St. Paul, Minn.: West Publishing Co., 1983.

''A Big Boon for Small Business.'' *Business Week,* November 1, 1982, 82.

''Goodies for Small Business.'' *Nation's Business,* December 1981, 84.

McQuown, Judith H. *Inc. Yourself: How to Profit by Setting Up Your Own Corporation.* New York: Macmillan Publishing Co., 1982.

Mancuso, Anthony, and Peter Jan Honigsberg. 2d ed. *The California Professional Corporation Handbook.* Berkeley, Calif.: Nolo Press, 1983.

"No Big Breaks for Small Business in the Tax Cuts." *Business Week,* August 24, 1981, 100.

Professional Report Editors and John Kirk. *Incorporating Your Business.* Chicago: Contemporary Books, 1981.

Weaver, Peter A. *You, Inc.: A Detailed Escape Route for Being Your Own Boss.* New York: Doubleday & Co., 1975.

A Description of Product or Service

B The Market and the Target Customer

C Competition

D Marketing Strategy

E Location

F Management

G Personnel

H Projected Income Statement

I Projected Cash Flow

J Projected Balance Sheet

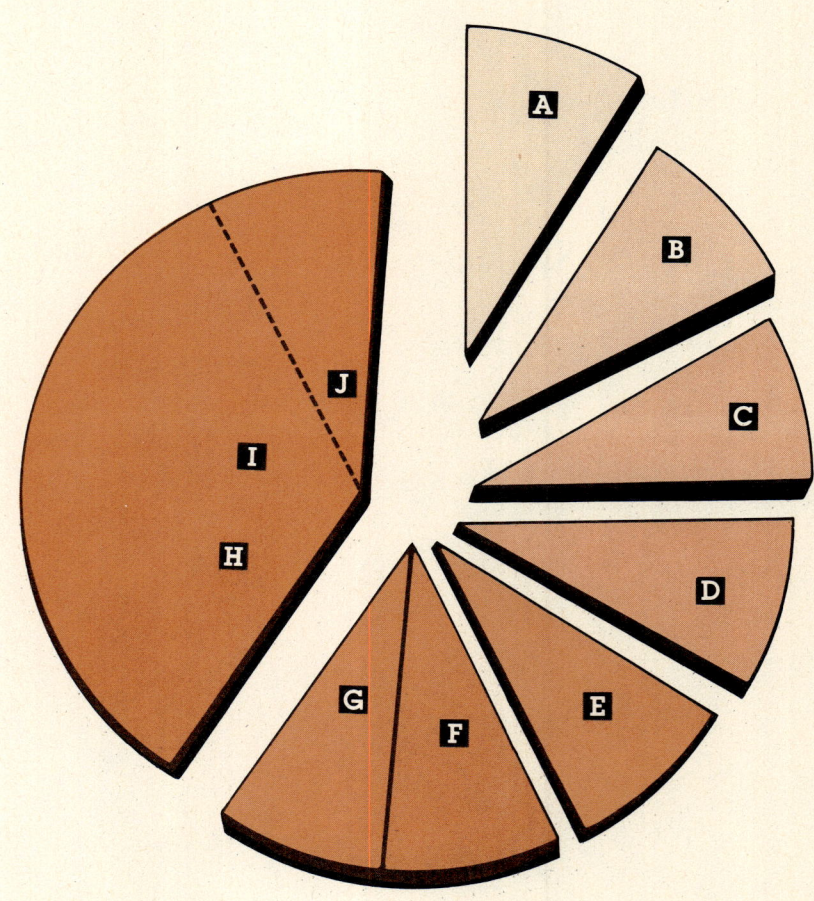

FIGURE 12.1 Chapter 12 allows you to complete the Management and Personnel sections of your Plan as you learn about the importance of a balanced team.

12

Fun-Time: Building Your Winning Team

LEARNING OBJECTIVES

To discover that, despite your entrepreneurial energies and tremendous creativity, you probably can't do it all.

To sense that balance in your business is another key to survival.

To take another look at yourself and identify dangerous shortcomings — shortcomings that can be dealt with through an objective view and positive action.

To explore new ways of putting together a Founder's Team.

To look back, over the way you've journeyed, and see if there's anyone you wish were working with you in this venture.

To use brainstorming techniques to pull together the perfect team.

To use the DISC Performax Personality Profile (or other systems) to help you identify who you are and what types of people you need for balance.

To survey your competitors and network your vendors for potential team members.

To brainstorm with your new team *before* you open the doors, so you can take advantage of the all-important resource, people.

 **B**uilding a winning team can be one of the most enjoyable tasks you face — if you can learn to see yourself objectively, and if you can learn to build your team around real business and psychological needs. Because that's just what the successful entrepreneur — the master architect of small business — does. The entrepreneur builds to win.

MASTER ARCHITECT

Entrepreneur means master architect, all right, but what does it bode for the rest of your team?

Take a moment to look inside yourself with New Eyes.
Do you see a bold entrepreneur?
Do you see a builder? A creator? A fearless innovator?

Looking Inside the Entrepreneur

Entrepreneur comes from *pre-hendere,* a Latin verb that's packed with power. *Hendere* itself means ''to get hold of,'' ''to seize,'' ''to grasp.'' The verb *hendere* comes up from *ghend,* meaning to *seize, take, get.* A close cousin in our time is *Apprehend.*

Way down the language line of word transformation, Latin *ghend* links up with an Anglo-Saxon verb *Bigetan* (to acquire) and also with *Beget,* which still means today what it meant in biblical times.

Beget. Begat. Begat. The power to create.

POWER. ENERGY. CLOUT.

Entrepreneur is, of course, French. The word arrived here by swimming into English on the back of ''enterprise.'' When the word crossed the English channel, our British language cousins, past masters of selling and marketing, cleverly repositioned the R and the E, to make it sound more clearly British.

From entREprise to entERprise.

Prise, waiting back there on the French coast, meant ''taken'' or ''captured'' or seized.'' Once on British soil, feminine *prise* is pronounced *prize.* And that's the way we entrepreneurial pirates like it.

If you like the historical tug of these words (grasp, beget, prize, apprehend, captured, seize, creator, builder), you're in the right business.

According to the dictionary, the word *enterprise* connotes industry, money, the readiness for adventure, initiative, and boldness. Remember *Star Trek?* The USS *Enterprise?* Kirk's mission in space?

To boldly go forth. . . .

So roll the words around for a minute. *Entrepreneur* means **master architect.** Builder. Creator.

If you like the sound of that, take a breather with Action Step 47.

This trip isn't over, and you've probably met some fascinating folks along the way. Remember?

Take a look at how far you've come. Relax. You owe it to yourself.

master architect
if you look at the origins of the word, entrepreneur, you see it means master architect

The Need to Balance Functions

This is a profile of an entrepreneur who needed a balanced team and didn't know it.

Case Study

Harry R. Marquez — B.S., Ph.D.

Harry was such a terrible student, his parents worried he'd never make it through high school. His grades in English were rotten. He couldn't spell. To Harry, history was a laugh, government a lie, and science an outmoded and unimaginative way of looking at the universe.

There were three courses Harry did all right in: Art, Physics (he liked electricity), and Latin. But you can't graduate from high school with three strong subjects and ten weak ones, so Harry joined the Army. He took some tests and the Army sent him to Germany, to drive tanks. One day, the tank broke down on maneuvers and Harry had it fixed in seven minutes.

Tanks were mostly metal and circuits, and electricity was always Harry's baby. Harry quickly became invaluable. He fixed tanks. The Army gave him weekend passes.

Harry already knew Spanish, because it had been spoken by his grandparents. He knew Latin. Now he met a German woman named Liliane. She was a model and her English was very good. Harry wanted to learn German, so he gave Liliane orders never to speak English when she was around him.

In six months, Harry was fluent in German.

At the end of his tour, Harry married Liliane and brought her back to the U.S. She got a job modeling while Harry looked up his old Physics teacher. After a lot of scrambling and maneuvering, Harry made it into a good university.

Here, he could choose courses he could handle. He even met an English teacher who taught him how to write. Harry finished his B.S. in Electrical Engineering in three years. At the end of two more, he had his doctorate. And along the way, he had discovered a field that looked hot: Industrial robots.

Harry landed a job with a *Fortune* 500 firm. The pay was good, but Harry hated the lack of freedom. When Harry couldn't create, his mind slowed down and he felt dead.

Working at night, Harry perfected an idea of his to make a two-armed robot. He took the idea upstairs, to a vice-president in a dark suit, but the guy wasn't interested.

So Harry formed his own company.

He didn't know the first thing about business, but he found a man who did. The man's name was Frederick S. Winslow and he had a sales background, a sincere smile, a warm handshake, and no money to help with the capitalization.

Winslow was a great talker. He had a way with words that could have made him a preacher or politician.

Harry wanted to locate in the East, where he was comfortable, but Winslow said the only place for this kind of firm was the Silicon Valley of California.

The name of the firm was Marquez Robotics. Harry and Liliane owned all the stock. Their first year, Marquez Robotics grossed just under a million. Harry loved it. He didn't understand a **balance sheet** and talk about cash flow put him right to sleep, but he loved having money to spend.

Continued

balanced team
a group of individuals with a complementary mix of skills, aptitudes, and strengths

ACTION STEP 47

View Mind Movies of the Fun Sights and People You Met Sizing up the Competition

Take a couple of minutes out from the rigors of your venture adventure to look back over your journey.

Just sit back, close your eyes, and enjoy the highlights of your trip. What have you learned so far? What was fun? Who did you meet that you found interesting or exciting or especially helpful?

Write down their names. If you can't remember a name, jot down the type of person (outgoing, sharp, detailed, energetic, and so on) and where you met.

Write a quick profile of the people you found most interesting. Ask yourself why.

Start with categories like age, sex, income, education, residence, and lifestyle; then slide over into personality.

How many on your list were bold, adventurous, industrious? How many were warm and pleasant? How many were inspiring?

How many would you consider using as part of your team?

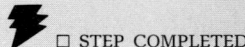 ☐ STEP COMPLETED

balance sheet
a financial tool which gives you a picture of your business at one point in time

He bought Liliane a Turbo Porsche. Crimson, with racing stripes. He bought himself an Eldorado. Grey, with everything on it. Harry was an artist. He had lived hard. Now he needed plush comfort. He also needed stimulation, and that meant people like himself, who were loaded with ideas, people who could work through the night on a project, then cap it off with a party.

So Harry hired a lot of people like himself, and he decorated the front office with attractive show girls on temporary leave from their acting careers, and lots of times the phones would ring like crazy and no one would answer them.

The second year, Winslow wanted a piece of the company.

But Harry didn't want to let go. He felt like a father. It was his company, built with his Army money plus the money he and Liliane had saved while he was breaking his back for the corporate world. And it was his two-armed robot.

So Harry said no.

Then two things happened.

Mrs. Liliane Marquez decided she wanted a divorce. And Mr. Frederick S. Winslow left the company.

Liliane drove her Turbo Porsche to San Francisco, where she leased an expensive townhome on Nob Hill. Winslow went down the road a half mile and founded a company called Winslow Electromagnetic. Like a lot of people, Winslow wanted his name on the front of the store. With him, he took two of Harry's key employees, both inventor-engineers, and 17 of Harry's largest customer accounts.

One by one, the attractive young women left Marquez Robotics to find their way back to the world of show business. One by one, the wild-and-crazy engineer-inventors left when Harry didn't have enough cash to meet his payroll.

Meanwhile, Harry was busy in his lab, working night and day on an electric motor that would take the place of the hydraulic engines used in most robots.

There was no one in the front office, no one to answer the phones. The books went from bad to worse. Harry was in a race with his creditors, who would ship only with a C.O.D., but he was so deep into his new invention he hardly noticed.

What Can Harry Marquez Teach Us?

We can learn at least two lessons from Harry's predicament. Number one, Harry could design great equipment, but he could not design a winning team. True, he did hire Winslow, who in many ways was a perfect complement to Harry. Winslow was a winning employee, but Harry couldn't read the man's drives for power and control.

Number two, Harry couldn't take the time to listen to his employees. The people he hired did not fill real business needs. In business, that's fatal.

We can suggest techniques to help people like Harry know themselves. **Self-analysis** is a must in small business.

But first, read Action Step 48. Then continue with the text, and we'll show you techniques you can use to get a better view of yourself — and to pick the right people for your team.

Some Street-Smart Advice.   If you hire good people, listen to them. A company is no more than its people. Successful businesses of whatever size view their employees as resources.

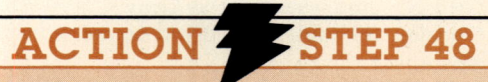

ACTION STEP 48

Brainstorm Your Ideal Team

What do you need to win at the game of small business? Money, of course. And energy, tremendous energy.

You've got that or you wouldn't have read this far.

You also need footwork, a terrific idea, intensity, the ability to concentrate, a sense of industry and thrift, and a nose for clues like Sherlock Holmes, the famous detective.

And you need . . . people.

People to support your effort. People to balance your skills. People to take up the slack. People to help you with tasks you find distasteful or don't understand.

So analyze yourself first. What do you like? What are you good at? What do you hate? What needs doing for the survival of your business?

If you can't do it, who will?

That one idea alone will get you started on building your ideal team.

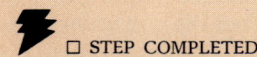 □ STEP COMPLETED

self-analysis
an introspective look at
your strengths and
weaknesses

BUILDING BALANCE INTO YOUR TEAM

To build a team, you need techniques. Balance is essential. You're probably thinking you already understand everything you need to know about balance. But if you're a creative entrepreneur-architect who enjoys solving every problem yourself, it will take time before you admit you need help. Fortunately, tools are available to give you perspective.

Analyzing the Team's Founder

Let's go back to Harry R. Marquez for a minute and try a **personality analysis.** We can say this about Harry:

Bright, creative.

Impatient with day-to-day operations.

A dreamer.

Quick learner, terrible student.

Could fix almost anything mechanical or electrical.

Liked pretty people (his model wife, the women from the theatre world).

Needed a certain amount of flash in the world (red Porsche, snazzy Eldorado).

Didn't want to give up piece of his company (he felt like a proud parent).

Didn't understand the power-drives of Frederick S. Winslow.

When the going got tough, Harry went back to his lab (womb, retreat from the world) to perfect yet another dazzling invention.

It's probably obvious to you that Harry needed balancing. But it wasn't obvious to him. He looked in the mirror and saw a hard-working guy. What kind of help did Harry need?

The DISC System

To answer, let's use a very revealing personality profile called **DISC.** The DISC system was developed in the seventies by John Geier, Ph.D. and it's owned by Performax Systems International. It's inexpensive and thorough, and it can give the impatient entrepreneur insight and quick perspective on people to balance the team. DISC takes about 25 minutes, and it's easy to analyze.

DISC is an acronym.

D = dominance.

I = influencing of others.

S = steadiness.

C = compliance.

Look at the grid on the following page. Where would you put Harry R. Marquez? Where would you put Frederick S. Winslow? Then check your answer with Figure 12.2 on page 221.

personality analysis
an enlightening way of looking at yourself and at the people around you

DISC
a system for profiling prospective or existing team members

D	I
Dominance	Influencing
S	C
Steadiness	Compliance

The DISC grid allows you to identify an individual's personality in relation to four different personality characteristics.

The Right Kind of Help

The beauty of the DISC grid is that it shows at a glance where you are. Harry's was a **top-heavy team.** He didn't have anyone to handle day-to-day operations. He didn't have anyone to answer the phones. In fact, when it came to phones, Harry was the caller, not the answerer. Harry needed help, but he didn't know it. What sort of help did he need?

top-heavy team
a team composed mostly of chiefs

Case Study

Mrs. Janet Ames — Compliant on the DISC Scale

Janet Ames is a capable woman in her mid-thirties. She has two well-behaved children. When her youngest reached the age of 10, Janet went back to work.

Janet came to work for Marquez Robotics three weeks after the previous vice-president for marketing, a Mr. Winslow, went off with several key employees and some very influential customers.

Janet went right to work as the new vice-president for marketing. It took her just two full working days to shape up the front office. The first thing she did was to hire a young man to handle the telephones. His name was Rudy. He was a fussy young man who kept a very tidy desk. Before noon on his first day, Rudy had established his own territory in

Continued

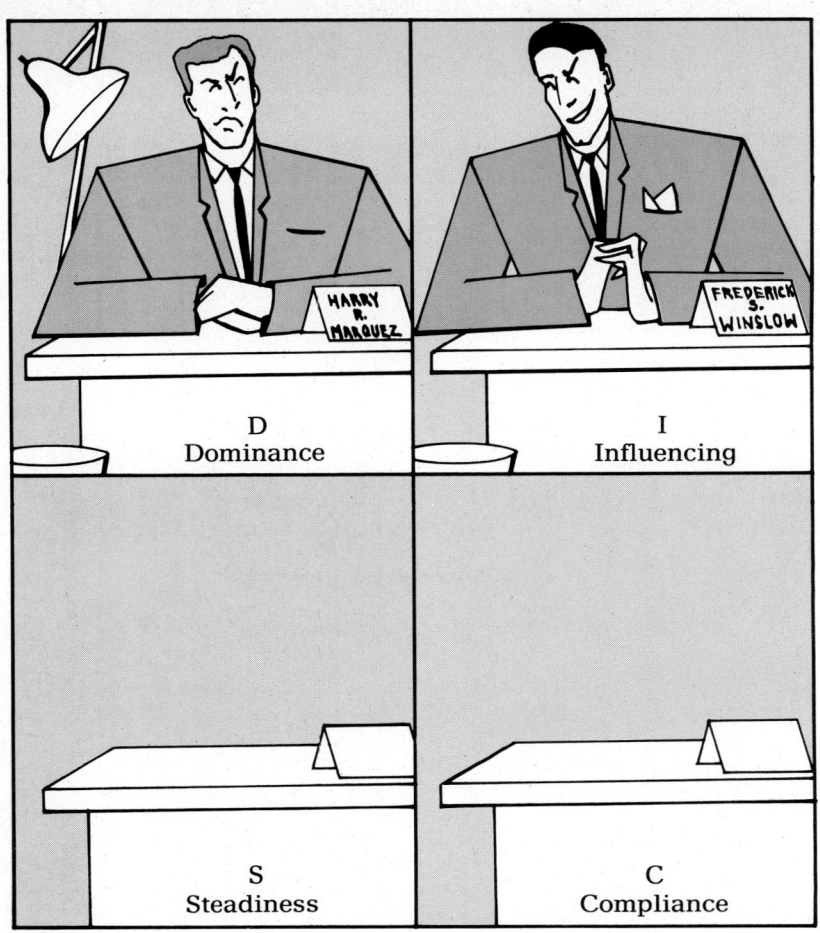

FIGURE 12.2 Harry's team was top-heavy.

one corner of the front office. He had his own desk, his own personalized nameplate, and his initials were monogrammed in large letters on his wastepaper basket.

Mrs. Ames liked that. It bespoke order.

Once she got the phone question settled, she began networking her contacts for someone to straighten out the books. Janet was a good bookkeeper, but she knew a mess when she saw one, and off in the distance she could smell tax problems for her new boss. In this instance, an expert was definitely called for.

Janet saw Dr. Marquez, the president and CEO, the day she was hired, and then she didn't see him again for eleven days.

While that might have bothered someone else, it suited the very stable Mrs. Ames just fine.

One of Mrs. Ames' philosophies was that it takes all kinds.

To her, Dr. Marquez and the men in the lab were just playful children. They needed their freedom to create. If they had been real children, of course, she would have applied some well-needed discipline. But they were adults, and you don't tell adults when it's time to scrub behind their ears. Especially if you are employed by them.

So Mrs. Ames worked hard at being diplomatic, at smoothing over rifts in the company surface, at helping and counseling and controlling.

Nine months after Mrs. Ames came to work for Marquez Robotics,

Continued

the company was again in the black. Mrs. Ames celebrated by hiring a young woman to help out in the front office. Her name was Sandra Star and she wanted to be an actress. Her smile made the customers happy and she took the office PR load off Rudy, who was promoted to Communications Chief.

Rudy spent three entire weekends personalizing his new office. And his name on the door was lettered in gold. He was delighted with his new title, Rudy Bowman, CC, and he felt a renewed loyalty and devotion to Mrs. Ames and the company.

Portrait of a Balanced Team

Turn back to the DISC grid on page 220. We have already placed Harry as a **Dominant.** Where would you put Mrs. Ames? Where would you put Rudy? Where would you put Sandra, the Secretary-Receptionist?

Now let's do a quick DISC analysis of Janet Ames:

Understands the need for control.

Is diplomatic with everyone.

Checks for accuracy.

Good at analysis, critical thinking, and sizing up a situation.

Complies with authority.

Gets the job done.

Likes standard operating procedures; if there aren't any, can establish.

Enjoys being part of a group.

Without too much effort, you can see that Mrs. Ames is probably a C **(Compliant)** on the grid. People like Mrs. Ames make good managers, and that's what Marquez Robotics needed.

Rudy Bowman, our classic S **(Steady),** is no slouch as a team member, either. Steadies love to sit in one place and control a very small turf. They are invaluable for specialized skills, listening, doing the books, security tasks. They get to work on time. They leave on time. Treat a Steady right and you'll be rewarded with tons of loyalty and fidelity.

And, finally, Sandra Star, the Secretary-Receptionist is an I **(Influencing).** She's the neon entertainment. Great for the front office as long as the working conditions are favorable. A ripple or two and she'll be off to another adventure.

See Figure 12.3 for the completed team picture.

Another Look at the Team's Founder

If you can, take a minute out to double-check the personality of Harry R. Marquez. As you read, try to explore the traits he has that remind you of yourself.

We can't reproduce all the DISC profiles here, but we can summarize briefly what's going on in Harry's personality. Harry is a Creative

Dominant
a person who shapes the environment by overcoming the opposition

Compliant
a person who works with existing circumstances to promote quality in products or services

Steady
a person who cooperates with others to carry out the task

Influencing
a person who shapes the environment by bringing others into alliance

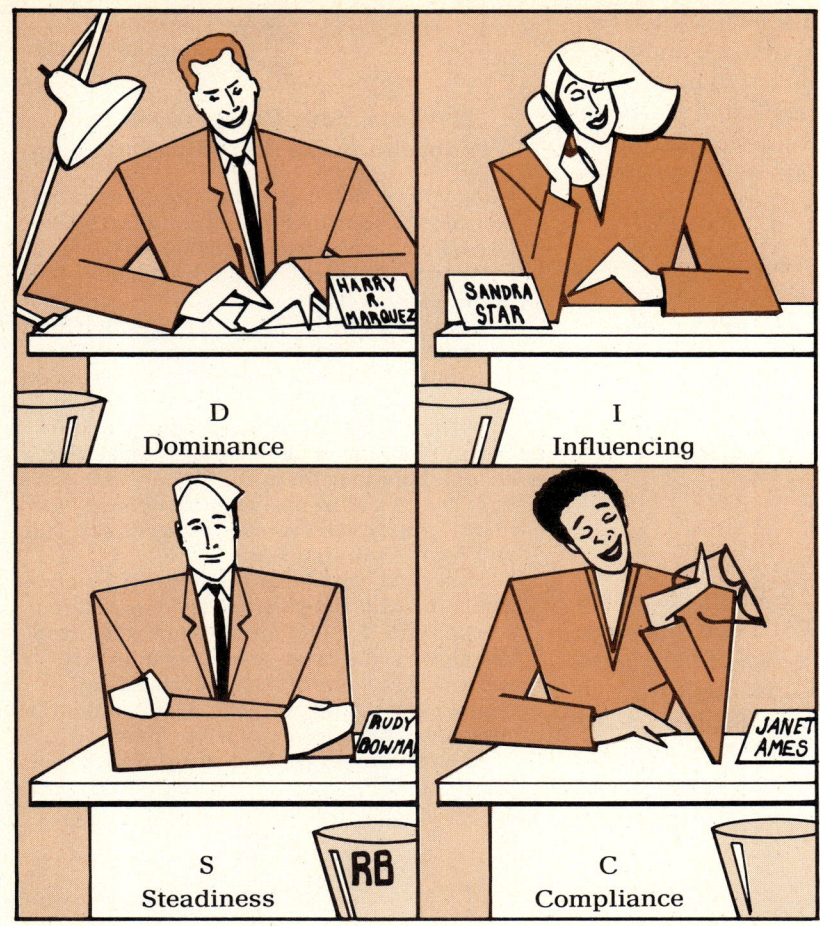

FIGURE 12.3 Janet Ames instinctively hired people who balanced Harry's team.

Achiever. He likes to dominate, control, and create. In many ways, he is the typical entrepreneur. How can you learn from Harry?

1. Operates from Internal Motivation and Deeply Felt Goals. Harry's main **joy in life** was to invent. He set his own goals and completed his tasks and he was surprised when others in the organization didn't do the same. He was unaware that some people need goals set for them. He did his work and expected everyone else to do theirs.

2. Bored with Routine Work. Harry couldn't believe that some people actually thrive on routine tasks. People like Harry are so busy setting their own pace that they seldom look back. Under pressure, they become aggressive and competitive. They like the limelight. When they don't get it, they can get sulky.

3. Judgment of Others by Concrete Results. Harry couldn't believe Frederick S. Winslow wanted a piece of the company because, to Harry the Creative Achiever, Winslow hadn't accomplished anything. To an inventor, sales is invisible and insubstantial. Money exists, but the sales and **marketing** functions of a business seem like mumbo jumbo and double-talk. From Harry's point of view, Frederick S. Winslow never really did anything except smile and glad-hand and take customers to lunch on company time. That shows Harry's limited point of view.

joy in life
where you get your main
reason for being

marketing
all the activities that take
place between
identification of the need
to the delivery of the
product or service

4. Super-Quick Thinker.   When he was on his own turf, Harry owned the fastest feet in the business. He was inventive, and if led along the right path, he could have invented a system to handle the problems of his organization. But business matters bored Harry, so the best thing for him to do was to bring someone on board who could manage the day-to-day affairs, negotiate, smooth over the rough spots, and pour oil on troubled waters.

> **Without a team, Harry R. Marquez would be out of business fast. Since he didn't want to work for someone else, he would have been in trouble. The smaller the organization, the more important the team.**

Team building is important.

SCOUTING AND HIRING

If you need help balancing your team, Appendix 12.1 lists addresses for three different kinds of personality profiles. DISC is among those listed. Action Step 49 teaches you how to use the idea of balance to scout potential team members. If you're able to imagine how each candidate would work out in your new business, you'll be well on your way to building a **winning team.** Look at Action Step 49 now.

And later, when you're hiring, we have one other piece of advice:

Keep the quality high.

If you're first rate, you'll hire first-rate people.
If you're second rate, you'll hire third-rate people.
If you're third rate, you'll hire fourth-rate people.

How long can you make it with anything but a first-rate team? As a master architect, what kind of materials do you want to build with?

Finally, you might want to consider additional tactics if you're putting together a fairly large team, one with departments that you can give names to (R & D, Administration, Finance, Marketing, Manufacturing, Quality Assurance, and so on). Take a look at Chapter 6 of Richard White's *The Entrepreneur's Manual.* White lays out a step-by-step grid for interviewing. He even tells you what to do when you meet a prospective employee for lunch. His six-step interactive program might be helpful to some of our readers — see the boxed article on the opposite page.

INTERNAL UNDERSTANDING MAKES A STRONGER TEAM

Entrepreneurs, while bright and intelligent and full of energy, can be short of self-knowledge.

In the case study that follows, we meet E. G. Bogard, a world-beater, CEO, adventurer — and an entrepreneur whose business is growing beyond the world of small business.

E. G. Bogard came up the hard way — a one-man shop, a disastrous

---

ACTION ⚡ STEP 49

Network Your Competitors and Vendors to Build that Winning Team

After you've taken the time to do some research into your own personality (your own strengths, your own weaknesses), you'll begin to get the feel for what kind of help you need in your venture.

Start with the list you made in Action Step 47, when you looked back over your adventure. Is there anyone there who can balance some of your skills?

Now make a list of the people you know. Out by the side of their names, make notes about where they fit on the DISC grid.

If you're a D-intensive entrepreneur, how many more D's can you take on your side and still have a winning team?

Now that you have the idea of balance firmly in mind, network you vendors and your competitors for potential team members. Whenever you meet someone new, try to apply DISC (or one of the other balancing systems). Keep asking yourself: "How would this person work out in my new business?"

Keep looking at your future team with New Eyes.

⚡   □ STEP COMPLETED

---

team building
the orderly procurement of people who together can achieve maximum results for the firm

winning team
what you've got to build to succeed in business

A Six-Step Interactive Program for Building Large Teams

Richard White, in *the Entrepreneur's Manual,* sets out a six-step program that lets the founders of a new business build their team by testing how well potential members interact. The program is designed for the start-up of a large organization: In White's scenario, the founders have the capital to set up team tests in an out-of-the-way spa.

Here are the six steps:

1. Begin with an **icebreaker.** Briefly tell everyone why you're here. Lay out the three main goals of the organization.
2. Introductions. Self-introductions are brief and to the point, but everyone can get a feel for who is in the room.
3. One-to-one interviews. Everybody interviews everybody else, to get a sense of the chemistry of the team. Use a large chalkboard to chart who has interviewed whom.
4. Divide everyone into departments (R & D, Finance, Marketing, and so on) to see who can work with whom.
5. Begin hypothetical negotiations *between* departments.
6. Secret ballot. Each prospective team member selects ideal teammates, using blackballs judiciously.

SOURCE: Adapted from Richard M. White, *The Entrepreneur's Manual* (Radnor, Pa.: Chilton Book Co., 1977). Copyright 1977 by the author. Reprinted with the permission of the publisher, Chilton Book Co., Radnor, Pa.

icebreaker
putting people at ease quickly

partnership, a small corporation. As we arrive on the scene, the growth of Bogard's company threatens to undermine his spectacular success. He has no idea how to handle it. He can barely admit there's a problem. And the problem is with Bogard.

Case Study

E. G. Bogard — CEO

E. G. Bogard's corporate family didn't understand him. If they did, they'd know better than to waste his valuable time.

Bogard was a self-made man. He'd started 14 years ago in his garage workshop in Skokie, and this year his Chicago manufacturing firm, which employed 200 people, was about to gross $17 million.

In his industry, Bogard had a reputation for running a **lean operation.** Three of his toughest competitors had gone down during the last recession, but Bogard had not only stayed afloat, but also managed to make a profit by trimming fat. By laying off employees and giving minimal raises, Bogard trimmed selling costs by 7% in one year.

Inc. magazine wrote him up as "Jack Sprat Bogard: The CEO with the Seven Per Cent Solution," but the article hadn't done much to help internal understanding.

Why, just yesterday, the **Executive Committee** had come in with a
Continued

lean operation
using the talents of a very few hardworking people to achieve business objectives

Executive Committee
advisers to the chief executive

recommendation about company cars, company blazers, and an all-ex-penses-paid tour to Hawaii.

The worst part was that it had taken them six pages, single-spaced, to get their message across.

Bogard hated waste.

Bogard was thinking about firing the lot when he went off for his regular game of Thursday handball. That was one ritual Bogard never missed. His opponent was Maury Applebaum. Maury was in advertis-ing, a dozen years younger than E. G. Bogard, and the only fellow around who could give Bogard a game. Bogard knew handball was out of style, but he didn't care. It gave him a chance to work up a good sweat. And he didn't have to worry about losing an eye from getting sideswiped with a metal racket.

That particular Thursday, Bogard was ferocious. He took his oppo-nent three straight games. After the match, Maury asked what was going on.

"It's nothing," Bogard snapped.

"Hey. Come on, E. G. This is Maury, remember? You were crazy out there today. You were wild."

"It's nothing," Bogard said.

But finally, over his one beer for the day, Bogard admitted what was going on. "It's my gang at the plant," he said. "They don't understand me. Maybe it's time to cash out and spend my days on the beach in Miami."

"You wouldn't last a week," Maury said.

"Probably not," Bogard said. "But lately I just can't seem to commu-nicate to my people."

"I may have an answer for you," Maury said. "Can you give me half an hour tomorrow morning?"

"Where would I find a half hour?"

"Fifteen minutes, then."

Reluctantly, Bogard agreed. He was the kind of man who carried his calendar in his head. It amazed his secretary.

The next morning, Maury Applebaum arrived, accompanied by a woman named Mary White. She was an intelligent, no-nonsense per-son. Mary White took one look at E. G. Bogard's desk, the high D's **paper jungle,** and went right to work.

"Mr. Bogard, I realize you're a busy man, so we'll get right to it. This is a **measurement tool** which can increase communication inside your company." Mary White held out a light blue folder. Bogard eyed it with suspicion.

"How long?" he asked. "And how much?"

"Fifteen minutes," she answered. "Eight dollars."

E. G. Bogard gave her a flinty smile. "Time me, Maury," he said, and dove into the folder.

The pale blue folder contained a personality measuring tool called DISC. Bogard turned out to be high in D (Dominance), low on I (In-fluencing others), medium high on S (Steady) and very low on C (Com-pliance).

Bogard's personality was categorized as Developer. A breakdown of the Developer showed:

Strong individuality.

Self-reliance.

Bypasses convention, comes up with innovative solutions.

Forceful behavior.

Continued

paper jungle
the mark of a Dominant
person on the DISC scale

measurement tool
any device that allows
management to assess
productivity

Can be shrewd at manipulating people and situations.

Hates boredom worse than anything.

Lacks empathy.

Wants to get things done.

"Hey," Bogard said, "that's me."

Mary White smiled at Maury Applebaum, who pointed at his watch. More than thirty minutes had passed since Bogard had begun his profile. But the CEO, intent on the DISC instrument, hadn't noticed.

He looked up. "How soon can we get a couple hundred of these?" he asked. "I want to shoot them down to my people."

"How about Monday?" she said.

"How about this afternoon. I'll have my comptroller issue a check now." Bogard reached for his phone.

Happiness is knowing who you are — and being able to exploit it.

Almost all Bogard's employees were delighted with the **profiling system.** At first, a few people felt threatened, but taking the test proved to be fun, and when the employees began to compare notes, they reached insights about themselves and about others.

The best thing to come out of the experience was a new understanding of the boss. All memos were now triple-spaced. They covered no more than one page. They were easy to read. The memos actually felt lean.

Bogard was happy. He was no longer misunderstood. He knew his family. They knew him. There were still differences among people. Nothing could do away with that. But somehow, everyone was working together with a lot more efficiency.

profiling system
a system that measures
differences between
people

ACTION STEP 50

Tap your People Resources by Brainstorming with Your New Team

Before you sign a lease or go into the hole for $50,000 worth of new equipment or hire a lot of folks or spend $1,000 for six-line telephone service, get your new team together and brainstorm the organization and objectives of your new business. A blackboard is a handy tool here, so that everyone can follow the track of the session. One way to begin is to ask each member of your team to write out objectives for the business.

You've found some good people, and it's taken some hard work. Make that work pay off by tapping your human resources.

Use brainstorming techniques to get ideas going. You'll be surprised at what develops.

If you have trouble narrowing down after the ideas start flowing, go back and review the seven-step procedure in Chapter 3.

  □ STEP COMPLETED

Now it's your turn. Action Step 50 is to be completed once you have built your team. It's your chance to brainstorm ways you're going to win. Make the most of all the creative human resources you've just brought on board! We think Action Step 50 is a great way to end a chapter on team building, and a great way to start your new business.

SUMMARY

It's fun being an entrepreneur. You're on your own, doing your own thing, running your own show. And one of the toughest things you have to admit is that you can't perform all business tasks with the same success.

This chapter helps you focus on what you can do and on where you need help.

This chapter provides tools to help you learn more about yourself, and about how you relate to people. One tool is the DISC Personality Profile. DISC is an acronym that combines the first letters of four major personality types:

D — Dominance.
I — Influencing.
S — Steadiness
C — Compliance.

We like the DISC Profile because it is relatively inexpensive and quick to take. Once you've spent 20–30 minutes with it, insights begin to flow, and there's enough explanatory material to guide you through your own interpretation. If you don't like DISC, there are two other profile systems listed in the Appendix to this chapter.

Another tool is the concept of balance. You want to construct a team where people's skills and personalities are complementary. The first two case studies (Harry R. Marquez and Janet Ames) illustrate the way different types of people can balance each other. Harry R. Marquez, a typical entrepreneur, is a D (energetic, creative, forceful, single-minded, and impatient with detail). Janet Ames, an excellent manager, is a C (calm, organized, supportive, and patient). She plans well and will see to it that the bills get paid and the phones get answered.

We touch on how to scout and hire the members of your team. We also stress the importance of internal understanding for a stronger team, as in the case study on E. G. Bogard.

Concepts of balance, proportion, the right materials, and the structural forces of personality — all of these are important to the master architect building a winning team.

ACTION STEP REVIEW

No matter what personality type you are, four Action Steps get you into the spirit of creative team building:

47 Look back across the paths you've taken to get this far and remember some of the people you met. Which of these people would you like to have working with you in your new venture? Ask yourself why? What qualities do they have that make you think about them?

48 Brainstorm your ideal team. What kind of help do you need to win at the game of small business? For example, if you've discovered that a lot of your promotion will be through personal selling, and you're the kind of person who has trouble meeting strangers and making cold calls, then you need to look for help in that area.

49 Network your competitors and vendors for team members. Now that you've developed the ideal team with your brainstorm, it's time to try to make that ideal team reality. There's a good chance you can find the kinds of people you need already working in your industry.

50 After you've assembled a winning team, set aside a couple of hours to brainstorm ways you're going to win. A blackboard is a handy tool here, so that everyone can follow the track of the session. One way to begin is to ask each member of your team to write out objectives for the business. If you need a launching place, refer to Action Step 12 in Chapter 3.

APPENDIX 12.1

The DISC system is not the only personality profile around. We like it for a couple of reasons:

1. Fun to take.

2. Quick. Easy. Accessible. You don't need a Ph.D. in Psychology and an expensive consultant to interpret the results for you.

3. Fast results. You use DISC and right away you start getting insights about yourself. (Some personality profiles require scoring by computer. That means you have to wait a couple of weeks, minimum, before you get help on team-building.)

4. Relatively inexpensive. A good personality profile can cost anywhere from $40 on up to $60. At the time of this writing, DISC runs around $8. For more information on DISC, contact:

Bill Rezmerski
Performax Systems
12755 State Highway 55
Minneapolis, MN 55441

If you don't like the sound of DISC. . . .

There are two other systems you might check out. One is the variation on the Firo-B profiling system developed by Anthony Alessandra in his book, *Non-Manipulative Selling.* Alessandra uses a cross-grid system, and four behavioral styles which he calls Amiable, Expressive, Analytical, and Driver. It's an interesting system, especially for sales situations. You can contact Dr. Alessandra through his publisher or at the following address:

Alessandra and Associates
P.O. Box 2767
La Jolla, CA 92038

The second instrument has been developed by Paul Hersey and Ken Blanchard (Blanchard is the co-author of *One-Minute Manager*), and you can get information on this and other tests by making contact with:

California American University
230 W. Third Avenue
Escondido, CA 92025

THINK POINTS

- Given the chance, people will hire themselves. How many more like you can the business take?
- There is a team lurking in your network.
- Look to your competitors and vendors for team members.
- People are the company.
- Balance the people on your team.
- Have each team member write out objectives for the business. Set up your own internal **MBO** (marketing by objectives) system.
- You can't grow until you have the right people.
- How much of your team can be built of part-timers and moon-lighters?

MBO
establishing measurable objectives over a specified time frame

REFERENCES

Alessandra, Anthony, Philip S. Wexler, and Jerry D. Dean. *Non-Manipulative Selling.* Englewood Cliffs, N.J.: Prentice-Hall, 1981.

Baty, Gordon B. *Entrepreneurship for the Eighties.* Reston, Va.,: Reston Publishing Co., 1981.

Connor, Tim. *The Soft Sell.* Alexandria, Va.: Sales Press, 1981.

David, Harry R. "Building a Winning Business Team." *Nation's Business,* August 1981.

Geier, John. *Personal Profile System.* Minneapolis, Minn.: Performax Systems International, n.d.

O'Brien, Roger T. "Blood and Black Bile: Four-Style Behavior Models in Training." *Training/HRD,* January 1983, 54–61. O'Brien explains the medieval, four-humors background of four-part profiling systems developed by Geier and Alessandra. Shows how far personality theory has evolved since the days of alchemy.

Ouchi, William G. *Theory Z: How American Business Can Meet the Japanese Challenge.* New York: Addison-Wesley Publishing Co., 1981.

Peters, Thomas J., and Robert H. Waterman, Jr. *In Search of Excellence: Lessons from America's Best-Run Companies.* New York: Harper & Row, Publishers, 1982. Not really in the area of small business, but has good advice for every business on action, autonomy, the customer, running lean, and so on.

Rhodes, Lucien. "The Un-Manager." *Inc.,* August 1982. Fascinating look at Bill Gore's lattice system of management. Inspiring reading for you denizens of the Information Society.

Riggs, Carol R. "Why Small Businesses Fail." *D & B Reports,* January/February 1983. Some very sharp insights on entrepreneurial failure due to pride, ego, and the God complex. Excellent reading.

Ward, Robert C. "Squaring Off on Quality Circles." *Inc.*, August 1982, 98–100.

Waters, Craig R. "Raiders of the Lost ARP." *Inc.*, November 1982. Echoes Riggs, preceding, on misplaced love of a glamorous corporate image.

White, Richard M. *The Entrepreneur's Manual.* Radnor, Pa.: Chilton Book Co., 1977.

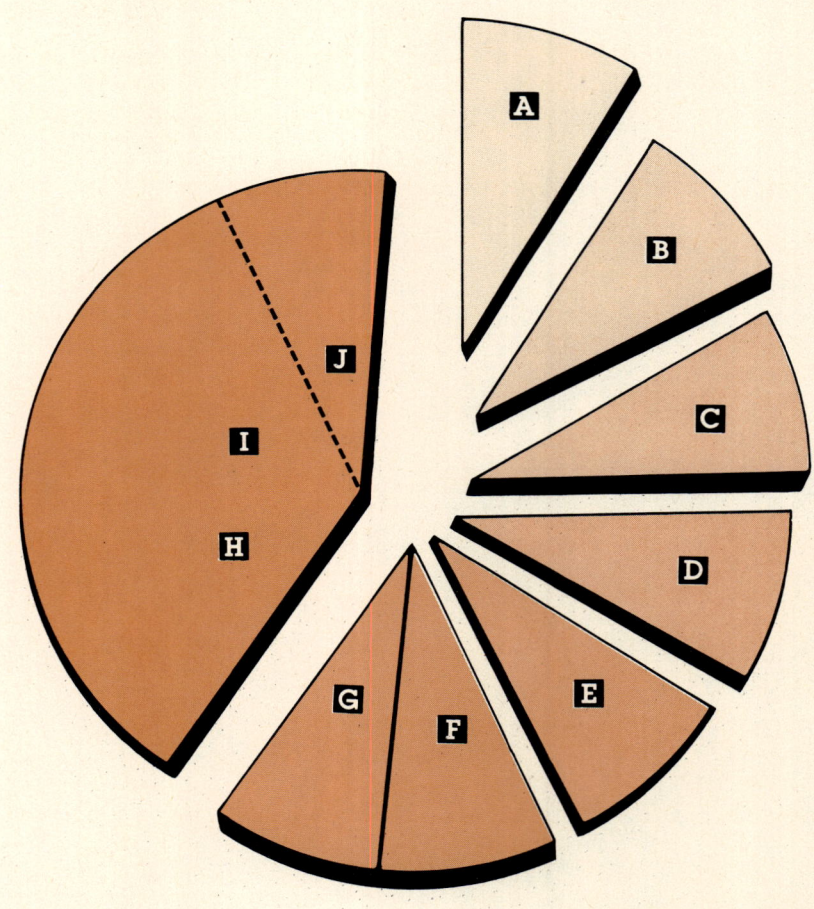

A Description of Product or Service

B The Market and the Target Customer

C Competition

D Marketing Strategy

E Location

F Management

G Personnel

H Projected Income Statement

I Projected Cash Flow

J Projected Balance Sheet

FIGURE 13.1 Chapter 13 gives you a time-out on your Business Plan as you investigate the alternatives of buying and franchising an existing business.

13

To Buy or to Franchise—There's the Rub

LEARNING OBJECTIVES

To learn what you can gain by looking at prospective businesses that are for sale.

To learn the pros and cons of purchasing a business.

To learn how to place a value on a business that's up for sale.

To develop your own method for examining a business that's up for sale from the inside.

To develop a sixth sense that will tell you when you need to hire yourself a professional Marketplace Detective.

To examine the value of intangibles like Goodwill by probing the depths of Ill Will and then turning the problem inside out.

To decide whether or not buying a franchise is the right step for you.

To develop techniques for examining franchises.

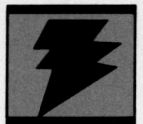 **I**n this chapter, we're looking at techniques for evaluating a business you might want to buy. The tactics are the same for a straight purchase or for a franchise.

In a straight purchase, you're buying an income stream. You could also be paying for inventory, location, Goodwill, and a covenant guaranteeing noncompetition.

In a franchise deal, you're paying a fee for the right to use a name. In some instances, your fee could also be paying for training, a business plan, help on your advertising, help negotiating your lease, and purchasing advantages.

We'll talk later about the special considerations required when buying a franchise. What follows applies equally to buying a business and buying a franchise.

WHY BUY A BUSINESS THAT'S ALREADY GOING?

The overwhelming reason for buying a business that's already going instead of building one with your own hands is — money.

1. **The Income Stream.** If you do your research and play detective thoroughly, you could start making money the day you take over a business that's already up and running. Since most start-ups have to plug along for months (even years) before making a **profit,** it's smart to think about buying a business.

2. **The Deal.** Money enters the picture here, too. If you find a **hungry seller,** you have the chance of negotiating **terms.** That means you might get into the business for less cash up front. You might also get a deal on fixtures and equipment. And if you're lucky, there might be a heavenly bargain in hidden inventory awaiting you in a warehouse somewhere.

These reasons are shown in Figure 13.2.

How to Buy and How Not to Buy

The smart buyer will play detective and go over everything in the business with microscope, geiger counter, computer analysis, clipboard, and sage advice from the taxi squad.

The smart buyer will not plunge into a business because of a sudden surge of raw emotion. Example: For a dozen years, you've eaten lunch around the corner at Millie's Cafeteria with your pals; when the place goes up for sale, nostalgia presses you into writing out a check and buying it for the wrong reasons.

Don't buy a business that way.

Every business in the country is for sale sometime. Deals are like buses: If you miss this one, another one will be along soon.

profit
what's left over after all expenses are paid

hungry seller
an owner who is marked by desperation

terms
a trade or quantity discount specified by seller

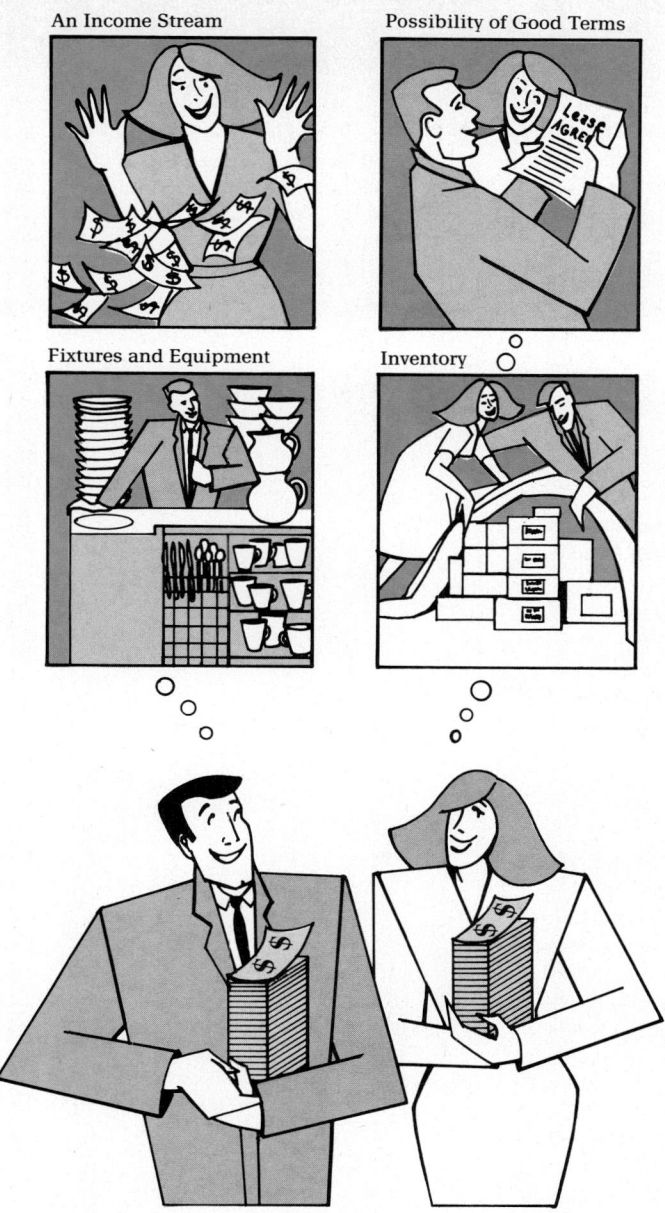

An Income Stream

Possibility of Good Terms

Fixtures and Equipment

Inventory

FIGURE 13.2 Four reasons why you might want to consider buying an ongoing business.

Start from the Outside

As you look at a business you think you want to buy, it's easier to start from the outside, with an Action Step that suggests techniques that will make you feel like a superspy. After checking the exterior, you then move inside, to check the books and talk to the owner while you psych out his or her reasons for selling.

But the first step is to get your telescope and your telephoto camera and to interview the **seller's customers** so that you can gather as much information as you can from the exterior. Action Step 51 tells you how (see page 237).

You'd be surprised how much is there.

seller's customers
if you're buying a business, they are about to become your customers

KNOW WHEN YOU NEED OUTSIDE HELP

We've already discussed the need for a taxi squad (see page 205) to help you realize your dream of owning and running a small business. But when you evaluate a small business for purchase, you may discover the need for a very special kind of outside support. If you have any lingering doubts about the business you are researching, you may need the perspective of someone more objective than one of your team players. Listen to Georgia Webster, and see what you can learn from her experiences.

If you're not the Sherlock Holmes type, find someone who is. You may get your dream shattered, but you will save money in the long run.

Case Study

Georgia Webster — Retailer

I'd worked for a large ad agency in New York for 12 years before I gave it up and moved west, to the Bay Area. I couldn't believe it. No snow. No grey-black winter slush. No icicles in April.

So I quickly became a sports freak, to make up for all the years I'd spent indoors. I took up tennis, then racquetball, then biking, then volleyball, then hiking.

I met Fred Webster on the tennis court. It was love at first sight, for both of us, and we were married six months later.

Fred is a very creative man who had always wanted to try something on his own. Since we both loved sports, we decided to look around for a sporting goods store that was up for sale.

We found **the perfect store** by networking our sports-minded friends. It was called The Sports Factory and it was located one block from a complex of tennis courts, three blocks from a new racquetball club, and a quarter of a mile from a park where they held bimonthly volleyball tournaments.

A friend of ours who's an accountant checked over the books. He said they looked perfect.

"Great P and L, Freddy," he said. "A lot better than the usual **industry ratios.** If you get the right terms, you could be clearing 50 Gs every quarter—and that's only the beginning. This guy doesn't even advertise."

"Why is he selling?" I asked.

"He's tired, dear," Fred said. "He's been here for a dozen years, and he wants to enjoy life."

But I'm from New York, and I wasn't so sure.

I sensed we needed help—some sort of Sam Spade of the business world—and all the time Fred was in a hurry to close the deal.

"This is an opportunity, Georgia," he kept saying. "A real opportunity. It won't come around again soon."

I knew Fred was unhappy in his job, but half the money we were going to invest was mine, and I still felt there was something not quite right. Frankly, the owner of The Sports Factory didn't look all that tired to me.

So I asked around, networking again, until I located a professor at
Continued

Stick to the Knitting

Advice: When you look at buying a business, stick to the knitting. That means you should think about buying a business in an industry you know something about. If you don't have experience in the business, the next best thing is to find work in this industry before you invest in it.

the perfect store |
an idealized vision of an idyllic business that runs itself and has no problems

industry ratios |
standards for an industry usually expressed as profit on sales or return on investment

one of the community colleges. His name was Harry Henkel, and he was the author of a small book called "Checklist for Going into Your Own Small Business." When I called him he listened patiently, and then we made an appointment to talk further, and at the end of 15 minutes he said he would check things out — for a small fee.

I told him to go ahead. But I didn't tell my husband.

Two days later, my Marketplace Detective called with some news.

"Mrs. Webster?"

"Yes. Speaking."

"This is Harry Henkel, over at the college. I have some news about your business venture."

"Oh?" I said. "So soon?"

"Yes. You remember that bulldozer that was working across the street?"

"No. I'm sorry. What bulldozer?"

"It just started grading last week. Right across the street from The Sports Factory."

"We were there on Sunday," I said. "I don't remember any bull-dozer."

"Well," he said. "I had a chance to talk to the driver on his lunch break. It seems one of the local developers is putting in a seven-store complex. And one of the stores will be a discount sporting goods store." He paused.

"Oh, no," I said. "Are you sure?" The store he mentioned was a monster **chain.** I knew they would compete with us for customers. Did the owner know? Was that why he was so "tired"?

"Yes," my detective said. "I double-checked at the city planners. Where they issue building permits." He paused again.

I was having trouble catching my breath. "Could I get this in writing?" I asked. "So that I could show my husband? He's the kind of man who likes everything documented."

My detective chuckled. "No problem, Mrs. Webster," he said. "It will be in the mail tomorrow. Let me know what you decide, okay?"

"Don't worry," I said. "And thank you. Thank you very much."

My Marketplace Detective cost me $175. But what he found out saved us thousands of dollars and years of heartache.

Armed with what we'd learned about The Sports Factory, we examined almost a hundred businesses before we found the right one for us.

It pays to investigate.

Georgia Webster came very close to purchasing the wrong business — and the only way she was able to avoid this mistake was by making the most of an outside perspective.

Now we'll concentrate on making the most of some inside perspectives.

LOOKING AT THE BUSINESS FROM THE INSIDE OUT

Only by looking at a business from the inside out will you be able to determine its real worth — and to determine what it would be like to own it. Action Step 52 (page 238) starts you on this process by having you cross the magic threshold of the business you want to buy —

chain
two or more stores operating under the same name

either on your own or with the help of a **business opportunity broker.** And so you won't get charmed out of your senses, we're also giving you a list of real-life instructions. Let this list be your amulet against magic spells.

In Action Step 52 we tell you to have fun. Does the thought of stepping into the business fill you with anxiety? It shouldn't. You *can* have fun if you're well-prepared. Which brings us to that list we promised you.

A LIST TO HELP YOU LOOK AT THE INSIDE OF A BUSINESS

Study the financial history.

Compare what you'd make if you bought this business to what you'd make if you invested the same money elsewhere.

Evaluate **tangible assets.**

Talk to suppliers (especially credit managers), employees, and so on.

Get an ironclad covenant from the seller not to compete.

Analyze the seller's motives.

Negotiate the cost of **Goodwill.** Plumb the depths of Ill Will. Some businesses are worth less than zero.

Insist on a bulk sales escrow. (Examine the Uniform Commercial Code.)

Let's look at the list in more detail.

Studying the Financial History

Ask to see all financial records, for at least five years back if they're available, and take time to study them. If you don't understand financial records, hire someone who does. Your aim in buying a business is to dip into an income stream. The financial records are a picture of that stream.

Where did the money come from and where did it go?

Look at the history of cash flow, of profit and loss, and of accounts receivable.

If your seller has a stack of accounts receivable a foot high, you'll want to remember that in three months a current-accounts dollar shrinks to 90 cents, in six months it's down to 50 cents, and in a year it's down to 30 cents.

Tip: You can use the seller's accounts receivable as a point for negotiation, but don't take over the job of collecting.

It's also a good idea to look at canceled checks, income tax returns (probably for the last 5 years), and at the salary the seller paid himself. If your seller was stingy with his own salary, make sure you can live on the same amount.

Comparing What Your Money Might Do Elsewhere

How much money are you putting into the business?

How long will it take you to make it back?

Have you figured in your time?

ACTION ⚡ STEP 52

Cross the Magic Threshold

Once you've learned all you can from the outside, it is time to cross the threshold for a look at the interior. This is an elaborate and time-consuming process, and there is a list following this Action Step to help you fasten onto what is important.

There are two ways of getting inside:

1. Contact the owner directly.

2. Get assistance from a business opportunity broker.

Brokers have lots of leads. You can locate them in the Yellow Pages under "Business Broker." You can also locate them in the classifieds.

Tip: Don't buy a business from the classifieds. Too many losers there.

After you've done your research, make contact with business brokers. Tell them what kind of business you're interested in. Make an appointment to go inside for a closer look. Have your list handy.

If you are asked to put down an "earnest money" deposit, handle it this way:

First, deposit the money in an escrow account. Second, include a stipulation that says your purchase of the business in question is subject to your inspection and approval of all financial records and all aspects of the business.

That gives you an escape hatch so you can get your deposit back.

Have fun in there.

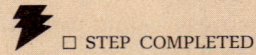 □ STEP COMPLETED

Let's say you put $50,000 into this business. Let's say you're making $25,000 a year.

Are there other investments you could make which would yield the same amount on your $50,000? In this case the business will give you a $33\frac{1}{3}$% return or full payback in three years.

If you're working in the business, you need to add in the cost of your time — $75,000 (assuming no raises over the three-year period). In three years the business needs to return $125,000 after expenses and taxes in order to cover the risks involved with your $50,000 investment and forgoing a $25,000 salary on the outside.

Evaluating Tangible Assets

If the numbers look good, move on to analyze everything that you can touch: real estate, equipment/fixtures, inventory.

1. Real Estate. Get an outside appraisal.
2. Equipment/Fixtures. This stuff is used, so you can get a good idea of values by checking with equipment dealers. Look in the want ads. Scour your area. You don't want to tie too much capital up in equipment that's outmoded or about to come apart. Suppliers have lots of leads on used equipment. Check with them.

   If you're not an expert in the equipment field, get help from someone who is.
3. Inventory. Count the **inventory** yourself. Make sure those boxes are packed with what you think they are. In your buyout agreement, make certain you specify the exact contents of shelves and cabinets. Don't get careless and write in something vague like "All shelves to be filled." Specify what goes on the shelves.

   Once you've got your count, double-check with the supplier to find out current prices.

   If you find merchandise that is damaged, out-of-date, out-of-style, soiled, worn, or not ready to sell as is, don't pay full price. Negotiate. This is **sacrificed merchandise** and should have a sacrifice price tag.

inventory
items carried in stock

sacrificed merchandise
distressed goods, usually sold at any cost

Talking to Insiders

Suppliers. Will suppliers agree to keep supplying you? Are there past difficulties between seller and supplier that will spill over to you as the new owner? You're dependent on your suppliers.

Employees. Identify key employees early. In small business, success can rest on the shoulders of one or two persons, and you don't want them to walk out the day you sign the papers and present your seller with a fat check.

The Noncompetition Covenant

Once you buy a business, you don't want the seller to set up the same business across the street.

Customers are hard to come by. You don't want to pay for them and have them spirited away by a cagey seller.

So you get an agreement, in writing, that says the seller won't set up in competition with you for the next five years.

You may need a lawyer to help you.

Whether you get a lawyer or do it yourself, be sure to specify the exact amount you're paying for the noncompetition covenant. That way, the IRS will allow you to deduct it against ordinary income over the life of the covenant.

Psyching out the Seller's Motives

People give all kinds of reasons for selling out.

Poor Health.
Restless. Wants to move on.
Creative. Wants to sell this and start something new.

Be wary of all reasons and try to unearth the real reasons. If the seller admits he's outfoxed the IRS, there's a good chance he'll try to outfox you, too.

Negotiating the Cost of Goodwill

A smart seller is going to ask you to pay him for building up Goodwill.

Your job is to play detective and find out how much Goodwill there is and where it's coming from.

You don't get something for nothing.

For example, maybe the seller plays it loose when he extends credit. Customers are responding, but there's no cash in the bank. If you continue that policy and keep granting easy credit, you could be in the red in a couple of months.

Or maybe he's one of those very special people, loved by everyone, who will take the Goodwill with him — like a halo — when he walks out the door.

So negotiate.

Let's say the asking price for the business is $100,000.

Let's say the tangible assets of the business (equipment, inventory, and so on) are worth $50,000.

In other words, the seller is trying to charge you $50,000 for Goodwill.

Before you negotiate:

1. Compare the Goodwill you're being asked to buy to the Goodwill of a similar business which is also on the market.
2. Figure out how long it will take you to pay for the Goodwill. Goodwill is intangible. You'll be unhappy stringing it out across the years. Remember: Even the best Goodwill comes out of profit.
3. Estimate how much you could be making if you invested that same $50,000 in T Bills.

You now have a context in which you can judge the seller's assessment of the value of Goodwill, and you can use the hard data you have generated to negotiate a realistic and more favorable price. (See also Action Step 53, ''Probe the Depths of Ill Will,'' on page 243.)

Bulk Sales Escrow and the U.C.C.

If you're thinking about buying a business, you'll want to make sure that the inventory you're buying is not tied up by creditors. The instrument you'll use to cut those strings is a bulk sales transfer or **bulk sales escrow** — moving a large volume of goods from the custody of the seller to your custody through a qualified third party. In most states, bulk sales transfer is specified under a series of regulations known as the Uniform Commercial Code (U.C.C.).

> **bulk sales escrow**
> an examination process to protect buyers from unknown liabilities

If there are no claims by creditors, the transfer of bulk sales should go smoothly. If there are claims, you'll want to be protected by law. Either consult an attorney who has experience in making bulk sales transfers, or locate an escrow company to act as a neutral party. (*Escrow* comes from *escroe,* an Old French word meaning ''parchment,'' ''deed,'' or ''scroll.'' The distant Indo-European root is *skeru-,* which means ''to cut,'' and you'll need an expert to help you cut creditors who have strings attached.)

(For a look at the jungle of documents involved in buying a business, see pages 169–221 in *Buying and Selling Business Opportunities* by Wilfred E. Tetreault.)

The quickest way to find an escrow company is to look in the yellow pages under ''escrow.''

CLOSE TO A DECISION?

A Checklist You Can't Afford to Ignore

After completing Action Steps 51 and 52, you will have reached a point where it's easy to make your final decision. But don't — at least not yet. We've included a helpful ''Final Checklist Before You Buy'' that reminds you of important details you might have overlooked. Even though you've found your dream business, complete this checklist (on page 242) before you decide.

Wrestling Holds for Your Negotiations

Let's go one more step. You know you're ready to buy. You've got the money. The numbers say you can't lose. You're ready to enter into negotiations. (If you're an experienced entrepreneur, you already know how to negotiate. If not, we refer you to an excellent book on the fine art of haggling in the References section at the end of this chapter.)

We're going to suggest two things about negotiations:

First, when it comes time to talk meaningful numbers, the most important area for you to concentrate on is terms — and not asking price. Favorable terms give you the cash flow you need to survive that first year, and then move from survival into success. Unfavorable terms can torpedo your chances for success, even when the total asking price is well below market.

Final Checklist Before You Buy

____ How long do you plan to own this business?

____ How old is this business? Can you sketch its history?

____ Is this business in the embryonic stage? The growth stage? The mature stage? Or the decline stage?

____ Has your accountant reviewed the books and made you a sales projection?

____ How long will it take for this business to show you a *complete* return on your investment?

____ What reasons does the owner offer for selling?

____ Will the owner let you see bank deposits? (If not, why not?)

____ Have you calculated utility costs for the next 3–5 years?

____ What does a review of tax records tell you?

____ How complete is the insurance coverage?

____ How old are receivables? (Remember: Age decreases the value of receivables.)

____ What is the seller paying himself? Is it low? High?

____ Have you interviewed your prospective landlord?

____ What happens when a new tenant takes over the lease?

____ Have you made spot checks on the currency of the customer list?

____ Who are your top 20 customers? Your top 50?

____ Is seller locked in to 1–3 major customers who control the business?

____ Are you buying inventory? What is seller asking?

____ Have you checked the value of the inventory with vendors?

____ Have you checked equipment value against used equipment from another source?

____ Whom does your seller owe money to?

____ Has your attorney checked for liens on seller's equipment?

____ Do you have maintenance contracts on the equipment you're buying?

____ Has your attorney or escrow company gone through bulk sales escrow?

____ Have you made certain that:

    ____ You're getting all brand names, logos, trade marks, and so on that you need?

    ____ Your seller has signed a non-competition covenant?

    ____ Your key lines of supply will stay intact once you take over?

    ____ Your key employees won't desert the business once you take over?

    ____ Your seller isn't leaving because of stiff competition?

    ____ You aren't paying for Goodwill but taking delivery on Ill Will?

    ____ You're getting the best terms possible?

    ____ You're buying an income-stream?

Second, when the seller starts talking Goodwill, you use your New Eyes to probe the depths of Ill Will. Goodwill is a slippery commodity. It can make the asking price soar. Naturally, Goodwill is what the seller is selling. Because you know that ahead of time, you can go in primed to deal. Action Step 53 lets you play the "intangible" game by turning the problem inside out. The seller wants to sell you Goodwill. You flip the coin over and explore **Ill Will,** which hangs on longer, like a cloud above the business.

An escrow company can help you evaluate inventory. But only you

Ill Will
all the minus factors of a business—the obvious opposite of Goodwill

can negotiate out the high cost of Goodwill—the intangible commodity.

Action Step 53 gets you started thinking about Ill Will in general and then gets you to zero in on the business you're about to buy.

Go for it!

Remembering Why You Started Out

Well, you've come a long way. You've worked hard at your research. You may be wondering if the digging was worth it. Only you can answer. There are bargains out there—especially if you are able to track down a buy like Woolett's Hardware.

For those hunter-buyers with vision and persistence, a beautiful business is lurking behind an ugly facade.

Case Study

Woolett's Hardware—Looking Beyond Cosmetics

I heard about Woolett's being up for sale more than a year ago. I'd just opened up my second store, also in the hardware line, and it took me just about a year—April to April—to streamline the paperwork.

A computer and a good manager saved my sanity.

When I finally got over there to check things out, I reckon Woolett's had been on the market a year and a half or so.

One look from the street, and you could see why.

Woolett's was a mess. The building was pre-war, and so was the paint. Out front, the sign was sagging. The parking lot needed grading badly, and there were pot holes six inches deep.

The entry way was littered with scraps of paper. The front door was boarded up.

Inside, things weren't much better.

The floor needed a good sweeping. The merchandise was covered with dust. And all around there was this feeling of mildew, age, disuse. Woolett's was dark, like a cave. It was tough finding a salesperson, and when you did, you couldn't get much help. Yet there were customers all over the store.

But after you've been in business awhile, you develop a sort of sixth sense about things. And the minute I stepped through that front door, I knew there was something special about Woolett's. Something hidden. Something the eye couldn't see right off.

I knew I had to dig deeper.

A visit to the local business realtor didn't help much.

"Make us an offer," he said. "We just dropped the price yesterday. To $400,000."

"What do the numbers look like?" I asked.

He dug into a slim manila folder. "Last year," he said, "they grossed just under $600,000. The net was around $200,000."

"What about inventory?" I asked. "What about loans and **liens** and accounts receivable? When can I interview the manager? And why is the owner selling?"

"Are you just asking?" he said. "Or is this for real?"

"This is for my son," I said. "He's new to the business. We aren't looking for a lot of surprises."

Continued

liens
legal obligations filed
against a piece of property

ACTION 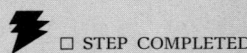 STEP 53

Probe the Depths of Ill Will

How many products have you vowed never to use again?

How many places of business have you vowed never to patronize again?

Why?

Make a list of the products you won't buy or use, ever again. Next to each item, write down the reason. Does it make you sick? Does it offend your sensibilities? Was the service too crummy to be beyond redemption?

After you finish with your list, ask some of your friends how they feel about certain businesses.

Study your lists. What are the common components of Ill Will? How long does Ill Will last? Is there a remedy for it? Or is a business plagued by Ill Will cursed forever after?

Now apply the list to the business you're about to buy. Survey target customers. How do they feel about this business?

Have fun with this step. Think about the nature of Ill Will when your seller starts asking you to pay for Goodwill.

☐ STEP COMPLETED

"Like I said, make us an offer."

"Let me check the books," I said.

I deposited $500 **earnest money** with an **escrow company.** And I made sure to include my usual **escape hatch** — a deposit receipt saying my offer on the business is contingent on my inspection and my approval of all financial records. It's a handy thing to do, and has saved me a lot of heartburn.

The minute that they got wind of a buyer, the manager and two of Woolett's best employees quit. The back office was a mess, and it took me three days of searching before I found something that made me know I was on the right track.

A supply of rolled steel. It was on the books at $12,000, but I knew it was worth $150,000.

I took that as a signal to buy.

The next day, I made an offer. Twelve thousand down, with the balance to be paid out of profits over the next five years.

They took the offer. We cleared escrow in thirty days.

The first thing we did was clean the place up. We surfaced the parking lot with asphalt, added a coat of paint, fixed the door, added lighting.

Business picked up right away. My son, newly married, was settling down, learning the business. He seemed to have managerial talents.

Then we found an extra set of records. They'd been hidden away in a safe.

The Woolett Corporation had a bank account containing $180,000. The corporation also owned five acres of land, mostly along the road leading to town.

And so there we were, right in the path of future growth.

That first year, we did just over a million dollars in sales. And there was every indication that we would do better from then on.

People walking into Woolett's hardly recognize the place. We spent some good money on lighting the store. We've added a large kitchen section, to appeal to our housewives. And in the summer we're generally open until eight.

If you're in the area, stop by.

earnest money deposit
money deposited by buyer in a neutral account to demonstrate interest to seller

escrow company
a neutral third party that holds deposits and deeds until all conditions agreed upon are met

escape hatch
a device that allows the purchaser to back out painlessly

WHY BUY A FRANCHISE?

The overwhelming reason for buying a franchise is — name recognition.

1. **Brand-Name Recognition.** If you ask the right questions and pick the right franchise, the marketing boost you get from the name of your franchise will be worth the effort.
2. **Support From Corporate.** Sometimes you buy more than brand-name recognition with your franchise. Sometimes you get additional services for your money: Corporate services could help with selecting a site, interior layout, inventory control, vendor connections, and a corporate-produced business plan.

These reasons are pictured in Figure 13.3.

Brand-Name Recognition

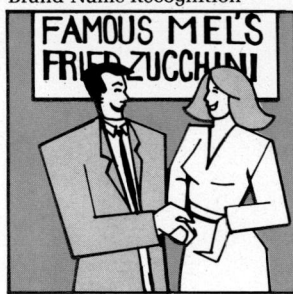

Help with Selecting a Site

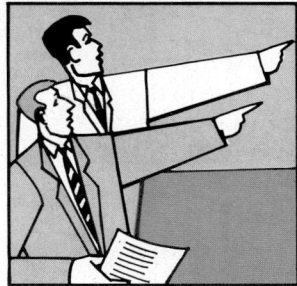

Help with Interior Layout

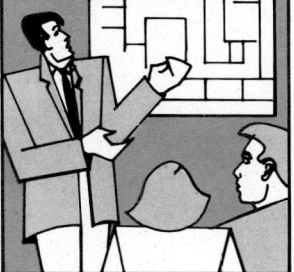

Help with Inventory Control

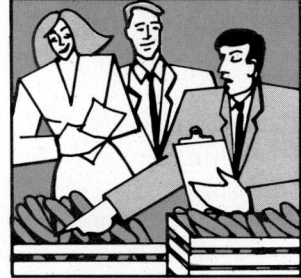

Vendor Connections

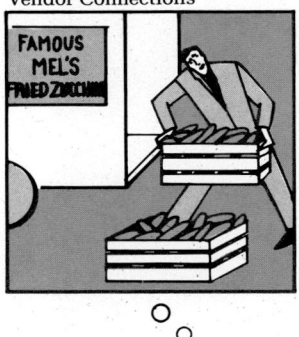

A Corporate-Produced
Business Plan

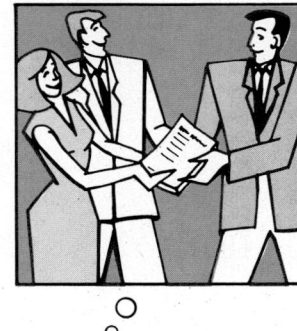

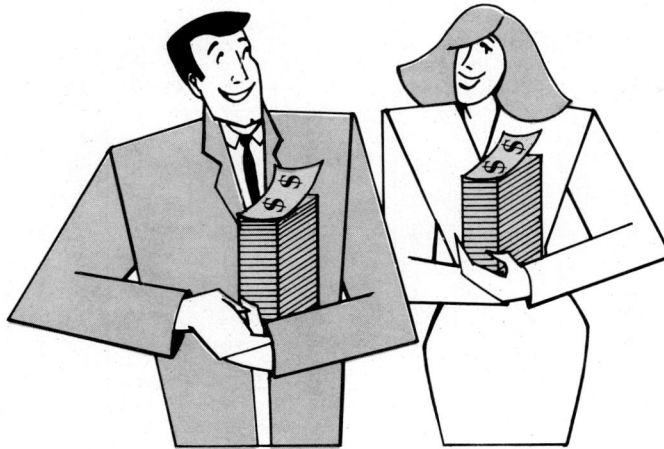

FIGURE 13.3 When you buy a franchise, you may be buying a number of things.

Franchises Made Simple

When you buy a **franchise,** you're really buying a license. If you wanted to bottle Coca-Cola, which is the most famous franchise in the world, you'd have to negotiate for a license from the Coca-Cola Bottling Company. You might find a bottler who wanted to sell you his license, but you'd still have to negotiate with Coke.

In some cases, buying a franchise is like buying a supplier for eternity. But many people have, because approximately 20% of the small businesses in the country are franchises. In Table 13.1 you can see the phenomenal growth of franchising from 1969 to 1982. In 1982, there were 466,000 franchise outlets providing a whopping $437 billion in annual revenues. If you compare that with only 384,000 outlets (generating a mere $116 billion) in 1969, you can see how franchising has mushroomed.

In Table 13.2 (pages 248–249), figures for individual industries help you add to your knowledge of trends, which you began thinking about in Chapter 2. If you're interested in becoming an auto or truck dealer, your window of opportunity has grown smaller (from 37,200 franchises down to 28,200). But if you're in business aids and services, the window has grown in size (from 10,500 to 50,200).

We're not asking you to memorize these tables. They were included to show you the vast range of opportunity in franchising, which seems to be moving from smokestacks and manufacturing to information and services.

Ask the Right Questions

Want a franchise? The evaluation process goes through the same steps, but you'll need to examine franchisors under a powerful microscope.

> **franchise**
> authorization granted by a manufacturer or distributor to sell products/services

---

TABLE 13.1 Franchising in the United States, 1969–1982

Item	Unit	1969	1970	1975	1976	1977	1978	1979	1980	1981[1]	1982[1]
Number of franchised establishments	1,000	384	396	435	443	451	452	452	442	447	466
Company-owned[2]	1,000	69	72	81	83	86	85	85	85	86	88
Franchisee-owned	1,000	315	324	354	360	365	367	367	357	361	378
Sales of products and services	Bil. dol.	116	120	191	222	253	287	312	336	380	437
Company-owned[2]	Bil. dol.	22	23	29	33	38	44	39	47	52	58
Franchisee-owned	Bil. dol.	94	96	162	189	215	243	273	289	328	379
Average sales per establishment	$1,000	302	302	439	500	562	635	690	760	611	667
Employment	1,000	(NA)	(NA)	3,511	3,792	4,151	4,496	4,605	4,668	(NA)	(NA)

NA Not available. [1]Estimated by respondents to annual survey of franchisors. [2]Represents establishments owned by the parent company.

SOURCE: *Statistical Abstract of the United States, 1982–83,* 103rd ed. (Washington, D.C.: U.S. Department of Commerce, 1983), 809.

Evaluating a franchise is like evaluating a business for sale, but because of the nature of **franchisors,** you need to ask some additional questions:

How long has this franchise been in business?

Who are the officers?

How many franchised operations like this one are there so far?

Where are they located?

What will this franchise do for me?

Even if You're Not Planning to Buy One

You can learn a lot about small business by probing franchises. As you can see from a glance at the tables, franchising is a major factor in the U.S. economy, and a look at several won't hurt you.

If you're an eager entrepreneur, however, there's a good chance you won't like the rules and regulations set down by franchisors.

In either case, it makes sense to check out "opportunities" offered by franchisors (especially in your industry) in order to get a better look at the marketplace. Action Step 54 starts you on this quest.

One warning: Beware of franchisors offering so-called "ground floor opportunities." You don't want to be the proud owner of a second or fifth franchise outlet. Anyone offering such an opportunity could be experimenting with your money. You want to buy a recognizable brand name, a proven business plan, excellent field support, and the certainty that this franchise will work in your location.

Susan J. Moore and her husband were lucky when it came time to investigate franchises: They had a source of inside information right in the family. They were also lucky because the franchisor they chose provided excellent support. Note that for Susan Moore, at least, corporate support was more important than name-brand recognition.

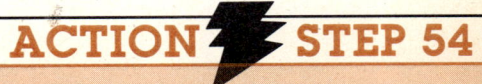

franchisors
the creators of the franchise

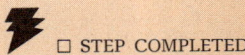

ACTION ⚡ STEP 54

Tackle the Franchise System

Franchises are everywhere. Big Mac, Roto-Rooter, Dale Carnegie, Holiday Inn, Exxon, Midas, and Hertz are only a few examples.

Before you sign up for one, you want to interview people on both sides of the franchise agreement.

Part A. Franchisors. Leave your checkbook at home and interview at least 3 franchisors. Here are some questions to start you off:

What's included in the franchise fee?

What's the duration of the agreement?

How can the agreement be bought back or canceled?

What are the royalty fees and other assessments?

What level of training and service can you expect?

Is the territory well defined?

What are the minimum volume requirements?

How much help can you expect on advertising and promotion?

Part B. Franchisees. Interview several franchisees in your industry. Ask them the same questions.

A handy Reference is the *Franchise Opportunities Handbook,* U.S. Dept. of Commerce.

⚡ ☐ STEP COMPLETED

Case Study

Susan J. Moore — Franchise Printer

My husband and I decided to buy a franchise rather than start a business from scratch for one reason — training.

We wanted a business of our own because he was traveling a lot and I was working very hard for a large company and while we were both drawing good salaries, we felt that we had what it took to succeed in small business.

We were both interested in the printing industry, and we chose a medium-sized national chain that seemed to have a franchise package we could live with.

We did have a little inside information on this particular franchisor: My brother had been with them for three years, up in the Pacific Northwest area, and he was able to make a good living.

I think it's important to mention that while we were interested in the quick-print industry, we weren't experts, so the two weeks of training came in very handy.

In addition, the people from corporate helped us in other areas:

Continued

TABLE 13.2   Number of Establishments and Sales, by Kind of Franchised Business, 1970–1982

Kind of Franchised Business	Number of Establishments (1,000)						Sales (mil. dol.)					
	1970	1975	1979	1980	1981[1]	1982[1]	1970	1975	1979	1980	1981[1]	1982[1]
All franchising, total	**396.3**	**434.5**	**452.5**	**442.4**	**447.1**	**465.6**	**119,758**	**190,931**	**312,188**	**336,220**	**379,919**	**437,440**
Auto and truck dealers[2]	37.2	31.8	33.0	29.4	28.9	28.2	58,812	94,497	155,738	143,861	164,789	194,295
Percent	9.4	7.3	7.3	6.6	6.5	6.1	49.1	49.5	49.9	42.8	43.4	44.4
Restaurants (all types)	32.6	43.0	58.9	60.0	63.5	69.1	4,602	12,262	24,766	27,867	31,567	36,484
Percent	8.2	9.9	13.0	13.6	14.2	12.2	3.8	6.4	7.9	8.3	8.3	8.3
Gasoline service stations[2]	222.0	189.5	164.8	158.5	151.3	147.0	29,340	47,387	71,894	94,470	105,145	117,762
Percent	56.0	43.6	36.4	35.8	33.8	31.6	24.5	24.8	23.0	28.1	27.7	26.9
Retailing (nonfood)	30.7	37.2	36.8	35.2	36.3	39.3	13,133	9,031	8,902	10,517	11,453	12,887
Percent	7.7	8.6	8.1	8.0	8.1	6.9	11.0	4.7	2.9	3.1	3.0	2.9
Auto, truck rental services	[3]10.7	6.5	7.5	7.3	7.6	8.0	[3]1,177	1,475	2,890	3,146	3,382	3,729
Automotive products and services[4]	20.4	47.5	45.1	40.2	40.7	43.2	1,936	5,0006	7,227	7,084	7,556	8,290
Business aids and services	10.5	22.2	41.0	40.7	44.3	50.2	723	1,397	6,280	6,749	7,624	9,081
Employment services	2.9	2.7	4.2	4.4	4.7	5.4	516	553	1,417	1,594	1,846	2,187
Tax preparation services	4.7	7.5	8.7	9.2	9.4	9.6	85	161	256	289	330	371
Accounting, credit, collection, and general	1.1	3.5	3.0	2.4	2.4	2.7	20	165	128	121	127	154
Other	1.7	8.3	25.1	24.7	27.8	32.5	101	518	4,479	4,745	5,321	6,369
Campgrounds	(NA)	1.0	1.0	(NA)	(NA)	(NA)	(NA)	61	97	(NA)	(NA)	(NA)
Construction, home improvement, maintenance, and cleaning	.7	10.8	14.1	14.3	15.0	16.4	63	639	1,382	1,475	1,659	1,959
Convenience stores	8.8	13.5	14.7	15.6	16.3	17.3	1,727	3,906	6,132	7,821	8,653	9,052

Please see notes on opposite page.

TABLE 13.2 Continued

Kind of Franchised Business	Number of Establishments (1,000)						Sales (mil. dol.)					
	1970	1975	1979	1980	1981[1]	1982[1]	1970	1975	1979	1980	1981[1]	1982[1]
Educational products and services........	4.9	1.3	2.7	3.2	3.6	4.1	86	173	267	339	389	450
Equipment rental services........	(3)	1.4	1.7	2.2	2.4	2.8	(3)	157	289	356	385	448
Food retailing[5]..	(NA)	11.8	14.5	15.5	16.3	17.4	(NA)	1,445	6,512	7,430	8,262	9,213
Hotels and motels..........	3.4	5.4	5.3	6.4	6.6	6.9	3,540	4,540	6,625	9,506	10,745	11,820
Laundry, dry cleaning services........	4.1	3.2	2.7	3.4	3.2	3.3	144	214	268	286	282	305
Recreation, entertainment, travel .	2.7	3.4	4.3	4.6	4.9	5.3	77	162	360	516	619	830
Soft drink bottlers [2,6]	2.7	2.4	2.0	1.9	1.8	1.7	4,102	8,165	12,194	14,352	16,831	20,089
Miscellaneous ..	4.8	2.7	2.5	3.6	4.3	5.2	295	414	363	447	578	746

NA   Not available.   [1] Estimated by respondents.   [2] Estimated by source on basis on Bureau of the Census and trade association data.   [3] Equipment rental services included with auto, truck rental services.   [4] Includes some establishments with significant sales of nonautomotive products such as household appliances, garden supplies, etc.   [5] Excludes convenience stores.   [6] Includes soft drinks, fruit drinks and ades, syrups, flavoring agents and bases. Excludes independent private label and contract-filler bottling companies, which accounted for 22 percent in recent years, of the value of shipments of the total industry.

SOURCE: *Statistical Abstract of the United States, 1982–83,* 103rd ed. (Washington, D.C.: U.S. Department of Commerce, 1983), 809.

1. Site selection
2. Market analysis
3. Negotiating the lease
4. Layout and Design
5. How to run the equipment

There are so many details to think of when you're starting a business, and we found it very helpful to have experts take over some of the tasks.

Another good feature is that corporate will allow you to finance up to 80% of your start-up costs. Since this particular franchise can run as high as $100,000 up front, we found that a nice feature.

We opened a second shop (different location) last January. Both stores are doing nicely. We print stationery, business cards, flyers, invitations — and we're developing a reputation for being on time in an industry which is perpetually late.

READY TO BUY A FRANCHISE?

A Checklist Just for Franchises

Earlier we gave you a checklist to look at before you made a final decision on buying a business. That checklist included considerations for franchises, too. But we've also provided you with a customized checklist for franchises (pages 251–253) with questions to help you generate a profile of the franchise. By using this checklist, you will be able to nail down most of the hard facts you need to make a wise decision.

A Final Word About Franchises

If you have few business skills, or perhaps little business experience, then your chances of succeeding are far greater by signing on as a franchisee. A franchisor with a well-developed Business Plan will keep you on track. Ask to see that Business Plan.

The key here is gut feeling. If you start feeling like an employee, strike out on your own, develop your own Plan, and give yourself that extra shot at success. A true entrepreneur will look at franchising as an option—an example to learn from—and then blend that knowledge into a unique business that explores the gaps exposed back in Chapter 3, ''Power Marketing.''

If you're not ready for that, franchising is one other way to start.

SUMMARY

There is one good reason to think about buying an existing business — money.

1. If you buy right, after months of playing Marketplace Detective, you could inherit a sweet income stream.
2. If you can locate a hungry seller, there's a chance that you can strike a deal and obtain some terrific terms.

Let's say you find a business for sale. The asking price is $1 million. Last year, the business had a profit of $50,000. So you set up these terms:

Down payment of $20,000.
A no-interest loan of $980,000.
Payments of 20% of profits each year until the loan is paid off.

Result: Each year you'd have an ROI (return on investment) of 200%. Your loan payment would be 20% of $50,000, or $10,000 a year. You'd have a profit of $40,000 left each year. At the end of 10

ACTION STEP REVIEW

We suggest you examine a business that's for sale in two steps—first, from the outside; second, from the inside.

51 Study the business you want to buy from the outside first, before you let the owner know you're interested. Where's the business on the arc of the life cycle? What's the location and how does it fit into the near future? Have you profiled the customers? Have you interviewed the neighbors? The mailman? The delivery people?

52 Once you're satisfied that the business is worth your time, take a trip inside. You can contact the owner directly, or you can deal with a Business Opportunity Broker. Here's where you look at the books and really dig beneath the surface of the business.

53 Evaluate Goodwill. Most sellers will want you to pay a hefty sum for the ''Goodwill'' they've built up over the years with their customers. One way to evaluate Goodwill is to look at its opposite, Ill Will. Start with yourself. How many products have you vowed never to use again? How many services? Once you've established the fluidity of Ill Will, interview some target customers. Find out how they feel about dealing with a new owner.

54 While the three Action Steps above apply to both existing business and franchises, you need to come in from a different angle if you're thinking about a franchise. Since approximately 20% of the small businesses in the country are franchises, the process gives you something to think about.

Interview franchisors first. You want to know what's included in the franchise fee, how long your agreement lasts, what kind of royalty fees there are, and so on.

After you interview franchisors, ask the same questions of franchisees.

Checklist for Evaluating a Franchise

General

	yes	no
1. Is the product or service:		
a. considered reputable?	_____	_____
b. part of a growing market?	_____	_____
c. needed in your area?	_____	_____
d. of interest to you?	_____	_____
e. safe,	_____	_____
protected,	_____	_____
covered by guarantee?	_____	_____
2. Is the franchise:		
a. local?	_____	_____
regional?	_____	_____
national?	_____	_____
international?	_____	_____
b. full-time?	_____	_____
part-time?	_____	_____
possible full-time in the future?	_____	_____

3. Existing franchises
  a. What date was the company founded and what date was the first franchise awarded? Company founded? _____ First franchise awarded? _____
  b. Number of franchises currently in operation or under construction. _____
  Information on those to contact:
  Franchise 1: owner _____
           address _____
           _____
           telephone _____
           date started _____
  Franchise 2: owner _____
           address _____
           _____
           telephone _____
           date started _____
  Franchise 3: owner _____
           address _____
           _____
           telephone _____
           date started _____
  Franchise 4: owner _____
           address _____
           _____
           telephone _____
           date started _____
  c. How many franchises are planned for the next 12 months (not including those awarded and not yet in operation)? _____

4. Why have franchises failed?
  a. How many franchises have failed? _____ How many of these have been in the last 2 years? _____
  b. Why have franchises failed?
  Franchisor reasons: _____
  _____
  _____
  Better Business Bureau reasons: _____
  _____
  _____

Checklist continued

Franchisee reasons: _____
_____
_____
_____

5. Franchise in local market area
   a. Has a franchise ever been awarded in this area? _____
      If so, and if it is still in operation:
      owner _____
      address _____
      telephone _____ date started _____
      If so, and if it is no longer in operation:
      person involved _____
      address _____
      date started _____ date ended _____
      reasons for failure _____
      _____

      How many inquiries have there been for the franchise from the
      area in the past 6 months? ____

6. What product or service will be added to franchise package:
   a. within 12 months? _____
      _____

   b. within 2 years? _____
      _____

   c. within 2 to 5 years? _____
      _____

7. Competition
   a. What is my competition? _____
      _____
      _____

8. Are all franchises independently owned?
   a. Of the total outlets, _____ are franchised, and _____ are
      company owned.
   b. If some outlets are company owned did they start out this way,
      _____ or were they repurchased from a franchisee? _____
      Date of most recent company acquisition. _____

9. Franchise operations:
   a. What facilities are required, and do I lease or build?

	build	lease
operated out of home	_____	_____
office	_____	_____
building	_____	_____
manufacturing facility	_____	_____
warehouse	_____	_____
_____	_____	_____

   b. Getting started—who is responsible for what?

	franchisor	franchisee
feasibility study	_____	_____
design	_____	_____
construction	_____	_____
furnishing	_____	_____
financing	_____	_____

Franchise company

1. The company:
   a. What is the name and address of the parent company, if different
      from the franchise company:
      name _____
      address _____
   b. Is the parent company public, ____ or private? ____

continued

c. If the company is public, where is the stock traded?

New York Stock Exchange _____

American Stock Exchange _____

over-the-counter _____

_____ _____

4. Forecast of income and expenses:

a. Is a forecast of income and expenses provided? _____

Is it:

based on actual franchisee operations? ___

based on a franchisor outlet? ___

purely estimated? ___

b. If a forecast is provided does it:

	yes	no
relate to your market area?	_____	_____
meet your personal goals?	_____	_____
provide adequate return on investment?	_____	_____
provide for adequate promotion and personnel?	_____	_____

5. What is the best legal structure for my company?

proprietorship _____

partnership _____

corporation _____

6. Are all details covered in a written franchise contract?

yes ___ no ___ (get copy for lawyer and accountant review)

a. What to look for—are these included:

	yes	no
franchise fee	_____	_____
termination	_____	_____
selling and renewal	_____	_____
advertising and promotion	_____	_____
patent and liability protection	_____	_____
home office services	_____	_____
commissions and royalties	_____	_____
training	_____	_____
financing	_____	_____
territory	_____	_____
exclusive vs non-exclusive	_____	_____
franchise	_____	_____

SOURCE: Adapted from C. R. Stigelman, *Franchise Index/Profile,* Small Business Management Series, No. 35 (Washington, D.C.: Small Business Administration, 1973), pp. 31–41.

years, you'd have paid the owner $100,000, and your profit would have been $400,000. With good terms, you don't need to think about paying off the loan, ever.

There is one good reason to think about buying a franchise — you want a marketing boost from the name. (Depending on the franchise, you may get other services for your money — help on site selection, help on interior layout, vendor connections, a business plan — but what you're buying is brand-name recognition.)

Whether you're investigating an existing business or a franchise, make sure you study the situation thoroughly.

Examine the financial history.

Compare what you'd make if you bought this business to what you'd make if you invested the same money elsewhere.

Evaluate tangible assets.

Talk to suppliers, employees, and others.

Get an ironclad covenant not to compete. (In the case of a franchise, make sure the franchisor won't set up competing franchisees in your area.)

Analyze the seller's motives.

Negotiate the cost of Goodwill. (You could be buying Ill Will.)

Insist on a bulk sales escrow.

THINK POINTS

⚡   Stick to what you know. Don't buy a business you know nothing about.

⚡   Don't let them rush you. A business is not a used car.

⚡   If your seller looks absolutely honest, check him out anyway.

⚡   Worry less about price. Work harder on terms.

⚡   Most good businesses are sold behind the scenes, before they reach the open market.

⚡   Make sure you're there when the physical inventory takes place. Look in those boxes yourself.

⚡   Get everything in writing. Be specific.

⚡   Always go through bulk sales escrow.

REFERENCES

Bank of America Marketing Publications Department. *How to Buy or Sell a Business.* Small Business Reporter Series. San Francisco: Bank of America. As this book goes to press, this publication was out of print. However, many B of A branches have some on hand; or, write to SBR Series, Bank of America, Department 3120, P.O. Box 37000, San Francisco, CA 94137, for its current status.

Burstiner, Irving. *The Small-Business Handbook.* Englewood Cliffs, N.J.: Prentice-Hall, 1979.

Buying and Selling a Small Business. Washington, D.C.: Small Business Administration, 1981.

Cohen, Herb. *You can Negotiate Anything: How to Get What You Want.* Secaucus, N.J.: Lyle Stuart, 1980. An intriguing look at the tactics of wheeling and dealing, with case studies and scenarios for working the marketplace.

Frost, Ted S. *Where Have All the Woolly Mammoths Gone?* West Nyack, N.Y.: Parker Publishing, 1976.

Jurek, Walter. *A Reference Manual on Buying and Selling a Business.* Santa Barbara, Calif.: Quality Services, n.d. If you cannot locate this book, it can be ordered through Quality Services, Inc., 3887 State Street, Santa Barbara, CA 93105.

Sullivan, Daniel, and Joseph Lane. *Small Business Management, a Practical Approach.* Dubuque, Iowa: William C. Brown Group, 1983.

Tetreault, Wilfred E. *Buying and Selling Business Opportunities: A Sales Transaction Handbook.* Reading, Mass.: Addison-Wesley Publishing Co., 1981. Contains an overwhelming set of documents needed to buy a business. One look at this book, and you'll decide to handle your own start-up.

U.S. Department of Commerce. *Franchise Opportunities Handbook.* Washington, D.C.: U.S. Department of Commerce, Office of Minority Business Enterprise, 1979.

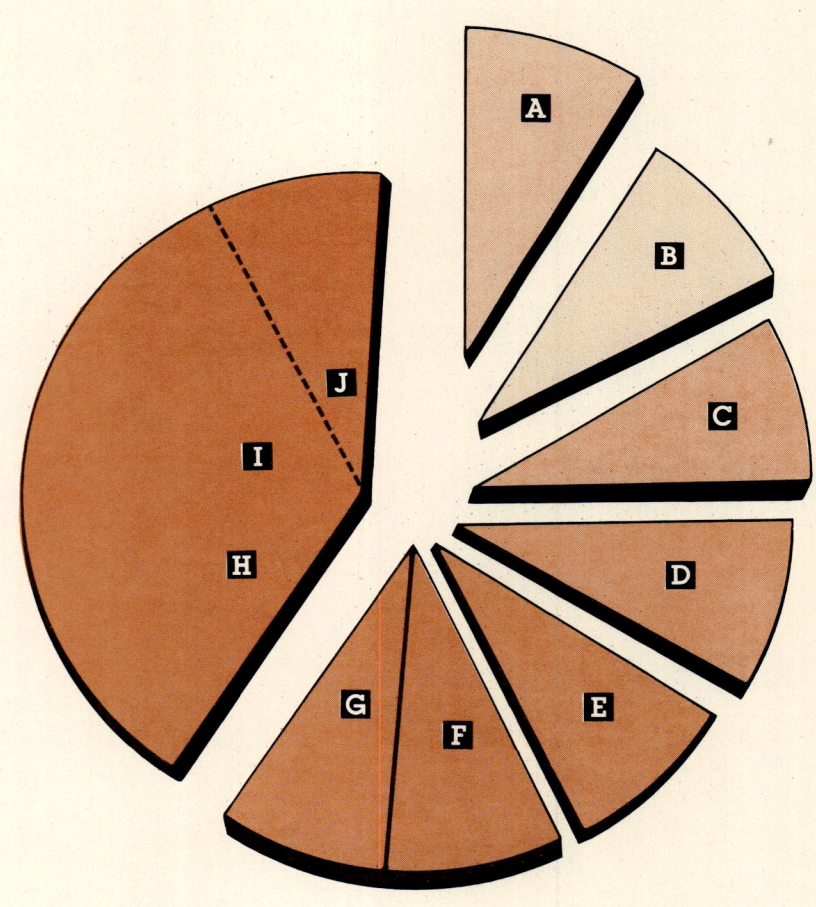

A Description of Product or Service

B The Market and the Target Customer

C Competition

D Marketing Strategy

E Location

F Management

G Personnel

H Projected Income Statement

I Projected Cash Flow

J Projected Balance Sheet

FIGURE 14.1 Chapter 14 lets you complete your preparations for the financial section of your Plan by celebrating the advantages offered by the small business computer.

14

Control: Your Small Business Computer

To determine how badly you need a computer for your small business.

To identify tasks in your business (such as high repetition or lots of numbers) that can be helped by a computer.

To develop a sense of what is going on in the computer industry and how it can affect your purchase of a small-business system.

To decide where to buy and who to buy from.

To know what questions to ask, and to distinguish who wants to help you from who is out to take your money and run.

To know what to read to get an overview of what is happening to information processing.

To use your New Eyes to forecast what will happen to computers in the next 5–10 years.

To tell yourself to keep learning in this field, even if the speed at which it changes makes you dizzy.

In many ways, the microcomputer is uniquely suited to the needs of small business. As we discuss what microcomputers mean to you, we want to emphasize that the computer is useful on two levels: As a signpost to the future, the computer helps you look at your daily activities and separate what brings you closer to the future from what shackles you to the past. As a tool, the computer can dramatically increase your effectiveness, even as it shortens the time between an idea and its realization.

WHAT MICROCOMPUTERS MEAN TO YOU

The Computer as Symbol

In his book, *The Third Wave*, futurist Alvin Toffler writes about the shift we're making, as a nation and as a people, from the Industrial Age to the Information Age.

The First Wave, Toffler says, was Agriculture: farms, livestock, harvest. The Second Wave was Industry: machinery, smokestacks, factories, robber barons. The Third Wave is electronic, the coming Age of Information based on the pulsing beat of the computer. And what's different about this Third Wave for us is how quickly it's coming. The shift from agriculture to industry took at least 100 years, but the shift between industry and the Information Society is taking place even as we write about it and try to pin it down. It's taking place here and now, in a few lightning-fast years.

If you hear strange and distant sounds but can't locate the source, it's just the future calling you from beyond the Third Wave.

If you sometimes feel the world is confused, one of the reasons is because we're all watching from **Toffler's Trough** — that low point or depression between the Second Wave and the Third.

It's hard to see from a trough, even with New Eyes.

We don't have a lot of choice about this wave. It's washing over us whether we like it or not.

The Third Wave is symbolized by the **computer,** a machine that has already reorganized our lives and our minds. If you have a digital watch, you're computerized. If you use a pocket calculator, you're computerized. If you receive a phone bill or a light bill or a personalized letter you know went to a million other folks — that's the computer talking.

When a computer talks, it hums and beeps.

Step back, if you can, to get some perspective on the sound. Isn't the computer the perfect symbol for the Age of Information? Quiet, unidirectional, unemotional, tireless, error-free.

And it's here to stay.

A Tool for Small Business

If you're in small business, or dreaming of going into one, this is your lucky day, because the **microcomputer** seems to have been created especially for the bold and adventurous entrepreneur.

Toffler's Trough
a low point or depression between the Second Wave and the Third

computer
a machine that processes information

microcomputer
a desk-top information processor that has created an entire industry

When they designed the microcomputer, it looks like they were thinking of putting more muscle into small business.

The right micro, hooked up with the right software, can put new strength into your small business.

How? By becoming an **electronic extension** of your mind and personality. (Figure 14.2, on page 262, pictures many of the tasks a microcomputer does well.)

It will take orders, handle details, print while you're doing something else, do your filing, cross-check other files, probe the future of profit and cash flow, print payroll checks, and put you in touch with business information that will help you survive.

The micro is amazing. It sits on a table or desktop. It doesn't cost an arm and a leg. If it needs moving, you can move it, in pieces. It can handle any repetitive detail in your business and thus leave your head free for entrepreneurial creativity. It will do accounting, word-processing, **general ledger,** mailing lists, customer (patient, client, student) files, flyers, newsletters, memos, and so on. And if it talks back, you can shut it down with the flick of a switch.

The mark of an entrepreneur is fast footwork. The reason you can succeed is not because your advertising budget can compete with the hefty purses of Madison Avenue. The reason is because you can spot an opportunity and get tooled up to deliver faster than the Big Guys.

With a micro on your desk top, you can be even quicker.

Who could ask for anything more?

WHERE TO BEGIN

Which Comes First, Hardware or Software?

There are three interlocking steps to using a micro in your business:

1. Identify the problem that needs solving, or the tasks you want done.
2. Locate software (the program that runs the computer) to solve the problem or do the task.
3. Find a piece of hardware that will:
   a. Listen to the software.
   b. Keep you happy punching keys and studying the screen.
   c. Not shatter your pocketbook.

Action Step 55 will start you on these three interlocking steps by having you list problems and tasks in your small business. The Action Step also provides a list of questions to help you focus on your business needs.

Before and After

If you talk to successful entrepreneurs who have computerized their small businesses, you soon learn that a going business concern often tells the entrepreneur why a business needs a computer. The information is after the fact. Business owners are often kicking themselves because they didn't act sooner — and with more strategic planning.

---

electronic extension
a link between the computer and the mind of the Heavy User

general ledger
a master collection of all accounting transactions

ACTION STEP 55

Identify Problems in Search of Solutions

Take a minute to list some problems and tasks in your small business.

You might think first about repetition. What do you do over and over? Think next about detail. What do you do that has to be precise? Think next about monitoring time. Where are the time lags in your business and where do they need to be tracked?

Use these questions to trigger your thoughts.

1. What are the demographic characteristics of your ten top customers? The top twenty? The top one hundred?
2. Is there a time lag between a sale and when you bill the customer?
3. Do you pay overtime? Do you pay hourly overtime to salaried employees?
4. Do you have a select list of active customers and a secondary list of customers who make fewer purchases but who are still important to your business?
5. Would you like to up-date your P & L (profit and loss statement) without having to consult your accountant?
6. Do you have trouble locating inventory?
7. Do you have 100 or more vendors? Does your buying produce more than 100 purchase orders per month?
8. Do you write more than 100 checks per month?
9. Would you like to do your own spreadsheet analysis just to break out your financial picture on your own?
10. When you up-date your Business Plan, would you like to be able to change a few numbers and have the new version printed while you're busy at something else?
11. Do you write the same business letter to several customers?
12. Would you like to be able to coordinate your customer mailing list with a program that corrected your typos and spelling errors?

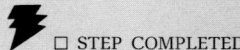 □ STEP COMPLETED

Listen to the entrepreneurs in the following case studies as they look back at their decisions concerning computer acquisition. You may be able to learn from them and avert the marketplace crises that forced them to rush into computerization.

Case Study

The Computer File

Arlene Jameson — Property Management

The reason we finally decided to computerize was because the business was exploding. We'd started it four years ago—just my husband and myself, doing property management—and we'd worked out of our home. As we expanded, we bought a trailer that we'd park at the construction site. Then we hired someone and bought another trailer, and by the fourth year we knew we'd either have to find a way to control the business or stop writing management contracts.

We really hated to lose all those customers. We could tell we were at a decision crossroads in our business.

So we consulted a **computer consultant.** He told us what kind of software we needed, and what kind of hardware would go best with the software, and we got our system.

For two weeks, I almost went crazy learning it. Converting our books was the hardest part. It took me three months, and all that time I was still doing books manually, with a pencil and a calculator.

But once I understood this electronic spreadsheet method, I'll never go back to the old way. Computers saved our business.

Paul Takahashi — Consultant

I had $500 in the bank when I was laid off. Like a lot of guys in that position, I went into the consulting business. After I'd been in business about a year, I knew I wasn't going to survive if I didn't get some help—especially with the repetitive parts of my business. That means numbers, of course, keeping the records straight. But it also means newsletters, flyers, printed invoices, that all-important letter that you've been meaning to revise that's sitting there, in the typewriter, waiting.

Well, the computer did all that, and more. I couldn't have survived without it. It gives my one-man show the **capabilities** of a much larger outfit.

Ron Terkel — Insurance Agent

The thing that sold me on computers was a file program called the Data Factory.

I'm an independent insurance agent, and one of the problems we have is **cross-filing.** We've got at least 20 different categories of claims and an incredible variety of possible adjustments and sometimes it takes hours for my staff to locate vital information.

Well, with this computer system, backed up by the Data Factory, we can search from one file to another.

It's great. It's like having x-ray vision and being able to see through a hundred manila folders all at once.

Now that we're on this system, I don't know how we ever did without it.

Free Help and Information

You can find lots of free offers of help and small business information in the ads in the *Wall Street Journal.* Here are two examples that were current as this book went to press:

1. Monroe Systems for Business offers a free demonstration of their Simon Says accounting system; write them at The American Road, Morris Plains, NJ 07950.

2. *LIST, the Software Resource Book* contains a guide to over 3,000 microcomputer programs, indexed by application, industry, and hardware. At this writing, *LIST* could be reached toll-free at 1-800-821-7700.

Ads like these are placed by firms that have something to sell—but companies are willing to give help and advice to gain customers. Hunt through the ads for the information you want. Good luck in your hunt!

computer consultant
a specialist who can help you solve problems with the computer

capabilities
defines the tasks possible

cross-filing
a dual reference system listed by two or more categories

HOW TO SHOP FOR YOUR MICROCOMPUTER

Inform Yourself

Once you have identified what tasks you need help with and what problems you want to solve, you are ready to learn more about available **computer systems.** A computer system includes both the hardware and the software that makes it go. If you think back to our three interlocking steps (page 259), you'll remember that you really want to focus on software first. This may not be an easy concept to master. Just remember that there are any number of machines out in the marketplace, and each is limited in the kinds of software it can use.

If you go out shopping for hardware before you have identified what software will be best for you, you're putting the cart before the horse.

To make the best decision, you have to inform yourself. And one of the best places to do that is the very marketplace where sales people are pushing computer systems. Action Step 56 gets you out into the market to shop for solutions to your business problems. You don't need to become an expert on computers. You just want to get one foot on the information treadmill. Action Step 56 shows you how.

Mentally Prepare Yourself

We're going to help you prepare yourself for your first visit to a computer systems store by having you imagine yourself in the following scenario. The action takes place in a large computer emporium. You play yourself as someone who is just beginning to investigate computer systems. Let's see how well you do.

"I'm in the market for a computer to help me in my business. What can you tell me?"

SALESPERSON: May I help you?

YOU: I'm in the market for a computer system.

SALES: You've come to the right place. What capabilities do you want?

YOU: Well, I'm in business for myself. Some of those ads in the *Journal* caught my eye, and I'd be interested in seeing the new Texas Instruments portable. [Reading from your list] I'm also interested in the IBM, the Apple Macintosh, the Televideo Personal, the Cromenco, the Kaypro, and the latest DEC Rainbow. I need help with accounting, mailing lists, data-base management, general ledger, and payroll.

SALES: Let me ask you something. If we can put you in a system today, one that will do everything you've ever dreamed of, would you be willing to take delivery this afternoon?

YOU: Hey! I just started looking!

SALES: Just asking. You look like a person who'd be interested in getting 27% off list.

YOU: [Looking around. Can this be true?]: This is the first store I've been in. I'm not sure what I want.

SALES: No problem. Take your time. But let me tell you, this is the deal of a lifetime.

computer systems
computer hardware, plus
the software that tells it
what to do

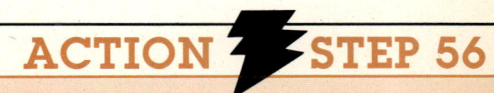
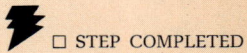

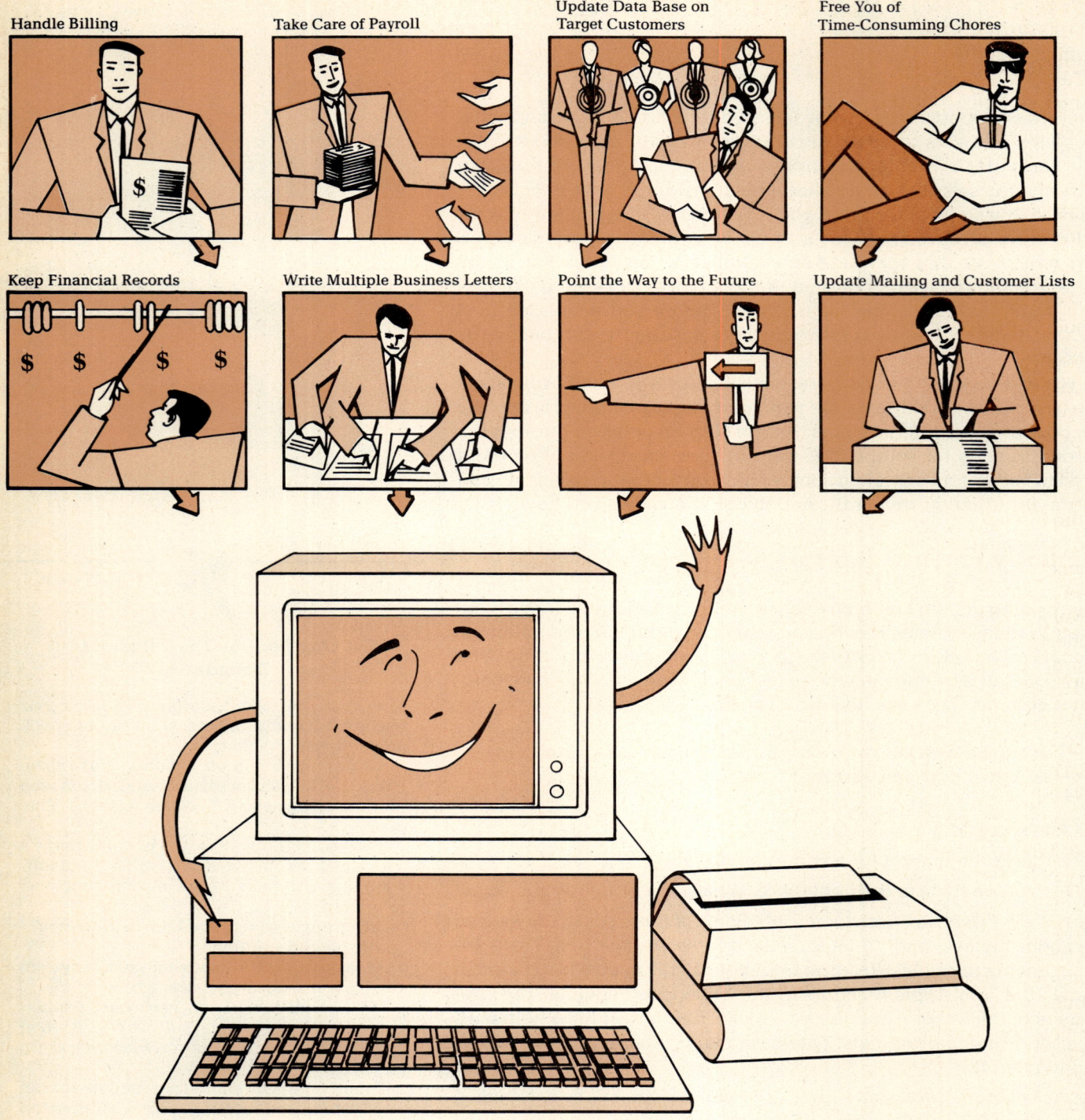

Handle Billing

Take Care of Payroll

Update Data Base on Target Customers

Free You of Time-Consuming Chores

Keep Financial Records

Write Multiple Business Letters

Point the Way to the Future

Update Mailing and Customer Lists

FIGURE 14.2 When you look at all the things a microcomputer does well, it seems like the micro was created especially for the bold and adventurous entrepreneur.

YOU: What kind of system is it?

SALES: My friend, we've got a factory authorization from the head office of Micro-Batics Ltd. — that's out in the Silicon Valley area of California — to discount their micro at 17%. Our distributor is adding another 10% on top of that. It's a super-buy. The sale's been going on for two weeks, and today's the last day. You've seen our ads in the paper? In the Business section?

YOU: Sorry. Who makes this system?

SALES: Like I said. It's a Micro-Batics 9000, the top of their line. It will do everything except chew bubble gum.

YOU: Micro-Batics? Never heard of it.

SALES: You will. Why not try it out? It's right over here.

[You sit down and stare at screen. You feel nervous, edgy.]

YOU: The screen is purple.

SALES: Compu-Mauve is the latest thing to protect VDT users against eyestrain. You haven't heard of Compu-Mauve?

YOU: There seem to be a lot of extra buttons.

SALES: We call this the keyboard. We call those function keys. Incidentally, this is an 8-bit machine, because our market research showed us that 16-bit was over-powered. This particular unit is CP/M based, with an optional add-on card that will give you modem capability. It comes, standard, with 128K of RAM and can be configured to any printer with a parallel port interface. The word-processing program is built right into the hardware here, so there's none of that changing disks when you want to do something simple like type a memo. All you do is hit a button, here, like this. [Hits button. Words appear on screen.]

YOU: How much does all of this cost, anyway?

SALES: Okay. I thought you'd never ask. The CPU goes for $1,500. The **VDT** — that's with the new Easy Eye Compu-Mauve screen — is $400. The monitor interface runs $500. You've got to have it anyway to interface with your printer. One drive or two?

YOU: I . . . uh . . . what's a drive?

SALES: We recommend two. Of course, if you'd like to go hard disk, I can get you a real deal on a Winchester-type Davong that holds up to 5M. I'd have to double-check that with my sales manager, but since I was the top salesman for the last two months, he'll probably see it my way. That hard disk retails for $1,995, but I can save you some bucks today, because of the sale. This system comes with a complimentary carton of paper, but diskettes are extra. Shall we write this up now?

YOU: I have to go. I'll come back some other time. Have you got anything to read on this stuff?

SALES [Miffed]: Sorry. We're fresh out.

Commentary. This salesperson is just off the used car lot. He's trapped back in the Industrial Age, where **pushing hardware** was the name of the game. You're making a purchase to hook you into the Information Society. There's someone out there to help. You may have to pay a consultant's fee, but a consultant will help you make a cleaner decision.

VDT
video display terminal

pushing hardware
an emphasis on the hardware sale over all other considerations

By the way, you did pretty well in the scenario. You didn't let yourself be intimidated.

Because we're still trapped in Toffler's Trough, we tend to shop for computers the same way we shopped for cars or stereos or refrigerators. In the scenario, you remembered to shop for solutions.

A computer may look like one more chunk of **Industrial Age hardware,** but it's really your key to unlock the door to the Age of Information.

One of the problems people face in computer-system selection is that the field changes fast. In 1982 Apple was the micro leader. In 1983 the IBM PC was the leader, and lots of companies began to copy the PC. In 1984 Apple demonstrated its staying power with increased Macintosh sales and by introducing its portable Apple IIc. There's a new language coming called C which will change the arena again. One way to keep up is to read all the popular computer magazines.

The future of the computer age is software.

BEFORE TEST–DRIVING YOUR MICROCOMPUTER

If you have found the computer system (software and hardware) for you, no doubt you're eager to test drive your micro. The only reason we want to give you a little advice first is so that you don't close a sale without thinking about some important considerations.

> **Industrial Age hardware**
> cars, stereos, refrigerators, boilers

Comdex: Where Industry Trends First Appear

The big show for the microcomputer industry occurs in late autumn of the year in Las Vegas. It's called Comdex, and it attracts people from all over the world. At Comdex/82, industry watchers noticed the Great Software Shift, which signalled a dramatic change in the industry.

Prior to 1982, software writers began aiming their programs at Apple.

In 1982, software writers began aiming their programs at the IBM-PC.

In less than a year after the discovery at Comdex, the IBM-PC had become the industry standard. By late 1983, the picture looked clear: "There are two kinds of companies in the industry," said a spokesman in the *Wall Street Journal* (December 12, 1983). "Those that make IBM compatibles and those that are slowly going out of business."

The fact that a large segment of the industry is following IBM has a bearing on what computer system you buy. For example, Compaq has built a portable copy cat computer, which is IBM compatible. Lotus 1-2-3, the integrated spread-sheet, was aimed at the IBM-PC from the start. Lotus shipped its first package in January, 1983. Microsoft, the creators of MS-DOS, sold its first version of an operating system to IBM. (An operating system makes the computer system go.) Now, 188 companies have licensed MS-DOS.

If you're looking for a microcomputer, IBM has given you something to think about.

1. Think Problem First, Software Second, Hardware Third. Invest a lot of time listing your problems and tasks. Invest a lot more locating software that will do the job. Work those computer salespeople.

2. Don't Buy Forever.   Once you've identified your immediate needs, buy a system for the next 18 months or so. This is the Age of Information and the computer will change your life, and a fancier system with more bells, more whistles, and more power, is already on its way from some new **Silicon Valley** somewhere.

3. Expand, Expand, Expand.   Buy a system you can expand. Research the components (things like printer and modem) you might need at some future date, and then check each system for the ports you plug into and the possibilities for **add-on memory** when you need more power.

4. Buy Local from a Reputable Dealer. You Get What You Pay For.   If it's your first computer system, buy from a local dealer who will throw in training, support, service, and hand-holding. During the first 200 hours of initiation into the World of Computers, the hand-holding is essential. (It's true — you can get some good deals out there, price-wise. But a dealer who's pulling in business with loss leaders is not going to help out when your computer says SYNTAX ERROR CAN'T READ DRIVE ONE NO FILE OPEN. Because you're in business, you don't want to be asking your computer for favors. Remember the movie *2001*? ''Open the pod door, Hal.'')

5. Hire a Consultant.   If this is your first system, you can save yourself lots of grief by hiring a computer consultant. A good consultant will help you identify what your problems are and how to solve them.

6. Thoughts on a Maintenance Contract.   If your system is under $6,000, you probably don't need to spend the extra dollars for an extended maintenance contract. Between $6,000 and $12,000, think it over carefully. Over $12,000, protect your investment with a maintenance contract.

7. Budget for software.   Budget at least 40% of your total system cost for **software cost.** The right software means the difference between happiness and despair.

8. ''Burning in'' the Machine.   Make sure your dealer ''burns in'' your machine. Average ''burn-in'' time is about 35 hours and gets the bugs out while the computer is still in the store.

9. Experience Pays, Innocence Hurts.   After you've learned thoroughly what your system can do, then you can start shopping around for discount software in the mail-order market. But remember, with mail order shopping you are on your own and without dealer support, so be careful.

10. Educate Yourself.   Keep taking computer classes. Knowledge will keep you on the Leading Edge and out of Toffler's Trough.

Silicon Valley
an area southeast of San Francisco, California, that is the heart of the microcomputer industry

add-on memory
a way of enlarging the memory-capacity of a computer system

software cost
you should budget at least 40% of you total system cost for software

burning in
the first 35 hours of operation of a computer-system, when things are likely to go wrong

Learning from Others

We all learn from our mistakes. What's even better than learning from our own mistakes is learning from the mistakes of others. That's why we think you'll appreciate the following case study. Because this true story involves a *Fortune* 500 company, we also think you'll appreciate the fact that you as a small business operator have the opportunity to be more astute than many of the Big Guys.

Case Study

A Well-Known *Fortune* 500 Company

In the early seventies, just before the Great Computer Boom, the management of a well-known *Fortune* 500 company decided to make the Grand Transformation from caveman bookkeeping to computer bookkeeping. They bought a mainframe plus terminals for the clerks who took telephone orders.

The caveman method was characterized by primitive tools: pencils, paper, carboned order blanks, typewriters, and an intricate network of grey tunnels (or chutes). The tunnels were about three inches in diameter, and they connected departments with other departments inside the giant megacorporation. The clerks taking orders would place the order blanks inside message cylinders, snap shut the little metal doors, and then insert the cylinders into an entry port, where they would be whisked away by air pressure.

Exciting.

Because of **bureaucratic lag,** it took several months of negotiation and research before management could agree on the proper system to replace the grey tunnels. The system that was finally chosen, a combination in-house mainframe computer with peripherals from other *Fortune* 500 giants, was magnificent.

"This system, without a doubt, will serve our firm until at least 1990," said one of the top managers.

"Yes," said another manager. "And perhaps beyond."

"Agreed," intoned a third. "Our system has great capacity. We'll interface with markets everywhere. For us, it's the perfect system."

bureaucratic lag
an almost endless span of time in the corporate world when things should get done but don't (drives entrepreneurs crazy)

Commentary. At the end of the first week, everyone was delighted with the system. Furthermore, everyone was using it like crazy because it was so useful. And it was fast.

At the end of the second week, the system was showing signs of minor overload. More and more people were standing in line to use it. They had discovered the computer could save them time which they could use for phone calls, conferences, thinking, and just being creative.

At the end of the third week, the system was overloaded beyond its capacity.

Moral: Even if you're a big hitter, the computer will change your life in ways you never imagined. Buy a system you can expand.

SOME LAST THOUGHTS

The microcomputer can help you complete your Business Plan in two ways: 1) If you create your Plan on a word processor, you'll be able to make changes easily, and 2) if you use an electronic spreadsheet, you will be able to speed up your financial projections. In Chapter 15, where we show you a sample Business Plan, there are several financial statements generated as an electronic spreadsheet.

As we end this chapter on microcomputers, we want to refer you to one of the best places to pick up on the latest trends in this fast-moving field: A yearly trade show called Comdex. Comdex shows are reported in the *Wall Street Journal* and other national business and computer magazines. See the boxed article, ''Comdex: Where Industry Trends First Appear,'' on page 264.

SUMMARY

Computers are here to stay. If you go into small business, you'll probably think about getting one. Two questions will arise:

1. How badly will you need a computer?
2. What model do you need and where should you buy it?

This chapter helps you focus on the computer as a small-business tool and to think of the computer as a symbol for the future. Here's some advice to think about before you start searching for your computer with New Eyes:

1. Think of computer acquisition as a three-step process — define your task(s) or problem(s); locate software to do the job; locate hardware to run the software.
2. Buy a good computer, but try not to lock yourself in with overpriced hardware. The computer industry changes fast. Improvements are the name of the game. Something fancier, and with more power, is coming along soon.
3. Buy a system you can expand.
4. Buy your first system locally, from a reputable dealer. You'll spend more money up front, but you're going to need dealer support during your first days, weeks, and months of operation.
5. Think about hiring a consultant.
6. If your system is under $6,000, you probably don't need a maintenance contract. Between $6,000–$12,000, give a maintenance contract serious thought. Over $12,000, get a maintenance contract.
7. Budget at least 40% of your total system cost for software.

ACTION STEP REVIEW

Action Steps for this chapter help you explore your relationship to the computer in small business.

55 List problems and tasks in your small business that might better be handled by a computer. The key here is repetition — what tasks do you do over and over? It could be anything from billing to sending out a monthly newsletter. Another key is quantity. Do you have 100 or more vendors, write more than 100 checks per month, or have a large customer list? Another key is efficiency. Would you like to update your Business Plan easily? When you write letters to customers, would you like a program to check spelling and style?

56 Once you've identified tasks where the computer might help, hit the streets and check out systems. System means software *plus* hardware. Don't let computer retailers sell you hardware the way they'd sell you a car or a stereo. Concentrate on software that will solve your problems.

Ask these questions:
Will this software help me?
Is it easy to use?
If I bring work home, will I be able to transfer it to a larger computer at work?
What will it cost if I want my computer to talk to another computer, in another city?
How many other computers will my computer be ''compatible'' with?

8. Make sure your dealer ''burns in'' your machine. The first 30–40 hours of operation should be in the shop, under the dealer's protection.

9. Wait until you're familiar with your machine and with software programs before you start buying discounted programs through the mail.

10. Keep taking computer courses. Keep reading.

THINK POINTS

⚡ A computer can be an extension of your entrepreneurial personality. What a treat for creative you!

⚡ Because it rises from the mists of the Industrial Age, the hardware for your computer system is easy to select — if you follow our advice of working back from problems to solutions to software. Let your software needs determine hardware needs.

⚡ Buy a microcomputer today. Learn what it can do.

⚡ Take a computer course. Educate yourself about the Information Society.

⚡ If you find yourself balking at computers because you don't know how they work, analyze your feelings about operating a car. You probably don't know how the internal combustion engine works either, but that doesn't mean you can't learn to drive.

⚡ You've got to compute to compete.

REFERENCES

Korngold, Bob. ''Building a Check Register into a General Ledger.'' *Small Business Computers,* March/April 1983, 50–53. Takes the beginner through a simple program in Visicalc.

The McWilliams Letter. Another Peter McWilliams project. (See also the following entries.) Ten issues a year of the latest computer nitty-gritty in a readable style. Newsletter format. From Prelude Press, P.O. Box 69773, Los Angeles, CA 90069.

McWilliams, Peter. *The Personal Computer Book.* Prelude Press: Los Angeles, 1982.

———. *The Word Processing Book.* Prelude Press: Los Angeles, 1982. Easy-to-read book about the art of word processing.

Mamis, Robert A. ''Unlocking Management Creativity.'' *Inc.,* June 1983.

Naiman, Arthur. *Word Processing Buyer's Guide.* New York: McGraw-Hill, 1983. Naiman has developed a 100-point checklist which he uses to evaluate 14 programs exhaustively and another 104 programs briefly. Naiman gives prices, addresses and sharp advice on word processors. He can't keep up with the industry, but who can?

Nevison, John. *Executive Computing.* Reading, Mass.: Addison-Wesley Publishing Co., 1981.

Trost, Stanley R. *Doing Business with SuperCalc.* Berkeley, Calif.: Sybex, 1983. One of a large line of books by Sybex. Step-by-step instructions on how to work a spreadsheet. Not overly imaginative, but at least it's written in English.

A Description of Product or Service

B The Market and the Target Customer

C Competition

D Market Strategy

E Location

F Management

G Personnel

H Projected Income Statement

I Projected Cash Flow

J Projected Balance Sheet

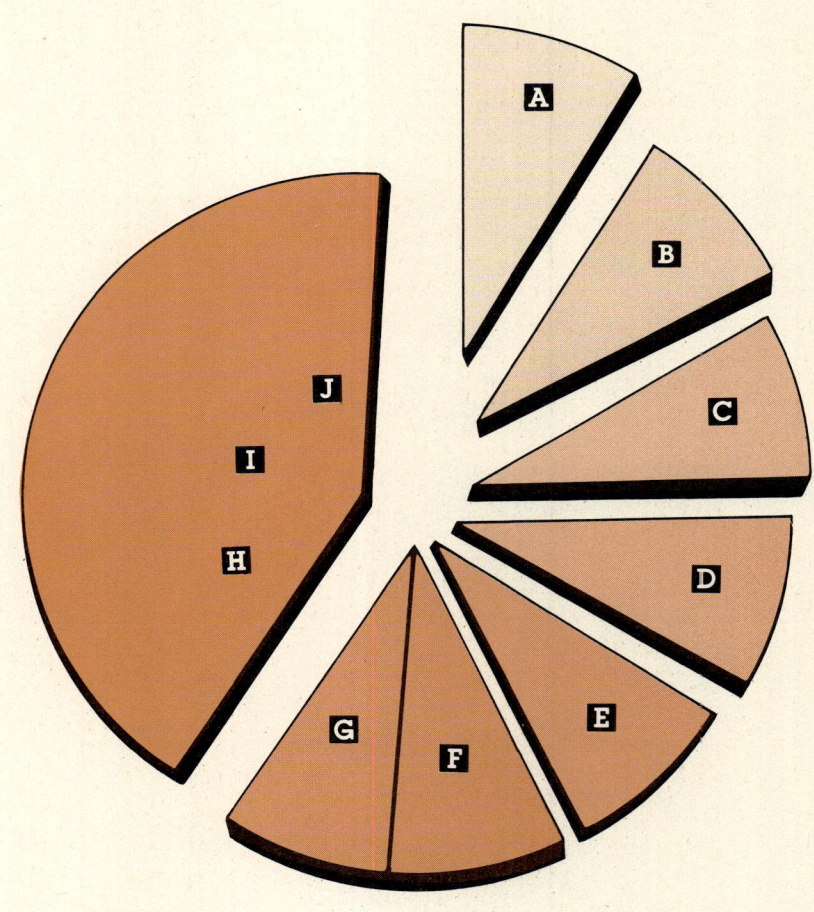

FIGURE 15.1 Chapter 15 tells you how to draw on all the materials you have generated to create your finished Business Plan.

15

Showcase: Pulling Your Plan Together

LEARNING OBJECTIVES

To pull all the information together into one coherent unit which becomes a portable show-case for your business.

To study a sample Business Plan to see how one group of entrepreneurs have defined and shown off their business.

To match or surpass the sample Business Plan in power and effectiveness.

To put your finished Business Plan to work.

**Y**our Business Plan could be the most important document you've ever pulled together.

While you're out there doing the work on your start-up, researching, finding the gaps, interviewing small business owners, profiling your target customers, a plan keeps you targeted. Because while you're out there hunting you're going to get a lot of distracting ideas for more new businesses.

You're an entrepreneur. Getting new ideas is easy for you.

You can't follow all of them to completion.

While you're out there, a Business Plan keeps your creativity on track and your power grooved. How? By being a constant reminder of who you are and where you are going.

A Business Plan is your roadmap to riches: Use it to keep your creativity on track. The finished Plan is a portable showcase for your business.

When you've finished your Business Plan, you've got something in writing to show to the people who are important to your business: your banker, lenders, relatives, venture capitalists, vendors, suppliers, key employees, friends, the SBA, and others.

The Plan is portable. You can make as many copies as you need to show the people who can help you succeed. You can mail it to your contacts across the country.

Planning is hard work. You'll stay up nights over this, maybe lose some sleep. But you'll save time in the end.

A pilot would not consider a long flight without a plan, and neither should you consider a business venture without a **Business Plan**.

Business Plan
a portable document
which becomes the
blueprint for your business

HOW TO WRITE YOUR BUSINESS PLAN

Two-Part Structure: Words and Numbers

Your Business Plan tells the world what kind of business you're in. For ease of handling, divide your plan in two sections, and document your Plan with Appendices.

Section I depends on your ability to use words to briefly introduce your strategies for Marketing and Management. Try to hook your reader with the excitement of creating a business, assessing the competition, designing a marketing plan, targeting customers, finding the right location, team-building — all those human things that most people can relate to, even if they're not in business.

Section II is Magic Numbers: income statement, cash flow projection, and projected balance sheet. This section of the Plan is aimed at bankers, credit managers, venture capitalists, vendors, SBICs, commercial credit lenders — and at the same time, you've got to make it accessible to the casual reader who searches for the bottom line.

Support the two sections with Appendices: resumes, maps, diagrams, photographs, tables, reprints from industry journals, letters from customers, letters from vendors, credit reports, personal financial statements, bids from contractors, and other documentation to support the viability of your plan. Note that in most cases, material in the Appendices comes from existing sources. You're not stating anything new, you're just supporting what you've already said. (Appendices vary according to each business, and for that reason sample Appendices are not included in this book.)

Just by following the Action Steps in this chapter, you will complete all the components you need to make a winning Business Plan. If you want to jump ahead for a quick overview of your Plan, take a look at our sample table of contents (Figure 15.3, page 276). Does it look familiar? That's because we structured this book to lead you to your Plan step by step.

The Relationship of Your Plan to This Book

You may be closer to having written your Business Plan than you think. If you have gone through the earlier chapters and completed the Action Steps, you already have the Building Blocks which are the foundation for your Plan. This chapter gives you the structure — earlier chapters gave you the materials.

Section I, the description of your business, draws directly from Chapters 2 – 7 and 13, which give you seven Building Blocks for your Plan. Each Building Block (see Figure 15.1) forms the base of a portion of Section I. For example, Building Block A (from Chapters 2 and 3) forms the base for subsection A, "Description of Product or Service."

Section II draws from Chapters 8 – 11 and 14, which give you the background and the skills to crunch numbers for the three financial statements that compose this section. The same chapters prepare you for writing good notes to each financial statement so that the statements mean something to your readers who can't relate to numbers.

How to Start Writing

If you're a creative thinker, chances are your thought processes don't always follow a linear sequence. That's great — it will help you as an entrepreneur! The Action Steps in this chapter *do* follow a linear sequence, because each Action Step is located next to the relevant portion of a finished Business Plan. This is a matter of convenience — you get to see an example of each component of the plan as it would appear in the finished product. But we don't expect you to write each section directly in sequence.

The best way to start writing a Business Plan is to begin with the material you feel most comfortable with. For example, if you really enjoyed interviewing Target Customers, you might begin with the Target Market and Target Customers subsection, referring back to Chapters 3 and 4 for boosts. Once you have a foothold in one section of the plan, the other sections will be closer to reach.

In this chapter you can treat the Action Steps as an expanded checklist to keep track of what parts of the Plan have been written and what parts haven't.

For example, in practice you would probably write the **cover letter** last of all, although that is the first Action Step that awaits you here. Think of the writing of this first cover letter as a valuable exercise. The more cover letters you write, the easier it becomes to write them effectively.

THE COVER LETTER

To aim your Plan to achieve the most good, you use a cover letter. Each time you send the Plan to a reader, you write a special cover letter and address it to that specific reader. The cover letter introduces the excitement of your Plan, and it tells the reader why you are sending it to that particular reader.

Action Step 57 gets you to write that letter. A sample cover letter appears in Figure 15.2.

What's Good About Our Sample Cover Letter?

1. The writer is making use of a previous contact.
2. The writer tells his reader — the manager of a national bank — that he is in the market for a loan. He does not put her on the spot by asking for money.
3. Instead, he asks for advice on where to find sources of capital.
4. The writer struck the right tone. To do that, he rewrote the letter several times.
5. You can do as well or better — it's worth the effort!

As you draft your cover letter, remember that the reader will pass judgment on your Business Plan (and on your business ability) on the basis of the letter. Do you want the entrance to your small business to look bright, attractive, and welcoming? Your Cover Letter is the doorway to your Business Plan.

A good cover letter will make your readers want to be a part of your venture.

SECTION I: WORDS

Preliminaries

Figure 15.3 provides a sample table of contents to give you a quick overview of a finished Business Plan. In practice, you would complete the table of contents last of all.

A. Description of Your Product or Service

Action Step 58 allows you to use the insights you gained in Chapters 2 and 3 to describe your business. Do you know your business? Prove it! By the time your reader finishes your description, you should have a

cover letter | a tailored introduction to your Business Plan

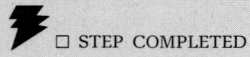

ACTION STEP 57

Write a Cover Letter for Your Plan

Address your letter to a specific person who can help your business. Be brief. You only need about two hundred words.

Tell your reader the reason you are sending the plan. If you are asking for money, tell the reader what you want it for and how much you want. Explain what it is going to be used for in the business.

Your purpose in writing the cover letter is to open the door gently to make way for further negotiations.

The cover letter is bait on your hook.

If you are putting money into the business, or if you have already donated, indicate how much.

The tone you are after in this opening move is confident and slightly formal. You want to appear neat, bright, organized, and in control of your venture.

As the cap-off, explain briefly how the money will be repaid.

A sample letter appears in Figure 15.2.

☐ STEP COMPLETED

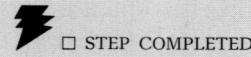

ACTION STEP 58

Describe Your Business

Excite your Reader about your business. Excitement is contagious. If you can get your reader going, there's a good chance you'll be offered money. Investors love hot ideas.

If this is a start-up, talk about your product or service. What makes it unique? What industry is it in? Where does the industry fit in the Big Picture?

Mention numbers wherever you can. Percentages and dollar amounts talk louder than words like "lots" and "many."

If this is a going business, you have a record of sales, costs, profit and loss, all of which need to dovetail into your needs for money.

Keep the words going and the typewriter smoking. At this point, you're still hooking the reader.

☐ STEP COMPLETED

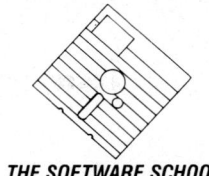

THE SOFTWARE SCHOOL

Mrs. Deborah Wallis
Manager, Franchise National Bank
1400 Market Circle
Anytown, USA

Dear Mrs. Wallis:

I've been meaning to write a formal thank you for the immense help you
provided on revising and updating the enclosed Business Plan. Your
input was helpful in the marketing area and invaluable on the Financial
Section. Everyone here at The Software School appreciates the care you
took reading over those early drafts.

Thanks very much.

We're now in the market for a loan of $50,000 (the figure you
suggested) to be used for capital expenditures--microcomputers, desks,
chairs, and upgrading our curriculum--and we'd appreciate any guidance
you could give us concerning sources of capital. (As I'm sure you'll
recall, our venture was launched without any equity debt whatsoever,
with each of our five principals putting up $20,000 apiece. And the
present Turbo Drive location already has space available for the second
classroom.)

We're planning to repay the loan out of new profit over the next three
years. (For more information, please refer to Financial Section,
beginning on page 14.)

Thank you very much for your help and advice. We couldn't have done it
without you.

Cordially,

Derek Campbell, CEO

47 TURBO DRIVE,
SUITES 108-110
NEWPORT BEACH
CALIFORNIA

FIGURE 15.2 This sample cover letter shows
how the CEO of The Software School sends his
company's Business Plan out to a potential lender.

TABLE OF CONTENTS

---

* The need for specific Appendices varies greatly from Business Plan to Business Plan. For that reason, Chapter 15 does not include sample Appendices. As you draft your own Plan, you will discover a number of opportunities to document and substantiate your business strategies, and this kind of documentation is best included as various Appendices.

convert to your side. To give you examples to follow, our text will reprint key sections from the Business Plan (newly revised and updated) for The Software School, an ongoing business that is seeking financing for acquiring more equipment.

Whether your business is ongoing or just starting up, the goals of Action Step 58 remain the same.

FIGURE 15.3 Here is the Table of Contents for The Software School's Business Plan.

Now let's see how The Software School tackled this portion of Section I.

┌─ **Business Plan** ─────────────────────

Description of the Business

The Software School, a California Corporation, is a microcomputer training facility located in Newport Beach, between Orange County's John Wayne Airport and a high-density executive business complex. It's the heart of Orange County's microcomputer users.

The school is now in its seventh month of operation, and we have a waiting list of 168 students (67% have put down deposits).

We train people in computer software systems from the Top Ten List of Best-Selling microcomputer software packages. Because of their power, these systems are complex. They provide a learning hurdle, especially at first.

Students are drawn to our teaching method because it gives them **hands-on experience** and also because it's fast. Working people are busy, and a student can upgrade a given software skill by 80% in eight hours. (For slower learners, we guarantee a second try, and a third, at no cost.) Most of our courses can be completed in one day or two evenings.

In contrast, the average college course (which teaches concepts instead of hands-on software systems) takes anywhere from 12 to 18 weeks. Our price is $100 for most courses, and so far no one has complained about the cost.

The Software School achieves this rather space-age learning speed with a sophisticated electronic teaching system adapted from flight-simulation techniques used by airlines in pilot training. We are constantly streamlining and upgrading the system, using funds already allocated in our start-up budget.

One especially bright note: We have done far better than we had hoped for. Actual income figures show us that our projections were conservative, and the actual figures have averaged 24% higher than originally projected. Projected income for the first six months, with an assumed **occupancy rate** of 50%, was just over $10,000 a month. The actual occupancy has not yet peaked, and for the last two months we have operated at 92% capacity.

In the service business, you're selling seats as well as skills and information, and as Appendix 1 shows, our promotion has generated a heavy demand for present courses like Computer Fundamentals, Wordstar, and Visicalc, while at the same time customers are asking for courses to meet their needs—for example, a course in Lotus 1-2-3, a second-generation data handler tailored for the IBM-PC.

Until the end of our fifth month, we were open six days a week, from 8 A.M. to 10 P.M. To meet demand with our current classroom facilities, we are now open on Sundays, from 9 A.M. to 6 P.M.

Sundays are full.

The demand increased dramatically when we contracted with some of Southern California's largest computer retailers to develop a training program. (See Appendix 2 for letters from specific sales managers.) These retailers sent their sales people for training; the sales people, in turn, refer customers to us. Computer retailers quickly discovered they could sell a better system to a buyer who was not afraid of computers. They were in the business of selling, not training.

Continued

hands-on experience
nonacademic exposure to real life, the real situation

occupancy rate
the percentage of a commercial property or development that is being occupied—used here in the sense of enrollments

Nothing impedes sales like fear of the product.

We combat that fear in a logical way, with knowledge. Our equipment (IBM-PCs) is top quality. Our staff combines excellent training skills with attention to people and their needs.

We have launched a solid start-up in a heated growth industry.

We plan to win.

Commentary: The Software School will get its funding because the writer of the Plan proves that his business is a winning concern.

Here's what the writer does:

1. Lets the facts speak for themselves.
2. Supports all claims with numbers.
3. Avoids hard-sell tactics.
4. Refuses to puff the product.

The writer does a terrific selling job without appearing to be selling at all!

B. The Market and the Target Customer

Action Step 59 gives you a chance to show just how you plan to win as you describe your market and your Target Customer. If you need a jolt to get started, review your work in Chapters 3 and 4. You'll also be able to review what the Business Plan for the Software School says about its market and TCs. Action Step 59 gives you good advice when it tells you to use secondary sources (like documents, tables, and quotes) to lend this portion credibility.

When you finish Action Step 59, see how The Software School's Business Plan handles the same situation.

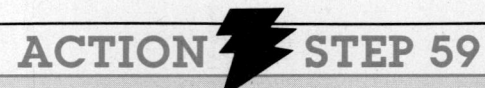

ACTION STEP 59

Describe the Market and the Target Customer

Bring all of your marketing research into this section and wow your reader with a picture of your target customer just sitting there waiting for your product or service.

Use data from secondary sources to lend credibility to the picture you are painting.

☐ STEP COMPLETED

Business Plan

The Market and the Target Customer

1. Industry Overview

Ten years ago, the personal computer did not exist in the U.S. marketplace. There were **mainframes,** of course, and terminals linked to invisible data banks—but nothing you could carry home in a suitcase.

Things have changed.

Approximately 200 firms are making personal computers. The lion's share of the market goes to Apple, IBM, Radio Shack, Texas Instruments, and so forth, and yet someone brings out a new PC (personal computer) almost every day of the year. The microcomputer industry is moving so fast that statistics can't keep pace. In 1981, the one

Continued

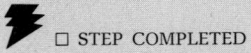

mainframes
massive hardware for
processing data

millionth computer was sold. The next year, 1982, one million computers were sold. By mid-1983, Kaypro's six-month sales were $26.1 million up from a previous $1.9 million and Kaypro had sold 47,500 units (*Wall Street Journal,* August 26, 1983). Estimates for future growth in this industry boggle the mind.

With all this sales flurry and emphasis on space-age speed, people can get left out. A computer can be your best friend, but only if you learn how to use it.

That means training.

Dataquest, Inc., market researchers in Cupertino, California, estimate that by 1986 the computer training industry will capture $3 billion of the $14 billion spent on personal computers.

It is a booming industry, and The Software School is on the **leading edge** of a major growth segment.

leading edge
the latest state of the art

2. Target Market

Our potential **total market** is Southern California, with a logical concentration in Orange County, which will show an increase in population from 1,970,000 in 1980 to 2,800,000 in the year 2000.

total market
every person or business that might need a product or service

Geographically, our target market encompasses Long Beach, La Habra, and Brea on the north; San Clemente on the south; Huntington and Newport Beaches on the west; and Orange, Fullerton, and Mission Viejo on the east. We are looking ahead to possible future expansion, from the heart of Orange County through the Southwestern United States.

For the moment, our focus will be Orange County.

Within this highly concentrated population area, our Target Customer is the small business person. Latest statistics show 76,000 small businesses in Orange County.

3. Target Customer

Our primary target customer is the small business, profiled below:

    Size: 1–30 employees
    Annual sales: $250,000 to $5 million
    Type of business: service industry
    Major output: paper (reports, letters, documents, etc.)

Our secondary target customer is the home user:

    Sex: 70% male
    Age: 18–35
    Education: some college
    Owns PC: 22%
    Access to Computer at Work: 52%
    Lives Near Computer Store: 73%
    Household Income: $35,000 plus
    Occupation: professional, managerial, executive, entrepreneurial

Commentary: Knowledge is power. In the Information Age, knowledge of your industry means Super-Power. The Software School, which is an information business, capitalized on expert knowledge to define the marketplace.

If your research is sound, it will show up in the writing.

Points to remember:

1. This is a revised Business Plan, so the writing is smooth. You will need to do several revisions in order to smooth out your Plan. How many revisions are you planning?

2. The reader of your Business Plan is a specialized Target Customer. How can you use your marketing abilities to look at this reader with New Eyes? Have you developed a profile of this very special Target Customer?

C. The Competition

Obviously if you know who your competitors are and how they fail to meet market needs, you are well on your way to strategic competition. Action Step 60 lets you persuade your reader how great your competitive tactics are. (If you need a reminder, reread Chapter 5. Competition changes according to where your business is in the life cycle, and a good way to begin your section on Competition is to place your industry in the proper life-cycle phase.)

How tough do your competitors look? As you go from Action Step 60 to read The Software School's assessment of its competition, note that the writer of the Plan takes a cool and objective look at his competition. He does not belittle them, and he certainly doesn't underestimate them. How did you handle your competition? The readers of your Business Plan will expect a business-like approach.

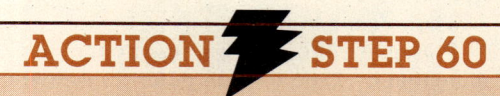

ACTION STEP 60

List Your Major Competitors

Briefly profile the businesses which compete with you directly. Try to be objective as you assess their operations.

What are their strengths? What are their weaknesses? What can you learn from them?

As you describe your competitors, use this opportunity to indicate how you're going to ace them out of the picture.

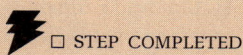 ☐ STEP COMPLETED

Business Plan

The Competition

The competition in Orange County in computer training is minimal at this time. The Software School has four main competitors:

1. Traherne Schools. Our oldest, most entrenched competitor. Three locations in Orange County: Brea, Garden Grove, and South Coast Plaza. Traherne's conducts a 6-hour course in Introduction to Microprocessors. The cost is $95. They currently run a course in VisiCalc for the Apple, and they have been planning to introduce a course in word processing for some time.

    Traherne's operates with a target market on the north rim of ours. Their South Coast Plaza Operation is closed on Saturdays.

2. *Big Micro* Computer Instruction. Excellent classroom facilities, located in El Toro, near the San Diego Freeway. All instruction is tied to Apple machines, and is free if you buy your hardware from Big Micro. Otherwise, courses usually cost around $95, and take 6–8 hours.

    The instructors try hard, but Big Micro is really in the business of pushing hardware.

3. Micro Hut Computer Center. Friendly salespeople with teaching skills double as teachers. Courses at Micro Hut are divided between Texas Instruments and Apple. Costs for Visicalc: $89. Costs for Word Processing: $149. (The Word-

Continued

Processing course takes about 12 hours of classroom time and is available only on Apple computers.)

Micro Hut is not in the education business. The courses are meant to help sell systems.

4. Your Micro and You. Local facility developed by professional educators. The atmosphere of YMAY is excellent. They offer a normal range of programs (BASIC, Pascal, Graphics, etc.) and also a course in using the computer in a small business.

Courses run around $125. All instruction is tied to the Apple. The market seems to be divided between adults with a casual interest in computers and children between the ages of 10–15.

These people have done it right.

Meeting the Competition

The Software School is in the computer education business. We are not selling hardware. We are not selling software.

Our program of instruction is geared to the times. We teach popular software, and we are constantly on the lookout for trends that will lead us to new markets.

According to reports from Comdex/Fall 1982 (the year's largest microcomputer show), software writers have switched from writing for the Apple to writing for the IBM-PC. (*Inc.,* March 1983). In a field of some 200 possible choices, the IBM-PC seems to be leading the way into the future. Our students train on the IBM.

Commentary: The Software School's Business Plan leaves no doubt that management is exploiting a market gap that is ignored by the competition — training people how to use popular software on the emerging industry leader, the IBM-PC. This is more than a matter of writing skill. Early on, the entrepreneurs who founded The Software School did the right research so they could make decisions ahead of time — just as you were asked to do in the earlier chapters.

How does it feel to have planned ahead?

D. Marketing Strategy

Action Step 61 gets you started on describing your marketing strategy. Need a reminder? Look back at your work in Chapter 6 — now you can make the most of it.

The following Marketing Strategy excerpt from The Software School's Business Plan demonstrates a carefully reasoned approach to every available form of marketing. The excerpt shows the importance of having conscious marketing policies so that your small business can retain a competitive edge. If you were reading a Business Plan where the writer did not demonstrate this careful and deliberate approach to marketing, how much faith would you have in the writer's business abilities?

As you read the excerpt, note that The Software School uses a three-pronged approach to reaching the public. This is one business that understands the importance of finding the right promotional mix.

ACTION ⚡ STEP 61

Describe Your Marketing Strategy

Now that you've profiled your Target Customer and assessed your competition, take some time to develop the thrust of your market strategy.

What techniques will you use to get the best and most cost-effective response?

Because a lot of consideration should be given to pricing, you might start with what your TC sees as a good value. Then develop your marketing mix.

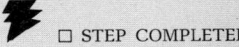 ☐ STEP COMPLETED

┌─ **Business Plan** ─┐

Marketing Strategy

An analysis of our competitors indicates that our price—$99 for a one-day course, $198 for a two-day course— is between two extremes.

Our price is competitive while it still maintains our image of quality. We're using a wide range of strategies to let our customers know where we are: **mass media advertising** (newspapers, television, and radio), special promotions (press releases, brochures, newsletter, etc.), and personal selling (commissioned sales people, networking, corporate contacts, trade shows, etc.).

1. Mass Media Advertising.

The Software School has been placing ads in the *LA Times* and in other local area newspapers to keep a continuous presence in front of our target customers. In the beginning, we used inducements (two-for-one, 15% reductions, etc.) but that is no longer necessary as our waiting lists grow.

As we continue to expand, we will develop advertising on radio and TV.

2. Creative Promotions/Ink/Free Ink.

In our first month of operation, we sponsored a scholarship contest in the local high schools, which resulted in some very positive press. In addition, the school has been featured in several of the local papers, and also in *Venture* magazine.

We are in the Information Business, and toward that end we are presently developing three different publications—a computer handbook, a newsletter, and a brief history of the founding of The Software School. In time, we hope that this history (a how-to for computer educators) will become a guide for the industry.

Our mailing list grows daily. We log all incoming calls with information on the callers and how they found out about us. This information helps us define our target market.

3. Personal Selling.

Personal contact has gained us our largest accounts so far. (Please refer to letters from computer retailers in Appendix 2.) We intend to intensify our efforts along these lines. Fortunately, our directors have experience and talent in the area of personal selling.

We maintain a booth at the major computer trade shows in the area, and approximately 17% of our hobbyist/home-user business comes from this source.

mass media advertising
reaching unselected hordes of people through print, sound, or visuals

Commentary: The writer lets you know how the entrepreneurs who run The Software School stay on top of the changing market picture:

1. They know when to drop two-for-one and other discount inducements from their continuous print campaign.

2. They are already looking ahead to radio and TV exposure.
3. They log all calls and gather information on the callers to maintain a base of up-to-date information on their target market.
4. They recognize how they have gained their largest accounts and they plan to intensify their efforts in that area.

E. Location

Action Step 62 leads you to the next part of your Business Plan, the subsection on location. Before tackling this Action Step, you may want to review your work in Chapter 7.

See how The Software School shows off its location to advantage.

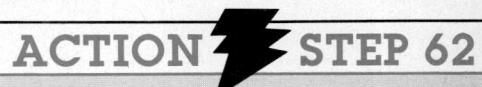

ACTION STEP 62

Show Off Your Location

The great thing about a location is that it's so *tangible.* A potential lender can visit your site and get a feel for what's going on.

A banker will often visit your business site. That's good news for you, because now the banker is on your turf.

Clean up the place before your banker arrives.

In this section, you want to persuade potential lenders to visit your site. Describe what goes on here. Use photographs and diagrams and illustrations to make it feel almost like home.

☐ STEP COMPLETED

Business Plan

Location

The Software School is currently in the first year of a three-year lease at 47 Turbo Drive, Newport Beach, California. The facility is all on the ground floor, and occupies 2100 square feet. The area, which is **zoned for business use,** is a hotbed of high-technology activity. Within the immediate area, there are two computer stores, one computer furniture store, one software dealer, an electronics store, and two printers, one of whom does typesetting work directly from software diskettes.

Within a 3–5 mile radius are 27 computer dealers.

During our lease negotiations, we persuaded the landlord to make extensive improvements in the interior, and to spread the cost out over the three-year term of the lease. The decor — blue carpet, white walls, orange furniture — gives the effect of a solid, logical, semi-plush business environment, where our target customer will be comfortable and learn fast.

The building is divided into: 1) reception area (300 square feet); 2) director's office (100 square feet); 3) classroom 1 (700 square feet); 4) lounge (200 square feet); and 5) storage area (800 square feet).

From the time of start-up, the principals had envisioned this area as a second classroom.

See diagram in Appendix 9.

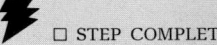

zoned for business use
property legally dedicated for applications of business use

Commentary: It's nice to paint an attractive picture of your business site, but at the same time, try to keep your reader interested by inspiring confidence in your choice. Location takes a tremendous amount of analysis. The writer gives himself a subtle pat on the back by describing the lease arrangements — upgrades by the landlord — and by identifying the need for a second classroom. If the reader needs more, he or she is referred to the Appendix. That's smart writing.

F. Management

The people at the top can make or break your small business. In almost every case, you are a member of the management team, and you want to use this Business Plan to inspire confidence in your team.

Writing this section will help you focus more closely on your management team members. Action Step 63 tells you how to introduce your team. (If you need a refresher, review your work in Chapter 13.)

Now let's see how The Software Shop introduces *its* management.

Business Plan

Management

Derek Campbell. Mr. Campbell was born in Shaker Heights, Ohio, in 19—. He took his B.S. degree in Industrial Engineering at Purdue University, then spent five years in the Marine Corps, where he was a flight instructor, a check pilot, and a maintenance officer. While in the service, Mr. Campbell completed an M.A. degree in Marketing, Management, and Human Relations.

Following military service, Mr. Campbell was employed as a pilot for United Airlines. He is currently the CEO of EuroSource, a software importing company.

Mr. Campbell is the author of several articles on computers and the Information Age.

He is listed in *Who's Who in California.*

Robert Jericho. Mr. Jericho was born in Dallas, Texas, in 19—. He took his B.S. degree in Geology and Physical Sciences at the University of Oklahoma, then served six years in the Marine Corps, where he was a flight instructor, flight operations officer, and schedules officer.

Following military service, Mr. Jericho was a pilot for Trans World Airlines.

He has completed training in the Nestar system managers course, the Apple computer maintenance course, and, for the last two years, has been working as an accountant and comptroller for EuroSource.

Business Plan

Directors

C. Hughes Smith. Mr. Smith was born in Corpus Christi, Texas, in 19—. He took his B.A. degree from Tulane University in Political Science and Philosophy, his M.A. degree in Business Administration from Stanford, and his Law degree from the University of Texas–Austin.

Mr. Smith is a Senior Vice President of Lowes and Lockwood, a residential home-building firm. He is a partner in Graebner and Ashe, a Houston law firm.

Mr. Smith is the author of numerous articles in the field of corporate planning and taxes. (Please see Personal Resumes in Appendix 4.)

Phil Carpenter. Mr. Carpenter was born in Duluth, Minnesota, in 19—. His B.A. degree is from the University of Kansas. His M.B.A., with a specialty in Marketing, is from the University of Wisconsin

Continued

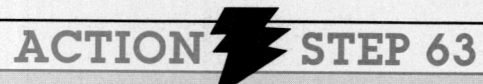

ACTION STEP 63

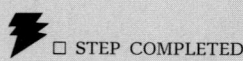

Introduce Your Management Team

Almost every study you read on small business failure puts the blame on management.

Use this section to highlight the positive qualities of your management team.

You want to focus on quality first—experience, accomplishments, education, training, flexibility, imagination, tenacity. Be sure you weave in experience that relates to your particular business.

Remember—dreamers make terrific master-builders, but they make lousy managers. Your banker knows this. Your potential investors will sense it. A great team can help you raise money.

The key to a great team is balance.

□ STEP COMPLETED

Mr. Carpenter spent 20 years in the corporate world (IBM, TRW, Inter-Comp, etc.), where he worked in marketing and industrial sales.

He is currently a Professor of Business at Huntington Beach Community College. Mr. Carpenter is the general partner in two going businesses, and is a small business consultant. He has written and lectured widely in the area of small business.

Dan Masters. Mr. Masters was born in Palo Alto, California, in 19—. His degrees (B.A., M.B.A.) are from Stanford, where he specialized in marketing and finance. Mr. Masters served his Army duty in Korea, where he worked on the United Nations Korean Civil Assistance Program, a long-term plan for making Korea economically independent. Following his military service, Mr. Masters was with Kodak and later with Sylvania (Senior Account Sales Executive, Sales Manager, etc.) for a total of 25 years.

Mr. Carpenter is currently Associate Professor of Business at San Juan Capistrano Institute of Business Science. He is active in several small businesses. He lectures widely on small business. He is the author of several articles in the field.

| Business Plan |

Other Available Resources

The Software School has retained the legal firm of Farney and Shields and the accounting firm of Hancock, Hancock, and Craig. Our insurance broker is Sharon Mandel, of Fireman's Fund. Our advertising agency is George Friend and Associates.

Commentary: This management team shows balance, diversity, experience (some interesting track records), the will to succeed, and, above all, a love of adventure. Robert Jericho and Derek Campbell were both flight instructors. Now they're using spage-age industrial training techniques in the computer classroom. In addition, pilots must plan and must take responsibility — good experience for running their own show.

Balance is important too, and this shows up in the short resumes. Jericho is the technician who handles systems management. Campbell is the marketeer and manager. Both have good people skills. Which do you suppose is the idea man?

Because The Software School is a corporation, it's smart to include directors of the corporation in the management subsection. In this case, the background of the directors completes the balancing of the team. All three directors have admirable depth in their business careers, with two of them sharing a combined 45 years of experience in the corporate world. Campbell very wisely uses his directors to assist him in the sales function.

The listing of the legal counsel and the insurance broker also adds to the impression of solid business practices. We know them as the ''taxi-squad.'' But in a Business Plan, where the language is more formal, they go by ''legal counsel'' and ''broker.''

G. Personnel

Action Step 64 gives you the chance to show off your personnel. For a start-up business, you're peering into the future with confidence, doing an informal job analysis for key employees who will help you succeed. For an ongoing business, you'll need to include people who are working for you now and what your personnel needs will be for the future. If you have five employees now, and you want to indicate growth, one easy way is to project how many jobs you'll be creating for the next five years.

When you start thinking about tasks and people to do them, it's handy to refer back to Chapter 13, where you worked with DISC and with finding the right person for the right job. This section on Personnel is important because it gives you one more chance to analyze job functions before you start interviews, hiring, and benefits—all of which are expensive.

You'll notice that The Software School gives a very brief rundown of its personnel situation.

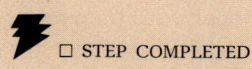

ACTION STEP 64

Introduce Your Personnel

Describe the kinds of people you need working for you and how they fit into your plan.

What skills will they need? How much will you have to pay them? Will there be a training period? How long? What fringe benefits will you offer? How will you handle overtime?

If you haven't written up job descriptions, now's a good time to do that. A job description will help you control the people who work for you.

☐ STEP COMPLETED

Business Plan

Personnel

At the end of six months of operation, The Software School has three full-time employees and 14 who are part-time.

The full-time employees are:

1. Manager, salaried at $2,000 per month.
2. Receptionist, salaried at $5 per hour.
3. Training Director, salaried at $1,500 per month.

The part-time employees include three directors, who assist in the marketing function, three outside commissioned sales people, and eight part-time instructors. According to our plan, one sales person is due to become full-time at the end of the seventh month.

We will continue to hold down overhead with part-time employees as long as it is feasible. We believe that a lean operation is one of the important parts of doing business.

Commentary: In describing their lean operation, the entrepreneurs who run The Software School keep their description lean as well. They show good sense when they express a commitment to hold down operating costs. Their decision underscores business discipline and foresight. If you were a potential investor in this business, wouldn't you appreciate some tight purse strings?

SECTION II: NUMBERS

Good Numbers

Section II, the ''financial'' section, is the heart of your Business Plan. This section is aimed at lenders — bankers, credit managers, venture capitalists, vendors, SBICs, commercial credit lenders — people who think in numbers. Lenders are professional. They are skeptics by trade, and they will not allow themselves to be swayed by your writing in Section I. Your job, therefore, is to let your numbers do the talking.

This is easier than you think.

You started jotting numbers down in Chapter 8, when you began thinking about money. You projected cash flow and income in Chapter 9. In Chapter 10, you tested your numbers on real lenders in the real world. Now, in Chapter 15, you're ready to organize your numbers into three standard instruments:

1. Projected income statement.
2. Projected cash flow statement (also called a ''pro forma'').
3. Projected balance sheet.

Model tables from The Software School follow. Use these models to set up your own financial categories. Create categories of your own, to fit your own business. You want to know where every nickel is going. You want to know when you'll make a profit. When you ask a lender for money, you want to appear neat, orderly, in control, and conservative. Would you want to lend money to a spendthrift?

You want to hear something like this from every skeptical lender who sees your Business Plan: ''You know, these numbers look good.''

Good Notes

One way to spot a professional lender is to hand over your Business Plan and then watch to see which section he or she reads first. Most lenders study the notes you have written to accompany income and cash flow projections. Knowing this allows you to be forewarned. Use these notes to tell potential lenders how you generated your numbers (''Advertising is projected at 5% of sales'') or what specific entries mean (''Leased Equipment — monthly costs on IBM microcomputers'').

Make these notes easy to read, with headings that start your readers off in the upper left hand corner and march them down the page, step-by-step, to the bottom line. (Some sample projection charts use tiny footnotes, on the same page. We prefer *large* notes, on a separate page. Notes are important, and they should be big.)

You spent time creating your Business Plan. You want lenders to read it, get excited, ask questions. These notes can help you accomplish that goal, even if you haven't started up and the numbers are projections into the future.

Good financial notes cap off a winning financial section for your Business Plan.

PROJECTED FINANCIAL STATEMENTS

H. Projected Income Statement

Your next Action Step has you put together your projected income statement (or profit and loss statement). With the information you've gathered so far, it shouldn't be too hard. In fact, Action Step 65 will be enjoyable — if the numbers look good.

The Software School's projected income statement is shown at Table 15.1, on pages 290–91. Your business structure may differ from The Software School's, but what shouldn't change is the careful documentation of each item with an appropriate note. For instance, if the professional lender wanted to see how figures for Commissions were generated in the projected statement, Note 6 would show that commissions average 10% of sales.

Business Plan

Notes for Projected Income Statement

1. **Instruction.** Based on 2.5% occupancy growth per month, starting at 35% (235 students) and growing to 60%. Students pay $99 per course.

2. **Books.** Revenue from books sold averages approximately 1% of instructional sales, rounded to bring total sales to an even $100 figure.

3. **Classroom Materials.** $7.50 per student.

4. **Instruction Personnel.** Instructor cost is $100 per 8 hour class, starting with 25 classes and growing to 30 classes by the end of the year.

5. **Books.** Cost of books is 70 percent of selling price.

6. **Commissions.** Average 10% of instructional sales.

7. **Advertising.** Projected at 5% of sales.

8. **Credit cards.** Approximately 50% of sales are paid with credit cards. The cost for charge cards is 2.5% of the sale.

9. **Salaries.** Start with 3 full-time employees. Bring on one additional person beginning the 10th month.

10. **Payroll Taxes.** The company's share of employee taxes averages 7% of commissions and salaries.

11. **Leased Equipment.** Monthly lease costs on IBM microcomputers.

12. **Licenses and Fees.** 10% of instruction sales paid for license (right to use copyrighted material).

13. **Accounting.** Average accounting and bookkeeping costs for the area and size of business.

14. **Rent.** Based on 3-year lease.

15. **Office Supplies.** Supplies equal .25% of sales.

16. **Dues and Subscriptions.** Estimated costs for magazines, newspapers, and organizations.

17. **Repair and Maintenance.** Projected to be 1% of sales.

Continued

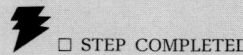

ACTION STEP 65

Project Your Income Statement

What you're driving at here is net profit. That's what's left in the kitty after you subtract expenses.

You figure your sales. Your first big bite is cost of goods sold. (In a service business, your big cost is labor.) That gives you a figure called gross margin.

Now you add up all your expenses (rent, utilities, insurance, etc.), then subtract that from gross margin.

You are almost now at a figure which is your net profit before taxes. (Businesses pay quarterly installments.) Subtract taxes.

You are now at net profit.

☐ STEP COMPLETED

18. **Insurance.** Based on current insurance contract for next 12 months, payable every 6 months.
19. **Telephone.** Figured at 1.5% of sales.
20. **Utilities.** Figured at 2% of sales.
21. **Depreciation.** Schedule established by accounting firm.
22. **Interest.** Loan at 13% with $5,000 payments due every 6 months until paid off.
23. **Miscellaneous.** Figured at 3% of sales.
24. **Reserve for Taxes.** State and federal taxes estimated at 20% of Net Profit.

I. Projected Cash Flow

Action Step 66 focuses all your attention on the projected cash flow. Remember, cash flow is the lifeblood of your business. By projecting cash flow figures out across the year, you get a month-by-month picture of just how healthy your business will be.

The Software School's cash flow projection is set out at Table 15.2 (pages 292–293). Notes for these numbers follow. If you quickly compare the projected income statement at Table 15.1 with the cash flow projection at Table 15.2, you will see that the same items are sometimes treated differently in each table. For example, expenses in the projected income statement are divided in monthly installments, but the same expenses in the cash flow projection are shown as bulk payments when due. Let's look at insurance expense. In the projected income statement we find a total expense of $960 shown as twelve monthly debits of $80 each. The same expense in the cash flow projection is shown as two payments of $480 each, falling due in the seventh and thirteenth months. If the entrepreneurs running the business had only $80 available to pay for insurance in the seventh month—because that is what is shown in the income statement—they would be in trouble.

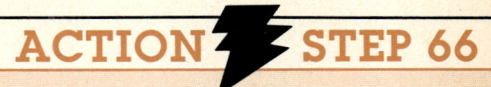

ACTION STEP 66

Project Your Cash Flow

Get used to doing cash flow. Once a month is not too often. If you prepared a cash flow for your business back in Chapter 9, bring those numbers forward. If you skipped that step, try it now.

Your banker will look here first.

1. Write down all the cash you will have for one year.
2. Add net profit.
3. Add any loans.
4. Figure your total cash needs for the year.
5. Spread these numbers out across the year. You may have a lot of cash at the start of the year. You want to make sure you have enough to get all the way through.
6. Now list all disbursements. Spread these out, too.
7. Now examine the figures. Is there any time during the year when you will run short of cash? It's better to know the truth now, when you're still working on paper.
8. If your cash picture looks good, drop in a couple of what-ifs. (Let's say you've budgeted $300 for utilities and an air conditioner goes out and it costs $200 to repair and the lease says it is your expense. Or let's say you see an opportunity for a sale, only you have to hire someone to handle it for you. Can your cash flow handle these surprises?)

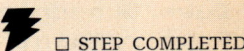 ☐ STEP COMPLETED

Business Plan

Notes for Cash Flow Projection

1. **Beginning of the Month.** Cash available as the month begins.
2. **Sales.** Includes all sales paid by cash, by check, or by credit card at the time the class is taken. Does not include accounts receivable.
3. **Credit Card Expense.** Fees of 2.5% paid to credit card companies. Approximately 50% of customers use charge cards.
4. **Loans.** Loan for new course development and audio-visual equiment.
5. **Total Cash Available.** Sum of all money available during the month.

Continued on page 294.

TABLE 15.1 The Software School's projected income statement shows profit and loss.

INCOME STATEMENT/SOFTWARE SCHOOL

	7th Month	8th Month	9th Month	10th Month	11th Month	12th Month
SALES						
Instruction	23285	24950	26630	28215	29900	31580
Books	215	250	270	285	300	320
TOTAL SALES	23500	25200	26900	28500	30200	31900
Cost of Instr/						
Clssrm Matrls	1765	1890	2020	2140	2265	2395
Inst/Personnel	2500	2500	2600	2600	2700	2700
Books	150	175	190	200	210	225
TOTAL COST/						
INSTR/BOOKS	4415	4565	4810	4940	5175	5320
GROSS PROFIT	19085	20635	22090	23560	25025	26580
EXPENSES						
SALES:						
Commissions	2330	2495	2665	2820	2990	3160
Advertising	1175	1250	1335	1410	1495	1580
Credit Cards	295	315	335	355	380	400
ADMINISTRATIVE:						
Salaries	3300	3300	3300	4500	4500	4500
Payroll taxes	570	580	600	695	715	725
Leased Equip	1270	1270	1270	1270	1270	1270
Licenses/fees	2330	2495	2665	2820	2990	3160
Accounting	500	500	500	500	500	500
Rent	3890	3890	3890	3890	3890	3890
Office Suppl	60	65	65	70	75	80
Dues/Subscrip	20	20	20	20	20	20
Repair/Maint	235	250	265	285	300	320
Insurance	80	80	80	80	80	80
Telephone	355	380	405	430	455	480
Utilities	470	505	540	570	605	640
Depreciation	1170	1170	1170	1335	1335	1335
Interest				650	650	650
Miscellaneous	705	755	805	855	905	955
TOTAL EXPENSES	18755	19320	19910	22555	23155	23745
NET PROFIT	330	1315	2180	1005	1870	2835
Reserve for taxes	65	265	435	200	375	565
NET PROFIT AFTER TAXES	265	1050	1745	805	1495	2270

INCOME STATEMENT/SOFTWARE SCHOOL

	13th Month	14th Month	15th Month	16th Month	17th Month	18th Month	TOTAL
SALES							
Instruction	33265	34945	37915	39600	42770	42770	395825
Books	335	355	435	500	530	530	4325
TOTAL SALES	33600	35300	38350	40100	43300	43300	400150
Cost of Instr/							
Clssrm Matrls	2520	2650	2875	3000	3240	3240	30000
Inst/Personnel	2800	2800	2900	2900	3000	3000	33000
Books	235	250	305	350	370	370	3030
TOTAL COST/ INSTR/BOOKS	5555	5700	6080	6250	6610	6610	66030
GROSS PROFIT	28045	29600	32270	33850	36690	36690	334120
EXPENSES							
SALES:							
Commissions	3325	3495	3790	3960	4275	4275	39580
Advertising	1660	1750	1895	1980	2135	2135	19800
Credit Cards	420	440	480	500	540	540	5000
ADMINISTRATIVE:							
Salaries	4500	4500	4500	4500	4500	4500	50400
Payroll taxes	745	755	785	795	825	825	8165
Leased Equip	1270	1270	1270	1270	1270	1270	15240
Licenses/fees	3325	3495	3790	3960	4275	4275	39580
Accounting	500	500	500	500	500	500	6000
Rent	3890	3890	3890	3890	3890	3890	46680
Office Suppl	85	90	95	100	110	110	1005
Dues/Subscrip	200	20	20	20	20	20	420
Repair/Maint	335	355	385	395	435	435	3995
Insurance	80	80	80	80	80	80	960
Telephone	505	530	575	600	650	650	6015
Utilities	670	705	765	800	865	865	8000
Depreciation	1335	1335	1335	1335	1335	1335	15525
Interest	650	650	650	595	595	595	5685
Miscellaneous	1010	1060	1150	1205	1300	1300	12005
TOTAL EXPENSES	24505	24920	25955	26485	27600	27600	284505
NET PROFIT	3540	4680	6315	7365	9090	9090	49615
Reserve for taxes	710	935	1265	1475	1820	1820	9930
NET PROFIT AFTER TAXES	2830	3745	5050	5890	7270	7270	39685

TABLE 15.2 The Software School's cash flow projection gives a monthly picture of the company's financial health.

CASH FLOW/SOFTWARE SCHOOL

	7th Month	8th Month	9th Month	10th Month	11th Month	12th Month
CASH—RECEIPTS						
Beginning of month	3970	7365	6015	51575	47060	35275
Sales	23500	25200	26900	28500	30200	31900
Less: credit card expense	(295)	(315)	(335)	(355)	(380)	(400)
Loan			60000			
TOTAL CASH AVAIL	27175	32250	92580	79720	76880	66775
DISBURSEMENTS						
Books	175	190	200	210	225	235
Instr/Materials		6000			7500	
Salaries:						
Instruction	2000	2000	2040	2080	2120	2160
Admnstrtn	2640	2640	2640	3120	3600	3600
Commissions	1730	1865	1995	2130	2255	2390
Payroll taxes	2045	2195	2250	2435	2690	2755
Advertising	1080	1175	1250	1335	1410	1495
Leased Equip	1270	1270	1270	1270	1270	1270
Licenses/fees	2160	2330	2495	2665	2820	2990
Legal/Accntng	500	500	500	500	500	500
Rent	3890	3890	3890	3890	3890	3890
Office Suppl	60	65	65	70	75	80
Dues/Subscrip	20	20	20	20	20	20
Repair/Maint	235	250	265	285	300	320
Insurance	480					
Telephone	325	355	380	405	430	455
Utilities	430	470	505	540	570	605
Interest				650	650	650
Loan Payback						
Miscellaneous	705	755	805	855	905	955
Income Tax Rsrv	65	265	435	200	375	565
TOTAL DISRSMNTS	19810	26235	21005	22660	31605	24935
Net Cash Before Capital Investment	7365	6015	71575	57060	45275	41840
Capital Equip			10000			
Contracted Crs Development			10000	10000	10000	10000
MONTHLY CASH FLOW	7365	6015	51575	47060	35275	31840

CASH FLOW/SOFTWARE SCHOOL

	13th Month	14th Month	15th Month	16th Month	17th Month	18th Month	TOTAL
CASH–RECEIPTS							
Beginning of month	31840	28645	27900	33115	43895	47800	364455
Sales	33600	35300	38350	40100	43300	43300	400150
Less: credit card expense	(420)	(440)	(480)	(500)	(540)	(540)	(5000)
Loan							60000
TOTAL CASH AVAIL	65020	63505	65770	72715	86655	90560	819605
DISBURSEMENTS							
Books	250	305	350	370	370	385	3265
Instr/Materials		9000			9000		31500
Salaries:							
Instruction	2200	2240	2280	2320	2360	2360	26160
Admnstrtn	3600	3600	3600	3600	3600	3600	39840
Commissions	2530	2660	2795	3030	3170	3420	29970
Payroll taxes	2805	2870	2925	3025	3075	3170	32240
Advertising	1580	1660	1750	1895	1980	2135	18745
Leased Equip	1270	1270	1270	1270	1270	1270	15240
Licenses/fees	3160	3325	3495	3790	3960	4275	37465
Legal/Accntng	500	500	500	500	500	500	6000
Rent	3890	3890	3890	3890	3890	3890	46680
Office Suppl	85	90	95	100	110	110	1005
Dues/Subscrip	200	20	20	20	20	20	420
Repair/Maint	335	355	385	395	435	435	3995
Insurance	480						960
Telephone	480	505	530	575	600	650	5690
Utilities	640	670	705	765	800	865	7565
Interest	650	650	650	595	595	595	5685
Loan Payback			5000				5000
Miscellaneous	1010	1060	1150	1205	1300	1300	12005
Income Tax Rsrv	710	935	1265	1475	1820	1820	9930
TOTAL DISRSMNTS	26375	35605	32655	28820	38855	30800	339360
Net Cash Before Capital Investment	38645	27900	33115	43895	47800	59760	480245
Capital Equip							10000
Contracted Crs Development	10000						50000
MONTHLY CASH FLOW	28645	27900	33115	43895	47800	59760	420245

6. **Books.** Books for sale are ordered and paid for one month in advance of projected sale.

7. **Instructional Materials.** Covers course materials purchased from licenser.

8. **Salaries.** Net salaries paid employees approximate 80% of gross salaries paid.

9. **Payroll Taxes.** Total of what was withheld from employees, plus payroll tax item on Income Statement.

10. **Advertising.** Established as 30-day accounts with all media companies where ads are placed.

11. **Leased Equipment.** Lease payments are due the first of each month.

12. **Licenses and Fees.** License fees are due the 15th of the following month.

13. **Legal and Accounting.** Due 30 days after bill is received.

14. **Rent.** Due at the first of each month.

15. **Office Supplies.** Paid at time of purchase or with subscription. No credit.

16. **Insurance.** Paid every 6 months in advance.

17. **Telephone and Utilities.** Paid within 30 days of receipt of bill.

18. **Interest.** Interest only, paid each month.

19. **Loan Payback.** $5,000 loan payment due every 6 months.

20. **Miscellaneous.** Paid in month expense occurs.

21. **Income Tax Reserve.** Paid into a special tax account at the bank.

22. **Total Disbursements.** Total cash expended during the month.

23. **Net Cash Before Capital Investment.** Cash balance before capital investment payments.

24. **Capital Equipment.** Purchase of additional audio-visual equipment.

25. **Contracted Course Development.** Contract payments due for new course development.

26. **Monthly Cash Flow** Cash balance after all payments at the end of the month.

J. Projected Balance Sheet

The professionals will look at your balance sheet (sometimes it's called a statement of financial position) to analyze the state of your finances at a given point in time. They are looking at things like liquidity (how easily your assets can be converted into hard cash) and capital structure (what sources of financing have been used, how much was borrowed, and so on). Professional lenders use such factors to evaluate your ability to manage your own business.

Action Step 67 gets you to project a balance sheet for your business. The sample in Table 15.3 (opposite page), shows the balance sheet at the end of the first six months of operation. These are projected figures. If you're just starting up, *all* figures will be projected. Action Step 67 refers to ROI, return on investment. ROI is a bottom-line figure which shows how much is earned on the total dollars invested in the business.

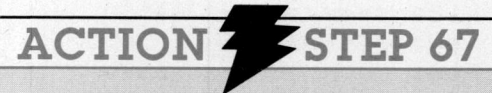

ACTION STEP 67

Project Your Balance Sheet

With a projected balance sheet, you are trying to predict, on paper, what your business will be worth at the end of a certain period of time. You also want to show your potential investors some good news about ROI.

1. Add up your assets. For convenience, divide these up into Current (cash, notes receivables, etc.), Fixed (land, equipment, buildings, etc.), and Other (intangibles like patents, royalty deals, copyrights, Goodwill, contracts for exclusive use, etc.). You'll need to depreciate fixed assets that wear out. As value, you show the net of cost minus the accumulated depreciation.

2. Add up your liabilities. For convenience, divide these into Current (accounts payable, notes payable, accrued expenses, interest on loans, etc.), and Long Term (trust deeds, bank loans, equipment loans, balloons, etc.).

3. Subtract the smaller figure from the larger. You now have a figure for your net worth.

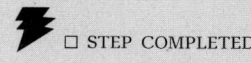 ☐ STEP COMPLETED

TABLE 15.2   The Software School's balance sheets show where the company is at the end of its first six months and where it will be at the end of its first 18 months.

	ACTUAL BALANCE SHEET/ SOFTWARE SCHOOL AS OF SEPTEMBER 30, 19XX (AFTER FIRST 6 MONTHS)			PROJECTED BALANCE SHEET/ SOFTWARE SCHOOL AS OF SEPTEMBER 30, 19XX (AFTER FIRST 18 MONTHS)		
ASSETS						
Cash	3970			59670		
Inst Mat & Bks	2500			4495		
TOTAL CORRECT			6470			64165
Lshld Imprvmnts	41000			41000		
Furniture	15100			15100		
Audio/Visual	10600			20600		
Office Equip	3600	70300		3600	80300	
Less Dep		7020	63280		22545	57755
License Agrmnt			25000	25000		
New Courses				50000		75000
TOTAL ASSETS			94750			196920
LIABILITIES						
Inst Salaries	1250			1500		
Admin "	1650			2250		
Commissions	2165			4275		
Accnts Payable	4495			9020		
Crrnt Lbltls		9560			17045	
Long Term Debt		-0-			55000	
Total Liabilities			9560			72045
NET WORTH						
Capital Stock	100000			100000		
Retained Earnings	(14810)		85190	24875		124875
TOTAL LIAB & NET WORTH			94750			196920

You have the same kind of information if you are a high roller and you invest money in bonds. The interest tells you your return on investment. If you had two funds, Bond A and Bond B, and Bond A paid you a 4% return and Bond B paid you 25%, which would have the better ROI?

You can compute ROI for a business by dividing net profit by investment dollars. For The Software School, take the profit from Table 15.1 (after taxes, it's $39,685) and divide by the owner's investment of $100,000 (from Table 15.3).

$$\frac{\$39,685}{\$100,000} = 39.7\%$$

Could you get 39.7% from a savings account or a bond fund? That's not a bad ROI. It would dazzle your lenders and probably get your business an appointment with a venture capitalist.

The Software School did not provide notes to its balance sheets, because in this case no notes are needed. In conjunction with the income statement and the cash flow projection, all the entries in the balance sheet will make sense to your professional readers. Under some circumstances, you would want to note unusual features of a balance sheet for an actual fiscal year, but in most cases—and in most projections—this won't be necessary.

PUTTING YOUR BUSINESS PLAN TO WORK

Well, do you feel like you're ready? You are. You have thoroughly researched your product or your service, your market and your Target Customer, your competition, your marketing strategy, and your location. You've discovered how to prepare for surprises you can't afford, how to handle numbers, how to pursue financing, when and why you should incorporate, how to build a winning team, and whether you should buy, franchise, or start on your own. You've surveyed the vistas that a small business computer can open up for you. And you've written it all up in a beautiful showcase: your winning Business Plan.

Before you're off and running, we have one last Action Step for you in a special Epilogue (see page 299). It tells you about a tool we think every entrepreneur should have—a tool to help you put your Business Plan to work.

SUMMARY

The long road is over, and you're ready to create your Business Plan. The Business Plan is a portable showcase for your business. When you visit vendors or bankers or potential lenders, you can take along a copy of your Business Plan to speak for you, to show the world you've got a blueprint for success.

Begin writing by starting with the material you feel most comfortable with. Once you have finished one section of the Plan, the other sections will fall into place more easily. Fortunately, your work in earlier chapters has prepared you for each section.

You'll probably write a cover letter for each copy of the Plan you send out. The cover letter personalizes the Plan and aims it so that it does the most good.

THINK POINTS

- Your Marketing and Management Section is the lure you use to get readers reading your Business Plan. Your Financial Section is the hook. Make sure you explain everything in the Financial Section with footnotes.
- Now that you have Plan A, have you thought about Plan B?

ACTION STEP REVIEW

57 With this Action Step you write the cover letter that acts as a mini-summary of your Business Plan and that opens the door for future business transactions.

58 Here, you describe your product or service against the backdrop of industry. You want to excite your reader without being flamboyant.

59 Using material gathered for your industry chronology (Action Step 13), you set the marketing background for your business. You lay out the boundaries of your Target Market; you also profile your Target Customer.

60 Here you list major competitors and how you will disarm them.

61 In this Action Step you describe your promotional strategies. What techniques will best serve your small business?

62 In discussing your site, emphasize how it will contribute to your success.

63 Brief biographies will best introduce your management team. In your Appendix, you can include more information. What you're trying to depict here, in a half page or so, is a great management track record in your industry.

64 In this Action Step you describe the kinds of people you need working for you. Emphasize the fact that you'll run lean.

65 Of the three financial statements in your Plan, you need to do the income statement first, so you'll have an idea about net profit for your first year—and then for the next three, if possible.

66 Cash flow tells you when you're going to need money. It's a handy tool, and it is the second financial statement you need.

67 Here, you show your potential investors and lenders what they can expect for an ROI. This financial statement completes the financial section of your Plan.

REFERENCES

Bangs, David J., and William R. Osgood. *Business Planning Guide.* Portsmouth, N.H.: Upstart Publishing Co., 1981. An excellent handbook for structuring a Business Plan. Clear writing, humorous examples. Their model business is Finestkind, a retail fish market located in York, Maine. Copies of the book can be ordered from Upstart Publishing Co., Portsmouth, NH, 03801.

Bank of America Marketing Publications Department. *Financing Small Business.* Small Business Reporter Series. San Francisco: Bank of America, 1980. A nicely detailed publication of the SBR Series, complete with a model Business Plan for Rainbow Liquors, a retail liquor store located in San Francisco. This particular model focuses on a husband-and-wife team named Cho, and the writers of the booklet list several government agencies that deal specifically with minority businesses. This booklet is worth a read. Available at a local Bank of America office or by writing SBR Series, Bank of America, Department 3120, P.O. Box 37000, San Francisco, CA, 94137.

TABLE A This is a sample PERT chart. Yours will need to be bigger and more detailed. You can use days, weeks, or months to plot the tasks ahead. (If you use years, reassess your industry.)

The Software School Marketing Plan						
Job Description	Week 1	Week 2	Week 3	Week 4	Week 5	Week 6
Befriend banker	x	x	x	x	x	x
Order letterhead		x				
Select site	x					
Get FNS (fictional name statement)	x					
Bulk mail payment			x			
Ad agency	x					
Lunch, lawyer			x			
Appointment, accountant				x		
Vendor statement					x	
Utility deposit						x
Review promotional material					x	
Survey phone system			x	x	x	
Order phone system						x
Open house						x

Epilogue
It's Time to Act on What You Know

Congratulations.

You have made it through 67 Action Steps. You have survived enough research to choke two IBM mainframes. You're on the brink of action. Now it's time to act.

Action Step 68 gives you a tool for planning your actions. It's called PERT, which is an acronym for Program Evaluation and Review Technique, and it's often used to establish schedules for large projects. Its use was pioneered in military research and development (maybe you heard about it in connection with the Polaris program for submarine-launched ballistics missiles). But it is such a useful tool—it lets you identify activities and their optimal sequence, and monitor their progress—that PERT was soon adapted by the aerospace industry, the construction industry, and other businesses that must plan complicated projects.

Beyond a planning tool, a PERT chart is like an extended Action Step. It's just the thing if you feel overwhelmed by the tasks in getting started up, and don't know where to begin; if you're a fast-track entrepreneur who can't wait to start doing everything at once, PERT is also recommended. It will make your scattered energies more effective by focusing them on the right job at the right time. A sample PERT chart is provided in Table A.

Are you ready?

On your mark, *get set*, GO!

What I hear, I forget.
What I see, I remember.
What I do, I understand.
— Old Entrepreneur's Proverb

ACTION ⚡ STEP 68

Construct Your Own PERT Chart and Go for It

You can plan your ears off, and that is what we have asked you to do. Rehearsal is over. Now you've got to step onto the stage and get the drama underway. You've got to move off the sidelines onto the playing field.

One way to shift from planning into action is to develop your own personal PERT chart. A PERT chart gives you timelines on when you should be taking action. It also tells you and the other members of your team how long certain jobs should take. Since it is yours, you fill it with whatever items your business needs: befriending a banker, choosing your fictitious name statement, taking a lawyer to lunch, ordering business letterheads, selecting a site, or contacting vendors—and attach deadlines.

As you already know, a successful package is made up of endless details. If you take the details one at a time, you'll get there without being overwhelmed.

For a model PERT chart, please see Table A.

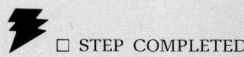 ☐ STEP COMPLETED

Appendix A:
A Test for Self-Starters

This self-administered test will indicate whether you have what it takes to run your own business.

Under each question, check the answer that says what you feel or comes closest to it. Be honest with yourself.

Are you a self-starter?

☑ I do things on my own. Nobody has to tell me to get going.

☐ If someone gets me started, I keep going all right.

☐ Easy does it. I don't put myself out until I have to.

How do you feel about other people?

☑ I like people. I can get along with just about anybody.

☐ I have plenty of friends — I don't need anyone else.

☐ Most people irritate me.

Can you lead others?

☑ I can get most people to go along when I start something.

☐ I can give the orders if someone tells me what we should do.

☐ I let someone else get things moving. Then I go along if I feel like it.

Can you take responsibility?

☑ I like to take charge of things and see them through.

☐ I'll take over if I have to, but I'd rather let someone else be responsible.

☐ There's always some eager beaver around wanting to show how smart he is. I say let him.

How good an organizer are you?

☑ I like to have a plan before I start. I'm usually the one to get things lined up when the group wants to do something.

☐ I do all right unless things get too confused. Then I quit.

☐ You get all set and then something comes along and presents too many problems. So I just take things as they come.

How good a worker are you?

☑ I can keep going as long as I need to. I don't mind working hard for something I want.

☐ I'll work hard for a while, but when I've had enough, that's it.

☐ I can't see that hard work gets you anywhere.

Can you make decisions?

☑ I can make up my mind in a hurry if I have to. It usually turns out O.K., too.

☐ I can if I have plenty of time. If I have to make up my mind fast, I think later I should have decided the other way.

☐ I don't like to be the one who has to decide things.

Can people trust what you say?

☐ You bet they can. I don't say things I don't mean.

☑ I try to be on the level most of the time, but sometimes I just say what's easiest.

☐ Why bother if the other fellow doesn't know the difference?

Can you stick with it?

☑ If I make up my mind to do something, I don't let *anything* stop me.

☐ I usually finish what I start—if it goes well.

☐ If it doesn't go [well] right away, I quit. Why beat your brains out?

How good is your health?

☐ I *never* run down!

☑ I have enough energy for most things I want to do.

☐ I run out of energy sooner than most of my friends seem to.

Now count the checks you made.

How many checks are there beside the *first* answer to each question?　　*6*

How many checks are there beside the *second* answer to each question?　　*2*

How many checks are there beside the *third* answer to each question?　　*0*

If most of your checks are beside the first answers, you probably have what it takes to run a business. If not, you're likely to have more trouble than you can handle by yourself. Better find a partner who is strong on the points you're weak on. If many checks are beside the third answer, not even a good partner will be able to shore you up.

SOURCE: Small Business Administration, *Checklist for Going into Business,* SBA Marketers Aid 71 (Washington, D.C.: Small Business Administration, 1977).

Appendix B:
Field Offices of the Small Business Administration

The Small Business Administration is closer than Washington, D.C.
The following list provides the addresses of many SBA field offices.

(RA: Regional Administrator; DD: District Director; BM: Branch Manager; OIC: Officer-in-Charge)

Region	Officer-in-Charge	Address
I Boston, Mass. 02110	James H. Angevine, RA	60 Batterymarch St.
Boston, Mass. 02114	John McNally, DD	150 Causeway St.
Springfield, Mass. 01101	Vincent Mineo, OIC	302 High St.
Augusta, Maine 04330	Thomas McGillicuddy, DD	40 Western Ave.
Concord, N.H. 03301	Bert F. Teague, DD	55 Pleasant St.
Hartford, Conn. 06106	(Vacancy) DD	1 Hartford Sq. W.
Montpelier, Vt. 05602	David Emery, DD	87 State St.
Providence, R.I. 02903	Jim Hauge, DD	40 Fountain St.
II New York, N.Y. 10278	Peter P. Neglia, RA	26 Federal Plaza
New York, N.Y. 10278	Harry Tishelman, DD	26 Federal Plaza
Melville, N.Y. 11747	Walter Leavitt, BM	35 Pinelawn Rd.
Hato Rey, P.R. 00919	Wilfred Benitez-Robles, DD	Carlos Chardon Ave.
St. Thomas, V.I. 00801	Lionel G. Baptiste, OIC	Veterans Dr.
Newark, N.J. 07102	Andrew Lynch, DD	970 Broad St.
Camden, N.J. 08104	Joseph T. Fernicola, OIC	1800 E. Davis St.
Syracuse, N.Y. 13260	J. Wilson Harrison, DD	100 S. Clinton St.
Buffalo, N.Y. 14202	Franklin J. Sciortino, BM	111 W. Huron St.
Elmira, N.Y. 14901	James Cristofaro, BM	180 Clemens Center Pkwy.
Albany, N.Y. 12207	Daniel S. O'Connell, OIC	445 Broadway
Rochester, N.Y. 14614	F. Peter Flihan, OIC	100 State St.
III Philadelphia, Pa. 19004	Peter Terpeluk, Jr., RA	231 St. Asaphs Rd., Bala Cynwyd
Philadelphia, Pa. 19004	William Gennetti, DD	231 St. Asaphs Rd., Bala Cynwyd
Harrisburg, Pa. 17101	Kenneth Olson, BM	100 Chestnut St.
Wilkes-Barre, Pa. 18701	John Sokolowski, BM	20 N. Penn Ave.
Wilmington, Del. 19801	John Williams, BM	844 Kind St.
Baltimore, Md. 21204	J. Arnold Feldman, DD	8600 LaSalle Rd., Towson
Clarksburg, W. Va. 26301	Marvin Shelton, DD	109 N. 3d St.
Charleston, W. Va. 25301	Edward Zimmerman, BM	Charleston National Plaza
Pittsburgh, Pa. 15222	Joseph Kopp, DD	960 Penn Ave.
Richmond, Va. 23240	M. Hawley Smith, DD	400 N. 8th St.
Washington, D.C. 20417	Bernard Layne, DD	1111 18th St. NW.

(RA: Regional Administrator; DD: District Director; BM: Branch Manager; OIC: Officer-in-Charge)

Region	Officer-in-Charge	Address
IV Atlanta, Ga. 30367	Miller A. Widemire, RA	1375 Peachtree St.
Atlanta, Ga. 30309	Clarence Barnes, DD	1720 Peachtree Rd.
Statesboro, Ga. 30458	Charles F. Henderson, OIC	127 N. Main St.
Birmingham, Ala. 35205	James Barksdale, DD	908 S. 20th St.
Charlotte, N.C. 28202	Larry Cherry, DD	230 S. Tryon St.
Greenville, N.C. 27834	Michael J. O'Callaghan, OIC	215 S. Evans St.
Columbia, S.C. 29201	Johne Patrick, DD	1835 Assembly St.
Jackson, Miss. 39201	(Vacancy) DD	100 W. Capital St.
Biloxi, Mass. 39530	D. Mike Shelton, BM	111 Fred Haise Blvd.
Jacksonville, Fla. 32202	Douglas E. McAllister, DD	400 W. Bay St.
Louisville, Ky. 40201	Billy Wells, DD	600 Federal Place
Miami, Fla. 33134	John L. Carey, DD	2222 Ponce de Leon Blvd.
Tampa, Fla. 33602	John W. Francis, OIC	700 Twigs St.
West Palm Beach, Fla. 33401	Roger Cosper, OIC	100 S. Narcissus St.
Nashville, Tenn. 37219	Robert M. Hartman, OIC	404 James Robertson Pkwy.
Knoxville,Tenn. 37902	(Vacancy) OIC	502 S. Gay St.
Memphis, Tenn. 38103	Richard A. Castilon, BM	167 N. Main St.
V Chicago, Ill. 60604	Richard D. Durkin, RA	219 S. Dearborn St.
Chicago, Ill. 60604	John L. Smith, DD	219 S. Dearborn St.
Springfield, Ill. 62701	Phil Ramos	4 North, Old State Capitol Plaza
Cleveland, Ohio 44199	S. Charles Hemming, Jr., DD	1240 E. 9th St.
Columbus, Ohio 43215	Frank Ray, DD	85 Marconi Blvd.
Cincinnati, Ohio 45202	Cecil G. Boatright, BM	550 Main St.
Detroit, Mich. 48226	Raymond Harshman, DD	477 Michigan Ave.
Marquette, Mich. 49855	(Vacancy) BM	220 W. Washington St.
Indianapolis, Ind. 46204	Robert General, DD	575 N. Pennsylvania St.
South Bend, Ind. 46601	(Vacancy) BM	501 E. Monroe St.
Madison, Wis. 53703	Curtis Charter, DD	212 E. Washington Ave.
Eau Claire, Wis. 54701	(Vacancy) OIC	500 S. Barstow St.
Milwaukee, Wis. 53202	Anthony J. McMahon, BM	517 E. Wisconsin Ave.
Minneapolis, Minn. 55403	Gelso C. Moreno, DD	100 N. 6th St.
VI Dallas, Tex. 75235	Reynaldo H. Lopez, RA	1720 Regal Row
Dallas, Tex. 75242	James S. Reed, DD	1100 Commerce St.
Marshall, Tex. 75670	George Lewis, OIC	100 S. Washington St.
Fort Worth, Tex. 76102	(Vacancy) BM	221 W. Lancaster
Albuquerque, N. Mex. 87110	(Vacancy) DD	5000 Marble Ave. NE.
Houston, Tex. 77054	Donald Grose, DD	2525 Murworth St.
Little Rock, Ark. 72201	Maurice Britt, DD	320 W. Capital Ave.
Lubbock, Tex. 79401	Philip O'Jibway, DD	1205 Texas Ave.
El Paso, Tex. 79902	Dick Valdez, BM	4100 Rio Bravo
Harlingen, Tex. 78550	Rodney Martin, DD	222 E. Van Buren St.
Corpus Christi, Tex. 78408	Miguel Cavazos, BM	3105 Leopard St.
New Orleans, La. 70113	Talon Aboussie, DD	1001 Howard Ave.
Shreveport, La. 71101	Jerry Tanner, DD	500 Fannin St.
Oklahoma City, Okla. 73102	Robert Ball, DD	200 NW. 5th St.
Tulsa, Okla. 74103	(Vacancy) OIC	333 W. Fourth St.
San Antonio, Tex. 78206	Julio Perez, DD	727 E. Durango Blvd.
Austin, Tex. 78701	Stan Rutland, OIC	300 E. 8th St.
VII Kansas City, Mo. 64106	William A. Powell, RA	911 Walnut St.
Kansas City, Mo. 64106	Patrick Smythe, DD	1150 Grande Ave.
Springfield, Mo. 65806	Shelby Slaughter, BM	309 N. Jefferson St.
Cape Girardeau, Mo. 63801	Jerry Martin, OIC	731A N. Main St.
Cedar Rapids, Iowa 52402	Ralph Potter, DD	373 Collins Rd. NE.
Des Moines, Iowa 50309	Conrad Lawlor, DD	210 Walnut St.
Omaha, Nebr. 68102	Rick Budd, DD	19th and Farnum St.
St. Louis, Mo. 63101	Robert Andrews, DD	815 Olive St.
Wichita, Kans. 67202	Clayton Hunter, DD	110 E. Waterman St.
VIII Denver, Colo. 80202	Carlos R. Suarez, RA	1405 Curtis St.
Denver, Colo. 80202	Doug Graves, DD	721 19th St.
Casper, Wyo. 82601	Paul Nemetz, DD	100 E. B St.
Fargo, N. Dak. 58102	Robert Pinkerton, DD	657 2d Ave.
Helena, Mont. 59601	John Cronholm, DD	301 S. Park Ave.
Salt Lake City, Utah 84138	Kent Moon, DD	125 S. State St.
Sioux Falls, S. Dak. 57102	Chester Leedom, DD	101 S. Maine Ave.

(RA: Regional Administrator; DD: District Director; BM: Branch Manager; OIC: Officer-in-Charge)

Region	Officer-in-Charge	Address
IX San Francisco, Calif. 94102	Irenemaree Castillo, RA	450 Golden Gate Ave.
San Francisco, Calif. 94105	(Vacancy) DD	211 Main St.
Fresno, Calif. 93721	Peter Bergin, DD	2202 Monterey St.
Sacramento, Calif. 95814	Walter W. Hill, OIC	660 J St.
Las Vegas, Nev. 89101	Robert Garrett, DD	301 E. Stewart
Reno, Nev. 89505	Robert L. Davis, OIC	50 S. Virginia St.
Honolulu, Hawaii 96850	David Nakagawa, DD	300 Ala Mona
Agana, Guam 96910	Jose M. L. Lujan, BM	Pacific Daily News Bldg.
Los Angeles, Calif. 90071	Gerald Morita, DD	350 S. Figueroa St.
Santa Ana, Calif. 92701	John S. Waddell, BM	2700 N. Main St.
Phoenix, Ariz. 85012	Walter Fronstin, DD	3030 N. Central Ave.
Tucson, Ariz. 85701	Richard A. Schulze, OIC	301 W. Congress St.
San Diego, Calif. 92188	George Chandler, DD	880 Front St.
X Seattle, Wash. 98104	Stephen Hall, RA	710 2d Ave.
Seattle, Wash. 98174	Maxine Wood, DD	915 2d Ave.
Anchorage, Alaska 99513	Frank Cox, DD	701 C St.
Fairbanks, Alaska 99701	Sprague Carter, BM	101 12th Ave.
Boise, Idaho 83702	Verne Leighton, DD	1005 Main St.
Portland, Oreg. 97204	Stewart Rollins, DD	1220 SW. 3d Ave.
Spokane, Wash. 99201	Valmer Cameron, DD	651 U.S. Courthouse

For further information, contact the Office of Information Services, Small Business Administration, 1441 I Street NW., Washington, D.C. 20416. Phone, 202-653-6365.

SOURCE: *1983/84 U.S. Government Manual* (Washington, D.C.: General Services Administration, 1983), 612–614.

Appendix C:
Trade Associations

Trade Associations help improve the health of the industries they represent by providing members with detailed industry information and by coordinating industry action as needed. Your library should have a current edition of The IMS Ayer Directory of Publications *and the* Encyclopedia of Associations *(see the References section in Chapter 2 for full bibliographic information), both good sources for locating trade associations. Some of the associations that are prominent in their fields are listed as follows:*

American Management Association
135 W. 5th Street
New York, NY 10020

Association of Management Consultants
811 E. Wisconsin Avenue
Milwaukee, WI 53202

National Association of Retail Grocers
2000 Spring Rd., Suite 620
Oak Brook, IL 60521

National Automatic Merchandising Association
7 S. Dearborn Street
Chicago, IL 60611

National Council for Small Business Management
  Development
c/o University of Wisconsin
Civic Center Campus
600 W. Kilborn Avenue
Milwaukee, WI 53203

National Federation of Independent Business
150 W. 20th Avenue
San Mateo, CA 94402

National Retail Hardware Association
964 N. Penn Street
Indianapolis, IN 46204

National Retail Merchants Association
100 W. 31st Street
New York, NY 10001

National Small Business Association
301-1225 15th Street NW
Washington, DC 20026

Sons of Bosses
53 E. Main Street
Morristown, NJ 08057

The Young President's Organization
375 Park Avenue
New York, NY 10022

Appendix D:
Sources of Census Information

Your local library may not be able to provide you with full census information, and that's why you'll want to know about the libraries listed below.

The Federal Depository Library Program provides Government publications to designated libraries throughout the United States. The Regional Depository Libraries listed below receive and retain at least one copy of nearly every Federal Government publication, either in printed or microfilm form for use by the general public. These libraries provide reference services and inter-library loans; however, they are *not* sales outlets. You may wish to ask your local library to contact a Regional Depository to help you locate specific publications, or you may contact the Regional Depository yourself.

Arkansas State Library
One Capitol Mall
Little Rock, AR 72201
(501) 371-2326

Auburn Univ. at Montgomery Library
Documents Department
Montgomery, AL 36193
(205) 279-9110 ext. 253

Univ. of Alabama Library
Documents Dept.—Box S
University, AL 35486
(205) 348-7369

Dept. of Library, Archives and Public Records
Third Floor—State Cap.
1700 West Washington
Phoenix, AZ 85007
(602) 255-4121

University of Arizona Lib.
Governments Documents Dept.
Tucson, AZ 85721
(602) 626-5233

California State Library
Govt. Publications Section
P.O. Box 2037
Sacramento, CA 95809
(916) 322-4572

Univ. of Colorado Lib.
Government Pub. Division
Campus Box 184
Boulder, CO 80309
(303) 492-8834

Denver Public Library
Govt. Pub. Department
1357 Broadway
Denver, CO 80203
(303) 571-2131

Connecticut State Library
Government Documents Unit
231 Capitol Avenue
Hartford, CT 06106
(203) 566-4971

Univ. of Florida Libraries
Library West
Documents Department
Gainesville, FL 32611
(904) 392-0367

Univ. of Georgia Libraries
Government Reference Dept.
Athens, GA 30602
(404) 542-8951

Univ. of Hawaii Library
Govt. Documents Collection
2550 The Mall
Honolulu, HI 96822
(808) 948-8230

Univ. of Idaho Library
Documents Section
Moscow, ID 83843
(208) 885-6344

Illinois State Library
Information Services Branch
Centennial Building
Springfield, IL 62706
(217) 782-5185

Indiana State Library
Serials Documents Section
140 North Senate Avenue
Indianapolis, IN 46204
(317) 232-3686

Univ. of Iowa Libraries
Govt. Documents Department
Iowa City, IA 52242
(319) 353-3318

University of Kansas
Doc. Collect.—Spencer Lib.
Lawrence, KS 66045
(913) 864-4662

Univ. of Kentucky Libraries
Govt. Pub. Department
Lexington, KY 40506
(606) 257-3139

Louisiana State University
Middleton Library
Govt. Docs. Dept.
Baton Rouge, LA 70803
(504) 388-2570

Louisiana Technical Univ. Library
Documents Department
Ruston, LA 71272
(318) 257-4962

University of Maine
Raymond H. Fogler Library
Tri-State Regional Doc. Depository
Orono, ME 04469
(207) 581-1680

University of Maryland
McKeldin Lib.—Doc. Div.
College Park, MD 20742
(301) 454-3034

Boston Public Library
Government Docs. Dept.
Boston, MA 02117
(617) 536-5400 ext. 226

Detroit Public Library
Sociology Department
5201 Woodward Avenue
Detroit, MI 48202
(313) 833-1409

Michigan State Library
P.O. Box 30007
Lansing, MI 48909
(517) 373-0640

University of Minnesota
Government Pubs. Division

409 Wilson Library
309 19th Avenue South
Minneapolis, MN 55455
(612) 373-7813

Univ. of Mississippi Lib.
Documents Department
University, MS 38677
(601) 232-5857

Univ. of Montana
Mansfield Library
Documents Division
Missoula, MT 59812
(406) 243-6700

Nebraska Library Comm.
Federal Documents
1420 P Street
Lincoln, NE 68508
(402) 471-2045
(In cooperation with University of
Nebraska-Lincoln)

University of Nevada Lib.
Govt. Pub. Department
Reno, NV 89557
(702) 784-6579

Newark Public Library
5 Washington Street
Newark, NJ 07101
(201) 733-7812

University of New Mexico
Zimmerman Library
Government Pub. Dept.
Albuquerque, NM 87131
(505) 277-5441

New Mexico State Library
Reference Department
325 Don GasparAvenue
Santa Fe, NM 87501
(505) 827-2033, ext. 22

New York State Library
Empire State Plaza
Albany, NY 12230
(518) 474-5563

**University of North Carolina at
Chapel Hill**
Wilson Library
BA/SS Documents Division
Chapel Hill, NC 27515
(919) 962-1321

University of North Dakota
Chester Fritz Library
Documents Department
Grand Forks, ND 58202
(710) 777-2617, ext. 27
(In cooperation with North Dakota
State Univ. Library)

State Library of Ohio
Documents Department
65 South Front Street
Columbus, OH 43215
(614) 462-7051

Oklahoma Dept. of Libraries
Government Documents
200 NE 18th Street
Oklahoma City, OK 73105
(405) 521-2502

Oklahoma State Univ. Lib.
Documents Department
Stillwater, OK 74078
(405) 624-6546

Portland State Univ. Lib.
Documents Department
P.O. Box 1151
Portland, OR 97207
(503) 229-3673

State Library of Penn.
Government Pub. Section
P.O. Box 1601
Harrisburg, PA 17105
(717) 787-3752

Texas State Library
Public Services Department
P.O. Box 12927—Cap. Sta.
Austin, TX 78753
(512) 471-2996

Texas Tech Univ. Library
Govt. Documents Department
Lubbock, TX 79409
(806) 742-2268

Utah State University
Merrill Library, U.M.C. 30
Logan, UT 84322
(801) 750-2682

University of Virginia
Alderman Lib.—Public Doc.
Charlottesville, VA 22901
(804) 924-3133

Washington State Library
Documents Section
Olympia, WA 98504
(206) 753-4027

West Virginia Univ. Lib.
Documents Department
Morgantown, WV 26506
(304) 293-3640

Milwaukee Public Library
814 West Wisconsin Avenue
Milwaukee, WI 53233
(414) 278-3000

St. Hist. Lib. of Wisconsin
Government Pub. Section
816 State Street
Madison, WI 53706
(608) 262-4347

Wyoming State Library
Supreme Ct. & Library Bld.
Cheyenne, WY 82002
(307) 777-6344

SOURCE: *U.S. Congress, Government Depository Libraries,* a Joint Committee publication, 98th
Cong. 1st sess., rev. May 1983.

Index
to Action Steps

Subject Index

Study Guide to Small Business: An Entrepreneur's Plan

Table of Contents

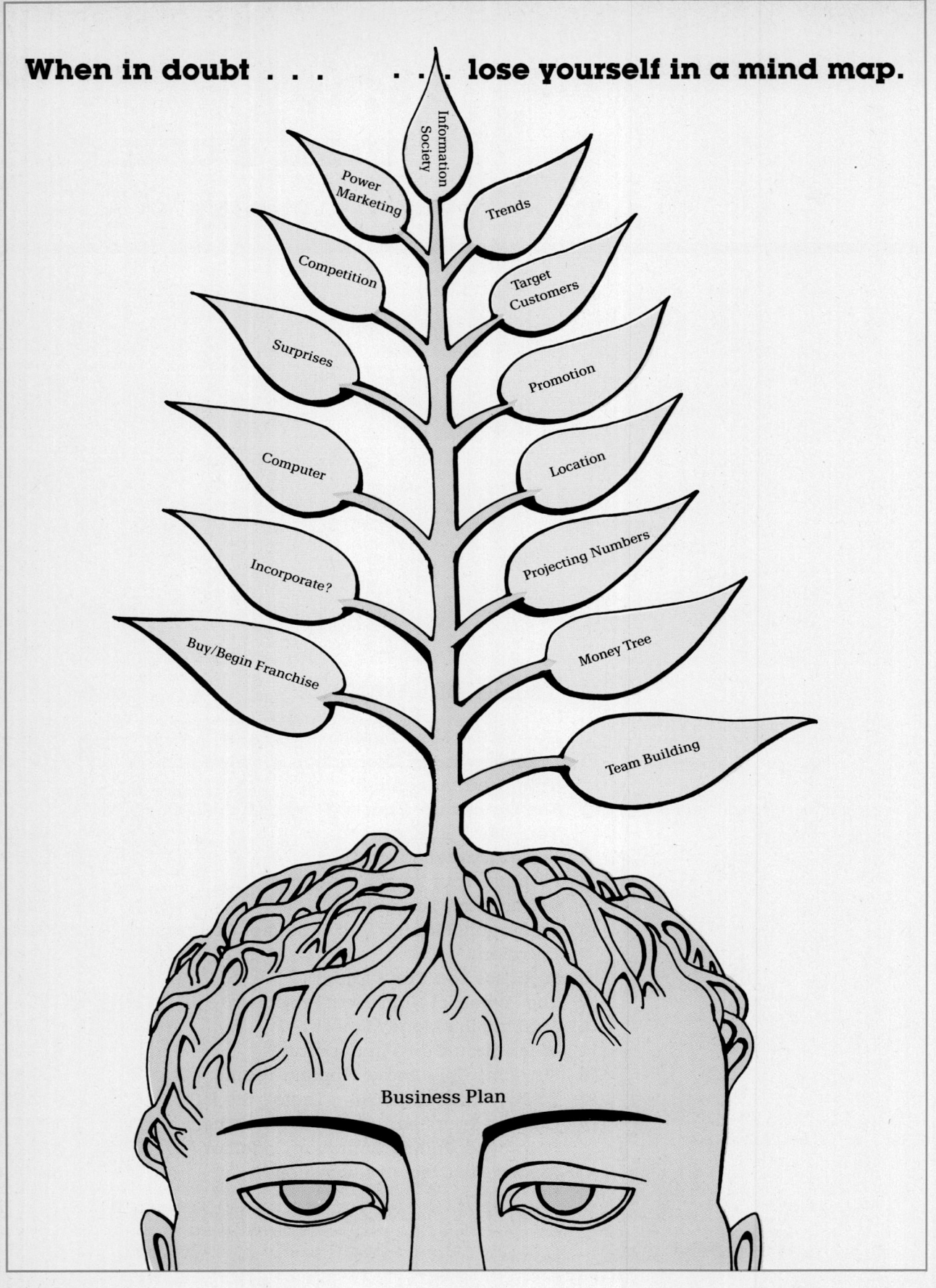

How to Use Mind Maps as You Study

Dear Creative Entrepreneur:

  You will see mind maps in various chapters of your text. They look like this:

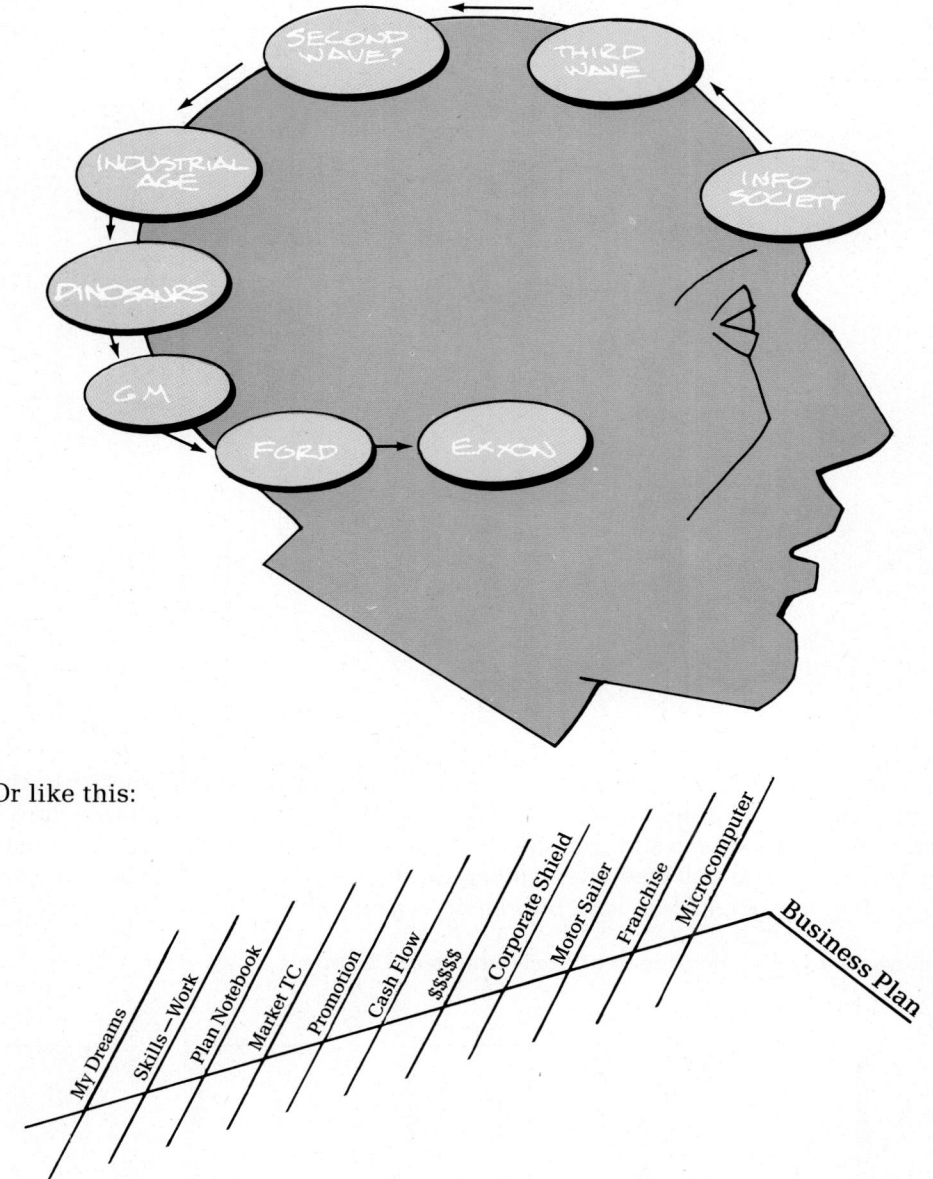

Or like this:

Mind maps are personal. You use them to loosen up your creative juices as they distract the logical, rational, numerical hemisphere of your brain. Use mind maps to explode ideas into insights. To read more about mind maps and how they work, see *Use Both Sides of Your Brain* by Tony Buzan, or *Writing the Natural Way* by Gabriele Rico. Both are cited in the Reference section of Chapter 1. Or look ahead to the section of Chapter 2 called "Working from Mind Maps." But before you start on anything else in this Study Guide, start on mind maps.

Mind maps allow you to have fun with information. All you need are pen and paper. You use simple boxes, triangles, circles, lines, and arrows. You can go anywhere or diagram any concept. There is no such thing as a wrong mind map. Try one now, on any subject:

Care to try another? Following is a baseline that you can use to mind map the large chunks of Chapter 1 of the text. You will notice that we have already drawn boxes for Action Steps and triangles for case studies. Add any additional mapping or comments you want. Remember, mind maps are not tests. When you are done, feel free to compare your mind map of Chapter 1 with ours on page SG-4.

Using this baseline, complete a mind map of the contents of Chapter 1 of text.

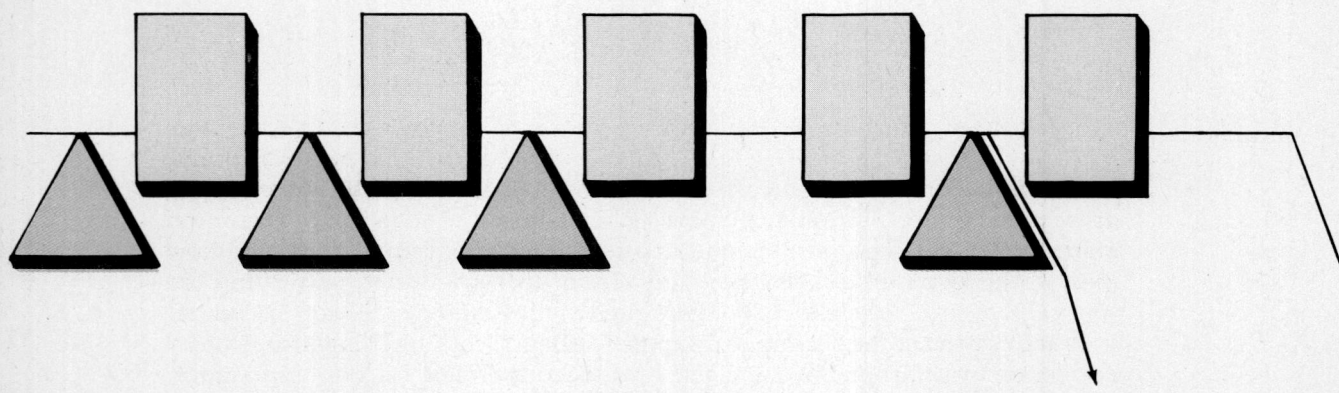

Learning isn't all questions (tough teacher) and answers (weary student). Learning is a growth process, necessary for survival in any culture, in any age. Learning is also fun.

The easy way to handle learning is to make knowledge visual. Images cling to the mind. For example, take the word *positioning*. It's a complex strategy of establishing a ladder inside the mind of your Target Customer. How do you remember positioning? You make a simple diagram.

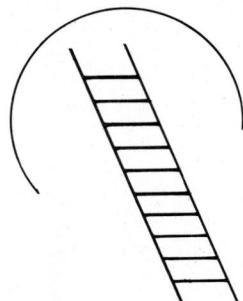

Then there's the term *life cycle* — a four-stage transition from birth to death. Products go through it. Services go through it. Industries and locations go through it. How do you remember the life cycle? You take the time to draw a diagram.

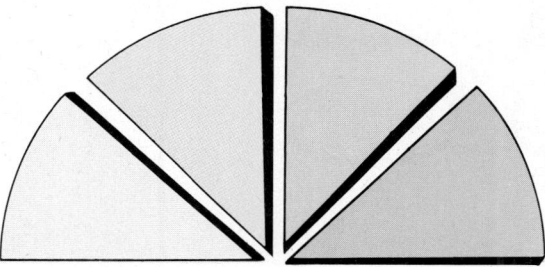

Later in the text we talk about *market segmentation.* A diagram can help you develop your thoughts on this abstract concept.

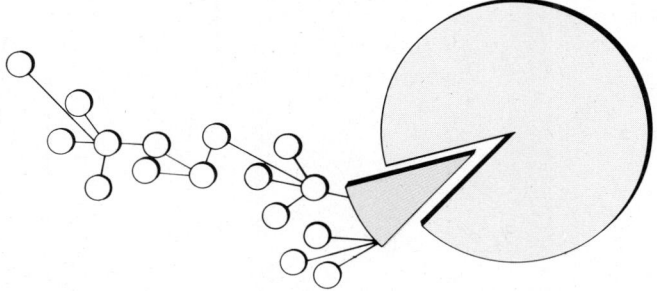

Both the text and the study guide are designed to let you use mind maps to explore this book. The text offers wide margins to allow you to make diagrams and mind maps as you read. At the beginning of each chapter of the study guide, we repeat the graph that is used to start each chapter of the text — only we provide extra blank space — so you can mind map how that chapter affects your ideas about your business and so you can diagram new ideas for your Business Plan.

Take the time to draw, to think, to observe with New Eyes. That's the way to use this study guide.

Our mind map of Chapter 1 of text looks like this.

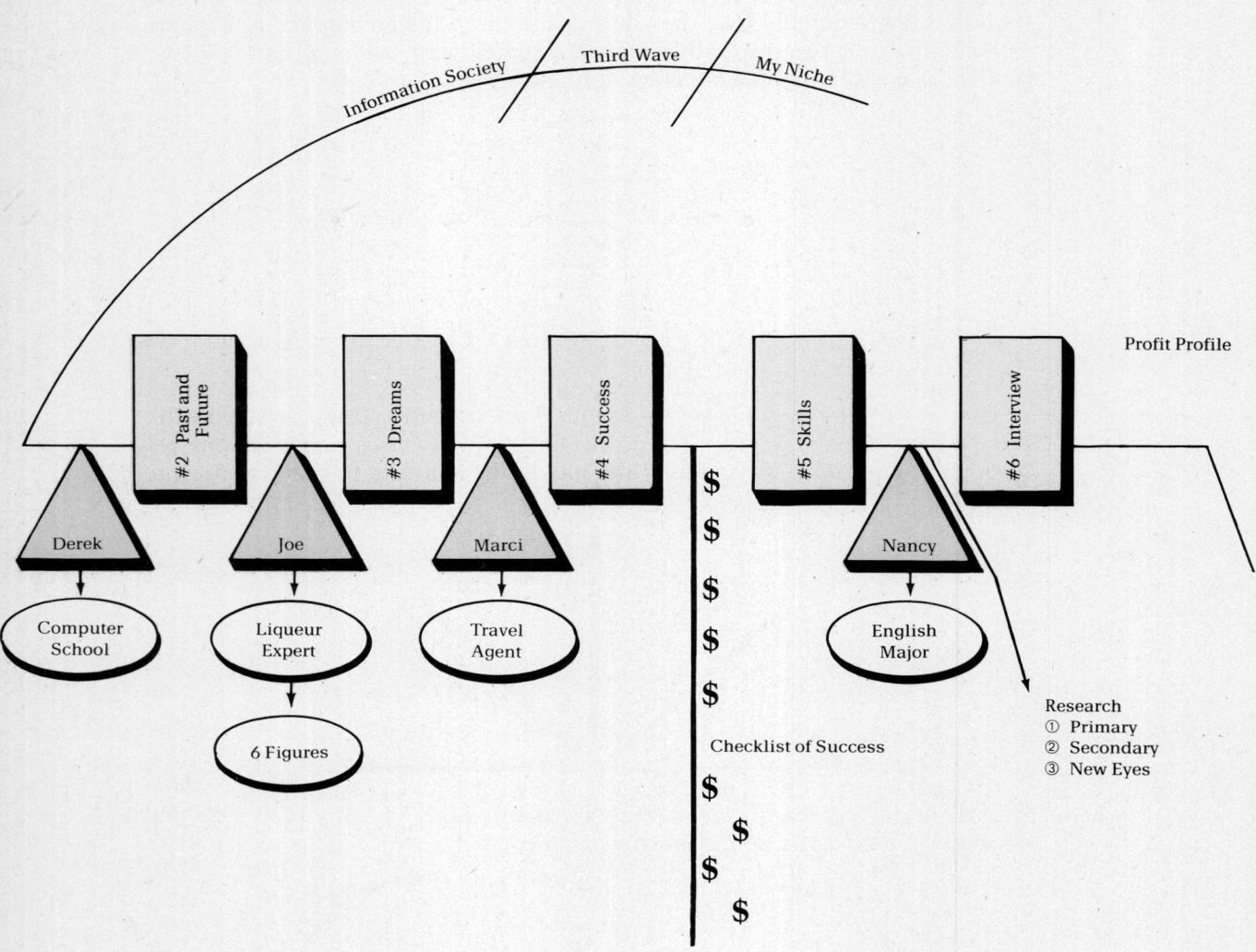

Doorways to the Information Society— Your Great Adventure

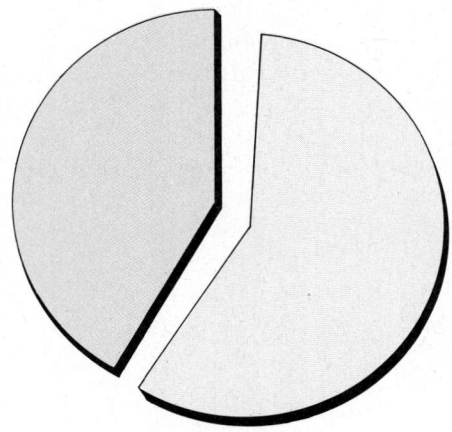

Draw a mind map of how Chapter 1 helps you in your business goals.

Objective Questions

Matching

Match each of the following numbered items with the lettered statement that best describes it by entering the number of the item in the space provided.

1. Target Customer
2. mind workers
3. gap
4. First Wave
5. Information Society

6. Business Plan
7. high growth industry
8. primary research
9. segment
10. production mind-set

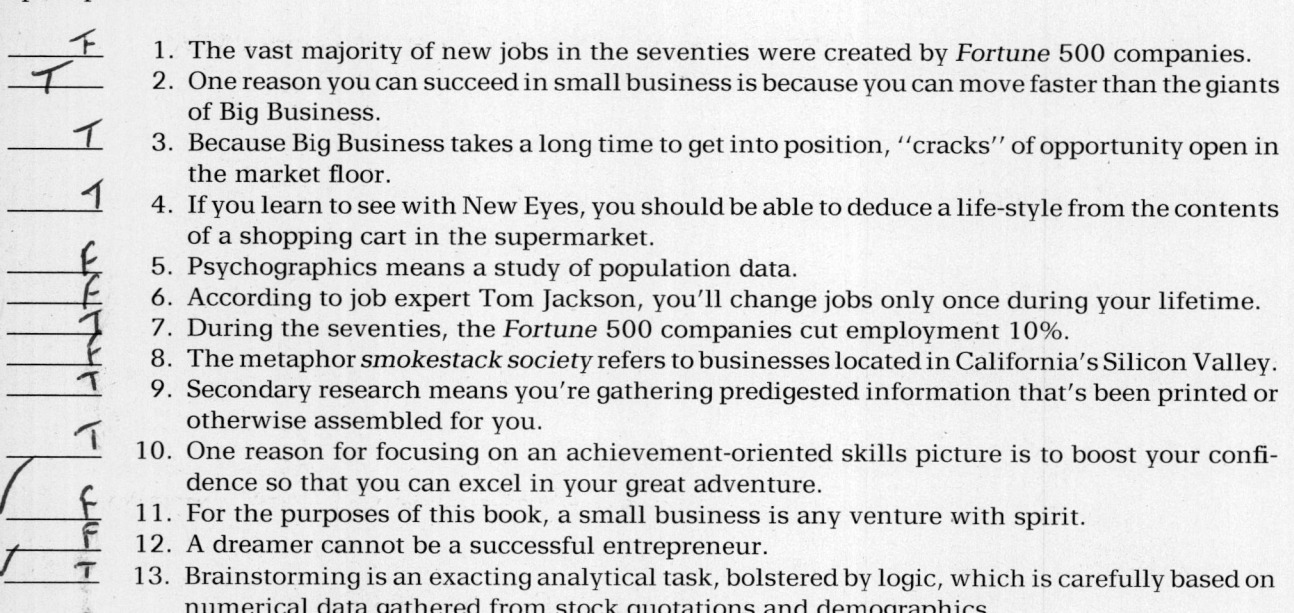

_5_____ A. Toffler's Third Wave
_8_____ B. gathering real information in the field
_1_____ C. the customer with the highest probability of buying your product or service
_10_____ D. Henry Ford displayed it by painting all cars black
_9_____ E. a slice of the total market
_4_____ F. Agriculture
_6_____ G. a blueprint for your business
_2_____ H. denizens of the Information Society
_2_____ I. an area in which emerging market demand exceeds supply
_3_____ J. where market needs are not being met

True – False

Determine whether each of the following statements is true or false and enter a T (True) or F (False) in the space provided.

_F_____ 1. The vast majority of new jobs in the seventies were created by *Fortune* 500 companies.
_T_____ 2. One reason you can succeed in small business is because you can move faster than the giants of Big Business.
_T_____ 3. Because Big Business takes a long time to get into position, "cracks" of opportunity open in the market floor.
_T_____ 4. If you learn to see with New Eyes, you should be able to deduce a life-style from the contents of a shopping cart in the supermarket.
_F_____ 5. Psychographics means a study of population data.
_F_____ 6. According to job expert Tom Jackson, you'll change jobs only once during your lifetime.
_T_____ 7. During the seventies, the *Fortune* 500 companies cut employment 10%.
_F_____ 8. The metaphor *smokestack society* refers to businesses located in California's Silicon Valley.
_T_____ 9. Secondary research means you're gathering predigested information that's been printed or otherwise assembled for you.
_T_____ 10. One reason for focusing on an achievement-oriented skills picture is to boost your confidence so that you can excel in your great adventure.
_F_____ 11. For the purposes of this book, a small business is any venture with spirit.
_F_____ 12. A dreamer cannot be a successful entrepreneur.
_T_____ 13. Brainstorming is an exacting analytical task, bolstered by logic, which is carefully based on numerical data gathered from stock quotations and demographics.
_F_____ 14. The father of brainstorming was Attila the Hun.
_T_____ 15. *Megatrends* was written from data assembled by information engineer Derek Campbell.

Multiple Choice

Select the best response for each of the following items and enter the corresponding letter in the space provided.

C 1. To do New Eyes research, you:
   a. research books and periodicals about information processing.
   b. see an optician.
   c. use your intuition to play Marketplace Detective.
   d. watch videotapes instead of reading texts.

D 2. Which one of the following jobs is not considered an information task?
   a. Teacher.
   b. Bureaucrat.
   c. Insurance broker.
   d. Coal miner.

D 3. The book that will give entrepreneurs a quick overview of the movement of society in the next 10–15 years is:
   a. *Up the Organization!*
   b. *The One-Minute Manager.*
   c. *In Search of Excellence.*
   d. *Megatrends.*

A 4. Which one of the following entrepreneurs from the case studies in Chapter 1 is the least enmeshed in the Information Society?
   a. Joseph Talmadge — liqueur expert.
   b. Derek Campbell — engineer.
   c. Nancy Tremaine — English major.
   d. Marci Reid — travel agent.

D 5. Interviewing small business owners in the field is an example of:
   a. secondary research.
   b. your definition of success.
   c. how you remember the Industrial Age.
   d. primary research.

C 6. The document which stands between you and small business failure is your:
   a. SBA management leaflet 6602.03.
   b. first year's ROI.
   c. Business Plan
   d. skills dossier.

B 7. The United States began moving toward a service economy in the year:
   a. 1984.
   b. 1945.
   c. 1918.
   d. 1929.

D 8. The Industrial Age is also referred to as:
   a. The Third Wave.
   b. The Information Economy.
   c. Toffler's Trough.
   d. The Second Wave.

B 9. You can generate a secret profit profile of a business if you know only certain key figures because:
   a. You can estimate some expenses with reasonable accuracy.
   b. Net profit always equals about 10% of Cost of Goods Sold.
   c. The IRS makes all business income tax returns available for public scrutiny.
   d. All small businesses have about the same return on investment.

_____ **D**   10. One of the best sources of up-to-date business information is:
   a. _Life_ magazine.
   b. _Redbook._
   c. _Ellery Queen's Mystery Magazine._
   d. the _Wall Street Journal._

Short-Answer Questions

1. What are your career plans? What industry do you want to be working in five years from now?
OWN MY OWN CELLULAR SERVICE BUS.
Why? _ENORMUS GROWTH POTENTIAL_
10 years from now? _BROADEN TO ALL COMMUNICATIONS_

2. What would you do if you had one year off, with no money worries?
1st priority _~~VACATION~~ BUY A HOME_
2nd priority _VACATION W/ MY FAMILY_
3rd priority _SPEND MORE TIME W/ MY FAMILY_

3. Name three small businesses in your immediate area which you think meet your criteria for success.
a. _ALREADY KNOW MY FIELD_
b. _____
c. _____

4. List four criteria for success in small business.
a. _PROPER CASH FLOW_
b. _ORGANIZED EFFECTIVE MARKETING_
c. _ORGAINIZED EFFECTIVE MANAGEMENT_
d. _COMPLETELY SATISFIED CUSTOMERS_

5. What skills do you have that will help you succeed in small business? (see Action Step 5)
a. _KNOWLEDGE OF CELLULAR_
b. _MANAGEMENT EXPERIENCE_
c. _MOTIVATION_
d. _IDEA THAT WILL FILL A GAP._
e. _CONTACTS & REFERENCES_

6. What do you need to learn to supplement the skills that you already have?
a. _WHERE I CAN GET MONEY._
b. _PROCESS CASH FLOW_
c. _MARKETING TECHNIQUES_

7. Following your field interviews from Action Step 6, summarize what you learned about the most outstanding of the businesses interviewed.
Name of business _CELLULAND_
Type of business _RETAIL CELLULAR PHONES_

Industry ___TELECOMMUNICATIONS___

Location ___PALO ALTO, EL CAMINO___

Owner's name ___GLENN LIU.___

Owner's personality ___VERY SERIOUS. CONCERNED W/ 100% CUST.___
___SATISFACTION___

Target Market:

    Sex ___LOTS OF !___

    Age ___ANY.___

    Income ___OVER $ 7000 MONTH.___

    Education ___VARIES___

    Residence ___VARIES___

    Occupation ___CONST, PRESIDENTS, SALESPERSONS,___

    Lifestyle Summary ___VARIES — SERIOUS PROFESSIONAL PEOPLE___
___ON THE GO.___

Owner's promotional strategy ___RADIO, T.V., NEWSPAPER. QUALITY___

Gross sales (if available) ___APPROX $100,000 MONTH.___

Profits (if available) ___APPROX 25,000 MONTH___

Marketing budget ___VARIES___

Rent ___5,000___

Salaries ___$7,000 FOR MANAGERS 25% PROFIT FOR SALES___

Anything that could be improved ___MOTIVATION OF SALES FORCE,___

Mistakes owner will admit to _____

Any recommendations on banker, attorney, accountant, etc?
___BE CAREFUL !___

Capsule Summary [in what way is this a helpful model for your business?]:

___2 YEARS OF WORKING EXP. CAN'T BE WRITTEN IN___
___1 PARAGRAPH.___

8. Profit profile. After you have interviewed three or four business owners, use your numbers to develop a profit profile. List what you know. Then try to figure out what each business was making.

   a. Gross sales ___ $75,000 _____

   Cost of goods sold _____

   Rent ___ 4,000 _____

   Salaries _____

   Marketing _____

   FICA/benefits (est. 20–30% of salaries) _____

   Other expenses (est. 8–12% of gross sales) _____

   b. Gross sales _____

   Cost of goods sold _____

   Rent _____

   Salaries _____

   Marketing _____

   FICA/benefits (est. 20–30% of salaries) _____

   Other expenses (est. 8–12% of gross sales) _____

   c. Gross sales _____

   Cost of goods sold _____

   Rent _____

   Salaries _____

   Marketing _____

   FICA/benefits (est. 20–30% of salaries) _____

   Other expenses (est. 8–12% of gross sales) _____

   d. Gross sales _____

   Cost of goods sold _____

   Rent _____

   Salaries _____

   Marketing _____

   FICA/benefits (est. 20–30% of salaries) _____

   Other expenses (est. 8–12% of gross sales) _____

The Big Picture: Charting Trends for Your Small Business

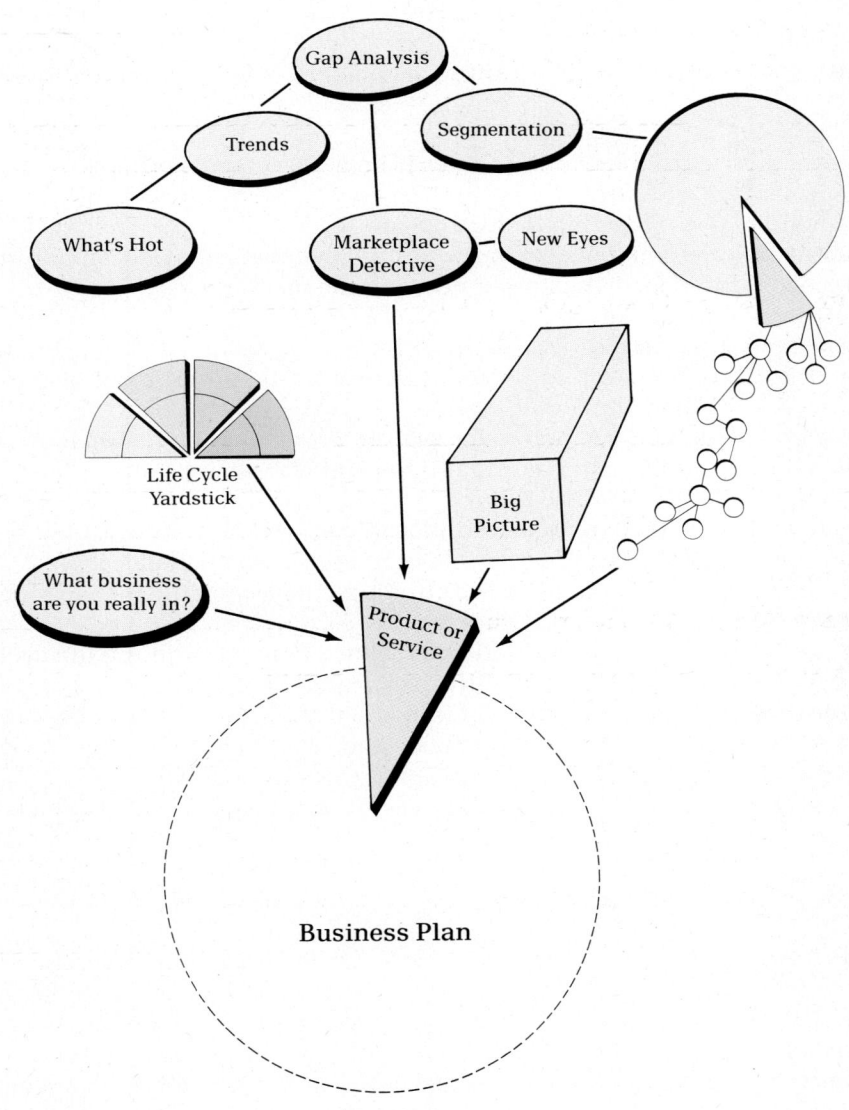

Here we start a mind map of how Chapter 2 of the text affects your Business Plan. What can you add to the map?

Objective Questions

Matching

Match each of the following numbered items with the lettered statement that best describes it by entering the number of the item in the space provided.

1. trend
2. life cycle
3. one-color stationery
4. singles
5. shelf velocity
6. New Eyes research
7. Deep Discount

8. designer jeans
9. market signal
10. high touch
11. target neighborhood
12. workaholic
13. Heavy User
14. Target Customer

15. fad
16. information
17. *Wall Street Journal*
18. trade journal
19. bank
20. gap analysis

_____ 11 A. the habitat of your Target Customer
_____ 12 B. a person whose chief joy in life comes from achievements at work
_____ 15 C. a trend that doesn't last
_____ 17-18 D. reading this gives you a Big Picture update
_____ 18 E. a publication written and distributed for the members of a particular industry or business
_____ 20 F. a procedure for identifying unmet needs in the marketplace
_____ 19 G. an institution that rents money
_____ 16 H. as you consume it, it grows
_____ 1 I. a large moving tendency that can be intuited and used to advantage by the entrepreneur who can see the handwriting on the wall
_____ 3 J. a smart purchasing move that helps save entrepreneurs money at start-up time
_____ 4 K. in 1982, they numbered 19 million in the United States
_____ 5 L. speed at which merchandise sells
_____ 6 M. a creative view of the marketplace that can be correlated with secondary sources
_____ 7 N. when the marketplace is flooded, this is what products sell at
_____ 10 O. society's attempt at balancing the electronic technology of the Information Age with human softness
_____ 9 P. they are everywhere, and they tell you where a product is on the life cycle
_____ 2 Q. A four-stage pathway of inevitability for virtually all industries, products, and services
_____ 13 R. a target customer who buys the lion's share of a particular product or service
_____ 14 S. the person most likely to buy your goods and/or services
_____ 8 T. a marketplace fad that lasted slightly longer than hula hoops

True–False

Determine whether each of the following statements is true or false and enter a T (True) or F (False) in the space provided.

_____ T 1. The life-cycle yardstick is important because it will give you a quick sense of what's happening in the world of business.
_____ F 2. Because of the positioning of designer jeans in the marketplace and also because of the HMUF (High Mark-Up Factor), manufacturing designer jeans would be a lucrative venture for the creative entrepreneur.
_____ T 3. You really don't need to decide what business you're really in until the doors of your business have been open for at least a year.
_____ F 4. Mary Clarke was really in the business of stabling horses.
_____ F 5. The automobile industry has been in a high-growth phase since the early 1980s.

_____T_____ 6. One reason the railroads went into decline was because they forgot what business they were really in.

_____T_____ 7. Hula hoops, designer jeans, Rubik's Cube, and spidery wall-walker toys are all examples of marketplace fads.

_____F_____ 8. *Megatrends* was based on research from 6,000 local papers over a period of a dozen years.

_____F_____ 9. Once you succeed in defining your business, you can sit tight and watch those dollars roll in because a definition is the final word.

_____F_____ 10. If you think you're in one kind of business, and your Target Customers think you're in something else, the obvious strategy is to show those customers the door, fast.

_____T_____ 11. Letterhead stationery is helpful to your information-gathering activities because it tells the world you're serious about going into business.

_____T_____ 12. Another way of talking about being in software sales is by saying you're in the problem-solving business.

_____F_____ 13. When you play Marketplace Detective, you can learn more about trends in small business by studying the national chains than by wasting time studying locally owned or regionally owned businesses.

_____T_____ 14. Market signals can be helpful indicators for workers in large industries as well as for small business owners.

_____T_____ 15. One reason a business like Private Screenings can exist is because certain segments of the marketplace are adopting a more relaxed attitude about sex.

_____F_____ 16. There is no need to ''walk the neighborhood'' and spy on strangers when you can find out everything you need to know by writing the appropriate U.S. government agency for the needed data.

_____F_____ 17. If you see a shopping cart loaded with baby food, disposable diapers, dog food, boxed cereal, large cartons of milk, you can assume that the shopper has a senior citizen life style, loves fishing, hunting, knitting, billiards, bingo, and dry martinis on the weekend.

_____F_____ 18. A full parking lot is absolute proof of a booming shopping center.

_____F_____ 19. If you're eager to try your wings in small business, there's no need to waste time taking a lot of personality tests.

_____T_____ 20. If you're in the baby bedding business, a child's nursery can be your marketplace.

Multiple Choice

Select the best response for each of the following items and enter the corresponding letter in the space provided.

_____D_____ 1. The life-cycle yardstick is an important tool because:
   a. it is an absolute mathematical instrument.
   b. it always correlates with the Dow-Jones averages.
   c. it can help you target a growth segment of a growth industry.
   d. it will prevent you from making foolish mistakes with your time and money.

_____B_____ 2. A good example of a hot growth industry would be:
   a. sedan-sized autos.
   b. robotics.
   c. tobacco.
   d. railroads.

_____B_____ 3. If you get into a business like toy retailing, your survival will depend on how well you can:
   a. keep one eye on the future.
   b. handle a 30-hour work week.
   c. forget you used to be a kid and concentrate on accounting controls.
   d. understand computer programming language.

_____C_____ 4. Gap analysis and segmentation:
   a. depend for their success on how close you are to getting your MBA in marketing.

b. are deeply mathematical in nature.

c. are fun because they allow you to be imaginative.

d. always correlate precisely with high-level entrepreneurial theory from the major universities.

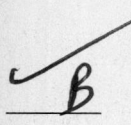 **B**

5. Knowing what business you're in is important because:

a. it will guarantee you an income of six figures in your first year.

b. it means you'll never have to waste time redefining your business goals.

c. it cuts down customer confusion.

d. it can be ascertained by amassing statistics from the files of the U.S. Census Bureau.

B   6. Railroads in the United States went into a decline for all the reasons below except which of the following?

a. The RRs forgot what business they were in.

b. The new plastic tracks became portable and flexible.

c. Jumbo jets carried people and goods faster.

d. The interstate highway system connected the country and made travel and shipping more flexible.

B   7. Which of the trends below was not much of a consideration in the intimate lingerie business?

a. Specialized consumer tastes.

b. A geographic shift from Frost Belt to Sunbelt.

c. High tech/high touch.

d. Relaxing national attitudes about sex.

C   8. You are out walking your target neighborhood. You see baby strollers, people walking dogs, four-year-old station wagons, bikes, newly planted lawns. The trees are small and supported with sticks. Some of the streets are still being put in. You can make the following marketplace assumption:

a. adult condo complex, restricted to retirees over 60.

b. singles condo complex catering to people of both sexes between 22–33.

c. family residential area, perhaps for first-time buyers.

d. old established residential area, heart of town.

D   9. One of the newest hot-growth industries may well be:

a. automobile manufacturing.

b. book publishing.

c. steel mills.

d. bio-genetics.

A   10. One of the many signals that a giant industry is in trouble would be:

a. layoffs, shrinking back orders, slow payment of bills, deferred maintenance.

b. sponsorship of rock concerts in the desert.

c. bringing in consultants on creativity, right hemisphere problem-solving, and the arts of Japanese management.

d. deciding what business they're in.

Short-Answer Questions

1. Where is your industry on the four-stage life-cycle yardstick? If you're in the decline stage, can you think of a related business that's in a different stage? Do any of your skills qualify you to move to a business venture in another stage? ___EMBRYONIC STAGE, NOT ANY THAT I'M INTERESTED OR QUALIFIED IN TO MOVE TO,___

_____

_____

2. Write down what business you're really in.

   CELLULAR — TELECOMMUNICATION INDUSTRY

   Now write down what *other* businesses you're in. (For example, if you want to open a camera shop where your major activity will be the memory business, you'll have several minibusinesses to be aware of: processing, camera rental, your photographer's school, retailing. List all your possible minibusinesses here.) _AUTO ELECTRICAL, WHOLESALING, RETAILING, INSURANCE, CONSULTING AND PURCHASING_

3. How old is your industry? How old is your particular segment? Below, list five to seven turning points in your industry. (For example, if you're thinking of going in the printing business, you should know that one major breakthrough came with Gutenberg, back in the 1400s. If you're in the computer service business, you know that your industry was born in the summer of 1969, when IBM let go of its profitable computer packages.)

Date	Turning Point/Trend
1. 1979	SCHAUMBURG ILL, CELLULAR WAS FIRST TESTED.
2. 1984	GTE BEGAN OPERATIONS IN THE BAY AREA.
3. 1985	PACTEL BOUGHT OUT 60% OF CELL ONE
4. 1985	BAY AREA — I WENT TO WORK IN CELLULAR.
5. 1985	BAY AREA — CELL ONE BECAME OPERATIONAL

4. **Model for a Shopping Cart Survey. Part I.** Your venture will be more fun if you train your mind to look for marketplace data. The following is a composite study, drawn from the marketplace. To prepare for Action Step 11, use this case as a model. Imagine you observe the following:

   A. Contents of cart:
      1. Imported beer, 2 cases.
      2. Mixed nuts, 4 cans.
      3. 16 steaks, porterhouse.
      4. Greens, tomatoes, imported olives, for salad.
      5. French bread.
      6. 17 Idaho potatoes, carefully selected.
      7. Cheese, imported Camembert.
      8. Cognac, 2 bottles.

   B. Shopper description:
      Clothes — Bermuda shorts, expensive shirt.
      Shoes — tennis, no socks.
      Jewelry — gold I.D. bracelet, gold watch, wedding band.
      Hair style — razor cut, medium.
      Eyeglasses — dark, prescription.
      General appearance — neat, careful dresser, excellent tan.

   The next step is to briefly summarize your observations. You should emerge with a pretty solid profile, as follows:

   Marketplace Observations: This upscale TC was observed on a Sunday afternoon at a food store located in an upper-middle class residential area. Census data for the area suggested a median household income of $65,000. The total bill came to $129.97, and was paid with cash from a large sheaf of bills. The TC was preparing for a party. Based on observation only, the following demographic profile can be assumed:
   Sex: male.
   Age: early 50s.
   Education: high probability for college degree.
   Occupation: executive.

Income: $50,000 +.
Residence: $170,000 +.

Part 2. When you move out into the arena to do your Shopping Cart Survey, use the case as a guide. First, list the contents of the cart. Second, describe the shopper. Third, summarize your observations.

A. Contents of cart:

1.   5.

2.   6.

3.   7.

4.   8.

B. Shopper description
   Clothes —
   Shoes —
   Jewelry —
   Hair-style —
   General appearance —
      Marketplace Observations:

Part 3. To develop your marketplace probe further, consider these questions:
Where is the location on the life-cycle yardstick?
Leaving the food store, how far would you have to drive to feel you're in a different economic customer base?
Did you make your study at rush hour? Lazy weekend afternoon? Early morning?
If you saw our upscale TC buying the same $129 worth of groceries at 2:30 P.M. on a weekday, what would you conclude about his occupation?
If a store is open 24 hours a day, what does it suggest about the Target Customers?
Is there any way you can sell your goods or services to any of the customers profiled?

5. Write down five business names that would tell your TC what business you're in. When you get your list, check with friends and fellow students. What do they think the names mean? (*Hint:* Quick Copy, Hamburger Hamlet, 1-Hr Foto, $1 Cleaner.)

1.

2.

3.

4.

5.

6. List your three most important information sources; on a separate sheet of paper write a brief paragraph about what you learned from each that will help you shape your Business Plan.

    1. _PACTEL MOBILE COMM. VICE PRESIDENT_
    2. _CELLULAND GLENN LIU PRESIDENT FRANCHISE_
    3. _CELLULAND KEN WILLIL PRESIDENT OF NETWORK._

Power Marketing

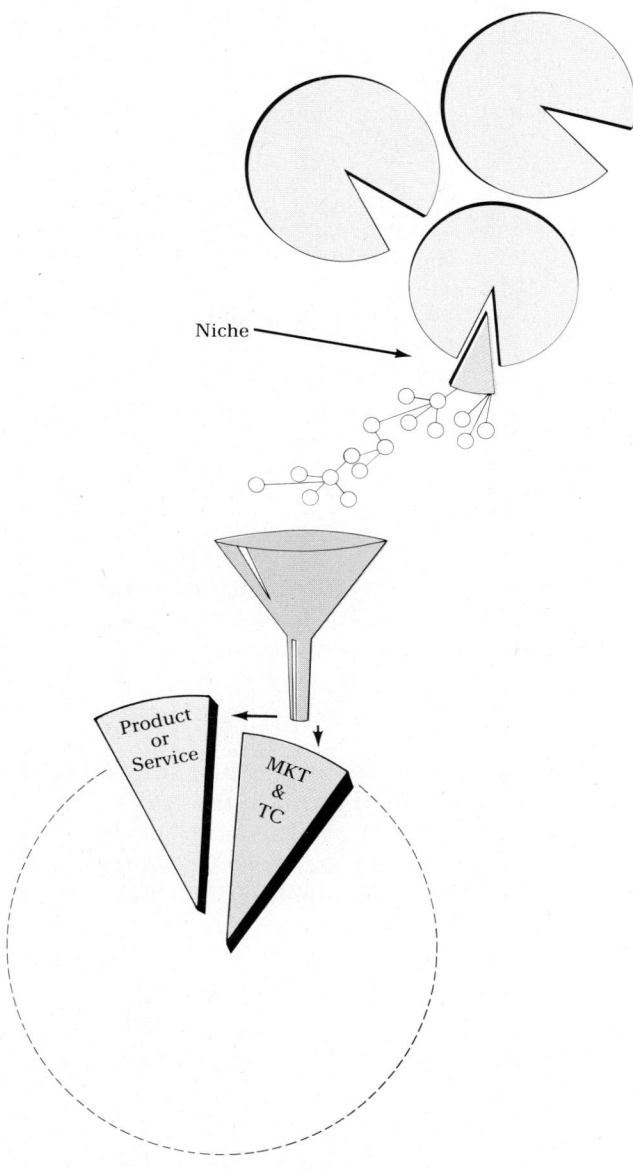

Niche

Product or Service

MKT & TC

Here we start a mind map of how Chapter 3 helps you refine your business idea. What can you add to the map?

Objective Questions

Matching

Match each of the following numbered items with the lettered statement that best describes it by entering the number of the item in the space provided.

1. Power Marketing
2. business objectives
3. psychological rewards
4. no competition
5. life cycle
6. positioning
7. industry breakthrough
8. component parts
9. Adam Osborne
10. forecasting
11. segment
12. demographics
13. psychographics
14. problems
15. support services
16. brainstorm
17. computerphobia
18. matrix grid
19. software
20. pricing

_____ 20   A. one of the four P's

18 → 1   B. screen or filter through which ideas are passed in order to form solutions

7 → 5   C. a new development in a particular product that changes the arena of competition

5 → 7   D. a four-stage yardstick that helps you look more carefully at business opportunities

_____ 19   E. the program that runs the computer

_____ 16   F. a free-for-all idea session that calls on creativity and flights of imagination for help in coping with problems

_____ 15   G. an activity that is usually trimmed with a product's price

_____ 13   H. a study of life-style — buying habits, dreams, attitudes, ambitions, and so on

_____ 11   I. a slice of the marketplace pie

_____ 9   J. entrepreneur who challenged the microcomputer industry with a portable machine the size of a sewing machine

_____ 10   K. a procedure practiced by market researchers that attempts to predict the future

1 → 18   L. a tool that helps you exploit gaps in the marketplace and connect your skills to your research

_____ 3   M. a feeling of satisfaction, hard to express, but quite real and powerful

_____ 17   N. irrational fear of a computer

_____ 2   O. an organized set of dreams that you are trying to translate into reality through hard work, tenacity, and information

_____ 4   P. means you're alone in your segment, like the first hunter arriving at the still and silent pond

_____ 8   Q. one example of an industry breakthrough in the microcomputer industry

_____ 6   R. a strategy for establishing yourself on a ladder in the mind of the prospect

_____ 14   S. can be turned into opportunities by the streetwise entrepreneur

_____ 12   T. a study of population involving measurable observables like sex, age, income, and education

True – False

Determine whether each of the following statements is true or false and enter a T (True) or F (False) in the space provided.

_____ T   1. Power Marketing is a tool that helps you aim your mind at a particular segment of the marketplace.

_____ F   2. All five members of the Info Team case study had technical or engineering backgrounds.

_____ T   3. Listing business objectives helps you focus and plan.

_____ F   4. The father of brainstorming was Alexander the Great of Persia.

_____ T   5. People get together in teams to balance their strengths and weaknesses.

_____ F   6. The average small business can get up and running in seven days.

_T_ 7. If you can locate an industry that really has magnetic pull for you, you'll be more interested and have more fun.

_F_ 8. When researching, you can do a much better job if you forget organization and just dive in.

_T_ 9. In the computer industry, the life cycle of a piece of hardware can be as short as 18 months.

_F_ 10. After the "shakeout" in the microcomputer industry in late 1983, there was no more competition in the hardware segment.

_T_ 11. Apple introduced the micro in the midseventies.

_T_ 12. Before 1982, most programmers had aimed their software at the Apple. In late 1982, the new "wrinkle" in the mircocomputer industry was that more people were developing software for the IBM-PC.

_F_ 13. The Info Team in the case study finally decided the best business to be in was retailing hot computer hardware.

_T_ 14. Once you begin to profile your Target Customer, you're on your way to finding your segment.

_T_ 15. An eager entrepreneur can transform a problem into a business opportunity.

_T_ 16. In the early micro days, when manufacturers were trying to market software, one of the obvious problems was user frustration.

_T_ 17. In marketing circles, "support" means there are services to backstop and expand the value of the sale.

_T_ 18. The obvious Target Customer for a school that teaches computer software techniques is an unhappy micro user who cannot understand the complicated documentation.

_T_ 19. Armonk is GHQ for IBM.

_F_ 20. One of the key moves in Power Marketing occurs when you use a little entrepreneurial alchemy to translate problems into solutions.

Multiple Choice

Select the best response for each of the following items and enter the corresponding letter in the space provided.

_C_ 1. Power Marketing convinced the Info Team to go into which of the following segments:
   a. Hardware repair.
   b. Software production.
   c. Computer school.
   d. None of the above.

_D_ 2. Which of the following are reasonable business objectives?
   a. Safety of investment.
   b. Psychological rewards.
   c. Fun and adventure.
   d. All of the above.

_B_ 3. The name of the grid used to sift data and correlate objectives is:
   a. Bernoulli's Sieve.
   b. matrix.
   c. Alchemist's Urn.
   d. Iacocca's Ladle.

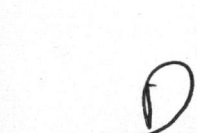 _C_ 4. Which of the following was not a problem that could be transformed into an opportunity by the Info Team?
   a. Unhappy, frustrated users.
   b. IBM declared bankruptcy in the summer of 1983.
   c. Minimal support from manufacturers.
   d. Confusion in the marketplace.

_D_ 5. Which of the following best describes the primary Target Customer discovered by the Info Team?
   a. Female, 45–57, college degree plus, income $55,000, suburban/rural, owns stable, rides six days a week.

b. Female, 18–34, some college, metro residence, $17,500, clerical/supervisory, reads *Cosmo, Glamour.*

c. Male, 18–34, some college, rural residence, $19,500, construction/crafts/artist/artisan.

d. Male, 18–35, some college, might own PC, access to computer at work, urban/suburban, $35,000, lives near computer store.

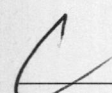

6. What year did Apple introduce the micro?
   a. 1485.
   b. 1977.
   c. 1945.
   d. 1984.

7. The phrase that best describes what was happening in the computer hardware marketplace in the early 1980s is:
   a. gentlemen's agreement not to compete.
   b. Bernoulli Effect.
   c. hot competition.
   d. Apple took over IBM HQ at Armonk.

8. According to the *Wall Street Journal* (August 19, 1983), the life cycle of a piece of computer hardware can be as short as:
   a. 9 months.
   b. 36 months.
   c. 3 months.
   d. 18 months.

9. Which of the following is not an accurate description of Power Marketing?
   a. A tool that helps you exploit gaps in the marketplace.
   b. A highly quantified system, firmly based in statistics.
   c. A technique that aims the power of your mind at a particular segment of the marketplace.
   d. A way to connect skills to a body of research.

10. One reason you need to be alert to industry breakthroughs:
    a. They give you the ammunition to jeer at your competitors.
    b. They prevent your key employees from selling company secrets.
    c. They give you the chance to change the competitive arena.
    d. They guarantee you a nonturbulent, debt-free start-up.

Short-Answer Questions

1. Describe your total market. (This is easier than it sounds. *Example:* The total market for the computer school would be everyone who owns, uses, or plans to own a micro.) Describe your total market briefly.

   _____

   _____

   _____

   _____

2. Segment your market, using logic combined with associative leaps. For help in starting segmentation, think of a large industry that's highly visible, like autos. You can segment according to *size* (Pinto, Cadillac limo), *price* (Mercedes, Chevette), *age* (Model T, Stutz Bearcat), *rarity* (Royale — there were only 6) *versus mass market* (Toyota), *country of origin* (Japan, Sweden, Germany, France, United States), *geographic distribution* (front-wheel drive Saabs in New England, Pacific Northwest; four-wheel drive Subarus in New Mexico; large sedans in the Midwest). Sometimes, it helps to create your own mind map. Use the space at the top of the opposite page for your map.

3. Profile your Target Customer.

Person	**Business**
Sex:	Size:
Age:	Industry:
Income:	Number of employees:
Occupation:	Type of employees:
Residence:	Branch offices:
Education:	Location:
Marital status:	Product/Service:
Geographic region:	SIC code:
Cultural origin:	Public/Private:
Religion:	

Leap into psychographics.

Buying habits:
Dreams:
Ambitions:
Attitudes:

For help on your psychographic leap, see the box in Chapter 4 of the text on *Nine American Lifestyles*, by Arnold Mitchell of SRI International (a research firm in Menlo Park, California). Mitchell segments life-style in groupings you can use for profiling your TC.

4. List major problems faced by the segments you discovered.

1. _____

2. _____

3. _____

4. _____

5. Brainstorm mad solutions to each major problem. Use the space provided to mind map your ideas.

6. Use the matrix grid that follows to squeeze some conclusions out of your data. Along the left hand side, list your business objectives. Along the top, list your solutions. In the boxes, place a +, 0, or — each time an objective clicks with a solution.

   + = 3
   0 = 2
   — = 1

   Total things up and see where you stand in your adventure.

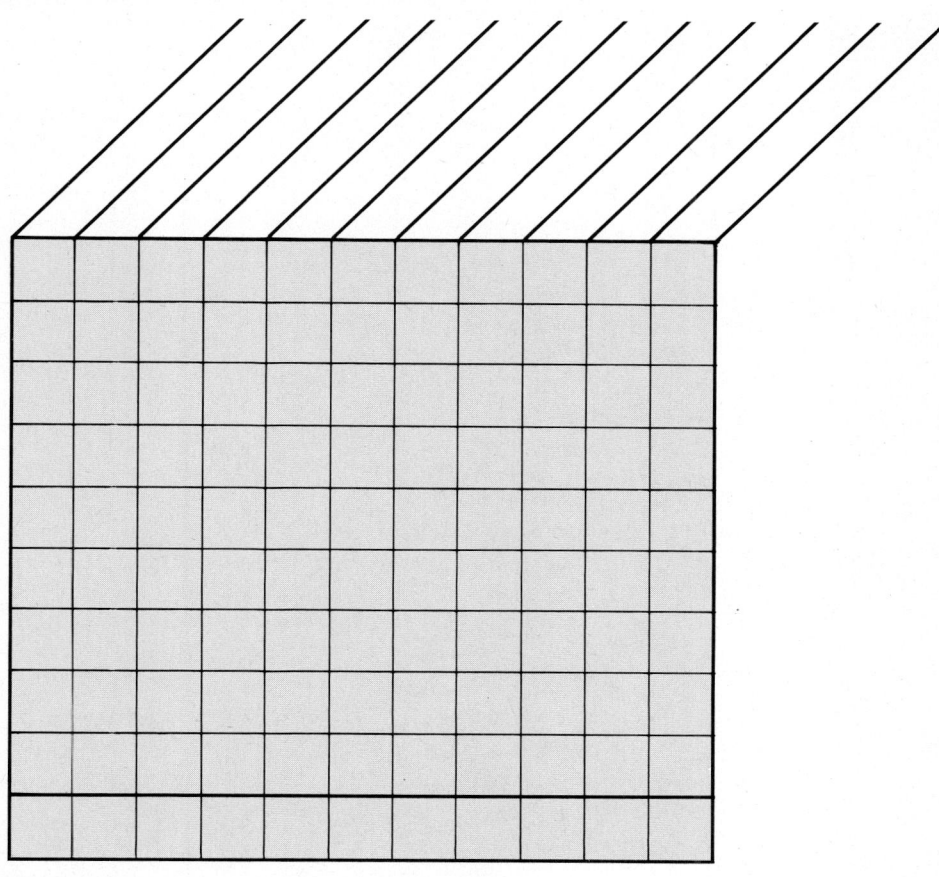

7. What has been the most fun so far in your adventure?

   _____

   Why was it fun? _____

   _____

   _____

4

Profiling Your
Target Customer

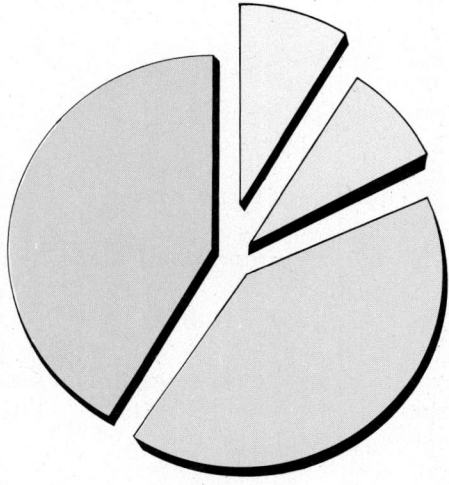

**Draw a mind map of how Chapter 4 helps you bring your business
idea into better focus.**

Objective Questions

Matching

Match each of the following numbered items with the lettered statement that best describes it by entering the number of the item in the space provided.

1. target market magazines	11. romance reader
2. Heavy User	12. competition
3. Hugh Hefner	13. baby boom
4. *Playboy* empire	14. primary Target Customer
5. demographic data	15. invisible Target Customer
6. newspaper	16. interview
7. *McCall's* reader	17. psychographics
8. magazine rack	18. profiling
9. display ad department	19. Business Plan
10. *Colliers, Coronet*	20. SIC codes

_____ A. a sudden increase in the number of births during a given period that results in a marketing phenomenon some 20 years later

_____ B. what develops when two or more hungry combatants decide they want the same slice of the marketplace pie

_____ C. drawing a magic circle around your customer

_____ D. a study of life-styles

_____ E. a customer who emerges, like magic, after you have been in business for awhile

_____ F. the most visible segment of your Target Market

_____ G. *McCall's, Cosmo, Playboy, Time*

_____ H. a blueprint for your business

_____ I. a Target Customer who accounts for a high percentage of sales of a certain product or service

_____ J. example of a Heavy User of a certain type of publication that is highly targeted

_____ K. an entrepreneur with a clear picture of his Target Customer

_____ L. general interest magazines that have vanished in this age of the special-interest reader

_____ M. the place you write to when asking for demographic information from magazines and newspapers

_____ N. a kingdom built on images and information

_____ O. an often overlooked guide to interest areas in a specific community

_____ P. female, 19–55, $27,000, metro-suburban, a high percentage are married, with children under 18; a high percentage are employed

_____ Q. facts and numbers relating to the study of population

_____ R. one good local source of marketing data

_____ S. an excellent technique for getting to know your Target Customer face-to-face

_____ T. federally sponsored standardized classification system of major industries and elements

True–False

Determine whether each of the following statements is true or false and enter a T (True) or F (False) in the space provided.

_____ 1. It is impossible for an entrepreneur to acquire new skills.

_____ 2. *Psychographics* refers to crazy people who write on walls with spray paint.

_____ 3. One of the best sources of customer profiles is the display ad departments of magazines.

_____ 4. If you can find out what your TC reads, watches, or listens to, you'll make your promotion task simpler.

_____ 5. When you go out for interviews, there's no real advantage to making up questions in advance if you just hit the street and wing it.

_____ 6. Interviewing Target Customers is a very useful technique when you're gathering information about the marketplace.

_____ 7. Once they heard about Fred's soccer shop, invisible customers began to appear.

_____ 8. If you've been in business before, there's no real need to waste time profiling your customers again and again. Just get to work and tell them how sharp you are.

_____ 9. A car driven by your Target Customer can be an indicator of income, self-image, and life-style.

_____ 10. Sarah Routledge is an example of a cagey entrepreneur because she learned how to survive by studying the needs and wants of the marketplace.

_____ 11. A habitual reader of romance fiction is one example of a Heavy User.

_____ 12. The Target Market for _Cosmopolitan_ magazine is predominantly male, 35–45, Master's degree or higher, $42,000 income, living in three metro areas: Los Angeles/San Diego; Seattle/Tacoma; Dallas/Fort Worth.

_____ 13. In the 1980s, we are surrounded by special-interest magazines advertising a host of special-interest products.

_____ 14. If a magazine goes under, one cause might be that, like the Railroads, it forgot what business it was in.

_____ 15. _McCall's_ is _Playboy's_ biggest competition for readers.

_____ 16. One reason to observe people at magazine racks is so you can begin to correlate life-style with reading behavior.

_____ 17. Advertising money is important for a magazine because it pays the bills.

_____ 18. A magazine cover is an important sales tool.

_____ 19. Hugh Hefner created his Target Customer out of thin air and imagination.

_____ 20. One way to begin market research is to start with what you read, listen to, watch, or buy — and then contrast your habits with habits of people from another life-style.

Multiple Choice

Select the best response for each of the following items and enter the corresponding letter in the space provided.

_____ 1. The visionary entrepreneur who built the Playboy Empire from a small business that started on a kitchen table in Chicago was:
a. Mayor Richard Joseph Daley.
b. Lee Iacocca.
c. Hugh Hefner.
d. Ray Kroc.

_____ 2. Which of the following pieces of data doesn't fit the _Playboy_ reader profile?
a. Male, 18–34.
b. Urban/suburban residence.
c. Housewife, five children, Heavy User of romances.
d. Consumer of alcoholic spirits.

_____ 3. Which of the following magazines is probably not vying for the same reader as _McCall's_?
a. _Redbook._
b. _EasyRiders._
c. _Ladies' Home Journal._
d. _Good Housekeeping._

_____ 4. A terrific book that profiles Target Customer is:
a. _Subliminal Seduction._
b. _The Great Gatsby._

    c. *Writing the Natural Way.*

    d. *Guerilla Tactics in the Job Market.*

_____ 5. Which of the following magazines is more special-interest than general interest?

    a. *Colliers.*   c. *Coronet.*

    b. *Look.*   d. *Runner's World.*

_____ 6. The letter from the romance publisher to Sarah Routledge:

    a. was a pink rejection slip.

    b. described a possible Target Reader.

    c. was an agreement to write a dictionary for gourmet cooks.

    d. contained several grammatical errors and misspelled words.

_____ 7. Competition in business can be defined as a situation that arises:

    a. when the world was young and green.

    b. in the Garden of Eden.

    c. when two hungry contestants go after the same slice of marketplace pie.

    d. when everyone leaves the arena.

_____ 8. Which of the following places should you avoid for help in launching a new business?

    a. The SBA.   c. Banks.

    b. SCORE.   d. Get-rich-quick magazine ads.

_____ 9. Which of the following was not a factor in the success of Fred Bowers' soccer shop?

    a. Investors liked his Business Plan.

    b. He knew soccer, had coached it.

    c. After he'd been open awhile, invisible customers began to appear.

    d. The tennis boom bubble burst, and a lot of people became overnight soccer players.

_____ 10. Which of the following questions would give you the least help when you interview potential Target Customers?

    a. How did you like the store?

    b. Look, when I open up a similar (and far superior) place next door, can I count on you to switch your business?

    c. Do you shop here often?

    d. How far did you drive to get here?

Short-Answer Questions

1. List five magazines or periodicals that you read regularly.

    1.   4.

    2.   5.

    3.

2. Ask two friends what magazines they read regularly.

Friend 1   **Friend 2**

    1.

    2.

    3.

    4.

    5.

How can you correlate what your friends read with life-styles and consumption patterns?

_____

_____

_____

_____

3. Select one magazine from your list for a quick market analysis:
   The cover is a sales tool. Describe cover or front page.

   Photo/Art. Layout:

   Words:
   What dominates?
   What attracts?
   What market does the cover or front page appeal to?

   _____

   _____

   _____

   Remember that ads pay for the magazine. Using Chapter 4 of your text as a guide, analyze the ads.
   Age-range of models:
   Dress/clothing:
   Major activity:

   Editorial content will usually support or extend the message of the advertisers. Describe editorial content. Range of topics covered:

   1.

   2.

   3.

   4.

   How does copy relate to ads? _____

   _____

   _____

4. In a list or brief paragraph, describe the life-style of your primary Target Customer. (Questions to get you started: What are your TC's ambitions? Attitudes? Activities? Dreams? Buying habits?) Remember you are trying to get under the skin of your TC.

   _____

   _____

   _____

   _____

   _____

   _____

   _____

5. List five publications probably read by your Target Customer. (Use one of the directories available in your library like *Ulrich's, Ayer's Directory, Standard Rate and Data.*)

   1.

   2.

   3.

   4.

   5.

6. Pay a visit to the market research department of your local newspaper. Tell them you're starting a new business and you're developing your promotion mix. Describe the Target Market you're trying to reach, then ask their market researchers for assistance and advice. Summarize what you learn here.

   _____

   _____

   _____

   _____

   _____

   _____

   _____

   _____

7. Census Bureau Data. Visit the nearest Federal Depository to locate the following information: List 10 items you purchased in the last six months, and then list the SIC Codes of at least five:

   Product   **SIC Code**

   1.

   2.

   3.

   4.

   5.

   6.

   7.

   8.

   9.

   10.

8. Using the latest *Survey of Buying Power* (published by *S & MM* magazine), select an area that would be most likely to contain the target customers for your product or service.

   Area: _____

9. Develop 10 – 15 interview questions you plan to use when you talk to Target Customers. For a start, see the questions from the Julia Gonzales case study in Chapter 4 of your text.

   1. _____

   2. _____

   3. _____

   4. _____

5. _____

6. _____

7. _____

8. _____

9. _____

10. _____

11. _____

12. _____

13. _____

14. _____

15. _____

10. List the names of 3 – 5 Target Customers you interviewed, and in a brief sentence state your conclusions from each interview.

1. _____   _____

   _____

2. _____   _____

   _____

3. _____   _____

   _____

4. _____   _____

   _____

5. _____   _____

   _____

5

Reading the Competition

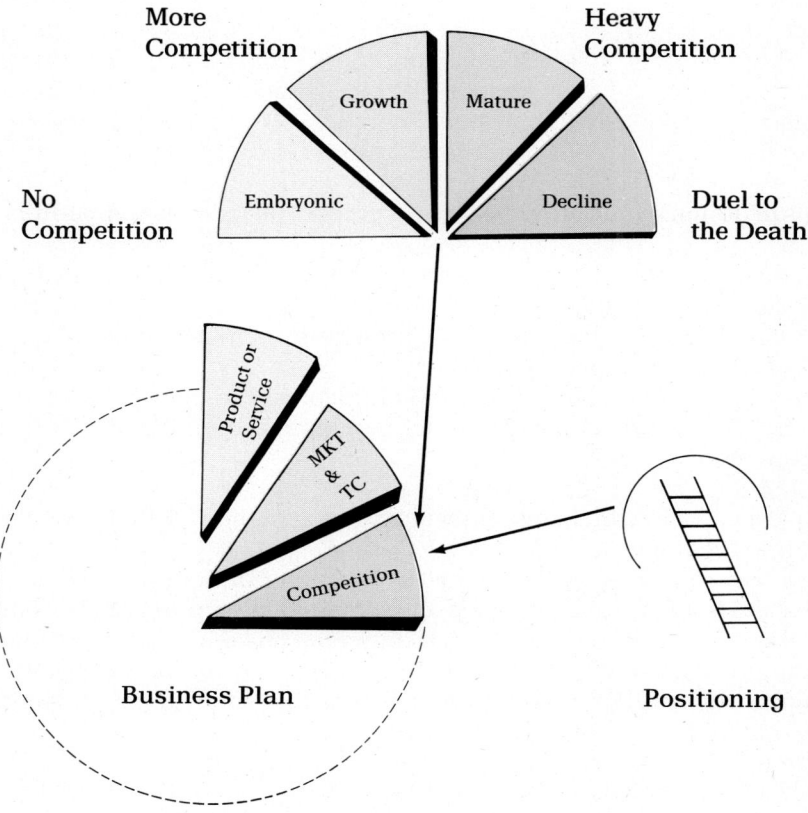

More Competition

Heavy Competition

Growth

Mature

No Competition

Embryonic

Decline

Duel to the Death

Product or Service

MKT & TC

Competition

Business Plan

Positioning

We have started a mind map of how Chapter 5 is helping you read your competition. How would you finish it?

Copyright © 1985 by Harcourt Brace Jovanovich, Inc. All rights reserved.

Objective Questions

Matching

Match each of the following numbered items with the lettered statement that best describes it by entering the number of the item in the space provided.

1. embryo
2. competition
3. Target Customer
4. arena
5. conglomerate
6. stealing customers
7. profit
8. product innovation
9. blind competition
10. decline stage
11. ladder
12. gasoline service station
13. Mystery Shopper
14. maintaining a presence
15. competing with yourself
16. competitor test-matrix
17. changing the arena
18. product differentiation
19. core market
20. positioning

_____ A. a focus of design which attempts to set a product off from its competitors by price, service, or repairs

_____ B. a metaphor for how a Target Customer ranks similar businesses; it also represents your step-by-step journey to the top

_____ C. a tool which allows you to rank your competitors in a number of areas including image, location, innovation, and flexibility

_____ D. establishing a ladder inside the mind of the prospect, or Target Customer

_____ E. when transforming a product or service by adding a simple benefit also transforms the nature of competition

_____ F. first stage of a business life cycle

_____ G. a heated contest in which the combatants have lost their ability to see clearly while they seek to destroy the other

_____ H. a fancy way of saying you've kept your image in front of the customer

_____ I. involves two steps: 1) you develop a first-class quality product; 2) when competitors smell money and try to penetrate your market with a cheapie, you've got one ready to ship

_____ J. an example of a service business in the mature stage of the life cycle

_____ K. a disguise adopted by cagey entrepreneurs as they study their competitors

_____ L. a form of technical breakthrough

_____ M. time to leave the arena

_____ N. one of your main reasons for being in business

_____ O. the person most likely to buy your product or service

_____ P. what ensues when two or more hungry combatants go after the same narrow slice of the marketplace pie

_____ Q. consumers whose perceived needs best fit the characteristics of a product

_____ R. a giant company composed of many diverse businesses

_____ S. a strategy for surviving in the mature stage of the life cycle

_____ T. a metaphorical battleground where business contests occur

True – False

Determine whether each of the following statements is true or false and enter a T (True) or F (False) in the space provided.

_____ 1. Competition is not affected in any way by the four-stage life-cycle.

_____ 2. Product innovation is not important enough for top management to worry about.

_____ 3. If you choose a business in the mature stage, you're going to have to steal more customers than you would have to steal in the growth stage.

_____ 4. There is more competition in the embryonic stage than in all of the other stages put together.

_____ 5. There has never been a business venture started over alcoholic beverages at lunchtime.

_____ 6. The team which developed skates for ducks was unbalanced by having too many technical people and engineers.

_____ 7. Pricing is very easy to establish in the embryonic stage.

_____ 8. The reason production runs get longer in the mature stage is because business owners want to take full advantage of capital equipment and experienced management.

_____ 9. If you spend dollars on advertising in the growth stage, and then can't follow up with distribution (getting the product to the consumer), you're going to lose sales and credibility.

_____ 10. In the embryonic stage, resellers and distributors clamor for your products.

_____ 11. One good way to promote is through contests.

_____ 12. Smaller firms rarely win price wars.

_____ 13. One signal that a product is in the mature stage occurs when manufacturers bring out several variations.

_____ 14. A faddish product can reach the decline stage in 90 days.

_____ 15. When a product such as rocking chairs enters the decline stage, there still might be opportunities for small entrepreneurs who sell to the core market.

_____ 16. A helpful definition for positioning is "establishing a ladder in the mind of the customer."

_____ 17. One good way of dealing with your competitors is to study their operations while you probe for strengths you can neutralize and weaknesses you can exploit.

_____ 18. If you're going into an industry in which you don't have much experience, your best strategy for disarming the competition is to dive in and scare them with the force of your splash.

_____ 19. When researching your competition, helpful tools include a camera and a map of the area.

_____ 20. Competing with your own products by developing Cheap Product B is dishonest.

Multiple Choice

Select the best response for each of the following items and enter the corresponding letter in the space provided.

_____ 1. The book that goes into detail about ladders in the mind of the customer or prospect is:
  a. *Guerilla Tactics in the Job Market*.
  b. *Nine American Lifestyles*.
  c. *Positioning: The Battle for Your Mind*.
  d. *The Third Wave*.

_____ 2. Which of the following is not a smart competitive strategy?
  a. Packing expensive lenses in popcorn.
  b. Being ready with Cheap Product B to follow Quality Product A.
  c. Changing the arena by product innovation.
  d. Fighting to the bitter end, to the final gasp of the decline stage.

_____ 3. A competitor test-matrix will help you to get a fix on:
  a. Image.
  b. Location.
  c. Flexibility.
  d. All of the above.

_____ 4. Which of the following is not a sound strategy for disarming the competition?
  a. Do it better.
  b. Treat your TCs like people.
  c. Do it faster.
  d. Start a price war the day you throw open your doors.

_____ 5. The arena that shifts a huge market can be the size of a:
  a. Quarter.
  b. TV screen.

c. Micro-chip.

d. All of the above.

_____ 6. Competing with yourself in business means:

a. you've got Cheap Product B ready to throw into the arena.

b. you wait for the decline stage before you advertise.

c. you argue with yourself about the 4 P's.

d. you enjoy playing both sides of the chessboard at once

_____ 7. If you're planning on opening a gasoline service station, you'll be in which stage of the life-cycle?

a. Embryo.

b. Growth.

c. Mature.

d. Decline.

_____ 8. Which of the following is not likely to occur in the embryo stage?

a. Not much competition.

b. Complete product acceptance.

c. Limited distribution.

d. Experimental pricing.

_____ 9. If you advertise your product, and get the TCs panting for it, and your distribution channels are not ready, what's likely to happen?

a. The competition will hold off shipping until you're ready.

b. Potential customers will keep clippings and videotapes of your ads and keep calling the retailers to check on availability.

c. You're going to lose sales and credibility.

d. Chase Manhattan will offer you an interest-free line of credit until you get your machinery rolling.

_____ 10. In what two stages of the life-cycle is your core market likely to be most visible?

a. Embryo, growth.

b. Growth, maturity.

c. Embryo, decline.

d. Maturity, decline.

Short-Answer Questions

1. Now you've got a good idea where your business will be on the life-cycle chart. Some segments of your business may be in different stages. For example, if you were to open a record store, you'd have 8-track tapes in decline, LPs in late maturity, cassettes in high growth, and video holograms on floating laser-driven bubble chips in the embryonic stage. Use the life-cycle chart below. Segment the various phases of your business and position each in its proper slot.

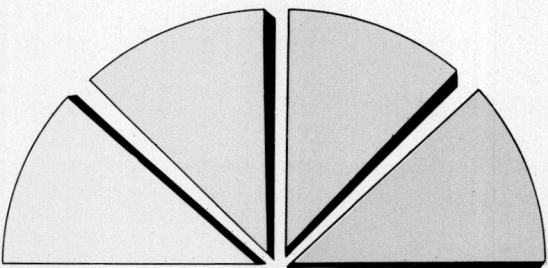

2. List three competitors you think will be tough for you to handle.

1. _____

2. _____

3. _____

3. Develop an analytical stance on each competitor. View them first from the outside. Then move inside. (In the next step, these notes will be transferred to your competitor test-matrix.)

Competitor A — from the outside
   Name:
   Location:
   Geographic proximity to market:
   Parking:
   Image
      perceived by you:
      perceived by TC:
      perceived by neighbors:
   Advertising:

If this were your business, and you had unlimited funds, what changes would you make?

_____

_____

_____

_____

Competitor A — from the inside
   Layout:
   Service:
   Atmosphere:
   Quality of merchandise:
   Cleanliness:
   Perceived sales volume:
   Pricing:

(What changes would you make?) _____

_____

_____

_____

Competitor B — from the outside
   Name:
   Location:
   Geographic proximity to market:
   Parking:
   Image
      perceived by you:
      perceived by TC:
      perceived by neighbors:
   Advertising:

If this were your business, and you had unlimited funds, what changes would you make?

_____

_____

_____

_____

Competitor B — from the inside
   Layout:
   Service:
   Atmosphere:
   Quality of merchandise:
   Cleanliness:
   Perceived sales volume:
   Pricing:

(What changes would you make?) _____

_____

_____

Competitor C — from the outside
   Name:
   Location:
   Geographic proximity to market:
   Parking:
   Image
      perceived by you:
      perceived by TC:
      perceived by neighbors:
   Advertising:

If this were your business, and you had unlimited funds, what changes would you make?

_____

_____

_____

_____

Competitor C — from the inside
   Layout:
   Service:
   Atmosphere:
   Quality of merchandise:
   Cleanliness:
   Perceived sales volume:
   Pricing:

(What changes would you make?) _____

_____

_____

_____

Name of Competitor	Location	Proximity to market	Parking	Image (you)	Image (TC)	Image (neighbors)	Advertising	Layout	Service	Atmosphere	Quality of merchandise	Cleanliness	Perceived sales volume	Pricing
A														
B														
C														
D														
E														
F														

Use this competitor test-matrix to compress the data from Short-Answer Question 3.

4. Use the competitor test-matrix provided on page SG-41 to compress the data from Question 3 into numbers on a 1 – 10 scale.

5. Networking your way in. Who do you know who knows someone who can give you inside information on your competition? Banker? Stock-broker? Librarian? List possibilities here.

   1.

   2.

   3.

6. Changing the arena. Once you study your competitors, you may have to make only one improvement to change the arena, thereby disarming your competition. Example 1: A manufacturer of baby bedding discovered that his competitors were slow on deliveries. By speeding up his own deliveries, he won the admiration of his customers. Example 2: An entrepreneur saw an increase in the number of two wage-earners per household, so he developed a door-to-door cleaning service. Again, delivery was the key. Example 3: At this writing, Hallmark has pilot stores testing the marketing of office products. Hallmark looked at the competition, discovered that most office stores were angled at the male buyer. A high percentage of office products, however, are bought by women (secretaries, managers, other professionals), so Hallmark is moving into that market.
   How will you change your arena? _____

   _____

   _____

7. Pretend you had unlimited funds. What's the wildest idea you can think of for disarming your competition? Mind map your thought processes here.

Promotion: Making that Customer Connection

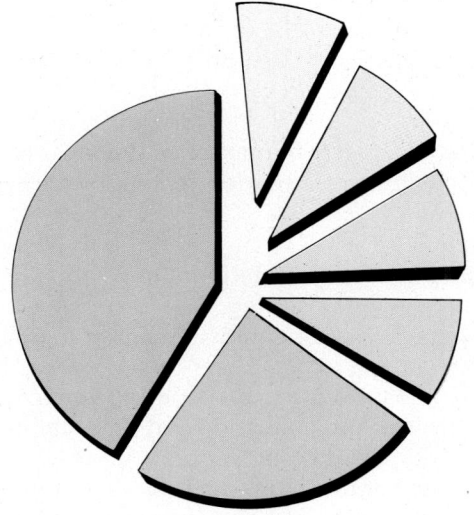

Draw a mind map showing how you plan to make your customer connection.

Objective Questions

Matching

Match each of the following numbered items with the lettered statement that best describes it by entering the number of the item in the space provided.

1. P-O-P display
2. trade show
3. personal selling
4. promotional mix
5. freebies
6. piggy back
7. co-op advertising
8. direct mail
9. free ink
10. news conference
11. grand opening
12. mailing list broker
13. Big Spender List
14. Lead Club
15. Chamber of Commerce

_____ A. All the elements that you blend to maximize the most effective communication to your TC
_____ B. they can grab your customer's attention, create interest in a new product, or allow you to gather market research
_____ C. should act as a silent sales clerk
_____ D. ties local promotional activities to national or regional advertising efforts
_____ E. can be a very expensive way of selling
_____ F. a place where denizens of the same industry gather to present their products and services to one another
_____ G. advertising costs are subsidized by participating vendors
_____ H. promotes local businesses and statewide and national business legislation
_____ I. a group of business and professional people who meet regularly to exchange sales clues
_____ J. a good way to keep track of those few customers that give you a big share of your business
_____ K. using the mail to attract individual customers
_____ L. print media attention — usually in response to effective news releases and personal cultivation
_____ M. firms who will sell you names of potential customers who fit your target market profile
_____ N. the big bang event to herald your arrival in the marketplace
_____ O. calling in members of the media to communicate a newsworthy event

True – False

Determine whether each of the following statements is true or false and enter a T (True) or F (False) in the space provided.

_____ 1. A contest drawing is a really easy way to build your mailing list.
_____ 2. Magazines will often rent you their subscriber lists.
_____ 3. Trade shows display your product or service in a high-intensity way.
_____ 4. The owner of a small firm is often its most effective salesperson.
_____ 5. If you listen, your target customers will tell you what it takes to induce them to buy.
_____ 6. The first step to gaining free ink (free publicity) is to probe your business and find something newsworthy.
_____ 7. Success in direct mail depends upon how well you have defined your target market.
_____ 8. P-O-P displays are usually very expensive.
_____ 9. Promotion is a pure science, and may be handled with numbers and rules.
_____ 10. A good ad will gain both the attention and interest of the target customer.
_____ 11. A smaller ad is likely to get lost on a page.

_____ 12. Newspapers often offer special supplements at reduced cost. The offer often includes free editorial copy.

_____ 13. A highly visible owner is often the best form of promotion.

_____ 14. Effective advertising is expensive, but you always get what you pay for.

_____ 15. Vendors often furnish tear sheets free of charge.

_____ 16. Leads Clubs are made up of people from the same profession, business, or industry.

Multiple Choice

Select the best response for each of the following items and enter the corresponding letter in the space provided.

_____ 1. Market Research is:
   a. asking your customers what they think.
   b. analyzing census data in the library.
   c. reviewing and analyzing appropriate secondary information.
   d. all of the above.

_____ 2. Promotion is:
   a. clawing you way up the corporate ladder.
   b. advancing one idea over another.
   c. all the things that you do to communicate your business message to your potential customers.
   d. limited to personal selling and paid advertising.

_____ 3. Display advertising is easy to spot because it is:
   a. usually sold by the column inch or fraction of a page.
   b. something that is put in your shop window.
   c. less graphic than classified advertising.
   d. most effective for products that require that they be in motion for demonstration purposes.

_____ 4. Point-of-purchase displays:
   a. always match your merchandising scheme.
   b. are silent salespeople.
   c. are never free.
   d. are primarily available to customers in the industrial and government markets.

_____ 5. Cooperative advertising:
   a. is usually more expensive than other forms of advertising.
   b. is always based on the national ad rate.
   c. rarely is subsidized by the vendor.
   d. none of the above.

_____ 6. A winning promotional mix:
   a. is the most effective blend of all elements to reach the target customer.
   b. consists of product development, distribution channels, and the four P's.
   c. is the same as the product mix, only with more flair.
   d. should be blended carefully to nullify the impact of random consumer perception.

_____ 7. A press kit should:
   a. include photographs of principals, the facility, and the product or service in use.
   b. relate newsworthy facts about the firm.
   c. be presented in an attractive folder to influential representatives of the media.
   d. all of the above.

_____ 8. Coupons:
   a. give you positive feedback on your promotion.
   b. should have an expiration date and multiple use disclaimers.

———   c. should be coded to identify the source and tested in small quantities before major use.
               d. all of the above.
———   9. Direct mail:
               a. is most effective when the potential customers are few in number and can be accurately located.
               b. must have a nine-digit zip code address.
               c. needs a response of at least 50% to justify its use.
               d. is the least sophisticated form of communication with your customers.
———   10. Commission sales representatives:
               a. are a fixed business cost.
               b. require no training or field assistance.
               c. should always be avoided because they lack motivation.
               d. none of the above.

Short-Answer Questions

1. Study the list in Chapter 6 on "The Right Promotional Mix," and then list three to five components of your promotional strategy.

   _____

   _____

   _____

   _____

2. Clip or copy three to five articles that got free ink for a small business in your area. List the titles below.

   1.

   2.

   3.

   4.

   5.

3. Free ink/free air (publicity) can save you a lot of advertising dollars. On a separate sheet of paper, use a mind map or list to brainstorm ways you can get free ink for your business.

4. A trade show can be important to your business. List the upcoming trade shows in your area. (Helpful hint: you can get information from trade associations and local convention centers; from *Exhibit Schedule,* published by Successful Meetings, 1422 Chestnut Street, Philadelphia, PA 19102; and from *Trade Show Convention Guide,* Budd Publications, Box 7, New York, NY 10004.

   _____

   _____

   _____

5. **At the Show.** What devices are people using to gather primary data on their potential customers?

   _____

   _____

   _____

   _____

6. **At the Show.** Look around. What surprised you?

_____

_____

_____

_____

7. **At the Show.** On a separate sheet of paper, draw a rough diagram of the main floor. Enter the names of exhibitors. Label eating areas, restrooms, entrances, exits. Then use arrows to indicate traffic flow. Where is the most traffic?

8. List three trade associations that deal with firms in your industry and in your market area that might be helpful to you:

_____

_____

_____

9. Develop two techniques for building a mailing list for a retail business:

1. _____

_____

_____

2. _____

_____

_____

10. List three sources that will help you do secondary market research:

1. _____

2. _____

3. _____

11. Finish this sentence: Proprietors of small firms are usually effective in the selling function because

_____

_____

_____

12. List three actions you can take to enhance your personal profile and call attention to your business:

1. _____

2. _____

3. _____

13. List three media kit sources that contain information on at least one segment of your market:

1. _____

2. _____

3. _____

14. What three ways can a map help you conduct market research?

1. _____

2. _____

3. _____

15. List three government agencies and/or public utilities that might have information on the projected growth of an area:

    1. _____

    2. _____

    3. _____

16. Describe how a Sales Leads Club works: _____

    _____

    _____

    _____

17. Brainstorm one crazy or off-the-wall promotion that would be appropriate for your business:

    _____

    _____

    _____

    _____

18. Rough out a promotional budget. Try to list your promotional tools (advertising, free ink, contest, direct mail, etc.) in priority order and estimate what each would cost.

    Tool   **Cost**

    1.

    2.

    3.

    4.

    5.

19. After you rough out your promotional budget, write down the first step you need to take to get things

    rolling: _____

    _____

    _____

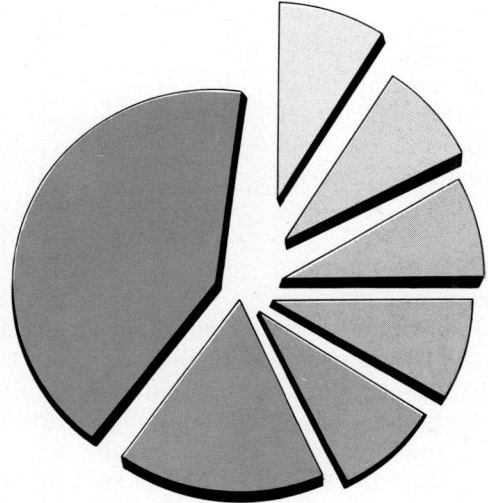

Draw a mind map of your search for your 100% location.

Objective Questions

Matching

Match each of the following numbered items with the lettered statement that best describes it by entering the number of the item in the space provided.

1. anchor tenant
2. food store
3. gross lease
4. 100% location
5. master plan
6. security factors
7. triple net lease
8. signage
9. census tracts
10. lease with option to purchase
11. cost per square foot
12. zoning
13. CC & Rs
14. traffic counts
15. labor pool
16. footprint
17. local newspapers

_____ A. One type of destination location
_____ B. major foot traffic draw for customers
_____ C. usually provided by police departments and insurance companies
_____ D. sign requirements and where sign may be placed
_____ E. useful to ensure rights of occupancy at the discretion of the tenant
_____ F. how monthly rent is often quoted on commercial or industrial buildings
_____ G. U.S. government data on demographics of a specific area
_____ H. a projected plan for growth or redevelopment of specific land use
_____ I. fixed rent without additional assessments
_____ J. mythical perfect site—a useful benchmark
_____ K. tenant can be charged for taxes, insurance, improvements in addition to base rental
_____ L. often a source of recent market data in specific areas
_____ M. covers conditions and restrictions that are a part of the deed
_____ N. how much space a building takes up on the lot
_____ O. provided by the department of highways or independent research firms
_____ P. regulation for use, policed by city or county government
_____ Q. available workers often listed by occupation

True–False

Determine whether each of the following statements is true or false and enter a T (True) or F (False) in the space provided.

_____ 1. A 100% location is mythical and probably doesn't exist.
_____ 2. A good location is more important for a brand new business than for an existing one.
_____ 3. A plumbing service business does not require a high traffic location.
_____ 4. A manufacturing business might play it smarter to locate near raw materials and a labor pool than near its customers.
_____ 5. A small retail merchant does not need to worry about drawing traffic generated by nearby stores.
_____ 6. Part of your location consideration should be to check on the level of municipal services.
_____ 7. If you have a great business, your customers will always find you.
_____ 8. High visibility can save you some advertising dollars.
_____ 9. Business locations have life cycles.
_____ 10. Real estate leasing agents are expensive, and you should do your best to avoid them.

_____ 11. An anchor tenant is found most commonly in boatyards.

_____ 12. Highway departments frequently do traffic flow studies.

_____ 13. Most local planning agencies will let you view their master plan for an area.

_____ 14. Public utility companies have no need to do long-range planning activities on population growth and energy needs.

_____ 15. Once you settle on your location, there is no need for you to double-check with municipal authorities on restrictions and land use.

_____ 16. Leases are drawn by landlords and their lawyers and there is little in a lease to protect the tenant.

_____ 17. The smartest way to break a lease is to throw a gigantic and obnoxious lease-breaking party.

_____ 18. Net and gross leases are exactly the same except that a gross lease is much less expensive.

_____ 19. A good lease, like a good contract, is fair to both parties and tells each what to expect from the other.

_____ 20. Newspapers and chambers of commerce have useful information on local markets.

Multiple Choice

Select the best response for each of the following items and enter the corresponding letter in the space provided.

_____ 1. A good example of a destination location is:
   a. a food store or doctor's office.
   b. a gift shop specializing in china.
   c. a flower shop.
   d. usually marked in red on your city map.

_____ 2. Gross leases are:
   a. usually based on cost per square yard.
   b. agreements that include everything in the monthly rate.
   c. less common today than in the 1970s.
   d. to make rent a variable cost for the tenant.

_____ 3. Generally speaking, a 100% location:
   a. has no competition within a ten-mile radius.
   b. costs twice as much as a 50% location.
   c. is the perfect place for your business.
   d. must be visible from the street.

_____ 4. A mall location:
   a. has more foot traffic.
   b. has the most restrictions.
   c. usually comes with a fixed plus percentage of sales rate.
   d. all of the above.

_____ 5. The best location:
   a. is away from all competition.
   b. is always the least expensive place for your business.
   c. makes you accessible to customers, suppliers, workers, transportation, and so on.
   d. demands a sharp building, expensively maintained and well-lighted for security reasons.

_____ 6. A gift shop, to be successful:
   a. needs to be close to high-traffic anchor retailers.
   b. is a destination location.
   c. will do well near hardware stores.
   d. will usually be leased on an industrial net basis.

_____ 7. A labor pool:
   a. is a place for workers to relax during inclement weather.
   b. is termed illegal under the Taft-Hartley Act.

      c. will affect the location of a manufacturing firm more than a service firm.

      d. is seldom a concern in a high-income area.

_____ 8. A cost of living cap or ceiling on the rent:

      a. will be of little help if hyperinflation occurs.

      b. will limit your annual rent increase.

      c. is standard on most commercial leases.

      d. tends to favor the landlord.

_____ 9. Restrictive covenants:

      a. are discriminatory and illegal.

      b. dictate what you can not do to a tenant.

      c. should be read and understood before you sign your lease.

      d. both a and b.

_____ 10. The commercial lease:

      a. is a standard legal form and, by statute cannot be modified.

      b. is designed by the building owner to protect the owner's interest.

      c. need not be shown to a prospective tenant's legal counsel because it has already been drawn up by a competent attorney and all lawyers are members of the same bar.

      d. is usually no more binding than the lease signed by apartment dwellers.

Short-Answer Questions

1. List the elements of a 100% location for your business:

_____

_____

_____

_____

2. List five kinds of businesses that are destination locations. Then list five that are not:

Destination Locations	**Not Destination Locations**
1. _____	1. _____
2. _____	2. _____
3. _____	3. _____
4. _____	4. _____
5. _____	5. _____

3. On a separate sheet of paper, make a rough drawing of your ideal site location in a commercial or industrial center. In your drawing, label the anchor tenant, your potential neighbors if there's a vacant building you're looking at, competitors (if any), parking (count the slots available to you), access, traffic, peak hours. If you're looking at a specific building, focus on suitability. For example, would you want a hearing aid store next to a record store? A book shop next to an auto body shop? Will your customers need a map to find you?

4. Develop a ranking of commercial or industrial centers in your area and arrange in order of priority (which is best for your firm?).

1. _____

2. _____

3. _____

4. _____

5. Information on local crime rates can be obtained from:

_____

6. Information on local labor pools can be obtained from:

_____

7. List variables that need to be weighed when you're considering certain types of leases:

    _____   _____

    _____   _____

    _____   _____

    _____   _____

    _____   _____

8. A high visibility location could save you money that would normally be spent on:

_____

9. List three ways you can determine the going market rate of a square foot of space in your area:

    1. _____

    2. _____

    3. _____

10. How much parking space will you need? At what times of day can you anticipate peak parking needs?
    Space:
    Peak needs:

11. Locations, like people and products and industries, go through life cycles. Where is your location on the life-cycle yardstick?

12. In what ways does the location affect a firm's image?

_____

_____

_____

_____

13. For your type of business, list some advantages of being
    1. Close to competitors:

_____

_____

_____

2. Away from competitors:

_____

_____

_____

14. A mature business might have less need for a 100% location. Explain.

_____

_____

15. A lease that allows the landlord to charge tenants for taxes, insurance, and improvements is often

called a _____ lease.

16. A lease that calls for a fixed rate of rent per month is often called a _____

lease.

17. An anchor tenant adds value to your location because:

_____

18. A CPI cap in a lease accomplishes the following:

_____

_____

_____

19. Only the following will legally release you from the obligations of a lease:

_____

_____

_____

Surprises You Can't Afford

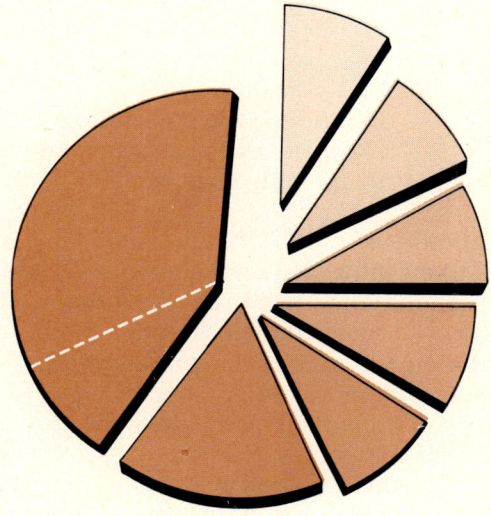

Draw a mind map of what surprises could affect your business and how you will protect yourself against them.

Objective Questions

Matching

Match each of the following numbered items with the lettered statement that best describes it by entering the number of the item in the space provided.

1. fringe benefits
2. partnerships
3. CC & Rs
4. workers disability insurance
5. opportunity cost
6. specific business experience
7. energy audit
8. fidelity bond

9. licenses, police permit
10. building inspector
11. flood, fire, earthquake, and so on
12. misuse of product
13. shrinkage
14. huge increases in the prime rate
15. major supplier going out of business
16. penalty clause

_____ A. have a high dissolution rate
_____ B. other payroll costs, like health plans, vacations, sick days, FICA
_____ C. covenants and restrictions contained in the deed that limit the use of real estate
_____ D. additional business cost, required in most states
_____ E. specific investment costs in terms of time and capital
_____ F. what creditors look for first in an entrepreneur
_____ G. insurance to protect you from dishonest employees
_____ H. supplied by most power companies
_____ I. although a nuisance, are there to protect you and the community
_____ J. may be required by city, county and state agencies before you open your doors
_____ K. will force contractors to finish job on schedule
_____ L. is a strong argument for secondary sources of supply
_____ M. should be factored into costs
_____ N. can become the problem of the manufacturer
_____ O. can eat your profit with high debt cost
_____ P. can be insured against

True–False

Determine whether each of the following statements is true or false and enter a T (True) or F (False) in the space provided.

_____ 1. It is better not to seek permission from building inspectors, because they'll just get in your hair and cause you tons of grief.
_____ 2. State and local controls are always in the best interests of small business.
_____ 3. Start-up costs for most small businesses usually run 47% under owner estimates.
_____ 4. A personal financial statement is a balance sheet.
_____ 5. Assets minus liabilities equal net worth.
_____ 6. People who keep a personal budget usually have less trouble understanding cash management.
_____ 7. Timing is a key planning ingredient.
_____ 8. Good planning includes a long list of what-ifs and optional strategies for dealing with changing circumstances.
_____ 9. An entrepreneur is as likely to underestimate the amount of time required to set up a small business as he is the amount of capital required.
_____ 10. Most entrepreneurs fail to calculate the true value of the time they invest in their firms.

———— 11. Job benefits for employees rarely exceed 10% of salary.

———— 12. Any new business is automatically exempted from Social Security (FICA) payments during its first 12 months of operation.

———— 13. Small businesses are more likely to be embezzled by dishonest employees than larger firms.

———— 14. It is much safer to have one giant customer than it is to nickel and dime yourself to death with a lot of smaller customers.

———— 15. Planning is a day-to-day matter because even the near term is impossible to anticipate.

Multiple Choice

Select the best response for each of the following items and enter the corresponding letter in the space provided.

———— 1. A personal financial statement:
   a. is a balance sheet.
   b. is totally unlike the financial statement of a business.
   c. often includes Goodwill.
   d. is seldom required if the owner is guaranteeing the debts of the firm.

———— 2. Public utility companies:
   a. usually request advance deposits.
   b. can help you estimate your bills.
   c. will tell you how to save energy.
   d. all of the above.

———— 3. City Hall:
   a. has no enforcement power if you violate city codes.
   b. will tell you what special permits are required for your business.
   c. is full of fools who have an interest only in stopping you from making a living.
   d. will never be influenced by other established businesses who don't want to see you open.

———— 4. Your first estimate of monthly expenses:
   a. will probably be lower than the real amount spent.
   b. will not be necessary, because estimating is a foolish waste of time (future profits are guaranteed to protect any overspending that occurs).
   c. will probably be much higher than you had planned.
   d. need not include minor details like office equipment and supplies.

———— 5. Advertising expenses:
   a. will be most needed in your early months of operation.
   b. should be divided equally among all available media.
   c. should be placed under the firm control of a major advertising agency.
   d. should be adjusted downward if sales lag.

———— 6. An insurance agent can provide you with the following types of protection:
   a. employee fidelity bond.
   b. partnership insurance.
   c. fire, theft, and liability.
   d. All of the above.

———— 7. Your competitors:
   a. will always treat you fairly.
   b. will do all they can to keep you from getting their customers.
   c. will shop you for weaknesses.
   d. B and C.

———— 8. The best way to minimize surprises is to:
   a. have lots of business experience.
   b. stay on top of your accounting reports.

        c. read trade journals, newspapers; attend trade shows.
        d. all of the above.
_____   9. Which of the following will help you identify missing inventory?
        a. Color coding.
        b. Weekly lie detector test for employees.
        c. Regular body search; regular inspection of employee homes.
        d. Frequent and random counting of inventory.
_____ 10. Most inventory shrinkage is caused by:
        a. sophisticated embezzlers.
        b. employees.
        c. organized crime figures.
        d. customers who pilfer.

Short-Answer Questions

1. List the agencies (if any) who will need to inspect or approve your business facility.

   1. _____   4. _____

   2. _____   5. _____

   3. _____   6. _____

2. Contact your local planning and zoning departments to learn what ordinances you will have to follow.
   Briefly note what you learn here: _____
   _____
   _____
   _____
   _____

3. When you interviewed small business owners (see Action Step 6), what unforeseen surprises did they
   encounter? _____
   _____
   _____

4. Contact your local public utility for a forecast of increased energy costs for the next five to ten years.
   Request energy-saving guidelines for your small business. Summarize the guidelines here.
   _____
   _____
   _____
   _____
   _____

5. List other investment options you could pursue with your money if you did not begin your own
   business. _____
   _____
   _____

6. Since you're thinking about starting your own business, devise an audit of your time for a realistic idea of how much time and energy you have to invest. Here's how. Use a two week period. In a separate notebook, divide each day into 15-minute slots. For two weeks, write down what you did every 15 minutes. Start with the last two hours. What did you do?

   Hour One   **Hour Two**
   1st quarter: _____   1st: _____
   2nd quarter: _____   2nd: _____
   3rd quarter: _____   3rd: _____
   4th quarter: _____   4th: _____

   When you finish your time audit, sit down and study it. Ask yourself what percentage of your time did you have to rest? Do you have the tenacity to do sustained work? Where were you most excited? Where did insights occur?

7. If you're thinking about forming a partnership, list special provisions you need to include in your partnership agreement. (For a probe into this area, see chapter 11, "When Should You Incorporate?")

   _____

   _____

   _____

   _____

   _____

   _____

8. List in priority the possible circumstances that could adversely affect your business.

   1. _____

   2. _____

   3. _____

   4. _____

9. List at least two reasons you should think about bonding your employees. (What circumstances might arise after you didn't bond your employees that would make you wish you had?)

   1. _____

   _____

   2. _____

   _____

10. Contact a security alarm company to discuss your security situation. Then list the systems they recommend for smaller businesses like yours. _____

    _____

    _____

    _____

    (Helpful hint: Before you buy a system, shop for prices.)

11. Identify a backup banker or capital source: _____

    _____

12. What techniques can be employed to evaluate the character and resources of a potential partner? (Helpful hint: to find out whether or not you and your partner are really meshing, see Chapter 12, on building a team.) _____

_____

_____

13. Contact an insurance agent who specializes in small business. On a separate sheet of paper, list the types of coverage you'll need, along with prices for premiums.

14. Contact some vendors and find out what percentage of your sales will be offset by returns of defective goods. Write the percentage down:
    Vendor 1:
    Vendor 2:
    Vendor 3:

15. List the areas where your business might be liable: _____

_____

_____

_____

_____

The Powers of Numerical Projection

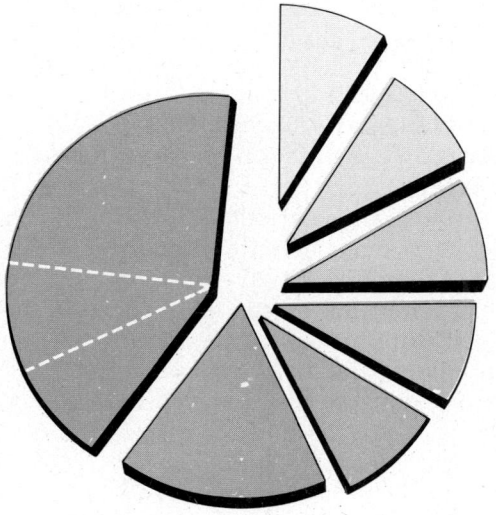

Draw a mind map of how Chapter 9 will help you open doors for your business.

Objective Questions

Matching

Match each of the following numbered items with the lettered statement that best describes it by entering the number of the item in the space provided.

1. turnover
2. projected profit and loss
3. cash-flow projection
4. projected sales forecast
5. return on investment
6. break-even point
7. cost of goods sold
8. fixed expenses
9. extended dating
10. net profit
11. gross profit

_____   A. sales minus cost of goods sold
_____   B. payment terms usually beyond 30 days
_____   C. that point where you make no profit and have no loss
_____   D. gross profit minus expenses
_____   E. anticipated sales for future time periods
_____   F. annual sales divided by average inventory investment
_____   G. how much profit you estimate you will earn
_____   H. the percentage rate of return on the capital invested in the business
_____   I. a projected analysis of working capital needs
_____   J. cost of inventory, including freight
_____   K. type of expenses required just to look like you're in business

True – False

Determine whether each of the following statements is true or false and enter a T (True) or F (False) in the space provided.

_____   1. High markup is usually needed for high-fashion items and items with a slow stock turn rate.
_____   2. For the small business owner, most seasonal purchasing is done 6 – 11 months ahead.
_____   3. Many seasonal vendors will extend credit well into the season.
_____   4. In the travel and printing businesses, it's common practice to collect money before the product or service is delivered.
_____   5. Because of slow receivables, the bed and breakfast business has slow cash flow problems.
_____   6. The quicker you can resupply inventory, the more stock you need to carry.
_____   7. Every business that extends credit should set aside a reserve for bad debt.
_____   8. The manufacturing business has much less need for working capital than a service business of the same magnitude.
_____   9. The only time you need to worry about doing a cash flow projection is when you are profitable every single month.
_____   10. Most trade associations publish information on monthly sales percentages for their members.
_____   11. Cash management means knowing where your cash is, and making sure you use it for maximum efficiency.
_____   12. An accurate sales forecast is one key to developing a winning Business Plan.
_____   13. A projected profit and loss statement will tell you when you're going to start making a profit.
_____   14. When you do project profit and loss, you may also find out what legal form you should choose for your business.
_____   15. One year of sales divided by the average inventory gives you the stock turnover rate.

_____ 16. As a general rule, the higher the stock turn, the higher your anticipated mark-up.

_____ 17. Gross profit minus expenses equals net profit.

_____ 18. No problems in a business are so serious that they can't be solved by giant increases in sales.

_____ 19. If a corporation anticipates a first-year loss, then the founders should consider starting out as a Subchapter S corporation.

_____ 20. Extended dating means a long courtship with your main vendor.

Multiple Choice

Select the best response for each of the following items and enter the corresponding letter in the space provided.

_____ 1. The term _break-even point_ signifies:
   a. piercing the corporate veil.
   b. that period in business which is prior to making a hefty profit.
   c. a theoretical point between profit and loss.
   d. a time when cash flow is equalized.

_____ 2. Extended dating means:
   a. a long courtship between the entrepreneur and one of the target customers.
   b. extended payment terms.
   c. a process used to develop plums for the fresh fruit industry.
   d. none of the above.

_____ 3. Return on investment means:
   a. the percentage of earnings based on amount of investment.
   b. finding lost capital.
   c. dividends paid by a _Fortune_ 500 corporation.
   d. retained earnings.

_____ 4. an income statement projected over months:
   a. traces the flow of cash through the business cycle.
   b. is a snapshot taken at an exact time in a business.
   c. requires an attorney to process it through the court system.
   d. is a moving picture of your business.

_____ 5. A balance sheet:
   a. consists of assets and liabilities.
   b. is very much unlike a personal financial statement.
   c. is no longer required by bankers when you apply for a loan.
   d. develops a finely tuned balance between profit and loss.

_____ 6. Turnover rate refers to:
   a. the timely rotation of dated stock.
   b. a figure you get when you divide annual sales by average inventory.
   c. rolling over bank assets worth more than $50,000.
   d. a ratio that, if reduced, will increase profitability by a specified percentage over the term specified.

_____ 7. Cost of goods sold:
   a. when deducted from sales will yield gross profit.
   b. shows cost less allowances of goods and materials.
   c. minus total expenses equals net profit before taxes.
   d. all of the above.

_____ 8. A cash flow statement:
   a. may include bank loans.
   b. shows total cash available for each month.
   c. allows you to identify cash needs.
   d. all of the above.

_____ 9. The income statement:
   a. tells you when you will make a profit.
   b. is a financial snap shot.
   c. gives you the net profit before taxes.
   d. both B and C.

_____ 10. A manufacturing business:
   a. is not capital intensive.
   b. will probably need cash for a long period of time.
   c. will have fewer cash flow problems than a bed and breakfast operation.
   d. none of the above.

Short-Answer Questions

1. Project your sales percentages by the month for a 12-month period for a model business in your industry. For example, if the model business does 3% in January, you write 3% in the box. What's the percentage in February? In March?

   Jan. _____ %   Apr. _____ %   July _____ %   Oct. _____ %
   Feb. _____ %   May _____ %   Aug. _____ %   Nov. _____ %
   Mar. _____ %   June _____ %   Sept. _____ %   Dec. _____ %

2. Which financial projection is the most important and becomes the basis for all other financial projections?

   _____

3. When do you expect to become profitable?

   _____

   At what point would you change the legal form of your business?

   _____

4. What is your industry standard for a stock-turn ratio?

   _____

   What is your source?

   _____

5. What will your average mark-up cost be?

   _____

6. When are your customers most likely to pay for services? Depending on the business, customers pay _before_ delivery, _at time of_ delivery, or _after_ delivery. Find out the payment standards, lags, and so on in your business.

   _____

7. If you offer credit, what percentage might be uncollectible?

   _____

8. List the reasons why you should use written and numbered purchase orders:

   _____

   _____

   _____

   _____

9. Describe accounts receivable.

   _____

   _____

10. Describe accounts payable.

_____

_____

11. Discuss briefly the reasons for using a cash-flow projection.

_____

_____

12. What is a break-even point? How do you determine it? Let's follow one example.
Your fixed expenses are $120,000.
Your variable expenses are $1.07 per unit.
You're selling the gizmo at $3.98 per unit.

$$\text{Break-even point (units)} = \frac{\$120,000}{\$2.91} = 41,237 \text{ (rounded)}$$

To figure break-even sales volume, multiply number or break-even units needed by selling price per unit.

$$41,237 \times \$3.98 = \$ \underline{\hspace{2cm}}$$

13. List three to five ways you can use your income statement.

_____

_____

_____

_____

_____

14. What is an electronic spreadsheet?

_____

_____

15. How are Subchapter S corporations taxed?

_____

_____

Shaking the Money Tree

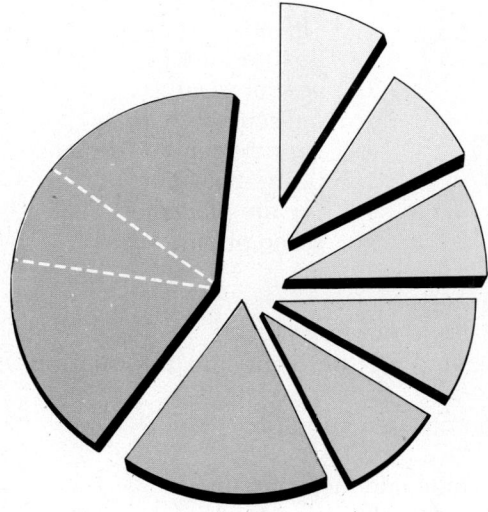

Draw a mind map of how you will go out to shake the money tree for your small business.

Objective Questions

Matching

Match each of the following numbered items with the lettered statement that best describes it by entering the number of the item in the space provided.

1. capital	11. capacity
2. banker	12. collateral
3. bank	13. SBICs
4. guaranteed loan	14. Business Plan
5. money guru	15. vendor form
6. possible source of money	16. unsecured credit
7. accounts receivable financing	17. venture capital firms
8. BDCs	18. limited partner
9. character	19. private placement
10. plastic money	20. going public

_____   A. shows you pay your bills on time
_____   B. one gateway to the world of money
_____   C. showcase for displaying all the ideas and information you've gathered in your venture adventure
_____   D. detailed information on each supplier
_____   E. life insurance
_____   F. provided by some banks and factoring firms
_____   G. knows more about money than you do
_____   H. goal is to increase employment within their specific state
_____   I. licensed by the SBA to provide money to small firms
_____   J. one type of SBA loan
_____   K. lenders who want equity participation
_____   L. regarded by some people as a formidable fortress or great modern cathedral
_____   M. tangible assets that can secure a loan
_____   N. your liquid cash
_____   O. earning power; ability to repay a loan
_____   P. a street-wise name for credit cards
_____   Q. guaranteeing loans and payments with your signature
_____   R. selling your securities in the open financial market
_____   S. investors who are not stockholders, have no liability
_____   T. capital stock sale to a limited group of investors

True – False

Determine whether each of the following statements is true or false and enter a T (True) or F (False) in the space provided.

_____   1. Money creates its own world, with its own customs, rules, myths.
_____   2. "Collateral" indicates that you have a visible money stream for lenders to dip into.
_____   3. Banks are conservative, and they probably won't want to lend you start-up money unless you sign over your house.
_____   4. People lend money to people.
_____   5. One good way to conserve cash is to persuade your customers to give you cash deposits when they place their orders.

_____ 6. When goods are moving slowly, the best strategy is to shelve them in the back room or warehouse and hold until next season.

_____ 7. It is best to avoid collateralizing your loans, unless you have no choice.

_____ 8. When you have to borrow money, you should shop around.

_____ 9. Buying smart is not nearly as important as raising money or selling.

_____ 10. When negotiating, you should use a lot of open-ended questions like: "What else can you do for me?"

_____ 11. When you're ready, it's a good idea to shake the money trees close to home first.

_____ 12. Borrowing on your life insurance can be a good source of money for your new business.

_____ 13. An unsecured personal line of credit from your bank is not a good source of money for a brand-new business.

_____ 14. Credit unions are considered nonbank lending sources.

_____ 15. The SBA has only one kind of loan program: "guaranteed."

_____ 16. The SBA makes fewer guaranteed loans than any other type.

_____ 17. SBICs (Small Business Investment Corporations) are privately operated companies that are licensed by the state within which they operate.

_____ 18. Venture capitalists come in lots of shapes—family firms (Rockefeller), industrial arms (GE), bank arms (B of A), and other arms (private groups of investors).

_____ 19. Venture capitalists will usually let you run the show if you give them a healthy ROI.

_____ 20. How well you buy is not nearly as important as how well you sell.

Multiple Choice

Select the best response for each of the following items and enter the corresponding letter in the space provided.

_____ 1. Before hunting the great money tree, you should:
   a. sit at the feet of a money guru.
   b. sketch out your Business Plan.
   c. befriend a banker, and befriend a backup banker.
   d. All of the above.

_____ 2. All of the following questions are good to ask your prospective banker except:
   a. What do you think of my Business Plan?
   b. Do you lend money to large businesses?
   c. Do you make SBA-guaranteed loans:
   d. What are your criteria for loans?

_____ 3. Which of the following is not a good strategy for dealing with bankers?
   a. Asking for money before you ask for advice and information.
   b. Luring a banker to your own turf.
   c. Negotiating for your line of credit or your loan while you're still working.
   d. Getting yourself a backup bank while you're negotiating with another bank.

_____ 4. Which of the following is not a good tip on saving?
   a. Work out of your home.
   b. Lease your equipment.
   c. Borrow money on goods (inventory) that aren't selling.
   d. Get your landlord to make onsite improvements and finance the cost over the term of the lease.

_____ 5. Which of the following items do you want to ask for on your Vendor Form?
   a. Amount of minimum purchase.
   b. Terms of dating or extended payment.
   c. Nearest competitor handling the same line.
   d. All of the above.

_____ 6. All of the following are reasons why lenders would want to lend you money for your business except:
   a. no competition.
   b. good marketing strategy.
   c. good profit picture.
   d. good ROI (return on investment).

_____ 7. Which of the following is not a good tip on saving?
   a. Use as little commercial space as you can.
   b. Keep your liquid cash in a safe place (like a lock box).
   c. Shop nonbank lenders.
   d. Look into R & D partnerships for product development funds.

_____ 8. The following are good sources of money for your new business, except:
   a. refinancing your car, boat, camper, or airplane.
   b. researching your assets (coin collections, old baseball cards, and so on).
   c. selling that crummy stock you've been holding.
   d. finding a competitor that's doing a good deal of business and borrowing from him.

_____ 9. Which of the following is not a good source of money for your small business?
   a. Venture capital firm.
   b. Stock brokerage house.
   c. Goodwill Industries.
   d. Credit union.

_____ 10. In 1982, the SBA began a program to award grants to high-tech firms for research. The first-year grants have a ceiling of:
   a. $25,000.
   b. $50,000.
   c. $75,000.
   d. $100,000.

Short-Answer Questions

1. Visit your local bank. Find out the following:
   A. Name of chief officer:

   _____

   B. Do they lend money to small businesses? _____

   C. Do they make SBA-guaranteed loans? _____

      1. If yes, do they lend money to start-ups? _____

      2. If yes, do they have a minimum and maximum loan amount? _____

      3. If yes, what are the time-periods for repayment?

         _____

      4. If yes, what's the percentage rate? _____
   D. What are their criteria for loan approval?

      _____

      _____

      _____

   E. Ask them to describe the loan approval process.

F. Do they offer lines of credit and if so under what conditions and what terms?

_____

_____

_____

G. Ask this question: "Would you review my business plan?"

Answer: _____

2. Now that you have found one bank that makes small business loans, phone some more until you locate two or three that make loans to start-ups.

Backup Bank 1

A. Name of bank: _____

B. Lending rate: _____

C. SBA-guaranteed loans: _____

D. Name of contact in bank: _____

Backup Bank 2

A. Name of bank: _____

B. Lending rate: _____

C. SBA-guaranteed loans: _____

D. Name of contact in bank: _____

Backup Bank 3

A. Name of bank: _____

B. Lending rate: _____

C. SBA-guaranteed loans: _____

D. Name of contact in bank: _____

3. When talking to bankers, try to get insight into how their various banks evaluate small business loans. Try these questions for probes:
A. What types of businesses are they most interested in?

_____

_____

B. Are there any they won't lend money to?

_____

_____

C. Ask your banker to rate each of the items below in relation to the loan-decision process. What's important? What's not important? Try to get your banker to use a 1–10 scale.
1. target customer
2. amount and type of competition
3. industry trends
4. product or service
5. marketing strategy
6. method of selling
7. profit picture, both gross and net
8. return on investment

9. founders team
10. personal assets or net worth

4. List friends or relatives who might be willing to invest in your business (or lend you money for the business):

_____

_____

_____

_____

5. Explore your list in Question 4, above. Select two or three people from that list to talk to. Let them see your Business Plan. Talk over the possibilities of getting them on board as investors.
   A. On a separate sheet of paper, list all their objections.
   B. Then list their positive comments.
   C. For each objection, come up with a solution. There's a good chance you'll get the same objections from bankers and venture capital people. On your sheet of paper, summarize your findings as shown:

Objection	Solution
1.	1.
2.	2.
3.	3.
etc.	etc.

6. Let's have some fun. If you're in a class, form several teams. If you're not in a class, get together some friends and relatives. Develop two lists. The first list contains the areas the federal government should get out of. The second list contains areas where the government could be of more help. Compile your findings, vote on the major suggestions and compose a class letter to your congressman, state senator, legislator, assemblyman, alderman, senator, or other representative.

   A. List areas where the government could be of more help:

   1. _____
   2. _____
   3. _____
   4. _____
   5. _____
   6. _____
   7. _____
   8. _____
   9. _____
   10. _____

   B. List areas the government should get out of:

   1. _____
   2. _____
   3. _____
   4. _____
   5. _____
   6. _____

7. _____

8. _____

9. _____

10. _____

When Should You Incorporate?

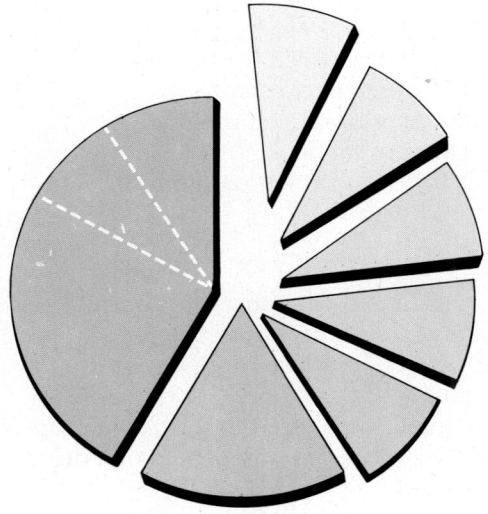

Draw a mind map charting the future of the legal status of your small business.

Objective Questions

Matching

Match each of the following numbered items with the lettered statement that best describes it by entering the number of the item in the space provided.

1. corporate shield
2. partnership agreement
3. lawyer
4. partnerships
5. corporation
6. limited partnership
7. sole proprietor
8. general partner
9. personal guarantee
10. corporate reports
11. form a Subchapter S corporation
12. corporate president
13. shareholders
14. offshore corporations
15. a corporate charter
16. minute book
17. do-it-yourself corporation

_____ A. unlimited liability
_____ B. a legal form which gives the owner absolute control
_____ C. limits liability of noncorporate investors
_____ D. a way of organizing your business so that you get the lowest tax rate
_____ E. taxed as an individual
_____ F. member of the taxi squad; not needed to form sole proprietorship
_____ G. a written contract between two or more people that describes duties, sharing of profits, and dissolution
_____ H. stands between you and your creditors
_____ I. are tricky and may not save you money
_____ J. another name for corporate owners
_____ K. must be an employee of the business
_____ L. if you are losing money
_____ M. a good source of secondary research material when you are studying legal forms of business
_____ N. often required by bankers to secure a corporate loan
_____ O. must be kept current
_____ P. may not provide the benefits you need
_____ Q. tells the state what your corporation will be doing

True–False

Determine whether each of the following statements is true or false and enter a T (True) or F (False) in the space provided.

_____ 1. A company which is incorporated in Delaware can only do business in California as a foreign corporation.
_____ 2. Most growth businesses do not need outside infusions of cash.
_____ 3. A Sub S corporation is limited to 75 owners.
_____ 4. Sub S corporate owners have unlimited liability.
_____ 5. A sole proprietor is limited to setting aside only $500 per year for retirement.
_____ 6. All corporate fiscal tax years must end on December 31.
_____ 7. Active owners of a corporation are known as employees.
_____ 8. A partnership agreement, drawn up by a lawyer, is required in order to establish a general partnership.
_____ 9. When setting up a corporation, you should secure the services of a "hot" trial attorney.

_____ 10. A corporation usually has more money-raising ability than other legal forms of business ownership.

_____ 11. In a limited partnership, one of the partners must be a general partner.

_____ 12. A corporation is said to have snob appeal.

_____ 13. To the consumer, the legal form of business ownership is often invisible.

_____ 14. You can form a partnership with a handshake.

_____ 15. In 1982, Congress changed the laws to discourage incorporation by professionals like lawyers and doctors.

Multiple Choice

Select the best response for each of the following items and enter the corresponding letter in the space provided.

_____ 1. A partnership:
   a. is a shield between you and trouble.
   b. will make you immortal.
   c. is taxed at the same rate as as individual.
   d. is very difficult to establish.

_____ 2. A sole proprietor has:
   a. absolute control; no need for written agreements; lots of money-raising ability; limited liability.
   b. divided control; no need for written agreements; limited money-raising ability; limited liability.
   c. absolute control; need for written agreements; limited money-raising ability; unlimited liability.
   d. absolute control; no need for written agreements; limited money-raising ability; unlimited liability.

_____ 3. A corporation has:
   a. shared control; a need for a lawyer to form; snob appeal; cancellation by death.
   b. shared control; lots of good reasons for a lawyer to form; snob appeal; an adjustable tax year.
   c. divided control; no need for written agreements; unlimited liability; adjustable tax year.
   d. absolute control; limited liability; adjustable tax year; no need for written agreements.

_____ 4. A limited partnership has:
   a. at least two partners; an overwhelming need for written agreements; moderate capital-raising ability.
   b. absolute control; no need for written agreements; a tax tier divided into four stages.
   c. shared control with limited partner; no need for written agreements; personal tax rate.
   d. control by general partner; no need for written agreements; a four-stage tax tier, graduated by increments of $25,000.

_____ 5. Which of the following questions is not helpful when you're dealing with a prospective lawyer?
   a. What kind of signals suggest that I should designate my company stock as IRS Section 1244?
   b. Can you give me a concrete example of how IRS Section 368 (a) (b) works?
   c. How does my corporation handle the ''depreciation recapture'' rule?
   d. Can you give me a concrete example of how the Bernoulli Effect relates to Cash Flow?

_____ 6. Which of the following would be least helpful when using your network to search for a good lawyer?
   a. Everyone you know.
   b. Local business associations.

c. Local bar association.

d. Local bankers.

_____ 7. All of the following are true about Paul Webber — Programmer/Entrepreneur except:

a. Paul was a computer programmer.

b. Paul sold out to Jerry.

c. Mildred became Paul's new partner.

d. Mildred didn't know the business.

_____ 8. You limit your personal liability when you:

a. form a corporation.

b. form a sole proprietorship.

c. become a general partner.

d. sign a personal guarantee.

_____ 9. As a sole proprietor, you:

a. upgrade your image.

b. control your fiscal year.

c. guarantee continuity.

d. none of the above.

_____ 10. What a corporation won't do:

a. limit your liability.

b. eliminate taxes altogether.

c. let you upgrade your image.

d. let you set aside more dollars for retirement.

Short-Answer Questions

Note: Items 1 to 4 below can be worked on as either an individual or class project.

1. Find a lawyer who has worked with several small businesses. Ask small business owners whom they have worked with and whom they would recommend to help you with your start-up.
   a. Find the owners at:
      1. Chamber of commerce (see if you can be invited to one meeting without being forced to join).
      2. Local bankers.
      3. Local accountants.
      4. Leads Clubs.
      5. Local shopping centers or business parks (entrepreneurs love to talk about business).
   b. On a separate sheet of paper, list the names you come up with. Use the following headings:

Name of Lawyer   **Source**   **Recommend?**

   c. Continue the above list until at least one name has been recommended three or four times.
2. Select a name from C, above. Give the lawyer a call. Say your're starting a new business and you're in the process of selecting an attorney and that his or her name has been recommended by several owners. You'd like to arrange a get-acquainted meeting. If there is no charge, set up a meeting. If there is a charge, go to the next name on the list.
3. Once you get a meeting set up, ask the following questions:
   a. Does working with small businesses provide the bulk of revenue for your practice.?
   b. Can you give me the names of small businesses you've worked with? Preferably one sole proprietor, one partnership, and one corporation?
   c. Could you give me a breakdown of different types of fees? What bases do you suggest for working with a new start-up like mine?

    d. What's the extent of your experience with real estate leases? What's a normal charge for reviewing a lease?

    e. Are there other small business professionals you would recommend who might help me?

       1. Accountant: _____

       2. Banker: _____

       3. Insurance agent: _____

       4. Tax person: _____

    f. Have you ever worked with a client who bought or sold a business?

    Name: _____

    Name: _____

    g. If yes, what are the major items to watch for in a buy-out? In a sale?

    _____

    _____

    _____

4. After your meeting, write down your reactions to the meeting. Do it ASAP, so you won't forget.
    a. Comfort-level — did you feel comfortable with this person?

    b. Confusion quotient — could you understand what he or she was saying?

    c. Expertise — did you feel he or she knew the ins and outs of the world of small business?

    d. Other — write down your reactions here.

5. Team Project. If possible, divide your group into three teams — sole proprietors, partners, and corporate types. Each team will then do in-depth research on the pros and cons of one type of legal form of business ownership.
    Select a spokesperson from each team to present findings. Develop a matrix grid (see Chapter Three, POWER MARKETING, for a model), and rate all three forms.
    a. Suggested sources:
       1. Books.
         Inc. Yourself, McQuown
         How to Form Your Own Corporation Without a Lawyer for Under $50, Nicholas
         Incorporating Your Business, Kirk
       2. Recent articles.
         Inc. magazine
         Venture magazine
         Wall Street Journal
       3. Interviews with local business owners — ask them the pros and and cons of their type of ownership.
       4. Attorneys, accountants, and other professsionals.

b. Categories for organizing your research:
   1. Ease of starting.
   2. Ability to raise capital.
   3. Liability.
   4. Costs.
   5. Lifespan.
   6. Government regulation or control.
   7. Personal interest.
   8. Decision-making process.
   9. Power to attract key employees.
   10. Strengths and weaknesses of management team.
   11. Taxes.
   12. Divided authority.
   13. Possible disagreements.
   14. General partnership.
   15. Limited partnership.
   16. General corporation.
   17. Sub S corporation.

Fun-Time: Building Your Winning Team

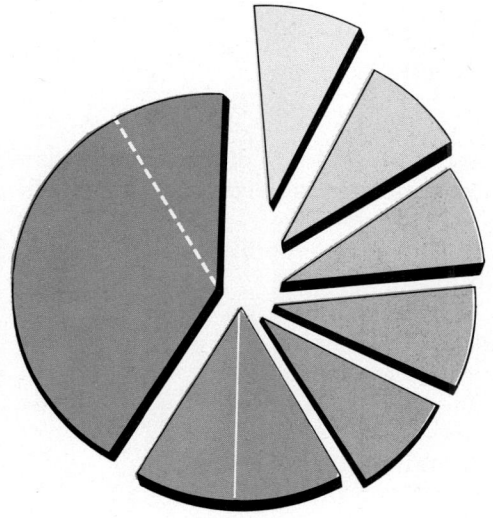

Draw a mind map showing how you will go about building your winning team.

Objective Questions

Matching

Matching each of the following numbered items with the lettered statement that best describes it by entering the number of the item in the space provided.

1. entrepreneur
2. enterprise
3. DISC
4. D
5. I
6. S
7. C
8. top-heavy team
9. brainstorming
10. Harry R. Marquez
11. successful team building
12. Janet Ames
13. balance
14. one-to-one interviews
15. secret ballot

_____ A. the last step in a large team-building process, when team members select teammates

_____ B. diplomatic, accurate, understands need for control, gets job done, can establish standard operating procedures

_____ C. a French word that means master architect, master builder

_____ D. industry, money, initiative

_____ E. the secret is to analyze yourself first

_____ F. DISC scale — stands for Influencing

_____ G. everybody interviews everybody else

_____ H. Dominance and Influence types all over the shop, competing like crazy, not answering the phones

_____ I. personality profile, useful for team-building

_____ J. DISC scale — stands for Dominance

_____ K. DISC scale — stands for Steadiness

_____ L. case study entrepreneur who was bright, quick, impatient, a dreamer

_____ M. one way to utilize your precious people-resources

_____ N. DISC scale — stands for Compliant

_____ O. the essential ingredient of a successful team

True – False

Determine whether each of the following statements is true or false and enter a T (True) or F (False) in the space provided.

_____ 1. The word entrepreneur comes from the Latin, *il miglior fabbro*, which means "the little craftsman."

_____ 2. Harry R. Marquez was a terrible student.

_____ 3. A company is no better than its people.

_____ 4. A small business management team doesn't need balance so much as it needs salespeople to clear out the inventory.

_____ 5. The DISC system was developed in the late Seventies by Jacob Bernoulli, a psychologist working in a lab with rats. The copyright is owned by Bernoulli Effect Inc.

_____ 6. The beauty of the DISC grid is that it shows at a glance where you are and what DISC types will help you get a balanced team together.

_____ 7. On the DISC grid, Harry R. Marquez is an I, or Influencing type of person.

_____ 8. Frederick R. Winslow, on the other hand, is a definite S, which stands for Steadiness.

———— 9. Janet Ames, the woman who came to work at Marquez Robotics as manager, was a C.

———— 10. The smaller the organization, the more important the team.

———— 11. Networking your competitors and vendors is a good way to build a winning team with people who know the business.

———— 12. If you're first-rate, you'll hire first-rate people.

———— 13. If you're second-rate, you'll also hire first-rate people because you'll realize you need them.

———— 14. Happiness is knowing who you are — and being able to exploit it.

———— 15. Given the chance, people will hire themselves.

———— 16. Your business can't grow until it has the right people.

Multiple Choice

Select the best response for each of the following items and enter the corresponding letter in the space provided.

———— 1. The word *entrepreneur* comes from the Latin verb:
   a. *bigetan.*
   b. *pre-hendere.*
   c. *prise.*
   d. *Star Trek.*

———— 2. Mind movies include:
   a. slides of your trip.
   b. sights.
   c. fun people you met along the way.
   d. all of the above.

———— 3. Harry R. Marquez started a company that built:
   a. hot sports cars.
   b. computers.
   c. robots.
   d. Lasers.

———— 4. Frederick S. Winslow was a good member of the Marquez Team because he had a solid background in:
   a. sales.
   b. inventing.
   c. designing.
   d. finance.

———— 5. In team building it is important to:
   a. build your team before it's too late.
   b. test them out before it starts costing you money.
   c. hire good people, then listen to them.
   d. all of the above.

———— 6. The Harry R. Marquez personality analysis concluded that Harry:
   a. understands need for procedures and controls.
   b. is a dreamer.
   c. is diplomatic with everyone.
   d. all of the above.

———— 7. Which of the following personality styles does *not* form part of the DISC acronym?
   a. Dominance.
   b. Sado-masochism.
   c. Influencing of others.
   d. Compliance.

_____ 8. Rudy Bowman, our classic S, is no slouch as a team member. Steadies are important to the team because they:
   a. are extremely creative.
   b. make good managers.
   c. love to control a very small turf.
   d. hog the spotlight and are good at entertaining the clients.

_____ 9. Richard White developed a step-by-step method of teambuilding, which involved everything below except:
   a. Carl Rogers encounter groups.
   b. ice-breaker.
   c. one-to-one interviews.
   d. secret balloting.

_____ 10. Case study personality E. G. Bogard turned out to be a Developer. Which of the descriptions below does not fit Mr. Bogard?
   a. Prefers innovative solutions.
   b. Displays lots of self-reliance.
   c. Loves to operate the telephone switchboard.
   d. Fears boredom.

Short-Answer Questions

1. Take a breather and do a couple of mind-movies of your trip.
   a. What have you learned so far?

   _____

   _____

   _____

   b. What was fun?

   _____

   _____

   _____

   c. Whom did you meet that you found interesting or exciting or especially helpful in your quest?

Name	**Personality Type**
1. _____	_____
	_____
2. _____	_____
	_____
3. _____	_____
	_____

2. Brainstorm your ideal team.
   a. Sit down with a few friends, relatives, or classmates who have a good feel for the type of business you plan to start. Ask everyone to list your strengths and weaknesses. (You can tell them briefly about the DISC scale and ask them whether you're a D, I, S, or C.) Compile their analyses here. Then thank them and go on to Part B alone.

Strengths	Weaknesses	DISC Type
_____	_____	_____
_____	_____	_____
_____	_____	_____
_____	_____	_____
_____	_____	

b. Once you discover how people perceive you, it's time to brainstorm the other members of your ideal team — people who will balance your strengths and weaknesses. What kind of people do you need for balance? Use the spaces provided to list your ideal team members.

Job Strengths	Personal Qualities	DISC Type
1. _____	_____	_____
2. _____	_____	_____
3. _____	_____	_____
4. _____	_____	_____
5. _____	_____	_____

Do any of the people who are helping you fit the ideal team?
Who?

_____

_____

Why?

_____

_____

What would it take to get them on your team?

_____

_____

3. Now that you have an idea what kind of team you need, take your thoughts out into the business arena and see how many players you can find.

Name	Team Position	Now Employed	DISC
a. _____	_____	_____	_____
b. _____	_____	_____	_____
c. _____	_____	_____	_____
d. _____	_____	_____	_____
e. _____	_____	_____	_____

4. Bring your new team together (or form a team with your classmates) and learn what they think of your organization. What should it look like? What image should it project? How can they help? Brainstorm some company objectives and organizational ideas. Keep track of your team's ideas on a separate sheet of paper.

To Buy or to Franchise— There's the Rub

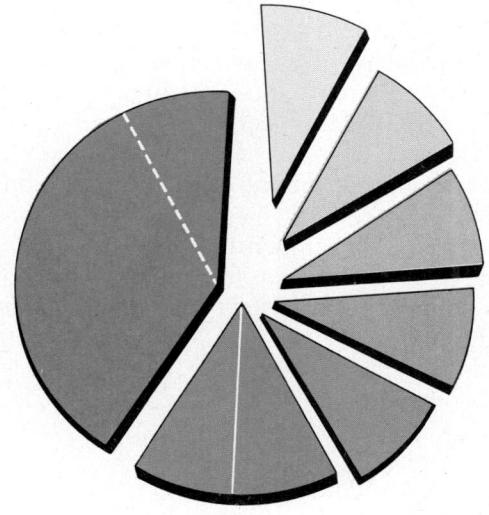

Draw a mind map investigating the pros and cons of buying an existing business or franchising.

Objective Questions

Matching

Match each of the following numbered items with the lettered statement that best describes it by entering the number of the item in the space provided.

1. income stream
2. the deal
3. taking on a franchise
4. Magic Threshold
5. business brokers
6. escape hatch
7. covenant not to compete
8. financial records
9. accounts receivable
10. tangible assets
11. Goodwill
12. Ill Will
13. franchisor
14. sacrificed goods
15. royalty fee
16. decision to buy a business
17. apparently honest seller
18. bulk sales escrow

_____ A. a must when buying a business; among other things it helps you make sure inventory is not tied up by creditors

_____ B. seller must do something else for awhile

_____ C. intangible asset that seller will use to raise asking price

_____ D. point for tough negotiation because they keep losing value

_____ E. everything you can touch

_____ F. picture of an income stream

_____ G. means unhappy customers

_____ H. like buying a supplier for eternity

_____ I. the creator of the franchise

_____ J. distressed goods, usually sold at any price

_____ K. should be handled with logic, not emotion

_____ L. a signal for you to be suspicious; check out motives anyway

_____ M. one good reason for buying an ongoing business

_____ N. a shorthand way of talking about negotiating terms

_____ O. buying the right to use a name

_____ P. what you cross to get inside a business

_____ Q. agents who sell businesses

_____ R. a device that allows you to back out of the purchase of a business painlessly

True – False

Determine whether each of the following statements is true or false and enter a T (True) or F (False) in the space provided.

_____ 1. The overwhelming reason for buying a business that's already going instead of building one with your own hands is money.

_____ 2. The smart buyer will plunge into a business because of a sudden surge of raw emotion.

_____ 3. Every business in the country is for sale sometime.

_____ 4. Deals are like buses. If you miss one, another one will be along soon.

_____ 5. The investigative and information-gathering tactics for buying a business or for buying a franchise are very different.

_____ 6. Your best bet for finding a business to buy is to search the classified section of your local paper under Business Opportunities.

_____ 7. An earnest money deposit is to show the seller you are an interested buyer and not a lookie-loo.

_____ 8. The main function of an offer with an escape hatch is to cheat the IRS.

_____ 9. Goodwill is an excellent example of a tangible asset.

_____ 10. The covenant not to compete is to keep the seller from opening a similar business in your market area.

_____ 11. A buyer should study the financial records for at least five years back if they are available.

_____ 12. Examples of tangible assets include real estate, equipment, fixtures, good will, and inventory.

_____ 13. In small business, success can rest on the shoulders of one or two key employees.

_____ 14. If you get it in writing, the IRS will allow you to deduct the cost of a covenant not to compete over the life of the covenant.

_____ 15. A smart seller is going to ask you to pay him for building up an invisible wealth of Goodwill.

_____ 16. Franchise means you're buying a license.

_____ 17. If you want to bottle Coca-Cola, you'll have to negotiate for a license.

_____ 18. When you're evaluating a franchise, you go through most of the same steps you would use to evaluate a business for sale.

_____ 19. Roto-Rooter is a franchise.

_____ 20. In the overall business-buying strategy, the terms for the deal are more important than the purchase price.

Multiple Choice

Select the best response for each of the following items and enter the corresponding letter in the space provided.

_____ 1. The overwhelming reason for buying a business that's already going instead of building one with your own hands is:
   a. attractive inventory.
   b. Goodwill.
   c. income stream.
   d. employees who need the work.

_____ 2. An advantage of buying an ongoing business is:
   a. less cash up front.
   b. a good deal on fixtures and equipment.
   c. a possible bargain in hidden inventory.
   d. all of the above.

_____ 3. The last place to look for a business to buy is:
   a. your own network of associates.
   b. classified ads in the newspaper.
   c. local bankers.
   d. business brokers.

_____ 4. If you are asked to make an "earnest-money" deposit, you should handle it with:
   a. a cashier's check, made out to seller.
   b. an offer with an escape hatch.
   c. a lawyer.
   d. a certified CPA.

_____ 5. When you explore the inner intricacies of a business, check the following:
   a. financial history.
   b. your suppliers.
   c. the seller's motives.
   d. all of the above.

_____ 6. Accounts receivable that are six months old are worth approximately:
  a. 90 cents on the dollar.
  b. 70 cents on the dollar.
  c. 50 cents on the dollar.
  d. 30 cents on the dollar.

_____ 7. When checking out all the tangible assets, your job is to evaluate all of the following except:
  a. real estate.
  b. Goodwill.
  c. equipment/fixtures.
  d. inventory.

_____ 8. All of the following can contribute to Ill Will except:
  a. delivery.
  b. cash.
  c. advertising.
  d. service.

_____ 9. When evaluating a franchisor, check out all the following except:
  a. noncompetitive franchises.
  b. how long this franchise has been in business.
  c. who are the officers.
  d. number of franchised operations like this one in existence.

_____ 10. All of the questions below except for one are good to ask franchisors:
  a. What's included in the franchise fee?
  b. What's the duration of the agreement?
  c. What level of training and service can you offer?
  d. Say I get tired of this business — can I relocate any time I wish?

Short-Answer Questions

1. Identify a business that you think is a real money machine.

   Type of business: _____

   Name: _____

   Address: _____
2. Where is it on the life cycle?

   _____

   _____

3. Once you've found the business and checked its position on the life cycle, gather more data about it. Visit your city or county planning office. What are the plans for the area for the next 5 – 10 years?

   Five years: _____

   _____

   _____

   Ten years: _____

   _____

   _____

4. Go to the site. On a separate sheet of paper, diagram everything you can.

   Traffic flow
   Major arterials
   Access
   Parking (Is parking lot a drop-off point for car-poolers?)
   Is building in good repair? (If not, what will it need before you move in?)
5. Take a good look at the customers.
   Describe what they're wearing:

   _____

   _____

   _____

   _____

   Describe what they're driving:

   _____

   _____

   _____

   _____

   What can you deduce about their life-style?

   _____

   _____

   _____

   _____

   How far do they travel to get here?

   Longest distance: _____

   Shortest distance: _____

   Average distance: _____

   Interview some customers. What do they have to say about this business?

   _____

   _____

   _____

   _____

   About the trading area?

   _____

   _____

   _____

   _____

Is there mostly Goodwill?

_____

Is there mostly Ill Will?

_____

6. Investigate your neighbors.
   Which neighbors will help you draw customers?

   a. _____

   b. _____

   c. _____

   Which neighbors won't help?

   d. _____

   e. _____

   Where is your major competition? How strong is the competition? Can competitors move in to this trading area?

   Location of Competitors: _____

   Strength: _____

   Assault probabilities: _____

7. Move inside the business. Either contact the owner directly or get the assistance of a business opportunity broker. Study the sales figures. Check profit percentages. Evaluate the tangible assets. Of special importance are:

   a. Sales. List the percentage of change for last five years.
      1.
      2.
      3.
      4.
      5.

   b. Profit. List the profit figures for the last five years.
      1.
      2.
      3.
      4.
      5.

   c. Tangible assets. Using the format that follows, list all assets. Look at the books and write down the accounting value. Then go out into the marketplace and get the current value.

Asset	Accounting Value	Current Value
1. _____	_____	_____
2. _____	_____	_____
3. _____	_____	_____
4. _____	_____	_____

   d. Terms. What kind of terms can you negotiate with the seller? (Try to get the seller to let you pay for the business out of profits you make after you take possession.)

   _____

   _____

8. You'll want to know whether or not vendors who have been supplying the seller will continue to supply you, as the new owner. Interview your vendors and suppliers.
   Will vendors continue to supply you?

   _____

   _____

   _____

   _____

   What suggestions do they have for improving the business?

   _____

   _____

   _____

   _____

   Can you get credit terms? (What are they?)

   _____

   _____

   _____

   _____

   (Use the same vendors application form you developed for Chapter 10, when you were trying to save money. The form works just as well when you're buying a business.)

9. Rethink your moves. Does it look as if you could do better by starting your own business from scratch instead of buying this business you're thinking about?

   _____

   _____

   _____

   _____

Control: Your Small Business Computer

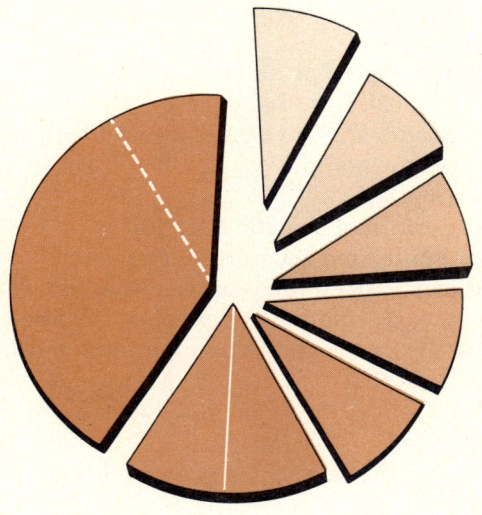

Draw a mind map of how a small business computer would help you control your small business operations.

Objective Questions

Matching

Match each of the following numbered items with the lettered statement that best describes it by entering the number of the item in the space provided.

1. defining problems and tasks
2. applications software
3. micro
4. burning in
5. electronic spreadsheet
6. word processing
7. computer hardware
8. memory
9. operating system
10. modem

_____ A. will fit on a desk; often called a personal computer
_____ B. should be done by your dealer, in the store
_____ C. the portion of the computer that you can see and touch
_____ D. the program that drives the computer
_____ E. capacity to store information
_____ F. program designed to perform a specific function
_____ G. a generic term for computerized accounting software
_____ H. the first step toward considering the purchase of a computer
_____ I. required in order to have a telephone connection between computers
_____ J. a highly efficient and flexible capacity for creating letters, documents, etc.

True–False

Determine whether each of the following statements is true or false and enter a T (True) or F (False) in the space provided.

_____ 1. It is a violation of copyright law to copy and sell proprietary software.
_____ 2. Computer hardware is the program that drives the computer.
_____ 3. A computer system is both hardware and software.
_____ 4. A modem will let your computer talk to another computer.
_____ 5. The most important consideration in buying your first computer system is dealing until you squeeze the price down to a respectable level.
_____ 6. A hard disk or Winchester drive is far less expensive than a floppy disk drive.
_____ 7. A floppy disk is a defective hard disk.
_____ 8. When a disk becomes "floppier" through exposure to humidity, and also through extended use, it is now in the "mature stage" and will allow hardware to interface with programs from any operating system whatsoever.
_____ 9. A new microcomputer should go through its burn-in period in a very warm office situation.
_____ 10. Forty percent or more of your computer budget should be allocated for software.
_____ 11. Computerphobia is a disease that occurs when a user-friendly program is debugged and the result is electric shock and information sickness.
_____ 12. The first step before purchasing a computer should be to define the problems that need solving in your business.
_____ 13. More and more, you need to understand programming languages (BASIC, Pascal, FORTRAN, COBOL) before purchasing a computer for business use.
_____ 14. Computers are useful in the performance of repetitive tasks.
_____ 15. There are good reasons for purchasing a small home computer before you need one in your business.

_____ 16. The experts say that when you're buying a computer, you should select the hardware on the basis of a well-known logo, then find software to fit, then begin developing applications to your particular type of business.

_____ 17. Microcomputers are of small value in spreadsheet analysis.

_____ 18. It can take 30–90 days to switch from a manual accounting system to a computerized system.

_____ 19. When shopping for a computer system, you should find a microcomputer store that has salespeople who understand small business problems and how to solve them.

_____ 20. There is a strong chance that word-processing software will make business use of the typewriter obsolete.

Multiple Choice

Select the best response for each of the following items and enter the corresponding letter in the space provided.

_____ 1. The first step in purchasing a computer should be:
   a. evaluating your physical space availability.
   b. learning a programming language.
   c. looking for a well-known company logo so you'll be assured of service and support.
   d. evaluating your needs.

_____ 2. Computers are most useful:
   a. in performing repetitive tasks.
   b. in digesting the inertial flow produced by AT & T's UNIX.
   c. in performing one-time functions.
   d. in developing antidotes to the Bernoulli Effect as it relates to corporate time management.

_____ 3. Powerful word processing programs can:
   a. speed up letter composition.
   b. personalize form letters.
   c. merge names and addresses from a mailing list.
   d. all of the above.

_____ 4. Some word processors have the capacity to:
   a. correct spelling.
   b. sign your name to letters.
   c. work without electrical power.
   d. both A and B.

_____ 5. A floppy disk:
   a. is warm and soft.
   b. contains instructions for the hardware.
   c. can be played at different rpms.
   d. is not subject to copyright laws.

_____ 6. Software:
   a. is often copyrighted.
   b. gives instructions to the hardware.
   c. is often for sale in retail stores.
   d. all of the above.

_____ 7. A microcomputer:
   a. is different from a personal computer.
   b. usually weighs over 200 pounds.
   c. costs more than a minicomputer.
   d. none of the above.

_____   8. A good way to learn about the micro for small business is to:
             a. read computer magazines.
             b. talk to people in similar businesses who are using computers.
             c. enroll in a course in microcomputer fundamentals.
             d. all of the above.

_____   9. A computer system:
             a. consists of software and hardware.
             b. is software alone.
             c. requires a CPU and a hard disk drive before it will operate.
             d. is required by the IRS for all retail firms incorporated after 1979, as result of the Berkman-Sterns Act.

_____ 10. A video display terminal:
             a. can be almost any color.
             b. is like a TV screen.
             c. can cause eye fatigue.
             d. all of the above.

Short-Answer Questions

1. What's the first step when you're thinking about buying a computer?

_____

2. What the 2nd step?

_____

3. The 3rd?

_____

4. Describe the routine functions of your business that might be handled by a computer. (Helpful hint: invoicing, accounting, mailing list, form letters, etc.)

_____

_____

_____

_____

_____

_____

_____

_____

5. What are the components of a computer system?

_____

_____

6. What 3 computer magazines would be most helpful for your type of business?

   1. _____

   2. _____

   3. _____

7. Name 2 more ways to keep up in computer developments:

    1. _____

    2. _____

8. Visit a computer store. Tell the salesperson what your business problems are. Ask for suggestions about solutions. What advice are you given?

    _____

    _____

    _____

    _____

    _____

    _____

    _____

9. Network your way to several computer consultants. What do they suggest in the way of a system? What is the value of using a consultant? Can they save you money on your system? Summarize their advice.

    _____

    _____

    _____

    _____

    _____

    _____

    _____

10. List your purchase options.

	Software	**Hardware**
Costs: Outright Purchase	_____	_____
Lease	_____	_____

11. On a separate sheet of paper, develop a time-line chart for installation or conversion to a micro system that will handle your business tasks. Events might include:
    Education
    Purchase evaluation/shopping
    Testing
    Consulting
    Info/file conversion
    Operator training
    Decision day

12. For comparative purposes, contact two accounting services in your area and find out what they would charge to handle some of your routine tasks. (If you check the *Wall Street Journal,* you'll see ads for free seminars for small business owners by large computerized companies like ADP.)

    Firm 1: _____

    Firm 2: _____

13. List sources in your area for computer education. Start with the yellow pages, under "Computer." You'll find courses at public schools, private colleges, specialized computer training centers, dealer-operated schools, weekend seminars, and so on.

_____

_____

_____

_____

_____

_____

14. Using your five-year growth plan, describe four or five functions that you would like a computer to perform after you've been in business awhile.

1. _____

2. _____

3. _____

4. _____

5. _____

Showcase: Pulling Your Plan Together

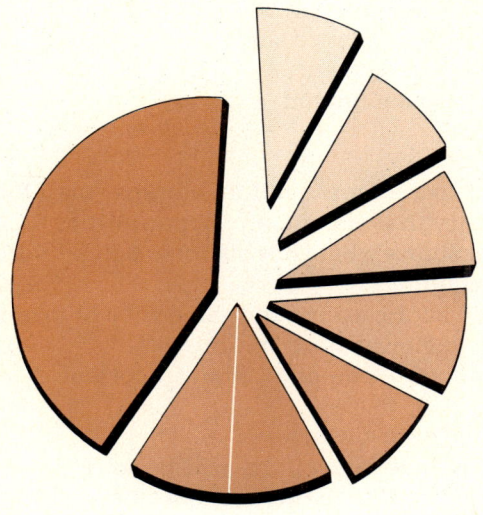

Draw a mind map of how you plan to showcase your business in your Business Plan.

Objective Questions

Matching

Match each of the following numbered items with the lettered statement that best describes it by entering the number of the item in the space provided.

1. Business Plan	10. demand
2. mini-summary	11. selling seats
3. Magic Numbers	12. industry overview
4. Appendices	13. your competitors
5. cover letter	14. information business
6. excitement	15. projected balance sheet
7. net profit	16. bad management
8. cash-flow section	17. leasing equipment
9. entrepreneur	

_____   A. the reason cited by experts for the failure of most small businesses

_____   B. a fast-growing industry that offers many opportunities for eager entrepreneurs

_____   C. a numerical tool that shows what your business will be worth after a certain period of time if your forecasts are accurate.

_____   D. hungry combatants who are eyeing the same slice of marketplace pie as you are

_____   E. a smart way to save money at start-up time

_____   F. a long look at an industry, compiled from important dates, breakthroughs, failures, and opportunities

_____   G. a portable blueprint of your business

_____   H. a way of talking about how many units will be sold

_____   I. a brief introduction to your Business Plan that summarizes what your business is and why it will succeed

_____   J. a major source of revenue for airlines, movie-theatres, and industrial schools

_____   K. income, cash flow, balance sheet

_____   L. a person who gets lots of ideas

_____   M. you fill these with resumes, photographs, location diagrams, product descriptions, or articles from industry journals

_____   N. helps you aim the plan at a specific reader

_____   O. what's left in the kitty after you subtract expenses

_____   P. your banker will probably look here first

_____   Q. a mystical response from your reader when he or she encounters your Business Plan

True – False

Determine whether each of the following statements is true or false and enter a T (True) or F (False) in the space provided.

_____   1. A Business Plan is your roadmap to riches.

_____   2. Your Business Plan could be the most important document you've ever pulled together.

_____   3. A Business Plan has nothing to do with keeping your entrepreneurial creativity on track.

_____   4. The Business Plan is portable.

_____   5. Good business planning is not hard work.

_____   6. Section I of the business plan is called "Magic Numbers" because of the sleight-of-hand you'll have to use to hypnotize prospective lenders.

_____ 7. The Magic Numbers section includes the income statement, cash flow projections, and projected balance sheet.

_____ 8. Sections I and II of the plan are followed by various appendices.

_____ 9. To aim the plan, you should begin with a cover letter.

_____ 10. Each time you send the plan to a different reader, all you need to do is pull out your old cover letter and change the address to that of your new reader.

_____ 11. The cover letter should be 5,000 words long, minimum.

_____ 12. The purpose of writing the cover letter is to open the door, gently, to make way for further negotiations.

_____ 13. The cap-off for the cover letter should not offend the reader by talking about how the money will be repaid. Save money talk for the appendices.

_____ 14. Investors love hot ideas.

_____ 15. Percentages and dollar amounts talk louder than words. Mention numbers whenever you can.

_____ 16. You should briefly profile the businesses which compete directly with you.

_____ 17. Save your ideas on how you're going to ace the competition for the appendices.

_____ 18. Since a lot of consideration should be given to pricing, you might start with what your TC sees as a good value.

_____ 19. The great thing about a location is that it's so tangible.

_____ 20. Almost every study you read on small business failure puts the blame on bad management.

_____ 21. A job description will help you control the people who work for you.

_____ 22. With the income statement, the main figure you are trying to bring out is gross sales.

_____ 23. Doing a cash flow projection once a year, with a casual six month update, is all that's required for most small firms.

_____ 24. With a projected balance sheet, you're trying to predict, on paper, what your business will be worth at the end of a certain period of time.

_____ 25. Your Business Section is the lure you use to get readers reading the Plan. The Financial Section is where you hook them.

Multiple Choice

Select the best response for each of the following items and enter the corresponding letter in the space provided.

_____ 1. When you are in business, a Business Plan can:
   a. keep your creativity on track.
   b. keep your power grooved.
   c. both A and B.
   d. none of the above.

_____ 2. When doing your plan, you will probably:
   a. work hard.
   b. stay up late and lose some sleep.
   c. save time in the end.
   d. all of the above.

_____ 3. Section I of your Plan includes all but which of the following?
   a. Assessments of the competition.
   b. Bids from contractors.
   c. Profiles of target customers.
   d. A look at your team.

_____ 4. Section II of your Plan should include all but which of the following?
   a. Management resumes.
   b. Balance sheet.

c. Cash flow projection.

d. Income statements.

_____ 5. Appendices to your Plan could include all but which of the following?

a. Detailed resumes.

b. Personal financial statements.

c. A design of your marketing plan.

d. Bids from contractors.

_____ 6. The cover letter should:

a. glorify your management team.

b. tell your reader why you're sending the Plan.

c. describe your TC with demographics and psychographics.

d. explain, in a minimum of 5,000 words, how you're going to disarm the competition.

_____ 7. In describing your business, you:

a. need to excite your reader about the business.

b. could include photographs of equipment and location in an appendix.

c. could refer to another appendix providing diagrams that show traffic flow, parking, access, transportation lines, and so on.

d. all of the above.

_____ 8. The target market for the Software School was:

a. the world.

b. bounded on the south by San Clemente, on the north by Long Beach, La Habra, and Brea.

c. too soft to profile.

d. diagrammed in detail by several movie studios who paid the school $2 million for rights to film a $40 million Compu-Kids movie in late 1983.

_____ 9. The primary Target Customer for the Software School was:

a. female, age 13 – 17, subscriber to _Seventeen_ magazine.

b. male, 55 – 67, poker player, resident of Leisure World

c. female, 22 – 54, $27,000 income, metro-suburban residence, married 73%, two children under 18 living at home, subscriber to _McCall's_ magazine.

d. small business, 1 – 30 employees, sales from $250,000 to $5 million, with a major output of paper.

_____ 10. When assessing your competition, you should look into all but which of the following?

a. Strengths.

b. Weaknesses.

c. Key employees.

d. Their private company books.

Short-Answer Questions

1. Write two cover letters for your business plan. Letter A should be addressed to your banker, or to a prospective lender. Letter B should be addressed to a person you'd like to have on your team — one of your key members. Use the following to prepare your letters.

Letter A

Name: _____

Position: _____

Address: _____

Goal for writing: _____

2 – 3 items you must include

1. _____

2. _____

3. _____

Letter B

Name: _____

Position: _____

Address: _____

Goal for writing: _____

2 – 3 items you must include

1. _____

2. _____

3. _____

2. Now turn loose your creative juices. Below, develop an outline or mind map that will turn into a paragraph or two describing your business. You want to excite your reader. Cover the following: What business you're in; description of product/service; what's unique about your business; what industry you're in. Whenever you can, use dollars or percentages to base your dream in reality.

3. Now put your marketing data into a free-flow description of your market and your Target Customer. Use the following categories to organize your thoughts.

Industry Overview. _____

_____

_____

_____

Target Market. _____

_____

_____

_____

Target Customer (Primary). _____

_____

_____

_____

Target Customer (Secondary). _____

_____

_____

_____

4. List your major competitors. Describe strengths and weaknesses.
   Competitor A

   Strengths: _____

   Weaknesses: _____
   Competitor B

   Strengths: _____

   Weaknesses: _____
   Competitor C

   Strengths: _____

   Weaknesses: _____
   Competitor D

   Strengths: _____

   Weaknesses: _____
   Competitor E

   Strengths: _____

   Weaknesses: _____

5. Develop your "attack plan" here. What techniques will you use to get the best, most cost-effective response from your market? How do you plan to disarm your competitors?

_____

_____

_____
_____
_____
_____
_____
_____
_____

6. Write a brief summary of why you picked your location. In your reader's mind, build the picture of the perfect location, the site that cannot fail.

_____
_____
_____
_____
_____
_____
_____

Now list all the benefits of this location to target customers.

_____
_____
_____

7. Let's hear it for the Management Team! List the team members in order of importance to the business. For each member, note experience, accomplishments, education, training, flexibility, imagination, tenacity, and finally, what they can do to help make your business a winner.

Team Member A: _____
_____
_____

Team Member B: _____
_____
_____

Team Member C: _____
_____
_____

Team Member D: _____
_____
_____
_____

8. Now that your management team is in place, list "shock troops"—other types of personnel you'll need. Cover the topics shown below.

Skills: _____
_____
_____
_____

Pay: _____
_____
_____

Training

   Kind: _____

   Length: _____

Fringe Benefits: _____
_____
_____
_____

Overtime: _____
_____
_____

Answers to Objective Questions

1 Doorways to the Information Society — Your Great Adventure

Matching

A. 5
B. 8
C. 1
D. 10
E. 9
F. 4
G. 6
H. 2
I. 3 or 7
J. 7 or 3

True–False

1. F	11. T
2. T	12. F
3. T	13. F
4. T	14. F
5. F	15. F
6. F	
7. T	
8. F	
9. T	
10. T	

Multiple Choice

1. C
2. D
3. D
4. A
5. D
6. C
7. B
8. D
9. A
10. D

2 The Big Picture: Charting Trends for Your Small Business

Matching

A. 11	K. 4
B. 12	L. 5
C. 15	M. 6
D. 17	N. 7
E. 18	O. 10
F. 20	P. 9
G. 19	Q. 2
H. 16	R. 13
I. 1	S. 14
J. 3	T. 8

True–False

1. T	11. T
2. F	12. T
3. F	13. F
4. F	14. T
5. F	15. T
6. T	16. F
7. T	17. F
8. T	18. F
9. F	19. F
10. F	20. T

Multiple Choice

1. C
2. B
3. A
4. C
5. C
6. B
7. B
8. C
9. D
10. A

3 Power Marketing

Matching

A.	20	K.	10
B.	18	L.	1
C.	7	M.	3
D.	5	N.	17
E.	19	O.	2
F.	16	P.	4
G.	15	Q.	8
H.	13	R.	6
I.	11	S.	14
J.	9	T.	12

True–False

1.	T	11.	T
2.	F	12.	T
3.	T	13.	F
4.	F	14.	T
5.	T	15.	T
6.	F	16.	T
7.	T	17.	T
8.	F	18.	T
9.	T	19.	T
10.	F	20.	T

Multiple Choice

1. C
2. D
3. B
4. B
5. D
6. B
7. C
8. D
9. B
10. C

4 Profiling Your Target Customer

Matching

A.	13	D.	17
B.	12	E.	15
C.	18	F.	14

G.	1	N.	4
H.	19	O.	6
I.	2	P.	7
J.	11	Q.	5
K.	3	R.	8
L.	10	S.	16
M.	9	T.	20

True–False

1.	F	11.	T
2.	F	12.	F
3.	T	13.	T
4.	T	14.	T
5.	F	15.	F
6.	T	16.	T
7.	T	17.	T
8.	F	18.	T
9.	T	19.	F
10.	T	20.	T

Multiple Choice

1. C
2. C
3. B
4. A
5. D
6. B
7. C
8. D
9. D
10. B

5 Reading the Competition

Matching

A.	18	K.	13
B.	11	L.	8
C.	16	M.	10
D.	20	N.	7
E.	17	O.	3
F.	1	P.	2
G.	9	Q.	19
H.	14	R.	5
I.	15	S.	6
J.	12	T.	4

True – False

1. F	11. T	13. T	
2. F	12. T	14. F	
3. T	13. T	15. T	
4. F	14. T	16. F	
5. F	15. T		
6. F	16. T		
7. F	17. T		
8. T	18. F		
9. T	19. T		
10. F	20. F		

Multiple Choice

1. C
2. D
3. D
4. D
5. D
6. A
7. C
8. B
9. C
10. C

Multiple Choice

1. D
2. C
3. A
4. B
5. D
6. A
7. D
8. D
9. A
10. D

6 Promotion: Making that Customer Connection

Matching

A. 4	K. 8
B. 5	L. 9
C. 1	M. 12
D. 6	N. 11
E. 3	O. 10
F. 2	
G. 7	
H. 15	
I. 14	
J. 13	

True – False

1. T	7. T
2. T	8. F
3. T	9. F
4. T	10. T
5. T	11. T
6. T	12. T

7 Location

Matching

A. 2	K. 7
B. 1	L. 17
C. 6	M. 13
D. 8	N. 16
E. 10	O. 14
F. 11	P. 12
G. 9	Q. 15
H. 5	
I. 3	
J. 4	

True – False

1. T	11. F
2. T	12. T
3. T	13. T
4. T	14. F
5. F	15. F
6. T	16. T
7. F	17. F
8. T	18. F
9. T	19. T
10. F	20. T

Multiple Choice

1. A
2. B
3. C
4. D
5. C
6. A
7. C
8. B
9. C
10. B

8 Surprises You Can't Afford

Matching

A. 2		K. 16
B. 1		L. 15
C. 3		M. 13
D. 4		N. 12
E. 5		O. 14
F. 6		P. 11
G. 8		
H. 7		
I. 10		
J. 9		

True – False

1. F	11. F
2. F	12. F
3. F	13. T
4. T	14. F
5. T	15. F
6. T	
7. T	
8. T	
9. T	
10. T	

Multiple Choice

1. A
2. D
3. B
4. C
5. A

6. D
7. D
8. D
9. D
10. B

9 The Powers of Numerical Projection

Matching

A. 11
B. 9
C. 6
D. 10
E. 4
F. 1
G. 2
H. 5
I. 3
J. 7
K. 8

True – False

1. T	11. T
2. T	12. T
3. T	13. T
4. T	14. T
5. F	15. T
6. F	16. F
7. T	17. T
8. F	18. F
9. F	19. T
10. T	20. F

Multiple Choice

1. C
2. B
3. A
4. D
5. A
6. B
7. A
8. D
9. D
10. B

10 Shaking the Money Tree

Matching

A. 9	K. 17	I. 14	O. 16
B. 2	L. 3	J. 13	P. 17
C. 14	M. 12	K. 12	Q. 15
D. 15	N. 1	L. 11	
E. 6	O. 11	M. 10	
F. 7	P. 10	N. 9	
G. 5	Q. 16		
H. 8	R. 20		
I. 13	S. 18		
J. 4	T. 19		

True – False

1. T	11. T	1. T	11. T
2. F	12. T	2. F	12. T
3. T	13. F	3. F	13. T
4. T	14. T	4. F	14. T
5. T	15. F	5. F	15. T
6. F	16. F	6. F	
7. T	17. T	7. T	
8. T	18. T	8. F	
9. F	19. T	9. F	
10. T	20. F	10. T	

Multiple Choice

1. D	1. A
2. B	2. D
3. A	3. B
4. C	4. A
5. D	5. D
6. A	6. C
7. B	7. B
8. D	8. A
9. C	9. D
10. B	10. B

11 When Should You Incorporate?

Matching

A. 8	E. 4
B. 7	F. 3
C. 6	G. 2
D. 5	H. 1

12 Fun-Time: Building Your Winning Team

Matching

A. 15	K. 6
B. 12	L. 10
C. 1	M. 9
D. 2	N. 7
E. 11	O. 13
F. 5	
G. 14	
H. 8	
I. 3	
J. 4	

True–False

1. F	11. T
2. T	12. T
3. T	13. F
4. F	14. T
5. F	15. T
6. T	16. T
7. F	
8. F	
9. T	
10. T	

Multiple Choice

1. B
2. D
3. C
4. A
5. D
6. B
7. B
8. C
9. A
10. C

13 To Buy or to Franchise — There's the Rub

Matching

A. 18	K. 16
B. 7	L. 17
C. 11	M. 1
D. 9	N. 2
E. 10	O. 15
F. 8	P. 4
G. 12	Q. 5
H. 3	R. 6
I. 13	
J. 14	

True–False

1. T	5. F
2. F	6. F
3. T	7. T
4. T	8. F

9. F	15. T
10. T	16. T
11. T	17. T
12. F	18. T
13. T	19. T
14. T	20. T

Multiple Choice

1. C
2. D
3. B
4. B
5. D
6. C
7. B
8. B
9. A
10. D

14 Control: Your Small Business Computer

Matching

A. 3
B. 4
C. 7
D. 9
E. 8
F. 2
G. 5
H. 1
I. 10
J. 6

True–False

1. T	11. F
2. F	12. T
3. T	13. F
4. T	14. T
5. F	15. T
6. F	16. F
7. F	17. F
8. F	18. T
9. F	19. T
10. T	20. T

Multiple Choice

1. D
2. A
3. D
4. A
5. B
6. D
7. D
8. D
9. A
10. D

True–False

1. T	11. F	21. T
2. T	12. T	22. F
3. F	13. F	23. F
4. T	14. T	24. T
5. F	15. T	25. T
6. F	16. T	
7. T	17. F	
8. T	18. T	
9. T	19. T	
10. F	20. T	

15 Showcase: Pulling Your Plan Together

Matching

A. 16	K. 3
B. 14	L. 9
C. 15	M. 4
D. 13	N. 5
E. 17	O. 7
F. 12	P. 8
G. 1	Q. 6
H. 10	
I. 2	
J. 11	

Multiple Choice

1. C
2. D
3. B
4. A
5. C
6. B
7. D
8. B
9. D
10. D